Mosby's

PARAMEDIC TEXTBOOK

About the Author and Contributors

Mick J. Sanders received his paramedic training in 1978 from St. Louis University Hospitals. He earned a Bachelor of Science degree in 1982 and a Master of Science degree in 1983 from Lindenwood College in St. Charles, Missouri. He has worked in various health care systems as a field paramedic, emergency department paramedic, and EMS instructor. For 12 years, Mr. Sanders served as Training Specialist with the Bureau of Emergency Medical Services, Missouri Department of Health, where he oversaw EMT and paramedic training and licensure in St. Louis city and the surrounding metropolitan area.

Kim McKenna, RN, BSN, CEN, EMT-P, is the Chief Medical Officer for the Florissant Valley Fire Protection District in Florissant, Missouri, and an Adjunct Instructor for St. Louis Community College in St. Louis, Missouri. Her past experiences include intensive care and emergency nursing. She has been involved in prehospital education since 1985, including 4 years as the primary instructor of a paramedic training program.

Gary Quick, MD, FACEP, is an Associate Professor in the Department of Emergency Medicine at the University of Oklahoma Health Sciences Center in Oklahoma City. Dr. Quick is a career emergency physician with over 25 years in clinical practice as well as extensive educational and research experience.

Lawrence M. Lewis, MD, FACEP, is Associate Professor of Emergency Medicine and Medicine and Chief of the Emergency Medicine Division at Washington University School of Medicine and Barnes-Jewish Hospital in St. Louis, Missouri. He completed his medical school training at the University of Miami School of Medicine before attending a residency at Washington University. He is an active researcher in emergency medicine with over 40 publications and serves on several national and state emergency medicine committees.

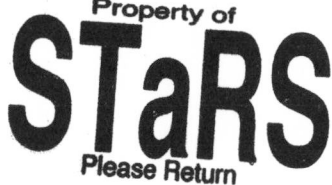

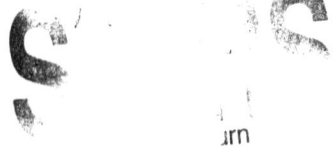

CONGRATULATIONS!

You now have access to MERLIN for

Mosby's Paramedic Textbook,
revised second edition,

by **Mick J. Sanders and Kim McKenna!**

sign on at:

http://www.mosby.com/MERLIN/

A website just for you as you learn prehospital emergency care with the new **revised second edition of *Mosby's Paramedic Textbook.***

what you will receive:

Whether you are a student, an instructor, or a clinician, you'll find information just for you. Things like:
- Content Updates
- Links to Related Products
- Author Information, Answers to Frequently Asked Questions, and more

plus:

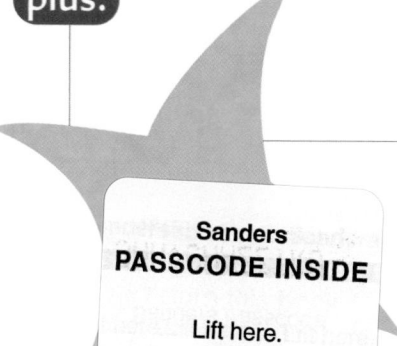

Sanders
PASSCODE INSIDE

Lift here.

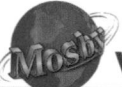 **WebLinks**

An exciting new program that allows you to directly access hundreds of active websites keyed specifically to the content of this book. The WebLinks are continually updated, with new ones added as they develop. **Peel the top layer only from the sticker on this page and register with the listed passcode.**

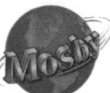 **Free access to Mosby's Virtual Classroom with NEW textbook purchase.**

Talk to your instructor about Mosby's Virtual Classroom! This instructor-driven, online learning environment allows your instructor to provide you with convenient access to course syllabuses, additional activities and review exercises, and a whole lot more. When your instructor chooses to take advantage of this powerful tool, your access to Mosby's Virtual Classroom is FREE for one year with the purchase of a NEW textbook. Purchase a NEW print workbook and you will receive FREE access to the interactive online workbook for an entire year! Find out more at MERLIN.

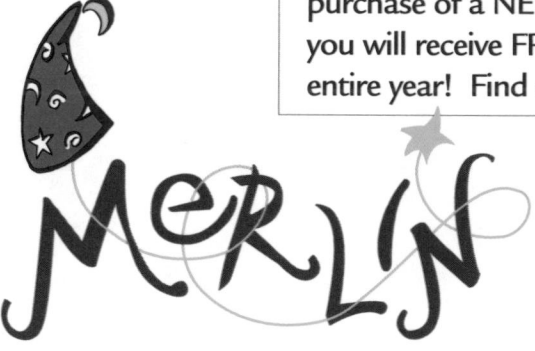

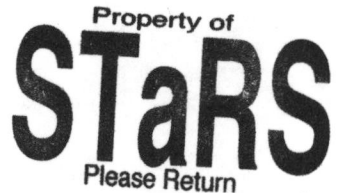
Property of
STaRS
Please Return

Mosby's **E**lectronic **R**esource **L**inks & **I**nformation **N**etwork

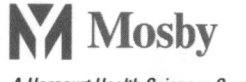 Mosby
A Harcourt Health Sciences Company

Mosby's PARAMEDIC TEXTBOOK

Revised Second Edition

Mick J. Sanders, EMT-P, MSA

PHYSICIAN ADVISERS

Lawrence M. Lewis, MD, FACEP
Associate Professor of Emergency Medicine
Chief, Emergency Medicine Division
Washington University School of Medicine/
   Barnes-Jewish Hospital
St. Louis, Missouri

Gary Quick, MD, FACEP
Associate Professor
Department of Emergency Medicine
University of Oklahoma
Oklahoma City, Oklahoma

CONTRIBUTING EDITOR

Kim McKenna, RN, BSN, CEN, EMT-P
Chief Medical Officer
Florissant Valley Fire Protection District
Florissant, Missouri

*with 900 illustrations
including 850 in color*

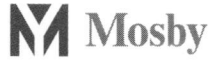 Mosby

A Harcourt Health Sciences Company

St. Louis   London   Philadelphia   Sydney   Toronto

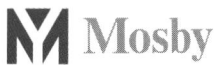

Publisher: Andrew Allen
Editor: Claire Merrick
Developmental Editor: Elaine Steinborn
Project Manager: Linda McKinley
Production Editor: Rich Barber
Designer: Stephanie Foley
Web Product Managing Editor: Kelly Trakalo

Second Edition
Copyright © 2001 by Mosby, Inc.

Previous edition copyrighted 1994

Pharmacology is an ever-changing field. Standard safety precautions must be followed, but as new research and clinical experience broaden our knowledge, changes in treatment and drug therapy may become necessary or appropriate. Readers are advised to check the most current product information provided by the manufacturer of each drug to be administered to verify the recommended dose, the method and duration of administration, and contraindications. It is the responsibility of the paramedic, relying on experience and knowledge of the patient, to determine dosages and the best treatment for each individual patient. Neither the Publisher nor the editor assume any liability for any injury and/or damage to persons or property arising from this publication.

The Publisher

Composition by Graphic World, Inc.
Lithography/color film by Graphic World, Inc.
Printing/binding by R.R. Donnelley & Sons Co.

Mosby, Inc.
11830 Westline Industrial Drive
St. Louis, Missouri 63146

International Standard Book Number 0-323-01416-X

01 02 03 04 / 9 8 7 6 5 4 3 2 1

To my family and in loving memory of my father

Foreword

We stand at the threshold of a new millennium. The "stuff" of which history is composed takes shape when an individual or a group looks back to determine where they have been and where they are going or should go. Conceiving and producing *Mosby's Paramedic Textbook, 2nd Edition* parallels in a microcosmic sense the production of such a history. The first edition was published in 1994 and reflected in detail the history of prehospital care and the development of EMS systems. In that first edition we discussed the importance of improving our efficiency in delivering time-dependent therapy to the patient such as thrombolytic therapy in acute myocardial infarction or stroke. Since 1994, we have witnessed the development of AMI and stroke treatment protocols, the use of which has been proven to reduce the "door to needle time" for these patients. New pharmacological interventions such as the use of amiodarone in ventricular fibrillation and the use of methylprednisolone therapy in spinal cord injuries have entered the paramedic's aramamentarium. Updating one's knowledge base has become a continuous challenge.

In this year of the millennium, let us take a moment to reflect on the difference EMS has made over the past century to ensure the nation's health, protection, and well-being. There are now 750,000 men and women wearing the EMS uniform laboring among our people to provide 24-hour care in the streets and in every nook that comprises the infrastructure of our complex society. For each of us, the retrospectroscope produces a discrete view of one small portion of the tapestry that EMS has been and is becoming. None of us enfolds the entire picture in our EMS mind. It remains important for us to realize whence we have come and by what route we have arrived so that we learn from the past. To fill in the details of the "big picture" of where we have been is one reason to embark upon this second edition.

To reflect upon how quickly scientific endeavor and application of technology have escorted change into our practice, consider the following observations. Thrombolytic therapy for stroke, once only a glimmer in the eye of the visionary neurologists, is now applied to certain identified subsets of stroke victims mandating that EMS providers recognize the signs and symptoms of potential stroke and then carry out an expeditious transfer to a capably equipped institution, which is able to obtain a head CT quickly and administer thrombolysis within the currently recommended 3-hour limit from onset of symptoms. The "stroke team" is now becoming more routine and brings rapid diagnosis and intervention as an expectation to the health care system for many stroke victims.

Hazardous materials management, always important to the paramedic, has acquired a deserved urgency and national ascendancy with the increasing threats of chemical and biological terrorism. Paramedic, police, fire, and emergency department services form the frontline of diagnosis and treatment for these events. The ability to recognize and address the possibility of a "chembio" exposure early in the event may save many lives.

Significant progress has occurred in the area of documentation of the prehospital medical record, but we are just now approaching the era of on-line, computer-generated charting. We will soon be empowered by immediate access to individual patient information in ways never before possible. When computer-generated records become widely available, outcome-based analysis of the EMS provider's practice will allow more focused and effective continuing education.

But changes in technology and therapy may be less profound than changes in the social aspects of health care. The transformation in how health care is delivered in this country impacts all health care professionals ethically, legally, and financially. These changes may have very profound effects on the role of the paramedic. In many places, paramedics "greet and treat" patients in their home without ever transporting the patient to the hospital, thus taking on a greater burden of medicolegal and ethical responsibility. Paramedics have also begun to fill a void as hospital-based providers of care. In this role, the paramedic often performs the function of triage evaluation and may initiate various diagnostic and treatment protocols. The scope and function of the paramedic is changing.

Mosby's Paramedic Textbook, 2ⁿᵈ Edition reflects the changes in the Department of Transportation National Standard Curriculum for EMT-Paramedic, but it reaches far beyond the strict requirements of that document. The text reflects a level of sophistication and professionalism for which we are very grateful and proud. We believe it to be the most complete, single reference source in the field and use it as a reference for emergency medicine residents and physicians as well. Whether you are a paramedic student or a seasoned veteran, *Mosby's Paramedic Textbook, 2ⁿᵈ Edition* continues to set the standard for excellence and should be a part of every paramedic's library. We hope and strongly believe that you will use it often. What better time to launch for the future than your first year of the new millennium?

Lawrence M. Lewis, MD FACEP
Gary Quick, MD, FACEP

Foreword

Emergency medical services is the modern way of obtaining help for the victim of a sudden illness or traumatic injury. Since the inception of EMS in the 1970s, the complexity and sophistication of these vital services have expanded rapidly. The 1980s were a time of growth and maturation for EMS providers. New skills, such as cardiac pacing, intraosseous infusion, and advanced airway techniques, were added to the repertoire and toolboxes of the early EMS providers. The 1990s was the decade of technological explosion, implementation of sophisticated patient monitoring systems, and advanced communications and transportation systems. Advanced treatments delivered in the prehospital setting for debilitating diseases, such as stroke and heart attack, changed the outcome of these devastating events for thousands of people.

Today, paramedics face the call for help armed with highly technical equipment, advanced pharmacological agents, and vast communications and transportation systems that could only be viewed as science fiction in the 1970s. Virtual hospitals, telehome care, Internet health care sites, and access to telemedicine exist in limited areas today but will probably be the norm in the next decade. Demands for timely and effective out-of-hospital care by a population better educated in every aspect of health care will force changes in all areas of our current EMS systems, including the providers, the types of services available, and the distribution of every type of resource needed to run an EMS system.

In the journey ahead, EMS will undergo a revolution. To date, this revolution in technology and knowledge has led to an expansion in the scope and complexity of the U.S. Department of Transportation's EMT-Paramedic national standard curriculum. The educational preparation needed to meet the roles and responsibilities of today's paramedic is becoming increasingly sophisticated, compared to what was required of our predecessors of the 1970s. The demand for an increase in our knowledge and competencies has in turn linked the professional paramedic to the health care education setting—the days of "on-the-job" training have passed. The EMS educational experience must facilitate the integration of the reality of "street practice" with the expanded educational preparation required of the paramedic.

The second edition of *Mosby's Paramedic Textbook* is the ideal source to facilitate the integration of "book knowledge" and "street practice." It is based on the 1998 national standard paramedic curriculum and is an excellent source of information. The textbook is appropriate and suitable for use in the primary classroom setting and also to bring the experienced EMS provider "up to the minute" with the latest information regarding prehospital emergency care. Areas of anatomy, physiology, and pathophysiology required to understand complex illness and injury have been expanded and cover both customary and fresh topics. Woven into the text is the author's well-thought-out rationale for how the new information included in the revised curriculum will assist paramedics as they become part of the EMS team.

As a professional educator, I know that each student learns in a different manner. However, it is a well-accepted tenet that the more senses involved in the learning process—the more likely it is that learning will take place. The innovative design of the second edition of *Mosby's Paramedic Textbook* is coupled with the latest in computer and interactive learning technologies to form a complete learning experience. Accompanying ancillaries include CD-ROM presentations, color slides, and Internet support to assist the students as they advance through the well-organized text. Practice examinations and case scenarios are provided to help both the instructor and student in bridging the gap between classroom experience and the world of work experience. Mick J. Sanders has taken his years of experience as a paramedic, educator, and author and brought together a text that will serve as a benchmark for excellence in paramedic education.

The promise of the future in EMS is exciting—fundamental changes, driven by new technology and medical advances, will occur. With these changes comes the opportunity for fulfillment in one of the most rewarding health care professions: EMS. For those of you willing to commit your talent, compassion, and experience to the tasks associated with completing the paramedic education program, an exciting and rewarding career awaits you.

Judith A. Ruple, PhD, RN, NREMT-P
Associate Professor
College of Health and Human Services
The University of Toledo
Toledo, Ohio

Foreword

A student walked into my office the other day and asked me a question I have answered many times before. "Which paramedic book is the best choice for me to use as I study for my refresher course?" In an automatic motion, I went to my bookshelf and pulled down the first edition of *Mosby's Paramedic Textbook*. I answered with my usual response, citing the strengths of the book compared to the others available. After copying the title and author, the student thanked me and left my office to go to class.

After she left, I pondered my response. Why is it that I automatically recommend Mick Sanders' book to anyone who asks? Is it because I have many friends who were involved in the process, and I have known the author since I started in this field many years ago? Is it because I have such great respect for Mick and his incredible knowledge of the EMS field? Is it because I was a reviewer for the workbook before publication? Is it because the book has been our primary text for the paramedic program since it was published?

Well, yes. But that alone isn't enough to get my recommendation. There has to be more than association. There has to be quality, accuracy, and something deep down that goes beyond just being a good book.

In today's changing world of EMS, being "good" just isn't enough. Do you know anybody who works hard to be "average," who strives to be called "adequate," who yearns to be told "Your medical performance during that clinical save was 'sufficient'?" If you needed advanced medical care, would you look around for someone who did the minimum required, or would you search for the most qualified, experienced, and excellent provider available? You wouldn't settle for anything less. When you go to work as an EMT, a nurse, a paramedic, do you not strive to provide excellent care to those whose lives you touch?

As I reviewed the chapters for this edition of the textbook, one theme came across as I pored over each page. Excellence. As chapters were rewritten and revised, that theme remained. Excellence. It needs to be a word in our daily vocabulary in EMS.

As our profession grows, so too must our body of knowledge. As reflected in the new D.O.T. guidelines, the EMS Education Agenda for the Future, and the National EMS Education and Practice Blueprint, more is being required from us as EMS professionals, both in knowledge base and in functional problem-solving ability. We must be able to *think*, and we must equally be able to *do*.

In order to be able to do our jobs both today and in the future, we need the tools to help us achieve excellence. But functioning equipment and state-of-the-art technology only meet half of our needs. A house built on a foundation of sand soon crumbles, while the house built on rock will withstand a thousand storms. In your hands, you hold the rock. The foundation of your education as a paramedic. The tool to fill in the gaps and to enhance an already strong foundation. This book is solid. It is complete. It is accurate. But more importantly, it is excellent.

In these pages, you, the student, will find a thorough discussion of every aspect of prehospital care presented in a logical, readable format. The objectives and chapter summaries will help you study, and the verbal and pictorial illustrations will help you understand. You, the instructor, will find not only a superb tool for your students, you will notice that this book follows and often, enhances, the latest D.O.T. curriculum and is very easy to work with as you teach. My initial anxieties about teaching the new curriculum vanished into thin air as I read through the pages of this text. This book has been the standard for paramedic education, and this second edition continues in that tradition of excellence.

I was excited when I read through the new T-method in Chapter 9. Mick's thoughtful consideration of students' math challenges has led to his creation of a new method for dosage calculations. To me, this is one more example of his dedication to quality in prehospital education, a commitment which he makes very seriously. In your hands rests the most excellent source of paramedic core material that is available today, a work I am proud to have been affiliated with.

This book took over 20 years in the making, as Mick Sanders brings his extensive background in EMS to the pages of this text. It is the culmination of his years as provider, educator, administrator, and writer. It is his personal commitment to excellence in prehospital care. I challenge you, the reader, to commit yourself likewise to excellence in whatever you choose to do, whether EMS is your career or avocation. You would want only the best EMS providers caring for you. Go and do likewise. Be the best. Be excellent!

Janet Fitts, RN, BSN, CEN, EMT-P
EMS Coordinator
East Central College
Union, Missouri

Preface

A revision to the 1978 Department of Transportation's National Standard Curriculum for EMT-Paramedic was a long time coming. For more than 20 years, paramedic instructors have had the hard task of augmenting the original curriculum to match the educational needs of paramedics—a profession that has changed in scope and practice at an unprecedented rate. The second edition of *Mosby's Paramedic Textbook* is a *single* and *complete* textbook that reflects and enhances the content of the new curriculum. It's all here in *one* book, and it's the *only* textbook the paramedic student will need to prepare for a career in EMS.

The second edition of *Mosby's Paramedic Textbook* was designed with today's paramedic student in mind—a student who can meet the educational demands of a profession that requires knowledge in anatomy and physiology, mathematics, pharmacology, advanced education in the health sciences, and physical skills in using highly technical and sophisticated equipment. In addition to academics and "hands-on" patient care, the textbook recognizes the importance of a paramedic who is always aware of personal safety; who realizes the value of caring for the emotional as well as the physical needs of a patient; who is involved in research, community education, and injury prevention; and who can make wise "street" judgments and appropriate life-and-death decisions in a split second. This describes today's paramedic—a member of a unique profession composed of highly-trained individuals dedicated to making a difference in people's lives.

Content and Organization

The second edition of *Mosby's Paramedic Textbook* has been extensively reviewed by physicians, nurses, paramedics, educators, and national and international experts in the field of emergency care—people who know and value the important role of the paramedic in health care delivery. The text follows the organization of the new curriculum, and meets *every* cognitive objective as defined by the Department of Transportation.

Like the curriculum, the textbook is divided into eight divisions. Division One explains the paramedic's role and the unique aspects of the profession, such as an overview of EMS systems, the importance of personal well-being, and an introduction to ethics and medical/legal issues. This division also introduces the paramedic student to general principles of pathophysiology, pharmacology, and medication administration, and the value of therapeutic communications in patient care. Division Two is devoted to basic and advanced methods of airway management and ventilation. Division Three focuses on patient assessment, including techniques of physical examination, clinical decision making, and the importance of documentation. Division Four is a thorough presentation of trauma, soft tissue injuries, and burns. Division Five addresses the many types of medical conditions that can lead to a medical emergency, including respiratory and cardiovascular emergencies, allergies and anaphylaxis, toxicology, and environmental conditions. This division also includes separate chapters on gastroenterology, hematology, behavioral and psychiatric disorders, gynecology, and obstetrics. Division Six describes special considerations for select patient groups, such as neonates, pediatrics, and geriatrics. It also addresses the needs of patients with special challenges, those who have been victims of abuse and neglect, and home care patients who may require acute interventions. Division Seven describes assessment based management and how to integrate treatment plans for patient care. And finally, Division Eight deals with the various aspects of advanced EMS systems, such as ambulance operations, medical incident command, rescue, Hazmat, and crime scene awareness. The textbook also is accompanied by a student workbook to help measure understanding of the core material.

Each chapter of the second edition of *Mosby's Paramedic Textbook* begins with an introduction and a list of objectives that provide an overview of the material to be presented. This allows the student to review the content and progression of each chapter in an easy-to-follow format. Key terms are included to highlight terminology and concepts critical to providing emergency care. Each chapter concludes with a bulleted summary that reviews the most important material presented in the chapter and references that can be used as a resource for supplemental reading. The second edition of *Mosby's Paramedic Textbook* also includes the following features that help make this textbook a leader in EMS education:

- Overview of Human Systems Chapter. An overview of human anatomy and physiology is presented early in the textbook. This chapter is an easily located reference to anatomical structures and their functions that can be reviewed throughout the course of study.
- Emergency Drug Index. The Emergency Drug Index (EDI) details specific information on more than 60 emergency drugs. It provides a quick source of reference for a drug's description, onset and duration, indications, contraindications, adverse reactions, drug interactions, packaging, dosage and administration for adult and pediatric patients, and special considerations. Drugs in the textbook that are found in the EDI are denoted with a bold italic font as a reminder to the reader of their importance and easy location of reference.
- Advanced ECG Rhythm Interpretation. All cardiac rhythms and dysrhythmias are presented in lead I, II, III, and MCL1 to enhance assessment of the cardiac patient. In addition, the text includes advanced electrophysiology, multi-lead ECG monitoring (including 12-lead monitoring), thrombolytic therapy, and current treatment modalities as recommended by the American Heart Association.
- Full-color Illustrations. More than 900 tables, charts, line drawings, and photographs are included in the text to illustrate anatomy, physiology, and patient management guidelines. State-of-the-art equipment and step-by-step demonstrations of practical skills also are presented in full color to demonstrate emergency care procedures.
- Sidebars. Sidebars expand on interesting and relevant information, such as unusual facts and figures, "nice-to-know" data, and "need-to-know" material, such as the rights of terminally ill patients and the possible effects of chemical warfare.
- Canadaian EMS Boxes. Information specific to Canadian EMS has been provided in the chapters to give an overview of education and certification requirements, EMS titles, and important Canadian EMS organizations.

- Critical Thinking Questions. Critical thinking questions are found in each chapter to aid in understanding concepts and how information presented in the text can impact day-to-day activities and "real-life" patient care.
- Box Notes. Box notes are presented in each chapter to highlight vital information and words of warning.
- Tricks of the Trade. Most chapters contain tricks of the trade that help apply technical, patient care information to "street level" practice to emphasize the paramedic's unique role in providing care in the out-of-hospital setting.
- Expanded Glossary. The glossary has been expanded to include definitions on more than 2400 medical terms presented in the textbook chapters.
- Appendix. New additions to the appendix include an easy reference table to map life-span development, a section on the origin of medical terminology, a detailed discussion of injury prevention and prevention strategies, a history of Canadian EMS, a listing of U.S. and Canadian EMS websites, and a bibliography of the information sources used to develop the new paramedic curriculum.
- Index. The thorough and detailed index makes it easy to find information that was presented in the text.

Finally, we chose to again include the division opener vignettes—a carry-over from the first edition. These portraits and quotations from paramedics around the United States and Canada are meant to illustrate a concept that lies at the very heart of this book: Behind all the high-tech equipment, the standards and protocols that guide our profession, and the quick, efficient skills that mark our patient care are *real people*—like you, who have chosen an important career that will make a difference in people's lives.

I hope reading this preface reinforces the decision you made to choose this textbook. Whether you're a paramedic student, practicing paramedic, nurse, administrator, or educator, I think you will find this textbook to be a valuable EMS resource.

Mick J. Sanders

Author Acknowledgments

Like the first edition of *Mosby's Paramedic Textbook*, the second edition resulted from the combined efforts of many talented individuals. In addition to my physician advisers, Larry Lewis and Gary Quick, and the many experts who reviewed the manuscript, I would like to make special note of the following people who helped to make this textbook possible:

Kim McKenna, RN, BSN, CEN, EMT-P, whose knowledge, expertise, and emotional support helped me bring this project to completion. She's been a colleague, a friend, a contributor, and a "can't-do-without" partner since the first edition of the text. She's the BEST!

Claire Merrick, executive editor, who over the years has become a good friend and ally. Writing a textbook is always a learning experience. Her insight, support, and sense of humor were invaluable in dealing with the complexities of this project.

Elaine Steinborn, developmental editor, who brought it all together and "made it happen." Her organization and attention to detail are reflected on every page of this text. I'm not sure how she found all the missing pieces but she did, and Kim and I are grateful for her involvement.

Rich Barber, senior production editor, whose patience, persistence, and low-key approach helped keep Kim and me sane and focused on the importance of the final product. Kim and I appreciate this opportunity to thank him.

Barb Aehlert, RN, for her excellent work on the ancillaries. Her experience as an author and educator, and her expertise were assets to the text.

Janice Ritchie Saia, RN, EMT-P, for her valuable review and input on Chapter 28.

Catherine Parvenski Barwell, for her review and contributions to the ancillaries.

Yavilah McCoy, who made sure the review process was complete. Her commitment to excellence, and her personal interest in this textbook will always be appreciated.

Derril Trakalo, marketing director, who had the insight and where-with-all to make us see the "big picture." Other "behind-the-scene" people at Mosby who played a major part in this project include Amy Buxton, Lin Dempsey, Jen Etling, Stephanie Foley, Dana Knighten, Tina Kult, Kelly Trakalo, Linda McKinley, Gayle Morris, Lana VanLaningham, and Kellie White. It was their contributions and hard work that enabled this text to be completed.

Janet Fitts, Larry Hatfield, and Rob Thriault for their careful review of the manuscript. Darrell Paranich and Jon King for their contributions to the Appendices. Karen Snyder for her "Tricks of the Trade" boxes. Don McKenna, for his excellent photography. Nadine Sokol, for the beautiful illustrations. Creve Coeur Fire Protection District, Eureka Fire Protection District, St. Louis City EMS, Tom Fitts, Rob Kuchick, Chris Shanks, and St. John's Mercy Medical Center for providing needed equipment and personnel. Models Diane Kaatman, Steve Tooley, Mark Flauter, Chris Arter, Larry Ashby, Tim Dorsey, Rosalyn Golden, Jason Herin, Julie Hull, Sue Lakebrink, Frank Lipski, Mindy McCoy, the McKenna family (Don, Becky, Ginny, Grant, Kim, Maggie, and Bill), Dan Peters, Steve Sanneman, Lance Varga, Joel Vanderploeg, and Monroe Yancie. Kimberly Davanzo, Bobbie Dilworth, Calvin Haupt, John MacLean, Robert McGraw, Melissa Napoli, Sam Thurmond, and Alberto Vazquez for providing portraits and quotes of "real life" paramedics. Also important to this project were the many EMS and fire agencies, physicians, hospitals, and equipment manufacturers who supplied emergency scene photos and illustrations to accompany the text (especially Larry Ashby, William Greenblatt, Ronald Olshwanger, James Silvernail, and Monroe Yancie).

I also want to thank those people who were instrumental in the success of the first edition, and for their contributions that carried over to this edition, especially Nancy Peterson, Mark Weiber, and Julie Long.

Finally, I want to mention a few people who were my "saving grace" during the many months I worked on this project: Dixie Allen (my mother), Ruby Hagood (my grandmother), Randy Sanders (my brother), and Will Denney (a great friend). I couldn't have done it without their personal interest and support.

Mick J. Sanders

Publisher Acknowledgments

The editors wish to acknowledge and thank the many reviewers of this book, who devoted countless hours to intensive review. Their comments were invaluable in helping develop and fine tune the revision of this textbook.

Organizations and individuals who took part in this extensive project were:

Joseph J. Acker, AHT, EMT-P
Northern Alberta Institute of Technology
Edmonton, Alberta, Canada

Richard Alcorta, MD, FACEP
State EMS Medical Director, MIEMSS
Surburban Hospital
Bethesda, Maryland

Chandra Aubin, MD
Emergency Medicine
Washington University School of Medicine/
    Barnes-Jewish Hospital
St. Louis, Missouri
(Chapter 35)

Alan J. Azzara, Esq, BA, JD, EMT-P
Quality Assurance Coordinator
North East Mobile Health Services
Topsham, Maine

Catherine A. Parvensky Barwell, RN/EMT-P, M.Ed.
College of Arts and Sciences
MCP Hahnemann University
Philadelphia, Pennsylvania

James P. Boedeker, MD
Assistant Clinical Professor
Department of Obstetrics and Gynecology
St. Louis University Medical School
St. Louis, Missouri

William Brandes
Fire Chief
Creve Coeur Fire Protection District
Creve Coeur, Missouri

David H. Brisson, RN, EMCA
Algonquin College
Ottawa, Ontario, Canada

Lawrence R. Brown, MD, PhD
Department of Emergency Medicine
Missouri Baptist Medical Center and
Washington University School of Medicine/
    Barnes-Jewish Hospital
St. Louis, Missouri

Roy Edward Cox, Jr., M.Ed., EMT-P
City of Pittsburgh Bureau of Emergency
    Medical Services
Pittsburgh, Pennsylvania

Kevin Cunningham, BS, EMT-P
Stamford Hospital
Stamford, Connecticut

John Czajkowski
Transportation Rescue Consultants, Inc.
Orlando, Florida

Heather Micholene Davis, MS, NREMT-P
UCLA-Daniel Freeman Hospital Paramedic
    Education
Inglewood, California

Jeff G. DeGraffenreid, M.Ed., Paramedic
Johnson County Medical Action Emergency
    Medical Services
Johnson County, Kansas

William H. Dribben, MD
Washington University School of Medicine/
    Barnes-Jewish Hospital
St. Louis, Missouri

William J. Dunne, MS, NREMT-P
UCLA Center for Prehospital Care
UCLA-Daniel Freeman Paramedic Education
    Program
Los Angeles, California

Lisa Susan Etzwiler, MD, FAAP
Director of Pediatric Emergency Services
St. Johns Mercy Medical Center
Assistant Clinical Professor of Pediatrics
St. Louis University School of Medicine
St. Louis, Missouri

Daryl Eustace
Director of EMS Education
Wallace State Community College
Hanceville, Alabama

Edward Ferguson, MD
Emergency Medicine
Washington University School of Medicine/
    Barnes-Jewish Hospital
St. Louis, Missouri
(Chapter 43)

Janet Fitts, RN, BSN, CEN, EMT-P
EMS Coordinator
East Central College
Union, Missouri

Ken Fowke, BSc, EMA-II
Paramedic Instructor
Algonquin College of Applied Arts and Sciences
Ottawa, Ontario, Canada

Timothy Gridley
Unit Hour Utilization Manager
MAST Ambulance
Kansas City, Missouri

Larry Hatfield
Creighton University
Omaha, Nebraska

Shirley A. Jones, MS Ed. MHA, EMT-P
Clarian Health Hospital
Indianapolis, Indiana

Antoinette Kanne, RN, MS
Trauma Coordinator
St. John's Mercy Medical Center
St Louis, Missouri

Lisa Keenly, MD
Emergency Medicine
Washington University School of Medicine/
    Barnes-Jewish Hospital
St. Louis, Missouri
(Chapter 27)

Anthony C. Kessels
Clinical Pharmacist
Barnes-Jewish Hospital
(Chapter 8)

J. Steven Kidd
Transportation Rescue Consultants, Inc.
Orlando, Florida

Jeffrey Levine, MD, FACS
Trauma Surgeon
St. John's Mercy Medical Center
St. Louis, Missouri

James Linardos, MS, EMT-I
Fire Chief, North Lake Tahoe Protection District
Lake Tahoe, Nevada

Michael Mullins, MD
Emergency Medicine
Washington University School of Medicine/
    Barnes-Jewish Hospital
St. Louis, Missouri
(Chapter 51)

Scott Mullins
Battalion Chief
Eureka Fire Protection District
Eureka, Missouri

Robert E. O'Connor, MD, MPH
Residency Program Director
Department of Emergency Medicine
Christiana Care Health System
Newark, Delaware

Nathan Piemann, MD
Emergency Medicine
Washington University School of Medicine/
Barnes-Jewish Hospital
St. Louis, Missouri
(Chapters 34, 46)

Denise S. Pope, RN, MSN, BSN, MSN
Instructor, Division of Nursing, College
    of Pharmacy
Nursing and Allied Health Sciences
Howard University
Washington, D.C.

John Eric Powell, MS, NREMT-P
Flight Paramedic
UT-Lifestar Aeromedical Service
University of Tennessee Medical Center-Knoxville
Roane State Community College
Knoxville, Tennessee

Chris Richter, MD
Emergency Medicine
Washington University School of Medicine/
    Barnes-Jewish Hospital
St. Louis, Missouri
(Chapter 8)

Becky Ridenhour, PharmD
St. Louis College of Pharmacy
St. Louis, Missouri

Cleeve Robertson, MD
Principal, Ambulance Training College
Provincial Administration of the Western Cape
South Africa

S. Rutherford Rose, PharmD, FAACT
Associate Professor of Emergency Medicine
Director, Virginia Poison Center
Medical College of Virginia Hospitals
Virginia Commonwealth University
Richmond, Virginia

Stanley Sakabu, MD, FACS
Associate Director, Trauma Service
St. John's Mercy Medical Center
St. Louis, Missouri

Robert J. Schappert III
Maryland Fire and Rescue Institute
University of Maryland
College Park, Maryland

Roberta J. Secrest, PhD, PharmD
Scientist/Manager
U.S. Medical Research
Hoechst Marion Roussel
Kansas City, Missouri

Sharon Smith, MD
Emergency Medicine
St. Louis Children's Hospital
St. Louis, Missouri
(Chapter 42)

Karen Snyder
University Hospital
Cincinnati, Ohio

Andrew W. Stern, NREMT-P, MPA, MA
Senior Paramedic and Flightmedic
Colonie Emergency Medical Services
Colonie, New York

Gail Stewart, BS, EMT-P, CHES
Educational Director
Florida Association of Professional EMTs
    and Paramedics
Tallahassee, Florida

Robert Thieriault, RCT (Adv.), CCP (F)
Registered Cardiology Technologist
Critical Care Flight Paramedic
The Michener Institute for Applied Health Sciences
Toronto, Ontario, Canada

Eric Thompson, MD
Emergency Medicine
Washington University School of Medicine/
    Barnes-Jewish Hospital
St. Louis, Missouri
(Chapter 28)

Bryan Troop, MD, FACS, FCCM
Director, Trauma Service
St. John's Mercy Medical Center
St. Louis, Missouri

Christina Wagner, MD
Emergency Medicine
Washington University School of Medicine/
    Barnes-Jewish Hospital
St. Louis, Missouri
(Chapter 41)

Bruce J. Walz, PhD
Department of Emergency Health Services
University of Maryland, Baltimore County
Baltimore, Maryland

Roxanne Ward, RN
Project Manager, HyP-HIT Study
Childrens Hospital of Eastern Ontario
    Research Institute
Woodlawn, Ontario, Canada

A. Keith Wesley, MD, FACEP
Sacred Heart Hospital
Eau Claire, Wisconsin

Brian S. Zachariah, MD, MBA
Emergency Department Medical Director
Los Colines Medical Center
President, The Prehospital Care Group
Dallas, Texas

And we offer a special thanks to those who helped on the first edition: National Association of EMTs Society of Paramedics Instructor/Coordinators Society; National Council of State EMS Training Coordinators; National Association of EMS Physicians; Thomas F. Anderson, PhD, RRT; Doug Austin, Jr.; Vatche H. Ayvazian, MD; John Barrett, MD; David S. Becker; John E. Blue, II, EMT-P, BS; Chip Boehm, RN, EMT-P; Kevin Brown, MD, MPH; Jeffrey A. Crill, RN, EMT-P; David DaBell, MD; Alice "Twink" Dalton; Theodore R. Delbridge, MD; Linda D. Dodge; Robert Elling, MPA, NREMT-P; Franklin E.Foster, JD; Bill Garcia, MICP; Mike Gray; Janet A. Head, RN, MS; Kenneth Hines; Steven Kidd; Mark A. Kirk, MD; Kevin Kraus, BS, EMT-P; Richard A. Lazar; Mark Lockhart, NREMT-P; Julie Long; Glenn H. Luedtke, NREMT-P; Mary Beth Michos, RN; Gary P. Morris; Keith Neely, EMT-P, MPA; Gregory Noll; Michael P. Peppers, PharmD; Dwight Polk, BA, NREMT-P; William Raynovich; Lou E. Romig, MD, FAAP; José V. Aalazar, BA, NREMT; Randy L. Sanders; Carol J. Shanaberger; JoAnn Shew, RN, CS, MSN; John Sinclair; Todd M. Stanford, BS, PA-C, MICP; Andrew W. Stern, NREMT-P, MPA; Mike Taigman; Vickie H. Taylor; Michael W. Turner; Patricia L. Westbrook, MS, CCC; Jason T. White; Sherrie C. Wilson, EMT-P, I/C; Monroe Yancie, NREMT-P; and Rodney C. Zerr.

Contents

Division One ——→

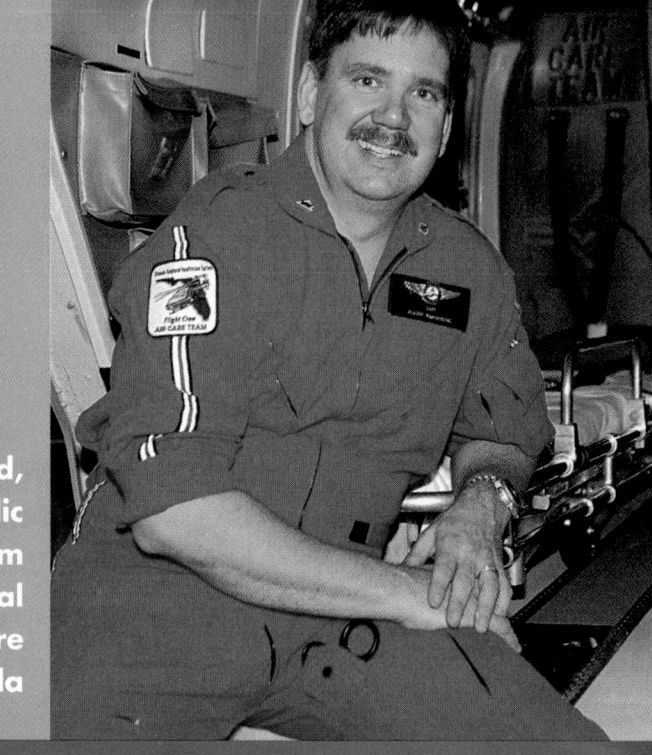

**Sam Thurmond,
Flight Paramedic
Air Care Team
Orlando Regional
Healthcare
Orlando, Florida**

"The most rewarding thing about being a paramedic is that everything you do is different. Days are never the same. You are always learning something and, every now and then, you get to make a difference."

Preparatory

IN THIS DIVISION

1 EMS Systems: Roles and Responsibilities

OBJECTIVES

Upon completion of this chapter, the paramedic student will be able to:

1. **Outline** key historical events that influenced the development of emergency medical services (EMS) systems.
2. **Identify** the key elements necessary for effective EMS systems operations.
3. **Differentiate** among training and roles and responsibilities of the four nationally recognized levels of EMS licensure/certification: first responder, EMT-Basic, EMT-Intermediate, and EMT-Paramedic.
4. **List** the benefits of membership in professional EMS organizations.
5. **Describe** the benefits of continuing education.
6. **Differentiate** among professionalism and professional licensure, certification, and registration.
7. **Describe** the paramedic's role in a patient care situation as defined by the U.S. Department of Transportation.
8. **Describe** the benefits of each component of off-line (indirect) and on-line (direct) medical direction.
9. **Outline** the role and components of an effective, continuous quality improvement program.
10. **Identify** the key components of prehospital research and its benefits to the EMS system.
11. **Describe** how to address ethical considerations related to research.

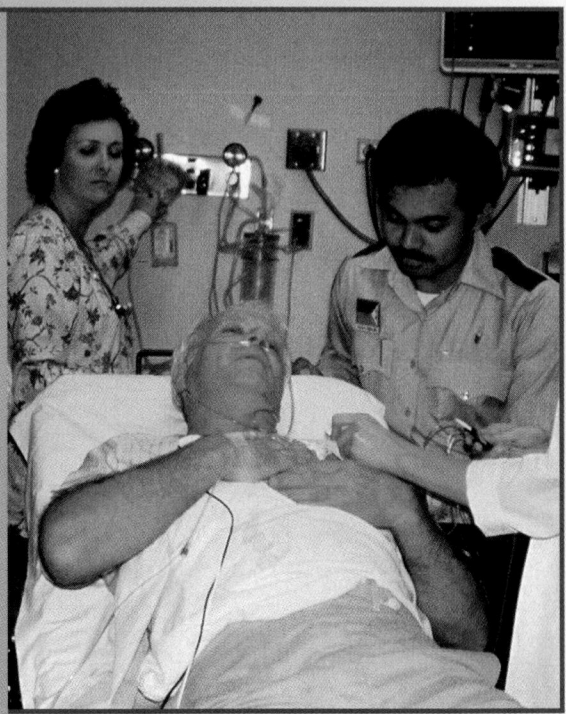

The role of the emergency medical technician–paramedic (**EMT-Paramedic**, or EMT-P) is different than that of the "ambulance driver" of the past. By comparison, today's paramedics work in sophisticated **emergency medical services** (EMS) systems. They are engaged in a variety of professional activities that enhance their ability to provide quality service and state-of-the-art patient care in the field and in less traditional health care settings where skills and knowledge of paramedics can be used.

KEY TERMS

advanced life support: The provision of care that paramedics or allied health professionals render, including advanced airway management, defibrillation, intravenous therapy, and medication administration.

basic life support: Care provided by persons trained in first aid, cardiopulmonary resuscitation, and other noninvasive care.

capitation: A method of payment to cover all health care expenses for each member of a managed care organization.

continuous quality improvement: A management approach to customer service and organizational performance that includes constant monitoring, evaluation, decisions, and actions.

emergency medical services: A national network of services coordinated to provide aid and medical assistance from primary response to definitive care; it involves personnel trained in rescue, stabilization, transportation, and advanced management of traumatic and medical emergencies.

EMT-Paramedic: A person who has completed training based on the *EMT-Paramedic National Standard Curriculum*, including advanced training in patient assessment, cardiac rhythm interpretation, defibrillation, drug therapy, and airway management.

extended scope of practice: The expansion of preventive health care services provided by EMTs and paramedics in the prehospital setting.

managed care organizations: Networks that provide patient care services to their members, including health maintenance organizations (HMOs) and preferred provider organizations (PPOs).

off-line (indirect) medical direction: The establishment and monitoring of all medical components of an EMS system, including protocols, standing orders, educational programs, and the quality and delivery of on-line (direct) medical direction.

on-line (direct) medical direction: The medical direction physician or designee who directly supervises prehospital care activities via radio or phone. On-line (direct) medical direction also is responsible for the activities of the emergency department staff and other designated physicians at the medical direction hospital.

reciprocity: The practice of granting an individual licensure or certification/registration based on licensure or certification/registration by another state, agency, or association.

standing orders: Specific treatment protocols that can be used by prehospital emergency care providers in the absence of on-line (direct) medical direction when delay in treatment would harm the patient.

treatment protocols: Guidelines that define the scope of prehospital intervention practiced by emergency care providers.

EMS System Development

Assignment of a specific time and place to the birth of organized prehospital emergency care is difficult. To understand EMS system development, one must consider events from ancient times to the present.

Before the Twentieth Century

Ancient writings indicate that regulation of the practice of medicine dates as far back as 1700 B.C. (see box on p. 4) in the civilizations of Mesopotamia, an ancient region of southwest Asia.[1] Medical documents, like the Edwin Smith papyrus of about the seventeenth century B.C., describe an instructional system of medical practice and reference the pulsation of the heart, palpation, and abnormal motor functions associated with brain injury.

Organized prehospital emergency care seems to have its roots in military history. Paintings of Roman battlegrounds suggest that certain warriors were charged with caring for the injured. The first "ambulance" is believed to have been a covered cart used by Jean Larry (one of Napoleon's surgeons) to transport wounded soldiers to treatment areas during the Napoleonic wars in the 1800s.[1] Clara Barton, an American nurse during the Civil War, coordinated emergency care services for the wounded and brought the American Red Cross (a Swiss organization) to the United States in 1905. The first civilian ambulance services were established in Cincinnati and New York City in the 1860s.

Twentieth Century

Medical care progressed rapidly during World War I, when it was necessary to care for soldiers who

CODE OF HAMMURABI (1700 B.C.)

- If a doctor has treated a freeman with a metal knife for a severe wound, and has cured the freeman, or has opened a freeman's tumor with a metal knife, and cured a freeman's eye, then he shall receive 10 shekels of silver.
- If the son of a plebeian, he shall receive five shekels of silver.
- If a man's slave, the owner of the slave shall give two shekels of silver to the doctor.
- If a doctor has treated a man with a metal knife for a severe wound, and has caused the man to die, or has opened a man's tumor with a metal knife and destroyed the man's eye, his hands shall be cut off.
- If the doctor has treated the slave of a plebeian with a metal knife for a severe wound and caused him to die, he shall render slave for slave.
- If he has opened his tumor with a metal knife and destroyed his eye, he shall pay half his price in silver.
- If a doctor has healed a freeman's broken bone or has restored diseased flesh, the patient shall give the doctor five shekels of silver.
- If he be the son of a plebeian, he shall give three shekels of silver.
- If a man's slave, the owner of the slave shall give two shekels of silver to the doctor.
- If a doctor of oxen or asses has treated either ox or ass for a severe wound, and cured it, the owner of the ox or ass shall give to the doctor one sixth of a shekel of silver as his fee.

were wounded by machine guns and massive bombardment. The military developed battlefield ambulance corps during this time. The military established air medical transportation systems during World War II and used helicopters to evacuate wounded soldiers during the Korean conflict. During Vietnam the military further expanded immediate care and rapid evacuation by well-trained corpsmen. These military efforts to care for wounded soldiers became the basis of current prehospital emergency care.

Through most of the early twentieth century and through the mid-1960s, urban hospital-based systems that later developed into municipal services, and funeral directors and volunteers untrained in emergency care provided prehospital care in the

United States. Most patients received only minimal stabilization at the scene and were hurriedly transported to the nearest hospital

? CRITICAL THINKING

How would you feel about moving to an area with this minimal level of EMS service?

Two landmarks in EMS development occurred in 1966:

1. The National Academy of Sciences–National Research Council's (NAS–NRC) Committee on Trauma and Shock published *Accidental Death and Disability: The Neglected Disease of Modern Society* (the "white" paper). This document provides a series of recommendations to improve care for injured victims, 11 of which were directly related to EMS (Box 1-1).
2. The U.S. Congress passed the Highway Safety Act of 1966. This act created the U.S. Department of Transportation (USDOT) and the National Highway Traffic Safety Administration (NHTSA) and provided legislative authority and financial assistance to improve EMS. The Highway Safety Act of 1966 directed states to develop an effective EMS program or be subject to loss of up to 10% of their federal highway construction funds. As a result of this act, states disbursed more than $142 million between 1968 and 1979 for the development of EMS and early **advanced life support** (ALS) pilot programs.

Early mortality rate comparisons from World War I to the Vietnam conflict also were an impetus for EMS to emerge as a nationwide system. Death rates for battlefield casualties were 8% in World War I, 4.5% in World War II, 2.5% in Korea, and less than 2% in Vietnam. This decline was due to advances in field care for trauma patients.[2] These and other factors helped formulate the blueprint for improving prehospital emergency medical care in the United States. During 1972 and 1973, federal and private sources provided $31 million to fund EMS programs in 37 states and Puerto Rico.

In 1973, Congress passed the Emergency Medical Service Systems (EMSS) Act and paved the way for states to benefit from federal funds by developing regional EMS organizations. This act identified 15

BOX 1-1

ELEVEN RECOMMENDATIONS FOR EMS IDENTIFIED IN THE WHITE PAPER

1. Extension of basic and advanced first aid training to greater numbers of the lay public
2. Preparation of nationally acceptable texts, training aids, and courses of instruction for rescue squad personnel, policeman, fireman, and ambulance attendants
3. Implementation of recent traffic safety legislation to ensure completely adequate standards for ambulance design and construction, ambulance equipment and supplies, and the qualifications and supervision of ambulance personnel
4. Adoption at the state level of general policies and regulations pertaining to ambulance services
5. Adoption at district, county, and municipal levels of ways and means of providing ambulance services applicable to the conditions of the locality, control and surveillance of ambulance services, and coordination of ambulance services with health departments, hospitals, traffic authorities, and communication services
6. Initiation of pilot programs to determine the efficacy of providing physician-staffed ambulances for care at the site of injury and during transportation
7. Initiation of pilot programs to evaluate automotive and helicopter ambulance services in sparsely populated areas and in regions where many communities lack hospital facilities adequate to care for seriously injured persons
8. Delineation of radio frequency channels and equipment suitable to provide voice communication between ambulances, emergency departments, and other health-related agencies at the community, regional, and national levels
9. Initiation of pilot studies across the nation for evaluation of models of radio and telephone installations to ensure effectiveness of communication facilities
10. Day-to-day use of voice communication facilities by the agencies serving emergency medical needs
11. Active exploration of the feasibility of designating a single nationwide telephone number to summon an ambulance

From National Academy of Sciences, National Research Council: *Accidental death and disability: the neglected disease of modern society,* Washington, DC, 1996, National Academy Press.

required components of the EMS system (Box 1-2) and mandated that emergency medical care programs funded by the U.S. Department of Health and Human Services (USDHHS) plan and implement a regional approach for emergency response and immediate care for trauma patients. This act

CANADIAN EMS STANDARDS

In Canada, the Canadian Health Act and its guiding principles were the impetus for provincial development of universally accepted prehospital care.

? CRITICAL THINKING

How does the "age" of the EMS profession compare with the "age" of your parents' or grandparents' professions?

played a major role in the development of regional EMS systems between 1974 and 1981.

In 1981, funding for EMS development changed with the Consolidated Omnibus Budget Reconciliation Act (COBRA), which consolidated EMS funding into state preventive health services block grants, thereby eliminating funding under the EMSS Act. These block grants were paid directly to state health departments instead of regional EMS organizations. Since these grants could be spent on projects other than EMS, they fell victim to political considerations and direct funding for EMS declined. Through cuts in funding and staff, the NHTSA's ability to support the USDHHS effort diminished. As a result, the responsibility for EMS system development and funding returned to individual states, and the momentous growth that EMS experienced in the 1960s and 1970s began to decline. The NHTSA continues to provide "10 System Elements" (the Statewide EMS Technical Assistance Program) as a recommended standard for EMS systems (Box 1-3). Other landmarks in EMS development are outlined in the box on p. 7.

BOX 1-2

FIFTEEN REQUIRED COMPONENTS OF THE EMS SYSTEM

1. Manpower
2. Training
3. Communications
4. Transportation
5. Facilities
6. Critical care units
7. Public safety agencies
8. Consumers
9. Access to care
10. Transfer of patients
11. Medical record-keeping
12. Consumer information and education
13. Review and evaluation
14. Disaster linkage
15. Mutual aid

BOX 1-3

THE NHTSA'S 10 SYSTEM ELEMENTS

1. Comprehensive EMS and trauma system legislation
2. Resource management and administration
3. Professional training
4. A communication system (911, communication centers, equipment, and the ability to communicate among ambulances, hospitals, fire, and police)
5. A transportation system (air, ground, and water)
6. Facilities (hospitals, trauma centers, specialty centers)
7. An inclusive trauma system fully integrated with EMS
8. Physician involvement (medical oversight)
9. Public information, education, and prevention
10. Data collection, quality improvement and evaluation, and research

From National Highway Traffic Safety Administration: *Emergency medical services: NHTSA leading the way*, Washington, DC, 1995, The Administration.

NOTE

The NHTSA and the Health Resources and Services Administration (HRSA), Maternal Child and Health Bureau, supported *EMS Agenda for the Future*, a federally funded consensus document. The National Association of EMS Physicians (NAEMSP) in conjunction with the National Association of State EMS Directors (NASEMSD) completed the document under contract.[3] They designed the *Agenda* for use by government and private organizations at the national, state, and local levels to help guide planning, decision making, and policy regarding EMS (Fig. 1-1). The *Agenda* recommended continued development of 14 attributes of EMS that focused on principles of public health and safety systems:

1. Integration of health services
2. EMS research
3. Legislation and regulation
4. System finance
5. Human resources
6. Medical direction
7. Education systems
8. Public education
9. Prevention
10. Public access
11. Communication systems
12. Clinical care
13. Information systems
14. Evaluation

CANADIAN EMS STANDARDS

In Canada, organization, funding, and service delivery are unique to each province. Each system is designed based on provincial needs and resources.

Recent developments in federal health care reform have begun to affect paramedics and the way health care, including emergency care, is provided. Most relevant to the EMS industry and to paramedics are the concepts of managed care and **extended scope of practice**. *Managed care* refers to patient care services that are provided to members by **managed care organizations** (MCOs) (e.g., health maintenance organizations [HMOs], preferred provider organizations [PPOs], and other provider networks). These plans, which now cover about 40% of the U.S. population, pay health care providers and some ambulance services a flat sum of money per member per month (PMPM) up front to cover all health care expenses

OTHER LANDMARKS IN THE DEVELOPMENT OF EMS

- 1958: Dr. Peter Safar demonstrates the efficacy of mouth-to-mouth ventilation.
- 1960: Cardiopulmonary resuscitation (CPR) is shown to be efficacious.
- 1967: Dr. Eugene Nagel trains Miami firefighters as "paramedics" at the University of Miami School of Medicine.
- 1968: The American Telephone and Telegraph Company designates "911" as the universal emergency telephone number.
- 1969: The USDOT and NHTSA develop the basic training course for EMTs.
- 1969: The Committee on Ambulance Design develops *Ambulance Design Criteria*, a report to the USDOT and the NHTSA to complement the NAS-NRC's *Medical Requirements for Ambulance Design and Equipment* (1968). This document recommends ambulance design standards and emergency equipment. The NHTSA agrees to issue matching federal funds to states that purchase vehicles meeting these standards.
- 1970: The National Registry of Emergency Medical Technicians (NREMT) is organized to standardize education, examinations, and certification of EMTs on a national level.
- 1972: President Nixon directs the U.S. Department of Health, Education, and Welfare to develop new ways to organize EMS, which results in $8.5 million in contracts being awarded to develop a model EMS system.
- 1972: The University of Cincinnati establishes the first residency program to train new physicians exclusively for the practice of emergency medicine.

- 1973: The "Star of Life" is adopted as the official symbol for EMS.
- 1974: President Gerald Ford proclaims the first National EMS Week.
- 1975: The National Association of Emergency Medical Technicians (NAEMT) is founded.
- 1975: The American Medical Association (AMA) accepts and approves the EMT-Paramedic role as an emergency health occupation.
- 1977: More than 40 EMT training agencies throughout the United States develop and test the national training standards for the paramedic for 2 years.
- 1980: The USDHHS releases the *Position Paper on Trauma Center Designation*, which describes trauma centers within EMS systems. Facilities are also categorized.
- 1984: The EMS for Children program, under the Public Health Act, provides funding for enhancing the EMS system to better serve pediatric patients.
- 1986: The 1979 Public Safety Officer's Act (SB 1479) is amended to expand the $50,000 compensation to include survivors of rescue squads, ambulance crew members, and public safety department volunteers killed in the line of duty (amended in 1990).
- 1990: President George Bush signs the Trauma Care Systems Planning and Development Act (HR 1602), which provides for annual grants to states based on geographical and population size to help establish and improve trauma systems. In 1995, Congress does not reauthorize funding for this act.
- 1991: Occupational Exposure to Blood-Borne Pathogens; Final Rule (CFR 29 1910.1030) establishes standards for workplace protection from blood-borne diseases.

(**capitation**). If patient care expenses are less than the monthly payment received, then the provider keeps the difference. If expenses exceed the monthly payment received, then the provider absorbs the costs. (Other types of reimbursement plans also can be used.) This reform affects EMS systems in the way that they provide patient care choices for their clients (e.g., emergency versus nonemergency response, resources, and personnel; transportation modes; health care facility options) and the type and amount of care provided at the scene for those patients whose condition does not mandate transportation to a hospital for physician evaluation.

NOTE

The federal government's insurance programs (Medicare and Medicaid) have guidelines that determine how patients qualify for EMS transportation and the conditions under which reimbursement for medical transportation will occur.

Extended scope of practice emerged from the cost-containment environment of managed care. As it pertains to EMS, *extended scope of practice* refers to expanding preventive health care services provided by EMTs and paramedics in the prehospital setting

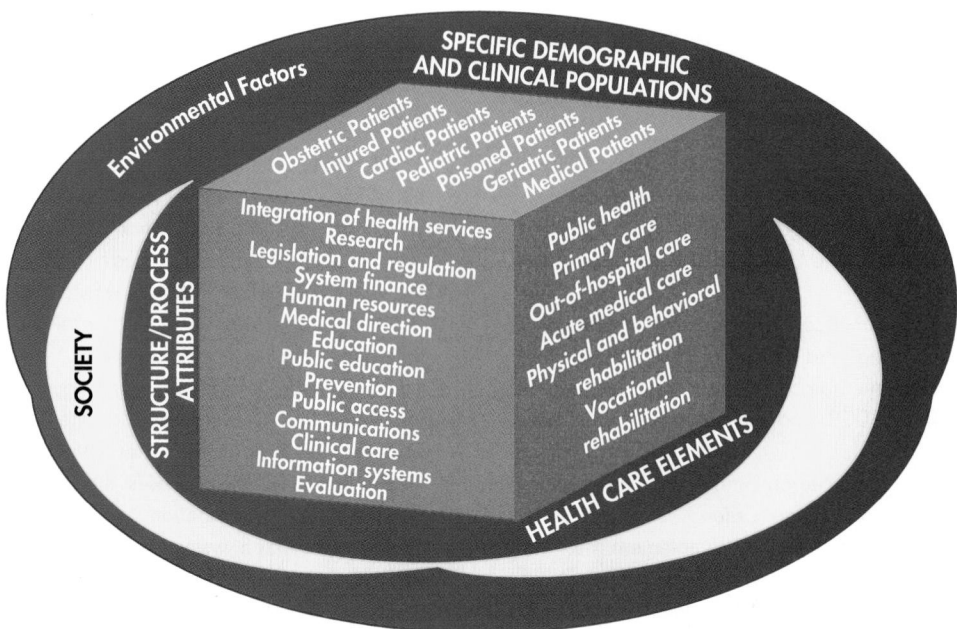

Fig. 1-1 EMS: Part of the health care system. (From National Highway Traffic Safety Administration, US Department of Transportation: *Emergency medical services: NHTSA leading the way,* Washington, DC, 1995, The Administration; accessed at www.nhtsa.dot.gov/people/injury/ems/ agenda/emsman.html#SERVICES.)

(EMS primary care). Examples include performing health screenings and physical examinations, triaging patients to an appropriate level of treatment, performing follow-up examinations, and providing immunizations. This expanded scope is driven not by what paramedics *can* do but rather by what they *should* do within a given system and the availability of other items (e.g., health care resources, transportation times). Expanded scope of practice for EMS providers will most likely continue to evolve as EMS agencies and managed care programs develop additional valuable patient services to enhance revenues, to further injury-prevention education programs, and to reflect changes in how medical care is delivered. Expanded scope also will ensure that EMS survives as a vital component of the health care system.

Current EMS Systems

Today's EMS system is a network of coordinated services that provides aid and medical care to the community. The NHTSA defines these services by the 10 components of the Technical Assistance Program Standards[4] (Fig. 1-2). The coordination of these services ensures that patients are quickly and properly treated and reduces health care costs by making the most efficient use of resources. All of this improves patient outcome and reduces hospital stays.[4]

EMS System Operations

The operations of an effective EMS system include citizen activation, dispatch, prehospital care, hospital care, and rehabilitation.

Citizen Activation

Although emergency public safety services are highly visible in the community, the public generally is not aware of the complexities involved in providing these services. Citizens expect police and fire protection and a quick response with qualified medical personnel when emergency care is needed. These expectations result from a reputation built on years of service, public relations activities, press coverage, and national media attention. Public expectations also arise from financial support in the form of taxes, donations, subscriptions for service, and user fees.

Emergency Medical Services System

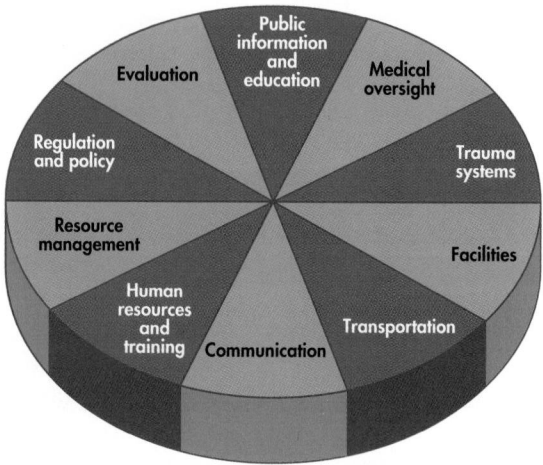

Fig. 1-2 Ten components of the EMS system. (From National Highway Traffic Safety Administration, US Department of Transportation: *Emergency medical services: NHTSA leading the way,* Washington, DC, 1995, The Administration; accessed at www.nhtsa.dot.gov/people/injury/ems/agenda/emsman.html#SERVICES.)

? CRITICAL THINKING

How is the EMS system funded in your community?

The public's involvement in EMS goes beyond funding. Citizens often are at the scene of an accident or illness and play an important role in recognizing the need for emergency services. Citizens sometimes administer first aid, help secure the scene and gain access to the patient, and can be instrumental in managing a crisis.

NOTE

Educating the public is fundamental to development of an effective EMS system. Paramedics help prepare the public to respond to a medical emergency and build support for EMS by participating in the development and presentation of public health care education and prevention programs (see Appendix C).

The 911 emergency telephone number provides easy access to public safety services, such as fire service, law enforcement, and EMS, throughout much

of the United States. The availability of emergency access via 911 continues to expand across the country as areas adopt the system. In areas that do not have 911, citizens should have easy access to emergency phone numbers. This can be accomplished through public awareness programs, telephone stickers, and telephone book covers. Other methods of activating an emergency response include firebox pull stations, citizen band radios, and cellular telephones. The 911 emergency number is further described in Chapter 16.

✓ TRICKS OF THE TRADE

A way to introduce EMS to school-age children and to ensure that they know how and when to call 911 is to visit elementary schools for a "show and tell" class.

Dispatch

An effective communications system coordinates an emergency response. After the emergency is recognized, communication centers are contacted through emergency telephone numbers or radio communications. The telecommunicator (dispatcher) serves as the primary contact with the public and directs the appropriate agencies (ground and air ambulances, fire departments, law enforcement, utility services, and others) to the scene. Some telecommunicators also are trained to provide emergency medical instructions by phone at the time of the call for help.

NOTE

A telecommunicator is trained in public safety telecommunications. The term applies to call takers, dispatchers, radio operators, data terminal operators, or any combination of such functions in a public service answering point (PSAP) located in a fire, police, or EMS communications center (see Chapter 16).

Prehospital Care

Seriously ill or injured patients may require prehospital intervention and stabilization involving both **basic life support** (BLS) and ALS skills. Depending on the circumstances (e.g., entrapment, distance to the hospital, availability of ALS), initial prehospital care may be limited to providing comfort and reassurance. It also could require spinal immobilization, airway protection, endotracheal intubation, intravenous cannulation, medication administration, defibrillation, and external cardiac pacing.

Hospital Care

When the patient is delivered to the emergency department, patient care resources expand to include physicians, physician assistants, nurse practitioners, nurses, technicians, ancillary support staff (allied health counselors, social workers, and others), secretaries, medical record staff, and diagnostic services such as those provided by laboratory, radiology, and cardiopulmonary departments. Resources available beyond the emergency department include surgery, intensive care, physical therapy, pharmacy, nutrition services, and many others.

Rehabilitation

After hospital delivery and definitive care, many patients receive some type of rehabilitation services before and after hospital discharge. Rehabilitation through education and physical and occupational therapy enables the patient to recover and maintain maximal independence. Examples range from helping patients and families adjust to necessary changes in lifestyle after heart attacks to retraining in activities of daily living and job rehabilitation to adapt to limb impairment or loss.

EMS Provider Levels

Various levels of providers and medical direction combine to make an effective prehospital EMS system, including dispatchers, first responders, EMT-Basics (EMT-Bs), EMT-Intermediates (EMT-Is), and EMT-Ps.

> **CANADIAN EMS STANDARDS**
>
> In some provinces in Canada, all EMS providers are called "paramedics" and are differentiated only by certain designated levels, such as EMA-I Paramedic for first responders and EMA-II Paramedic for personnel providing care similar to paramedics in the United States.

> **NOTE**
>
> An effective EMS system is a "team" concept that is composed of communications specialists, EMS personnel, fire and rescue personnel, law enforcement, and other public and private service agencies.

> ✓ **TRICKS OF THE TRADE**
>
> You are only one "link" in the chain of a team, and the team is only as strong as the weakest link. Cooperation and respect among all team members are essential.

Dispatcher

A dispatcher (telecommunicator) is the primary contact with those who call for emergency assistance and directs the appropriate agencies (ground and air ambulances, fire departments, law enforcement, etc.) to the scene. An effective EMS dispatch communications system includes the following functions:

- *Receive and process calls for EMS assistance.* The dispatcher receives and records calls for EMS assistance and selects an appropriate course of action for each call. This function involves obtaining as much information as possible about the emergency event, including name, call back number, and address, and may include dealing with distraught callers.
- *Dispatch and coordinate EMS resources.* The dispatcher directs the appropriate emergency vehicles to the correct address. In addition, the dispatcher coordinates the movements of emergency vehicles while en route to the scene, to the medical facility, and back to the operations base.
- *Relay medical information.* The dispatch center can provide a telecommunications channel among appropriate medical facilities and EMS personnel, fire, police, rescue workers, and private citizens. The channel can consist of telephone, radio, or biomedical telemetry.
- *Coordinate with public safety agencies.* The dispatcher provides for communications between public safety units (fire, law enforcement, rescue) and elements of the EMS system to facilitate coordination of services such as traffic control, escort, fire suppression, and extrication. For all of these events to take place in an integrated, well-

coordinated system, the dispatcher must know the location and status of all EMS vehicles and the availability of support services. In larger systems, computer-aided dispatching can be used. This advanced technology provides for one or more of the following capabilities or functions:

- Automatic entry of 911
- Automatic interface to vehicle location with or without map display
- Automatic interface to mobile data terminal
- Computer messaging among multiple radio operators, call takers, or both
- Dispatch note taking, reminder aid, or both
- Display of call information
- Emergency medical dispatch review
- Manual or automatic updates of unit status
- Manual entry of call information
- Radio control and display of channel status
- Standard operating procedure review
- Telephone control and display of circuit status

Many EMS and public service agencies require specialized training for their dispatch personnel so that emergency instructions can be given to the caller while waiting for EMS arrival. This training can include the USDOT's training program for EMD, which is further described in Chapter 16.

? CRITICAL THINKING

What type of dispatching is done in your community? Are dispatchers trained to the level of emergency medical dispatcher (EMD)?

First Responder

First responders are the first trained personnel of the EMS system to arrive at the scene of an emergency. Examples of trained first responders include fire department personnel, law enforcement officers, designated industrial or commercial medical response teams, and athletic trainers. The first responder has completed training based on the *First Responder National Standard Curriculum* and is capable of the following:

1. Recognizing the seriousness of the patient's condition or extent of injuries
2. Assessing requirements for emergency medical care

3. Administering appropriate emergency medical care for life-threatening injuries relative to airway, breathing, and circulation
4. Performing safely and effectively the expectations of the job description as defined in the national curriculum

Because they are often the first to arrive at the scene of an injury or an illness, first responders are an integral part of an effective EMS response team.

NOTE

A curriculum is a specific blueprint for learning that is derived from content and performance standards.

EMT-Basic

The EMT-B has completed training based on the *EMT-Basic National Standard Curriculum* and is trained in all phases of BLS, including the use of automated external defibrillators (AEDs) and assistance of a patient with the administration of some emergency medications. Some EMT-Bs also are trained in advanced airway procedures (nasogastric tube insertion and orotracheal intubation). In addition to patient care education, EMT-Bs receive training in emergency vehicle operations (emergency driving responses, tactics, techniques, and maintenance) and play an ancillary role in public education and health promotion programs that the community deems appropriate.

NOTE

A discussion of public education and health promotion programs can be found in the appendices.

EMT-Intermediate

The EMT-I is an EMT-B who has completed training based on the *EMT-Intermediate National Standard Curriculum*, which is derived from the training curriculum for EMT-Paramedics. The degree of training and skills that the EMT-I practices varies between states and EMS systems and can include ALS procedures such as advanced airway adjuncts, intravenous therapy, defibrillation, cardiac rhythm interpretation, and administration of some emergency medications. Like the EMT-B, the EMT-I participates in public education and health promotion programs in the community.

EMT-Paramedic

The EMT-P is an EMT-B or EMT-I who has completed training based on the *EMT-Paramedic National Standard Curriculum*. Paramedics are trained in all aspects of BLS and ALS procedures relevant to prehospital emergency care. The paramedic has advanced training in patient assessment, cardiac rhythm interpretation, defibrillation, drug therapy, and airway management (see box below). Specific roles and responsibilities of the paramedic are discussed later in this chapter.

National EMS Group Involvement

There are many groups and organizations at the national, state, regional, and local levels that are involved in development, education, implementation, and setting standards of EMS (Box 1-4). Membership and participation in professional organizations help promote the professional status of the paramedic by exposing the paramedic to current trends in emergency care, to continuing education, and to resource experts. They also provide for national representation and a means for a unified voice in other health care organizations and issues of national matters.

One such organization is the National Registry of EMTs (NREMT). The NREMT contributes to the development of professional standards in the EMS industry. This organization verifies competency for EMTs and paramedics by preparing and conducting examinations and by simplifying the process of state-to-state mobility and **reciprocity** for its members. The NREMT can spread the cost of examination development and validation across a large user base.

? CRITICAL THINKING

What issue do you think your national EMS association should work on to enhance patient care in your area?

There are many roles of EMS standard-setting groups. Their primary role, however, is to establish standards with input from the profession and the community. By doing so, they help ensure that the general public is protected from individuals and agencies who do not meet professional standards for licensure or certification.

DESCRIPTION OF THE PARAMEDIC PROFESSION

The description of the paramedic profession provides the philosophy and rationale for the depth and breadth of coverage:

- Paramedics have fulfilled requirements prescribed by a credentialing agency to practice the art and science of out-of-hospital medicine in conjunction with medical direction. Through performing assessments and providing medical care, their goal is to prevent and reduce mortality and morbidity caused by illness and injury. Paramedics primarily provide care to emergency patients in an out-of-hospital setting.
- Paramedics possess knowledge, skills, and attitudes consistent with the expectations of the public and the profession. Paramedics recognize that they are an essential component of the continuum of care and serve as linkages among health resources.
- Paramedics strive to maintain high-quality, reasonable-cost health care by delivering patients directly to appropriate facilities. As an advocate for patients, paramedics seek to be proactive in affecting long-term health care by working with other provider agencies, networks, and organizations. The emerging roles and responsibilities of the paramedic include public education, health promotion, and participation in injury- and illness-prevention programs. As the scope of service continues to expand, the paramedic will function as a facilitator of access to care and as an initial treatment provider.
- Paramedics are responsible and accountable to medical direction, the public, and their peers. Paramedics recognize the importance of research and actively participate in the design, development, evaluation, and publication of research. Paramedics seek to take part in lifelong professional development, perform peer evaluation, and assume an active role in professional and community organizations.

From US Department of Transportation, National Highway Transportation Administration: *EMT-Paramedic national standard curriculum*, Washington, DC, 1998, The Department.

Paramedic Education

Initial Education

The national standard curriculum for paramedics was revised in 1998. The *National EMS Education and Practice Blueprint* outlines a diagram of an education model that culminated from this revision (Fig. 1-3).[5] Based on this model, the paramedic student must demonstrate "competencies" in math, reading, and writing before enrollment in a paramedic training program. Prerequisites or corequisites (education classes to be taken before or simultaneously with the paramedic program) include EMT-B training and human anatomy and physiology. The model further defines minimum content for a standardized program of study, which averages 1000 to 1200 hours of instruction[6] depending on state requirements and local needs, current practices, individual training sites, and clinical programs. New to this revision is the definition of cognitive (knowledge), psychomotor (skills), and affective (attitude) objectives.

When choosing a training site for paramedic education, the student should consider the program's educational resources, including accreditation, facilities, quality of instructors, equipment, clinical experiences, references from past students, text requirements, and other instructional materials.

Continuing Education

Continuing education provides a way for all health care providers to maintain fundamental technical and professional skills and to learn new and/or advanced skills and knowledge. Some skills learned during the primary course of study will infrequently be used, and new information, procedures, and resources that enhance patient care are continuously being developed.

Continuing education can take many forms, including the following:

- Conferences and seminars
- Lectures and workshops
- Quality-improvement reviews
- Skill laboratories
- Certification and recertification programs
- Journal studies
- Multimedia presentations
- Internet-based learning
- Case presentations
- Independent study

✓ TRICKS OF THE TRADE

Another way to participate in continuing education is to become a topic "expert." Share your knowledge and expertise with your colleagues.

BOX 1-4

SAMPLING OF NATIONAL EMS ORGANIZATIONS AND ASSOCIATIONS

American Organizations
American Ambulance Association (AAA)
American College of Emergency Physicians (ACEP)
Association of Air Medical Services (AAMS)
Emergency Nurses' Association (ENA)
National Association of EMS Educators (NAEMSE)
National Association of EMS Physicians (NAEMSP)
National Association of Emergency Medical Technicians (NAEMT)
National Association of Search and Rescue (NASAR)
National Association of State EMS Directors (NASEMSD)
National Council of State EMS Training Coordinators (NCSEMSTC)
National Flight Nurses' Association (NFNA)

National Flight Paramedic Association (NFPA)
National Registry of Emergency Medical Technicians (NREMT)

Canadian Organizations
Canadian Confederation of Ambulance Service Associations (CCASA)
Canadian Association of Critical Care Nurses (CACCN)
Society of Prehospital Care Educators (SPCE)
Paramedic Association of Canada (PAC)
Shock Trauma Air Rescue Society (STARS)
Canadian Association of Emergency Physicians (CAEP)
Major Industrial Accident Control of Canada (MIACC)
Canadian Medical Association's Conjoint Committee for Accreditation of Educational Programs in EMS Technology

PARAMEDIC: NATIONAL STANDARD CURRICULUM
DIAGRAM OF EDUCATIONAL MODEL

COMPETENCIES
Mathematics, reading, and writing

PRE- or CO-REQUISITE
EMT or EMT-Basic Human anatomy and physiology

PREPARATORY
EMS systems/The roles and responsibilities of the paramedic The well-being of the paramedic Illness and injury prevention Medical/legal issues Ethics General principles of pathophysiology Pharmacology Medication administration Therapeutic communications Lifespan development

AIRWAY MANAGEMENT AND VENTILATION

MEDICAL	PATIENT ASSESSMENT	TRAUMA
Pulmonary Cardiology Neurology Endocrinology Allergies and anaphylaxis Gastroenterology Urology Toxicology Hematology Environmental conditions Infectious and communicable diseases Behavioral and psychiatric disorders Gynecology Obstetrics	History taking Techniques of physical examination Patient assessment Clinical decision making Communications Documentation	Trauma systems/mechanism of injury Hemorrhage and shock Soft-tissue trauma Burns Head and facial trauma Spinal trauma Thoracic trauma Abdominal trauma Musculoskeletal trauma

SPECIAL CONSIDERATIONS
Neonatology Pediatrics Geriatrics Abuse and assault Patients with special challenges Acute interventions for the home care patient

ASSESSMENT-BASED MANAGEMENT

OPERATIONS
Ambulance operations Medical incident command Rescue awareness and operations Hazardous materials incidents Crime scene awareness

LIFELONG LEARNING
Continuing education

Fig. 1-3 Diagram of Department of Transportation (DOT) education model. (From US Department of Health and Human Services, Health Resources and Services Administration, Maternal and Child Health Bureau: *Emergency medical services agenda for the future,* Washington, DC, 1999, The Administration.)

Licensure, Certification, and Registration

Licensure, certification, and registration are processes by which the paramedic is granted permission to practice his or her skills. The exact terminology of granting this permission varies by state.

Licensure

Licensure is a process of occupational regulation in which a license is granted to practice a profession. With licensure, permission is granted by a competent authority (a government body) to engage in any business, profession, or activity that would otherwise be unlawful. Some states and local authorities require that paramedics be licensed.

Certification

Certification grants authority to an individual who has met predetermined qualifications to participate in an activity. Through certification, the person receives a document from a government or nongovernment entity verifying the fulfillment of requirements to practice in a particular field. Some states or local authorities require certification of paramedics.

> **NOTE**
>
> There is an unfounded general belief that "licensed professionals" have greater status than those who are "certified" or "registered." A certification, granted by a state, conferring a right to engage in a trade or profession is in fact a "license."

Registration

Registration is the act of enrolling one's name in a "register," or book of record. For example, a paramedic can be licensed or certified in his or her state and be registered with the NREMT.

Professionalism

Rigorous training and performance standards have helped establish EMTs and paramedics as health care professionals. The term *profession* refers to the existence of a specialized body of knowledge or expertise, and the practitioners of a profession generally are self-regulated through a license or certification that verifies competence. In addition, most professions maintain standards, including initial and continuing education requirements. *Professionalism* refers to the way in which a person follows the standards of conduct and performance established by the profession. This usually includes adherence to a "code of ethics" approved by the profession (see box on p. 16).

Health Care Professional

Health care professionals conform to the standards of their profession. They instill pride in the profession and earn the respect of others by providing quality patient care and striving for high standards. EMS professionals occupy positions of public trust and are highly visible role models. As such, the public has high societal expectations of EMTs and paramedics while they are both on and off duty. Therefore professional conduct at all times and a commitment to excellence in daily activities complement the image of the EMS professional. Image and behavior are vital to establishing credibility and instilling confidence.

> ✓ **TRICKS OF THE TRADE**
>
> Even though the public cannot gauge the "quality" of medical care that you provide, most are "experts" at judging professionalism.

> **NOTE**
>
> The professional paramedic represents his or her employer; the EMS agency; the state, county, city, or district EMS office; and his or her peers.

Attributes of the Professional Paramedic

Many attributes of professionalism can be applied to the role of the paramedic. Eleven of these attributes are as follows[6]:

1. *Integrity.* Integrity (honesty in all actions) is perhaps the most important behavior for EMS pro-

EMT CODE OF ETHICS

Professional status as an Emergency Medical Technician and Emergency Medical Technician-Paramedic is maintained and enriched by the willingness of the individual practitioner to accept and fulfill obligations to society, other medical professionals, and the profession of Emergency Medical Technician. As an Emergency Medical Technician at the basic level or an Emergency Medical Technician-Paramedic, I solemnly pledge myself to the following code of professional ethics:

- A fundamental responsibility of the Emergency Medical Technician is to conserve life, to alleviate suffering, to promote health, to do no harm, and to encourage the quality and equal availability of emergency medical care.
- The Emergency Medical Technician provides services based on human need, with respect for human dignity, unrestricted by consideration of nationality, race, creed, color, or status.
- The Emergency Medical Technician does not use professional knowledge and skills in any enterprise detrimental to the public well-being.
- The Emergency Medical Technician respects and holds in confidence all information of a confidential nature obtained in the course of professional work unless required by law to divulge such information.
- The Emergency Medical Technician, as a citizen, understands and upholds the law and performs the duties of citizenship; as a professional, the Emergency Medical Technician has the never-ending responsibility to work with concerned citizens and other health care professionals in promoting a high standard of emergency medical care to all people.
- The Emergency Medical Technician shall maintain professional competence and demonstrate concern for the competence of other members of the Emergency Medical Services health care team.
- An Emergency Medical Technician assumes responsibility in defining and upholding standards of professional practice and education.
- The Emergency Medical Technician assumes responsibility for individual professional actions and judgment, both in dependent and independent emergency functions, and knows and upholds the laws which affect the practice of the Emergency Medical Technician.
- An Emergency Medical Technician has the responsibility to be aware of and participate in matters of legislation affecting the Emergency Medical Technician and the Emergency Medical Services System.
- The Emergency Medical Technician adheres to standards of personal ethics, which reflect credit upon the profession.
- Emergency Medical Technicians, or groups of Emergency Medical Technicians, who advertise professional services, do so in conformity with the dignity of the profession.
- The Emergency Medical Technician has an obligation to protect the public by not delegating to a person less qualified any service which requires the professional competence of an Emergency Medical Technician.
- The Emergency Medical Technician will work harmoniously with, and sustain confidence in, Emergency Medical Technician associates, the nurse, the physician, and other members of the emergency medical services health care team.
- The Emergency Medical Technician refuses to participate in unethical procedures and assumes the responsibility to expose incompetence or unethical conduct of others to the appropriate authority in a proper and professional manner.

fessionals and is assumed by the public. Examples of behavior that demonstrate integrity are being truthful, not stealing, and providing complete and accurate documentation.

2. *Empathy.* Empathy is the identification with and understanding of the feelings, situations, and motives of others. It must always be demonstrated to patients, families, and other health care professionals. Examples of behavior demonstrating empathy include showing caring, compassion, and respect for others; understanding the feelings of the patient and family; being calm and helpful to those in need; and being supportive and reassuring of others.

3. *Self-motivation.* Self-motivation is the internal drive for excellence and self-direction. Examples include taking the initiative to complete assignments, to improve and correct behavior, and to follow through on tasks without constant supervision. Some marks of self-motivation include showing enthusiasm for learning, being committed to **continuous quality improvement** (CQI) (described later in this

chapter), accepting constructive feedback, and taking advantage of all learning opportunities.

4. *Appearance and personal hygiene*. Paramedics are aware of how they present themselves as a representative of their profession. They ensure that their clothing and uniforms are clean and in good repair, and they are aware of the importance of personal hygiene and good grooming.

✓ **TRICKS OF THE TRADE**

You should always have an extra uniform available "just in case."

5. *Self-confidence*. Paramedics must trust and rely on themselves, often in difficult circumstances. Therefore an accurate assessment of personal and professional strengths and limitations is important. The ability to trust personal judgment demonstrates self-confidence.

6. *Communications*. The exchange of information and the ability to convey this information to others verbally and in writing is vital to the paramedic's job. For example, the paramedic must demonstrate communication skills by speaking clearly, writing legibly, listening actively, and adjusting communication strategies to various situations.

7. *Time management*. Time management refers to organizing and prioritizing tasks to make optimal use of time. Examples include being punctual and completing tasks and assignments on time.

8. *Teamwork and diplomacy*. The ability to work with others using tact and interpersonal skills to achieve a common goal describes teamwork and diplomacy. As a member of the EMS team, the paramedic must place the success of the team above personal success by supporting and respecting other team members, being flexible and open to change, and communicating with co-workers to resolve problems.

9. *Respect*. Having regard for others and showing consideration and appreciation are examples of respect. Paramedics are polite to others and avoid the use of derogatory or demeaning terms. They know that showing respect brings credit to themselves, their association, and their profession.

10. *Patient advocacy*. The paramedic must always act as the patient's advocate, even when the patient disagrees with patient-care recommendations. Paramedics should not attempt to impose their personal beliefs on patients or allow personal biases (religious, ethical, political, social, legal) to influence patient care. The paramedic must always place the needs of the patient above self-interests and protect the patient's confidentiality.

11. *Careful delivery of service*. Paramedics deliver the highest quality of patient care with careful attention to detail and appropriate prioritization of care, and they critically evaluate their performance and attitude on every call. As part of the careful delivery of service, paramedics master and refresh their skills; perform complete equipment checks; ensure careful and safe ambulance operations; follow established policies, procedures, and protocols; and comply with the orders of their supervisors.

? **CRITICAL THINKING**

Which of these professional attributes represent your strengths? Which ones do you think you need to work on?

Roles and Responsibilities of the Paramedic

The roles and responsibilities of the paramedic can be divided into two categories: primary responsibilities and additional responsibilities[6] (Box 1-5).

Primary Responsibilities

The paramedic must be physically, mentally, and emotionally prepared for the job of providing emergency care. This includes a daily commitment to positive health practices (see Chapter 2), having the appropriate equipment and supplies, and maintaining adequate knowledge and skills of the profession. The paramedic must respond to the scene in a safe and timely manner. During scene assessment the paramedic must consider personal safety; safety

BOX 1-5

ROLES AND RESPONSIBILITIES OF THE PARAMEDIC

Primary Responsibilities
Preparation
Response
Scene assessment
Patient assessment
Recognition of injury or illness
Patient management
Appropriate patient disposition
Patient transfer
Documentation
Returning to service

Additional Responsibilities
Community involvement
Support of primary care efforts
Advocation of citizen involvement in EMS
Participation in leadership activities
Personal and professional development

BOX 1-6

SAMPLING OF SPECIALIZED CARE FACILITIES

Emergency department
Operating suite
Postanesthesia recovery room or surgical intensive care unit
Intensive care unit for trauma patients
Cardiac treatment center
Neurology center
Facility with acute hemodialysis capability
Burn specialization center
Facility with acute spinal cord or head injury management capability
Facility with special radiological capabilities
Rehabilitation facility
Clinical laboratory service
Toxicology (including HAZMAT or decontamination) service
Hyperbaric treatment center
Facility with reperfusion capability
Pediatric facility
Psychiatric facility
Trauma center
High-risk obstetrical facility

of the crew, patients, and bystanders; and the mechanism of injury or probable cause of illness.

The paramedic must perform patient assessment quickly to recognize the injury or illness so that priorities of care and transportation can be established. Managing the emergency often involves following protocols and interacting with medical direction as needed. After stabilizing the patient in the field, the paramedic should provide appropriate transportation by ground or air to a proper receiving facility based on the patient's condition. Selection of the receiving facility for optimal patient care requires a knowledge of available facilities, hospital designation, and categorization (Box 1-6). Knowledge of transfer agreements and payers insurance systems also can be a factor in arranging for patient transportation.

The paramedic is the patient's advocate as care is transferred to the staff at the receiving facility. Transfer of the patient includes briefing the hospital staff about the patient's condition at the scene and during transportation and providing thorough and accurate documentation in the patient care report (PCR). The paramedic should complete required documentation in a timely manner so that the EMS crew can return to service. The crew should prepare the ambulance for return to service by replacing equipment and supplies (per agency protocol). The crew also should openly review the call to see if there are ways to improve the patient care services that were provided at the scene and during transportation.

Additional Responsibilities

Other responsibilities of the paramedic include community involvement, supporting primary care efforts, advocating citizen involvement in the EMS system, participating in leadership activities, and personal and professional development.

Community involvement for the paramedic includes being a role model for the profession, advocating injury prevention programs (see Appendix C), and participating as a leader in community activities. Teaching CPR, first aid, and injury prevention programs are ways to improve the health of the community and can enhance compliance with treatment regimens. These activities also help ensure appropriate use of EMS resources and improve the integration of EMS with other health care and public safety agencies.

A few communities and their health care organizations use paramedics to support primary care efforts and prevention and wellness agendas. In addition, paramedics can play a role in educating the public about appropriate use of prehospital and other non-EMS health care resources (e.g., alternatives to ambulance transportation, nonhospital emergency department clinical providers, freestanding emergency clinics). These programs that teach when, where, and how to use EMS and emergency departments appropriately encourage better use of community resources.

Advocating citizen involvement in EMS improves the EMS system as a whole. Citizens who are active in establishing needs and parameters for using EMS in their community offer an objective view into quality improvement and problem resolution. In addition, citizen involvement creates informed, independent advocates for the EMS system.

There are many ways that paramedics can participate in leadership activities in their communities, such as conducting primary injury prevention initiatives (activities and risk surveys), assisting media campaigns to promote EMS issues, and distributing informational materials about EMS and other health programs.

The paramedic has a responsibility for personal and professional development. Methods to accomplish this include continuing education, student mentoring, membership in professional organizations, becoming involved in work-related issues that affect career growth, exploring alternative career paths in the EMS profession, conducting and supporting research initiatives, and being actively involved in legislative issues related to EMS.

Medical Direction for EMS

Many services provided by paramedics are derived from medical practices whereby paramedics func-

tion as "physician extenders." This is made possible through medical direction (medical control or medical oversight). The medical direction physician serves as the medical leader, resource, and patient advocate for the EMS system. This relationship between the physician and paramedic permits delivery of advanced prehospital care. The ideal medical direction physician is properly educated as an EMS medical director and is motivated to provide the following[6]:

- EMS system design and operations
- Education and training of EMS personnel
- Participation in personnel selection
- Participation in equipment selection
- Development of clinical protocols in cooperation with expert EMS personnel
- Participation in CQI and problem resolution
- Direct input into patient care
- Interface between EMS systems and other health care agencies
- Advocacy within the medical community
- Guidance as the "medical conscience" of the EMS system (advocating for quality patient care)

Types of Medical Direction

There are two types of medical direction—**on-line (direct) medical direction** and **off-line (indirect) medical direction.**[7] Both are equally important in ensuring that the components of quality medical care are in place in an EMS system. When the paramedic crew contacts the hospital by radio or telephone, patient information is transmitted and orders are received through direct on-line communication with a physician or physician designee, such as a registered nurse, physician assistant, or paramedic trained to provide ALS orders in the medical direction system. On-line (direct) medical direction provides for immediate and patient-specific care, telemetry, and CQI while paramedics are on the scene.

> **NOTE**
> As a rule, on-line medical direction supercedes off-line medical direction.[8]

An advisory group or medical director who has full medical direction authority and responsibility for EMS system operations often provides administrative off-line (indirect) medical direction. This type of medical direction is further classified as *prospective* and *retrospective*.[6] Prospective off-line medical direction includes the authority to establish **treatment protocols, standing orders** (see box below), and training for treatment and triage of prehospital patients (see Chapters 13 and 48). It also can involve the selection of equipment, supplies, and personnel. *Retrospective off-line medical direction* refers to activities performed after the EMS call has been completed (e.g., reviewing the patient care report and providing CQI).

> **NOTE**
>
> Paramedics must follow established protocols unless otherwise advised by medical direction.

On-Scene Physicians

Although some of the first ambulance personnel were physicians (see box in right column), it is rare for a medical direction physician to be on the scene providing direct field supervision of EMS personnel. There are times, however, when a physician (physician intervenor) who witnesses the accident or illness (or sometimes the patient's private physician) is present at the emergency scene. When this occurs, interaction between the on-scene physician and the EMS crew is necessary.

> **NOTE**
>
> A physician intervenor may or may not be familiar with EMS function and training in medical oversight responsibilities. The lines of authority and responsibility for these physicians vary from state to state.

If a nonmedical direction physician or the patient's private physician is present at the scene of an emergency, EMS personnel should follow established protocols or, if none are in place, immediately contact on-line medical direction. Written policies developed by many EMS agencies require that the scene physician establish communication with the

---

PROTOCOLS

Treatment protocols are written guidelines that define the scope of prehospital intervention for EMS providers. The medical director of the ALS service or representatives of a regional EMS advisory group develop treatment protocols. *Standing orders* are more specific than treatment protocols and normally are included in a protocol when a delay in treatment would harm the patient. Most protocols and standing orders comply with national standards (e.g., the American Heart Association standards for advanced cardiac life support or the American College of Surgeons standards for advanced trauma life support), state EMS medical practice acts, and regional guidelines. Written protocols define the standard of care for paramedic crews and on-line physicians. Situations in which the paramedic crew functions strictly by standing orders usually are limited (e.g., intubation of a nonbreathing patient, first-line medication administration in cardiac arrest, or situations in which radio contact has failed and a delay in treatment could compromise patient outcome).

HISTORY OF THE PHYSICIAN-STAFFED AMBULANCE

Until World War II, ambulances staffed by an "ambulance surgeon" (a physician or intern) were common in the United States. This practice still exists in some countries. Physician-staffed ambulances were obsolete by the 1950s as emergency out-of-hospital care became the duty of fire departments and private ambulance providers.

In the 1960s, the work of J. Frank Pantridge reintroduced physicians to on-scene care. Dr. Pantridge headed the Department of Cardiology at Belfast's Royal Victoria Hospital and was Professor of Cardiology at the city's Queens University. He introduced the concept of managing out-of-hospital episodes of acute myocardial infarction by sending mobile coronary care units, staffed by nurses and physicians, to the scene. The successful results of his work prompted a similar program in the United States, headed by Dr. William J. Grace, Director of Medicine at St. Vincent's Hospital and Medical Center in New York City. Although both of these programs used only physicians and nurses to provide care, they had a major influence on the evolution of the paramedic profession.

on-line medical direction physician so that they can make decisions regarding legal responsibility for the patient's care. With the approval of medical direction, an on-scene physician can assume responsibility for patient management. However, if a scene physician attempts to direct patient care in opposition to medical direction, other EMS providers on the scene should request law enforcement to ensure scene safety and uninterrupted emergency care.

Improving System Quality

A major goal of any EMS system is to continually evaluate and improve care. One way to accomplish this goal is through a modified form of quality assurance (QA) known as *continuous quality improvement* (CQI) (see box below).

QUALITY ASSURANCE AND CONTINUOUS QUALITY IMPROVEMENT

Quality assurance (QA) is a system of quality management that traditionally was associated with identifying deviations from a standard (e.g., protocols) and correcting these deviations through some type of punitive action. Continuous quality improvement (CQI) is a modified form of QA that focuses on the system and not the individual, thereby removing much of the punitive aspect associated with a QA program. CQI is less rigid than QA and considers many factors that often apply to EMS. It encompasses the entire medical direction system and involves all health providers in the problem-solving process.

The EMS provider should use information obtained from CQI activities to modify treatment protocols and educational activities where appropriate. The goal of CQI is to identify and correct problems in a positive environment and to improve the overall system. Example CQI activities include a review of the following:

- Outcome measures of prehospital care (e.g., scene times, procedure completion rates, mortality reviews)
- Care while treatment is ongoing (concurrent reviews)
- Written EMS patient care paperwork (retrospective reviews)
- Random or selected radio communication tapes
- New procedures, equipment, or therapies

NOTE

CQI is the continuous study and improvement of a process, system, or organization.

Continuous Quality Improvement

A CQI program identifies and attempts to improve problems in areas such as medical direction, financing, training, communication, prehospital management and transportation, interfacility transportation, receiving facilities, specialty care units, dispatch, public information and education, audit and quality assurance, disaster planning, and mutual aid. CQI is a multidisciplinary process that involves all caregivers in the problem-solving aspect and emphasizes the importance of enabling "front-line" personnel to effectively perform their jobs. With this group approach, all parties can be involved in elaborating on the cause of the problem, developing remedies, designing a course of action to correct the problem, enforcing the plan of correction, and reexamining the issue to see if the problem has been satisfactorily resolved.

✓ TRICKS OF THE TRADE

CQI programs should not be viewed as a "waste of time." They *will* improve the system.

? CRITICAL THINKING

There has been an increased number of needle-stick injuries in your agency. How could the CQI process affect this situation?

Key actions or categories for EMS leaders to improve quality within their organization are as follows[8]:

1. *Leadership* involves efforts by senior leadership and management leading by example to integrate CQI into the strategic planning process and throughout the entire organization and to promote quality values and CQI techniques in work practices.

2. *Information and analysis* concerns managing and using the data needed for effective CQI. Since CQI is based on management by fact, information and analyses are critical to CQI success.
3. *Strategic quality planning* involves three major components: (a) development of long- and short-term organizational objectives for structural, performance, and outcome quality standards; (b) identification of ways to achieve those objectives; and (c) measurement of the effectiveness of the system in achieving quality standards.
4. *Human resource development and management* involves working to develop the full potential of the EMS workforce. This effort is guided by the principle that the entire EMS workforce is motivated to achieve new levels of service and value.
5. *EMS process management* concerns the creation and maintenance of high-quality services. Within the context of CQI, process management refers to the improvement of work activities and work flow *across* functional or department boundaries.
6. *EMS system results* entail assessment of the quality results achieved and examination of the organization's success at achieving CQI.
7. *Satisfaction of patients and other stakeholders* involves ensuring ongoing satisfaction by those internal and external to the EMS system with the services provided.

Benefits that can be gained by applying these seven guidelines and recommendations include improvements in service and patient care delivery, economic efficiency and/or profitability, patient and community satisfaction and loyalty, and health outcomes.

EMS Research

EMS research is a desirable activity for an EMS system and is essential to the continued evolution of EMS. Quality EMS research helps shed light on the efficacy, effects, and cost-effectiveness of EMS interventions based on experimental data and can lead to changes in professional standards, training, equipment, and procedures. In the health care climate of managed care and reduced spending by government agencies, future EMS funding probably will be dependent on scientifically proving the

value of EMS services. Therefore outcome studies are needed to ensure continued funding for EMS. Today's paramedic must have a fundamental knowledge of research principles to interpret published studies and to determine their value to EMS practice. The paramedic also must demonstrate a willingness to participate in the collection of research data required for the continued development of EMS care.

NOTE

EMS research enhances recognition and respect for EMS professionals.

? CRITICAL THINKING

How do you feel about research?

Basic Principles of Research

Quality EMS research begins with identification of a specific problem or question. The research is then carried out through standard research methods (Box 1-7) and reviewed by peers. The findings are published in a reputable professional journal for peer evaluation (Box 1-8). There are many applications for EMS research. Examples include gathering research to draw conclusions about which proce-

BOX 1-7

TYPES OF RESEARCH

Descriptive (observational). A research design in which events are monitored and analyzed without an attempt to manipulate or alter the outcome

Experimental. A research design in which an intervention is introduced and the effects are monitored for an outcome

Prospective. A research design in which the specific question, hypothesis, and data collection are defined before the study begins

Retrospective. A research design in which the specific question, hypothesis, and data collection are defined after the data already exists

Cross-sectional. A research design in which a group of subjects is studied during a specified (usually short) period of time

dures, techniques, and equipment are scientifically sound; answer clinically important questions; and find results that lead to system improvements (see box in lower right column).

> **NOTE**
>
> Research should be important to every EMS professional. Through understanding the basic principles of research, the EMS provider can make decisions regarding the merit of a research study and its implications for an EMS system.

> ✓ **TRICKS OF THE TRADE**
>
> EMS research should not be thought of as "someone else's job." It is important to every EMS service and every EMS provider.

After identifying a specific problem or question to be studied (e.g., the ability of a drug to lower a patient's blood pressure more effectively than another), the hypothesis (the statement to be tested by the study) must be defined. A hypothesis for the drug study might be that drug A lowers blood pressure more effectively and with fewer side effects than drug B.

> **BOX 1-8**
>
> ## STEPS IN CONDUCTING RESEARCH
>
> 1. Prepare a question.
> 2. Write a hypothesis.
> 3. Decide what to measure and the best way to measure it.
> 4. Define the population.
> 5. Identify study limitations.
> 6. Seek study approval.
> 7. Obtain informed consent.
> 8. Gather data after conducting pilot trials.
> 9. Analyze the data with an awareness of the pitfalls in interpreting the data.
> 10. Determine what to do with the research product (publish, present, perform follow-up studies).

From Menegazzi J: *Research: the who, what, why, when and how,* Wilmington, Ohio, 1994, Ferno-Washington.

> **NOTE**
>
> A hypothesis states the relationship between two or more variables. A variable is anything that varies in amount or type.

The next step in the research process is to define the population for the study. This can be any group of people (for example, all patients with a diastolic pressure above 100 mm Hg), places, or things. If the population group is very large, the researcher can use a sample of the population (e.g., all patients over 50 years of age who have a diastolic pressure above 100 mm Hg). The researcher should draw the sample *randomly* so that the patients in the study have an equal chance of being assigned to either one group (Drug A Study) or the other (Drug B Study).

Randomization prevents selection bias (systematically placing the best or worst patients in a study group). The researcher can accomplish randomization using computer software programs, using a statistical table of random digits, or by flipping a coin. Another way to limit bias is through systematic sampling. Using this method, patients are assigned to groups in the order in which they are encountered in the prehospital setting. For example, the first patient seen is assigned to group A, the second to group B, the third to group A, and so on. The researcher also can use alternative time sampling to prevent bias

> **THE UTSTEIN STYLE: REPORTING OUTCOMES OF OUT-OF-HOSPITAL CARDIAC ARRESTS**
>
> Historically, EMS research on out-of-hospital cardiac arrest has been difficult to gather on a national level since there are many differences in terminology and definitions between EMS systems. For example, do the data that the EMS system reports differentiate among arrests in which bystander CPR was initiated before EMS arrival? The Utstein Style is a collection of uniform guidelines (templates) for reporting outcomes of prehospital cardiac arrest. These guidelines define several terms and activities used by EMS systems so that all participants reporting data in a study are "speaking the same language." Using these templates, researchers can conduct appropriate comparisons between the results published by EMS systems.

by assigning a treatment group based on the day, week, or month in which they are encountered in the study. With convenience sampling (the least preferred method of randomization), patients are assigned to groups when a particular person or crew is working.

> **NOTE**
>
> Even with carefully designed randomization, unavoidable sampling errors occur. They result from the fact that even the "best" sample will not work perfectly to represent its population because of the chance inclusion of one person in the study group rather than the chance inclusion of someone else.

> **NOTE**
>
> A *parameter* is a characteristic of a population that is difficult or impossible to measure. For example, it would be nearly impossible to determine the "exact" age (hour of birth) of all patients in a group. Nuisance variables (e.g., the use of audible and visual warning devices that can contribute to a rise in a patient's blood pressure) also can make it difficult to draw accurate conclusions from a study. Parameters and nuisance variables are difficult to identify, control, avoid, or completely eliminate.

In addition to the bias of the researcher, there can be bias on the part of the participants in the study as a result of their expectations. To lessen this possibility, the researcher can use blinding (either single, double, or triple). In a single-blind method, one party (the patient, the health care provider, or the person gathering the data) is unaware (blinded) of the treatment at the time that it is given and of the effect to be measured during the study. In a double-blind study, two parties are blinded. A triple-blind study occurs when all parties are blinded. *Unblinding* refers to all parties being made aware of the study, treatment, and outcome to be measured.

Statistics

Statistics refers to numerical facts or data that are classified and tabulated to present significant information about a given subject. Statistics can be either descriptive or inferential.

Descriptive statistics. Descriptive statistics does not attempt to infer anything that goes beyond the data.

Descriptive statistics can be either qualitative or quantitative. Qualitative analysis is the nonnumerical organization and interpretation of observations for discovering important underlying dimensions and patterns of relationships (e.g., age and gender of a sample). Qualitative analysis is not as precise as quantitative analysis.

Quantitative analysis in descriptive statistics uses *mean, median,* and *mode* to describe the most commonly occurring values within a sample. The mean is the arithmetic "average" of the group (e.g., the average age of the person in the sample). The median is obtained by first arranging the measurement according to size from smallest to largest and then choosing the one in the middle (or the mean of the two that are nearest to the middle). The median sometimes is referred to as the *fiftieth percentile* and frequently is used to divide a sample into two halves. The mode is the number that occurs more often than any other number in a set of data.

The following is an example of quantitative analysis:

There are 13 people in your sample. Their ages are 53, 53, 53, 54, 55, 55, 56, 57, 59, 60, 64, 71, and 79. The mean (average) age of the group is 59.15 years, the median (middle) age is 56, and the mode age is 53.

> **NOTE**
>
> A *standard deviation* describes how much the scores in a set of numbers differ from the mean, or how much the group varies from the average. A standard deviation is a single number, derived through mathematical equations, that tells how much deviation from the mean is typical of a given group. In a standard distribution, about 65% (two thirds) of all the numbers in the sample will be within 1 standard deviation of the mean, and about 95% will be within 2 standard deviations of the mean. If the standard deviation is large, it indicates an "abnormal" or skewed distribution of variability in the data or population under study.

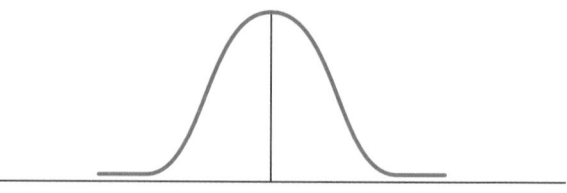

Bell curve.

Inferential statistics. Inferential statistics provides a means to infer whether the relationships observed in a sample are likely to occur in the larger population. The researcher can use inferential statistics to decide whether the results of the study support or contradict the initial hypothesis. To do this, one must assume the opposite of what one may want to prove by stating a null hypothesis, or a precise statement that the results are a chance of variation. This is done in a court proceeding where the accused is assumed to be innocent until proven guilty beyond a reasonable doubt. The assumption that the accused is not guilty is a null hypothesis; if it cannot be rejected, the accused will go free, but this does not necessarily mean that the accused is really innocent. A research hypothesis is the opposite of the null hypothesis (e.g., the accused is guilty until proven innocent).

> **NOTE**
>
> A *null hypothesis* states that there is no difference between two or more treatments. The sureness with which a null hypothesis can be rejected is called *confidence.*

Inferential statistics requires that one specify the probability with which one is willing to risk rejecting the hypothesis about the population mean even though it is true (or rejecting the null hypothesis when it actually is true, and failing to reject the null hypothesis when it actually is false). This probability is known as the *level of significance,* the acceptable risk of sampling errors. The level of significance, established through mathematic equations, usually is 0.05 (1 chance in 20) or 0.01 (1 chance in 100) that the difference between two groups is larger than expected as a result of chance alone. The results are considered statistically significant (too large to be "reasonably" attributed to chance) if the difference between the two groups is larger than the level of significance.

> **NOTE**
>
> In statistics, rejecting the null hypothesis when it is true (a false alarm) is referred to as a *Type I error.* Accepting the null hypothesis when it is false (failing to detect a real phenomenon) is a *Type II error.* A Type II error occurs when it is "too" small to see.

Research Ethics

When planning research, the researcher should consider involving an institution review board (IRB). The widespread use of IRBs resulted from a mandate in 1966 by the U.S. Public Health Services, which required a review by a "committee of institutional associates" for any federally funded research involving human subjects. Today, most IRBs involved in EMS research consist of physicians, attorneys, psychologists, allied health professionals, and lay members of the community. Their purpose is to minimize the risk of patients unknowingly entering into research that could harm them in any way. In 1981, the USDHHS adopted regulations for research practice with three basic tenets[9] that are followed by most IRBs:

1. The risks to the subjects are so outweighed by the sum of the benefit to the subject and the importance of the knowledge to be gained as to warrant a decision to allow the subjects to accept the risks.
2. Legally effective informed consent will be obtained by adequate and appropriate methods.
3. The rights and welfare of any such subjects will be protected adequately.

> **? CRITICAL THINKING**
>
> *Why do you think the development of IRBs was needed for research?*

> **NOTE**
>
> Many peer-reviewed EMS journals require documentation that the research was authorized by an IRB.

Consent. Traditional informed consent requires that the subject voluntarily (without coercion) agrees to participate in the research project, is legally competent, and completely understands what is being presented. With respect to EMS research and the problems associated with obtaining informed consent in emergency situations, alternatives to informed consent have been developed,[9] including the following:

- *Consent at a distance.* The base-station physician administers informed consent to the subject via radio or telephone.
- *Consent by proxy.* The paramedic administers informed consent to the subject.

BOX 1-9

FIFTEEN STEPS IN EVALUATING AND INTERPRETING RESEARCH

1. Was the research peer reviewed?
2. What was the research hypothesis?
3. Was the study approved by an institutional review board and conducted ethically?
4. What was the population being studied?
5. What were the inclusion and exclusion criteria for the study?
6. What method was used to draw a sample of patients?
7. How many patient groups participated?
8. How were patients assigned to groups?
9. What type of data were gathered?
10. Does it appear that the study had a sufficient number of patients enrolled?
11. Do there appear to be any potential confounding variables that are not accounted for?
12. Were the data properly analyzed?
13. Is the author's conclusion logical and based on the data?
14. Could the results apply in local EMS systems?
15. Are patients in the study similar to those in the local EMS system?

- *Stepped consent.* The paramedic provides the subject with a brief overview of the experimental therapy. Full informed consent is obtained at the hospital.
- *Cohort consent.* Permission is obtained to enter into the study at some future time (e.g., during an asthma exacerbation or sickle cell crisis).
- *Deferred consent.* This is used during resuscitation, whereby the subject is stabilized and receives experimental therapy without permission, after which the family is approached for traditional informed consent.
- *Surrogate consent.* Lay persons are presented with the experimental protocol and are asked to rule if they feel that the treatment is appropriate.
- *Consent jury.* A lay panel determines certain aspects of the experimental protocol, particularly potential risks and complications that must be presented during a request for consent.

Research Format

The format for writing a manuscript for scientific literature has five basic sections:

1. The introduction provides a brief, historic background of the research, previously published research, a rationale for the study, and the research hypothesis.
2. The methods section describes exactly how the experiment was done so that it can be replicated by others. This section also should define the inclusion or exclusion criteria for the study (how patients were chosen) and the statistical methods used to analyze the data.
3. The results section provides answers to study questions and data (e.g., tables and figures) that briefly support the research findings.
4. The discussion section allows the author to interpret the research findings. Limitations of the project and suggestions for improving the study through follow-up research usually are presented in this section.
5. The *conclusion* section provides a brief and succinct summary of the four previous sections (Box 1-9).

SUMMARY

- Organized prehospital care has its roots in military history.

- Through most of the early twentieth century and up to the mid-1960s, urban hospital-based systems that later developed into municipal services and funeral directors and volunteers who often were untrained in emergency care provided prehospital care in the United States.

- The operations of an effective EMS system include citizen activation, dispatch, prehospital care, hospital care, and rehabilitation.

- Various levels of providers with their own distinct roles and responsibilities, including telecommunicators (dispatchers), first responders, EMT-Basics, EMT-Intermediates, and EMT-Paramedics, combine to make an effective prehospital EMS system.

- Membership and participation in professional organizations help promote the professional status of the paramedic.

- Continuing education provides a way for all health care providers to maintain fundamental technical and professional skills.

- Professionalism refers to the way in which a person follows the standards of conduct and performance established by the profession.

- The roles and responsibilities of the paramedic can be divided into two categories: primary responsibilities and additional responsibilities.

- There are two types of medical direction—on-line (direct) medical direction and off-line (indirect) medical direction. Both types are equally important in ensuring that the components of quality medical care are in place in an EMS system.

- A continuous quality improvement (CQI) program identifies and attempts to resolve problems in areas such as medical direction, financing, training, communication, prehospital management and transportation, interfacility transfer, receiving facilities, specialty care units, dispatch, public information and education, audit and quality assurance, disaster planning, and mutual aid.

- Quality EMS research helps shed light on the efficacy, effects, and cost-effectiveness of EMS interventions based on experimental data and can lead to changes in professional standards, training, equipment, and procedures.

- When planning research, the researcher should consider involving an institutional review board (IRB).

REFERENCES

1. Lyons A, Petrucelli J: *Medicine: an illustrated history*, New York, 1987, Harry N. Abrams.
2. McNeil E: *Airborne care of the ill and injured*, New York, 1983, Springer-Verlag.
3. National Highway Traffic Safety Administration, US Department of Health and Human Services, Health Resources and Services Administration, Maternal and Child Health Bureau: *Emergency medical services agenda for the future*, Washington, DC, 1999, The Administration.
4. National Highway Traffic Safety Administration, US Department of Transportation: *Emergency medical services: NHTSA leading the way*, Washington, DC, 1995, The Administration.
5. National Registry of Emergency Medical Technicians: *National emergency medical services education and practice blueprint*, Columbus, Ohio, 1993, The Registry.
6. US Department of Transportation National Highway Traffic Safety Administration: *EMT-Paramedic national standard curriculum*, Washington, DC, 1998, The Department.
7. National Association of EMS Physicians, National Highway Traffic Safety Administration, Maternal and Child Health Bureau: *National standard curriculum for medical direction*, Washington, DC, 1998, The Administration.
8. National Highway Traffic Safety Administration: *A leadership guide to quality improvement for emergency medical services (EMS) systems*, Washington, DC, 1997, The Administration.
9. Menegazzi J: *Research: the who, what, why, when and how*, Wilmington, Ohio, 1994, Ferno-Washington.

2 The Well-Being of the Paramedic

OBJECTIVES

Upon completion of this chapter, the paramedic student will be able to:

1. **Describe the components of wellness and associated benefits.**

2. **Discuss the paramedic's role in promoting wellness.**

3. **Outline the benefits of specific lifestyle choices that promote wellness, including proper nutrition, weight control, exercise, sleep, and smoking cessation.**

4. **Identify risk factors and warning signs of cancer and cardiovascular disease.**

5. **Identify preventive measures to minimize the risk of work-related illness or injury associated with exposure, lifting and moving patients, hostile environments, vehicle operations, and rescue situations.**

6. **List signs and symptoms of addiction and addictive behavior.**

7. **Distinguish between normal and abnormal anxiety and stress reactions.**

8. **Give examples of stress-reduction techniques.**

9. **Outline the 10 components of critical incident stress management.**

10. **Given a scenario involving death or dying, identify therapeutic actions you may take based on your knowledge of the dynamics of this process.**

11. **List measures that may be taken to reduce the risk of infectious disease exposure.**

12. **Outline actions that should be taken following a significant exposure to a patient's blood or other body fluids.**

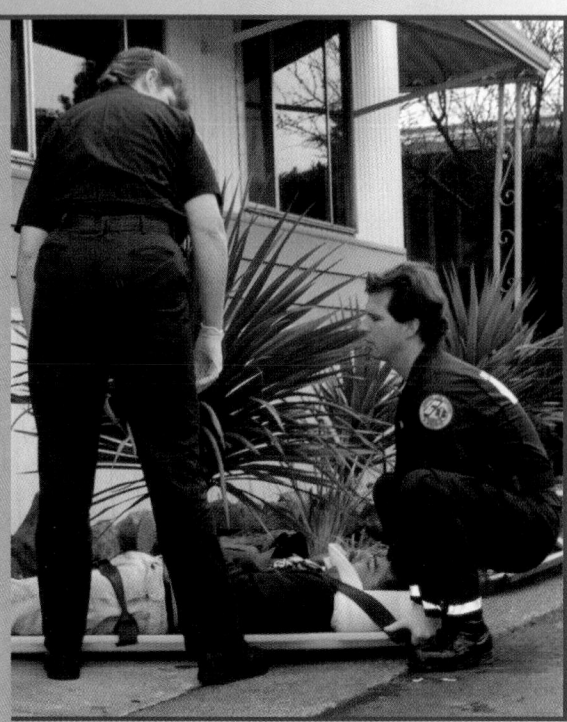

The paramedic has a demanding job that requires physical and mental well-being. By adopting a lifestyle that enhances personal wellness, paramedics can improve their health and serve as role models and coaches for others.

KEY TERMS

addiction: A compulsive, uncontrollable dependence on a substance, habit, or practice to such a degree that cessation causes severe emotional, mental, or physiological reactions.

adrenaline: An endogenous adrenal hormone.

anxiety: A state or feeling of apprehension, uneasiness, agitation, uncertainty, or fear resulting from the anticipation of some threat or danger.

autonomic nervous system: The part of the nervous system that regulates involuntary vital functions, including the activity of cardiac muscle, smooth muscle, and glands.

Circadian rhythm: A pattern based on a 24-hour cycle, especially repetition of certain physiological phenomena, such as sleeping and eating.

distress: Negative, debilitating, or harmful stress.

eustress: Positive, performance-enhancing stress.

stress: A nonspecific mental or physical strain caused by any emotional, physical, social, economic, or other factor that initiates a physiological response.

universal precautions: Infection control practices in health care that are observed with every patient and procedure and that prevent exposure to blood-borne pathogens.

Wellness Components

Wellness has two main components: physical well-being and mental and emotional health. Both are essential to the paramedic's personal health to safely deliver emergency care and manage stressful situations inherent in the profession.

Physical Well-Being

Several factors play a major role in maintaining physical health. These include good nutrition, physical fitness, adequate sleep, and the prevention of disease and injury.

Nutrition

Nutrients are foods that contain the elements necessary for body function. The six categories of nutrients are carbohydrates, fats, proteins, vitamins, minerals, and water.

Carbohydrates are composed of carbon, hydrogen, and oxygen and are obtained primarily from plant foods. The only important source of animal carbohydrate is lactose (milk sugar). Plants store carbohydrates as starch. Starch is made up of granules enclosed by cellulose walls that swell and burst when cooked, making them easier to digest than raw, uncooked starchy foods.

Fats in food are mixtures of three types of fatty acids (saturated, polyunsaturated, and monounsaturated) that differ in chemical makeup and in the types of foods in which they appear. Saturated fats are found primarily in meat and dairy products and in some vegetable fats. These fats raise the cholesterol levels in the blood by shutting down the process that normally removes excessive cholesterol from the body. Polyunsaturated fats are found in safflower, sunflower, corn, soybean and cottonseed oils, and some fish. These fats help rid the body of newly formed cholesterol. Monounsaturated fats are liquid vegetable oils such as canola and olive. Like polyunsaturated fats, these also may decrease blood cholesterol levels (Box 2-1).

> **NOTE**
>
> Cholesterol is present in all foods of animal origin and is heavily concentrated in fat and in poultry skin. It is a white, waxy substance found in every cell and is needed by the body for normal functioning. Not all cholesterol is harmful; an adequate amount of cholesterol is needed for body functions. It is manufactured in the liver and is carried through the bloodstream. Adding cholesterol to the diet can raise blood cholesterol levels and increases the risk of heart disease and stroke.

Proteins are composed of hydrogen, oxygen, carbon, and nitrogen (and most contain sulfur and phosphorus). They are essential to building body tissue during growth, maintenance, and repair. When proteins are digested, they break down into amino acids (classified as either *essential* or *nonessential*). Essential amino acids are necessary for body

BOX 2-1

FAT AND CHOLESTEROL CONTROL

Tips for a Healthful Eating Plan

- Select lean cuts of meat, such as loin and round cuts, and trim all visible fat.
- Buy lower-fat versions of your favorite dairy products, such as skim milk and skim-milk–based cheeses.
- For added flavor, use herbs and spices in place of high-fat flavorings or sauces on vegetables, meats, poultry, and fish.
- Chill soups and stews and skim off the fat that collects on the surface.
- Choose low-fat or nonfat versions of your favorite salad dressings, mayonnaise, yogurt, and sour cream.
- Use low-fat or fat-free marinades to tenderize and add flavor to leaner cuts of meat.

To Reduce Saturated Fats

- Use polyunsaturated or monounsaturated oil whenever a recipe calls for melted shortening or butter.
- Use vegetable-oil margarine in place of butter or lard. Look for whipped, lower-fat tub margarine.

Be "Fat" Smart

- Saturated fats usually are solid at room temperature and primarily come from animal foods such as meat, poultry, butter, and whole milk. Coconut, palm, and palm kernel oils are also high in saturated fat. Saturated fat is responsible for raising blood cholesterol levels.
- Polyunsaturated fats usually are liquid at room temperature and are found in vegetable oils. Safflower, sunflower, corn, and soybean oils contain the highest amounts of polyunsaturated fats. Polyunsaturated fats can help decrease high blood cholesterol levels when part of a healthful diet.
- Monounsaturated fats also are liquid at room temperature and are found in vegetable oils, such as canola and olive. Monounsaturated fats can help decrease high blood cholesterol levels if they are part of a lower-fat diet.
- Dietary cholesterol comes only from animal sources such as the fat in dairy products, egg yolks, meats, poultry, and seafood. Vegetables, fruits, and grains do not contain cholesterol.
- Hydrogenation is a process that makes an oil more solid at room temperature. Hydrogenated vegetable oils give some processed foods, such as margarine and crackers, a longer shelf life.

From The American Dietetic Association. National Center for Nutrition and Dietetics. The ABCs of fat, oil, and cholesterol. www.eatright.org, Chicago, Ill.

growth and cellular life. They must be obtained in food, because they are not produced in the body. Nonessential amino acids are *not* necessary for body health and growth and can be manufactured in the body. Proteins that contain all the essential amino acids are complete proteins and are found in meats and dairy products. Proteins that are missing one or more essential amino acids are incomplete proteins (e.g., those in grains and vegetables). Proteins can be used as a source of energy but should be spared for their more important role in body health by the sufficient intake of carbohydrates.

Vitamins are organic substances that are present in minute amounts in foods. Because they are essential for metabolism and cannot be produced in adequate amounts by the body, they must be obtained in food or through vitamin supplements. (An adequate intake of vitamins through a balanced diet should make vitamin supplements unnecessary in healthy individuals.) Vitamins are classified as water soluble and fat soluble. Vitamins C and B complex contain eight water-soluble vitamins. Water-soluble vitamins cannot be stored in the body and must be provided by the daily diet. Fat-soluble vitamins (vitamins A, D, E, and K) can be stored in the body; therefore a daily dietary intake of these vitamins is not required.

Minerals are inorganic elements that play an essential role in biochemical reactions in the body. They include calcium, chromium, iron, magnesium, potassium, selenium, sodium, and zinc. Like vitamins, minerals are obtained through the diet (Table 2-1).

NOTE

Diseases caused by vitamin deficiency (e.g., scurvy, rickets, beriberi) are rare in the United States and Canada and can be prevented by making proper food choices.

TABLE 2-1	THE ABCs OF NUTRITION	
	FUNCTION	**SOURCE**
Vitamins		
A	Proper eye function; keeps skin, hair, and nails healthy; helps maintain healthy gums, glands, bones, teeth; helps ward off infection; may protect against lung cancer	Liver,* dairy products,* fish, carrots, yellow squash, dark-green leafy vegetables, corn, tomatoes, papaya
B_1 (thiamine)	Helps convert carbohydrates into biological energy; promotes proper nerve function	Pork,* unrefined and enriched cereals, organ meats,* legumes, nuts*
B_2 (riboflavin)	Crucial in the production of body energy	Milk,* cheese,* yogurt,* green leafy vegetables, fruits, bread, cereals, meats*
B_3 (niacin)	Lowers cholesterol levels in blood only in very high doses; may protect against cardiovascular disease	Yeast, meats* including liver,* cereals, legumes, seeds*
B_6	Essential for protein breakdown and absorption	Beef,* poultry,* fish, pork,* bananas, nuts,* whole grains, vegetables
B_{12}	Essential for the healthy function of nerve tissue	Meats,* meat products,* shellfish, fish, poultry,* eggs*
Biotin	Needed for breakdown of glucose (a type of sugar) and formation of certain fatty acids necessary for several important body functions	Meats,* poultry,* fish, eggs,* nuts,* seeds,* legumes, vegetables
C (ascorbic acid)	Strengthens blood vessel walls; keeps gums healthy; promotes healing of cuts and wounds	Strawberries, citrus fruits, tomatoes, cabbage, cauliflower, broccoli, greens
D	Helps build and maintain teeth and bones; needed for body to absorb calcium	Egg yolks,* fish and cod liver oil,* fortified milk and butter*
E	Helps form red blood cells, muscle tissue, and other tissues; may protect against heart disease	Poultry,* seafood, seeds,* nuts,* cooked greens, wheat germ, fortified cereals, eggs*
K†	Needed for normal clotting of blood	Spinach, broccoli, brussels sprouts, kale, turnip greens
Minerals		
Calcium	Helps build strong bones and teeth; promotes proper muscle and nerve function; helps blood to clot; helps activate enzymes needed to convert food to energy; may protect against the development of fragile, porous bones	Milk,* cheese,* yogurt,* buttermilk, other dairy products,* green leafy vegetables
Chromium	Works with insulin to maintain normal blood sugar	Whole-grain cereals, condiments (black pepper, thyme), meat products,* cheeses*
Iron	Essential to make hemoglobin, the oxygen-carrying component of red blood cells	Red meat* and liver,* shellfish and fish, legumes, dried apricots, fortified breads and cereals
Magnesium	Activates enzymes needed to release energy in body; promotes bone growth; needed to make cells and genetic material	Green leafy vegetables, beans, nuts,* fortified whole-grain cereals and breads, oysters, scallops
Potassium	With sodium, helps to regulate body's fluid balance; plays a major role in muscle contraction, nerve conduction, beating of the heart	Bananas, citrus fruits, dried fruits, deep yellow vegetables, potatoes, legumes, milk,* bran cereal

U.S. Department of Agriculture's Center for Nutrition Policy and Promotion, Washington, D.C. www.usda.gov.
*These foods are high in fat and/or cholesterol. Use sparingly or substitute low-fat versions, where possible.
†Green leafy vegetables and other foods rich in vitamin K can contribute to blood clotting. If you take a drug that prevents blood clotting, talk to your physician before changing your diet.

Continued

TABLE 2-1	THE ABCs OF NUTRITION—cont'd	
	FUNCTION	**SOURCE**
Minerals—cont'd		
Selenium	Interacts with vitamin E to prevent breakdown of cells in body	Organ meats,* seafood, meats,* cereals and grains, egg yolks,* mushrooms, onions, garlic
Sodium	Helps maintain body fluid balance	Salt, processed foods, foods in brine, salted crackers and chips, cured meats, soy sauce (Note: sodium is so prevalent that low intake is very rare. The problem is avoiding excessive intake of sodium.)
Zinc	Boosts the immune system and helps fight disease; element in more than 100 enzymes—proteins that are essential to digestion and other functions	Red meats,* some seafoods, grains

Water is the most important nutrient, because cellular function depends on a fluid environment. Water composes 50% to 60% of our total body weight. (Infants have the greatest percentage of body water; older adults have the least.) Water is obtained through consumption of liquids and fresh fruits and vegetables. It also is produced when food is oxidized during digestion.

Food groups. The U.S. Department of Agriculture (USDA) defines five major food groups: meat, fish, and poultry; grains; dairy products; fruits; and vegetables. These can be cast into a Food Guide Pyramid (Fig. 2-1). The base of the pyramid comprises breads, cereals, rice, and pasta. The second level is made up of vegetables and fruits. The third level is dairy products (milk, yogurt, and cheese). The fourth level is meat, poultry, fish, dry beans, eggs, and nuts. The top of the pyramid is for fats, oils, and sweets (the "sixth" food group). When planning a healthy diet, individuals should use the pyramid and eat "from the bottom up." The foods nearest to the base should be eaten in greater quantity to obtain proper nutrition; the items toward the top should be consumed more sparingly (see the box in the right column).

? CRITICAL THINKING

Does your average diet meet these guidelines? If not, in what areas do you need to make changes?

FIBER

The human body requires fiber to maintain good health and to fight disease. Fiber (found only in plant foods) may be either soluble or insoluble. Soluble fiber (e.g., fiber obtained from peas, beans, oats, barley, and some fruits and vegetables) helps control the level of blood sugar and may lower the level of blood cholesterol. Insoluble fiber (found in whole grains and many vegetables) helps hold water in the colon and can reduce or prevent constipation. This type of fiber also may help prevent intestinal disease (e.g., diverticulosis, hemorrhoids, and certain cancers). Many authorities recommend a dietary intake of 20 to 35 g of fiber each day.

Principles of weight control. Guidelines for ideal weight (*Dietary Guidelines for Americans*) established by the U.S. Department of Agriculture and Health and Human Services are controversial and should be used only as a guide (Box 2-2). People who are overweight tend to be at greater risk for developing high blood pressure, diabetes mellitus, heart disease, some cancers, and other illnesses. The principles of weight control are to eat the right balance of foods in moderation, limit fat consumption to no more than 65 g of fat per day in a 2000-calorie diet, and exercise regularly (see the box at the top of p. 34).

Anyone committed to weight control for a healthier life should set realistic goals. For example, it generally is recommended that a steady weight

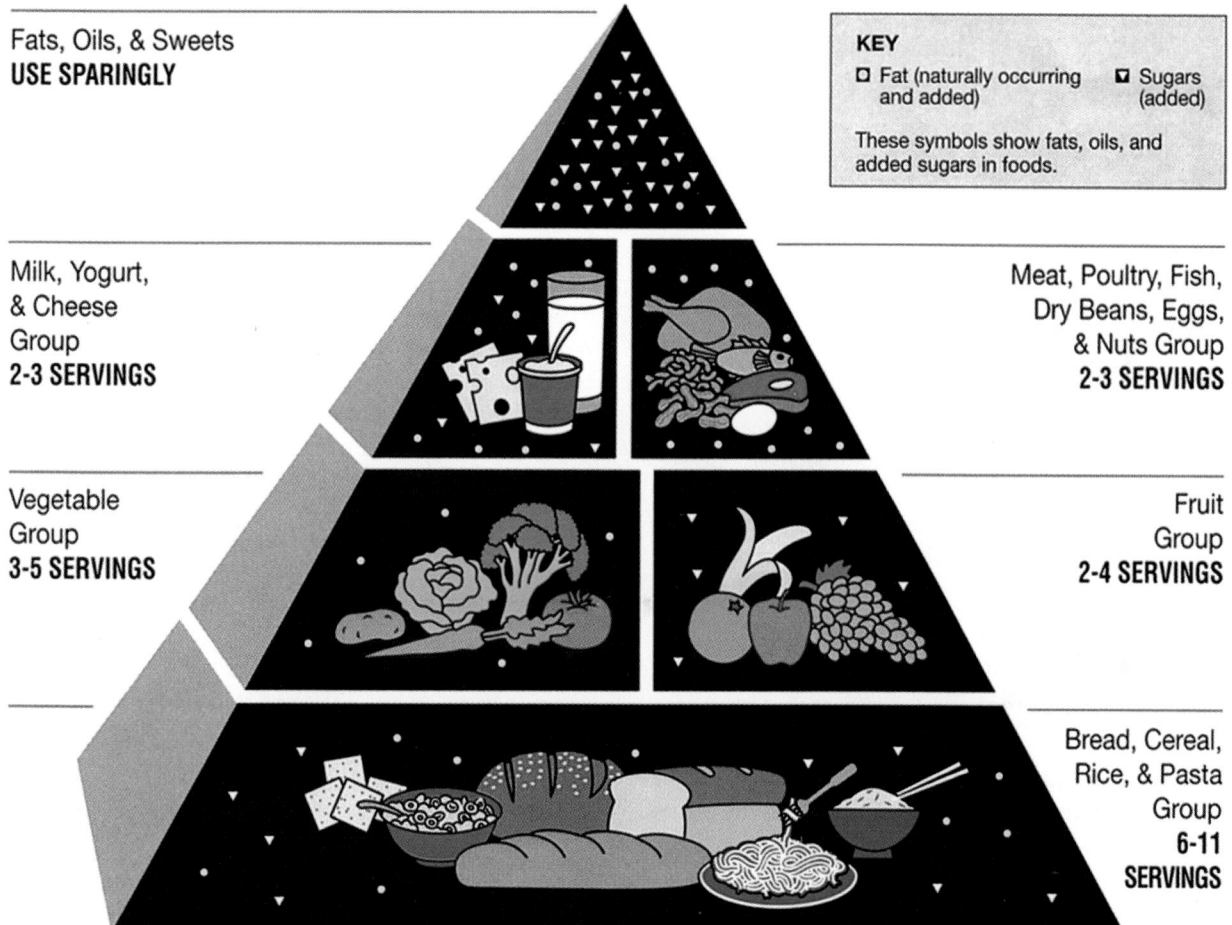

Fats, Oils, & Sweets
USE SPARINGLY

KEY
☐ Fat (naturally occurring   ☑ Sugars
  and added)   (added)

These symbols show fats, oils, and
added sugars in foods.

Milk, Yogurt,
& Cheese
Group
2-3 SERVINGS

Meat, Poultry, Fish,
Dry Beans, Eggs,
& Nuts Group
2-3 SERVINGS

Vegetable
Group
3-5 SERVINGS

Fruit
Group
2-4 SERVINGS

Bread, Cereal,
Rice, & Pasta
Group
**6-11
SERVINGS**

Fig. 2-1 The USDA Food Pyramid. (From U.S. Department of Agriculture: *USDA's food guide pyramid,* USDA Human Nutrition Information Pub. No. 249, Washington, D.C., 1992, U.S. Government Printing Office.)

loss of ½ to 1 pound per week should be the goal. A healthy lifestyle is balanced with proper nutrition and physical activity. A healthy diet includes a variety of foods that are low in fat, saturated fat, and cholesterol in addition to plenty of grain products, vegetables, and fruit. A diet also should be moderate in simple sugars, salt, and sodium. Alcoholic beverages should be avoided or consumed only in moderation. Finally, a system for analyzing weight control progress is essential. Adjustments and professional advice sometimes may be needed to achieve weight-control goals.

Physical Fitness

Physical fitness can be described as a condition that helps people look, feel, and do their best. It is individual and varies from person to person. It also is

BOX 2-2

DIETARY GUIDELINES FOR AMERICANS

Eat a variety of foods.
Balance the food you eat with physical activity—
  maintain or improve your weight.
Choose a diet with plenty of grain products, vegetables, and fruits.
Choose a diet low in fat, saturated fat, and cholesterol.
Choose a diet moderate in sugars.
Choose a diet moderate in salt and sodium.
If you drink alcoholic beverages, do so in moderation.

From U.S. Department of Agriculture and U.S. Department of Health and Human Services: *Nutrition and your health: dietary guidelines for Americans,* Home and Garden Bulletin No. 232, Washington, D.C., December 1995, U.S. Government Printing Office.

GETTING A HANDLE ON FAT

Eat foods that are less than 30% fat. Try to aim for no more than 3 g of fat per 100 calories, which provides about 27% of the total calories from fat. This is important for the following reasons:

- Each gram of fat has more than double the calories of a gram of protein or carbohydrate.
- The body uses less calories to "store" the fat as excess weight.
- 23% of the calories in complex carbohydrates are burned to make them into a usable form in the body; only 3% of fat calories are burned before they are "worn" on the hips or abdomen.
- Decreasing fat intake to less than 30% of daily calories helps reduce cholesterol, decreases risk of heart disease, helps with weight loss, and reduces risk of diabetes.

More than 90% fat: whipped cream, pork sausage, cooking oils, margarine, butter, gravy, mayonnaise

More than 80% fat: spare ribs, bologna, cream cheese, salad dressing, high-fat steaks (T-bone, Porterhouse, tenderloin, filet mignon)

More than 70% fat: half and half, peanuts, hot dogs, pork chops, most cheeses and nuts, sirloin steak, bacon, lamb chops

More than 60% fat: potato and corn chips, regular ground beef, ham, eggs

More than 50% fat: round steak, pot roast, creamed soup, ice cream, sweet rolls

More than 40% fat: whole milk, cake, doughnuts, french fries

More than 30% fat: muffins, cookies, fruit pies, lowfat milk, cottage cheese, tuna, chicken, turkey

More than 20% fat: lean fish, beef liver, ice milk

More than 10% fat: bread, pretzels, whole grains, legumes

Less than 10% fat: sherbet, nonfat milk, most fruits and vegetables, baked potato

---

influenced by age, sex, heredity, personal habits, exercise, and eating habits. Being physically fit offers many benefits, which include the following:

- Decreased resting heart rate and blood pressure
- Increased oxygen-carrying capacity
- Enhanced quality of life
- Increased muscle mass and metabolism
- Increased resistance to injury
- Improved personal appearance and self-image
- Maintenance of motor skills throughout life

Cardiovascular endurance. A smart prerequisite to any fitness program is a physical examination performed by a physician and a fitness assessment performed by a certified physical trainer. The purpose of these assessments is to evaluate a person's present physical condition and to make a baseline assessment for weight, including body mass index or BMI (see the box in the right column); high blood pressure; heart trouble (including family history); arthritis or other bone problems; muscular, ligament or tendon problems; and other known or suspected diseases. These assessments also will help to establish a heart rate target zone, a measure used to improve cardiovascular endurance through exercise. Ideally, the heart rate target zone should be maintained during exercise for 20 minutes to increase cardiovascular endurance.

THE BODY MASS INDEX

The Body Mass Index (BMI) is a widely used measurement of body fat that corrects for height. It is the only body fat index that conveys the risk of disease or death. A healthy BMI is 19 to 25. A BMI of 25 to 29 indicates "moderately overweight." A BMI of 30 or more indicates "severely overweight." To calculate your body mass index, use the following formula:

Step 1: Multiply your weight in pounds by 0.45
Example: 150 pounds $\times$ 0.45 = 67.5

Step 2: Multiply your height in inches by 0.025
Example: 5'9", or 69 inches $\times$ 0.025
= 1.725

Step 3: Square the answer from step 2
Example: 1.725 $\times$ 1.725 = 2.976

Step 4: Divide the answer in step 1 by the answer in step 3
Example: $\dfrac{67.5}{2.976}$
= BMI of 22.7

? CRITICAL THINKING

Calculate your BMI. Does it fall within the recommendations?

NOTE

A simple way to determine the heart rate target zone is to multiply the established maximum heart rate of 220 minus a person's age in years, and then multiply this number by 70%.

Example for a 25-year-old:
Maximum heart rate (220-25) =
195 × 70% = 136 beats per minute

Muscle strength. Another part of the fitness assessment evaluates muscular strength and endurance. Muscular strength is the ability of a muscle to exert force for a brief period. Muscle endurance is the ability of a muscle, or a group of muscles, to sustain repeated contractions or to continue applying force against a fixed object. Many exercises improve muscle strength and endurance.

The principles of training for muscle strength and endurance should consider isometric and isotonic exercises, resistance, repetitions, sets, and frequency. *Isometric* exercises are those that do not result in any movement of a joint (e.g., contraction performed against an immovable object such as a wall or door frame). These exercises do not increase muscle bulk significantly, but they do strengthen the muscle at the joint angle at which the contraction is performed. *Isotonic* exercises move a joint through a range of motion against resistance of a fixed weight (e.g., lifting a barbell). These exercises increase muscle bulk by developing tension within the muscle. *Resistance* refers to the amount of weight moved or lifted during isotonic exercises. A *repetition* ("rep") refers to the complete execution of an exercise from start to finish. A *set* is the specified number of times an exercise (rep) is executed start to finish, one after another, without any rest time. *Frequency* refers to the minimal number of workouts that will have a positive effect on muscle strength and endurance.

Muscular flexibility. Flexibility refers to the ability to move joints and use muscles through their full range of motion. During the fitness assessment, flexibility is measured in a number of ways. A lack of normal flexibility may lead to muscle strains and other injuries.

Muscular flexibility can be improved by stretching exercises, performed slowly, without a bounc-ing motion. The intensity of stretching exercises to increase flexibility should be mild (no straining or breath holding, no pain or discomfort). The frequency of flexibility exercises should be tailored to the individual's specific level of activity. For example, if daily work on an ambulance requires lifting patients into and out of the ambulance, regular stretching exercises specific to the paramedic's arms, back, thighs, calves, and hips would be beneficial (see the box at the top of p. 36).

? CRITICAL THINKING

How many minutes per week do you perform physical activities that raise your heart rate? What benefits does a paramedic gain by maintaining a high level of personal fitness?

The Importance of Sleep

Sleep plays an important role in being physically fit, because it helps to rejuvenate a tired body. The average adult needs 7 to 8 hours of sleep each day. In EMS, where rotating shifts and 24-hour work shifts are common, sleep deprivation may occur and interrupt the normal **Circadian rhythm**.

The Circadian (Latin for "about a day") rhythm is the body's physiological ebb and flow as it relates to the earth's orbit. This timing system is based roughly on the solar day as the earth revolves around the sun. For example, a person grows hungry or tired, energetic or irritable, at fairly predictable intervals each day as the body's internal systems fluctuate. Periods of sleepiness and wakefulness are influenced by the level of melatonin (secreted by the pineal gland) and cortisol (secreted by the adrenal glands). Release of these hormones is stimulated by darkness and suppressed by light. Therefore when the normal and regular division between night and day is disrupted on an ongoing basis (e.g., working rotating work shifts or responding to emergency calls in the early morning hours during a 24-hour work shift), irritability, depression, and physical illness can result (see the box on p. 36). Research is underway to help shift workers and their employers modify work schedules so that alterations in normal "biorhythms" will have minimal adverse effects on employee health and productivity.

PREVENTION AND REHABILITATION OF LOW BACK PAIN

The back is a complex system of ligaments, muscles, bones, nerves, and intervertebral discs, all of which can be injured by improper lifting techniques. EMS workers are highly vulnerable to low back pain and injury. An area of the back that frequently is a source of low back pain and injury is the lordosis (an inward curvature in the lumbar spine that is normally present to some degree). Abnormal curvature in this area can result from poor posture and from being overweight with associated weak abdominal muscles. Back injury can be prevented or lessened to a significant degree by being physically fit, performing regular stretching exercises, and following some general rules of lifting:

1. Know the weight (ask the patient's weight if you can, and add the weight of the equipment). Two people should work together to lift objects that weigh more than 60 pounds.

2. Know your physical ability and limitations.
3. Keep your back positioned with a normal curvature.
4. Use your legs and abdominal muscles to support the weight; use your back muscles to maintain balance.
5. Keep the weight close to your body.
6. Communicate clearly and frequently with your partner.

If back pain or injury occurs while lifting, pushing, pulling, or stretching, immediately report the situation to your supervisor. Treatment for back pain usually begins with rest, the application of ice or cold packs to minimize swelling, and sometimes pain medication and muscle relaxants. A rehabilitation program will normally follow the initial injury and often includes exercises to improve abdominal muscle strength and control of the pelvis and flexibility of the lower back.

From *EMT: injury free*, Wilmington, Ohio, 1991, Ferno-Washington.

GETTING YOUR Zs

Working nights, 24-hour shifts, and rotating shifts can inhibit getting enough rest. Here are some helpful tips:

- Allow some time to "unwind" and relax before trying to go to sleep.
- Consider exercise before sleeping as a way to reduce stress.
- Avoid stimulants (e.g., caffeine in coffee, soda, tea, chocolate) during the last few hours of your work shift.
- Eat simple carbohydrates (e.g., cookies or candy bar) to release serotonin (a hormone that may help induce sleep).
- Keep your sleeping area cool and dark so that your body will "think" it's nighttime.
- Make sure your family and friends know about your work shifts and your sleeping schedule to minimize interruptions.
- Try to maintain a "normal" period of dedicated sleep time each day.
- Consult a physician about your sleep difficulties when needed.

? CRITICAL THINKING

Do you get enough sleep? If not, which of these strategies should you try in an attempt to increase your hours of sleep?

NOTE

The Circadian rhythm is responsible for the "jet lag" that occurs during air travel to a distant time zone. Studies suggest that the symptoms of jet lag may be relieved by the administration of melatonin.

Disease Prevention

A paramedic can do much to help prevent personal serious illness. As health care professionals, paramedics have a responsibility to serve as role models in disease prevention.

Cardiovascular disease. Cardiovascular disease accounts for more than 1 million deaths each year in the United States.[1] For most, this disease process can be altered through healthy living. In addition to improving cardiovascular endurance, several

CANADIAN EMS STANDARDS

Cardiovascular disease (heart disease and stroke) is Canada's number one killer, accounting for about 36% of all deaths each year.

BOX 2-3

UNDERSTANDING THE CHOLESTEROL NUMBERS

Cholesterol circulates through the body attached to different size fat-carrying proteins called *lipoproteins*. Low-density lipoproteins (LDLs) are more common and are thought to carry cholesterol to the cells where they can promote blood vessel disease. Smaller high-density lipoproteins (HDLs) are believed to carry cholesterol to the liver and help prevent or slow down blood vessel disease. Very low-density lipoproteins (VLDLs) consist mostly of triglycerides (the main fatty substance in the fluid portion of blood) that are absorbed by the intestines and are therefore affected by fasting (abstaining from all or certain foods).

Cholesterol
High blood cholesterol: 240 mg/dL or higher
Borderline high blood cholesterol: 220–239 mg/dL
Desirable blood cholesterol: below 200 mg/dL

LDL Cholesterol: The "Bad" Cholesterol
Very high LDL cholesterol: 189 mg/dL or higher
High LDL cholesterol: 160–189 mg/dL or higher
Borderline high LDL cholesterol: 130–159 mg/dL
Desirable LDL cholesterol: below 100 mg/dL

HDL Cholesterol: Higher Is Better
Low HDL cholesterol: less than 40 mg/dL
Desirable HDL cholesterol: above 60 mg/dL

VLDL Triglyceride: Lower Is Better
Should not exceed 200–300 mg/dL

BOX 2-4

THE SEVEN WARNING SIGNS OF CANCER (CAUTION) AS DESIGNATED BY THE AMERICAN CANCER SOCIETY

Change in bowel or bladder habits
A sore throat that does not heal
Unusual bleeding or discharge
Thickening or lump in the breast or elsewhere
Indigestion or difficulty swallowing
Obvious change in a wart or mole
Nagging cough or hoarseness

---

are potentially life threatening. The fundamental cause of all cancer is a change or mutation in the nucleus of a cell. Most common cancers are linked to one of three environmental risk factors: smoking, sunlight, or diet. Dietary factors are associated with some cancers of the gastrointestinal tract and may be linked to others, such as cancer of the breast, prostate, or uterus. A lack of dietary fiber is believed to be a risk factor for these cancers. Steps in cancer prevention include the following:

- Elimination of smoking
- Dietary changes
- Limitation of sun exposure; using sunscreen
- Regular physical examinations
- Attention to the warning signs (Box 2-4)
- Periodic risk assessment

Infectious disease. Most infectious diseases can be avoided by practicing good personal hygiene (including hand washing) and by following **universal precautions** and other guidelines in the workplace as established by the Centers for Disease Control and Prevention (CDC), the Occupational Safety and Health Administration (OSHA), the National Fire Protection Association (NFPA), the Federal Emergency Management Agency (FEMA), the United States Fire Administration (USFA), and others (Table 2-2). If potential exposure to an infectious disease occurs, it should be reported immediately to the receiving hospital and the appropriate designated officer in the local agency so that communications can be coordinated between the hospital and emergency response organization (see Chapter 37). As an additional safeguard against infectious diseases, OSHA requires that a periodic

other steps are necessary in preventing this disease. These include the following:

- Eliminating cigarette smoking
- Controlling high blood pressure
- Maintaining a favorable body-fat composition through regular exercise
- Maintaining a good total cholesterol/HDL ratio (Box 2-3)
- Monitoring triglyceride levels
- Estrogen therapy for postmenopausal women
- Reducing stress
- Periodic risk assessment

Cancer

The term *cancer* encompasses more than 100 diseases affecting nearly every part of the body, and all

TABLE 2-2	PERSONAL EQUIPMENT FOR PROTECTION AGAINST TRANSMISSION OF HIV AND HEPATITIS B VIRUS			
ACTIVITY	**DISPOSABLE GLOVES**	**GOWN**	**MASK**	**PROTECTIVE EYEWEAR**
Bleeding control (spurting blood)	Yes	Yes	Yes	Yes
Bleeding control (minimal blood)	Yes	No	No	No
Emergency childbirth	Yes	Yes	Yes*	Yes*
Intravenous therapy	Yes	No	No	No
Endotracheal intubation	Yes	No	Yes*	Yes*
Oral or nasal suctioning	Yes	No	No	No
Administration of an injection	No	No	No	No

*If splashing is likely.

risk assessment be made available to employees, including regular testing for tuberculosis and vaccinations for infectious diseases (e.g., hepatitis B).

Injury Prevention

Job-related injuries can be minimized by being knowledgeable about body mechanics during lifting and moving; being alert for hostile environments; prioritizing personal safety during rescue situations; practicing safe vehicle operations; and by utilizing safety equipment and supplies.

Body mechanics during lifting and moving. In addition to the general rules for lifting previously described, the paramedic should consider the following guidelines when lifting and moving patients or equipment:

- Only move a victim you can safely handle; get additional help if needed.
- Look where you're walking or crawling.
- Move forward rather than backward when possible.
- Take short steps, if walking.
- Bend at the hips and knees.
- Lift with the legs, not the back.
- Keep the load close to the body.
- Keep patient's body in line when moving.

Hostile environments. Responding to violent crimes of murder, rape, robbery, acts of terrorism, and aggravated assault (and often, the associated use of illegal drugs) may place paramedics in an unavoidable

hostile environment that threatens their personal safety. When these situations occur, paramedics should do the following:

- Carefully evaluate the scene for safety concerns and not enter the scene until it is safe.
- Coordinate all activities with law enforcement personnel.
- Follow protocols for establishing a Medical Incident Command (see Chapter 49).
- Plan an entrance and escape route(s).
- Above all else, stay alert and be prepared for the unexpected.

Safely managing a violent scene requires specialized training and organization among many emergency response agencies. As a member of the emergency response team, paramedics should participate in organized planning, training, and practice sessions designed to ensure emergency provider safety in hostile environments (see Chapter 52).

Rescue situations. Rescue situations also can present many personal safety issues. Examples include exposure to hazardous materials, inclement weather, temperature extremes, fire, toxic gases, unstable structures, heavy equipment, road hazards, and sharp edges and fragments. Initial scene assessment for hazards, personal protective measures, and constant monitoring throughout the operation is essential for every rescue response. A safe rescue requires appropriate use of protective gear, specialized training, and safe rescue practices (see Chapter 50).

Safe vehicle operation. Proper operation of an emergency vehicle is important for personal safety and the safety of the crew and patient (see Chapter 48). Many factors affect safe vehicle operations, including the following:

- Safe driving of the vehicle
- Safe and appropriate use of escorts to and from emergency scenes
- Adverse environmental conditions (e.g., inclement weather)
- Appropriate use of audible and visual warning devices
- Proceeding through intersections safely
- Parking at the emergency scene
- Maintaining "due regard" for the safety of all others

? CRITICAL THINKING

Is there any patient situation that would justify using unsafe vehicle operations that could jeopardize the safety of those in the ambulance or in other vehicles?

Some EMS agencies require their employees to receive specialized driver's training such as the United States Department of Transportation's (USDOT) *Emergency Vehicle Operation Course* (EVOC). These supervised programs allow EMS providers to practice emergency driving maneuvers in a safe and controlled setting.

Safety equipment and supplies. Appropriate use of safety equipment and supplies is an important aspect of injury prevention for EMS providers. Standards for protective clothing and equipment are required by OSHA. These and other standards (such as those established by NFPA) are used by many states, municipalities, and fire and EMS agencies to ensure employee safety (see Chapter 50). Safety equipment and supplies include the following:

- Body substance isolation equipment
- Head protection
- Eye protection
- Hearing protection
- Respiratory protection
- Gloves
- Boots

BOX 2-5

COMMON DRUGS AND SUBSTANCES THAT ARE MISUSED OR ABUSED

- Alcohol
- Central nervous system stimulants (e.g., cocaine and amphetamines)
- Cigarettes and other tobacco products
- Hallucinogens
- Inhalants
- Marijuana
- Narcotics and related drugs
- Sedative-hypnotics
- Tranquilizers
- Nonprescription substances:
  Sedatives
  Appetite suppressants
  Laxatives
  Cough and cold preparations
  Nasal sprays
  Analgesics

- Coveralls
- Turnout coat and pants
- Specialty equipment

Mental and Emotional Health

Many factors contribute to mental and emotional health. An important factor is to be aware of "warning signs" that could indicate a potential problem (e.g., signs of substance misuse and health disorders caused by anxiety and stress). Also important to maintaining good emotional health is realizing the value of having personal time; being connected with family, peers, and the community; and accepting the personal differences that make people unique.

Substance Misuse and Abuse Control

The misuse and abuse of drugs and other substances may lead to chemical dependency (**addiction**) with a wide range of effects on physical and mental health (Box 2-5). Warning signs of addiction and addictive behavior include the following:

- Using a substance to relieve tension
- Using an increasing amount of the substance
- Lying about using the substance

- Experiencing guilt about using the substance
- Avoiding discussion about using the substance
- Interfering with daily activities as a result of substance abuse

<table>
<tr><td>**?** CRITICAL THINKING</td></tr>
</table>

Do you know anyone with these behaviors?

Methods used to manage substance abuse depend on the type of substance being misused. Substance misuse/abuse control may include a combination of professional counseling, physician-controlled drug therapy, and support programs.

Smoking cessation. Cigarette smoking is a major health hazard that is responsible for more than 400,000 deaths each year in the United States.[1] The health ramifications of cigarette smoking are numerous, including an increased risk of the following:

- Coronary heart disease (CHD)
- Myocardial infarction (MI)
- Sudden death
- Dying from a variety of diseases
- Miscarriage, premature birth, and birth defects

Regardless of the reasons cigarette smokers give for smoking (peer pressure, relief of stress, weight control, and others), most people continue to smoke because of the addictive properties of nicotine (the stimulant in tobacco). Other harmful chemicals in cigarette smoke include hydrocarbons ("tar") and carbon monoxide. Exposure to these chemicals also is considered a health hazard for nonsmokers who have an increased risk of developing smoking-related illnesses through "passive smoking" (secondhand smoke).

Many resources and smoking cessation programs are available to those who want to quit smoking. Examples include support groups and "quit smoking campaigns" sponsored by the American Heart Association, the American Cancer Society, the American Red Cross, government health agencies, and local health care organizations. Other techniques that may be used alone or in conjunction with these health programs include the use of prescription and nonprescription drugs (e.g., bupropion [Zyban], dermal patches, nicotine chewing

gum) that decrease the physical effects of smoking cessation and help to "wean" the smoker off of nicotine (Box 2-6).

Anxiety and Stress

Anxiety can be defined as the uneasiness or dread about future uncertainties. **Stress** can result from the interaction of events that cause anxiety and the coping abilities of the individual. Although stress can be positive (described later in this chapter), it usually is associated with generating a negative effect (e.g., fear, depression, guilt). Recognizing and effectively coping with anxiety and stress is important for career longevity in the EMS profession.

> **NOTE**
>
> The term *stress* was coined in its medical usage by Austrian-born Hans Seyle, a professor at the University of Montreal, who published a book by that title in 1950.

Personal Time for Meditation and Contemplation

Setting aside some "personal time" for meditation and contemplation can greatly enhance mental and perhaps even physical health. *Meditation* is a form of relaxation whereby individuals limit their awareness to a repeated or constant focus that holds some attraction (e.g., controlled breathing, a pleasant site, fragrance, or a mantra). This quiet time of meditation provides an uninterrupted period for thoughtful introspection (contemplation) of important things in a person's life. Most who practice meditation do so once or twice a day for 10 to 20 minutes.

> **NOTE**
>
> Spirituality is a unique characteristic of human existence and should not be overlooked as an effective means for some to achieve mental and physical well-being.

Family, Peer, and Community Connections

Belonging to groups can affect a person's motivation and performance in positive ways. People tend to associate with others most like themselves (e.g., family members, co-workers, members of community and religious organizations). These groups provide a "connection" with people who share similar values and interests. As a rule, these relationships

---

BOX 2-6

BODY CHANGES WHEN YOU STOP SMOKING

Within 20 minutes of your last cigarette:

Pulse and blood pressure drop to normal
Body temperature of hands and feet increases to normal

Within 8 hours of your last cigarette:

Carbon monoxide level in blood drops to normal
Oxygen level in blood increases to normal

Within 24 hours of your last cigarette:

Chance of heart attack decreases

Within 48 hours of your last cigarette:

Nerve endings begin to regenerate
Ability to smell and taste is enhanced

Within 72 hours of your last cigarette:

Bronchial tubes relax, making breathing easier
Lung capacity increases

Within 2 weeks to 3 months:

Circulation improves
Walking becomes easier
Lung function increases up to 30%

Within 1 to 9 months after your last cigarette:

Coughing, sinus congestion, fatigue, and shortness of breath decrease
Cilia regrow in lungs, increasing the ability to handle mucus, clean the lungs, and reduce infection

Within 5 years of your last cigarette:

Lung cancer death rate for the average smoker (one pack/day) decreases

Within 10 years of your last cigarette:

Lung cancer death rate drops to 12 deaths per 100,000—almost the rate of nonsmokers
Precancerous cells are replaced
Risk for other cancers—such as those of the mouth, larynx, esophagus, bladder, kidney, and pancreas—decreases (20 chemicals in tobacco smoke cause cancer)

From the American Cancer Society.

---

are healthy and raise self-esteem by providing a way to contribute to group activities and goals and to interact in decision making, communication, and cooperative work.

Freedom from Prejudice

Accepting cultural differences allows individuals to learn about other cultures, to see cultural variations in a positive light, and to affirm the values of these differences. The four major ethnic minority groups in the United States are Hispanic/Latinos (Mexican-American, Puerto Rican, Cuban, Central and South American), Asians (Chinese, Korean, Japanese), Southwest Asians (Vietnamese, Laotians, Cambodians), and African-Americans. Providing health care to patients of some cultures may require special communication skills and additional education to understand their customs and beliefs. Obtaining this education can be personally fulfilling and worthwhile. It allows the paramedic to see life from another "view."

Stress

As previously stated, stress can be both positive and negative. "Good" stress (**eustress**) is a positive response to stimuli and is considered "protective." "Bad" stress (**distress**) is a negative response to environmental stimuli and is the source of anxiety and stress-related disorders.

Phases of the Stress Response

The responses to stress may be physical, emotional, or both. The three stages of the stress response are the alarm reaction, resistance, and exhaustion (Fig. 2-2).[2] Dr. Seyle called these phases of the stress response the general adaption syndrome (GAS) to describe the attempt of body and mind to deal with stressful events.

Alarm Reaction

The human body can quickly prepare itself to do battle or run from danger. This "fight or flight"

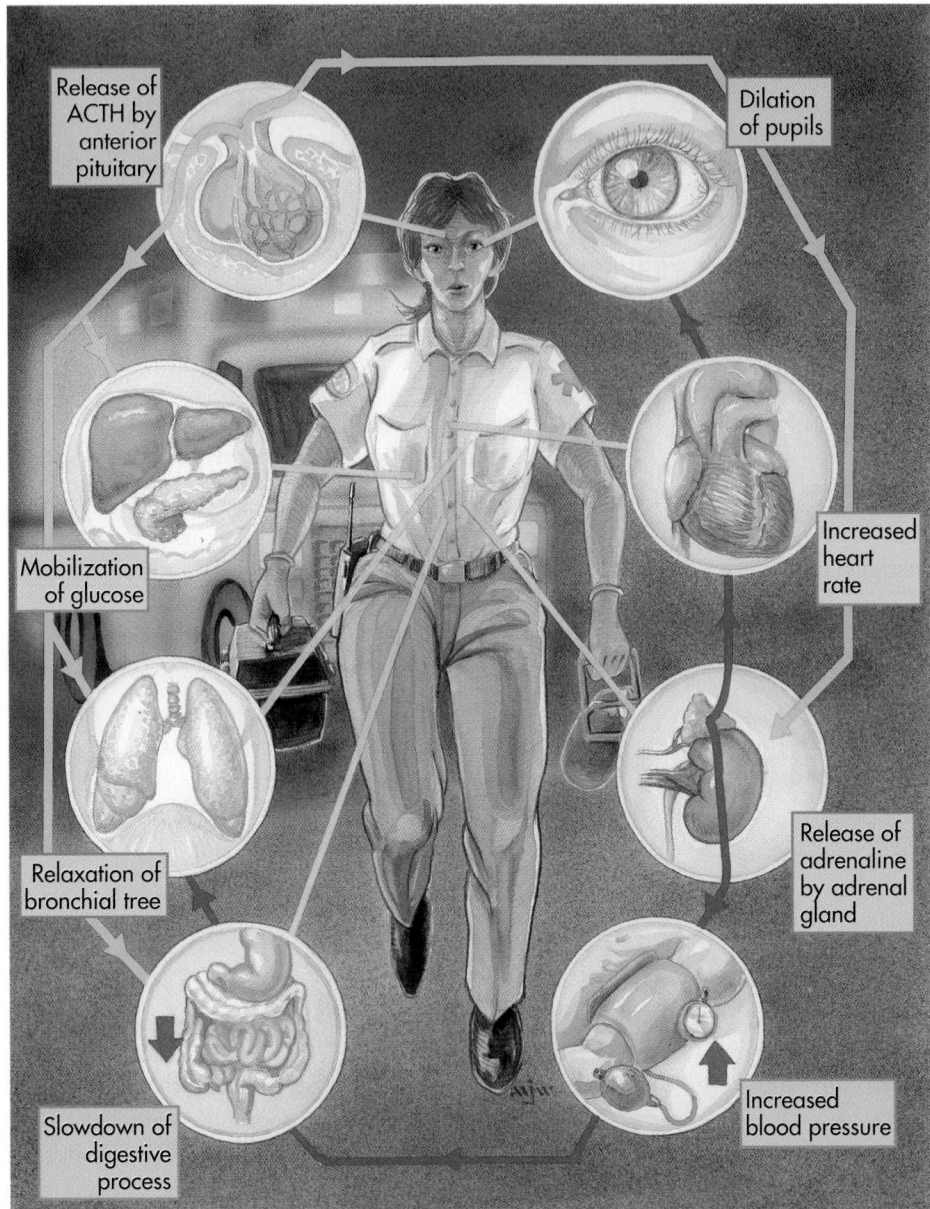

Fig. 2-2 Physiological response to stress. During the alarm reaction, the release of adrenocorti-cotropic hormone *(yellow)* results in a sympathetic discharge of adrenaline *(red)*. These "stress hormones" stimulate glucose production and cause the heart rate to increase, blood pressure to rise, and pupils to dilate. The bronchial tree relaxes for deep breathing, the digestive process slows, and the blood supply shifts to accommodate clotting mechanisms in case the body is wounded.

phenomenon occurs when any emergency situation threatens one's safety or comfort. This reaction is considered positive (eustress) in that it prepares individuals to be alert and to defend themselves. Initially, the body's response to stress is unaffected by the type of situation. It reacts equally to events that are pleasant or unpleasant, dangerous or exciting, happy or sad. The purpose of the response is to

rapidly achieve top physical preparedness to cope with the event. Examples would be an argument with a co-worker, performing an unfamiliar patient care procedure, and participating in the delivery of a healthy infant.

The alarm reaction is mediated by the **autonomic nervous system** (ANS) and coordinated by the hypothalamus. The hypothalamus triggers the pituitary gland to release adrenocorticotropic hormone (ACTH) into the bloodstream. This "stress hormone" stimulates glucose production and increases the blood's concentration of energy-providing nutrients necessary for the response to stress. ACTH also activates the adrenal glands for an intense sympathetic discharge of **adrenaline** and noradrenaline, which cause heart rate to increase, blood pressure to rise, and the pupils of the eyes to dilate, thereby improving vision. The combination of these hormones relaxes the bronchial tree for deeper breathing, increases blood sugar for maximal energy, slows the digestive process, and shifts blood supply to accommodate the clotting mechanism in case the body is wounded. After these physiological events, the body becomes ready for an emergency (fight or flight) and can perform feats of strength and endurance far beyond its normal capacity (see Fig. 2-2). The alarm reaction takes only seconds and occurs to some extent at the body's first exposure to a stressor. When the body realizes that a particular event is not dangerous or does not require the alarm reaction, the response stops. The individual begins to adapt to the situation, and bodily functions return to normal.

Resistance

The stress response raises the level of resistance to the agent that provoked it and others like it. That is, if a particular stress persists long enough, a person's reactions change. For example, as a paramedic becomes accustomed to responding to emergency scenes in an ambulance using audible and visual warning devices, the alarm reaction that once occurred is no longer elicited. Therefore reactions to stressors may change over time.

Exhaustion

As stress continues, coping mechanisms become exhausted and resistance fails. For example, paramedics may appear to be unaffected by the stress of life-threatening emergencies, when in fact all of their adaptive resources have been used to reach this stage of resistance. When any "reservoir" of adaptive resources no longer exists, resistance to other types of stress tends to decline as well, and the body may become susceptible to physical and psychological ills. Rest and recovery usually are needed before individuals are ready for another "emergency."

Factors That Trigger the Stress Response

Each person has unique capabilities to deal with stressful situations. Individual reactions to stress are "customized" based on previous exposure to a specific type of stress, perception of the stressful event, and personal coping skills. Many factors can trigger the stress response. Examples include the following:

- Loss of something that is of value
- Injury or threat of injury
- Poor health or nutrition
- Frustration
- Ineffective coping skills

Physiological and Psychological Effects of Stress

Anxiety is a common symptom of stress. Feeling anxious in certain situations or unusual circumstances is considered normal and healthy. This response provides a warning system that protects us from being overwhelmed by a sudden stimulation and prepares us for action in critical situations. This adaptive response to stress prepares the paramedic to make quick, appropriate decisions regarding the emergency and to perform at maximal efficiency.

Stress that is not effectively reduced by a solution to the conflict or emergency event may lead to an abnormally continued state of vigilance and alertness beyond the existing state of the emergency. The paramedic may then begin to experience chronic anxiety. Chronic anxiety fails to stimulate effective coping behavior, and a person may respond to conflict or stress by anxious behavior alone. Anxiety interferes with thought processes, personal relationships, and work performance. A person may develop problems in concentration, lose the ability to trust other people, or become isolated or withdrawn.

Individuals who frequently are exposed to stressful situations or who are unable to cope effectively with stressful events may experience a chronic state of anxiety leading to physical, emotional, cognitive, and behavioral effects (Box 2-7). Some warning signs, such as chest pain and difficulty breathing, may require immediate evaluation and medical care; others require less immediate action. The presence of one or more warning signs is an indicator of distress; however, absence of warning signs does not preclude the possibility of a stress reaction.

WARNING SIGNS AND SYMPTOMS OF STRESS

Physical
- Cardiac rhythm disturbances
- Chest pain
- Difficulty breathing
- Nausea
- Profuse sweating
- Sleep disturbances
- Vomiting

Emotional
- Anger
- Denial
- Fear
- Feeling of being overwhelmed
- Inappropriate emotions
- Panic reactions

Cognitive
- Confusion
- Decreased level of awareness
- Difficulty making decisions
- Disorientation
- Distressing dreams
- Memory problems
- Poor concentration

Behavioral
- Changes in eating habits
- Crying spells
- Excessive silence
- Hyperactivity
- Increased alcohol consumption
- Increased smoking
- Withdrawal

Causes of Stress in EMS

A variety of sources can produce stress in EMS work. Environmental stress includes noise, inclement weather conditions, confined work spaces, poor scene lighting, spectators, rapid response to the scene, and life-and-death decision making. Psychosocial stress arises from family relationships, conflicts with co-workers, abusive patients, and similar sources. Personality stress is the human element that relates to the way a person thinks and feels (e.g., the need to be liked, personal expectations, and feelings of guilt and anxiety). Choosing a career in EMS requires developing an understanding of job-related stress and effective stress management.

Reactions to Stress

Perhaps certain personalities are attracted to certain types of careers.[3] Many believe that EMS providers, firefighters, police officers, and others in public safety professions are predisposed to stressful and demanding jobs. However, no personality is immune from potential conflicts in managing stress.

Adaptation

Adaptation is a dynamic process involving "learning" successful ways to deal with stressful situations. This process usually begins with using defense mechanisms, then developing coping skills, followed by problem solving, and culminating in mastery.

Defense mechanisms are adaptive functions of the personality (see the box on p. 45). They assist a person in adjusting to stressful situations and help a person to avoid dealing with problems. Denial, for example, is a defense mechanism that might be used to emotionally separate a person from the event long enough to adequately deal with a problem that normally would be overwhelming.

Coping is an active, confronting process involving gathering information and using it to change or adjust to a new situation. Some beneficial coping mechanisms include engaging in regular physical exercise and dealing with stress by being involved in work activity that results in financial rewards and enhanced productivity. Other positive coping mechanisms include the ability to find humorous aspects in personal crises and "talking through" stressful situations with family members, friends, and co-workers.

People also may use harmful or negative coping mechanisms. An individual may become withdrawn or use alcohol or other drugs. Some have angry outbursts toward family members and co-workers, whereas others may become silent. These negative coping mechanisms threaten interpersonal relationships with co-workers and loved ones and should be considered as signs that an individual is having trouble dealing with stress.

COMMON DEFENSE MECHANISMS

Repression: Repression is believed to be the mechanism underlying all other defense mechanisms. Repression is the involuntary attempt to keep certain feelings or memories from reaching conscious awareness. Traumatic events, intolerable and dangerous impulses, and other unacceptable ideas are forced out of consciousness. This defense mechanism may be viewed as a result of an approach-avoidance conflict, which is a conflict between trying to remember or think about something and trying to avoid the topic because it produces fear. Once repressions form, they usually are difficult to abolish. The individual must be reassured that no danger exists in remembering the event. For example, an EMS co-worker is killed while on duty. The partner has no recall of the event from the time they arrived at the scene until after the event.

Regression: Regression is characterized by a return to earlier levels of emotional adjustment. Of all the reactions to anxiety and danger, extreme regression may be the most dramatic and debilitating. The individual returns to an earlier developmental phase of life when tension and conflict could be avoided. For example, an EMS worker throws a "temper tantrum" because he was assigned driver status on a work shift when he thought he would have direct patient-care duties.

Projection: Projection involves attributing one's own undesirable characteristics, feelings, motives, or desires to someone else. It may appear as aggression toward others when the problem is actually self-anger. Often, individuals are incorrect in labeling their own motives and the motives of others. For example, a paramedic crashes an emergency vehicle en route to a call. Because of guilt, she feels that others blame her for the crash when in fact she is blaming herself.

Rationalization: Rationalizations occur when, as a result of social training, people feel the need to logically explain their behavior because acceptance of the true explanation would provoke anxiety or guilt. The individual is trying to prove that the behavior is "rational" and therefore worthy of the approval of self and others. Rationalization is a commonly used defense mechanism. For example, a paramedic performs a poor physical examination on a trauma patient and fails to discover a femur fracture. When questioned by medical direction, she justifies her actions by stating that the police were hurrying her to clear the scene.

Compensation: Compensation is an attempt to substitute or cover up for a real or imagined weakness by emphasizing a more positive trait, skill, or attribute. Compensatory mechanisms disguise and conceal frustration and consequent anxiety by focusing attention on other behavior. For example, an EMS crew member has weak clinical skills and feels inadequate at emergency scenes. He compensates by becoming an instructor in water rescue.

Reaction formation: Reaction formation is a defensive behavior that prevents unacceptable desires from being expressed by exaggerating opposing attitudes and behavior and thereby expressing the opposite of the true motive. The original impulse is still subconsciously present but is masked by actions or attitudes that do not cause anxiety or stress. For example, a paramedic is outwardly friendly to a co-worker whom she dislikes.

Sublimation: Sublimation (a form of substitution) is the modification of unacceptable urges so that they become socially acceptable. Sublimation is considered a defense mechanism, but its functions are believed to extend beyond that of protection. It requires an energy transformation in which instinctual drives are substituted in activities that may produce a higher cultural achievement. For example, a paramedic who is angered from seeing people die in drunk-driving crashes establishes a public awareness program on the hazards of drinking and driving.

Denial: Denial is a defense mechanism in which elements of reality that consciously would be intolerable are rejected. Protection from unpleasant reality is obtained by refusing to perceive it. There may be denial of the experience itself or the memory of it. For example, an individual who has just lost a loved one may be unable to accept the reality of death. (Denial differs from repression in that individuals who use repression as a defense mechanism seem to "deliberately" keep their feelings or memories at a distance from the conscious mind.)

Substitution: This defense mechanism substitutes an alternative activity or goal for an originally desired but unobtainable one. It may involve the redirection of an emotion from the original object to a more acceptable substitute object. Substitution often results from frustration. For example, a co-worker is experiencing marital problems and feels that it is unacceptable to argue with his spouse. He substitutes and displaces his anger at work by being irritable and hostile toward other crew members.

Isolation: Isolation involves the separation of unacceptable impulses, acts, or ideas from their origin in memory. This defense mechanism removes the emotional charge from the event and prevents feelings from accompanying the memory. Isolation probably is helpful to the EMS providers who must "turn off" feelings until after the emergency call has been completed. For example, an EMS provider who also is a parent renders emergency care to a dying child without being overwhelmed by personal emotions.

Problem solving involves analyzing a problem situation and generating options to deal with the issue immediately and in the future. Problem solving allows a person to clearly identify the problem and determine a course of action. This is a healthy approach to everyday concerns.

Mastery refers to the ability to see multiple options and potential solutions for challenging situations. It results from extensive experience and the use of effective coping mechanisms with situations that are very similar. Mastery may be difficult to achieve.

Stress Management Techniques

To manage stress effectively, a person must recognize the early warning signs of anxiety. Some of the physical effects of anxiety an individual may notice include the following:

- Heart palpitations
- Difficult or rapid breathing
- Dry mouth
- Chest tightness or pain
- Anorexia (lack of appetite), nausea, vomiting, diarrhea, abdominal cramps, flatulence, "butterflies"
- Flushing, diaphoresis, body temperature fluctuation
- Urgency and frequency in urination
- Dysmenorrhea (painful menstruation), decreased sexual drive or performance
- Aching muscles, joints

Physical effects that may not be as noticeable include the following:

- Increased blood pressure and heart rate
- Blood shunting (diversion of the flow) to muscles
- Increased blood glucose levels
- Increased adrenaline production by adrenal glands
- Reduced gastrointestinal peristalsis
- Pupillary dilation

Many warning signs appear during the emergency response or within 24 hours after the event. Some responses, however, may be delayed for quite some time and may not appear for months or years after the event. If signs and symptoms of stress-related illness appear, the person should seek appropriate medical or psychological help.

Intervening to alleviate stress is as important as recognizing its warning signals. Methods that may be used to initially manage stress include reframing, controlled breathing, progressive relaxation, and guided imagery. All of these methods require practice to perform them properly. Reframing involves looking at the situation from a different emotional viewpoint and then placing it in a different "frame" that fits the facts of another situation equally well, thereby changing its meaning. Controlled breathing is a natural stress control technique whereby a person concentrates on his or her depth and rate of breathing to achieve a calming effect. It may begin with very deep breathing, followed by less deep breathing, and finally normal breathing. Progressive relaxation is a stress reduction strategy in which the person systematically "tightens and relaxes" particular muscle groups (from head-to-toe or toe-to-head), thereby "fooling" the brain into initiating muscle relaxation throughout the body. Guided imagery is used in conjunction with meditation. Another person familiar with the technique acts as a "guide" during a stress response so that the individual experiencing stress can concentrate on an image that helps relieve stress. (Once guided imagery is learned, a person can use the technique without prompting.)

Other stress interventions include being aware of personal limitations; peer counseling and group discussions; proper diet, sleep, and rest; and pursuit of positive activities outside of EMS to balance work and recreation. Although the responsibility for personal health and well-being belongs to the individual, intervention programs may be available through EMS agencies, hospitals, and other groups.

Critical Incident Stress Management

Critical incident stress management (CISM) evolved from the early 1970s concept of critical incident stress debriefing (CISD), a program developed to assist emergency personnel exposed to a major incident. Pioneered by Jeff Mitchell, CISM is based on a partnership of mental health professionals and peer group support. The program is designed to allow emergency workers an opportunity to vent their feelings relating to a particular call or situation that had a powerful emotional impact (Box 2-8).

NOTE

Defusing usually takes place within 8 hours after an event to allow an initial release of feelings and an opportunity for people to share their experiences. It is an informal gathering of the people involved in the event and two-person CISM-trained teams who are also peers. A defusing usually lasts less than 1 hour.

Debriefing is more formal than defusing. It is conducted in a confidential setting and usually takes place 24 to 72 hours after the event. The debriefing is conducted by a specially trained CISM team of other emergency services personnel and mental health workers. Only those present at the incident are allowed to attend a debriefing.

Components of CISM

CISM is designed to help emergency personnel understand their reactions and reassures them that what they are experiencing is normal and may be common to others involved in the incident. The process may be initiated for a particular individual or may include various members of the emergency team (e.g., police, EMS crew members, firefighters, and emergency department staff). The 10 components of CISM include the following[4]:

1. Preincident stress training for all personnel
2. On-scene support for obviously distressed personnel
3. Individual consults when only one or two personnel are affected by an incident
4. Defusing services immediately after a large-scale incident
5. Mobilization services after a large-scale incident
6. Critical incident stress debriefing 24 to 72 hours after an event for any emergency personnel involved in a stressful incident
7. Follow-up services to ensure personnel are recovering
8. Specialty debriefings to nonemergency groups when no other timely resources are available within the community
9. Support during routine discussions of an incident by emergency personnel
10. Advice to command staff during large-scale events

In addition to CISM, other approaches can help manage stress. These include employee assistance programs, counseling, spouse support programs, family life programs, pastoral services, and periodic stress evaluations. These and other techniques can be valuable resources to the paramedic in understanding and dealing with job-related stress (Box 2-9).

? CRITICAL THINKING

Imagine which type of call would be a critical incident for you personally.

BOX 2-8

POTENTIAL SITUATIONS FOR CISM

- Line-of-duty injury or death
- Disaster
- Emergency worker suicide
- Infant/child death
- Extreme threat to emergency worker
- Prolonged incident that ends in loss or success
- Victims known to operations personnel
- Death/injury of civilian caused by operations
- Other significant event

BOX 2-9

TECHNIQUES FOR REDUCING CRISIS-INDUCED STRESS

- Allow adequate rest for emergency workers
- Provide food and fluid replacement
- Limit exposure to the incident
- Change assignments
- Provide post-event defusing/debriefing

Dealing with Death, Dying, Grief, and Loss

Death and dying will always be part of health care delivery. Even though medical science has given society the ability to postpone death in some instances and perhaps lessen its physical pain, the fight for self-preservation is inevitably lost.

Patient and Family Needs

In the delivery of EMS, paramedics will provide care to a dying person surrounded by loved ones. In these situations, the emotional needs of the dying patient, family, and loved ones should be of utmost importance. Both the patient and their significant others will need to be comforted, given privacy, and treated with respect and dignity. Loved ones may need to express feelings of rage, anger, despair, and guilt, and they may need the paramedic to provide control and direction for this solemn event. The paramedic's role in this scenario is important and may be a determining factor in the way survivors adjust to their loss (see the box below).

Stages of the Grieving Process

In 1968 Elizabeth Kubler-Ross began her work on the psychological aspects of death and dying. Her studies identified five predictable stages of dying: denial, anger, bargaining, depression, and acceptance. Kubler-Ross found that patients and loved ones dealing with the death process generally experience the following five stages[5]:

1. Denial, characterized by the feeling "No, not me," is a predictable response to news of a life-threatening illness or situation. The news is so overwhelming that it must be absorbed slowly. The patient seeks other opinions, verifies the accuracy of medical reports, or simply seems to ignore what he or she has been told. Denial is a valuable defense mechanism and is troubling only when no indication exists that the patient understands the seriousness of the situation. Most patients, families, and friends deny death to some degree to continue with the daily business of living.

2. Anger, the "Why me?" phase, is probably the most difficult for persons who care about or are trying to help the dying person. In this phase, all efforts to help or console the person are rejected. This anger is really the anger of the dying person toward all the people who continue to live, or more accurately, anger directed toward God because He does not appear to have acted fairly or justly with the dying person.

3. Bargaining is reflected in a "Yes, me, but. . ." frame of mind. The reality of being very sick and of probably dying is admitted, but the person tries to bargain for extension or quality of life. These bargains usually are secret, frequently made with God, and rarely kept. For example, a father promises to be a "perfect patient" if only he can live to see his son's wedding.

4. Depression is the "Yes, me" reaction to anticipated death. It involves preparing to say and saying goodbye to everything and everyone a person has known and loved. The inherent sadness of this phase is appropriate and should be respected.

5. Acceptance, the simple and quiet "Yes," grows out of individuals' convictions that they have done what is possible to be ready to die. Personal energy and interpersonal interests decrease significantly. During this phase, relatives and friends usually need more help than the dying person, whose most important wish is not to die alone.

HOSPICE PROGRAMS

Hospice programs began in England in 1967 and have since become a standard service of many health care institutions in the United States and Canada. The purpose of these programs is to help the terminally ill patient, family, and loved ones cope with anticipated death. The hospice philosophy encourages home care for the patient to provide for a more natural environment. In addition, volunteers and health care professionals provide counseling and other psychological support to the patient and family throughout the death process. Hospice programs are well respected in the medical community and play an important role in helping many patients and their families accept death as a natural event in life.

Dying patients and their loved ones may fluctuate between these stages and may or may not experience all five stages.

Although paramedics seldom are involved in a particular patient's process of accepting death, they frequently are exposed to the various reactions of patients and families experiencing the death process. For example, denial may be apparent in some family members who do not appear to recognize or acknowledge the seriousness of a situation in which decisions about resuscitation must be made; anger may be directed at the paramedic crew or other health care workers; and bargaining may occur in the form of a mother who says, "Please save my child, and I promise that I'll always make her wear her seat belt!" The paramedic must understand the psychological aspects of the stages of grief (see the box in the right column).

NOTE

When it is necessary to convey news of a sudden death to family members, the paramedic's initial contact with the family can significantly influence the grief response. The paramedic should gather the family in a private area and advise them of the patient's death, with a brief description of the circumstances causing the death. The words "death" or "dead" should be used and euphemisms such as "he's passed on," or "she's no longer with us" should be avoided. The paramedic should be compassionate and allow time for the news to be absorbed and for questions to be asked. (Not all silent moments need to be filled with words; silent contemplation should be allowed.) The family should be permitted to see their relative if they choose; they should be advised in advance if resuscitation equipment is still connected to the patient. These efforts, combined with empathic communication with the family, help relatives deal with the loss of a loved one.

Common Needs of the Paramedic When Dealing with Death and Dying

Dealing with death is difficult for everyone, and the paramedic's feelings and emotions also must be considered. The paramedic may experience some of the same stages of grief previously described. These reactions are normal, and a great deal of effort may be required to disguise or suppress these emotions at the scene or while rendering care. However, the paramedic should discuss these feelings as soon as possible with friends, co-workers, and family in a constructive way that will lessen the emotional burden. Like others, the paramedic will need an opportunity to process the specific incident and obtain closure. Available resources, such as employee assistance programs and counseling and pastoral services, help avoid the effects of cumulative stress.

? CRITICAL THINKING

What personal experiences have you had with death? How did you or others who were close to the deceased react to the initial news of the death?

RECOMMENDED COMMUNICATION STRATEGIES

It is uncomfortable to be in a situation involving death and dying, and communication with the patient and loved ones may be difficult. The following recommendations for communications and activities may help a paramedic deal with dying patients and their families:

- Answer questions honestly for the patient and family, and explain all activities.
- Do not initiate the subject of dying; let it come from the patient or family.
- If the patient or family asks you if the patient is going to die, advise that you are doing everything you possibly can but that the situation is critical. This allows a brief time for the patient and family to prepare themselves.
- Do not falsely reassure the patient or family (e.g., "everything's going to be okay").
- Use compassionate, nonverbal communication (facial expression, touching).
- Offer to contact someone if the patient is alone.
- If family is not present, assure the patient that emergency department personnel will notify them. If they are nearby, encourage the family to come to the patient immediately or to meet the patient at the emergency department.
- Allow the family to stay with the patient when appropriate.

Developmental Considerations When Dealing with Death and Dying

The way people cope with their own death or the death of a loved one depends on their age, maturity, and understanding of death. The paramedic should be particularly sensitive to the emotional needs of all age groups during this crisis. The following guidelines may be helpful when offering advice to family members who will be helping the young or elderly cope with the death of a loved one.[4]

Children up to age 3 will probably sense that something "has happened" in the family. They will realize that people are sad and crying. They also may be aware of increased activity in the household. The family should be urged to watch for changes in eating or sleeping patterns and for an increase in irritability. In addition, the family should be sensitive to the child's needs and try to maintain consistency in their routines and with significant people in the child's life.

Children 3 to 6 years of age do not have a concept of the finality of death. They may believe that the person will return and may continually ask "when." This age group believes in "magical thinking" and may feel that they are responsible for the death. They also may believe that everyone else they love will die too. The family should watch for changes in the child's behavior patterns with friends and at school, difficulty sleeping, and changes in eating habits. The family should emphasize that the child is not responsible for the death. Reinforce the fact that crying is normal when people are sad; encourage children to talk about their feelings.

Children 6 to 9 years of age are beginning to understand the finality of death. They want detailed explanations for the death and can differentiate fatal illness from just "being sick." Like the 3- to 6-year-olds, these children may be afraid that other loved ones will die too. This age group may be uncomfortable with expressing their feelings and may act silly or embarrassed when talking about death. The paramedic should suggest to the family that they talk about the normal feelings of anger, sadness, and guilt, and that they share their own feelings about death with the child. The family should not be hesitant to cry, because it will let the child know that expression of feelings is acceptable.

Children 9 to 12 years of age are aware of the finality of death and may want to know the details surrounding the event. They will be concerned with practical matters involving their lifestyle and may try to "act like an adult." (Most, however, will show regression to an earlier stage of emotional response.) The paramedic should suggest to the family that they set aside time to talk to the child about feelings and encourage the sharing of memories to facilitate the grief response.

Older adults usually show concern about other family members. In addition, they may be concerned about their further loss of independence and about impending financial matters. Family members should be sensitive and understanding about these issues as they are very "real" concerns for this age group.

Preventing Disease Transmission

Because emergency workers often manage ill and injured patients, preventing disease transmission must be a priority in daily practice. Specific concerns for personal health and safety include being aware of common sources of exposure, using personal protection, and knowing what to do if a significant exposure has occurred (Box 2-10).

BOX 2-10

DISEASE TRANSMISSION TERMINOLOGY

Air-borne and *blood-borne pathogens* are organisms carried through air or blood (and other body fluids) that create disease processes in the human body or host. Some pathogens (e.g., certain bacteria) can survive outside a host, whereas others (such as viruses) can survive only in the human cell (see Chapter 37). Exposure occurs in cases of contact with a potentially infectious body fluid substance or other infectious agent. Cleaning, disinfection, and sterilization are methods used to destroy infectious organisms that may have come in contact with equipment and instruments. Body substance isolation ("universal precautions") refers to practices designed to prevent or reduce contact with body substances and other infectious agents.

Common Sources of Exposure

Common exposure to infectious agents in the pre-hospital setting include needle sticks and broken or scraped skin. Mucous membranes such as those that line the eyes, nose, and mouth also are a source for entry of infectious agents or microorganisms. Therefore, the paramedic should practice the universal precautions described earlier during all patient-care encounters. (See Table 2-2 for a review of universal precautions.)

Protection from Air-Borne and Blood-Borne Pathogens

The following list contains some general guidelines to help prevent exposure to infectious diseases. (A more complete discussion of infectious disease is presented in Chapter 37.)

1. Follow engineering and work practices and maintain good personal health and hygiene habits (including frequent hand washing and general cleanliness).
2. Maintain immunizations for tetanus, diphtheria, polio, hepatitis B, MMR (measles, mumps, and rubella), and influenza.
3. Conduct periodic tuberculosis screening.
4. Practice body substance isolation (universal precautions) in all patient encounters.
5. Appropriately clean, disinfect, and/or dispose of used materials and equipment immediately.
6. Use puncture-resistant containers to dispose of needles and other sharp objects.
7. Separate and label all soiled laundry (clothes, bed linens, etc.) and equipment until the items can be appropriately cleaned and disinfected.
8. Conduct periodic health-risk assessment.

Documenting and Managing an Exposure

The paramedic is responsible to be familiar with laws, regulations, and national standards that address issues of infectious disease and to take personal protective measures against exposure. In the event of a potential exposure to an infectious disease or a significant exposure to a patient's blood or body fluids, the paramedic should do the following:

1. Wash the area of contact thoroughly and immediately
2. Immediately document the situation in which the exposure occurred
3. Describe actions taken to reduce chances of infection
4. Comply with all required reporting responsibilities and time frames
5. Cooperate with incident investigation
6. Be screened for tuberculosis and other potential diseases
7. Obtain proper immunization boosters
8. Obtain a complete medical follow-up

S U M M A R Y

- Wellness has two main components: physical well-being and mental and emotional health.

- As health care professionals, paramedics have a responsibility to serve as role models in disease prevention.

- Physical fitness can be described as a condition that helps individuals look, feel, and do their best.

- Sleep helps to rejuvenate a tired body.

- Steps to reduce cardiovascular disease include the following: improving cardiovascular endurance, eliminating cigarette smoking, controlling high blood pressure, maintaining a normal body-fat composition, maintaining good total cholesterol/HDL ratio, monitoring triglyceride levels, using estrogen therapy for postmenopausal women, reducing stress, and making a periodic risk assessment.

- Most common cancers are linked to one of three environmental risk factors: smoking, sunlight, and diet.

- Job-related injuries can be minimized by being knowledgeable about body mechanics during lifting and moving, being alert for hostile environments, prioritizing personal safety during rescue situations, practicing safe vehicle operations, and by utilizing safety equipment and supplies.

- The misuse and abuse of drugs and other substances may lead to chemical dependency (addiction) with a wide range of effects on physical and mental health.

- "Good" stress (eustress) is a positive response to stimuli and is considered "protective." "Bad" stress (distress) is a negative response to environmental stimuli and is the source of anxiety and stress-related disorders.

- Adaptation is a dynamic process whereby we "learn" successful ways to deal with stressful situations. This process usually begins with using defense mechanisms, then developing coping skills, followed by problem solving, and culminating in mastery.

- CISM is designed to help emergency personnel understand their reactions and reassures them that what they are experiencing is normal and may be common to others involved in the incident.

- When it is necessary to convey news of a sudden death to family members, the paramedic's initial contact with the family can significantly influence the grief process.

- It is the paramedic's responsibility to be familiar with laws, regulations, and national standards that address issues of infectious disease and to take personal protective measures against exposure.

- Actions to take after significant exposure include disinfection, documentation, incident investigation, screening, immunization, and medical follow-up.

◼ REFERENCES

1. American Heart Association, *Basic life support for health-care providers*, Dallas, 1997, The Association.
2. Seyle H: *The stress of life*, New York, 1956, McGraw-Hill.
3. Mitchell J, Bray G: *Emergency services stress: guidelines for preserving the health and careers of emergency services personnel*, Englewood Cliffs, NJ, 1990, Brady.
4. US Department of Transportation National Highway Traffic Safety Administration, *EMT-Paramedic national standard curriculum*, Washington, DC, 1998, The Department.
5. Bassuk E et al: *Behavioral emergencies*, Boston, 1983, Little, Brown.

3 Injury Prevention

OBJECTIVES

Upon completion of this chapter, the paramedic student will be able to:

1. **Identify roles of the EMS community in injury prevention.**

2. **Describe the epidemiology of trauma in the United States.**

3. **Outline the aspects of the EMS system that make it a desirable resource for involvement in community health activities.**

4. **Describe community leadership activities that are essential to enable the active participation of EMS in community wellness activities.**

5. **List areas that paramedics should be familiar with to participate in injury prevention.**

6. **Evaluate a situation to determine opportunities for injury prevention.**

7. **Identify resources necessary to conduct a community health assessment.**

8. **Relate how alterations in the epidemiological triangle can influence injury and disease patterns.**

9. **Differentiate among primary, secondary, and tertiary health prevention activities.**

10. **Describe strategies to implement a successful injury prevention program.**

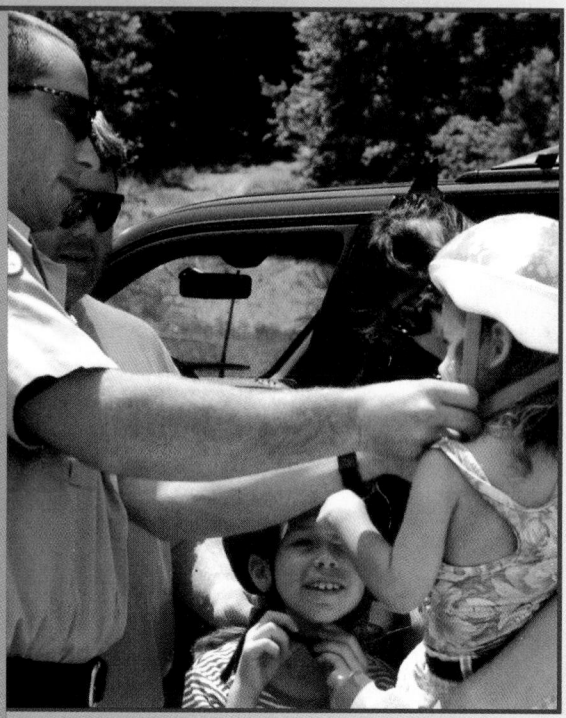

Every community has a responsibility to provide injury prevention through leadership and educational activities. The objectives of injury prevention are to decrease the incidence of preventable illness and injury, to preserve life and function, and to prevent people from requiring costly medical care. As a member of the community's health care system, the EMS provider can be an important resource in injury prevention programs (Box 3-1).

KEY TERMS

community health assessment: An assessment of a target community to identify needs and resources required to provide prevention and wellness promotion activities.

injury risk: Real or potentially hazardous situations that put individuals at increased risk for sustaining an injury.

injury surveillance: The ongoing systematic collection, analysis, and interpretation of injury data essential to the planning, implementation, and evaluation of public health practice.

primary injury prevention: The practice of preventing an injury from occurring.

teachable moment: The time after an injury has occurred when the patient and observers remain acutely aware of what has happened and may be more receptive to being taught ways that the event or illness could have been prevented.

> **NOTE**
>
> The reader should refer to Appendix C to review various injury prevention programs.

> **NOTE**
>
> Public health issues should be a concern for every health care professional. Paramedics have a professional responsibility to be involved in injury prevention initiatives and to promote wellness.

Injury Epidemiology

Unintentional injuries are the leading cause of death among all persons 1 to 33 years of age and the fifth leading cause of death overall, exceeded only by heart disease, cancer, stroke, and chronic obstructive pulmonary disease.[1] In 1998, more than 92,000 injury-related deaths occurred in the United States.

Incidence, Morbidity, and Mortality

Unintentional injuries result in more years of potential life lost before 65 years of age than any other cause of death. From a financial viewpoint, the economic effect of fatal and nonfatal unintentional injuries amounted to $480,500,000,000 in 1998, or about $5000 per household (Fig. 3-1). The lost quality of life from these injuries is valued at an additional $1,087,700,000, making the comprehensive cost $1,568,200,000 in 1998[1] (Table 3-1). About 42% of all hospital emergency department visits in the United States are injury related. In

---

BOX 3-1

INJURY AND ILLNESS PREVENTION TERMINOLOGY

Injury: Intentional or unintentional damage to the person resulting from acute exposure to thermal, mechanical, electrical, or chemical energy or the absence of such essentials as heat and oxygen

Injury risk: Real or potentially hazardous situations that put individuals at increased risk for sustaining an injury

Injury surveillance: The ongoing collection, analysis, and interpretation of injury data essential to the planning, implementation, and evaluation of public health practice, closely integrated with the timely dissemination of these data to those who need to know, with the final link in the chain being the application of these data to prevention and control

Primary injury prevention: The practice of preventing an injury from occurring

Secondary and tertiary prevention: The care and rehabilitation activities, respectively, that are intended to prevent further problems from an event that has already occurred

Teachable moment: The time after an injury has occurred when the patient and observers remain acutely aware of what has happened and may be more receptive to being taught ways that the event or illness could be prevented

Years of productive life: The calculation obtained by subtracting the age of the victim's death from 65 (the average age of retirement)

TOTAL COST $480.5 BILLION

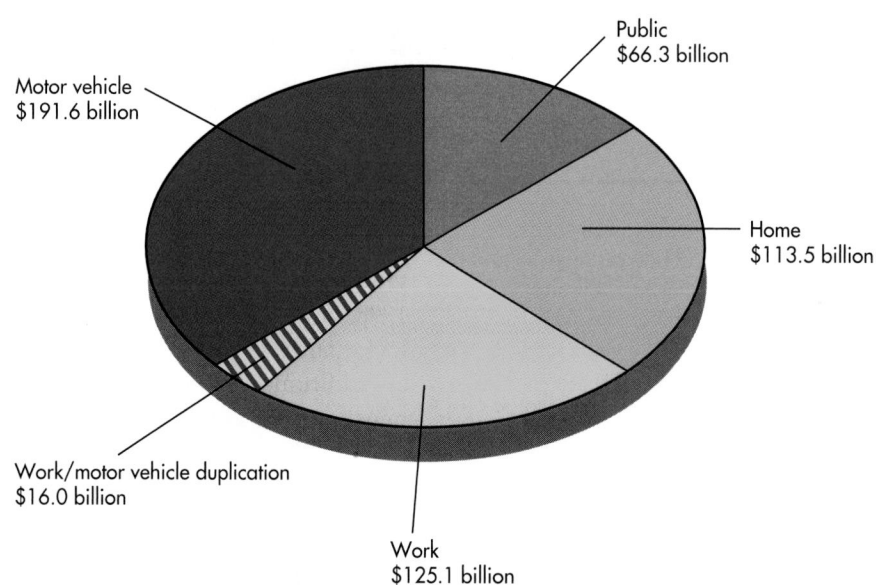

Fig. 3-1 Cost of unintentional injuries by class in 1998. (From National Safety Council: *Injury facts,* Itasca, Ill, 1999, The Council.)

addition, an estimated 19 hospitalizations and 254 emergency department visits occur for each injury-related death.

> **NOTE**
>
> While you are reading this chapter, at least 4 people will be killed by unintentional injury and another 390 will be disabled. A death caused by unintentional injury occurs in the United States every 6 minutes.

Feasibility of EMS Involvement

More than 600,000 EMS providers in the United States are widely distributed amid the population. As noted in *Emergency Medical Services: Agenda for the Future,* "People attracted to the EMS service are among society's best, and desire to contribute to their community's health. The composition of the EMS workforce reflects the diversity of the population it serves."[2] Therefore this valuable human resource playing a role in public education as a component of health promotion seems only fitting. The following considerations support the feasibility of EMS involvement in community health and injury prevention.

- EMS providers are often the most medically educated individuals in rural settings.
- EMS providers are high-profile role models.
- EMS providers are often considered as the champion of the customer.
- EMS providers are welcome in homes, schools, and other environments.
- EMS providers are considered authorities on injury and prevention.
- EMS providers are often the first to identify situations that pose a risk for illness or injury (e.g., unsanitary conditions, unsafe home environments).

> **? CRITICAL THINKING**
>
> *Can you remember any program that a firefighter or paramedic taught you when you were a child? How did you feel about the firefighters and paramedics?*

TABLE 3-1	COST EQUIVALENTS
THE COST OF . . .	**IS EQUIVALENT TO . . .**
. . . All Injuries ($480.5 billion)	. . . 58 cents of every dollar paid in 1998 federal personal income taxes, **or** . . . 59 cents of every dollar spent on food in the United States in 1998.
. . . Motor-Vehicle Crashes ($191.6 billion)	. . . purchasing 840 gallons of gasoline for each registered vehicle in the United States **or** . . . more than 19 times greater than the combined profits reported by Exxon, Mobil, and Chevron in 1998.
. . . Work Injuries ($125.1 billion)	. . . 45 cents of every dollar of 1998 corporate dividends to stockholders, **or** . . . 17 cents of every dollar of 1998 pre-tax corporate profits, **or** . . . nearly triple the combined profits reported by the top five Fortune 500 companies in 1998.
. . . Home Injuries ($113.5 billion)	. . . an $89,300 rebate on each new single-family home built in 1998, **or** . . . 52 cents of every dollar of property taxes paid in 1998.
. . . Public Injuries ($66.3 billion)	. . . a $6.9 million grant to each public library in the United States **or** . . . a $79,900 bonus for each police officer and firefighter.

From National Safety Council: *Injury facts,* Itasca, Ill., 1999, The Council.

NOTE

As managed care evolves, a demand on EMS services for supportive care and intervention will increase. Paramedics and EMS agencies must adapt to their new role in the health care delivery system (see the box in the right column).

✓ TRICKS OF THE TRADE

Think about your role in community health and education as an *opportunity* to serve your community and a way to ensure your job security.

Essential Community Leadership Activities

For EMS providers and other public-service personnel to play active roles in community health and injury prevention programs, the community must take measures to ensure successful participation (Box 3-2).

Protect the EMS Provider from Injury

A logical first step for the development of injury prevention and wellness promotion within the community is to protect the well-being of the EMS

EFFECTS OF HEALTH CARE REFORM ON EMS SERVICES

To control costs, managed care reduces the number and duration of hospitalizations. Because sicker patients are discharged from hospitals earlier, the likelihood for repeated EMS calls to the same homes or locations is increased. These calls are for emergencies and nonemergency transportations to convalescent care or for readmission to or follow-up services at hospitals. The need to provide some supportive medical care and intervention in the patient's home is also growing (see Chapter 46). Examples of services that paramedics and other health care professionals provide to patients in their homes include the following:

- Caring for patients on monitors, ventilators, infusion pumps, and other complex medical equipment
- Drawing blood samples
- Providing wound care
- Measuring blood pressure
- Performing 12-lead electrocardiograms (ECGs)
- Peforming other duties traditionally done before patients were released from the hospital

Many patients now self-administer IV antibiotics and other IV medications at home. Premature infants ("premie graduates") often go home with advanced monitoring and life support equipment. Paramedics must be prepared to assist these patients with their special needs

ESSENTIAL COMMUNITY LEADERSHIP ACTIVITIES

- Protect the EMS provider from injury.
- Provide primary injury prevention education to EMS providers.
- Support and promote collection and use of injury data.
- Obtain support and resources for primary injury prevention activities.
- Empower individual EMS providers to conduct primary injury prevention activities.

NOTE: EMS, through expanded scope of practice, will be performing these leadership activities for both injury prevention and wellness.

workforce. Policies should help ensure EMS provider safety during an emergency response, while at the scene, and during patient transportation. This can be accomplished through traffic safety ordinances, public education, and cooperation with law enforcement, fire service personnel, and other public service agencies.

NOTE

Several states have enacted legislation that makes assaulting a prehospital provider a felony.

Personal protective equipment (PPE) must be provided to minimize eye, back, and skin injury. Other safety measures include protection from exposure to communicable diseases and hazardous chemicals. Communities can reduce work-related injuries by implementing personal safety programs and by establishing a wellness program for EMS providers (see Chapter 2).

✔ TRICKS OF THE TRADE

Little in life is more important than your health and well-being. Personal safety and protection is *your* responsibility.

Provide Education to EMS Providers

EMS primary and continuing education programs should incorporate the fundamentals of primary injury prevention. Community leaders should help establish a liaison relationship between EMS programs with public and private specialty groups (e.g., hospitals, other public health and safety agencies, safety councils, social services, religious organizations, colleges, and universities) for specific education and training. Cooperation with these groups can help identify targets for prevention activities and encourages sharing the tasks of program implementation.

Support and Promote Collection and Use of Injury Data

Communities should develop policies that promote injury documentation by EMS providers. They should evaluate and sometimes modify the tools for data collection so that prompt recording of data is feasible and realistic. The data collected should contribute to local, state, and national surveillance programs (e.g., head and spinal cord injury registries).

Obtain Support and Resources for Primary Injury Prevention Activities

The community will need to establish internal budgetary support for the injury prevention programs. In addition, the community may need to seek other financial resources for fees and equipment, publicity, networking with other injury prevention organizations, and initiating or attending meetings of local organizations that are involved or are requesting involvement in injury prevention. The community can obtain grants to support these initiatives from state and national organizations (e.g., the Centers for Disease Control and Prevention [CDC], Emergency Medical Services for Children [EMSC]), private donations, community block grants, and institutions.

NOTE

Regardless of available funding, EMS providers have an obligation to provide prevention initiatives on any call where a preventable event has occurred.

Empower Individual EMS Providers to Conduct Primary Injury Prevention Activities

The community must establish internal budgetary support to identify and encourage interest and support for injury prevention activities from EMS providers. This support can influence individual EMS provider participation in the following ways:

- Providing rotating assignments to prevention programs
- Providing salary for off-duty injury prevention activities
- Rewarding and/or remunerating participation for on- and off-duty prevention activities

Essential Provider Activities

Essential EMS provider activities are based on education. These activities include the knowledge and practice of the personal injury prevention strategies listed in Box 3-3. The EMS provider also needs to be knowledgeable about illnesses and injuries com-

mon to various age groups, recreational activities, workplaces, and other facilities in the community (Box 3-4). These essential provider activities are presented throughout this text by subject matter and in Appendix C.

Implementation and Prevention Strategies

In addition to the primary personal injury prevention strategies described in Box 3-3, the EMS provider needs to implement other prevention strategies for patient care considerations, recognizing signs and symptoms of exposure to danger, recognizing the need for outside assistance, documentation of primary care and injury data, and on-scene education.

Patient Care Considerations

The EMS provider needs to recognize signs and symptoms of suspected abuse and potentially abusive situations to ensure the safety of the EMS crew and the patient (see Chapter 44). The goal is to resolve (in a nonjudgmental way) any conflict without violence. Preplanning for these situations should identify outside resources such as support programs sponsored by municipal, community, and religious organizations (Box 3-5).

✓ **TRICKS OF THE TRADE**

Being judgmental is not part of the job. Document your findings and report them.

Recognizing Signs and Symptoms of Exposure to Danger

With personal safety being the priority, EMS providers should stay alert for signs of potentially dangerous situations. These include recognizing both general and specific environmental parameters that will help assess a patient's need for preventive information and direction. Examples include the following:

- Safety hazards in the home
- Inadequate housing conditions
- Inadequate food and clothing
- Absence of protective devices (e.g., smoke detectors)
- Hazardous materials (e.g., lead-based paint, dangerous chemicals)
- Communicable disease (and potential for transmission)
- Signs of abuse and/or neglect

? CRITICAL THINKING

Do you know an EMS provider who was injured on the job? How did the injury occur? Can you identify any measures that could have prevented it?

Recognizing the Need for Outside Resources

Most communities have several outside resources that can be of assistance to members of the community. Providers of these resources and services usu-

BOX 3-5

SAMPLING OF OUTSIDE RESOURCES AND SERVICES

Municipal
Animal control services
Child protective services
Fire service personnel
Law enforcement personnel
Social services

Community
Abuse support groups for spouses, children, and older adults
Alternative health care services (e.g., free clinics)
Alternative means of transportation
Alternative modes of education
Assistance for food, shelter, and clothing
Day care services
Disaster services (e.g., American Red Cross)
Immunization programs
Managed care organizations
Mental health resources and counseling
Rape or crisis intervention
Rehabilitation programs
Services for the disabled
Work-study programs

Religious
Family counseling
Grief support
Pastoral services
Support groups

ally are eager to assist or collaborate with developing injury prevention strategies.

Documentation

Documenting patient care and primary injury data is important for several reasons. Patient care documentation provides a record of the events involved in the patient encounter and is valuable to others who will be involved in the patient's care during the health care episode (see Chapter 17). Gathering primary injury data can be helpful in designing injury prevention strategies. For example, studying a large number of patients who received head injuries during horseback riding incidents may identify that helmet use was notably absent in all seriously injured patients. Primary injury data include the following:

- Scene conditions
- Mechanism of injury
- Use of protective devices
- Absence of protective devices
- Risks at the scene
- Other factors as noted by the EMS agency

> **NOTE**
>
> EMS providers can use patient care information and injury data for EMS research.

On-Scene Education

If the reason for the EMS response is likely to be repeated (e.g., an older adult patient fell from slipping on a floor rug), the paramedic should take time for on-scene education. In this situation, on-scene education can consist of advising the patient or family members to ensure that all floor rugs have a nonslip backing and to remove those that do not. For on-scene education to be effective, the EMS provider must recognize the teachable moment, be nonjudgmental and objective, and have a sense of good "timing." Informing people about how to prevent a recurrence and how to use protective devices (e.g., working smoke detectors) to improve safety is a way to employ injury prevention on many EMS calls. Other methods of on-scene education for injury prevention are described in Appendix C.

> **NOTE**
>
> The paramedic must consider ethnic, religious, and social diversities when providing on-scene education. For education to be effective, communication must be appropriate for the patient's age and vocabulary.

> **? CRITICAL THINKING**
>
> *The next time you visit an older adult family member or friend, see if you can identify any potential hazards that exist in his or her home.*

Participation in Prevention Programs

Effective prevention programs require a **community health assessment** before intervention and education can take place.

Community Health Assessment

Paramedics may likely have limited time and resources to provide prevention and wellness promotion activities. To maximize available time and resources, the EMS provider should perform a community health assessment to identify the target for community health education (Fig. 3-2). This assessment often is a large undertaking and may be more effectively conducted through a group effort with other health agencies (Box 3-6) to evaluate the following:

- Population demographics
- Morbidity statistics
- Mortality statistics
- Crime and fire information
- Community resource allocation
- Hospital data (e.g., emergency department visits, length of stay)
- Senior citizen needs
- Education standards
- Recreational facilities
- Environmental conditions
- Other factors

This "landscape" view of the community's health can yield valuable, and sometimes unexpected, information about the target population. It also can identify factors that interrelate or contribute to specific health risks. After the assessment, the EMS provider should choose the target for community health education carefully and employ an appropriate intervention.

> **NOTE**
>
> Ideally, the EMS provider should compare the data collected during the community health assessment with those of another population with similar demographics (e.g., a city of similar size within the state).

Injury requires that the host (patient) interact with the agent causing the disease (illness or injury)

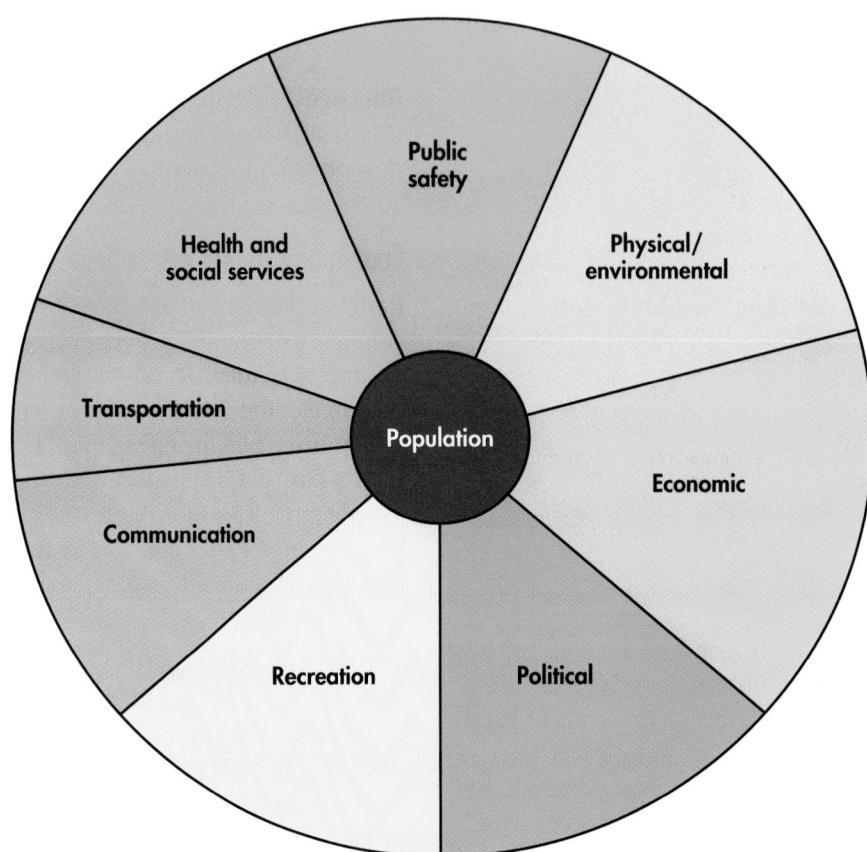

Fig. 3-2 Community health assessment.

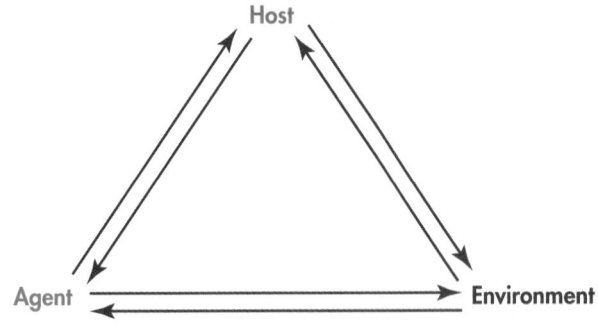

Fig. 3-3 Epidemiological triangle.

in an environment conducive to exposure of the host to the agent (Fig. 3-3). Changing one or more of the factors in the epidemiological triangle can alter disease or injury patterns.[3] For example, it is well known that the use of a personal restraint system while operating or riding in an automobile can save lives in some car crashes. In response to government regulation, car manufacturers designed automobiles with air bags, automatic shoulder belts, and alert devices that changed the environment of the host and increased the exposure to safety measures and the likelihood that occupants would use a personal restraint system (see Appendix C).

Community Health Intervention

Once a health risk has been identified, the EMS provider must implement a plan that will attempt to reduce or eliminate the risk and improve the health of the community. The three levels of health prevention activities are primary, secondary, and tertiary (Box 3-7). Primary prevention activities prevent problems before they occur (e.g., seat belt education, legislation to require helmets while bicycling). Secondary prevention activities find problems and intervene early (e.g., blood pressure screenings to detect hypertension). Tertiary prevention activities correct and

---

BOX 3-6

SAMPLING OF COMMUNITY HEALTH INFORMATION SOURCES

Census data (public library, Internet)
    Population demographics
    Distribution of age, sex, race, ethnicity
    Socioeconomic status
Health departments (city, county, state, Internet)
    Births and deaths (including cause)
    Infectious disease statistics
    Environmental hazards (sanitation, air quality)
    State trauma registry statistics
Law enforcement
    Crime rate statistics
    Response times
Emergency medical services
    Call types and response times
    Geographic distribution
    Clustering of illnesses and injuries
Fire service
    Location and frequency of fires
    Response times
    Fire-related injuries and fatalities
Communication
    Newspapers, radio, and television stations

Local government
    Housing and tax information
    Form of government
    Distribution of grant monies
    Parks and recreation
Federal government
    Federal Emergency Management Agency (FEMA)
    Centers for Disease Control and Prevention (CDC)
National Safety Council
Hospitals
School board
    Education and literacy rates
    Health services and school lunch programs
Chamber of Commerce
    Industry and economic figures
    Employment statistics
    Religious organizations
Disaster planning
    Emergency coordinating council
    American Red Cross

---

prevent further deterioration of a disease or problem (e.g., providing EMS services in a community).

TRICKS OF THE TRADE

A good primary prevention activity is to be a good role model in your community. Wear your seat belt when on and off duty.

Community Health Education

A successful injury prevention program must serve the entire target population within a community. The community must make efforts to improve education and training for EMS and other public service agencies so that special groups can be included in the prevention program. Examples include train-

BOX 3-7

THREE LEVELS OF HEALTH PREVENTION ACTIVITIES

Primary: Prevent problems before they occur
Secondary: Find problems and intervene early
Tertiary: Correct and prevent further deterioration of a disease or problem

ing EMS providers to communicate effectively with the following:

- Various ethnic, cultural, and religious groups
- Non–English-speaking populations
- Those with learning disabilities
- Those who are physically challenged

The EMS provider must consider the reading level and age of the target population when preparing educational materials so that communication is effective. Before implementation of any type of large-scale educational program, the EMS provider should "test" the program on a target audience to evaluate its appeal and to ensure that the message is understood. The EMS provider can provide community health education to promote wellness and injury prevention in numerous ways, including the following:

- Verbal
  Lectures
  Informal discussions
  Informal teaching on an EMS call
  Audio tapes
  Radio programs
- Written/static visual
  Bulletin boards, exhibits
  Flyers, pamphlets, posters
  Models
  Slides, photographs
- Dynamic visual
  Videotapes
  Television
  Internet resources

? CRITICAL THINKING

What method of health education is most likely to change your personal behaviors? Would that same method be equally effective for a 5-year-old or a 70-year-old person?

SUMMARY

- EMS providers, as members of the community's health care system, can be an important resource in injury prevention.

- Unintentional injuries are the fifth leading cause of death overall, exceeded only by heart disease, cancer, stroke, and chronic obstructive pulmonary disease.

- More than 600,000 EMS providers in the United States are widely distributed amid the population. This valuable human resource playing a role in public education as a component of health promotion seems only fitting.

- For EMS personnel to play an active role in community health, the community must protect the EMS provider from injury, provide education to EMS providers, support and promote collection and use of injury data, obtain resources for primary injury prevention activities, and empower EMS providers to conduct primary injury prevention.

- EMS providers should have essential knowledge about personal injury prevention and about maladies and injuries common to various age groups, recreation activities, workplaces, and other facilities in the community.

- In addition to the primary personal injury prevention strategies, the paramedic should recognize signs and symptoms of abuse and abusive situations and exposure to danger, identify and use outside community resources, appropriately document primary injury data, and identify and appropriately use the teachable moment.

- To maximize available time and resources, the EMS provider should identify targets for community health education by performing a community health assessment.

- Identification of the goals for community education requires an understanding that illness or injury is related to the extent or exposure to an agent; the strength of the agent; the susceptibility of the individual (host); and the biologic, social, and physical environment.

- Primary injury prevention involves preventing an injury from occurring. Secondary and tertiary prevention prevent further problems from an event that has already occurred.

- A successful injury prevention program should consider the entire target population, reading level, and age. The EMS provider can provide community health education in diverse ways, including verbal, written/static material, and dynamic visual.

REFERENCES

1. National Safety Council: *Injury facts*, Itasca, Ill, 1999, The Council.
2. National Highway Traffic Safety Administration: *Emergency medical services: agenda for the future*, Washington, DC, 1996, The Administration.
3. Swanson J, Nies M: *Community health nursing: promoting the health of aggregates*, ed 2, Philadelphia, 1977, WB Saunders.

4 Medical/Legal Issues

OBJECTIVES

Upon completion of this chapter, the paramedic student will be able to:

1. **Describe the basic structure of the legal system in the United States.**
2. **Relate how laws affect the paramedic's practice.**
3. **List situations that the paramedic is legally required to report in most states.**
4. **Describe the four elements involved in a claim of negligence.**
5. **Describe measures paramedics may take to protect themselves from claims of negligence.**
6. **Describe the paramedic's responsibilities with regard to patient confidentiality.**
7. **Outline the process for obtaining expressed, informed, and implied consent.**
8. **Describe legal complications relating to consent.**
9. **Describe actions to be taken in a refusal-of-care situation.**
10. **Describe legal considerations related to patient transportation.**
11. **Outline legal issues related to specific resuscitation situations.**
12. **List measures the paramedic should take to preserve evidence when at a crime or accident scene.**
13. **Detail the components of the narrative report necessary for effective legal documentation.**
14. **Define common medical-legal terms that apply to prehospital situations involving patient care.**

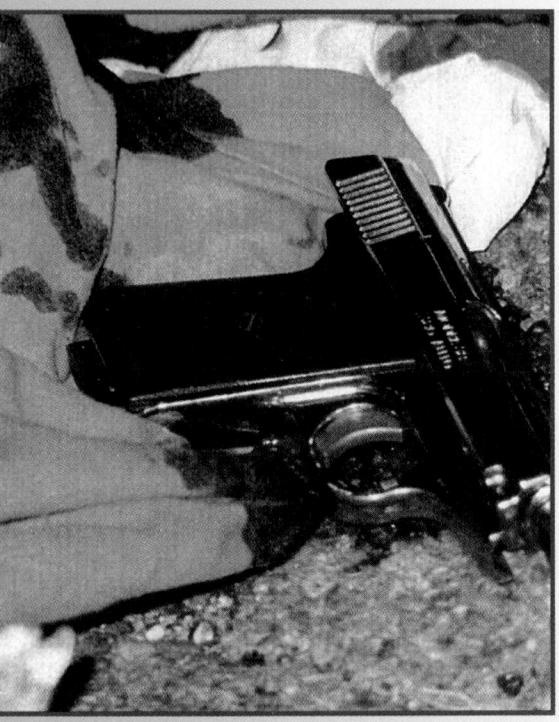

Historically, only hospitals and physicians were affected by medical malpractice because EMS personnel were not expected to meet professional standards of patient care. However, with today's state and national certification, licensure, and the paramedic's role as a health care professional, medical liability for EMS personnel is now a real concern.

KEY TERMS

abandonment: Terminating medical care without legal excuse or turning care over to personnel who do not have training and expertise appropriate for the medical needs of the patient.

assault: Creating apprehension, or unauthorized handling and treatment of a patient.

battery: Physical contact with a person without consent and without legal justification.

expressed consent: Verbal or written consent to the treatment.

false imprisonment: Intentional and unjustifiable detention of a person.

implied consent: The presumption that an unconscious or incompetent person would consent to lifesaving care.

informed consent: Consent obtained from a patient after explaining all facts necessary for the patient to make a reasonable decision.

involuntary consent: Treatment that is granted by authority of law.

negligence: Failure to use such care as a reasonably prudent EMS provider would use in similar circumstances.

Legal Duties and Ethical Responsibilities

The paramedic's legal duties are to the patient, the employer, the medical director, and the public. These legal duties are defined by statutes and regulations and are based on generally accepted standards of medical care. In addition to legal duties, paramedics, like other health care professionals, have ethical responsibilities that include:

- Responding with respect to the physical and emotional needs of every patient
- Maintaining mastery of skills
- Participating in continuing education/refresher training
- Critically reviewing performance and seeking improvement
- Reporting honestly
- Respecting confidentiality
- Working cooperatively and with respect for other emergency workers and health care professionals
- Staying current with new concepts and modalities

> **NOTE**
>
> The *NAEMT Code of Ethics* in Chapter 1 exemplifies ethical guidelines for the paramedic.

Failing to perform EMS duties appropriately can result in civil or criminal liability. As described in this chapter, the best legal protection is providing appropriate assessment and care coupled with accurate and complete documentation.

> **NOTE**
>
> Laws pertaining to patient care delivery vary by state. Every paramedic should be aware of his or her state's Medical Practice Act and other regulatory statutes. If necessary, consult with a private attorney experienced in EMS law or the state Attorney General's office (or its equivalent) to clarify state laws and their application to EMS activities. The information contained in this chapter is *general* information and is not intended to be a complete guide to any state's legislative system, EMS laws, or regulations.

The Legal System

The structure of the legal system in the United States is composed of five types of law. These are legislative law, administrative law, common law, criminal law, and civil law.

Legislative law is made by legislative branches of government, such as city councils, district boards, general assemblies, and Congress. The power of these bodies to make law is defined by statutes, state constitutions, and in the case of Congress, the U.S. Constitution.

Administrative law refers to regulations that are developed by a governmental agency to provide details about the function and process of the law (e.g., general requirements for paramedic licensure). These regulations may address areas such as examinations, licenses, and maintenance of records. Regulatory agencies may hold disciplinary hearings regarding revocation or suspension of licenses. An example of a regulatory agency is a state EMS bureau.

Common law (case or judge-made law) is derived from society's acceptance of customs or norms over time and is based on the decisions of the state and federal judicial systems. With reference to patient care activities, these court decisions may offer guidance in defining acceptable conduct and **negligence** and interpreting statutes and regulations applicable to EMS.

Criminal law is a type of law in which the federal, state, or local government prosecutes individuals for violating the laws enacted to protect society (a "public" complaint). Violation of criminal law may be punishable by fine, imprisonment, or both.

Civil law (tort law) is an area of law that deals with "private" complaints brought by a plaintiff against another person (defendant) for an illegal act or wrong-doing (tort) for which the plaintiff requests the court to award damages. Most EMS activities that result in litigation are civil suits.

How Laws Affect the Paramedic

As previously stated, the U.S. legal system has been active on issues pertaining to medical malpractice. To safeguard against litigation, the paramedic must be knowledgeable of these issues and how they can affect patient care activities.

Scope of Practice

Scope of practice refers to the range of duties and skills that a paramedic is allowed and expected to perform when necessary. These usually are set by state law or regulation and by local medical direction. For example, the scope of practice for most paramedics in most states would include endotracheal intubation, defibrillation, the administration of medications, and other BLS and ALS procedures.

? CRITICAL THINKING

Why is it necessary to define the scope of practice for a profession?

Medical Direction

As described in Chapter 1, medical direction is a required component for paramedic practice. Depend-

ing on state and local requirements, medical direction may be provided through on-line (direct) medical direction and/or off-line (indirect) medical direction. EMS systems should also have a policy in place to guide paramedics in dealing with on-scene (bystander) physicians. Some states, for example, provide cards for paramedics to issue to on-scene physicians officially prohibiting interference with paramedics performing their duties. (Use of these cards often requires legislative or regulatory support.)

Medical Practice Act

A *medical practice act* refers to legislation that governs the practice of medicine. This legislation varies by state, but it prescribes how and to what extent a physician may delegate authority to paramedics to perform medical acts.

Licensure and/or Certification

As described in Chapter 1, paramedic licensure and/or certification may be required by state or local authorities. Licensure is a process of occupational regulation whereby a governmental agency (e.g., a state medical board) grants permission for a person who meets established qualifications to engage in the profession or occupation. Certification may be granted by a governmental body (e.g., city, county, state) or a nongovernmental certifying agency or professional association (e.g., the National Registry of EMTs) to a person who has met predetermined qualifications to participate in an activity.

? CRITICAL THINKING

How does licensure/certification help to ensure the safety of your community?

Motor Vehicle Laws

Motor vehicle codes usually define standards for equipping and operating emergency vehicles[1] (see Chapter 48). Like most laws, these codes vary by state.

NOTE

Criminal statutes do not always require proof of intent or intentional conduct for an activity to be considered criminal in nature. For example, an emergency vehicle crash from reckless driving may result in civil and criminal lawsuits. Excessive speed, failure to consider road and weather conditions, and inappropriate use or nonuse of audible and visual warning devices are important areas of potential liability for all emergency drivers. The paramedic should be well aware of state motor vehicle codes and laws pertaining to emergency vehicle operations.

Mandatory Reporting Requirements

Paramedics and other health care professionals may be required by law to report cases of abuse or neglect of children and older adults, spouse abuse, and cases involving rape, sexual assault, gunshot wounds, stab wounds, animal bites, and certain communicable diseases (Box 4-1). The content of the report and to whom it must be made is set by law, regulation, or policy. Local protocols established by medical direction and the EMS agency give direction in these areas. Some states provide for penalties when mandatory reporting requirements are not satisfied.

> **? CRITICAL THINKING**
>
> *What will you do if your state requires the reporting of gunshot wounds and your patient, who has a small-caliber flesh wound, refuses care and begs you not to tell anyone so that her privacy will be protected?*

> **NOTE**
>
> Many mandatory reporting statutes provide for immunity for the reporting individual to help minimize the fear of legal consequences associated with such reporting should the report be false or unfounded. These statutes either prohibit lawsuits against individuals who file reports or offer a defense in court in the event of a lawsuit.

Protection for the Paramedic

Some state and federal regulations provide protection for the paramedic with respect to notification of infectious disease exposure, immunity statutes, and special crimes against EMS personnel. Some of these regulations vary by state and local jurisdictions.

Notification of infectious disease exposure

The *Ryan White Comprehensive AIDS Resources Emergency Act of 1990* (PL 101-381) requires that emergency responders be advised if they have been exposed to infectious diseases, including hepatitis, tuberculosis, bacterial (meningococcal) meningitis, rubella (German measles), and HIV. The act also requires that employers name a designated officer to coordinate communications between the hospital and the emergency response organization in case there is an exposure. Notification must be made within 48 hours of disease determination so that postexposure management procedures can be initiated (see Chapter 37).

> **? CRITICAL THINKING**
>
> *Why would some health care facilities not report significant infectious disease exposures to EMS personnel before the Ryan White law of 1990?*

Immunity statutes. Protecting state and other governmental entities from litigation (governmental immunity) originated from an ancient English common law based on the concept that "the king can do no wrong." In modern law, this means that governmental agencies cannot be held liable for the negligent acts of their employees. Since the 1950s, the trend in many states has been to discard this doctrine or limit the extent of its application. In some states, for example, immunity, if exercised, may only apply to the governmental agency and not to the individual employee or operator of an emergency vehicle. Because governmental immunity

> **BOX 4-1**
>
> **CASES REPORTABLE UNDER LAW IN MOST STATES**
>
> - Neglect or abuse of children
> - Neglect or abuse of older adults
> - Spouse abuse
> - Rape, sexual assault
> - Gunshot wounds
> - Stab wounds
> - Animal bites
> - Certain communicable diseases

statutes vary throughout the country, individual EMS providers may or may not be protected by this statute.

Good Samaritan legislation exists in some form in all 50 states. The intent of these laws is to encourage people to help others without fear of litigation when an emergency arises. As a rule, a person who provides emergency first aid in good faith and without expectation of compensation and in a manner that another person with similar training would provide is covered by these laws. However, these laws generally do not protect health care professionals from acts of gross negligence, reckless disregard, or willful or wanton misconduct. They also generally do not apply to paid, on-duty EMS employees.

TRICKS OF THE TRADE

Don't rely on protection from Good Samaritan laws. They were designed to protect the lay public who acted in good faith to the best of their abilities.

? CRITICAL THINKING

Would the absence of Good Samaritan laws affect your decision about whether to stop and render aid to an ill or injured stranger while off-duty?

Special crimes against a paramedic. Paramedics may become victims of assault or battery while performing their duties. To deter crimes against paramedics, some localities have enacted ordinances that provide the same level of protection for EMS providers as for law enforcement personnel. These ordinances make it illegal to harm or threaten to harm EMS crews or to obstruct patient care activities. The paramedic should use good judgment and work closely with the dispatch center and police so that dangerous situations can be avoided.

NOTE

If the scene is not safe, and it cannot be made safe, the EMS crew should retreat from the scene and not enter the area until it is properly secured.

The Legal Process

The anatomy of an injury lawsuit against a paramedic includes a series of specific steps[1] (Fig. 4-1). It begins when an incident occurs where a person (plaintiff) feels he or she has been injured as a result of negligent patient care. The plaintiff then hires an attorney who conducts a case investigation to determine whether the plaintiff's complaint has merit. The investigation may include examining patient care reports, textbooks, journal articles, and local protocols. If the attorney believes the plaintiff's case has merit, a complaint is prepared and filed in court outlining the negligent conduct that resulted in the alleged injury. After the complaint is filed in court, the complaint and a summons are served on the defendant and the litigation process is initiated. The summons (usually served by a sheriff or other authorized person) requires that the defendant answer the complaint or risk automatically losing the case. At this point, the defendant and all parties involved (e.g., the paramedic, ambulance service, hospital) usually will retain an attorney to defend against the lawsuit.

Anatomy of an Injury Lawsuit

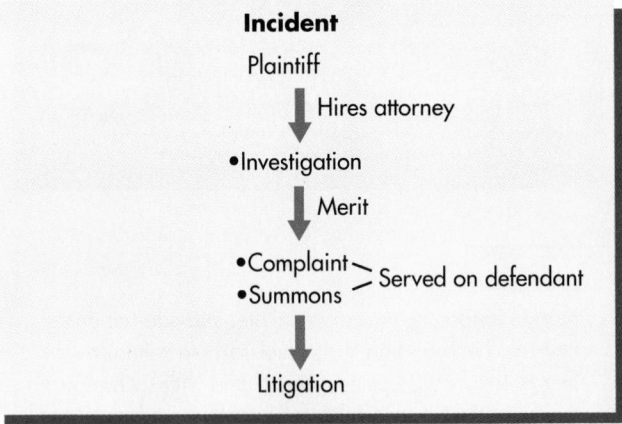

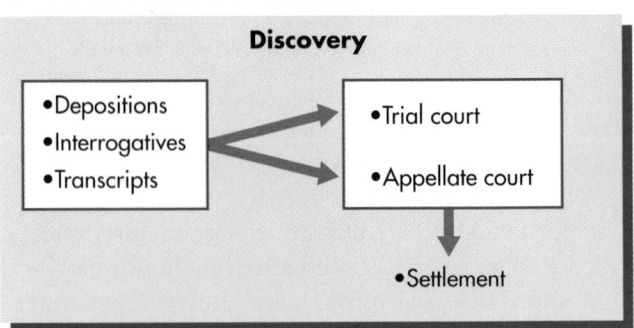

Fig. 4-1 Anatomy of a lawsuit.

The next step in the legal process is known as *discovery*. Discovery usually involves the exchange of documents and the taking of depositions and interrogatives. Depositions are testimonies taken under oath outside of a courtroom. The person giving the deposition answers questions from the other side's attorney about the lawsuit, and a court reporter types the questions and answers to prepare a transcript that may be used during the trial. When giving a deposition, the attorney should always be present. An interrogative is a questionnaire about the lawsuit that is answered in consultation with the party's lawyer and then returned to the other side's lawyer when completed. During discovery, each side is entitled to receive all relevant information pertaining to the lawsuit. Other documents that may be gathered during discovery include any patient care reports (PCRs). Following discovery, the case will either be settled out of court or it will go to trial.

> **NOTE**
>
> The legal process may involve both trial and appellate courts. A trial court determines the outcome of individual cases. The outcome may be determined by a judge or by a jury. The appellate court hears appeals of decisions by trial courts or other appeals courts. Decisions that are reached in appellate court may set precedent for later cases of a similar nature.

> ✓ **TRICKS OF THE TRADE**
>
> At some point in your EMS career, you probably will be asked to give a deposition. It comes with the territory.

> **? CRITICAL THINKING**
>
> *How important will your written documentation be regarding a case that occurred 5 years ago?*

> **NOTE**
>
> Quality improvement (QI) materials are "discoverable" in some states.

During the trial, each party presents its side of the case. Based on the evidence, a judge or jury determines liability and any damages to be awarded to the plaintiff. The decision of the trial court may be appealed by either side, but the appeal usually can only be based on errors in law made by the trial court.

Settlement may occur at any stage during the litigation. In settlement, the plaintiff agrees to accept an amount of money in exchange for a promise not to pursue the claim. After the case is settled, it is dismissed.

Legal Accountability of the Paramedic

Paramedics are responsible for acting in a reasonable and prudent manner and for providing a level of care and transportation consistent with their education, training, and local protocol. Failure to meet these responsibilities can result in legal liability.

> **NOTE**
>
> Nearly anyone can be sued, regardless of the legitimacy of the complaint. A lawsuit itself is not an indication of guilt or wrongdoing unless the allegations are proven.

Components of Negligence

Lawsuits involving patient care usually result from civil claims of negligence: the failure to act as a reasonable, prudent paramedic would act in similar circumstances. In most states, four elements must be proved for negligence to exist: (1) There was a duty to act; (2) there were actions performed at a level below the standard of care (a breach of duty); (3) there was damage to the patient or other individual (plaintiff); and (4) the breach was the proximate cause of the damage.

> **? CRITICAL THINKING**
>
> *What ALS interventions do you think that you will perform as a paramedic that have an increased risk of doing harm to the patient compared to BLS skills?*

Duty to Act

Paramedics assume a "duty" to provide emergency care when requested while working for an EMS service. This duty may be formal (contractual) or informal (volunteer). Once a paramedic undertakes the duty to act, he or she must *continue to act* until patient care responsibilities have been transferred to another health care worker who has training and experience appropriate to the needs of the patient, or it is abundantly clear that the patient no longer needs assistance. Duties include the following:

- To respond and render care
- To obey laws and regulations
- To operate emergency vehicles reasonably and prudently
- To provide care and transportation to the expected standard
- To provide care and transportation consistent with the scope of practice and local medical protocols
- To continue care and transportation through to its appropriate conclusion

> **NOTE**
>
> The delegation of scope of practice between a physician and a paramedic usually is only effective when the paramedic is on duty. Therefore an off-duty paramedic who provides emergency care usually must act in a BLS capacity unless there is specific authorization from medical direction for ALS procedures to be performed while off-duty.

Breach of Duty

For negligence to exist, plaintiffs must prove that the paramedic had a duty to act and that the duty was breached or violated. The paramedic must exercise the degree of care, skill, and judgment that any other similarly trained paramedic would provide under similar circumstances. This standard of

> **NOTE**
>
> Standard of care is a measure of competence of a professional. It differs from scope of practice, which identifies specific medical practices that are permitted by licensure and/or certification.

care is established by court testimony and referenced to published codes, standards, criteria, and guidelines applicable to the situation.

> **NOTE**
>
> Many states consider national standards when defining acceptable care. If written national or state standards have been violated, it may be easier for the plaintiff to prove breach of duty.

Breach of duty may occur by malfeasance (performing a wrongful or unlawful act); misfeasance (performing a legal act in a manner that is harmful or injurious); or nonfeasance (failure to perform a required act or duty). In some cases, negligence may be so obvious that it does not require extensive proof. *Res ipsa loquitur* is a Latin phrase that means "the thing speaks for itself" and implies that the facts are so clear, that without a doubt, the injury could only have been caused by negligence; *negligence per se* means that negligence is shown by the fact that a statute or ordinance was violated and injury resulted.

Damage to the Patient or Other Individual (Plaintiff)

The third element of negligence is proof that the plaintiff suffered compensable damages. Examples include medical expenses, lost earnings, conscious pain and suffering, and wrongful death. Punitive damages may also be awarded in excess of compensable damages to punish the wrongdoer and to deter others from causing similar harm in the future. Punitive damages generally are not covered by malpractice insurance (described later in this chapter).

Proximate Cause

Finally, the plaintiff must prove that the negligent act or inaction caused the injury or worsened an already present injury and that the injury or additional harm was foreseeable to the paramedic. The element of proximate cause sometimes is difficult to establish and often involves expert witnesses who address issues of duty, standard of care, and conflicting views of causation. For example, was a cervical spine injury caused by the motor vehicle crash, or was it the result of rescue efforts by the EMS crew?

Areas for potential negligent conduct other than direct patient care activities include (1) patient transportation to a medical facility contrary to medical direction advice, trauma center designation, or other known special patient care needs and facility capabilities; (2) failure to maintain equipment, supplies, or vehicles; and (3) driving negligently or recklessly.

Defenses to Negligence Claims

Most authorities stress that the best protection for health care professionals against such claims of negligence is training, competent patient care skills, and thorough documentation of all patient care activities. Other defenses to negligence and their pros and cons are provided in the following list:

? CRITICAL THINKING

Do you think that an effective quality management program can decrease the risk for negligence law suits? How?

1. Good Samaritan laws
   • Generally do not protect providers from acts of gross negligence, reckless disregard, or willful or wanton misconduct
   • Generally do not prohibit the filing of a lawsuit
   • May provide coverage for paid or volunteer providers
   • Vary from state to state
2. Governmental immunity
   • Trend is toward limiting protection
   • May only protect governmental agency, not provider
   • Varies from state to state
3. Statute of limitations
   • Limit the number of years after an incident during which a lawsuit can be filed
   • Set by law and may differ for cases involving adults and children
   • Varies from state to state
4. Contributory negligence
   • Plaintiff may be found to have contributed to his or her own injury
   • Damages awarded may be reduced or eliminated based on the plaintiff's contribution to the injury

✓ TRICKS OF THE TRADE

Remember the saying: *If it wasn't written down, it wasn't done.* In addition to providing good patient care, thorough documentation is your best defense against litigation.

Liability Insurance

Adequate professional liability (malpractice) insurance should be carried by all practicing health care professionals. Policies provide coverage for legal defense and potential judgments against the policyholder. Malpractice insurance policies fall into two categories: primary policies and umbrella policies. Primary policies are personal policies that offer certain limits of coverage for the types of risks insured against. For example, a policy with a $100,000 policy limits pays up to that amount for covered damages caused by the insured.

? CRITICAL THINKING

What kind of liability insurance protects you now as an EMT and as a student paramedic in your clinical sites?

Umbrella policies are professional liability insurance policies carried by a paramedic employer, such as an ambulance service or hospital. These policies usually offer additional limits of coverage for on-duty employees who perform activities within the scope of practice that the employer authorizes in policy or protocol. A $1,000,000 umbrella policy, for example, covers damages caused by the insured in excess of those limits contained in the underlying primary policy of insurance. The amount of coverage of these umbrella policies varies by hospital and EMS agency. If the umbrella policy does not cover the individual employee's liability, then separate individual insurance coverage may be desirable. Individual insurance coverage can be obtained from a variety of companies. Group insurance plans usually are less expensive and may provide better coverage than the more expensive individual policies.

Special Liability Concerns

Several liability concerns are unique to prehospital care. These include liability of the paramedic medical director, liability for "borrowed servants," and considerations for issues relating to civil rights.

Liability of the Paramedic Medical Director

In delegating patient care to paramedics, the medical direction physician assumes vicarious liability for the treatment rendered in the out-of-hospital setting. This liability may hold true for actions performed through both on-line (direct) medical direction and off-line (indirect) medical direction where care is provided by use of protocols and standing orders. Therefore negligence on the part of a paramedic may become the responsibility of the medical direction physician, even in the absence of direct supervision, in addition to the paramedic's employer.

> **NOTE**
>
> Vicarious liability arises by virtue of the employer-employee relationship and by being a principal agent who is authorized to perform for the benefit of another. Even though the paramedics are not employees of the medical direction physician, they act as agents in place of the medical direction physician. As such, the law may view the actions of the paramedic as an indirect legal responsibility of the medical direction physician.

Liability for Borrowed Servants

Borrowed servants is another legal doctrine in which a servant serves two "masters." An example of this is an EMT-Basic who is employed by a municipality but who works under the supervision of a paramedic. This doctrine can create liability for the supervising paramedic as well as the employer and the medical direction physician (through vicarious liability). The amount of liability for the supervising paramedic depends on the degree of supervision and control given to the paramedic by the employer.

> **NOTE**
>
> The borrowed servant doctrine is based on the theory that when a person has control over someone else's employee, he or she should be responsible for their acts, even though there is no employer-employee relationship. Paramedics who normally have complete supervisory responsibilities over EMT-Bs must protect the interest of the patient by making sure the EMT-Bs perform properly.

Civil Rights

The first civil rights law was enacted in 1866 to prohibit discrimination based on race. Since that time, these laws have been modified several times to make it illegal to discriminate by reason of race, color, sex, religion, national origin, and in the case of health care, the ability to pay (see the box below). In the case of a municipal ambulance service, a patient could bring claim under the civil rights act for a number of possible violations such as treatment and transport without proper consent.

COBRA/OBRA

The *Consolidated Omnibus Budget Reconciliation Act* (COBRA) (now known as *Emergency Medical Treatment and Active Labor Act* [EMTALA]) became effective in 1986. This act addressed the medical screening, stabilization, and transfer of patients with emergency medical conditions or who are in active labor for Medicare-participating hospitals. It also addressed the issue of "patient dumping" (the transfer, diversion, or premature discharge of patients from a hospital because of their inability to pay) and established penalties of up to $20,000 for each violation. COBRA was amended as the *Omnibus Budget Reconciliation Act* (OBRA '89 and '90) to provide clarity and greater en-

forcement to the COBRA regulations. It also increased the potential fine to $50,000 per infraction. The major provisions of OBRA include:

- Medical screening as it relates to the sending and receiving hospitals' capabilities
- Stabilization of the patient at a referring hospital (legal and financial responsibility)
- Provision of appropriate transfer methods, ensuring that the patient is stable and has consented to the transfer
- Definition of "appropriate transfer" as the provision of the needed level of care and resources available during the transfer
- Whistle-blower protection for physician and hospital staff

Another law, the *Rehabilitation Act of 1973*, prohibits discrimination against handicapped individuals solely based on a person's handicap. This act applies to any program or activity receiving federal financial assistance and may include EMS agencies that receive Medicare or Medicaid reimbursement. Title II of the *Americans with Disabilities Act* (ADA) also provides for equal accessability for public services by individuals with disabilities, including receiving appropriate patient care regardless of disease condition (e.g., AIDS, HIV, TB, and other communicable diseases).

Protection Against Negligence Claims

Paramedics must be aware of how patient care activities can pose a threat of litigation for negligence. The best protection against such claims are:

- Education/training/continuing education and skills retention
- Appropriate quality improvement
- Appropriate medical direction, on- and off-line
- Accurate, thorough documentation (see Chapter 17)
- Professional attitude and demeanor

Paramedic-Patient Relationships

The relationship formed between the paramedic and the patient during a patient care encounter is a legal one. Legal issues that may arise from providing patient care include confidentiality, consent, transportation, and the occasional use of force.

Confidentiality

Many states prohibit physicians from revealing patient information without the patient's consent. In some states, paramedics do not have this legal obligation but rather an ethical obligation to protect a patient's privacy. Information obtained from a patient (e.g., a patient history of communicable disease) usually can be conveyed without the patient's permission to other health care providers involved in the patient's care. Similarly, information obtained from a patient regarding an accident or crime may be reported to law enforcement personnel and testified to in court. There is, however, a potential liability for invasion of privacy and defamation (libel or slander, described on p. 76) if personal information is released with malicious intent or reckless disregard or to people not legally entitled to the information.

Defining Confidentiality

Information related to a patient's history, assessment findings, and any treatment rendered generally is considered confidential information. As a rule, the release of this information requires written permission from the patient or legal guardian, with the following exceptions:

- When other care providers have a "need to know" (e.g., communicable diseases)
- When required by law (e.g., child abuse, gunshot wounds)
- When required for third-party billing (e.g., Medicare/Medicaid)
- When required in response to a proper subpoena

When releasing confidential information without the patient's written permission is necessary, the paramedic must follow all reporting requirements and procedural policies established by state/local laws, the EMS agency, and medical direction.

Improper Release of Information

The improper release of confidential information or the release of inaccurate information can result in liability. Two areas in which liability may be incurred are invasion of privacy and defamation (libel and/or slander).

Invasion of privacy. Invasion of privacy is the release, without legal justification, of information regarding a patient's private life that might reasonably expose the person to ridicule, notoriety, or embarrassment. For example, a paramedic is caring for a public official who was involved in a motor vehicle crash. After the call, the paramedic tells everyone at the ambulance base that the official had a tattoo of a Nazi insignia on his left shoulder. A custodian at the base overhears the conversation and tells his wife, who works at the official's office building. The next day, a flyer is distributed with a caricature of the official in the back of an ambulance with a descriptive tattoo. Within a few days, the EMS agency is contacted by the official's attorney claiming an invasion of privacy.

TRICKS OF THE TRADE

Remember the saying: "What you hear here, what you see here, when you leave here, let it stay here."

? CRITICAL THINKING

Have you ever been in a situation where you or a colleague said something about a patient that you think may have violated confidentiality? What did you do about it?

NOTE

The fact that the information released is true is not a defense for invasion of privacy.

Defamation. *Defamation* refers to making an untrue statement about someone's character or reputation without legal privilege or consent of the individual.

Libel refers to false statements about a person made in writing or through the mass media with malicious intent or reckless disregard for the falsity of the statements. *Slander* refers to false verbal statements about a person made with malicious intent or reckless disregard for the falsity of the statements. If the paramedic in the previous example had lied about the official's tattoo, he and the office worker who prepared and distributed the flyer could be sued for libel and slander.

Consent

Patient rights have been defined and clarified by legislation and the judicial system through malpractice litigation. A competent patient's right to choose what medical care and transportation to receive is a fundamental concept of law and medical practice.

? CRITICAL THINKING

Imagine being called to care for a patient who is clearly having signs and symptoms of a heart attack but is alert and refusing care. How will you feel? What strategies will you use to try to persuade the patient to allow your care and transport?

For consent to be given, the patient must be of legal age and able to make a reasoned decision regarding:

- Nature of the illness or injury
- Treatment recommended
- Risks and dangers of treatment
- Alternative treatments and associated risks
- Dangers of refusing treatment (including transport)

Types of Consent

Informed consent is patient consent signifying that he or she knows, understands, and agrees to the care rendered—a consent given based on full disclosure of the information. Verbal or written consent to the treatment is called **expressed consent.** (Consent also can be expressed nonverbally by actions or simply by the patient allowing care to be rendered.)

Implied consent presumes that unconscious or mentally impaired persons needing immediate emergency care would consent to lifesaving treatment if they were able to do so. Unconscious patients and victims of shock, head injury, and alcohol or other drug intoxication are examples of patients to whom emergency care should be delivered in the absence of informed consent. It should be noted, however, that a competent adult patient who regains consciousness can revoke consent at any time during care and transport. This commonly is seen in situations involving diabetic patients and those with seizure disorders who may choose to refuse *insulin* or anticonvulsant medications.

Involuntary consent refers to treatment that is granted by authority of law. Examples include caring for patients who are held involuntarily for mental health evaluation, and patients who may be held under arrest or in protective custody by law enforcement personnel. The paramedic must follow established policies and procedures when providing care for these patients.

Special Consent Situations

Situations may occur where obtaining consent for treatment is difficult (e.g., emergencies involving minors, mentally incompetent adults, institutionalized patients, or prisoners). In these cases, consent for medical care may need to be obtained from a parent, legal guardian, representative of a state agency, or another legal authority. If a delay in obtaining consent would be life threatening, how-

ever, the patient should be treated. EMS personnel should be familiar with state laws governing these unique circumstances, and EMS systems should have protocols covering such situations.

Minors. In most states, a person is considered a minor until age 18, unless emancipated (legally released from parental control and supervision). Emancipation may include minors who are married, parents, or in the armed forces, and those living independently who are self-supported (e.g., college students not living at home or not receiving financial aid).

Unemancipated minors (those under parental control and supervision) are not legally able to give *or* withhold consent, although consent should be sought before treatment. Therefore consent of a parent, legal guardian, or court-appointed custodian usually is required. If a delay in obtaining consent would be life threatening, however, the emergency doctrine of treating and transporting the patient without consent applies. Although the courts will assume that the parents would have consented to treatment, the paramedic should thoroughly document the nature of the emergency and the reason the child required immediate care.

Mentally incompetent adults. Providing emergency care for mentally incompetent adults is similar to providing emergency care for minors with reference to obtaining consent, since these patients may not be legally able to give or withhold consent. Competence may be impaired by a number of factors, including disease, injury, anxiety, mental illness, mental retardation, and alcohol or other drug use. If the patient is not mentally or emotionally able to make rational and appropriate decisions about the care received, the emergency doctrine of treating and transporting without consent should be applied.

Prisoners or arrestees. As a rule, incarceration or detention does not deny a person the right to make decisions about medical treatment. However, if a prisoner or arrestee has a limb- or life-threatening injury or illness and refuses to give consent, the court or police who have the patient in custody may (in some cases) authorize treatment. The authority of law provides consent through the emergency doctrine. Paramedics who routinely provide care in prison settings should be aware of local and state laws regarding consent for this population.

Refusal of care or transport. A mentally competent adult has the right to refuse medical care, even if the decision could result in death or permanent disability. Refusal of care may be based on religious beliefs, inability to pay for medical care, fear, or lack of understanding of medical procedures. The paramedic should be sensitive to these concerns and carefully explain a procedure and answer any questions the patient has. Documentation of this explanatory effort on the patient care report is prudent.

Involving medical direction, law enforcement, family members, and friends at the scene may help persuade the patient to accept care and transportation. Despite these efforts, however, some patients still refuse treatment. If this occurs, the paramedic should leave the patient with the understanding that he or she can call again for help, despite the initial refusal. In addition, family members or friends should be encouraged to stay with the patient, if possible.

> **NOTE**
>
> Cases involving refusal of care are a significant cause of lawsuits against EMS agencies. The paramedic should always consult with medical direction.

When dealing with any patient who refuses care, the paramedic should thoroughly document the event. Names and addresses of others who wit-

nessed the event should be obtained, and all attempts made to obtain consent should be recorded. In addition, the patient should be advised of the medical risks associated with refusal of care, and this advice should be recorded on the patient care report (PCR). Law enforcement officers and other allied health professionals at the scene should be asked to make similar documentation of the event. Many EMS systems will require the paramedic to obtain a "release of liability" signed by the patient and a disinterested witness documenting the refusal of care, transportation, or both.

Some EMS systems require EMS crews to contact medical direction while at the scene and review the case with the physician or physician designee. Medical direction personnel may discuss the situation with the patient while the call is recorded. This policy may be useful in suppressing legal action, but the most critical legal document of refusal is the written PCR prepared by the paramedic.

Legal Complications Related to Consent

Four other legal complications related to consent may result in a civil or criminal violation. Definitions and examples of these areas of liability are provided below:

Abandonment: Inappropriate termination of care or turning care over to personnel who do not have training and expertise appropriate for the medical needs of the patient. Abandonment may occur at the scene or when the patient is delivered to the emergency department. Examples include allowing a first responder to provide care for a patient who requires ALS care and placing a critical patient in the care of an unlicenced emergency department "tech" at the receiving hospital.

False imprisonment: Intentional and unjustifiable detention of a person. Examples include charges brought by a patient who was transported without consent or who was restrained without proper cause or authority.

Assault: Creating apprehension, or unauthorized handling and treatment of patients. An example is threatening to restrain a patient unless he or she "quiets down."

Battery: Physical contact with persons without their consent and without legal justification. An example is drawing a patient's blood without permission.

The paramedic can avoid these additional areas of liability by using good judgment and by being sensitive to any special needs of the patient who is experiencing a crisis. The paramedic should always document any unusual situations or actions on the PCR and involve medical direction and law enforcement personnel when necessary.

Use of Force

It occasionally may be necessary to employ "reasonable" force or to use restraints when dealing with unruly or violent patients who are not able to make rational, informed decisions regarding their care. Examples include patients with behavioral emergencies and those with altered levels of consciousness caused by injury, substance abuse, or illness.

Most law enforcement agencies have the authority to place patients in "protective custody," thereby permitting treatment. EMS personnel should become involved in restraining patients only when it can be done safely and there is reason to suspect that patients are a threat to themselves or others (see Chapter 38). Most EMS agencies have specific protocols that should be followed when it is necessary to restrain patients. Some protocols require that violent patients be placed in protective custody by law enforcement personnel before paramedics become involved in patient care.

> **NOTE**
>
> Using reasonable force to restrain a patient must always be humane and never punitive in nature.

> **NOTE**
>
> Chemical restraint refers to the use of sedative drugs to help subdue a patient (e.g., violent patients or combative patients with head injuries who are being transported by helicopter). The use of these agents in the prehospital setting to restrain a patient is controversial. The paramedic should consult with medical direction and follow established protocols.

Transportation

Legal responsibilities for the patient continue until patient care is transferred to another component of the health care system (or it is abundantly clear that the patient no longer requires care). Important aspects of this continuum of care are issues related to patient transport.

> **? CRITICAL THINKING**
>
> *Your supervisor decides that exceeding the posted speed limit (even with audible and visual warning devices) is too dangerous to the community and disallows it on all but cardiac arrest calls. What will you do?*

Level of Care During Transportation

As previously stated, once patient care has been initiated, care must be continued until the patient is transferred to another health care professional who has training and expertise appropriate for the medical needs of the patient. Once the duty to act is assumed, the paramedic must continue to act until patient care has been appropriately transferred.

Use of Emergency Vehicle Operating Privileges

The driver of the emergency vehicle must operate the vehicle in conformity to laws, regulations, and policies and in a manner that safeguards the patient, crew, and public. "Right-of-way" privileges that usually are given to operators of emergency vehicles include allowing the driver to:

- Travel slightly faster than the posted speed limit
- Move safely from one lane into the opposite lane of traffic
- Safely enter and pass through red-light intersections
- Appropriately use audible and visual warning devices
- Park in unauthorized areas

> **NOTE**
>
> Paramedics should be aware of specific laws in their state regarding right-of-way privileges.

> **NOTE**
>
> As a rule, emergency vehicles should not exceed 10 miles per hour above posted speed limits during emergency response or patient transport.

Excessive speed and inappropriate use or nonuse of audible and visual warning devices are examples of ways in which vehicle operating privileges are abused. Drivers of emergency vehicles are responsible for the safety of all during emergency response and patient transport (see Chapter 48).

Choice of Patient Destination

Hospital selection should be based on patient needs and hospital capability. As a rule, the patient's choice of hospital destination should be honored unless situations or the patient's condition dictates otherwise. Examples of hospital selection include hospitals that are on "diversion status" due to patient load, and the need for speciality care that only can be provided at designated facilities (see the box below). Protocols for hospital selection must be established, and medical direction should be involved in cases when a patient's choice of hospital cannot be honored.

TRICKS OF THE TRADE

In many ways, EMS is a business. In a business sense, patients are your *clients*. Their wishes should be honored when possible.

NOTE

Some EMS services use a "nearest hospital rule" for transporting patients, even if the nearest hospital is not the patient's choice of facility.

Payer Protocols

There may be times when restrictions established by health care plans affect when and where a patient can be transported for medical care. For example, Medicare, the largest single payer of ambulance services in the United States, has complex regulations as to what types of services and patient transports are eligible for reimbursement (see the box on p. 81). Paramedics need a basic understanding of these programs so that the EMS agency can be paid for their services and to help the patient determine what services are likely to be covered by their insurance policies.

NOTE

The majority of patients transported by ambulance are covered by Medicare, Medicaid, Blue Shield, or a combination of the three.[2]

In limb- or life-threatening emergencies, payer protocols should not be a factor in providing patient care or transportation to the closest appropriate facility. However, a complete description of patient care activities must be provided on the patient care report, since some claims are rejected for reimbursement because of poor documentation.

Resuscitation Issues

Issues regarding resuscitation are complex and often involve certain legal and ethical considerations

CATEGORIZATION OF HOSPITAL RESOURCE CAPABILITIES

Categorization of hospital emergency services was recommended by the American Medical Association in the early 1970s. In 1990, *Resources for Optimal Care of the Injured Patient* was published by the Task Force of the American College of Surgeons (ACS) Committee on Trauma. It described three levels of trauma centers based on resources, admissions, staff, research, and education involvement.

A level I institution can provide total care for every aspect of injury and is uniquely qualified to care for the most severely injured patient, especially in the surgical critical care setting, followed by level II and *level III* facilities. Categorization of hospital resources identifies hospitals capable of handling trauma patients and en-

ables EMS providers to rapidly transport patients to appropriate medical facilities. Based on ACS guidelines, some state governmental agencies have designated certain institutions as trauma centers. Other specialized care facilities, such as pediatric trauma centers, burn centers, hyperbaric centers, and poison treatment centers, provide care for critically ill or injured patients with special needs. (NOTE: A level IV facility [primarily a referral center] also has been designated by ACS and is recognized by some states.)

In 1991, the Department of Health and Human Services and EMS Division provided financial grants for states to develop comprehensive statewide trauma systems as part of the 1990 Trauma Systems Planing and Development Act (PL 101-590). These grants were last awarded in 1994.

for the patient, family, EMS crew, and medical direction. Resuscitation issues that relate directly to EMS include withholding or stopping resuscitation, advance directives, potential organ donation, and death in the field.

Withholding or Stopping Resuscitation

As previously stated, competent and informed adult patients have the right to refuse medical care, including cardiopulmonary resuscitation (CPR). This right does not depend on the presence or absence of terminal illness, the agreement of family members, or approval of physicians. As a rule, patients who are pulseless should be resuscitated (unless directed otherwise by a physician), unless one or more of the following is present[3]:

- Obvious clinical signs of death
- Resuscitation attempts that would place the rescuer at significant risk of personal injury
- The presence of documentation in the form of "No-CPR" orders, "Do Not Resuscitate" (DNR) orders, or "Do Not Attempt Resuscitation" (DNAR) orders, or another reliable reason to believe that CPR is not indicated, warranted, or in the patient's best interest (Box 4-2).

At times, it may be difficult for the paramedic to determine whethere resuscitation should be initiated. An example would be a family member who requests CPR for a patient despite the presence of a No-CPR order. In this situation (or if the paramedic suspects that the No-CPR order is invalid), resus-

> **? CRITICAL THINKING**
>
> *You are called to care for a debilitated older adult patient in full cardiac arrest. The family tells you that they want nothing done, and are sobbing and begging you not to resuscitate him. They do not have the written documentation needed by your agency to permit the do-not-resuscitate order. What will you do? How will you feel about your decision?*

> **NOTE**
>
> According to the American Heart Association, unwitnessed deaths in the presence of known serious, chronic, debilitating disease or in the terminal state of fatal illness may be a reliable criterion in some settings to believe that CPR is not indicated. CPR also is not indicated for traumatic arrests with extended response or transport times after a patient's airway is ensured.

citation should be initiated and medical direction should be contacted. Paramedics generally should err in the direction of providing resuscitation and life support in most circumstances in which any issue is unclear. If evidence later indicates that resuscitation should be withheld, life-support measures can be stopped.

Procedures for determining when to stop resuscitation should be established by local protocols. The

---

MEDICARE MEDICAL POLICY: COVERED AMBULANCE SERVICES

Ambulance service must be medically necessary and reasonable. Medical necessity is established when the patient's clinical condition is such that the use of any other method of transportation would endanger the patient's medical condition. The patient's condition at the time of the transport is the determining factor in whether ambulance transport will be covered. Reimbursement may be made for expenses incurred by a patient for ambulance services that meet the following conditions:

1. Was transported in an emergency situation (e.g., as a result of an accident, injury, or acute illness), or
2. Needed to be restrained, or
3. Was unconscious or in shock, or
4. Required oxygen or other emergency treatment on the way to his or her destination, or
5. Had to remain immobile because of a fracture that had not been set or the possibility of a fracture, or
6. Sustained an acute stroke or myocardial infarction, or
7. Was experiencing severe hemorrhage, or
8. Was bed confined (unable to get up from bed without assistance *and* unable to ambulate *and* unable to sit in a chair or wheelchair), or
9. Could be moved only by stretcher

Source: Xact Medicare Services, Medicare Medical Policy Bulletin, Freedom of Information: Covered ambulance services, (T-2D). http://www.xact.org/policy/t2.html

BOX 4-2

DEFINITIONS

Orders for No-CPR, Do Not Resuscitate (DNR), and Do Not Attempt Resuscitation (DNAR) represent a decision made between the patient and his or her physician that CPR should be withheld in the event of cardiac arrest. These orders carry no limitation for other forms of treatment such as oxygen, fluid replacement, and drug administration. Some nursing home orders will specify "levels of care/support" to be provided (e.g., no intubation).

BOX 4-3

DEFINITIONS (see Chapter 28 for more discussion)

Countershock: A high-intensity, short-duration electric shock applied to the area of the heart.

Ventricular fibrillation: A pulseless, cardiac rhythm of the heart.

Asystole: The absence of mechanical and electrical activity in the heart.

Agonal: A cardiac rhythm frequently seen as the last rhythm in an unsuccessful resuscitation, otherwise known as "dying heart" rhythm.

role of medical direction also should be clearly delineated in these situations. As a model, it has been recommended by the AHA that resuscitation be discontinued in the prehospital setting when the patient is nonresuscitable after an adequate trial of BLS in conjunction with advanced cardiac life support (ACLS). This determination should be made by EMS authorities and ambulance medical directors, who generally should ensure that[3]:

- Endotracheal intubation has been successfully accomplished
- Intravenous access has been achieved and rhythm-appropriate medications and countershocks for ventricular fibrillation (VF) have been administered according to ACLS protocols
- Persistent asystole or agonal electrocardiographic patterns are present and no reversible causes are identified (Box 4-3)

Advance Directives

In 1991, a federal law known as the *Patient Self-Determination Act of 1990* required all institutions that accept Medicare or Medicaid to recognize any kind of "advance directive," such as durable power of attorney for health care or a "do not resuscitate" order[4] (Fig. 4-2). These legal documents are executed to inform health care practitioners of an individual's wishes for treatment or withholding of treatment in the event that the person becomes incapacitated and unable to communicate those wishes directly. Many states also have enacted legislation regarding "living wills" and the "right to die with dignity" for patients suffering from a terminal ill-

ness. The EMS service must work closely with medical direction to develop procedures and protocols that help EMS providers contend with these laws and policies.

NOTE

No-CPR orders should not be confused with advance directives. Advance directives require interpretation by a physician and need to be formulated into a treatment plan (which may include No-CPR orders) consistent with the patient's wishes. Medical direction must establish and implement policies for dealing with advance directives.

If the EMS crew is dispatched to a dying patient who has requested that he or she not be resuscitated, medical direction should be immediately contacted so that decisions can be made regarding any patient care activities. If it is determined that the patient is not to receive medical intervention to prolong life, reasonable measures of comfort should be provided to the patient as well as emotional support to family members and loved ones.

✓ TRICKS OF THE TRADE

Issues like this represent the "downside" of EMS. As you provide care and emotional support to the patient and family, remember to "take care" of yourself too. Your mental well-being is important for a long and rewarding career.

DO NOT RESUSCITATE (DNR) REQUEST

MISSOURI DEPARTMENT OF HEALTH
BUREAU OF EMERGENCY MEDICAL SERVICES

OUTSIDE THE HOSPITAL DO NOT RESUSCITATE (DNR) REQUEST

DNR #   13132

I, _____, request limited emergency care as herein described.
      (name)

I understand DNR means that if my heart stops beating or if I stop breathing, no medical procedure to restart breathing or heart functioning will be instituted.

I understand this decision will <u>not</u> prevent me from obtaining other emergency medical care by outside the hospital care providers and/or medical care directed by a physician prior to my death.

I understand I may revoke this directive at any time.

I give permission for this information to be given to the outside the hospital care providers, doctors, nurses, or other health personnel as necessary to implement this directive.

I hereby agree to the "Do Not Resuscitate" (DNR) order.

Patient/Appropriate Surrogate Signature **(Mandatory)**	Date
Witness **(Mandatory)**	Date

REVOCATION PROVISION

I hereby revoke the above declaration.

Signature	Date

I AFFIRM THIS DIRECTIVE IS THE EXPRESSED WISH OF THE PATIENT/PATIENT'S APPROPRIATE SURROGATE, IS MEDICALLY APPROPRIATE, AND IS DOCUMENTED IN THE PATIENT'S PERMANENT MEDICAL RECORD.

In the event of a cardiac or respiratory arrest, no cardiopulmonary resuscitation will be initiated.

Physician's Signature **(Mandatory)**	Date
Physician - Printed Name	Physician's Telephone Number
Address	Facility or Agency Name

MO 580-1936 (8-94)   EMS-21

THIS DNR REQUEST FORM SHOULD BE KEPT WITH THE PATIENT IN A VISIBLE LOCATION AT ALL TIMES.
THIS FORM WILL NOT BE ACCEPTED IF IT HAS BEEN AMENDED OR ALTERED IN ANY WAY.

DO NOT RESUSCITATE (DNR) REQUEST

Fig. 4-2 Advance directive. (Courtesy Missouri Department of Health, Bureau of Emergency Medical Services, Jefferson City, Mo.)

EMS and medical direction should work closely with the families and private physicians of terminally ill patients in private homes and hospice programs so that they will make appropriate use of the EMS system (i.e., when to call 911). Even though resuscitation may not be indicated, EMS may be needed to manage pain, treat acute medical illness or traumatic injury, and provide transportation to a hospital. Policies need to be established and adopted by local or state EMS authorities to allow persons to decline resuscitation attempts but still have access to other emergency medical treatments and ambulance transport.

Potential Organ Donation

Each day about 55 people receive organ transplants, and another 10 people on the waiting list die because not enough organs are available[5] (Box 4-4). The donation of organs and tissues and the subsequent transplantation process is complex and requires the involvement of many health care professionals. Paramedics can play an important role in the evaluation of potential donors by identifying a patient as a potential donor (Box 4-5), establishing communication with medical direction, and providing emergency care that will help maintain viable organs.

Identifying potential donors who are dead or near dead is a vital role for EMS in organ procurement. This can be done by searching for information such as a donor card and by talking with next-of-kin about the patient's intent to donate tissue or organs at his or her death. Even if there is no donor card or other document, the family still has the right to make the decision to donate (see the box on p. 85).

NOTE

A patient's intent to be a donor or *not* to be donor may be noted on his or her driver's license.

NOTE

Special training should be obtained by EMS personnel through tissue procurement organizations in how to approach the family about organ donation.

BOX 4-4

UNOS TRANSPLANT STATISTICS

Every 16 minutes a new name is added to the national transplant waiting list.

On January 23, 2000, the UNOS national patient waiting list for organ transplant included the following:

Type of Transplant	Patients Waiting for Transplant
Kidney	44,031
Liver	14,514
Pancreas	8233
Pancreas islet cell	182
Kidney-pancreas	961
Intestine	117
Heart	4063
Heart-lung	224
Lung	3590
TOTAL	67,050*

NOTE: UNOS policies allow patients to be listed with more than one transplant center (multiple listing); therefore the number of registrations is greater than the actual number of patients.
*Some patients are waiting for more than one organ; therefore the total number of patients is less than the sum of patients waiting for each organ.

BOX 4-5

GENERAL GUIDELINES FOR VITAL ORGAN DONATION

- Declaration of brain death by a licensed physician
- Stable blood pressure and heart rate with minimal use of dopamine (less than 10 to 20 μg/kg/min)*
- Age: newborn to 70 years
- No active infection (sepsis or communicable disease)
- No malignancies (except primary brain tumors)

General Guidelines for Nonvital Tissue Donation

- Donation possible from 6 to 24 hours after heartbeat has ceased
- Age: 3 months to 70 years
- No active infection (sepsis or communicable disease)
- No malignancies (except primary brain tumor)

From *The Manual for Organ and Tissue Donation*, Intermountain Organ Recovery System, 1990.
*See Chapters 8 and 28.

Once the patient has been identified as a potential organ donor, medical direction should be contacted so they can notify the appropriate organ procurement agencies. These organizations are staffed 24 hours each day by trained personnel who will assist in all aspects of the donation, including gathering the appropriate documentation. The paramedic should carefully and thoroughly record all patient care activities, vital sign assessments, and scene events (e.g., presence of drug paraphernalia) that may affect the agencies' evaluation of the potential donor.

Donations usually are separated into two categories: vital, or heart-beating, donors, and the more common donor who has no heartbeat (nonvital tissue donor). Vital donors may donate the heart, liver, kidneys, lungs, and pancreas. These donors must meet the criteria for brain death (Box 4-6), and the donor's heartbeat and circulation must be maintained until the vital organs are harvested. The nonvital (no heartbeat) tissue donor can donate corneas, skin, bones, tendons, heart valves, and saphenous veins up to 24 hours after cardiac death.

The paramedic's role in helping to maintain viable organs in the prehospital setting is to preserve organ function. This is best accomplished by airway management and appropriate fluid resuscitation to maintain blood pressure and organ perfusion (see Chapter 7). Eye care should be provided to all nontransported scene deaths with lubrication/saline solution or a commercial product (e.g., Lacri-Lube), and the eyes taped closed so that donation of the cornea can continue to be an option for the family.

Death in the Field

In the field, determination of death usually is confirmed by the following signs:

- No spontaneous electrical activity in the heart as confirmed by electrocardiogram (ECG) in several leads
- No spontaneous respirations
- Absent cough and gag reflex
- No spontaneous movement
- No response to painful stimuli
- Fixed and dilated pupils

Other signs that are used in determining death include the presence of dependent lividity and rigor mortis (see the box on p. 86). When an apparent death is encountered in the field, the paramedic should:

- Contact medical direction for guidance and follow established state and/or local protocols
- Document any observations or unusual findings at the scene
- Notify appropriate authorities per protocol (e.g., police, coroner)
- Disturb the scene as little as possible
- Provide emotional support to surviving family and friends at the scene

---

LEGAL NEXT OF KIN

When a patient death occurs in the prehospital setting, organ and tissue donation should be offered as the final option for the surviving family, regardless of the decision to transport the patient to the hospital. Obtaining consent for organ or tissue donation is, of course, a very delicate subject and should be approached with compassion and in a positive manner. When approaching a family for organ donation, consent must be obtained from the next-of-kin as defined by law. The accepted legal order is:

1. Spouse (even if separated but not divorced)
2. Adult son or daughter (over age 18)
3. Parents (for any unmarried child)
4. Siblings (in the event both parents are deceased and the donor is unmarried or divorced with no adult children)
5. Legal guardian

BOX 4-6

BRAIN DEATH CRITERIA

Brain death is defined as the loss of all brain function, including that of the brainstem.[6] These patients are ventilator-dependent, make no spontaneous respiratory effort, and have lost all spontaneous movement. The clinical findings are usually confirmed in the hospital by electroencephalogram (EEG) or a brain-flow scan. In most states, brain death must be declared by two separate physicians, neither of whom can be involved in the removal or transplantation of the organs.

PHYSIOLOGICAL CHANGES THAT OCCUR AFTER DEATH

Within minutes after death, postmortem changes begin to occur in the body. The surface of the skin becomes pale and yellowish; body temperature falls and reaches that of the environment within 24 hours; blood pressure and muscle tension decrease; and the pupils become dilated. Blood and fluids begin to drain away from the face, nose, and chin and gravity causes blood to settle in the most dependent, lowest tissues. This results in a bluish-purple discoloration in the tissues known as *postmortem lividity*.

Within 6 hours after death, muscle stiffening (rigor mortis) occurs from chemical changes in the body. Smaller muscles in the face are usually affected first, followed by a stiffening of the entire body within 12 to 14 hours. Signs of tissue decay are usually obvious within 24 to 48 hours after death (depending on environmental temperatures). The rigor mortis diminishes and the body becomes flaccid within 12 to 14 hours. As the body decays, the skin loosens from the underlying tissues and swelling and bloating become evident.

Crime and Accident Scene Responsibilities

Paramedics play two important roles when managing crime and accident scenes: (1) providing patient care (the primary focus) and (2) helping to preserve evidence at the scene when possible.

> **NOTE**
>
> The paramedic should never enter a crime or accident scene until it has been determined safe. *Personal safety is always the first priority in any emergency response.* If the scene is not safe, the paramedic should not enter until it has been secured.

> **? CRITICAL THINKING**
>
> *At the scene of a shooting, you can see a patient with slow, gasping respirations, but the police will not let you enter the crime scene. How will you feel?*

BOX 4-7

SCENE SAFETY CONSIDERATIONS

- Do not approach the crime scene until it has been secured.
- Approach the scene from a direction that appears safe and allows for easy egress.
- Maintain constant radio contact with police or dispatch.
- Survey and assess the scene before approaching the patient.
- Keep all unnecessary people away from the patient.
- Do not initiate unnecessary conversations with bystanders.

Crime and Accident Scene Considerations

When responding to a crime scene, it is best to be in direct radio communication with law enforcement personnel at the scene. This will provide the paramedic with information regarding scene safety and the number of patients (Box 4-7). If police are not on the scene or if the EMS crew is the first to respond, contact with the dispatch center should be maintained so that appropriate information can be relayed to law enforcement personnel. In addition to providing patient care, the paramedic should observe and document the overall scene and make an effort to protect potential evidence (Box 4-8).

> **NOTE**
>
> Law enforcement is in charge of the crime scene, and EMS is in charge of patient care. EMS should work closely with police, who will be providing protection for the EMS crew as well.

Responding to an accident scene requires the same commitment to personal safety and preservation of possible evidence (see Chapter 52). In addition, accident scenes and crime scenes often require additional personnel and resources. Examples include:

- Additional emergency vehicles for large numbers of patients
- Aeromedical service

BOX 4-8

CRIME SCENE PRESERVATION

Lifesaving procedures always take precedence over forensic considerations. However, the paramedic should disturb the scene as little as possible to help preserve evidence. Some forensic considerations include:

- Park the ambulance away from skid marks, tire prints, or other evidence.
- Follow the same path to and from the ambulance and patient.
- Avoid stepping on blood stains.
- Do not touch or move weapons or other environmental clues unless it is absolutely necessary for patient care.
- Document the exact condition of the patient and wound appearance on arrival at the scene, including environment of the patient and body position in relation to objects and doorways.

- If possible, cut or tear clothing along a seam to avoid altering tears made by a penetrating object. Avoid cutting through a hole made in the clothing by a wounding object.
- Do not shake clothing; keep all clothing in a paper bag rather than a plastic bag that may alter evidence; do not give it to the victim's family members.
- Save any avulsed tissue for forensic pathology.
- If a bullet is retrieved, place it in a padded container to prevent marring and secure the evidence until it is delivered to the authorities; obtain a receipt.
- Document any dying declarations made by patients.
- Report all actions and alterations made to the crime scene to the police.

- Law enforcement
- Fire service for auto extrication, fire suppression, and lighting
- Specialized rescue units
- Hazardous materials teams

Documentation

The PCR serves several functions. Of particular importance is that it provides a legal record of the patient care delivered in the field. It also becomes a permanent part of the patient's hospital record.

NOTE

A paramedic might view documentation as a chance to write good and appropriate future evidence. The opportunity should be seized enthusiastically and effectively.

The PCR as a Legal Record

In the legal professions, the general belief is that "if it was not written down, it was not done." The paramedic's documentation of an emergency call will be one of the first items reviewed in the case of a lawsuit for negligence or malpractice. Memory is fallible, and claims may not be filed until years after

an event. As a result, EMS personnel may be expected to testify to events years after they occurred. The paramedic will be allowed to refer to written reports to refresh his or her memory about details while testifying. Therefore thoroughness and attention to detail are absolutely essential in documentation (see Chapter 17). Characteristics of an effective PCR include the following:

- Completed promptly. It is a record made "in the course of business" not long after the event. Timely completion is essential to the PCR becoming part of the hospital record.
- Completed thoroughly. It should cover assessment, treatment, and other relevant facts and "paint" a complete, clear picture of the patient's condition and the care provided.

? CRITICAL THINKING

Think back to the first call you were on when a patient refused medical care. Can you remember exact details about their level of consciousness, what you told them about the risks of refusing care, and what you told them to do if the problem got worse? Do you think all of those facts are in the written documentation of that call in the event of litigation?

- Completed objectively. The paramedic should make observations rather than assumptions or conclusions and should avoid the use of emotional and value-laden words or phrases.
- Completed accurately. Descriptions should be as precise as possible, and the paramedic should avoid using abbreviations or jargon not commonly understood.
- Written with confidentiality maintained. The paramedic should follow established policy for release of patient information, and whenever possible, obtain patient consent before releasing information.

All patient care records need to be maintained at least for the extent of the statute of limitations. This statute varies by state from 2 to 6 years for personal injury suits. Patient records involving minors may need to be kept for a longer time since the statute of limitations may not begin until the minor is 18 years of age. (This also will vary from state to state.)

S U M M A R Y

- The structure of the legal system in the United States is composed of five types of law. These are legislative law, administrative law, common law, criminal law, and civil law.

- To safeguard against litigation, the paramedic must be knowledgeable of legal issues and the effects they may have.

- Paramedics and other health care professionals may be required by law to report cases of abuse or neglect of children and older adults, spouse abuse, and cases involving rape, sexual assault, gunshot wounds, stab wounds, animal bites, and certain communicable diseases.

- Lawsuits involving patient care usually result from civil claims of negligence: the failure to act as a reasonable, prudent paramedic would act in similar circumstances.

- Most authorities stress that the best protection against claims of negligence is training, competent patient care skills, and thorough documentation of all patient care activities.

- Some state and federal regulations provide protection for the paramedic with respect to notification of infectious disease exposure, immunity statutes, and special crimes against EMS personnel.

- Information related to a patient's history, assessment findings, and any treatment rendered generally is considered confidential information. As a rule, the release of this information requires written permission from the patient or legal guardian, with certain exceptions.

- A mentally competent adult has the right to refuse medical care, even if the decision could result in death or permanent disability.

- Four other legal complications related to consent are abandonment, false imprisonment, assault, and battery.

- A competent patient's right to decide what medical care (and transportation) to receive is a fundamental concept of law and medical practice.

- Legal responsibilities for the patient continue until patient care is transferred to another component of the health care system (or it is abundantly clear that the patient no longer requires care). Legal issues related to patient transport include: level of care during transportation, use of the emergency vehicle operating privileges, choice of patient destination, and payer protocols.

- Resuscitation issues that relate directly to EMS include withholding or stopping resuscitation, advance directives, potential organ donation, and death in the field.

- EMS plays two important roles when responding to crime and accident scenes: (1) focusing on patient care; (2) preserving evidence at the scene when possible.

- In the legal profession, the general belief is that "if it was not written down, it was not done." Therefore thoroughness and attention to detail are absolutely essential in documentation.

REFERENCES

1. U.S. Department of Transportation National Highway Traffic Safety Administration: *EMT-paramedic national standard curriculum*, Washington, DC, 1998, The Department.
2. Fitch J et al: *EMS management beyond the street*, ed 2, Carlsbad, Calif., 1993, JEMS.
3. American Heart Association: *Advanced cardiac life support*, Dallas, Tex, 1997, The Association.
4. Hall S: New act compels EMS to define new roles, *JEMS* 17(1):19, 1992.
5. Information accessed from http://www.organdonor.gov on April 7, 1998.
6. Winmill D, Clawson J: Seize the moment: the EMS role in organ donation, *JEMS* 15(11):48, 1990.

5 Ethics

Upon completion of this chapter, the paramedic student will be able to:

1. *Define ethics and bioethics.*
2. *Distinguish between professional, legal, and moral accountability.*
3. *Outline strategies that may be used to resolve ethical conflicts.*
4. *Describe the role of ethical tests in resolving ethical dilemmas in health care.*
5. *Discuss specific prehospital ethical issues including allocation of resources, decisions surrounding resuscitation, confidentiality, and consent.*
6. *Identify ethical dilemmas that may occur related to care in futile situations, obligation to provide care, patient advocacy, and the paramedic's role as physician extender.*

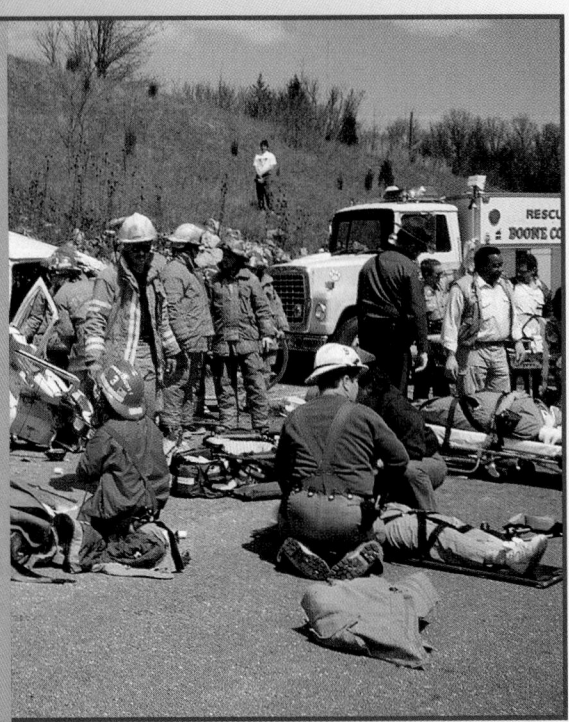

Ethical dilemmas will always be present in prehospital care, and there will be times when paramedics will be expected to perform duties that may involve conflicts in moral judgment. Examples include issues involving patient confidentiality, patient rights, field testing of experimental drugs or procedures, and honoring a Do Not Resuscitate (DNR) order. Ethical issues are dynamic ones, and the ethical dilemmas of today may be decided by law tomorrow.

KEY TERMS

bioethics: The systematic study of moral dimensions—including moral vision, decisions, conduct, and policies—of the life sciences and health care.

ethics: The discipline relating to right and wrong, moral duty and obligation, moral principles and values, and moral character; a standard for honorable behavior designed by a group with expected conformity.

morals: Social standards or customs; dealing with what is right or wrong in a practical sense.

unethical: Conduct that fails to conform to moral principles, values, or standards.

Ethics Overview

Ethics is the discipline relating to right and wrong, moral duty and obligation, moral principles and values, and moral character[1]; it is a standard for honorable behavior designed by a group with expected conformity. **Morals** refers to social standards or customs; dealing with what is right or wrong in a practical sense. The term **unethical** refers to conduct that fails to conform to these moral principles, values, or standards.[2]

> **NOTE**
>
> Ethical decisions are based on a systematic appraisal of moral judgments—a concept that places responsibility on individuals.

The concept of ethics dates back to the ancient Greek philosophers, such as Hippocrates, Socrates, Plato, Aristotle, and others who turned Greek atten-

> **NOTE**
>
> Bioethics is the systematic study of moral dimensions—including moral vision, decisions, conduct, and policies—of the life sciences and health care, using a variety of ethical methodologies in an interdisciplinary setting.

tion toward questions of ethics and virtue ("how should one live?") for moral accountability and away from choice and fate that traditionally had been guided by astrology (see the box at the top of p. 95). These philosophers laid the basis for a science of medical ethics (**bioethics**), the analysis of choice in medicine.[3]

Many ethical and other value choices can be made instinctively, drawing on personal long-standing beliefs, commitments, and habits. For example, most people believe it is wrong to steal, be deceitful, or to commit murder. In health care, however, paramedics will be faced with life issues that involve a patient with beliefs, commitments, and habits that may be quite different from the paramedic's personal experience. Throughout history, guidance in these situations has been provided through a variety of professional "codes" that represent the collective wisdom of a group. *The EMT Code of Ethics*, the *Code for Nurses with Interpretative Statements*, the *American Medical Association's Principles of Medical Ethics*, and the *Principles of Ethics for Emergency Physicians* are examples of professional codes (see the boxes on pp. 92–94).

In addition to professional codes, an individual's personal code of ethics is comprised of principles of appropriate conduct that provide guidance when making moral choices. A personal code is an important reflection on one's life. For the paramedic, a personal code of ethics must consider professional, legal, and moral accountability.

> **NOTE**
>
> The professional paramedic is accountable to the patient, the medical director, and the EMS system for fulfilling the standard of care.

Professional Accountability

As professionals, paramedics conform to a standard established by their level of training and regional practice. Responsibilities include commitment to

THE HIPPOCRATIC OATH (FOURTH CENTURY BC)

The *Oath of Hippocrates* is a brief statement of principles thought to be conceived during the fourth century B.C. The oath protected the rights of the patient and addressed the moral character of the physician as a healer. The Hippocratic oath was modified in the tenth or eleventh century to eliminate reference to pagan gods and remains an expression of ideal conduct for the physician.

I swear by Apollo Physician and Asclepius and Hygieia and Panaceia and all the gods and goddesses, making them my witnesses, that I will fulfill according to my ability and judgment this oath and this covenant:

To hold him who has taught me this art as equal to my parents and to live my life in partnership with him, and if he is in need of money to give him a share of mine, and to regard his offspring as equal to my brothers in male lineage and to teach them this art—if they desire to learn it—without fee and covenant; to give a share of precepts and oral instruction and all the other learning to my sons and to the sons of him who has instructed me and to pupils who have signed the covenant and have taken an oath according to the medical law, but to no one else.

I will apply dietetic measures for the benefit of the sick according to my ability and judgment; I will keep them from harm and injustice.

I will neither give a deadly drug to anybody if asked for it, nor will I make a suggestion to this effect. Similarly I will not give to a woman an abortive remedy. In purity and holiness I will guard my life and my art.

I will not use the knife, not even on sufferers from stone, but will withdraw in favor of such men as are engaged in this work.

Whatever houses I may visit, I will come for the benefit of the sick, remaining free of all intentional injustice, of all mischief and in particular of sexual relations with both female and male persons, be they free or slaves.

What I may see or hear in the course of treatment or even outside of the treatment in regard to the life of men, which on no account one must spread abroad, I will keep to myself holding such things shameful to be spoken about.

If I fulfill this oath and do not violate it, may it be granted to me to enjoy life and art, being honored with fame among all men for all time to come; if I transgress it and swear falsely, may the opposite of all this be my lot.

THE EMT CODE OF ETHICS

Professional status as an Emergency Medical Technician and Emergency Medical Technician–Paramedic is maintained and enriched by the willingness of the individual practitioner to accept and fulfill obligations to society, other medical professionals, and the profession of Emergency Medical Technician. As an Emergency Medical Technician at the basic level or an Emergency Medical Technician–Paramedic, I solemnly pledge myself to the following code of professional ethics:

A fundamental responsibility of the Emergency Medical Technician is to conserve life, to alleviate suffering, to promote health, to do no harm, and to encourage the quality and equal availability of emergency medical care.

The Emergency Medical Technician provides services based on human need, with respect for human dignity, unrestricted by consideration of nationality, race, creed, color, or status.

The Emergency Medical Technician does not use professional knowledge and skills in any enterprise detrimental to the public well-being.

The Emergency Medical Technician respects and holds in confidence all information of a confidential nature obtained in the course of professional work unless required by law to divulge such information.

The Emergency Medical Technician, as a citizen, understands and upholds the law and performs the duties of citizenship; as a professional, the Emergency Medical Technician has the never-ending responsibility to work with concerned citizens and other health care professionals in promoting a high standard of emergency medical care to all people.

The Emergency Medical Technician shall maintain professional competence and demonstrate concern for the competence of other members of the Emergency Medical Services health care team.

An Emergency Medical Technician assumes responsibility in defining and upholding standards of professional practice and education.

The Emergency Medical Technician assumes responsibility for individual professional actions and judgment, both in dependent and independent emergency functions, and knows and upholds the laws which affect the practice of the Emergency Medical Technician.

An Emergency Medical Technician has the responsibility to be aware of and participate in matters of legislation

THE EMT CODE OF ETHICS—cont'd

affecting the Emergency Medical Technician and the Emergency Medical Services System.

The Emergency Medical Technician adheres to standards of personal ethics which reflect credit upon the profession.

Emergency Medical Technicians, or groups of Emergency Medical Technicians, who advertise professional services, do so in conformity with the dignity of the profession.

The Emergency Medical Technician has an obligation to protect the public by not delegating to a person less

qualified any service which requires the professional competence of an Emergency Medical Technician.

The Medical Technician will work harmoniously with, and sustain confidence in, Emergency Medical Technician associates, the nurse, the physician, and other members of the emergency medical services health care team.

The Emergency Medical Technician refuses to participate in unethical procedures and assumes the responsibility to expose incompetence or unethical conduct of others to the appropriate authority in a proper and professional manner.

NURSES CODE OF ETHICS
AMERICAN NURSES ASSOCIATION CODE OF ETHICS

- The nurse provides services with respect for human dignity and the uniqueness of the client unrestricted by considerations of social or economic status, personal attributes, or the nature of health problems.
- The nurse safeguards the client's right to privacy by judiciously protecting information of a confidential nature.
- The nurse acts to safeguard the client and the public when health care and safety are affected by the incompetent, unethical, or illegal practice of any person.
- The nurse assumes responsibility and accountability for individual nursing judgments and actions.
- The nurse maintains competence in nursing.
- The nurse exercises informed judgment and uses individual competence and qualifications as criteria

in seeking consultation, accepting responsibilities, and delegating nursing activities to others.
- The nurse participates in activities that contribute to the ongoing development of the profession's body of knowledge.
- The nurse participates in the profession's efforts to implement and improve standards of nursing.
- The nurse participates in the profession's efforts to establish and maintain conditions of employment conducive to high-quality nursing care.
- The nurse participates in the profession's effort to protect the public from misinformation and misrepresentation and to maintain the integrity of nursing.
- The nurse collaborates with members of the health professions and other citizens in promoting community and national efforts to meet the health needs of the public.

From American Nurses Association: *Code for nurses with interpretive statements,* Kansas City, Mo, 1985, The Association.

AMERICAN MEDICAL ASSOCIATION'S PRINCIPLES OF MEDICAL ETHICS
(ALSO ADOPTED BY THE AMERICAN COLLEGE OF EMERGENCY PHYSICIANS)

Preamble: The medical profession has long subscribed to a body of ethical statements developed primarily for the benefit of the patient. As a member of this profession, a physician must recognize responsibility not only to patients, but also to society, to other health professionals, and to self. The following principles adopted by the American Medical Association are not laws, but standards of conduct which define the essentials of honorable behavior for the physician.
- A physician shall be dedicated to providing competent medical service with compassion and respect for human dignity.

- A physician shall deal honestly with patients and colleagues, and strive to expose those physicians deficient in character or competence, or who engage in fraud or deception.
- A physician shall respect the law and also recognize a responsibility to seek changes in those requirements which are contrary to the best interests of the patient.
- A physician shall respect the rights of patients, of colleagues, and of other health professionals, and shall safeguard patient confidences within the constraints of the law.

high-quality patient care; continuing education; skill proficiency; and licensure, certification, or both. The paramedic is accountable by law to that level of training and that standard of care. A paramedic who is accountable to the profession is more likely to provide good patient care and make decisions that are ethically acceptable.

✓ TRICKS OF THE TRADE

One way to measure professional accountability is to ask yourself "Would I want this paramedic taking care of my mother?"

Legal Accountability

Through patient care activities, the paramedic also assumes a distinct role in the health care legal system (see Chapter 4). Legal issues frequently are entwined with ethical issues; however, ethics is not synonymous with law. (Ethics deals with moral behavior; law deals with legal behavior.) Many ethical decisions occur outside the boundaries of the law, and many legal decisions may not be ethical. (An example is a patient who has a living will in a state in which the legality of advance directives has not been resolved.) The paramedic should consider the importance of legal accountability as it relates to medical ethics and abide by the law when ethical conflicts occur.

STATEMENTS FOR ETHICAL LIVING

Socrates: The unexamined life is not worth living. Know thyself. Morality is the necessity of the heart. The soul is that which is.

Plato: Justice is the harmony of all virtues. Truth belongs to the mind.

Aristotle: Sense reveals only individual existence. The universal is immanent in the individual. Man finds his ethic only in his natural self realization.

Zoroastrianism and Parsis: Good thoughts, good words, good deeds. The Reality is one, the wise by many men call it.

Buddhism: Let a man lift himself up by his own self; let him not depress himself; for he himself is his friend and he himself is his enemy.

Confucianism: Seek to be in harmony with all your neighbors.

Taoism: Being in one's inmost heart in kindly sympathy with all things.

Christianity: Love thy neighbor as thyself.

Judaism: Perform righteousness on earth that ye may find treasures in heaven.

Islam: Do what God likes, and avoid what He dislikes.

? CRITICAL THINKING

Which of these statements of ethical living best represents your personal philosophy?

Moral Accountability

Moral accountability refers to *personal* ethics (personal values and beliefs). Combining moral, legal, and professional accountability may be difficult in emergency settings, and at times the paramedic will have to draw on personal ethics to resolve conflicts among these roles and responsibilities and to decide on a course of action. When dealing with ethical questions, the paramedic should remember the following key points[4,5]:

1. Emotion may not be a reliable determinant for ethical decision making. Conscience should be monitored because it can be a reasonably good guide if one's conscience is well-informed concerning right or wrong. Rational decision making (decisions that rely on research and prudence regarding what is right) also is useful, but some knowledge deficit may permit the paramedic to come to a flawed decision.

2. Decisions must not be based solely on the opinions of others or global protocols that were designed to guide, not dictate, practice (e.g., codes of the profession). If paramedics encounter a situation that they have never confronted before, a poor, or even unethical, decision is likely to be made. In these circumstances, paramedics should consult with medical direction, a supervisor, or a set of guidelines or other resources rather than limit themselves to their own knowledge base or principles. Sometimes, input from patients and their loved ones can be a key source of information and can lead to a better decision.

3. Once the ethical question has been answered, the answer becomes a "rule" to guide behavior, at least in the particular setting. Once the rule has been identified, it should become a barrier to acting in opposition to the rule. Paramedics are expected not to break the rule without a strong explanation for their actions.

NOTE

With reference to answering ethical questions, no one knows all the answers, and none of the tools or techniques available to use is sufficient in every case to arrive at the "right" decision. Nonetheless, health care providers are accountable for personal and professional actions and decisions. Seeking counsel and guidance with such decisions is always prudent.

A Rapid Approach to Emergency Ethical Problems

A method of ethical case analysis has been designed as a way to rapidly approach emergency ethical problems.[6] The "rules of thumb" process involves the following steps:

1. Ask yourself if you have experienced a similar ethical problem in the past. If so, use that experience as a precedent for this problem and

"follow the rule." (These "rules" must be periodically evaluated.)

2. If you have not experienced a similar ethical problem in the past, buy time for deliberation and for consulting with co-workers and medical direction.

3. If there is no option to buy time for deliberation, use a set of three tests to help you make a decision[7] (Fig. 5-1):

   • Test 1: Impartiality Test–Would you accept the action if you were in the patient's place?
   • Test 2: Universalizability Test–Would you feel comfortable having this action performed in all relevantly similar circumstances?
   • Test 3: Interpersonal Justifiability Test–Are you able to provide good reasons to justify and defend your actions to others?

TRICKS OF THE TRADE

A final question you might ask yourself is "Will I be able to sleep tonight if I perform this action?"

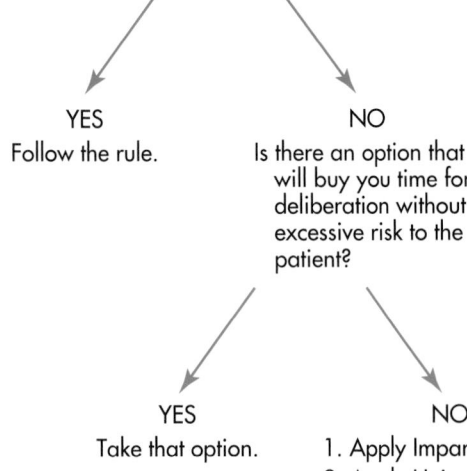

Is this a type of ethical problem for which you have already worked out a rule or is it at least similar enough so that the rule could reasonably be extended to cover it?

YES
Follow the rule.

NO
Is there an option that will buy you time for deliberation without excessive risk to the patient?

YES
Take that option.

NO
1. Apply Impartiality Test.
2. Apply Universalizability Test.
3. Apply Interpersonal Justifiability Test.

Fig. 5-1 A rapid approach to emergency ethical problems. (Modified from Iserson KV: An approach to ethical problems in emergency medicine. In Iserson KV et al: *Ethics in emergency medicine*, Baltimore, 1986, Williams & Wilkins.)

The first test is a good way to correct partiality or personal bias. The second test helps eliminate moral decision difficulty (shortsightedness). The final test requires that the paramedic has reasons for proceeding and that others would approve of the reasons. If all three tests can be answered in the affirmative, then the paramedic has a reasonable probability that the proposed action falls within the scope of being ethically acceptable.

Ethical Tests in Health Care

The fundamental question of ethical tests in health care is, "What is in the patient's best interest?" However, doing what is best, or what one thinks is best, is not sufficient to justify actions. Determining what the patient wants must first be defined by patient statements (if the patient is mentally competent), written statements, and family input (if the patient demonstrates altered mental status or incompetence). The role of "good faith" in making ethical decisions ("Am I doing my best to help and not harm my patient?") should be balanced with the wishes of the patient and the patient's family. The global concept of health care (providing patient benefit and avoiding harm) recognizes and respects the patient's autonomy, as well as the various legal issues that affect the delivery of health care (Box 5-1).

Resolving Ethical Dilemmas

Resolving ethical dilemmas when global concepts of health care are in conflict can be guided by the health

---

BOX 5-1

GLOBAL CONCEPTS OF ETHICAL HEALTH CARE

Therapeutic activity of the Greek doctor was subject to the following rules:

• To help the patient, or at least to do no harm
• To refrain from interfering if the illness were incurable and inevitably mortal
• Insofar as possible, to attack the cause of the disease therapeutically

Today, these global concepts of ethical health care can be stated as:

• Provide patient benefit
• Do no harm

care community and by the public. The health care community's role in resolving ethical conflicts is to establish standards of care, to provide research and treatment protocols, and to make prospective and retrospective reviews of decisions and policies with the intent of educating the paramedic and improving the quality of patient care. The public's role in managing ethical conflicts in medicine includes creating laws, setting public policy, allocating resources to protect patient rights, and participating in the use of advance directives and other self-determination documents to make patient wishes known.

Ethical Issues in Contemporary Paramedic Practice

Paramedics will face several ethical issues during the course of their careers. Most will deal with the patient's right to self-determination (autonomy) and the paramedic's obligation to provide patient care (beneficence) (Box 5-2). Some of the more common issues (and sample case studies) are described in this section. For each case study, the paramedic should apply the rapid approach to emergency medical problems (described earlier in this chapter) and answer the following ethical questions:

1. What is the patient's best interest?
2. What are the patient's rights?
3. Does the patient understand the issues at hand?
4. What is the paramedic's professional, legal, and moral accountability?

> **NOTE**
>
> Even though there may be disagreement about a specific set of values, there often is general agreement over what may constitute ethically wrong actions.

Allocation of Resources

Fairness in the allocation of resources and obligations is a commonly accepted bioethical value that is incorporated into society-wide health care policies. This perceived "right" to universal access to an adequate level of health care is a complex economic issue that is affected by the need to contain health care costs. Factors that affect true parity in the allocation of resources include a person's access to health insurance (which may define what medical services are covered or excluded) and treatment decisions that are made when resources are inadequate to meet patient care needs (e.g., during a multiple-casualty disaster). When rationing of care is required, it should be based on ethically oriented criteria.[8]

The allocation of resources is more of a policy rather than a clinical concept. It can, however, pose ethical dilemmas in prehospital care, as illustrated in the following case study:

Case Study 1

A paramedic crew has been dispatched to the home of a 74-year-old man complaining of chest pain and shortness of breath. The patient is in obvious

---

BOX 5-2

COMMONLY ACCEPTED BIOETHICAL VALUES

Autonomy: Self-determination; a person's ability to make moral decisions, including those affecting personal medical care. The three components of autonomy are agency (awareness of onself as having desires and intentions and acting on them); independence (absence of influences that so control what a person does that it cannot be said he or she wants to do it); and rationality (rational decision making).

Beneficence: A duty to confer benefits. The practice of good deeds. Obligation to benefit others or seek their good.

Confidentiality: The presumption that confidential information will not be revealed to others without the patient's permission. Confidentiality, like privacy, is valued because it protects individual preferences and rights.

Allocation of resources: The consistent access to quality medical services. Distributing health-related services among various people and uses.

Nonmaleficence: The prevention of harm; from Hippocratic tradition that established *primum non nocere* ("Above all, do no harm"). A prohibition on actions with foreseeable harmful effects.

Personal integrity: Adhering to a personal set of values and moral standards.

distress and provides a significant cardiac history. He requests to be transported to the Veteran's Hospital (30 miles away) where he had heart surgery several years ago. Based on the patient's history, physical exam, and ECG findings, the paramedic crew (in consultation with medical direction) elects to transport the patient to the closer, medical direction hospital to be stabilized. The patient becomes very anxious and complains of increasing chest pain. He advises the paramedic crew that he has no medical insurance and demands to be transported to the VA hospital.

Decisions Surrounding Resuscitation

Advance directives, living wills, and other self-determination documents can help the paramedic make decisions about the appropriateness of resuscitation in the prehospital setting. The presence of appropriate documents and knowledgeable family members often will make resuscitation decisions much easier. In other cases, however, the decision to initiate or withhold resuscitation measures will not be so clear, as illustrated in the following case study:

Case Study 2

The paramedic crew has been dispatched to a restaurant where an elderly woman has collapsed. She has suffered cardiac arrest, and a waiter is performing CPR. The ECG monitor reveals ventricular fibrillation. Defibrillatory shocks are delivered, but the rhythm remains unchanged. As resuscitation measures are continued, the woman's husband says to the paramedics "She said she didn't want this; her living will is at home. Please stop what you're doing and let her go."

Confidentiality

Most people are considered to have a fundamental right to privacy as control over personal information. The principle of confidentiality states that private and personal information will not ordinarily be disclosed by a health care professional to other persons without the patient's consent. In some cases, the release of confidential information is required by law (e.g., the disclosure of positive HIV status to others involved in the patient's care). Conflict between ethics and confidentiality

may arise, however, particularly if the public health would benefit from the disclosure of confidential information, as described in the following case study:

> **? CRITICAL THINKING**
>
> *Your partner contacts a former patient to ask for a date using the phone number from the patient care report. Do you think that action violates any ethical principles? If so, which ones?*

Case Study 3

The paramedic crew has been dispatched to a motor vehicle crash in which a young man has struck another car head on, killing the driver of the other vehicle. The patient is shaken but has only minor injuries. While preparing the patient for transport, he confides to the paramedic that he had used cocaine shortly before the crash occurred, but asks the paramedic to keep the information confidential and not tell the law enforcement officers at the scene.

Consent

As described in Chapter 4, competent patients have a legal right to decide what medical care they will receive. This right to make decisions regarding health care is a fundamental element of the patient-physician relationship, as described in the *AMA's Principles of Medical Ethics*. It also can be inferred from the *EMT Code of Ethics*. Cases in which patients refuse lifesaving care can produce legal and ethical conflicts, as illustrated in the following case study:

Case Study 4

The paramedic crew has been dispatched to an office building where a 55-year-old woman collapsed at a business meeting. She is alert and oriented, complains of chest pain, and is pale and diaphoretic. The paramedics advise the patient of the possibility of a heart attack and the need for immediate care and transport for physician evaluation. She insists on waiting until after the meeting has concluded to seek medical care on her own, and she asks the EMS crew to leave.

Other Ethical Principles for Patient Care Situations

Other ethical principles for patient care situations relate to care in futile situations, legal obligations to provide care, patient advocacy and paramedic accountability, and the paramedic's role as a physician extender.

Care in Futile Situations

An action is considered *futile* if it serves no purpose or is completely ineffective. When emergency care is being provided in situations that may be futile, the paramedic should consult with medical direction to determine a course of action. Examples of futile situations in health care include continuing resuscitation initiated by bystanders when the patient has obviously expired and providing life support measures for a patient who has fatal injuries. The definition of futility may pose an ethical dilemma when there is disagreement or lack of agreement about the goals of treatment.

? CRITICAL THINKING

You arrive at a home where you find a 3-month-old baby who has obviously been dead for several hours. The mother is screaming, "Help her, help her." Your partner decides to proceed with ALS care even though it is clearly futile. Is this decision ethical?

NOTE

Not all futility judgments are controversial. For example, it generally is recommended that CPR is futile and should not be attempted on patients with obvious signs of death (e.g., decapitation, rigor mortis, tissue decompensation, or extreme dependent lividity).[8]

Obligation to Provide Care

In the prehospital setting, the paramedic's obligation to provide care seldom is an issue. (The patient's request for emergency service presents a legal duty to act.) In other areas of the health care arena, however, an obligation to provide care (other than emergency care) may be affected by the patient's ability to pay for service, the patient's health insurance, and other economic factors. Legislation is in place to protect well-meaning caregivers from liability (e.g., Good Samaritan legislation), and to protect patients from unethical health care practices, such as "economic triage" and "patient dumping" (see Chapter 4).

Patient Advocacy and Paramedic Accountability

While providing care, the paramedic will serve as the patient's advocate. This advocacy may at times conflict with the paramedic's accountability to the patient, the physician medical director, and the health care system (e.g., health maintenance organization protocols). In these situations, the paramedic should discus all options with medical direction. *As a rule, it is prudent and ethical to err on the side of providing the needs of the patient when conflict arises.* Examples of ways in which a paramedic can serve as the patient's advocate include:

- Educating patients on the delivery of health care and the role that they can play to effect change in the nation's health care system
- Ensuring that health care decisions are made by patients and their doctors and are based on the medical needs of patients, not financial considerations
- Informing patients of federal, state, and private sector health care reform initiatives
- Promoting patient access to reliable information about state-of-the-art medical technologies and treatments
- Promoting fairness and equality in America's health care system

Role as Physician Extender

As a physician extender, the paramedic generally is responsible for following orders of the medical director or his or her designee. There may, however, be occasions when orders received from medical direction seem inappropriate. An example is a medication order that the paramedic believes:

- Is contraindicated for the patient
- Is medically acceptable, but not in the patient's best interest
- Is medically acceptable, but morally wrong

The converse also occurs. For example, a paramedic might request treatment for a situation in which the field impression is unsure or the physician is lacking information to approve the request. In these or similar situations where there is conflict between medical direction and the paramedic, communication is the key to resolving short-term and long-term concerns.

✓ TRICKS OF THE TRADE

You are the "eyes and ears" of the physician. The physician's understanding of the patient's condition and the emergency scene will only be as good as the information you provide.

? CRITICAL THINKING

Your patient is critical and you cannot secure the airway. Medical direction tells you to divert because they have no ICU beds. You repeat the urgency of your patient's condition and are still told to divert. You elect to override the physician's order and transport to that hospital. Can you justify disobeying the physician's order?

SUMMARY

- Ethics is the discipline relating to right and wrong, moral duty and obligation, moral principles and values, and moral character. Bioethics is the science of medical ethics. Morals refers to social standard or customs.

- As a professional, the paramedic must conform to a standard established by his or her level of training and regional practice. Paramedics must abide by the law when ethical conflicts occur.

- A paramedic's actions must be morally acceptable.

- The rapid approach to emergency ethical problems is a step-by-step process that involves reviewing past experiences; deliberation (if possible); and performing the impartiality test, universalizability test, and interpersonal justifiability test to reach an acceptable decision.

- Two concepts of ethical health care are to provide patient benefit and do no harm.

- Fairness in the allocation of resources is a commonly accepted bioethical value.

- Advance directives, living wills, and other self-determination documents can help the paramedic make decisions about the appropriateness of resuscitation in the prehospital setting.

- The principle of confidentiality states that a health care professional may not reveal information provided by the patient to others without the patient's consent.

- Cases in which patients refuse lifesaving care can produce legal and ethical conflicts.

- Other areas that are likely to raise ethical questions in the prehospital setting include providing care in futile situations, the paramedic's obligation to provide care, patient advocacy, and the paramedic's role as physician extender.

REFERENCES

1. Sanderson B: *Ethics of civilization: ancient wisdom and folly,* http://www.west.net/~beck/EC1-Ethics.html, 1996.
2. American Medical Association, Council on Ethical and Judicial Affairs: *Code of medical ethics: current opinions with annotations,* Chicago, Ill., 1997, The Association.
3. Veatch R: *Medical ethics,* ed 2, Sudbury, Mass, 1997, Jones and Bartlett.
4. U.S. Department of Transportation National Highway Traffic Safety Administration: *EMT-Paramedic national standard curriculum,* 1998, Washington, DC, The Department.
5. Bourn S: Through traffic keep right, *JEMS* 21(5):26, 1996.
6. Rosen P, Barkin R: *Emergency medicine: concepts and clinical practice,* ed 4, St Louis, 1998, Mosby.
7. Iserson K et al: *Ethics in emergency medicine,* ed 2, Tucson, Ariz., 1995, Galen Press.
8. American Heart Association: *Advanced cardiac life support,* 1997, Dallas, Tex, The Association.

6 Overview of Human Systems

OBJECTIVES

Upon completion of this chapter, the paramedic student will be able to:

1. Discuss the importance of human anatomy as it relates to the paramedic profession.

2. Describe the anatomical position.

3. Properly interpret anatomical directional terms and body planes.

4. List the structures that compose the axial and appendicular regions of the body.

5. Define the divisions of the abdominal region.

6. List the three major body cavities.

7. Describe the contents of the three major body cavities.

8. Discuss the functions of the following cellular structures: the cytoplasmic membrane, the cytoplasm (and organelles), and the nucleus.

9. Describe the process by which human cells reproduce.

10. Differentiate and describe the following tissue types: epithelial tissue, connective tissue, muscle tissue, and nervous tissue.

11. For each of the 11 major organ systems in the human body, label a diagram of anatomical structures; list the functions of the major anatomical structures; and explain how the organs of the system interrelate to perform the specified functions of the system.

12. For the special senses, label a diagram of the anatomical structures of the special senses, list the functions of the anatomical structures of each sense, and explain how the structures of the senses interrelate to perform their specialized functions.

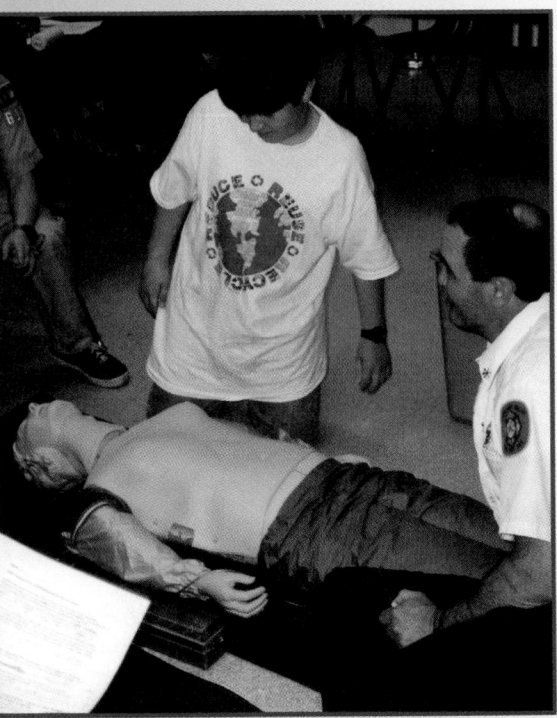

Human anatomy is the study of how the human body is structurally organized. The paramedic must thoroughly understand human anatomy to organize a patient assessment by body region and to communicate effectively with medical direction and other members of the health care team.

KEY TERMS

anatomical position: A position standing erect with the feet and palms facing the examiner.

anterior: The front, or ventral, surface.

capillaries: Tiny vessels that connect arterioles to venules.

central nervous system: The brain and spinal cord.

homeostasis: A state of equilibrium in the body with respect to functions and composition of fluids and tissues.

inferior: Toward the feet; below a point of reference in the anatomical position.

integumentary system: The largest organ system in the body, consisting of the skin and accessory structures.

limbic system: The part of the brain involved with emotions and olfaction.

lymphatic system: The network of vessels, ducts, nodes, valves, and organs involved in protecting and maintaining the body's internal fluid environment.

organ: A structure made up of two or more kinds of tissues, organized to perform a more complex function than any one tissue alone.

parasympathetic nervous system: The subdivision of the autonomic nervous system usually involved in activating vegetative functions such as digestion, defecation, and urination.

peripheral nervous system: A subdivision of the nervous system consisting of nerves and ganglia.

plasma membrane: The outer covering of a cell that contains the cellular cytoplasm; also known as the *cell membrane.*

prone: The position in which the patient is lying on the stomach (face down).

reticular activating system: A functional system in the brain essential for wakefulness, attention, concentration, and introspection.

somatic nervous system: The part of the nervous system composed of nerve fibers that send impulses from the central nervous system to skeletal muscle.

superior: Situated above or higher than a point of reference in the anatomical position.

supine: The position in which the patient is lying on the back (face up).

system: Interconnected functions or organs in which a stimulus or an action in one area affects all other areas.

Terminology

Directional terms used by the medical profession refer to the human body in the **anatomical position,** which is a person standing erect with the feet and palms facing the examiner. A patient in the **supine** position is lying on the back (face up). A patient in the **prone** position is lying on the stomach (face down). A patient in the lateral recumbent position is lying on the right or left side. Regardless of the patient's actual position, the paramedic should always communicate patient information with reference to the anatomical position (Fig. 6-1).

Directional terms, such as *up* or *down, front* or *back,* and *right* or *left,* also are communicated in anatomical terminology and always refer to the patient, not the examiner (e.g., the patient's left arm). (Important directional terms are listed in Table 6-1.)

Anatomical Planes

Internal body structure relationships are classified into anatomical planes, or imaginary straight-line divisions of the human body (Fig. 6-2). The sagittal plane runs vertically through the middle of the body, producing right and left sections. A plane that is to one side of the midline is said to be parasagittal. The transverse, or horizontal, plane divides the body into top and bottom, or **superior** and **inferior,** sections. The frontal, or coronal, plane divides the body into front and back, or **anterior** and posterior, positions.

Body Regions

The human body is divided into several regions for the purpose of organizing anatomical structures. The appendicular region includes the limbs, or extremities. The axial region consists of the head, neck, thorax, and abdomen. The abdomen usually

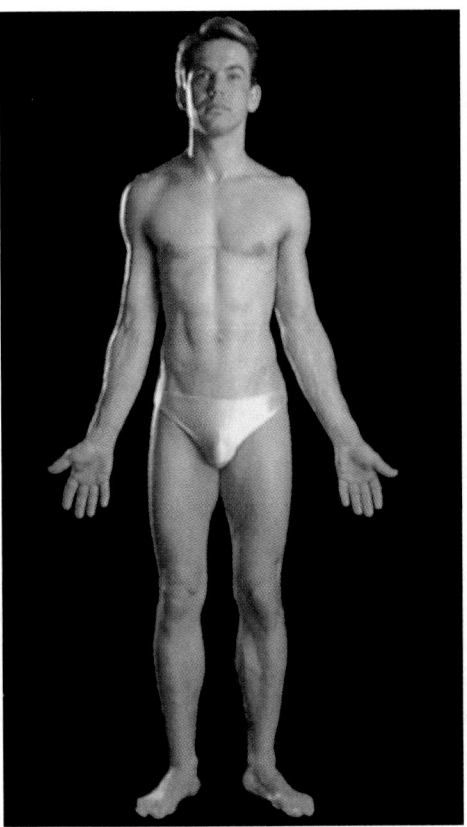

Fig. 6-1 Anatomical position. A human in the anatomical position is standing with the feet and palms of the hands facing forward with the thumbs to the outside.

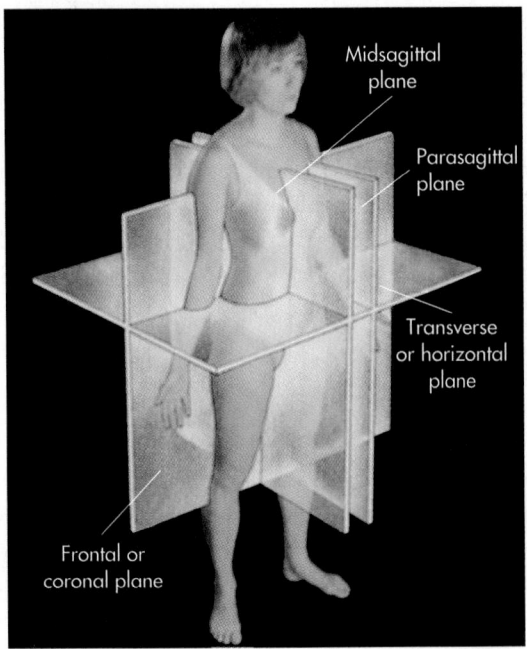

Fig. 6-2 Body planes.

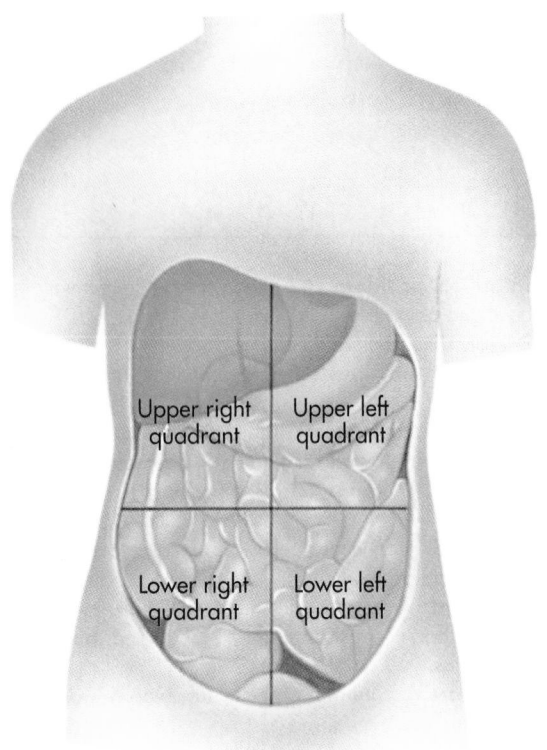

Fig. 6-3 Abdominal quadrants.

is divided into four quadrants: the upper right, lower right, upper left, and lower left. The dividing lines consist of two imaginary divisions that run horizontally through the umbilicus and vertically from the xiphoid process through the symphysis pubis (Fig. 6-3).

Body Cavities

The three major cavities of the human body are the thoracic cavity, abdominal cavity, and pelvic cavity. The thoracic cavity is divided into two portions by a midline structure known as the mediastinum. The mediastinum includes the trachea, esophagus, thymus, heart, and great vessels. The lungs are located on either side of this midline structure. The thoracic cavity is surrounded by the rib cage and separated from the abdominal cavity by the diaphragm. The thorax contains two pleural cavities (which contain the lungs) and a pericardial cavity (which contains the heart). These cavities are lined with a serous

TABLE 6-1 — DIRECTIONAL TERMS

TERM	DEFINITION	TERM	DEFINITION
Left	Toward the left side	Distal	Farther than another structure from the point of attachment to the trunk
Right	Toward the right side	Medial	Toward the midline of the body
Superior	Situated above another structure (usually synonymous with "cephalic")	Lateral	Away from the midline of the body
Inferior	Situated below another structure (usually synonymous with "caudal")	Anterior	The front of the body (synonymous with "ventral")
Cephalic	Toward the head of the body	Posterior	The back of the body (synonymous with "dorsal")
Caudal	Toward the distal end of the spine	Ventral	Pertaining to the front
Proximal	Closer than another structure to the point of attachment to the trunk	Dorsal	Pertaining to the back

membrane. The serous membrane that comes in contact with the organ is visceral, and the serous membrane that comes in contact with the cavity wall is parietal. A thin, lubricating film of fluid is produced by these membranes and reduces the friction that occurs during movement of organs against other organs or body cavities.

An imaginary plane separates the abdominal cavity from the pelvic cavity. The division is drawn between the symphysis pubis and the sacral promontory (the projecting portion of the pelvis at the base of the sacrum). The abdominal and pelvic cavities are lined with a thin sheet of membranous tissue that secretes serous fluid. The serous membrane that

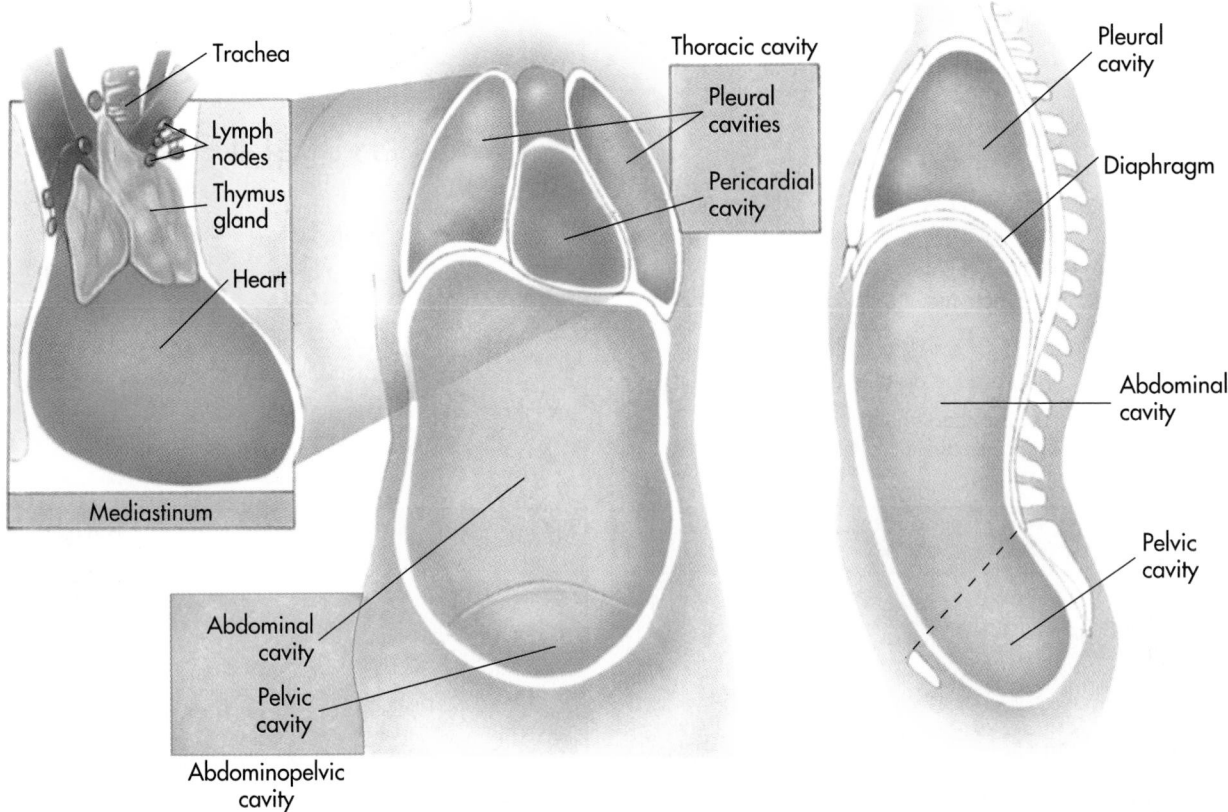

Fig. 6-4 Body cavities. The thoracic cavity includes the two pleural cavities and the pericardial cavity. Some of the contents of the mediastinum are shown on the left. The abdominopelvic cavity contains the abdominal cavity and the pelvic cavity.

covers the abdominal organs is known as visceral peritoneum. The serous membrane that covers the body cavity wall is known as the parietal peritoneum. Peritoneal organs are held in place by connective tissue called mesentery. The mesentery anchors some of the abdominal organs to the body wall and provides a pathway for nerves and vessels to reach the organs. Abdominopelvic organs that do not have mesentery or peritoneum are said to be retroperitoneal (behind the peritoneum); they include the kidneys, adrenal glands, pancreas, portions of the colon, and the urinary bladder. The pelvic cavity is enclosed by the bones of the pelvis. The abdominal and pelvic cavities are often referred to collectively as the peritoneal or abdominopelvic cavity (Fig. 6-4).

Cell Structure

Cells are the most basic unit of life. They are highly organized units that are composed of protoplasm,

or living matter. The three main parts of all human cells are the cytoplasmic membrane (**plasma membrane**), cytoplasm, and nucleus.

Cytoplasmic Membrane

The cytoplasmic membrane encloses the cytoplasm, forming the outer boundary of the cell. It is believed to have two layers of phosphate-containing fat molecules known as phospholipids that form a fluid framework for the cytoplasmic membrane (Fig. 6-5). Substances outside this membrane are considered extracellular (outside of cells) or intercellular (between cells), and substances inside this membrane are intracellular. The functions of the cytoplasmic mem-

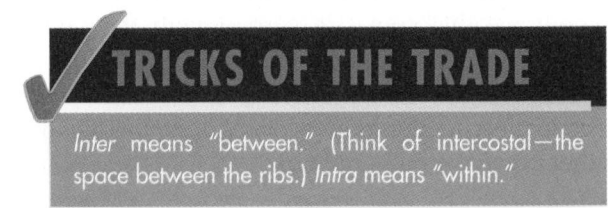

TRICKS OF THE TRADE

Inter means "between." (Think of intercostal—the space between the ribs.) *Intra* means "within."

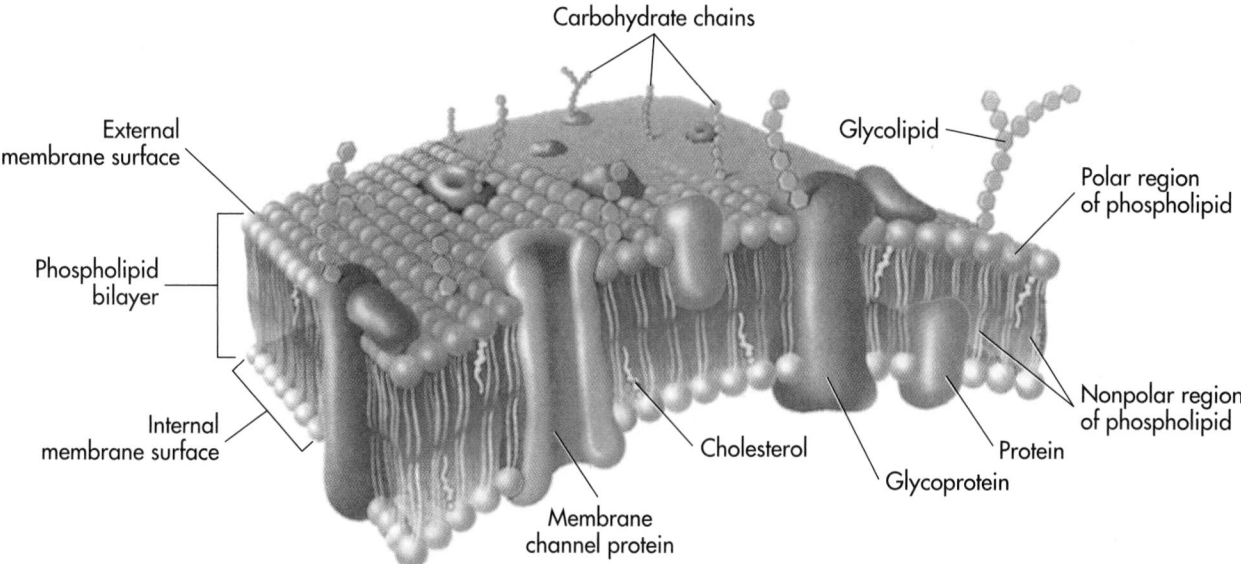

Fig. 6-5 Fluid mosaic model of the plasma membrane.

brane are to enclose and support the cell contents and regulate what moves into and out of the cell.

The central layer of the cytoplasmic membrane is a lipid bilayer composed of a double layer of lipid molecules. The lipid bilayer has a liquid quality, and protein molecules "float" on both the inner and the outer surfaces. Some of these proteins have carbohydrate molecules bound to them and are thought to function as membrane channels, carrier molecules, receptor molecules, enzymes, or structural supports in the membrane (see Chapter 7).

Cytoplasm

The cytoplasm lies between the cytoplasmic membrane and the nucleus. The nucleus can be viewed as a round or spherical structure in the center of the cell. Specialized structures in the cell, known as organelles, are located in the cytoplasm and perform functions important to the cell's survival (Table 6-2 and Fig. 6-6).

The endoplasmic reticulum is a network of connecting sacs or canals that winds through a cell's cytoplasm, serving as a miniature circulatory system for the cell. The tubular passageways or canals in the endoplasmic reticulum carry proteins and other substances through the cytoplasm of the cell from one area to another. The two types of endoplasmic reticulum are smooth and rough. Smooth endoplasmic reticulum is found in cells that handle or manufacture fatty substances; it also participates in

detoxification processes through the chemical action of enzymes. Rough endoplasmic reticulum is found in cells that manufacture proteins to be secreted for use outside the cell.

Ribosomes are the "factories" in the cells where protein is synthesized. Ribosomes are macromolecules of protein composed of thousands of atoms. They usually are bound to the endoplasmic reticulum but also are found free in cytoplasm. Ribosomes form complexes with strands of ribonucleic acid (RNA), which through the genetic code provide the blueprint for the new protein. Individual amino acids are attached in long chains with peptide bonds to form the new proteins.

The Golgi apparatus concentrates and packages materials for secretion from the cell. It consists of tiny sacs composed of smooth endoplasmic reticulum that are stacked one on the other near the nucleus. The Golgi apparatus concentrates and in some cases chemically modifies the proteins by synthesizing and attaching carbohydrate molecules to the proteins to form glycoproteins or attaching lipids to the proteins to form lipoproteins. These concentrated globules move slowly outward to and

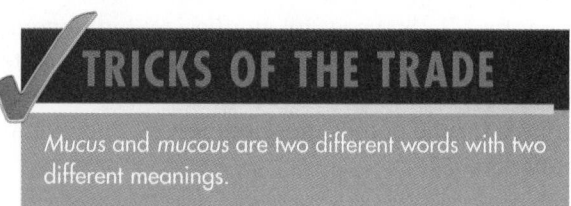

TRICKS OF THE TRADE

Mucus and *mucous* are two different words with two different meanings.

TABLE 6-2	SOME MAJOR CELL STRUCTURES AND THEIR FUNCTIONS

CELL STRUCTURE	FUNCTION
Plasma membrane	Serves as the boundary of the cell; protein and carbohydrate molecules on the outer surface of plasma membrane perform various functions; for example, they serve as markers that identify cells of each individual or as receptor molecules for certain hormones
Endoplasmic reticulum	Ribosomes attached to rough endoplasmic reticulum synthesize proteins; smooth endoplasmic reticulum synthesizes lipids and certain carbohydrates
Ribosomes	Synthesize proteins; a cell's "protein factories"
Mitochondria	Synthesize adenosine triphosphate; a cell's "powerhouses"
Lysosomes	A cell's "digestive system"
Golgi apparatus	Synthesizes carbohydrate, combines it with protein, and packages the product as globules of glycoprotein
Centrioles	Function in cell reproduction
Cilia	Short, hairlike extensions on the free surfaces of some cells capable of movement
Flagella	Single and much larger projections of cell surfaces than cilia; the only example in humans is the "tail" of a sperm cell
Nucleus	Dictates protein synthesis, thereby playing an essential role in other cell activities, namely active transport, metabolism, growth, and heredity
Nucleoli	Play an essential role in the formation of ribosomes

through the cell membrane, at which point they break open and spill their contents. An example of a Golgi apparatus product is mucus.

Lysosomes are membranous-walled organelles that contain enzymes enabling them to function as intracellular digestive systems. These enzymes include those that digest nucleic acids, proteins, polysaccharides, and lipids. Certain white blood cells (leukocytes) have large numbers of lysosomes that contain enzymes to digest phagocytotic bacteria. If tissues are damaged, these powerful enzymes may escape from ruptured lysosome sacs into the cytoplasm, digesting both damaged and healthy cells. Lysosomes also digest organelles of the cell that are no longer functional (autophagia).

The mitochondria ("power plants of the cell") are found throughout the cell and are the site of aerobic oxidation. It is here that energy, derived from the efficient metabolism of nutrients and oxygen via the Krebs' cycle (further described in Chapter 7), is used to synthesize high-energy triphosphate bonds (e.g., adenosine triphosphate, or ATP). These triphosphate bonds are the energy source for the body's muscles, nerves, and overall function.

? CRITICAL THINKING

Your patient has bad lung disease and poor oxygenation. What effect will this have on cellular energy production?

Centrioles are paired, rod-shaped organelles that lie at right angles to each other in a specialized zone of cytoplasm known as the centrosome. Each centriole is composed of microtubules that play an important role in the process of cell division. At some point in their existence, all human cells contain a nucleus in which the genetic material of the cell is located. The nucleus is a large, membrane-bound organelle that ultimately controls all other organelles in the cytoplasm. It may be spherical, elongated, or lobed, depending on the type of cell in which it is found. The nucleus usually is located near the center of the cell, but some cells, such as red blood cells (RBCs), or erythrocytes, lose their nucleus as they develop. Other cells, such as certain bone cells, have more than one nucleus.

Nucleus

The nucleus is a relatively large structure that is not always located near the center of the cell. The cell

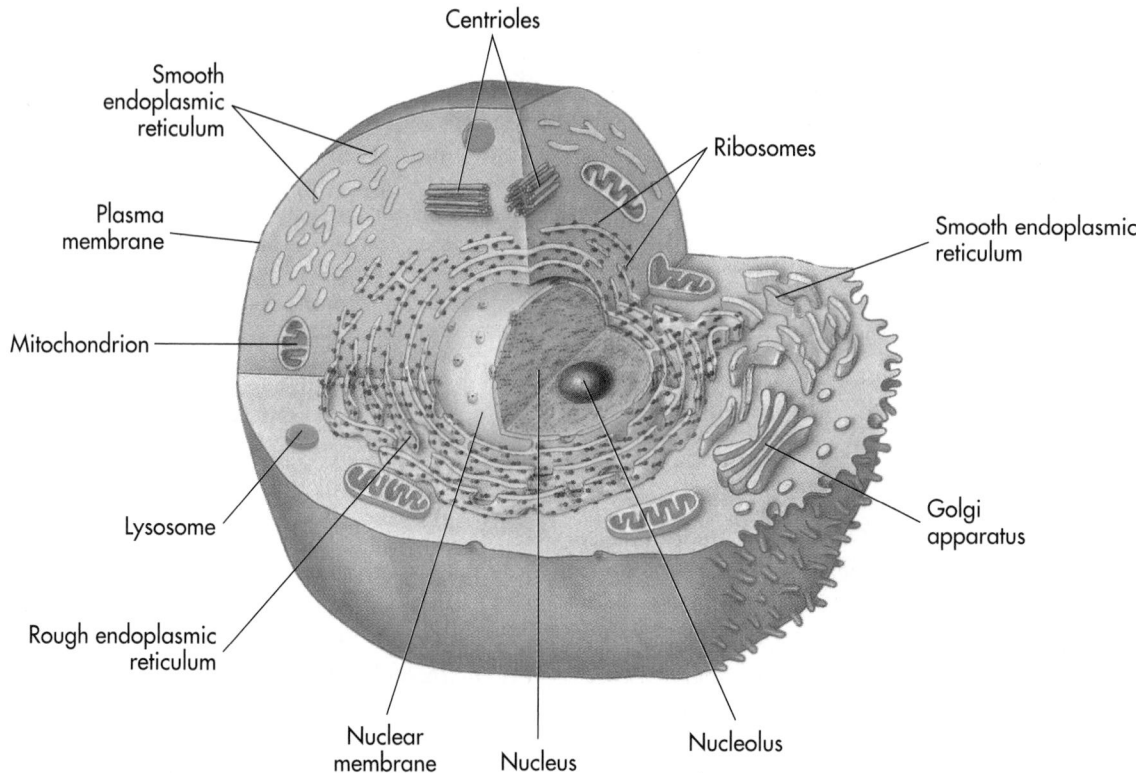

Fig. 6-6 Artist's interpretation of cell structure. (From Thibodeau GA: *Structure and function of the body,* ed 9, St Louis, 1992, Mosby.)

nucleus is surrounded by a nuclear membrane, which encloses a special type of protoplasm known as nucleoplasm. The nucleoplasm contains a number of specialized structures, two of which are the nucleolus and the chromatin granules. The nucleolus consists of deoxyribonucleic acid (DNA), which "programs" the formation of RNA, and protein, which makes ribosomes. These ribosomes then migrate through the nuclear membrane into the cytoplasm of the cell and produce proteins. Chromatin granules are threadlike structures made up of proteins and DNA. During cell division, the chromatin condenses to form the 23 pairs of chromosomes characteristic of human cells. The information contained within nuclear DNA determines most of the chemical events that occur within the cell. The primary functions of the nucleus are cell division and control of genetic information.

Major Classes of Cells

Free-living cells of multicellular "social" organisms are subdivided into two major classes by the way genetic material is organized inside them. The two main types are eukaryotes ("true nucleus") and prokaryotes ("before nucleus").

Eukaryotes are larger than prokaryotes and have more extensive intracellular anatomy. They have a separate membrane-bound nucleus that contains the genetic material (chromosomes, DNA, and so on). The fluid filling of the eukaryotes is divided into the nucleoplasm, situated inside the nuclear membrane, and the cytoplasm, placed outside the nuclear membrane. Nearly all human body cells are eukaryotes, as are those of all living organisms except for bacteria, cyanobacteria (blue-green algae), and mycoplasms, which are prokaryotes.

> **NOTE**
>
> Bacteria and mycoplasms cause a number of diseases in humans and other animals. Viruses have an intimate association with cells but are not classified as cells.

In the simpler prokaryote cells, the genetic material and enzymes required for energy production, cell growth, and cell division are contained in the jellylike cytoplasm, which is surrounded by the plasma membrane. Unlike eukaryotes, these cells have a simple internal organization and no nucleus that is bound by a plasma membrane. Their DNA is attached to the plasma membrane.

> **NOTE**
>
> The most significant categorizing feature of cells is the presence or absence of a nucleus.

Chief Cellular Functions

Cells have evolved in myriad ways to fulfill specific tasks in the human body. Through differentiation (maturation), cells become "specialized" in one type of function or act in concert with other cells to perform a more complex task. For example, RBCs only carry out one function (transporting respiratory gases around the body), and the cells in the pancreas synthesize and secrete large quantities of the digestive enzymes required to break down foods. The seven chief cellular functions are as follows[1]:

1. Movement (muscle cells)
2. Conductivity (nerve cells)
3. Metabolic absorption (kidney and intestinal cells)
4. Secretion (mucous gland cells)
5. Excretion (all cells)
6. Respiration (all cells)
7. Reproduction (most cells)

> **NOTE**
>
> Not all cells are capable of continuous division, and some cells (e.g., nerve cells) cannot reproduce.

> **NOTE**
>
> An estimated 200 different specialized types of cells exist in the human body.

Cell Reproduction

All human cells, with the exception of reproductive (sex) cells, reproduce by a process known as mitosis. In this process, cells divide to multiply—one cell divides to form two cells. Many cell types in the body (e.g., epithelial, liver, bone marrow cells) undergo cell division throughout an individual's life. Other cell types (e.g., nerve, skeletal muscle cells) divide until near the time of birth.

Tissues

Characteristics of cell structure and composition are used to classify tissue types. The four main types of tissue that make up the body's many organs are epithelial, connective, muscle, and nervous tissue.

Epithelial Tissue

Epithelial tissue covers surfaces or forms structures (e.g., glands) derived from body surfaces. This tissue consists almost entirely of cells that have little or no intercellular material between them, and they form continuous sheets that contain no blood vessels. Epithelium covers the outside of the body and lines the digestive tract, the vessels, and many body cavities.

Epithelial tissues can be subdivided according to the shape and arrangement of the cells found in each type. If classified according to shape, epithelial cells are squamous (flat and scalelike), cuboidal (cube-shaped), or columnar (more tall than wide). If classified according to arrangement, epithelial cells are simple (a single layer of cells of the same shape), stratified (multiple layers of cells of the same shape), or transitional (several layers of cells of differing shapes).

> **?   CRITICAL THINKING**
>
> *Think about the role of each of the tissue types. Compare that with the types of materials used in the construction of a building. Imagine each tissue type as a component of building a body.*

Connective Tissue

Connective tissue is the most abundant and widely distributed type of tissue in the body. It consists of cells separated from each other by intercellular material known as the extracellular matrix. This nonliving matrix gives most connective tissue its fundamental characteristics and is the basis for separating connective tissue into the following seven subgroups:

1. Areolar connective tissue is a loose tissue that consists of delicate webs of fibers and a variety of cells embedded in a matrix of soft, sticky gel. It is the "loose packing" material of most organs and other tissues and attaches the skin to the underlying tissues. The areolar connective tissue contains three major types of protein fibers: *collagen, reticulum,* and *elastin.*

2. Adipose, or fat, tissue is a specialized connective tissue that stores lipids. Lipids take up less space per calorie than either carbohydrates or proteins. Therefore adipose tissue not only functions as an insulator and protector but also is a site of energy storage.

3. Fibrous connective tissue consists mainly of bundles of strong, white collagenous fibers arranged in parallel rows. Tendons are composed of this type of connective tissue, which is characterized by strength and inelasticity.

4. Cartilage is composed of cartilage cells (chondrocytes) that are located in tiny spaces and distributed throughout a relatively rigid matrix. The composition of cartilage varies somewhat by its anatomical location and ultimate function. For example, hyaline cartilage, which is present at articulating surfaces, is firm and smooth, whereas fibrocartilage is more flexible and supple. Cartilage constitutes part of the human skeleton and covers the articulating surfaces of bones. In addition, cartilage forms the major skeletal tissue of the embryo before it is replaced by bony tissue.

   The type of cartilage depends on the relative amounts of collagen, elastin, and ground substance, which is composed of nonfibrous protein and other organic molecules and fluid. Increased amounts of collagen or elastin function to allow cartilage to spring back after being compressed. Blood vessels do not penetrate the substance of cartilage, so cartilage heals slowly after injury.

5. Bone is a highly specialized form of hard, connective tissue that consists of living cells and mineralized matrix. The strength and rigidity of this matrix allow bone to support and protect other tissues and organs.

Bones are classified according to their shape. Long bones are longer than they are wide. Examples of long bones are the humerus, ulna, radius, femur, tibia, fibula, and phalanges. Short bones are about as broad as they are long. Examples of short bones are the carpal bones of the wrist and the tarsal bones of the ankle. Flat bones have a thin, flattened shape. Examples of flat bones are certain skull bones, ribs, sternum, and scapulae. Irregular bones are those that do not fit the other three categories. Examples of irregular bones include vertebrae and facial bones.

Each growing long bone consists of a diaphysis (shaft), an epiphysis at the end of each bone, and an epiphyseal or growth plate. The epiphyseal plate is the site of bone elongation. When bone growth stops, the epiphyseal plate becomes ossified and is called the *epiphyseal line.* Injury to this area can impair bone growth if not recognized and treated properly (see Chapter 26).

? CRITICAL THINKING

Intraosseous infusion is a critical lifesaving intervention for children that involves the insertion of a needle into the bone of the leg to give fluids and drugs. Why could the failure to correctly identify anatomical landmarks or placement of the needle in the epiphysis be harmful?

Bones contain large cavities, such as the medullary cavity in the diaphysis, and smaller cavities, such as in the epiphyses of long bones and throughout the interior of other bones. These spaces are filled with yellow marrow (mainly adipose tissue) or red marrow (the site of blood formation). Blood supply to most bones is excellent, so some bones, such as the tibia and sternum, are suitable choices for venous access via intraosseous infusion (described in Chapter 9).

Bones can be further classified as cancellous or spongy bone and compact bone. Cancellous bone has spaces between the plates of the bone and resembles a sponge. Compact bone is essentially solid. Unlike cartilage, bone has a rich blood supply and can repair itself much more readily than cartilage.

6. Blood is a unique connective tissue because the matrix between the cells is liquid. The liquid matrix of blood allows it to flow rapidly through the body, carrying nutrients, oxygen, waste products, and other materials.

7. Hemopoietic tissue is the connective tissue found in the marrow cavities of bones and in such organs as the spleen, tonsils, and lymph nodes. This connective tissue is responsible for the formation of blood cells and **lymphatic system** cells that are important in the body's defense against disease.

Muscle Tissue

Muscle tissue is a contractile tissue responsible for movement. It is highly specialized to contract or shorten forcefully. Muscle tissue is responsible for all mechanical processes providing motion for the body. Muscle tissue is classified as skeletal, cardiac, and smooth or visceral muscle, according to both anatomical location and function. When classified according to its appearance, muscle is either striated or nonstriated. When classified according to its function, muscle is either voluntary (consciously controlled) or involuntary (not normally consciously controlled). The three types of muscles are striated voluntary (skeletal) muscle, striated involuntary (cardiac) muscle, and nonstriated involuntary (smooth) muscle.

Skeletal muscle attaches to bones and represents a large portion of the human body's total weight. Contraction of these muscles is responsible for body movement. Cardiac muscle is the muscle of the heart. Contraction of the cardiac muscle pumps blood throughout the body. Smooth muscle is widespread throughout the body and is responsible for a variety of functions. Examples include movement in the digestive, urinary, and reproductive systems.

Nervous Tissue

The nervous tissue is characterized by the ability to conduct electrical signals, which are known as action potentials. The nervous tissue consists of two basic kinds of cells: neurons and neuroglia.

Neurons, or nerve cells, are the actual conducting cells of nervous tissue. They are composed of three major parts: cell body, dendrite, and axon. The cell body contains the nucleus and is the site of general cell functions. Dendrites and axons are nerve cell processes (projections of cytoplasm surrounded by membrane). Dendrites receive electrical impulses and conduct them toward the cell body. Axons usually conduct impulses away from the cell body. Neurons have many different sizes and shapes, especially in the brain and spinal cord.

Neuroglia are the support cells of the brain, spinal cord, and peripheral nerves. These cells are divided into several subgroups that nourish, protect, and insulate neurons.

Organ Systems

An **organ** is a structure made up of two or more kinds of tissues organized to perform a more complex function than any one tissue can. A **system** is a group of organs arranged to perform a more complex function than any one organ can (Fig. 6-7). The human body contains 11 major organ systems:

1. Integumentary
2. Skeletal
3. Muscular
4. Nervous
5. Endocrine
6. Circulatory
7. Lymphatic
8. Respiratory
9. Digestive
10. Urinary
11. Reproductive

Integumentary System

The **integumentary system** is the largest organ system of the body. It consists of the skin and accessory structures such as hair, nails, and a variety of glands. The functions of the integumentary system include protection of the body against injury and dehydration, defense against invading microorganisms, and temperature regulation.

? CRITICAL THINKING

Based on your knowledge of the functions of the skin, what signs, symptoms, or complications would you expect in a patient with burns covering half the body?

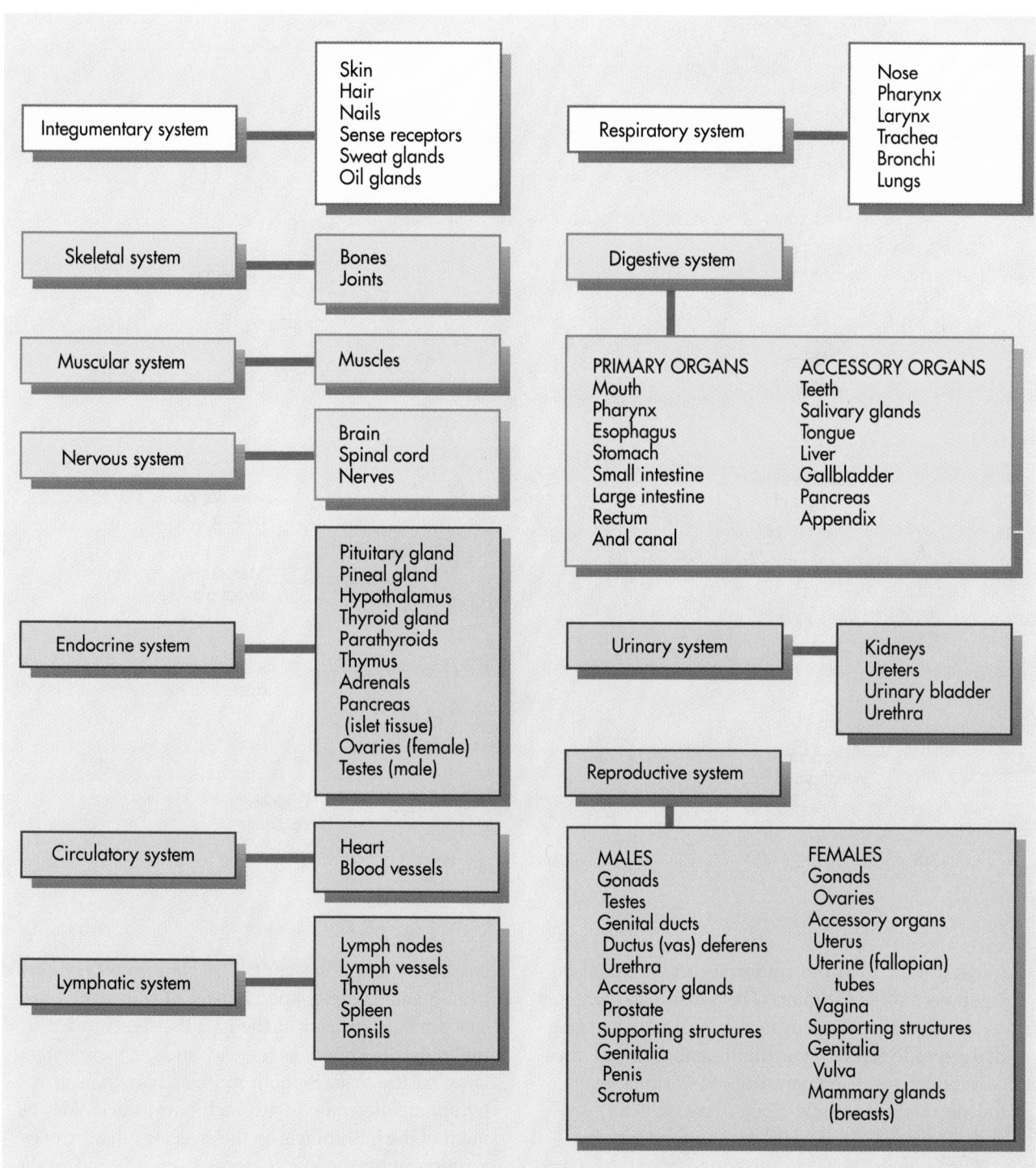

Fig. 6-7 Body systems and their organs.

Skin

The skin is a sheetlike organ composed of two distinct layers of tissue: the epidermis and the dermis (Fig. 6-8). The epidermis is the outermost layer of skin, consisting of tightly packed epithelial cells. Cells of the innermost layer of the epidermis can undergo mitosis and can repair themselves if injured. Because of this characteristic, the body can maintain an effective barrier against infection, even when subjected to injury and normal wear and tear.

The dermis is the deeper of the two layers of skin and is made up largely of connective tissue. It is

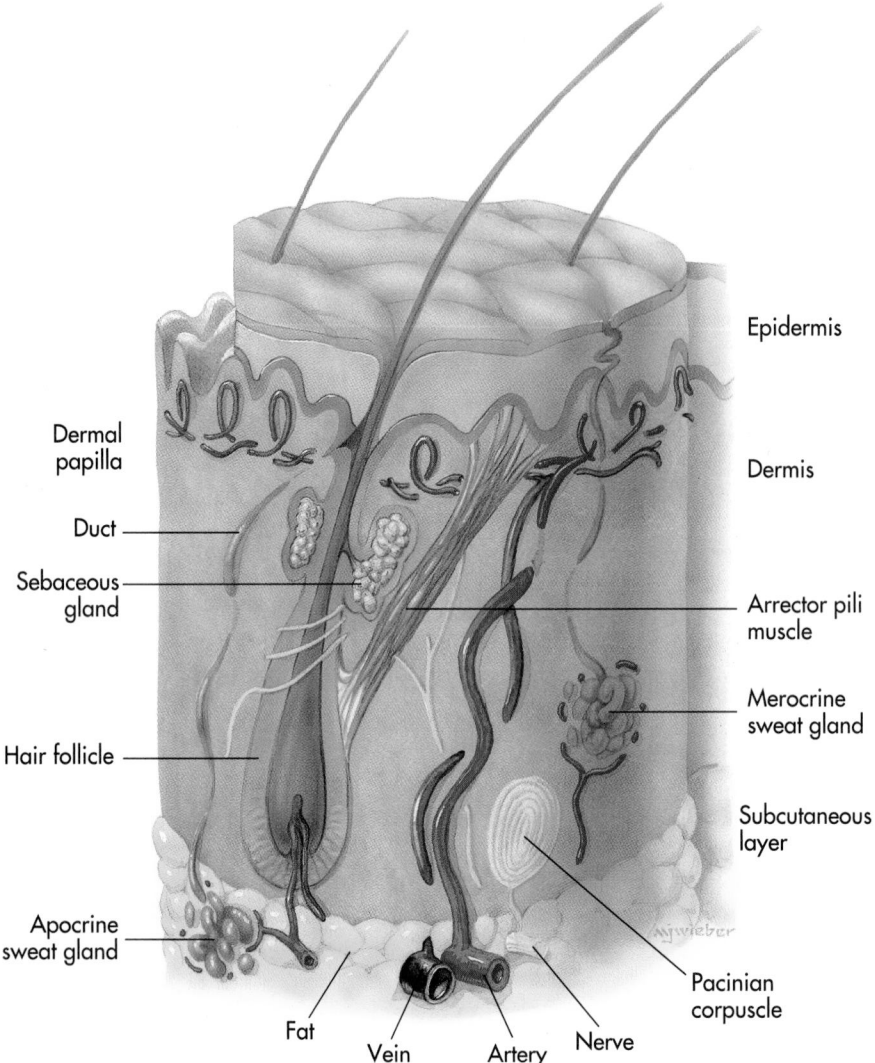

Epidermis

Dermal papilla

Dermis

Duct

Sebaceous gland

Arrector pili muscle

Merocrine sweat gland

Hair follicle

Subcutaneous layer

Apocrine sweat gland

Pacinian corpuscle

Fat   Vein   Artery   Nerve

Fig. 6-8 Microscopic view of the skin.

much thicker than the epidermis and contains collagenous and elastic fibers. The dermis also contains a specialized network of nerves and nerve endings that provide sensory information about pain, pressure, touch, and temperature. At various levels of the dermis are muscle fibers, hair follicles, sweat and sebaceous glands, and many blood vessels.

The layers of skin are supported by a thick layer of loose connective tissue and fat known as subcutaneous tissue. Subcutaneous tissue insulates the body from temperature extremes, serves as a source of stored energy, and acts as a shock absorber to protect underlying tissue from injury.

Hair

Hair growth begins when cells of the epidermal layer of the skin grow into the dermis, forming a small tube called the *hair follicle*. Hair growth begins from a small, cap-shaped cluster of cells called the *hair papilla*. The part of the hair that lies hidden in the follicle is known as the *root*, and the visible part is called the *shaft*. Smooth muscles known as *arrector pili* are associated with each hair follicle. Movement of the hair follicle by the arrector pili produces a pressure on the skin ("goose bumps") and pulls the hairs upward.

Nails

Nails are produced by cells in the epidermis. The visible part of the nail is the nail body. The root of the nail lies in a groove and is hidden by a fold of skin known as the *cuticle*. The crescent-shaped white area of the nail is called the *lunula* and is most visible on the thumbnail. The nail bed that lies under the nail contains many blood vessels. In healthy individuals, this layer of epithelium appears pink through the translucent nail body.

Glands

The major glands of the skin are the sebaceous and sweat glands. Most sebaceous glands are located in the dermis and secrete oil (sebum) for the hair and skin. This oil prevents drying and protects against some bacteria. Sebum secretion increases during adolescence, stimulated by increased blood levels of the sex hormones. Other skin glands include the ceruminous glands of the external auditory meatus, which produce cerumen (earwax), and the mammary glands.

Sweat (sudoriferous) glands are the most numerous skin glands. They usually are classified as merocrine or apocrine according to their mode of secretion. Merocrine sweat glands are the most common and open directly onto the surface of the skin through sweat pores. The coiled portion of the gland produces a fluid that is mostly water but also contains some salts (mainly sodium chloride) and small amounts of ammonia, urea, uric acid, and lactic acid. As the body temperature rises, the sweat glands produce sweat, which evaporates and cools the body. Apocrine glands usually open into hair follicles. These glands are found in the axillae and genitalia and around the anus. They become active at puberty through the influence of sex hormones. Apocrine glands secrete an organic substance that is odorless when released but is quickly metabolized by bacteria to cause body odor.

> **? CRITICAL THINKING**
>
> *The ability to sweat is impaired in the elderly. What implications does this have?*

Skeletal System

The skeletal system consists of bones and associated connective tissues, including cartilage, tendons, and ligaments. The skeletal system provides a rigid framework for support and protection and provides a system of levers on which muscles act to produce body movements. The skeletal system contains 206 individual bones. Bones are divided into two categories: the axial skeleton and the appendicular skeleton (Fig. 6-9).

Axial Skeleton

The axial skeleton consists of the skull, hyoid bone, vertebral column, and thoracic cage. The skull is composed of 28 separate bones divided into the following groups: the auditory ossicles, cranial vault, and facial bones (Fig. 6-10). The 6 auditory ossicles (three on each side of the head) are located inside the cavity of the temporal bone. The auditory ossicles function in hearing.

The cranial vault consists of 6 bones that surround and protect the brain. They are the parietal, temporal, frontal, occipital, sphenoid, and ethmoid bones.

The 14 facial bones form the structure of the face in the anterior skull but do not contribute to the cranial vault. The bones include the maxilla, mandible, zygomatic, palatine, nasal, lacrimal, vomer, and inferior nasal concha bones. The frontal and ethmoid bones contribute to both the cranial vault and the face.

The hyoid bone is attached to the skull by muscles and ligaments and "floats" in the superior aspect of the neck, just below the mandible. The hyoid bone serves as the attachment point for several important neck and tongue muscles.

The vertebral column consists of 26 bones, which can be divided into five regions: 7 cervical vertebrae, 12 thoracic vertebrae, 5 lumbar vertebrae, 1 sacral bone, and 1 coccygeal bone (Fig. 6-11). A total of 34 vertebrae originally form during development, but the 5 sacral vertebrae fuse to form 1 bone, as do the 4 or 5 coccygeal bones.

The weight-bearing portion of the vertebrae is a bony disk called the *body*. Intervertebral disks, located between the bodies of adjacent vertebrae, serve as shock absorbers for the vertebral column, provide additional support for the body, and prevent the vertebral bodies from rubbing against each other. The spinal cord is protected by the vertebral arch and the dorsal portion of the body. A transverse process extends laterally from each side of the arch, and a single spinous process is present at the point of junction. Much vertebral movement is accomplished by the contraction of skeletal muscles attached to the transverse and spinous processes.

The thoracic cage protects vital organs within the thorax and prevents the collapse of the thorax during respiration. It consists of the thoracic

Axial skeleton   **Appendicular skeleton**   **Axial skeleton**

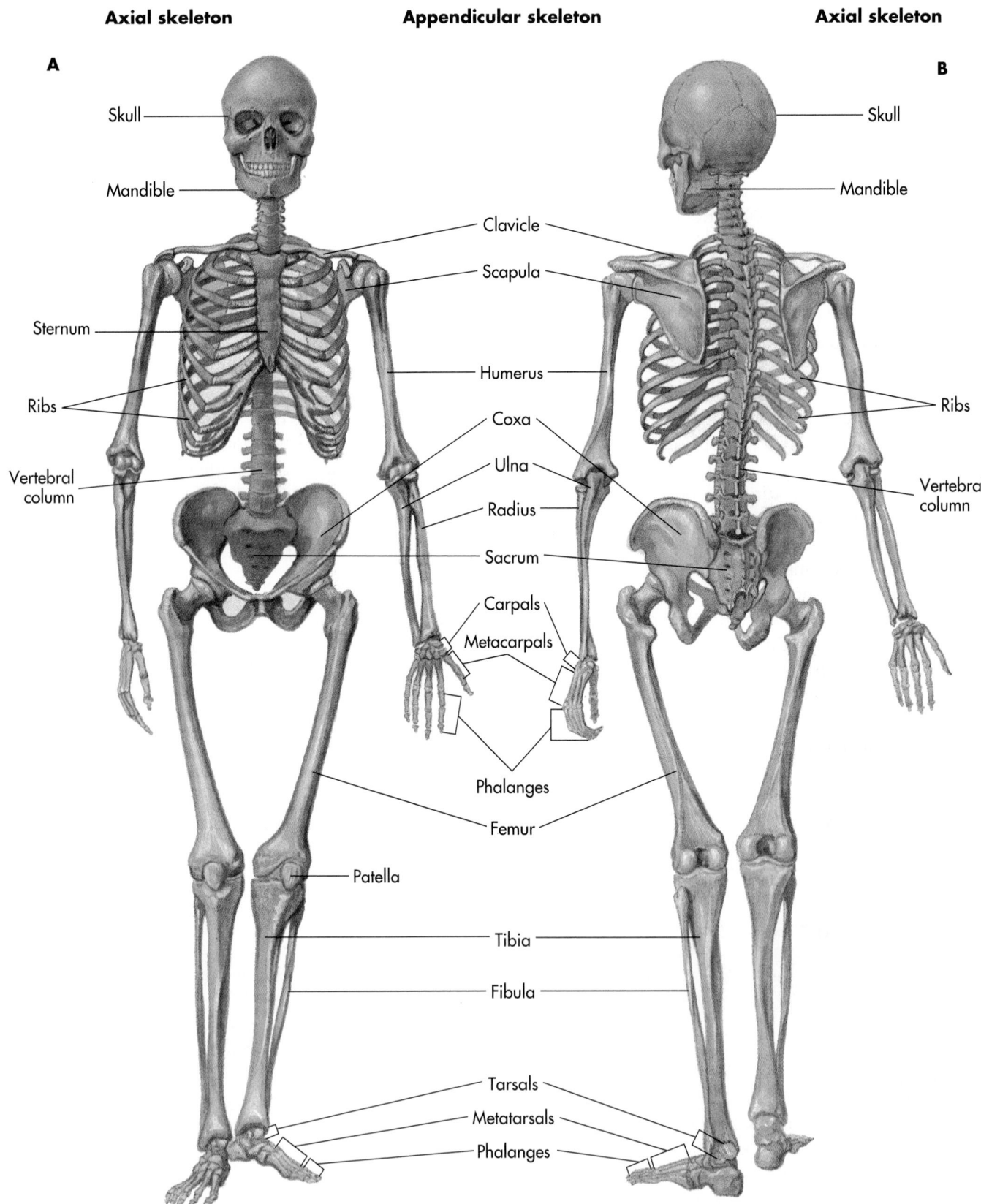

Fig. 6-9 Anterior (**A**) and posterior (**B**) view of the skeleton.

A

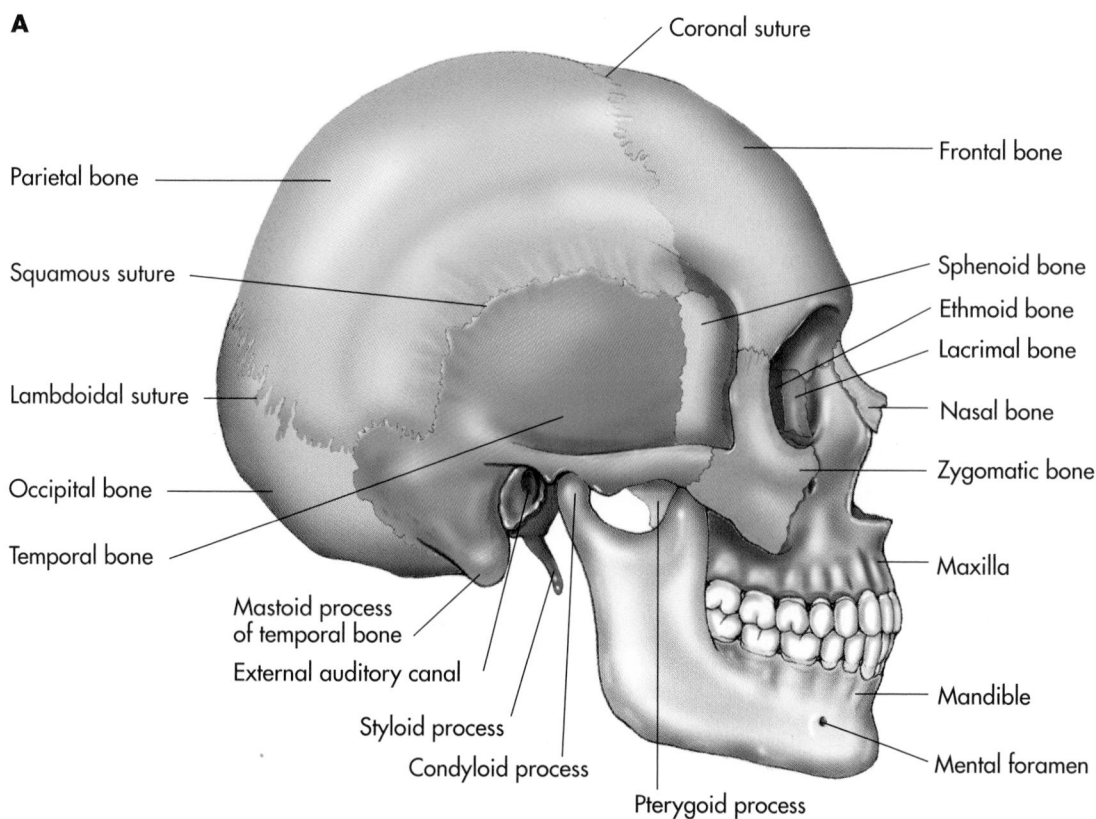

B

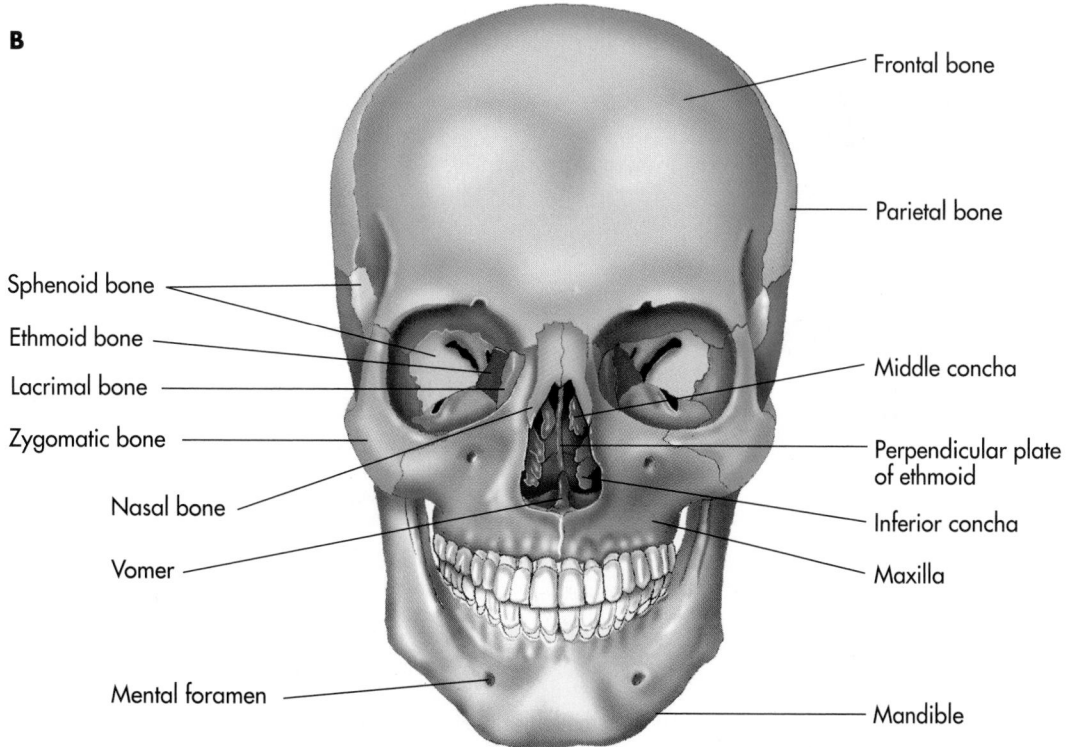

Fig. 6-10 Skull viewed from the right side (**A**) and the front (**B**).

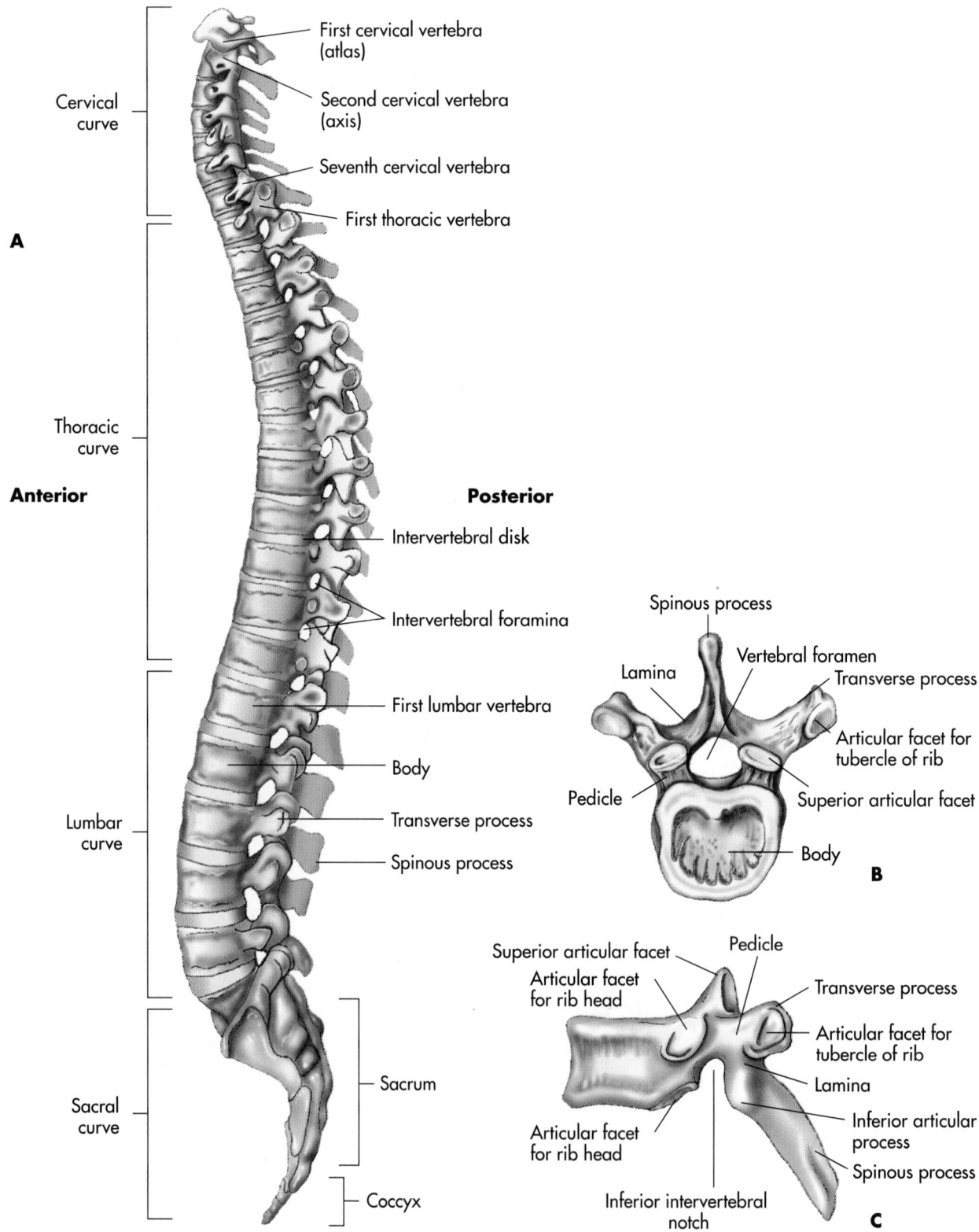

A

Cervical curve

First cervical vertebra (atlas)

Second cervical vertebra (axis)

Seventh cervical vertebra

First thoracic vertebra

Thoracic curve

Anterior   **Posterior**

Intervertebral disk

Intervertebral foramina

First lumbar vertebra

Body

Transverse process

Spinous process

Lumbar curve

Sacrum

Sacral curve

Coccyx

B

Spinous process

Lamina   Vertebral foramen

Transverse process

Pedicle   Articular facet for tubercle of rib

Superior articular facet

Body

C

Superior articular facet   Pedicle

Articular facet for rib head   Transverse process

Articular facet for tubercle of rib

Lamina

Inferior articular process

Spinous process

Articular facet for rib head

Inferior intervertebral notch

Fig. 6-11 A, Vertebral column viewed from the left side. **B,** Superior view of the vertebrae. **C,** Lateral view of the vertebrae.

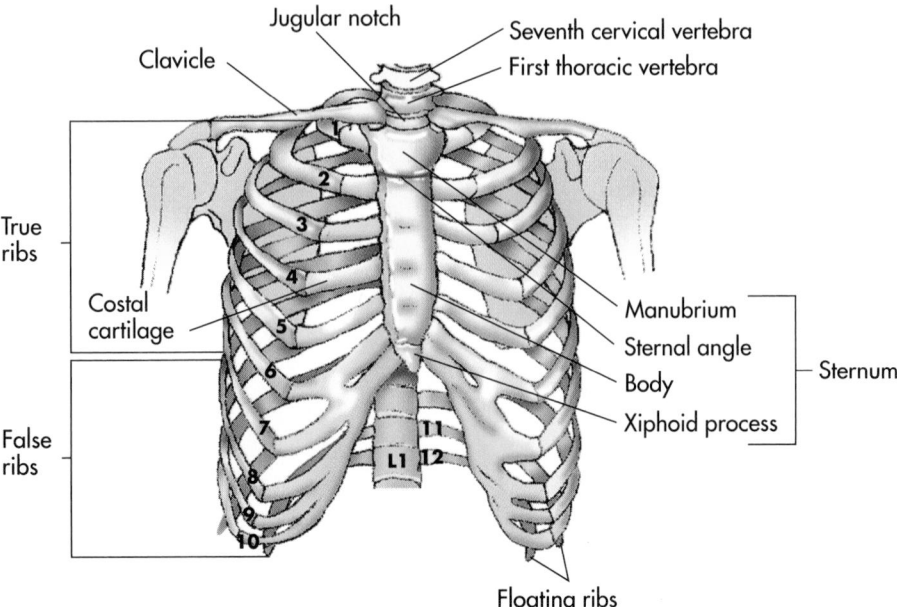

Fig. 6-12 Entire rib cage as seen from the front.

vertebrae, ribs with their associated costal cartilages, and sternum (Fig. 6-12).

The 12 pairs of ribs can be divided into *true* or *false* ribs. The superior 7 (the true ribs) articulate with the thoracic vertebrae and attach directly through their costal cartilages to the sternum. The inferior 5 (the false ribs) articulate with the thoracic vertebrae but do not attach directly to the sternum. The eighth, ninth, and tenth ribs are joined to a common cartilage, which is attached to the sternum. The eleventh and twelfth ribs are "floating" ribs that have no attachment to the sternum.

The sternum is divided into three parts: the manubrium, body, and xiphoid process. At the superior margin of the manubrium is the jugular notch, which can easily be palpated at the anterior base of the neck. The point at which the manubrium joins the body of the sternum is the sternal angle (also known as the angle of Louis). The second rib is found lateral to the sternal angle and is used clinically as a starting point for counting the other ribs.

✓ TRICKS OF THE TRADE

The first rib is buried under the clavicle and is difficult to palpate. That is why the second rib is the starting point for counting other ribs.

Appendicular Skeleton

The appendicular skeleton consists of the bones of the upper and lower extremities and their girdles, by which they are attached to the body.

The scapula and clavicle constitute the pectoral girdle, which attaches the upper limbs to the axial skeleton. The direct point of attachment between the bones of the appendicular and axial skeleton occurs at the sternoclavicular joint between the clavicle and the sternum.

The humerus is the second longest bone in the body. The head of the humerus articulates with the scapula. The greater and lesser tubercles are on the lateral and anterior surfaces of the proximal end of the humerus, where they function as sites of muscle attachments. The humerus articulates with the radius and ulna at its distal end. The capitulum (lateral aspect of the humerus) articulates with the head of the radius, and the trochlea (medial aspect of the humerus) articulates with the ulna. Proximal to the trochlea and capitulum are the medial and lateral epicondyles, respectively, which function as muscle attachments for the muscles of the forearm. (Fig. 6-13 illustrates the bones of the upper extremity.)

The large bony process of the ulna (the *olecranon process*) can be felt at the point of the elbow. This process fits in a large depression on the posterior surface of the humerus known as the *olecranon*

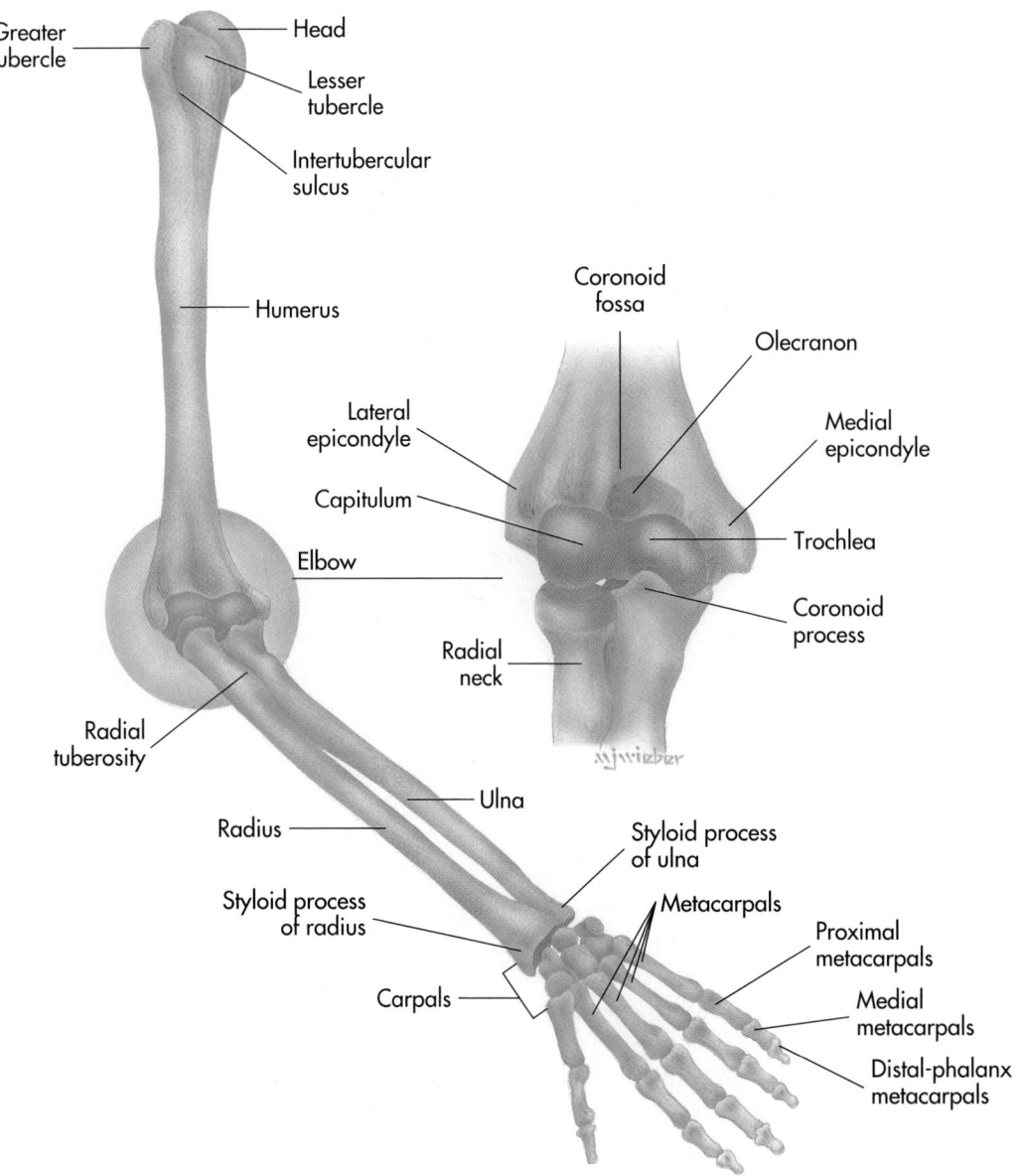

Fig. 6-13 Bones of the upper extremity.

fossa. The structural relationship between these two processes makes movement of the joint possible. The distal end of the ulna has a small head that articulates with the radius and wrist bones. The posterior-medial side of the head has a small styloid process to which the ligaments of the wrist are attached. The proximal end of the radius articulates with the humerus, and the medial surface of the head constitutes a smooth cylinder where the radius rotates against the radial notch of the ulna. Major anterior arm muscles (biceps brachii) are attached to the radial tuberosity.

The wrist is composed of 8 carpal bones, which are arranged in two rows of 4 each. A total of 5 metacarpals are attached to the carpal bones and constitute the bony framework of the hand. A total of 28 phalanges make up the 10 digits of the hands. There are 2 phalanges for each thumb and 3 for each finger.

The pelvic girdle attaches the legs to the trunk (Fig. 6-14). The girdle consists of 2 coxae (hip bones), 1 located on each side of the pelvis. Each coxa surrounds a large obturator foramen, through which muscles, nerves, and blood vessels pass to the leg. A

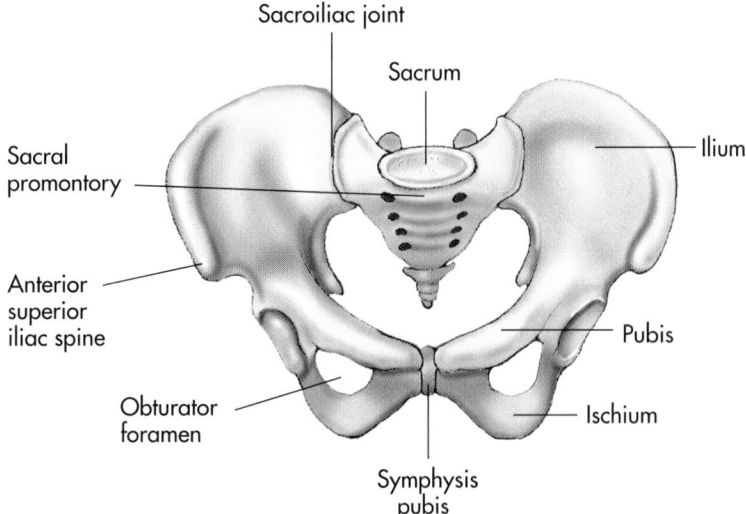

Fig. 6-14 Complete pelvic girdle, anterior view.

fossa called the acetabulum is located on the lateral surface of each coxa and is the point of articulation of the lower limb with the girdle. During development, each coxa is formed by the fusion of 3 separate bones: the ilium, ischium, and pubis. The superior portion of the ilium is the iliac crest. The crest ends anteriorly as the anterior-superior iliac spine and posteriorly as the posterior-superior iliac spine.

The femur is the longest bone in the body. It has a well-defined neck and a prominent rounded head that articulates with the acetabulum. The proximal shaft has 2 tuberosities: a greater trochanter lateral to the neck and a smaller or lesser trochanter inferior and posterior to the neck. Both trochanters are attachment sites for muscles that attach the hip to the thigh. The distal end of the femur has medial and lateral condyles that articulate with the tibia. Located laterally and proximally to the condyles are the medial and lateral epicondyles, which are sites of muscle and ligament attachment. (Fig. 6-15 illustrates the bones of the lower extremity.)

? CRITICAL THINKING

Why should you anticipate blood loss when large bones are fractured?

Distally, the femur also articulates with the patella, which is located in a major tendon of the thigh muscle. The patella allows the tendon to turn the corner over the knee.

The 2 bones of the leg are the tibia and the fibula. The tibia is the largest of the 2 and supports most of the weight of the leg. A tibial tuberosity can be seen and palpated just inferior to the patella. The proximal end of the tibia has flat medial and lateral condyles that articulate with the condyles of the femur. The distal end of the tibia forms the medial malleolus, which helps to form the medial side of the ankle joint.

The fibula does not articulate with the femur but does have a small proximal head that articulates with the tibia. The distal end of the fibula forms the lateral malleolus to create the lateral aspect of the ankle joint.

The foot consists of 7 tarsal bones (Fig. 6-16). The talus articulates with the tibia and the fibula to form the ankle joint. The calcaneus is located inferior and just lateral to the talus, supporting the bone. It protrudes posteriorly where the calf muscles attach to it and is easily identified as the heel. The foot consists of tarsals, metatarsals, and phalanges, which are arranged in a manner similar to the metacarpals and phalanges of the hand, the great toe being analogous to the thumb. The ball of the foot is the junction between the metatarsals and the phalanges. Strong ligaments and leg muscle tendons normally hold the foot bones firmly in their arched position.

Biomechanics of Body Movement

With the exception of the hyoid bone, every bone in the body connects to at least 1 other bone.

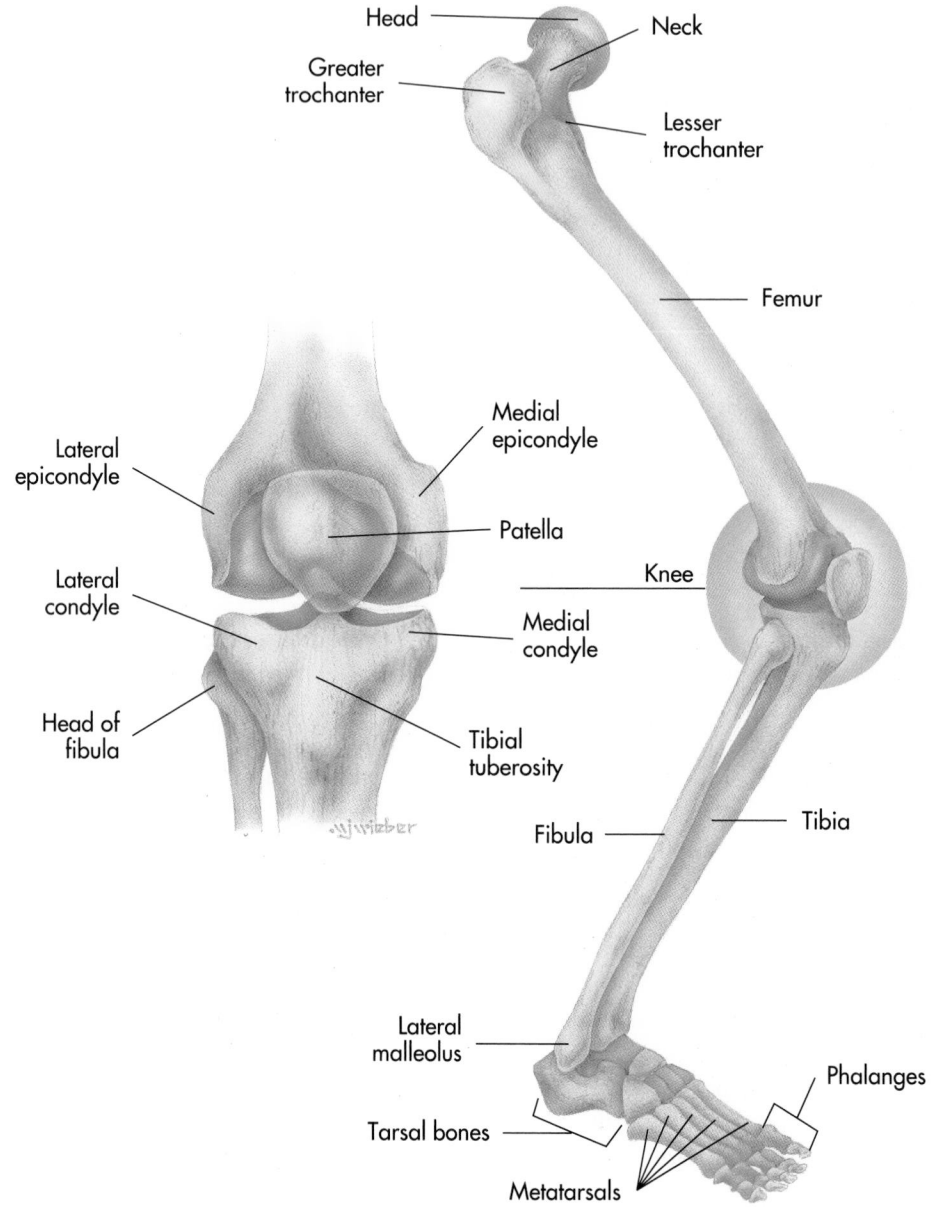

Fig. 6-15 Bones of the lower extremity.

The connections or joints commonly are named according to the bones or portions of bones that are united at the joint. The three major classifications of joints are fibrous, cartilaginous, and synovial.

Fibrous joints

Fibrous joints consist of 2 bones united by fibrous tissue that have little or no movement. The joints are further divided on the basis of structure into sutures, syndesmoses, or gomphoses. Sutures (seams between flat bones) are located in the skull bones

and may be completely immobile in adults. In newborns, the sutures have gaps between them, called fontanels; these gaps are fairly wide to allow "give" to the skull during birth and allow growth of the head during development (Fig. 6-17).

> **? CRITICAL THINKING**
>
> *Why might the structure of the skull sutures be a disadvantage after trauma to the head of an adult?*

A

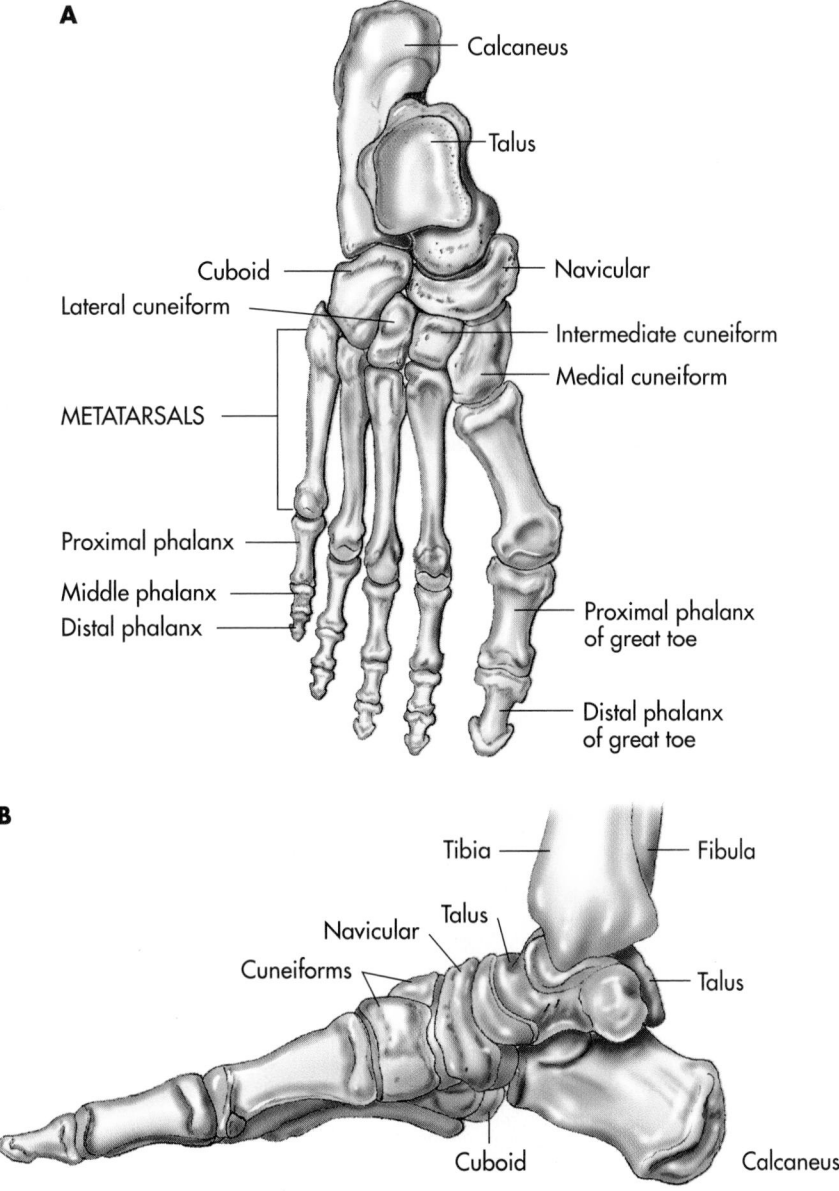

Calcaneus

Talus

Cuboid

Lateral cuneiform

METATARSALS

Navicular

Intermediate cuneiform

Medial cuneiform

Proximal phalanx

Middle phalanx

Distal phalanx

Proximal phalanx
of great toe

Distal phalanx
of great toe

B

Tibia

Fibula

Navicular

Talus

Cuneiforms

Talus

Cuboid

Calcaneus

Fig. 6-16 Bones of the right ankle and foot. **A,** Dorsal view. **B,** Medial view.

A syndesmosis is a fibrous joint in which the bones are separated by a greater distance than in a suture and are joined by ligaments. These ligaments may provide some movement of the joint. An example of this joint is the radioulnar syndesmosis that binds the radius and ulna together (Fig. 6-18).

A gomphosis joint consists of a peg that fits into a socket. The peg is held in place by fine bundles of collagenous connective tissue. The joints between the teeth and the sockets along the processes of the mandible and maxillae are examples of gomphoses joints.

Cartilaginous joints

Cartilaginous joints unite two bones by means of hyaline cartilage (synchondroses) or fibrocartilage (symphyses). A synchondrosis allows only slight movement at the joint. Common examples of this type of joint are the epiphyseal plate of a growing bone and the cartilage rod between most of the ribs and the sternum. Symphysis joints are slightly moveable because of the flexible nature of the fibrocartilage. Symphyses include the junction between the manubrium and the body of the sternum in adults, the symphysis pubis of the coxae, and the intervertebral disks.

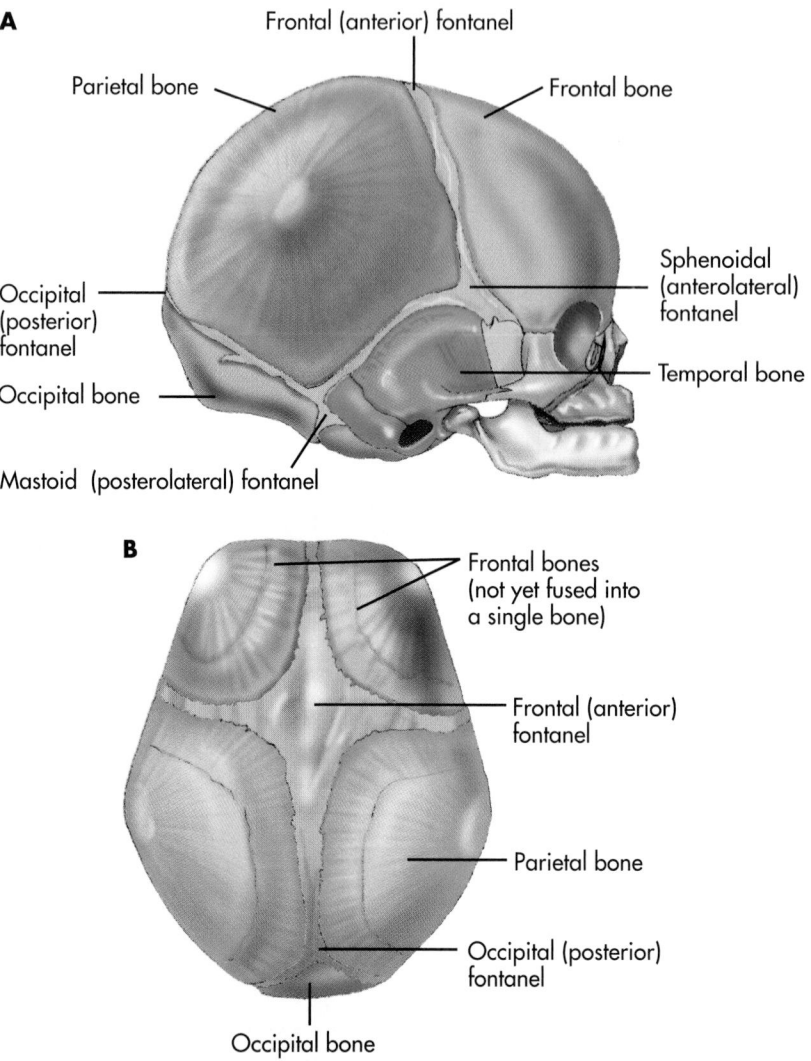

Fig. 6-17 Fetal skull showing fontanels. **A,** Lateral view. **B,** Superior view.

Synovial joints

Synovial joints contain synovial fluid, a thin, lubricating film that allows considerable movement between articulating bones. Most joints that unite the bones of the appendicular skeleton are synovial. The articular surfaces of bones within synovial joints are covered with a thin layer of hyaline cartilage, which provides a smooth surface where the bones meet. The joint is enclosed by a joint capsule, which consists of an outer fibrous capsule and an inner synovial membrane. The synovial membrane lines the joint and produces synovial fluid. Synovial joints are classified into six divisions according to the shape of the adjoining articular surfaces (Fig. 6-19):

1. Plane or gliding joints consist of two opposed flat surfaces that are about equal in size. Examples of

these joints are the articular processes between vertebrae.

2. Saddle joints consist of two saddle-shaped articulating surfaces oriented at right angles to one another. Movement in these joints can occur in two planes. An example of a saddle joint is the carpometacarpal joint of the thumb.

3. Hinge joints consist of a convex cylinder in one bone applied to a corresponding concavity in another bone. These joints permit movement in one plane only. Examples of hinge joints are those of the elbow and knee.

4. Pivot joints consist of a relatively cylindrical bony process that rotates within a ring composed partly of bone and partly of ligament. An example of a pivot joint is the head of the radius articulating with the proximal end of the ulna.

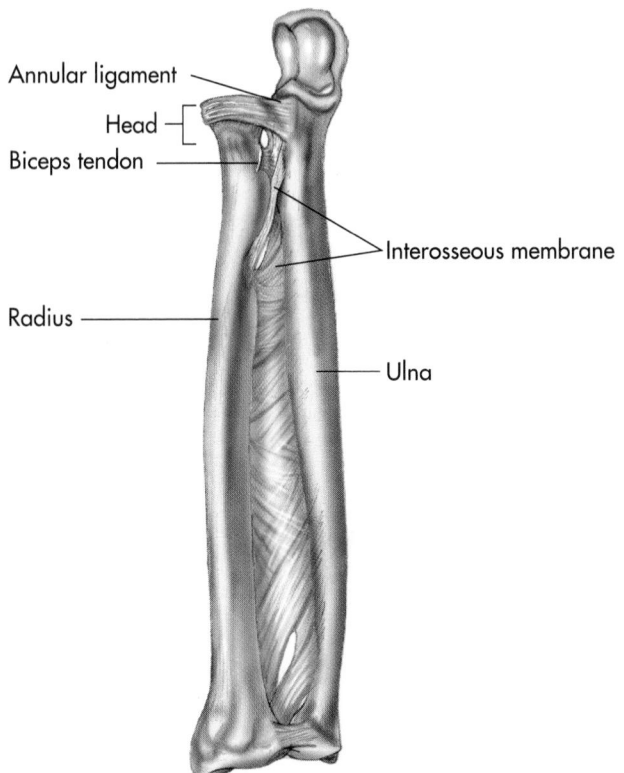

Annular ligament

Head

Biceps tendon

Interosseous membrane

Radius

Ulna

Fig. 6-18 Radioulnar syndesmosis of right forearm.

5. Ball-and-socket joints consist of a ball (head) at the end of one bone and a socket into an adjacent bone into which a portion of the ball fits. These joints allow wide ranges of movement in almost any direction. Examples are the shoulder and hip joints.

6. Ellipsoid joints are modified ball-and-socket joints where the articular surfaces are ellipsoid rather than spherical in shape. The shape of the joint limits movement, making it similar to a hinge motion, but the motion occurs in two planes. The atlantooccipital joint is an ellipsoid joint.

Types of movement

Body movement may be described in relation to the anatomical position; that is, movement away from the anatomical position and movement toward it. (Examples of each are listed in Table 6-3; also see Figs. 6-20 through 6-24.)

> ? CRITICAL THINKING
>
> *Why would it be an advantage to use these body movement terms in your radio report or written patient care report?*

Muscular System

The three primary functions of the muscular system are movement, postural maintenance, and heat production. As previously discussed, the major types of muscles are skeletal, cardiac, and smooth muscle. Skeletal muscle is far more common than other types of muscle in the body and is the focus of this section. Cardiac and smooth muscle are presented later in this text. (These muscle types are compared in Table 6-4.)

Physiology of Skeletal Muscle

Muscle tissue consists of specialized contractile cells or muscle fibers. Skeletal muscle contracts in response to electrochemical stimuli. Nerve cells regulate the function of skeletal muscle fibers by controlling the series of events that result in muscle contraction.

Each skeletal muscle fiber is filled with thick and thin myofilaments, which are fine, threadlike structures. The thick myofilaments are formed from the protein myosin, and the thin myofilaments are composed of the protein actin. The sarcomere is the contractile unit of skeletal muscle, containing thick and thin myofilaments. During the contraction process, energy obtained from ATP molecules enables the two types of myofilaments to slide toward each other and shorten the sarcomere and eventually the entire muscle.

Neuromuscular junction

A nervous impulse enters the muscle fiber through a specialized nerve known as a motor neuron. The point of contact between the nerve ending and the muscle fiber is the neuromuscular junction or synapse (Fig. 6-25). Each muscle fiber receives a branch of an axon, and each axon innervates more than a single muscle fiber. When a nerve impulse passes through this junction, specialized chemicals are released, causing the muscle to contract.

> ? CRITICAL THINKING
>
> *What might you find in your examination of the eye if exposure to a chemical nerve weapon caused too much chemical stimulation at the synapse for the muscles of the eye?*

Skeletal Muscle Movement

Most muscles extend from one bone to another and cross at least one joint. Muscle contraction causes

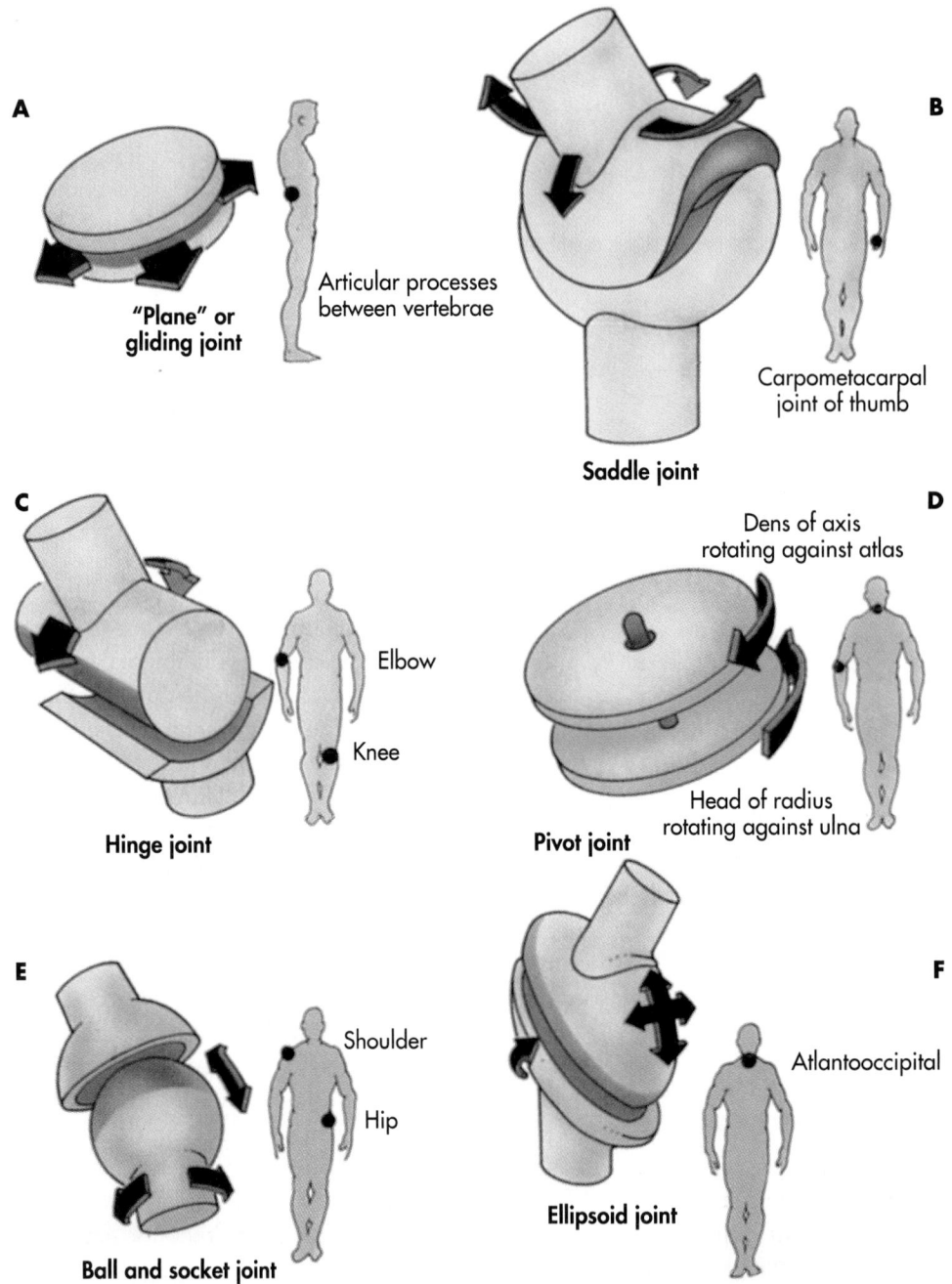

Fig. 6-19 Types of synovial joints and selected examples. **A,** Plane. **B,** Saddle. **C,** Hinge. **D,** Pivot. **E,** Ball-and-socket. **F,** Ellipsoid.

most body movements by pulling one of the bones toward the other across the moveable joint. The points of attachment of each muscle are the origin and insertion. The origin is the end of the muscle attached to the more stationary of the two bones. The insertion is the end of the muscle attached to the bone undergoing the greatest movement. Some muscles of the face are not attached to bone at both ends but attach to the skin, which moves when muscles contract.

The contraction of some muscles with the simultaneous relaxation of others produces movement. Muscles that work in cooperation with one another to cause movement are called *synergists,* and a muscle working in opposition to another muscle (moving the structure in an opposite direction) is called

TABLE 6-3	BODY MOVEMENT TERMINOLOGY
TERM	**DEFINITION**
Flexion	Bending
Extension	Stretching out
Protraction	Movement in the anterior direction
Retraction	Movement in the posterior direction
Abduction	Movement away from the midline
Adduction	Movement toward the midline
Inversion	Turning inward
Eversion	Turning outward
Excursion	Movement from side to side
Rotation	Movement of a structure about its axis
Circumduction	Movement in a circular motion
Pronation	Rotation of the forearm so that the anterior surface is down
Supination	Rotation of the forearm so that the anterior surface is up
Elevation	Movement of a structure in a superior direction
Depression	Movement of a structure in an inferior direction
Opposition	Movement of the thumb and little finger toward each other
Reposition	Movement of a structure to its original position

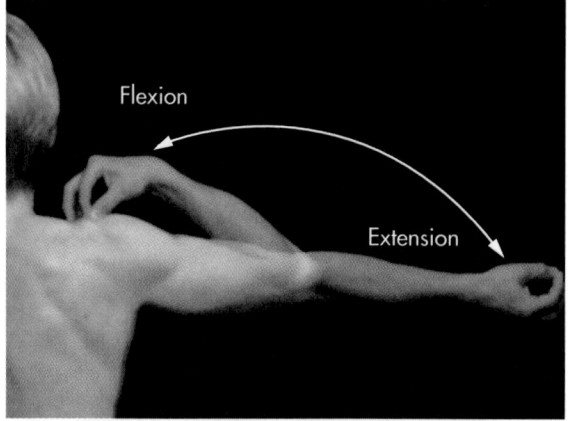

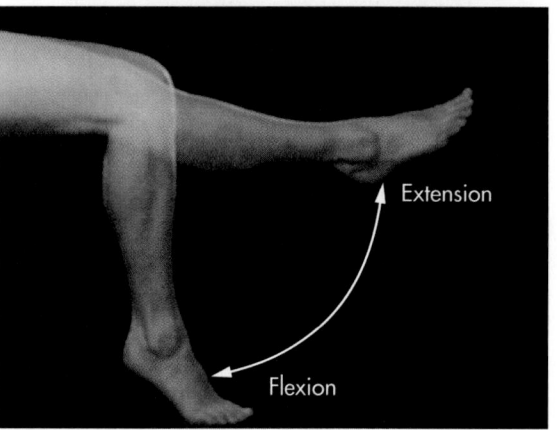

Fig. 6-20 Flexion and extension of the elbow (**A**) and the knee (**B**).

an *antagonist*. The muscle that is primarily responsible for a particular movement is called the *prime mover*. For example, the biceps brachii, brachialis, and triceps brachii muscles are all involved in flexion and extension of the forearm at the elbow joint. The biceps brachii is the prime mover during flexion, and the brachialis is the synergistic muscle. When the biceps brachii and the brachialis muscles flex the forearm, the triceps brachii relaxes (antagonistic muscle). During extension of the forearm, the triceps brachii becomes the prime mover, and the biceps and brachialis become the antagonistic muscles. The coordinated activity of synergists and antagonists is what makes muscular movement smooth and graceful (Fig. 6-26).

Types of muscle contraction

Muscle contractions are classified as either *isometric* or *isotonic*, depending on the type of contraction that predominates. In isometric contractions, the length of the muscle does not change, but the amount of tension increases during the contraction process. Isometric contractions are responsible for the constant length of the postural muscles of the body. During isotonic contractions, the amount of tension produced by the muscle is constant during contraction, but the length of the muscle changes. An example of isotonic contraction is the movement of the arms or fingers. Most muscle contractions are a combination of isometric and isotonic contractions.

Postural maintenance

Postural maintenance is a result of muscle tone, the constant tension produced by muscles of the body for long periods. This tone is responsible for keeping the back and legs straight, the head in an

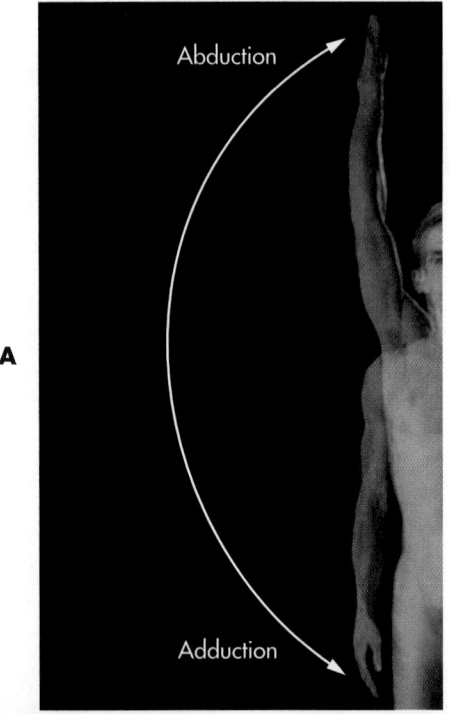

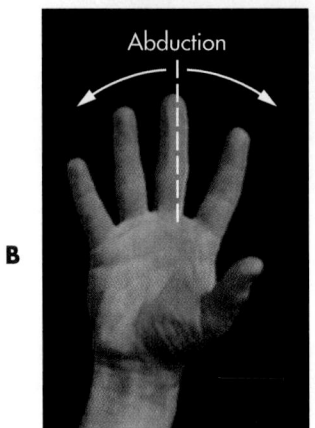
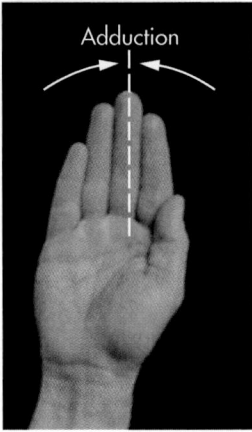

Fig. 6-21 Abduction and adduction of the upper extremity (**A**) and the fingers (**B**).

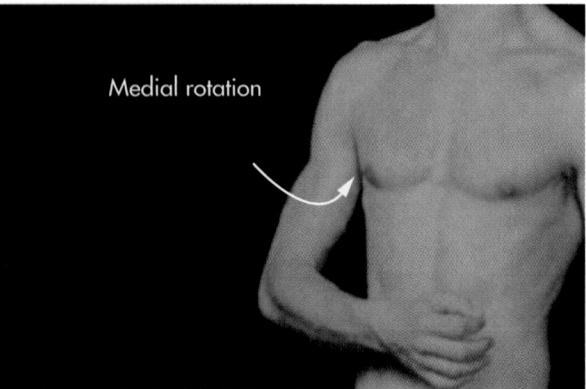

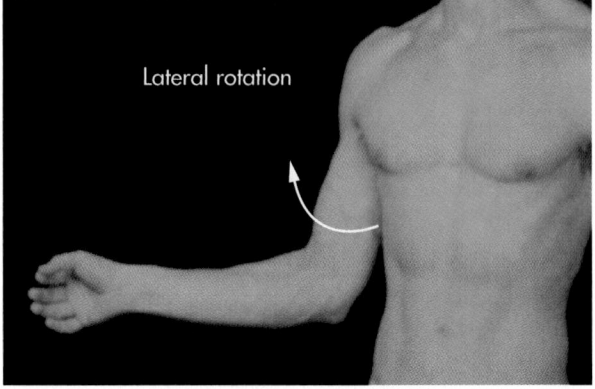

Fig. 6-22 Medial and lateral rotation of the humerus.

upright position, and the abdomen from bulging. These positions balance the distribution of weight and therefore put less strain on muscles, tendons, ligaments, and bones.

Heat production

The energy required to produce muscle contraction is obtained from ATP. Most of the energy released in the breakdown of ATP during a muscular contraction is used to shorten the muscle fibers, but some energy is lost as heat during the chemical reaction. The normal body temperature results in large part from this metabolism in skeletal muscle. If the body temperature declines below a certain level, the nervous system responds by inducing shivering. Shivering involves rapid contractions of skeletal muscle that produce shaking rather than coordinated movements. The muscle movement increases heat production up to 18 times that of resting levels. The heat produced during shivering can exceed that produced during moderate exercise, helping to raise the body temperature to its normal range.

> **? CRITICAL THINKING**
>
> *Children under 3 months cannot shiver. How will you account for that in your pre-hospital care for patients in this age group?*

Nervous System

The nervous system and the endocrine system are the major regulatory and coordinating systems of the body. The nervous system rapidly transmits in-

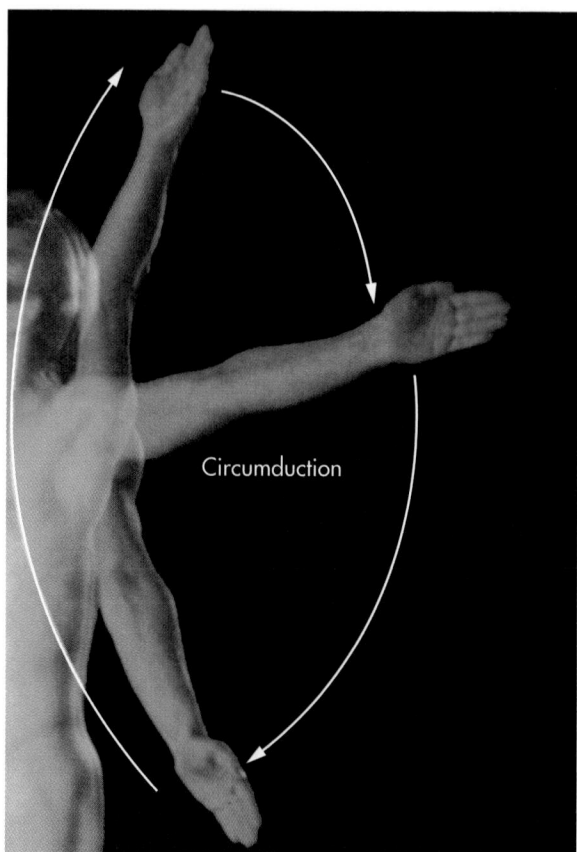

Fig. 6-23 Circumduction of the shoulder.

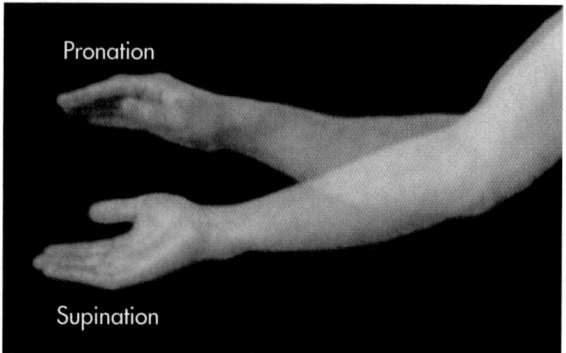

Fig. 6-24 Pronation and supination.

formation by means of nerve impulses conducted from one body area to another. The endocrine system transmits information more slowly by means of chemicals secreted by ductless glands into the bloodstream. These chemicals and hormones are then circulated to other parts of the body. The constancy of the internal environment of the body (**homeostasis**) is maintained to a large degree by these regulatory and coordinating activities.

Divisions

The human body has a single nervous system, even though some of its subdivisions are referred to as separate systems. Each subdivision has structural and functional features that separate it from the other subdivisions (Fig. 6-27).

The **central nervous system** (CNS) consists of the brain and spinal cord, which are encased in and protected by bone. The brain and spinal cord are continuous with each other. The **peripheral nervous system** (PNS) consists of the nerves and ganglia (collections of nerve cell bodies located outside the CNS). A

total of 43 pairs of nerves originate from the CNS to form the PNS; 12 pairs, the cranial nerves, originate from the brain, and the remaining 31 pairs, the spinal nerves, originate from the spinal cord. The afferent division transmits action potentials from the sensory organs to the CNS. The efferent division transmits action potentials from the CNS to effector organs such as muscles and glands (Fig. 6-28). The efferent division is further divided into the **somatic nervous system** and the autonomic nervous system (described in Chapter 2). The somatic nervous system transmits impulses from the CNS to skeletal muscle. The autonomic nervous system transmits action potentials from the CNS to smooth muscle, cardiac muscle, and certain glands.

? CRITICAL THINKING

How are the cranial nerves like the Supreme Court?

Central nervous system

The CNS consists of the brain and spinal cord. The major regions of the adult brain are the brain stem (consisting of the medulla, pons, and midbrain), the diencephalon (which includes the thalamus and hypothalamus), the cerebrum, and the cerebellum (Fig. 6-29). (The functions of these divisions are described in Table 6-5.)

Brain stem. The medulla, pons, and midbrain constitute the brain stem. The brain stem connects the spinal cord to the remainder of the brain and is responsible for many essential functions. All but 2 of the 12 cranial nerves enter or exit the brain through the brain stem.

TABLE 6-4	COMPARISON OF MUSCLE TYPES		
FEATURES	**SKELETAL MUSCLE**	**CARDIAC MUSCLE**	**SMOOTH MUSCLE**
Location	Attached to bones	Heart	Walls of hollow organs, blood vessels, eyes, glands, and skin
Cell shape	Very long and cylindrical (1-40 mm in length and may extend the entire length of a muscle, 10-100 μm in diameter)	Cylindrical and branched (100-500 μm in length, 100-200 μm in diameter)	Spindle-shaped (15-200 μm in length, 5-10 μm in diameter)
Nucleus	Multiple, peripherally located	Single, centrally located	Single, centrally located
Special features		Intercalated disks join the cells to each other	
Striations	Yes	Yes	No
Control	Voluntary	Involuntary	Involuntary
Capable of spontaneous contraction	No	Yes	Yes
Function	Body movement	Pumps blood	Food movement through the digestive tract, emptying of the urinary bladder, regulation of blood vessel diameter, change in pupil size, contraction of many gland ducts, movement of hair, and many other functions

? CRITICAL THINKING

What will be the initial prehospital management priority in a patient with an injury that affects the medulla? Why?

The medulla, also known as the *medulla oblongata*, is the most inferior portion of the brain stem. It acts as a conduction pathway for both ascending and descending nerve tracts. Several body functions, such as regulation of heart rate, blood vessel

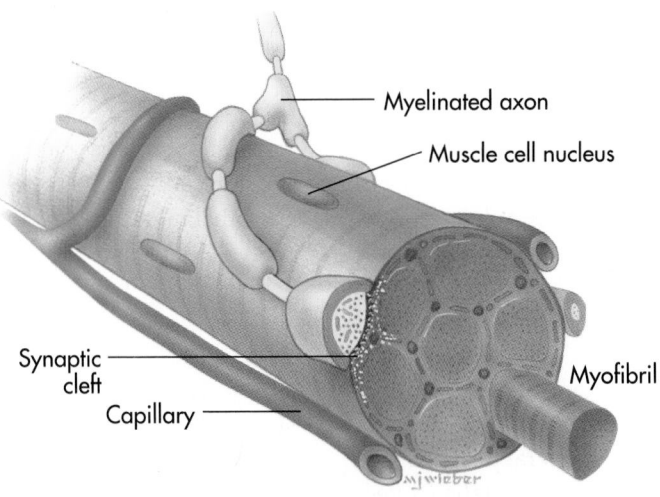

Fig. 6-25 Neuromuscular junction.

Myelinated axon

Muscle cell nucleus

Synaptic cleft

Capillary

Myofibril

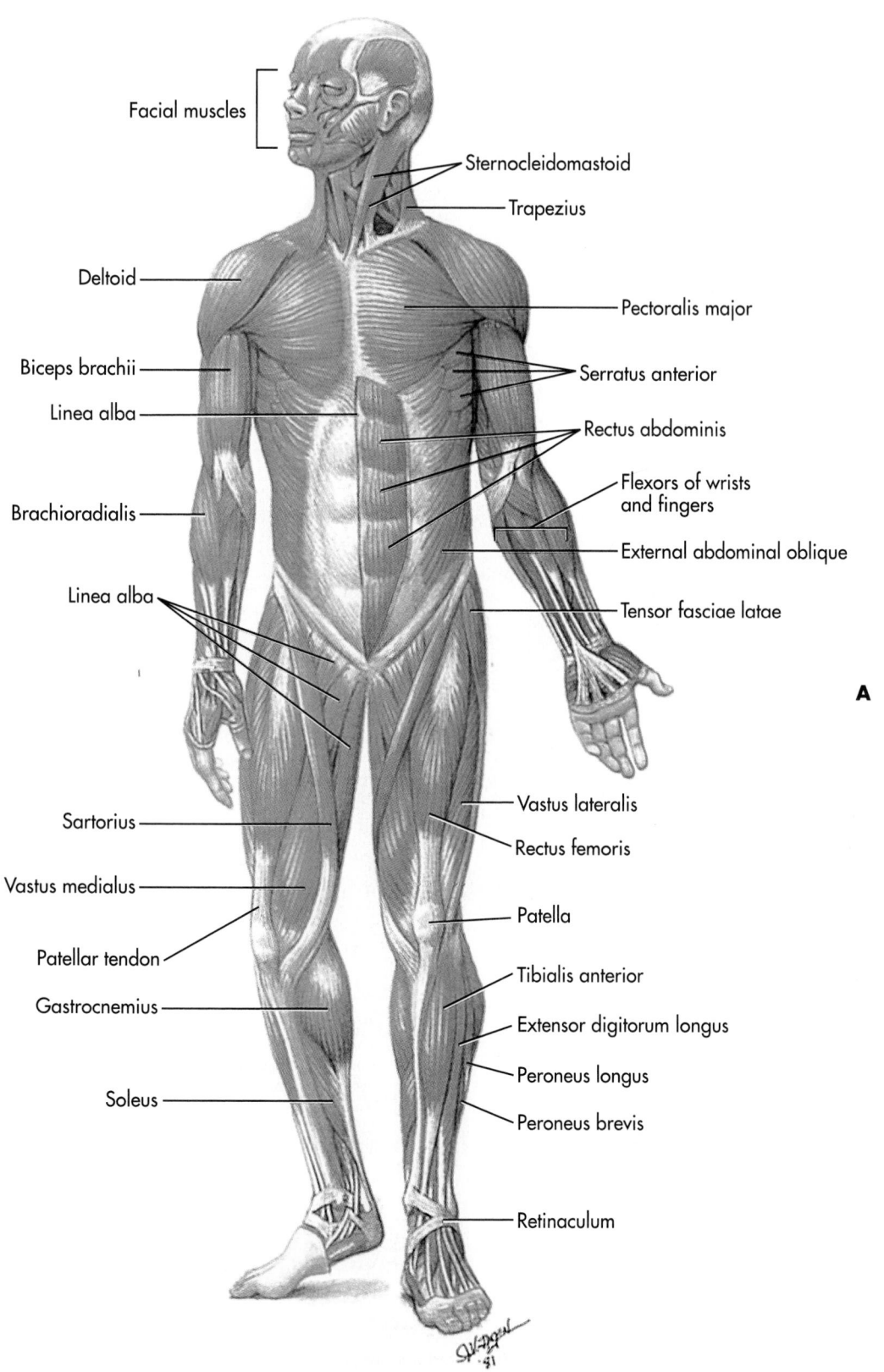

Facial muscles

Sternocleidomastoid

Trapezius

Deltoid

Pectoralis major

Biceps brachii

Serratus anterior

Linea alba

Rectus abdominis

Flexors of wrists
and fingers

Brachioradialis

External abdominal oblique

Linea alba

Tensor fasciae latae

Vastus lateralis

Rectus femoris

Sartorius

Vastus medialus

Patella

Patellar tendon

Tibialis anterior

Gastrocnemius

Extensor digitorum longus

Peroneus longus

Soleus

Peroneus brevis

Retinaculum

A

Fig. 6-26 A, Anterior view of body musculature.

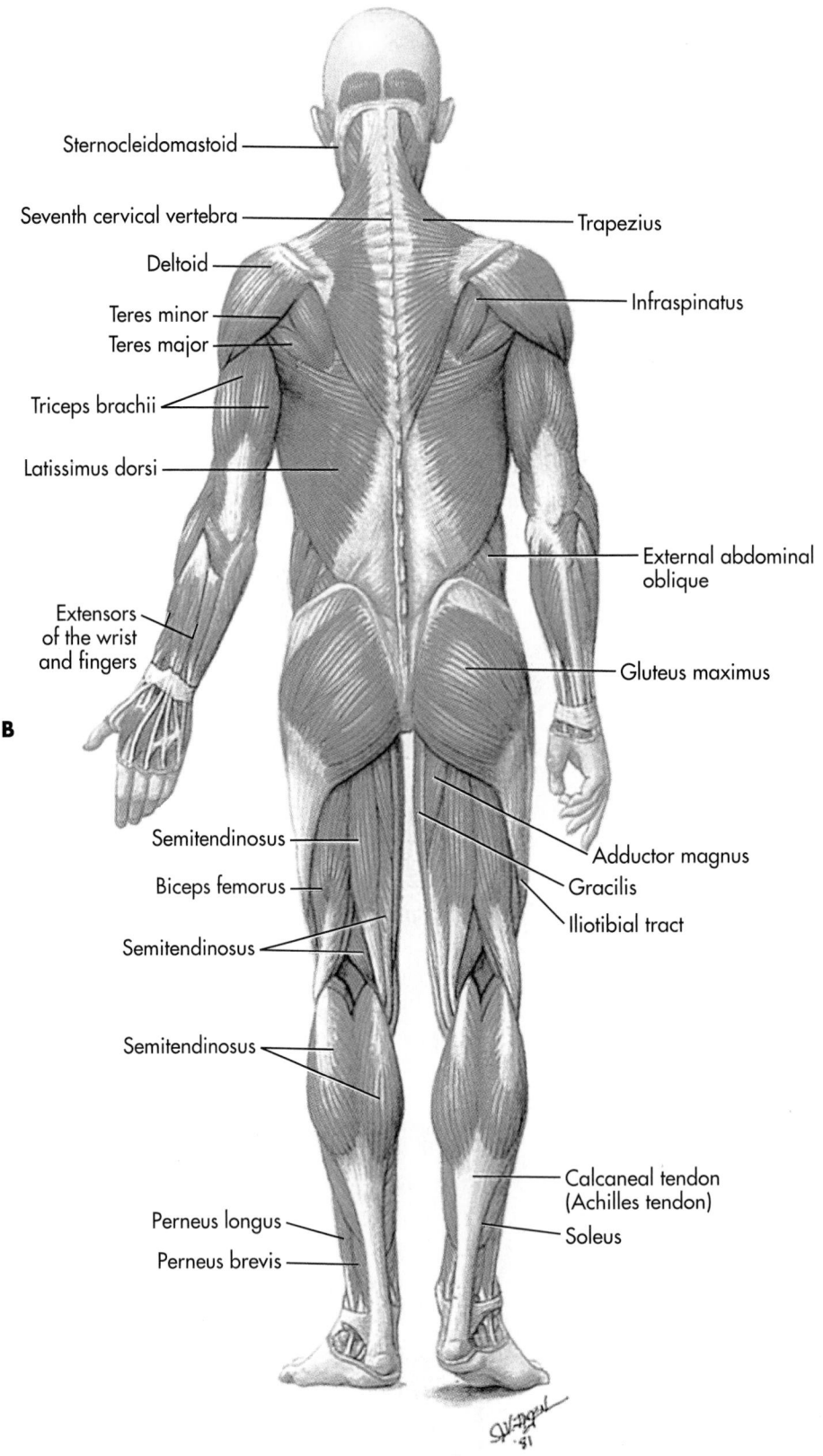

Sternocleidomastoid

Seventh cervical vertebra

Deltoid

Teres minor
Teres major

Triceps brachii

Latissimus dorsi

Extensors
of the wrist
and fingers

B

Semitendinosus

Biceps femorus

Semitendinosus

Semitendinosus

Perneus longus

Perneus brevis

Trapezius

Infraspinatus

External abdominal
oblique

Gluteus maximus

Adductor magnus
Gracilis
Iliotibial tract

Calcaneal tendon
(Achilles tendon)
Soleus

Fig. 6-26, cont'd B, Posterior view of body musculature.

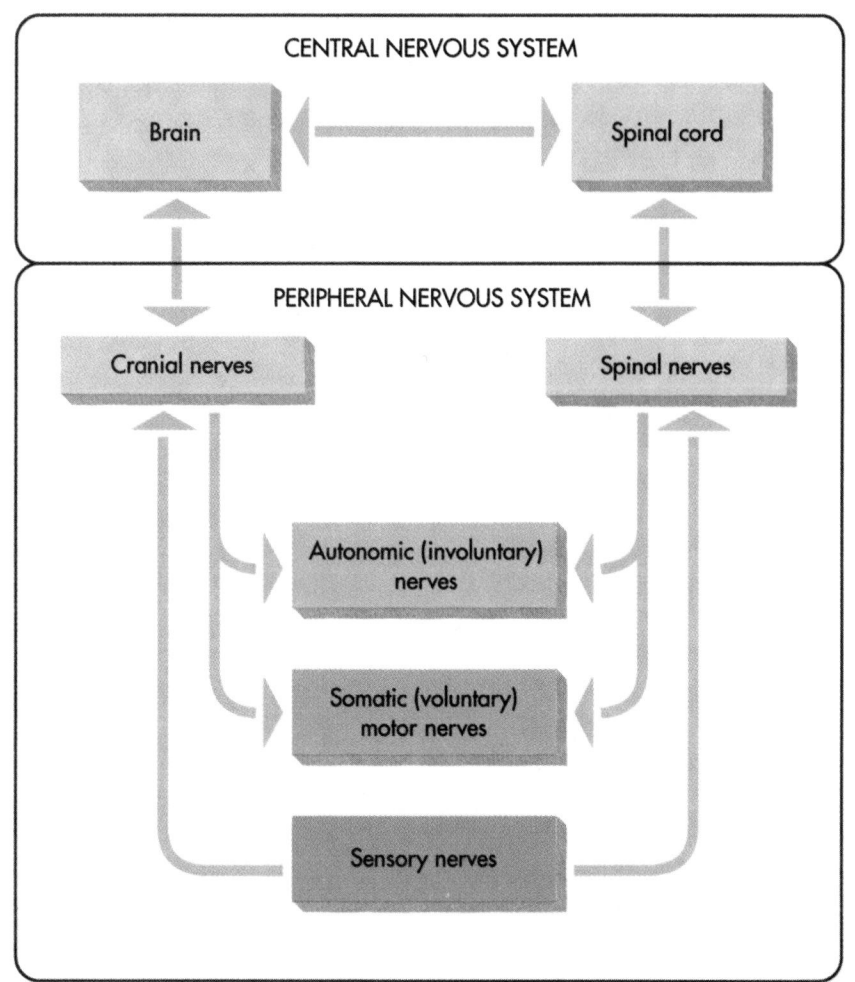

CENTRAL NERVOUS SYSTEM

Brain ⟷ Spinal cord

PERIPHERAL NERVOUS SYSTEM

Cranial nerves   Spinal nerves

Autonomic (involuntary) nerves

Somatic (voluntary) motor nerves

Sensory nerves

Fig. 6-27 Divisions of the nervous system. (From Thibodeau GA: *Structure and function of the body,* ed 9, St Louis, 1992, Mosby.)

diameter, breathing, swallowing, vomiting, coughing, and sneezing, are controlled by the medulla.

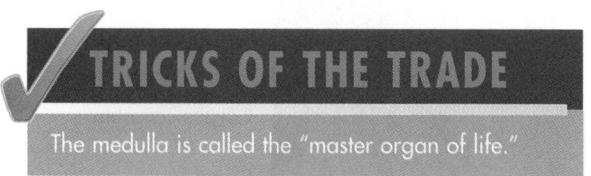

TRICKS OF THE TRADE

The medulla is called the "master organ of life."

The pons contains ascending and descending nerve tracts and relays information from the cerebrum to the cerebellum. In addition, the pons houses the sleep center and respiratory center that, along with the medulla, help control breathing.

The midbrain, or mesencephalon, is the smallest region of the brain stem. It is involved in hearing through audio pathways in the CNS and in visual reflexes such as visual tracking of moving objects and turning of the eyes. Other parts of the midbrain help regulate the automatic functions that require no conscious thought (e.g., coordination of motor activities, muscle tone).

The reticular formation is a group of nuclei scattered throughout the brain stem that receives axons from a large number of sources, especially from the nerves that innervate the face. The reticular formation and its connections are known as the **reticular activating system.** This system is involved in the sleep-wake cycle and is important in arousing and maintaining consciousness. Coma after head injury results from damage to the reticular activating system.

Diencephalon. The diencephalon is the part of the brain between the brain stem and the cerebrum. Major components of this organ include the thalamus

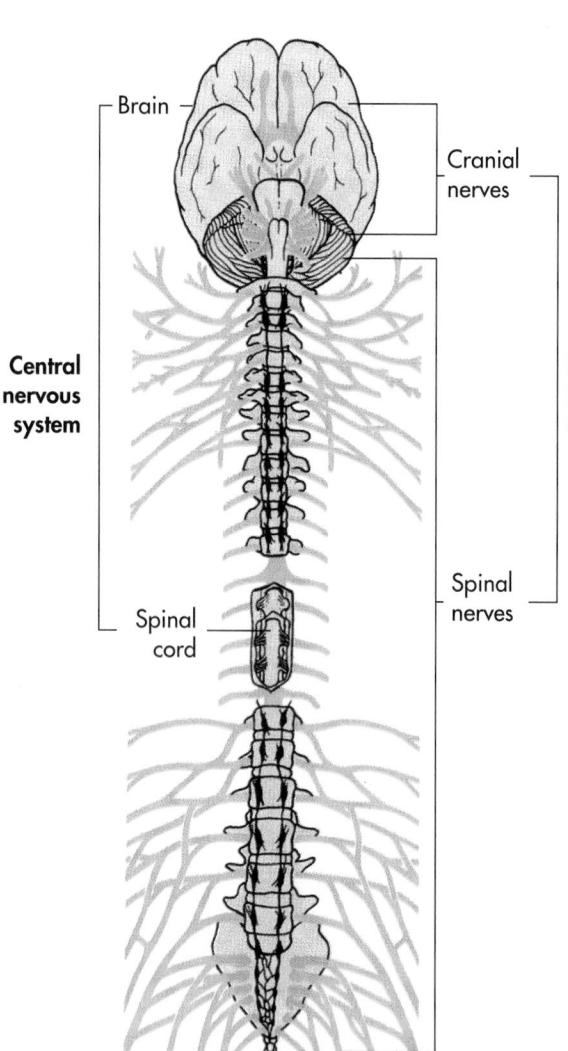

Brain

Cranial
nerves

**Central
nervous
system**

**Peripheral
nervous
system**

Spinal
nerves

Spinal
cord

Fig. 6-28 The central nervous system consists of the brain and spinal cord. The peripheral nervous system consists of cranial nerves, which arise from the brain, and spinal nerves, which arise from the spinal cord.

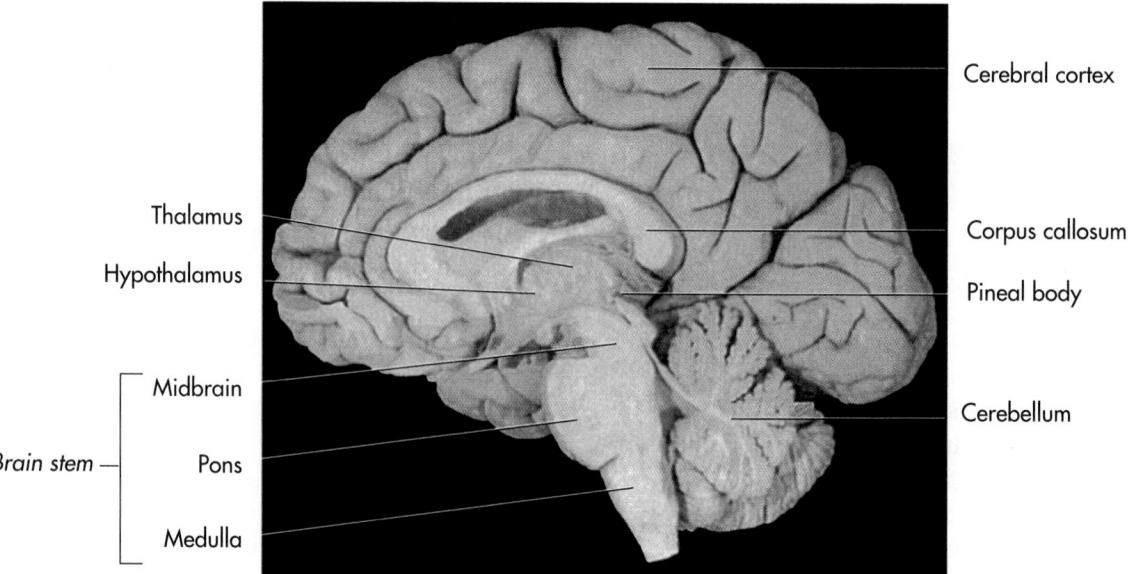

Cerebral cortex

Thalamus

Hypothalamus

Corpus callosum

Pineal body

Brain stem

Midbrain

Pons

Medulla

Cerebellum

Fig. 6-29 Section of preserved brain. (From Thibodeau GA: *Structure and function of the body,* ed 9, St Louis, 1992, Mosby.)

TABLE 6-5	FUNCTIONS OF MAJOR DIVISIONS OF THE BRAIN

BRAIN AREA	FUNCTION
Brain stem	
Medulla	Two-way conduction pathway between the spinal cord and higher brain centers; cardiac, respiratory, and vasomotor control centers
Pons	Two-way conduction pathway between areas of the brain and other regions of the body; influences respiration
Midbrain	Two-way conduction pathway; relay point for visual and auditory impulses
Diencephalon	
Hypothalamus	Regulation of body temperature, water balance, sleep-cycle control, appetite, and sexual arousal
Thalamus	Sensory relay station from various body areas to cerebral cortex; emotions and alerting or arousal mechanisms
Cerebellum	Muscle coordination; maintenance of equilibrium and posture
Cerebrum	Sensory perception, emotions, willed movements, consciousness, and memory

TABLE 6-6	HYPOTHALAMIC FUNCTIONS

FUNCTION	DESCRIPTION
Autonomic	Helps control heart rate, urine release from the bladder, movement of food through the digestive tract, and blood vessel diameter
Endocrine	Helps regulate pituitary gland secretions and influences metabolism, ion balance, sexual development, and sexual functions
Muscle control	Controls muscles involved in swallowing and stimulates shivering in several muscles
Temperature regulation	Promotes heat loss when the hypothalamic temperature increases by increasing sweat production (anterior hypothalamus) and promotes heat production when the hypothalamic temperature decreases by promoting shivering (posterior hypothalamus)
Regulation of food and water intake	Hunger center promotes eating, and satiety center inhibits eating; thirst center promotes water intake
Emotions	Large range of emotional influences over body functions; directly involved in stress-related and psychosomatic illnesses and with feelings of fear and rage
Regulation of the sleep-wake cycle	Coordinates responses to the sleep-wake cycle with other areas of the brain (e.g., the reticular activating system)

and hypothalamus. The thalamus is the largest portion of the diencephalon. The thalamus receives sensory input from various sense organs of the body and relays these impulses to the cerebral cortex. The thalamus also has other functions, such as influencing mood and general body movements associated with strong emotions such as fear or rage.

The hypothalamus is a major controller in the brain. It serves as a "gatekeeper" to determine what information is passed along to the cerebrum and is an active participant in emotions, hormonal cycles, and sexuality. (A summary of the various hypothalamic functions appears in Table 6-6.)

Cerebrum. The cerebrum is the largest portion of the brain. It is divided into left and right hemispheres, and each cerebral hemisphere is divided into lobes named for the bones that lie over them (Fig. 6-30).

The frontal lobe is important in voluntary motor function, motivation, aggression, and mood. The

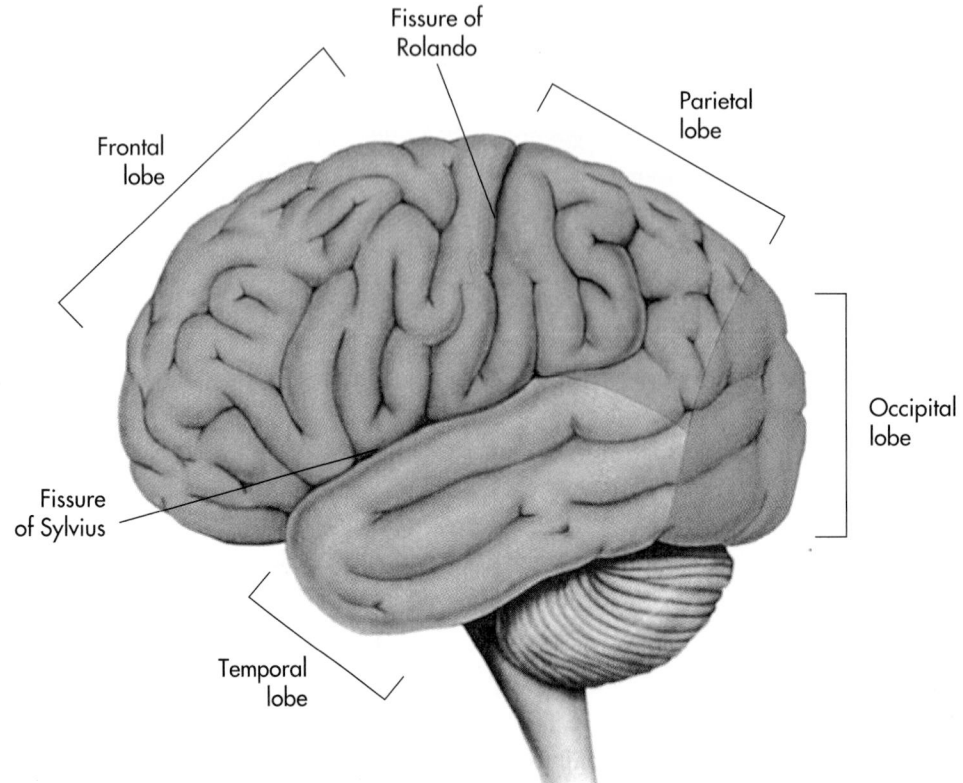

Frontal
lobe

Fissure of
Rolando

Parietal
lobe

Occipital
lobe

Fissure
of Sylvius

Temporal
lobe

Fig. 6-30 Lobes of the cerebrum. (From Thibodeau GA: *Structure and function of the body,* ed 9, St Louis, 1992, Mosby.)

parietal lobe is the major center for the reception and evaluation of most sensory information (excluding smell, hearing, and vision). The occipital lobe functions in the reception and integration of visual input and is not distinctly separate from other lobes. The temporal lobe receives and evaluates olfactory and auditory input and plays an important role in memory. A thin layer of gray matter made up of neuron dendrites and cell bodies composes the surface of the cerebrum (cerebral cortex).

The **limbic system** consists of portions of the cerebrum and diencephalon. It influences emotions, visceral responses to those emotions, motivation, mood, and sensations of pain and pleasure.

? CRITICAL THINKING

An older adult patient has a new onset of staggering gait. What area of the brain do you suspect has altered function?

Cerebellum. The cerebellum is the second largest part of the human brain. It is involved in gross mo-

tor coordination, and the production of smooth, flowing movements. A major function of the cerebellum is to compare impulses from the motor cortex with those from moving structures (e.g., position of the body or body parts that innervate the joints and tendons of the structure being moved). The cerebellum compares the intended movement with the actual movement. If a difference is detected, the cerebellum sends impulses to the motor cortex and the spinal cord to correct the discrepancy. Loss of cerebellum functioning results in an inability to make precise movements.

Spinal cord. The spinal cord lies within the spinal column and extends from the occipital bone to the level of the second lumbar vertebrae. The spinal cord has a central gray portion and a peripheral white portion. The white matter consists of nerve tracts, and the gray matter consists of nerve cell bodies and dendrites. The dorsal root conveys afferent nerve processes to the cord, and the ventral root conveys efferent nerve processes away from the cord. Spinal ganglia, or dorsal root ganglia, contain the cell bodies of sensory neurons (Fig. 6-31).

Spinal cord   Posterior (dorsal) roots

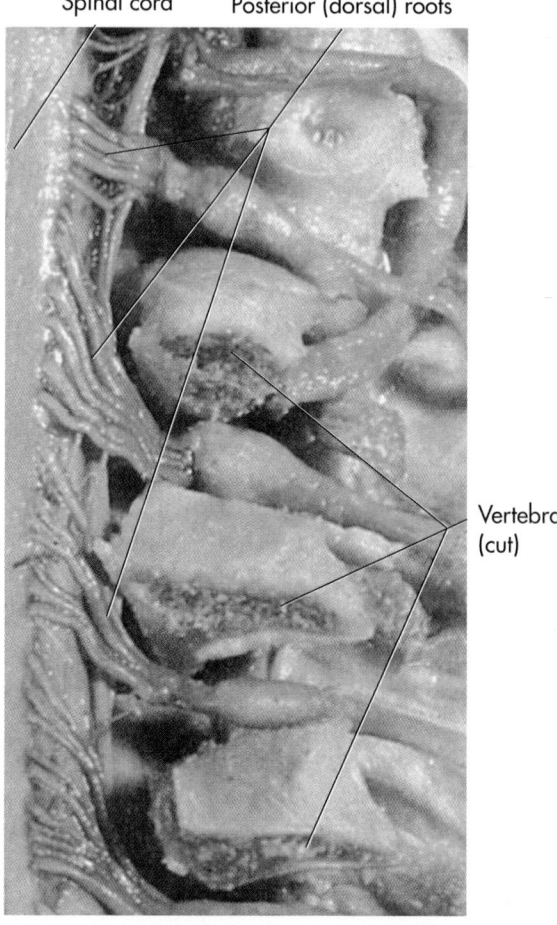

Vertebrae
(cut)

Fig. 6-31 Dissection of the cervical segment of the spinal cord. (From Thibodeau GA: *Structure and function of the body,* ed 9, St Louis, 1992, Mosby.)

The spinal cord is the primary reflex center of the body. Many of these reflexes are autonomic or visceral (e.g., increased heart rate in response to decreased blood pressure). Other reflexes include the stretch reflex ("knee-jerk reflex") and withdrawal reflexes (removing a limb or other body part from a painful stimulus). In addition to functioning as a primary reflex center, the spinal cord tracts carry impulses to the brain in afferent, ascending tracts, and they carry motor impulses from the brain in efferent, descending tracts. (Ascending and descending pathways are further addressed in Chapter 29.)

The organs of the nervous system are surrounded by a tough, fluid-containing membrane known as the meninges. The meninges are surrounded by bone and have three connective tissue layers. The most superficial and thickest layer is the dura mater, consisting of two layers around the brain and one layer around the spinal cord. The two layers of the dura mater are fused around most of the brain but are separate in several places. The dura mater of the brain is tightly attached and continuous with the periosteum of the cranial vault, whereas the dura mater of the spinal cord is separated from the periosteum of the vertebral canal by the epidural space.

The arachnoid layer is the second meningeal layer. The space between this layer and the dura mater is known as the subdural space, which contains a small amount of serous fluid. The third meningeal layer is the pia mater. It lies external to a basement membrane formed by special cells called the *glia limitans*, which completely envelops the CNS. The space between the pia mater and the arachnoid layer is the subarachnoid space. This space is filled with blood vessels and cerebrospinal fluid (CSF) (Fig. 6-32).

The CSF is similar to plasma and interstitial fluid (fluid that occupies the space outside the blood vessels). It serves to bathe the brain and spinal cord and act as a protective cushion around the CNS. Cerebrospinal fluid is formed continually from fluid filtering out of the blood in a network of brain capillaries and cells known collectively as the choroid plexus. This special fluid fills the ventricles of the brain, the subarachnoid space, and the central canal of the spinal cord.

Peripheral nervous system

The PNS collects information from numerous sources, both inside the body and on the body surface. This information is relayed by way of afferent fibers to the CNS, where it is evaluated. Efferent fibers in the PNS relay information from the CNS to various parts of the body, primarily to muscles and glands.

Spinal nerves. The spinal nerves arise from numerous *rootlets* along the dorsal and ventral surfaces of the spinal cord. All of the 31 pairs of spinal nerves, except for the first pair of spinal nerves and the spinal nerves in the sacrum, exit the vertebral column though adjacent vertebrae. The first pair of spinal nerves exits between the skull and the first cervical vertebrae. The spinal nerves in the sacrum exit through the bone. A total of 8 spinal nerve pairs exit the vertebral column in the cervical region, 12 in the thoracic region, 5 in the lumbar region, 5 in the sacral region, and 1 in the coccygeal region (Fig. 6-33).

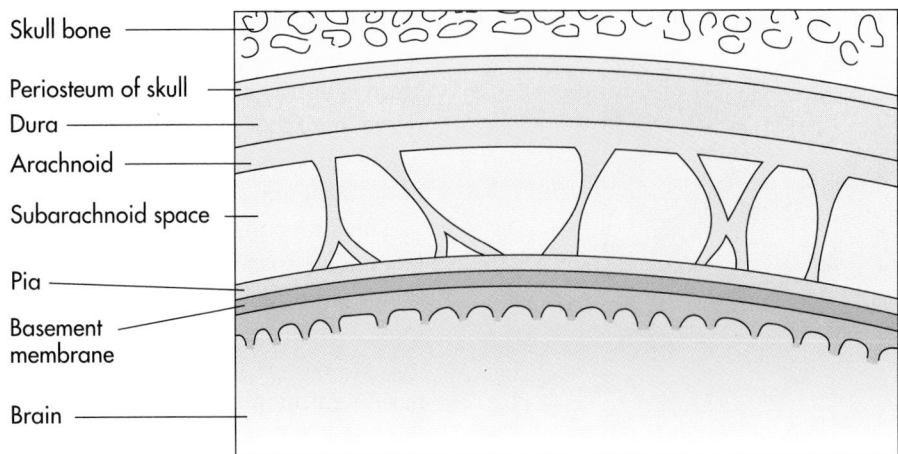

Skull bone

Periosteum of skull

Dura

Arachnoid

Subarachnoid space

Pia

Basement membrane

Brain

Fig. 6-32 Meningeal coverings of the brain and spinal cord.

Each spinal nerve except C1 has a specific cutaneous sensory distribution. Detailed mapping of the skin surface reveals a close relationship between the source on the cord of each spinal nerve and the level of the body it innervates. (An understanding of this relationship is important when examining a patient with a spinal cord injury.) The skin surface areas supplied by a single spinal nerve are known as dermatomes. (A dermatome "map" of the body is illustrated in Fig. 6-34.)

? CRITICAL THINKING

Will the person with a spinal cord injury at the level of C5 have movement in his or her hands?

Cranial nerves. The 12 cranial nerves are divided into three general categories: sensory, somatomotor and proprioception, and parasympathetic. Sensory functions include the special senses, such as vision, and the more general senses, such as touch and pain. Somatomotor functions control the skeletal muscles through motor neurons, and proprioception provides the brain with information about the position of the body and its various parts, including joints and muscles. Parasympathetic function involves the regulation of glands, smooth muscle, and cardiac muscle (functions of the autonomic nervous system). Some cranial nerves have only one of the three functions, whereas others have more than one (Table 6-7). (Fig. 6-35 illustrates the origin of cranial nerves.)

Autonomic nervous system

As previously stated, the PNS is composed of afferent and efferent neurons. Afferent neurons carry action potentials from the periphery to the CNS, and efferent neurons carry action potentials from the CNS to the periphery. Afferent neurons provide information to the CNS that may stimulate both somatomotor and autonomic reflexes. Therefore they cannot be easily divided into functional groups. In contrast, efferent neurons differ structurally and functionally. They can be clearly separated into either the somatomotor nervous system or the autonomic nervous system.

Somatomotor neurons innervate skeletal muscles and play an important role in locomotion, posture, and equilibrium. The movements controlled by the somatomotor nervous system usually are considered to be conscious movements. Their effect on skeletal muscle is always excitatory. Neurons of the autonomic nervous system innervate smooth muscle, cardiac muscle, and glands and usually are unconsciously controlled. The effect of autonomic neurons on their target tissue is either inhibitory or excitatory.

The autonomic nervous system is composed of sympathetic and parasympathetic divisions. Both of these divisions, in turn, consist of autonomic ganglia and nerves. The action potentials in sympa-

? CRITICAL THINKING

What would happen to a person's heart rate if you administer a drug that blocks the action of the parasympathetic nervous system?

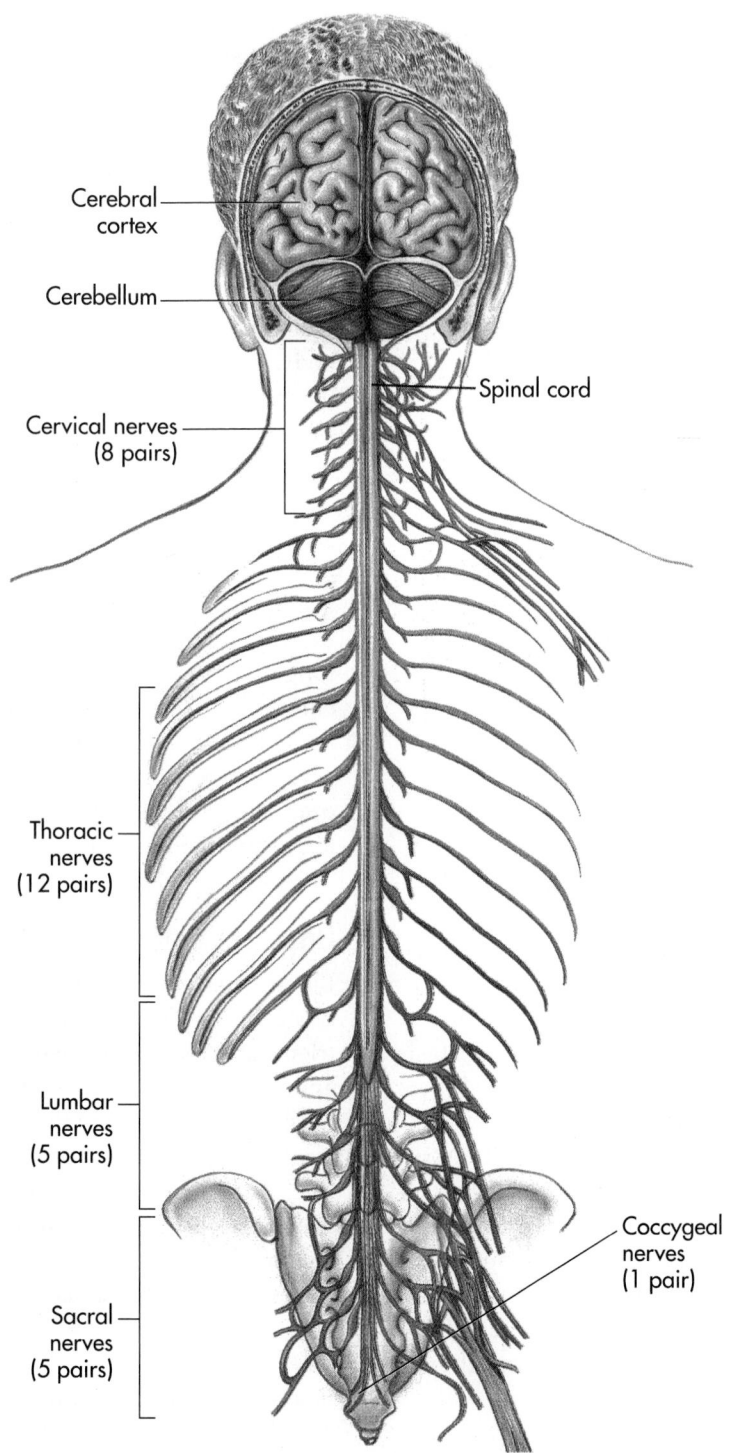

Fig. 6-33 Spinal cord and spinal nerves. (From Thibodeau GA: *Structure and function of the body,* ed 9, St Louis, 1992, Mosby.)

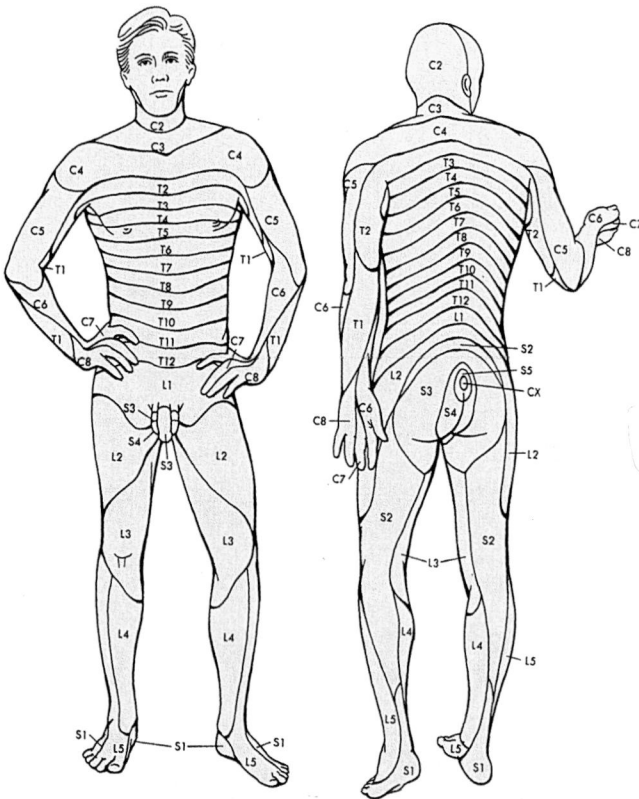

Fig. 6-34 Dermatome map. Letters and numbers indicate the spinal nerves innervating a given region of the skin.

thetic neurons generally prepare an individual for physical activity, whereas parasympathetic stimulation activates vegetative functions such as digestion, defecation, and urination.

The functions of the autonomic nervous system serve to maintain or quickly restore homeostasis (Table 6-8). Many internal organs receive fibers from parasympathetic and sympathetic divisions (Fig. 6-36). Therefore sympathetic and parasympathetic impulses continually bombard them, influencing their function in opposite or antagonistic ways. For example, the heart receives sympathetic impulses that increase the heart rate and parasympathetic impulses that decrease the heart rate. The ratio between these two forces determines the actual heart rate.

Endocrine System

The endocrine system is composed of glands that secrete hormones into the circulatory system (Fig. 6-37). The endocrine and nervous systems have a signifi-

cant amount of functional and anatomical overlap. Some neurons secrete regulatory chemicals (neurohormones) that function as hormones, such as antidiuretic hormone (ADH), into the circulatory system. Other neurons innervate endocrine glands and influence their secretory activity. Conversely, some hormones secreted by the endocrine glands affect the nervous system.

Hormones, including neurohormones, are classified as proteins, polypeptides, derivatives of amino acids, or lipids. Lipid hormones are either steroids or derivatives of fatty acids. Hormones are dissolved in blood plasma and quickly distributed throughout the body. In general, the amount of hormone that reaches the target tissue directly correlates with the concentration of the hormone in the blood. (Table 6-9 lists endocrine glands, hormones, and their functions.)

Some hormones are present in relatively constant levels in the circulatory system; others change suddenly in response to certain stimuli; still others change in relatively constant cycles. For example, thyroid hormones in the blood vary within a small range of concentrations, so their concentration is chronically maintained. Epinephrine is released in large amounts in response to stress or physical exercise, so its concentration changes acutely. Reproductive hormones increase and decrease in cyclic fashion in women during their reproductive years.

Circulatory System

Blood vessels extend throughout the body, carrying blood to and from all tissues. Blood transports nutrients and oxygen to tissues, carries carbon dioxide and waste products away from tissues, and carries hormones produced in the endocrine glands to their target tissues. In addition, blood plays an important role in temperature regulation and fluid balance and protects the body from bacteria and foreign substances. These and other functions of blood help to maintain homeostasis.

Blood Components

Blood is a special form of connective tissue consisting of cells and cell fragments (formed elements) surrounded by a liquid intercellular matrix (plasma). About 95% of the volume of formed elements consists of RBCs (erythrocytes). The remaining 5% consists of white blood cells (leukocytes) and cell fragments called platelets.

TABLE 6-7		CRANIAL NERVES	
	NERVE	**CONDUCTS IMPULSES**	**FUNCTIONS**
I	Olfactory	From nose to brain	Sense of smell
II	Optic	From eye to brain	Vision
III	Oculomotor	From brain to eye muscles	Eye movements
IV	Trochlear	From brain to external eye muscles	Eye movements
V	Trigeminal	From skin and mucous membranes of head and from teeth to brain; also from brain to chewing muscles	Sensations of face, scalp, and teeth; chewing movements
VI	Abducens	From brain to external eye muscles	Turning eyes outward
VII	Facial	From taste buds of tongue to brain; from brain to face muscles	Sense of taste; contraction of muscles of facial expressions
VIII	Acoustic	From ear to brain	Hearing; sense of balance
IX	Glossopharyngeal	From throat and taste buds of tongue to brain; also from brain to throat muscles and salivary glands	Sensation of throat, taste, swallowing movements; secretion of saliva
X	Vagus	From throat, larynx, and organs in thoracic and abdominal cavities to brain; also from brain to muscles of throat and to organs in thoracic and abdominal cavities	Sensations of throat and larynx and of thoracic and abdominal organs; swallowing, voice production, slowing of heartbeat, acceleration of peristalsis
XI	Spinal accessory	From brain to certain shoulder and neck muscles	Shoulder movements, turning movements of head
XII	Hypoglossal	From brain to muscles of tongue	Tongue movements

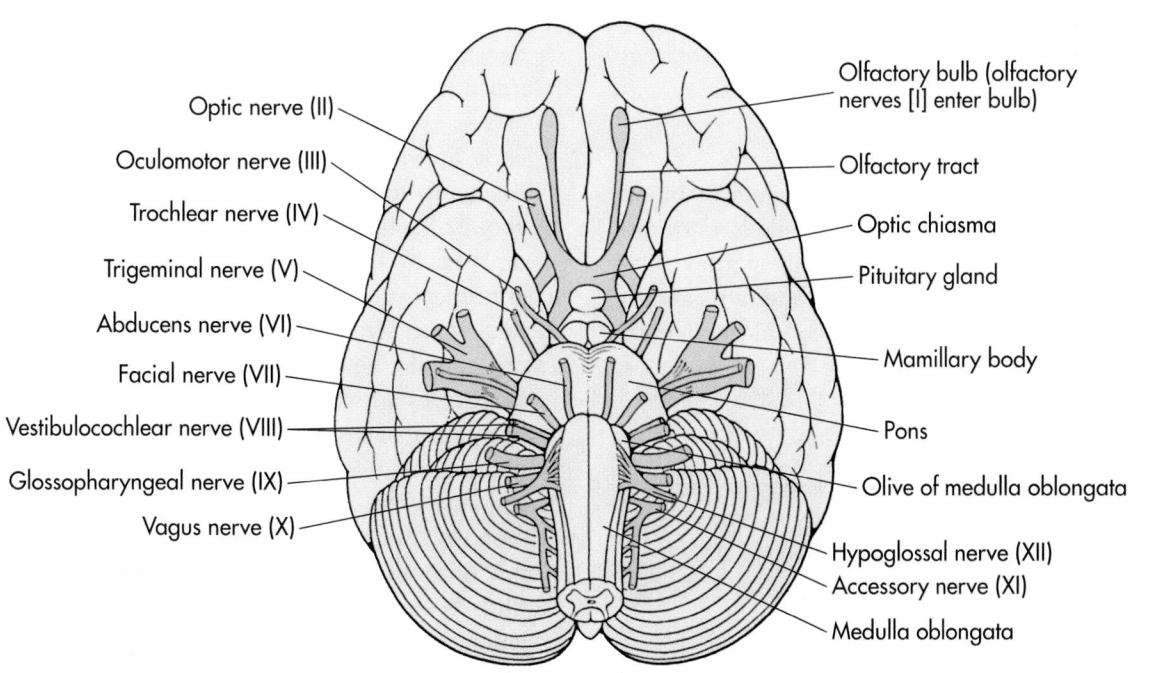

Fig. 6-35 Origin of cranial nerves.

TABLE 6-8   FUNCTIONS OF THE AUTONOMIC NERVOUS SYSTEM

VISCERAL EFFECTORS	SYMPATHETIC CONTROL	PARASYMPATHETIC CONTROL
Heart muscle	Accelerates heartbeat	Slows heartbeat
Smooth muscle		
Of most blood vessels	Constricts blood vessels	None
Of blood vessels in skeletal muscles	Dilates blood vessels	None
Of the digestive tract	Decreases peristalsis; inhibits defecation	Increases peristalsis
Of the anal sphincter	Stimulates—closes sphincter	Inhibits—opens sphincter for defecation
Of the urinary bladder	Inhibits—relaxes bladder	Stimulates—contracts bladder
Of the urinary sphincters	Stimulates—closes sphincter	Inhibits—opens sphincter for urination
Of the eye		
Iris	Stimulates radial fibers—dilation of pupil	Stimulates circular fibers—constriction of pupil
Ciliary	Inhibits—accommodation for far vision (flattening of lens)	Stimulates—accommodation for near vision (bulging of lens)
Of hairs (pilomotor muscles)	Stimulates—"goose bumps"	No parasympathetic fibers
Glands		
Adrenal medulla	Increases epinephrine secretion	None
Sweat glands	Increase sweat secretion	None
Digestive glands	Decrease secretion of digestive juices	Increase secretion of digestive juices

Plasma

Plasma is a pale yellow fluid composed of about 92% water and 8% dissolved or suspended molecules. Plasma contains proteins such as albumin, globulins, and fibrinogen. When the proteins that produce clots are removed from the plasma, the remaining fluid is called serum.

Formed elements Three formed elements of blood are erythrocytes, leukocytes, and platelets, or thrombocytes (cell fragments) (Table 6-10). Formed elements are produced in the embryo and fetus and in tissues such as the liver, thymus, spleen, lymph nodes, and red bone marrow.

? CRITICAL THINKING

If the number of erythrocytes drops, a person may become short of breath during mild exertion. Why will this happen?

1. Erythrocytes are the most numerous of the formed elements. There are about 5.2 million erythrocytes in one drop of male blood and about 4.5 million in one drop of female blood. The major erythrocyte contents include lipids, ATP, and the enzyme carbonic anhydrase. The main component of erythrocytes is hemoglobin, the protein that gives blood its red color. The primary functions of erythrocytes are to transport oxygen from the lungs to the various tissues of the body and to transport carbon dioxide from the tissues to the lungs. Under normal conditions, about 2.5 million erythrocytes are destroyed and replaced by the body each second. The average erythrocyte circulates for 120 days.

2. Leukocytes are clear white blood cells that do not contain hemoglobin. The several types of leukocytes are all involved in protecting the body against invading microorganisms and removing dead cells and debris. Some leukocytes are classified according to their appearance, based on the presence or absence of cytoplasmic granules. Classifications include neutrophils, eosinophils, and basophils. Other types of leukocytes are nongranular and are named according to nuclear morphology and major site of proliferation. These include lymphocytes and monocytes.

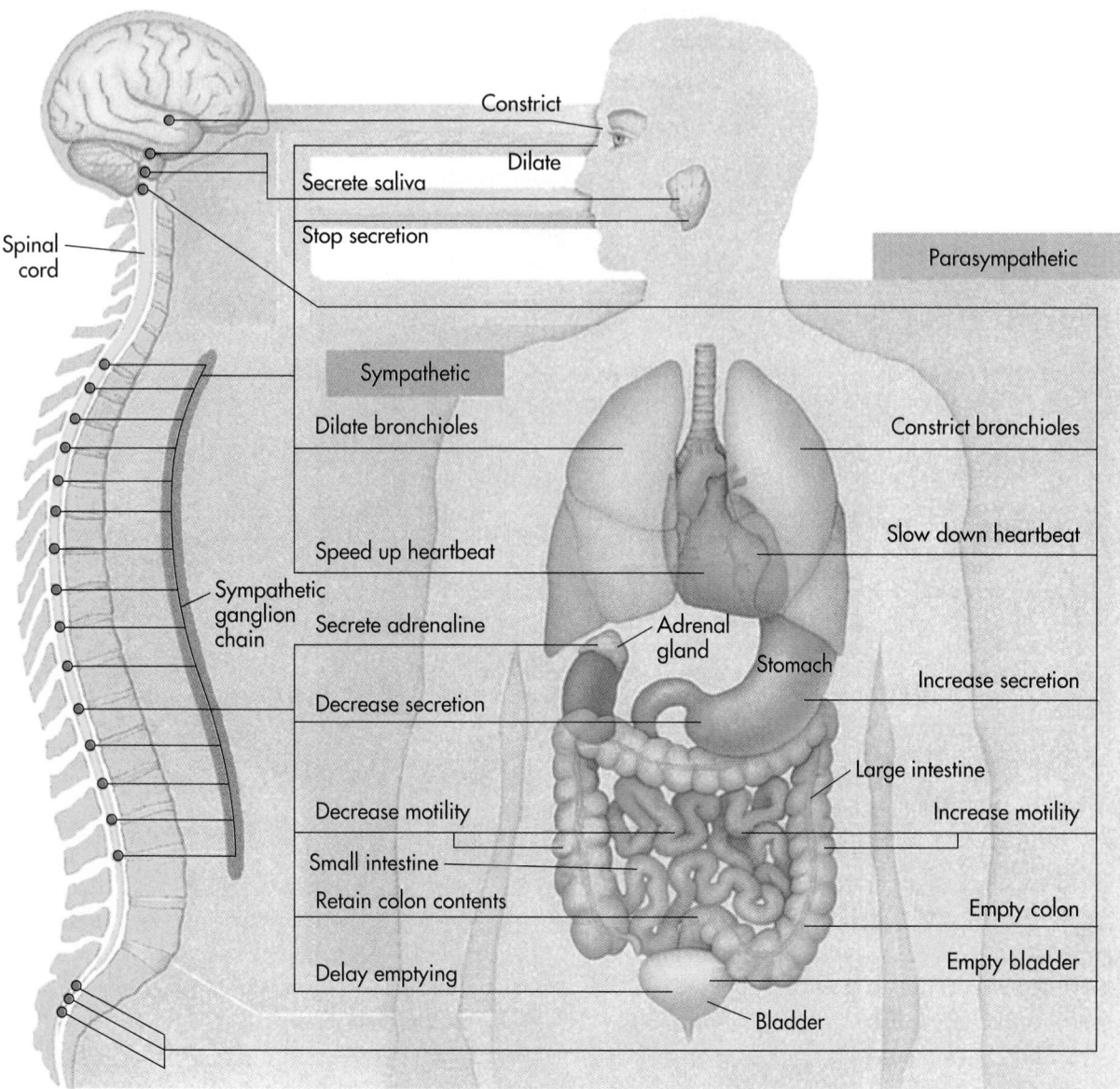

Fig. 6-36 Innervation of major target organs by the ANS. The sympathetic fibers are highlighted with red, and the parasympathetic are highlighted with blue. (From Thibodeau GA: *Structure and function of the body,* ed 9, St Louis, 1992, Mosby.)

Neutrophils are the most common type of leukocyte in the blood. These cells normally remain in the circulation for 10 to 12 hours, after which they move into tissue to seek out and destroy bacteria and other foreign matter (phagocytosis). They also secrete lysosomes that can destroy certain bacteria. Neutrophils usually survive for 1 to 2 days after leaving the circulation.

Eosinophils leave the circulation to enter the tissues during an inflammatory reaction. Their numbers usually are elevated in the blood of people who have allergies and certain parasitic infections. Although these cells have phagocytic properties, they are not thought to be as important in this function as neutrophils.

Basophils are the least common of all leukocytes. Like eosinophils, basophils leave the circulation and migrate through tissues to play a role in allergic and inflammatory reactions. They also release heparin, which inhibits blood clotting.

Lymphocytes are the smallest of all leukocytes and are capable of migrating through the cytoplasm of other cells. The many different types of lymphocytes play a major role in immunity,

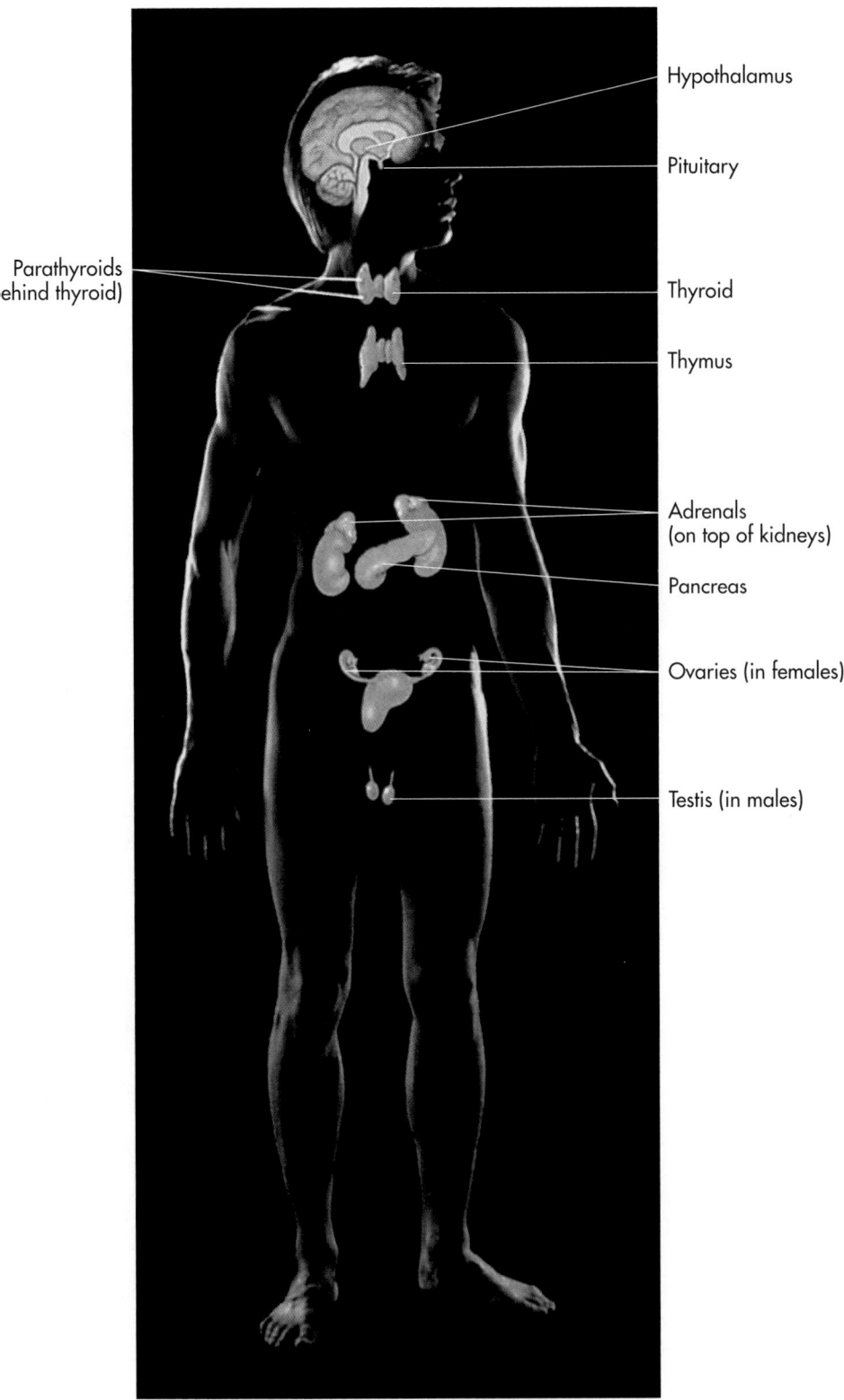

Fig. 6-37 Endocrine system.

TABLE 6-9	ENDOCRINE GLANDS, HORMONES, AND THEIR FUNCTIONS

GLAND/HORMONE	FUNCTION
Anterior Pituitary	
Thyroid-stimulating hormone (TSH)	Tropic hormone Stimulates secretion of thyroid hormones
Adrenocorticotropic hormone (ACTH)	Tropic hormone Stimulates secretion of adrenal cortex hormones
Follicle-stimulating hormone (FSH)	Tropic hormone *Female:* stimulates development of ovarian follicles and secretion of estrogens *Male:* stimulates seminiferous tubules of testes to grow and produce sperm
Luteinizing hormone (LH)	Tropic hormone *Female:* stimulates maturation of ovarian follicle and ovum; stimulates secretion of estrogen; triggers ovulation; stimulates development of corpus luteum (luteinization) *Male:* stimulates interstitial cells of the testes to secrete testosterone
Melanocyte-stimulating hormone (MSH)	Stimulates synthesis and dispersion of melanin pigment in the skin
Growth hormone (GH)	Stimulates growth in all organs; mobilizes food molecules, causing an increase in blood glucose concentration
Prolactin (lactogenic hormone)	Stimulates breast development during pregnancy and milk secretion after pregnancy
Posterior Pituitary*	
Antidiuretic hormone (ADH)	Stimulates retention of water by the kidneys
Oxytocin	Stimulates uterine contractions at the end of pregnancy; stimulates the release of milk into the breast ducts
Hypothalamus	
Releasing hormones (several)	Stimulate the anterior pituitary to release hormones
Inhibiting hormones (several)	Inhibit the anterior pituitary's secretion of hormones
Thyroid	
Thyroxine (T_4), triiodothyronine (T_3)	Stimulate the energy metabolism of all cells
Calcitonin	Inhibits the breakdown of bone; causes a decrease in blood calcium concentration
Parathyroid	
Parathyroid hormone (PTH)	Stimulates the breakdown of bone; causes an increase in blood calcium concentration
Adrenal Cortex	
Mineralocorticoids: aldosterone	Regulate electrolyte and fluid homeostasis
Glucocorticoids: cortisol (hydrocortisone)	Stimulate gluconeogenesis, causing an increase in blood glucose concentration; also have antiinflammatory, antiimmunity, and antiallergy effects
Sex hormones (androgens)	Stimulate sexual drive in the female but have negligible effects in the male
Adrenal Medulla	
Epinephrine (adrenaline), norepinephrine	Prolong and intensify the sympathetic nervous response during stress
Pancreatic Islets	
Glucagon	Stimulates liver glycogenolysis, causing an increase in blood glucose concentration
Insulin	Promotes glucose entry into all cells, causing a decrease in blood glucose concentration

*Posterior pituitary hormones are synthesized in the hypothalamus but released from axon terminals in the posterior pituitary.

TABLE 6-9	ENDOCRINE GLANDS, HORMONES, AND THEIR FUNCTIONS—cont'd
GLAND/HORMONE	**FUNCTION**
Ovary	
Estrogens	Promotes development and maintenance of female sexual characteristics
Progesterone	Promotes conditions required for pregnancy
Testis	
Testosterone	Promotes development and maintenance of male sexual characteristics
Thymus	
Thymosin	Promotes development of immune-system cells
Placenta	
Chorionic gonadotropin, estrogens, progesterone	Promote conditions required during early pregnancy
Pineal	
Melatonin	Inhibits tropic hormones that affect the ovaries; may be involved with the body's internal clock
Heart (atria)	
Atrial natriuretic hormone (ANH)	Regulates fluid and electrolyte homeostasis

including antibody production. Lymphocytes originate in bone marrow and are most abundant in lymphoid tissues: the lymph nodes, spleen, tonsils, lymph nodules, and thymus.

Monocytes are the largest of the leukocytes. They remain in the circulation for about 3 days before transforming into macrophages, large "eating" cells that migrate through various tissues. An increase in the number of monocytes is common in patients with chronic infections.

3. Platelets are produced within bone marrow and are 40 times as common in blood as leukocytes. Platelets play an important role in preventing blood loss by forming "plugs" that seal holes in small vessels and by forming clots that seal off larger wounds in the vessels.

Cardiovascular System

The heart and cardiovascular system are responsible for circulating blood throughout the body. (The cardiovascular system is discussed more thoroughly in Chapters 19 and 28.)

Anatomy of the heart

The heart is a muscular pump consisting of four chambers: two atria and two ventricles. The adult heart is shaped like a blunt cone and is about the size of a closed fist. It is located in the medi-astinum of the thoracic cavity in the pericardial cavity. The blunt, rounded point of the heart is the apex, and the larger, flat portion at the opposite end is the base.

The heart lies obliquely in the mediastinum, with the base directed posteriorly and slightly superiorly. The apex is directed anteriorly and slightly inferiorly. Two thirds of the heart's mass lies to the left of the midline of the sternum (Figs. 6-38 and 6-39).

Pericardium. The pericardium, or the pericardial sac, has a fibrous outer layer (fibrous pericardium) and a thin inner layer (serous pericardium) that surrounds the heart. The portion of the serous pericardium that lines the fibrous pericardium is the parietal pericardium; the portion that covers the heart surface is the visceral pericardium or the epicardium. The cavity between the parietal pericardium and the visceral pericardium normally contains a small amount of pericardial fluid that reduces friction as the heart moves within the pericardial sac.

? CRITICAL THINKING

Why would a sudden increase in the amount of pericardial fluid be harmful?

TABLE 6-10	CLASSES OF BLOOD CELLS
BLOOD CELL	**FUNCTION**
Erythrocyte	Oxygen and carbon dioxide transport
Neutrophil	Immune defenses (phagocytosis)
Eosinophil	Defense against parasites
Basophil	Inflammatory response
B lymphocyte	Antibody production (precursor of plasma cells)
T lymphocyte	Cellular immune response
Monocyte	Immune defenses (phagocytosis)
Platelet	Blood clotting

Coronary vessels. Seven large veins normally carry blood to the heart: four pulmonary veins carry blood from the lungs to the left atrium, the superior and inferior venae cavae carry blood from the body to the right atrium, and the coronary sinus carries blood from the walls of the heart to the right atrium. Two arteries, the aorta and pulmonary trunk, exit the heart. The aorta carries blood from the left ventricle to the body, and the pulmonary trunk carries blood from the right ventricle to the lungs. The right and left coronary arteries exit the aorta near the point where the aorta leaves the heart and supply the heart muscle with oxygen and nutrients (Fig. 6-40).

Heart chambers and valves. The right and left chambers of the heart are separated by a septum. The *interatrial septum* separates the right and left atria, and the *interventricular septum* separates the two ventricles. The atria open into the ventricles through the *atrioventricular canals.* An atrioventricular valve on each atrioventricular canal is composed of cusps or flaps. These valves allow blood to flow from the atria into the ventricles but prevent blood from flowing back into the atria. The atrioventricular valve between the right atrium and right ventricle has three cusps and is called the tricuspid valve. The atrioventricular valve between the left atrium and left ventricle has two cusps and is called the bicuspid, or mitral, valve.

The aorta and pulmonary trunk possess aortic and pulmonary semilunar valves, which meet in the center of the artery to block blood flow. Blood flowing out of the ventricles pushes against each valve, forcing it open, but when blood flows back from the aorta or pulmonary trunk toward the ventricles, the valves close.

Conduction system of the heart

The heart's specialized muscle tissue has the unique capability for spontaneous, rhythmic self-excitation by way of four specialized structures embedded in the wall of the heart. These structures are the sinoatrial node (SA node), the atrioventricular node (AV node), the bundle of His, and the Purkinje fibers (Fig. 6-41).

An impulse conduction normally begins in the SA node. From there it spreads in all directions through both of the atria, causing an atrial contraction. As the electrical impulses reach the AV node, they are relayed to the ventricles through the bundle of His and the Purkinje fibers. This impulse conduction causes both of the ventricles to contract shortly after the atrial contraction.

Route of blood flow through the heart

This text presents blood flow through the heart with a discussion of right heart and left heart circulation (Fig. 6-42). It is important to remember that both atria contract at the same time, followed shortly thereafter by essentially simultaneous contraction

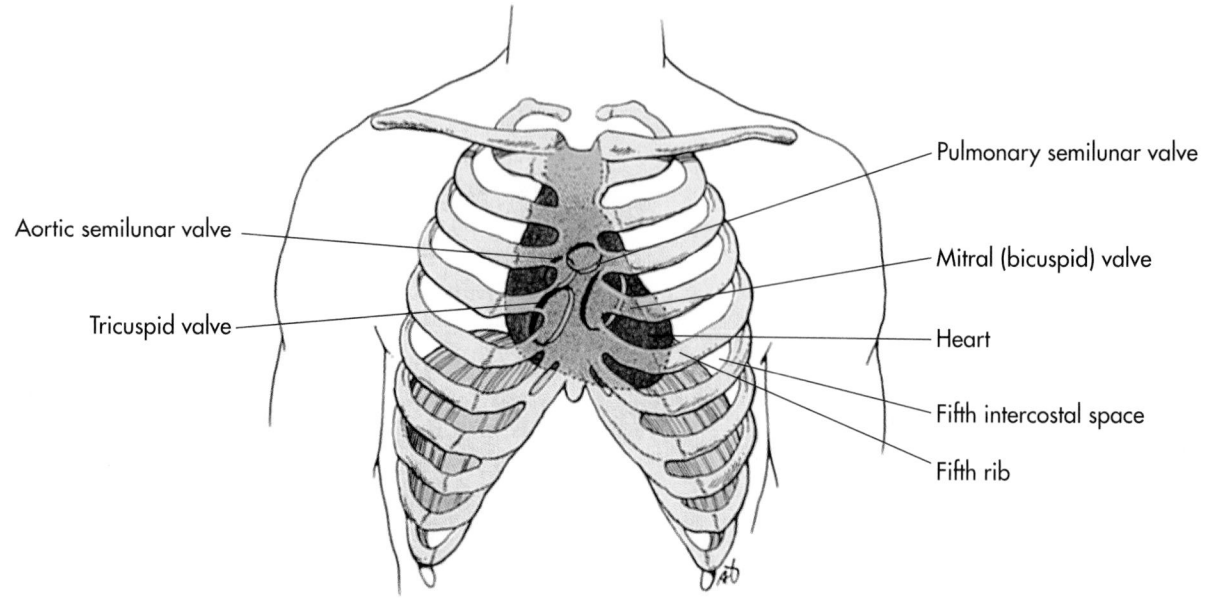

Fig. 6-38 Location of the heart in the thorax.

of both ventricles, to clearly understand electrical impulses of the heart, pressure changes, and heart sounds, which are discussed in other chapters.

? CRITICAL THINKING

A clot forms in the right atria of the heart. Will it be circulated to the extremities? Why?

Blood enters the right atrium from the systemic circulation via the inferior and superior venae cavae and from the heart via the coronary sinus. Most of this blood passes into the right ventricle as the ventricle relaxes after the previous contraction. When the right atrium contracts, the blood remaining in the atrium is pushed into the ventricle. The contraction of the right ventricle pushes blood against the tricuspid valve, forcing it closed, and against the pulmonary semilunar valve, forcing it open. This flow allows blood to enter the pulmonary trunk. The pulmonary trunk divides into left and right pulmonary arteries that carry blood to the lungs, where carbon dioxide is released and oxygen is picked up.

Blood returning from the lungs enters the left atrium through four pulmonary veins. The blood passing from the left atrium to the relaxed left ventricle opens the bicuspid valve. The contraction of the left atrium completes the filling of the left ventricle.

Contraction of the left ventricle pushes blood against the bicuspid valve, closing it. The pressure of the blood against the aortic semilunar valve causes it to open, allowing blood to enter the aorta. Blood flowing through the aorta is distributed to all parts of the body except for the pulmonary vessels in the lungs.

Peripheral Circulation

Blood is pumped from the ventricles of the heart into large elastic arteries, which branch repeatedly to form many progressively smaller arteries. As these vessels become smaller, the amount of elastic tissue in the arterial wall decreases, and the amount of smooth muscle increases.

Blood flows from the arterioles into **capillaries** and from capillaries into the venous system. Compared with artery walls, vein walls are thinner and contain less elastic tissue and fewer smooth muscle cells. As veins approach the heart, the walls increase in diameter and thickness.

Capillary network

Arterioles supply blood to each capillary network (Fig. 6-43). Blood flows through this network and into the venules. The ends of the capillaries closest

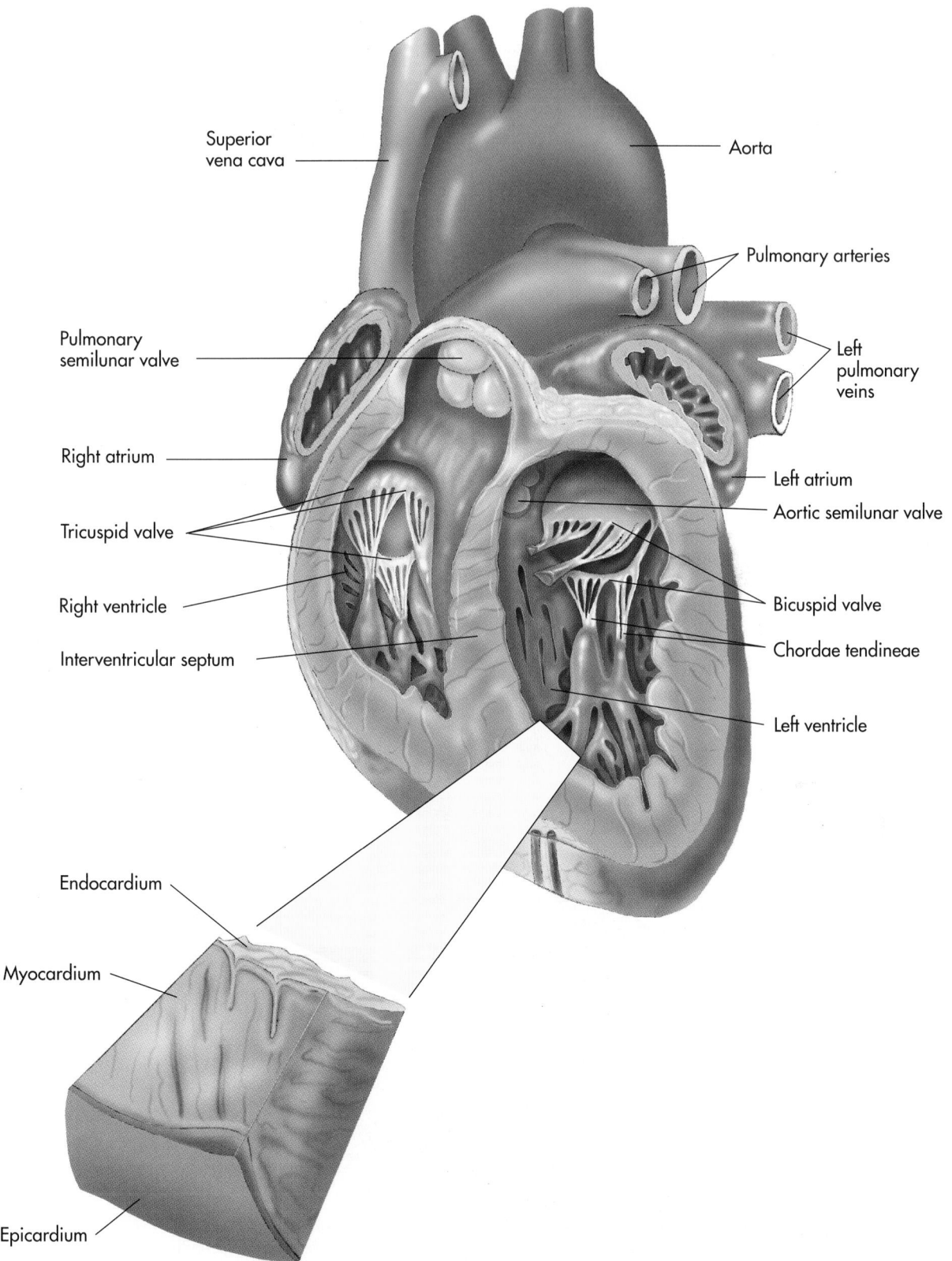

Fig. 6-39 Internal view of the heart.

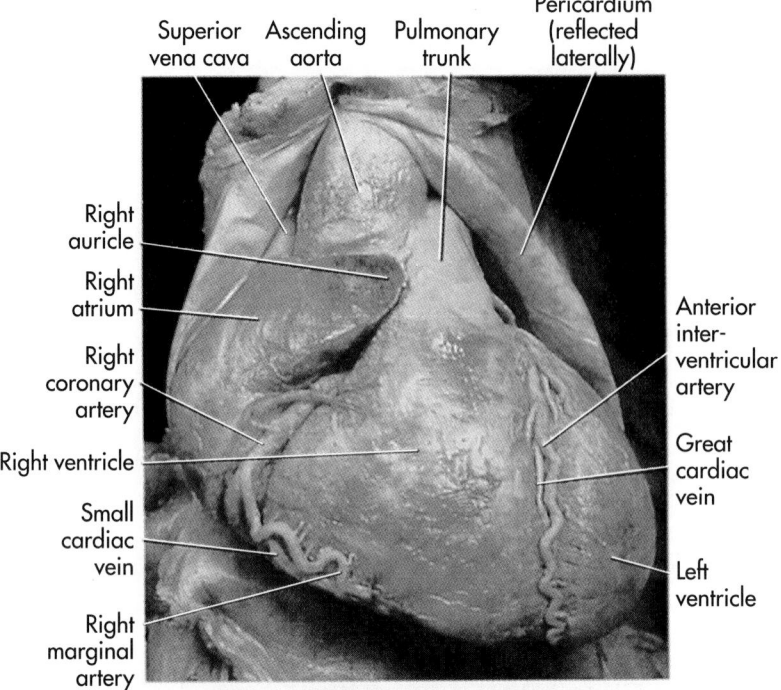

Fig. 6-40 Anterior surface of the heart.

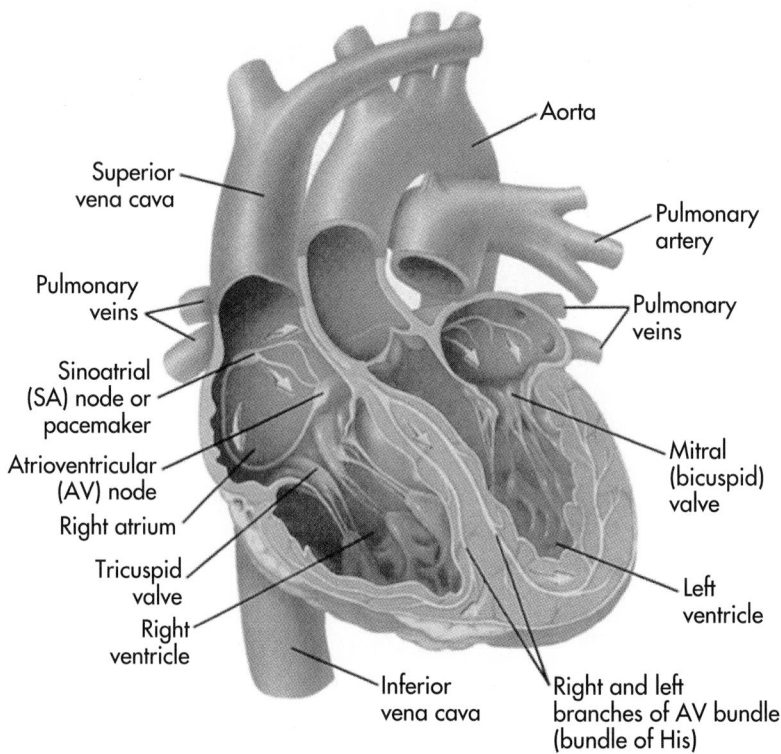

Fig. 6-41 Conduction system of the heart. (From Thibodeau GA: *Structure and function of the body,* ed 9, St Louis, 1992, Mosby.)

Normal blood flow

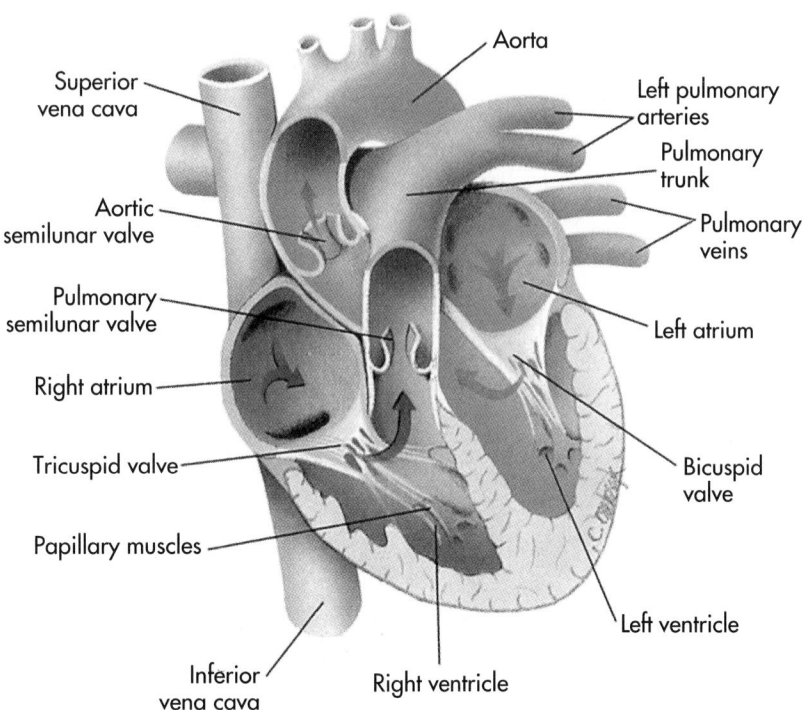

Fig. 6-42 Frontal section of the heart revealing the four chambers and direction of blood flow through the heart.

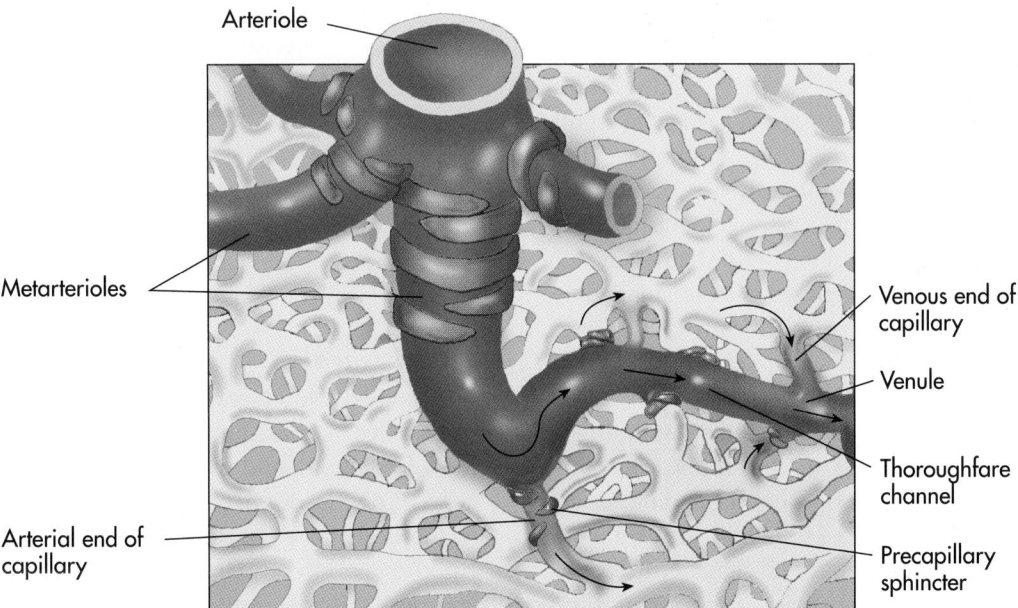

Fig. 6-43 Capillary network. The metarteriole, giving rise to the network, feeds directly from the arteriole into the thoroughfare channel, which feeds into the venule. The network forms numerous branches that transport blood from the thoroughfare channel and may return to the thoroughfare channel.

to arterioles are arterial capillaries; the ends closest to venules are venous capillaries.

Blood flow through arterioles may continue through metarterioles and into a thoroughfare channel to a venule in a relatively constant way, or it may enter the capillary circulation. Flow in the capillaries is regulated by smooth muscle cells known as precapillary sphincters. Nutrient and product waste exchange is the major function of capillaries.

> **NOTE**
>
> This *shunting* process may effectively bypass tissues when capillaries are closed and thoroughfare channels are open.

Arteries and veins

With the exception of capillaries and venules, blood vessel walls are composed of three distinct layers (tunics) of elastic tissue and smooth muscle: the tunica intima (inner layer), the tunica media (middle layer), and the tunica adventitia (outer layer). The thickness and composition of each layer vary with the type and diameter of the blood vessel.

Large elastic arteries are often called *conducting arteries* because they are the arteries largest in diameter. These vessels have more elastic tissue and less smooth muscle than other arteries. Medium-sized and small arteries have relatively thick muscular walls and well-developed elastic membranes. These vessels are called *distributing arteries* because the smooth muscle allows these vessels to partially regulate blood supply to various body regions by constriction or dilation. Arterioles are the smallest arteries in which the three tunics can be identified. Like small arteries, arterioles are capable of vasodilation and vasoconstriction.

Venules have only a few isolated smooth muscle cells and are very similar in structure to the capillaries. Venules collect blood from the capillaries and transport it to small veins, which in turn transport the blood to the medium-sized veins. Nutrient exchange occurs across the walls of the venules, but as the small veins increase in thickness, the degree of nutrient exchange decreases.

As venules increase in diameter, the vessels become veins, whose walls are a continuous layer of smooth muscle cells. Medium-sized and large veins

collect blood from small veins and deliver it to the large venous trunks. Large veins transport blood from the medium-sized veins to the heart.

Veins with large diameters have valves that allow blood to flow to but not from the heart. There are many valves in medium-sized veins, and more valves in the veins of the lower extremities than of the upper extremities. They help prevent the backflow of blood, especially in dependent tissues.

Arteriovenous anastomoses (AV shunts) allow blood to flow from arteries to veins without passing through capillaries. Natural AV shunts occur in large numbers in the sole of the foot, palm, and nail bed, where they regulate body temperature. Pathological shunts can result from injury or tumors and cause a direct flow of blood from arteries to veins. Severe shunts may lead to "high output" heart failure from increased venous return to the heart and its resultant demand on cardiac output.

Pulmonary Circulation

Blood from the right ventricle is pumped into the pulmonary trunk, which bifurcates into the right and left pulmonary arteries (which transport blood to the respective lungs). After the exchange of oxygen and carbon dioxide, two pulmonary veins exit each lung and enter the left atrium.

> **TRICKS OF THE TRADE**
>
> Pulmonary veins are the only veins in the body that carry oxygenated blood, and pulmonary arteries are the only arteries in the body that carry deoxygenated blood.

Systemic Circulation

Oxygenated blood enters the heart from the pulmonary veins, passing through the left atrium into the left ventricle and from the left ventricle into the aorta. From the aorta, blood is distributed to all parts of the body. The arteries of systemic circulation include the aorta, coronary arteries, arteries of the head and neck, arteries of the upper and lower limbs, the thoracic aorta and its branches, the abdominal aorta and its branches, and arteries of the pelvis (Fig. 6-44).

The veins of systemic circulation include coronary veins, veins of the head and neck, veins of the upper and lower limbs, veins of the thorax, veins of

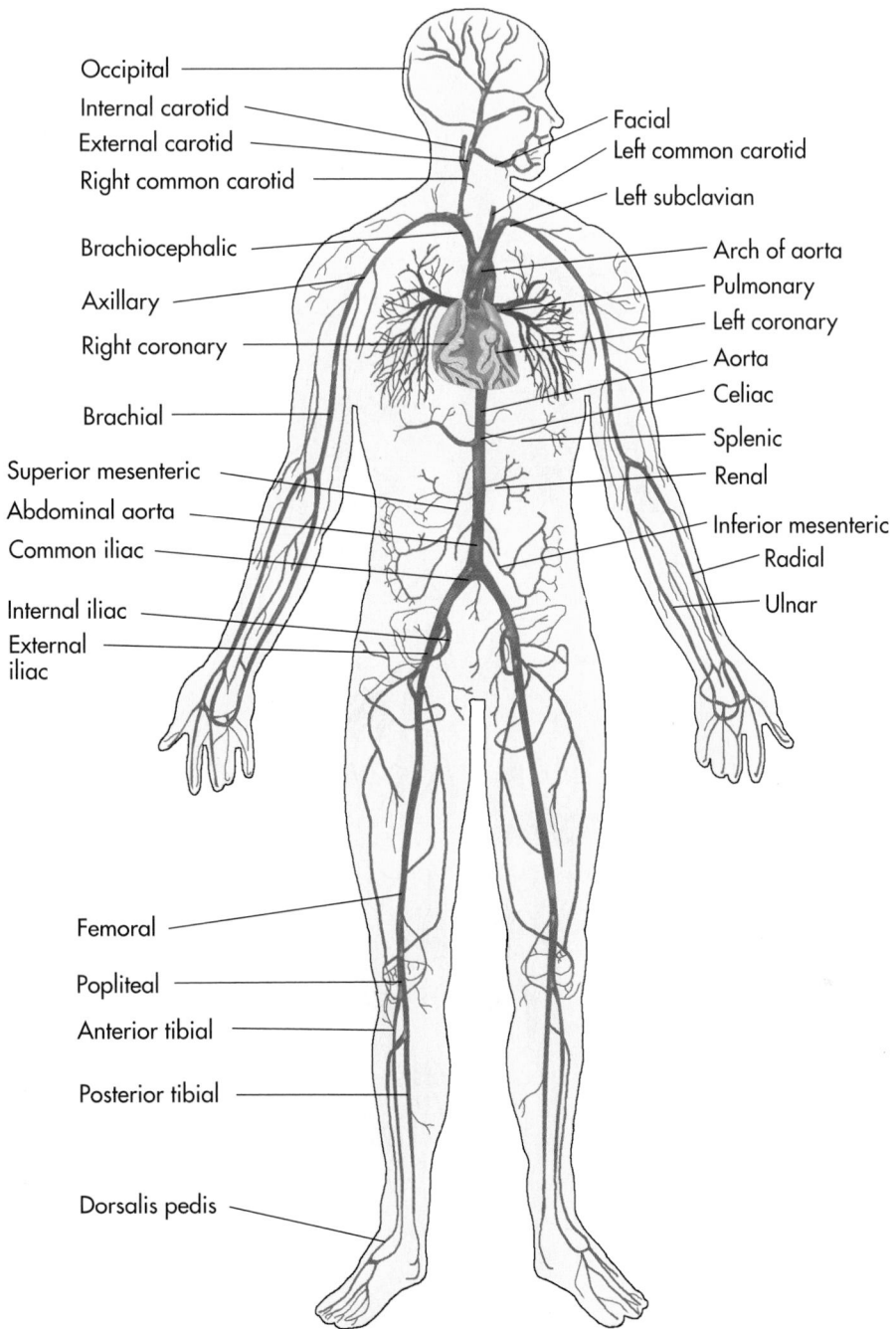

Occipital

Internal carotid

External carotid

Right common carotid

Brachiocephalic

Axillary

Right coronary

Brachial

Superior mesenteric

Abdominal aorta

Common iliac

Internal iliac

External iliac

Femoral

Popliteal

Anterior tibial

Posterior tibial

Dorsalis pedis

Facial

Left common carotid

Left subclavian

Arch of aorta

Pulmonary

Left coronary

Aorta

Celiac

Splenic

Renal

Inferior mesenteric

Radial

Ulnar

Fig. 6-44 Principal arteries of the body.

the abdomen and pelvis, and the hepatic portal system, which transports blood from the digestive tract to the liver (Fig. 6-45).

Lymphatic System

The lymphatic system is considered part of the circulatory system because it consists of a moving fluid that comes from the body and returns to the blood. Unlike the circulatory system, the lymphatic system only carries fluid away from the tissues.

The lymphatic system includes lymph, lymphocytes, lymph nodes, tonsils, spleen, and the thymus gland. The three basic functions of the lymphatic system are to help maintain fluid balance in tissues,

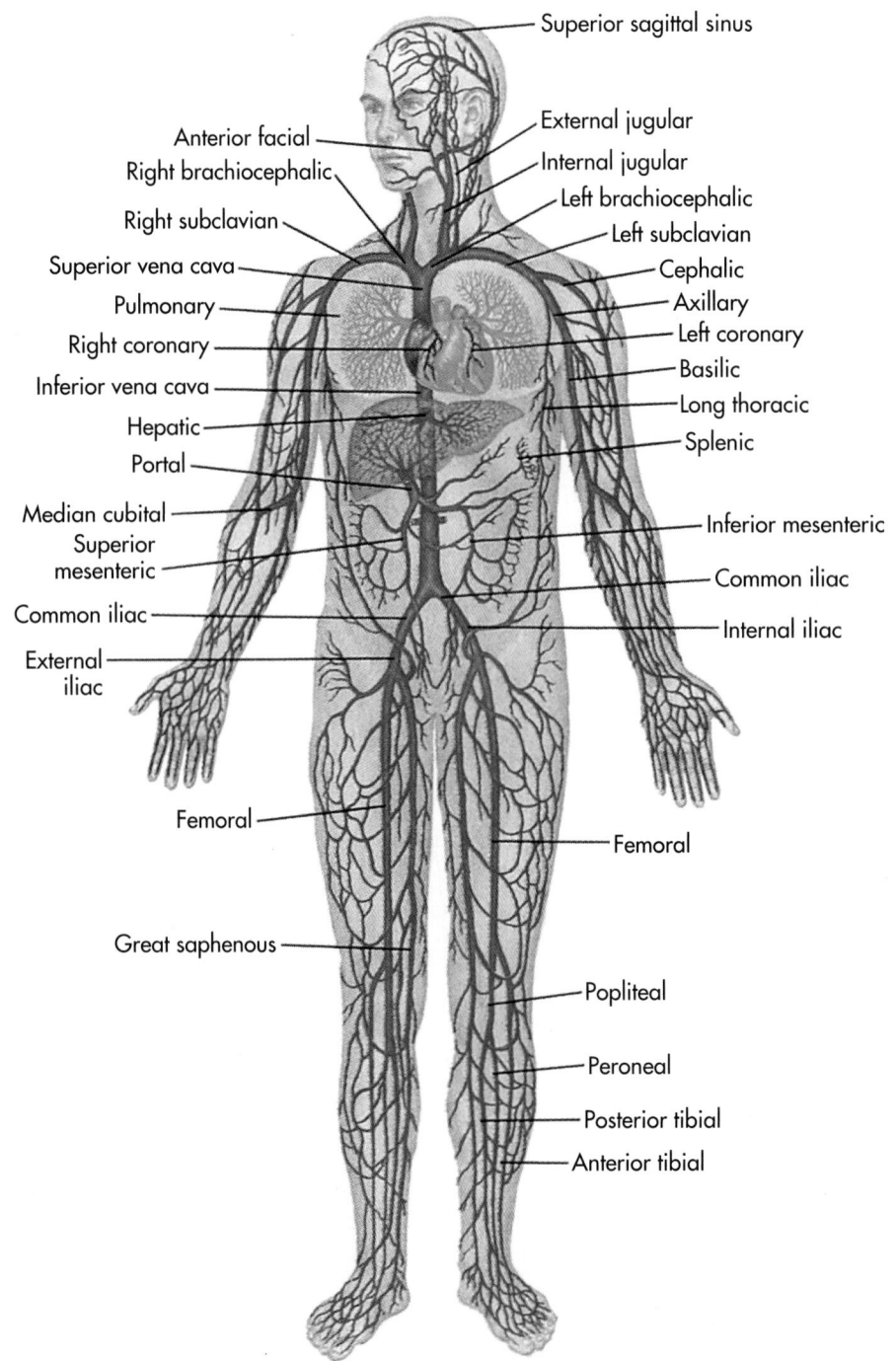

Fig. 6-45 Principal veins of the body. (From Thibodeau GA: *Structure and function of the body,* ed 9, St Louis, 1992, Mosby.)

absorb fats and other substances from the digestive tract, and play a role in the body's immune defense system.

The lymphatic system begins in the tissues as lymph capillaries. Lymph capillaries differ structurally from blood capillaries in that lymph capillaries have a series of one-way valves that allow fluid to enter the capillary but prevent fluid from passing back into the interstitial spaces. Lymph capillaries are present in almost all tissues of the body with the exception of the CNS, bone marrow, and tissues without blood vessels (e.g., cartilage, epidermis, cornea). Lymph capillaries join to form larger lymph capillaries that resemble small veins.

Lymph nodes are distributed along various lymph vessels, and most lymph passes through at least one node before entering the blood. Passing through the node filters the lymph, removing microorganisms and foreign substances to prevent them from entering the general circulation. Three major collections of lymph nodes are located on each side of the body: inguinal nodes, axillary nodes, and cervical nodes. If a part of the body is inflamed or otherwise diseased, the nearby lymph nodes become swollen and tender as they limit the spread of microorganisms and foreign substances.

After passing through lymph nodes, lymph vessels converge toward either the right or left subclavian vein. Vessels from the upper right limb and the right side of the head enter the right lymphatic duct. Lymph vessels from the rest of the body enter the larger thoracic duct. The right lymphatic duct drains the right thorax, right upper limb, and right side of the head and neck and opens into the right subclavian vein. The thoracic duct drains the left thorax, the left upper extremity, and the left side of the head and neck. The duct ends by entering the left subclavian vein. Thus all fluid drained from the tissue spaces eventually returns to the venous circulation.

Lymph serves a unique transport function by returning tissue fluid, proteins, fats, and other substances to the general circulation. The lymphatic system does not form a closed ring or circuit like the "true" circulatory system. Once lymph is formed, it flows only once through its system of lymphatic vessels before draining into the right and left subclavian veins.

? CRITICAL THINKING

Why might a woman who has had a radical mastectomy (removal of breast and lymph tissue) have a chronically swollen arm?

Respiratory System

Oxygen is an essential requirement for normal cell metabolism, from which carbon dioxide is a major waste product. The organs of the respiratory system and the cardiovascular system transport oxygen to individual cells and transport carbon dioxide from individual cells to the lungs, where it is released into the air.

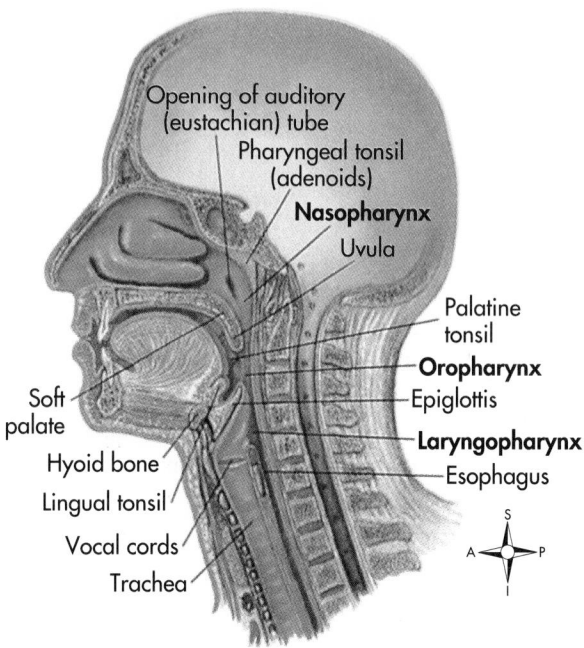

Fig. 6-46 Airway structures. (From Thibodeau GA: *Structure and function of the body,* ed 9, St Louis, 1992, Mosby.)

The respiratory system is a very complex component of the human body. The purpose of this section is to familiarize the reader with respiratory anatomy. (Further discussions of the respiratory system are presented in Chapters 11 and 27.)

Airway Anatomy

The structures of the respiratory system are divided into upper airway and lower airway by their locations relative to the glottic opening (the vocal cords and the space between them). For the purpose of this discussion, all airway structures located above the glottis are considered to be upper airway, and all structures located below the glottis are considered to be lower airway (Fig. 6-46).

Upper airway structures

The entrance to the respiratory tract begins with the nasal cavity and includes the nasopharynx, oropharynx, laryngopharynx, and larynx.

? CRITICAL THINKING

Why might a chronic cocaine abuser have a higher risk of sinus infection?

Nasopharynx. Air passes into the nasal cavity through the nostrils or *nares.* The right and left nasal cavities are separated by the nasal septum, a bony partition covered with a mucous membrane. This membrane has a rich blood supply that warms and humidifies the nasal lining and the inspired air as it passes through the nose. Inside each nostril, a slight enlargement known as the *vestibule* is lined with coarse hairs that trap foreign substances carried into the nasal cavity by inspired air. The floor of the nasal cavity is composed of the hard palate; the lateral walls are formed by bony ridges coated with respiratory mucosa. These ridges are known as *conchae*, or *turbinates*.

Two patches of yellow-gray tissue lie just beneath the bridge of the nose and compose the olfactory membranes. Located in the roof of the nasal cavity, these membranes contain the receptors for the sense of smell. The nasal cavities also connect to the middle-ear cavities through the auditory (or eustachian) tubes.

Sinuses are cavities in the bones of the skull that connect to the nasal cavities by small channels (Fig. 6-47). Four groups of sinuses, each named for the skull bone in which it lies, are: the frontal sinuses, above the eyebrows; maxillary sinuses (the largest sinuses), in the cheekbones; ethmoid sinuses, just behind the bridge of the nose; and sphenoid sinuses, in a bone that cradles the brain, slightly anterior to the pituitary gland. These hollow chambers are lined with mucous membranes that secrete mucus into the nasal cavities. They are thought to aid in adding resonance to the voice and decreasing the weight of the skull.

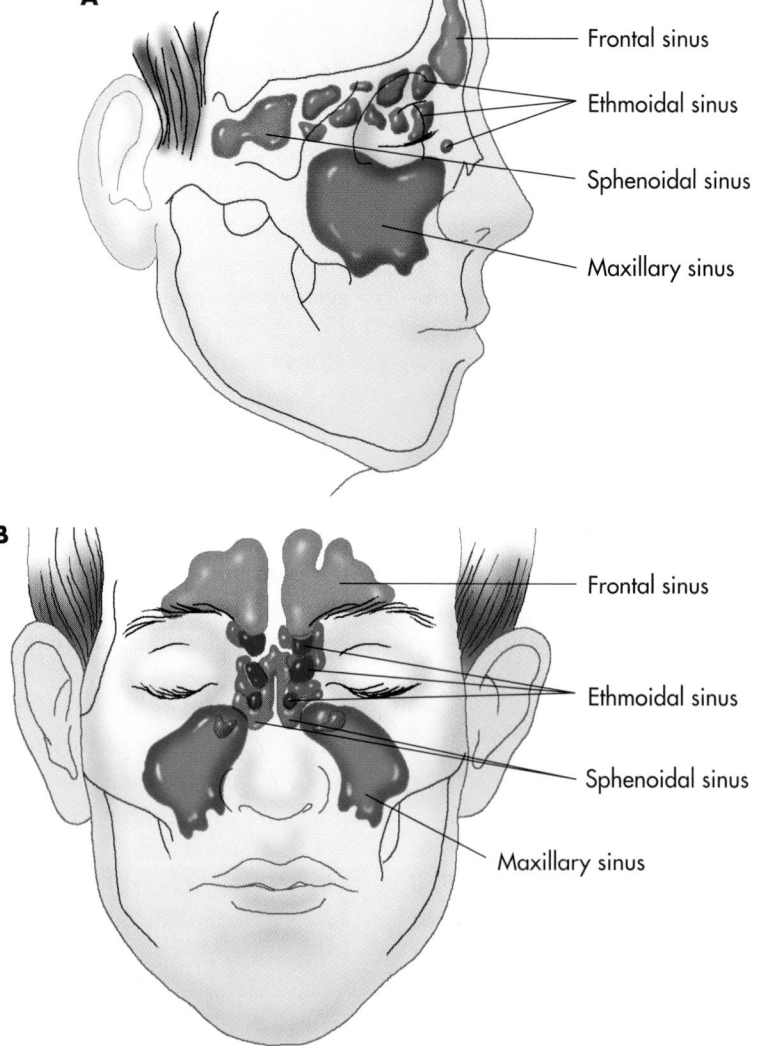

Fig. 6-47 Paranasal sinuses. Side (**A**) and front (**B**) views.

The back of each nasal cavity opens into the nasopharynx, the superior part of the pharynx, which extends from the internal nares to the level of the uvula. Like the nasal cavity, the nasopharynx is lined with mucous membrane.

Oropharynx. At the level of the uvula, the nasopharynx ends and the oropharynx begins, extending downward to the level of the epiglottis. Anteriorly, the oropharynx opens into the oral cavity, which contains the lips, cheeks, teeth, tongue (which is attached to the mandible), hard and soft palates, and palatine tonsils. The palatine tonsils and the pharyngeal tonsils (located in the roof and posterior wall of the nasopharynx) form a partial ring of lymphoid tissue surrounding the respiratory tract. This ring is completed by the lingual tonsils, which lie on the floor of the oropharyngeal passageway at the base of the tongue.

Laryngopharynx. The laryngopharynx extends from the tip of the epiglottis to the glottis and the esophagus. The laryngopharynx is lined with mucous membrane that protects internal surfaces from abrasion.

Larynx. The laryngopharynx opens into the larynx, which lies in the anterior neck (Fig. 6-48). The larynx serves three main functions: it is the air passageway between the pharynx and the lungs, it is a protective sphincter to prevent solids and liquids from passing into the respiratory tree, and it is involved in producing speech.

The larynx consists of an outer casing of nine cartilages connected to each other by muscles and ligaments. Six of the nine cartilages are paired; three are unpaired. The largest, most superior of the cartilages is the unpaired thyroid cartilage, or Adam's apple. This prominence is hardly visible in children or adult females but is marked in males after puberty.

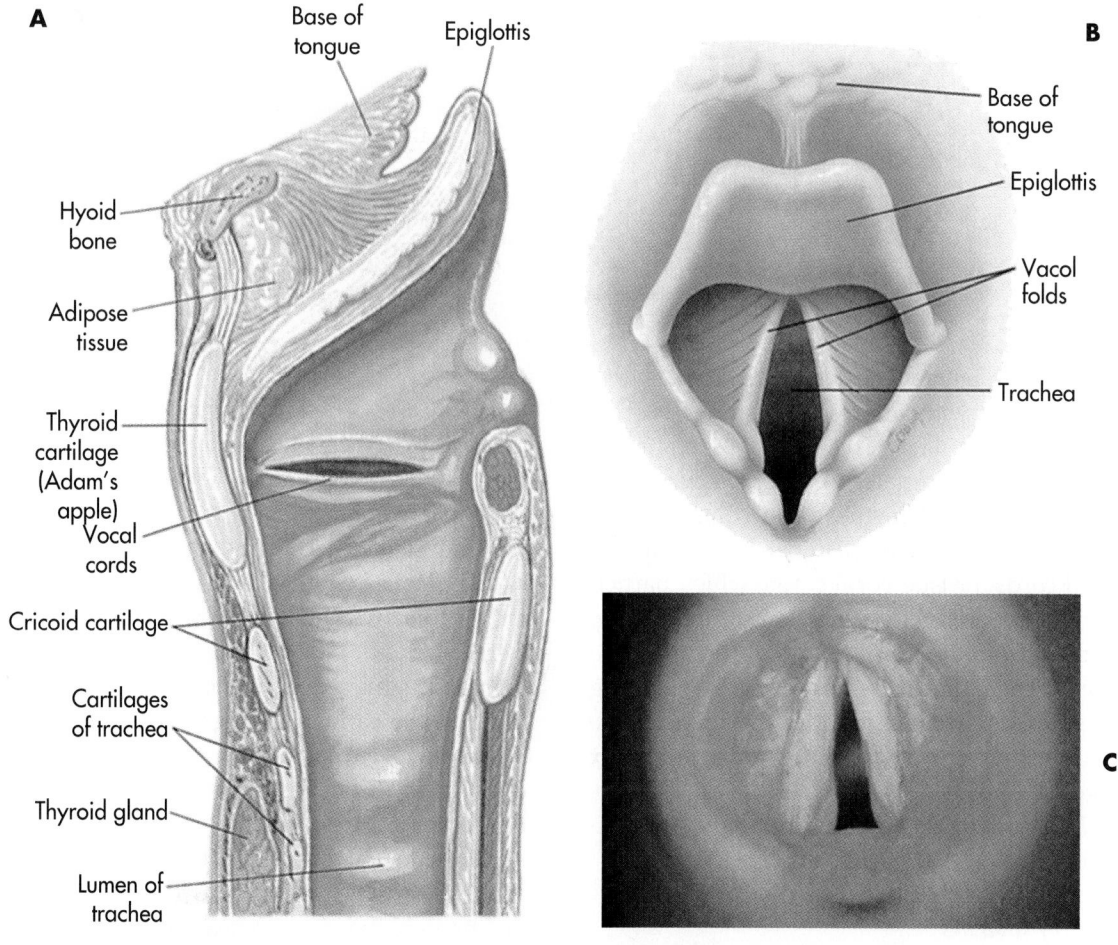

Fig. 6-48 Larynx. **A,** Sagittal section. **B,** Superior view. **C,** Photograph taken with an endoscope. (From Thibodeau GA: *Structure and function of the body,* ed 9, St Louis, 1992, Mosby.)

The most inferior cartilage of the larynx is the unpaired cricoid cartilage (the only complete cartilaginous ring in the larynx). This cartilage forms the base of the larynx on which all other cartilages rest. The third unpaired cartilage is the epiglottis.

The six paired cartilages are stacked in two pillars between the cricoid cartilage and the thyroid cartilage. The largest inferior cartilages are ladle shaped and are known as the *arytenoid cartilages*. The middle pair are horn shaped and are known as *corniculate cartilages*. The smallest, most superior cartilages are wedge shaped and are known as *cuneiform cartilages*.

The U-shaped hyoid bone is tucked beneath the mandible. As previously mentioned, it is the only bone of the human body that does not articulate with another bone. The hyoid bone helps to suspend the airway by anchoring the muscles (particularly those of the tongue) to the jaw. The fibrous membrane that joins the hyoid and the thyroid cartilage is called the *thyroid membrane*. The membrane joining the thyroid and cricoid cartilages is called the cricothyroid membrane.

? CRITICAL THINKING

Why can't a person talk when an endotracheal tube is correctly positioned in the trachea?

Two pairs of ligaments extend from the anterior surface of the arytenoid to the posterior surface of the thyroid cartilage. The superior pair forms the vestibular folds, or false vocal cords, which are not directly involved in the production of voice sounds. The inferior pair of ligaments composes the vocal cords, or true vocal cords, which participate directly in producing voice sounds. In talking, air expelled from the lungs rushes up the throat to the larynx. There the air creates sound by vibrating the vocal cords. Muscles tighten the folds of the cords to produce the high-pitched tones and relax the cords to produce the deeper tones. The lip, tongue, and jaw further modify the sounds into intelligible words.

Lower airway structures

Below the glottis are the structures of the lower airway and lungs. These structures include the trachea, the bronchial tree (primary bronchi, secondary bronchi, and bronchioles), the alveoli, and the lungs (Fig. 6-49).

Trachea. The trachea is the air passage from the larynx to the lungs. It is composed of dense connective tissue and smooth muscle reinforced with 15 to 20 C-shaped pieces of cartilage that form an incomplete ring. This ring protects the trachea and maintains an open passage for air. The adult trachea is about 1.5 centimeters (cm) in diameter and 9 to 15 cm in length. The trachea is located anterior to the esophagus and extends from the larynx to the fifth thoracic vertebrae.

NOTE

A cm is equal to 0.4 inch. One inch is equal to 2.54 cm.

The trachea is lined with ciliated epithelium that contains many goblet cells. These cilia protect the lower airway by sweeping mucus, bacteria, and other small particles toward the larynx. There they may be expelled through coughing or enter the esophagus, where they are swallowed and digested. Constant exposure to some irritants (e.g., cigarette smoke) may produce a tracheal epithelium that lacks cilia and goblet cells. When this protective mechanism is disrupted, the mucus and bacteria may contribute to disease.

Bronchial tree. The lower airway may be thought of as an inverted tree; the many subdivisions become narrower and shorter until they terminate at the alveoli. The large branches are primary bronchi; they divide into smaller secondary bronchi and bronchioles.

The trachea divides into the right and left primary bronchi at the level of the angle of Louis (the sternomanubrial joint). The point of bifurcation of the trachea into the right and left mainstem bronchi is called the carina. The right primary bronchus is shorter, wider, and more vertical. Like the trachea, the primary bronchi are lined with ciliated epithelium and are supported by C-shaped cartilage rings. As the bronchi sequentially branch into smaller subdivisions, the amount of cartilage decreases and the bronchi become increasingly muscular until there is no cartilage. The primary bronchi extend from the mediastinum to the lungs.

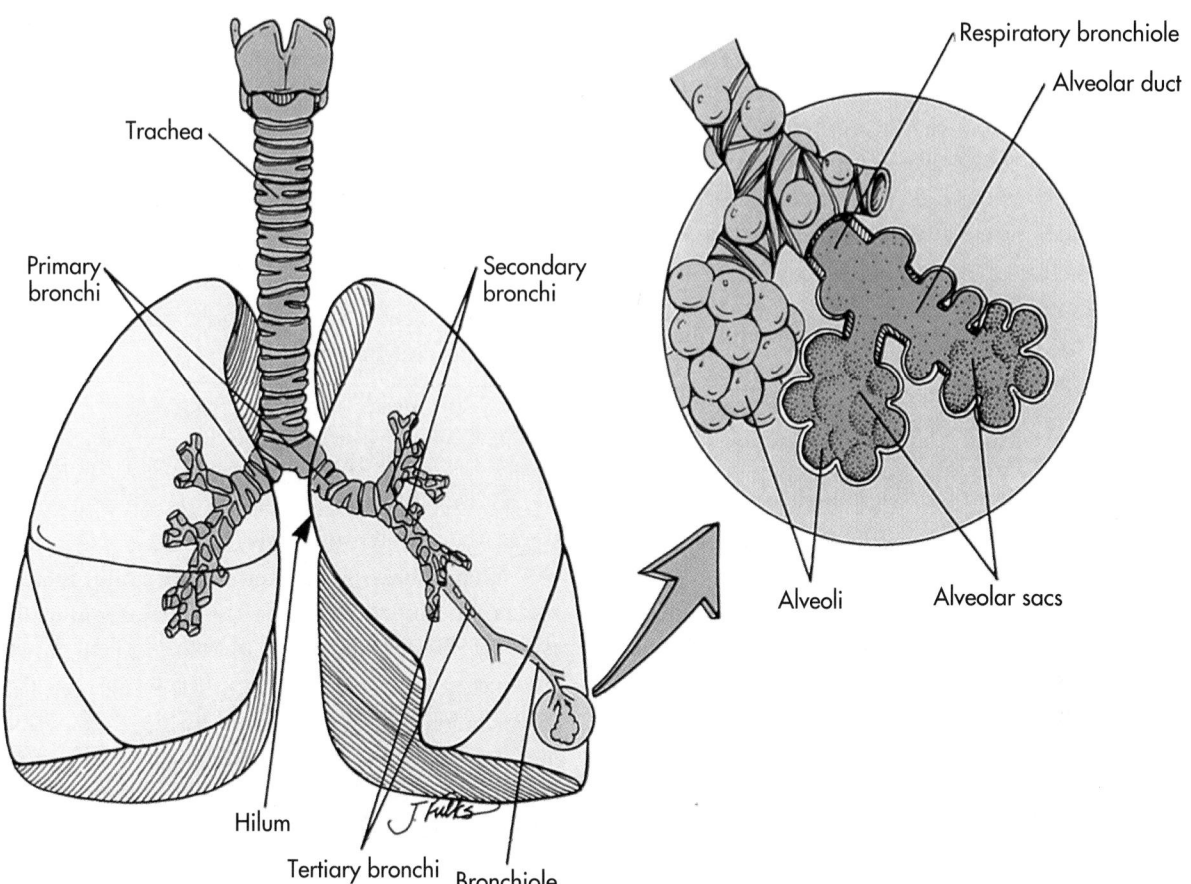

Fig. 6-49 Anatomy of the trachea and lungs. Inset shows enlargement of a terminal bronchiole and its associated alveoli. (From Thibodeau GA: *Structure and function of the body,* ed 9, St Louis, 1992, Mosby.)

? CRITICAL THINKING

What is the advantage of having multiple bronchiole branches?

The primary bronchi divide into the secondary bronchi as they enter the right and left lungs. Two secondary lobar bronchi in the left lung conduct air to its two lobes; three in the right lung conduct air to its three lobes. From there, the secondary bronchi divide into the tertiary segmental bronchi, of which there are 10 in the right lung and 9 in the left. The tertiary bronchi extend to the individual segments of each

NOTE

A mm is equal to 0.04 inch. One inch is equal to 25.40 mm.

lobe of the lung (lobule). The bronchial tree continues to branch several times. As the cartilage continues to decrease and the diameter is reduced to about 1 millimeter (mm), the bronchi become bronchioles.

The bronchiole walls are devoid of cartilage, and their muscles are sensitive to certain circulating hormones, such as epinephrine. Contraction and relaxation of these muscles alter resistance to air flow. The bronchioles can constrict if the smooth muscle contracts forcefully. (An example of this phenomenon is an asthma exacerbation.) Bronchioles continue to divide, eventually becoming terminal bronchioles and finally respiratory bronchioles. Each respiratory bronchiole divides to form alveolar ducts. These ducts end as grapelike clusters of tiny, hollow air sacs called alveoli. It is here that the majority of respiratory gas exchange takes place.

Alveoli. The alveoli are the functional units of the respiratory system and are the prominent constituent of lung tissue. Some 300 million alveoli exist in the two lungs. The wall of an alveolus consists of a single layer of epithelial cells and elastic fibers that permit it to stretch and contract during breathing. The exchange of oxygen and carbon dioxide in the lungs takes place in the alveoli (see Chapter 11).

Each alveolus is surrounded by a fine network of blood capillaries arranged so that air within the alveolus is separated by a thin respiratory membrane from the blood contained within the alveolar capillaries. The large surface area of the respiratory membrane may be decreased by respiratory diseases, such as emphysema and lung cancer, which significantly restrict the exchange of oxygen and carbon dioxide.

Alveoli are coated with pulmonary surfactant, a thin film produced by alveolar cells. This fluid prevents the alveoli from collapsing. In addition, pores in the alveolar membrane allow for a limited flow of air between alveoli. This collateral ventilation provides some protection for the alveolus that is occluded by disease.

? CRITICAL THINKING

One effect of toxic smoke inhalation is destruction of pulmonary surfactant. Why won't oxygen therapy alone always help? What do you think might help?

Lungs. The lungs are large, paired, spongy organs whose principal function is respiration. Although there is smooth muscle in the bronchioles of the lungs, the lungs expand and contract during the respiratory cycle as a result of the expansion of the thoracic cavity during inspiration and elastic recoil during expiration. The lungs are attached to the heart by the pulmonary artery and veins. The two lungs are separated by the mediastinum and its contents (the heart, blood vessels, trachea, esophagus, lymphatic tissues, and vessels). The point of entry for the bronchi, vessels, and nerves of each lung is known as the *hilum*, or root, of each lung. At birth, the color of the lungs is rose pink. However, by adulthood, the color of the lungs changes to slate gray with dark patches as particulate matter is inhaled and deposited in the tissues. An adult lung weighs less than 2 pounds.

Each lung is conical in shape, with its base resting on the diaphragm and its apex extending to a point about 2.5 cm superior to each clavicle. The right lung is divided into three lobes. The left lung is slightly smaller than the right and is divided into two lobes. Each lobe is divided into lobules separated by connective tissue. Major blood vessels and bronchi do not cross this connective tissue, allowing for a diseased lobule to be surgically removed, leaving the remaining lung relatively intact. There are 9 lobules in the left lung and 10 lobules in the right lung.

Both lungs are surrounded by a separate pleural cavity and are attached to each other only at the point of entry of the bronchi, vessels, and nerves of each lung (Fig. 6-50). The two layers of pleura (*visceral* and *parietal*) are so close that they are virtually in contact with each other. They are separated by a thin fluid that acts as a lubricant to allow the pleural membranes to slide past each other during respiration.

Between the two pleurae there is a potential space known as the pleural space. When there is significant chest wall injury or pulmonary pathology, the pleural space may become filled with air (pneumothorax) or blood (hemothorax). Other fluid collections that may accumulate in the pleural space include transudates, most commonly from congestive heart failure (CHF), and exudates, which can result from infectious or malignant etiologies.

Digestive System

The digestive system provides the body with water, electrolytes, and other nutrients used by cells. To accomplish this function, the digestive system is specialized to ingest food, propel the food through the gastrointestinal (GI) tract (digestive tract), and absorb nutrients across the wall of the lumen of the GI tract.

The GI tract is an irregular-shaped tube associated with accessory organs (primarily glands) that secrete fluid into the digestive tract. The first section of the digestive tract is the oral cavity. The salivary glands and tonsils are accessory organs of the oral cavity. The oral cavity opens posteriorly into the pharynx and inferiorly into the esophagus. The esophagus opens inferiorly into the stomach (through the muscular *cardiac sphincter*), where small glands secrete acids and enzymes to assist with digestion. The cardiac sphincter prevents food from reentering the esophagus when the stomach contracts.

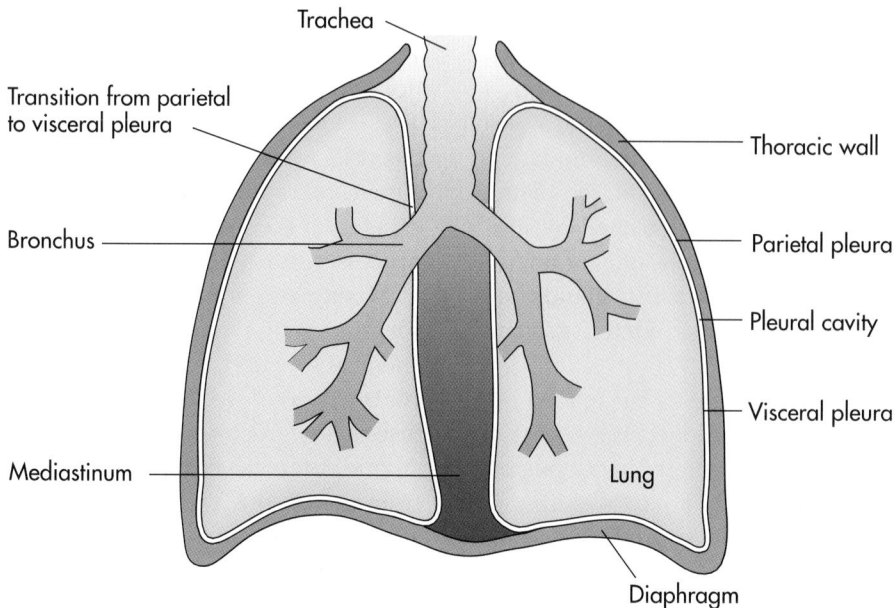

Trachea

Transition from parietal to visceral pleura

Bronchus

Mediastinum

Thoracic wall

Parietal pleura

Pleural cavity

Visceral pleura

Lung

Diaphragm

Fig. 6-50 Lungs surrounded by pleural cavities.

The stomach opens into the duodenum, the first section of the small intestine. Important accessory structures in this segment of the GI tract are the liver, the gallbladder, and the pancreas. The jejunum, the major site of absorption, is the next segment of the small intestine. The last segment of the small intestine is the ileum. It is similar in function to the jejunum but has fewer digestive enzymes and provides less absorption.

The last section of the digestive tract is the large intestine, whose major functions are to absorb water and salts and concentrate undigested food into feces. Its major accessory glands secrete mucus. The first segment of the large intestine is the cecum with its attached appendix. The cecum is followed by the ascending, transverse, descending, and sigmoid portions of the colon and the rectum. The rectum joins the anal canal, which ends at the anus.

Functions of the Digestive Tract

As food moves through the digestive system, secretions are added to liquefy and digest the food and to provide lubrication. The processes of secretion, movement, and absorption are regulated by nervous and hormonal mechanisms.

Oral cavity

Saliva contains a digestive enzyme called salivary amylase that begins the chemical digestion of carbohydrates. In addition, saliva prevents bacterial infection in the mouth by washing the oral cavity with substances that provide a weak antibacterial action. Salivary gland secretion is stimulated by the parasympathetic and sympathetic nervous systems, with the parasympathetic controlling salivation in the relaxed state.

Food in the mouth is chewed (masticated) by the teeth to physically break it up to facilitate swallowing and processing. Food is then swallowed by voluntary and involuntary mechanisms. The pharynx elevates to receive the food from the mouth. As the pharyngeal muscles contract, the upper esophageal sphincter relaxes, the esophagus opens, and food is pushed into the esophagus. During this phase of swallowing, the vocal folds are moved medially and the epiglottis is tipped posteriorly to close the entrance of the airway and prevent aspiration.

Muscular contractions in the esophagus occur in peristaltic waves, pushing the food through the esophagus toward the stomach. These contractions cause relaxation of the cardiac sphincter (also known as the *lower esophageal sphincter*) and allow food to enter the stomach.

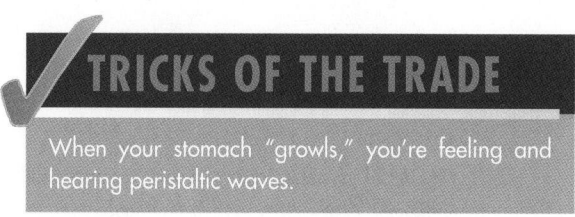

✓ TRICKS OF THE TRADE

When your stomach "growls," you're feeling and hearing peristaltic waves.

Stomach

The stomach functions primarily as a storage area and mixing chamber for ingested food. Although some digestion and absorption occur in the stomach, these are not its major functions. The stomach secretes mucus to protect the surface of the stomach wall and duodenum. It is lined by mucous membranes that contain thousands of microscopic gastric glands. These gastric glands secrete hydrochloric acid, intrinsic factor, gastrin, and pepsinogen.

About 2 to 3 liters (L) of gastric secretions are produced by the stomach each day; the process is regulated by nervous and hormonal mechanisms. The ingested food is thoroughly mixed with the secretions of the stomach glands to produce a semisolid mixture called chyme. Movements resembling peristalsis slowly force chyme toward the pyloric sphincter, through the pyloric opening, and into the duodenum (Fig. 6-51).

Small intestine

The mucosa of the small intestine produces secretions that contain mucus, electrolytes, and water. These substances lubricate and protect the intestinal wall from the acidic chyme and digestive enzymes. In addition, secretions of the liver and pancreas enter the small intestine to aid in the digestive process.

Mixing and propulsion of chyme along with absorption of fluid and nutrients are the primary mechanical functions of the small intestine. Peristaltic contractions move the chyme through the small intestine toward the ileocecal sphincter, where the chyme enters the cecum. When the cecum distends from the chyme, the sphincter closes. This closure slows the rate of movement of chyme from the small intestine into the large intestine and prevents material from returning to the ileum from the cecum.

> **NOTE**
>
> A L is equal to 1.06 quarts. One gallon is equal to 3.79 L.

> **? CRITICAL THINKING**
>
> *What might happen if the excretion of protective mucus in the small bowel was impaired?*

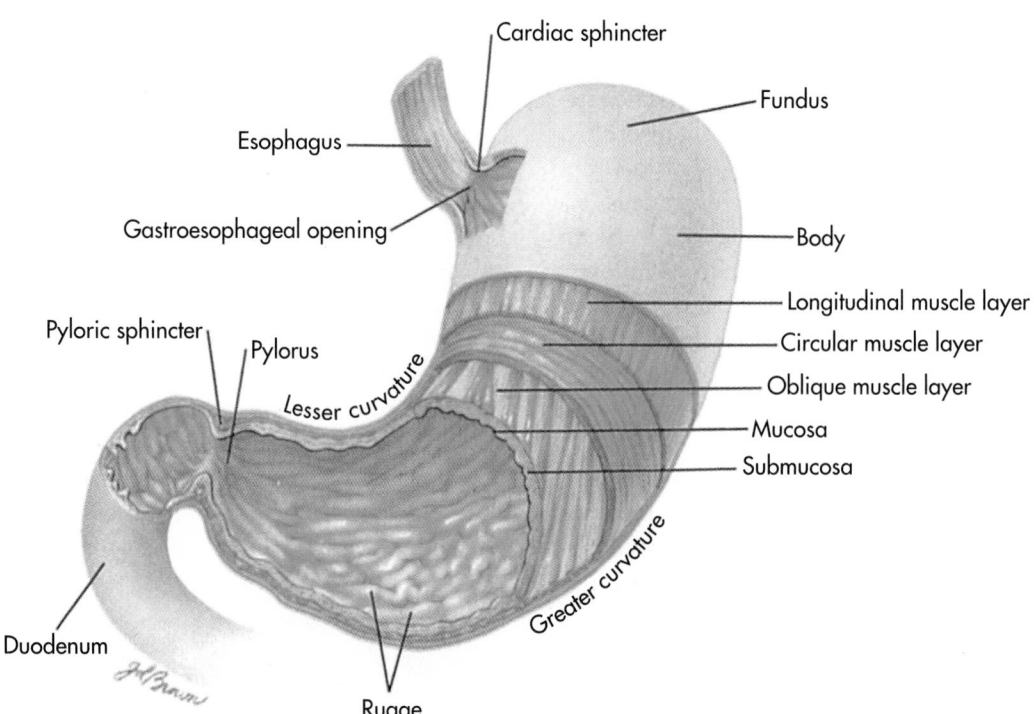

Fig. 6-51 Muscle layers of the stomach wall. (From Thibodeau GA: *Structure and function of the body,* ed 9, St Louis, 1992, Mosby.)

Liver

The liver is the largest internal organ and serves a myriad of biochemical functions. It lies just under the diaphragm in the upper regions of the abdominal cavity. It is a very vascular organ that receives a blood supply from two sources, the hepatic artery and the portal vein. The liver plays a major role in iron metabolism, plasma-protein production, detoxification of drugs and other substances circulating in plasma, and numerous other biochemical pathways.

About 600 to 1000 milliliters (mL) of bile are secreted by the liver each day. Bile contains no digestive enzymes, but it dilutes stomach acid and emulsifies fats. Most bile salts are reabsorbed in the ileum and carried back to the liver in the blood. Other bile salts are lost through feces.

NOTE

A mL is equal to 0.5 teaspoon volume. One tablespoon volume is equal to 15 mL.

In addition to secreting bile, the liver performs other functions necessary for healthy survival. It plays a major role in the metabolism of certain foods and helps maintain a normal blood glucose concentration. The liver is also a line of defense against many byproducts of metabolism that are toxic if accumulated in the body. Blood proteins (e.g., albumin, fibrinogen, globulins, clotting factors) also are produced and released into the circulation by the liver.

Gallbladder

Bile is continuously secreted by the liver and stored in the gallbladder. When chyme containing lipid or fat enters the duodenum, the gallbladder is stimulated by the hormones cholecystokinin and secretin, which are secreted by the intestinal mucosa. This stimulation causes the gallbladder to contract, forcing concentrated bile into the small intestine. The

? CRITICAL THINKING

When is the person who suffers from gallstones (cholelithiasis) most likely to have pain? Why?

gallbladder's only function is to concentrate and store the bile produced by the liver.

Pancreas

The pancreas is both an exocrine gland that secretes pancreatic juice and an endocrine gland that secretes hormones (e.g., insulin) into the blood. Pancreatic juice is the most important digestive juice. It contains digestive enzymes, sodium bicarbonate, and alkaline substances that neutralize the hydrochloric acid in the digestive juices entering the small intestine. Pancreatic juice also contains amylase, which continues digestion initiated in the oral cavity.

Large intestine

Chyme moves through the small intestine in 3 to 5 hours, but passage through the large intestine takes 18 to 24 hours. Processes involving the absorption of water and salts, the secretion of mucus, the action of microorganisms, and the conversion of chyme produce feces. Feces remain in the colon until eliminated through defecation.

The contents of the large intestine are propelled toward the anus by peristaltic contractions three to four times each day. During movement through the large intestine, material that escaped digestion in the small intestine is acted on by bacteria. As a result of this bacterial action, additional nutrients may be released and absorbed. Some of the bacteria also synthesize vitamin K, which is needed for normal blood clotting to produce the B-complex vitamins. Once formed, these vitamins are absorbed from the large intestine, where they enter the blood.

Distention of the rectal wall by feces initiates the defecation reflex, causing weak contractions and relaxations of the internal anal sphincter. The external anal sphincter (under conscious cerebral control) prevents the movement of feces out of the rectum until it is relaxed. During defecation, pressure in the abdominal cavity increases and forces the contents of the colon through the anal canal and out of the anus.

Urinary System

The urinary system works with other body systems to maintain homeostasis by removing waste products from the blood and helping to maintain a constant body fluid volume and composition. The kidneys also are involved in the control of RBC production and in vitamin D metabolism. The contents of the urinary system include two kidneys, two ureters, the urinary bladder, and the urethra.

? CRITICAL THINKING

Why should you anticipate anemia and decreased calcium levels in patients with renal failure?

Kidneys

The kidneys, each shaped very much like a kidney bean, lie on the posterior abdominal wall behind the peritoneum. They are located on either side of the vertebral column near the lateral border of the psoas muscles. The superior pole of each kidney is protected by the rib cage. The right kidney is slightly lower than the left because of the superior position of the liver. A fibrous renal capsule surrounds each kidney, as does a dense deposit of adipose tissue that protects the kidney from injury.

The kidney is divided into an outer cortex and an inner medulla. The medulla consists of a number of triangular divisions, called the *renal pyramids*, that extend into the cortex (Fig. 6-52). The papilla is the innermost end of a pyramid. Several large urinary tubes (calyces) extend to the renal pelvis from the kidney tissue.

The basic functional unit of the kidney is the nephron. The nephron consists of a large terminal end (called a *renal corpuscle*) a proximal convoluted tubule, the loop of Henle, and a distal convoluted tubule. The distal convoluted tubule empties into a collecting duct, which carries the urine from the cortex of the kidney to the calyces. The terminal end of the nephron is enlarged to form Bowman's capsule. The wall of Bowman's capsule is indented to form a double-walled chamber occupied by a network of blood capillaries known as the glomerulus. Together, the glomerulus and Bowman's capsule form the renal corpuscle.

Ureters, Urinary Bladder, and Urethra

The ureters extend from the renal pelvis to the urinary bladder. The triangular area of the bladder wall between the two ureters and the urethra is called the *trigone*. (Fig. 6-53 depicts the male urinary bladder.) This region differs from the rest of the bladder wall in that it does not expand during bladder filling.

The urinary bladder is a hollow, muscular organ that lies in the pelvic cavity just posterior to the pubic symphysis. The size of the bladder depends on the volume of urine.

? CRITICAL THINKING

Why is the bladder more susceptible to injury when full versus empty?

At the junction of the urethra and the urinary bladder, smooth muscle of the bladder forms the internal urinary sphincter. The external urinary sphincter surrounds the urethra as the urethra extends through the pelvic floor. These sphincters control the flow of urine through the urethra. In the male, the urethra extends to the end of the penis, where it opens to the outside (see Fig. 6-53). The female urethra is much shorter than the male urethra and opens into the vestibule anterior to the vaginal opening.

Urine Production

Nephrons are the structural components of the kidney and are where urine is produced. The more than two million nephrons form urine in a three-step process that includes filtration, reabsorption, and secretion.

1. The first step of urine formation is the passage of fluid from the glomerular capillaries into Bowman's capsule. Blood flowing through the glomeruli exerts pressure, and this glomerular blood pressure pushes water and small molecular dissolved substances out of the glomeruli into the Bowman's capsule. Simply stated, glomerular blood pressure causes filtration through the glomerular capillaries. Glomerular filtration normally occurs at the rate of 125 mL/minute or 180 L/day (glomerular filtration rate), of which 90% is reabsorbed. Healthy people produce 1 to 2 L of urine each day.

2. The filtrate leaves the renal capsule and flows through the proximal convoluted tubule, the loop of Henle, the distal convoluted tubule, and into the collecting duct. During this process, many substances in the filtrate are reabsorbed by the blood capillaries around the tubules and reenter the general circulation. Substances reabsorbed include water, glucose and other nutrients, and most of the sodium and other ions.

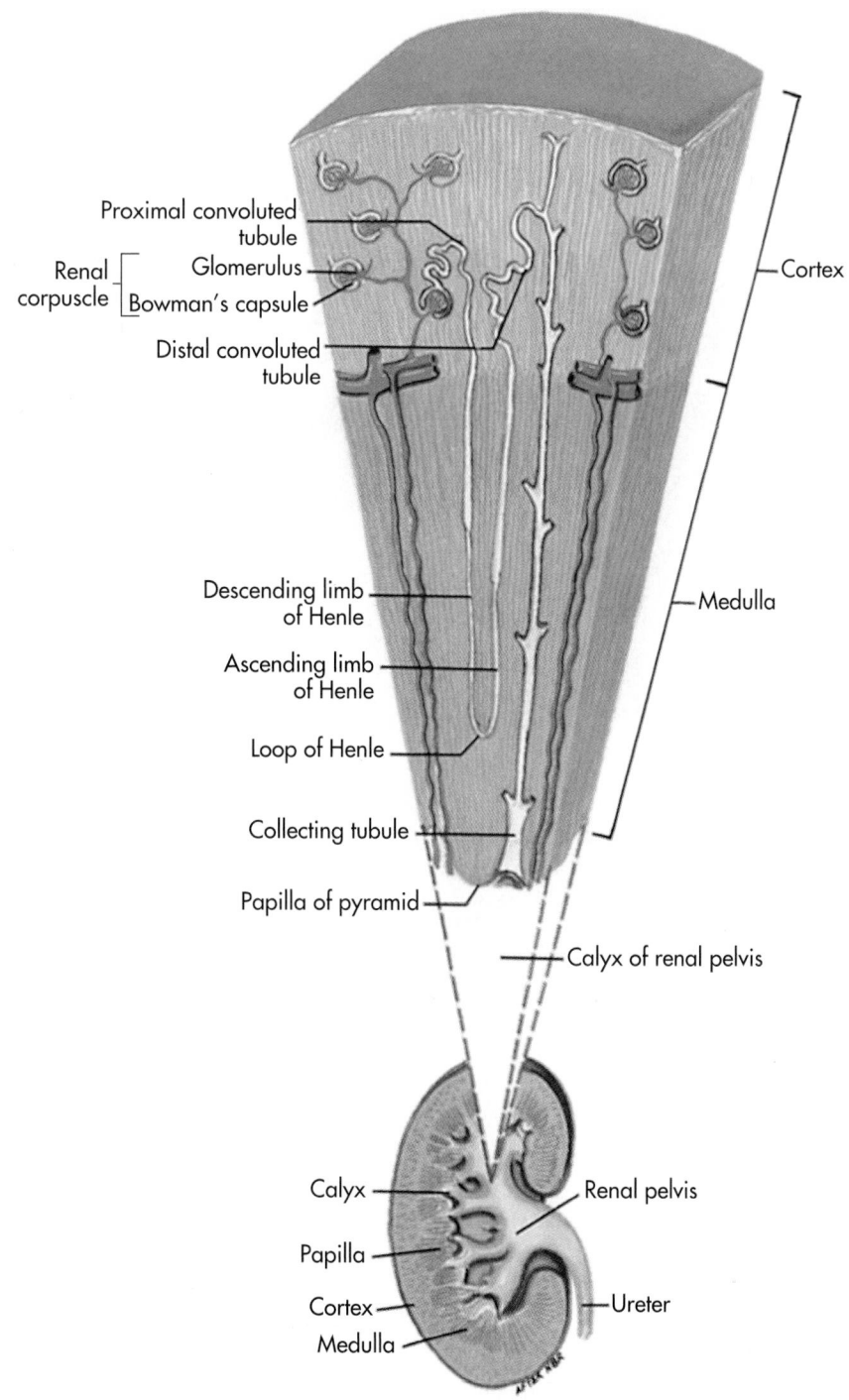

Proximal convoluted tubule

Renal corpuscle
Glomerulus
Bowman's capsule

Distal convoluted tubule

Cortex

Descending limb of Henle

Ascending limb of Henle

Loop of Henle

Collecting tubule

Papilla of pyramid

Medulla

Calyx of renal pelvis

Calyx

Papilla

Cortex

Medulla

Renal pelvis

Ureter

Fig. 6-52 Magnified wedge cut from a renal pyramid. (From Thibodeau GA: *Structure and function of the body,* ed 9, St Louis, 1992, Mosby.)

3. Secretion is the process by which substances move into urine in the distal convoluted tubule and collecting duct from blood in the capillaries around these structures. Unlike reabsorption, which moves substances out of the urine and into the blood, secretion moves substances out of the blood and into the urine. Secreted substances include hydrogen and potassium ions, ammonia, and certain drugs. (Fig. 6-54 depicts the formation of urine.)

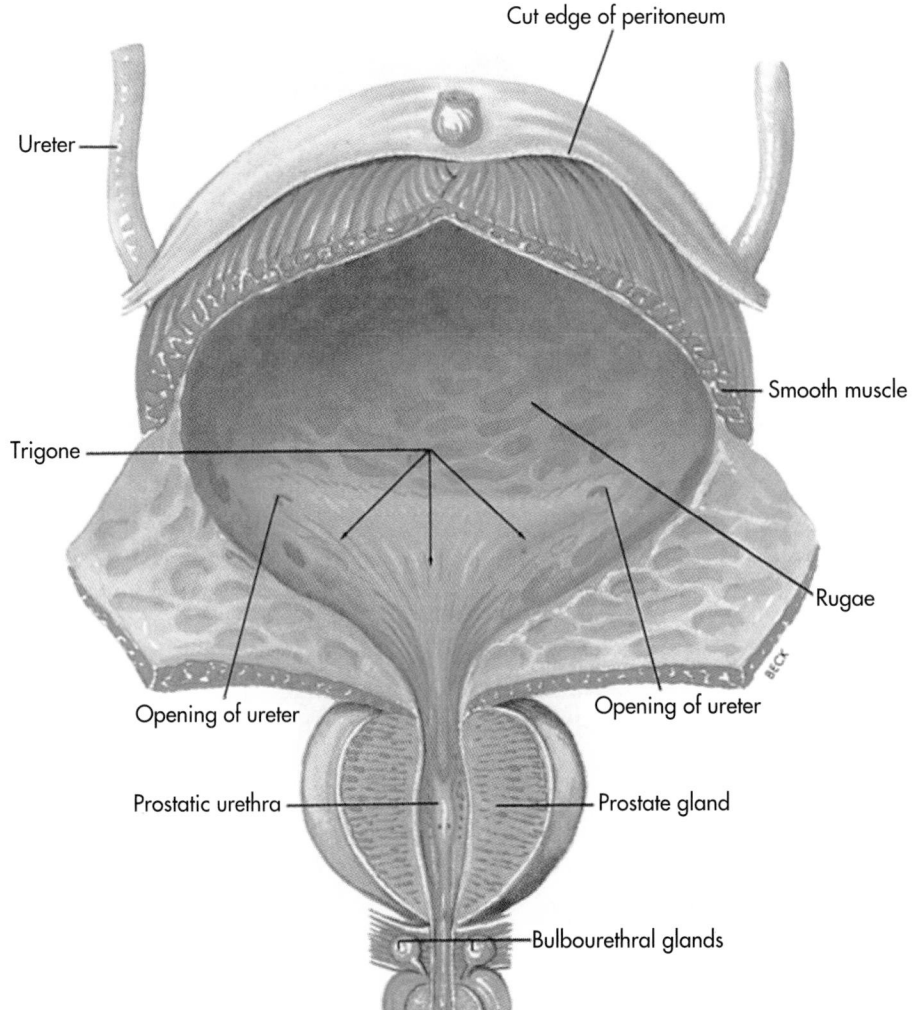

Fig. 6-53 Male urinary bladder. (From Thibodeau GA: *Structure and function of the body,* ed 9, St Louis, 1992, Mosby.)

Urine Regulation

The body usually can control both the amount and composition of urine it secretes. This involves hormonal mechanisms, autoregulation, and sympathetic nervous system stimulation.

Aldosterone is a steroid hormone secreted by the adrenal gland. The hormone passes through the circulatory system from the adrenal gland to the kidney and stimulates the tubules to reabsorb sodium salts and water.

ADH secreted by the posterior pituitary gland tends to decrease the amount of urine produced by making distal and collecting tubules permeable to water, thus increasing water reabsorption. As a result, water is retained by the body in the presence of ADH.

Atrial natriuretic factor is a hormone secreted from the cells in the right atrium of the heart when the pressure in the right atrium increases. This hormone inhibits ADH secretion and reduces the ability of the kidney to concentrate urine. As a result, the body produces a large volume of dilute urine.

Prostaglandins and kinins are substances formed in the kidneys that affect kidney function. These substances are believed to influence the rate of filtrate formation and sodium ion reabsorption.

Autoregulation is the ability of the kidneys to regulate a stable glomerular filtration rate over a wide range of systemic blood pressures. When there are small increases in glomerular capillary pressure, the rate of filtrate formation increases substantially. Therefore large increases in arterial blood pressure increase the rate of urine production. Conversely, when arterial blood pressure decreases, urine production decreases. Through autoregulation, the kid-

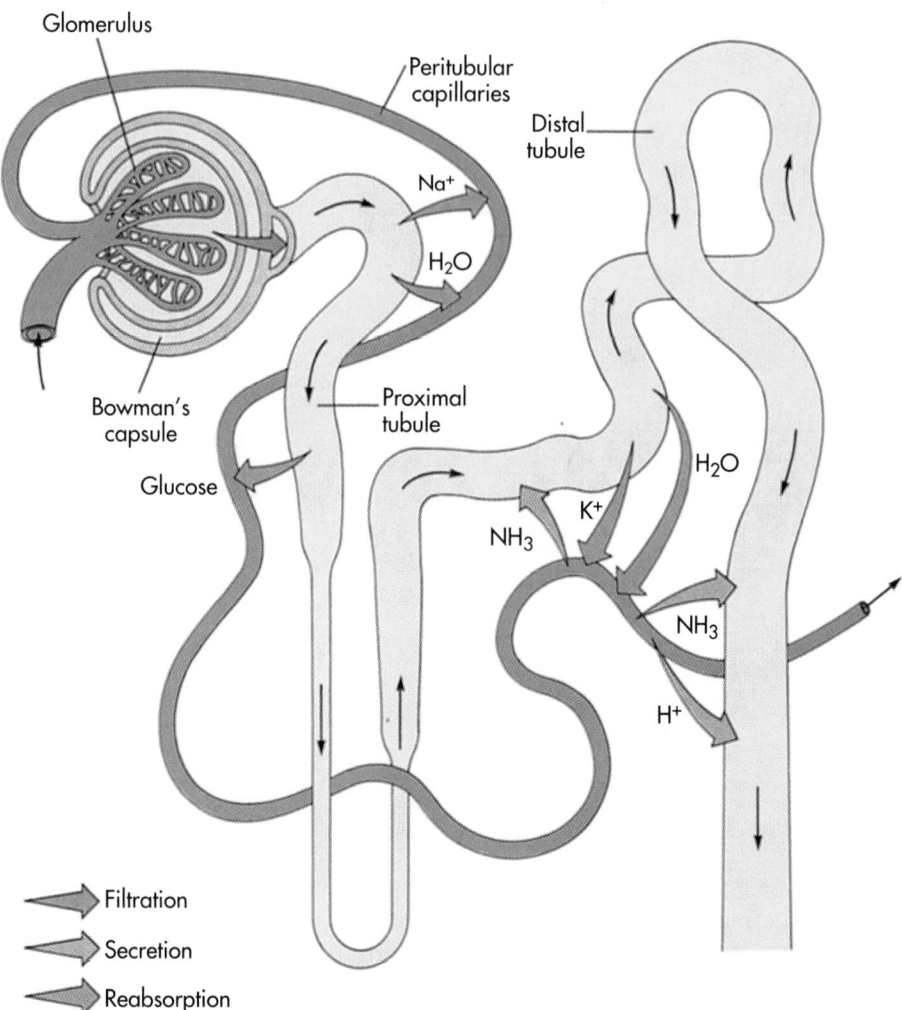

Glomerulus

Peritubular capillaries

Distal tubule

Bowman's capsule

Proximal tubule

Glucose

Na⁺

H_2O

NH_3

K^+

H_2O

NH_3

H^+

Filtration

Secretion

Reabsorption

Fig. 6-54 Formation of urine. Steps in urine formation in successive parts of a nephron: filtration, reabsorption, and secretion. (From Thibodeau GA: *Structure and function of the body,* ed 9, St Louis, 1992, Mosby.)

neys change the degree of constriction or dilation of the arterioles in the renal capsule to maintain glomerular capillary pressure and urine production within normal limits over a rather wide range of arterial blood pressures.

Sympathetic neurons innervate the blood vessels of the kidney. The sympathetic stimulation in response to severe stress, intense exercise, or circulatory shock constricts the small arteries and the afferent arterioles, decreasing renal blood flow.

Reproductive System

Unlike many other organs and systems of the human body, the male and female reproductive systems are very different. The purpose of the male reproductive system is to produce and transfer spermatozoa to the female, and the purposes of the female reproductive system are to produce oocytes and to receive the spermatozoa for fertilization, conception, gestation, and birth.

Male Reproductive System

The male reproductive system consists of the testes, epididymis, ductus deferens, urethra, seminal vesicles, prostate gland, bulbourethral glands, scrotum, and penis (Fig. 6-55).

The testes are ovoid organs within the scrotum that develop as retroperitoneal organs in the abdominopelvic cavity. They move from the abdominal cavity to the scrotum by way of the inguinal canal, a canal common to both men and women. Normally the inguinal canal is closed, but it persists as a weak spot in the abdominal wall where the

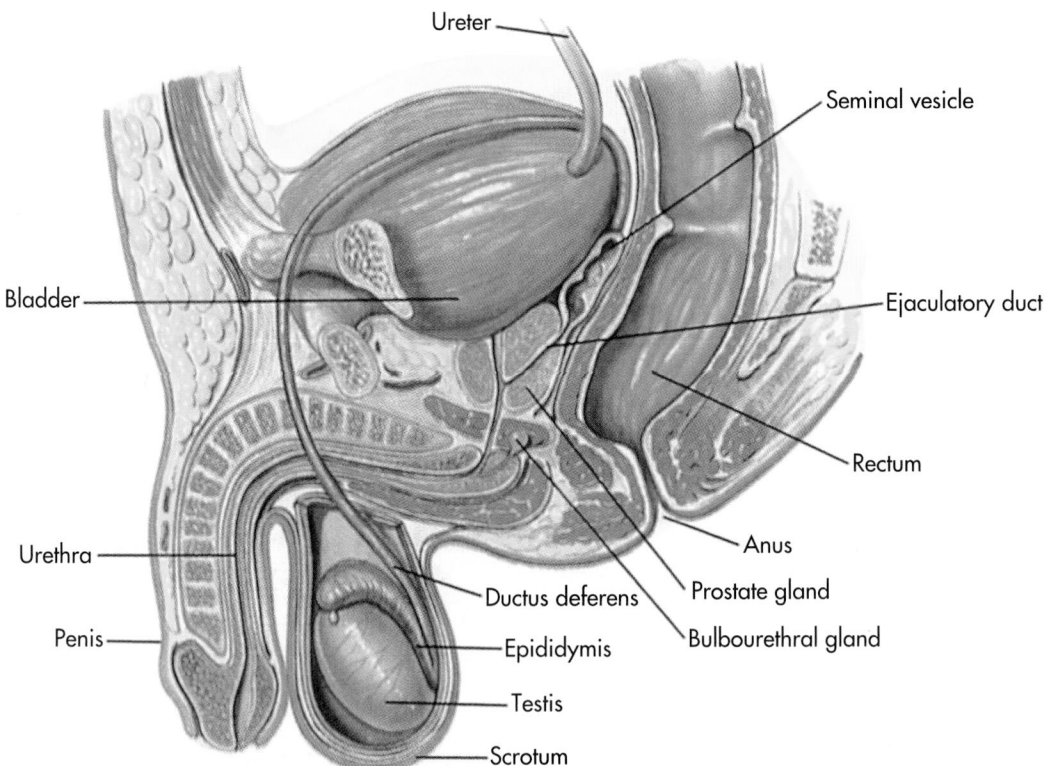

Fig. 6-55 Sagittal section of the male pelvis.

testes pass through it. If the inguinal canal weakens or ruptures, an inguinal hernia may result. Interstitial cells of the testes secrete the male hormone testosterone. Before puberty (12 to 14 years of age), the testes remain relatively simple and unchanged. At the time of puberty, however, the interstitial cells increase in number and size, and spermatozoa production begins. The testes contribute about 5% of the seminal fluid (semen).

The final maturation of spermatozoa occurs within the epididymis, a convoluted comma-shaped structure on the posterior side of the testis. Infection or injury can block one epididymis or both, resulting in infertility.

The ductus deferens, or vas deferens, emerges from the tail of the epididymis and ascends to the seminal vesicle, finally associating with the blood vessels and nerves that supply the testis. These structures and their coverings constitute the spermatic cord. The ductus deferens and the spermatic cord structures ascend and pass through the inguinal canal to enter the abdominal cavity. The ductus deferens crosses the lateral wall of the cavity, travels over the ureter, and loops over the posterior surface of the urinary bladder to approach

the prostate gland. The ductus deferens is surrounded by smooth muscle that helps to propel sperm through this duct.

The urethra is a passageway for both urine and male reproductive fluids. The urethra can be divided into three portions: the prostatic portion (the part of the urethra that passes through the prostate gland), the membranous portion (extending from the prostatic urethra through the muscular floor of the pelvis), and the spongy portion (extending the length of the penis).

The seminal vesicle is a sac-shaped gland that lies adjacent to each ductus deferens. A short duct from the seminal vesicle joins the ductus deferens to form the ejaculatory duct. These ducts project into the prostate gland and end by opening into the urethra. Seminal vesicles produce about 60% of seminal fluid.

? CRITICAL THINKING

What symptoms would you anticipate in patients with prostate glands greatly enlarged by either benign or malignant disease?

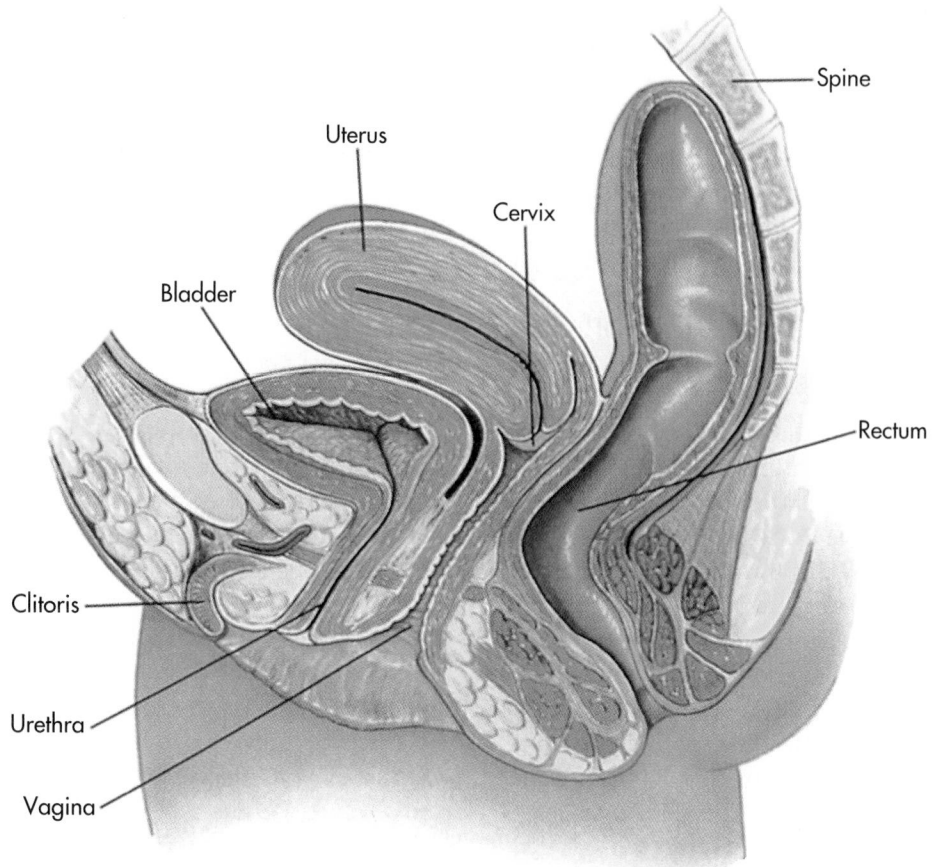

Fig. 6-56 Sagittal section of the female pelvis.

The prostate gland consists of both glandular and muscular tissue and is about the size and shape of a walnut. It is located dorsal to the symphysis pubis at the base of the bladder, surrounding the prostatic urethra and the two ejaculatory ducts. A total of 20 to 30 small prostatic ducts secrete prostatic fluid into the prostatic urethra. The prostate gland contributes about 30% of seminal fluid.

The bulbourethral glands are a pair of small glands located near the membranous portion of the urethra. In young adults they are each about the size of a pea, but they decrease in size with age. The gland is a compound mucous gland with small ducts that unite to form a single duct from each gland. The two bulbourethral glands enter the spongy urethra at the base of the penis. The bulbourethral glands add secretions to semen, contributing about 5% of seminal fluid.

The scrotum is divided into two internal compartments by a connective tissue septum. Beneath the skin of the scrotum is a layer of superficial fascia (loose connective tissue) and a layer of cuta-neous muscle called the *dartos muscle*. The dartos and the cremaster muscles of the abdomen are important for regulating temperature in the testes (required for spermatogenesis). They pull the testes near the body in cold temperatures and allow the testes to descend away from the body in warm temperatures and during exercise.

The penis consists of three columns of erectile tissue. Engorgement of this tissue with blood causes the penis to enlarge and become firm, producing an erection. The penis is the male organ of copulation and functions in the transfer of spermatozoa from the male to the female.

Female Reproductive System

The female reproductive organs consist of the ovaries, uterine (or fallopian) tubes, uterus, vagina, external genital organs, and mammary glands. The internal reproductive organs lie within the pelvis between the urinary bladder and the rectum and are held in place by a group of ligaments (Fig. 6-56).

The small ovaries are attached to the posterior of the broad ligament called the *mesovarium*. Two other ligaments associated with the ovary are the suspensory ligament and the ovarian ligament. The ovarian arteries, veins, and nerves traverse the suspensory ligament and enter the ovary through the mesovarium. Each ovary consists of a dense outer portion called the *cortex* and a looser inner portion called the *medulla*. Numerous small vesicles, called ovarian follicles (each of which contains an oocyte), are distributed throughout the cortex.

The uterine tubes are ducts for the ovaries. Each tube is located along the superior margin of the broad ligament and opens directly into the peritoneal cavity to receive the oocyte. Once inside the uterine tube, the oocyte is transported by cilia and peristaltic contractions of the smooth muscle within the uterine tube.

The uterus is the size and shape of a medium-sized pear. It is oriented in the pelvic cavity with the larger rounded portion (the fundus) directed superiorly. The narrower portion (the cervix) is directed

inferiorly. The main portion of the uterus (the body) is positioned between the fundus and the cervix. The major ligaments holding the uterus in place are the broad ligament, round ligaments, and uterosacral ligaments (Fig. 6-57).

The vagina is the female organ of copulation and functions to receive the penis during intercourse. It extends from the uterus to the outside of the body and provides a passage for menstrual flow and childbirth. The smooth muscle layer of the vagina allows the organ to increase in size to accommodate the penis during intercourse and to greatly stretch during delivery. The vaginal orifice is covered by a thin mucous membrane called the *hymen*. The openings in the hymen usually are enlarged during the first sexual intercourse but also may be perforated or torn during strenuous exercise.

The external genitalia, referred to as the vulva, consists of the vestibule and its surrounding structures (Fig. 6-58). The vestibule is the space into which the vagina and urethra open. It is bordered by a pair of thin, longitudinal skin folds called the *labia minora*. A small erectile structure, called the

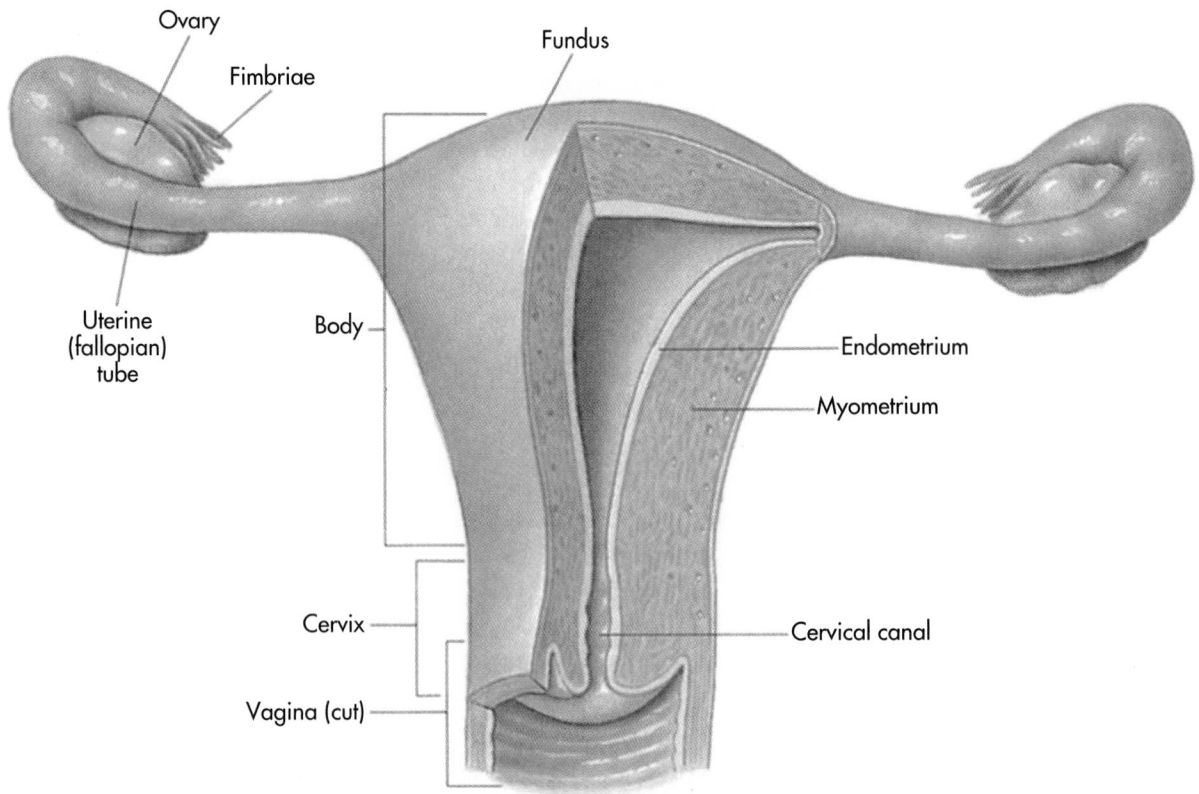

Fig. 6-57 Internal anatomy of the female pelvis. (From Thibodeau GA: *Structure and function of the body,* ed 9, St Louis, 1992, Mosby.)

clitoris, is located in the anterior margin of the vestibule. The two labia minora unite over the clitoris to form a fold of skin known as the *prepuce*. Lateral to the labia minora are two prominent folds of skin called the *labia majora*, which unite anteriorly in an elevation over the pubic symphysis to form the mons pubis. Most of the time, the labia majora are in contact with each other, concealing the deeper structures within the vestibule.

The perineum is divided into triangles by perineal muscles. The urogenital triangle contains the external genitalia, and the posterior anal triangle contains the anal opening. The region between the vagina and the anus is called the *clinical perineum* (an area that sometimes tears during childbirth).

The mammary glands are the organs of milk production located within the breasts or *mammae*. Externally, the breasts of both males and females have a raised nipple surrounded by a circular pigmented areola. Nipples are very sensitive to tactile stimulation and may become erect in response to sexual arousal. The areolae normally have a slightly bumpy surface because of the presence of areolar

glands just below their surface. Secretions from these glands protect the nipple and areola from chafing during nursing.

The female breasts begin to enlarge during puberty (usually between age 12 and 13) under the influence of estrogen and progesterone. Each adult female mammary gland consists of 15 to 20 glandular lobes covered by adipose tissue. Each lobe possesses a single lactiferous duct, which subdivides to form smaller ducts, each of which supplies a lobule. These ducts expand at their ends to form secretory sacs called *alveoli*, which secrete milk during nursing (Fig. 6-59).

Special Senses

Senses provide the brain with information about the outside world. Four senses are recognized as "special senses": smell, taste, sight, and hearing and balance. (The sense of touch is now considered to be a "general sense," which consists of several types of nerve endings scattered throughout the body and not localized to a specific area.)

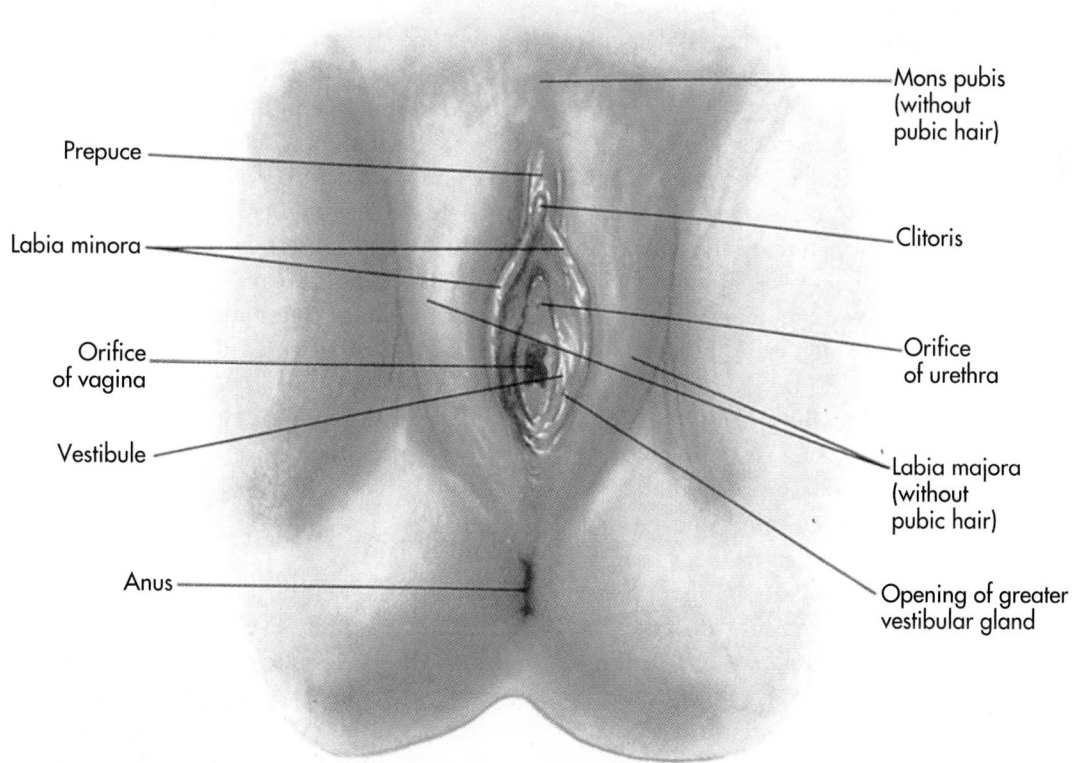

Fig. 6-58 Female external genitalia. (From Thibodeau GA: *Structure and function of the body,* ed 9, St Louis, 1992, Mosby.)

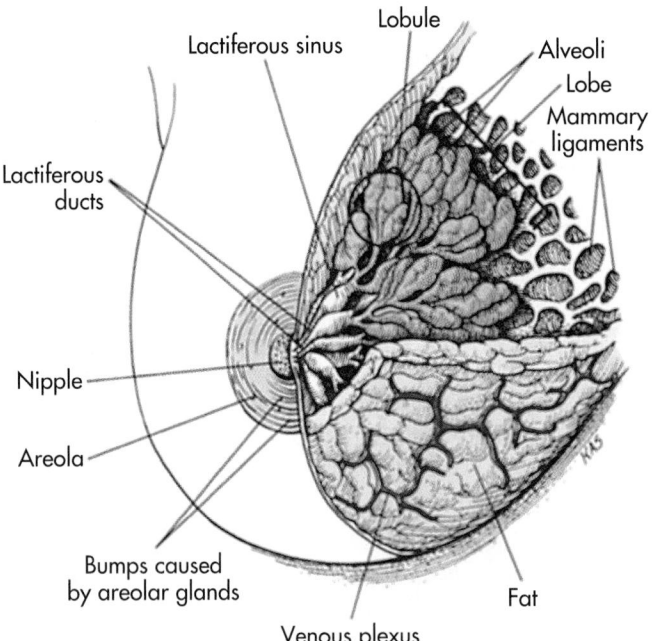

Fig. 6-59 Blood supply, mammary glands, and duct system of the right mamma.

Olfactory Sense Organs

The receptors for the fibers of the olfactory or first cranial nerves lie in the mucosa of the upper part of the nasal cavity (Fig. 6-60). Most of the nasal cavity is involved with respiration; only a small portion is devoted to olfaction.

The dendrites of olfactory neurons extend to the epithelial surface of the nasal cavity, where they form vesicles. These vesicles possess extremely long cilia that lie in a thin, mucous film on the epithelial surface. When olfactory cells are stimulated by airborne molecules, the resulting nerve impulses travel through the olfactory nerves in the olfactory bulb and olfactory tract. There they enter the thalamic and olfactory centers of the brain, where the nervous impulses are interpreted as specific odors.

The exact mechanism of olfactory stimulation is not clearly understood. It is generally believed that the variety of detectable smells are actually combinations of seven primary odors: (1) camphoraceous, (2) musky, (3) floral, (4) pepperminty, (5) ethereal, (6), pungent, and (7) putrid. Although olfactory receptors are extremely sensitive (even to slight odors), they also are easily fatigued. The olfactory system quickly adapts to continuous stimulation, and a particular odor may cease to be noticed in a short time. This is an important factor to consider when dealing with hazardous materials incidents (see Chapter 51).

Taste

The sensory structures that detect taste stimuli are called the *taste buds*, and the receptors for the taste nerve fibers are in the seventh and ninth cranial nerves. Most taste buds are associated with specialized portions of the tongue. However, taste buds also are located on other areas of the tongue, palate, lips, and throat.

Taste detected by taste buds can be divided into four basic types: bitter, sour, salty, and sweet. The tip of the tongue rèacts more strongly to sweet and salty tastes, the back of the tongue to bitter taste, and the sides of the tongue to sour taste (Fig. 6-61). All the other taste sensations result from a combination of taste bud and olfactory receptor stimulation.

Visual System

The visual system includes the eyes, the accessory structures (eyelids, eyebrows, eyelashes, and tear glands), and the optic nerve, tracts, and pathways. The second cranial nerve (optic nerve) conducts impulses from the eye to the brain, where these impulses produce the sensation of vision. The third cranial nerve (oculomotor nerve) conducts impulses from the brain to the muscles of the eye, where they cause contractions that move the eye.

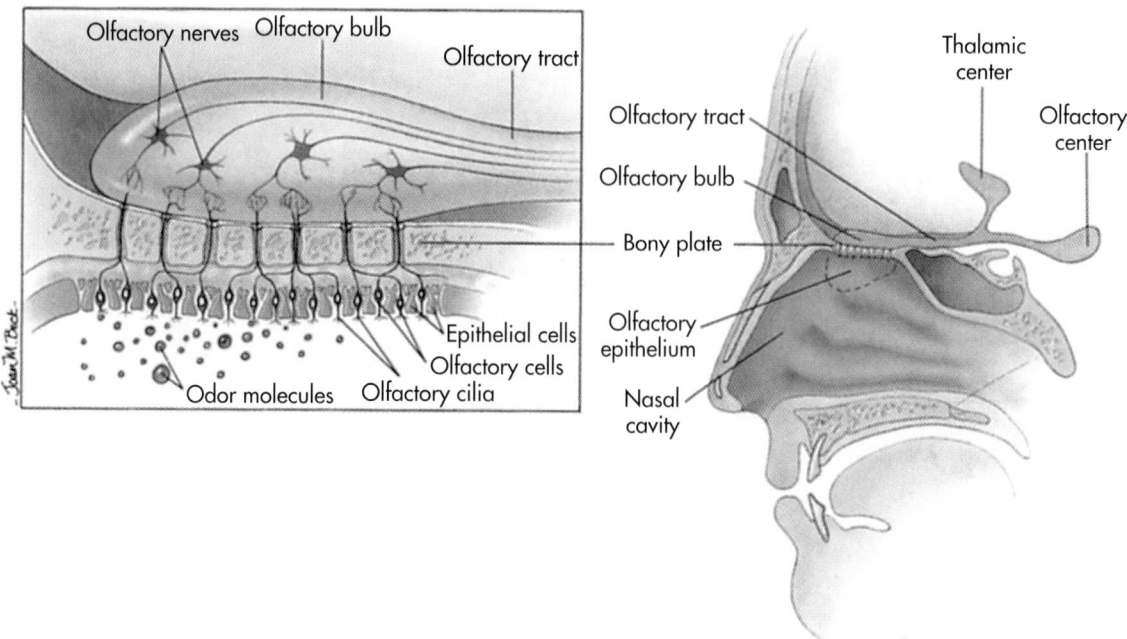

Fig. 6-60 Olfactory structures. Gas molecules stimulate olfactory cells in the nasal epithelium. Sensory information is then conducted along nerves in the olfactory bulb and olfactory tract to sensory-processing centers in the brain. (From Thibodeau GA: *Structure and function of the body,* ed 9, St Louis, 1992, Mosby.)

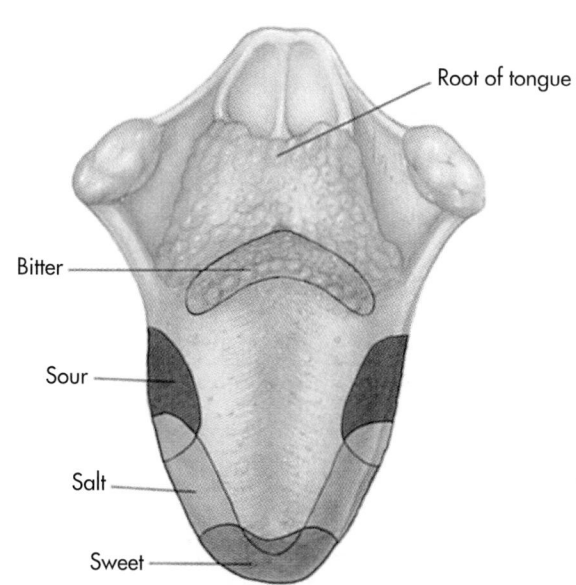

Fig. 6-61 Tongue. Dorsal surface and regions sensitive to various tastes. (From Thibodeau GA: *Structure and function of the body,* ed 9, St Louis, 1992, Mosby.)

? CRITICAL THINKING

Why is examination of the eyes a key component of the neurological evaluation?

Anatomy of the Eye

The eye is composed of three layers: the fibrous tunic, consisting of the sclera and cornea; the vascular tunic, consisting of the choroid, ciliary body, and iris; and the nervous tunic, consisting of the retina (Fig. 6-62).

1. The sclera is the firm, opaque, white outer layer of the eye. The sclera helps to maintain the shape of the eye, protects the internal structures of the eye, and provides an attachment point for the muscles that move the eye. The sclera is continuous with the meningeal layers of the brain that extend along the optic nerve. The cornea is continuous with the sclera. It is an avascular and transparent structure that permits light to enter the eye. The cornea also bends and refracts entering light.

2. The vascular tunic contains most of the blood vessels of the eyeball. The part of this layer associated with the sclera is the choroid. Anteriorly, the vascular tunic consists of the ciliary body and the iris. The ciliary body consists of ciliary muscles that can change the shape of the lens and of complex capillaries involved in producing aqueous humor. The iris is the colored part of the eye. It consists mainly of smooth muscle that surrounds the pupil. Light enters through the

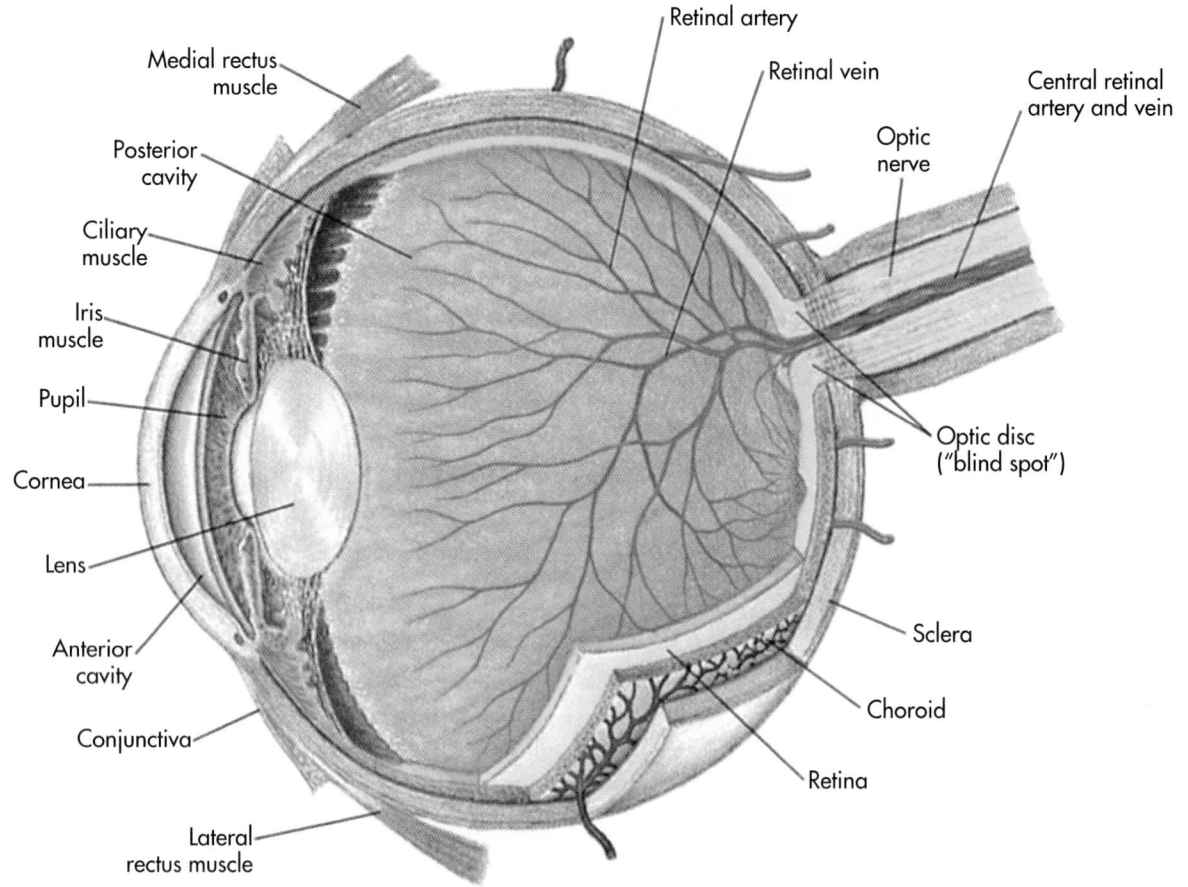

Fig. 6-62 Horizontal section through the left eyeball. The eye is viewed from above. (From Thibodeau GA: *Structure and function of the body,* ed 9, St Louis, 1992, Mosby.)

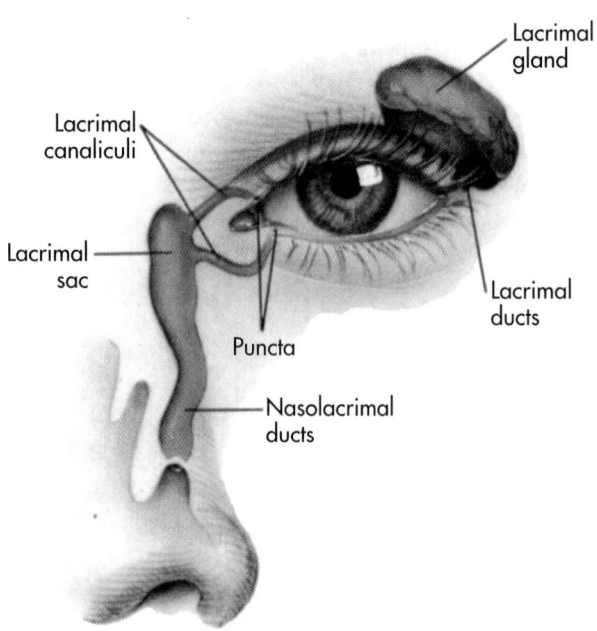

Fig. 6-63 Lacrimal structures of the eye.

pupil, and the iris regulates the amount of light by controlling the size of the pupil.

3. The retina consists of an outer pigmented retina and an inner sensory layer, which responds to light. The sensory retina contains photoreceptor cells, called *rods* and *cones*, and numerous relay neurons. (Rods are the receptors for night vision, and cones are the receptors for daytime and color vision.)

Compartments of the eye

The two compartments of the eye are separated by a lens, which is suspended between the two eye compartments by ligaments. These two compartments are known as the *anterior* and *posterior chambers*. The anterior chamber is filled with aqueous humor, which helps maintain intraocular pressure (pressure within the eye that keeps the eye inflated), refract light, and provide nutrition for the anterior chamber.

The posterior chamber of the eye is almost completely surrounded by the retina. It is filled with a

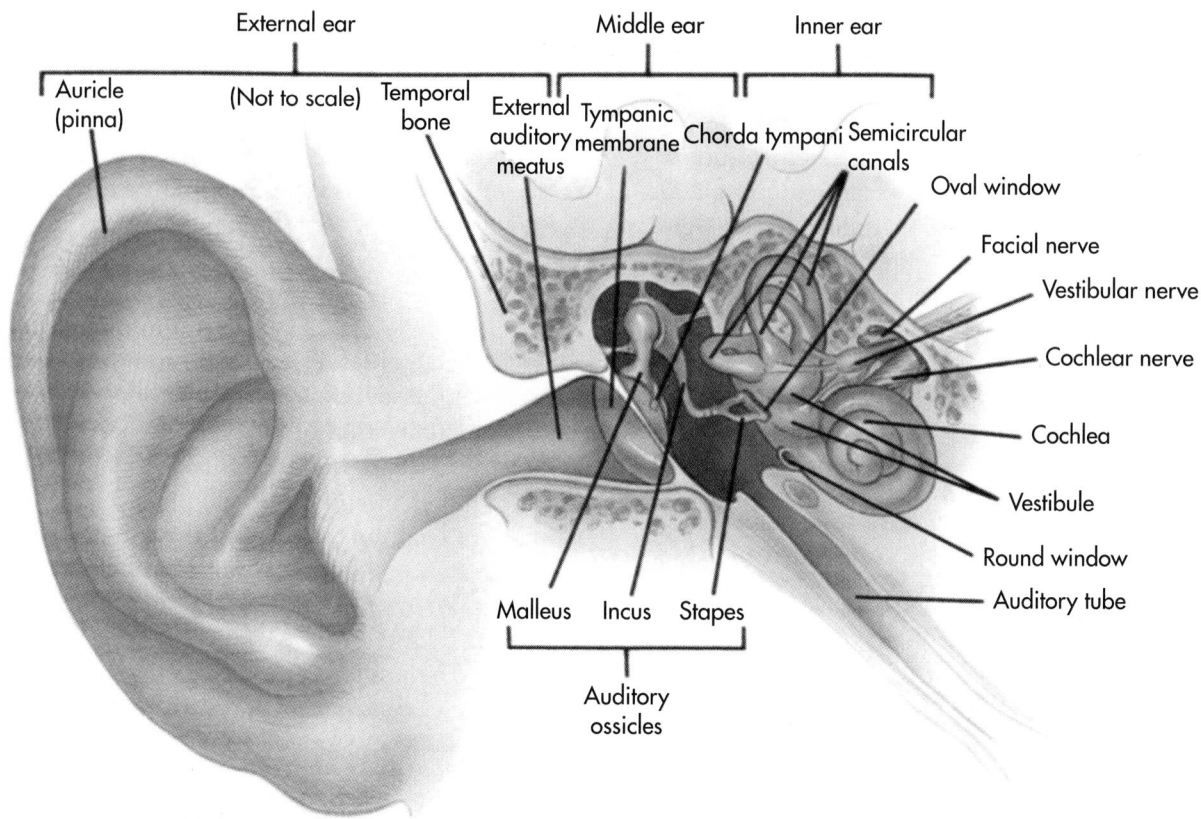

Fig. 6-64 External, middle, and inner ear.

transparent, jellylike substance called vitreous humor. Like aqueous humor, the vitreous humor helps maintain intraocular pressure. In addition, it helps to hold the retina in place and functions in the refraction of light in the eye.

Accessory structures

The eye's accessory structures protect, lubricate, move, and aid in the function of the eye. These structures include the eyebrows, eyelids, conjunctiva, and lacrimal gland.

Eyebrows protect the eyes by providing shade from direct sunlight and preventing perspiration from running into the eyes.

Eyelids protect the eyes from foreign objects. Blinking, which normally occurs about 25 times per minute, helps to lubricate the eyes by spreading tears over their surfaces. Eyelids also help to regulate the amount of light entering the eyes.

The conjunctiva is a thin, transparent mucous membrane that covers the inner surface of the eyelids and the outer surface of the sclera.

The lacrimal gland produces lacrimal fluid (tears) that leaves the gland through several ducts, passing over the anterior surface of the eyeball. The gland is situated in the superolateral corner of the orbit. Tears constantly are produced by this gland to moisten the surface of the eye, lubricate the eyelids, and wash away foreign objects. Tears also contain lysosomes that destroy some forms of bacteria.

Most tears evaporate from the surface of the eye. Excess fluid is collected in the medial corner of the eye by the lacrimal canals through a punctum (the opening of each canal). The lacrimal canals open into a lacrimal sac, which in turn continues into the nasolacrimal duct (Fig. 6-63).

Hearing and Balance

The organs of hearing can be divided into three portions: external, middle, and inner ear (Fig. 6-64). The external and middle ear are involved in hearing only, and the inner ear functions in both hearing and balance. The special senses of hearing and balance are both transmitted by the vestibulocochlear nerve (eighth cranial nerve).

The external ear includes the auricle, or pinna, and the external auditory meatus, which opens into the external auditory canal. The external auditory canal is lined by hairs and ceruminous glands, which produce cerumen. It terminates medially at the eardrum, or tympanic membrane. The middle ear is an air-filled space within the temporal bone, which contains the auditory ossicles.

? CRITICAL THINKING

Besides pain and impaired hearing, what other symptom would you anticipate in a patient with an inner ear problem?

The inner ear contains the sensory organs for hearing and balance. It consists of interconnecting tunnels and chambers within the *bony labyrinth.* Inside the bony labyrinth is another set of membranous tunnels and chambers called the *membranous labyrinth,* which is filled with a clear fluid called *endolymph.* The space between the membranous and bony labyrinth is filled with a fluid called *perilymph.* These fluids are similar to cerebrospinal fluid.

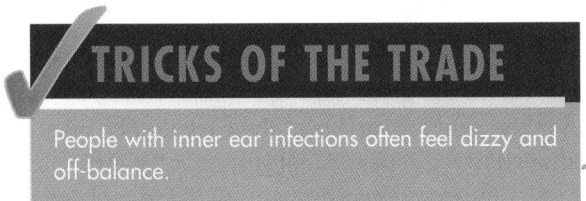

TRICKS OF THE TRADE

People with inner ear infections often feel dizzy and off-balance.

The auricle is shaped to collect sound waves and direct them toward the external auditory meatus. From the external auditory meatus, sound waves travel through the auditory canal to the tympanic membrane, causing the membrane to vibrate.

The middle ear is connected to the inner ear by two membrane-covered openings, the round and oval windows. Two other openings that are not covered by membranes provide a passage for air from the middle ear. One opens into the mastoid air cells. The second opening, the auditory (or eustachian) tube, opens into the pharynx and permits the equalization of air pressure between the outside air and middle ear cavity. (The shorter eustachian tubes in children make it easier for bacteria to travel from infected areas in the throat to the middle ear. This anatomical difference between children and adults is responsible for the increased frequency of pediatric earaches and infections.) The auditory ossicles of the middle ear (called the *malleus, incus,* and *stapes*) transmit vibrations from the tympanic membrane to the oval window.

The bony labyrinth of the inner ear is divided into three regions, called the *vestibule, cochlea,* and *semicircular canals.* The vestibule and semicircular canals are involved primarily in balance, and the cochlea is involved in hearing. The hearing sense organ, which lies inside the cochlea, is called the *organ of Corti.* In young, healthy people, the frequencies that can be detected by the ear range (over octaves) from 20 to 20,000 cycles per second.

SUMMARY

- The paramedic must thoroughly understand human anatomy to organize a patient assessment by body region and communicate effectively with medical direction and other members of the health care team.

- The anatomical position refers to a patient standing erect with palms facing the examiner.

- Directional terms, such as up or down, front or back, and right or left, are communicated in anatomical terminology and always refer to the patient, not the examiner. Internal body structure is classified into anatomical planes, or imaginary straight-line divisions, of the human body.

- The appendicular region of the body includes the limbs, or extremities. The axial region consists of the head, neck, thorax, and abdomen.

- The abdomen usually is divided into four quadrants: the upper right, lower right, upper left, and lower left.

- The three major cavities of the human body are the thoracic cavity, the abdominal cavity, and the pelvic cavity.

- The thoracic cavity contains the trachea, esophagus, thymus, heart, great vessels, lungs, and cavities and membranes that surround them. The abdominopelvic cavity is surrounded by membranes and contains organs and blood vessels.

- The cytoplasmic membrane encloses the cytoplasm, forming the outer boundary of the cell.

- Cytoplasm lies between the cytoplasmic membrane and the nucleus. Specialized structures in the cell (organelles) are located in the cytoplasm and perform functions important to the cell's survival. The nucleus is a large, membrane-bound organelle that ultimately controls all other organelles in the cytoplasm.

- All human cells, with the exception of the reproductive (sex) cells, reproduce by a process known as mitosis. In this process, cells divide to multiply.

- The four main types of tissue that compose the body's many organs are epithelial, connective, muscle, and nervous tissue. Epithelial tissue covers surfaces or forms structures. Connective tissue consists of cells separated from each other by intercellular material known as the extracellular matrix. Muscle tissue is contractile tissue that is responsible for movement. The nervous tissue is characterized by the ability to conduct electrical signals, which are known as action potentials.

- A system is a group of organs arranged to perform a more complex function than can any one organ alone. The eleven major organ systems in the body are the integumentary, skeletal, muscular, nervous, endocrine, circulatory, lymphatic, respiratory, digestive, urinary, and reproductive.

- The integumentary system consists of the skin and accessory structures such as hair, nails, and a variety of glands. The functions of the integumentary system include protecting the body against injury and dehydration, defense against infection, and temperature regulation.

- The skeletal system consists of bone and associated connective tissues, including cartilage, tendons, and ligaments. The skeletal system provides a rigid framework for support and protection and provides a system of levers on which muscles act to produce body movements.

- The three primary functions of the muscular system are movement, postural maintenance, and heat production.

- The nervous system and the endocrine system are the major regulatory and coordinating systems of the body. The nervous system rapidly transmits information by means of nerve impulses conducted from one body area to another. The endocrine system transits information more slowly by means of chemicals secreted by ductless glands into the bloodstream.

- The heart and cardiovascular system are responsible for circulating blood throughout the body. Blood transports nutrients and oxygen to tissues, carries carbon dioxide and waste products away from tissues, and carries hormones produced in endocrine glands to their target tissues. In addition, blood plays an important role in temperature regulation and fluid balance and protects the body from bacteria and foreign substances.

- The lymphatic system includes lymph, lymphocytes, lymph nodes, tonsils, spleen, and thymus gland. The three basic functions of the lymphatic system are to help maintain fluid balance in tissues, absorb fats and other substances from the digestive tract, and play a role in the body's immune defense system.

- The organs of the respiratory system and the cardiovascular system transport oxygen to individual cells and transport carbon dioxide from individual cells to where it is released into the air. The entrance to the respiratory tract begins at the nasal cavity and includes the nasopharynx, oropharynx, laryngopharynx, and larynx. Below the glottis are the structures of the lower airway and lungs. These structures include the trachea, the bronchial tree, the alveoli, and the lungs.

- The digestive system provides the body with water, electrolytes, and other nutrients used by cells. The GI tract is an irregularly shaped tube associated with accessory organs (primarily glands) that secrete fluid into the digestive tract.

- The urinary system works with other body systems to maintain homeostasis by removing waste products from the blood and helping to maintain a constant body fluid volume and composition. The contents of the urinary system include two kidneys, two ureters, the urinary bladder, and the urethra.

- The purpose of the male reproductive system is to produce and transfer spermatozoa to the female; the purpose of the female reproductive system is to produce oocytes and to receive the spermatozoa for fertilization, conception, gestation, and birth. The male reproductive system consists of the testes, epididymis, ductus deferens, urethra, seminal vesicles, prostate gland, bulbourethral glands, scrotum, and penis. The female reproductive organs consist of the ovaries, uterine (or fallopian) tubes, uterus, vagina, external genital organs, and mammary glands.

- Senses provide the brain with information about the outside world. Four senses are recognized as "special senses": smell, taste, sight, and hearing and balance.

REFERENCE

1. McCance K, S Huether: *Pathophysiology: the biologic basis for disease in adults and children*, ed 2, St Louis, 1994, Mosby.

7 General Principles of Pathophysiology

OBJECTIVES

Upon completion of this chapter, the paramedic student will be able to:

1. Describe the normal characteristics of the cellular environment and the key homeostatic mechanisms that strive to maintain a fluid and electrolyte balance.

2. Outline pathophysiological alterations in water and electrolyte balance and their effect on body functions.

3. Describe the treatment of patients who have selected fluid or electrolyte imbalances.

4. Describe the mechanisms within the body that maintain normal acid-base balance.

5. Outline pathophysiological alterations in acid-base balance.

6. Describe the management of a patient with an acid-base imbalance.

7. Describe alterations in cells and tissues related to cellular adaptation, injury, neoplasia, aging, or death.

8. Outline the effects of cellular injury on local and systemic body functions.

9. Describe alterations in body functions related to genetic and familial disease factors.

10. Outline the causes, adverse systemic effects, and compensatory mechanisms associated with hypoperfusion.

11. Describe how the body's inflammatory and immune responses respond to cellular injury or antigenic stimulation.

12. Explain how alterations in immunity and inflammation can cause harmful effects on body functions.

13. Describe the impact of stress on the body's response to illness or injury.

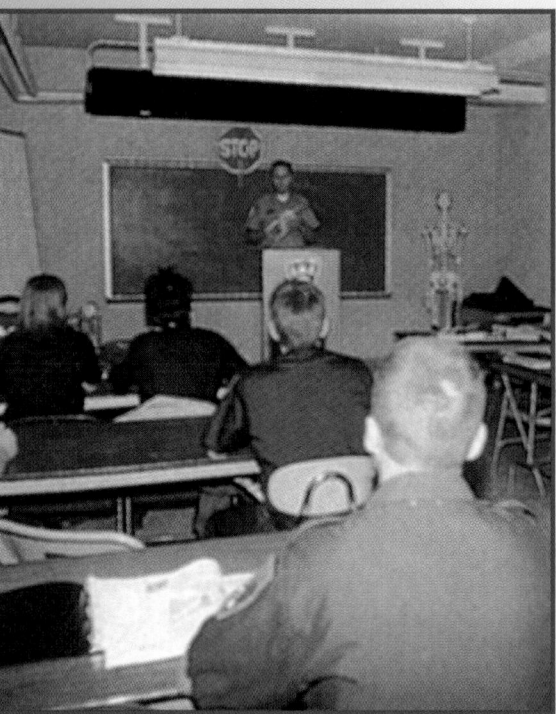

Paramedics should appreciate the correlation of pathophysiology with disease process so that they can better understand, anticipate, direct, and provide appropriate care to patients. With knowledge of physical and biological principles, paramedics can apply these to the mechanisms and complications of disease.

KEY TERMS

acidosis: A condition in which the blood is abnormally acidic (arterial pH below 7.35); an abnormal increase in hydrogen ion concentration.

active transport: A carrier-mediated process that can move substances against a concentration gradient.

aerobic: Of or pertaining to the presence of air or oxygen.

afterload: The total resistance against which blood must be pumped. Also known as peripheral vascular resistance.

alkalosis: A condition in which the blood is abnormally basic (pH greater than 7.0 in water or solution).

allergens: Substances that can produce hypersensitivity reactions in the body.

anaerobic: Of or pertaining the absence of oxygen.

antigens: Substances (usually proteins) that cause the formation of an antibody and react specifically with that antibody.

atrophy: A decrease or shrinkage in cellular size that adversely affects cell function.

B lymphocytes: Lymphocytes that are responsible for antibody-mediated immunity.

cation: An ion with a positive charge.

diffusion: The process in which solid, particulate matter in a fluid moves from an area of higher concentration to an area of lower concentration, resulting in an even distribution of the particles in the fluid.

dysplasia: Abnormal cellular growth.

edema: The accumulation of fluid within the interstitial spaces.

extracellular fluid: The water found outside the cells; includes the intravascular and interstitial compartments.

facilitated diffusion: A carrier-mediated process that moves substances into or out of cells from a high to a low concentration.

hypercalcemia: A greater-than-normal concentration of calcium in the blood.

hyperkalemia: A greater-than-normal concentration of potassium in the blood.

hypermagnesemia: A greater-than-normal concentration of magnesium in the blood.

hyperplasia: An excessive increase in cell number.

hypersensitivity reactions: Altered immunological responses to an antigen that result in a pathological immune response after reexposure.

hypertonic: A solution that causes cells to shrink.

hypertrophy: An increase in cell size.

hypokalemia: A lower-than-normal concentration of potassium in the blood.

hypomagnesemia A condition that results from an abnormally low concentration of magnesium in the blood plasma.

hyponatremic: A condition caused by a less-than-normal concentration of sodium in the blood.

hypoperfusion: Inadequate circulation that results in insufficient delivery of oxygen and nutrients necessary for normal tissue and cellular function. Also known as shock.

hypotonic: A solution that causes cells to swell.

hypoxemia: Inadequate cellular oxygenation.

immune response: A defense function of the body that produces antibodies to destroy invading antigens and malignancies.

interstitial fluid: Fluid that occupies the space outside the blood vessels.

intracellular fluid: The fluid found in all body cells.

ischemia: Insufficient perfusion of oxygenated blood to a body organ or part.

isotonic: A solution that causes cells to neither shrink nor swell.

lactic acidosis: A disorder characterized by an accumulation of lactic acid in the blood, resulting in a lowered pH in muscle and serum.

mediated transport mechanisms: Mechanisms that use carrier molecules to move large, water-soluble molecules or electrically charged molecules across cell membranes.

metaplasia: A change from one cell type to another that is better able to tolerate adverse conditions; a conversion into a form that is not normal for that cell.

multiple organ dysfunction syndrome: The progressive failure of two or more organ systems after a very severe illness or injury.

necrosis: Death of a cell or group of cells as the result of disease or injury.

negative feedback mechanisms: Any mechanism that tends to balance a change in a system.

osmolality: The osmotic concentration of a solution.

osmosis: Diffusion of solvent (water) through a membrane from a less concentrated solution to a more concentrated solution.

partial pressure: The pressure exerted by a single gas.

peripheral vascular resistance: The total resistance against which blood must be pumped. Also known as afterload.

pH: An inverse logarithm of the hydrogen ion concentration.

preload: The amount of blood returning to the ventricle.

semipermeable membranes: Membranes that are pervious such that fluids and other substances can pass through them.

solutes: Substances dissolved in solution.

Starling's law: The hypothesis used to describe the movement of fluid back and forth across the capillary wall (net filtration).

stroke volume: The volume of blood ejected from one ventricle in a single heartbeat.

T lymphocytes: Thymus-derived lymphocytes of immunological importance; responsible for cell-mediated immunity.

virulence: The relative strength of a pathogen.

SECTION ONE
CELLULAR PHYSIOLOGY

Basic Cellular Review

As described in Chapter 6, the cell is the fundamental unit found in higher life forms. All cells require various key components and structures: a cell membrane to hold them together and separate the internal (cellular) environment from the external environment, enzymes to bring about biochemical processes, internal membranes to encapsulate chemicals, and genetic material for producing components for their own replication. Cells form the four basic tissue types, which include the following:

1. Epithelial
2. Connective (including hematological tissue)
3. Muscle
4. Nervous

NOTE

Refer to Chapter 6 to review basic cellular function and tissue types.

The Cellular Environment

The cells of the body live in a fluid environment of which water is the main component. The importance of body water is highlighted by two facts. First, it is the medium in which all metabolic reactions occur; and secondly, the precise regulation of the volume and composition of body fluid is essential to health. The human body can be viewed as containing two fluid compartments: the **intracellular fluid** (ICF) and **extracellular fluid** (ECF) (Fig. 7-1).

Intracellular and Extracellular Fluid

ICF is the fluid found in all body cells. It accounts for 40% of total body weight. ECF is the water found outside the cells and includes the intravascular and interstitial compartments. This fluid accounts for about 20% of total body weight, the intravascular component (blood plasma) composing about one third of this. **Interstitial fluid** (IF) is the extracellular fluid between the cells and outside the vascular bed (i.e., connective tissue, cartilage, and bone). This category also includes special fluids, such as cerebrospinal fluid and intraocular fluid, and accounts for about 15% to 16% total body weight.

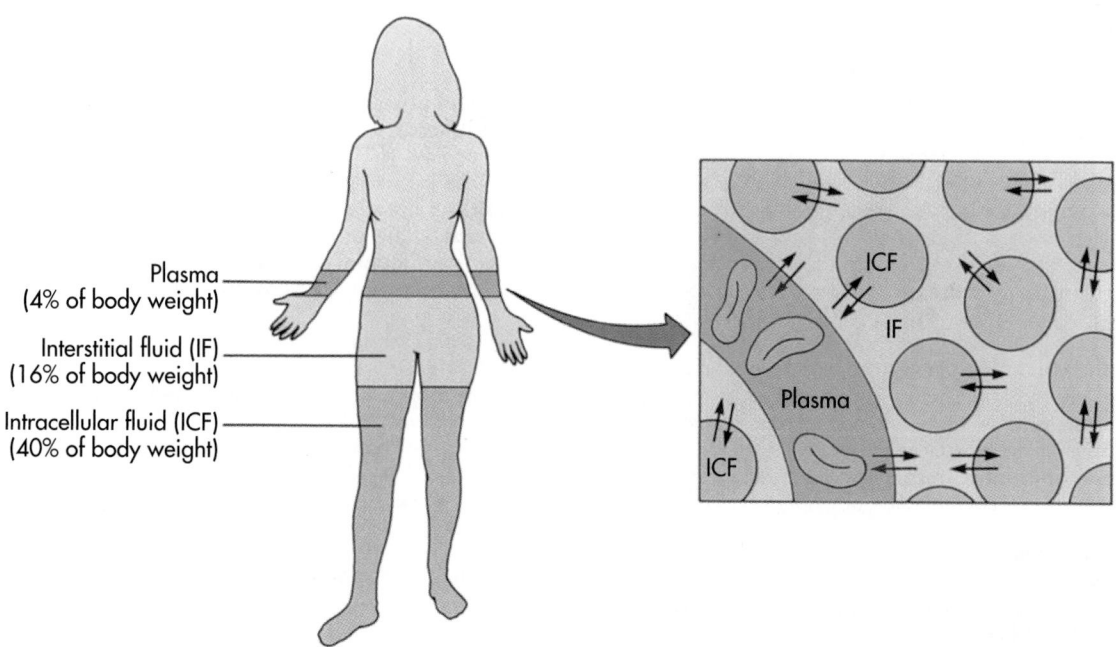

Plasma
(4% of body weight)

Interstitial fluid (IF)
(16% of body weight)

Intracellular fluid (ICF)
(40% of body weight)

Fig. 7-1 Fluid compartments of the body.

Aging and the Distribution of Body Fluids

Water is the main component of body mass, accounting for 50% to 60% of total body weight in adults. The distribution and amount of total body water (TBW) change with age. For example, TBW in newborn infants accounts for about 80% of their body weight. During childhood, TBW decreases to 60% to 65% of body weight, and further declines with age (Table 7-1).

> **NOTE**
>
> The normal reduction in TBW in older adults is clinically important in the presence of fever or dehydration. Loss of body fluids with illness or injury can be severe or life threatening.

Water Movement Between ICF and ECF

Body fluids constantly move from one compartment to another. In healthy individuals, the volume of fluid in each compartment remains about the same. To keep the volume stable, the body uses **osmosis, diffusion**, and **mediated transport mechanisms**.

> **NOTE**
>
> Knowledge about the movement of fluids in the body and possible alterations in body fluids is important in understanding illness and disease.

Osmosis

The movement of molecules within a cell or across cell membranes is essential for normal body functioning. Fluid compartments are separated by membranes, most of which allow water to pass freely but regulate or restrict the flow of **solutes** (substances dissolved in solution) on the basis of their size, shape, electrical charge, or other chemical proper-

ties. These membranes are referred to as **semipermeable membranes.** Channels in membranes permit passage of solutes; they may be open at all times to specific solutes, or closed at times, depending on the physiology of the cell. The ability of the cell membrane to selectively regulate solute transition enables the cell to maintain homeostasis (a relative constancy in the internal environment of the body).

Osmosis is functionally defined as the flow of fluid across a semipermeable membrane from a lower solute concentration to a higher solute concentration (Fig. 7-2). With gases, the driving force of osmosis is produced by the **partial pressure** of the dissolved gases (osmotic pressure). These include oxygen, nitrogen, carbon dioxide, and water. With nongaseous particles (e.g., electrolytes), osmotic pressure depends

> **NOTE**
>
> In any mixture of gases, the combination of the pressures exerted by all the gases is referred to as the *total pressure*, and the pressure exerted by a single gas is referred to as the *partial pressure*. The partial pressure of a gas in a mixture is denoted by a P preceding the gas (e.g., PO_2, PCO_2) (see Chapter 11).

> **NOTE**
>
> Electrolytes are salt substances whose molecules dissociate into charged components when in water, producing positively and negatively charged ions. An ion with a positive charge is called a **cation**, and an ion with a negative charge is called an *anion*. Sodium is the most abundant ECF cation and is responsible for the osmotic balance of the ECF space. Potassium is the most abundant ICF cation and maintains the osmotic balance of the ICF space. The body also contains nonelectrolytes (substances with no electrical charge), such as glucose and urea.

TABLE 7-1	TOTAL BODY WATER IN RELATION TO BODY WEIGHT		
TBW (%) BODY BUILD	**TBW (%) ADULT MALE**	**TBW (%) ADULT FEMALE**	**INFANT**
Normal	60	50	70
Lean	70	60	80
Obese	50	42	60

From McCance KL, Huether SE: *Pathophysiology: the biologic basis for disease in adults and children*, ed 3, St Louis, 1998, Mosby.

Fig. 7-2 Osmosis. **A,** The end of a tube containing 3% salt solution is closed at one end with a semipermeable membrane that allows water molecules to pass through it but retains the salt molecules within the tube. **B,** The tube is immersed in distilled water. Because the tube contains salt and water molecules, the tube has proportionately less water than the beaker, which contains only water. The water molecules diffuse with their concentration gradient into the tube. Because the salt molecules cannot leave the tube, the total fluid volume inside the tube increases, and fluid moves up the glass tube as a result of osmosis. **C,** Water continues to move into the tube until the weight of the column of the water in the tube (hydrostatic pressure) exerts a downward force equal to the osmotic force moving water molecules into the tube. The hydrostatic pressure that prevents net movement of water into the tube is called the *osmotic pressure* of the solution in the tube.

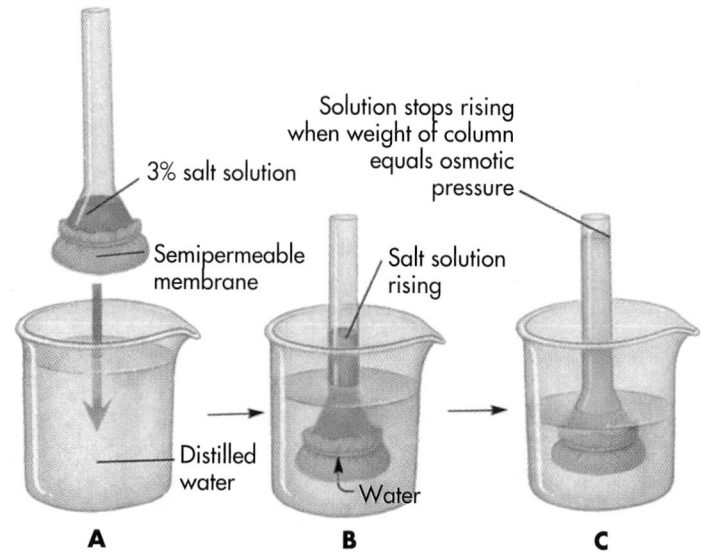

Fig. 7-3 Effects of hypotonic, isotonic, and hypertonic solutions on red blood cells. **A,** Hypotonic solutions with low ion concentrations result in swelling and lysis of cells. **B,** Isotonic solutions with normal ion concentrations result in normal-shaped cells. **C,** Hypertonic solutions with high ion concentrations result in shrinkage (crenation) of the cell.

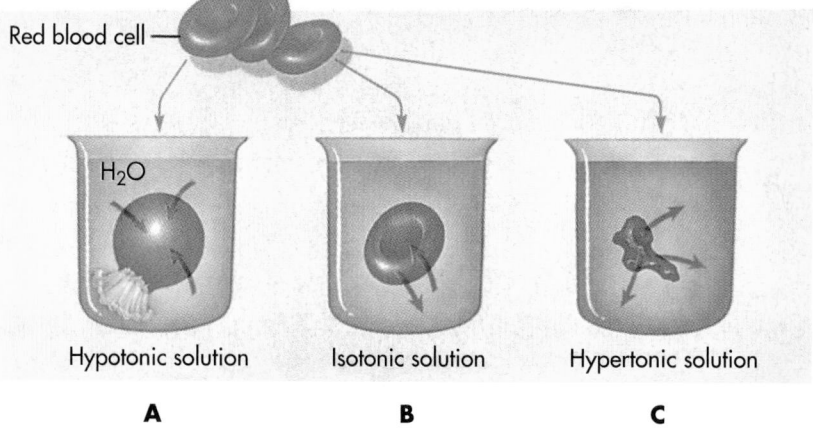

on the number and molecular weights of particles on each side of the membrane and the permeability of the membrane to these particles.

When a living cell is placed in a solution that has a higher solute concentration (and thus a lower water concentration) than that inside the cell, the solution is referred to as **hypertonic** with respect to the cell. The osmotic pressure exerted on the cell produces a net movement of water molecules out of the cell. This net movement causes the cell to dehydrate, shrink (crenate), and, if severe enough, leads to cellular death.

When a living cell is placed in a solution that has a lower solute concentration (and thus a higher water concentration) than that inside the cell, the solution is referred to as **hypotonic** with respect to the cell. In this situation, osmotic pressure draws water molecules from the surrounding solution into the cell. The net movement of water molecules into the cell causes it to swell and perhaps burst, or lyse.

When a living cell is placed in a solution in which the solute concentration (and water concentration) is the same as the solution inside the cell, the solution is referred to as **isotonic.** Isotonic solutions have no net movement of water molecules (Fig. 7-3) (see the box on the following page).

Diffusion

Diffusion results from the constant, random motion of all the atoms, molecules, or ions in a solution.

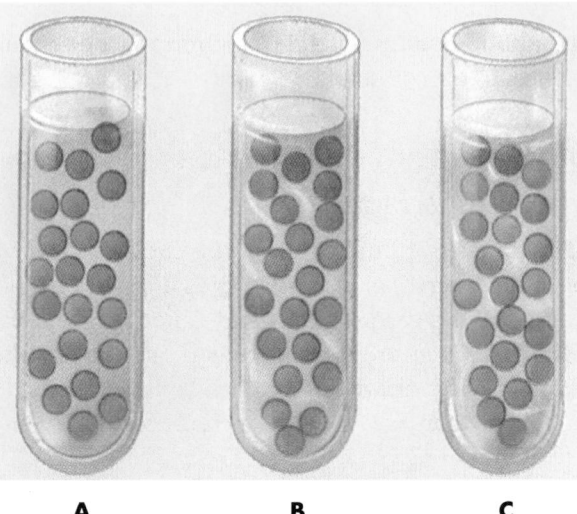

A   **B**   **C**

Fig. 7-4 Diffusion. **A,** One solution (*red,* representing one type of molecule) is layered onto a second solution (*blue,* representing a second type of molecule). A concentration gradient for the red molecules from the red solution into the blue solution exists because there are no red molecules in the blue solution. A concentration gradient for the blue molecules from the blue solution into the red solution also exists because there are no blue molecules in the red solution. **B,** Red molecules move with their concentration gradient into the blue solution, and the blue molecules move with their concentration gradient into the red solution. **C,** Red and blue molecules are distributed evenly throughout the solution. Even though the red and blue molecules continue to move randomly and equilibrium exists, no net movement occurs because no concentration gradient exists.

FLUID REPLACEMENT THERAPY

Intravenous therapy is based on hypertonic, hypotonic, and isotonic properties.

Hypertonic Solutions

A hypertonic solution has a higher concentration of solute molecules than that inside normal cells. When this solution is infused into a normally hydrated patient, it draws water from the cells into the vascular space. Examples of hypertonic solutions are mannitol (Osmitrol), sodium bicarbonate, and 50% dextrose (D_{50}).

These solutions are often used to treat cerebral edema (mannitol), metabolic acidosis (bicarbonate), and profound hypoglycemia (50% dextrose). In addition, recent studies have suggested the use of some hypertonic solutions (for example, dextran, hetastarch, and NaCl [3%, 5%, and 7.5%]), for volume restoration after trauma.[3] By drawing tissue fluid into the vascular space, hypertonic solutions may reduce the volume of infusion and post-resuscitation pulmonary problems.

Hypotonic Solutions

A hypotonic solution has a solute concentration lower than that of the cells. When this solution is infused into a normally hydrated patient, water moves from the solution into the cells. These solutions supply calories and replenish salt and water and are used to hydrate patients or to prevent dehydration. Examples of hypotonic solutions include 2.5% dextrose in water and 0.45% normal saline (½NS). Although technically isotonic, D_5W acts physiologically as a hypotonic solution because the solute (glucose) is actively transported into cells, leaving excess free water behind.

Isotonic Solutions

In an isotonic solution, the concentration of solute molecules equals that inside most normal cells. When this solution is infused into a normally hydrated patient, it neither draws water out of the cells nor moves water into the cells but rather stays in the vascular space. Isotonic solutions are usually prescribed to replace extracellular fluid lost from blood loss, severe vomiting, or any situation in which the chloride loss equals or exceeds the sodium loss. Examples of isotonic solutions are 0.9% normal saline and lactated Ringer's solution.

This passive process moves molecules or ions from an area of higher concentration to an area of lower concentration (Fig. 7-4). Because more solute particles are in an area of high concentration than in an area of low concentration and because the particles move randomly, more solute particles move from the higher to the lower concentration than in the opposite direction. At equilibrium, in contrast, the net movement of solute stops. The random molecular motion continues, but the movement of solutes in one direction is balanced by equal movement in the opposite direction.

? CRITICAL THINKING

> *What happens to a raisin when it is placed in a cup of water for an hour? Why does this change occur? Is the water hypotonic, hypertonic, or isotonic relative to the inside of the raisin? Does a concentration gradient exist?*

If a solute concentration is greater at one point than at another point in the solvent, a concentration gradient exists. Solutes diffuse down their concentration gradients from high to low concentration until equilibrium is achieved. Some nutrients enter and some waste products leave the cell by diffusion. The maintenance of appropriate intracellular concentrations of certain substances depends on this process.

Mediated Transport Mechanisms

A number of essential molecules (e.g., glucose) cannot enter most cells by diffusion, and a number of products (e.g., some proteins) cannot exit most cells by diffusion. To move large water-soluble molecules or electrically charged molecules across the cell membranes, mediated transport mechanisms are necessary. These transport mechanisms use carrier molecules, proteins that combine with solutes on one side of a membrane and transport the solute to the other side (Fig. 7-5).

Mediated transport can be divided into two categories: **active transport** and **facilitated diffusion**. Active transport is a carrier-mediated process that can move substances against a concentration gradient from areas of lower concentration to areas of higher concentration. To work against this concentration gradient, energy is expended by the cell. Active transport occurs at a faster rate than diffusion.

Facilitated diffusion is a carrier-mediated process that moves substances into and out of cells from a high to a low concentration. For these substances, the direction of movement is *with* the concentration gradient, but like active transport, the movement is faster than that for which ordinary diffusion can account. Facilitated diffusion is distinguished from active transport in that it does not require an expenditure of energy. Its moving force is a downhill concentration gradient.

Water Movement Between Plasma and Interstitial Fluid

The transfer of fluid between the circulating blood and the interstitial fluid occurs as a result of pressure changes at the arterial and venous ends of the capillary. There are about 10 billion capillaries in the human body, and few functional cells of the body are more than 5/1000 of an inch (20 to 30 microns) away from one.

Anatomy of the Capillary Network

The typical capillary is a thin-walled tube of endothelial cells without elastic tissue, connective tissue, or smooth muscle that would impede the transfer of water and solutes. Blood enters the capillary network from the arterioles and flows through the capillary network into the venules. The ends of the capillaries closest to the arterioles are called *arteriolar capillaries*, and the ends closest to the venules are called *venous capillaries*.

The exchange of nutrients and metabolic end products takes place at the capillary level. The arterioles give rise directly to capillaries or in some tissues to metarterioles, which then give rise to capillaries. As described in Chapter 6, most tissues appear to have two distinct types of capillaries: true capillaries and thoroughfare channels. From a metarteriole, blood may flow into a thoroughfare channel that connects arterioles and venules directly, bypassing the true capillaries. Blood flow through thoroughfare channels is relatively constant. From these thoroughfare channels, fluid commonly exits and reenters the network of true capillaries.

The capillaries of some tissues contain small cuffs of smooth muscle that encircle their proximal and distal portions, known as *capillary sphincters*. The sphincter at the arterial end is known as the *precapillary sphincter*, and that at the venous end is known as the *postcapillary sphincter*. These sphincters control capillary blood flow by opening and closing the entrance and exit to the capillary. Blood flow in true capillaries is not uniform and depends on the contractile state of the arterioles

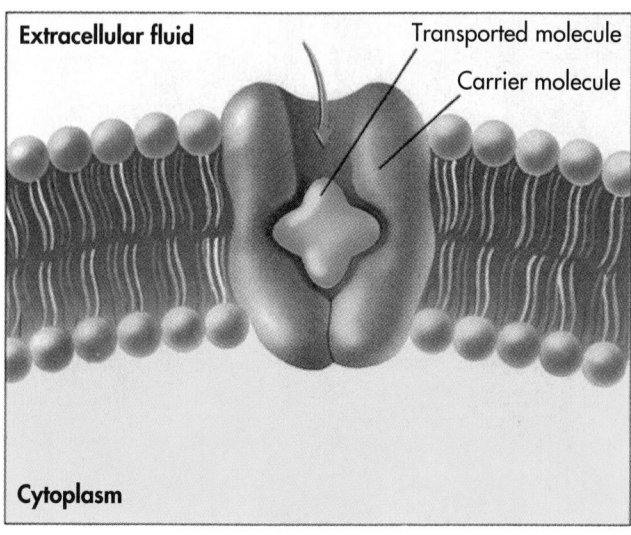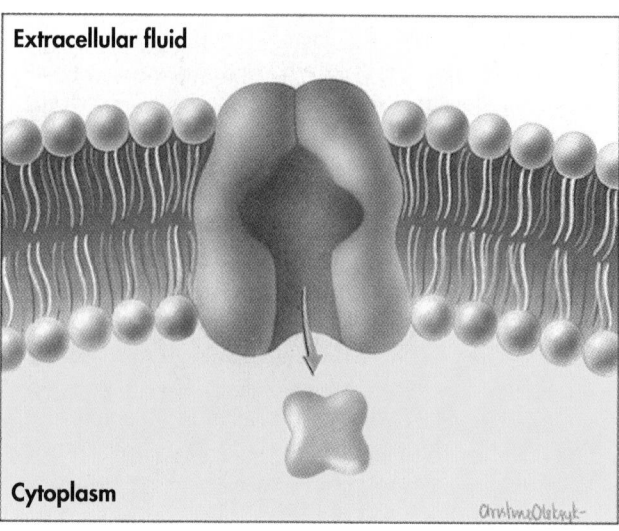

A   **B**

Fig. 7-5 Mediated transport by a carrier molecule. **A,** The carrier molecule binds with a molecule on one side of the plasma membrane and changes shape. **B,** The molecule is released on the other side of the plasma membrane.

and the precapillary and postcapillary sphincters (if present).

The blood flow through the capillaries that provides the exchange of gases and solutes between blood and tissue is referred to as *nutritional flow.* Blood that bypasses the capillaries in traveling from the arterial to the venous side of the circulation is known as *nonnutritional* or *shunt flow.* True arteriovenous anastomoses (AV shunts), which occur naturally in the sole of the foot, the palm of the hand, the terminal phalanges, and the nail bed, are important in regulating body temperature. Some evidence also suggests the presence of AV shunts upstream from the capillary sphincters.

Sympathetic fibers innervate all blood vessels of the body except the capillaries, capillary sphincters, and most metarterioles. Sympathetic innervation of blood vessels includes both vasoconstrictor and vasodilator (vasomotor) fibers. However, the sympathetic vasoconstrictor fibers are the most important in regulating blood flow. During normal circulation in the healthy body when arterial blood pressure is adequate, arterioles are open (though with some vasomotor tone), AV shunts are closed, and about

20% of the capillaries are open at any given time (Fig. 7-6).

Diffusion across the capillary wall. Tissue cells do not exchange material directly with blood. The interstitial fluid always acts as a middle man. Nutrients must diffuse across the capillary wall into the interstitial fluid to enter cells, and metabolic end products must first move across cell membranes into interstitial fluid to diffuse into the plasma.

At the arteriole end of the capillary, the forces moving fluid out of the capillary are greater than the forces attracting fluid into it. At the venous end, these forces are reversed, so more fluid is attracted into the capillary. Hydrostatic and osmotic pressure are the two forces responsible for this movement of fluid. The osmotic pressure results from the presence of plasma proteins (mostly albumin), which are too large to pass through the wall of the capillary; this pressure is referred to as *blood colloid osmotic pressure* or *oncotic pressure.*

At the venous end of the capillary, the hydrostatic pressure is lower. The concentration of proteins in the capillary increases slightly because of the movement of fluid out of the arteriolar end, resulting in a

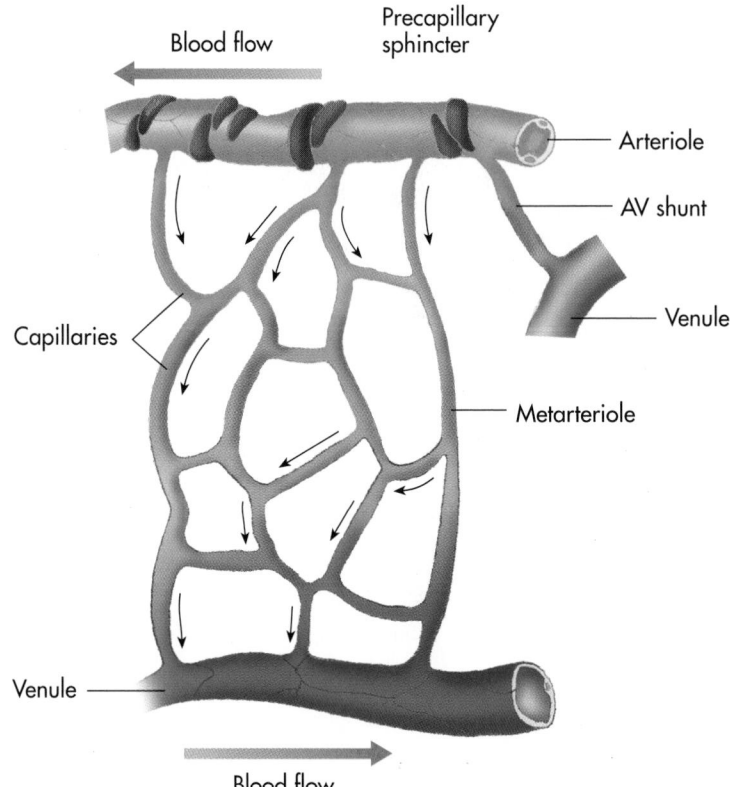

Fig. 7-6 Microcirculation. The circular structures on the arteriole and venule represent smooth muscle fibers; branching solid lines represent sympathetic nerve fibers. The arrows indicate the direction of blood flow.

greater plasma protein concentration and a greater colloid osmotic pressure. As a result, nearly all of the fluid that leaves the capillary at its arteriolar end reenters the capillary at its venous end. The remaining fluid enters the lymphatic capillaries and eventually is returned to the general circulation.

NOTE

The movement of fluid back and forth across the capillary wall is called *net filtration* and is best described by **Starling's hypothesis:**

Net filtration = forces favoring filtration −
forces opposing filtration

The forces favoring filtration include capillary hydrostatic pressure and the interstitial oncotic pressure. The forces opposing filtration are the plasma oncotic pressure and the interstitial hydrostatic pressure.

Fluid also may be exchanged across the capillary wall as a result of the cyclic dilation and constriction of the capillary sphincter. When this sphincter dilates, the pressure rises in the capillary, forcing fluid to move into the interstitial spaces. When the capillary sphincter constricts, the pressure in the capillary drops, and fluid moves into the capillary (Fig. 7-7).

Capillary and Membrane Permeability
An important factor in the movement of fluid back and forth across the capillary wall is the integrity of the capillary membrane. Changes in membrane permeability may permit the escape of plasma proteins into the interstitial space. The resultant increase in interstitial oncotic pressure alters the relationship defined by Starling's law and leads to osmotic movement of water into the interstitial space, causing tissue **edema**.

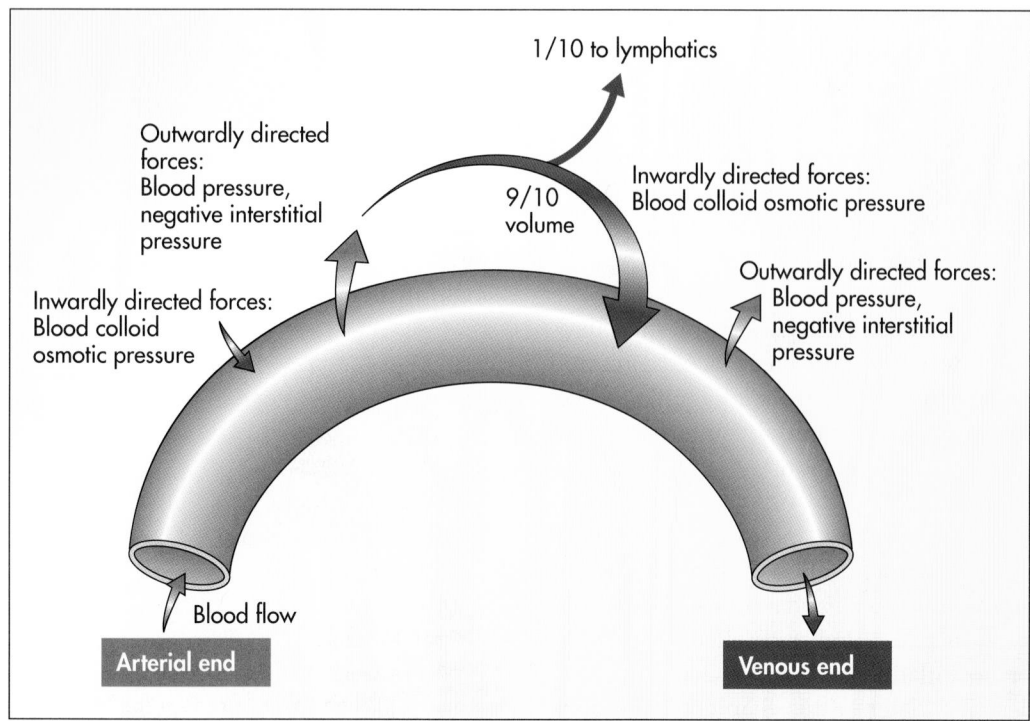

1/10 to lymphatics

Outwardly directed forces:
Blood pressure, negative interstitial pressure

9/10 volume

Inwardly directed forces:
Blood colloid osmotic pressure

Inwardly directed forces:
Blood colloid osmotic pressure

Outwardly directed forces:
Blood pressure, negative interstitial pressure

Blood flow

Arterial end

Venous end

Fig. 7-7 Total pressure differences between the inside and the outside of the capillary at its arteriolar and venous ends. At the arteriolar end, the sum of the forces causes fluid to move from the capillaries into the tissues. At the venous end, the sum of the forces attracts fluid into the capillary.

Alterations in Water Movement

Edema is the accumulation of fluid within the interstitial spaces. It results from any condition that leads to a net movement of fluid out of capillaries and into the interstitial tissues.

> **NOTE**
>
> Edema is a problem of fluid distribution and does not necessarily indicate a fluid excess.

Pathophysiology of Edema

The normal flow of fluid through the interstitial space depends on four factors:

1. The capillary hydrostatic pressure that filters fluid from the blood through the capillary wall
2. The oncotic pressure exerted by the proteins in the blood plasma, which attracts fluid from the interstitial space back into the vascular compartment

3. The permeability of the capillaries, which determines the ease with which fluid can pass through the capillary wall
4. The presence of open lymphatic channels, which collect some of the fluid forced out of the capillaries by the hydrostatic pressure of the blood and return the fluid to the circulation

When this process is disturbed, alterations in water movement can develop. The most common mechanisms responsible for edema are increased hydrostatic pressure, decreased plasma oncotic pressure, increased capillary permeability, and lymphatic obstruction.

Increased capillary hydrostatic pressure. An increase in hydrostatic pressure can result from venous obstruction or sodium and water retention. Venous obstruction can cause the hydrostatic pressure of fluid within the capillaries to become great enough to cause fluid to escape into the interstitial spaces.

Conditions that can lead to venous obstruction and edema include thrombophlebitis, hepatic obstruction, tight clothing around an extremity, and prolonged standing.

Sodium and water retention can cause a volume overload and edema. Congestive heart failure (CHF) and renal failure are two conditions associated with sodium and water retention.

Decreased oncotic pressure. Decreases in plasma albumin lead to a decrease in plasma oncotic pressure and cause fluid to move into the interstitial space. This condition most commonly results from liver disease or protein malnutrition.

Increased capillary permeability. Increases in capillary permeability cause the filtration of fluid into the interstitial space to be greater than normal. This condition usually is associated with allergic reactions in addition to inflammation and the **immune response** (described later in this chapter) that results from trauma (e.g., burns, crushing injuries). Proteins escape from the vascular bed and produce edema through a loss of capillary oncotic pressure and a gain in interstitial fluid oncotic pressure.

Lymphatic vessel obstruction. When lymphatic channels become blocked from infection or are surgically removed, proteins and fluid accumulate in the interstitial space. The obstruction blocks the normal pathway by which fluid is returned from the interstitial space into the circulation and leads to edema in the region that normally is drained by the lymphatic channels. Conditions that can cause obstruction in the lymphatic channels include certain malignancies, parasitic infections, and the surgical removal of lymphatics, as often performed after radical mastectomy (axillary lymph node dissection).

Clinical Manifestations of Edema

Edema may be localized or generalized. Localized edema usually is limited to an injury site (e.g., a sprained ankle) or organ system (e.g., cerebral edema, pulmonary edema). Edema of specific organs such as the brain, lungs, or larynx can be life threatening.

Generalized edema is more widespread and is most conspicuous in dependent parts of the body. It usually is noted first in the legs and ankles when standing or sitting and the sacrum and buttocks when lying down (gravity-dependent areas of the body). Generalized edema usually is associated with weight gain, swelling, and puffiness. It often is associated with other symptoms from the underlying illness. The most common diseases in industrialized countries that cause generalized edema are heart disease, kidney disease, and liver disease. In developing countries, the most common causes are malnutrition and parasitic disease.

> **? CRITICAL THINKING**
>
> *Why does the RICE (rest, ice, compression, elevation) treatment for swelling from a sprained ankle decrease tissue edema?*

> **NOTE**
>
> When edematous tissue is compressed with a finger, the fluid is pushed aside, leaving a "pit" or indentation that gradually refills with fluid. This condition is referred to as *pitting edema*.

> **NOTE**
>
> Fluid that accumulates in the peritoneal cavity is called *ascites*.

Water Balance, Sodium, and Chloride

Water follows the osmotic gradient established by changes in sodium concentration. Therefore sodium and water balance are closely related.

Water Balance

Water balance primarily is regulated by antidiuretic hormone (ADH) (see Chapter 6). It is the secretion of ADH and the perception of thirst that help regulate water balance. The release of ADH is initiated by an increase in plasma **osmolality** (the osmotic pressure of a solution) or a decrease in circulating blood volume and a lowered venous and arterial pressure. Increased plasma osmolality stimulates hypothalamic neurons (osmoreceptors) to cause the perception of thirst and to increase the release of ADH from the posterior pituitary gland.

In response to ADH release, water is reabsorbed into the plasma from the distal renal tubules and collecting ducts of the kidneys. This decreases the amount of water lost in the urine and results in a decrease in plasma osmolality (returning it to normal) as the water is reabsorbed. Volume-sensitive receptors and baroreceptors (found in the heart and great vessels) also can stimulate the release of ADH when body fluids are depleted from conditions such as vomiting, diarrhea, or excessive sweating.

> **NOTE**
>
> Volume-sensitive receptors and baroreceptors are nerve endings that are sensitive to changes in volume or pressure. Volume-sensitive receptors are located in the right and left atrium and thoracic vessels. Baroreceptors are found in the aorta, pulmonary arteries, and carotid sinus.

Sodium and Chloride Balance

Sodium (the major ECF cation) balance is regulated by aldosterone, a hormone secreted from the adrenal cortex. Along with chloride and bicarbonate, sodium regulates osmotic forces and therefore regulates water balance. (Chloride, the major ECF anion, provides electroneutrality in relation to sodium. Increases or decreases in chloride are proportional to changes in sodium.)

The secretion of aldosterone is initiated when sodium levels are decreased or potassium levels are increased. Aldosterone increases the reabsorption of sodium and secretion of potassium by the distal tubules of the kidneys.

The enzyme renin also is secreted by the kidneys when circulating blood volume or water balance is reduced. Renin stimulates the formation of angiotensin I, which is then converted to angiotensin II. Angiotensin II is a potent vasoconstrictor and acts to stimulate the secretion of ADH. This results in reabsorption of sodium and water and an elevation in the systemic blood pressure (described later in this chapter). This mechanism to regulate sodium and water is known as the *renin-angiotensin system* (Fig. 7-8). Natriuretic hormone helps regulate sodium by promoting urinary secretion of sodium. The result is a decrease in tubular reabsorption of sodium and a subsequent loss of sodium and water (Table 7-2).

> **NOTE**
>
> Atrial natriuretic factor, a substance released from the atrial cells of the heart (described in Chapter 6 and later in this chapter), also helps control the balance of sodium and water by promoting renal elimination of sodium.

Alterations in Sodium, Chloride, and Water Balance

In the healthy body, homeostatic mechanisms maintain a constant balance between intake and excretion of water. The water gained each day approximately equals the water lost. The body gains water primarily by drinking fluids, by ingesting food containing moisture, and by forming water through the oxidation of hydrogen in food during the metabolic process. The body loses water through the kidneys as urine, through the bowel as feces, through the skin as perspiration, through exhaled air as vapor, and by the excretion of tears and saliva. Two abnormal states of body-fluid balance can occur. If the water lost exceeds the water gained, a water deficit, or dehydration, occurs. If the water gained exceeds the water lost, a water excess, or overhydration, occurs.

Dehydration

Dehydration may be classified as isotonic (excessive loss of sodium and water in equal amounts), **hypernatremic** (loss of water in excess of sodium), and **hyponatremic** (loss of sodium in excess of water).

TABLE 7-2	ELECTROLYTE CONCENTRATIONS OF INTRACELLULAR AND EXTRACELLULAR FLUID	
	Predominant Cations Intracellular Potassium (K^+) Calcium (Ca^{++}) Magnesium (Mg^{++}) Extracellular Sodium (Na^+)	Predominant Anions Intracellular Phosphate (PO_4^{3-}) Extracellular Chloride (Cl^-) Bicarbonate (HCO_3^-)

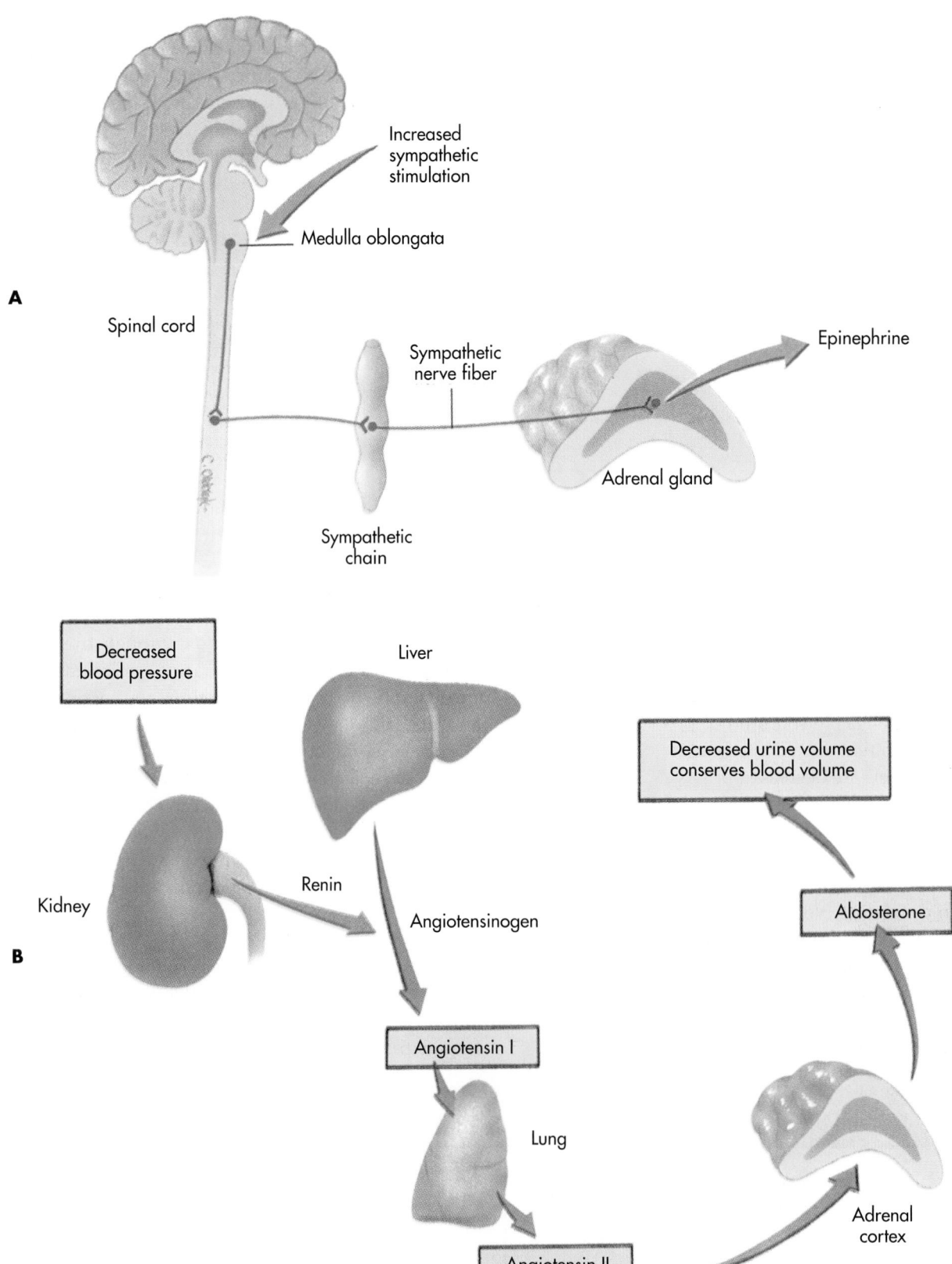

Fig. 7-8 Role of the adrenal medulla, **A,** and renin-angiotensin-aldosterone mechanism, **B,** in regulating blood pressure.

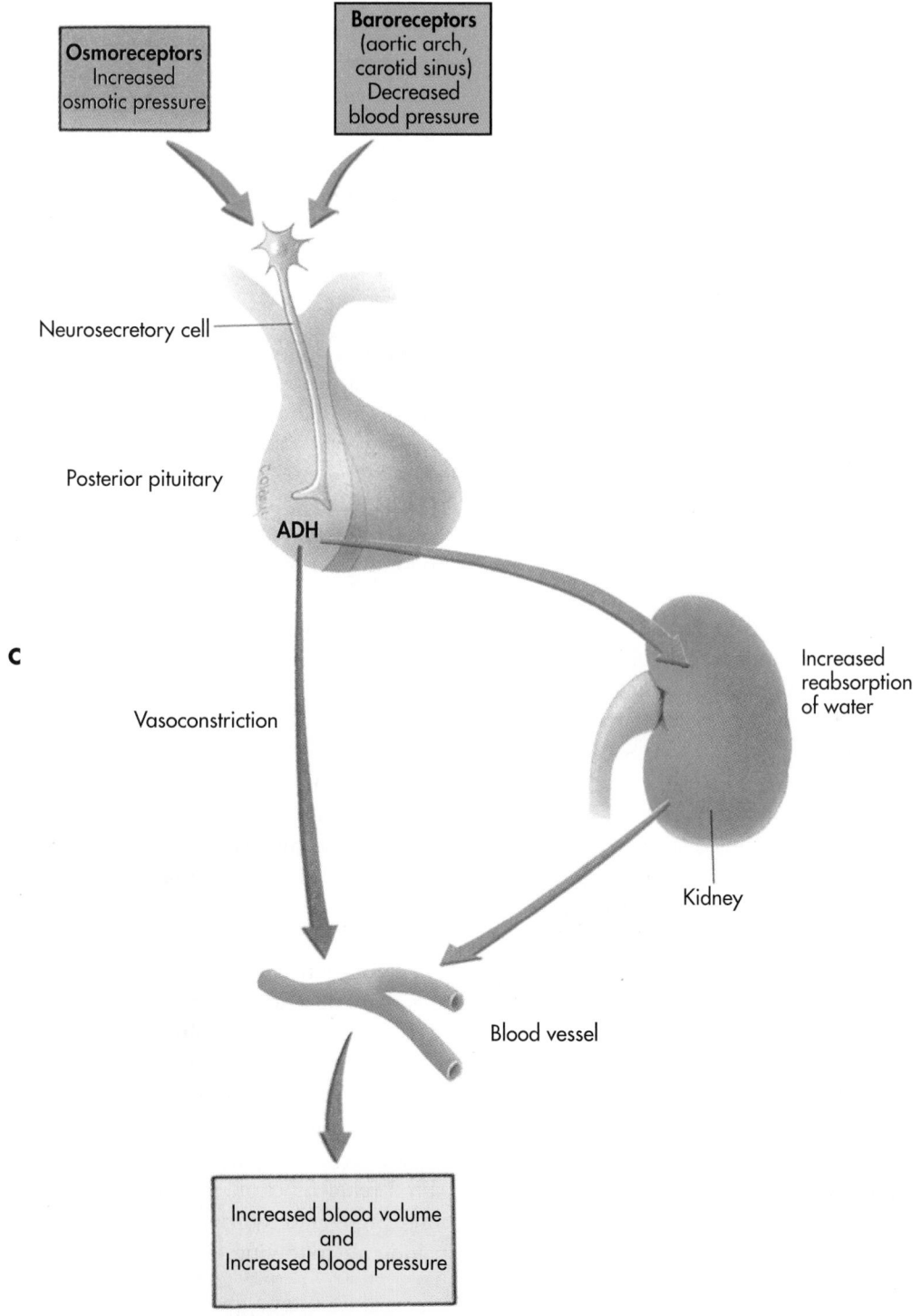

Fig. 7-8, cont'd Role of vasopressin (ADH) mechanism, **C,** in regulating blood pressure.

? CRITICAL THINKING

Based upon the causes of dehydration and your knowledge of anatomy and physiology, what two age groups do you think are at highest risk for dehydration? Why?

Isotonic dehydration
Causes
Usually severe or long-term vomiting or diarrhea
Systemic infection
Intestinal obstruction

Signs and symptoms
Dry skin and mucous membranes
Poor skin turgor
Longitudinal wrinkles or furrows of the tongue
Oliguria (decreased urinary output)
Anuria (essentially no urinary output—100 mL or less in 24 hours)
Acute weight loss
Depressed or sunken fontanelles in infants

Treatment
Intravenous infusion of an isotonic solution that has a solute concentration equal to that of blood (typically 0.9% sodium chloride or normal saline)

Hypernatremic dehydration
Possible causes
Excessive use or misuse of diuretics
Continued intake of sodium in the absence of water consumption
Excessive loss of water with little loss of sodium
Profuse, watery diarrhea

NOTE

Inhalation or ingestion of saltwater (e.g., near-drowning), may cause hypernatremia without dehydration.

Signs and symptoms
Dry, sticky mucous membranes
Flushed, doughy skin
Intense thirst
Oliguria or anuria
Increased body temperature
Altered mental status

Treatment
Volume replacement usually begins with isotonic fluids, because the patient often is both salt- and water-depleted, with the water supply being more depleted. (Isotonic fluids are relatively "hypotonic" in these patients.)

Hyponatremic dehydration
Possible causes
Use of diuretics
Excessive perspiration (heat-related illness)
Salt-losing renal disorders
Increased water intake (e.g., excessive use of water enemas)

NOTE

Inhalation or ingestion of fresh water (e.g., near-drowning) and compulsive water drinking may cause hyponatremia without dehydration.

Signs and symptoms
Abdominal or muscle cramps
Seizures
Rapid, thready pulse
Diaphoresis
Cyanosis

Treatment
Intravenous fluid replacement with normal saline or lactated Ringer's solution
Occasionally, hypertonic saline (e.g., in seizures caused by hyponatremia)

Overhydration
Overhydration is an increase in body water with a resultant decrease in solute concentration. (The total body amount of solute actually may be increased, but because body water is increased more, the solute concentration is decreased.) This water excess may result from parenteral administration of excessive fluids, impaired cardiac function, impaired renal function, or some endocrine dysfunctions. Signs and symptoms of overhydration may include the following:

- Shortness of breath
- Puffy eyelids
- Edema

- Polyuria (voiding a large volume of urine in a given time)
- Moist crackles (on pulmonary examination)
- Acute weight gain

The treatment of overhydration depends on the cause. For excessive water administration and certain endocrine problems, water restriction is the primary treatment. For patients with cardiac or renal impairment, a diuretic may be indicated. When profound hyponatremia is associated with overhydration (serum sodium level less than 120 milliequivalent [mEq] per liter and associated seizures or altered consciousness), administration of saline may be indicated.

NOTE

A milliequivalent (see Chapter 9) is the number of grams of solute dissolved in 1 mL of a normal solution.

Electrolyte Imbalances

In addition to water and sodium imbalances, disturbances in the balance of electrolytes (other than sodium) may occur. These include potassium, calcium, and magnesium.

Potassium. Potassium is the major positively charged ion in ICF. The body must maintain potassium levels within a narrow range (serum level of 3.5 to 5 mEq/L) for normal nerve, cardiac, and skeletal muscle function. Obligate potassium losses (those that cannot be avoided) usually are minimal and normally can be replenished through dietary intake. Excess potassium usually is excreted normally by the kidneys. Potassium plays an important role in muscle contraction, enzyme action, nerve impulses, and cell membrane function. Potassium imbalances interfere with neuromuscular function and may cause cardiac rhythm disturbances (dysrhythmias), including sudden cardiac death.

Hypokalemia (potassium deficit) can be caused by reduced dietary intake (rare), poor potassium absorption by the body, increased gastrointestinal losses that result from vomiting or diarrhea, renal disease, infusion of solutions poor in potassium, and medications (most commonly diuretics, but steroids, theophylline, and others have also been implicated). The most common cause in the United States is diuretic use. Signs and symptoms of hypokalemia may include the following:

- Malaise
- Skeletal muscle weakness
- Cardiac dysrhythmias
- Decreased reflexes
- Weak pulse
- Faint or distant heart sounds
- Shallow respiration
- Low blood pressure
- Anorexia
- Vomiting
- Gaseous distention
- Excessive thirst (rare)

In-hospital treatment of hypokalemia is intravenous or oral potassium replacement.

? CRITICAL THINKING

What common illness mimics many of the signs and symptoms of fluid and electrolyte imbalance?

Hyperkalemia is defined as an increase in serum potassium levels. This condition may be caused by acute or chronic renal failure, burns, crush injuries, severe infections or other conditions in which large amounts of potassium are released, excessive use of potassium salts, and a shift of potassium from the cells into the extracellular fluid (such as occurs in **acidosis**). Signs and symptoms of hyperkalemia may include the following:

- Cardiac conduction disturbances
- Irritability
- Abdominal distention
- Nausea
- Diarrhea
- Oliguria
- Weakness (an early sign) and paralysis (a late sign of severe hyperkalemia)

In-hospital treatment for hyperkalemia involves restricting potassium and administering a cation exchange resin, either orally or by a nasogastric tube. In emergencies, particularly life-threatening cardiac dysrhythmias, the use of *calcium* intravenously can be lifesaving. Other important therapeutic efforts include intravenous administration of glucose and *insulin* (25 g of *50% dextrose* and 10 units regular *insulin*), which helps lower the serum potassium level by forcing potassium intracellularly along with the glucose. *Sodium bicarbonate* also causes potassium to shift intracellularly.

Calcium. Calcium, a bivalent cation (an ion with two positive charges), is essential for a variety of body functions, including neuromuscular transmission, cell membrane permeability, hormone secretion, growth and ossification of bones, and muscle contraction (including smooth, cardiac, and skeletal muscle). Calcium intake in a balanced diet usually is sufficient for normal body needs, although growing evidence suggests that certain groups (e.g., pregnant and lactating women) may be calcium deficient in their diet. Calcium is excreted through urine, feces, and perspiration.

A decrease in serum calcium (hypocalcemia) may result from endocrine dysfunction (mostly underactivity of the parathyroid gland), renal insufficiency, decreased intake or malabsorption of calcium, or deficiency, malabsorption, or inability to activate vitamin D (which is responsible for calcium absorption). Signs and symptoms of hypocalcemia may include the following:

- Paresthesia
- Tetany
- Abdominal cramps
- Muscle cramps
- Neural excitability
    Personality changes
    Abnormal behavior
    Convulsions

In-hospital treatment for hypocalcemia is intravenous administration of calcium ions. Calcium salt and vitamin D may be given orally for maintenance.

Hypercalcemia may be caused by various tumors. Other common causes include parathyroid overactivity, thyroid dysfunction, diuretic therapy, and excessive administration of vitamin D (as in the treatment of osteoporosis). Calcium can be deposited in various body tissues, including many organ systems. Examples include the gastrointestinal system, central nervous system, renal system, neuromuscular system, and the cardiovascular system. Signs and symptoms of hypercalcemia include the following:

- Hypotonicity of the muscles (decreased muscle tone or tension)

- Renal stones
- Altered mental status
- Deep bone pain

The treatment of hypercalcemia is aimed at controlling the underlying disease, hydration, and, occasionally, drug therapy to lower calcium. In-hospital therapy for severe hypercalcemia may include forced diuresis with normal saline and *furosemide* (Lasix), as well as the administration of calcium-lowering drugs such as thyrocalcitonin, steroids (glucocorticoids), and plicamycin (a cytotoxic drug that inhibits bone reabsorption of calcium).

NOTE

Alterations in serum phosphate levels also can occur, resulting in hypophosphatemia and hyperphosphatemia. Low serum phosphate levels may be caused by intestinal malabsorption and increased renal excretion of phosphate. Elevated serum phosphate levels are associated with acute or chronic renal failure or low activity of the parathyroid gland.

Magnesium. Magnesium is a bivalent cation that activates many enzymes. About 50% of the body's magnesium exists in an insoluble state in bone, 45% as an intracellular cation, and 5% in extracellular solution. Magnesium is excreted by the kidneys and has physiological effects on the nervous system similar to those seen with calcium.

Magnesium deficit (hypomagnesemia) may be encountered in alcoholism, diabetes, malabsorption, starvation, diarrhea, diuresis, and diseases causing hypocalcemia and hypokalemia. The condition is characterized by increased irritability of the central nervous system. Signs and symptoms of hypomagnesemia include the following:

- Tremors
- Nausea or vomiting
- Diarrhea
- Hyperactive deep reflexes
- Confusion (including hallucinations)
- Seizures or myoclonus
- Cardiac dysrhythmias, which may lead to cardiac arrest

In-hospital treatment for significant symptomatic hypomagnesemia is intravenous fluid administration of a solution that contains magnesium, most commonly *magnesium sulfate*.

Magnesium excess (**hypermagnesemia**) occurs primarily in patients with chronic renal insufficiency. It also can occur in patients ingesting large amounts of magnesium-containing compounds such as cathartics (e.g., magnesium citrate, *magnesium sulfate*) or antacids (e.g., magnesium hydroxide). Hypermagnesemia causes central nervous system depression, profound muscular weakness, and areflexia; it also causes cardiac rhythm disturbances, which may lead to sudden death. Signs and symptoms include the following:

- Sedation
- Confusion
- Muscle weakness
- Respiratory paralysis

The most effective treatment for hypermagnesemia is hemodialysis, which can return blood levels to normal in about 4 hours. In addition, calcium salts that act as an antagonist to magnesium may be given parenterally. Administration of intravenous glucose and *insulin* also drive magnesium back into the cells and can be used in emergencies when respiratory depression or cardiac conduction defects are present.

Acid-Base Balance

Acids and bases are produced by the body through normal metabolism. For physiological functioning, a balance of these acids and bases must be maintained in a narrow range. Acids are substances that release, or donate, hydrogen ions (protons with a positive charge); bases receive, or absorb, hydrogen ions. A solution increases in acidity as the hydrogen ion concentration increases and increases in alkalinity (basicity) when the hydrogen ion concentration falls.

Hydrogen ion concentration (moles/L) is expressed by the term **pH,** which is the negative logarithm (base 10) of the concentration of hydrogen ions. A mole (in chemistry) is 6.023 multiplied by 10^{23} molecules (Avogadro's number). Although grasping the meaning of a number this large in real terms is not necessary, the significance of a small change in pH should be understood: *the strength of an acid or base changes by 10 times with **each** unit change of pH* (Box 7-1 and Fig. 7-9).

NOTE

10^{-7}moles/L = pH 7.0

Buffer Systems

The healthy body is sensitive to changes in the concentration of hydrogen ions and tries to maintain the pH of extracellular fluid at 7.4. This is accomplished through three interrelated compensatory mechanisms: carbonic acid-bicarbonate buffering, protein buffering, and renal buffering. These compensatory mechanisms are stimulated by changes in pH and require normal organ function to be effective in maintaining acid-base balance.

1. *Carbonic acid-bicarbonate buffering.* Bicarbonate, carbon dioxide, and carbonic acid are always present in a dynamic balance in the blood. Bicarbonate (HCO_3^-) arises from the transport of carbon dioxide in the blood. Under the influence of the enzyme carbonic anhydrase, carbon dioxide dissolves in the water of blood and reacts with water in red blood cells to form carbonic acid (H_2CO_3). Carbonic acid breaks down into hydrogen and bicarbonate ions. At a physiological pH of 7.4, the normal ratio of carbonic acid to bicarbonate is 1:20, respectively, and is summarized by the chemical equation:

$$CO_2 + H_2O \rightleftharpoons H_2CO_3 \rightleftharpoons H^+ + HCO_3^-$$

Bicarbonate (HCO_3^-) may link up with a cation to form base bicarbonate (e.g., $NaHCO_3$).

BOX 7-1

pH

A solution of pH 1 is 1,000,000 times as acidic as a solution of pH 7.

pH 2 is 100,000 times as acidic as pH 7.

pH 3 is 10,000 times as acidic as pH 7.

pH 4 is 1000 times as acidic as pH 7.

pH 5 is 100 times as acidic as pH 7.

pH 6 is 10 times as acidic as pH 7.

A pH of 7 is neutral (distilled water).

A pH of 8 is 1/10 as acidic as a pH of 7, or 10 times as alkaline.

pH 9 is 1/100 as acidic and 100 times as alkaline as pH 7.

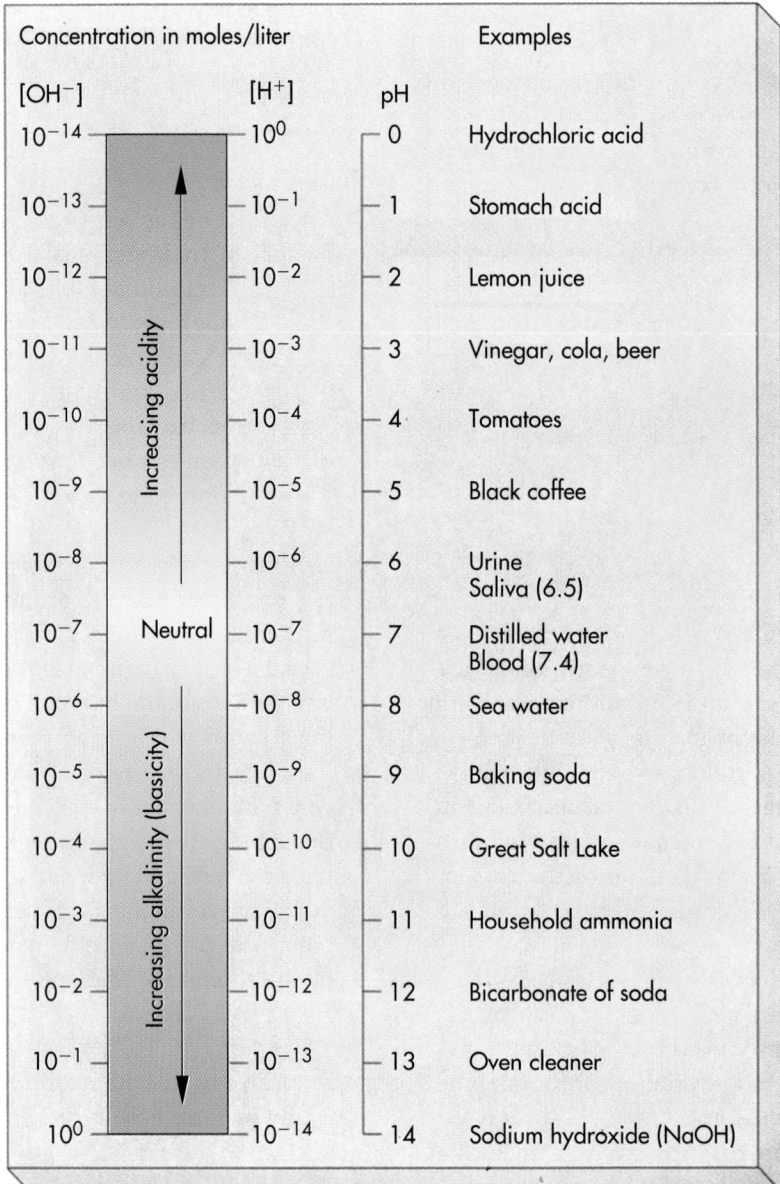

Concentration in moles/liter			Examples
[OH⁻]	[H⁺]	pH	
10^{-14}	10^{0}	0	Hydrochloric acid
10^{-13}	10^{-1}	1	Stomach acid
10^{-12}	10^{-2}	2	Lemon juice
10^{-11}	10^{-3}	3	Vinegar, cola, beer
10^{-10}	10^{-4}	4	Tomatoes
10^{-9}	10^{-5}	5	Black coffee
10^{-8}	10^{-6}	6	Urine Saliva (6.5)
10^{-7}	10^{-7}	7	Distilled water Blood (7.4)
10^{-6}	10^{-8}	8	Sea water
10^{-5}	10^{-9}	9	Baking soda
10^{-4}	10^{-10}	10	Great Salt Lake
10^{-3}	10^{-11}	11	Household ammonia
10^{-2}	10^{-12}	12	Bicarbonate of soda
10^{-1}	10^{-13}	13	Oven cleaner
10^{0}	10^{-14}	14	Sodium hydroxide (NaOH)

Increasing acidity · Neutral · Increasing alkalinity (basicity)

Fig. 7-9 pH scale. A pH of 7 is considered neutral. Values less than 7 are acidic (the lower the number, the more acidic the substance). Values greater than 7 are basic (the higher the number, the more basic the substance). Representative fluids and their approximate pH values are listed.

It is the ratio of carbonic acid to base bicarbonate that determines the concentration of hydrogen ions. As long as there is 1 mEq of carbonic acid for each 20 mEq of base bicarbonate in the extracellular fluid, the hydrogen ion concentration stays within normal limits. This compensatory mechanism occurs immediately in response to changes in pH with the respiratory rate in maintaining this balance (Fig. 7-10).

2. *Protein buffering.* Both intracellular and extracellular proteins have negative charges and can serve as buffers for alterations in hydrogen ion concentration. However, because most proteins are inside cells, this primarily is an intracellular buffer system. Hemoglobin (Hb) is an excellent intracellular buffer because of its ability to bind with hydrogen ions (forming a weak acid) and carbon dioxide.

After oxygen is released in the peripheral tissues, hemoglobin binds with carbon dioxide and

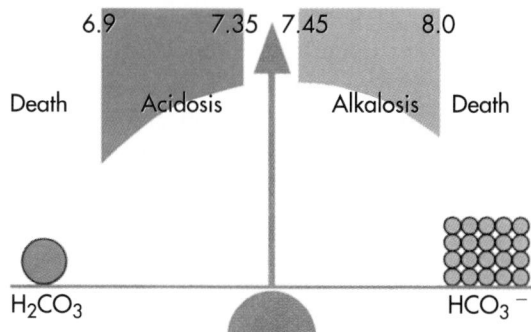

Fig. 7-10 Bicarbonate buffer system. When body fluids are in acid-base balance, the ratio of HCO_3 to H_2CO_3 is normally 20:1, and the pH is between 7.35 and 7.45.

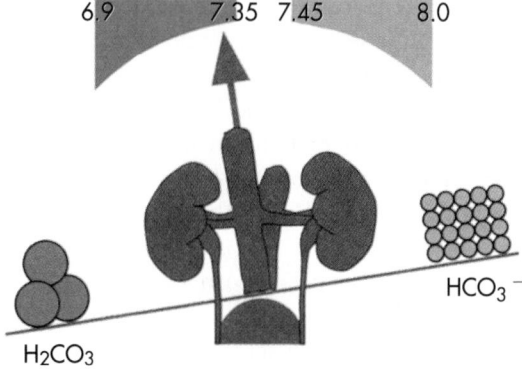

Fig. 7-11 Metabolic acidosis. An excess of metabolic acids consumes bicarbonate and liberate hydrogen ions, resulting in acidosis.

hydrogen ions. As the blood reaches the lungs, these actions reverse themselves. Hemoglobin binds with oxygen, releasing carbon dioxide and hydrogen ions. The hydrogen ions released combine with bicarbonate ions, forming carbonic acid. The carbonic acid breaks down into carbon dioxide and water, and the lungs expire the carbon dioxide. Therefore in normal circumstances, respirations help maintain pH. Because the respiratory centers are more responsive to pH changes than oxygen, it is the amount of carbon dioxide (and hence the pH) in the blood, rather than the need for oxygen in the tissues, that controls the rate of breathing in healthy individuals. Increasing alveolar ventilation to lower carbon dioxide concentrations occurs within minutes in response to decreases in pH.

3. *Renal buffering.* The kidneys help maintain acid-base balance through three mechanisms. The first is recovery of bicarbonate, which is filtered into the tubules. The second is excretion of hydrogen ions against a gradient to acidify the urine. (Normally, the kidney can acidify urine to a pH of about 5.0.) The third is excretion of ammonium ions (NH_4), each of which carries a hydrogen ion with it. The renal system compensates for acid-base imbalances slowly in comparison with the

protein and bicarbonate buffer systems. The kidneys can take from several hours to days to restore the pH to within the normal physiological range.

Acid-Base Imbalance

Any condition that increases the carbonic acid or decreases the base bicarbonate causes acidosis. Any condition that increases base bicarbonate or decreases carbonic acid causes **alkalosis**. Metabolic disturbances tend to affect the bicarbonate side of the equation, whereas respiratory disturbances through changes in the partial pressure of carbon dioxide tend to affect the carbonic acid side.

Metabolic acidosis. Metabolic acidosis results from an accumulation of acid or a loss of base. When excessive acid is produced by the body, the acid spills into the extracellular fluid, consuming some bicarbonate buffers. This results in an increase in acid and a decrease in available base (Fig. 7-11). Metabolic acidosis can be summarized by the equation:

$$\uparrow H^+ + HCO_3^- \rightarrow \uparrow H_2CO_3 \rightarrow H_2O + \uparrow CO_2$$

This increase in available hydrogen ions forces the reaction to the right, decreasing the amount of base bicarbonate.

NOTE

The concentration of carbonic acid (dissolved carbon dioxide) is controlled by the lungs. The concentration of bicarbonate is controlled by the kidneys.

NOTE

Metabolic acidosis occurs when the amount of acid generated exceeds the body's buffering capacity.

The healthy respiratory system immediately attempts to compensate for the acidosis by increasing the rate and depth of ventilation to reduce carbon dioxide. As the carbon dioxide level falls, so does the concentration of carbonic acid, returning pH toward normal. In addition, the kidneys excrete more hydrogen ion to equilibrate the excess acid in the extracellular fluid.

The four most common forms of metabolic acidosis encountered in the prehospital setting are **lactic acidosis**, diabetic ketoacidosis, acidosis resulting from renal failure, and acidosis from ingestion of toxins.

1. *Lactic acidosis*. Lactic acid is produced when a large number of cells are inadequately perfused, resulting in a shift from **aerobic** (with oxygen) to **anaerobic** (without oxygen) metabolism. The end product of anaerobic metabolism is lactic acid, which releases hydrogen ions, creating systemic acidosis. Normally, lactate is converted by the liver back to glucose or is oxidized to carbon dioxide and water. When the rate of lactic acid production exceeds the rate of its metabolism, lactic acidosis occurs. The most common causes of systemic lactic acidosis are extreme exertional states (e.g., seizures), **ischemia** (reduced blood supply) to large muscles or organs (e.g., mesenteric ischemia), circulatory failure, and shock. Specific complications associated with lactic acidosis are thought to include the following:

   • Decreased force of cardiac contraction
   • Decreased peripheral response to catecholamines
   • Hypotension and shock
   • Cardiac muscle that is refractory to defibrillation

? CRITICAL THINKING

Think about the last time you ran so fast you had a muscle cramp. What acid-base changes were going on inside your body? How did your body compensate for those changes?

The treatment for lactic acidosis is to reestablish tissue perfusion and cardiac output. This permits the liver to regenerate bicarbonate by metabolizing lactate to carbon dioxide and water. Medical direction may recommend hyperventilation to induce respiratory alkalosis, vigorous rehydration to support circulation, and perhaps the intravenous administration of **sodium bicarbonate** for immediate compensation (if the patient is in cardiac arrest). Correction of lactic acidosis frequently depends on identification and correction of the underlying cause.

2. *Diabetic ketoacidosis*. Ketoacidosis usually is a complication of diabetes mellitus but also can be seen in alcoholics (alcoholic ketoacidosis). It usually results when a patient fails to take adequate **insulin** or when the need for insulin increases (e.g., in cases of infection or trauma). With impaired glucose utilization (insulin is required for many cells to absorb glucose), fatty acids are metabolized with the production of ketone bodies and release of hydrogen ions. Large quantities of ketone bodies exceed the ability of the body's buffering system to compensate, resulting in acidosis and a decrease in blood pH. The pathophysiology of this disorder is further addressed in Chapter 30.

NOTE

Prehospital care for patients with diabetic ketoacidosis is the administration of normal saline for volume repletion.

3. *Renal failure*. The kidneys help maintain acid-base balance by reabsorbing or secreting either bicarbonate or hydrogen ions as needed to keep the pH constant. Renal failure affects the compensatory mechanisms of the kidneys to varying degrees. Patients with moderate-to-severe renal failure frequently have mild-to-moderate acidosis. Acidosis results because the failing kidneys are unable to efficiently excrete the acid waste products that are produced by normal metabolic processes.

4. *Ingestion of toxins*. The ingestion of some toxins, such as ethylene glycol, methanol, and salicylate, can cause metabolic acidosis. These and other toxins lead to the production of toxic metabolites and may result in acid-base disorders characterized by metabolic acidosis and compensatory respiratory alkalosis. Treatment for various toxic ingestions frequently includes gastrointestinal

evacuation but also may entail hemodialysis, diuresis, hydration to promote excretion, and specific antagonistic or antidotal therapy.

Metabolic alkalosis. Metabolic alkalosis (rare) most often results from loss of hydrogen ions (primarily from the stomach), ingestion of large amounts of absorbable base sodium bicarbonate (baking soda) or calcium carbonate (Tums, other antacids), or excessive intravenous administration of alkali (e.g., intravenous injection of *sodium bicarbonate*). Diuretic use also may contribute to development of metabolic alkalosis (Fig. 7-12). Metabolic alkalosis can be summarized by the chemical equation:

$$\downarrow H^+ + HCO_3^- \rightarrow \downarrow H_2CO_3^- \rightarrow H_2O + \downarrow CO_2$$

Decreased hydrogen ions drive the reaction to the left, resulting in increased bicarbonate concentration.

Loss of hydrogen ions is the initial cause of metabolic alkalosis. This may result from vomiting (hydrochloric acid loss), gastric suction, or increased renal excretion of hydrogen ion in urine. When vomiting occurs, not only is gastric acid lost but volume is also depleted.

Chronic diuretic use can result in volume depletion. The loss of sodium chloride and potassium causes a relative increase in bicarbonate. (The kidney defends against volume depletion by increasing its reabsorption of sodium and thus water.) When sodium is reabsorbed, either potassium or hydrogen ions must be excreted to maintain electrical neutrality. Excretion of hydrogen ions can lead to a net increase in bicarbonate and subsequent metabolic alkalosis.

Initially, the respiratory system tries to compensate by retaining carbon dioxide. However, this compensatory mechanism is limited by the development of **hypoxemia**. (The rise in P_{CO_2} and decrease in P_{O_2} as a result of hypoventilation will stimulate respiration.) The treatment for metabolic alkalosis is directed at correcting the underlying condition. Volume depletion, if present, should be corrected with isotonic solutions, and hypokalemia may require correction with potassium replacement.

Respiratory acidosis. Respiratory acidosis is caused by the retention of carbon dioxide, leading to an increase in P_{CO_2}. This state usually is caused by an imbalance in the production of carbon dioxide and its elimination through alveolar ventilation (Fig. 7-13). Respiratory acidosis can be summarized by the chemical equation:

$$\downarrow Respiration = \uparrow CO_2 + H_2O \rightarrow \uparrow H_2CO_3 \rightarrow \uparrow H^+ + HCO_3^-$$

Reductions in alveolar ventilation may occur as a result of the following:

- Respiratory depression
- Respiratory arrest
- Cardiac arrest
- Neuromuscular impairment
- Medications (sedatives, hypnotics)

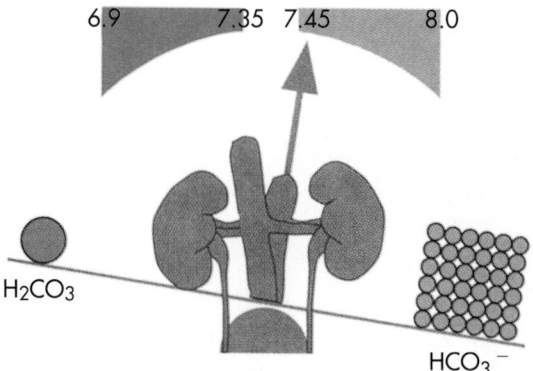

Fig. 7-12 Metabolic alkalosis. An excess of bicarbonate results in alkalosis.

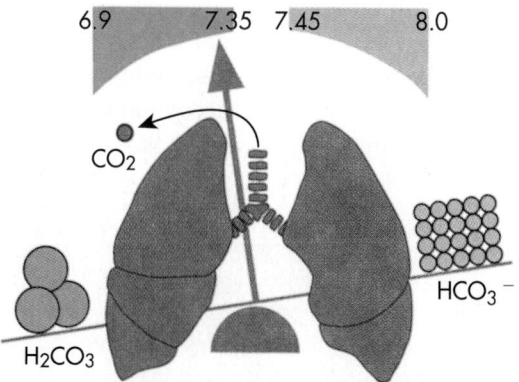

Fig. 7-13 Respiratory acidosis. An excess of carbon dioxide in the body results in acidosis.

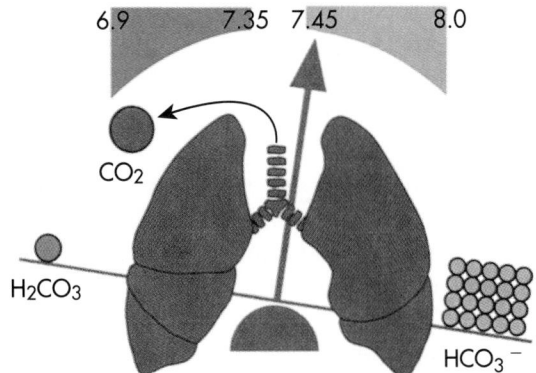

Fig. 7-14 Respiratory alkalosis. A deficit of carbon dioxide results in alkalosis.

- Chest wall injury
    Flail chest
    Pneumothorax
- Pulmonary processes
    Obstructed airway
    Chronic obstructive pulmonary disease
    Pulmonary edema

> **NOTE**
>
> In respiratory acidosis, the primary abnormality is failure of the lungs to excrete carbon dioxide efficiently.

When the respiratory system cannot continue as a compensatory mechanism to correct the acidosis, the body's renal system must conserve bicarbonate and excrete more hydrogen ions to help bring the pH into normal limits. Because the kidneys take some time to restore pH, the patient in respiratory acidosis should be treated by improving ventilation to quickly eliminate carbon dioxide. This may be accomplished by assisting ventilations to decrease P_{CO_2}. Supplemental oxygen also should be administered to help correct any accompanying hypoxemia (which can itself lead to acidosis).

> **? CRITICAL THINKING**
>
> *What kind of acid-base imbalance exists in a patient you have just defibrillated and resuscitated from cardiac arrest? How are you going to correct that imbalance?*

Respiratory alkalosis. Hyperventilation may produce respiratory alkalosis by decreasing P_{CO_2} (Fig. 7-14).

> **ACID-BASE DETERMINANTS AND OTHER LABORATORY STUDIES**
>
> **Blood Gas Analysis**
> Blood gases are obtained for two reasons: to determine if the patient is well oxygenated and to determine the patient's acid-base status. Most often, blood gases are measured on arterial blood obtained from the patient in a heparinized syringe. Arterial samples more commonly are obtained for this test than venous samples, because arterial samples give more direct information about the lungs' ability to oxygenate blood and remove carbon dioxide.
>
> The acid-base status of a patient is assessed by measuring arterial P_{CO_2} and pH level. The pH level indicates whether an acid or base state is present. The P_{CO_2} level indicates whether a respiratory component exists to the acidosis or alkalosis (i.e., whether alveolar hypoventilation or hyperventilation is present). Table 7-3 summarizes the abnormalities that occur in the mixed acid-base disturbances.
>
> At present, determining pH by blood gas analysis is not considered part of the duty of paramedics in the prehospital setting. The use of pulse oximetry provides a continuous reading of arterial oxygen saturation without invasive procedures. (Under normal circumstances, a saturation of 90% correlates with a P_{O_2} of 60 mm Hg.)

Hyperventilation is common in patients who are acutely ill and frequently is seen in the early stages of sepsis, peritonitis, shock, and respiratory ailments. Respiratory alkalosis can be summarized by the chemical equation:

$$\uparrow \text{Respiration} = \\ \downarrow CO_2 + H_2O \rightarrow \downarrow H_2CO_3 \rightarrow \downarrow H^+ + HCO_3^-$$

> **NOTE**
>
> Respiratory alkalosis is due to hyperventilation, which lowers the alveolar P_{CO_2}, and subsequently the level of P_{CO_2} in the blood.

When carbonic acid is lacking because of excessive carbon dioxide elimination, the blood pH rises. Therefore the kidneys must excrete bicarbonate ions and retain hydrogen ions in an effort to return the pH to normal. The treatment for

ACID-BASE DISTURBANCE	HCO₃⁻	Pco₂	pH
TABLE 7-3 — **SIMPLE ACID-BASE DISTURBANCES**			
Metabolic acidosis	↓	↓	↓
Respiratory acidosis	↓	↑	↓
Metabolic alkalosis	↑	↑	↑
Respiratory alkalosis	↑	↓	↑

respiratory alkalosis is directed at treating the underlying cause of the hyperventilation. Initial interventions include placing the patient on low-concentration oxygen and providing calming measures to assist the patient with slow, controlled breathing.

Mixed acid-base disturbances. Many conditions, including various forms of shock, may produce mixed abnormalities of acid-base regulation. In these patients, simultaneous respiratory and metabolic alterations commonly are seen because of pathology and physiological changes in both the respiratory and metabolic components of the acid-base system (see the box on p. 202). Examples of mixed acid-base disturbances include the following:

• Combined respiratory and metabolic acidosis
• Metabolic acidosis and respiratory alkalosis
• Respiratory acidosis and metabolic alkalosis
• Combined respiratory and metabolic alkalosis

SECTION TWO
CELLULAR INJURY AND DISEASE

Alterations in Cells and Tissues

Knowledge of the structural and functional reactions of cells and tissues to injurious agents is important to understanding disease processes. Alteration in cells and tissues can result from adaptation, injury, neoplasia (actual formation of a tumor), aging, or death.

Cellular Adaptation

Cells adapt to their environment to escape and protect themselves from injury. (An adapted cell is neither normal nor injured.) Cellular adaptations are common and are a central part of the response to changes in physiological condition. In many instances, the adaptation enables cells to function more efficiently. Therefore determining a pathological response versus an extreme adaptation to changing conditions is difficult. The five most significant adaptive changes in cells include the following:

1. Atrophy (a decrease in cell size)
2. Hypertrophy (an increase in cell size)
3. Hyperplasia (an excessive increase in cell number)
4. Metaplasia (a change from one cell type to another that is better able to tolerate adverse conditions; a conversion into a form that is not normal for that cell)
5. Dysplasia (abnormal cellular growth)

Atrophy is a decrease or shrinkage in cellular size that adversely affects cell function. It can affect any organ, but it is most common in skeletal muscle, the heart, secondary sex organs, and the brain. Causes of atrophy include decreased use, chronic inflammation, inadequate nutrition or starvation, inadequate hormonal or nervous stimulation, and reduced blood supply. An example of atrophy is a skeletal muscle that is reduced in size because of prolonged immobilization in a cast. Atrophy may be reversed (in some conditions) when normal function is restored.

Hypertrophy is an increase in the size of cells (without an increase in numbers) and a subsequent increase in the size of the affected organ. Hypertrophy results when cells are required to do more work to accomplish a task. Examples of "normal" or physiological hypertrophy are a weight lifter's large muscles, increased growth of the uterus during pregnancy, and the development of sexual organs in adolescence (initiated by sex hormones). Examples of pathological hypertrophy are enlargement of the heart (myocardial hypertrophy) and the kidneys (which also can be physiological).

Hyperplasia is an excessive increase in the number of cells that results in an increase in the size of a tissue or organ. Hyperplasia occurs in response to increased demand and may be a pathological event or a normal adaptive mechanism that allows certain organs to regenerate (compensatory hyperplasia). Examples of compensatory hyperplasia are the formation of a callus or increased red blood cell formation at high altitudes. An example of pathological hyperplasia is endometrial hyperplasia, which can cause excessive menstrual bleeding. Hyperplasia and hypertrophy often occur together.

> ### ? CRITICAL THINKING
>
> **What would happen to muscle strength if there was hyperplasia, hypertrophy, or atrophy of the muscle cells?**

Metaplasia is the conversion into a form that is not normal for that cell, or the reversible replacement of normal tissue cells by other cells that may be better able to tolerate adverse environmental conditions. An example of metaplasia is the conversion that occurs in the bronchial lining as a result of cigarette smoking. The normal ciliated epithelial cells are replaced by nonciliated squamous epithelial cells, which are more resistant to irritation. (Bronchial metaplasia can be reversed when one quits smoking cigarettes.) Chronic inflammation of the cervix also can result in metaplasia.

Dysplasia refers to abnormal changes of mature cells. The individual cells vary in size, shape, and color, and their relationship to one another also is abnormal. Dysplastic changes often are considered precancerous and are seen most frequently in epithelial tissue. The changes often result from chronic irritation or inflammation and frequently are found adjacent to cancerous cells.

> ### NOTE
>
> Dysplasia is not considered a true cellular adaptation, but rather an atypical hyperplasia.

Cellular Injury

Numerous processes can cause cellular injury. The mechanisms involved in cellular injury are complex. The specific site of injury often is characteristic of a particular pathological process. As a rule, cellular injury occurs if the cell is unable to maintain homeostasis as a result of the following:

1. Hypoxic injury
2. Chemical injury
3. Infectious injury (i.e., bacteria, viruses)
4. Immunological and inflammatory injury
5. Genetic factors
6. Nutritional imbalances
7. Physical agents

Hypoxic Injury

Hypoxic injury is the most common cause of cellular injury. It may result from decreased amounts of oxygen in the air, loss of hemoglobin or altered hemoglobin function, decreased number of red blood cells, diseases of the respiratory or cardiovascular systems, external compression (e.g., in trauma), or poisoning and loss of cytochromes. Hypoxic injury commonly is a result of atherosclerosis (narrowing of arteries) and thrombosis (complete blockages of anatomy by blood clots). Prolonged ischemia leads to infarction or cell death (see Chapter 28). Atherosclerosis and thrombosis are the leading causes of myocardial infarction and stroke.[1]

> ### NOTE
>
> If cells do not have an adequate supply of oxygen, they cannot generate enough energy to maintain the mechanisms (ion pumps) required to move some substances across the cell membrane, which results in a loss of electrostatic potential and cellular swelling.

Chemical Injury

Many chemical agents can cause cellular injury. Examples of injurious chemicals include heavy metals (lead), carbon monoxide, ethanol, drugs, and complex toxins. Some chemicals injure cells directly (e.g., curare, cyanide); others are metabolized and yield a toxin that affects the cells (e.g., carbon tetrachloride [CCl_4]).

The injury begins with a biochemical interaction between a toxic substance and an integral part of the cellular structure. Some drugs and toxins (e.g., salicylate, certain venoms) affect the cellular membrane. This interaction can damage the plasma membrane and lead to increased permeability, cellular swelling, and irreversible cellular injury (see Chapter 34). Other toxins, such as carbon monoxide, primarily affect the cytochrome system found in the mitochondria, which leads to a halt in oxidative metabolism. Still others affect the genetic material (a primary target for chemotherapy drugs).

Infectious Injury

The **virulence** of microorganisms depends on their ability to survive and reproduce in the human body, where they injure cells and tissues. The disease-producing potential of microorganisms depends on their ability to do the following:

- Invade and destroy cells
- Evade the defense of the organism
- Produce toxins
- Produce **hypersensitivity reactions**

Bacteria. The survival and growth of bacteria depend on the effectiveness of the body's defense mechanisms and the bacteria's ability to resist these mechanisms (see Chapter 37). Many bacteria that survive and proliferate in the body produce poisons or toxins that can injure or destroy cells and tissues. These toxins take two forms: exotoxins and endotoxins.

Bacteria make exotoxins (toxins that have highly specific effects) when they have been identified by viruslike particles called *bacteriophages,* which carry the necessary genetic material to make the toxin. Exotoxins are produced by a microorganism and excreted into the medium surrounding it. Their effects are produced by their release as metabolic products during bacterial growth. Examples of exotoxins include those produced by several streptococci (which cause sore throats and rheumatic fever) and by *Clostridium botulinum*, a bacterium that causes a particularly severe type of food poisoning.

> **NOTE**
>
> Toxoids are modified (harmless) toxins used as vaccines so that the body develops specific antibodies against them. The best-known toxoid is tetanus toxoid, made from tetanus toxin.

Endotoxins are contained in the cell walls of some bacteria and are released during treatment with antibiotics or when the cell walls disintegrate. Examples of bacteria that produce endotoxins are gonococci and meningococci (the bacteria that cause gonorrhea and meningitis).

> **NOTE**
>
> Because endotoxins do not stimulate strong antibodies, developing vaccines against endotoxin-bearing bacteria has not been possible. Instead, the body uses a group of proteins collectively called the *complement system*. This system coats bacteria and helps to kill them directly or assists in having them taken up by neutrophils in the blood or by macrophages in the tissues. The reticuloendothelial system (composed of cells in the spleen, lymph nodes, liver, bone marrow, lungs, and intestines) works in conjunction with the lymphatic system to dispose of debris that results from the immune system's attack on invading organisms.

Bacteria that produce endotoxins are also called *pyrogenic bacteria,* because they not only activate the inflammatory process but also produce fever directly through the release of cell-membrane toxins. As part of the inflammatory process, white blood cells are released from the bone marrow, causing the increased white blood cell count in the blood commonly found with infection. Inflammation also increases capillary permeability and allows substances that destroy bacteria to migrate from capillaries to the site of infection (see Chapter 37). Fever is caused by the release of endogenous pyrogens (proteins that act on the thermoregulatory centers of the hypothalamus) from macrophages or circulating white blood cells that are attracted to the injury site (Fig. 7-15).

> **?**   **CRITICAL THINKING**
>
> *Will treating a fever with antipyretic drugs cause the body to rid itself of the toxin that caused the fever?*

The ability to produce hypersensitivity reactions is a rare but life-threatening pathogenic mechanism of bacterial toxins. The hypersensitivity develops after reexposure to a toxin, causing an inflammatory response. Occasionally, the response is so extreme that the host is killed instead of the bacteria. For example, the complement system can activate blood clotting and cause white cells to aggregate and form "clumps."

The net effect of overactivation of the complement system by endotoxins is the blockage of small

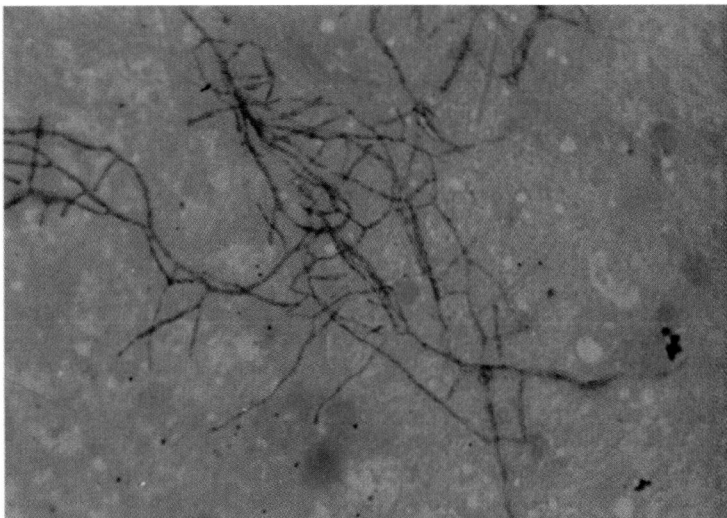

Fig. 7-15 Nocardia in lesion of lower leg, stained with Gomori methenamine-silver stain. (From Baron EJ, Peterson LR, Finegold SM: *Bailey & Scott's diagnostic microbiology,* ed 9, St Louis, 1994, Mosby.)

blood vessels in the lungs (with the clumps) and the formation of small blood clots in small arteries elsewhere in the body. Fortunately, this life-threatening reaction is infrequent, and the complement system normally acts as an efficient defense against most bacterial toxins without causing any damage. (Hypersensitivity reactions are also described later in this chapter and in Chapter 31.)

> **NOTE**
>
> When the body's defense mechanisms fail and the microorganisms proliferate in the blood, bacteremia (septicemia) develops. The endotoxins (along with a number of proteins involved in the inflammatory response) cause vasodilation that reduces blood pressure and oxygen delivery, leading to shock. Other signs of bacteremia may include chills, fever, and an altered level of consciousness. Rashes or red streaks (lymphangitis) also may be associated with bacteremia.

? CRITICAL THINKING

In septic shock, toxins affect the cell membrane permeability, allowing fluids to leak out of the blood vessels more freely. How could that affect cardiac output?

Viruses. Viruses are responsible for many human diseases, including the common cold, influenza, chick-enpox, smallpox, hepatitis, herpes, and acquired immunodeficiency syndrome (AIDS). They are intracellular parasites that work very differently from bacteria (Fig. 7-16). Viruses lack much of the machinery that allows bacterial and other cells to grow rapidly and multiply. They can reproduce only by infecting the living cells of host tissue (often destroying the host cell).

> **NOTE**
>
> Viruses usually consist of a protein coat (capsid) that encloses a core of nucleic acid. They have no organelles and therefore have no metabolism. They do not produce endotoxins or exotoxins.

Viruses require nucleic acid (either DNA or RNA) to replicate. (Unlike all other cellular forms of life, viruses never contain both DNA and RNA.) Cells are thought to engulf the virus particles by surrounding them with part of the cell membrane. Once inside the cell, the virus loses its capsid and begins to replicate viral nucleic acids. Some viruses cause the cell to burst, and others replicate without destroying the cell. The capsid allows the virus to resist phagocytosis but often evokes a very strong immune response. Viruses, however, can rapidly produce irreversible and lethal injury in susceptible hosts, whether they are immunosuppressed or not.

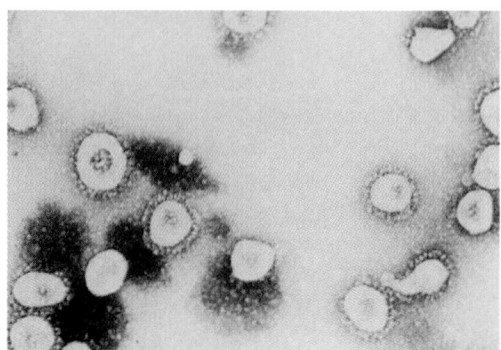

Fig. 7-16 Coronavirus. (From U.S. Department of Health, Education and Welfare; Public Health Service, Centers for Disease Control, Atlanta, Georgia.)

Rabies, smallpox, and influenza are examples of viral illnesses, which are highly infectious and associated with significant mortality and morbidity. Viral infections are easier to prevent than treat. Vaccines have proven to be the best safeguard against viral disease (see the box in the right column).

✓ TRICKS OF THE TRADE

Observing universal precautions and being up-to-date with vaccinations are your best defenses against viruses.

NOTE

Viral infections usually cause active illness; the signs and symptoms are based on the type and location of cells infected. Therefore certain viruses tend to cause respiratory illness (e.g., influenza), whereas others cause gastroenteritis (enteroviruses), CNS disease (e.g., St. Louis B encephalitis, rabies), or liver disease (hepatitis).

Immunological and Inflammatory Injury

Cellular membranes are injured by direct contact with cellular and chemical components of the immune and inflammatory responses, such as phagocytic cells (monocytes, neutrophils, and macrophages) and such substances as antibodies, lymphokines, complements, and proteases (see Chapters 35 and Chapter 37). If the cell membrane is injured or the transport mechanism (responsible for moving potassium into the cell and moving sodium out) be-

INFLUENZA VACCINES

Influenza viruses fall into three major types: A, B, and C. Type A mutates every 2 to 3 years, and Type B every 3 to 6 years. (Type C apparently does not mutate.) The mutations allow the virus to escape containment by the immune system, even if the person has had previous influenza infection. (Type A influenza viruses have caused worldwide epidemics, killing tens of thousands of people.) Each year, virologists and epidemiologists analyze cultures from the southern hemisphere (where the flu season falls during the northern hemisphere's summer) to determine which strains are likely to appear in the upcoming flu season and thereby prepare effective vaccines. If the expected strain strikes, the vaccine can provide protection to about 75% of those who have been vaccinated.

gins to fail, an increase in intracellular water will occur, causing cellular swelling. If cellular swelling continues, the cell may eventually rupture.

Injurious Genetic Factors

Genetic disease results from a chromosomal abnormality or a defective gene. These genetic defects may be inherited (e.g., sickle cell anemia) or may result from spontaneous mutations (e.g., Down syndrome). Some genetic disorders can alter the cell's structure and function. For example, genetic disorders that cause alterations in the structural or metabolic component of the specific target cells include Huntington's disease and muscular dystrophy (see Chapter 35).

NOTE

The term *congenital* refers to any abnormality that is present at birth, even though it may not be detected until some time after birth.

Injurious Nutritional Imbalances

Cells require adequate amounts of essential nutrients to function normally. If required nutrients are not provided through diet and transported to cells (or if excessive amounts are consumed and transported to cells), pathophysiological cellular effects can occur. Examples include protein-calorie malnutrition, obesity, hyperglycemia, scurvy, and rickets.

Injurious Physical Agents

Many physical agents can injure cells and tissues. Examples of physical agents (including environmental agents) that can cause cellular or tissue injury include the following:

- Temperature extremes (hypothermic and hyperthermic injury)
- Changes in atmospheric pressure (blast injury, decompression sickness)
- Ionizing radiation (radiation injury)
- Nonionizing radiation
- Illumination (light injury, [e.g., vision injury, skin cancer])
- Mechanical stresses (e.g., noise-induced hearing loss, overuse syndromes)

Manifestations of Cellular Injury

An injured cell may exhibit various morphological (form and structure) abnormalities. The two most common changes are cellular swelling and fatty change. Cellular injury has both local and systemic manifestations.

Cellular Manifestations

Injured cells (and some healthy cells) experience cellular accumulations of substances such as fluids and electrolytes, triglycerides (lipids), glucose, calcium, uric acid, protein, melanin, and bilirubin. These substances normally are present in certain cells of the body, but abnormal intracellular accumulation may lead to cellular damage. Also, injured cells may be unable to rid themselves of excessive amounts of water, sodium, or calcium, which leads to increased injury. If water, sodium, or calcium continue to accumulate, the cells become irreversibly damaged.

Some substances, such as lipids, also can accumulate in cells. The macrophage can ingest excessive extracellular lipids and cellular debris from injured cells. Some macrophages circulate throughout the body, whereas others remain fixed in tissues (such as the liver and spleen). Phagocytes migrate to injured tissue and engulf dying cells and abnormal extracellular substances. As more phagocytes migrate to injured tissue to engulf the metabolites, the affected tissue begins to swell.

NOTE

Phagocytosis by the fixed macrophages of the reticuloendothelial system causes enlargement of the liver (hepatomegaly) or the spleen (splenomegaly), seen with many diseases associated with abnormal accumulation of various metabolic products (amyloidosis) or abnormal cells (hemolytic disease).

Cellular swelling. As previously described, the swelling in injured cells results from membrane alterations associated with rapid leakage of potassium out of the cell and the influx of sodium and water. The increase in intracellular sodium increases osmotic pressure, which draws more water into the cell. If the swelling affects all cells in an organ, the organ increases in weight and becomes distended. Cellular swelling usually is reversible.

NOTE

Inflammation, whether due to infection, trauma, or autoimmune reactions, is associated with cellular swelling, often accompanied by fever.

Fatty change. Fatty change occurs if the enzyme systems that metabolize fat are impaired or overwhelmed, leading to intracellular lipid accumulation. This condition is common in liver cells (fatty liver) because they are actively involved in fat metabolism. Because hepatic metabolism and secretion of lipids are crucial to proper body function, deficiencies in these processes lead to major pathological changes.

NOTE

Alcohol abuse is a common cause of fatty liver, which usually is a precursor to cirrhosis.

Systemic Manifestations

Many systemic manifestations are associated with cellular injury. These include fever, malaise, a loss of well-being, altered appetite, altered heart rate, leukocytosis, and pain. In addition, cellular enzymes may be present in extracellular fluid from injured cells or tissue.

Cellular Death/Necrosis

A cell dies if it has been irreparably damaged. Shortly after cell death, structural changes begin to occur within the nucleus and cytoplasm. The lysosome (a sac of digestive enzymes found in many cells) begins to have membrane breakdown, releasing lysosomal enzymes that begin to digest the cell. The nucleus shrinks and dissolves or breaks into fragments (see the box in the right column).

Necrosis is the death of cells or tissues through injury or disease. It also can occur by cellular self-destruction (autolysis). Different types of necrosis tend to occur in different organs or tissues and may indicate the cause of cellular injury. Necrotic changes take several hours to develop and are recognized easily on histological examination by their structure and staining characteristics.

Genetics and Familial Diseases

People are born with a genetic predisposition to the development of certain diseases. The genetics of some diseases, such as hemophilia or sickle cell anemia, are well understood. Patients either have no genetic predisposition, are carriers of the disease, or have the disease. Other disease processes (such as arthritis, diabetes, and hypertension) certainly are linked to genetics but also are strongly associated with environmental factors. The medical profession continues its attempts to decrease the incidence or severity of these inherited medical conditions through environmental manipulation.

Factors Causing Disease

Factors that cause disease may be simplistically classified as *genetic* or *environmental*. However, a strong interaction occurs between the two. For example, genes cannot exert their effects without an environment in which to operate, and environmental factors act differently on different people. Conversely, the environment may be the same, but people have unique genetic compositions. Therefore the interaction between genetics and environment is very complex.

Genetic

Heredity is governed by the laws of chance and probability, because each pair of chromosomes is

---

NORMAL CELLULAR AGING AND DEATH

Cellular aging and death are common processes and are natural parts of the cell cycle. As the cell ages, it becomes less efficient in carrying out its functions and more susceptible to harmful environmental influences. With progressive damage, cells lose their ability to repair themselves and eventually begin to malfunction. Cellular changes that occur in immunological cells slowly lead to decreased immunity and enhanced susceptibility to infectious disease. Malignancies increase with age as a result of decreased immunity as well as an increased incidence of malignant transformation of various cells. Other examples of the manifestations of aging cells include gray hair, reduced muscle mass, menopause, arteriosclerosis, memory and vision impairment, and arthritis.

---

sorted at random when packaged into eggs and sperm. With more than 100,000 genes involved in our genetic makeup, the range of variation is enormous. Different types of genetic diseases can arise, either by individual genetic changes or by virtue of entire chromosomal abnormalities.

Mistakes sometimes are made when chromosomes are packaged, resulting in chromosomes that are rearranged. Entire chromosomal abnormalities lead to such diseases as Down syndrome or Turner's syndrome. More commonly, it is simply a single gene on the chromosome that is passed on, resulting in an abnormal protein. This is the type of genetic defect responsible for sickle cell anemia and hemophilia. Finally, some conditions are polygenic and multifactional, but with a strong inherited component. These diseases include coronary artery disease (CAD), hypertension, and cancer.

NOTE

Genes are not entirely unchangeable units of inheritance. They sometimes can change or be changed by environmental influences (see the box on p. 210).

Environmental

Many common chronic diseases may occur because of a mismatch between genetic and environmental

EXAMPLE OF HOW GENES CAN BE CHANGED BY ENVIRONMENTAL INFLUENCES

The gene responsible for sickle cell anemia was recognized to be much more common in environments in which malaria was prevalent. People with sickle cell disease have sickle-shaped red blood corpuscles that clog the capillaries, often proving fatal. However, in people who are carriers of the sickle cell trait, less than one percent of the red corpuscles are abnormal. These individuals do not die from sickle cell anemia and are more resistant to malaria than noncarriers of the sickle cell trait. Thus the trait proved protective and was increased as a result of normal selection.

factors (Tables 7-4 and 7-5). Important environmental factors include the following:

- Microorganisms and immunological exposures
- Personal habits and lifestyle
- Chemical substances
- Physical environment
- Psychosocial environment

The goal in preventing disease is to identify the genetic and environmental influences that lead to major diseases. This knowledge will help people with specific susceptibilities to modify environmental factors to decrease their risk of developing illness (see Appendix C).

Age and Gender

Age and gender also appear to play a major role in the occurrence of familial (hereditary) diseases. This is particularly true for diseases that are not due to a single genetic defect. In the polygenic disorders, cumulative effects of genes and environment over time lead to diseases associated with age-related changes in metabolism. This may explain why heart disease, hypertension, and cancer are more common in people over age 40 than in those who are younger.

Gender is associated with sex-specific diseases from hormonal and anatomical differences. Examples include breast cancer in women and testicular cancer in men. Lifestyle and environmental differences in gender-related activities also may be responsible for the predisposition to some diseases. Examples of gender/lifestyle/environmental combinations

include the higher rate of lung cancer and coronary artery disease in men who smoke cigarettes.

Analyzing Disease Risk

Epidemiologists who study disease use disease "rates" and risk factor analysis. Rates help describe the occurrence of disease; risk factors are indicators of a person's predisposition to developing a disease.

Disease Rates

Three commonly used statistics to assess the societal impact of disease are incidence rate, prevalence rate, and mortality rate. Incidence rate is the number of new cases detected during a given period of time (usually 1 year) per number of persons in a population surveyed. The prevalence rate refers to the number of persons *living* with the disease per number of persons in the population. The mortality rate is the number of persons who have died from the disease during an interval (often 1 year) per number of persons in the surveyed population. An example of a study using disease rates to evaluate coronary artery disease in American men aged 50 to 64 years showed an incidence rate of 2.2%, a prevalence rate of 9.7%, and an annual mortality rate of 0.92% in this population.[2]

Risk Factor Analysis

The presence of particular risk factors in any group of individuals is associated with an increased disease rate in that group. *Causal risk factors* are those that, when removed or eliminated, will result in the delay or prevention of the disease. *Noncausal risk factors* are helpful in predicting a person's chances of developing the disease but have no direct effect on the underlying cause of the disease (Fig. 7-17).

NOTE

Risk factors cannot precisely predict whether a person will develop a disease but can provide clues about the probability of developing a disease.

Combined Effects and Interactions Among Risk Factors

When one or more risk factors interact, the individual effects of risk factors may be greatly magnified.

TABLE 7-4	ENVIRONMENTAL FACTORS AFFECTING THE OCCURRENCE OF DISEASE	
TYPE	**EXAMPLES**	
Microorganisms and immunological exposures	Bacteria Viruses Fungi Protozoa Vectors (e.g., insects and animals) Allergens	
Personal habits and lifestyle	Smoking Physical exercise Dietary intake	
Chemical substances	Toxins Pollutants Medications Solvents, fumes Contaminants	
Physical environment	Climate Radiation Physical trauma Geographic location (e.g., sun exposure, altitude) Community (e.g., water and food supplies)	
Psychosocial milieu	Family status (e.g., bereavement, loss, status change) Stress Coping skills Social isolation Ethnic and racial customs Religious customs	

For example, some risk factors alone may present little or no risk for disease, but in the presence of another factor, the risk increases substantially.

Familial Disease Tendency

Family members (siblings, parents with offspring, spouse pairs, twins) are sometimes predisposed to develop certain diseases more often than individuals of the general population. Often, the familial risk factors are genetic or shared environmental factors. Examples include certain illness, such as heart disease and pulmonary disease, which result from choices such as smoking and consumption of dietary fat.

> **? CRITICAL THINKING**
>
> *Think about how many risk factors you have for heart disease. Which of these factors are genetic and which ones could you eliminate by modifying your habits or environment?*

Aging and Age-Related Disorders

Increased age is a risk factor for many diseases such as heart attack, stroke, and cancer. It probably represents the cumulative effects of genetics and environmental factors. Age-related disorders occur throughout life. Some disorders such as dental cavities or strep throat are more common in younger age groups, whereas the degenerative disorders (e.g., arthritis) are more common in older age groups (Table 7-6).

Common Familial Diseases and Associated Risk Factors

High-risk individuals can take steps to avoid many familial diseases. Examples include coronary heart disease and colorectal cancer. These conditions are described in detail throughout this text. Table 7-7 lists some known familial diseases and environmental factors that might play a role in causing and eventually preventing the development of disease.

TABLE 7-5	POPULATIONS WITH SHARED DISEASE TENDENCIES (DUE TO SHARED ENVIRONMENTAL FACTORS, COMMON GENE POOL, OR BOTH)		
DISEASE	**POPULATIONS**	**SUGGESTED ENVIRONMENTAL FACTORS**	**SHARED GENE POOL**
Early coronary heart disease	Very high in Finland (very low in Japan)	Animal fat intake	Genes for high blood cholesterol
Colon cancer	Low in developing countries (e.g., Africa); high in "westernized" countries (e.g., United States, Europe)	Dietary fiber and fat intake	
Thalassemia (type of anemia)	High in persons of Mediterranean descent; low in other areas		Major dominant gene for thalassemia
Malaria (many other infectious diseases)	High in some parts of Africa and Asia; low in United States and Europe	Trypanosomes, mosquitoes, disease control measures	
Early noninsulin dependent diabetes and obesity	Native Americans	Change from scarce food supply to plenty	Apparent shared gene pool among various Native American tribes
Lung cancer	Low rates in Mormons and Seventh Day Adventists	Health code against use of tobacco	
Skin cancers	Higher rates among whites than blacks; higher rates in "sun belt" than in other locations	Ultraviolet light	Inherited level of skin pigmentation

From McCance KL, Huether SE: *Pathophysiology: the biologic basis for disease in adults and children,* ed 2, St Louis, 1994, Mosby.

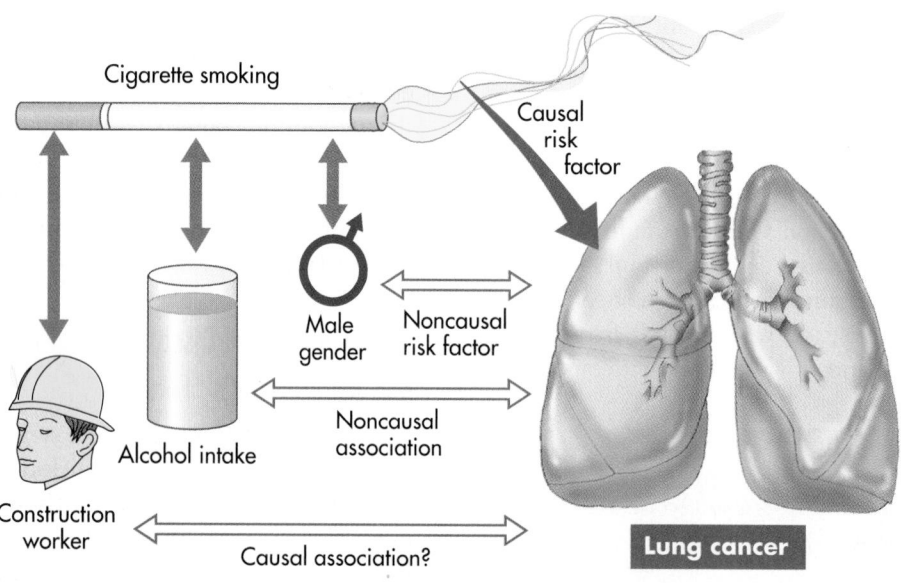

Fig. 7-17 Causal and noncausal risk factors and associations.

TABLE 7-6	AGE-RELATED DISORDERS	
AGE	**DISORDERS CORRELATED WITH AGE RANGE**
Birth-14 years	Congenital disorders Allergy Infection Cancer (leukemia, Wilms' tumor, medulloblastoma, retinoblastoma) Trauma or injury Diabetes (early onset)
15-30 years	Allergy (asthma) Endocrine Trauma or injury (suicide) Venereal disease
30-40 years	Ulcer Hypertension Breast cancer Homicide Suicide Complications of pregnancy Alcoholism
40-60 years	Heart disease (hypertension, rheumatic, infarction) Kidney disease (glomerular nephritis) Liver disease (cirrhosis) Cancer (lung, colon, breast, ovary)
60-80 years	Cardiovascular Cancer (lung, colon, prostate)
80-100 years	Cancer (leukemia, lymphoma, prostate) Dementia (Alzheimer's, Parkinson's) Osteoporosis Infection Cardiovascular Trauma or injury (fracture)

Modified from King DW, Fenoglio CM, Lefkowitch JH: *General pathology: principles and dynamics,* Philadelphia, 1988, Lea & Febiger.

Hypoperfusion

The term **hypoperfusion** is used to describe inadequate circulation of blood and nutrients to tissues. Hypoperfusion can result from a number of medical and traumatic conditions.

Pathogenesis

Hypoperfusion often is the result of decreased cardiac output. Decreased cardiac output, if prolonged, leads to shock (a continued state of hypoperfusion), **multiple organ dysfunction syndrome** (MODS), and other disease states associated with impaired cellular metabolism.

Decreased Cardiac Output

Cardiac output (minute volume) is the total amount of blood pumped by the ventricles per minute, usually expressed in liters per minute. Cardiac output is a crucial determinant of organ perfusion and depends on several factors. These include the strength of contraction, rate of contraction, and amount of venous return available to the ventricle (**preload**).

> **NOTE**
>
> Cardiac output is determined by multiplying the heart rate by the volume of blood ejected by the ventricles during each beat (**stroke volume**). For example, if the ventricle contracts 72 times per minute and ejects 42 mL of blood with each contraction, the cardiac output would be 72 beats per minute multiplied by 42 mL per beat, or 3.02 L/min. Decreased cardiac output usually is associated with a decrease in blood pressure, tissue perfusion, and impaired cellular metabolism.

Compensatory Mechanisms

Compensatory mechanisms used by the body to manage blood pressure and cardiac output include a number of **negative feedback mechanisms** (any mechanism that tends to balance a change in a system). Negative feedback mechanisms important in maintaining cardiac output and tissue perfusion are baroreceptor reflexes, chemoreceptor reflexes, central nervous system ischemic response, hormonal mechanisms, reabsorption of tissue fluids, and the splenic discharge of stored blood (seen in animals, but minimal in humans).

Baroreceptor reflexes. Baroreceptors (Fig. 7-18, *A*) help maintain blood pressure and cardiac output in two ways (both of which are negative feedback mechanisms): (1) by lowering blood pressure in response to increased arterial pressure, and (2) by increasing blood pressure in response to decreased arterial

TABLE 7-7	COMMON FAMILIAL DISEASE AND ASSOCIATED ENVIRONMENTAL RISK FACTORS

IMMUNOLOGICAL DISORDERS	ASSOCIATED ENVIRONMENTAL RISK FACTORS
Asthma and Other Allergies	Fur, dust, pollen, mold (other allergens)
Rheumatic fever	Group A-strep bacterial infection
Cancer	
Breast cancer	Obesity, high dietary fat, alcohol, hormones
Colorectal cancer	Inadequate fiber intake, high dietary fat
Lung cancer	Cigarette smoke, environmental pollutants
Endocrine Disorders	
Diabetes mellitus-insulin dependent	Viral infection, blood sugar control problems over years
Diabetes mellitus-non-insulin dependent	Obesity, dietary sugar and fiber, blood sugar control problems over years
Hypertension	Diet, obesity, inadequate exercise
Hematological Disorders	
Drug-induced hemolytic anemia	Aspirin, antibiotics, infection
Sickle cell anemia	Precipitated by cold weather, infection
Hemochromatosis	Ingestions, transfusions
Cardiovascular Disorders	
Coronary artery disease	Exercise, alcohol, diet, smoking, obesity, and stress can affect all cardiovascular disorders
Cardiac myopathies	Infection, alcohol or other drugs
Mitral valve prolapse	Infection
Hypertension and stroke	Diet, obesity
Renal Disorders	
Gout	Poor diet, injury, stress
Kidney stones	Decrease water intake
Gastrointestinal Disorders	
Malabsorption disorders	
Lactose intolerance	Milk product ingestion
Ulcerative colitis	Stress, dietary intake of "trigger" foods
Crohn's disease	Stress, dietary intake of "trigger" foods
Peptic ulcers	Stress, diet, infection
Gallstones	Dietary fat, obesity
Obesity	Dietary fat, sugar, total calories, stress affecting appetite, cultural perceptions
Neuromuscular Disorders	
Multiple sclerosis	Virus, warm environment, stress
Alzheimer's disease	Decreased mental stimulation later in life
Psychiatric Disorders	
Schizophrenia	Uncertain influence, dramatic success with drug treatment
Manic-depression	Uncertain influence, dramatic success with drug treatment

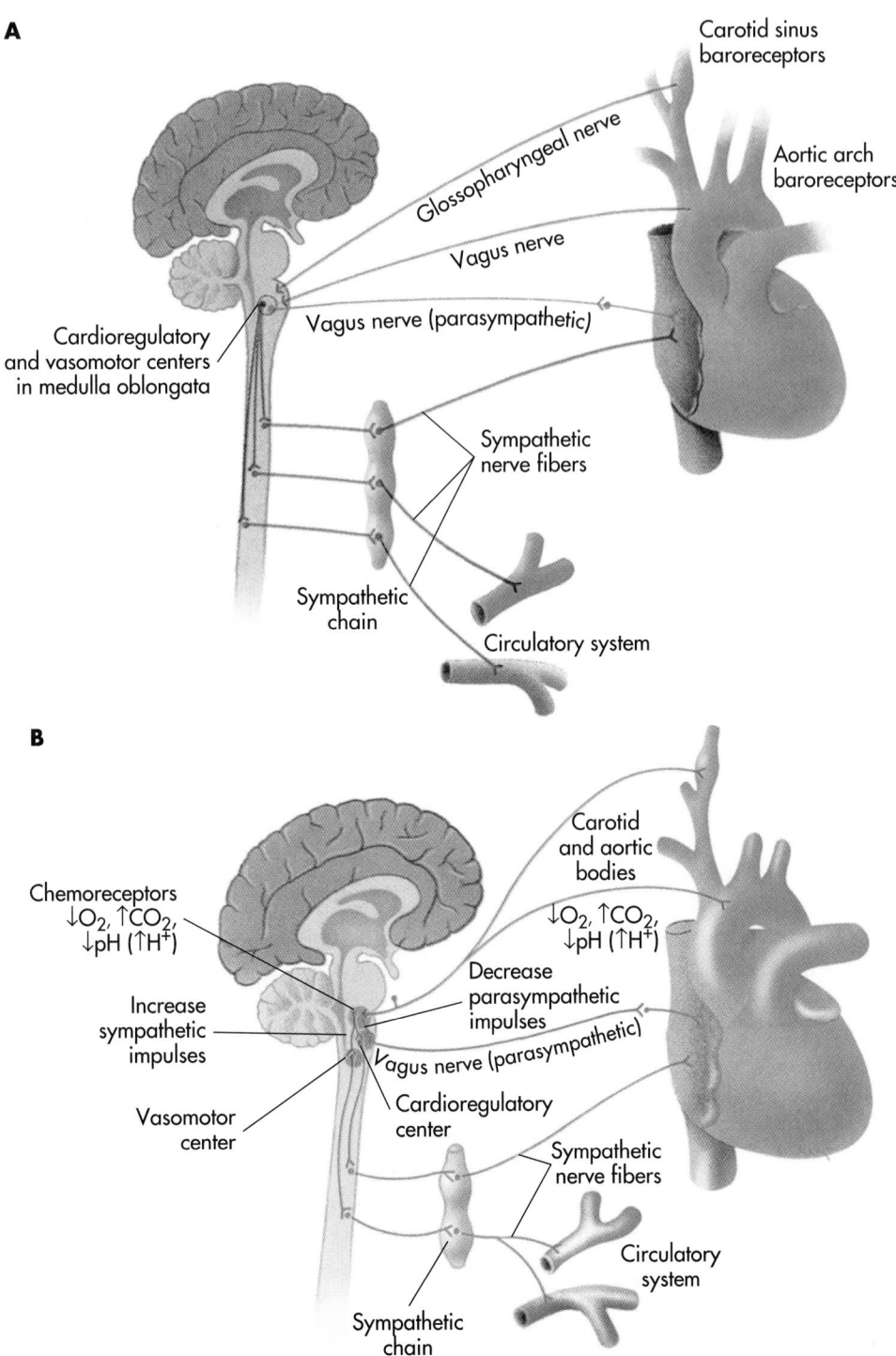

Fig. 7-18 A, Baroreceptor reflexes. Baroreceptors located in the carotid sinuses and the aortic arch detect changes in blood pressure. Impulses are conducted to the cardioregulatory and vasomotor centers. The heart rate can be decreased by the parasympathetic system; the heart rate and stroke volume can be increased by the sympathetic system. The sympathetic system can also constrict or dilate blood vessels. **B,** Chemoreceptor reflexes. Chemoreceptors located in the medulla and carotid and aortic bodies detect changes in blood oxygen, carbon dioxide, or pH levels. Impulses are conducted to the medulla. In response, the vasomotor center can cause vasoconstriction or dilation of blood vessels by the sympathetic system, and the cardioregulatory center can cause changes in the pumping activity of the heart through the parasympathetic and sympathetic system.

pressure. Normal blood pressure partially stretches the arterial walls so that the baroreceptors produce a constant, low-level frequency stimulation. This stimulation increases progressively from a lower pressure limit of 60 mm Hg, reaching a maximum at 180 to 200 mm Hg. Impulses from the baroreceptors travel through the vagus and Herring's nerve to the glossopharyngeal nerve, where they inhibit the vasoconstrictor center of the medulla and excite the vagal center. These impulses result in vasodilation in the peripheral circulatory system and a decrease in the heart rate and strength of contraction. The combined effect is a decrease in arterial pressure.

> **NOTE**
>
> Baroreceptors adapt in 1 to 3 days to the ambient pressure in the immediate locale. Therefore the baroreceptors are not responsible for modulating the average blood pressure on a long-term basis.

Baroreceptors are not stimulated when the blood pressure is less than 60 mm Hg. When baroreceptor stimulation ceases because of a fall in arterial pressure, the negative feedback mechanism evokes several cardiovascular responses (Box 7-2). Vagal (parasympathetic) stimulation is reduced, and sympathetic response is increased. The increase in sympathetic impulses results in increased **peripheral vascular resistance** (PVR) and an increase in heart rate and stroke volume. Sympathetic discharges also produce generalized arteriolar vasoconstriction, which decreases the size of the vascular compart-

ment. Constricting capacitance vessels shift blood into the central circulation. This, coupled with the constriction of blood vessels in skin, muscles, and viscera, helps maintain perfusion of the central organs. The vasoconstriction in these peripheral vascular beds results in the characteristic pale, cool skin of patients suffering from hypovolemic shock.

> **NOTE**
>
> Peripheral vascular resistance is the resistance to blood flow in the systemic circulation (small arteries, arterioles, venules, veins). **Afterload** (the systemic vascular resistance on the left side of the heart) is the pressure against which the ventricle has to contract to eject its contents.

Chemoreceptor reflexes. Low arterial pressure (if it leads to hypoxemia, acidosis, or both) also may stimulate peripheral chemoreceptor cells that lie within the carotid and aortic bodies. Because of the location of these bodies, the chemoreceptor cells have an abundant blood supply. When the PO_2 or pH decreases, these cells stimulate the vasomotor center of the medulla. At the same time, the rate and depth of ventilation are increased to help eliminate excess carbon dioxide and maintain acid-base balance. Chemoreceptors are more involved in regulation of respiration than in cardiovascular rate and rhythm or blood pressure regulation. During profound hypotension or acidosis, however, they can and do lead to vasoconstriction. This vasomotor stimulation results in enhanced peripheral vasoconstriction, which is initiated by the baroreceptors (Fig. 7-18, *B*).

Central nervous system ischemic response. When blood flow to the vasomotor center of the medulla is decreased sufficiently to cause ischemia, the neurons in the vasomotor center become excited, raising arterial pressure. This is known as the *central nervous system ischemic response*. The degree of sympathetic vasoconstriction can be so intense that it elevates arterial pressure for as long as 10 minutes, sometimes to more than 200 mm Hg. If the ischemia lasts longer than a few minutes, the vagal centers are activated, resulting in vasodilation in the periphery and bradycardia. Like the chemoreceptor reflex, the cerebral ischemic response functions only in emergency situations and does not become active until blood pressure falls below 50 mm Hg.

BOX 7-2

BARORECEPTOR RESPONSES TO LOW BLOOD PRESSURE: SYMPATHETIC NERVOUS SYSTEM

Cardiac Effects
Increased strength of contraction
Increased rate of contraction

Peripheral Effects
Arteriolar constriction
Decreased container size
Increased peripheral resistance

Hormonal mechanisms. Several hormonal mechanisms also help control arterial pressure through negative feedback. These include the adrenal medullary mechanism, the renin-angiotensin-aldosterone mechanism, and the vasopressin mechanism.

Adrenal medullary mechanism. When sympathetic stimulation of the heart and blood vessels increases, stimulation of the adrenal medulla also increases. The hormones secreted by the adrenal medulla, epinephrine and norepinephrine, affect the cardiovascular system in a way very similar to the sympathetic nervous system. As a result heart rate, stroke volume, and vasoconstriction increase.

Renin-angiotensin-aldosterone mechanism. As previously described, renin is an enzyme released by the kidneys into the circulatory system. Renin acts on a plasma protein (angiotensinogen) by altering its structure to produce angiotensin I, which is in turn cleaved by angiotensin-converting enzyme (mostly in the lungs) to angiotensin II (active angiotensin).

> **NOTE**
>
> Angiotensin-converting enzyme (ACE) inhibitors are drugs that block the conversion of the precursor angiotensin I to the active molecule angiotensin II, thereby lowering blood pressure and putting less stress on the heart. Examples of ACE inhibitors include captopril (Capoten), enalapril (Vasotec), and lisinopril (Prinivil).

Angiotensin II causes vasoconstriction in arterioles and to a lesser degree in veins. This vasoconstriction results in increased peripheral resistance, increased venous return to the heart, and a resultant increase in blood pressure. In addition, angiotensin II stimulates the release of aldosterone, which acts on the kidneys to conserve sodium and water.

The renin-angiotensin-aldosterone mechanism is an important regulatory loop to increase blood pressure in circulatory shock. It requires about 20 minutes to become effective in hypovolemia caused by hemorrhagic shock and remains active for about 1 hour.

Vasopressin mechanism. When the blood pressure drops or the concentration of solutes in the plasma increases (increased serum osmolality), the hypothalamic neurons are stimulated. This stimulation causes the anterior pituitary to increase its secretion of vasopressin, or antidiuretic hormone (ADH). ADH acts directly on the blood vessels, causing vasoconstriction within minutes after a rapid fall in the blood pressure. ADH also decreases the rate of urine production (by enhancing reabsorption of water), helping maintain the blood volume and the blood pressure.

> **NOTE**
>
> The atrial natriuretic factor also helps control arterial pressure through negative feedback. Its release is initiated by elevated atrial pressure (usually a sign of volume overload), and it increases the rate of urine production. Loss of water through the urine decreases blood volume, thus decreasing the atrial pressure. This is the only hormonal system actively used to decrease volume and pressure.

Reabsorption of tissue fluids. Arterial hypotension, arteriolar constriction, and reduced venous pressure during hypovolemia lower the blood pressure in the capillaries (hydrostatic pressure). This decrease promotes reabsorption of interstitial fluid into the vascular compartment. Considerable quantities of fluid may be drawn into the circulation during hemorrhage. It has been estimated that about 0.25 mL/min/kg of body weight, or 1 L/hr in the adult male, can be autoinfused from the interstitial spaces after acute blood loss.

Splenic discharge of blood. Some of the blood that circulates through the spleen continues through the microcirculation and is stored in an area called the *venous sinuses.* The venous sinuses are capable of storing more than 300 mL of blood. Sudden reductions in blood pressure cause the sympathetic nervous system to stimulate constriction of these sinuses. Constriction can expel as much as 200 mL of this blood into the venous circulation to help restore blood volume or pressure in the circulation.

> **? CRITICAL THINKING**
>
> *What compensatory changes can you evaluate while assessing your patient's radial pulse?*

Types of Shock

Shock is classified based on the primary cause (Box 7-3). Although these classifications are separate and distinct, two or more types may be combined. Below is a brief description of the five types of shock. A more thorough discussion of shock is presented in Chapter 19.

- Hypovolemic shock is most frequently caused by hemorrhage but also may be caused by severe dehydration. In either case, circulating volume is lost.
- Cardiogenic shock results when cardiac action cannot deliver adequate circulation for tissue perfusion.
- Neurogenic shock results most often from spinal cord injury with resultant loss of sympathetic vasomotor tone.
- Anaphylactic shock occurs when the body is exposed to a substance that produces a severe allergic reaction.
- Septic shock most often results from a serious systemic bacterial infection.

BOX 7-3

COMMON ETIOLOGICAL CLASSIFICATION OF SHOCK

Hypovolemic shock
Cardiogenic shock
Neurogenic shock
Anaphylactic shock
Septic shock

Multiple Organ Dysfunction Syndrome

Multiple organ dysfunction syndrome (MODS) is the progressive failure of two or more organ systems after a very severe illness or injury. Sepsis and septic shock are common causes of MODS, although it may follow any period of prolonged shock, regardless of the cause (see Chapter 19).

Pathophysiology

Any process that triggers the body's inflammatory response has the potential to initiate MODS, including traumatic, septic, and burn injury. The syndrome begins with vascular endothelial damage that results from endotoxins and inflammatory mediators that are released into the circulation. When this occurs, the vascular endothelium becomes permeable, allowing fluid and cells to leak into the interstitial spaces, contributing to hypotension and hypoperfusion. The release of mediators activates three major plasma enzyme cascades: complement, coagulation, and kallikrein/kinin.

Complement activates phagocytes and induces further inflammation and damage to the endothelium. As a result of the endothelial damage, coagulation becomes uncontrolled, resulting in microvascular thrombus formation and tissue ischemia. Activation of the kallikrein/kinin system releases bradykinin (a potent vasodilator), which contributes to low systemic vascular resistance. The overall effect of these three systems is a hyperinflammatory and hypercoagulable state that leads to edema formation, cardiovascular instability (hypotension), and clotting abnormalities. These inflammatory processes cause maldistribution of systemic and organ blood flow that results in a hyperdynamic circulation with increased venous return. The shunting of blood past selected regional capillary beds and the formation of interstitial edema from changes in permeability cause a decrease in oxygen delivery to the tissues. In addition, capillary obstruction occurs from microvascular thrombi and the aggregation of inflammatory cells. Resultant ischemia contributes to MODS.

The same hormonal responses that help conserve volume in shock also cause the body to enter into a hypermetabolic (catabolic) state, altering carbohydrate, fat, and lipid metabolism to meet the increased demand for energy. Over time, the sympathetic drive and the hyperdynamic circulation places excessive demands on the heart, and the net result is depletion of oxygen and fuel supplies. The decrease in oxygen delivery to the cells, hypermetabolism, and the associated myocardial depression create an imbalance in oxygen supply and demand. Tissue hypoxia with cellular acidosis and impaired cellular function soon follow, and multiple organ failure ensues (the box below and Fig. 7-19).

NOTE

No specific therapy exists for MODS. Early detection is critical so that supportive measures can be initiated immediately.

CLINICAL MANIFESTATIONS OF MODS

Following resuscitation (within 24 hours), the patient develops a low-grade fever, tachycardia, dyspnea, and altered mental status. The lungs begin to fail, resulting in adult respiratory distress syndrome (ARDS). After 7 to 10 days, bacteremia is common and signs of kidney and liver failure appear. During days 14 to 21, renal and liver failure become severe, and the GI and immune systems fail, followed by cardiovascular collapse. If the patient does not improve by the end of the third week, survival is unlikely. Death usually occurs between day 21 and 28.

Cellular Metabolism Impairment

Virtually all cellular activities on which life depends require energy. Active transport pumps within the cellular membrane require a substantial percentage of the cell's energy production to maintain normal fluid and electrolyte composition within the cell. Adenosine triphosphate (ATP) and other high-energy phosphate molecules provide the fuel for all of the energy-related functions of the cell. Most cellular metabolism in the healthy body is accomplished through aerobic metabolism. Anaerobic metabolism occurs when the metabolic requirement for energy outstrips the oxygen supply. However, it can supply only a small fraction of the energy produced by aerobic metabolism (2 ATP molecules per molecule of glucose rather than the 36 ATP molecules generated per molecule of glucose in aerobic metabolism) and cannot meet the body's energy requirements alone.

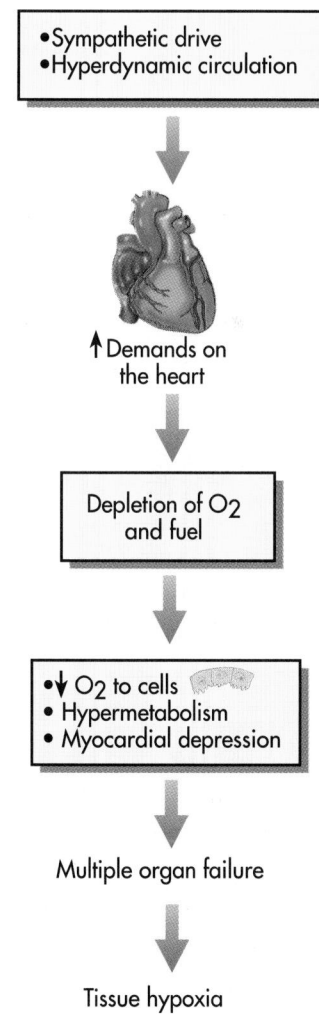

Fig. 7-19 Multiple organ dysfunction syndrome.

Glucose is an important fuel for producing energy and is essentially the only fuel that can be used anaerobically under conditions of cellular hypoxia (as occurs in a state of shock). Under these conditions, glucose is metabolized to lactate and pyruvate, producing a net sum of 2 ATP molecules. If oxygen is present (aerobic metabolism), pyruvate enters the Krebs cycle, a sequence of reactions that breaks down a molecule of pyruvic acid into molecules of carbon dioxide and water (Fig. 7-20). The Krebs cycle, which is 18 times more efficient in producing ATP than glycolysis (the breakdown of glucose to lactate), cannot occur in the absence of oxygen. Because anaerobic ATP production is so inefficient, the rate of glycolysis must be greatly increased to meet the body's energy requirements. This leads to an increase in production of lactic acid and a resultant metabolic acidosis.

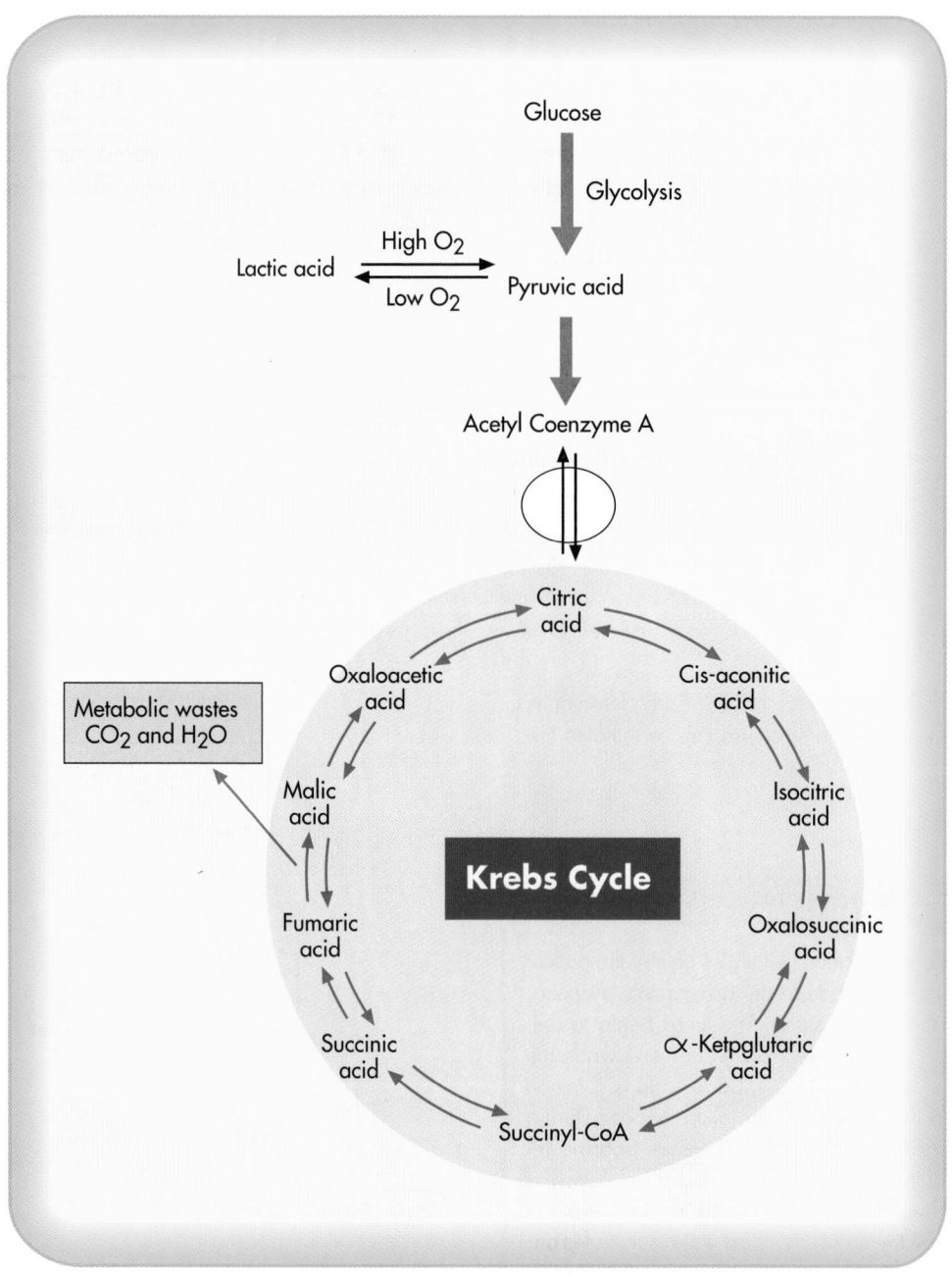

Fig. 7-20 Krebs cycle.

As tissue metabolites (and hydrogen ions) continue to accumulate, they stimulate vasodilation. This vasodilation opposes the previously described hormonally regulated constriction of the precapillary sphincters, thereby decreasing the body's ability to continue vital tissue perfusion by maintaining the proper size of the vascular compartment. (The postcapillary sphincters are more resistant to the vasodilatory effects of tissue metabolites and stay constricted long after the precapillary sphincters dilate.) This in turn increases the capillary hydrostatic pressure, causing a fluid loss from the vascular space into the interstitial space. In addition, the insufficient energy production from anaerobic metabolism affects the cells' ability to maintain a normal sodium-potassium differential across the cell membrane. Intracellular potassium leaks out of the cell, and sodium leaks into the cell, producing cellular swelling and decreased transmembrane potential. Energy production is further impaired until finally the cells are irreversibly damaged.

Self-Defense Mechanisms

The body's first lines of defense against illness and injury are external barriers that include the skin and the mucous membranes of the digestive, respiratory, and genitourinary tract. These surfaces form a continuous closed barrier between the internal organs and the environment (see Chapter 37). Once these external barriers have been breached, permitting harmful chemicals, foreign bodies, or microorganisms to penetrate cells and tissues, the second and third lines of defense are activated. In order, these are the inflammatory response and the immune response.

Inflammatory Response

Inflammation is a local reaction to cellular injury. The response may be initiated by physical, thermal, or chemical damage or by microbial infection. When invasion occurs, this line of defense is activated to prevent further invasion of the pathogen by isolating, destroying, or neutralizing the microorganism. As a rule, the inflammatory response is protective and beneficial. However, if the response is sustained or directed toward the host's own **antigens**, healthy tissue may be destroyed.

NOTE

An antigen is a substance that can be recognized as "foreign material" by the antibody system and bound by specific antibodies (protective protein substances developed by the body for this purpose). Specific antibodies bind to specific antigens when the two fit together. The attachment of antibodies facilitates antigen neutralization and removal from the body.

Stages of the Inflammatory Response

The inflammatory response may be divided into three separate stages: cellular response to injury, vascular response to injury, and phagocytosis.

Cellular response to injury. Metabolic changes occur with any type of cellular injury. The most common primary effect of injury on the cell's aerobic respiration and ATP-generating process (oxidative phosphorylation) leads to decreasing energy reserves. When the energy sources are depleted, the sodium-potassium pump can no longer function effectively; the cell swells because of the accumulation of sodium ions. The organelles within the cell also swell. This swelling, along with increasing acidosis, leads to further impairment of enzyme function and further deterioration in the integrity of membranes. Eventually the membranes of the cellular organelles begin to leak. Release of hydrolytic enzymes by the lysosomes contributes further to cellular destruction and autolysis. As the cellular contents are dissolved by enzymes, the inflammatory response is stimulated in surrounding tissues.

Vascular response to injury. After cellular injury, localized hyperemia develops as the surrounding arterioles, venules, and capillaries dilate. The associated increase in filtration pressure and capillary permeability causes fluid to leak from the vessels into the interstitial space, producing edema. Leukocytes (particularly neutrophils and monocytes) begin to collect along the vascular endothelium and, as a result of release of chemotactic factors, eventually migrate to the injured tissue.

Phagocytosis. Phagocytosis is the process by which leukocytes engulf, digest, and destroy pathogens. The circulating macrophages are also responsible for clearing the injured area of dead cells and other debris. Intracellular phagocytosis (ingestion of bacteria and dead cell fragments) occurs at the site of tissue invasion and may extend into the general circulation if the infection becomes systemic. Intracellular phagocytosis stimulates the release of chemicals that induce lysis of the leukocytes. These leukocytes combine with dead organisms and fluid to form an inflammatory exudate, commonly known as *pus*. The function of exudate is to deliver leukocytes, plasma protein, and other chemicals to the site of injury.

? CRITICAL THINKING

What pathophysiological inflammatory response causes each of these signs or symptoms: heat, redness, pain, and swelling?

NOTE

Exudate may be watery (serous exudate), as seen with blisters; thick and clotted (fibrinous exudate), as seen with lobar pneumonia; or pus filled (purulent exudate), as seen with cysts or abscesses. If bleeding occurs, the exudate is described as *hemorrhagic exudate*.

Mast Cells

Mast cells are specialized cells that are widely distributed throughout connective tissues. Their cytoplasm is filled with granules containing vasoactive amines (histamine, serotonin) and chemotactic factors. When tissue is injured, the mast cells discharge their granules (degranulation) as part of the inflammatory response. Mast cell degranulation is stimulated by physical injury (e.g., thermal or mechanical trauma), chemical agents (e.g., toxins, snake and bee venoms), hypersensitivity reactions, or as a direct result of complement components.

Local and Systemic Response to Acute Inflammation

Acute inflammation may be characterized by both local and systemic effects (Fig. 7-21). Local responses include vascular changes (vasodilation and increased vascular permeability) and the formation of exudate. Systemic responses include fever, leukocytosis, and an increase in circulating plasma proteins. The characteristic signs of localized inflammation are heat, redness, tenderness, swelling, and pain.

Chronic Inflammation Responses

Chronic inflammation (inflammation lasting 2 weeks or longer) can result from an unsuccessful acute inflammatory response due to bacterial contamination by a foreign body (e.g., wood splinter, glass), persistent infection, or continued exposure to an antigen. If the inflammatory process is severe or prolonged, the body will attempt to repair or replace tissue that has been damaged. This tissue repair occurs as cells produce connective tissue fibers and new blood vessels. If the area of tissue destruction is large, scar tissue will be formed.

Immune Response

The first two lines of defense against injurious agents respond to each agent using the identical nonspecific mechanism, but the immune response is specific to individual pathogens. Immunity may be natural, present at birth, or acquired, resulting from exposure to a specific antigenic agent or pathogen. Acquired immunity includes that resulting from inoculation (immunization) against certain infectious diseases (e.g., measles). Acquired immunity is further classified as humoral immunity and cell-mediated immunity. Humoral immunity is associated with the production of antibodies that combine with and eliminate foreign material. Cell-mediated immunity is characterized by the formation of a population of lymphocytes that attack and destroy foreign material (see Chapter 37).

NOTE

Cell-mediated immunity is the body's best defense against viruses, fungi, parasites, and some bacteria. It also is responsible for the body rejecting transplanted organs.

? CRITICAL THINKING

What kind of immunity protects you from each of the following: hepatitis, feline leukemia, and chickenpox?

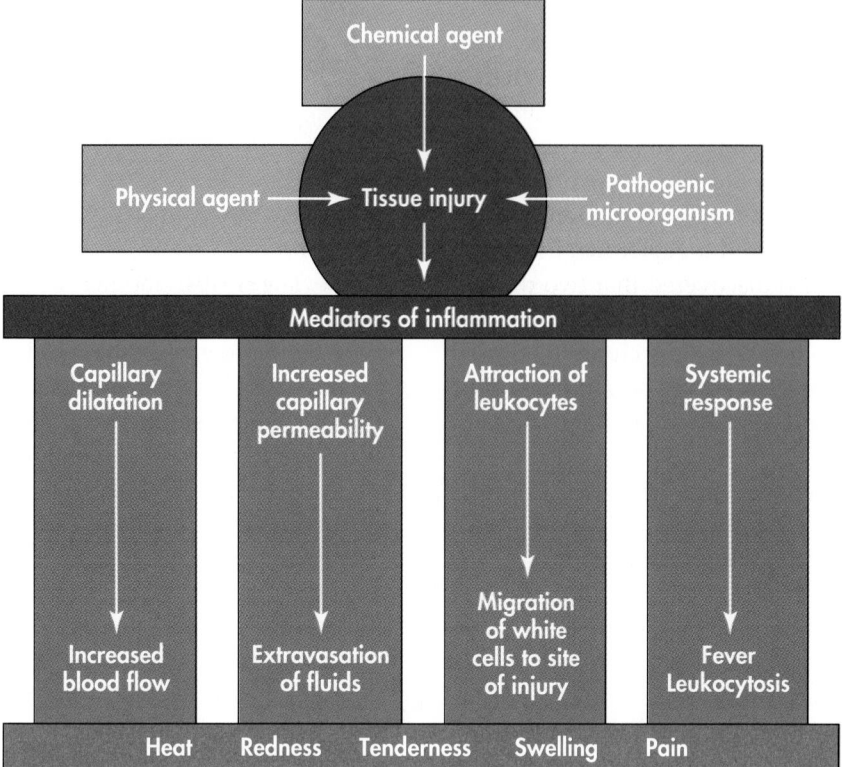

Fig. 7-21 Inflammation. (Redrawn from Crowley L: *Introduction to human disease,* ed 3, Boston, 1992, Jones and Bartlett.)

> **NOTE**
>
> The immune response is affected by age. For example, most infants are born with enough natural immunity from disease to protect them until they have made their own antibodies. On the other hand, cells of the immune system become less efficient with age, and older persons become more susceptible to diseases. The aging immune system also becomes less able to eliminate abnormal cells that may arise within the body.

Induction of the Immune Response

As previously defined, an antigen is a substance (molecule or molecular complex) that *reacts* with preformed components of the immune system (e.g., lymphocytes and antibodies). An immunogen is an antigen that can also *induce* the formation of antibodies. Therefore some antigens are not able to induce the immune response. To be immunogenic, the antigenic molecule must be

• Sufficiently foreign to the host
• Sufficiently large

• Sufficiently complex
• Present in sufficient amounts

The immune response is triggered after foreign materials have been cleared from the area of inflammation. After phagocytes digest the pathogens, antigenic material appears on their surface. When the antigen is recognized by receptors on lymphocytes as foreign or "non-self," a chain of events is set into play to destroy or neutralize the antigen. Briefly, this involves lymphocytes either maturing into plasma cells (derived from **B lymphocytes**), which produce antibody, or into sensitized lymphocytes that are capable of interacting directly with the foreign antigen (**T lymphocytes**) to neutralize or destroy the agent. (The immune response is presented in depth in Chapter 37.)

> **NOTE**
>
> Immune *tolerance* refers to the immune system's ability to allow self-antigens (vs. non-self–antigens) to exist by preventing their recognition by lymphocytes and antibodies.

Blood Group Antigens

In the early 1900s, it was found that there were individual differences in human blood. When a donor's blood was separated into plasma and red blood cell components and mixed with separated blood samples from another donor, two reactions were noted. When combined with foreign plasma, the red cells either clumped together (agglutinated) or did not. It was also discovered that two distinct agglutinins (substances on red blood cells acting as antigens) were responsible for the clumping. Based on possible combinations of these antigens, four types of human blood were identified: A, B, AB, and O (Fig. 7-22).

Type A blood has anti-B antibodies in the plasma and would therefore clump type B blood. Type B blood has anti-A antibodies and would clump Type A blood. Type AB blood has neither antibody and can therefore receive any of the four types of blood (*universal recipient*). Type O blood has both anti-A and anti-B antibodies, so it cannot receive any type of blood other than Type O. Type O blood has neither antigen, however, and can therefore be given to patients with any blood type. Type O blood has become known as the *universal donor*.

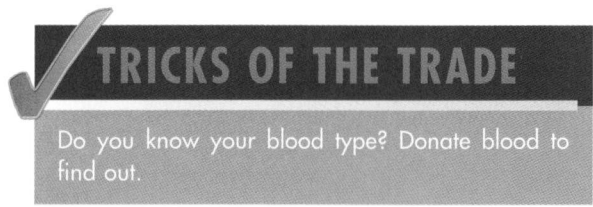

Rh Factor

In the late 1940s, another determinant in human blood was discovered: the Rh factor. (Rh was taken from the word *rhesus*, the monkey species used for the research.) It was found that when the blood of a rhesus monkey was injected into a rabbit, the rabbit's immune system developed antibodies; when a sample of the rabbit's plasma was mixed with a sample of human red blood cells, the human cells usually clumped (Rh-positive). About 85% of Americans have Rh-positive blood. The percentages in the population of ABO and Rh blood groups are as follows:

O positive	38.4%	B positive	9.4%
O negative	7.7%	B negative	1.7%
A positive	32.3%	AB positive	3.2%
A negative	6.5%	AB negative	0.7%

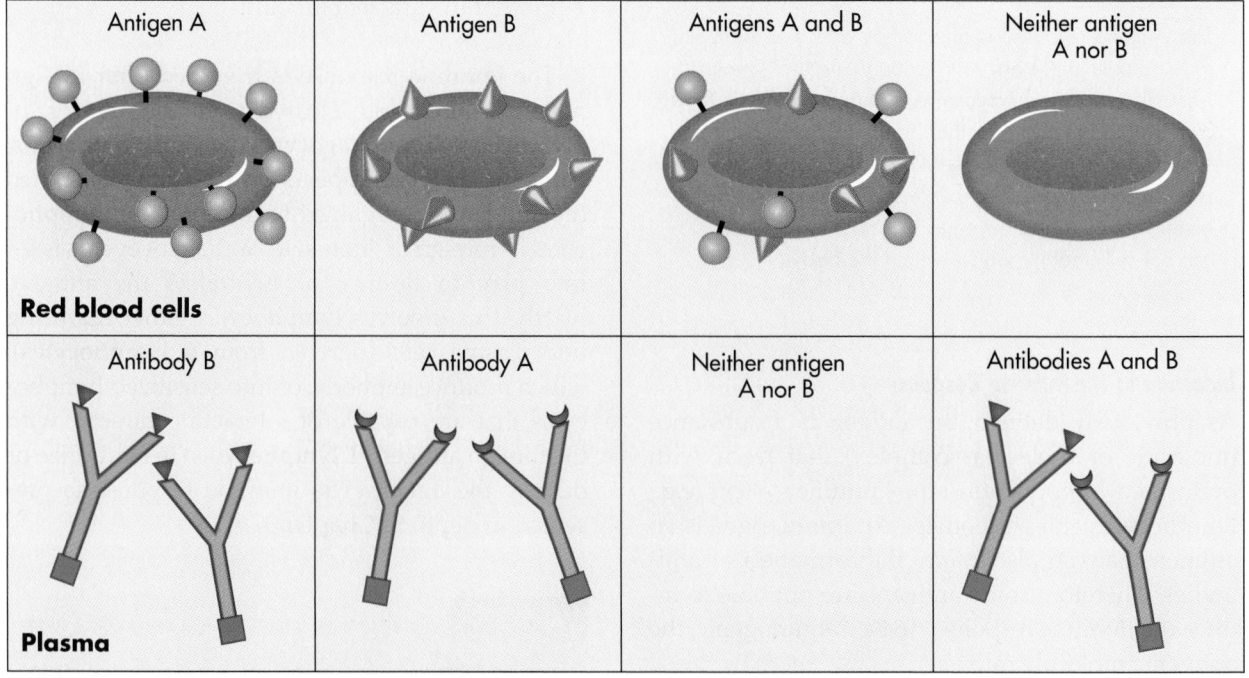

Fig. 7-22 ABO blood groups. Type A blood has red blood cells with type A surface antigens and plasma with type B antibodies. Type B blood has type B surface antigens and plasma with type A antibodies. Type AB blood has types A and B surface antigens and no plasma antibodies. Type O blood has no ABO surface antigens but A and B plasma antibodies.

Variances in Immunity and Inflammation

Immune responses are normally protective mechanisms against harmful microorganisms and other injurious agents. However, these responses may sometimes be inappropriate and have undesirable effects.

Hypersensitivity: Allergy, Autoimmunity, and Isoimmunity

Hypersensitivity is an altered immunological reactivity to an antigen that results in a pathological immune response after reexposure. These abnormal responses include allergy, autoimmunity, and isoimmunity (Box 7-4). *Allergy* refers to an exaggerated immune response to environmental **allergens**; autoimmunity is an immune response against the host's own cells (self-antigens); isoimmunity is an immune response directed against beneficial foreign tissues (e.g., blood transfusions and transplanted organs). Of these, allergy is the most common and least life threatening (see Chapter 31).

Mechanisms of Hypersensitivity

Hypersensitivity reactions may be immediate or delayed. Immediate hypersensitivity is associated with the presence of antibodies in the serum that, with reexposure, lead to an antigen-antibody reaction. Mild reactions associated with immediate hypersensitivity include itching and hives. Severe reactions may include life-threatening respiratory distress and anaphylaxis.

Delayed hypersensitivity reactions are a product of cell-mediated immunity whereby the body develops hypersensitivity after exposure to a foreign antigen from bacteria, parasites, or other microorganisms. These reactions may take from several hours up to 1 to 2 days to appear and are at a maximum severity days after reexposure to the antigen. An example of delayed hypersensitivity reaction is the response against grafted tissue. A more common example is poison ivy.

IgE reactions. Antibodies or immunoglobulins (Ig), are produced by plasma cells in response to antigenic stimulation. Five distinct classes of immunoglobulins are produced in humans (Box 7-5). IgE

BOX 7-4

AUTOIMMUNE AND ISOIMMUNE DISEASES

Graves' disease
Rheumatoid arthritis
Myasthenia gravis
Immune thrombocytopenic purpura
Isoimmune neutropenia
Systemic lupus erythematosus (SLE)
Rh and ABO isoimmunization

BOX 7-5

CLASSES OF IMMUNOGLOBULINS

IgG

IgG accounts for 70% to 75% of antibodies in normal serum. IgG is most abundant in blood but is also found in lymph, cerebrospinal, synovial, and peritoneal fluid and breast milk. It is the major antibody involved in secondary immune responses and the only antitoxin antibody developed. IgG is also the only immunoglobulin that crosses the placenta, providing temporary immunity in neonates.

IgM

IgM accounts for approximately 5% to 10% of antibodies in normal serum and is the dominant antibody in ABO incompatibilities. IgM triggers the increased production of IgG in acute infections and the complement fixation required for an effective antibody response.

IgA

IgA accounts for approximately 15% of antibodies in normal serum. This immunoglobulin is found in blood, secretions such as tears and saliva, and the respiratory tract, stomach, and accessory organs. IgA combines with a protein in the mucosa and defends body surfaces against invading microorganisms.

IgE

IgE accounts for less than 1% of antibodies in normal serum. It is found in some tissues and on the surface membranes of basophils and mast cells; it is responsible for immediate hypersensitivity reactions.

IgD

IgD accounts for less than 1% of antibodies in normal serum. Its precise biological function is unknown.

accounts for less than 1% of antibodies in normal serum; it is responsible for immediate (type I) hypersensitivity reactions. With type I reactions, the response is mediated through IgE, which is bound to mast cells or basophils. When an antigen reacts with an IgE molecule bound to a mast cell or circulating basophil, these cells promptly release a host of chemical mediators into the extracellular space. The target organs and the manifestations of the reaction vary from hives to hay fever to asthma to life-threatening anaphylaxis (see Chapter 31).

NOTE

Hypersensitivity reactions are divided into four distinct types: type I (IgE-mediated allergic reactions), type II (tissue-specific reactions), type III (immune-complex-mediated reactions), and type IV (cell-mediated reactions). These types are further described in Chapters 8 and 31.

Immunity and Inflammation Deficiencies

Deficiencies in immunity and inflammation refer to the failure of these mechanisms of self-defense to function at their normal capacity. The source of the deficiency may be congenital (caused by an anomaly present at birth) or acquired. Acquired immune deficiencies may be caused by infection (the human immunodeficiency virus [HIV] being the prime example), cancer (in particular leukemias), immunosuppressive drugs, and aging. Whether congenital or acquired, the cause of the deficiency is usually the disruption of lymphocyte function, although neutrophil dysfunction also has been described.

Acquired Deficiencies

Acquired immune deficiencies are far more common than congenital forms (Box 7-6). They may be classified in the following groups:

- Nutritional deficiencies (e.g., severe deficits in calorie or protein intake)
- Iatrogenic deficiencies (caused by some form of medical treatment)
- Deficiencies caused by trauma (e.g., bacterial infection, burns)
- Deficiencies caused by stress (depressed immune function)
- Acquired immunodeficiency syndrome (AIDS)

NOTE

AIDS is currently the best-known example of acquired dysfunction of the immune system. HIV causes AIDS and results in a debilitating illness that is manifested by various opportunistic infections and malignancies that until recently were almost always fatal. Since the disease was first identified in 1981, it has become a global health problem, affecting between 5 and 10 million people worldwide (see Chapter 37).

? CRITICAL THINKING

Think about a time when you or someone close to you became ill because of an acquired immune deficiency. What kind of deficiency caused it? Was it preventable?

Stress and Disease

Prolonged emotional or psychological stress can result in physical illness with a triad of manifestations that include disturbances in cognition, emotion, and behavior. In recent years, the links between stress and its relation to disease have created a new field of science called *psychoneuroimmunology*.

BOX 7-6

ACQUIRED DEFICIENCIES

The following physiological or pathophysiological conditions are known to be associated with acquired deficiencies:

Pregnancy

Infancy

Infections such as rubella (congenital), cytomegalovirus (congenital), measles, leprosy, tuberculosis

Down syndrome

Malignancies such as Hodgkin disease, leukemia, myeloma

Stress caused by surgery or emotional trauma

Malnutrition

Aging

Diabetes

Alcoholic cirrhosis

Sickle cell anemia

Immunosuppressive treatment

Anesthesia

From McCance K, Heuther S: *Pathophysiology: the biologic basis for disease in adults and children,* ed 2, St Louis, 1994, Mosby.

Psychoneuroimmunology is the study of the interaction of the emotional state with the central nervous system and the body's defense against external infection and abnormal cell division.

Neuroendocrine Regulation of Stress

As described in Chapter 2, the sympathetic nervous system is activated during the stress response, causing the adrenal gland to release catecholamines (epinephrine, norepinephrine, and dopamine) into the blood stream. At the same time, the hypothalamus stimulates the pituitary gland to release hormones that include ADH, prolactin, growth hormone, and ACTH. In turn, ACTH stimulates the cortex of the adrenal gland to release cortisol (Tables 7-8 and 7-9).

Catecholamines

Catecholamines act by stimulating two major classes of receptors: α-adrenergic receptors and β-adrenergic receptors. These two classes are further divided into two subclasses: α_1 and α_2, and β_1 and β_2. The α_1 receptors are postsynaptic and are located on the effector organs. The primary role of the α_1 receptor is to stimulate contraction of smooth muscle. The α_2 receptors are found on the presynaptic nerve endings. Stimulation of the α_2 receptors inhibit the further release of norepinephrine in a negative feedback mechanism. The β_1 receptors are located primarily in the heart; β_2 receptors are located predominantly in the bronchiolar and arterial smooth muscle. The β receptors stimulate the heart; dilate bronchioles; dilate blood vessels in the skeletal muscle, brain, and heart; and aid in glycogenolysis. (Chapter 8 further describes α and β receptors.) Epinephrine

TABLE 7-8	PHYSIOLOGICAL EFFECTS OF CORTISOL
FUNCTIONS AFFECTED	**PHYSIOLOGICAL EFFECTS**
Carbohydrate and lipid metabolism	Diminishes peripheral uptake and utilization of glucose; promotes gluconeogenesis in liver cells; enhances the gluconeogenic response to other hormones; promotes lipolysis in adipose tissue
Protein metabolism	Increases protein synthesis in the liver and depresses protein synthesis (including immunoglobulin synthesis) in muscle, lymphoid tissue, adipose tissue, skin, and bone; increases plasma level of amino acids; stimulates deamination in the liver
Inflammatory effects	Decreases circulating eosinophils, lymphocytes, and monocytes; increases release of polymorphonuclear leukocytes from the bone marrow; decreases accumulation of leukocytes at the site of inflammation; delays healing; permissive for vasoconstrictive action of norepinephrine
Lipid metabolism	Lipolysis in the extremities and lipogenesis in the face and trunk
Immune reserve	Decreases the tissue mass of all lymphoid tissues (e.g., decreases protein synthesis); promotes rapid decrease in circulating lymphocytes, eosinophils, basophils, and macrophages; inhibits the production of interleukin-1 and interleukin-2; consequently, also blocks cell-mediated immunity and the generation of fever
Digestive function	Promotes gastric secretion
Urinary function	Enhances urinary excretion
Connective tissue function	Decreases proliferation of fibroblasts in connective tissue (thus delaying healing)
Muscle function	Maintains normal contractility and maximal work output for skeletal and cardiac muscle
Bone function	Decreases bone formation
Vascular system and myocardial function	Maintains normal blood pressure; permits increased responsiveness of arterioles to the constrictive action of adrenergic stimulation; optimizes myocardial performance
Central nervous system function	Somehow modulates perceptual and emotional functioning, essential for normal arousal and initiation of daytime activity

From McCance KL, Huether SE: *Pathophysiology: the biologic basis for disease in adults and children,* ed 3, St Louis, 1998, Mosby.

| TABLE 7-9 | PHYSIOLOGICAL EFFECTS OF THE CATECHOLAMINES* |

ORGAN	PROCESS OR RESULT
Brain	Increased blood flow Increased glucose metabolism
Cardiovascular system	Increased rate and force of contraction Peripheral vasoconstriction
Pulmonary system	Increased oxygen supply Bronchodilation Increased ventilation
Muscle	Increased glycogenolysis Increased contraction Increased dilation of skeletal muscle vasculature
Liver	Increased glucose production Increased gluconeogenesis Increased glycogenolysis Decreased glycogen synthesis
Adipose tissue	Increased lipolysis Increased fatty acids and glycerol
Skin	Decreased blood flow
Skeleton	Decreased glucose uptake and utilization (decreases insulin release)
Gastrointestinal and genitourinary tracts	Decreased protein synthesis
Lymphoid tissue	Increased protein breakdown (lymphoid tissue shrinks)

From Granner, 1988.
*Some of these responses require glucocorticoids (e.g., cortisol) for maximal activity.

activates both α and β receptors; norepinephrine primarily excites α receptors (Table 7-10).

Cortisol

Cortisol (hydrocortisone) circulates in the plasma and mobilizes substances needed for cellular metabolism. The primary metabolic effect of cortisol is the stimulation of gluconeogenesis. It also enhances the elevation of blood glucose by decreasing glucose utilization. In addition, cortisol acts as an immunosuppressant by causing lymphocyte reproduction to decrease, particularly the T-lymphocyte population. This in turn leads to decreased cellular immunity. Cortisol also decreases migration of macrophages into the inflamed area and decreases phagocytosis, in part by stabilizing lysosomal membranes. This decrease in immune cell activity may be beneficial, because it prevents immune-mediated tissue damage. Whether cortisol's effects are adaptive or destructive varies by the type of stress event and the duration of exposure to the stressor.

Role of the Immune System

Many immunological conditions and diseases appear to be triggered by stress, although the exact mechanisms linking stress to these conditions is not clearly defined. It is believed, however, that the immune, nervous, and endocrine systems communicate through complex pathways and are potentially affected by factors involved in the stress reaction (Table 7-11).

Stress, Coping, and Illness Interrelationships

As described in this chapter and in Chapter 2, the ill effects of stress are affected by the nature, intensity, and duration of the stressors and by the perception and coping skills of the individual. It is important to recognize signs and symptoms of stress and to incorporate stress management techniques such as meditation and imagery to reduce the stressful event. In healthy persons, these interventions help avoid harmful physiological and psychological illness associated with stress.

TABLE 7-10	SUMMARY OF THE PHYSIOLOGICAL ACTIONS OF THE α AND β RECEPTORS
RECEPTOR	**PHYSIOLOGICAL ACTIONS**
α_1	Increased glycogenolysis; smooth muscle contraction (blood vessels, genitourinary tract)
α_2	Smooth muscle relaxation (gastrointestinal tract); smooth muscle contraction (some vascular beds); inhalation of lipolysis, renin release, platelet aggregation, and insulin secretion
β_1	Stimulation of lipolysis, myocardial contraction (increased rate, increased force of contraction)
β_2	Increased hepatic gluconeogenesis; increased hepatic glycogenolysis; increased muscle glycogenolysis; increased release of insulin, glucagon, and renin; smooth muscle relaxation (bronchi, blood vessels, genitourinary tract, gastrointestinal tract)

From Granner, 1988.

TABLE 7-11	EXAMPLES OF STRESS-RELATED DISEASES AND CONDITIONS
TARGET ORGAN OR SYSTEM	**DISEASE OR CONDITION**
Cardiovascular system	Coronary artery disease Hypertension Stroke Disturbances of heart rhythm
Muscles	Tension headaches Muscle contraction backache
Connective tissues	Rheumatoid arthritis (autoimmune disease) Related inflammatory diseases of connective tissue
Pulmonary system	Asthma (hypersensitivity reaction) Hay fever (hypersensitivity reaction)
Immune system	Immunosuppression or deficiency Autoimmune diseases
Gastrointestinal system	Ulcer Irritable bowel syndrome Diarrhea Nausea and vomiting Ulcerative colitis
Genitourinary system	Diuresis Impotence Frigidity
Skin	Eczema Neurodermatitis Acne
Endocrine system	Diabetes mellitus Amenorrhea
Central nervous system	Fatigue and lethargy Type A behavior Overeating Depression Insomnia

From McCance KL, Huether SE: *Pathophysiology: the biologic basis for disease in adults and children,* ed 3, St Louis, 1998, Mosby.

SUMMARY

- The importance of body water is highlighted by two facts: it is the medium in which all metabolic reactions occur, and the precise regulation of the volume and composition of body fluids is essential to health. Water follows osmotic gradients established by changes in sodium concentrations. Therefore sodium and water balance are closely related.

- Two abnormal states of body-fluid balance can occur. If the water gained exceeds the water lost, there is a water excess or overhydration. If the water lost exceeds the water gained, there is a water deficit or dehydration.

- In addition to the possibility of fluid imbalances, disturbances in the balance of electrolytes (other than sodium) may occur. These include potassium, calcium, and magnesium. Imbalances of these electrolytes can interfere with neuromuscular function and may cause cardiac rhythm disturbances.

- Treatment of isotonic dehydration may include volume replacement with isotonic or occasionally hypotonic solutions. Hypotonic dehydration management may involve intravenous replacement with normal saline or lactated Ringer's solution or occasionally hypertonic saline (e.g., in seizures caused by hyponatremia). Interventions for overhydration depend on the cause and may include water restriction, diuretic administration, or if hyponatremia is present, administration of saline. In-hospital treatment of hypokalemia is intravenous or oral potassium replacement. Management of hyperkalemia may involve potassium restriction, enteral administration of a cation exchange resin, or intravenous administration of glucose and insulin, sodium bicarbonate, or calcium.

- Treatment of hypocalcemia is intravenous administration of calcium ions. Hypercalcemia management may include controlling the underlying disease, hydration, and occasionally, drug therapy such as furosemide and other calcium-lowering drugs.

- Significant magnesium deficit typically is corrected by administration of intravenous magnesium sulfate. The most effective treatment for magnesium excess is hemodialysis. Calcium salts that antagonize magnesium may also be given.

- The healthy body is sensitive to changes in the concentration of hydrogen ions and tries to maintain the pH of extracellular fluid at 7.4. This is accomplished through three interrelated compensatory mechanisms: carbonic acid–bicarbonate buffering, protein buffering, and renal buffering.

- Metabolic acidosis occurs when the amount of acid generated exceeds the body's buffering capacity. The four most common forms of metabolic acidosis encountered in the prehospital setting are lactic acidosis, diabetic ketoacidosis, acidosis resulting from renal failure, and acidosis from ingestion of toxins.

- Loss of hydrogen is the initial cause of metabolic alkalosis. This may result from vomiting (hydrochloric acid loss), gastric suction, or increased renal excretion of hydrogen ion in urine. Respiratory acidosis is caused by the retention of carbon dioxide, leading to an increase in P_{CO_2}. This state usually is caused by an imbalance in the production of carbon dioxide and its elimination through alveolar ventilation. Hyperventilation may produce respiratory alkalosis by decreasing P_{CO_2}.

- Treatment for metabolic acidosis is aimed at correcting the underlying cause of the acidosis. For metabolic alkalosis, treatment is directed at correcting the underlying condition. Volume depletion, if present, should be corrected with isotonic solutions, and hypokalemia may require correction with potassium replacement. The patient in respiratory acidosis should be treated by improving ventilation quickly to eliminate carbon dioxide. The treatment for metabolic alkalosis is aimed at treating the underlying cause of the hyperventilation.

- Knowledge of the structural and functional reactions of cells and tissues to injurious agents is important to understanding disease processes. Altered cells and tissues can result from adaptation, injury, neoplasia, aging, or death.

- An injured cell may exhibit abnormal physical shape or size. Cell injury has both cellular and systemic manifestations.

- Factors that cause disease may be simplistically classified as genetic or environmental. However, a strong interaction occurs between the two.

- The term hypoperfusion is used to describe inadequate tissue circulation. Hypoperfusion may result from decreased cardiac output. Decreased cardiac output can lead to shock, multiple organ dysfunction syndrome (MODS), and other disease states associated with impaired cellular metabolism. Negative feedback mechanisms important in maintaining cardiac output and tissue perfusion are baroreceptor reflexes, chemoreceptor reflexes, central nervous system ischemia response, hormonal mechanisms, reabsorption of tissue fluids, and the splenic discharge of stored blood.

- The body's first lines of defense against illness and injury are external barriers that include the skin and mucous membranes of the digestive, respiratory, and GU tract. Once these barriers have been breached, permitting harmful chemicals, foreign bodies, or microorganisms to penetrate cells and tissues, the second and third lines of defense are activated. In order, these are the inflammatory response and the immune response. Both the external barriers and inflammatory response respond to all organisms using the identical nonspecific mechanism, but the immune response is specific to individual pathogens.

- Immune responses normally are protective mechanisms against harmful microorganisms and other injurious agents. These responses may sometimes be inappropriate and have undesirable effects. Examples of inappropriate responses include hypersensitivity and immunity or inflammation deficiencies.

- Many immune-related conditions and diseases are associated with stress, although the exact mechanisms causing these illnesses are not clearly defined. It is believed, however, that the immune, nervous, and endocrine systems communicate through complex pathways and are potentially affected by factions involved in the stress reaction.

REFERENCES

1. *Advanced cardiac life support*, Dallas, 1997, American Heart Association.
2. *EMT-Paramedic national standard curriculum*, Washington, DC, 1998, US Department of Transportation National Highway Traffic Safety Administration.
3. McCance K, Heuther S: *Pathophysiology: the biologic basis for disease in adults and children*, ed 2, St Louis, 1994, Mosby.

8 Pharmacology

OBJECTIVES

Upon completion of this chapter, the paramedic student will be able to:

1. Explain what a drug is.
2. Identify the four types of drug names.
3. Outline drug standards and legislation and the enforcement agencies pertinent to the paramedic profession.
4. Describe the paramedic's responsibilities in drug administration.
5. Distinguish among drug forms.
6. Differentiate among the four types of allergic reactions to drugs.
7. Outline autonomic nervous system functions that may be changed with drug therapy.
8. Discuss factors that influence drug absorption, distribution, and elimination.
9. Describe how drugs react with receptors to produce their desired effects.
10. List variables that can influence drug interactions.
11. Identify special considerations for administering pharmacological agents to pregnant patients, pediatric patients, and older patients.
12. Outline drug actions and care considerations for a patient who is given drugs that affect the nervous, cardiovascular, respiratory, endocrine, and gastrointestinal systems.
13. Explain the meaning of drug terms that are necessary to safely interpret information in drug references.

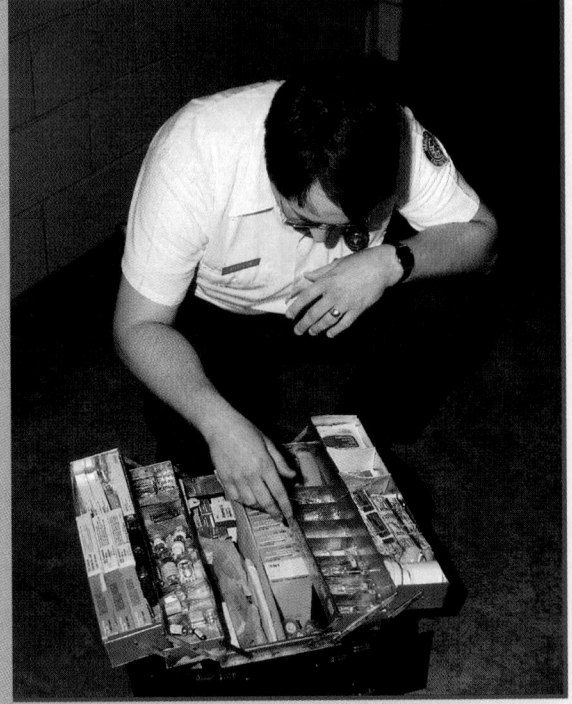

Pharmacology *can be defined as the science of drugs used to prevent, diagnose, and treat disease. It deals with the interactions between living systems and chemical molecules. To ensure maximum effectiveness and reduce the potential for harm, the paramedic must have a thorough understanding of a drug and its actions before it is administered.*

KEY TERMS

absorption: The process by which drug molecules are moved from the site of entry into the body into the general circulation.

adrenergic: Of or pertaining to the sympathetic nerve fibers of the autonomic nervous system, which use epinephrine or epinephrine-like substances as neurotransmitters.

agonists: Drugs that combine with receptors and initiate a sequence of biochemical and physiological changes.

antagonists: Agents designed to inhibit or counteract the effects of other drugs or undesired effects caused by normal or hyperactive physiological mechanisms.

anticholinergic: Of or pertaining to the blocking of acetylcholine receptors, resulting in inhibition of transmission of parasympathetic nerve impulses.

biological half-life: The time required to metabolize or eliminate half the total amount of a drug in the body.

biotransformation: The process by which a drug is chemically converted to a metabolite.

chemical name: The exact designation of a chemical structure as determined by the rules of chemical nomenclature.

cholinergic: Of or pertaining to the effects produced by the parasympathetic nervous system or drugs that stimulate or antagonize the parasympathetic nervous system.

contraindications: Medical or physiological factors that make it harmful to administer a medication that would otherwise have a therapeutic effect.

controlled substance: Any drug defined in the categories of the Comprehensive Drug Abuse Prevention and Control Act (also known as the *Controlled Substances Act*) of 1970.

cumulative action: The effect that occurs when several doses of a drug are administered or when absorption occurs more quickly than removal by excretion or metabolism or both.

distribution: The transport of a drug through the bloodstream to various tissues of the body and ultimately to its site of action.

drug: Any substance taken by mouth; injected into a muscle, blood vessel, or cavity of the body; or applied topically to treat or prevent a disease or condition.

drug interaction: Modification of the effects of one drug by the previous or concurrent administration of another drug, thereby increasing or diminishing the pharmacological or physiological action of one or both drugs.

drug receptors: Parts of a cell (usually an enzyme or large protein molecule) with which a drug molecule interacts to trigger its desired response or effect.

excretion: The elimination of toxic or inactive metabolites, primarily by the kidneys; the intestines, lungs, and mammary, sweat, and salivary glands also may be involved.

first-pass metabolism: The initial biotransformation of a drug during passage through the liver from the portal vein that occurs before the drug reaches the general circulation.

generic name: The official, established name assigned to a drug.

idiosyncrasy: An abnormal or peculiar response to a drug.

loading dose: A large quantity of drug that temporarily exceeds the body's capacity to excrete it.

maintenance dose: The amount of a drug required to keep a desired steady state of drug concentration in tissues.

official name: The name of a drug that is followed by the initials USP or NF, denoting its listing in one of the official publications; usually the same as the generic name.

parenteral: Pertains to any medication route other than the alimentary canal.

pharmacodynamics: The study of how a drug acts on a living organism.

pharmacokinetics: The study of how the body handles a drug over a period of time, including the processes of absorption, distribution, biotransformation, and excretion.

placental barrier: A protective biological membrane that separates the blood vessels of the mother and the fetus.

potentiation: Enhancement of the effect of a drug, caused by concurrent administration of two drugs in which one drug increases the effect of the other.

summation: The combined effects of two drugs that equal the sum of the individual effects of each agent.

synergism: The combined action of two drugs that is greater than the sum of each agent acting independently.

therapeutic action: The desired, intended action of a drug.

therapeutic index: A measurement of the relative safety of a drug.

tolerance: A physiological response that requires that a drug dosage be increased to produce the same effect formerly produced by a smaller dose.

trade name: The copyright name of a drug, designated by the drug company that sells the medication.

untoward effects: Side effects that prove harmful to the patient.

NOTE

This chapter introduces the paramedic to general principles of pharmacology and emergency medications commonly used in the prehospital setting. A more complete description of the emergency drugs discussed in this chapter can be found in the *Emergency Drug Index.* Medications described in this text that are included in the *Index* are denoted by bold italic type.

NOTE

The drug information presented in this section conforms to current medical literature, to manufacturers' monographs, and to the clinical practice of the general medical community at the time of publication. Although every effort has been made to ensure accuracy and completeness, the authors, editors, medical advisers, and publisher disclaim liability for any discrepancies, incongruities, undetected errors, omissions in content, or reader misunderstanding. Local protocol for drug administration may vary from the information presented in this chapter. The paramedic should follow the guidelines established by medical direction.

SECTION ONE
DRUG INFORMATION

Historical Trends in Pharmacology

The science of pharmacology may date back as early as 10,000 to 7000 BC[1] It is thought that medicinal herbs were among the plants grown by humans in the Neolithic period, but it is not known if they were recognized to possess healing properties. A number of medications are mentioned in the Bible, such as gums, spices, oils, and possibly narcotics. Drugs derived from plants were heavily used throughout the Middle Ages as digestives, laxatives, and diuretics.

The concept of "chemical medicine" was born in the seventeenth century, and some preparations introduced during the seventeenth and eighteenth centuries, such as opium and *syrup of ipecac,* are still in use today. Accurate studies of drug dosage in the nineteenth century led to the development of manufacturing plants to produce drugs, and knowledge of their expected actions became more precise.

Modern Health Care

Modern health care and pharmaceutics are experiencing a period of change, with the focus on the expansion of consumer health education and research. These changes have resulted from the consumers' motivation to take responsibility for health and disease prevention and from the need to discover new treatments, cures, or methods to prevent the disease processes that limit growth, everyday living, or average life span. Research also is being expanded to provide new incentives to develop drugs, known as *orphan drugs,* that are used to treat people suffering from rare, chronic diseases such as hemophilia, leprosy, Cushing's syndrome, and Tourette's syndrome.

Drug Names

A **drug** may be defined as "any substance taken by mouth, injected into a muscle, blood vessel, or cavity of the body, or applied topically to treat or prevent a disease or condition."[2] Drugs have been identified or derived from five major sources: plants (alkaloids, glycosides, gums, and oils), animals and humans, minerals or mineral products, microorganisms, and chemical substances made in the laboratory (Box 8-1).

Drugs can be identified by the following four types of names:

1. **Chemical name:** A drug's chemical name is a precise description of the drug's chemical composition and molecular structure.
2. **Generic name** (nonproprietary name): This name often is a markedly abbreviated form of the chemical name, and it is used more commonly than the chemical name. Generic medications usually have the same therapeutic efficacy as nongeneric drugs but generally are less expensive. This is the official name approved by the U.S. Food and Drug Administration (FDA).
3. **Trade name** (brand or proprietary name): The trade name is a copyright name designated by the drug company that sells the medication. Trade names are proper nouns, and the first letter is capitalized. This text shows the trade name in parentheses after the generic name of the drug. The trade name usually is suggested by the first manufacturer of the drug.

EXAMPLES OF DRUGS AND THEIR SOURCES

Plant Sources
Digoxin
Morphine sulfate
Atropine sulfate

Animal and Human Sources
Epinephrine
Insulin
Adrenocorticotropic hormone (ACTH)

Mineral or Mineral Product
Iron
Iodine
Sodium bicarbonate
Calcium chloride

Microorganism Sources
Penicillin
Streptomycin

Laboratory-Produced Chemicals
Lidocaine (Xylocaine)
Midazolam (Versed)
Diazepam (Valium)

4. **Official name:** The official name of a drug is followed by the initials *United States Pharmacopeia* (*USP*) or *National Formulary* (*NF*), which denote its listing in one of the official publications. In most cases the official name is the same as the generic name.

An example of the four names for a drug would be:

Chemical name: ethyl 1-methyl-4-plenylisoni-pecotate hydrochloride

Generic name: ***meperidine hydrochloride***

Trade name: Demerol

Official name: meperidine hydrochloride USP

Drug Standards and Legislation

Before 1906 little control was exercised over the use of medications. Drugs often were sold or distributed by traveling medicine men, drugstores, mail order companies, and legitimate and self-proclaimed physicians. Listing the ingredients of the medications was not required, and many drug products contained opium *(morphine)*, heroin, and alcohol.

Effects of Drug Legislation

In 1906 Congress passed the Pure Food and Drug Act to protect the public from mislabeled or adulterated drugs. This act prohibited the use of false and misleading claims for medications and restricted the sale of drugs with a potential for abuse (Table 8-1). The Pure Food and Drug Act also designated the USP and the NF as official standards and empowered the federal government to enforce them. In 1980 the United States Pharmacopeial Convention purchased the *National Formulary,* making the USP the only official book of drug standards in the United States. Other drug standards and legislation are listed in Box 8-2.

NOTE

Standardization is necessary because drugs may vary significantly in strength and activity. The technique for measuring a drug's strength, purity, or effectiveness through chemical analysis and chemical observation is known as *assay. Bioassay* is a subset of assay in which the concentration of a drug is determined by comparing its effect on an organism, animal, or isolated tissue with that of a drug that produces a known effect.

NOTE

A **controlled substance** is any drug defined in the categories of the *Controlled Substances Act (CSA)* of 1970. These categories include opium and its derivatives, hallucinogens, depressants, and stimulants. It is illegal for any person to possess a controlled substance unless it has been obtained by a valid prescription or order or unless its possession is pursuant to actions in the course of professional practice. The authority for use of controlled substances and other prescription medications is a function of state agencies operating under government restrictions provided by the federal Drug Enforcement Agency (DEA). Paramedics and other allied health professionals who administer medications should be familiar with state laws governing the administration and storage of drugs and record-keeping requirements. Violations of the CSA are punishable by fine or imprisonment, or both.

TABLE 8-1	CONTROLLED SUBSTANCES	
CHARACTERISTICS	**DISPENSING RESTRICTIONS**	**EXAMPLES**
Schedule I Has high abuse potential Has no accepted medical use; for research, analysis, or instruction only May lead to severe dependence	Approved protocol is required.	Heroin, marijuana (cannabis), tetrahydrocannabinols, lysergic acid diethylamide (LSD), mescaline, peyote, psilocybin, methaqualone
Schedule II Has high abuse potential Has accepted medical uses May lead to severe physical or psychological dependence, or both	Written prescription is necessary (signed by the practitioner); only emergency dispensing is permitted without written prescription (only required amount may be prescribed for emergency period). No prescription refills are allowed. Container must have warning label.*	Opium, **morphine sulfate,** hydromorphone, **meperidine,** codeine, oxycodone, methadone, secobarbital, pentobarbital, amphetamine, methylphenidate, cocaine, and others
Schedule III Has less abuse potential than drugs in schedules I and II Has accepted medical uses May lead to moderate to low physical dependence or high psychological dependence	Written or oral prescription is required. Prescription expires in 6 months. No more than five refills are allowed in a 6-month period. Container must have warning label.*	Preparations containing limited quantities of or combined with one or more active ingredients that are noncontrolled substances (codeine, hydrocodone, **morphine sulfate,** dihydrocodeine, or ethylmorphine) and nonnarcotic drugs such as derivatives of barbituric acid, except those that are listed in another schedule, glutethimide, methyprylon, chlorphentermine, paregoric, and others
Schedule IV Has lower abuse potential compared with schedule III drugs Has accepted medical uses May lead to limited physical or psychological dependence	Written or oral prescription is required. Prescription expires in 6 months, with no more than five refills allowed. Container must have warning label.*	Barbital, phenobarbital, chloral hydrate, meprobamate, fenfluramine, chlordiazepoxide, **diazepam,** oxazepam, clorazepate, flurazepam, **lorazepam,** dextropropoxyphene, pentazocine, mazindol, alprazolam, and others
Schedule V Has low abuse potential compared with schedule IV drugs Has accepted medical uses May lead to limited physical or psychological dependence	Drug may require written prescription or be sold without prescription (check state law).	Medications (generally for relief of coughs or diarrhea) that contain limited amounts of certain opioid controlled substances

*The warning must read: "Caution: Federal law prohibits the transfer of this drug to any person other than the patient for whom it was prescribed."

BOX 8-2

DRUG STANDARDS AND LEGISLATION

1912: Congress passed the Sherley Amendment prohibiting fraudulent therapeutic claims.

1914: The Harrison Narcotic Act was passed to control the sale of narcotics and to help curb drug addiction or dependence. This was the first narcotic act to be passed by any nation, and it established the word *narcotic* as a legal term.

1938: Prompted by more than 100 deaths in 1937 from ingestion of a diethylene glycol solution of sulfanilamide, the federal Food, Drug, and Cosmetic Act was passed. This act contained a provision to prevent marketing of a new drug before it was properly tested. In addition, the act required that the label list all ingredients used in preparing the drug and the directions for drug use.

1952: The Durham-Humphrey Amendment changed the 1938 drug act, restricting the dispensing of legend (prescription) drugs. Legend drugs must bear the legend, "Caution: Federal law prohibits dispensing without prescription."

1962: The Kefauver-Harris Amendment required that a new drug's safety and efficacy be proved before it could be approved for use.

1970: The Comprehensive Drug Abuse Prevention and Control Act (also known as the *Controlled Substances Act [CSA]*) superseded the Harrison Narcotic Act of 1914. The CSA classifies a controlled substance by its use and abuse potential. Drugs are classified into number schedules from schedule I (drugs with highest abuse potential) to schedule V (drugs with lowest abuse potential); see Table 8-1.

Drug Regulatory Agencies

In July 1973 the Drug Enforcement Agency, a subsidiary of the Department of Justice, became the nation's sole legal drug enforcement body. Other regulatory bodies or services include the following:

? CRITICAL THINKING

News stories often feature "miracle" drugs that are used in other countries but that are not yet available in the United States because they lack FDA approval. Why wouldn't the FDA automatically approve drugs already known to be helpful in the international market?

- Food and Drug Administration (FDA): The FDA is responsible for enforcing the federal Food, Drug, and Cosmetic Act of 1937. The FDA may seize offending goods and criminally prosecute individuals involved.
- Public Health Service: The Public Health Service is an agency of the U.S. Department of Health and Human Services. One of the Public Health Service's duties is to regulate biological products, which include viruses, therapeutic serums, antitoxins, or analogous products applicable in the prevention or cure of human diseases or injuries. The agency examines and licenses these products and inspects and licenses the establishments that produce them.
- Federal Trade Commission (FTC): The FTC is an agency of the federal government directly responsible to the president of the United States. Its principal action with respect to drugs lies in its power to suppress false or misleading advertising aimed at the public.
- Canadian Drug Control: In Canada, the Health Protection Branch of the Department of National Health and Welfare is responsible for administering and enforcing the Food and Drugs Act, the Proprietary or Patent Medicine Act, and the Narcotics Control Act.
- International Drug Control: International control of drugs began in 1912 when the first "Opium Conference" was held at The Hague. Various international treaties were adopted, obligating governments to control narcotic substances. These treaties were consolidated in 1961 into one document, known as the *Single Convention on Narcotic Drugs*, which became effective in 1964. Later the International Narcotics Control Board was established to enforce this law.

Drug References

Several publications provide information on various drugs, their preparation, and recommended administration. These references include the *American Medical Association Drug Evaluation*, the *American Hospital Formulary Service* (AHFS) *Drug Information*, medication package inserts, the *Physician's Desk Reference* (PDR), and the *Nursing Drug Reference* (NDR) (Box 8-3). Paramedics should be familiar with these publications and other emergency pharmacology manuals, particularly regarding drugs commonly administered in the prehospital setting.

BOX 8-3

DRUG REFERENCES

American Medical Association (AMA) Drug Evaluation: The *AMA Drug Evaluation* provides information on drug groups, dosages, prescribing information, and usage. It also covers valid clinical applications of drug use that differ from those approved by the FDA thus far.

Hospital Formulary: The *Hospital Formulary,* a manual published by the American Society of Hospital Pharmacists, provides an overview in monograph form of nearly every available (approved and unapproved) drug in the United States. It is updated regularly and is available in all hospital pharmacies and in many emergency departments. The *Hospital Formulary* is considered by many to be the most reliable source of information on medications and drugs.

Medication package inserts: Most medications are packaged with written literature describing product use. These inserts provide valuable information as new drugs are introduced, and the health care professional should consult them to become familiar with the product.

Physician's Desk Reference: The *PDR,* published yearly by the Medical Economics Company, is a concise compilation of drug information, including FDA-approved indications, contraindications, and adverse effects. In addition to providing product information through several cross-referenced indices, it serves as an identification guide by showing actual-size, color pictures of commonly prescribed medications. The *PDR* also lists emergency telephone numbers for poison control centers throughout the United States.

Nursing Drug Reference: The *NDR* is published yearly and includes nursing considerations, side effects, adverse reactions, precautions, interactions, and contraindications for drug and IV therapy. It contains an alphabetical listing of commonly prescribed drugs and detailed monographs for drugs recently approved by the FDA.

NOTE

The Internet also can be a valuable source of information about pharmacotherapeutics and often is the most current source of information. The findings of current research also can be sought on the Internet for information about particular drug studies and treatments.

NOTE

Paramedics are held responsible for safe and therapeutically effective drug administration, and they are personally responsible—legally, morally, and ethically—for each drug they administer. As part of the professional scope of patient management, paramedics must:

- Use correct precautions and techniques when administering medications
- Observe and document the effects of drugs
- Keep their knowledge base current regarding changes in trends in pharmacology
- Establish and maintain professional relationships
- Understand pharmacology
- Carefully evaluate patients to identify drug indications and contraindications
- Take a drug history from patients that includes:
  Prescribed medications (name, strength, daily dosage)
  Over-the-counter medications
  Vitamins
  Alternative drug therapies (homeopathic medicines, herbal medicines)
  Any adverse drug reactions
- Seek medical direction

? CRITICAL THINKING

Your patient is acutely ill and reports taking only an herbal medicine, which is not found in standard drug reference materials. Where can you or the medical staff find information about these alternative therapies?

Drug Forms and Preparations and Routes of Administration

Drugs and drug preparations are available in many forms (Box 8-4), and each has specific indications, advantages, and disadvantages, which are explained throughout the chapter and in the *Emergency Drug Index.*

Overview of Routes of Administration

The mode of drug administration affects the rate at which onset of action occurs and may affect the therapeutic response that results. The routes of drug administration are categorized as *enteral* (administration along any portion of the gastrointestinal tract), **parenteral** (administration by any route other

BOX 8-4

VARIOUS FORMS OF DRUG PREPARATIONS

Preparations for Oral Use

Liquids

Aqueous solution—substance dissolved in water and syrups

Aqueous suspension—solid particles suspended in liquid

Emulsion—fat or oil suspended in liquid with an emulsifier

Spirits—alcohol solution

Elixir—aromatic, sweetened alcohol and water solution

Tincture—alcohol extract of plant or vegetable substance

Fluid extract—concentrated alcoholic liquid extract of plant or vegetables

Extract—syrup or dried form of pharmacologically active drug, usually prepared by evaporating a solution

Solids

Capsule—soluble case (usually gelatin) that contains liquid, dry, or beaded drug particles

Tablet—compressed, powdered drugs in the form of a small disk

Troche or lozenge—medicated tablets that dissolve slowly in the mouth

Powder or granules—loose or molded drug substance for administration with or without liquids

Preparations for Parenteral Use

Ampule—sealed glass container for liquid injectable medication

Vial—glass container with rubber stopper for liquid or powdered medication

Cartridge or Tubex—single-dose unit of parenteral medication to be used with a specific injecting device

Intravenous infusions (suspended on hanger at bedside)

Flexible collapsible plastic bags (150 to 1000 mL)—used for continuous infusion of fluid replacement with or without medications

Intermittent intravenous infusions—usually secondary intravenous setup of a small plastic bag (50 to 250 mL) to which medication is added. It runs as a "piggyback," hung separately from the primary intravenous infusion via a secondary administration tubing set usually for 20 to 120 minutes. The primary intravenous solution is run between medication doses.

Heparin lock—a port site for direct administration of intermittent intravenous medications without the need for primary intravenous solution

Preparations for Topical Use

Liniment—liquid suspension for lubrication that is applied by rubbing

Lotion—liquid suspension that can be protective, emollient, cooling, astringent, antipruritic, or cleaning

Ointment—semisolid medicine in a base for local protective, soothing, astringent, or transdermal application for systemic effects (nitroglycerin, scopolamine, estrogen)

Paste—thick ointment primarily used for skin protection

Plasters—solid preparations that are adhesive, protective, or soothing

Cream—emulsion that contains aqueous and oily bases

Aerosol—fine powder or solution in a volatile liquid that contains a propellant

Preparations for Use on Mucous Membranes

Drops for eyes, ears, or nose—aqueous solutions with or without gelling agent to increase retention time in the eye

Topical instillation of aqueous solution of medications—usually for topical action but occasionally for systemic effects (enema, douche, mouthwash, throat spray, gargle)

Aerosol sprays, nebulizers, and inhalers—aqueous solutions of medication delivered in droplet form to the target membrane, such as the bronchial tree (bronchodilators)

Foam—powder or solution of medication in volatile liquid with propellant (vaginal foams for contraception)

Suppositories—usually medicinal substances mixed in a firm but malleable base (cocoa butter) to facilitate insertion into a body cavity (rectum or vagina)

Miscellaneous Drug Delivery Systems

Intradermal implants—pellets that contain a small deposit of medication that are inserted into a dermal pocket; they are designed to allow medication to leach slowly into tissue and are usually used to administer hormones such as testosterone or estradiol

Micropump system—small, external pump attached by belt or implanted that delivers medication via a needle in a continuous steady dose (insulin, anticancer chemotherapy, opioids)

Membrane delivery systems—drug-laden membranes are instilled into the eye to deliver a steady flow of medication (pilocarpine or corticosteroids)

than the alimentary canal), *pulmonary* (administration by inhalation or through an endotracheal tube), and *topical* (administration by application to the skin and mucous membranes). The various routes of drug administration are described in detail later in this chapter and in Chapter 9.

Pharmacological Terminology

Drugs may act in the body in many ways. Some of these actions are desirable (therapeutic effects), and others are undesirable or even harmful (side effects). Drugs also may interact with other drugs to produce uncommon and frequently unpredictable effects. Box 8-5 presents some pharmacological definitions.

Allergic Reactions to Drugs

Allergic reactions, which account for 6% to 10% of all drug reactions, usually do not occur with the first exposure to a drug. As described in Chapter 7, at least one previous exposure is required for the immune system to develop the antibodies that cause the clinical reactions. Because previous exposure is required, patients at risk of developing drug allergies sometimes can be identified in interviews. However, patients do not always know the names of drugs they have received, and they may have been unknowingly exposed to a drug through food or milk products (e.g., penicillin, which is commonly used in livestock medicine). Another unusual circumstance is cross-reactivity, in which a drug can trigger an allergic reaction in a patient who has never taken that drug but who is allergic to a chemically similar drug. For example, some patients with an allergy to penicillin may also be allergic to cephalosporins, although they have not previously taken a cephalosporin; some patients with an allergy to *aspirin* may also be allergic to *ketorolac* (Toradol).

Allergic reactions are caused by the drug in its original form or by a metabolite of the drug that is formed when the drug is broken down in the body. Most drugs are not very allergenic, but some drugs elicit strong immune system reactions. Drug allergies can be divided into four classifications (types I through IV), based on the mechanism of the body's immune reaction.

Type I reactions, or anaphylactic reactions, occur soon after exposure to a drug. They are caused by a specific type of antibody (IgE) attached to mast cells. When a specific antigen attaches to these IgE antibodies, the chemical substances in the mast cell (including histamine and slow reactive substance of anaphylaxis) are released. These reactions commonly produce urticaria (hives) accompanied by severe itching. Type I reactions usually are not serious. However, they can progress to severe reactions that involve the cardiovascular and respiratory systems (anaphylaxis). Drugs frequently associated with type I reactions include penicillins, cephalosporins, and iodides.

Type II reactions, or cytotoxic reactions, are delayed reactions that involve certain cytotoxic antibodies of the IgG class. These antibodies are capable of lysing cells and commonly cause hemolytic reactions and destruction of platelets. Examples of type II reactions include drug-induced hemolytic anemia and conditions resembling systemic lupus erythematous. Drugs associated with type II reactions include quinidine (Quinaglute Dura Tabs, and others), *procainamide* (Pronestyl), and *hydralazine* (Apresoline).

Type III reactions are delayed reactions frequently described as *serum sickness.* Like type II reactions, specific antibodies usually are involved. These antibodies (usually IgG) bind the antigen in the bloodstream and form complexes. These complexes filter out in various anatomical locations and produce an inflammatory reaction. Symptoms include urticaria, joint pain, swollen lymph nodes, and fever. Drugs associated with type III reactions include penicillins, iodides, sulfonamides, *phenytoin* (Dilantin), and some antitoxins that use horse serum (e.g., tetanus antitoxin).

Type IV reactions are those in which contact dermatitis is produced by topical application of a drug. Type IV reactions are produced by the T-lymphocytes, not the hormonal antibodies. They usually require more than 24 hours to become evident. Poison ivy rash is a prototypical example of a

---

BOX 8-5

PHARMACOLOGICAL TERMINOLOGY

Antagonism: the opposition of effects between two or more medications that occurs when the combined (conjoint) effect of two drugs is less than the sum of the drugs acting separately

Contraindications: medical or physiological factors that make it harmful to administer a medication that would otherwise have therapeutic value

Cumulative action: The tendency for repeated doses of a drug to accumulate in the blood and organs, causing increased and sometimes toxic effects; it occurs when several doses are administered or when absorption occurs more quickly than removal by excretion or metabolism

Depressant: a substance that decreases a body function or activity

Drug allergy: a systemic reaction to a drug resulting from previous sensitizing exposure and the development of an immunological mechanism

Drug dependence: a state in which withdrawal of a drug produces intense physical or emotional disturbance; previously known as *habituation*

Drug interaction: beneficial or detrimental modification of the effects of one drug by the prior or concurrent administration of another drug that increases or decreases the pharmacological or physiological action of one or both drugs

Idiosyncrasy: abnormal or peculiar responses to a drug (accounting for 25% to 30% of all drug re-

actions) thought to result from genetic enzymatic deficiencies or other unique physiological variables and leading to abnormal mechanisms of drug metabolism or altered physiological effects of the drug

Potentiation: the enhancement of effect caused by the concurrent administration of two drugs in which one drug increases the effect of the other drug

Side effect: undesirable and often unavoidable effect of using therapeutic doses of a drug; action or effect other than those for which the drug was originally given

Stimulant: a drug that enhances or increases body function or activity

Summation: the combined effect of two drugs such that the total effect equals the sum of the individual effects of each agent:

$$(1 + 1 = 2)$$

Synergism: the combined action of two drugs such that the total effect exceeds the sum of the individual effects of each agent:

$$(1 + 1 = 3 \text{ or more})$$

Therapeutic action: the desired, intended action of a drug

Tolerance: decreased physiological response to the repeated administration of a drug or chemically related substance, possibly necessitating an increase in dosage to maintain a therapeutic effect (tachyphylaxis)

Untoward effect: a side effect that proves harmful to the patient

---

type IV reaction. Drugs associated with type IV reactions include sunscreens, acne preparations, antiinflammatory agents (e.g., topical corticosteroids), and antibiotic powders and ointments. Hand and skin rashes from wearing latex gloves may signal a type IV reaction to latex (see Chapter 31).

SECTION TWO
AUTONOMIC PHARMACOLOGY

Review of Anatomy and Physiology

The nervous system may be divided into the central nervous system and peripheral nervous system. Following is a review of the anatomy and physiol-

ogy of the autonomic division of the peripheral nervous system as it pertains to pharmacology.

Autonomic Division of the Peripheral Nervous System

Anatomical and physiological differences within the autonomic division of the peripheral nervous system are the basis for its further subdivision into sympathetic and parasympathetic components. The cell bodies of the neurons in these two divisions are located in different areas of the central nervous system and leave at different levels. The sympathetic fibers exit from the thoracic and lumbar regions of the spinal cord, and the parasympathetic fibers exit from the cranial and sacral portions of the spinal cord. Although the two divisions leave at different levels, the heart, many glands, and smooth muscles are innervated by both sympathetic and parasympathetic nerve fibers.

Preganglionic and Postganglionic Neurons

Autonomic innervation by the sympathetic and parasympathetic nervous system may be viewed as involving a two-neuron chain that exists in a series between the central nervous system and the effector organs (Fig. 8-1). This two-neuron chain is composed of a preganglionic neuron, located in the central nervous system, and a postganglionic neuron, located in the periphery. The preganglionic fibers pass between the central nervous system and the ganglia. The postganglionic fibers pass between the ganglia and the effector organ. Many of the sympathetic ganglia lie close to the spinal cord, whereas others lie about midway between the spinal cord and the effector organ. The parasympathetic ganglia lie close to or within the walls of the effector organ. The anatomical area that serves as a functional junction between these two neurons is known as a *synapse* (Fig. 8-2).

Cholinergic and Adrenergic Fibers

In the sympathetic and parasympathetic divisions, the neurotransmitter for the preganglionic fiber at the junction between the preganglionic fiber and the synapse is acetylcholine. The neurotransmitter at the junction between the parasympathetic postganglionic fiber and the effector cell also is acetylcholine. Fibers that release acetylcholine are known as **cholinergic** fibers. All preganglionic neurons of the autonomic division and all postganglionic neurons of the parasympathetic division are cholinergic.

The neurotransmitter between the sympathetic postganglionic fiber and the effector cell is norepinephrine, a member of the catecholamine family. Fibers that release norepinephrine are known as **adrenergic** fibers (a term derived from *noradrenalin*, the British name for norepinephrine). Most postganglionic neurons of the sympathetic division are adrenergic, but a few are cholinergic. The actions of the autonomic nervous system depend on the interaction between the neurotransmitter released by the ganglionic cells and the receptor effector cells. For example, stimulation of the sympathetic nerves causes excitatory effects in some organs and inhibitory effects in others. Likewise, parasympathetic stimulation causes excitation in some organs but inhibition in others.

Because the parasympathetic and sympathetic systems function continuously and simultaneously innervate many of the same organs, the opposing actions of the two systems balance one another. (Most organs, however, are predominantly controlled by one or the other of the two systems.) In general, the sympathetic system dominates during stressful events, and the parasympathetic system is most active during periods of emotional and physical calm.

Transmission of Nerve Impulses

The variety among neurotransmitters and receptors provides the basis for the variability in response to stimulation of sympathetic and parasympathetic nerves (excitatory or inhibitory) (Fig. 8-3). For cholinergic synapses, acetylcholine molecules combine with cholinergic receptor molecules. These cholinergic receptors exist in two structurally different forms, nicotinic receptors and muscarinic receptors. Although acetylcholine binds to and activates both types of receptor molecules, nicotine (an alkaloid substance found in tobacco) specifically binds to and activates nicotinic receptors but not muscarinic receptors. Muscarine, an alkaloid extracted from some poisonous mushrooms, specifically binds to and activates muscarinic receptors but not nicotinic receptors. Although nicotine and muscarine are not naturally present in the human body, they allow differentiation between the two classes of cholinergic receptors.

When acetylcholine binds to nicotinic receptors, an excitatory response occurs. When it binds with muscarinic receptors, it results in excitation or inhibition, depending on the target tissue in which the receptors are found. When acetylcholine binds to muscarinic receptors in cardiac muscle, the heart rate slows; when it binds to muscarinic receptors in smooth muscle cells of the gastrointestinal (GI) tract, the rate and amplitude of contraction increase. *Atropine* blocks muscarinic but not nicotinic receptor sites (thereby affecting the heart rate without causing paralysis). In contrast, curare, a nicotinic receptor blocker, causes paralysis.

? CRITICAL THINKING

What signs or symptoms related to pulse rate, gastrointestinal tract activity, and pupil diameter would you expect if your patient has eaten some poisonous mushrooms containing muscarine?

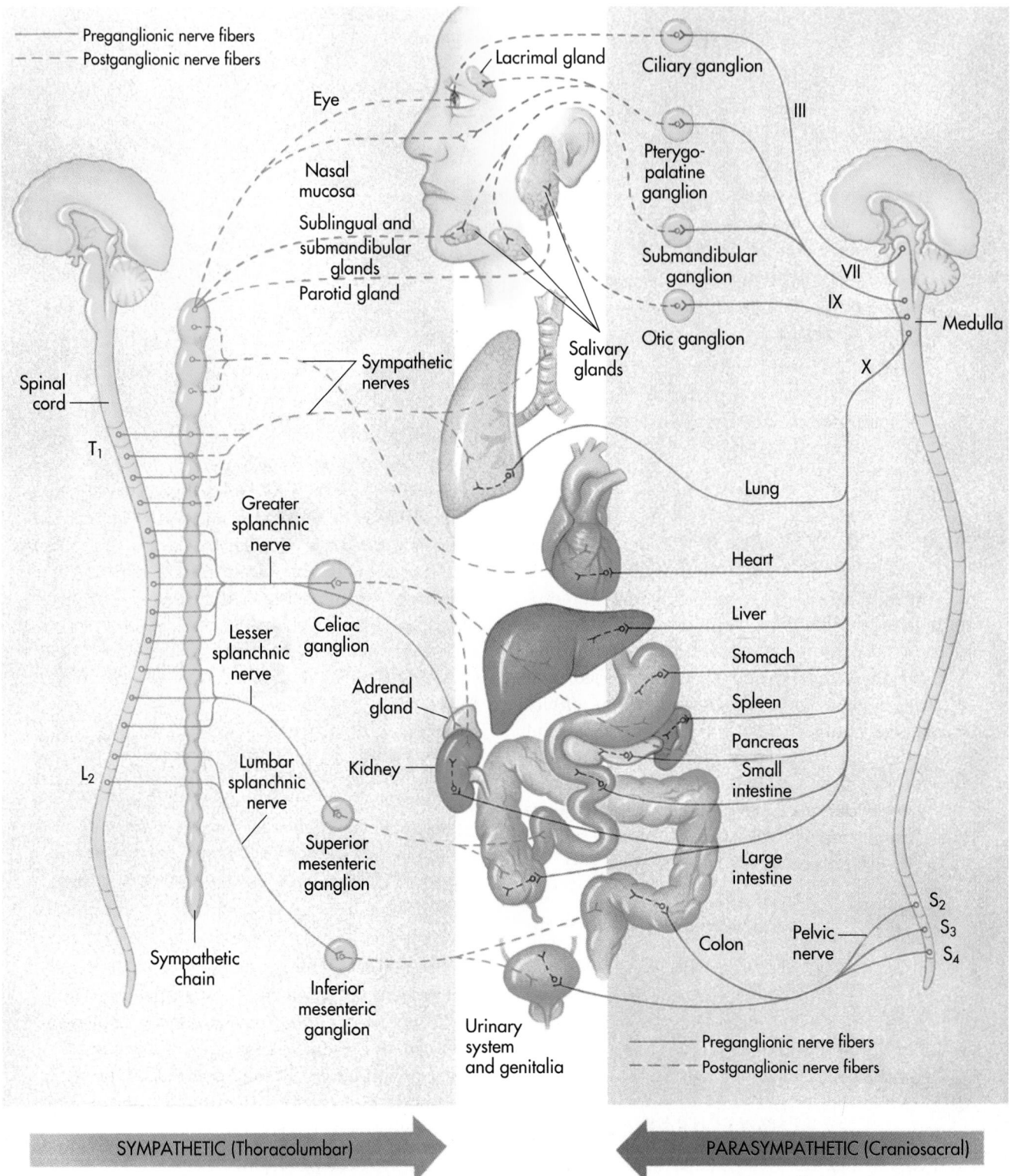

Fig. 8-1 Innervation of major target organs by the autonomic nervous system, showing preganglionic fibers *(solid lines)* and postganglionic fibers *(broken lines).*

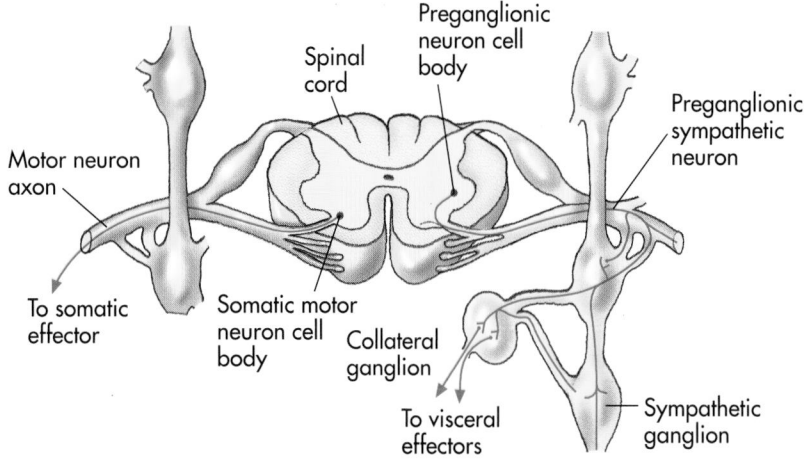

Fig. 8-2 Autonomic conduction pathways.

For adrenergic synapses, norepinephrine molecules combine with adrenergic receptor molecules within the membranes of the effector organ. These receptors belong to two structural categories, the alpha adrenergic receptors (alpha receptors) and the beta adrenergic receptors (beta receptors). Norepinephrine binds to and activates both types of receptor molecules, although it has more affinity for alpha receptors. The hormone epinephrine, which is produced by the adrenal medulla, also is classified as an adrenergic substance and has nearly equal affinity for both receptors. In tissues containing alpha and beta receptor cells, one type is more abundant and therefore has a predominant effect. Both receptors can be excitatory or inhibitory. For example, beta receptors are stimulatory in cardiac muscle but inhibitory in intestinal smooth muscle (Table 8-2).

> **NOTE**
> The neuroactive peptides (e.g., endorphins), another chemical class of neurotransmitters, have important pain-relieving effects on the body.

SECTION THREE
MECHANISMS OF DRUG ACTION

General Properties of Drugs

Drug actions are achieved by a biochemical interaction between the drug and certain tissue components in the body (usually receptors). *Drugs do not confer any new functions on a tissue or organ; they only modify existing functions.* In addition, drugs generally exert several effects rather than a single one. To produce the desired effect, a drug must enter the body and reach appropriate concentrations at its site of action. This process is influenced by three phases of drug activity: the pharmaceutical phase, the pharmacokinetic phase, and the pharmacodynamic phase.

> **NOTE**
> It is important for the paramedic to perform a thorough patient assessment and to obtain a complete medical (and drug) history from the patient. Integrating pathophysiological principles of pharmacology with patient assessment allows the paramedic to form a field impression and to implement a pharmacological management plan.

Pharmaceutical Phase

Pharmaceutics is the science of dispensing drugs. One component of this field is the study of the ways in which various forms of drugs (solid or liquid) influence pharmacokinetic and pharmacodynamic activities (described later). The term *dissolution* refers to the rate at which a solid drug goes into solution after ingestion. The faster the rate of dissolution, the more quickly the drug is absorbed.

> **NOTE**
> All drugs must be in solution to cross the biological membrane to achieve absorption.

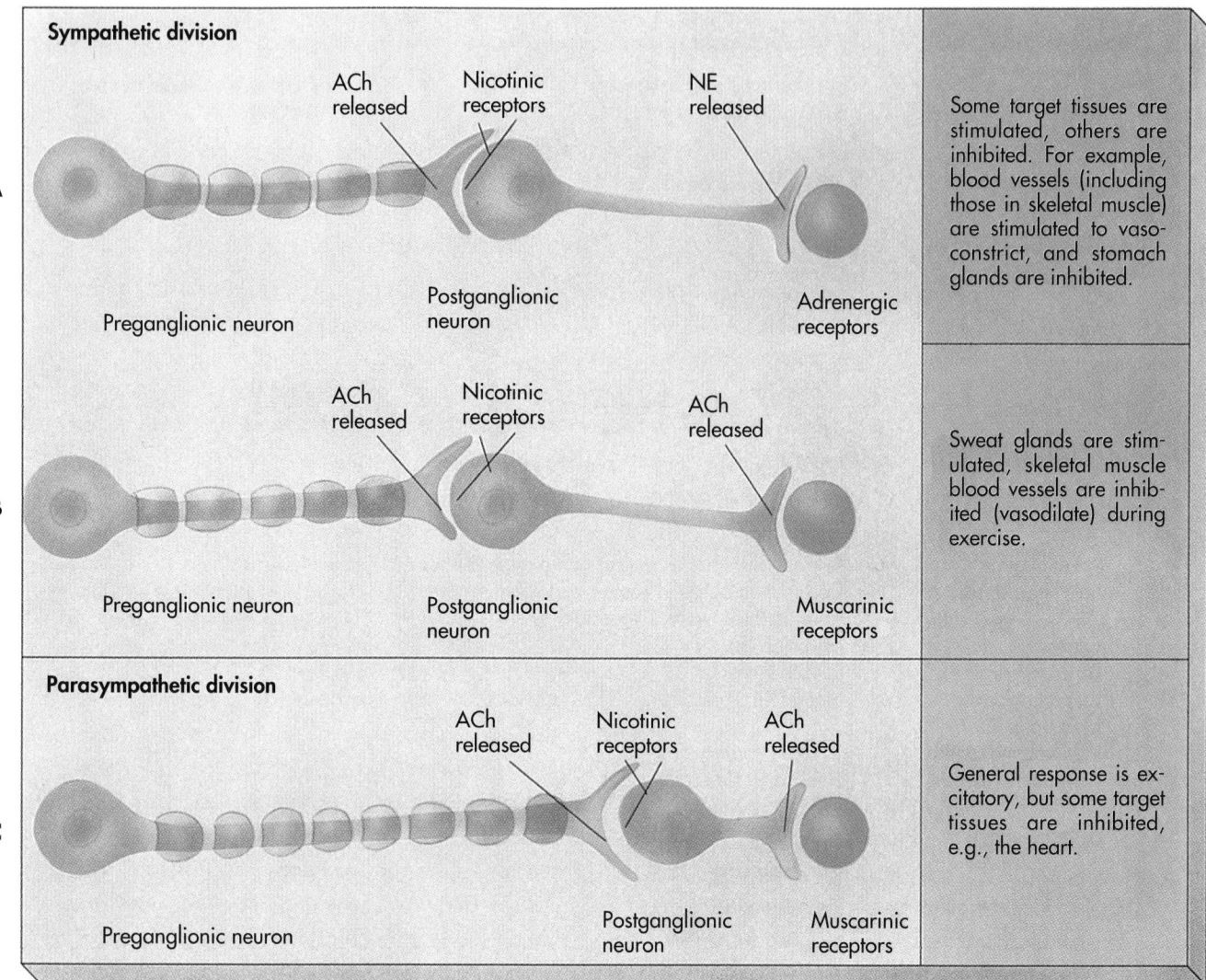

Fig. 8-3 Location of the nicotinic, muscarinic, and adrenergic receptors in the autonomic nervous system. Nicotinic receptors are found on the cell bodies of sympathetic and parasympathetic postganglionic cells in the autonomic ganglia. **A,** Adrenergic receptors are found in most target tissues innervated by the sympathetic division. **B,** Some sympathetic target tissues have muscarinic receptors. **C,** All parasympathetic target tissues have muscarinic receptors. *NE,* Norepinephrine; *ACh,* acetylcholine.

Pharmacokinetic Phase

Pharmacokinetics is the study of how the body handles a drug over a period of time, including the processes of **absorption**, **distribution**, **biotransformation**, and **excretion**. These factors affect a patient's response to drug therapy.

Drug Absorption

Absorption involves the movement of drug molecules from the entry site to the general circulation. The degree to which drugs attain pharmacological activity depends partly on the rate and extent to which they are absorbed, which in turn depend on the drug's ability to cross the cell membrane. The drug crosses the membrane through the processes of passive diffusion and active transport (described in Chapter 7). Although most drugs enter the cell by passive diffusion, some require a carrier-mediated mechanism to assist them across the membrane.

The cell membrane consists of a lipid bilayer throughout which protein molecules are irregularly dispersed. The protein molecules may act as a carrier, enzyme, receptor, or antigenic sites (an antigenic

TABLE 8-2	AUTONOMIC INNERVATION OF TARGET TISSUES

ORGAN	EFFECT OF SYMPATHETIC STIMULATION	EFFECT OF PARASYMPATHETIC STIMULATION
Heart		
Muscle	Increased rate and force (b)	Slowed rate (c)
Coronary arteries	Dilated (b),* constricted (a)*	Dilation (c)
Systemic blood vessels		
Abdomen	Constricted (a)	None
Skin	Constricted (a)	None
Muscle	Dilated (b, c), constricted (a)	None
Lungs		
Bronchi	Dilated (b)	Constriction (c)
Liver	Release of glucose into blood (b)	None
Skeletal muscles	Breakdown of glycogen to glucose (b)	None
Metabolism	Increase of up to 100% (a, b)	None
Glands		
Adrenal glands	Release of epinephrine and norepinephrine (c)	None
Salivary glands	Constriction of blood vessels and slight production of thick, viscous secretion (a)	Dilation of blood vessels and thin, copious secretion (c)
Gastric glands	Inhibition (a)	Stimulation (c)
Pancreas	Inhibition (a)	Stimulation (c)
Lacrimal glands	None	Secretion (c)
Sweat glands		
Merocrine glands	Copious, watery secretion (c)	None
Apocrine glands	Thick, organic secretion (c)	None
Gut		
Wall	Decreased tone (b)	Increased motility (c)
Sphincter	Increased tone (a)	Decreased tone (c)
Gallbladder and bile ducts	Relaxation (b)	Contraction (c)
Urinary bladder		
Wall	Relaxation (b)	Contraction (c)
Sphincter	Contraction (a)	Relaxation (c)
Eye		
Ciliary muscle	Relaxation for far vision (b)	Contraction for near vision (c)
Pupil	Dilation	Constriction (c)
Errector pili muscles	Contraction (a)	None
Blood	Increased coagulation (a)	None
Sex organs	Ejaculation (a)	Erection (c)

a, Mediated by alpha receptors; *b*, mediated by beta receptors; *c*, mediated by cholinergic receptors.
*Normally blood flow through coronary arteries increases as a result of sympathetic stimulation of the heart because of increased demand by cardiac tissue for oxygen. In experiments that isolate the coronary arteries, however, sympathetic nerve stimulation, acting through alpha receptors, causes vasoconstriction. The beta receptors are relatively insensitive to sympathetic nerve stimulation but can be activated by drugs.

site is capable of binding to and reacting with an antibody). Lipid-soluble drugs can pass through the lipid membrane, but water-soluble drugs cannot. Water-soluble substances such as urea, alcohol, and electrolytes must enter the cell through membrane pores.

Absorption begins at the site of administration. The rate and extent of absorption depend on the following factors[3]:

1. *The nature of the absorbing surface (cell membrane) the drug must traverse:* If a drug must pass through a

single layer of cells (intestinal epithelium), transport is faster than if it must pass through several layers of cells (skin). In addition, the greater the surface area of the absorbing site, the greater the absorption and the quicker the drug takes effect. For example, the small intestine offers a large absorption area, whereas the stomach has a relatively small absorption surface area.

2. *Blood flow to the site of administration:* A rich blood supply enhances absorption (e.g., the sublingual route), and a poor blood supply delays it (e.g., the subcutaneous route). For example, a patient in shock may not respond to intramuscular administration of a drug because diminished circulation reduces absorption. In contrast, intravenous administration of a drug immediately places the drug in the circulatory system, where it is completely absorbed and delivered to its target tissue.

3. *The solubility of the drug:* The more soluble the drug, the more rapidly it is absorbed. Parenterally administered nonintravenous drugs prepared in oily solutions are absorbed more slowly than drugs dissolved in water or in isotonic sodium chloride.

4. *The pH of the drug environment:* In solution, many drugs exist in an ionized (charged) and nonionized (uncharged) form. How and to what extent a drug ionizes depend on whether the drug is an acid or a base and on its relative strength. A nonionized drug is lipid soluble and readily diffuses across the cell membrane. An ionized drug is lipid insoluble and nondiffusable. An acidic drug (e.g., **aspirin**) is relatively undissociated (nonionized) in an acidic environment such as the stomach. The drug then readily diffuses across the membranes into the circulation. A drug that is basic in the same acidic environment tends to ionize and is not easily absorbed through the gastric membrane. The reverse occurs when the drug is in an alkaline medium (Fig. 8-4).

5. *The drug concentration:* Drugs administered in high concentrations tend to be absorbed more rapidly than those administered in low concentrations. In some situations it is necessary to administer a large dose (**loading dose**) that temporarily exceeds the body's capacity for excretion of the drug. This rapidly establishes a therapeutic drug level at the receptor site. A smaller dose (**maintenance dose**) can then be administered to replace the amount

of drug excreted. Thus loading doses are based more on the volume of distribution (of which body size is an important component) and less on capacity for excretion (e.g., renal failure). Maintenance doses are exactly the opposite.

? CRITICAL THINKING

What common condition encountered in the prehospital setting requires that drugs be administered at higher than usual doses to achieve therapeutic levels?

6. *The form of the drug dosage:* Drug absorption can be manipulated by pharmaceutical processing. An example is a combination of an active drug with another substance that is slowly released or a drug that resists digestive action (enteric coatings).

Routes of Drug Administration

As a rule, drugs are administered for local or systemic effects. Some drugs given locally produce local and systemic effects if they are partly or entirely absorbed. Other drugs are applied for local absorption and yet are targeted solely for systemic effects (e.g., **nitroglycerin paste** and ointment hormones). The route of administration greatly influences drug absorption (Table 8-3). These routes can be classified as *enteral, parenteral, pulmonary,* and *topical* (see Chapter 9).

Enteral route. Drugs administered along any portion of the GI tract (either orally, rectally, or through a nasogastric tube) are said to use the enteral route (Box 8-6). The enteral method of giving drugs is the safest, most convenient, and most economical route of administration. It also is the least reliable and slowest of the common routes because of the frequent changes in the gastrointestinal environment (e.g., with food contents, emotional state, physical activity). This route allows for four types of absorption: oral absorption, gastric absorption, absorption from the small intestine, and rectal absorption.

Oral absorption. Although the oral cavity has a rich blood supply, little absorption normally occurs in the mouth. Certain drugs, such as **nitroglycerin** (Nitrostat) tablets and some hormones, are prepared to be absorbed orally. When administered by sublingual or buccal routes, these drugs rapidly dissolve in the salivary secretions and are absorbed by

pH effects on drug molecules

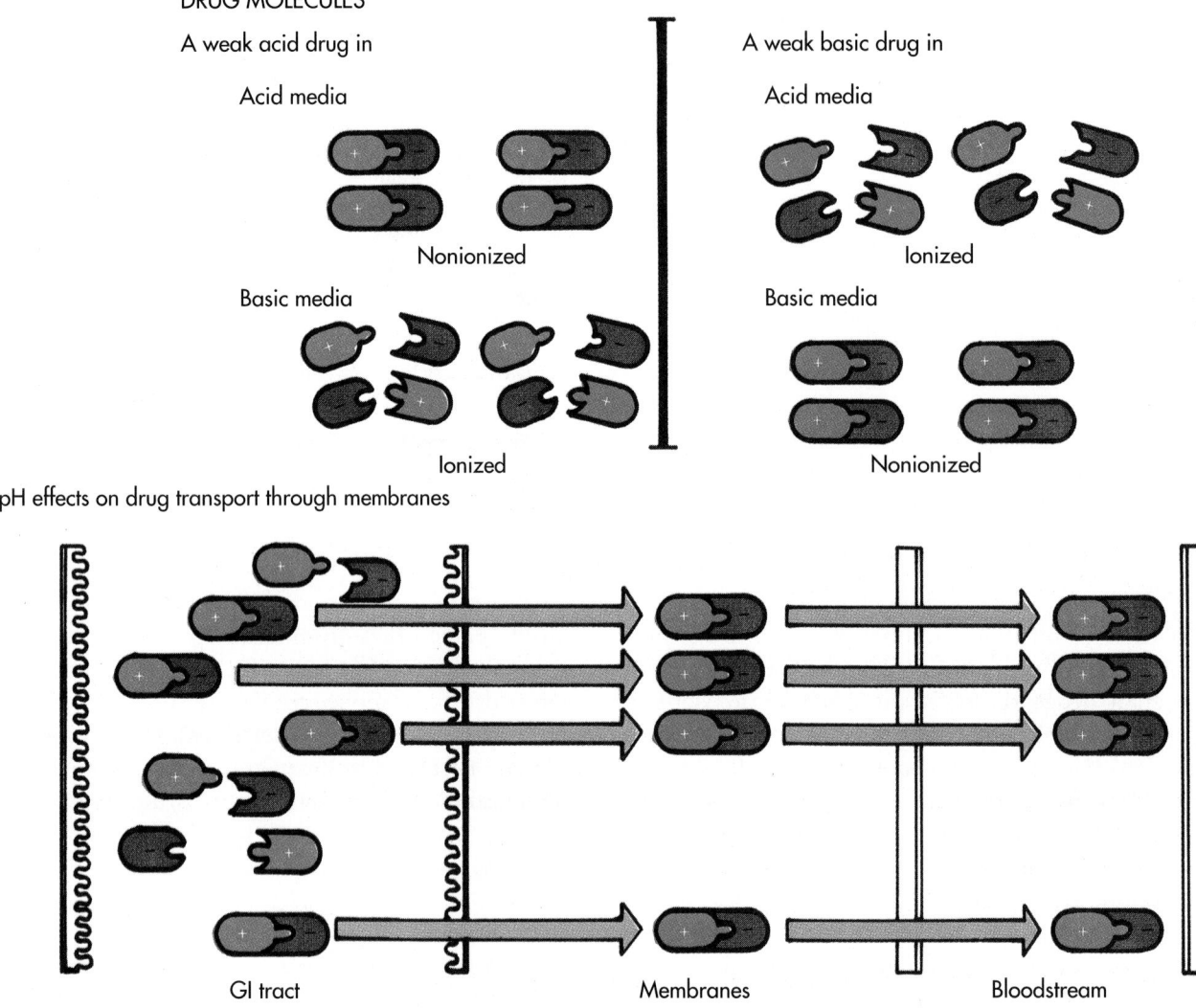

Fig. 8-4 Effect of pH on drug ionization and transport.

the oral mucosa. Drugs that are absorbed in the upper GI tract enter the systemic circulation, initially bypassing gastrointestinal fluids and the liver. Drugs absorbed in the stomach and intestines are absorbed into the portal vein system and are subject to **first-pass metabolism** (described later) in the liver. In sublingual administration, the medication is placed under the tongue, and the tablet or spray dissolves in the salivary secretions. The effects of sublingual medication usually are apparent within a few minutes. With buccal administration, the drug is placed between the teeth and mucous membrane of the cheek. As in sublingual administration, absorption by buccal administration usually is rapid.

? CRITICAL THINKING

Why is nitroglycerin spray, rather than the tablet form, likely to be more effective in geriatric patients?

Gastric absorption. The stomach also has a rich blood supply but is not considered an important site of drug absorption. The length of time a medication remains in the stomach varies, depending on the pH of the environment and gastric motility. For example, the pH of the stomach is about 1.4. Weakly acidic drugs tend to remain nonionized and

TABLE 8-3	COMPARISON OF DRUG ABSORPTION RATES BY COMMON ROUTES OF ADMINISTRATION			
ROUTE	**RATE OF ABSORPTION**		**ROUTE**	**RATE OF ABSORPTION**
Enteral	Slow		Endotracheal	Rapid
Sublingual	Rapid		Intraosseous	Immediate
Subcutaneous	Slow		Pulmonary	Rapid
Intramuscular	Moderate		Topical	Moderate
Intravenous	Immediate (no absorption required)			

are readily absorbed into the circulation. In comparison, basic drugs ionize in the stomach and are poorly absorbed. Altering the gastric emptying rate may alter the rate and extent of drug absorption. Many drugs are administered on an empty stomach with sufficient water (8 ounces) to ensure rapid passage into the small intestine. Other drugs cause gastric irritation and usually are given with food.

Absorption from the small intestine. The small intestine has a rich blood supply and thus a larger absorption area than the stomach. Most drug absorption occurs in the upper part of the small intestine. The pH of intestinal fluid is alkaline (7.0 to 8.0), which increases the rate of absorption of basic drugs. Prolonged exposure allows more time for drug absorption. An increase in intestinal motility (e.g., diarrhea) decreases exposure to the intestinal membrane and diminishes absorption.

Rectal absorption. Although the surface area of the rectum is not large, it is very vascular and capable of drug absorption. Drugs administered rectally are subject to erratic absorption because of rectal contents, local drug irritation, and the uncertainty of drug retention. It is estimated that 50% of a drug that has been rectally administered will bypass the liver after absorption, making first-pass metabolism by the liver less than that of an orally given dose.

? CRITICAL THINKING

The drugs given rectally in emergency situations usually are anticonvulsants. Why do you think this route would be selected over the oral or intravenous route?

BOX 8-6

SOME EMERGENCY DRUGS ADMINISTERED VIA THE ENTERAL ROUTE

Activated charcoal
Aspirin
Nitroglycerin
Syrup of ipecac

NOTE

The way in which rectal medications are absorbed depends on whether there is passage through the superior or inferior hemorrhoidal veins.

Parenteral route. Drugs administered by injection are said to use the parenteral route (Box 8-7). The commonly used parenteral routes for administering medications include the following:

1. Subcutaneous (SQ, SC) route: A subcutaneous injection is given beneath the skin into the connective tissue or fat immediately beneath the dermis. This route is used only for small volumes of drugs (0.5 mL or less) that do not irritate tissue. The rate of absorption usually is slow and can provide a sustained effect.
2. Intramuscular (IM) route: An intramuscular injection is given into the skeletal muscle. Absorption generally occurs more rapidly than with a subcutaneous injection because of greater tissue blood flow.
3. Intravenous (IV) route: An intravenous injection is given directly into the bloodstream, bypassing

---

BOX 8-7

EXAMPLES OF EMERGENCY DRUGS ADMINISTERED VIA THE PARENTERAL ROUTE

Adenosine (Adenocard)
Amiodarone (Cordarone)
Atropine
Dextrose 50%
Diazepam (Valium)
Diphenhydramine (Benadryl)
Epinephrine (Adrenalin)
Furosemide (Lasix)
Labetalol (Normodyne)
Lidocaine (Xylocaine)
Midazolam (Versed)
Morphine
Naloxone (Narcan)
Oxytocin (Pitocin)
Vasopressin (Pitressin)
Verapamil (Isoptin)

---

the absorption process. This route produces an almost immediate pharmacological effect. Most intravenous drugs should be administered slowly to help prevent adverse reactions.

4. Intrathecal route: Intrathecal injection refers to a drug that is administered directly into the spinal subarachnoid space, bypassing the blood-brain barrier (described later in this chapter). This route sometimes is used to achieve rapid drug effects during anesthesia (spinal block) and in the treatment of acute central nervous system (CNS) infections.

5. Intradermal route: An intradermal injection is made just below the epidermis. This route primarily is used for allergy testing and to administer local anesthetics.

6. Endotracheal (ET) route: Access to the endotracheal route generally is through an endotracheal tube, which allows drug delivery into the pulmonary alveoli and systemic absorption via the capillaries of the lungs. Because of the large surface area of the alveolar sacs, the rate of absorption by this route is almost as rapid as that of the intravenous route. Administration of drugs via an endotracheal tube usually is reserved for situations in which an intravenous line cannot be established. Medications that can be administered

by the ET tube include *lidocaine* (Xylocaine), *epinephrine* (Adrenalin), *atropine*, and *naloxone* (Narcan). This route is somewhat erratic and may be less reliable than intravenous or intraosseous delivery and should therefore be used in adult patients only if these first-line methods are unavailable. It is recommended that 2 to 2½ times the recommended intravenous dose (diluted in 10 mL normal saline) be administered when giving medication by this route.[4]

NOTE

A mnemonic for the four medications that may be administered by the ET route is L-E-A-N (*l*idocaine, *e*pinephrine, *a*tropine, and *n*aloxone).

---

7. Intraosseous (IO) route: An intraosseous injection is given directly into the bone marrow cavity of pediatric (and occasionally adult) patients through an established, free-flowing IO infusion system. Agents infused by this method are thought to circulate via the medullary cavity of the bone. Through the numerous venous channels of long bones, fluids or drugs rapidly enter the central circulation. The length of time from injection to entry into the systemic circulation is thought to equal that of the intravenous route.[5] Emergency medications known to be effective when administered via the IO route are *epinephrine* (Adrenalin), *atropine, sodium bicarbonate, dexamethasone* (Decadron), *dopamine* (Intropin), and *dobutamine* (Dobutrex).

Pulmonary route. Medication can be administered by inhalation in the form of gas or fine mist (aerosol). The most commonly used inhalation medications are bronchodilators (Box 8-8), but the pulmonary circulation can absorb a number of other medications if necessary, such as drugs for ET administration.

Because of the large surface area and the rich capillary network adjacent to the alveolar membrane, absorption into the bloodstream is rapid. Drugs such as bronchodilators and steroids can be given by various inhalation devices, such as a nebulizer, propelling the agent into alveolar sacs. This produces primarily local effects but occasionally results in unwanted systemic effects (e.g., elevated heart rate).

BOX 8-8

EMERGENCY DRUGS ADMINISTERED VIA THE PULMONARY ROUTE

Albuterol (Proventil, Ventolin)
Amyl nitrite
Epinephrine racemic (Micronefrin)
Metaproterenol (Alupent)
Nitrous oxide/oxygen (Nitronox)
Oxygen

BOX 8-9

EMERGENCY DRUGS ADMINISTERED VIA THE TOPICAL ROUTE

Nitropaste (Nitro-Bid Ointment)
Lidocaine (viscous solution)

Topical route. In most cases drugs applied topically to the skin and mucous membranes are rapidly absorbed and are intended to produce a local effect (Box 8-9). Only lipid-soluble compounds are absorbed through the skin, which acts as a barrier to most water-soluble compounds. To prevent adverse systemic effects, intact skin surfaces should be used as an administration site. Massaging the skin promotes drug absorption as the capillaries dilate and local blood flow increases.

Drug Distribution

Distribution is the transport of a drug through the bloodstream to various tissues of the body and ultimately to its site of action. After a drug has entered the circulatory system, it is rapidly distributed throughout the body. The rate at which this occurs depends on the permeability of capillaries to the drug molecules.

To review, lipid-soluble drugs readily cross capillary membranes to enter most tissues and fluid compartments. Lipid-insoluble drugs require more time to arrive at their point of action. Cardiac output and regional blood flow also affect the rate and extent of distribution into body tissues. Generally, a drug is first distributed to organs that have a rich blood supply (the heart, liver, kidneys, and brain). Then, depending on its composition, the drug enters tissue with a lesser blood supply, such as muscle and fat.

Drug reservoirs. Drugs may accumulate at certain locations that function as storage sites, forming reservoirs by binding to specific tissues. As serum levels decline, tissue-bound drug is released from its storage site into the bloodstream. The released drug maintains significant serum drug levels and may

permit sustained release of the agent, allowing continued pharmacological effect at the receptor site. The two general processes that create drug reservoirs are plasma protein binding and tissue binding.

As drugs enter the circulatory system, they may attach to plasma proteins (mainly albumin), forming a drug-protein complex.

The extent to which this binding occurs affects the intensity and duration of the drug's effect. The albumin molecule is too large to diffuse through the membrane of the blood vessel, so it traps the bound drug in the bloodstream. A drug bound to plasma protein is pharmacologically inactive and becomes a circulating drug reservoir. The free drug (unbound drug) exists in proportion to the protein-bound fraction and is the only portion of the drug that is biologically active. As the free drug is eliminated from the body, the drug-protein complex dissociates, and more drug is released to replace the free portion that was metabolized or excreted. This process is summarized in the following equation:

$$\text{Free drug} + \text{Protein} \rightleftharpoons \text{Drug-protein complex}$$

Although albumin and other plasma proteins provide a number of binding sites, it is possible for two drugs to compete for the same site and displace each other. If certain combinations of drugs are administered simultaneously, this competition can have serious consequences. For example, if a patient taking the anticoagulant medication warfarin (Coumadin) is given quinidine (e.g., Quinaglute Dura Tabs), the quinidine may displace some of the protein-bound warfarin, causing warfarin toxicity, which can be manifested as severe hemorrhage.

Other factors that influence a drug's binding ability include the concentration of plasma proteins (especially albumin), the number of binding sites on the protein, the affinity of the drug for the protein, and the acid-base balance of the patient. Various disease states, such as liver disease, alter the body's ability to handle many medications. These alterations result from a decrease in serum albumin levels (albumin is manufactured by the liver) and a decrease in hepatic metabolism. These and other factors may result in more free drug being available for distribution to tissue sites (increased free drug fraction and enhanced pharmacological response).

A second type of "drug pooling" occurs in fat tissue and bone. Lipid-soluble drugs have a high affinity for adipose tissue, where these drugs are stored. Because fat tissue has relatively low blood flow, it serves as a stable reservoir for drugs. Some lipid-soluble drugs can remain in body fat for as long as 3 hours after administration. Other drugs (e.g., tetracycline) have an unusual affinity for bone. These drugs accumulate in bone after being absorbed onto the bone crystal surface.

? CRITICAL THINKING

Tetracycline typically is not given to pregnant women because of the harmful effects it has on the development of the baby's teeth. Why would it affect the teeth?

Barriers to drug distribution. The blood-brain barrier and the **placental barrier** are protective biological membranes that prevent the passage of certain drugs into these body sites. The blood-brain barrier consists of a single layer of capillary endothelial cells that line the blood vessels entering the central nervous system. These cells are tightly joined at common borders by continuous intercellular junctions. This special anatomical arrangement permits only lipid-soluble drugs (e.g., general anesthetics, barbiturates) to be distributed into the brain and cerebrospinal fluid. Drugs that are poorly soluble in fat (e.g., many antibiotics) have trouble passing this barrier and cannot enter the brain.

The placental barrier consists of membrane layers that separate the blood vessels of the mother and the fetus. Like the blood-brain barrier, the placental barrier is not permeable to many lipid-insoluble drugs, so it provides some protection to the fetus. However, it does allow the passage of certain non-lipid-soluble drugs (e.g., steroids, narcotics, anesthetics, and some antibiotics). If these drugs are administered to the pregnant mother, they may affect the developing embryo or fetus or the neonate.

Biotransformation

After absorption and distribution, the body eliminates most drugs, first by biotransformation and then by excretion. Biotransformation (metabolism) is a process whereby the drug is chemically converted to a metabolite. The purpose of biotransformation usually is to "detoxify" a drug and render it less active; in some cases, however, this process produces active or even toxic metabolites. An example is the production of toxic metabolites that results from an acetaminophen overdose. The liver is the primary site of drug metabolism, but other tissues (plasma, kidneys, lungs, and the intestinal mucosa) also can be involved.

Orally administered drugs absorbed through the gastrointestinal tract normally travel to the liver before entering the general circulation. When this occurs, a significant amount may be metabolized (first-pass metabolism) before the drug reaches the systemic circulation, reducing the amount of drug available for distribution. Medications affected by this initial biotransformation can be given orally in high dosages or administered parenterally to initially bypass the liver.

Individuals metabolize drugs at variable rates. For example, patients with liver, renal, or cardiovascular dysfunction are expected to have prolonged drug metabolism. Infants with immature metabolic capacity and older adults with degenerative metabolic function experience depressed biotransformation. If drug metabolism is delayed, drug accumulation and cumulative drug effects may occur. Therefore the paramedic may need to consider dosage reductions (particularly maintenance doses) for patients in these categories (Fig. 8-5).

Excretion

Excretion is the elimination of toxic or inactive metabolites. The kidney is the primary organ for excretion, but the intestine, lungs, and mammary, sweat, and salivary glands also may be involved.

Excretion by the kidneys. A drug can be excreted in the urine unchanged or as a chemical metabolite of its previous form. Renal excretion consists of three mechanisms: passive glomerular filtration, active tubular secretion, and partial reabsorption (Fig. 8-6).

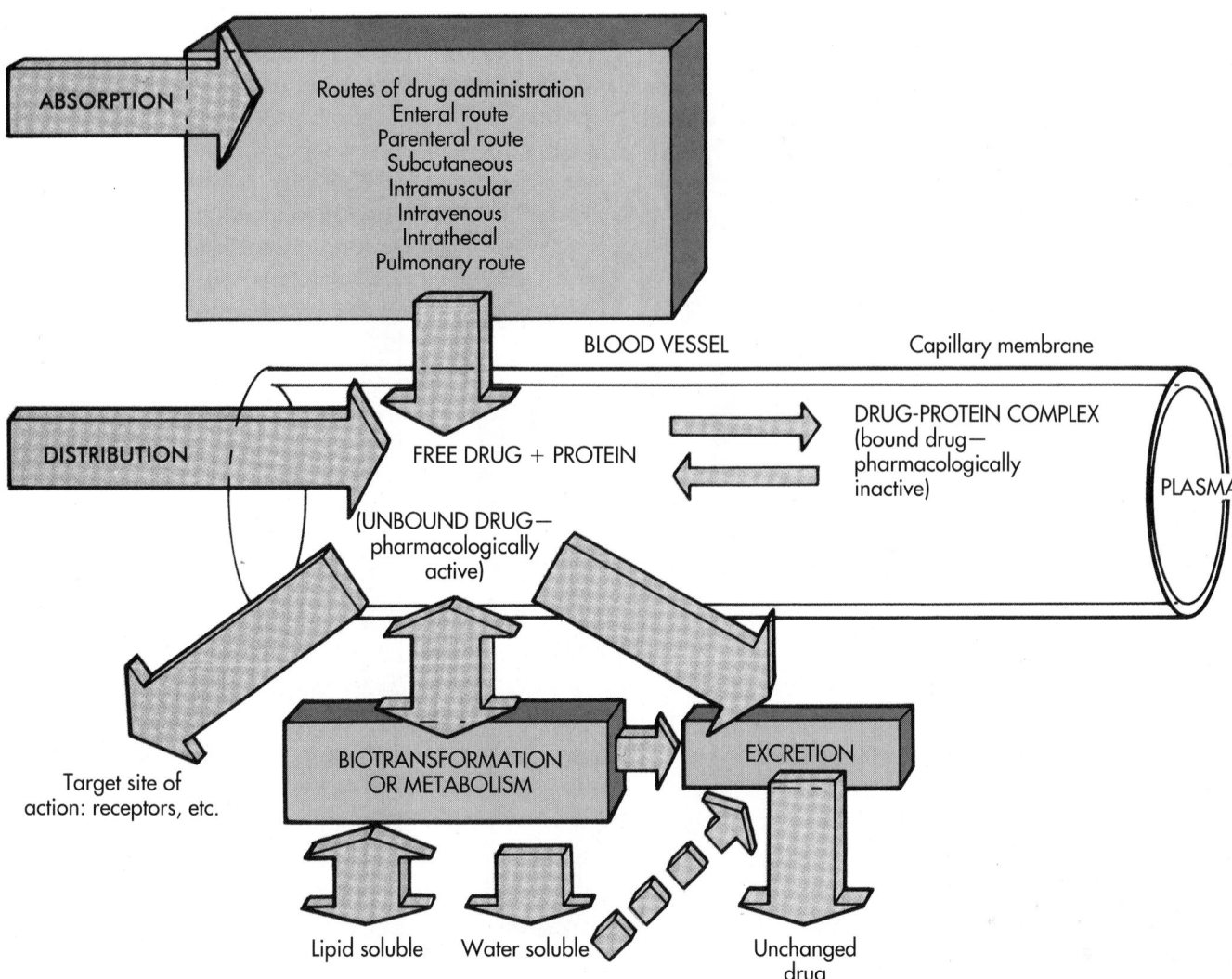

Fig. 8-5 Pharmacokinetic phase of drug action, showing absorption, distribution, biotransformation, and excretion of drugs. Only free drug is capable of movement for absorption, distribution to the target site of action, biotransformation, and excretion. The drug-protein complex represents bound drugs; because the molecule is large, it is trapped in the blood vessel and serves as a storage site for the drug.

Passive glomerular filtration is a simple filtration process that can be measured as the glomerular filtration rate (GFR) (described in Chapter 6). The GFR is the total quantity of glomerular filtrate (usually expressed in milliliters) formed each minute in all nephrons of both kidneys. The availability of a drug for glomerular filtration depends on its free concentration in plasma. Unbound drugs and water-soluble metabolites are filtered by the glomeruli. Drugs highly bound to protein do not pass through this structure.

After filtration, lipid-soluble compounds are reabsorbed by the renal tubules and thus reenter the systemic circulation. Water-soluble compounds are not reabsorbed and are therefore eliminated from the body. Because of the proportional relationship between free and bound drug, as free drug is filtered from the blood, bound drug is released from its binding sites into the plasma. The rate of excretion and the drug's **biological half-life** (described later in this chapter) depend on how quickly bound drug is released.

? CRITICAL THINKING

You pick up your patient at the renal dialysis center. How will you know which medicines you can safely administer?

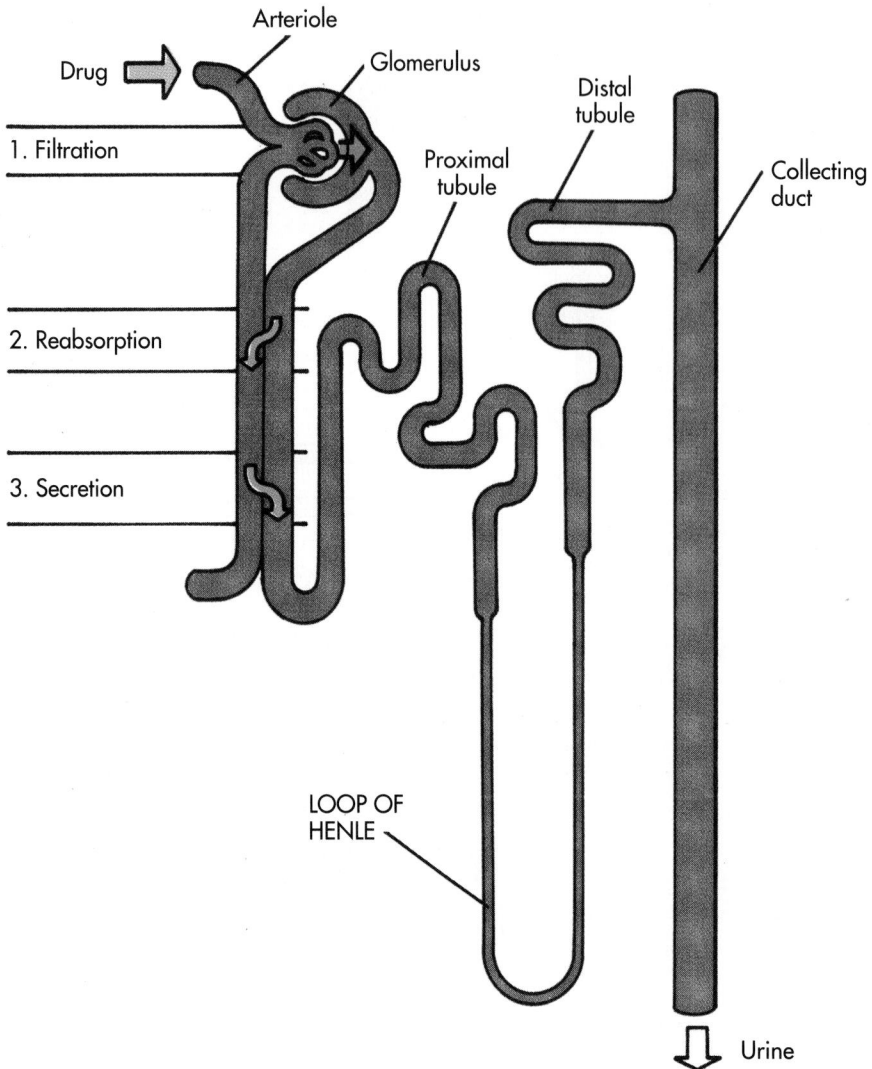

Fig. 8-6 Drug excretion process.

Active tubular secretion involves the transport of free drug from the blood across the proximal tubular cell and into the tubular urine by an active process against a concentration gradient. Drugs actively secreted by the renal tubules can be affected by other drugs that compete for the same active transport process. An example of competitive **drug interaction** is that between *amiodarone* (Cordarone) and *digoxin* (Lanoxin), in which the first drug reduces the clearance (complete removal by the kidneys) of the second drug, with a resultant increase in the plasma concentration of the second drug.

Partial resorption is resorption from the renal tubule by passive diffusion. This resorption can be

greatly influenced by the pH of the tubular urine, which can vary between 5.0 and 8.0. Weak acids are excreted more readily in alkaline urine and more slowly in acidic urine because they are ionized (water soluble) in alkaline urine but nonionized (lipid soluble) in acidic urine. The reverse is true for weak bases. For example, an increase in urinary pH decreases the resorption and increases the clearance of weak acids such as *furosemide* (Lasix) and *aspirin*, whereas a decrease in urinary pH increases the clearance of weak bases such as amphetamine and tricyclic antidepressants.

As a rule, substances that are completely or almost completely excreted by the normal kidney can be removed by an artificial process resembling glomerular filtration. This process, hemodialysis, can be used to remove a wide variety of substances. It is not very effective for drugs that are highly tissue or protein bound and is of limited benefit with rapidly acting toxins.

Excretion by the intestine. Drugs are eliminated through the intestine by biliary excretion. After liver metabolism, the metabolites are carried in bile and passed into the duodenum. The metabolites are then eliminated with the feces. Some drugs are reabsorbed by the bloodstream, returned to the liver, and later excreted by the kidneys.

Excretion by the lungs. Some drugs can be eliminated by the lungs (e.g., general anesthetics, volatile alcohols, inhaled bronchodilators). Factors that can alter drug elimination via the lungs include the rate and depth of respiration and cardiac output. Deep breathing and an increase in cardiac output (which increases pulmonary blood flow) promote excretion. Conversely, the respiratory compromise and decreased cardiac output that may occur during illness or injury can prolong the period required to eliminate drugs through the lungs.

Excretion by the sweat and salivary glands. Sweat is a relatively unimportant means of drug excretion. However, elimination of drugs and their metabolites, or both, via this route can produce some side effects. (Examples include various skin reactions and discoloration of sweat.) Drugs excreted in saliva usually are swallowed and eliminated in the same manner as other orally administered medications. Certain substances given intravenously can be excreted into saliva, causing the individual to describe or complain about the taste of the drug.

Excretion by the mammary glands. Many drugs or their metabolites cross the epithelium of the mammary glands and are excreted in breast milk. Because breast milk is acidic (pH 6.5), basic compounds that ionize at this pH (e.g., narcotics) achieve high concentrations in this fluid. In contrast, weak acids, such as diuretics and barbiturates, are less concentrated. Nursing mothers are cautioned not to take any medication except under the supervision of a physician. Mothers usually are advised to take prescribed medications immediately after breast feeding to diminish any risk to the infant.

Factors that Influence the Action of Drugs

Many factors can alter the response to drug therapy, including age, body mass, gender, pathological state, genetic factors, psychological factors, environment, and time of administration. The paramedic should recognize these factors and consider individual responses and complications that may result from drug therapy.

Age. It generally is accepted that pediatric and geriatric patients are highly responsive to drugs. This results in part from the immature hepatic and renal systems of the child and the natural deterioration of these systems in the older adult. These variations in body function can reduce the effectiveness of excretory and metabolic mechanisms. The older patient also may have underlying disease processes that can produce unexpected variations in response to drug therapy. Medication doses for children usually are modified on the basis of body weight or surface area (see Chapter 42).

Body mass. Many drugs are given according to body mass (kilograms). An indirect relationship exists between body mass and the final concentration of drug in a particular patient for any given dosage (i.e., the larger the patient, the lower the concentration for any given dose of drug). The average adult drug dose is calculated on the basis of drug quantity that produces a particular effect in 50% of the population between the ages of 18 and 65 and who weigh about 150 pounds (68 kg). The administration of drugs in children is always based on body mass.

Gender. The differences in drug effects on men and women result partly from size differences. Because women usually are smaller than men, they may have higher concentrations of drugs administered without consideration of size. Differences in the relative proportions of fat and water in the bodies of men and women also can cause variations in drug distribution.

Environment. Drugs that affect mood and behavior may be susceptible to the individual's environment and the personality of the user. For example, sensory deprivation and sensory overload may affect a person's response to a drug. The physical environment also can affect the actions of some drugs for certain people. For example, temperature extremes and changes in altitude may increase sensitivity to some drugs.

Time of administration. The presence or absence of food in the GI tract affects the manner in which drugs are tolerated and absorbed. Other factors that may influence drug activity and reactions to drug therapy include an individual's biological rhythms (e.g., sleep-wake cycles and circadian rhythms).

Pathological state. Illness or injury and the severity of symptoms can affect the type and amount of drug needed to achieve a desired effect. In addition, underlying disease processes such as circulatory, hepatic, or renal dysfunction can interfere with the physiological processes of drug action and elimination.

Genetic factors. Genetics can alter the response of some individuals to a number of medications through inherited metabolic (enzymatic) deficiencies or altered receptor site sensitivities. These pharmacogenetic abnormalities may manifest as idiosyncrasies or may be mistaken for drug allergies.

Psychological factors. A patient's belief in the effects of a drug may strongly influence and potentiate drug effects. For example, a placebo can have the same result as a pharmacological agent if the patient believes the placebo will have the desired effect. In contrast, patient hostility and mistrust can diminish the perceived effects of a drug.

NOTE

The paramedic can enhance the action of a drug by telling the patient that the drug is going to be effective and when it will take effect.

Pharmacodynamic Phase

Pharmacodynamics is the study of how a drug acts on a living organism, including the pharmacologi-

cal response observed relative to the concentration of the drug at an active site in the organism. As previously stated, drugs do not confer any new function on a tissue or organ of the body; rather, they modify existing functions. Although there are numerous theories of drug action, most drug actions are thought to result from a chemical interaction between the drug and various receptors throughout the body. The most common form of drug action is the drug-receptor interaction.

Drug-Receptor Interaction

It generally is believed that most drugs bind to **drug receptors** to produce their desired effect (Box 8-10). According to this theory, a specific portion of the drug molecule (the active site) selectively combines or interacts with some molecular structure (the reactive site on the cell surface or within the cell) to produce a biological effect. These reactive cellular sites are known as *receptors.*

The relationship of a drug to its receptor may be thought of as a key fitting into a lock (Fig. 8-7). The drug represents the key, and the receptor represents the lock. The drug molecule with the best fit to a receptor produces the best response. After absorption, a drug is believed to gain access to a receptor after it leaves the bloodstream and is distributed to tissues that contain receptor sites. Drugs that bind to a receptor and cause a physiological response are referred to as **agonists.** Conversely, drugs that bind to a receptor and whose presence prevents a physiological response or other drugs from binding are referred to as **antagonists.**

Drug-Response Assessment

In the prehospital setting, the response to drug therapy often can be assessed by observing the pharmacological effect of the drug on specific physiological parameters. Examples include monitoring blood pressure after administration of an antihypertensive medication and pain relief after administration of an analgesic.

Each drug has its own characteristic rate of absorption, distribution, biotransformation, and excretion. Therefore the effectiveness of some drugs cannot be monitored solely by the patient's response. For example, medications such as theophylline, *digoxin* (Lanoxin) and *phenytoin* (Dilantin) must reach a certain concentration at the target site to achieve the desired effect. Tissue concentrations often are proportional to and can be estimated from

DRUG-RECEPTOR INTERACTION TERMS

Affinity: a drug's propensity to bind or attach itself to a given receptor site

Efficacy (intrinsic activity): the drug's ability to initiate biological activity as a result of binding to a receptor site

Agonist: a drug possessing affinity and efficacy that combines with receptors and initiates a sequence of biochemical and physiological changes

Antagonist: an agent that inhibits or counteracts effects produced by other drugs or undesired effects caused by normal or hyperactive physiological mechanisms

Competitive antagonist: an agent with an affinity for the same receptor site as an agonist. (The competition with the agonist for the site inhibits the action of the agonist; increasing the concentration of the agonist tends to overcome the inhibition. Competitive inhibition responses are usually reversible.)

Noncompetitive antagonist: an agent that combines with different parts of the receptor mechanism and inactivates the receptor so that the agonist cannot be effective regardless of its concentration (Noncompetitive antagonist effects are considered to be irreversible or nearly so.)

Partial antagonist: an agent with affinity and some efficacy but that may antagonize the action of other drugs with greater efficacy (Frequently antagonists share some structural similarities with their agonists.)

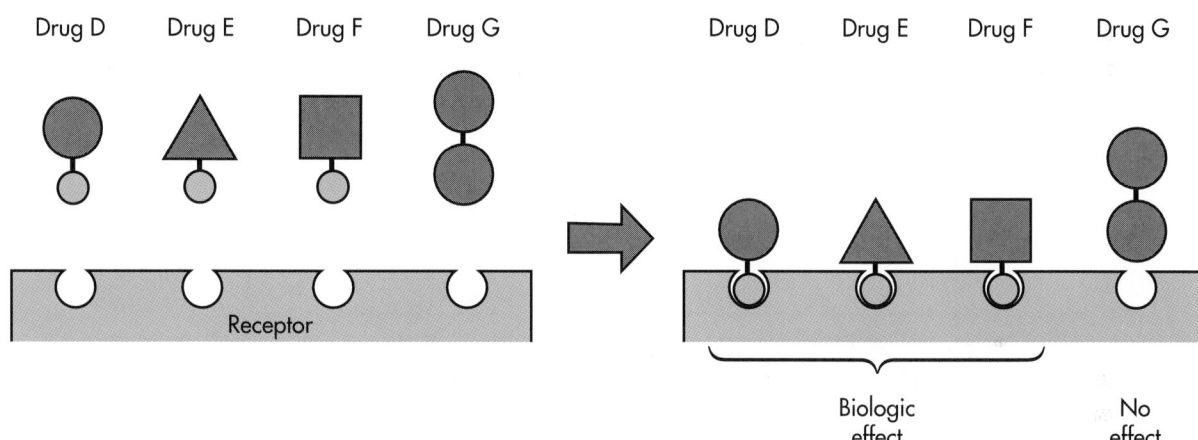

Fig. 8-7 Lock-and-key fit between a drug and the receptors through which it acts. The site on the receptor that interacts with a drug has a definite shape. A drug that conforms to that shape can bind and produce a biological response. In this example, only the shape along the lower surface of the drug molecule is important in determining if the drug binds to the receptor.

serum drug levels. Therapeutic drug levels generally reflect ranges in tissue concentration that relate to a therapeutic response.

Plasma-level profiles (Box 8-11) demonstrate the relationship between the plasma concentration and the level of the therapeutic effectiveness over time (Fig. 8-8). These profiles depend on the rate of absorption, distribution, biotransformation, and excretion after drug administration.

The therapeutic range for most drugs is based on the concentration that provides the highest probability of response with the least risk of toxicity. The dosage (loading and maintenance) required to achieve a therapeutic concentration varies because of the previously described factors that influence the actions of drugs: age, body mass, gender, pathological state, and genetic and psychological factors. Although doses in the therapeutic range have a high probability of efficacy and a low probability of toxicity in most patients, some patients fail to respond to these doses, and others may develop toxicity.

Biological Half-Life

The rate of biotransformation and excretion of a drug determines its biological half-life (t½). Biological half-life is defined as the time required to metabolize or eliminate half the total amount of drug in the body (Fig. 8-9). For example, if a 100-mg

BOX 8-11

PLASMA-LEVEL PROFILE TERMS

Duration of action: the period from onset of drug action to the time when a drug effect is no longer seen

Loading dose: a bolus of a drug given initially to rapidly attain a therapeutic plasma concentration

Maintenance dose: the amount of drug necessary to maintain a steady therapeutic plasma concentration

Minimum effective concentration: the lowest plasma concentration that produces the desired drug effect

Onset of action or **latent period:** the interval between the time a drug is administered and the first sign of its effects

Peak plasma level: the highest plasma concentration attained from a dose

Termination of action: the point at which a drug's effect is no longer seen

Therapeutic range: the range of plasma concentrations most likely to produce the desired drug effect with the least likelihood of toxicity (the range between minimum effective concentration and toxic level)

Toxic level: the plasma concentration of which a drug is likely to produce serious adverse effects

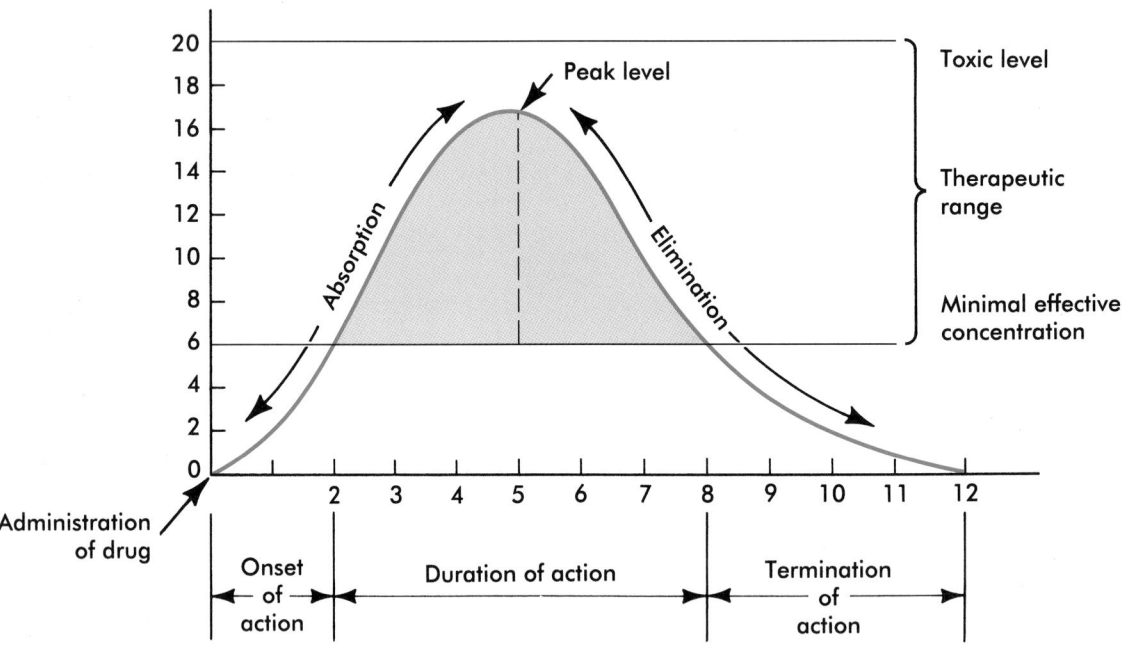

Fig. 8-8 Plasma-level profile of a drug.

injection of *meperidine* (Demerol) is administered and its half-life is 4 hours, 50 mg will be eliminated in the first 4 hours, 25 mg (half of the remaining 50 mg) will be eliminated in the second 4 hours, and

so on. A drug is considered gone from the body after five half-lives have passed.

The half-life of a drug is important when determining the rate of administration. A drug that has a short half-life (e.g., 2 to 3 hours) must be administered more often to maintain a therapeutic range than a drug with a long half-life, such as 12 hours. The half-life of a drug may be markedly lengthened in individuals with hepatic dysfunction or renal disorders. These and other disease processes may require a reduction in drug dosage or a longer interval between doses.

? CRITICAL THINKING

Adenosine, an intravenous antidysrhythmic medicine, has a half-life of only 1 to 3 seconds. How will this brief half-life influence the speed and frequency of administration of this drug?

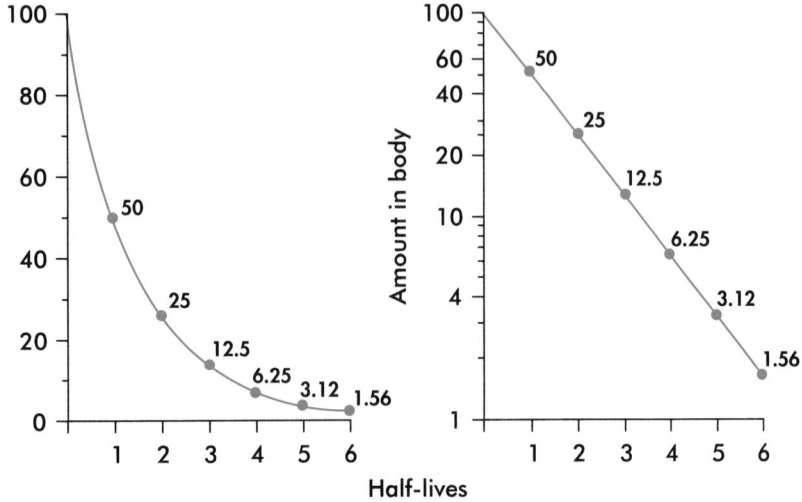

Fig. 8-9 Plotting the amount of drug in the body at each half-life. When the amount is plotted on a cartesian scale *(left)*, an exponential decline is seen. When the amount is plotted on a logarithmic scale *(right)*, a straight line is used to determine the half-life.

Therapeutic Index

The **therapeutic index** (TI) is a measurement of the relative safety of a drug. It represents the ratio between two factors: lethal dose 50 (LD_{50}), the dose of a drug that is lethal in 50% of laboratory animals tested, and effective dose 50 (ED_{50}), the dose that produces a therapeutic effect in 50% of a similar population. The TI is calculated as follows:

$$TI = \frac{LD\ 50}{ED\ 50}$$

The closer the ratio to 1, the greater the danger in administering the drug to human beings. In certain drugs, such as *digoxin* (Lanoxin), the difference between the ED and the LD is small. These drugs are said to have a low TI. In contrast, drugs such as *naloxone* (Narcan) have a wide margin between the ED and LD (a high TI). Great caution must be taken to avoid toxicity caused by medications administered in the field.

Drug Interactions

Many variables can influence drug interactions, including intestinal absorption, competition for plasma-protein binding, biotransformation, action at the receptor site, renal excretion, and alteration of electrolyte balance. Not all drug interactions are dangerous; some may even be beneficial.

Drug-Drug Interactions

Some drug-drug interactions are clinically significant and can be dangerous. The paramedic should be aware of common drug-drug interactions and seek medical direction before giving medications concurrently (see the *Emergency Drug Index*). The drugs listed below are associated with clinically significant drug-drug interactions:

- Blood thinners
- Tricyclic antidepressants (TCAs)
- Monoamine oxidase (MAO) inhibitors
- Amphetamines
- Digitalis glycosides
- Diuretics
- Antihypertensives

Other factors that can influence drug interactions include:

- Drug-induced malabsorption of food and nutrients
- Food-induced malabsorption of drugs
- Enzyme alterations that affect the metabolism of food or drugs

> **NOTE**
>
> Grapefruit and grapefruit juice can boost blood levels of some drugs as much as 1000% through liver enzyme inhibition. Emergency drugs that can be affected include **verapamil** (Isoptin) and **midazolam** (Versed).

- Alcohol consumption
- Cigarette smoking that affects drug metabolism or excretion
- Food-initiated alteration of drug excretion

Drug Storage

Certain precepts should guide the manner in which drugs are secured, stored, distributed, and accounted for. The paramedic should follow agency protocol and local and state regulations. Emergency medical service (EMS) personnel also should be aware that drug potency and the effectiveness of some diluents can be affected by temperature, light, moisture, and shelf-life.

Drug Profiles and Special Considerations in Drug Therapy

Paramedics should be familiar with the drug profiles of any drug they administer (Box 8-12). Realizing that not all components of drug profiles can be committed to memory, the paramedic should make regular use of pharmacology references and seek medical direction as needed.

Special Considerations in Drug Therapy

Special considerations in drug therapy must be taken into account when caring for pregnant patients, pediatric patients, and older adult patients. These considerations are described below, throughout this text by subject matter, and in the *Emergency Drug Index.*

Pregnant Patients

Before using any drug during pregnancy, the expected benefits should be considered against the possible risks to the fetus. Drugs given to a pregnant patient may cross the placental barrier and harm the fetus or may be communicated to a newborn during breast-feeding. The FDA has established a scale to indicate drugs that may be harmful to a fetus during pregnancy (Box 8-13).

Pediatric Patients

Pharmacological considerations for pediatric patients are presented here and throughout the text. Following is a summary of the pharmacokinetics

---

BOX 8-12

COMPONENTS OF A DRUG PROFILE

Drug name
Classification
Mechanisms of action
Indications
Pharmacokinetics
Side/adverse effects
Dosages
Contraindications
Considerations for:
    Pediatric patients
    Geriatric patients
    Pregnant patients
    Other special groups
Storage requirements

---

that influence dosing principles in the neonate, infant, and pediatric populations.

Age. The effects of drugs are rather unpredictable among infants because of the variation in the development and maturation of the different organ systems.

? CRITICAL THINKING

Drug doses vary for pediatric and neonatal patients and are almost always weight related. How can you ensure accuracy of dosing for these patients during life-threatening situations when seconds count—even though you know the wrong dose calculation could be lethal?

Absorption. Drug absorption in infants and children follows the same general principles as in adults. Factors that influence drug absorption include blood flow at the site of intramuscular or subcutaneous administration as determined by the patient's physiological status and, for orally administered drugs, the underlying gastrointestinal function. Physiological conditions that might reduce blood flow to the muscle and subcutaneous tissue include shock, vasoconstriction, and heart failure. The smaller muscle mass of the infant further complicates drug absorption because of diminished peripheral perfusion to these areas.

BOX 8-13

PREGNANCY CATEGORY RATINGS FOR DRUGS

Drugs have been categorized by the Food and Drug Administration (FDA) according to the level of risk to the fetus. These categories are listed for each drug herein under *Pregnancy Safety* and are interpreted as follows[1]:

Category A: Controlled studies in women fail to demonstrate a risk to the fetus in the first trimester, and there is no evidence of risk in later trimesters; the possibility of fetal harm appears to be remote.

Category B: Either (1) animal reproductive studies have not demonstrated a fetal risk but there are no controlled studies in pregnant women or (2) animal reproductive studies have shown an adverse effect (other than decreased fertility) that was not confirmed in controlled studies on women in the first trimester and there is no evidence of risk in later trimesters.

Category C: Either (1) studies in animals have revealed adverse effects on the fetus and there are no controlled studies in women or (2) studies in women and animals are not available. Drugs in this category should be given only if the potential benefit justifies the risk to the fetus.

Category D: There is positive evidence of human fetal risk, but the benefits for pregnant women may be acceptable despite the risk, as in life-threatening diseases for which safer drugs cannot be used or are ineffective. An appropriate statement must appear in the "Warnings" section of the labeling of drugs in this category.

Category X: Studies in animals or humans have demonstrated fetal abnormalities, there is evidence of fetal risk based on human experience, or both; the risk of using the drug in pregnanct women clearly outweighs any possible benefit. The drug is contraindicated in women who are or may become pregnant. An appropriate statement must appear in the "Contraindications" section of the labeling of drugs in this category.

Liquids and suspensions disperse quickly in gastrointestinal fluids and are therefore more readily absorbed than tablet or capsule medications. Increases in peristalsis (e.g., diarrheal conditions) and lowered gastrointestinal enzyme activities tend to decrease overall absorption of orally or rectally administered medications.

Distribution. Because most drugs are distributed in body water, increases in total body water and extracellular volume can increase the volume of drug distribution. Compared with adults, infants have proportionately higher volumes of total body water (70% to 75% compared to 50% to 60%) and a higher ratio of extracellular to intracellular fluid (40% compared to 30%); higher dosages of water-soluble drugs may be needed to achieve effective blood levels in the newborn.

Another major factor that affects drug distribution is drug binding to plasma proteins. In general, protein binding of drugs is reduced in the infant; therefore the concentration of free drug in plasma is increased. This can result in a greater drug effect or toxicity. Regarding CNS effects, the blood-brain barrier in the infant is much less effective than in adults, allowing drugs greater access to this area.

Biotransformation. Various liver enzyme systems for metabolism generally mature unevenly. Because of the infant's decreased ability to metabolize drugs, many drugs have slow clearances and prolonged half-lives in the body. This predisposes the infant to developing toxicity from drugs metabolized by the liver unless doses are adjusted accordingly.

Elimination. The GFR is much lower in newborns than in older infants, children, and adults. Therefore drugs eliminated through renal function are cleared from the body very slowly in the first few weeks of life. Renal excretory mechanisms progress to maturity after 1 year of age. Before that age, excretion of some substances through the renal system may be delayed because of immaturity, resulting in higher serum levels and a longer duration of action than intended.

Older Adult Patients

Important changes in drug responses occur with increasing age in most individuals. Factors associated with aging that significantly affect pharmacokinetics include increased incidence of multiple diseases with a concomitant use of medications, nutritional problems, decreasing clearance efficiency, and the possibility of decreased dosing compliance for a variety of reasons. This summary is intended to serve as a review of the pharmacokinetics that influence dosing principles in the older adult.

Age. Declines in the functional capacity of most major organ systems begin in young adulthood and continue throughout life. Thus older adults do not lose specific function at an accelerated rate compared with young and middle-aged adults, but rather experience a depleting physiological reserve. It generally is accepted that a linear decrease in physiological function (GFR, cardiac function, maximal breathing capacity) begins no later than age 45. Decreased renal function has the greatest impact on medication administration.

Absorption. Although little evidence exists of major alterations in drug absorption with age, conditions associated with age may alter the rate at which some drugs are absorbed. Examples of these conditions include altered nutritional habits, greater consumption of nonprescription drugs (e.g., antacids, laxatives), and changes in gastric emptying. Reduced production of gastric acid and slowed gastric motility may result in unpredictable rates of dissolution and absorption of weakly acidic drugs.

Distribution. Changes in body composition, such as reduced lean body mass, reduced total body water, and increased fat as a percentage of body mass, have been noted in the older adult. Levels of serum albumin, which binds many drugs, especially weak acids, also usually decline. This affects drug distribution by decreasing protein binding of drugs, which results in an increase in the amount of free drug in the circulation. Thus the ratio of bound to free drug in these patients may be significantly altered.

Biotransformation. The capacity of the liver to metabolize drugs does not appear to decline consistently with age for all drugs. However, disorders common with aging, such as congestive heart failure, can impair liver function. In addition, hepatic recovery from injury, such as that caused by alcohol or viral hepatitis, declines.

It generally is believed that certain drugs are metabolized more slowly in older adults because of decreased liver blood flow. This decrease may lead to drug accumulation and toxicity. The paramedic should exercise caution when administering medication metabolized primarily in the liver to a patient with a history of liver disease. Older patients with severe nutritional deficiencies also may have impaired hepatic function.

Elimination. Renal function is the most important factor for clearance of most drugs from the body. The natural reduction in function associated with aging usually is caused by loss of functioning nephrons and a decrease in blood flow, both of which result in a decreased GFR. A decrease in renal function caused by decreases in renal blood flow also may occur secondary to congestive heart failure. The practical result of renal impairment is a marked prolongation of the half-life of many drugs and the possibility of accumulation to toxic levels. Other reversible conditions (e.g., dehydration) can cause additional reduction in renal clearance of drugs.

Drug administration problems. Intentional and unintentional noncompliance with medication therapy may be common in older patients. Although this rarely influences the administration of emergency medications, the paramedic should be familiar with the most common factors that contribute to drug administration problems in older adults, particularly because noncompliance or medication errors may be a precipitating factor in the patient's condition. Following are some common causes of noncompliance and medication errors:

- The expense of drugs may lead to noncompliance in patients with fixed incomes. Older patients may not routinely take prescribed medications or may be unwilling to receive medications in emergency situations.
- Noncompliance in taking prescribed medications may result from forgetfulness or confusion, especially if the patient has several prescriptions and different dosing intervals.
- Older patients may forget instructions on the need to complete medication because symptoms have disappeared. Disappearance of symptoms often is regarded as the best reason to stop the therapy.
- Errors in self-administered medications may result from physical disabilities such as arthritis or visual impairment.

• Noncompliance may be deliberate. A patient may be opposed to taking a drug because of past experiences. A careful drug history is especially important when caring for older adults. The paramedic should remember that a patient has the right to refuse medication.

SECTION FOUR
DRUGS THAT AFFECT THE NERVOUS SYSTEM

Review of Anatomy and Physiology

The components of the nervous system include the central nervous system and the peripheral nervous system (Fig. 8-10). The paramedic should refer to the earlier discussion in this chapter and to Chapter 6 to review the anatomy and physiology of the nervous system (Box 8-14).

Narcotic Analgesics and Antagonists

Narcotic analgesics relieve pain. Narcotic antagonists reverse the effects of some narcotic analgesics. Pain has two components: the sensation of pain, which involves the nerve pathways and the brain, and the emotional response to pain, which

may be a result of the individual's anxiety level, previous pain experience, age, gender, and culture. Classifications of pain are listed and defined in Box 8-15.

Opiates are drugs that contain or are extracted from opium. The term *opioid* designates synthetic drugs that have pharmacological properties similar to those of opium or **morphine,** the chief alkaloid of opium. Opioids work by binding with opioid receptors in the brain and other body organs, altering the patient's pain perception and emotional response to a pain-provoking stimulus. Opioid analgesics include **morphine**, codeine (Methylmorphine), hydromorphone (Dilaudid, Dilaudid-HP), **meperidine** (Demerol), methadone (Dolophine, Methadose), oxycodone (Percodan, Tylox, Percocet), hydrocodone (Lortab), and propoxyphene (Darvon, Dolene).

> **NOTE**
>
> Endorphins serve as the body's own supply of opiates by binding to opiate receptors, thereby blocking pain.

Opioid analgesics may produce undesirable effects such as nausea and vomiting, constipation, urinary retention, cough reflex suppression, orthostatic hypotension, respiratory depression, and CNS depression (including respiratory depression). Most of

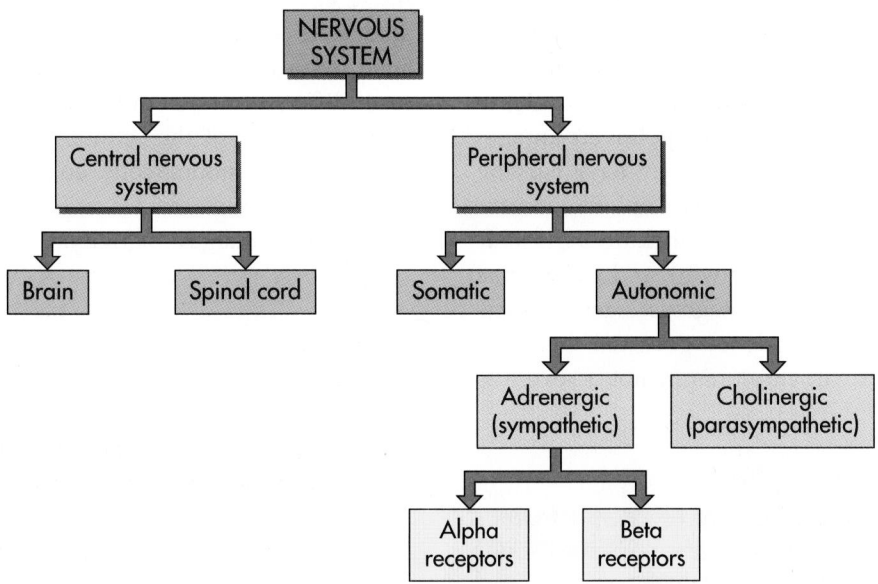

Fig. 8-10 Overview of the nervous system.

BOX 8-14

EMERGENCY DRUGS: NERVOUS SYSTEM

Atropine (Atropine)
Diazepam (Valium)
Dopamine (Dobutrex)
Epinephrine (Adrenalin)
Isoproterenol (Isuprel)
Labetalol (Normodyne)
Magnesium sulfate
Meperidine (Demerol)
Morphine (Astramorph/PF)
Naloxone (Narcan)
Norepinephrine (Levophed)
Pancuronium (Pavulon)
Phenytoin (Dilantin)
Physostigmine (Antilirium)
Propranolol (Inderal)
Succinylcholine (Anectine)

BOX 8-15

CLASSIFICATIONS OF PAIN

Acute pain: pain sudden in onset that usually subsides with treatment (e.g., pain associated with acute myocardial infarction, acute appendicitis, renal colic, or traumatic injuries)

Chronic pain: persistent or recurrent pain that is difficult to treat (e.g., pain that accompanies cancer and rheumatoid arthritis)

Referred pain: visceral pain felt at a site distant from its origin (e.g., pain from a myocardial infarction felt in the arm)

Somatic pain: pain arising from skeletal muscles, ligaments, vessels, or joints

Superficial pain: pain arising from the skin or mucous membrane

Visceral pain: "deep" pain arising from smooth musculature or organ systems that may be difficult to localize and is often described as *dull* or *aching.*

these effects can be overcome by careful administration of the analgesic and careful patient monitoring.

Opioid antagonists "block" the effects of opioid analgesics (e.g., opioid-induced respiratory depression and sedation) by displacing the analgesics from their receptor sites. *Naloxone* (Narcan), naltrexone (Trexan), and *nalmefene* (Revex) are opioid antagonists.

Opioid agonist-antagonist agents have analgesic and antagonist effects. Although the exact mechanism of action is unknown, these medications have pharmacokinetic and adverse effects similar to those of *morphine.* They may competitively antagonize some opioid receptors but may have varying degrees of agonist effect at other opioid receptor sites. Examples of these drugs include *butorphanol* (Stadol), pentazocine (Talwin), and *nalbuphine* (Nubain). Opioid agonist-antagonist agents generally have a lower dependency potential than opioids, and withdrawal symptoms are not as severe as

those of the opioid agonist medications. They may precipitate withdrawal symptoms in addicts.

Nonnarcotic Analgesics

Nonnarcotic analgesics act by a peripheral mechanism that interferes with local mediators released when tissue is damaged; these mediators stimulate nerve endings and cause pain. When nonnarcotic analgesics are present, the nerve endings in damaged tissues are stimulated less often. This mechanism differs from that of narcotic analgesics, which act at the level of the central nervous system. An example of a nonnarcotic analgesic is *ketorolac* (Toradol), a nonsteroidal antiinflammatory drug that exhibits analgesic activity.

Anesthetics

Anesthetic drugs are CNS depressants that have a reversible action on nervous tissue. The three major categories of anesthesia are general, regional, and local. General anesthesia is achieved by intravenous or inhalation routes and is the most common type of anesthesia used during surgery to induce unconsciousness (see the box on p. 265). Regional anesthesia is obtained by inject-

? CRITICAL THINKING

Why would a nonnarcotic analgesic be selected instead of a narcotic for a paramedic returning to work on the ambulance?

STAGES AND SIGNS OF GENERAL ANESTHESIA

Stage I: Stage of Analgesia

The patient initially experiences analgesia without amnesia and then a combination of the two. Speech becomes difficult, auditory or visual hallucinations may occur, and the sense of hearing is lost. This stage ends with the patient's loss of consciousness.

Stage II: Stage of Excitement

The patient appears to be delirious, excited, and amnestic and may laugh, swear, or sing. Respirations become irregular in volume and rate (retching and vomiting may occur). The patient may become incontinent and struggle. This stage ends with reestablishment of regular breathing. This stage has become rare since the introduction of balanced anesthesia.

Stage III: Stage of Surgical Anesthesia

This stage begins with the reestablishment of regular respirations and extends to complete cessation of spontaneous breathing. Changes in ocular movements, eye reflexes, and pupil size indicate the various planes of this stage and increasing depth of anesthesia.

Stage IV: Stage of Medullary Depression (Toxic Stage)

Stage IV begins with the cessation of spontaneous breathing, indicating severe depression of the vasomotor centers of the medulla and respiratory center. Full circulatory and respiratory support is required to lighten the anesthetic state should the patient progress to this stage.

BOX 8-16

EXAMPLES OF ANESTHETICS

Inhalation Anesthetics
Gases
Cyclopropane
Nitrous oxide; oxygen (Nitronox)

Volatile liquids
Halothane (Fluothane)
Methoxyflurane (Penthrane)
Enflurane (Ethrane)
Isoflurane (Forane)

Intravenous Anesthetics
Ultrashort-acting barbiturates
Thiopental sodium (Pentothal)
Thiamylal sodium (Surital)
Methohexital sodium (Brevital Sodium)

Nonbarbiturates
Etomidate (Amidate)
Fentanyl (Sublimaze)

Sufentanil (Sufenta)
Alfentanil (Alfenta)

Dissociative anesthetics
Ketamine (Ketalar)

Neuroleptic anesthetics
Droperidol-fentanyl (Innovar injection)

Local Anesthetics
Topical
Benzocaine (Anbesol)
Cocaine
Ethyl chloride
Lidocaine (Xylocaine)

Injectable
Lidocaine (Xylocaine)
Procaine (Novocain)

---

ing a local anesthetic drug near a nerve trunk or at specific sites in a large region of the body (e.g., spinal block). Local anesthesia is achieved topically to produce a loss of sensation or by injection to "block" an area surrounding an operative field, making it insensitive to pain (e.g., minor wound repair) (Box 8-16).

Antianxiety and Sedative-Hypnotic Agents and Alcohol

Antianxiety and sedative-hypnotic agents and alcohol are presented together because of their similarities in pharmacological action. Antianxiety agents are used to reduce feelings of apprehension, nervousness, worry, or fearfulness.

Sedatives and hypnotics are drugs that depress the central nervous system, produce a calming effect, and help induce sleep (see the box below). The major difference between a sedative and a hypnotic is the degree of CNS depression induced by the agent. For example, a small dose of an agent administered to calm a patient is called a *sedative*; a larger dose of the same agent sufficient to induce sleep would be called a *hypnotic*. Therefore an agent may be a sedative or a hypnotic, depending on the dose used.

As previously stated, alcohol has actions characteristic of sedative-hypnotic or antianxiety drugs. Socially, alcohol is used mainly as a self-prescribed antianxiety agent; it is considered a major source of drug abuse and dependency.

Scattered throughout the brain stem is a group of nuclei collectively called the *reticular formation.* The reticular formation and its neural pathways constitute a system known as the *reticular activating system* (described in Chapter 6), which is involved with the sleep-wake cycle. Through these pathways incoming signals from the senses and viscera are collected, processed, and passed to the higher brain centers. The reticular activating system determines the level of awareness to the environment and therefore governs actions and responses to it. Antianxiety and sedative-hypnotic agents and alcohol act by depressing this system.

Classifications

Two prototypical groups of drugs used to treat anxiety or induce sleep are the benzodiazepines and barbiturates, respectively. Benzodiazepines comprise the drug class most commonly used today to treat anxiety and insomnia. Barbiturates constitute an older drug class with many uses, from sedation to anesthesia.

Benzodiazepines. Benzodiazepines were introduced in the 1960s as antianxiety drugs. Currently they are among the most widely prescribed drugs in clinical medicine. This popularity is partly because of their very high therapeutic index. Overdoses of 1000 times the therapeutic dose have been reported not to result in death unless taken in conjunction with other CNS depressants, such as alcohol.[6] Benzodiazepines are thought to work by binding to specific receptors in the cerebral cortex and limbic system (a major integrating system that governs emotional behavior). These drugs are highly lipid soluble and are widely distributed in the body tissues. They also are highly bound to plasma protein, usually more than 80%. Benzodiazepines have four actions: anxiety reducing, sedative-hypnotic, muscle relaxing, and anticonvulsant. All benzodiazepines are schedule IV drugs because of their potential for abuse. Commonly prescribed benzodiazepines are alprazolam (Xanax), chlordiazepoxide (Librium), clorazepate (Tranxene), *diazepam* (Valium), flurazepam (Dalmane), prazepam (Centrax), *midazolam* (Versed), *lorazepam* (Ativan), and triazolam (Halcion).

> ### THE PHYSIOLOGY OF SLEEP
>
> Sleep can be viewed as a series of rhythms, each with its own brain-wave patterns. These rhythms can be divided into two major categories: *rapid eye movement* (REM) and *non-rapid eye movement* (non-REM). During sleep, a person moves through REM sleep and then through four stages of non-REM sleep. REM, or active sleep, is the time of irregular body activity, vivid dreaming, and rapid eye movements. During REM the eyes move back and forth under the closed lids as they follow the action of a dream, and the heart rate, blood pressure, and respirations may become irregular. During non-REM the person drifts out of wakeful awareness, the muscles relax, and the blood pressure, heartbeat, and breathing begin to decline. The brain sends signals to the arms, legs, and other large muscles to stop moving, and "sleep paralysis" occurs. The first REM period lasts nearly 10 minutes, and the whole cycle repeats itself usually four to five times each night. Each cycle lasts an average of 90 minutes. As the night wears on, REM periods lengthen, and non-REM periods grow shorter. The final REM period of the night may last as long as 1 hour.

> ### ? CRITICAL THINKING
>
> *Why would a benzodiazepine be preferred over a narcotic when preparing to reduce a dislocated shoulder?*

> ### NOTE
>
> ***Flumazenil*** (Romazicon) is a specific benzodiazepine receptor antagonist and has been shown to be effective in reversing benzodiazepine-induced sedation and coma[7] (see Chapter 34 and the *Emergency Drug Index*).

Barbiturates. Barbiturates were once the most commonly prescribed class of medications for sedative-hypnotic effects, but they have been virtually replaced by the benzodiazepines. Barbiturates are divided into four classes according to their duration of action: ultra short acting, short acting, intermediate acting, and long acting. The differences in onset and duration of action depend on their lipid solubility and protein-binding properties. Ultra-short-acting barbiturates commonly are used as intravenous anesthetics. These drugs act rapidly and can produce a state of anesthesia in a few seconds. An example of an ultra-short-acting barbiturate is thiopental sodium (Pentothal).

Short-acting barbiturates produce an effect in a relatively short time (10 to 15 minutes) and peak over a relatively short period (3 to 4 hours). This class of drugs rarely is used to treat insomnia; it more commonly is used for preanesthesia sedation and in combination with other drugs for psychosomatic disorders. Examples include pentobarbital (Nembutal) and secobarbital (Seconal).

Intermediate-acting barbiturates have an onset of 45 to 60 minutes and peak in 6 to 8 hours. Short-acting and intermediate-acting agents have similar patient responses in the clinical setting. Examples of intermediate-acting barbiturates include amobarbital (Amytal) and butabarbital (Butisol Sodium).

Long-acting barbiturates require over 60 minutes for onset and peak over a period of 10 to 12 hours. These agents are used to treat epilepsy and other chronic neurological disorders and to sedate patients with severe anxiety. Examples of long-acting barbiturates include mephobarbital (Mebaral) and phenobarbital (Luminal).

Miscellaneous Sedative-Hypnotic Drugs. A number of antianxiety and sedative-hypnotic drugs that occasionally are used do not fall into the previously discussed drug classes. These agents are more similar to barbiturates than benzodiazepines in that they are generally shorter acting. Examples of miscellaneous drugs with antianxiety and sedative-hypnotic effects are chloral hydrate (Noctec), ethchlorvynol (Placidyl), and *etomidate* (Amidate). In addition to these drugs, antihistamines such as *hydroxyzine* (Vistaril, Atarax) have pronounced sedative effects.

Alcohol Intake and Behavioral Effects

Alcohol is a general CNS depressant that can produce sedation, sleep, and anesthesia. In addition, alcohol enhances the sedative-hypnotic effects of other drug classes, including all general CNS depressants, antihistamines, phenothiazines, narcotic analgesics, and tricyclic antidepressants. If alcohol is taken with other drugs, this enhancement could result in coma or death. Blood alcohol is measured in milligrams per deciliter (mg/dL). Based on the amount of alcohol consumed and blood alcohol levels, characteristic behavioral effects can be predicted. Behavioral effects associated with alcohol intake are further described in Chapter 34.

Anticonvulsants

Anticonvulsant drugs are used to treat seizure disorders, most notably epilepsy. Epilepsy is a neurological disorder characterized by a recurrent pattern of abnormal neuronal discharges within the brain. These discharges result in a sudden loss or disturbance of consciousness, sometimes associated with motor activity, sensory phenomena, or inappropriate behavior. It is estimated that epilepsy occurs in 0.5% to 1% of the population. In 50% of these cases, the cause is unknown (primary or idiopathic epilepsy). Secondary epilepsy is epilepsy that can be traced to trauma, infection, a cerebrovascular disorder, or some other illness. (Epilepsy is further discussed in Chapter 29.)

The exact mode and site of action of anticonvulsant drugs are not understood. In general, these drugs depress the excitability of neurons that fire to initiate the seizure or suppress generalization of the small focal depolarization that occurs, thus preventing the spread of seizure discharge. Anticonvulsants are presumed to modify the ionic movements of sodium, potassium, or calcium across the nerve membrane, thereby reducing the response to incoming electrical or chemical stimulation. Benzodiazepines also stimulate major inhibitory neurotransmitters in the central nervous system. Many patients require drug therapy throughout their lives to control seizure disorders.

Classifications

Several drugs are available for control of seizure disorders. The choice of drug depends on the type of seizure disorder (generalized, partial, or status) and the patient's tolerance and response to the prescribed medication. Classes of anticonvulsant drugs are presented in Box 8-17.

CLASSES OF ANTICONVULSANT DRUGS

Hydantoins
Ethotoin (Peganone)
Mephenytoin (Mesantoin)
Phenytoin (Dilantin)
Fosphenytoin (Cerebyx)

Barbiturates
Mephobarbital (Mebaral)
Phenobarbital (Luminal)

Succinimides
Ethosuximide (Zarontin)
Methsuximide (Celontin)
Phensuximide (Milontin)

Benzodiazepines
Clonazepam (Klonopin)
Diazepam (Valium)
Lorazepam (Ativan)

Other
Carbamazepine (Tegretol)
Gabapentin (Neurontin)
Lamotrigine (Lamictal)
Magnesium sulfate
Topiramate (Topamax)
Valproic acid (Depakene)

NOTE

A new class of drugs (GI lipase inhibitors, or "fat blockers") block the absorption of about 30% of dietary fat. These drugs sometimes are used in the management of obesity in conjunction with a reduced-calorie diet. An example of a GI lipase inhibitor is orlistat (Xenical).

NOTE

A two-drug combination of fenfluramine and phentermine ("fen-phen") that was used to manage obesity was withdrawn from the market in 1997. It was found to produce serious complications, including potentially fatal primary pulmonary hypertension and valvular heart disease.

Central Nervous System Stimulants

CNS stimulants are classified by where they exert their major effects in the nervous system—on the cerebrum, the medulla and brain stem, or in the hypothalamic limbic regions. All CNS stimulants work to increase excitability by blocking activity of inhibitory neurons or their respective neurotransmitters or by enhancing the production of the excitatory neurotransmitters. Some of the more common CNS stimulant drugs are anorexiants and amphetamines.

Anorexiants

Anorexiants are appetite suppressants used to treat obesity. They work by producing a direct stimulant effect on the hypothalamic and limbic regions and perhaps other areas of the nervous system. Examples of anorexiants include phendimetrazine (Plegine) and mazindol (Mazanor, Sanorex).

Amphetamines

Amphetamines stimulate the cerebral cortex and reticular activating system, thereby increasing alertness and responsiveness to environmental surroundings. They primarily are used in the treatment of attention deficit disorder (ADD) with hyperactivity and narcolepsy. ADD with hyperactivity primarily is seen in children and adolescents and is characterized by a short attention span and impulsive behavior. Individuals with narcolepsy experience excessive drowsiness, sudden sleep attacks during daytime hours, and sometimes sleep paralysis. Medications used to treat these disorders include methamphetamine (Desoxyn) and dextroamphetamine tablets and elixir. Nonamphetamine CNS stimulants used to treat ADD with hyperactivity include methylphenidate (Ritalin) and pemoline (Cylert).

NOTE

Amphetamines and other stimulants have a paradoxical effect of calming children with ADD with hyperactivity, probably by increasing neurotransmitter levels of dopamine.

Psychotherapeutic Drugs

Psychotherapeutic drugs include antipsychotic agents, antidepressants, and lithium. These drugs are used to treat psychoses and affective disorders, especially schizophrenia, depression, and mania (see Chapter 38).

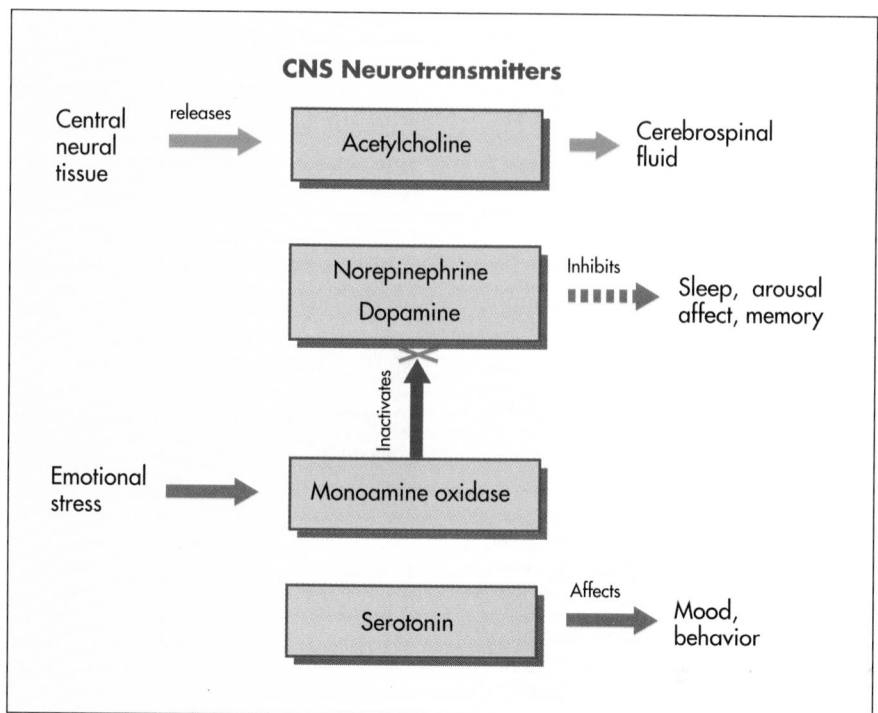

Fig. 8-11 Neurotransmitters in the brain and their effects on emotion.

Central Nervous System and Emotions

Neurotransmitters in the CNS that have major effects on emotion include acetylcholine, norepinephrine, dopamine, serotonin, and monoamine oxidase (Fig. 8-11). Alterations in the levels of these neurotransmitters are associated with changes in mood and behavior. Drug therapy alleviates symptoms by temporarily modifying unwanted behavior.

> **NOTE**
>
> Acetylcholine is released from central neural tissue into the cerebrospinal fluid during activity. Norepinephrine and dopamine have widespread inhibitory effects on functions such as sleep and arousal, affect, and memory. Serotonin levels affect mood and behavior. Monoamine oxidase is an enzyme that inactivates dopamine and serotonin, which are produced during intense emotional states.

Antipsychotic Agents

The primary use of antipsychotic drugs is to treat schizophrenia. This class of drugs represents the only clearly effective treatment for this condition. Other psychiatric indications for the use of antipsy-

chotic drugs include Tourette's syndrome and controlling disturbed behavior in patients with senile dementia associated with Alzheimer's disease. Effective antipsychotic (neuroleptic) drugs block dopamine receptors in specific areas of the central nervous system. These drugs can be classified into the following groups:

- Phenothiazine derivatives
    Chlorpromazine (Thorazine)
    Thioridazine (Mellaril)
    Fluphenazine (Prolixin)
- Butyrophenone derivatives
    Haloperidol (Haldol)
- Dihydroindolone derivatives
    Molindone (Moban)
- Dibenzoxazepine derivatives
    Loxapine (Loxitane)
- Thienbenzodiazepine derivatives
    Olanzapine (Zyprexa)
- Atypical agents
    Clozapine (Clozaril)
    Risperidone (Risperdal)

With continued use of antipsychotics, some patients develop supersensitivity of dopamine receptors that leads to tardive dyskinesia. Tardive dyskinesia is a potentially irreversible neurological disorder characterized by involuntary repetitious movements of the muscles of the face, limbs, and trunk. Other identifying features include excessive blinking of the eyelids, lip smacking, tongue protrusion, foot tapping, and rocking side-to-side.

Antidepressants

Antidepressants are used to treat affective disorders (mood disturbances), including depression, mania, and elation. Tricyclic antidepressants (TCAs) and monoamine oxidase (MAO) inhibitors are prescribed for depression; lithium (an antimanic drug) is the preferred treatment for mania.

> **NOTE**
>
> Depression may be exogenous, resulting from a person's response to a loss or disappointment (e.g., "the blues"). Exogenous depression is considered "normal" and usually is temporary and remits without the use of drug therapy. Endogenous depression lasts 6 months or longer and is characterized by the absence of external causes; it may be the result of genetic or biochemical alterations. Antidepressants often are needed to treat this disorder. Depression may be defined as a unipolar (continued or recurrent episodes) or a bipolar (manic-depressive) disorder (see Chapter 38).

Tricyclic antidepressants. TCAs are thought to treat depression by increasing levels (blocking reuptake) of the neurotransmitters norepinephrine and serotonin. Examples include imipramine (Tofranil) and amitriptyline (Elavil). Newer classes of antidepressants (second-generation drugs) also have been developed. These include bupropion (Wellbutrin), fluoxetine (Prozac), trazodone (Desyrel), and sertraline (Zoloft).

> **? CRITICAL THINKING**
>
> *Knowing that tricyclic antidepressants increase levels of norepinephrine, what side effects might you expect in an overdose situation?*

MAO inhibitor antidepressants. Central-acting monoamines, especially norepinephrine and serotonin, are thought to cause depression and mania. Monoamine oxidase (an enzyme found in nerve cells

thought to be produced during tense emotional states) is responsible for metabolizing norepinephrine within the nerve. MAO inhibitors block this enzyme, leading to increased levels of norepinephrine. Examples of MAO inhibitors used to treat depression include isocarboxazid (Marplan), phenelzine (Nardil), and tranylcypromine (Parnate). MAO inhibitors also are used as antihypertensive agents (described later in this chapter).

> **NOTE**
>
> MAO inhibitors can cause life-threatening reactions when taken with other drugs and certain foods (see the Emergency Drug Index).

Lithium. Lithium is a monovalent cation that is closely related to sodium. They are both actively transported across cell membranes, but lithium cannot be as effectively pumped out of the cell as can sodium. It therefore accumulates in the cells, which results in a decrease in intracellular sodium and perhaps an improvement in a manic state. In addition, lithium appears to enhance some of the actions of serotonin and may decrease levels of norepinephrine and dopamine. It also appears to block the development of dopamine receptor supersensitivity that may accompany long-term therapy with antipsychotic agents. Lithium carbonate, which is used to treat manic disorders, is available in capsule, tablet, and syrup form (e.g., lithium citrate).

Drugs for Specific Central Nervous System—Peripheral Dysfunction

Several movement disorders result from an imbalance of dopamine and acetylcholine. Two of the most common are Parkinson's disease (including parkinsonism syndromes) and Huntington's disease.

Parkinson's Disease

Parkinson's disease is a chronic disabling disease characterized by rigidity of voluntary muscles and tremor of the fingers and extremities (Box 8-18). The disease most often affects people over age 60 but may occur in younger people, especially after acute encephalitis or cases of carbon monoxide or metallic poisoning, or from the use of some illicit drugs. It is thought to result from an abnormally low concentration of dopamine.

BOX 8-18

SYMPTOMS OF PARKINSON'S DISEASE

Immobile facial expression (parkinsonism facies)
Bobbing of the head
Resting tremor
"Pill-rolling" of the fingers
Shuffling gait
Forward flexion of the trunk
Loss of postural reflexes

NOTE

Parkinsonism syndromes mimic the characteristics of Parkinson's disease. They usually are idiopathic but may result from treatment with antipsychotic drugs (drug-induced parkinsonism) that block dopaminergic receptors (e.g., **haloperidol,** metoclopramide, and phenothiazines).

Huntington's Disease

Huntington's disease is an inherited disorder characterized by progressive dementia and involuntary muscle twitching (chorea). Like Parkinson's disease, Huntington's disease is thought to be related to an imbalance of dopamine, acetylcholine, and perhaps other neurotransmitters.

Drugs with Central Anticholinergic Activity

Drugs that inhibit or block acetylcholine are referred to as **anticholinergic.** They work by restoring the normal dopamine-acetylcholine balance in the brain. Common anticholinergic agents include benztropine (tablets and injections) and ethopropazine hydrochloride.

Drugs That Affect Brain Dopamine

Three classifications of drugs affect brain dopamine: those that release dopamine, those that increase brain levels of dopamine, and dopaminergic agonists (Box 8-19). Levodopa (L-Dopa), a drug that increases brain levels of dopamine, is the current drug of choice in the treatment of movement disorders associated with dopamine-acetylcholine imbalance.

BOX 8-19

DRUGS THAT AFFECT BRAIN DOPAMINE

Levodopa (Larodopa)
Carbidopa-levodopa (Sinemet)
Amantadine (Symmetrel)
Bromocriptine (Parlodel)
Pergolide (Permax)

MAO inhibitors. Two types of monoamine oxidase have been identified: monoamine oxidase A, which metabolizes norepinephrine and serotonin, and monoamine oxidase B, which metabolizes dopamine. Selegiline (Deprenyl) is a selective inhibitor of monoamine oxidase B that retards the breakdown of dopamine. It often is used in conjunction with levodopa because it enhances and prolongs the antiparkinsonism effects of levodopa (allowing the dose of levodopa to be reduced).

Drugs That Affect the Autonomic Nervous System

The nervous and endocrine systems are the major means of controlling and integrating body functions. These two systems share three characteristics: a high-level integration in the brain, the ability to influence processes in distant regions of the body, and the extensive use of negative feedback mechanisms (described in Chapter 7). The major difference between the nervous and endocrine systems is the mode of transmission of information.

Endocrine system transmission primarily is chemical via blood-borne hormones. The hormones are not targeted for a particular organ but instead diffusely affect many cells and organs concurrently. In contrast, the nervous system primarily relies on rapid electrical transmission of information over nerve fibers, with chemical impulses carrying signals only between nerve cells and their effector cells in a very localized manner, perhaps affecting only a few cells. (Drugs that affect the endocrine system are presented later in this chapter.)

Classifications

The autonomic drugs mimic or block the effects of the sympathetic and parasympathetic divisions of the autonomic nervous system (see the box below). These drugs can be classified into four groups:

1. Cholinergic (parasympathomimetic) drugs, which mimic the actions of the parasympathetic nervous system

2. Cholinergic blocking (parasympatholytic) drugs, which block the actions of the parasympathetic nervous system
3. Adrenergic (sympathomimetic) drugs, which mimic the actions of the sympathetic nervous system or the adrenal medulla
4. Adrenergic blocking (sympatholytic) drugs, which block the actions of the sympathetic nervous system or adrenal medulla

Cholinergic drugs. Acetylcholine plays an important role in the parasympathetic and sympathetic divisions of the nervous system. It has two major effects in the nervous system: (1) a stimulant effect on the ganglia, adrenal medulla, and skeletal muscle (the "nicotinic effect" of acetylcholine) and (2) stimulant effects at postganglionic nerve endings in cardiac muscle, smooth muscle, and glands (the "muscarinic effect" of acetylcholine) (Table 8-4). Drugs that affect nicotinic or cholinergic receptor sites on autonomic ganglia are ganglionic-stimulating drugs (e.g., nicotine and nicotine gum) and ganglionic-blocking drugs (e.g., trimethaphan).

Cholinergic drugs act directly (choline esters) by combining with cholinergic receptors in postsynaptic membranes or indirectly by inhibiting the en-

---

ANATOMICAL AND FUNCTIONAL TERMS FOR THE AUTONOMIC NERVOUS SYSTEM

The anatomical names and functional terms for the autonomic nervous system are often used interchangeably: sympathetic or adrenergic, and parasympathetic or cholinergic. The terms *parasympathomimetic* and *sympathomimetic* mean to mimic or to produce an effect similar to activation of either system. The words *parasympatholytic* and *sympatholytic* mean to block the normal effects seen with activation of either system. The term *anticholinergic* is synonymous with *parasympatholytic*.

Anatomical name	Functional term	Primary neurotransmitter
Sympathetic	Adrenergic	Norepinephrine
Parasympathetic	Cholinergic	Acetylcholine

TABLE 8-4	SITES FOR MUSCARINIC AND NICOTINIC ACTIONS OF ACETYLCHOLINE	
SITE	**MUSCARINIC ACTION***	**NICOTINIC ACTIONS**
Cardiovascular		
Blood vessels	Dilation	Constriction ⎫
Heart rate	Slowed	Increased ⎬ With large doses after atropine
Blood pressure	Decreased	Increased ⎭
Gastrointestinal		
Tone	Increased	Increased
Motility	Increased	Increased
Sphincters	Relaxed	—
Glandular secretions	Increased salivary, lacrimal, intestinal, and sweat secretion	Initial stimulation and then inhibition of salivary and bronchial secretions
Skeletal muscle	—	Stimulation
Autonomic ganglia	—	Stimulation
Eye	Pupil constriction Decreased accommodation	—
Blocking agent	Atropine	Tubocurarine
Remarks	Above effects increase as dosage increases.	Increased dosage inhibits effects and causes receptor blockade.

*Usual sites for therapeutic effects.

zyme that normally degrades acetylcholine. This inhibition results in accumulation of acetylcholine, which causes a prolonged and intensified response at various effector sites. Cholinergic drugs have little therapeutic value and generally are not considered emergency medications. The major exception to this is *physostigmine* (Antilirium), an indirect-acting cholinergic drug that may be used to manage extreme cases of poisoning resulting from atropine-type drugs.

NOTE

Indirect-acting cholinergic drugs are used to treat myasthenia gravis, a condition characterized by weakness of the skeletal muscles. These drugs work to elevate the concentration of acetylcholine at myoneural junctions, thereby increasing muscle strength and function.

Cholinergic blocking (anticholinergic) agents have many uses in emergency medicine. These drugs work by blocking the muscarinic effects of acetylcholine, thereby decreasing acetylcholine's action on its effector organ.

The best-known cholinergic blocking drug used in emergency care is *atropine,* a belladonna alkaloid that functions as a competitive antagonist. It works by occupying muscarinic receptor sites, preventing or reducing the muscarinic response to acetylcholine. Large doses dilate the pupils, inhibit accommodation of the eyes, and increase the heart rate by blocking the cholinergic effects of the heart. Synthetic substitutes for *atropine* have been developed to obtain only the antispasmodic effects of the drug (e.g., in the treatment of gastric and duodenal ulcers). These synthetic drugs include dicyclomine (Bentyl) and glycopyrrolate (Robinul).

Adrenergic drugs. Adrenergic drugs are designed to produce activities like those of neurotransmitters. The three types of adrenergic agents are direct acting, indirect acting, and dual acting (direct and indirect).

Direct-acting drugs. Three naturally occurring catecholamines are present in the body: epinephrine, norepinephrine, and dopamine. Epinephrine acts mainly as an emergency hormone released by the adrenal medulla, and norepinephrine acts as an important transmitter of nerve impulses. Dopamine is a precursor of epinephrine and norepinephrine and

has a transmitter role of its own in certain parts of the central nervous system. Examples of synthetic catecholamine drugs and the three endogenous catecholamines are *epinephrine* (Adrenalin), *norepinephrine* (Levophed), *dopamine* (Intropin), and *dobutamine* (Dobutrex).

Catecholamines depend on their ability to act directly with alpha and beta receptors. Two subgroups of alpha receptors have been identified, alpha$_1$ and alpha$_2$. Alpha$_1$ receptors are postsynaptic receptors located on the effector organs. The primary role of the alpha$_1$ receptor is to stimulate contraction of smooth muscle. In the vasculature, this results in an increase in blood pressure. Alpha$_2$ receptors are found on presynaptic and postsynaptic nerve endings. When stimulated, presynaptic receptors inhibit the further release of norepinephrine. Like alpha$_1$ receptors, alpha$_2$ postsynaptic receptors mediate vasoconstriction to increase resistance and thus increase blood pressure.

Beta receptors are subdivided into beta$_1$ and beta$_2$ receptors. This classification is based on their response to drugs but also follows anatomical distinctions. Beta$_1$ receptors are located primarily in the heart, whereas beta$_2$ receptors are located predominantly in the bronchiolar and arterial smooth muscle. Beta receptors stimulate the heart; dilate bronchioles; dilate blood vessels in the skeletal muscle, brain, and heart; and aid in glycogenolysis (Table 8-5).

NOTE

A memory aid that may be useful for differentiating the physiological effects of beta receptors is: a person has one heart (beta-$_1$ effects) and two lungs (beta-$_2$ effects).

Norepinephrine acts mainly on alpha receptors and causes almost pure vasoconstriction. Epinephrine acts on alpha and beta receptors and produces a mixture of vasodilation and vasoconstriction, depending on the relative number of alpha and beta receptors present in the target tissue. The following are the most important alpha and beta activities in human beings:

- Alpha activities
  Vasoconstriction of arterioles in the skin and splanchnic area, resulting in a rise in blood pressure and peripheral shunting of blood

TABLE 8-5	ADRENERGIC RECEPTOR STIMULATION

EFFECTOR ORGANS	RECEPTOR TYPE	ADRENERGIC RESPONSE
Heart		
Cardiac muscle (atria, ventricles)	$Beta_1$	Increased force of contraction
Sinoatrial node	$Beta_1$	Increased heart rate
Atrioventricular node	$Beta_1$	Increased conduction velocity, shortened refractory period
Conduction tissue	$Beta_1$	
Blood vessels		
Arterioles (smooth muscle)		
Coronary	Alpha, $beta_2$, dopaminergic	Constriction, dilation
Cerebral	Alpha	Constriction
Pulmonary	Alpha, $beta_2$	Constriction, dilation
Mesenteric visceral	Alpha, $beta_2$, dopaminergic	Constriction, dilation
Renal	Alpha, $beta_2$, dopaminergic	Constriction, dilation
Skin, mucosa	Alpha	Constriction
Skeletal muscle	Alpha, $beta_2$	Constriction, dilation
Veins	Alpha, $beta_2$	Constriction, dilation
Lungs		
Bronchial smooth muscle	$Beta_2$	Bronchodilation (relaxation)
Bronchial glands	$Alpha_2$, $beta_2$	Inhibition
Gastrointestinal tract		
Smooth muscle (motility, tone)	$Alpha_2$, $beta_2$	Decrease
Sphincter	Alpha	Contraction
Secretion	?	Inhibition
Gallbladder and ducts	—	Relaxation
Liver	$Beta_2$	Glycogenolysis, gluconeogenesis
Spleen capsule	Alpha, $beta_2$	Contraction, relaxation
Pancreas: insulin secretion	Alpha	Decrease
Adipose tissue	$Beta_1$	Lipolysis
Urinary bladder		
Detrusor muscle	$Beta_1$	Relaxation
Sphincter	Alpha	Contraction
Kidney ureter	Alpha	Contraction
Kidney secretion (renin)	$Beta_2$	Increase
Uterus		
Pregnant	Alpha	Contraction
Nonpregnant	$Beta_2$	Relaxation
Sex organs, male	Alpha	Ejaculation
Skin		
Pilomotor muscles	Alpha	Contraction
Sweat glands	Cholinergic	Increased secretion
Eye		
Radial muscle, iris (pupil size)	Alpha	Contraction–pupil dilation (mydriasis)
Ciliary muscle	Beta	Relaxation for far vision

to the heart and brain from the shifting of blood volume

Pupil dilation

Relaxation of the gut

- Beta activities

Cardiac acceleration and increased contractility

Vasodilation of arterioles supplying the skeletal muscle

Bronchial relaxation

Uterine relaxation

Indirect-acting and dual-acting drugs. Indirect-acting adrenergic drugs act indirectly on receptors by triggering the release of the catecholamines, norepinephrine and epinephrine, which then activate the alpha and beta receptors. Dual-acting adrenergic drugs have indirect and direct effects. An example of a drug in this classification is ephedrine (ephedrine sulfate).

Adrenergic blocking agents may be classified into alpha- and beta-blocking drugs. Alpha-blocking drugs block the vasoconstricting effect of catecholamines. They are used in certain cases of hypertension and to help prevent necrosis when *norepinephrine* (Levophed) or *dopamine* (Intropin) has extravasated into the tissues. They have limited clinical application in the prehospital setting.

> **NOTE**
>
> Because of the possibility of extravasation and tissue necrosis, all drugs with alpha effects should be administered through a secure intravenous line well positioned in a large vein.

Beta-blocking agents have greater clinical application and frequently are used in emergency care. These drugs block beta receptors, thereby inhibiting their action at the effector site. Beta-blocking agents are grouped into selective blocking agents, which block beta$_1$ or beta$_2$ receptors, and nonselective beta blocking agents, which block beta$_1$ or beta$_2$ receptor sites. Selective beta$_1$ blocking agents also are known as *cardioselective blockers* because they block the beta$_1$ receptors in the heart. Examples of important selective beta$_1$ blocking agents are *metoprolol* (Lopressor) and *atenolol* (Tenormin). These drugs are antihypertensives and antidysrhythmics and are used in managing hypertension and select patients with suspected MI and high-risk unstable angina.

> **? CRITICAL THINKING**
>
> *Why will physicians typically not prescribe a nonselective beta blocker such as propranolol (Inderal) for patients with a history of asthma?*

Nonselective beta-blocking agents inhibit beta$_1$ receptors in the heart and beta$_2$ receptors in the smooth muscle of the bronchioles and blood vessels. Examples include the antianginal antihypertensives nadolol (Corgard) and *propranolol* (Inderal), and the antihypertensive *labetalol* (Normodyne, Trandate). (*Labetalol* also has some alpha-blocking activity.)

Skeletal Muscle Relaxants

Skeletal muscle contraction is evoked by a nicotinic cholinergic transmission process. It is therefore subject to the same types of pharmacological modification as autonomic ganglionic transmission. Skeletal muscle relaxants can be classified as central-acting, direct-acting, and neuromuscular blockers.

Central-Acting Muscle Relaxants

Central-acting drugs are used to treat muscle spasms. They are thought to work by producing CNS depression in the brain and spinal cord. Antispastic agents include baclofen (Lioresal), cyclobenzaprine (Flexeril), and *diazepam* (Valium).

Direct-Acting Muscle Relaxants

Direct-acting muscle relaxants work directly on skeletal muscles to produce muscle relaxation, resulting in a decrease in muscle contraction. Dantrolene (Dantrium) is an example of a direct-acting muscle relaxant.

Neuromuscular Blockers

Neuromuscular blocking drugs produce complete muscle relaxation and paralysis by binding to the nicotinic receptor for acetylcholine at the neuromuscular junction. Neuromuscular transmission is thus inhibited and remains so for a variable period, depending on the type and amount of neuromuscular blocker used.

Neuromuscular blockers are sometimes used to achieve total paralysis before ET intubation (described in Chapter 11), to relieve muscle spasms of the larynx, to suppress tetany, during electroconvulsive therapy (ECT) for depression, and to allow for breathing control by a respirator. Because these blocking agents produce complete paralysis, ventilatory support must be provided and the efficacy of ventilation and oxygenation closely monitored. (These muscle relaxants do not inhibit pain or seizure activity.) Examples of neuromuscular blockers include *pancuronium* (Pavulon), vecuronium (Norcuron), and *succinylcholine* (Anectine).

SECTION FIVE
DRUGS THAT AFFECT THE CARDIOVASCULAR SYSTEM

Review of Anatomy and Physiology

The heart is composed of many interconnected branching fibers or cells that form the walls of the two atria and two ventricles. Some of these cells are specialized to conduct electrical impulses. Others have contraction as their primary function. All of these cells are nourished through a profuse network of blood vessels (coronary vasculature). Cardiac drugs are classified by their effects on these tissues. Boxes 8-20 and 8-21 list cardiac drugs and pharmacological terms that describe their actions.

Cardiac Glycosides

Cardiac glycosides are naturally occurring plant substances that have characteristic effects on the heart. These compounds contain a carbohydrate molecule (sugar) that, when combined with water, is converted into a sugar plus one or more active substances. Glycosides may work by blocking certain ionic pumps in the cellular membrane, which indirectly increases the calcium concentration to the contractile proteins. An important cardiac glycoside is *digoxin* (Lanoxin), which is used to treat heart failure and to manage certain tachycardias.

Digitalis glycosides can affect the heart in two different ways: (1) they increase the strength of contraction, which is a positive inotropic effect, and (2) they have a dual effect on the electrophysiological properties of the heart. They have a modest negative chronotropic effect (causing slight slowing) and a more profound negative dromotropic effect, decreasing conduction velocity.

Side Effects

Many patients who take cardiac glycosides develop side effects at one time or another because of the small therapeutic index. The symptoms may be neurological, visual, gastrointestinal, cardiac, or psychiatric. These symptoms often are vague and can be easily attributed to a viral illness; therefore a high index of suspicion must be maintained in patients taking cardiac glycosides. The most common side effects of cardiac glycosides are anorexia, nausea or vomiting, visual disturbances (flashing lights, altered color vision), and cardiac rhythm disturbances (usually slowing with varying degrees of blocked conduction).

The toxic effects of cardiac glycosides are dose related. These effects may be increased by the presence of other drugs, such as diuretics, which may predispose the patient to cardiac rhythm disturbances. Dysrhythmias may include bradycardias, tachycardias, and even ventricular fibrillation. For these reasons, patients taking these drugs require close monitoring. Treatment for digitalis toxicity may include correction of electrolyte imbalances, neutralization of the free drug, and use of antidysrhythmics.

NOTE

Proarrhythmias are serious dysrhythmias seemingly generated by antidysrhythmic agents. All antidysrhythmics have some degree of proarrhythmic effects, and the sequential use of two or more antidysrhythmics compounds these effects. As a rule, it is best not to use more than one agent to manage dysrhythmias (unless absolutely necessary).

Antidysrhythmics

Antidysrhythmic drugs are used to treat and prevent disorders of cardiac rhythm. The pharmacological agents that suppress dysrhythmias may do so by direct action on the cardiac cell membrane *(lidocaine)*, by indirect action that affects the cell *(propranolol)*, or both.

Cardiac rhythm disturbances may be caused by ischemia, hypoxia, acidosis or alkalosis, electrolyte abnormalities, excessive catecholamine exposure, autonomic influences, drug toxicity, or scarred and diseased tissue. Dysrhythmias result from disturbances in impulse formation, disturbances in impulse conduction, or both.

Classifications

Antidysrhythmic drugs have been classified into categories based on their fundamental mode of ac-

BOX 8-20

EMERGENCY DRUGS: CARDIOVASCULAR SYSTEM

Drugs Used to Treat Dysrhythmias
Adenosine (Adenocard)
Amiodarone (Cordarone)
Atropine
Beta-Adrenergic Blockers
  Atenolol (Tenormin)
  Metoprolol (Inderal)
Calcium-Channel Blockers
  Diltiazem (Cardizem)
  Verapamil (Isoptin)
Dopamine (Intropin)
Isoproterenol (Isuprel)
Lidocaine (Xylocaine)
Magnesium
Procainamide (Pronestyl)

Drugs Used to Optimize Cardiac Output and Blood Pressure
Calcium Chloride
Digoxin (Lanoxin)
Dobutamine (Dobutrex)
Dopamine (Intropin)
Epinephrine (Adrenalin)
Furosemide (Lasix)
Nitroglycerin (Nitrostat, Tridil)
Norepinephrine (Levophed)
Sodium Bicarbonate
Vasopressin (Pitressin)

BOX 8-21

PHARMACOLOGICAL TERMS TO DESCRIBE ACTIONS OF CARDIOVASCULAR DRUGS

Chronotropic: Chronotropic drugs affect heart rate. If the drug accelerates the heart rate (e.g., ***isoproterenol*** [Isuprel]), it is said to have a *positive* chronotropic effect. A drug that decreases the heart rate (e.g., **verapamil** [Isoptin]) is said to have a *negative* chronotropic effect.

Dromotropic: Dromotropic drugs affect conduction velocity through the conducting tissues of the heart. If a drug speeds conduction, it is said to have a *positive* dromotropic effect. Examples of drugs with positive dromotropic effects include **isoproterenol** (Isuprel) and **phenytoin** (Dilantin). Drugs with negative dromotropic effects delay conduction (e.g., **verapamil** [Isoptin] and **adenosine** [Adenocard]).

Inotropic: Inotropic drugs strengthen or increase the force of cardiac contraction (a positive inotropic effect). Some examples include **digoxin** (Lanoxin), **dobutamine** (Dobutrex), **epinephrine** (Adrenalin), and **isoproterenol** (Isuprel). A drug that weakens or decreases the force of cardiac contraction has a negative inotropic effect. An example of such a drug is **propranolol** (Inderal).

tion on cardiac muscle.[8] Drugs that belong to the same class do not necessarily produce identical actions. However, all antidysrhythmic drugs have some ability to suppress automaticity.

NOTE

Local protocols and standing orders often are established to allow paramedics to administer certain drugs in specific situations before seeking medical direction. Examples include antidysrhythmics for a patient with specific cardiac conduction disturbances and first-line cardiac life support drugs for a patient in cardiac arrest.

Class I. Class I drugs are sodium channel blockers, which work to slow conduction. They are further divided into subclasses (Ia, Ib, and Ic) based on the extent of sodium-channel blockade. Examples of Class Ia drugs include quinidine (Quinaglute, Duraquin),

disopyramide, and *procainamide* (Pronestyl). Class Ib drugs decrease or have no effect on conduction velocity. Examples include *lidocaine* (Xylocaine) and *phenytoin* (Dilantin). Class Ic drugs profoundly slow conduction and are indicated only for control of life-threatening ventricular dysrhythmias. An example of a Class Ic drug is flecainide (Tambocor).

Class II. Class II drugs are beta-blocking agents, which reduce adrenergic stimulation of the heart. An example is *propranolol* (Inderal).

? CRITICAL THINKING

How might the signs of shock in a patient taking digoxin or propranolol vary from what might normally be expected?

Class III. Class III drugs produce potassium channel blockade, which increases contractility. Unlike other antidysrhythmic agents, drugs in this class do not suppress automaticity and have no effect on conduction velocity. These drugs are thought to terminate dysrhythmias that result from the reentry of blocked impulses. An example is *amiodarone* (Cordarone).

Class IV. Class IV drugs are also known as *calcium channel blockers*. These drugs are thought to work by blocking the inflow of calcium through the cell membranes of the cardiac and smooth muscle cells. This action depresses the myocardial and smooth muscle contraction, decreases automaticity, and in some cases decreases conduction velocity. Examples of calcium channel blockers include *verapamil* (Isoptin) and *diltiazem* (Cardizem).

Antihypertensives

High blood pressure affects as many as 50 million adults and children in the United States[9] and has been directly related to an increased incidence of stroke, cerebral hemorrhage, heart and renal failure, and coronary heart disease. The exact mechanism of action of many antihypertensive drugs is unknown. The ideal antihypertensive drug should accomplish the following:

- Maintain blood pressure within normal limits for various body positions
- Maintain or improve blood flow without compromising tissue perfusion or blood supply to the brain
- Reduce the workload of the heart
- Have no undesirable side effects
- Permit long-term administration without intolerance

Classifications

Antihypertensive drugs used to reduce blood pressure are classified into four major categories: diuretics, sympathetic blocking agents (sympatholytic drugs), vasodilators, and angiotensin-converting enzyme (ACE) inhibitors. Calcium channel blockers are also used to treat people with hypertension who do not respond to other drug therapies.

> **NOTE**
>
> Calcium channel blockers work as antihypertensives by limiting the flow of calcium into the small muscles wrapped around arteries that would normally cause arterial constriction.

Diuretics. Diuretics once were considered the initial drug of choice in managing mild hypertension. They also frequently were used with other antihypertensives when hypertension could not be controlled by diuretics alone. Use of these medications results in a loss of excess salt and water from the body by renal excretion. The decrease in plasma and extracellular fluid volume (which decreases preload and stroke volume), plus a direct effect on arterioles, results in lowered blood pressure. This response causes an initial decline of cardiac output, followed by a decrease in peripheral vascular resistance and a lowering of the blood pressure.

Thiazides are diuretics that are moderately effective in lowering blood pressure. Many antihypertensive agents cause retention of sodium and water, and thiazides may be given concomitantly to help prevent this side effect. An example of a thiazide diuretic is hydrochlorothiazide (HCTZ).

Loop diuretics are powerful, short-acting agents that inhibit sodium and chloride reabsorption in the loop of Henle. These medications cause excessive loss of potassium and an increase in the excretion of sodium and water. Loop diuretics produce fewer side effects than most other antihypertensives, although hypokalemia and profound dehydration can result from their use. These agents are prescribed to patients who have renal insufficiency or who cannot take other diuretics. An example of a loop diuretic is *furosemide* (Lasix).

> **NOTE**
>
> Many drugs are excreted by the kidneys, and patients with renal system dysfunction (acute or chronic renal failure) may accumulate drugs in their systems. These patients often require modifications in drug doses and dosing intervals in addition to diet modification and fluid restriction.

Potassium-sparing agents do not cause the potassium loss seen with other diuretics. These medications promote sodium and water loss without an accompanying loss of potassium. Potassium-sparing agents are used to treat hypertensive patients who become hypokalemic with other diuretics or who are apparently resistant to the antihypertensive effects of other diuretics. Potassium-sparing agents also can be used to treat some edematous states such as cirrhosis of the liver with ascites. An example of a potassium-sparing agent is spironolactone (Aldactone).

Combinations of diuretic agents also may be prescribed to lower blood pressure. These combination diuretics usually include hydrochlorothiazide (HCTZ). Examples include Aldactazide, a combination agent with HCTZ and spironolactone, and Dyazide, which contains HCTZ and triamterene. Other agents (e.g., calcium channel blockers, beta blockers, and ACE inhibitors) commonly are prescribed for therapy of hypertension. ACE inhibitors and carvedilol (Coreg, a beta blocker) often are used to manage patients with hypertension and congestive heart failure.

Sympathetic blocking agents.

Sympathetic blocking agents may be classified as beta-blocking agents and adrenergic-inhibiting agents. Beta-blocking agents are used to treat cardiovascular disorders, including patients with suspected MI, high-risk unstable angina, and hypertension. These drugs work by decreasing cardiac output and inhibiting renin secretion from the kidneys. Both actions result in lower blood pressure. In addition, beta-blocking drugs compete with epinephrine for available beta receptor sites, inhibiting tissue and organ response to beta stimulation. Examples of beta-blocking agents include the following:

- Beta$_1$-blocking agents (cardioselective)
  Acebutolol (Sectral)
  Atenolol (Tenormin)
  Metoprolol (Lopressor)
- Beta$_1$- and beta$_2$-blocking agents (nonselective)
  Labetalol (Normodyne, Trandate) (also has alpha$_1$-blocking properties)
  Nadolol (Corgard)
  Propranolol (Inderal)

Adrenergic-inhibiting agents work by modifying the sympathetic nervous system and are effective antihypertensive drugs. Arterial pressure is influenced through various mechanisms of the heart, blood vessels, and kidneys. Sympathetic stimulation increases the heart rate and force of myocardial contraction, constricts arterioles and venules, and causes the release of renin from the kidneys. Blocking this sympathetic stimulation can reduce blood pressure.

Adrenergic-inhibiting agents are classified as centrally acting adrenergic inhibitors or peripheral adrenergic inhibitors. The mechanism by which many of these agents work is unknown. It generally is believed that most have multiple sites of action. Examples include the following drugs:

- Centrally acting adrenergic inhibitors
  Clonidine hydrochloride (Catapres)
  Methyldopa (Aldomet)
- Peripheral adrenergic inhibitors
  Guanethidine sulfate (Ismelin)
  Reserpine (Sandril, Serpasil)
  Prazosin hydrochloride (Minipress)
  Phentolamine (Regitine)
  Phenoxybenzamine (Dibenzyline)

Vasodilator drugs.

Vasodilator drugs act directly on the smooth muscle walls of the arterioles, veins, or both, lowering peripheral resistance and blood pressure. This stimulates the sympathetic nervous system and activates the baroreceptor reflexes, leading to an increase in heart rate, cardiac output, and renin release. Combined therapy usually is prescribed to inhibit the sympathetic response.

In addition to their use as antihypertensives, some vasodilator drugs are effective for treating angina pectoris (ischemic chest pain). For example, nitrates dilate veins and arteries. Their dilating effects on veins lead to venous pooling and a diminished blood return to the heart, thus reducing left ventricular end-diastolic volume and pressure. The subsequent decrease in wall tension helps reduce myocardial oxygen demand and the chest pain associated with myocardial ischemia. Vasodilator drugs are classified as arteriolar dilators and arteriolar and venous dilators. Examples of each include the following:

- Arteriolar dilator drugs
  Diazoxide (Hyperstat IV)
  Hydralazine (Apresoline)
  Minoxidil (Loniten)
- Arteriolar and venous dilator drugs
  Sodium nitroprusside (Nipride, Nitropress)
  Nitrates and nitrites
  Amyl nitrite inhalant
  Isosorbide dinitrate (Isordil, Sorbitrate)
  Nitroglycerin sublingual tablet (Nitrostat)
  Nitroglycerin paste (Nitro-Bid, Nitrostat, Nitrol)
  Intravenous *nitroglycerin* (Tridil)

Angiotensin-converting enzyme (ACE) inhibitor drugs. As described in Chapter 7, the renin-angiotensin-aldosterone system plays an important role in maintaining blood pressure and sodium and fluid balance. A disturbance in this system can result in hypertension. In addition, kidney damage can result in an inability to regulate the release of renin through normal feedback mechanisms, causing elevated blood pressure in some patients.

Angiotensin II is a powerful vasoconstrictor. It raises blood pressure and causes the release of aldosterone, which contributes to sodium and water retention. By inhibiting conversion of the precursor angiotensin I to the active molecule angiotensin II (which is brought about through ACE), the renin-angiotensin-aldosterone system is suppressed and blood pressure is lowered. Examples of ACE inhibitors include captopril (Capoten), enalapril (Vasotec), and lisinopril (Prinivil).

> **NOTE**
>
> Popular antiinflammatory drugs such as Advil, Motrin, Naprosyn, and Indocin can blunt the actions of ACE inhibitors.

Other antihypertensive agents. Other antihypertensive drugs include calcium channel blocking drugs and ganglionic-blocking agents. Calcium channel blocking agents such as *verapamil* (Isoptin), and *diltiazem* (Cardizem) reduce peripheral vascular resistance by inhibiting the contractility of vascular smooth muscle. They dilate coronary vessels through the same mechanism. The effects of these drugs are important in treating hypertension, decreasing the oxygen requirements of the heart (through decreased afterload), and increasing oxygen supply (by abolishing coronary artery spasm), thus relieving the causes of angina pectoris. The various drugs in this class differ in degree of selectivity for coronary (and peripheral) vasodilation or decreased cardiac contractility.

Ganglionic-blocking agents block sympathetic and parasympathetic ganglia. These drugs decrease peripheral vascular resistance, cardiac output, and stroke volume and are considered less safe than those previously described. They rarely are used today. Their major contribution in the past was to treat hypertension in patients who had dissecting aortic aneurysms. Today, these patients would most likely be treated with a combination beta-blocking agent and sodium nitroprusside (Nipride, Nitropress). Examples of these ganglionic-blocking agents include trimethaphan (Arfonad), pargyline hydrochloride (Eutonyl), and metyrosine (Demser).

Monoamine oxidase inhibiting drugs work to lower blood pressure by blocking the release of norepinephrine at the sympathetic junction, thereby interfering with vasoconstriction. Because these drugs affect sympathetic impulses, they reduce peripheral vascular resistance and decrease blood pressure. MAO inhibitors may adversely interact with many over-the-counter medications, prescription drugs, and some foods and may cause life-threatening side effects. They are not widely used to treat hypertension.

Antihemorrheologic Agents

Antihemorrheologic agents are used to treat peripheral vascular disorders caused by pathological or physiological obstruction (e.g., arteriosclerosis). These drugs improve blood flow (and the delivery of oxygen) to ischemic tissues by restoring red-blood-cell flexibility and lowering blood viscosity. An example of an antihemorrheologic agent is pentoxifylline (Trental).

SECTION SIX
DRUGS THAT AFFECT THE BLOOD

Anticoagulants, Fibrinolytics, and Blood Components

Bleeding and thrombosis are altered states of hemostasis. Understanding the drugs that affect blood coagulation and the use of fibrinolytic agents and blood components is necessary in prehospital patient management.

Anticoagulants

As described in Chapter 6, platelets are small cell fragments in the blood that provide the initial step in normal repair of blood vessels. Blood coagulation is a process that results in the formation of a stable fibrin clot that entraps platelets, blood cells, and plasma. The end result of this process is called a blood clot, or thrombus. Abnormal thrombus formation (i.e., intravascular clotting) is the major cause of myocardial infarction (from coronary thrombosis) and stroke (from cerebral vascular thrombosis).

The coagulation process also occurs in the venous system, although the underlying mechanisms responsible for the thrombosis differ. Arterial thrombi commonly are associated with atherosclerotic plaques, hypertension, and turbulent blood flow that damages the endothelial lining of blood vessels. Damage to the endothelium causes platelets to stick and aggregate in the arterial system. Arterial thrombi are composed mostly of platelets but also involve the chemical substances that contribute to the coagulation process (in particular, fibrinogen and fibrin). Myocardial infarctions and strokes are frequently the result of arterial thrombi.

The three major risk factors for various thromboses are stasis, localized trauma, and hypercoagulable states. Stasis, or reduced blood flow, results from immobilization or venous insufficiency. It is responsible for the increased incidence of deep vein thrombosis (DVT) in most bedridden patients. Localized trauma may initiate the clotting cascade and cause arterial and venous thrombosis. Hypercoagulability is the mechanism behind the increased incidence of DVT in women who take birth control pills and is also responsible for many of the familial thrombotic disorders (see Chapter 28).

Agents That Affect Blood Coagulation

Drugs that affect blood coagulation may be classified as antiplatelet, anticoagulant, and fibrinolytic agents.

Antiplatelet agents. Drugs that interfere with platelet aggregation are known as *antiplatelet* or *antithrombic* drugs. These drugs sometimes are prescribed prophylactically for patients at risk of developing arterial clots and those who have suffered myocardial infarction or stroke. Antiplatelet agents also are used to treat certain valvular heart diseases, valvular prostheses, and various intracardiac shunts. Among the most common antiplatelet drugs are *aspirin*, dipyridamole (Persantine), clopidrogrel (Plavix), ticlopidine (Ticlid), and abciximab (ReoPro).

Anticoagulant agents. Anticoagulant drug therapy is designed to prevent intravascular thrombosis by decreasing blood coagulability. It commonly is used to prevent postoperative thromboembolism; it also is used during hemodialysis and in reperfusion

therapy for select patients with acute coronary syndromes. This therapy primarily is prophylactic against future clot formation and has no direct effect on a blood clot that has already formed or on ischemic tissue injured by inadequate blood supply as a result of a thrombus. The major side effect of anticoagulant therapy is hemorrhage, and patients taking anticoagulants are prone to bleeding complications. Examples of anticoagulant agents include warfarin (Coumadin) and *heparin* (Liquaemin).

> **NOTE**
>
> Platelet adhesion, activation, and aggregation that result in the formation of an arterial thrombus are pivotal in the pathogenesis of acute coronary syndromes (acute myocardial infarctions). Recent studies indicate that the administration of a glycoprotein (GP) IIb/IIIa receptor antagonist may reduce ischemic complications after plaque fissure or rupture by inhibiting GP receptors in the membrane of platelets (thereby inhibiting platelet aggregation). These drugs may be included along with **aspirin, heparin,** and beta blockers during in-hospital reperfusion therapy for select patients. Examples of GP IIb/IIIa inhibitors include abciximab (ReoPro), eptifbatide (Integrilin), and tirofiban (Aggrastat).

Fibrinolytic Agents

Fibrinolytic drugs dissolve clots after their formation by promoting the digestion of fibrin. Fibrinolytic therapy has become the treatment of choice for treating acute myocardial infarction in certain groups of patients and in the management of some stroke patients. The goal is to reestablish blood flow and prevent ischemia and tissue death. Fibrinolytic therapy also has been used in acute pulmonary embolism, DVT, and peripheral arterial occlusion. Fibrinolytics are used in the prehospital setting in several areas of the United States. These drugs include *streptokinase* (Streptase), *tissue plasminogen activator* (t-PA, Activase), *retivase* (Retavase), reteplase, alteplase, anistreplase, and tenectaplase (see Chapter 28 and the Emergency Drug Index).

> **? CRITICAL THINKING**
>
> *If fibrinolytics have the potential to dissolve clots and reverse the catastrophic effects of myocardial infarction and stroke, why aren't they given to everyone suspected of having these conditions?*

Antihemophilic Agents

Hemophilia (further described in Chapter 35) is a group of hereditary bleeding disorders in which the individual is deficient in one of the factors necessary for coagulation of blood. These conditions are characterized by persistent and uncontrollable hemorrhage after even minor injury. Bleeding may occur into joints, the urinary tract, and on occasion the central nervous system. Hemophilia A (classic hemophilia) is caused by a deficiency of factor VIII. Hemophilia B (the "Christmas disease") results from a deficiency in factor IX complex. Replacement therapy of the missing clotting factor can be effective in the management of hemophilia. These include factor VIII (Factorate), factor IX (Konyne), and anti-inhibitor coagulant complex (Autoplex).

> **NOTE**
>
> Coagulation factors refer to the 13 proteins contained in blood plasma that interact to produce a blood clot.

Hemostatic Agents

Hemostatic agents hasten clot formation to reduce bleeding. Systemic hemostatic agents (e.g., Amicar, Cyklocapron) generally are used to control rapid blood loss after surgery by inhibiting fibrinolysis. Topical hemostatic agents (e.g., Gelfoam, Novocell) are used to control capillary bleeding during surgical and dental procedures.

Blood and Blood Components

The healthy body maintains a normal balance of blood and its components. However, illness and injury, such as hemorrhage, burns, and dehydration, may impair this balance and require replacement therapy.

Replacement Therapies

The usual treatment of choice in managing an imbalance of blood or blood components is to replace the sole blood component that is deficient. Replacement therapy may include transfusing the following:

- Whole blood (rarely used)
- Packed red blood cells
- Fresh-frozen plasma
- Plasma expanders (Dextran)
- Platelets
- Coagulation factors
- Fibrinogen
- Albumin
- Gamma globulins

Antihyperlipidemic Drugs

Hyperlipidemia refers to an excess of lipids in the plasma. There are several types of hyperlipidemia, and all are associated with elevated levels of cholesterol and triglycerides. Because this condition is thought to play a role in the development of atherosclerosis, anithyperlipidemic drugs are sometimes used in conjunction with diet and exercise to control serum lipid levels (Box 8-22).

> **NOTE**
>
> Antihyperlipidemic drugs do not reverse existing atherosclerosis.

BOX 8-22

EXAMPLES OF ANTIHYPERLIPIDEMIC DRUGS

Atorvastatin (Lipitor)
Cerivistatin (Baycol)
Cholestyramine (Questran)
Niacin (Nicobid)
Pravastatin (Pravachol)
Lovastatin (Mevacor)
Simvastatin (Zocor)

BOX 8-23

EMERGENCY DRUGS: RESPIRATORY SYSTEM

Albuterol (Proventil, Ventolin)
Dexamethasone (Decadron)
Diphenhydramine (Benadryl)
Epinephrine (Adrenalin) 1:1000
Promethazine (Phenergan)
Racemic epinephrine (Micronephrin)

Review of Anatomy and Physiology

The respiratory system includes all structures involved in the exchange of oxygen and carbon dioxide. Serious narrowing of any portion of the respiratory tract may be an indication for pharmacological therapy (Box 8-23). Emergencies involving the respiratory system usually are caused by reversible conditions such as asthma, emphysema with infection, and foreign body airway obstruction (see Chapter 11).

Smooth muscle fibers of the tracheobronchial tree are arranged along the length of the tubular air passage and directly influence the diameter of the airways. The bronchial smooth muscle tone is maintained by impulses from the autonomic nervous system. Parasympathetic fibers from the vagus nerve innervate bronchial smooth muscle through the release of acetylcholine. This neurotransmitter interacts with the muscarinic receptors on the membranes of the cell, producing bronchoconstriction.

Sympathetic fibers primarily affect beta$_2$ receptors in the lungs through the release of epinephrine from the adrenal medulla and the release of norepinephrine from the peripheral sympathetic nerves. The epinephrine reaches the lungs by way of the circulatory system and interacts with beta$_2$ receptors to produce smooth muscle relaxation and bronchodilation. Thus the beta$_2$ receptor plays the dominant role in bronchial muscle tone. (Although beta$_1$ receptors also are found on bronchial smooth muscle, their ratio to beta$_2$ receptors is 1:3.)

Bronchodilators

Bronchodilator drugs are the primary treatment modality for obstructive pulmonary disease such as asthma, chronic bronchitis, and emphysema. These drugs may be classified as sympathomimetic drugs and xanthine derivatives. Many of these agents are administered by inhalation via a nebulizer or pressure cartridge (see Chapter 27).

Sympathomimetics

Sympathomimetic drugs are grouped according to their receptor action: nonselective adrenergic drugs have alpha, beta$_1$ (cardiac), and beta$_2$ (respiratory) activity. Nonselective beta adrenergic drugs have both beta$_1$ and beta$_2$ effects. Selective beta$_2$ receptor drugs act primarily on beta$_2$ receptors in the lungs (bronchial smooth muscle). Box 8-24 summarizes the alpha, beta$_1$, and beta$_2$ activities of the adrenergic drugs used as bronchodilators.

Nonselective adrenergic drugs stimulate alpha and beta receptors. The alpha activity mediates vasoconstriction to reduce mucosal edema. Beta$_2$ activity produces bronchodilation and vasodilation. Undesirable beta$_1$ effects include an increase in heart rate and force of contraction. Undesirable beta$_2$ effects include muscle tremors and central nervous system stimulation. Examples of nonselective adrenergic drugs include epinephrine inhalation aerosol (Bronkaid Mist, Primatene Mist), epinephrine inhalation solution (Adrenalin), and *racemic epinephrine* inhalation solution (micro-Nephrin).

Because nonselective beta adrenergic drugs are not selective for beta$_2$ receptors, they have a wide range of effects (previously described). Examples of nonselective beta adrenergic drugs include *epinephrine* (Adrenalin, Asmolin, and others), ephedrine (Ephed II), and ethylnorepinephrine (Bronkephrine), which each have some alpha activity; isoproterenol inhalation solution (Aerolone, Vapo-Iso, Isuprel); and isoproterenol inhalation aerosol (Isuprel Mistometer, Norisodrine Aerotrol).

The selective action of beta$_2$ selective drugs lessens the incidence of unwanted cardiac effects caused by beta$_1$ adrenergic agents. Patients with hypertension, cardiac disease, or diabetes can better tolerate this group of bronchodilators. Examples of selective beta$_2$ receptor drugs include *albuterol* (Proventil, Ventolin), bitolterol (Tornalate), and isoetharine (Bronkosol, others).

Xanthine Derivatives

The xanthine group of drugs includes caffeine, theophylline, and theobromine. These drugs relax smooth muscle (particularly bronchial smooth muscle), stimulate cardiac muscle and the central nervous system, increase diaphragmatic contractility, and promote diuresis through increased renal perfusion. The action of various theophylline compounds depends on

BOX 8-24

ALPHA, BETA₁, AND BETA₂ ACTIVITIES OF ADRENERGIC DRUGS USED AS BRONCHODILATORS

Alpha Effects (Vasoconstriction)
Systemic effects
Vasoconstriction
Increased blood pressure

Inhalation
Decreased bronchial congestion
Increased duration of action for coadministered beta₂ drugs

Beta₁ Effects
Systemic effects
Cardiac stimulation
  Increased heart rate
  Increased force of contraction
  Possible palpitations and dysrhythmias
Relaxation of gastrointestinal tract

Inhalation
Some bronchodilation and increased heart rate
Fewer effects than with subcutaneous administration

Beta₂ Effects
Systemic effects
Bronchiole dilation
Stimulation of skeletal muscles (tremors)
Vasodilation (mainly in blood vessels supplying muscle)
Glycogenolysis

Central Nervous System Effects
Nervousness
Anxiety
Insomnia
Irritability
Dizziness
Sweating

Inhalation
Lower incidence of systemic effects than with subcutaneous administration

the content of theophylline, which is the active constituent. Theophylline products vary in their rate of absorption and therapeutic effects. There are many theophylline-containing preparations, including aminophylline (Amoline, Somophyllin, Theo-Dur, Aminophyllin), dyphylline (Dilor, Droxine, Lufyllin), and theophylline (Bronkodyl, Elixophyllin, Somophyllin-T, others).

> **NOTE**
> Theophylline preparations generally are not considered a first-line drug in the treatment of acute reactive airway disease.

Other Respiratory Drugs

A variety of other pharmacological agents can be used to treat asthma and other obstructive pulmonary diseases. These drugs include prophylactic asthmatic agents, such as cromolyn sodium (Intal, Sodium Cromoglycate); aerosol corticosteroid agents, such as beclomethasone dipropionate (Vanceril Inhaler, Beclovent); *dexamethasone* (Decadron); and

muscarinic antagonists (anticholinergics), such as *ipratropium* (Atrovent) and glycopyrrolate (Robinul). These medications reduce the allergic or inflammatory response to a variety of stimuli or have an effect on bronchial smooth muscle. In the acute care setting, intravenous steroids (e.g., *methylprednisolone* [Solu-Medrol]) may be given in an attempt to decrease the inflammatory response and improve airflow.

Mucokinetic Drugs

Mucokinetic drugs are used to move respiratory secretions, excessive mucus, and sputum along the tracheobronchial tree. These agents work by altering the consistency of these secretions so that they can more easily be removed from the body. Individ-

> **NOTE**
> Mucus is a normal secretion produced by the surface cells in the mucous membranes. Sputum is an abnormal viscous secretion (that consists mainly of mucus) originating in the lower respiratory tract.

uals with chronic pulmonary disease often use mucokinetic drugs to clear their respiratory passages and to improve ciliary activity.

Mucokinetic drugs include diluents (water, saline solution), aerosols, and mucolytic drugs or expectorants (Mucomyst).

Oxygen and Miscellaneous Respiratory Agents

Oxygen is chiefly used to treat hypoxia and hypoxemia. It is a colorless, odorless, and tasteless gas that is essential for sustaining life. (Oxygen and oxygen delivery are described in detail in Chapter 11.)

Direct Respiratory Stimulants

Direct respiratory stimulants (analeptics) act directly on the medullary center of the brain to increase the rate and depth of respirations. These drugs are considered inferior to mechanical ventilatory measures to treat respiratory depression and to counteract drug-induced respiratory depression caused by anesthetics. An example of a direct respiratory stimulant is doxapram (Dopram).

Reflex Respiratory Stimulants

Spirits of ammonia is the only drug given by inhalation as a reflex respiratory stimulant. The noxious vapor is administered in cases of fainting and works by irritating sensory nerve receptors in the throat and stomach. After inhalation, respirations are stimulated through afferent messages to the control centers of the brain.

Respiratory Depressants

Respiratory depressants include those of the opium and barbiturate groups of drugs previously described. Respiratory depression is a common side effect for these useful drugs, but they seldom are given to intentionally inhibit rate and depth of respiration.

Cough Suppressants

The cough is a protective reflex to expel harmful irritants. It may be productive when removing irritants or secretions from the airway, or nonproductive (dry and irritating). When the cough is prolonged or secondary to an underlying disorder, treatment with antitussive drugs may be indicated. Box 8-25 presents a few narcotic and nonnarcotic antitussive agents.

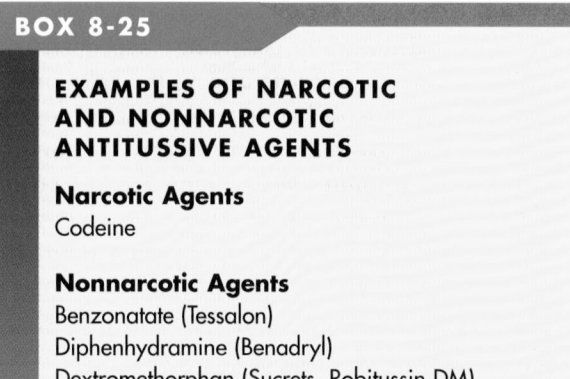

BOX 8-25

EXAMPLES OF NARCOTIC AND NONNARCOTIC ANTITUSSIVE AGENTS

Narcotic Agents
Codeine

Nonnarcotic Agents
Benzonatate (Tessalon)
Diphenhydramine (Benadryl)
Dextromethorphan (Sucrets, Robitussin DM)

Antihistamines

Histamine is a chemical mediator found in almost all body tissues. The concentration is highest in the skin, lungs, and gastrointestinal tract. The body releases histamine when exposed to an antigen, such as pollen or insect stings. This results in increased localized blood flow, increased capillary permeability, and swelling of the tissues. In addition, histamine produces contractile action on bronchial smooth muscle.

Allergic responses involving histamines and other chemical mediators include local effects such as angioedema, eczema, rhinitis, urticaria, and asthma. Systemic effects from the release of histamine and certain other mediators may result in anaphylaxis (see Chapter 31).

Antihistamines compete with histamine for receptor sites, thereby preventing the physiological action of histamine. The two types of histamine receptors are H_1 receptors (acting primarily on the blood vessels and the bronchioles) and H_2 receptors (acting mainly on the gastrointestinal tract). In addition to blocking some actions of histamine, antihistamines also have anticholinergic or atropine-like action. This may result in tachycardia, constipation, drowsiness, sedation, and inhibition of secretions. Most antihistamines also have a local anesthetic effect that may soothe the skin irritation caused by an allergic reaction. The primary clinical use of antihistamines is for allergic reactions, but they also are sometimes prescribed to control motion sickness or as a sedative or antiemetic. Examples of antihistamines are dimenhydrinate (Dramamine), *diphenhydramine* (Benadryl), *hydroxyzine* (Vistaril), *promethazine* (Phenergan, others), and the newer H_1 receptor antagonists, loratadine (Claritin) and fexofenadine (Allegra).

Serotonin

Serotonin is a naturally occurring vasoconstrictor material found in platelets and in the cells of the brain and intestine. It has several pharmacological actions that are exerted on various smooth muscles and nerves. Serotonin is not administered as a drug but has a major influence on other drugs and some disease states. It is helpful in repairing damaged blood vessels, stimulates smooth muscle contraction, and acts as a neurotransmitter in the central nervous system, where it has an effect on sleep, pain perception, and some mental illnesses.

Antiserotonins

Antiserotonins (serotonin antagonists) work to inhibit responses to serotonin and its influence on other drugs and disease states. Specific antiserotonins block smooth muscle contraction and vasoconstriction and inhibit the action of serotonin in the brain. Some antiserotonins are used to treat vascular headaches and allergic disorders. Examples of these drugs include cyproheptadine (Periactin), lysergic acid diethylamide (LSD), and methysergide maleate (Sansert).

SECTION EIGHT
DRUGS THAT AFFECT THE GASTROINTESTINAL SYSTEM

Review of Anatomy and Physiology

The GI system is comprised of the digestive tract, the biliary system, and the pancreas (see Chapter 6). The primary function of the GI system is to provide the body with water, electrolytes, and other nutrients used by cells. Drug therapy for the GI system can be divided into drugs that affect the stomach and drugs that affect the lower GI tract. In emergency care, conditions of the stomach or gastrointestinal tract that may require drug therapy usually are limited to nausea and vomiting (Box 8-26.)

Drugs That Affect the Stomach

Conditions of the stomach that may require drug therapy include hyperacidity, hypoacidity, ulcer disease, nausea, vomiting, and hypermotility.

Antacids

Antacids buffer or neutralize hydrochloric acid in the stomach and are prescribed for the relief of symptoms associated with hyperacidity. These conditions include peptic ulcer, gastritis, esophagitis, heartburn, and hiatal hernia. Common over-the-counter antacids include Alka-Seltzer, Gaviscon, and Rolaids.

Antiflatulents

Antiflatulents prevent the formation of gas in the GI tract. Gas retention is a common condition with diverticulitis, ulcer disease, and spastic or irritable colon. These drugs sometimes are used in combination with antacids. Simethicone (Mylicon) is an example of an antiflatulent.

Digestants

Digestant drugs promote digestion in the GI tract by releasing small amounts of digestive enzymes in the small intestine. Examples of digestants include pancreatin and pancrelipase (Pancrease).

Emetics and Antiemetics

Vomiting is an involuntary action coordinated by the emetic center of the medulla. It may be initiated through the central nervous system as a secondary reaction to emotion, pain, or disequilibrium (motion sickness); through irritation of the mucosa of the gastrointestinal tract or bowel; or through stimulation from the chemoreceptor trigger zone of the medulla by circulating drugs and toxins (e.g., opiates or digitalis).

Emetics. Drugs used to induce vomiting are rarely administered today as part of the treatment for

---

BOX 8-26

EMERGENCY DRUGS: GASTROINTESTINAL SYSTEM

Activated charcoal
Diphenhydramine (Benadryl)
Hydroxyzine (Vistaril)
Prochlorperazine (Compazine)
Promethazine (Phenergan)
Syrup of ipecac

drug overdoses and poisonings. These drugs include apomorphine and *syrup of ipecac.* The treatment of drug overdoses and poisoning is further addressed in Chapter 34.

Antiemetics. Drugs used to treat nausea and vomiting include antagonists of histamine, acetylcholine, and dopamine, and other drugs whose actions are not clearly understood. These drugs are most effective when administered before rather than after nausea and vomiting have begun. For example, drugs used to treat motion sickness or vertigo should be taken 30 minutes before traveling. Common antiemetics include scopolamine (Transderm-Scop), dimenhydrinate (Dramamine), *diphenhydramine* (Benadryl), *hydroxyzine* (Vistaril), meclizine (Antivert), *promethazine* (Phenergan), prochlorperazine (Compazine), and ondansetron (Zofran).

> **NOTE**
>
> Cannabinoids are drugs derived from hemp plants. They have been used experimentally as an antiemetic in patients receiving cancer chemotherapy. Examples of these drugs include dronabinol (Marinol) and nabilone (Cesamet). These drugs use a synthetic derivative of the active ingredient in marijuana.

Cytoprotective Agents

Cytoprotective agents are drugs that protect cells from damage. They are used along with other drugs to treat peptic ulcer disease by protecting the gastric mucosa. Examples of these drugs include sucralfate (Carafate) and misprostol (Cytotec).

H₂-Receptor Antagonists

As previously described, the action of histamine is mediated through H_2 receptors and has been associated with gastric acid secretion. H_2-receptor antagonists block the H_2 receptors and reduce the volume of gastric acid secretion and its acid content. Examples of H_2-receptor antagonists include cimetidine (Tagamet), ranitidine (Zantac), and famotidine (Pepcid).

Drugs That Affect the Lower Gastrointestinal Tract

Constipation and diarrhea are two common conditions of the lower GI tract that may require drug therapy. Drugs used to manage these conditions include laxatives and antidiarrheals.

Laxatives

Laxatives produce defecation. They are used to evacuate the bowel and to soften hardened stool for easier passage. Situations that may indicate the need for laxative use include the following:

- Constipation
- Neurological diseases (e.g., multiple sclerosis, Parkinson's disease)
- Pregnancy
- Rectal disorders
- Drug poisoning
- Surgery and endoscopic examination

> **NOTE**
>
> Regular or excessive use of laxatives is common in older adults and in those with eating disorders. Laxative abuse may result in permanent bowel damage and electrolyte imbalance.

Numerous types of laxatives are available, and many can be bought without a prescription. Examples include saline laxatives (Epsom salt, Milk of Magnesia), stimulant laxatives (Dulcolax, castor oil, Ex-Lax), bulk-forming laxatives (Mitrolan, Metamucil), lubricant laxatives (mineral oil), fecal moistening agents (Colace, glycerin suppositories), and those used for bowel evacuation (GoLYTELY, Chronulac).

Antidiarrheal Drugs

Antidiarrheal drugs are used to reduce an abnormal frequency of bowel evacuation. Common causes of acute and chronic diarrhea include bacterial or viral invasion, drugs, diet, and numerous disease states (e.g., diabetes insipidus and inflammatory bowel syndromes). Drugs used to treat diarrhea include the following:

- Adsorbents
  Bismuth subsalicylate (Pepto-Bismol)
- Anticholinergics
  Donnatal
- Opiates
  Paregoric
  Codeine
- Other agents
  Diphenoxylate (Lomotil)
  Loperamide (Imodium)

SECTION NINE
DRUGS THAT AFFECT THE EYE AND EAR

Drugs That Affect the Eye

Drugs used to treat eye disorders include antiglaucoma agents, mydriatics and cycloplegics, antiinfective/antiinflammatory agents, and topical anesthetics.

Antiglaucoma Agents

Glaucoma is an eye disease in which the pressure of the fluid in the eye is so abnormally high that it causes compression or obstruction of the eye's small internal blood vessels or the fibers of the optic nerve, or both. The result is nerve fiber destruction and partial or complete loss of vision. Glaucoma is a common eye disorder in people over age 60 and is responsible for 15% of blindness in adults in the United States.[10] Agents used to reduce the pressure in chronic glaucoma include cholinergic and anticholinesterase drugs. Some of these drugs (e.g., pilocarpine) dilate the pupil of the eye, and some constrict the pupil; others (e.g., acetazolamide) slow the secretion of aqueous fluid. If these drug therapies fail, surgery may be indicated.

> **NOTE**
>
> If glaucoma is diagnosed early, drugs can control it for a lifetime. Most physicians recommend testing for glaucoma every 2 years after age 35.

Mydriatic and Cycloplegic Agents

Mydriatic and cycloplegic agents are applied topically to cause dilation of the pupils and paralysis of accommodation to light. They are used to treat inflammation and to relieve ocular pain by putting the eye to rest. These drugs are also used during routine eye examinations and in ocular surgery. Examples of these drugs include atropine ophthalmic solution, cyclopentolate hydrochloride ophthalmic solution (Cyclogyl), homatropine ophthalmic solution (Isopto Homatropine), epinephrine, and oxymetazoline (OcuClear).

> **? CRITICAL THINKING**
>
> *You are caring for an older adult patient who had mydriatic eye drops instilled by an ophthalmologist. If you didn't know this history, what might you consider after your physical examination of this patient?*

Antiinfective/Antiinflammatory Agents

Antiinfective and antiinflammatory agents are used to treat eye conditions such as conjunctivitis, sty, and keratitis (corneal inflammation caused by bacterial infection). Examples of these drugs include bacitracin (Baciguent), chloramphenicol (Chloroptic), erythromycin (Ilotycin), and natamycin (Natacyn).

Topical Anesthetic Agents

Local anesthetics are used to prevent pain during surgical procedures and eye examinations and in the treatment of some eye injuries (e.g., a corneal abrasion). These drugs usually have a rapid onset (within 20 seconds) and last 15 to 20 minutes. Examples of these drugs include proparacaine HCl (Opthaine) and *tetracaine HCl* (Pontocaine).

> **NOTE**
>
> Other eye medications include artificial tear solutions and lubricants to provide additional moisture, irrigation solutions, and antiallergic agents to relieve symptoms of itching, tearing, and redness. Many of these drugs and solutions are available without prescription.

Drugs That Affect the Ear

Drugs used to treat disorders of the external ear canal include antibiotics, steroid/antibiotic combinations, and miscellaneous preparations. These drugs include the following:

- Antibiotics used to treat infections
  Chloramphenicol (Chloromycetin Otic)
  Gentamicin sulfate (Garamycin)

- Steroid/antibiotic combinations used to treat superficial bacterial infections

    Neomycin sulfate/polymyxin B sulfate/ hydrocortisone (Cortisporin Otic)

    Neomycin/colistin/hydrocortisone (Coly-Mycin S Otic)

- Miscellaneous preparations used to treat ear wax accumulation, inflammation, pain, fungal infections, and other minor conditions

    Boric acid in isopropyl alcohol (Aurocaine 2)

    Triethanolamine with chlorbutanol in propylene glycol (Cerumenex)

NOTE

Persons with inner ear infections or serious illness associated with hearing impairment may require systemic antibiotics and a thorough evaluation by a physician to prevent complications.

SECTION TEN
DRUGS THAT AFFECT THE ENDOCRINE SYSTEM

Review of Anatomy and Physiology

The endocrine system is a major means of controlling and integrating body functions. (Emergency drugs that affect the endocrine system are presented in Box 8-27.) Information from various regions in the body is transmitted via blood-borne hormones to distant sites. Hormones are natural chemical substances that act after secretion into the bloodstream from endocrine glands (ductless glands that secrete internally). These glands include the anterior and posterior pituitary, thyroid, parathyroid, and adrenal glands and the thymus, pancreas, testes, and ovaries. Hormones from the various endocrine glands work together to regulate vital processes, including the following:

- Secretory and motor activities of the digestive tract
- Energy production
- Composition and volume of extracellular fluid
- Adaptation (e.g., acclimatization and immunity)
- Growth and development
- Reproduction and lactation

Drugs That Affect the Pituitary Gland

The hormones of the anterior and posterior pituitary gland exert an important effect in regulating the secretion of other hormones (see Chapter 6). Box 8-28 lists drugs that affect the anterior and posterior pituitary. (Disorders of the endocrine glands are further described in Chapter 30.)

Drugs That Affect the Thyroid and Parathyroid Glands

The thyroid hormone controls the rate of metabolic processes and is required for normal growth and development. Parathyroid hormone regulates the level of ionized calcium in the blood through the release of calcium from bone, the absorption of calcium from the intestine, and the rate of excretion of calcium by the kidneys.

BOX 8-27

EMERGENCY DRUGS: ENDOCRINE SYSTEM

Dexamethasone (Decadron)
Dextrose 50%
Glucagon
Insulin
Methylprednisolone (Solu-Medrol)
Oxytocin (Pitocin, Syntocinon)

BOX 8-28

DRUGS THAT AFFECT THE ANTERIOR AND POSTERIOR PITUITARY GLAND

Anterior Pituitary Gland Drugs
Used to treat growth failure in children caused by growth hormone (GH) deficiency:
    Somatrem (Protropin)
    Somatropin (Humatrope)

Posterior Pituitary Gland Drugs
Used to treat the symptoms of diabetes insipidus resulting from antidiuretic hormone (ADH) deficiency:
    Vasopressin (Pitressin)

Disorders of the thyroid gland include goiter (enlargement of the thyroid gland), hypothyroidism (thyroid hormone deficiency), and hyperthyroidism (thyroid hormone excess). Disorders of the parathyroid include hypoparathyroidism and hyperparathyroidism. The drugs used to treat these disorders are listed in Box 8-29.

Drugs That Affect the Adrenal Cortex

The adrenal cortex secretes three major classes of steroid hormones: glucocorticoids (cortisol), mineralocorticoids (primarily aldosterone), and sex hormones. Glucocorticoids raise blood glucose, deplete tissue proteins, and suppress the inflammatory reaction. Mineralocorticoids regulate electrolyte and water balance. Sex hormones (small amounts of estrogen, progesterone, and testosterone produced in both men and women) have little physiological effect under normal circumstances. Drugs that affect the adrenal cortex are listed in Box 8-30.

> **NOTE**
>
> Two disorders of the adrenal cortex are Addison's disease (adrenal cortical hypofunction) and Cushing's disease (adrenal cortical hyperfunction) (see Chapter 30).

Drugs That Affect the Pancreas

The pancreas is an exocrine gland (providing digestive juices to the small intestine) and an endocrine gland. The endocrine portion of the pancreas consists of pancreatic islets (islets of Langerhans), which produce the hormones that enter the circulatory system.

Hormones of the Pancreas

The pancreatic hormones play an important role in regulating the concentration of certain nutrients in the circulatory system. The two major hormones secreted by the pancreas are insulin and glucagon.

Insulin is the primary hormone that regulates glucose metabolism. In general, it increases the ability of the liver, adipose tissue, and muscle to take up and use glucose. Glucose not immediately needed as an energy source is stored in the skeletal muscle, liver, and other tissues as glycogen.

Glucagon primarily influences the liver, although it has some effect on skeletal muscle and adipose tissue. In general, glucagon stimulates the liver to break down glycogen so that glucose is released into the blood. Glucagon also inhibits the uptake of glucose by muscle and fat cells. The balancing action of these two hormones protects the body from hyperglycemia and hypoglycemia.

This balance of hormonal actions is important when considering the metabolic derangements that can occur in diabetes mellitus. The relationship of glucagon and insulin to other hormones and substances such as *dextrose 50%* (D50) and *thiamine* (vitamin B$_1$) is addressed in Chapter 30. Box 8-31 lists drugs that affect the pancreas.

BOX 8-29

DRUGS THAT AFFECT THE THYROID AND PARATHYROID GLANDS

Thyroid Drugs
Used to treat hypothyroidism and to prevent goiters:
   Thyroid
   Iodine products
   Levothyroxine

Parathyroid Drugs
Used to treat hyperparathyroidism:
   Vitamin D
   Calcium supplements

BOX 8-30

DRUGS THAT AFFECT THE ADRENAL CORTEX

Glucocorticoids
Betamethasone (Celestone)
Dexamethasone (Decadron)
Methylprednisolone (Solu-Medrol)

Mineralocorticoids
Desoxycorticosterone acetate (DOCA)
Fludrocortisone (Florinef)

Adrenal Steroid Inhibitors
Aminoglutethimide (Cytadren)
Metyrapone (Metopirone)

Drugs That Affect the Female Reproductive System

Drugs that affect the female reproductive system include synthetic and natural substances such as hormones, oral contraceptives, ovulatory stimulants, and drugs used to treat infertility.

Female Sex Hormones

Two main types of hormones are secreted by the ovary: estrogen and progesterone. Supplemental estrogen is indicated for estrogen deficiency or replacement, treatment of breast cancer, and as prophylaxis for osteoporosis in postmenopausal women. Progesterone (and synthetic progestins) may be used to treat hormonal imbalance, endometriosis, and specific cancers, and to prevent pregnancy when used properly.

Oral Contraceptives

Oral contraception is the most effective form of birth control. It commonly is known as "the pill" and is a combination of estrogen and progesterone that results in suppression of ovulation (see Chapter 39). Several different types of oral contraceptives and their drug combinations are available. All are nearly 100% effective in preventing pregnancy.

Ovulatory Stimulants and Infertility Drugs

The absence of ovulation (anovulation) may be a pathological condition in women with abnormal bleeding or infertility. The condition is sometimes treated with gonadotropins, thyroid preparations, estrogen, and synthetic agents. One example of a drug used to induce ovulation and increase fertility is clomiphene citrate (Clomid).

> **NOTE**
>
> Drugs used during labor and delivery to increase or decrease uterine contractility include **oxytocin** (Pitocin) and ritodrine (Yutopar), respectively. In prehospital care **oxytocin** (Pitocin) is used to control postpartum hemorrhage after infant and placental delivery (see Chapter 40).

Drugs That Affect the Male Reproductive System

Adequate amounts of the male sex hormone testosterone are needed for normal development and maintenance of male sex characteristics.

BOX 8-31

DRUGS THAT AFFECT THE PANCREAS

Insulin Preparations
Rapid acting
Humulin 70/30
Regular insulin
Semilente

Intermediate acting
Humulin
Lente insulin
NPH insulin

Long acting
Ultralente
PZI

Oral Hypoglycemic Agents
Dymelor - acetohexamide
Diabinese - chlorpropamide
Glucophage - metformin
Glucotrol - glipizide
Micronase - glyburide
Tolinase - tolazamide
Orinase - tolbutamide

Hyperglycemic Agents
Glucagon
Proglycem - diazoxide
Dextrose
Oral glucose (Glutose, Insta-Glucose)

Testosterone Therapy

Testosterone therapy is indicated for the treatment of hormone deficiency (e.g., testicular failure), impotence, delayed puberty, female breast cancer, and anemia. The choice of dosage and length of therapy depend on the diagnosis, age of the patient, and intensity of side effects/adverse reactions. An example of an oral testosterone drug is methyltestosterone (Metandren).

> **NOTE**
>
> Impotence is the inability of a man to achieve or maintain an erection, leading to decreased sexual function. The condition afflicts as many as 20 million Americans on a continuing basis.[11]

Drugs That Affect Sexual Behavior

Sexual drive (libido) can be affected by psychological, social, and physiological factors (and oftentimes a combination of these). Negative effects of these factors can result in a lack of interest in sexual activity in both men and women and impotence in men.

Drugs That Impair Libido and Sexual Gratification

Some drugs interfere with sympathetic nervous stimulation and occasionally cause sexual dysfunction by inactivating nervous mechanisms (both directly and indirectly) that are responsible for sexual arousal. Some of these drugs include antihypertensives, antihistamines, antispasmodics, sedatives and tranquilizers, antidepressants, alcohol, and barbiturates.

> **BOX 8-32**
>
> ### EXAMPLES OF ANTINEOPLASTIC AGENTS
>
> Fluorouracil (Adrucil)
> Mechlorethamine (Mustargen)
> Methotrexate (Amethopterin)
> Streptozocin (Zanosar)
> Doxorubicin (Adriamycin)

Drugs That Enhance Libido and Sexual Gratification

In addition to changing medications (under a physician's supervision) to avoid drug-induced sexual dysfunction, a patient may be prescribed drugs to enhance libido and sexual gratification. Drugs that enhance sexual function include levodopa (L-Dopa) and sildenafil citrate (Viagra).

> **NOTE**
>
> The administration of **nitroglycerin** (Nitrostat) or nitrate/nitrite medications may be contraindicated in patients taking Viagra because the combination can cause a lethal drop in blood pressure. Other drugs that may produce untoward effects in patients taking Viagra include some antibiotics, cimetidine, and some blood pressure–lowering medications.[12] The paramedic should always question the patient about Viagra use before administering any of these medications. Nitroglycerin usually is contraindicated if Viagra has been taken in the previous 24 hours.

SECTION TWELVE
DRUGS USED IN NEOPLASTIC DISEASES

Antineoplastic Agents

Antineoplastic agents are used in cancer chemotherapy to prevent the proliferation of malignant cells (Box 8-32). These drugs do not directly kill tumor cells but rather interfere with cell reproduction or replication through various mechanisms.

> **NOTE**
>
> Any individual who handles antineoplastic agents should be properly trained in safety procedures. These drugs are considered cytotoxic (toxic to human cells).

Antineoplastic agents are nonselective and are injurious to all cells in the body. Side effects from these drugs may include infection, hemorrhage, nausea and vomiting, and changes in bowel habits. Short-term toxicity from these agents may affect the pulmonary, cardiovascular, renal, and integumentary systems. Prehospital care for these patients primarily is supportive and is aimed at providing comfort measures and emotional support.

SECTION THIRTEEN
DRUGS USED IN INFECTIOUS DISEASE AND INFLAMMATION

Antibiotics

Antibiotics are used to treat local or systemic infection. They kill or suppress the growth of microorganisms by disrupting the bacterial cell wall, by disturbing the functions of the cell membrane, or by interfering with the cell's metabolic functions. This group of drugs includes penicillins, cephalosporins and related products; macrolide antibiotics; tetracyclines; and miscellaneous antibiotic agents (e.g., metronidazole [Flagyl] and spectinomycin [Trobicin]).

NOTE

Antibiotics are much more toxic to bacteria than they are to a patient. Some antibiotics, however, may produce marked hypersensitivity that can lead to a fatal reaction if the drug is later administered to a sensitized patient.

NOTE

Some bacteria that are initially sensitive to antibiotics eventually become resistant by developing methods to circumvent a drug's effect. The widespread use and misuse of antibiotics leads to the development of resistant strains and may complicate treatment when a person is infected with an antibiotic-resistant organism.

Penicillins

Penicillins are considered the most effective and least toxic of all available antimicrobial drugs. They are very active against gram-positive and some gram-negative bacteria (see the box in the right column). Penicillins are used in the treatment of many infections, including tonsillitis, pharyngitis, bronchitis, and pneumonia. Examples of penicillins include amoxicillin (Amoxil), ampicillin (Amcill), dicloxacillin (Dynapen), and penicillin V potassium (Pen Vee K).

Cephalosporins

Cephalosporins (and related products) resemble penicillins but are active against both gram-positive and gram-negative bacteria. They are widely used to treat ear, throat, and respiratory infections. They also are particularly useful in the treatment of urinary tract infection (UTI), which often is caused by bacteria resistant to penicillin-type antibiotics. Examples of cephalosporins and related products include cefazolin (Ancef), cephalothin (Keflin), cefoxitin (Mefoxin), and cefotaxime (Claforan).

NOTE

About 6% to 10% of those allergic to penicillins are also allergic to cephalosporins.

Macrolide Antibiotics

Macrolides (erythromycins) are used to treat infections of the skin, chest, throat, and ears. They are particularly useful in the treatment of pertussis ("whooping cough") and legionnaires' disease. Examples of erythromycin drugs include Eryc, E-Mycin, E.E.S, and Erythrocin. Other antibacterial agents include azithromycin (Zithromax) and clarithromycin (Biaxin).

GRAM'S STAIN

Gram's stain is an iodine-based stain used to differentiate various types of bacteria. Basically, a specimen is stained with gentian violet, followed by Gram's solution, and then treated with a decolorizing agent such as acetone. The specimen is then counterstained with a red dye (safranin). Specimens that retain the dark violet stain are known as gram-positive; those that lose the violet stain after decolorization but take up the counterstain (causing them to appear pink) are gram-negative. Examples of gram-positive bacteria are staphylococci, streptococci, and pneumococci. Examples of gram-negative bacteria are gonococci and meningococci.

Tetracyclines

Tetracyclines are active against many gram-negative and gram-positive organisms ("broad-spectrum"). They commonly are used to treat conditions such as acne, bronchitis, syphilis, gonorrhea, and certain types of pneumonia. Examples of tetracyclines include demeclomycin (Declomycin), doxcycline (Vibramycin), and tetracycline (Achromycin).

NOTE

Tetracyclines may discolor developing teeth and are therefore not usually prescribed for children under the age of 12 or for pregnant women.

Antifungal and Antiviral Drugs

In addition to infection from bacterial organisms, people can be infected by fungi and viral diseases.

Antifungal Drugs

Some fungi are harmlessly present at all times in areas of the body such as the mouth, skin, intestines, and vagina. These are prevented from multiplying through competition from bacteria and from the actions of the immune system. Fungal infections are more common and serious in individuals taking long-term antibiotics (which destroy the bacterial competition), in those who are immunosuppressed as a complication of illness (e.g., infection with the human immunodeficiency virus), and in those who are taking corticosteroids or immunosuppressant drugs (described later in this chapter). Fungal infections can be broadly classified into superficial infections, subcutaneous infections, and deep infections (Box 8-33). Examples of antifungal drugs include tolnaftate (Tinactin), fluconazole (Diflucan), and nystatin (Mycostatin).

NOTE

There are about 50 species of fungi that can cause illness and sometimes fatal disease in human beings.

Antiviral Drugs

To date, few effective drugs exist to treat minor viral infections, such as colds. In fact, very few drugs exist for use in any viral infections. This is due partly to the relative delay in the onset of symptoms that occurs in viral diseases, making drug therapy difficult once the disease is established. Viral infections range from trivial and harmless (e.g., warts) to

NOTE

A few drugs offer symptomatic relief from flu viruses. These include oseltamivir (Tamiflu) and zanamivir (Relenza), which are effective against A and B flu viruses, and amantadine (Symmetrel) and rimantadine (Flumadine), which are effective against flu virus A (see Chapter 37).

BOX 8-33

CATEGORIES OF FUNGAL INFECTIONS

Examples of Superficial Infections
Candidiasis (*thrush*): Affects the genitals or inside of the mouth and vaginal and intertriginous areas
Tinea (including *ring worm, athlete's foot, jock itch*): Affects external areas of the body

Examples of Subcutaneous Infections (rare)
Sporotrichosis: May follow inoculation of spores through a puncture or scratch
Mycetoma ("Madura foot"): Occurs in tropical countries

Examples of Deep Infections
Aspergillosis
Histoplasmosis
Cryptococcosis
Blastomycosis
Candidiasis (that spreads from its usual site to the esophagus, urinary tract, or other internal sites)

extremely serious diseases such as influenza, rabies, acquired immunodeficiency syndrome (AIDS), and probably some types of cancers (Table 8-6).

Many agents have been tested as antiviral drugs, but few have been proven effective against specific virus-infected cells without toxic effects to uninfected cells. Examples of specific antiviral drugs include acyclovir (Zovirax), which is effective against herpes infection, and zidovudine (Retrovir, AZT, ZDV) and lamivudine (Epivir), which are currently used to treat human immunodeficiency (HIV) infection.

Protease Inhibitors

Although the complete mechanism of action of protease inhibitors is not clearly understood, they appear to inhibit the replication of retroviruses (e.g., HIV) in both acute and chronically infected cells. Side effects and adverse reactions of these drugs include nausea and vomiting, headache, malaise, fever, and flulike symptoms. Examples of protease inhibitors include indinavir (Crixivan), ritonavir (Norvir), and saquinavir (Invirase).

> **NOTE**
>
> The administration of antiviral drugs and protease inhibitors for a health care worker who has been exposed to body fluids that may contain HIV or another virus known or suspected to be resistant to antiviral drugs is important and is a postexposure prophylaxis (PEP) recommendation by the Centers for Disease Control and Prevention (CDC).[13]

Other Antimicrobial Drugs and Antiparasitic Drugs

Various drugs are used to treat "atypical" microbial infection (e.g., *Mycobacterium tuberculosis*, *Mycobacterium leprae*) and infection and disease caused by parasite and insect vector (e.g., trichomoniasis, malaria). Classifications and examples of these drugs are listed in Box 8-34.

> **NOTE**
>
> Malaria is still a prevalent disease in tropical areas and may be carried into the United States by refugees and immigrants. Tuberculosis is on the rise in individuals with AIDS and in the homeless, drug abusers, and those taking immunosuppressant drugs.

Antiinflammatory and Nonsteroidal Antiinflammatory Drugs

Inflammation

Inflammation is a defense mechanism of body tissues in response to physical trauma, foreign biological and/or chemical substances, surgery, radiation, and electricity. Regardless of the event producing inflammation, the inflammatory response is very similar. For example, if bacterial infection or an injury to the tissues occurs, chemical mediators are released or activated. These mediators cause vasodilation and increased blood flow (localized warmth

TABLE 8-6	COMMON VIRUSES AND VIRAL DISEASES OR CONDITIONS
VIRAL FAMILY	**DISEASES OR CONDITIONS**
Papovavirus	Warts
Adenovirus	Cold sores, genital herpes, chickenpox, herpes zoster (shingles), congenital abnormalities (cytomegalovirus)
Picornavirus	Poliomyelitis, viral hepatitis A and B, respiratory infections, myocarditis, rhinovirus (common cold)
Togavirus	Yellow fever, encephalitis
Orthomyxovirus	Influenza
Paramyxovirus	Mumps, measles, rubella
Coronavirus	Common cold
Rhabdovirus	Rabies
Retrovirus	AIDS, degenerative brain disease, possibly cancer

BOX 8-34

EXAMPLES OF ANTIMICROBIAL AND ANTIPARASITIC DRUGS

Antimalarial Agents
Quinine (Quinamm)
Quinacrine (Atabrine)
Pyrimethamine (Daraprim)

Antitubercular Agents
Aminosalicylate (Nemasol)
Capreomycin (Capastat)
Isoniazid (Izonid, INH))
Rifampin (Rifadin)
Streptomycin

Antiamebic Agents
Emetine HCl
Iodoquinol (Yodoxin)
Paromomycin (Humatin)

Antihelminthic Agents
Diethylcarbamazine (Hetrazan)
Mebendazole (Vermox)

Leprostatic Agents
Dapsone (DDS)
Clofazimine (Lamprene)

Cephalosporins
Cefazolin (Ancef)
Cephalexin (Keflex)
Cephradine (Anspor)
Cefaclor (Ceclor)
Ceftriaxone (Rocephin)

Fluoroquinolones
Ciprofloxacin (Cipro)
Enoxacin (Penetrex)
Norfloxacin (Noroxin)

Penicillins
Amoxicillin (Amoxil)
Ampicillin (Polycillin)
Dicloxacillin (Dynapen)
Penicillin G
Penicillin V

and redness at the site). This process brings phagocytes and other leukocytes to the area and prevents the spread of infection by walling off the infected site. Finally, phagocytes clean the area, and the damaged tissues are repaired.

Inflammation can be localized or systemic. Local inflammation is confined to a specific area of the body. Symptoms include redness, heat, swelling, pain, and loss of function. Systemic inflammation occurs in many parts of the body. In addition to local symptoms at the inflammation site, red bone marrow produces and releases large numbers of neutrophils that promote phagocytosis, pyrogens stimulate fever production, and increased vascular permeability in severe cases may result in decreased blood volume. Drugs used to treat inflammation or its symptoms may be classified as analgesic-antipyretic drugs and nonsteroidal antiinflammatory drugs (NSAIDs). A number of medications have both properties.

Analgesic-Antipyretic Drugs

An antipyretic drug is one that reduces fever. The body's thermoregulatory mechanism is located in the anterior hypothalamus (the "thermostat" of the body). Normally, the "set point" of this hypothalamic center is about 98.6° F (37° C). When an inflammatory response occurs in the body, endogenous pyrogens are released by the phagocytic leukocytes, producing fever. Analgesic-antipyretic drugs work by reversing the effect of the pyrogen on the hypothalamus so that the set point of the hypothalamus is returned to normal. The analgesic effects of these drugs act on peripheral pain receptors to block activation. Examples of these drugs include the following:

- Acetaminophen (Datril, Tylenol, Panadol, and others)
- *Aspirin*/acetylsalicylic acid (A.S.A, Aspergum, Bayer Aspirin, and others)
- *Aspirin* (buffered) (Aluprin, Bufferin, Alka-Seltzer, and others)

Nonsteroidal Antiinflammatory Drugs

Aspirin is the prototype of the nonsteroidal antiinflammatory drug. New drugs also have been developed, which, like *aspirin*, are analgesic, antipyretic, and antiinflammatory. These drugs often are prescribed for patients with various inflammatory conditions, such as rheumatoid arthritis, and especially for those who cannot tolerate *aspirin.* In addition, these drugs may be used to treat painful joint disorders (with or without inflammation), such as osteoarthritis, low back pain, and gout. It should be noted that like *aspirin,* the other non-steroidal antiinflammatory agents may decrease platelet activity and may cause gastrointestinal bleeding.

> **NOTE**
>
> Gout is a metabolic disease associated with high levels of uric acid in the blood (hyperuricemia) that is characterized by attacks of acute pain, swelling, and tenderness of joints. The condition is treated with uricosuric drugs, colchicine, and NSAIDs.

Nonsteroidal antiinflammatory drugs are thought to act by inhibiting specific enzymes so that prostaglandins (substances that promote inflammation and pain) are not formed. Examples of these drugs include the following:

- *Aspirin* (Bayer Timed-Release, Bufferin, and others)
- Diflunisal (Dolobid)
- Ibuprofen (Advil, Motrin, Nuprin, and others)
- Indomethacin (Indocin and others)
- Naproxen (Anaprox, Aleve, Naprosyn)
- Sulindac (Clinoril)
- *Ketorolac* (Toradol)

SECTION FOURTEEN
DRUGS THAT AFFECT THE IMMUNOLOGICAL SYSTEM

Review of Anatomy and Physiology

As described earlier in this chapter and in Chapter 6, the immunological system is comprised of cells and organs that defend the body against invasion by foreign substances. Organs and tissues of the immune system include the spleen, tonsils, lymph nodes, and thymus (Fig. 8-12).

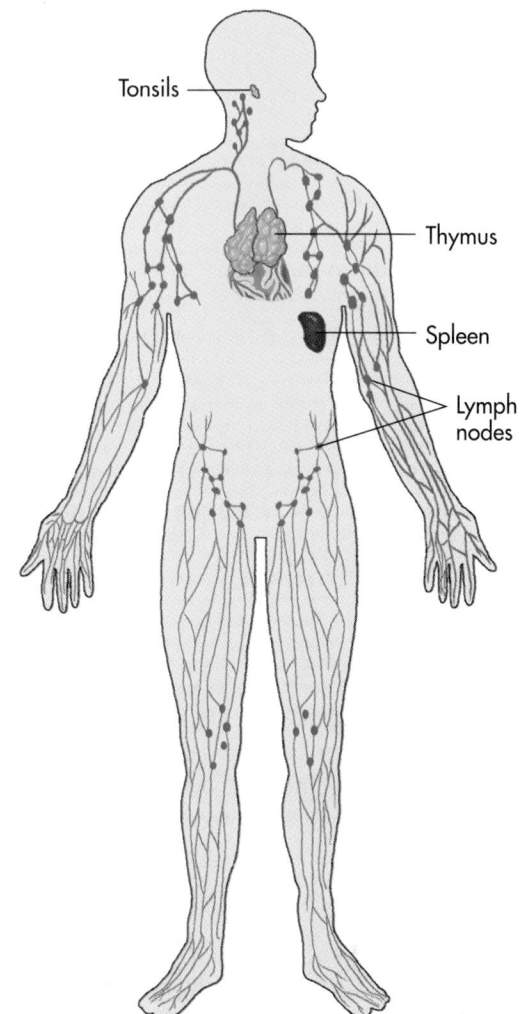

Fig. 8-12 Organs and tissues of the immune system.

> **? CRITICAL THINKING**
>
> *Why would it be important to know that a patient with altered level of consciousness is taking an immunosuppressant drug?*

Immunosuppressants

Immunosuppressant drugs reduce the activity of the body's immune system by suppressing the production and activity of lymphocytes. They are prescribed after transplant surgery to prevent the rejection of foreign tissues and are sometimes given to halt the progress of autoimmune disorders when other treatments are ineffective. Examples of immunosuppressant drugs include antirejection drugs (used in organ transplantation), anticancer drugs, and corticosteroids.

Immunomodulating Agents

Immunomodulating agents are drugs that increase the efficiency of the body's immune system by activating the immune defenses or by modifying a biological response to an unwanted stimulus. These drugs include vaccines that protect against specific infectious agents. Two drugs belonging to this group are the interferons (used to treat viral infections such as hepatitis C and certain types of cancer) and zidovudine (used to treat AIDS). Some immunomodulating agents enhance the ability of a vaccine to stimulate the immune system and are added to the vaccine for this reason.

Serums and Vaccines

Serum is the clear fluid that separates from blood when it clots. Serum contains salts, glucose, and other proteins (including antibodies formed by the body's immune system to protect against infection). Serum can be prepared from the blood of a person (or in rare cases an animal) infected with a microorganism that usually contains antibodies that can protect against that organism if the serum is injected into someone else. This forms the basis for passive immunization (see Chapter 37).

> **NOTE**
>
> There are two main types of immunization. In passive immunization, antibodies are injected and provide immediate but short-lived protection against specific disease-causing bacteria, viruses, or toxins. Active immunization primes the body to make its own antibodies against such microorganisms and confers longer-lasting immunity.

Vaccines contain killed or modified microorganisms ("live attenuated organisms") that usually do not cause the disease. They are administered to a person to produce specific immunity to a disease-causing bacterial toxin, virus, or bacterium (active immunization). If the particular infectious agent invades the body at a later time, the sensitized immune system quickly produces antibodies to destroy the agent or the toxin it produces. Examples of live attenuated vaccines are those given to protect against measles, mumps, rubella, yellow fever, and polio. Diphtheria and tetanus vaccines contain inactivated bacterial toxins. Cholera, typhoid fever, pertussis, rabies, viral hepatitis B, influenza, and Salk injected polio vaccines contain killed organisms. (In the case of hepatitis B, the vaccine contains only part of the hepatitis B virus.)

> **NOTE**
>
> Smallpox was declared extinct by the World Health Organization in 1980 because of near-universal vaccination. Polio has virtually been eliminated from the United States, Canada, and Europe since the development of effective vaccines in the 1950s, but it is still a risk for anyone who has not been vaccinated and who lives in or travels to southern Europe, Africa, or Asia. Measles is another disease that has been nearly eradicated in the United States and Canada.

> **NOTE**
>
> A newborn child is, to some extent, protected against infection by barriers (e.g., the skin); by substances in the mouth, in the urinary tract, or on the eye surface that destroy microorganisms; and by antibodies that have been passed to the child from the mother (including those received in breast milk). This "natural" immunity does not guard against all diseases, however, and active immunization against specific disease-causing microorganisms that cause childhood illness should be provided to the child beginning at birth (see Chapter 42).

S U M M A R Y

- A drug may be defined as "any substance taken by mouth; injected into a muscle, blood vessel, or cavity of the body; or applied topically to treat or prevent a disease or condition.

- Drugs can be identified by the following four types of names: chemical name; generic or nonproprietary name; trade, brand, or proprietary name; and official name.

- The Drug Enforcement Agency (DEA) is the nation's sole legal drug enforcement body. Additional regulatory bodies or services include the Food and Drug Administration (FDA); the Public Health Service; the Federal Trade Commission (FTC); in Canada, the Health Protection Branch of the Department of National Health and Welfare; and for international drug control, the International Narcotics Control Board.

- Paramedics are held responsible for safe and therapeutically effective drug administration, and they are personally responsible—legally, morally, and ethically—for each drug they administer.

- Drug allergies can be divided into four classifications based on the mechanism of the body's immune reaction. They are type I (anaphylactic), type II (cytotoxic), type III (serum sickness), and type IV (contact dermatitis) reactions.

- The parasympathetic and sympathetic nervous systems function continuously and simultaneously innervate many of the same organs; the opposing actions of the two systems balance one another. In general, the sympathetic system dominates during stressful events, and the parasympathetic system is most active during periods of emotional and physical calm.

- The degree to which drugs attain pharmacological activity depends partly on the rate and extent to which they are absorbed, which in turn depends on the drug's ability to cross the cell membrane. The rate and extent of absorption depend on the nature of the cell membrane the drug must cross, blood flow to the site of administration, solubility of the drug, pH of the drug environment, drug concentration, and drug dosage form.

- The route of drug administration greatly influences drug absorption. These routes can be classified as enteral, parenteral, pulmonary, and topical.

- Distribution is the transport of a drug through the bloodstream to various tissues of the body and ultimately to its site of action. After absorption and distribution, the body eliminates most drugs, first by biotransformation and then by excretion. The kidney is the primary organ for excretion; however, the intestine, lungs, and mammary, sweat, and salivary glands may also be involved.

- Many factors can alter the response to drug therapy, including age, body mass, gender, pathological state, genetic factors, and psychological factors.

- Most drug actions are thought to result from a chemical interaction between the drug and various receptors throughout the body. The most common form of drug action is the drug-receptor interaction.

- Many variables can influence drug interactions, including intestinal absorption, competition for plasma-protein binding, biotransformation, action at the receptor site, renal excretion, and alteration of electrolyte balance.

- Narcotic analgesics relieve pain. Narcotic antagonists reverse the narcotic effects of some analgesics. Nonnarcotic analgesics act by a peripheral mechanism that interferes with local mediators released when tissue is damaged; these mediators stimulate nerve endings and cause pain.

- Anesthetic drugs are CNS depressants that have a reversible effect on nervous tissue. Antianxiety agents are used to reduce feelings of apprehension, nervousness, worry, or fearfulness. Sedatives and hypnotics are drugs that depress the central nervous system and that produce a calming effect and help induce sleep. Alcohol is a general CNS depressant that can produce sedation, sleep, and anesthesia.

- Anticonvulsant drugs are used to treat seizure disorders, most notably epilepsy.

- All CNS stimulants work to increase excitability either by blocking activity of inhibitory neurons or their respective neurotransmitters or by enhancing the production of the excitatory neurotransmitters.

- Psychotherapeutic drugs include antipsychotic agents, antidepressants, and lithium. These drugs are used to treat psychoses and affective disorders, especially schizophrenia, depression, and mania.

- Several movement disorders can result from an imbalance of dopamine and acetylcholine. Drugs that inhibit or block acetylcholine are referred to as *anticholinergic*. Three classes of drugs affect brain dopamine: those that release dopamine, those that increase brain levels of dopamine, and dopaminergic agonists.

- The autonomic drugs mimic or block the effects of the sympathetic and parasympathetic divisions of the autonomic nervous system. These drugs are classified into four groups: cholinergic (parasympathomimetic) drugs, cholinergic blocking (parasympatholytic) drugs, adrenergic (sympathomimetic) drugs, and adrenergic blocking (sympatholytic) drugs.

- Skeletal muscle relaxants can be classified as central acting, direct acting, and neuromuscular blockers.

- Cardiac drugs are classified by their effects on specialized cardiac tissues. Cardiac glycosides are used to treat congestive heart failure and certain tachycardias. Antidysrhythmic drugs are used to treat and prevent disorders of cardiac rhythm. The pharmacological agents that suppress dysrhythmias may do so by direct action on the cardiac cell membrane (lidocaine), by indirect action that affects the cell (propranolol), or both.

- Antihypertensive drugs used to reduce blood pressure are classified into four major categories: diuretics, sympathetic blocking agents (sympatholytic drugs), vasodilators, and angiotensin-converting enzyme (ACE) inhibitors. Calcium channel blockers also are used to treat people with hypertension who do not respond to other drug therapies.

- Antihemorrheologic agents are used to treat peripheral vascular disorders caused by pathological or physiological obstruction (e.g., arteriosclerosis) by improving blood flow to ischemic tissues.

- Drugs that affect blood coagulation may be classified as *antiplatelet, anticoagulant,* or *fibrinolytic agents.* Drugs that interfere with platelet aggregation are known as *antiplatelet* or *antithrombic drugs.* Anticoagulant drug therapy is designed to prevent intravascular thrombosis by decreasing blood coagulability. Fibrinolytic drugs dissolve clots after their formation by promoting the digestion of fibrin.

- Hemophilia is a group of hereditary bleeding disorders involving a deficiency of one of the factors necessary for coagulation of blood. Replacement therapy of the missing clotting factor can be effective in the management of hemophilia.

- Hemostatic agents hasten clot formation to reduce bleeding. Systemic hemostatic agents generally are used to control rapid blood loss after surgery by inhibiting fibrinolysis. Topical hemostatic agents are used to control capillary bleeding during surgical and dental procedures.

- The treatment of choice in managing an imbalance of blood or blood components is to replace the sole blood component that is deficient. Replacement therapy may include transfusing whole blood (rare), packed red blood cells, fresh-frozen plasma, plasma expanders, platelets, coagulation factors, fibrinogen, albumin, or gamma globulins.

- Hyperlipidemia refers to an excess of lipids in the plasma. Antihyperlipidemic drugs are sometimes used in conjunction with diet and exercise to control serum lipid levels.

- Bronchodilator drugs are the primary treatment modality for obstructive pulmonary disease such as asthma, chronic bronchitis, and emphysema. These drugs may be classified as sympathomimetic drugs and xanthine derivatives.

- Mucokinetic drugs are used to move respiratory secretions, excessive mucus, and sputum along the tracheobronchial tree.

- Oxygen is used chiefly to treat hypoxia and hypoxemia.

- Direct respiratory stimulant drugs (analeptics) act directly on the medullary center of the brain to increase the rate and depth of respiration.

- Spirits of ammonia is the only drug given by inhalation as a reflex respiratory stimulant.

- When a cough is prolonged or occurs secondary to an underlying disorder, treatment with antitussive drugs may be indicated.

- The primary clinical use of antihistamines is for allergic reactions, but they also are sometimes prescribed to control motion sickness or as a sedative or antiemetic.

- Drug therapy for the GI system can be divided into drugs that affect the stomach and drugs that affect the lower GI tract. Antacids buffer or neutralize hydrochloric acid in the stomach. Antiflatulents prevent the formation of gas in the GI tract. Digestant drugs promote digestion in the GI tract by releasing small amounts of hydrochloric acid in the stomach. Drugs used to induce vomiting may be administered as part of the treatment of certain drug overdoses and poisonings. Drugs used to treat nausea and vomiting include antagonists of histamine, acetylcholine, and dopamine and other drugs whose actions are not clearly understood.

- Cytoprotective agents and other drugs are used to treat peptic ulcer disease by protecting the gastric mucosa. H_2-receptor antagonists block the H_2 receptors and reduce the volume of gastric acid secretion and its acid content.

- Constipation and diarrhea are two common conditions of the lower GI tract that may require drug therapy. Drugs used to manage these conditions include laxatives and antidiarrheals.

- Drugs used to treat eye disorders include antiglaucoma agents, mydriatics, and cyloplegics, antiinfective/antiinflammatory agents, and topical anesthetics.

- Drugs used to treat disorders of the ear include antibiotics, steroid/antibiotic combinations, and miscellaneous preparations.

- The endocrine system is a major means of controlling and integrating body functions. A number of drugs are used to treat disorders of the anterior and posterior pituitary, the thyroid and parathyroid glands, and the adrenal cortex.

- The pancreatic hormones play an important role in regulating the concentration of certain nutrients in the circulatory system. The two major hormones secreted by the pancreas are insulin and glucagon. Imbalances in either of these hormones may necessitate drug therapy to correct metabolic derangements.

- Drugs that affect the female reproductive system include synthetic and natural substances such as hormones, oral contraceptives, ovulation stimulants, and drugs used to treat infertility.

- Adequate amounts of the male sex hormone (testosterone) are needed for normal development and maintenance of male sex characteristics.

- Antineoplastic agents are used in cancer chemotherapy to prevent the proliferation of malignant cells.

- Antibiotics are used to treat local or systemic infection. This group includes penicillin, cephalosporins, and related products; macrolide antibiotics; tetracyclines; and miscellaneous antibiotic agents.

- In addition to infection from bacterial organisms, people can be infected by fungi and viral diseases. Examples of antifungal drugs include tonaftate (Tinactin), fluconazole (Diflucan), and nystatin (Mycostatin).

- Very few drugs exist for use in any viral infections. Specific antiviral drugs include acyclovir (Zovirax), which is effective against herpes infection, and zidovudine (Retrovir, AZT), which currently is used to treat HIV infection.

- Drugs used to treat inflammation or its symptoms may be classified as analgesic-antipyretic drugs and nonsteroidal antiinflammatory drugs (NSAIDs). A number of medications have both properties.

- Immunosuppressant drugs reduce the activity of the body's immune system by suppressing the production and activity of lymphocytes. They are prescribed after transplant surgery to prevent the rejection of foreign tissues and are sometimes given to halt the progress of autoimmune disorders.

- Immunomodulating agents are drugs that increase the efficiency of the body's immune system by activating the immune defenses or by modifying a biological response to an unwanted stimulus.

- Serum that contain antibodies that can protect against that organism if injected into someone else form the basis for passive immunization. Vaccines contain killed or modified microorganisms that are administered to a person to produce specific immunity to a disease-causing bacterial toxin, virus, or bacterium (active immunization).

REFERENCES

1. Lyons A, Petrucelli R: *Medicine: an illustrated history,* New York, 1987, Abradale Press.
2. Glanze W, editor: *Mosby's medical, nursing, and allied health dictionary,* ed 4, St Louis, 1994, Mosby.
3. McKenry L, Salerno E: *Mosby's pharmacology in nursing,* ed 18, St Louis, 1992, Mosby.
4. American Heart Association: Guidelines for cardiopulmonary resuscitation and emergency cardiac care, *JAMA* 268(16):2172, 1992.
5. Pratt J: Intraosseous infusion, *Int Pediatr* 4(1):19, 1989.
6. Syverud S et al: Prehospital use of neuromuscular blocking agents in a helicopter ambulance program, *Ann Emerg Med* 17(3):237, 1988.
7. Rosen P, Barkin R: *Emergency medicine: concepts and clinical practice,* ed 4, St Louis, 1998, Mosby.
8. Gonzalez E et al: Intravenous amiodarone for ventricular arrhythmias: overview and clinical use, *Resuscitation* 39:33, 1998.
9. American Heart Association: *Basic life support for healthcare providers,* Dallas, 1997, The Association.
10. American Medical Association: *The American Medical Association home medical encyclopedia,* New York, 1989, The Association.
11. *The medical advisor: the complete guide to alternative and conventional treatments,* Alexandria, Va, 1996, Time-Life Books.
12. Hazinski et al: 2000 Handbook of Emergency Cardiovascular Care for Healthcare providers, American Heart Association, 2000.
13. US Department of Health and Human Services, Centers for Disease Control: Public Health Service guidelines for the management of health care worker exposures to HIV and recommendations for postexposure prophylaxis, No RR-7, *MMWR* 47, 1998.

9 Venous Access and Medication Administration

OBJECTIVES

Upon completion of this chapter, the paramedic student will be able to:

1. Convert selected units of measurement between the household, apothecary, and metric systems.

2. Identify steps used to perform drug dosage calculations.

3. Calculate the correct volume of drug to be administered in a given situation.

4. Compute the correct rate for an infusion of drugs or intravenous fluids.

5. List measures that should be employed to ensure safe administration of medications.

6. Describe actions the paramedic should take if a medication error occurs.

7. Relate measures that should be taken to preserve asepsis during parenteral drug administration.

8. Explain techniques of drug administration by enteral and parenteral routes.

9. Describe the steps to safely initiate an intravenous infusion.

10. Identify complications and adverse effects associated with intravenous access.

11. Describe the steps to safely initiate intraosseous infusion.

12. Explain techniques of drug administration by percutaneous routes.

13. Identify special considerations for administering pharmacological agents to pediatric patients.

14. Explain the technique for obtaining a venous blood sample.

15. Describe how to safely dispose of contaminated items and sharps.

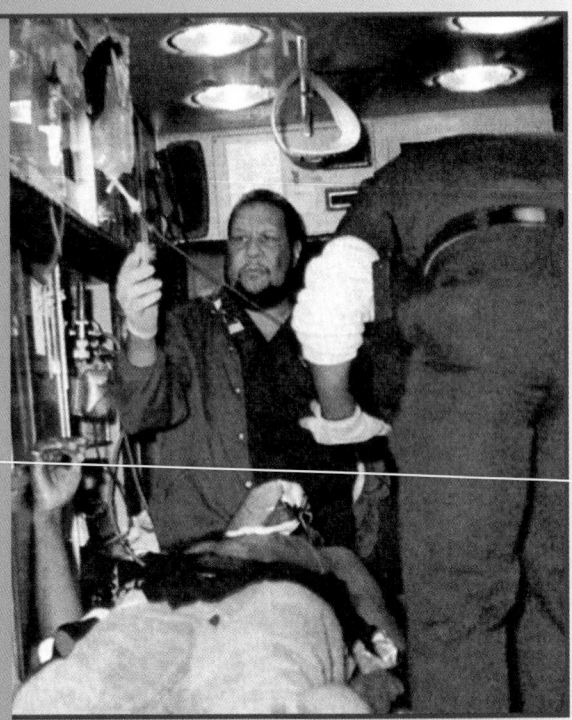

The ability to safely gain venous access and to administer prescribed medications is an important part of professional paramedic practice. This chapter addresses techniques in medication administration and emphasizes the paramedic's patient care responsibilities associated with medication therapy.

KEY TERMS

gram: A metric unit of mass equal to one thousandth of a kilogram.

kilogram: A metric unit of mass equal to 1000 grams or 2.2046 pounds.

liter: A metric unit of capacity equal to 1 cubic decimeter, 61.025 cubic inches, or 1.0567 liquid quarts.

medical asepsis: The removal or destruction of disease-causing organisms or infected material.

meter: A metric unit of length equal to 1000 millimeters.

microgram: A metric unit of mass equal to one millionth of a gram.

milligram: A metric unit of mass equal to one thousandth of a gram.

milliliter: A metric unit of capacity equal to one thousandth of a liter.

NOTE

Mathematical principles used in administering drugs include multiplication and division, Roman numerals, fractions, decimal fractions, proportions, and percent. The paramedic must have a good working knowledge of these principles and must be adept with math calculations.

Mathematical Equivalents Used in Pharmacology

Three systems for measuring drug dosage are in common use today—the metric system, the apothecary system, and the common household system. Each system deals with units of mass and volume, and a physician may use any of these three systems in ordering drugs.

Metric System

The French developed the metric system of weights and measures in the latter part of the eighteenth century, and Congress declared it to be the official measurement system in the United States in 1866.[1] Although the use of the metric system in the United States is not mandatory, it has been adopted by the medical sciences and pharmacies, in weighing currency at the federal mints, and in the armed forces. About 92% of the countries of the world use the metric system.

Definitions of Units

The basic metric units of measurement are the **meter,** the **liter,** and the **gram.** The meter is the unit for linear measurement, the liter for capacity or volume, and the gram for weight. A meter is slightly longer than a yard; a liter, slightly more than a quart; and a gram, slightly more than the weight of a steel paper clip.

The basic units of the metric system can be divided or multiplied by 10, 100, or 1000 parts to form secondary units that differ from each other by 10 or some multiple of 10. Subdivisions of these basic units are made when the decimal point is moved to the left, and multiples of the basic unit are made when the decimal point is moved to the right. The names of the secondary units are formed by joining Greek or Latin prefixes to the primary unit (Table 9-1).

The meter (m) is the unit of length from which the other metric units of length are derived (Fig. 9-1). Centimeters (cm) and millimeters (mm) are the primary linear measurements used in medicine. They are used, for example, to measure the size of body organs and to measure blood pressure.

The liter (L) is the unit of capacity or volume (Fig. 9-2). Fractional parts of a liter are expressed

TABLE 9-1	COMMON METRIC PREFIXES	
	PREFIX	**MEANING**
	kilo-	1000 times greater
	deci-	10 times less
	centi-	100 times less
	milli-	1000 times less
	micro-	1,000,000 times less

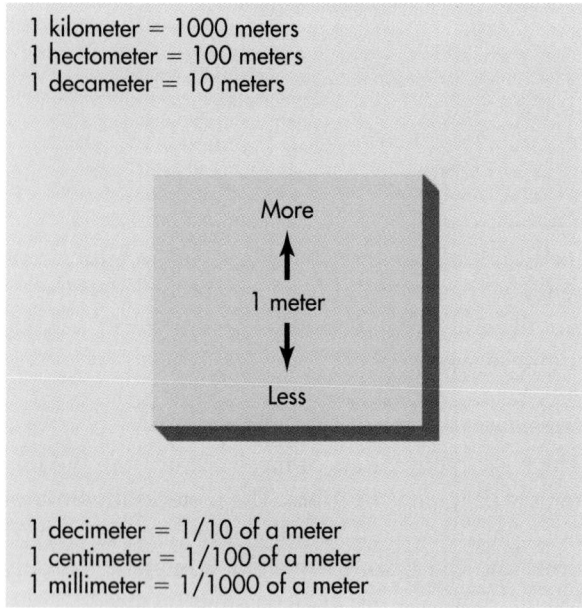

Fig. 9-1 The meter for measuring length.

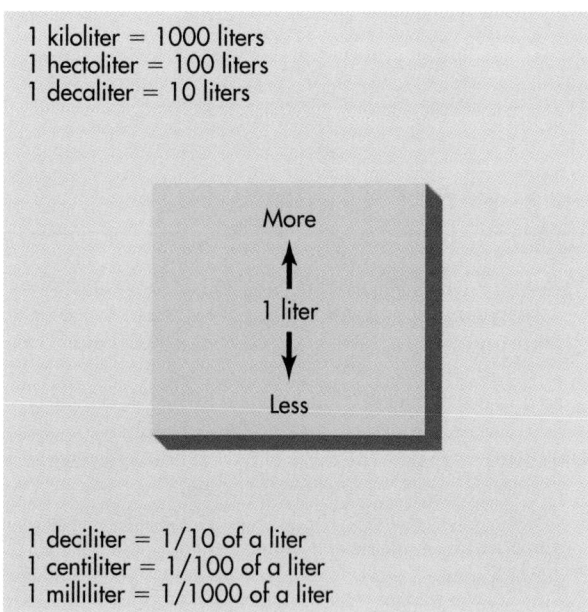

Fig. 9-2 The liter for measuring capacity.

in **milliliters** (mL) or cubic centimeters (cc). The liter is equal to 1000 mL or 1000 cc. The National Bureau of Standards recommends that the abbreviation ml or mL be used to express fractional parts of a liter.

The gram (g) is the metric unit of weight used in weighing drugs and various pharmaceutical preparations (Fig. 9-3). The gram equals the weight of 1 mL of distilled water at 4° C. A **kilogram** (kg) is equal to 1000 grams or 2.2 pounds. A **milligram** (mg) is equal to one thousandth of a gram. A **microgram** (µg) is equal to one millionth of a gram.

Metric Style of Notation

The National Bureau of Standards has recommended the following style of metric notation, except when it conflicts with use of proper English language[2]:

- Units are not to be capitalized (gram, not Gram).
- Periods should not be used with unit abbreviations (mL, not m.L. or mL.).
- A single space should be left between the quantity and the symbol (24 kg, not 24kg).
- Abbreviations should not be pluralized (kg, not kgs).
- As a rule, fractions should not be used, only decimal notation (0.25 kg, not 1/4 kg).
- Numerical quantities less than 1 should have a 0 placed to the left of the decimal point (0.75 mg, not .75 mg).

? CRITICAL THINKING

Why does the placement of a 0 to the left of the decimal place reduce the likelihood of making a drug dosing error?

Apothecary System

The apothecary system is considered less precise and less convenient than the more widely adopted metric system. Only a few medications are now available in units of the apothecary system (e.g., *aspirin*).

The primary unit of mass in the apothecary system is the grain (gr). The grain was derived from the age-old standard of the weight of a single grain of wheat (about 60 to 65 mg). Other units of mass used in the apothecary system are the dram (dr), ounce (oz), and pound (lb). A total of 60 gr constitutes 1 dram, and 8 drams equals 1 ounce.

NOTE

Aspirin (gr v) contains 325 milligrams of medication (5 grain × 65 mg = 325 mg).

The primary unit of volume in the apothecary system is the minim (m). The minim equals the volume of water that would weigh a grain (about 0.005

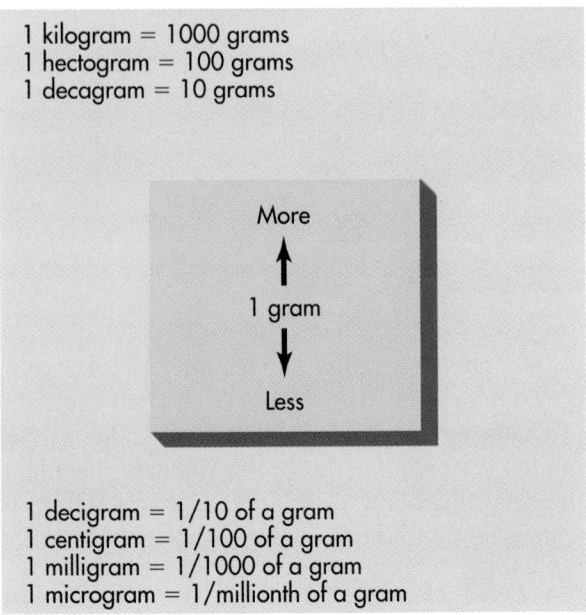

1 kilogram = 1000 grams
1 hectogram = 100 grams
1 decagram = 10 grams

1 decigram = 1/10 of a gram
1 centigram = 1/100 of a gram
1 milligram = 1/1000 of a gram
1 microgram = 1/millionth of a gram

Fig. 9-3 The gram for measuring weight.

or 0.006 mL). The equivalent of 60 m is 1 fluid dram (f dr), and 8 f dr equals 1 fluid ounce (f oz).

In written prescriptions, the apothecary system places abbreviations before the numeral. Whole numerical quantities are usually expressed in lower case Roman numerals (e.g., 10 grains would be written as "grains x"). Fractional quantities are usually expressed by Arabic numerals rather than by decimals (e.g., 1/4 grain would be written as "grain 1/4" rather than "0.25 grain").

> **NOTE**
>
> The only apothecaries' conversion necessary in emergency drug therapy is the conversion of pounds to kilograms. (1 kilogram is equal to 2.2 lb.) When one is converting the weight of the adult patient from pounds to kilograms, it is acceptable to round the whole number up when the number to the right of the decimal point is 5 or greater. For example, 70.90 kg could be rounded up to 71 kg.

Household System

Household measures include the glass, cup, tablespoon, teaspoon, drop, quart, and pint. Standard measures of the household system usually are not available in most homes. For example, the average coffee cup may hold 5 to 9 oz or more, and the average household teaspoon may hold 4 to 6 mL of

---

BOX 9-1

SYSTEMS OF EQUIVALENTS

Metric System
1.0 g = 0.001 kg
1.0 g = 1000 mg
1.0 L = 1000 mL

Apothecary System
1.0 gr = 1/60 dram (dr or l) = 1/480 oz
60 gr = 1 dr
8 dr = 1 oz (or K)
1.0 minim (m) = 1/60 f dr = 1/480 f oz
60 m = 1 f dr (or f l)
8 f dr = 1 f oz (or f K)

Household System
1.0 lb = 16 oz
1.0 pt = - quart (qt) = 1/8 gallon (gal)
1.0 pt = 16 f oz = 32 tablespoons (T)
1.0 T = 3 teaspoons (t)
1.0 t = 5 mL
1.0 T = 15 mL
1.0 pt = 480 mL
1.0 qt = 960 mL
1.0 gal = 3.84 L

---

liquid. Household measurements are only approximations (Box 9-1).

> **NOTE**
>
> Not all drops are the same size. As a rule, one average-size drop is equal to one minim.

Temperature Conversions

Normal body temperature is 37° Celsius (centigrade) or 98.6° Fahrenheit. A simple formula can be used to convert between the two readings. To convert a Celsius reading to Fahrenheit, multiply the Celsius reading by 9/5 and then add 32. To convert from Fahrenheit to Celsius, subtract 32 from the Fahrenheit reading and then multiply by 5/9 (Fig. 9-4).

> **NOTE**
>
> To convert Celsius to Fahrenheit multiply *first*, then add 32. To convert Fahrenheit to Celsius subtract 32 *first*, then multiply.

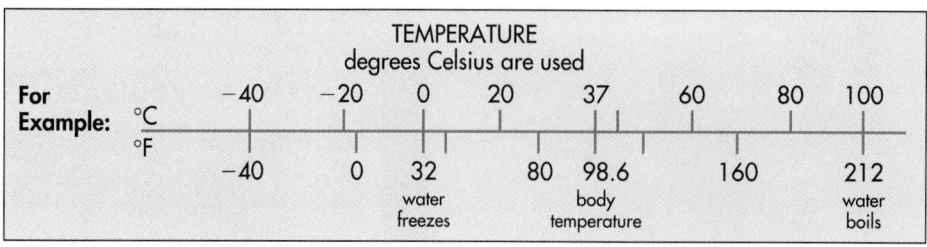

Fig. 9-4 Temperature conversions.

Drug Calculations

While providing emergency care, the paramedic is required to calculate adult and pediatric drug dosages, infusion rates, and the strength of drug solutions and diluted solutions. To perform these tasks, one must apply common mathematical skills in a logical sequence. These skills include a working knowledge of decimals, fractions, and ratios and proportions. This text presents common equations for drug calculations that are accepted within the medical community. Other methods of drug calculations may work as well (see the box on pp. 310-311).

Calculation Methods

The paramedic should choose a calculation method that is precise and reliable. To perform drug calculations:

• Convert all units of measure to the same unit and system.
• Assess the computed dosage to determine whether it is reasonable.
• Use one method of dose calculation consistently.

Conversion of All Units of Measure

Conversions usually are not necessary with most emergency drug preparations since most drugs are packaged in milligrams and administered in milligrams. Some drugs, though (e.g., *dopamine* [Intropin]), are packaged in milligrams but administered in micrograms, and therefore must be converted to "like units." When conversion to like

? CRITICAL THINKING

Would you overdose or underdose your patient if you failed to convert the 800 μg of dopamine to 0.8 mg in this example?

units is necessary, the conversion must be completed before the drug dose is calculated.

Example: You are to administer 800 μg per minute of *dopamine* (Intropin). You have 200 mg of the drug in 250 mL of solution. Convert 800 μg to 0.8 mg so that both measures of weight are in the same units.

$$800 \ \mu g \div 1000 = 0.8 \ mg$$

NOTE

Math Tip: Move the decimal point to the right when multiplying (converting the measurement to smaller units) and to the left when dividing (converting the measurement to larger units).

When the dose is given per unit of weight (kg), it will be necessary to convert the patient's weight from pounds to kilograms before calculating the total dose of drug to be given.

Example: You are to administer 1 mg/kg of *lidocaine* (Xylocaine) to a patient who weighs 132 lb. Divide 132 by 2.2 to convert pounds to kilograms (132 lb equals 60 kg). Total dose equals 1 mg/kg multiplied by 60 kg, which equals 60 mg.

$$132 \ lb \div 2.2 = 60 \ kg$$
$$1 \ mg \times 60 \ kg = 60 \ mg$$

Assessment of Computed Doses

Many emergency drugs are supplied in units that contain enough drug for a normal adult dose. After computations are performed, the paramedic should determine whether the answer is reasonable.

Example: You are to administer 8 mg of *diazepam* (Valium). It is supplied in a 2-mL ampule that contains 10 mg of the drug. Therefore, a "reasonable" calculation of volume would be less than 2 mL.

Methods of Calculation

Many drug calculations can almost be performed intuitively, because many drugs are packaged to supply one adult dose. However, a paramedic should never rely on intuitive calculations no matter how simple the drug dose may seem. There are three methods of calculation in common use:

Method 1: Basic Formula ("Desire Over Have")

Method 1 requires that information be substituted in the following formula:

$$\frac{D}{H} \times Q = X$$

Where *D* is the desired dose to be administered, *H* is the known dose on hand, *Q* is the unit of measure or volume on hand, and *X* is the unit of measure to be administered.

> **NOTE**
>
> Math Tip: "Desire over have" is considered by many to be the easiest formula to use and will work for nearly all emergency drug calculations.

Example: You are to administer 25 mg of *diphenhydramine* (Benadryl). You have a 10-mL vial that contains 50 mg of the drug. How many milliliters will you give? Using the desire-over-have formula, calculate the dose.

$$\frac{25 \text{ mg}}{50 \text{ mg}} \times 10 \text{ mL} = X$$
$$\frac{25}{5} \times 1 \text{ mL} = X$$
$$5 \times 1 \text{ mL} = X$$
$$X = 5 \text{ mL}$$

> **NOTE**
>
> Math Tip: When using the basic formula, *always* divide the bottom number into the top number; that is, divide the top number by the bottom number.

Method 2: Ratios and Proportions

Method 2 uses ratios and proportions to calculate the drug dosage. A ratio compares two numbers and is the same as a fraction. When used to calculate drug doses, a ratio refers to the weight or quantity of a drug in solution. For example, the ratio of 10 mg of *morphine* in 1 mL of solution is 10 mg to 1 mL. A proportion is an equation made up of two ratios, and states that the two ratios are equal. For example 2/3 is equal to 4/6 (2 : 3 :: 4 : 6), therefore the ratios are equivalent and the proportions are true.

To use this method, the equation must be set up ensuring that the same units of measure are stated in the same sequence (e.g., mg : mL = mg : xmL). x will be the quantity (e.g., mL) to be solved.

Dose on Hand : Volume on Hand :: Desired Dose : Desired Volume

Example: You are to administer 40 mg of *furosemide (Lasix).* You have 100 mg of the drug in 10 mL of solution. How many mL will you give? Calculate the dose using ratios and proportions.

100 mg : 10 mL :: 40 mg : xmL

Multiply inside numbers (means) and outside numbers (extremes), and drop the unit of measurement terms.

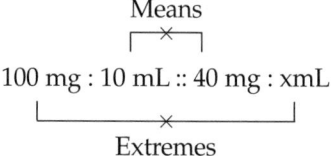

> **NOTE**
>
> Math Tip: Remember the phrases "middle for means" and "end for extremes." In a proportion, the product of the means is always equal to the product of the extremes.

Solve the proportion by dividing both sides of the equation by the number before x (100).

$$\frac{100x}{100} = \frac{400}{100} = 4 \text{ mL}$$

To check your answer, multiply the means and then multiply the extremes. The sum product will be equal if the proportion is true.

$$100 \times 4 = 400 \left. \right\} \text{Sum parts}$$
$$10 \times 40 = 400 \left. \right\} \text{are equal}$$

Method 3: Dimensional Analysis

Dimensional analysis is useful for complex drug calculations that require multiple conversions of a

THE "T" METHOD

The "T" method is a method for calculating conversions, drug doses, and IV flow rates that does not require advanced mathematical skills. Guidelines for using the T method for calculating a drug dose are listed below:

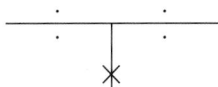

1. One T is required for every step in the calculation. (To use the T method, you must know two things: (1) the prescribed dose, and (2) the gram or milligram or microgram per mL concentration of the drug.)
2. The number entered on the lower *right* side of the T is always a "given in 1" (a known factor, such as *known in 1 mL* or *known in 1 kg*), or a multiple of 10 when converting within the metric system, that will never have to be solved for. The answer solved for in the equation will always be on *top* of the T in the lower *left* side. The number on top of the T is always the *larger* number (either a known number or one to be solved for). The number in the lower left side is always the *smaller* number (either a known number or one to be solved for).

	Larger Number	
Smaller number		Given in 1

3. If a number is placed on top of the T, it will always be *divided* by the other number in the T to find the answer.

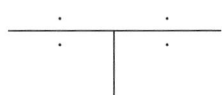

4. If both numbers are in the bottom of the T, *multiplication* must be performed to find the answer.

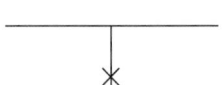

Example 1: You are to administer meperidine 25 mg IM. You have 50 mg of the drug in 1 mL of solution. How many milliliters will you give?

Step 1:
Place the "given" (50 mg/in 1 mL) in the lower right corner of the T.

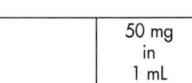

Step 2:
Place the larger number (the desired dose of 25 mg) on top of the T.

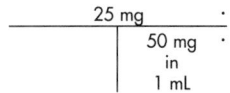

Step 3:
Divide 25 by 50 (basic formula) to obtain the smaller number (the required dose of 0.5 mL).

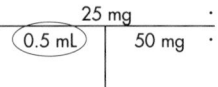

Example 2: You are to administer lidocaine 1 mg/kg IV to a 177-pound man. You have 100 mg in 5 mL of solution. How many milliliters will you give? This calculation will require four steps (four Ts).

Step 1:
Convert the patient's weight to kilograms:

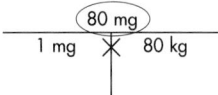

Step 2:
Calculate the prescribed dose in milligrams:

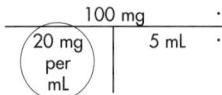

Step 3:
Determine the mg/mL concentration of the drug. (Remember, in this example, there are 5 mL of solution, not 1 mL.)

Step 4:
Use the basic formula to calculate the dose:

THE "T" METHOD—cont'd

Example 3: You are to administer atropine 0.02 mg/kg IV to a pediatric patient who weighs 30 pounds. You have 1 mg of the drug in 10 mL of solution. How many milliliters will you give? This calculation will require four steps (four Ts).

Step 1:

Convert the patient's weight to kilograms:

$$\dfrac{30 \text{ lb}}{\boxed{13.6 \text{ kg}}\ \bigg|\ \begin{array}{c} 2.2 \text{ kg} \\ \text{in} \\ 1 \text{ kg} \end{array}}$$

Step 2:

Calculate the prescribed dose in milligrams:

$$\dfrac{\boxed{0.27 \text{ mg}}}{0.02 \text{ mg} \ \times\ 13.6 \text{ kg}}$$

Step 3:

Determine the mg/mL concentration of the drug.

$$\dfrac{1 \text{ mg}}{\boxed{0.1 \text{ mg/mL}}\ \bigg|\ 10 \text{ mL}}$$

Step 4:

Use the basic formula to calculate the dose:

$$\dfrac{0.27 \text{ mg}}{\boxed{2.7 \text{ mL}}\ \bigg|\ \begin{array}{c} 0.1 \text{ mg/in} \\ 1 \text{ mL} \end{array}}$$

---

similar basic dimensional unit so that all units of measure are converted to like units (e.g., milligrams). It is based on the same principle as the basic formula, but does not require memorization of the desire-over-have equation. All conversion factors are set up in one equation and separated by multiplication signs.

NOTE

Math Tip: When using dimensional analysis, convert all units to the easiest math operation to lessen the possibility of error.

Example: You are to administer 0.8 mg of *naloxone* (Narcan). The drug is packaged in 1 mL of solution containing 0.4 mg of the drug.

Step 1: Set up the equation, placing the desired unit of measure in the answer to the left of the equal sign: Place the first factor to the right of the equal sign, making sure it is the same unit as the answer. Place the nonratio factor (5 mg) over 1 without the unit label:

$$\text{mL} = \dfrac{1 \text{ mL}}{0.4 \text{ mg}} \times \dfrac{0.8 \text{ mg}}{1}$$

Step 2: Cancel like units of measure in the numerator and denominator, and reduce the fraction:

$$\text{mL} = \dfrac{1 \text{ mL}}{0.4 \text{ mg}} \times \dfrac{0.8 \text{ mg}}{1}$$

NOTE

Math Tip: The only unit remaining after canceling the like units should be the unit of the answer. If this is not the case, the equation is set up incorrectly.

Step 3: Multiply the numerators and then the denominators.

$$\text{mL} = \dfrac{1 \text{ mL}}{0.4 \text{ mg}} = \dfrac{0.8 \text{ mg}}{1}$$

Step 4: Divide the numerator by the denominator to solve the equation.

$$\text{mL} = \dfrac{0.8 \text{ mL}}{0.4} = 2 \text{ mL}$$

Calculating IV Flow Rates

To calculate IV flow rates, the paramedic must know the volume to be infused, the period of time in minutes over which the fluid is to be infused, and the number of drops (gtt) per mL the infusion set delivers (drop factor). The flow rate can then be calculated with the following equation:

$$\text{gtt/min} = \frac{\text{Volume to be infused} \times \text{Drop factor}}{\text{Time of infusion in minutes}}$$

Example: You are to administer 250 mL of normal saline over 90 minutes. Your infusion set delivers 10 gtt/mL. Calculate drops per minute using the above formula:

$$\text{gtt/min} = \frac{250 \text{ mL} \times 10 \text{ gtt/mL}}{90 \text{ minutes}} = \frac{2500 \text{ gtt}}{90 \text{ min}} =$$

$$27.7 \text{ or } 28 \text{ gtt/min}$$

NOTE

The two most common IV infusion sets used in emergency care are microdrip tubing (which delivers 60 gtt/mL), and macrodrip tubing (which delivers 10, 15, or 20 gtt/mL).

? CRITICAL THINKING

When would it be an advantage to use a microdrip tubing? When would it be better to use a macrodrip tubing?

NOTE

Math Tip: When a drop factor of 60 is used, the gtt/min will always equal the mL/hr infusion.

Calculating IV Infusions

It may be necessary to administer medications via a continuous IV infusion. Calculating the correct drip rate is essential to avoid overdosing or underdosing the patient (see the box on page 313). In order to calculate and administer a prescribed drug by continuous infusion, the paramedic must know the prescribed dose, the concentration of the drug in 1 mL of solution, and the drop factor of the IV in-

fusion set. The calculation is then made using the following IV drip formula:

$$\text{gtt/min} = \frac{\text{Prescribed dose} \times \text{Drop factor}}{\text{Concentration of drug in 1 mL}}$$

Example: You are to administer a *procainamide* (Pronestyl) infusion at 3 mg/minute. You have 1 g of the drug in 250 mL of D5W. The infusion set delivers 60 gtt/mL. How many drops per minute will you deliver?

Convert all units to like measurements and calculate the concentration of the drug in 1 mL.

THE "CLOCK" METHOD FOR CALCULATING FLOW RATES

Visualize a clock to calculate flow rates of IV medications. For example, if the concentration of a drug in solution is 4 mg/mL and microdrip tubing is used that delivers 1 mL in 60 drops, and 60 drops are delivered in 1 minute, then 4 mg will be delivered with every 60 drops of solution. Visualizing a clock where 4 mg and 60 drops are at the 12:00 position, you can calculate that 15 drops/minute will deliver 1 mg/minute; 30 drops will deliver 2 mg/min; and 45 drops will deliver 3 mg/min. You can employ this same method with any drug in solution when microdrip is being used to deliver the medication.

LIDOCAINE INFUSION CLOCK

- Mix 2 g of lidocaine in 500 mL D₅W or NS (or 1 g in 250 mL) = 4 mg/mL
- Infusion dose range = 2–4 mg/min
- When administered with a minidrip (60 gtts/mL) intravenous administration set, lidocaine drip rates resemble a seconds "clock"

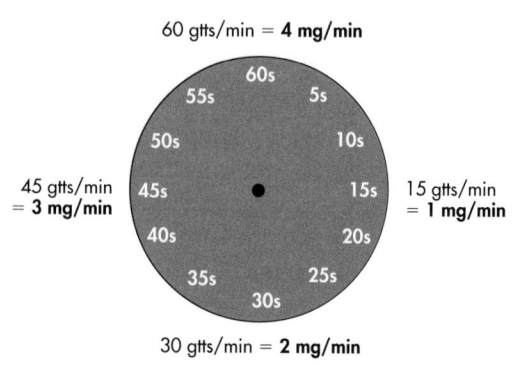

$$1 \text{ g} \times 1000 = 1000 \text{ mg}$$
$$1000 \text{ mg} \div 250 \text{ mL} = 4 \text{ mg/mL}$$

Calculate drops/min using the IV drip formula:

$$\text{gtt/min} = \frac{3 \text{ mg/min} \times 60 \text{ gtt/mL}}{4 \text{ mg in 1 mL}} = \frac{180}{4} = 45 \text{ gtt/min}$$

NOTE

Math Tip: Most ACLS drugs (with the exception of **dopamine** [Intropin] and **magnesium sulfate**) that are administered by continuous IV infusion are mixed "1 in 250" (1 gram of drug in 250 mL of solution) to yield a concentration of 4 mg/mL.

Calculating Drugs Dosages for Infants and Children

The doses of some medications for infants and children are administered in the same proportion to body weight as the doses used for adults. Other medications are given in greatly reduced doses because of differences in the child's ability to metabolize the drug. Pediatric drug doses are often cal-culated in the prehospital setting by use of memory aids (e.g., charts, tapes, dosage books, dosage wheels) or with the advice of medical direction (Fig. 9-5). Drugs used in the management of pediatric emergencies are further described in the *Emergency Drug Index* and in Chapters 41 and 42.

NOTE

The most accurate method for calculating a pediatric drug dose is based on the child's body surface area. Body surface area as a function of weight is described in Chapter 42.

NOTE

Paramedics who administer medication do so by the authority provided through on-line/direct or off-line/indirect medical direction. It is the paramedic's professional and legal responsibility to follow all patient management protocols, policies, and procedures that specify regulations of medication administration, including policies that establish the stocking and supply of drugs.

SHORTCUT FOR CALCULATING DOPAMINE DRIPS

Dopamine (Intropin) is a very potent drug, and calculating the correct dose can intimidate the best mathematician. The following is a shortcut for calculating **dopamine** infusions using 60 drop/minute IV tubing and a standard mixture of drug in solution (e.g., 400 mg in 250 mL; 800 mg in 500 mL).
Formula:

$$\frac{\text{Dose} \times \text{weight in kg} \times 60 \text{ drops/min}}{1600} = \text{Drops per minute}$$

Example:

You are to administer 5 μg per kg of dopamine per minute to a 75-kg patient.

$$\frac{5 \ \mu\text{g} \times 75 \text{ kg} \times 60 \text{ drops/min}}{1600} = \text{14 drops per minute}$$

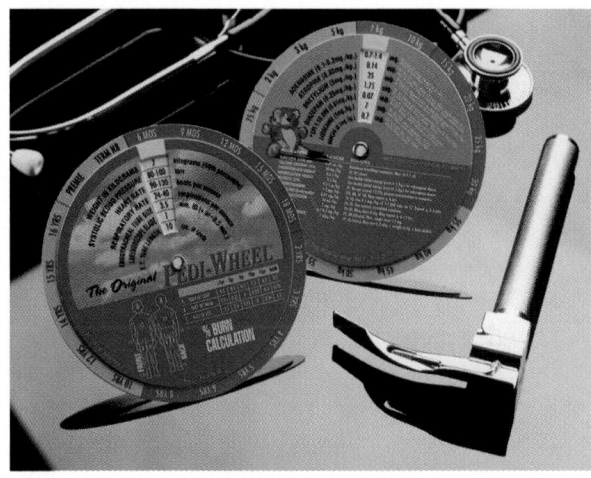

Fig. 9-5 PediWheel.

Drug Administration

Safety considerations and procedures should be a high priority during administration of any medication.

Safety Considerations and Procedures

The paramedic should observe the following guidelines when administering drugs to patients:

- When preparing or giving medicines, concentrate on the procedure and avoid distractions.
- In the prehospital setting, ensure that medication orders received from medical direction are clearly understood. Repeat all orders back to medical direction for confirmation before administering a drug. In the emergency department or other patient care areas, make certain that you have a written order for every medication you administer. Verify the patient's name on the armband or identification tag and verify that the patient has no allergy to the medication. Be sure that the *right* patient receives the *right* dose of the *right* drug via the *right* route at the *right* time (the "five patient rights" of drug administration). Also ensure that correct and thorough documentation occurs (the sixth patient right of drug administration).

> **NOTE**
>
> The "five patient rights" of drug administration
>   Ensure that the *right* patient receives the *right* dose of the *right* drug via the *right* route at the *right* time.

- Make a habit of reading the label of the medicine and comparing it to the medication order at least three times before administration: (1) when removing the drug from the drug kit or supply area, (2) when preparing the medication for administration, and (3) just before administering it to the patient (before the container is discarded).
- Always verify the route of administration. Some medications can be prepared for administration by several routes (e.g., intramuscular or intravenous).

- Make certain that the information on the medication label corresponds exactly to the prescriber's order.
- Never give a medicine from an unlabeled container or from a container on which the label is not legible.
- If you are uncertain of your drug calculation, have a co-worker check your calculation or contact medical direction for verification.
- Handle multidose vials carefully and with aseptic technique, so that medicines are not wasted or contaminated.
- When preparing multiple injections, always label the syringe immediately. Keep the medication container with the syringe. Do not rely on memory to determine which solution is in which syringe.
- Never administer an unlabeled medication prepared by another person. In doing so, you accept the responsibility for accuracy, dose, and correct medication.
- Never administer a medication that is outdated or that appears discolored, cloudy, or in any other way unusual or tampered with.
- If the patient or your co-workers express doubt or concern about a medication or dose, recheck to make certain that there is no error before administering the medication. Be aware that the patient has the right to refuse medication.
- Carefully monitor the patient for any adverse effects for at least 5 minutes after administration of any medication. (A longer observation time may be required for intramuscular and oral medications.)
- Document all medications given. This documentation should include the name of the drug, the dosage, and the time and route of administration. When recording parenteral medications, note the site of injection. The patient's response, adverse as well as intended, should be recorded.
- Follow governmental guidelines and local EMS policies regarding the return and disposal of any unused medication.

> **? CRITICAL THINKING**
>
> *Your clinical preceptor hands you an unlabeled syringe of medication and tells you to give it IV push. What will you do?*

Medication Errors

Medication errors occur with astonishing frequency. More than 700,000 patients receive the wrong medicine or the incorrect dose of medicine in U.S. hospitals each year.[3] Common causes of medication errors are as follows:

- A wrong medication dose was ordered by the prescriber.
- Drug calculations were in error.
- Drugs were administered via the wrong route.
- The wrong patient received the drug.

If an incident involving a medication error occurs, the paramedic should:

- Accept professional responsibility for his or her actions.
- Immediately advise medical direction or the prescriber.
- Assess and carefully monitor the patient for effects of the drug.
- Document the medication error as required by local and state drug administration policies and those of the medical direction institution.
- Modify personal practice to avoid a similar error in the future.
- Follow EMS agency procedures for documentation and quality improvement activities.

Medical Asepsis

Medical asepsis is the removal or destruction of disease-causing organisms or infected material. Medical asepsis is accomplished by using "clean" technique (versus sterile technique) that includes hygienic measures, cleaning agents, antiseptics, disinfectants, and barrier fields.

> **NOTE**
>
> Sterile technique (surgical asepsis) employs the use of sterile equipment and sterile fields that are free from all forms and types of life. Clean technique focuses on destroying or inhibiting only the pathogens (not all forms and types of life).

Antiseptics and Disinfectants

Antiseptics and disinfectants are chemical agents used to kill specific groups of microorganisms. They generally are not very effective against spores of bacteria and fungi, many viruses, and some resistant bacterial strains. Disinfectants are used only on nonliving objects and are toxic to living tissue. Antiseptics are applied only to living tissue and are more dilute to prevent cell damage. Some chemical agents (e.g., alcohol and some chlorine compounds) have both antiseptic and disinfectant properties (Box 9-2 and Table 9-2).

Universal Precautions in Medication Administration

Universal precautions (described in the Appendix of this chapter) should be part of every patient encounter. When administering drugs, the paramedic should observe handwashing and gloving procedures if indicated; face shields are indicated during the administration of endotracheal drugs (see table on inside cover).

> **NOTE**
>
> Handwashing is frequently called the most important measure to reduce the risk of transmitting organisms from one person to another or from one site to another on the same patient.[4] Handwashing offers protection for both the paramedic and the patient. If soap and water are not readily available, a waterless sanitizing solution should be used.

> **BOX 9-2**
>
> ### SAMPLING OF ANTISEPTICS AND DISINFECTANTS
>
> **Antiseptics**
> Hexachlorophene
> Silver nitrate
> Benzoyl peroxide
>
> **Disinfectants**
> Cresol
> Carbolic acid
> Lysol

TABLE 9-2	REPROCESSING METHODS FOR EQUIPMENT USED IN THE PREHOSPITAL HEALTH CARE SETTING*

ORGANISMS DESTROYED	METHODS	USE
Sterilization		
All forms of microbial life, including high numbers of bacterial spores	Steam under pressure (autoclave), gas (ethylene oxide), dry heat, or immersion in EPA-approved chemical "sterilant" for prolonged period (e.g., 6 to 10 hours or according to manufacturer's instructions. NOTE: Liquid chemical sterilants should be used *only* on instruments impossible to sterilize or disinfect with heat).	For instruments or devices that penetrate skin or contact normally sterile areas of the body (e.g., scalpels, needles) (Disposable invasive equipment eliminates the need to reprocess these types of items. When indicated, however, arrangements should be made with a health care facility for reprocessing of reusable invasive instruments.)
High-Level Disinfection		
All forms of microbial life *except* high numbers of bacterial spores	Hot water pasteurization (80° to 100° C, 30 minutes) or exposure to an EPA-registered sterilant chemical, except for a short exposure time (10 to 45 minutes or as directed by the manufacturer)	For reusable instruments or devices that come into contact with mucous membranes (e.g., laryngoscope blades, endotracheal tubes)
Intermediate-Level Disinfection		
Mycobacterium tuberculosis, vegetative bacteria, most viruses, and most fungi, but *not* bacterial spores	EPA-registered "hospital disinfectant" chemical germicides that have a label claim for tuberculocidal activity, commercially available hard-surface germicides, or solutions containing at least 500 ppm free available chlorine (a 1:100 dilution of common household bleach—approximately 1 cup bleach per gallon of tap water)	For surfaces that come into contact only with intact skin (e.g., stethoscopes, blood pressure cuffs, splints) *and* have been visibly contaminated with blood or bloody body fluids (Surfaces *must* be precleaned of visible material before the germicidal chemical is applied for disinfection.)
Low-Level Disinfection		
Most bacteria, some viruses, some fungi, but not *Mycobacterium tuberculosis* or bacterial spores	EPA-registered hospital disinfectants (no label claim for tuberculocidal activity)	For routine housekeeping or removal of soiling in the *absence* of visible blood contamination
Environmental Disinfection		
	Any cleaner or disinfectant agent intended for environmental use	For environmental surfaces that have become soiled and that should be cleaned and disinfected (e.g., floors, woodwork, ambulance seats, countertops)

Important: To ensure the effectiveness of any sterilization or disinfection process, equipment and instruments must first be thoroughly cleaned of all visible soil.
*EPA, Environmental Protection Agency.

Enteral Medication Administration

As described in Chapter 8, enteral medications refer to those drugs that are administered and absorbed through the gastrointestinal tract. These methods include oral, gastric, and rectal drug administration.

Oral Route

The oral route is the most frequently used method of drug administration. The patient should be in an upright or sitting position. The pill, tablet, or capsule should be placed in the patient's mouth and

BOX 9-3

SOLID AND LIQUID ORAL MEDICATIONS

Caplets
Capsules
Time-released capsules
Lozenges
Pills
Tablets
Elixirs
Emulsions
Suspensions
Syrups

swallowed with enough fluid (4 to 8 ounces) to ensure that the drug reaches the stomach.

? CRITICAL THINKING

Think of some clinical situations where oral medication administration would not be appropriate. Why?

Many oral drugs are available in solid and liquid forms (Box 9-3). If the medication is in a suspension, the stock bottle or unit dose should be shaken thoroughly before the drug is poured for administration. A drug not packaged as a unit dose should be measured in a medicine cup, medicine dropper, or by syringe.

Administration of Medications by Gastric Tube

Most drugs that can be administered orally can also be administered via a gastric tube (orogastric tube, nasogastric tube). Before administering a drug through this route, verify correct placement of the tube by injecting 30 mL to 50 mL of air into the tube and auscultating the epigastric region for sound of air movement. Once the correct position is confirmed, administer the drug through the tube, followed by a small amount of water (about 30 mL) to flush the drug and to help maintain the patency of the tube. An emergency drug that is administered through this route is *activated charcoal*. (Nasogastric and orogastric tube insertion are described in Chapter 32.)

BOX 9-4

PROCEDURE FOR ADMINISTRATION OF RECTAL DRUGS

1. Carefully restrain the child. If possible, place the child in a knee-chest or lateral recumbent position with legs flexed at hip and knee.
2. Draw the drug dose into a syringe and remove the needle. (A slightly higher dose may be required because absorption will be incomplete. Consult with medical direction.)
3. Introduce the lubricated syringe just beyond the external sphincter (aiming just above the junction of the skin and mucous membranes and directed toward the rectal wall).
4. Inject the solution into the rectum.
5. Facilitate drug retention by squeezing the buttocks together with manual pressure.

NOTE: This same procedure also is appropriate for adult patients.

Rectal Administration of Medications

Some drugs (e.g., suppositories) are designed for rectal administration. Other drugs can be given through the rectal route when vascular access cannot be established. Emergency drugs that can be administered rectally include *diazepam* (Valium) and *lorazepam* (Ativan). Box 9-4 describes the procedure for administering rectal drugs to a child.

Parenteral Administration of Medications

Parenteral drugs are administered outside the gastrointestinal tract and usually refer to injections.

NOTE

Parenteral administration of drugs can be especially hazardous because the drugs given by injection are usually considered irretrievable. In addition, there is a slight chance of infection because the integrity of the skin is broken. Other potential hazards associated with parenteral administration include lipodystrophy, cellulitis or abscess formation, necrosis, skin slough, nerve injury, prolonged pain, and periostitis. Aseptic technique, accurate drug dosage, proper rate of injection, and proper site of injection are essential to minimize the risk of harm.

Parenteral routes for drug administration include intradermal, subcutaneous, intramuscular, intravenous, and intraosseous. (Percutaneous medications will also be presented in this section.)

Equipment Used for Injections

Syringes and Needles

The choice of syringe and needle depends on the route of administration, characteristics of the fluid (e.g., aqueous, oil-based), and volume of medication. Syringes in common use today are made of disposable plastic. Sizes range from 1-mL tuberculin and insulin syringes to 60-mL irrigation syringes. Tuberculin syringes are marked in 0.01-mL gradients and should be used when the volume to

be administered is small. Insulin syringes are available in 0.5- and 1-mL volumes and are marked in 1-unit increments. When used with the specified strength of insulin, this syringe allows

> **NOTE**
>
> Some IV catheters provide additional protection against accidental need sticks by retracting the needle into case as the catheter is advanced. Needleless IV tubings and connectors also have been developed with built-in puncturing devices made of plastic that are sharp enough to pierce the rubber medication port on IV tubing. Other IV devices have locking ports with blunt ends or no puncturing device at all (see the box on p. 319).

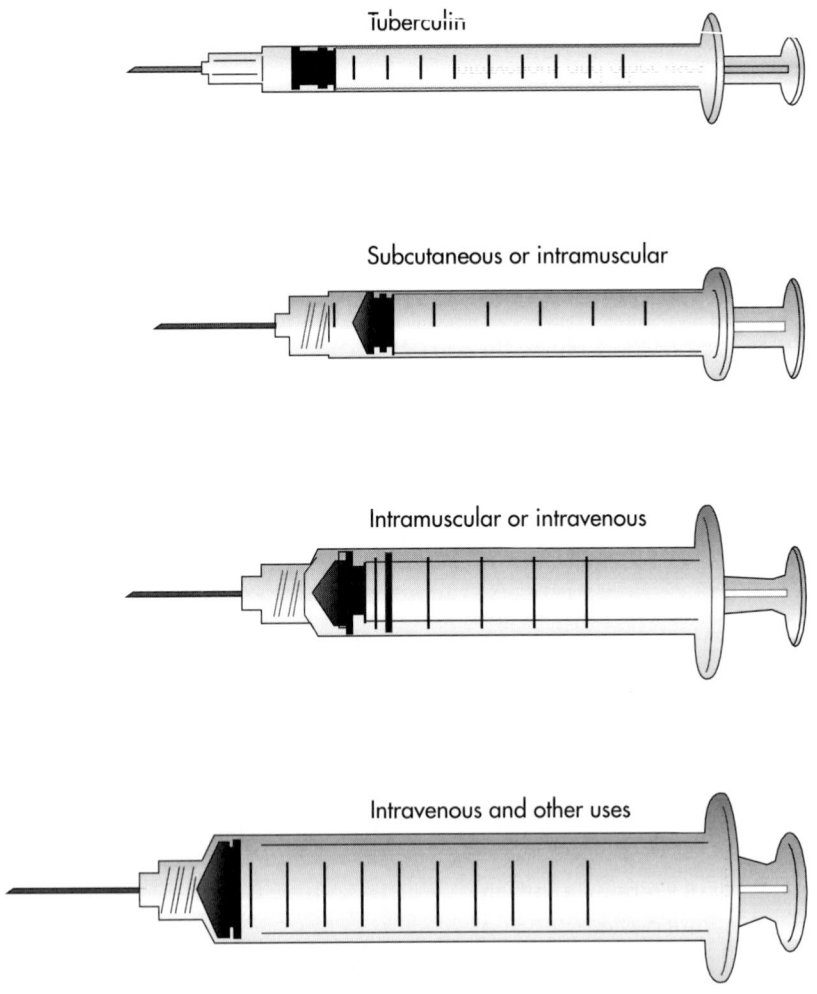

Fig. 9-6 Syringes.

the patient to easily draw up the correct dose without performing calculations. Tuberculin and insulin syringes should not be substituted for each other. Fig. 9-6 illustrates syringes used to accurately measure varying amounts of liquids and liquid medications.

Needles vary in length and gauge from 3/8 inch to 3 or more inches in length and from 12 gauge (large lumen) to 30 gauge (small lumen). Smaller-lumen (larger gauge) needles are usually used for intradermal injections. Subcutaneous injections are usually given with a 5/8-inch, 23- or 25-gauge needle. Intramuscular injections are usually given with a 19- or 21-gauge, 1- to 2-inch needle; occasionally a 16- or 18-gauge needle is used.

Parenteral Medication Containers

Medications used for injection are usually supplied in single-dose ampules, multidose vials, or prefilled syringes. Single-dose ampules are glass containers that hold one dose of a medication for injection, after which the ampule is discarded. Multidose vials are glass containers equipped with rubber stoppers that permit several medication doses to be withdrawn for injection.

To prepare a prescribed medication for injection, the paramedic should choose the appropriate needle and syringe. The size of the syringe should be in proportion to the volume of solution to be administered. To withdraw medication from an ampule or vial, the paramedic should do the following (Fig. 9-7):

1. Assemble the necessary equipment (alcohol swab or gauze, syringe, 18-gauge needle to withdraw medication if using an ampule, and appropriate-gauge needle for injection).

NEEDLE AND SHARPS INJURIES

Injuries to health care workers from conventional needles and sharps account for between 600,000 and one million injuries each year.* Although infection with the hepatitis C virus (HCV) is the most frequent infection resulting from needle stick and sharps injury,† the transmission of other diseases also is possible. These diseases include HIV, hepatitis B, syphilis, herpes simplex, herpes zoster, Rocky Mountain spotted fever, and tuberculosis. The following measures should be taken to avoid such exposures:

- Health care personnel should obtain assistance when administering infusion therapy or injections to uncooperative patients.
- Needles should not be recapped, purposely bent or broken by hand, removed from disposable syringes, or otherwise manipulated by hand. If recapping or needle removal is necessary because no alternative is feasible or a specific medical procedure requires it, use of a mechanical device or a one-handed technique is recommended. Needleless products should be used when available.
- Disposable syringes and needles, scalpel blades, and other sharp items should be placed in puncture-resistant containers for disposal.

*Evaluation of safety devices for preventing percutaneous injuries among healthcare workers during phlebotomy procedures, *MMWR* 46, 1997.
†Recommendations for prevention and control of hepatitis C virus (HCV) infection and HCV-related chronic disease, *MMWR*, 47, 1998.

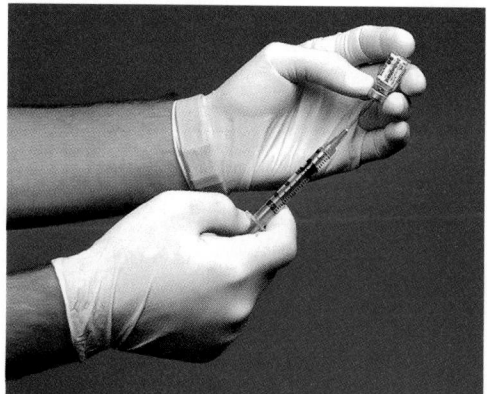

Fig. 9-7 Withdrawing medication from a vial.

2. Compute the desired volume of medication to be administered.
3. If using a vial:
    a. Clean the rubber stopper with alcohol.
    b. Using the needle chosen for the injection, inject a volume of air into the vial equivalent to the amount of solution to be withdrawn; this prevents a vacuum in the vial, which can make the solution difficult to withdraw. Withdraw the volume required and remove the syringe from the vial.
    c. Gently advance the plunger of the syringe to expel air from the solution.
4. If using an ampule:
    a. Lightly tap or shake the ampule to dislodge any solution from the neck of the container.
    b. Wrap the neck of the glass ampule with an alcohol swab or gauze dressing for protection.
    c. Grasp the ampule, snap off the top, and discard the top in an appropriate medication disposal container. (The ampule is designed to break easily when pressure is exerted at the neck.)
    d. Carefully insert an 18-gauge needle into the solution without allowing it to touch the edges of the ampule and draw the solution into the syringe.
    e. Carefully remove the 18-gauge needle and discard it in the appropriate container. Attach the needle to be used for injection.
    f. Gently advance the plunger of the syringe to expel air.

Mixing medications. Two compatible drugs (e.g., *meperidine* [Demerol] and *hydroxyzine* [Vistaril]) can be mixed together into one injection if the total volume of the dosage is within accepted limits. When mixing medications, it is important not to contaminate one medication with another and to maintain aseptic technique. To mix medications, the paramedic should follow these steps:

> **NOTE**
>
> Some hospitals and EMS services require that a filter needle be used as a precaution for glass particles when withdrawing medications from an ampule. An additional precaution is the use of in-line tubing filters for intravenous injections.

> **NOTE**
>
> Some medications (e.g., **streptokinase** [Streptase], and **Reteplase** [Retavase]) are dry powders that must be reconstituted before administration. Carefully read the manufacturer's information and use the correct amount of the diluent prescribed for this purpose. Always mix the diluent and powder in the closed vial before withdrawing the dose. Some drugs are packaged in a vial that contains the diluent and powder in two compartments (Mix-o-vial).

Mixing Medications From Two Vials

1. Use only one syringe to mix the drugs.
2. Aspirate the volume of air equivalent to the first drug's dosage. Inject the air into vial A, ensuring that the needle does not touch the solution. Withdraw the needle.
3. Aspirate air equivalent to the second drug's dose and inject the volume of air into vial B. Withdraw the required medication from vial B.
4. Apply a new sterile needle to the syringe and insert it into vial A. Be careful not to push the plunger or expel the drug from the syringe into the vial.

> **NOTE**
>
> The paramedic should never inject medication back into a vial from a syringe. To do so introduces risk of infection or mixing drugs. The top of the vial or bottle is a "one-way street."

5. Withdraw the desired amount of the drug from vial A into the syringe.
6. Apply a new sterile needle and administer the injection.

Mixing Medications From One Vial and One Ampule

1. Withdraw the desired drug dose from the vial first.
2. Use the same syringe and needle to withdraw medication from the ampule.

> **NOTE**
>
> If there is any uncertainty about drug compatibility, the paramedic should consult with medical direction.

3. Apply a new sterile needle and administer the drug.

Prefilled syringes. There are several manufacturers of prefilled syringes (Fig. 9-8), and the techniques for activating and using the products vary. The paramedic should be familiar with the devices used by particular EMS systems. The technique for activating a common type of prefilled syringe follows:

1. Calculate the desired volume of medication to be administered.
2. Pop off the protective caps from the syringe barrel and medication cartridge.
3. Screw the cartridge into the syringe barrel.

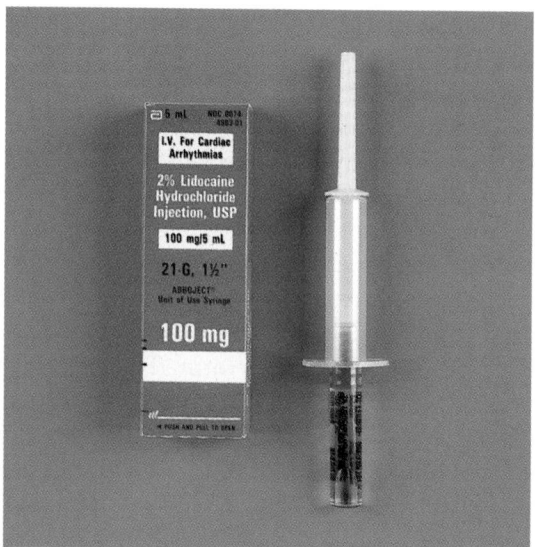

Fig. 9-8 Prefilled syringe for injection of medication.

4. Gently advance the plunger of the syringe to expel air.

Preparing the Injection Site

The injection site should be prepared by cleansing the area with alcohol, iodine swabs, or both (per local protocol), using aseptic technique:

1. Thoroughly scrub the site with alcohol to remove dirt, dead skin, and other surface contaminants.
2. Disinfect the site with overlapping concentric circles, moving outward from the site.
3. Allow the site to dry.

Intradermal Injections

An intradermal injection is made just below the epidermis or outer layer of skin (Fig. 9-9). This site is commonly used for allergy testing and for administration of local anesthetics. The syringe used for intradermal injection is usually a tuberculin syringe, and the volume injected is usually less than 0.5 mL. Common sites for intradermal injections are the medial surface of the forearm and the back. The procedure for these injections is as follows:

1. Choose the injection site and cleanse the skin surface.
2. Hold the skin taut with one hand.
3. With the other hand, hold the syringe with the needle bevel up at a 10- to 15-degree angle from injection site.
4. Gently puncture the skin until the bevel is completely under the skin surface and inject the prescribed medication. The injection will usually

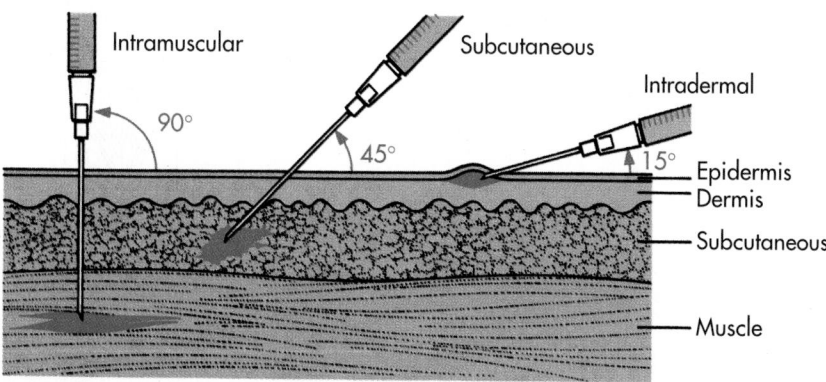

Fig. 9-9 Comparison of angle of injection and location of deposition of medication for intramuscular, subcutaneous, and intradermal injections. (From Clark JBF: *Pharmacological basis of nursing,* ed 4, St Louis, 1993, Mosby.)

produce a raised wheal resembling a mosquito bite.
5. Withdraw the needle and appropriately discard the equipment.

Subcutaneous Injections

Subcutaneous injections are given to place medication below the skin into the subcutaneous layer. The volume of a subcutaneous injection is usually less than 0.5 mL, administered through a ½ or ⅝-inch, 23- or 25-gauge needle. The most common drug administered via this route in the prehospital setting is *epinephrine* (Adrenalin). Common sites for subcutaneous injections are illustrated in Fig. 9-10. The procedure for subcutaneous injections follows:

1. Choose the injection site.
2. Elevate the subcutaneous tissue by "pinching" the injection site.
3. With the needle bevel up, insert the needle at a 45-degree angle in one quick motion.
4. Pull back slightly on the plunger (aspirate) to ensure needle placement. If no blood is aspirated, gently but smoothly inject the medication. If blood is present on aspiration, withdraw the needle, discard the medication and equipment, and begin again.
5. After the injection, withdraw the needle at the same angle it was inserted. Use an alcohol swab to massage the site. This helps distribute medication and promote absorption by dilating blood vessels in the area and increasing blood flow.

Intramuscular Injections

Deeper injections are made into muscular tissue, passing through the skin and subcutaneous tissue, when a drug is too irritating to be given subcutaneously (although irritation may occur via this route as well) or when a greater volume or faster absorption is desired. A volume up to 5 mL may be given by intramuscular injection.

The type of needle used depends on the site of the injection, condition of the tissue, size of the patient, and nature of the drug to be injected (small lumens for thin solutions and larger lumens for suspensions and oils). Because the muscle layer is below the subcutaneous layer, a longer needle is generally used (usually 1½ inches and 19 or 21 gauge). The procedures for intramuscular injections are the same as those previously described, but the needle is inserted at a 90-degree angle and the skin is held taut, not pinched.

Several muscles are commonly used for intramuscular injections, including the deltoid muscle, dorsogluteal site, vastus lateralis muscle, rectus femoris muscle, and ventrogluteal muscle. The deltoid muscle is located in the upper arm. It forms a triangular shape, with the base of the triangle along the acromion process and the peak of the triangle ending approximately a third of the way down the lateral aspect of the upper arm (Fig. 9-11). This muscle is used primarily for vaccinations with small volumes of injection, because the muscle is small and can accommodate only small doses of injection (1 mL or less). When injections are made in this location, care should be taken to avoid hitting

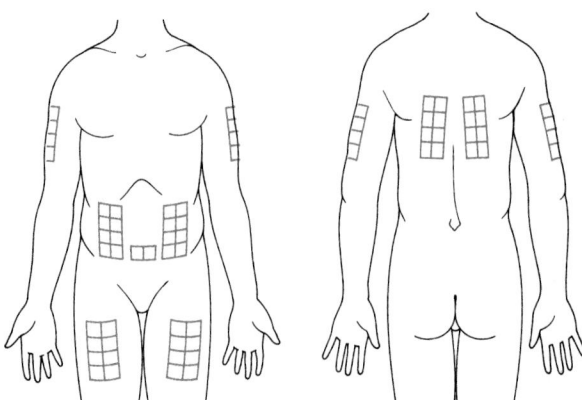

Fig. 9-10 Commonly used subcutaneous injection sites. (From Clark JBF: *Pharmacological basis of nursing*, ed 4, St Louis, 1993, Mosby.)

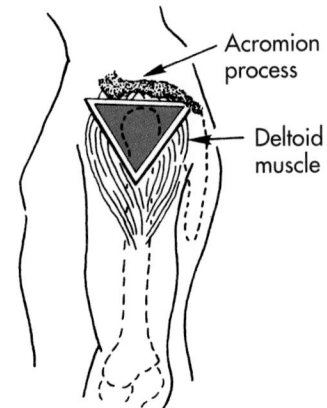

Fig. 9-11 Deltoid muscle injection site roughly forms an inverted triangle, with the acromion process as the base. The muscle may be visible in well-developed patients. (From Clark JBF: *Pharmacological basis of nursing*, ed 4, St Louis, 1993, Mosby.)

the radial nerve. The patient should be sitting upright or lying flat and should be told to relax the arm muscles.

The dorsogluteal site consists of several gluteal muscles, although the gluteus medius muscle is most commonly used for injection. There are two ways to define this site: (1) divide the buttocks on one side into imaginary quadrants, and administer the medication into the upper outer quadrant, or (2) locate the posterior superior iliac spine and the greater trochanter of the femur, drawing an imaginary line between the two landmarks. Then give the injection up and out from this line (Fig. 9-12). This site should not be used for children under age 3 because the muscles are not yet well developed and because of the proximity of the sciatic nerve (the largest nerve in the body). Large, well-developed muscles can accommodate an injection up to 5 mL, but anything over 3 mL may be uncomfortable for the patient. When an injection is being administered via this route, the patient should be lying prone, with the toes pointing inward to promote muscle

relaxation. Another complication resulting from gluteal injections is injection into the hip joint, although the risk of this is minimized by attention to anatomical landmarks.

The vastus lateralis and the rectus femoris muscles are located in the thigh and lie side by side. To identify necessary landmarks, the paramedic should place one hand on the patient's upper thigh and one hand on the lower thigh. The area between the paramedic's hands is the middle third of the thigh and the middle third of the underlying muscle (Fig. 9-13). The vastus lateralis lies lateral to the midline and is the preferred injection site for children. It is well developed in all patients and has few major blood vessels and nerves that can be injured. The rectus femoris is most often used for self-injection because of its accessibility. Acceptable volumes for injection vary with the age of the patient and the size of the muscle. Up to 5 mL may be injected into a well-developed adult. The patient should be sitting upright or lying supine and should be advised to relax his or her muscles.

The ventrogluteal muscle is accessible when the patient lies in a supine or lateral recumbent position. The greater trochanter should be palpated with the palm, with the index finger pointing to the anterior superior iliac spine. The paramedic's remaining three fingers should extend toward the

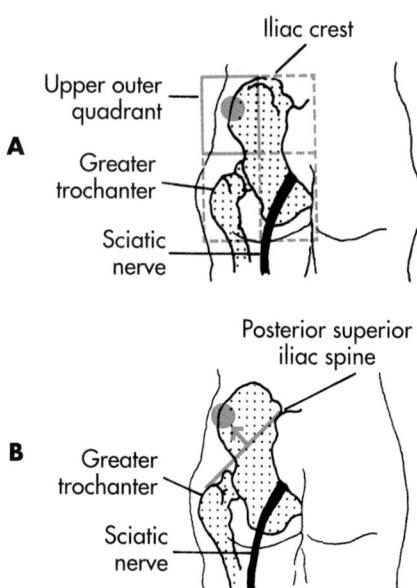

Fig. 9-12 Two accepted methods for defining the dorsogluteal injection site. **A,** The patient's buttocks can be divided on one side into imaginary quadrants. The center of the upper outer quadrant should be used as the injection site. **B,** The paramedic locates by palpation the posterior superior iliac spine and the greater trochanter and then draws an imaginary line between the two. An injection site up and out from that line should be used. (From Clark JBF: *Pharmacological basis of nursing,* ed 4, St Louis, 1993, Mosby.)

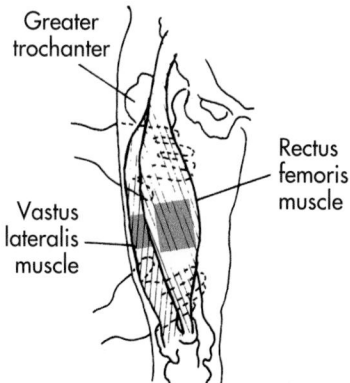

Fig. 9-13 To define the vastus lateralis muscle injection site and the rectus femoral muscle site, place one hand below the patient's greater trochanter and one hand above the knee. The space between the two hands defines the middle third of the underlying muscle. The rectus femoris is on the anterior thigh; the vastus lateralis is on the lateral side. (From Clark JBF: *Pharmacological basis of nursing,* ed 4, St Louis, 1993, Mosby.)

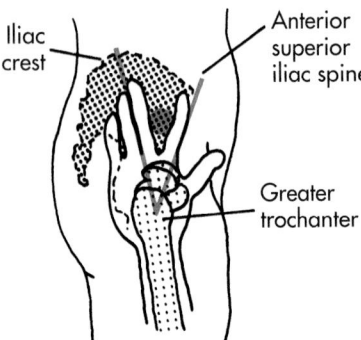

Fig. 9-14 To locate the ventrogluteal muscle injection site, place the palm of one hand on the trochanter of the femur. Make a V with the fingers of that hand, with one side running from the greater trochanter to the anterior-superior iliac spine and the other side running from the greater trochanter to the iliac crest. (From Clark JBF: *Pharmacological basis of nursing,* ed 4, St Louis, 1993, Mosby.)

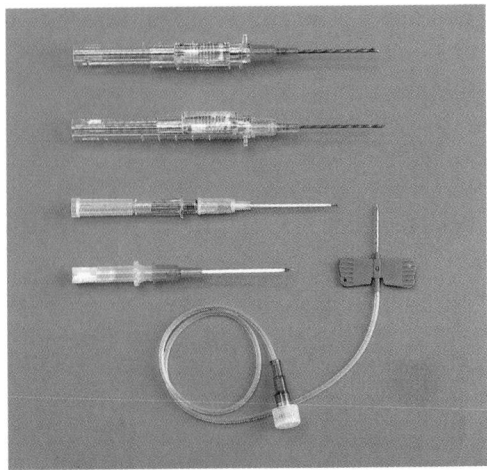

Fig. 9-15 Various types of IV catheters.

iliac crest. The injection is then made into the center of the V formed between the fingers (Fig. 9-14). This injection site may be used for all patients. It is desirable because the site is free of large nerves and fat tissue. In the adult, this muscle may accommodate up to 5 mL of drug.

Intravenous Therapy

Intravenous cannulation is used to gain access to the body's circulation. Intravenous cannulation is indicated (1) to administer fluids, (2) to administer drugs, and (3) to obtain specimens for laboratory determinations.

> **NOTE**
>
> The intravenous route of drug administration places the drug directly into the bloodstream, bypassing all barriers to drug absorption.

> **? CRITICAL THINKING**
>
> *What are the advantages to selecting the upper extremity for intravenous access in an adult?*

IV Fluid Administration

The route of choice for fluid therapy in the prehospital setting is through a peripheral vein in an ex-

tremity. Provided that the arms have no major injury, upper extremity veins should be used. (Some EMS services advise to avoid upper extremity sites when a major injury to the neck or upper thorax has occurred on that side.) When upper extremity sites are inappropriate, lower extremity sites may be used.

> **NOTE**
>
> IV fluids (described in Chapter 8) commonly used in the prehospital setting include normal saline, lactated Ringer's solution, and mixtures of glucose and water. Normal saline and lactated Ringer's solution generally are used to provide fluid replacement and as a vehicle for drug administration.

Choice of intravenous catheters. There are three main types of intravenous catheters: (1) hollow needles ("butterfly" type), (2) indwelling plastic catheters *over* a hollow needle (e.g., Angiocath or Jelco), and (3) indwelling plastic catheters inserted *through* a hollow needle (e.g., Intracath; seldom used in the prehospital setting) (Fig. 9-15).

Hollow needles are not recommended for intravenous fluid replacement in the prehospital setting because of the difficulty in stabilizing the needle. Occasionally, the paramedic chooses the "butterfly" type needle for the pediatric patient if adequate stabilization can be maintained through the use of armboards or other immobilization devices. The over-the-needle catheter is generally preferred for

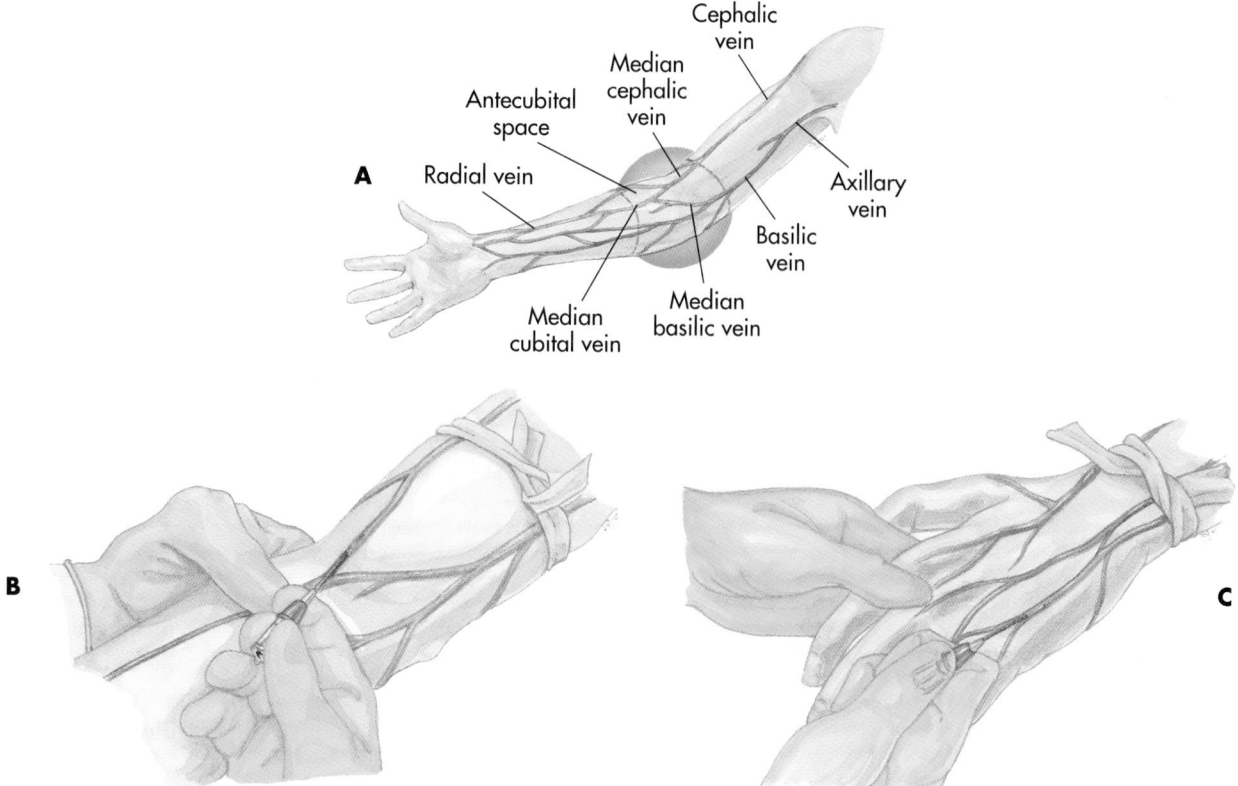

Fig. 9-16 A, Veins of the upper extremity. **B,** Antecubital venipuncture. **C,** Dorsal hand venipuncture.

use in the prehospital setting. It is easily secured and more comfortable for the patient.

Peripheral intravenous insertion. Common areas used for peripheral intravenous therapy are the hands and arms, including the antecubital fossae (AC space). Alternative sites include the long saphenous veins and the external jugular veins. However, the incidence of embolism and infection is higher at these alternative sites. Figs. 9-16 through 9-18 illustrate sites and techniques for peripheral cannulation.

Another consideration in choosing a puncture site for intravenous therapy is the clinical status of the patient. Injuries or diseases involving an extremity interfere with the use of veins in the affected area for venipuncture or venous cannulation. Examples include trauma, dialysis fistula, and a history of mastectomy.

Steps
1. If the patient is conscious, explain the procedure. This explanation should include why intravenous therapy is necessary and what the procedure entails.

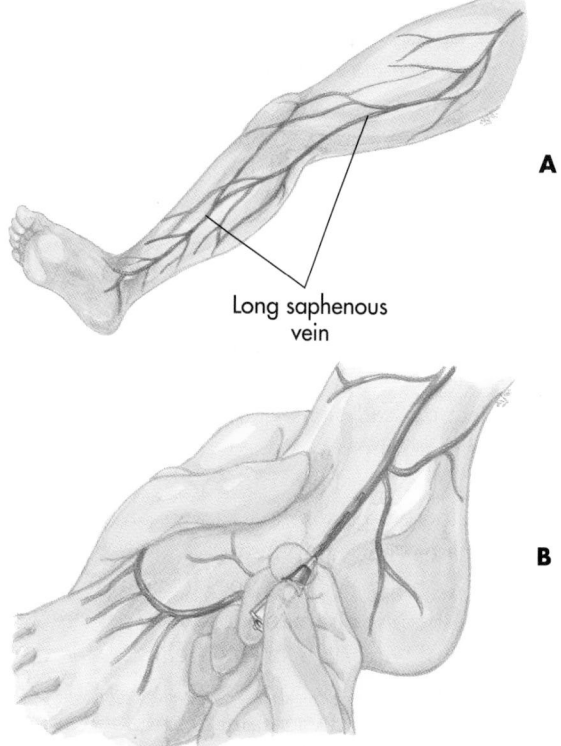

Fig. 9-17 A, Long saphenous vein. **B,** Venipuncture of the long saphenous vein.

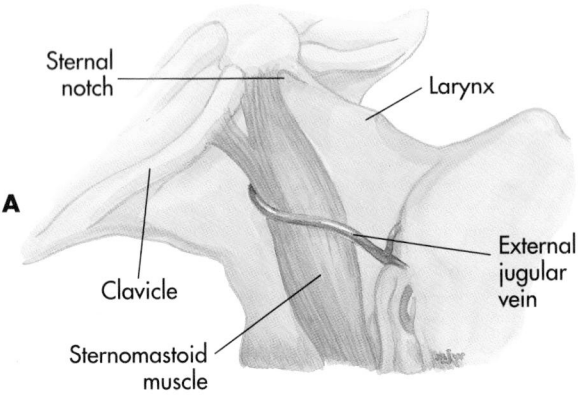

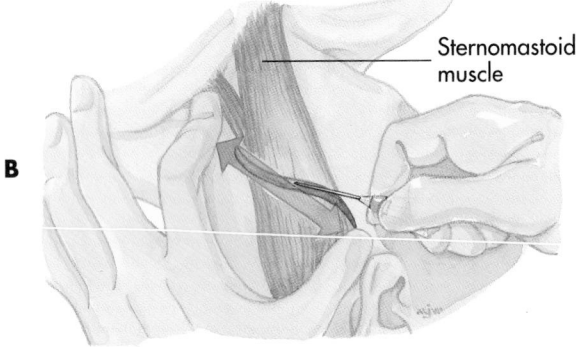

Fig. 9-18 A, Anatomy of the external jugular vein. **B,** External jugular venipuncture.

2. Assemble the necessary equipment.
   a. Inspect the prescribed fluid for contamination, appearance, and expiration date. Never use fluids that are cloudy, outdated, or in any other way suspected of contamination.
   b. Prepare the microdrip or macrodrip infusion set, and attach the infusion set to the bag of solution.
3. Clamp the tubing and squeeze the reservoir on the infusion set until it fills half way. Then open the clamp and flush the air from the tubing. Close the clamp.
4. Select the catheter. A large-bore catheter (14 to 16 gauge) should be used for fluid replacement, and a smaller-bore catheter (18 to 20 gauge) should be used for "keep open" lines.
5. Prepare other equipment:
   a. Alcohol or iodine wipes to cleanse the skin
   b. Antibiotic ointment or cream (per protocol)
   c. Sterile dressings or 4 × 4 gauze pads
   d. Adhesive tape, torn or cut into several strips
   e. Syringes and vacutainers for blood samples
   f. Tourniquet (rubber drain tubing or blood pressure cuff may be used)

6. Apply gloves for personal and patient protection.
7. Select the puncture site. If using an upper extremity, allow the patient's arm to hang dependent, and apply the tourniquet above the antecubital space. (The tourniquet should be just tight enough to tamponade venous vessels but not occlude arterial flow.) When selecting a suitable vein, begin by looking at the dorsum of the hand and forearm. Choose a vein that is fairly straight and easily accessible. The forearm is better than the hand because it allows hand movement and is more easily secured after cannulation. If a second puncture attempt is necessary, the second puncture should always be *proximal* to the first puncture. Therefore the vein selected for initial cannulation should be the most suitable distal vein. Avoid veins near joints, where immobilization will be difficult, and veins near injured areas. If the long saphenous vein is chosen, begin site selection near the medial malleolus of the foot. To locate the external jugular vein, place the patient in a supine head-down position, and turn the patient's head toward the opposite side.
8. Prepare the puncture site. Cleanse the area with alcohol or iodine wipes (per protocol):
   a. Thoroughly clean the site with alcohol to remove dirt, dead skin, blood, and other surface contaminants.
   b. Disinfect the site with overlapping concentric circles, moving outward.
9. Stabilize the vein by applying distal pressure and tension to the point of entry (Fig. 9-19, *A*). With the bevel of the needle up in adults (down in infants and children), pass through the skin and into the vein from the side or directly on top. Advance the needle and catheter about 2 mm beyond the point where blood return in the hub of the needle was first encountered. Slide the catheter over the needle and into the vein (Fig. 9-19, *B*). Withdraw the needle while stabilizing the catheter (Fig. 9-19, *C*). Apply pressure on the proximal end of the catheter to stop escaping blood. Obtain blood samples, if needed, with a syringe or vacutainer.
10. Release the tourniquet and attach tubing (Fig. 9-19, *D*). Open the tubing clamp and allow fluid infusion to begin at the prescribed flow rate (Fig. 9-19, *E*).

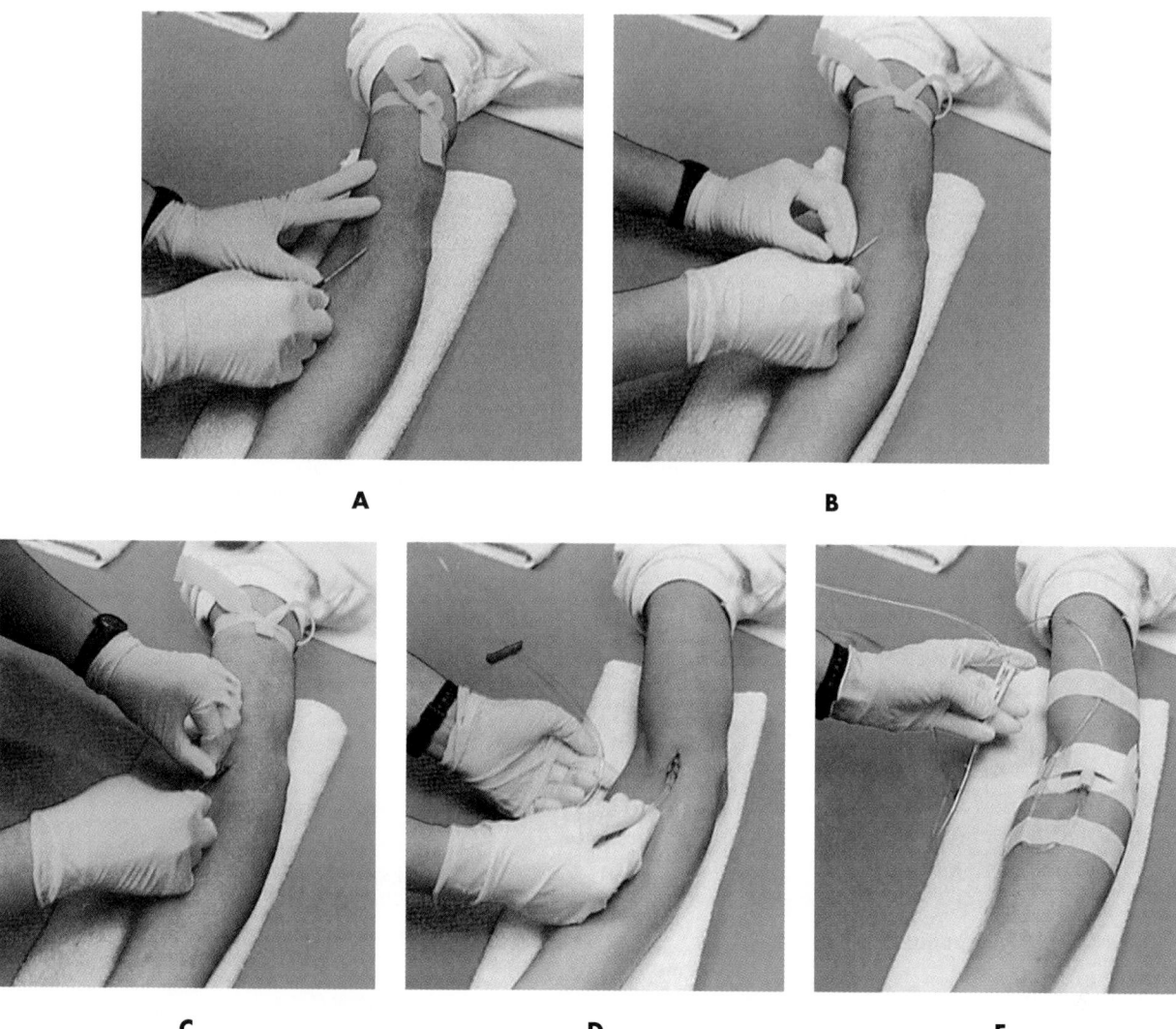

Fig. 9-19 A, Stabilize the vein by applying distal pressure and tension to the point of entry. **B,** With the bevel of the needle up, pass into the vein from the side or directly on top. **C,** Slide the catheter over the needle and into the vein and withdraw the needle while stabilizing the vein. **D,** Release the tourniquet and attach intravenous tubing. **E,** Open the tubing clamp and allow fluid infusion to begin at the prescribed flow rate. Cover the puncture site with antibiotic ointment and dressing.

11. Cover the puncture site with antibiotic ointment and dressing to ensure asepsis and to secure the line. Anchor the tubing, and secure the catheter. Catheter movement can increase the risk of phlebitis and cause migration of pathogens along the cannula into the vein.
12. Document the infusion procedure.

Central venous cannulation. Central venous cannulation may be within the scope of paramedic practice in some advanced life support systems. However, central venous infusion should never be considered as a means of rapid fluid replacement in the prehospi-

tal setting. Sites for central venous cannulation include the femoral vein, internal jugular vein, and subclavian vein. Figs. 9-20 through 9-22 illustrate sites and techniques for central venous cannulation.

Steps. Preparation for cannulation of the central vessels is the same as for peripheral veins. The patient's body position and the paramedic's knowledge of anatomy and familiarity with the procedure are important in determining the success of this procedure. Central vein cannulation requires special training and authorization from medical direction.

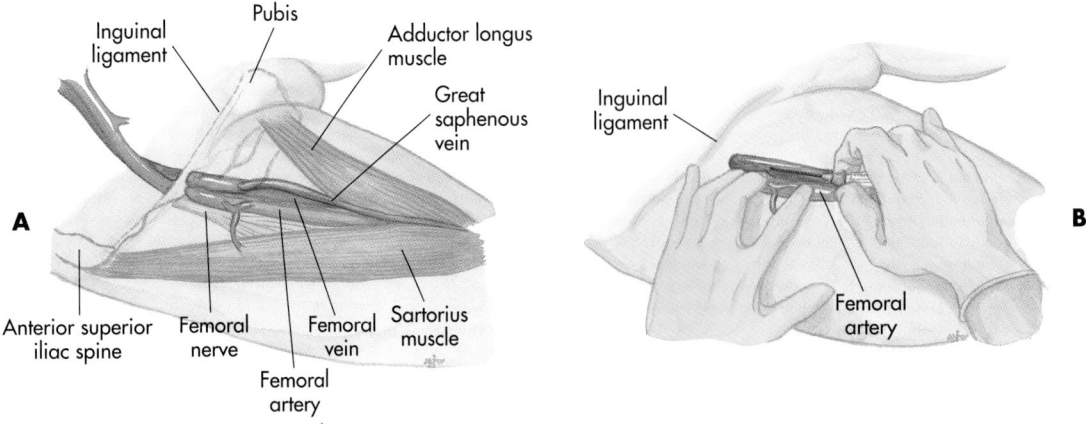

Fig. 9-20 A, Anatomy of the femoral vein. **B,** Femoral venipuncture.

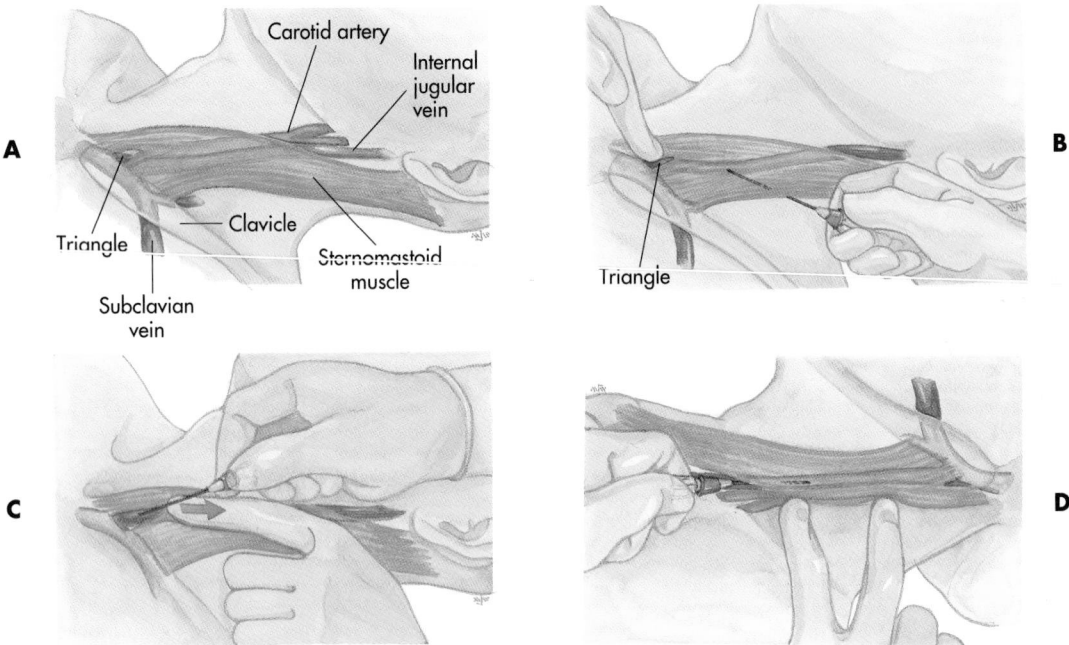

Fig. 9-21 A, Anatomy of the internal jugular vein. **B,** Posterior approach for internal jugular venipuncture. **C,** Central approach for internal jugular venipuncture. **D,** Anterior approach for internal jugular venipuncture.

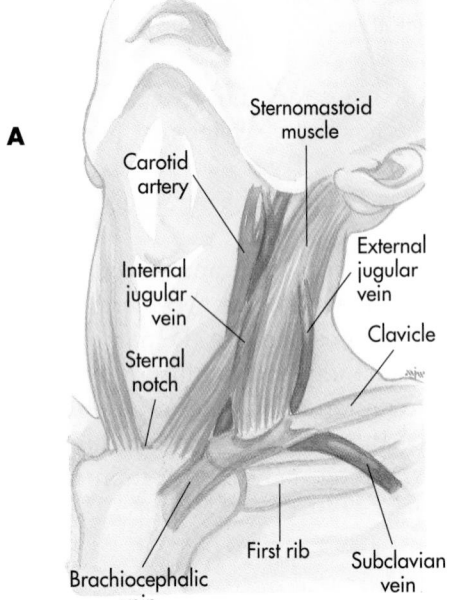

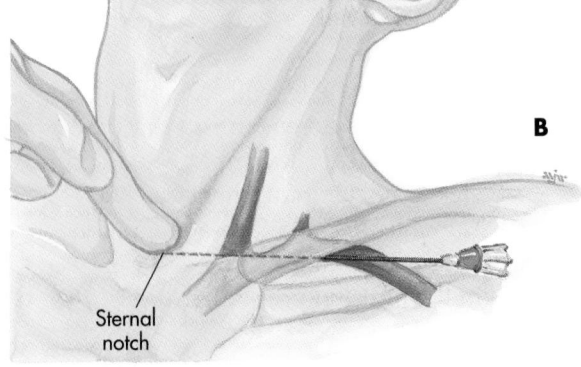

Fig. 9-22 A, Anatomy of the subclavian vein. **B,** Infraclavicular subclavian venipuncture.

Complications of all IV techniques. There are several possible complications associated with all intravenous techniques. These include local complications, systemic complications, infiltration, and air embolism.

Local and Systemic Complications. Local complications may involve hematoma formation, thrombosis, cellulitis, and phlebitis. Systemic complications include the following:

• Sepsis
• Pulmonary embolism
• Catheter fragment embolism
• Fiber embolism originating from cotton or paper fibers contained in the catheter irrigation solution, leading to foreign body reactions
• Arterial puncture

Infiltration. Infiltration may occur when the needle or catheter has been displaced or when blood or fluid leaks from around the catheter. Signs and symptoms include the following:

• Coolness of skin at the puncture site
• Swelling at the puncture site, with or without pain
• Sluggish or absent flow rate

If infiltration is suspected, the fluid reservoir should be lowered to a dependent position to check for the presence of backflow of blood into the tubing. (The absence of backflow suggests infiltration.) If any of these signs and symptoms are present, the intravenous flow should be discontinued, the needle or catheter immediately removed, and a pressure dressing applied to the site (Box 9-5). An alternative puncture site should be chosen and the infusion restarted with new equipment. In addition, the incident should be documented.

Air Embolism. Air embolism is uncommon but can be fatal. Although the volume of air that the human bloodstream can tolerate has not been firmly established, fatalities have been reported after 100 mL of air entering the cardiovascular system.[5] A total of 10 mL of air can be fatal in a critically ill patient.

The embolism is caused by air entering the bloodstream via the catheter tubing. The risk of air embolism is greatest when a catheter is passed into the central circulation, where negative pressure may actually pull in air. Air can enter the circulation either on insertion of the catheter or when the tubing is disconnected to replace solutions or add new extension tubing (Box 9-6). With subsequent pumping, blood foaming occurs in the heart. If enough air enters the heart chamber, it can impede the flow of blood, leading to shock.

Signs and symptoms of air embolism include hypotension; cyanosis; weak, rapid pulse; and loss of

BOX 9-5

DISCONTINUING AN IV INFUSION

To discontinue or remove an IV infusion, follow these steps:
1. Put on gloves.
2. Carefully remove any securing tapes and dressings.
3. Close the drip chamber to stop the flow of fluid.
4. Place sterile gauze over the insertion site, and apply gentle pressure with one hand. With the other, swiftly withdraw the catheter, pulling straight back from the angle of insertion.
5. Apply firm pressure to the insertion site for 2 to 5 minutes to prevent bleeding or bruising.
6. Cover the insertion site with a bandage.
7. Appropriately dispose of all equipment.

BOX 9-6

REPLACING IV SOLUTIONS

At times, replacing a bag of IV fluids during infusion will be necessary. To do so, prepare all equipment in advance and follow these steps:
1. Hold the infusing bag upside down in one hand and remove the spike chamber. Discard the old bag.
2. Quickly insert the spike chamber into the new bag, and squeeze the chamber.
3. Insert an 18-guage needle in an injection port in the IV tubing to allow air to be expelled from the tubing before it reaches the patient.
4. After the air has been expelled, remove the needle and adjust the flow rate of the infusion.
5. Document the time the IV fluids were replaced.

consciousness. If air embolism is suspected, the following steps should be taken:

1. Close the tubing.
2. Turn the patient on his or her left side with head down. (If air has entered the heart chambers, this position may keep the air in the right side of the heart and away from the cardiac valves. The pulmonary artery may absorb small air bubbles.)
3. Check tubing for leaks.
4. Administer high-concentration oxygen.
5. Notify medical direction.

The possibility of an air embolism can be minimized by ensuring that all tubing connections are secure and that fluid containers are changed before they are empty.

Complications specific to central venous cannulation. Cannulation of the central veins presents specific dangers in addition to the complications common to all intravenous techniques. The paramedic must be alert to these dangers because they can be fatal if unrecognized. (Although the femoral vein is not truly a central vein because the catheter is inserted in an area below the diaphragm, it will be included in this section.)

Complications from Femoral Vein Cannulation
- Local complications:
  Hematoma may occur from the vein itself or the adjacent femoral artery.
  Thrombosis may extend to the deep veins and lead to edema of the leg.
  Phlebitis may extend to the deep veins.
  Use of the femoral vein frequently precludes subsequent use of the saphenous vein.
- Systemic complications:
  Thrombosis or phlebitis that may extend proximally to the iliac veins or even the inferior vena cava.

Complications from Internal Jugular and Subclavian Cannulation
- Local complications:
  Hematoma may occur, either from the vein itself or from an adjacent artery.

Damage may occur to an adjacent artery, nerve, or lymphatic duct. Inadvertent puncture of the carotid artery is not uncommon when attempting jugular cannulation.

- Systemic complications:
  Pneumothorax is common.
  Hemothorax can occur.
  Air embolism can occur.
  Fluid may infiltrate into the mediastinum or the pleural cavity from an extruded catheter.

Intravenous Medications

Medications can be given directly into the vascular system via the intravenous route by injection or infusion. An intravenous injection can be administered through a previously established intravenous infusion line, heparin or saline lock, or implantable port (e.g., Port-A-Cath, Hickman catheter), or directly into the vein with a sterile needle or butterfly device. An intravenous infusion is administered by adding a drug to an infusing intravenous solution (e.g., normal saline), diluting the drug in a larger volume of fluid and administering the medication through a volume-control in-line device (e.g., burette, Volutrol, infusion pump), or intermittent infusion ("intravenous piggyback" or "secondary set").

Intravenous injections generally consist of a small amount of medication (usually less than 5 mL) and are called *intravenous push* or *intravenous bolus medications*. To administer an intravenous injection, the injection port of the intravenous line should be cleansed with alcohol or the cap from the needleless port removed. The prescribed medication is then injected slowly (usually from 1 to 3 minutes). The rate of injection depends on the type of medication and patient response. Most intravenous tubing is equipped with one-way valves to prevent backflow of medication. If such a valve is not present or cannot be identified, the tubing above the injection site should be clamped during drug administration. After the injection, the infusion of fluids is continued.

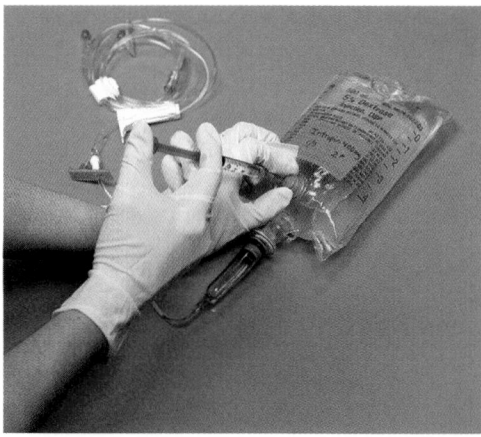

Fig. 9-23 Adding medication to an intravenous reservoir.

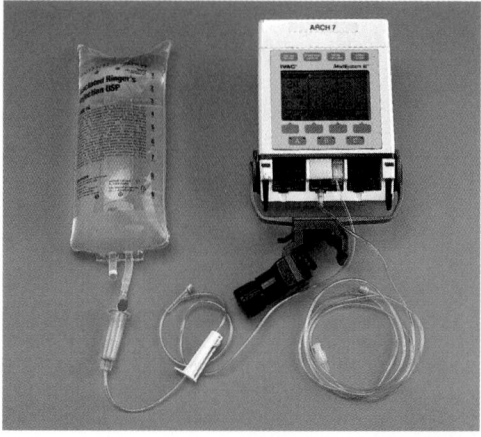

Fig. 9-24 Intravenous infusion pump.

Intravenous infusions for drug administration can take several forms. To add a medication to the fluid reservoir of an established intravenous line, the paramedic should follow these steps (Fig. 9-23):

1. Compute the volume of the drug to be added to the fluid reservoir.
2. Draw up the prescribed dose in a syringe. If prefilled syringes are used, note the volume of medication in the syringe and the dose to be used.
3. Cleanse the rubber sleeve of the fluid reservoir with an alcohol swab.
4. Puncture the rubber sleeve and inject the prescribed medication into the fluid reservoir.
5. Withdraw the needle and discard the needle and syringe. Gently mix the medication with the fluid by agitating the reservoir.
6. Label the fluid reservoir with the name of the medication added, amount of the medication added, resultant concentration of the medication in the reservoir, and date, time, and name of the paramedic who prepared the infusion.
7. Calculate the rate of administration in drops per minute as prescribed.

A number of in-line, volume-control devices allow more accurate delivery of medication diluted in precise amounts of fluids than is possible by simply setting the drip rate. They are often used to administer intravenous medications to children and adults who need precise doses of medication that can readily cause toxicity when administered too rapidly (e.g., antidysrhythmics, vasopressors). In-line devices include electronic flow-rate regulators that regulate fluid passage by a magnetically acti-

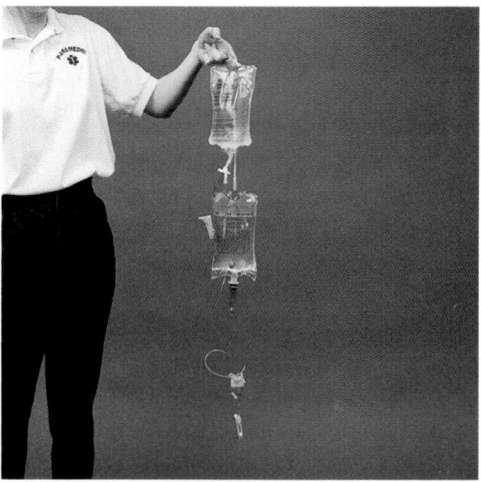

Fig. 9-25 Intravenous piggyback setup.

vated metal ball valve and infusion pumps that exert pressure on tubing or fluid by pumping against pressure gradients. The paramedic should follow the instructions of the equipment manufacturer and become familiar with these devices before using them (Fig. 9-24).

NOTE

Other mechanical (nonelectric) devices (e.g., Dial-A-Flow) are available and are used by some EMS systems to prevent an unnoticed increase in flow rate.

Intermittent infusions are given via a setup that is secondary to the primary intravenous infusion. The piggyback medication is hung in tandem and connected to the primary setup (Fig. 9-25). Most intermittent diluted drug infusions are meant to have a total infusion time of 20 or 30 minutes to 1 hour (depending on the drug and patient response). To prepare an intermittent infusion, the paramedic should follow these steps:

1. Prepare the prescribed medication and add it to the secondary fluid as described above.
2. Bleed the air out of the secondary administration set and attach a 1-inch, 18-gauge needle.

3. Cleanse the medication port of the primary infusion tubing and insert the needle or access pin of the piggyback medication.
4. Tape the needle (if present) securely to the medication port.
5. Calculate the flow rate of the secondary infusion in drops per minute.
6. Lower the primary infusion reservoir so that its center of gravity is lower than the secondary infusion reservoir.

BOX 9-7

INDWELLING VASCULAR DEVICES

Heparin or Saline Lock

A heparin or saline lock is a peripheral intravenous cannula that has no attached intravenous tubing (Fig. 9-26). These vascular access devices are used to have ready access to peripheral veins for the brief administration of medications or for frequent intravenous therapy on an outpatient basis (e.g., chemotherapy). The cannula is filled with 0.5 to 1.0 mL of a heparin or saline solution to prevent clotting while it is not in use.

To gain access to the peripheral vein, 4 mL of normal saline should be drawn into a syringe. Aseptic technique is used; 2 mL of the normal saline is used to flush the heparin lock reservoir before and after the prescribed medication or intravenous fluid infusion. After intravenous therapy, 0.5 to 1.0 mL of heparin or 3 mL of 0.9% normal saline should be injected into the reservoir to keep the lock patent.

Atrial Catheters

An atrial catheter (Fig 9-27) is a long, Silastic indwelling catheter sometimes used by patients with cancer, gastrointestinal dysfunction, or debilitating diseases and by those who need intermittent intravenous administration of antibiotics, nutritional supplements, or other intravenous medications. Patients are sometimes discharged from the hospital with the catheter in place and are taught to maintain it and to administer various medications and fluid therapies through the device.

The atrial catheter is approximately 90 mm long and 1.6 mm in diameter. It is surgically placed in the right atrium under fluoroscopy and local anesthesia. When seen on the patient's chest, the catheter looks like a thin, white cord with a Luer plug attached on the end. It protrudes from a small incision near the clavicle, which is usually covered with a dressing. Atrial catheters should only be used for venous access in emergency situations such as acute fluid loss, pulmonary edema, or cardiac arrest. Connecting intravenous lines to the catheter increases the chance of infection and embolism; therefore the catheter should not be used in stable patients. When it is necessary to gain access to an atrial catheter, the following procedure should be followed[3]:

1. Gather needed material:
   20-mL, 5-mL, and 3-mL syringes
   18-gauge needle
   30-mL multidose vial of bacteriostatic 0.9% normal saline solution; povidone-iodine (Betadine); and intravenous administration set
2. Draw up 3 mL of normal saline and set it aside.
3. Apply gloves for patient and personal protection.

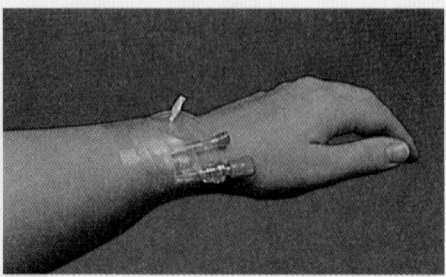

Fig. 9-26 Heparin lock.

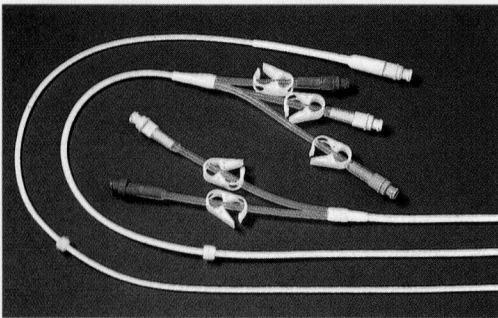

Fig. 9-27 Single-, dual-, and triple-lumen right atrial catheters.

7. Open the piggyback line flow clamp, and adjust the flow rate to the desired dose. Clamp the tubing of the primary infusion to allow the piggyback medication to infuse. After administration of the piggyback medication, restart the primary infusion, and discard the piggyback equipment.
8. Always label the bag with the medication.

Another device for intravenous drug administration is a drug "pump." Drug pumps are used by patients who need a slow injection of medication in the home (e.g., patients undergoing cancer chemotherapy). These devices usually consist of a syringe with a battery attachment that regulates the injection of medication. Drug pumps are used to administer medication subcutaneously or can be attached to indwelling vascular devices such as the Port-A-Cath or Hickman catheter (Box 9-7).

BOX 9-7

INDWELLING VASCULAR DEVICES—cont'd

NOTE: Most patients with an atrial catheter are immunosuppressed or severely debilitated, so they are susceptible to routine pathogens. Special care should be taken by the paramedic to avoid contamination.
4. Explain the procedure to the patient.
5. Clamp the catheter with a padded smooth shunt clamp to prevent nicking or severing the catheter.
NOTE: Because the atrial catheter is a central line catheter, an air embolism is possible when changing tubing or changing syringes.
6. Remove and discard the intermittent infusion device. (Connections are usually taped to avoid disconnection and air embolism.)
7. Wipe the connection site with povidone-iodine and allow it to dry.
8. Connect the 5-mL syringe. Remove the clamp and withdraw 5 mL of blood. (Do not use heparinized blood for the specimen.)
9. Replace the clamp.
10. Attach the 3-mL syringe of normal saline to the catheter, remove the clamp, and flush to prevent clot formation within the catheter.
11. Replace the clamp and remove the syringe.
12. Connect the intravenous tubing to the catheter, making sure that the tubing is free of air.
13. Remove the clamp and begin infusion.
14. Tape the connection site between the intravenous tubing and the catheter. Use like any other peripheral intravenous line.

Implantable Ports

Implantable ports are venous access devices that are surgically implanted, with the distal end of the catheter inserted into a large central vein. An example of such a device is the Port-A-Cath (Fig. 9-28). The injection end of the catheter is implanted subcutaneously, often on the chest wall, and has a self-sealing septum over a small chamber or reservoir. The tubing extends from the side of the reservoir to the venous insertion point. Each time the implantable port is accessed, the skin must be punctured with a needle, but no daily cleansing is required as it is with partially implanted ports such as the Hickman catheter. Implantable ports should not be used in stable patients. To use implantable ports, use the following procedure:
1. Locate the device and stabilize it with one hand.
2. Puncture the skin and septum with a Huber needle attached to a 3-mL syringe containing sterile saline. (Huber needles are special stainless-steel needles; they may be straight for injections or angled 90 degrees for intravenous infusion.)
3. Aspirate blood to determine patency and then inject the saline to flush the system.
4. Connect intravenous tubing to the reservoir, making sure that the tubing is free of air.
5. Tape the connection site between the intravenous tubing and the reservoir.
6. After use, flush the device with a heparinized solution.

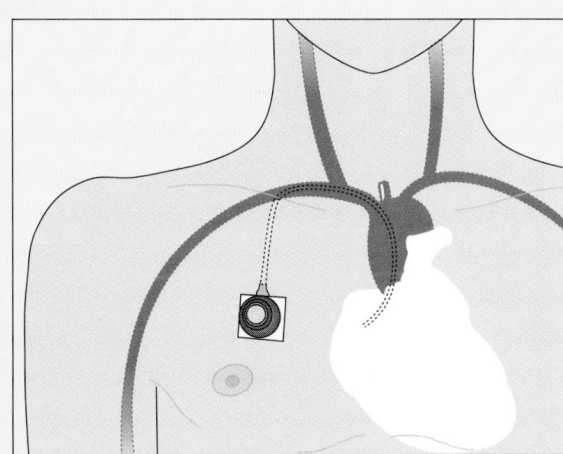

Fig. 9-28 Port-A-Cath.

Intraosseous Medications

Studies have shown that IO infusion is relatively safe and effective when initiated in children. The procedure is currently being used by EMS services in many areas of the United States for vascular access in critically ill children when peripheral cannulation is unavailable. (Other methods of obtaining vascular access in children will be discussed in Chapters 41 and 42.)

Fluids and drugs infused through IO access pass quickly from the marrow cavities into the sinusoids, to large venous channels and emissary veins, and then to the systemic circulation. Normal saline, lactated Ringer's solution, 5% dextrose in water, plasma, blood, and most ALS medications may be infused quickly through this route (Figs. 9-29 and 9-30).

IO infusion generally should be considered only for unconscious children and *only* when peripheral cannulation is unobtainable. Example

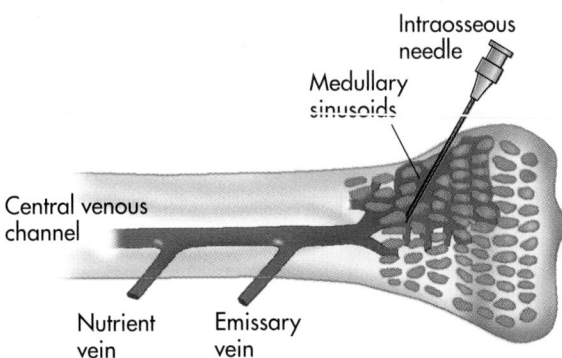

Fig. 9-29 Sites for intraosseous access.

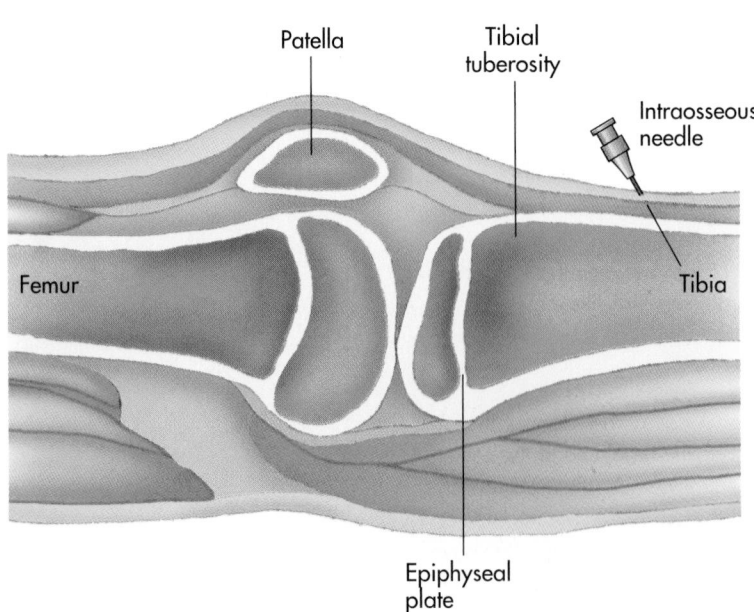

Fig. 9-30 Obtaining intraosseous access.

scenarios include cardiopulmonary arrest and peripheral vascular collapse (as in shock, major trauma, or burns). In addition, IO infusion is recommended in critically ill children in whom vascular access is impaired by obesity or edema, when other sites for venous access fail, and in children with life-threatening status asthmaticus. Special training and authorization for this procedure must be provided by medical direction.

> **NOTE**
>
> IO access may be difficult to obtain in adults and is associated with delayed circulation and may be complicated by marrow emboli.[7]

The site of choice for initiating this procedure in children is the tibia, one to two fingerbreadths below the tubercle on the anteromedial surface. An alternative choice would be the femur, two to three fingerbreadths above the lateral condyles in the midline, or just proximal to the medial malleolus.

Necessary equipment
- Alcohol wipes
- Povidone-iodine (Betadine) wipes
- Antibiotic ointment
- Tape
- Bone marrow needle
- IV tubing (pediatric infusion set)
- IV fluids (specified by medical direction): normal saline, lactated Ringer's solution, or special pediatric fluids

Method of insertion
1. Apply gloves for personal and patient protection.
2. Cleanse the site as previously described for peripheral and central cannulation.
3. Prepare bone marrow needle for proper depth during insertion. Insert needle pointing away from epiphyseal plate, advancing to periosteum.
4. Using a boring or screwing motion, advance the needle until it penetrates bone marrow (usually noted by decreased resistance and a slight "pop" sound).
5. Remove stylet.

6. Aspirate bone marrow into saline-filled syringe. (Bone marrow may not always be aspirated.)
7. Infuse saline by syringe to ensure placement and to clear clots.
8. Secure needle with tape and securing screw if so equipped (although needle is usually well stabilized by the bone).
9. Attach standard IV tubing and fluids to infuse under gravity or pressure as prescribed by medical direction.
10. Document procedure.

Contraindications
- Fracture of the site or proximal to the site
- Traumatized extremity
- Cellulitis
- Burns that may be infected by the technique
- Congenital bone disease

Potential complications
Technical
- Subperiosteal infusion from improper placement
- Penetration of posterior wall of medullary cavity, resulting in soft-tissue infusion
- Slow infusion from clotting of marrow

Systemic
- Osteomyelitis (less than 0.6%, usually with prolonged infusion)
- Fat embolism (not yet reported in children)
- Slight periostitis at the injection site (usually clearing in 2 to 3 weeks)
- Infection (acceptably low rate; comparable with that of other infusion techniques)
- Fracture

Administration of Percutaneous Medications

Percutaneous routes for drug administration refer to those drugs that are absorbed through the mucous membrane or skin. These include topical drugs; sublingual drugs and buccal drugs; inhaled drugs; endotracheal drugs; and drugs for the eye, nose, and ear.

Topical Drugs

In addition to the various emollients and antibiotic ointments, the most commonly used transdermal emergency medication is *nitroglycerin*. Two types

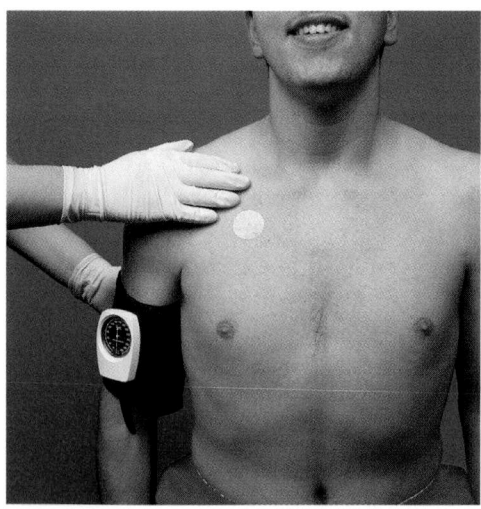

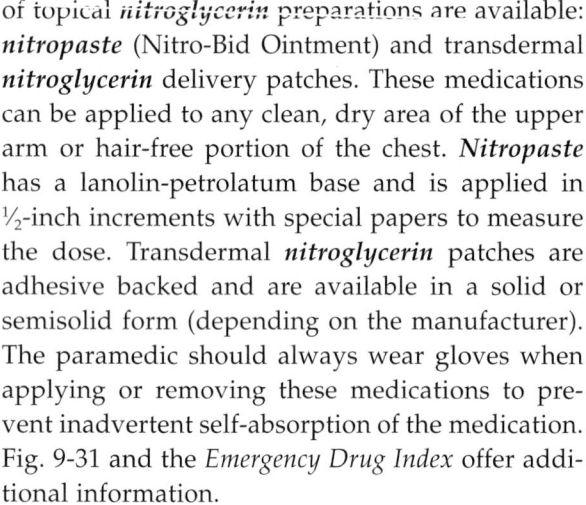

Fig. 9-31 Application of nitroglycerin paste and a nitro-glycerin patch.

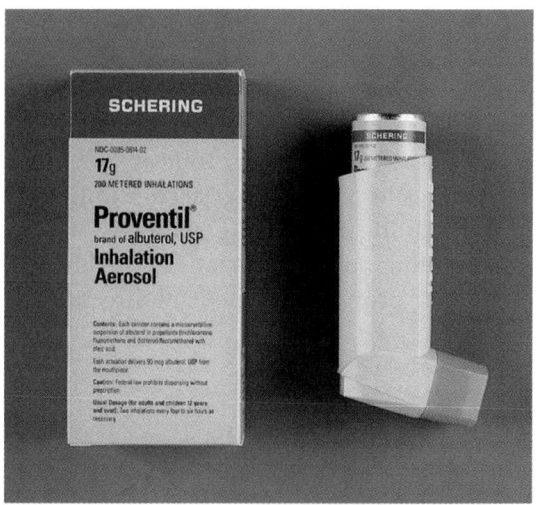

Fig. 9-32 MDI.

of topical *nitroglycerin* preparations are available: *nitropaste* (Nitro-Bid Ointment) and transdermal *nitroglycerin* delivery patches. These medications can be applied to any clean, dry area of the upper arm or hair-free portion of the chest. *Nitropaste* has a lanolin-petrolatum base and is applied in ½-inch increments with special papers to measure the dose. Transdermal *nitroglycerin* patches are adhesive backed and are available in a solid or semisolid form (depending on the manufacturer). The paramedic should always wear gloves when applying or removing these medications to prevent inadvertent self-absorption of the medication. Fig. 9-31 and the *Emergency Drug Index* offer additional information.

Drugs such as scopolamine, clonidine, and estrogen are also used in patch form. These drug patches can influence the patient unfavorably during illness. They should be recognized by the paramedic and removed if indicated. Usual sites are postauricular areas and the chest, back, and upper arms.

Sublingual Drugs

The most frequently prescribed sublingual drugs are nitrates (e.g., *nitroglycerin* [Nitrostat]), which are used to treat angina pectoris. The tablet should be placed under the tongue, where it dissolves. Drinking fluids should be avoided while the drug is being absorbed. If the patient inadvertently swallows the tablet, the effects will be diminished and delayed.

Buccal Drugs

Buccal drugs are held between the patient's cheek and gum, where they dissolve to achieve their desired effects. As with the sublingual route, drinking fluids should be avoided while the drug is being absorbed. Glucose gel preparations are an example of emergency medication administered via the buccal route.

Inhaled Drugs

In addition to oxygen and *nitrous oxide* (Nitronox), several other drugs may be administered via inhalation. These include bronchodilators, corticosteroids, antibiotics, and mucokinetic agents delivered through aerosolization.

Aerosols are liquid or solid particles of a substance dispersed in gas or solution. The effectiveness of aerosolization therapy depends on the number of droplets that can be suspended in the gas or solution, particle size (diameter in microns), output (cc/min), and rate and depth of the patient's breathing. Rapid, shallow breathing decreases the number and retention of droplets reaching the deep bronchioles of the lungs. Delivery of medications by aerosolization offers certain advantages over other routes, including rapid onset and reduced systemic side effects.

Aerosols are produced by devices called *nebulizers*. The most common nebulizers are intermittent positive pressure breathing (IPPB) devices (de-

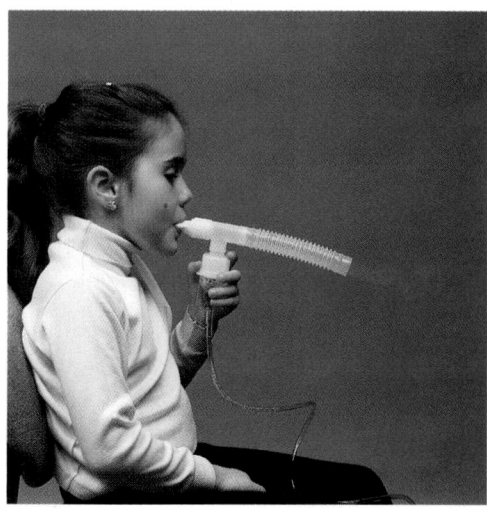

Fig. 9-33 Administration of medication via a hand-held nebulizer.

signed for in-hospital use), metered-dose inhalers (pressure cartridges), and hand-held nebulizers that operate by a compressed air or oxygen source regulated by a flowmeter.

Metered-Dose Inhaler

The metered-dose inhaler (MDI) (Fig. 9-32) has emerged as the most commonly used device in aerosol therapy. It is convenient and delivers a measured dose with each push of the cartridge. MDIs are typically prescribed for self-treatment of asthma. Other medications prepared in MDIs include *albuterol* (Proventil, Ventolin), and *isoetharine* (Bronkosol). To prepare a medication for inhalation by this method, the paramedic should follow these steps:

1. Remove the mouthpiece and protective cap from the canister (the drug container).
2. Carefully snap off the cap and turn the mouthpiece sideways.
3. Insert the canister stem into the hole inside the mouthpiece.
4. Shake the canister and mouthpiece well.
5. Invert the MDI and hold it close to the patient's mouth. Advise the patient to exhale, pushing as much air from the lungs as possible.
6. Place the mouthpiece in the patient's mouth and instruct the patient to close his or her lips loosely around it with the tongue underneath the mouthpiece. As the patient inhales deeply over

5 seconds, press down on the canister quickly and then release it.

? CRITICAL THINKING

What will happen to the medication if the patient does not use the MDI properly?

> **NOTE**
>
> Most MDI medications are administered using aero chambers (spacers). These are beneficial devices for children and other patients who might need additional time to inhale the medication; who lack coordination; or who have increased anxiety or a decreased ability to inhale for 5 seconds. Aero chambers permit the patient to receive the maximum benefit of the drug and do not require exact synchronization.

7. Instruct the patient to hold his or her breath 5 to 10 seconds before exhaling.
8. Repeat the procedure in 5 to 10 minutes to take advantage of possible deeper penetration by a second round of therapy (if required).

Hand-Held Nebulizers

Hand-held nebulizers are another method of administering some medications via inhalation in the prehospital setting. Disposable nebulizer kits are available from various manufacturers and usually include a mouthpiece or aerosol mask, oxygen tubing, and reservoir tubing (Fig. 9-33). These devices are attached to a nonhumidified portable or onboard oxygen source and use the Bernoulli principle to create an aerosol mist (sometimes referred to as a *jet* or *pneumatic nebulizer*). Medications

> **NOTE**
>
> The specific procedure may vary slightly, depending on the patient's ability to tolerate the treatment by mouthpiece or mask. A tight seal around the mouthpiece is required, so the patient must be able to cooperate during treatment. (Medication aerosolization may be administered by mouthpiece or mask. Each has an advantage, in that treatment by mouthpiece lessens the amount of medication wasted, but patients with severe dyspnea who are mouth breathers tolerate mask administration much better.)

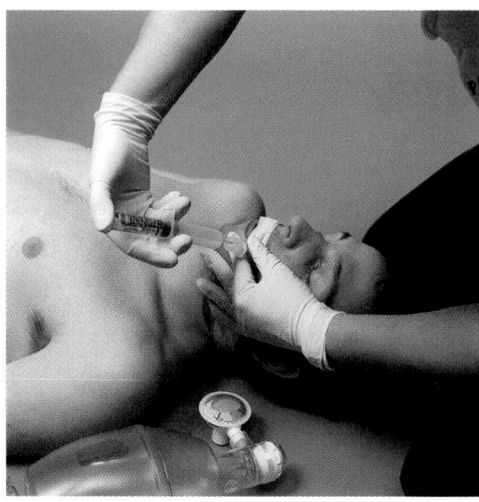

Fig. 9-34 Drug administration via an ET tube.

appropriate for nebulization therapy include *albuterol* (Proventil, Ventolin), *metaproterenol* (Alupent), *isoetharine* (Bronkosol), and *atropine*.

To administer a medication via a hand-held nebulizer, the paramedic should follow these steps:

1. The prescribed drug is mixed (using aseptic technique) with a specified amount of normal saline and instilled in the nebulizer. Some medications are available in a packaged unit dose and contain a fixed amount of diluent (usually 0.9% normal saline).
2. The nebulizer is then attached to a T-piece and mouthpiece and connected to the unit delivering nonhumidified oxygen (for the hypoxic patient) or compressed gas with connecting tubing. (If a patient is unable to use the mouthpiece, a simple face mask may be used in its place.)
3. The oxygen flowmeter should be adjusted to 4 to 6 L/min to produce a steady, visible mist. (A flow rate of 4 to 6 L usually provides a steady production of mist without excessive medication waste. The higher the flow rate, the greater the medication use.) If an aerosol mask is used, the flow rate of oxygen should be maintained at 6 to 10 L/min to prevent potential build-up of exhaled carbon dioxide in the mask.
4. When the mist is visible, the patient should begin treatment. Instruct the patient to inhale slowly and deeply by mouth and to hold a breath 3 to 5 seconds before exhaling. This technique causes topical deposition of the aerosol particles deep

within the tracheobronchial tree. Inhalation and exhalation should be continued until the aerosol canister is depleted of the medication. Repeat treatments usually are not given more often than every 15 to 20 minutes (usually to a maximum of three). Management for severe asthma, however, may incorporate continuous nebulized beta agonists, tailored to the patient's response.

Nebulization therapy requires a cooperative patient who can be instructed to breathe deeply so that the drug can be absorbed. If the patient cannot inhale the drug or if the bronchospasm is severe enough to make nebulization therapy ineffective, administration of medication via another route should be considered. If during the course of management by aerosolization significant changes in heart rate or dysrhythmias are noted, the treatment should be stopped, and medical direction should be contacted for further orders. Paramedics and ambulance crew should avoid the medication vapor stream during nebulization therapy.

Endotracheal Drugs

The endotracheal route of drug administration is an alternative that may be used when intravenous access cannot be established. The emergency drugs typically administered by this route include *lidocaine* (Xylocaine), *epinephrine* (Adrenalin), *atropine,* and *naloxone* (Narcan). When administering medication via this route, the paramedic should follow these steps (Fig. 9-34):

1. Ensure proper tube placement by direct visualization and auscultation (see Chapter 11).
2. Ensure adequate oxygenation and ventilation of the patient's lungs.
3. Prepare the medication (per medical direction) so that it is 2 to 2½ times the intravenous dose, and dilute the dose to 10 mL with normal saline (or prepare a 10-mL normal saline flush, per protocol).
4. Hyperventilate the patient's lungs.
5. Remove the air source from the ET tube and inject the medication through a catheter deep into the tube, or inject directly into the tube followed by a normal saline flush (per protocol).
6. Resume ventilations with several large ventilations to help ensure that the medication gets as

deep into the pulmonary tree as possible (to enhance absorption).

7. Monitor the patient for the desired therapeutic effect and any possible side effects.

Drugs for the Eye, Nose, and Ear

Eye medications are usually in the form of drops or ointments. To administer these drugs, the patient should be lying down or sitting with the head tilted back. While stabilizing the patient's head with one hand, use the thumb or fingers of the other hand to gently pull down the lower lid. The medication should be applied into the conjunctival sac of the lower lid, never onto the eyeball.

Nose drops are best administered with the patient lying down with the head over the edge of a bed. With the head in a midline position, instill the drops into each nostril. Advise the patient to refrain from blowing his or her nose for several minutes so that the drug can be absorbed. Administering nasal sprays requires that the patient inhale via one nostril while occluding the other and squeezing the spray applicator. The patient's head should be upright or tilted back during administration of the drug.

Ear medications are usually in the form of drops. The patient should lie down with the affected ear up. In adults or children over age 3, pull the top of the ear up and back to straighten the ear canal before instilling the prescribed number of drops. In children under age 3, pull the ear down and straight back. The patient should remain in the ear-up position for about 10 minutes to allow the medicine to disperse.

Special Considerations for Pediatric Patients

Administering drugs to infants and children can be quite difficult, particularly in emergency situations. The following guidelines for drug administration will help the paramedic:

- Try to establish a positive relationship and accept the child's fearful or anxious behavior as a natural response.
- Be honest when a medication or procedure will be unpleasant or painful.
- If appropriate, allow the child to help administer the medication (e.g., holding the medicine cup or placing a pill in the mouth).
- Use only mild physical restraint if it is required, and explain to the child why it is necessary.
- Enlist the assistance of parents or other caregivers when the situation allows.
- When parenteral medications are required, make certain the injection site is well stabilized and that the injection is given quickly. Two or more persons should be available to hold children over 4 years of age despite promises that they will "be still."
- Remember when administering medications that the younger and smaller the child, the narrower the margin for error.

Obtaining a Blood Sample

Venous blood samples are often obtained in the prehospital setting for glucose testing and for laboratory determinations performed in the hospital. If possible, these samples should be obtained at the time an IV is established and, if they are obtained from the IV, always prior to the infusion of any fluids. When obtaining a blood sample from an IV site, the paramedic should follow these steps.

1. Have all equipment prepared in advance.
2. After removing the needle from the IV catheter, put manual pressure above the IV site to prevent the free flow of blood from the catheter.

? **CRITICAL THINKING**

Why should a venous blood sample never be drawn above an IV infusion site?

3. Insert the vacutainer into the hub of the IV catheter while stabilizing the site.
4. Push vacuum blood collection tubes into the barrel of the vacutainer to draw blood from the IV catheter (see the following box).

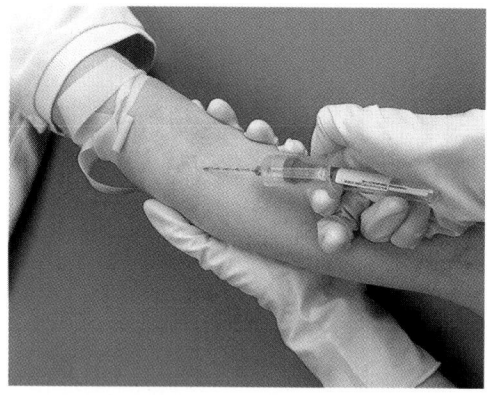

Fig. 9-35 Obtaining a blood sample with a Vacutainer.

5. After obtaining the required specimens, attach the IV tubing and begin infusion.
6. Label the sample with the patient's name and the time and date it was obtained.

If a blood sample is required in the absence of an IV, the paramedic will need to obtain the sample using a vacutainer (Fig. 9-35) or a needle and syringe and then transfer the sample to an evacuation tube. Follow these steps to obtain a blood sample using a needle and syringe:

1. Apply a tourniquet above the selected site.
2. Cleanse the site as previously described for venipuncture.
3. With an 18- or 20-gauge needle attached to a 10- or 12-cc syringe, enter the vein.
4. Withdraw the plunger using an even, steady motion to obtain the sample.
5. After the sample has been obtained, release the tourniquet, withdraw the needle, and apply manual pressure to the site.

THE DIFFERENCES BETWEEN BLOOD SAMPLE TUBES

TUBE STOPPER COLOR	ADDITIVES/ PRESERVATIVES	LABORATORY TESTS	COMMENTS
Green	Heparin	Electrolytes, glucose—not enzymes	Invert tube several times. Heparin prevents clotting of blood without killing cells.
Lavender	EDTA anticoagulant	Blood cell count, hemoglobin (Hgb), hematocrit (Hct), erythrocyte sedimentation rate (ESR)	Invert tube several times to prevent clotting. Used for whole-blood hematology determinations.
Light Blue	Sodium citrate	Prothrombin time (PT), activated partial thrombin time (PTT), fibrinogen levels	Invert tube several times to prevent clotting. Be sure to fill tube completely. Used primarily for coagulation studies, so it is often needed for patients with bleeding problems (in the abdomen, brain, or elsewhere).
Red	None	Serum electrolytes, liver and other enzymes, therapeutic drug levels, blood-banking	No inversions are needed, since the objective is to produce a clot. Some companies make tubes with clot activators, which hasten clotting to speed testing—check with your local lab.

From Miller CD: *EMS Pocket Guide, JEMS.*

6. Immediately transfer the sample to the appropriate evacuation tube.

7. Label the sample with the patient's name and the time and date it was obtained.

Disposal of Contaminated Items and Sharps

Needles and other sharp objects can injure the patient, paramedic, co-workers, and other allied health professionals and can be the source of hepatitis or HIV infection. The Centers for Disease Control and Prevention recommends that needles should *not* be capped before disposal, nor be bent or broken. Rather, they should be discarded with the syringe intact into a clearly marked, appropriate container (Fig. 9-36). These containers should be puncture- and leak-proof. When full (indicated by the "full line," which is usually no more than ¾ full) these containers should be discarded according to established policies for disposition of contaminated items and sharps.

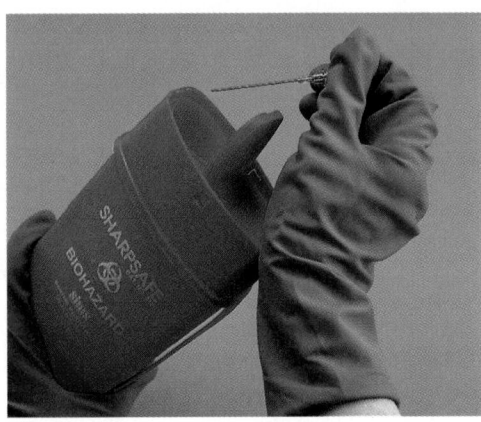

Fig. 9-36 Disposal of needle/syringe in sharps container.

SUMMARY

- Three systems for measuring drug dosage are in common use today—the metric system, the apothecary system, and the common household system. Each system deals with units of mass and volume, and any of these three systems may be used by a physician when ordering drugs.

- The paramedic should choose a calculation method that is precise and reliable. To perform drug calculations:

  - Convert all units of measure to the same size and system

  - Assess the computed dosage to determine whether it is reasonable

  - Use one method of dose calculation consistently

- Many drug calculations can be performed almost intuitively; however, paramedics should never rely on intuitive calculations. Methods of calculation include: basic formula (desire over have); ratios and proportions; and dimensional analysis.

- IV flow rates can be calculated using the following formula:

$$\text{Drops/min} = \frac{\text{volume to be infused} \times \text{drops/mL of infusion set}}{\text{Total time of infusion in minutes}}$$

- Safety considerations and procedures should be a high priority during administration of any medication. Ensure that the right patient receives the right dose of the right drug via the right route at the right time.

- If an incident involving a medication error occurs, paramedics should accept responsibility for their actions; immediately advise medical direction; assess and monitor the patient for effects of the drug; document the medication error as required by local, state, and medical direction policies; and modify personal practice to avoid a similar error in the future.

- Medical asepsis is accomplished by using "clean" technique that includes hygienic measures, cleaning agents, antiseptics, disinfectants, and barrier fields.

- Enteral medications refer to those drugs that are administered and absorbed through the gastrointestinal tract. These methods include oral, gastric, and rectal drug administration. Parenteral drugs are administered outside the intestines and usually refer to injections. Parenteral routes for drug administration include intradermal, subcutaneous, intramuscular, intravenous, and intraosseous.

- The route of choice for fluid replacement in the prehospital setting is through a peripheral vein in an extremity. The over-the-needle catheter generally is preferred for use in the prehospital setting.

- There are several possible complications associated with all intravenous techniques. These include local complications, systemic complications, infiltration, and air embolism.

- Cannulation of the central veins presents specific dangers in addition to the complications common to all intravenous techniques.

- Fluids and drugs infused through intraosseous (IO) access pass from the marrow cavities into the sinusoids, to large venous channels and emissary veins, and then to the systemic circulation. The site of choice for initiating this procedure in children is the tibia, one to two fingerbreadths below the tubercle on the anteromedial surface.

- Percutaneous routes for drug administration refer to absorption of drugs through the mucous membrane or skin. These include topical drugs; sublingual drugs and buccal drugs; inhaled drugs; endotracheal drugs; and drugs for the eye, nose, and ear.

- Administering drugs to infants and children can be quite difficult, particularly in emergency situations. Pediatric drug doses often are calculated in the prehospital setting using memory aids (e.g., charts, tapes, dosage books) or with the advice of medical direction.

- If possible, venous blood samples should be obtained at the time an IV is established and prior to the infusion of any fluids. Should a blood sample be required in the absence of an IV, the paramedic will need to obtain the sample using a needle and syringe (or a special vacuum needle and sleeve).

- The Centers for Disease Control and Prevention recommends that needles should not be capped before disposal, nor bent or broken. Rather, they should be discarded with the syringe into a into a clearly marked, appropriate, puncture- and leak-proof container.

Appendix

Precautions to Prevent Transmission of HIV: Universal Precautions

Universal precautions ("universal blood and body fluid precautions") were initially developed by the Centers for Disease Control in 1987 and are now the minimum standard of practice recommended by the Occupational Safety and Health Act of 1991 and all health care agencies. Universal precautions are intended to be used in the care of *all* patients, especially those in emergency-care settings in which the risk of blood exposure is increased and the infection status of the patient is usually unknown. Universal precautions include the following:

1. All health care workers should routinely use appropriate barrier precautions to prevent skin and mucous-membrane exposure when contact with blood or other body fluids of any patient is anticipated. Gloves should be worn for touching blood and body fluids, mucous membranes, or nonintact skin of all patients; for handling items or surfaces soiled with blood or body fluids; and for performing venipuncture and other vascular access procedures. Gloves should be changed after contact with each patient. Masks and protective eyewear or face shields should be worn during procedures that are likely to generate droplets of blood or other body fluids, to prevent exposure of mucous membranes of the mouth, nose, and eyes. Gowns or aprons should be worn during procedures that are likely to generate splashes or spray of blood or other body fluids.

2. Hand and other skin surfaces should be washed immediately and thoroughly if contaminated with blood or other body fluids. Hands should be washed immediately after gloves are removed.

3. All health care workers should take precautions to prevent injuries caused by needles, scalpels, and other sharp instruments or devices during procedures, when cleaning used instruments; during disposal of used needles, and when handling sharp instruments after procedures. To prevent needle-stick injuries, needles should not be recapped, purposely bent or broken by hand, removed from disposable syringes, or otherwise manipulated by hand. After they are used, disposable syringes and needles, scalpel blades, and other sharp items should be placed in puncture-resistant containers for disposal; the puncture-resistant containers should be located as close as practical to the use area. Large-bore reusable needles should be placed in a puncture-resistant container for transport to the processing area.

4. Although saliva has not been implicated in HIV transmission, to minimize the need for emergency mouth-to-mouth resuscitation, mouthpieces, resuscitation bags, or other ventilation devices should be available for use in areas in which the need for resuscitation is predictable.

5. Health care workers who have exudative lesions or weeping dermatitis should refrain from all direct patient care and from handling patient-care equipment until the condition resolves.

6. Pregnant health care workers are not known to be at a greater risk of contracting HIV infection than health care workers who are not pregnant; however, if a health care worker develops HIV infection during pregnancy, the infant is at risk of infection resulting from perinatal transmission. Because of this risk, pregnant health care workers should be especially familiar with and strictly adhere to precautions to minimize the risk of HIV transmission.

Implementation of universal blood and body fluid precautions for all patients eliminates the need for the isolation category of "Blood and Body Fluid Precautions" previously recommended by the CDC for patients known or suspected to be infected with bloodborne pathogens. Isolation precautions (e.g., enteric, acid-fast bacillus ["AFB"]) should be used as necessary if associated conditions, such as infectious diarrhea or tuberculosis, are diagnosed or suspected.

Source: Precautions to Prevent Transmission of HIV: Universal Precautions, Centers for Disease Control. Recommendations for prevention of HIV transmission in health care settings. MMWR 1987;36 (suppl no. 2S), http://aepo-xdv-www.epo.cdc.gov/wonder/prevguid/p0000318/body0006.htm.

◼ REFERENCES

1. Moseley R: *Everything you always wanted to know about metrics,* Valdese, N.C., 1978, R&R Enterprises.
2. Salerno E: *Pharmacology for health professionals,* St Louis, 1999, Mosby.
3. Institute for Healthcare Improvement: *Healthplan,* Boston, 1998, The Institute.
4. Hospital Infection Control Practices Advisory Council: Part II. *Recommendations for isolation precautions in hospitals,* 1997, www.cdc.gov/ncidod/hip/isolat/isopart2.htm.
5. *Needle and cannula technique,* Chicago, 1977, Abbott Laboratories.
6. American Heart Association: *Pediatric advanced life support,* Dallas, 1997, The Association.
7. Rosen P, Barkin R: *Emergency medicine: concepts and clinical practice,* ed 4, vol 1, St Louis, 1998, Mosby.

10 *Therapeutic Communications*

OBJECTIVES

Upon completion of this chapter, the paramedic student will be able to:

1. **Define therapeutic communications.**
2. **Outline the elements in effective therapeutic communications.**
3. **Identify internal factors for effective communications.**
4. **Describe external factors for effective communications.**
5. **Outline the elements of an effective patient interview.**
6. **Summarize strategies to gather appropriate patient information.**
7. **Discuss methods to assess mental status during the interview.**
8. **Describe techniques to enhance communications when interviewing patients unmotivated to talk; hostile patients; children; older adults; hearing-impaired patients; blind patients; patients under the influence of drugs or alcohol; sexually aggressive patients; or patients with different cultural traditions.**

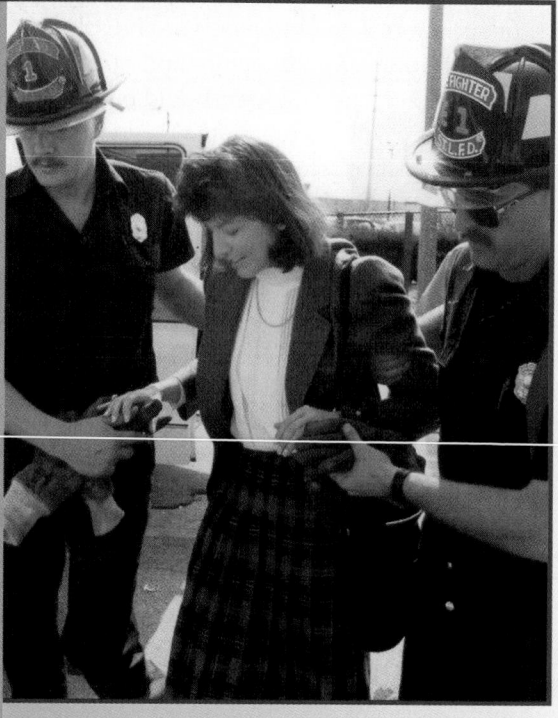

Therapeutic communications *is a planned, deliberate, professional act that uses communications techniques to achieve a positive relationship and shared understanding of information for desired patient-care goals. Therapeutic communications can facilitate positive patient interaction, improve patient care, diffuse or prevent escalation of potentially violent situations, and reduce the risk of litigation.*

decoding: The act of interpreting symbols and format.

encoding: The act of placing a message in an understandable format (either written or verbal).

therapeutic communications: A planned, deliberate, professional act that uses communications techniques to achieve a positive relationship and shared understanding of information for desired patient-care goals.

Communications

Communications is the basic element of human interaction. It refers to nonverbal and verbal behavior and includes all symbols and clues used by persons when giving and receiving meaning.[1] The process of communications incorporates several elements. The paramedic must be conscious and aware of each element to interact effectively with a patient. Each element is crucial, and information and meaning can be gained or lost if any one of the elements is altered (Fig. 10-1).

Elements of the Communications Process

Communications is a dynamic process. The elements of this process include the source, encoding, the message, decoding, the receiver, and feedback.

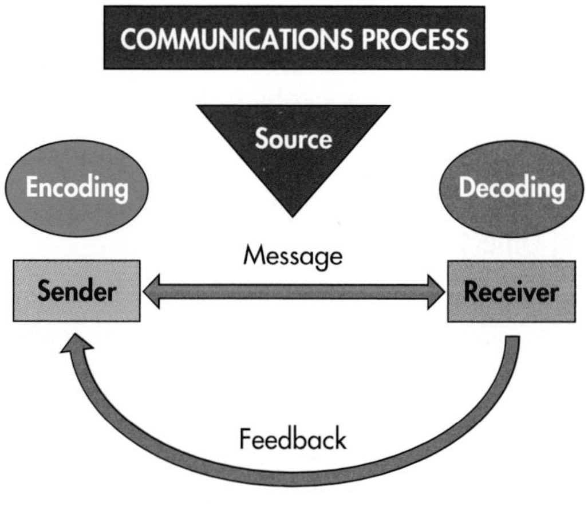

Fig. 10-1 The communications process.

Source

Verbal communications uses spoken or written words (common symbols) to express ideas or feelings. These common symbols should be simple, short, and direct to avoid confusion. Box 10-1 lists methods that can be used to achieve clarity in verbal communications.

? CRITICAL THINKING

Think about the last time you had a misunderstanding with someone. Would any of the communications techniques listed in Box 10-1 have improved the situation?

NOTE

Language is only effective when each person clearly understands the message.

Encoding

Encoding is the act of placing a message in a format (either written or verbal) which, when translated, is understood by the sender and receiver. Encoding is

BOX 10-1

EFFECTIVE VERBAL COMMUNICATIONS TECHNIQUES

1. Use fewer words to avoid confusion.
2. Use words that express an idea simply.
3. Avoid vague phrases.
4. Use examples (including demonstrations) if the message will be easier to understand.
5. Repeat important parts of a message.
6. Avoid technical jargon.
7. Use an appropriate speed or pace; avoid long pauses or rapid shifts to another subject.

the responsibility of the sender (the encoder), because the sender defines the content and emotional tone of the message. During communications, the sender role may change as parties exchange information. For example, the paramedic may initially be the sender of the message when asking a patient for information. When the patient responds to the paramedic, the patient will assume the role of the sender.

Message

The message is the information that is sent or expressed by the sender. It should be clear and organized and should be communicated in a manner familiar to the person receiving it. The message may include verbal and nonverbal symbols (e.g., spoken words, facial expressions, gestures). As a rule, the more ways (or formats) a message is communicated, the more likely the receiver will understand it. For example, combining soothing words and a reassuring touch to a patient experiencing pain will communicate the message of compassion better than spoken words alone.

> **NOTE**
>
> Not all symbols have universal meaning. The paramedic should consider cultural differences and language barriers before sending a message.

Decoding

Decoding is the act of interpreting symbols and format. It prompts the receiver to respond to the sender's message. The decoding process can fail when symbols or words sent in the message are uncommon to both parties or when interpretation of the message is based on different understandings of symbols or format. For example, the word *pain* may mean a horrific discomfort to one person, but a mild annoyance to another. Therefore, when communicating with a patient, the paramedic must carefully select words that cannot easily be misinterpreted.

Receiver

The receiver (the decoder) is the person intended to understand the message. Like the role of the sender, the role of the receiver will switch back and forth between participants during the communications process.

> **? CRITICAL THINKING**
>
> *Did you ever attend a class where nothing made sense? Reflect back on the reason that you didn't understand the content. Was it an encoding or decoding problem?*

Feedback

Feedback is the receiver's response to the sender's message. The quality of the feedback helps reveal if the intended meaning of the message was received. If the message was not received, the sender must further clarify the message by modifying its content and assessing the new feedback. Feedback (like the message) may be verbal or nonverbal.

> **NOTE**
>
> Communications is an ongoing process that requires equal responsibility from both parties to make it effective.

> **NOTE**
>
> Medical conditions, such as a stroke, can impair a person's ability to encode or decode information.

Internal Factors for Effective Communications

To effectively communicate with patients, paramedics must genuinely like people, must be able to empathize with others, and must have the ability to listen (see the box on p. 347). These internal factors each play an important role in therapeutic communications.

Liking Others

As a "helping profession," health care is dependent on the relationships forged between patients and health care providers. These relationships are based on trust and caring and cannot be achieved without a genuine concern for others and an understanding of human strengths and weaknesses. Patients must trust and believe that a paramedic *wants* to care for

ACTIVE LISTENING ATTITUDES AND GUIDELINES

1. Listen to understand, not to ready yourself to reply, contradict, or refute. This attitude is extremely important.
2. Remember that understanding involves more than knowing the dictionary meaning of the words that are used. It involves paying attention to the tone of the voice, facial expressions, and overall behavior of the patient.
3. Observe all this and be careful not to interrupt too quickly. Look for clues to what the other person is trying to say, putting yourself (as best you can) in the patient's shoes, seeing the world as the patient sees it, accepting the patient's feelings as facts that have to be taken into account—whether you share them or not.
4. Put aside your own views and opinions for the time being. Realize that you cannot listen to yourself inwardly, and at the same time listen outwardly to the patient.
5. Control your impatience. Listening is faster than talking. The average person speaks about 120 words per minute, but can listen to about 400 words per minute. The paramedic who is an effective listener does not jump ahead of the patient, but gives the person time to tell the story. What the patient says next may not be what the paramedic expects to hear.

6. Do not prepare your answer while you listen. Get the whole message before deciding what to say. The last sentence of the patient may give a new slant to what was said before.
7. Show interest and alertness. This stimulates the patient and improves communications.
8. Do not interrupt. When you ask questions, it is to secure more information not to trap or force the patient into a corner.
9. Expect the patient's language to differ from yours. Do not quibble about words; try to get at what was meant.
10. Your purpose is opposite that of a debater. Look for areas of agreement and not for weak spots that you plan to attack and blast with an artillery of counterarguments.
11. Before giving an answer in a particularly difficult discussion, summarize what you understand the patient said. If your interpretation is not accepted by the patient, clarify the contested points before proceeding with your own views.
12. Let the patient characterize his or her own self, interests, position, and opinions.

Adapted with permission from Legal Advocates for Abused Women.

their needs. Paramedics can convey this trust to patients by accepting them for who they are and by respecting them as individuals.

Empathy

Empathy is the ability to view the world from another inner frame or reference point of view while remaining yourself. It is widely accepted as a clinical component of a helping profession. Unlike sympathy (expressing one's own feelings about another person's predicament), empathy uses sensitive and objective communications to help patients explain and explore their feelings, so that problem solving can occur (see the box on p. 348).

Ability to Listen

Listening is an active process that requires complete attention and practice. To be an effective listener, the paramedic should use the following skills[2]:

1. Face patients while they speak.
2. Maintain natural eye contact to show willingness to listen.

✓ TRICKS OF THE TRADE

Keep in mind that your patient's age and background can affect their ability to comprehend what you say. Add anxiety into the situation and chaos can rule. Use simple terminology that you can expect the patient to understand.

✓ TRICKS OF THE TRADE

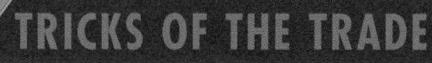

If a patient tells you he believes he is going to die— BELIEVE HIM!

EMPATHY VS. SYMPATHY

The following scenario demonstrates the difference between empathy and sympathy and how empathy can have a positive effect on the paramedic-patient relationship:

Your crew has been dispatched to the home of a 60-year-old male with substernal chest pain. On your arrival, the patient is sitting on the living room sofa with his wife. They are obviously distraught and fearful for his life. The EMS crew initiates standard procedures for chest pain, per protocol, and begins to transport the patient to the emergency department. This conversation occurs between the paramedic and the patient while en route to the hospital:

Paramedic: Even though you're feeling better, I can tell you're worried and afraid.

Patient: Yes, I am. I'm afraid I'm going to die.

Paramedic: Would you like me to explain to you and your wife what will happen after we arrive in the emergency department, and what the doctors and nurses will do to make sure you get the best possible care?

Patient: Yes, my wife and I would like that very much.

In this conversation, the paramedic's use of empathy after sensing the patient's frame of mind calmed the patient and his wife, gave them useful information, and partly addressed their concerns. Using sympathy alone (e.g., saying "I understand how you feel, but don't worry, everything will be okay") would have ignored the patient's fears and prevented any problem solving to occur.

3. Assume an attentive posture. Avoid crossing the legs and arms because this may convey a defensive attitude.
4. Avoid distracting body movements, such as wringing hands, tapping feet, or fidgeting with an object in the hands.
5. Nod in acknowledgment when patients talk about important points or look for feedback.
6. Lean toward the speaker to communicate involvement.

NOTE

Good listening is an active, learned process that requires practice.

External Factors for Effective Communications

Effective communications requires a suitable physical environment. Issues such as privacy, interruption, eye contact, and personal dress are external factors that can be controlled by the paramedic to enhance communications during the paramedic-patient encounter.

Privacy, Interruptions, and the Physical Environment

When possible, the paramedic should ensure privacy during the encounter to help eliminate any inhibitions and distractions. Interruptions should be few except when patient care information is being received from crew members or is critical in nature. When possible, lighting should be adequate, noise and interference minimized, and the patient interview should be initiated away from distracting equipment.

The paramedic should be aware of the patient's "private space" (a comfortable distance of 4 to 5 feet from the patient's body[3]), or twice the patient's arm length away. Entering this space usually will cause the patient to back away.

NOTE

A person's "private space" is a form of subconscious personal protection that varies by individual and by culture. Some patients may become defensive if this space is invaded.

Eye Contact

The paramedic should maintain eye contact with the patient as much as possible, even when taking notes. Eye contact is a type of nonverbal communications that can help express gentleness, sincerity, and authority and can help make the patient feel safe and secure. If possible, the paramedic should be positioned at eye level (equal seating) with the patient.

Personal Dress

Communications with a patient begins with first impressions. The paramedic's appearance should be professional, and his or her clothing should be clean and meet conventional professional standards. These standards help the patient immediately identify an EMS provider and help set the tone of the paramedic-patient encounter.

The Patient Interview

The patient interview may be as important as physical assessment skills because the information gathered during the patient interview often helps determine the direction of the physical examination. The patient interview should be initiated early and should continue throughout the patient encounter.

> **NOTE**
>
> Because of the nature of emergency medical care, EMS personnel often think in terms of specific illness and injury, grouping patients into general classifications such as trauma or medical cases. Good emergency care, however, involves viewing each patient as a total individual and attending to patient needs in a caring, concerned, and receptive manner.

Communications Techniques

The paramedic should approach the conscious patient and make a personal introduction by name and title: "Hello. My name is [name], and I am a paramedic with [name of EMS agency]. What's your name?" A verbal exchange with the patient will provide information regarding the patient's level of consciousness, sensorium, any hearing or speech impediments, and language barriers. During the introduction, the paramedic should be positioned to achieve eye contact with the patient.

Nonverbal communications can convey negative feelings or the insecurities of both the patient and paramedic. Voice inflection, facial expression, and body position, for example, may reflect feelings of anger, fear, or impatience. Similarly, initiating intravenous therapy with trembling, sweaty hands will make the patient question the paramedic's skills. The paramedic should use nonverbal communications to gain the trust and cooperation necessary to care effectively for the patient.

Touch is a form of communication that conveys compassion and reassurance. Small gestures such as holding a patient's hand, squeezing a shoulder, or wiping tears from the patient's eyes will help comfort an individual in distress. Experience and familiarity with patient-care activities will help determine the appropriateness of these gestures.

Conversing with patients requires listening to what is said and to interpreting what is said. Patients may say that they feel fine, but their appearance and tone of voice may indicate that they are ill and afraid. If the paramedic is unsure of the message in a patient's response, a line of questioning should be pursued to better understand what the patient is trying to communicate.

Most patients do not converse in medical terminology, and many have only a vague understanding of their bodies. The patient interview should accordingly consist of common words and phrases that can be clearly understood. The paramedic should guide and direct the patient interview without manipulating the patient's response and should avoid using leading questions (questions that can only be answered with "yes" or "no"). Open-ended questions encourage a free-form response. For example, the paramedic should ask "When did this pain begin?" rather than "Did the pain begin this morning?"

> **NOTE**
>
> Open-ended questions:
> • Are asked in a narrative form
> • Encourage the patient to talk
> • Do not restrict the areas of a response

The paramedic should ask only one question at a time, and the patient should be given ample time to answer the question before the paramedic asks another. If the patient responds with something that does not appear relevant to the question, the response should be clarified. The paramedic should be flexible and should not discount the patient's experiences or information.

Paramedics should try to answer all questions posed by the patient. This does not mean that a full explanation is required for each inquiry, but rather a sensitive response that addresses the question. The paramedic should carefully choose an answer and should attempt to avoid any response that increases the patient's anxiety.

Responses

The paramedic can use many different responses to facilitate a good patient interview. These include:

- Silence—Gives patients more time to gather their thoughts
- Reflection—By echoing (paraphrasing) patients' words, they can clarify or expound on the information provided
- Empathy—Encourages patients to talk more openly
- Clarification—Lets patients rephrase a word that is confusing to the paramedic
- Confrontation—Focuses patients' attention on one specific factor of the interview
- Interpretation—Links events; makes associations or implies a cause; is based on observation or conclusion
- Explanation—Provides information to patients; encourages sharing of factual or objective information
- Summary—Provides for a review of the interview by asking open-ended questions that allows patients to clarify details

Traps of Interviewing

Some communications techniques can result in "traps" that can be damaging to the patient interview. These include:

- Providing false assurance or false reassurance
- Offering poor or unwanted advice
- Showing approval or disapproval
- Giving an opinion that takes away the patient's decision making
- Changing the subject inappropriately
- Stereotyping the patient or complaint
- Using professional jargon
- Talking too much
- Asking leading or biased questions
- Interrupting the patient

- Asking the patient "why" questions (viewed as accusations)
- Being defensive in response to criticism

Developing a Good Patient Rapport

Techniques used to develop good patient rapport require experience and practice. Some general guidelines can be applied to most patient encounters to help establish good rapport.

1. Put patients at ease by letting them know that you are "on their side"; that you respect their comments; and that you are there to help them.
2. Recognize and respond to visual clues that they need help.
3. Find the suffering and show compassion.
4. Assess their level of understanding and insight, and become their ally.
5. Show expertise.

> **? CRITICAL THINKING**
>
> *What techniques could you use to promote effective communications with a suicidal patient who is telling you that you don't care about him?*

Strategies to Get Information

Patients generally communicate with health care providers in three ways: (1) by "pouring out" the information in the form of complaints; (2) by revealing some problems while concealing others they think are embarrassing; or (3) by hiding the most embarrassing parts of their problem from the paramedic (and personally denying the issue). Obtaining information from the patient is best accomplished based on techniques of open-ended and closed (direct) questions. These techniques include resistance, shifting focus, recognizing defense mechanisms, and distraction.

> **NOTE**
>
> Closed questions let the paramedic gain specific information that focuses on a particular aspect of the patient's condition. "What part of your back hurts?" and "When was your last meal?" are examples of closed questions.

Resistance

Resistance from the patient to provide information often occurs for one of two reasons: (1) The patient wants to maintain a personal image and is fearful of losing that image or (2) the patient is uncertain if the paramedic will respond with rejection and ridicule. Therefore the paramedic should be nonjudgmental to obtain information from these patients (Box 10-2). Paramedics must be willing to talk to patients about *any* condition in a professional manner to develop a trusting relationship.

> **NOTE**
>
> Patient must believe that they can trust the paramedic before personal information is revealed.

Shifting Focus

The paramedic may have to shift the focus of questioning away from an obvious problem that the patient is hesitant to discuss. For example, a male patient who is experiencing groin pain may initially describe the pain (especially to a female paramedic) as occurring in the "lower back." By shifting the focus of questioning to low back pain, the paramedic can use another "angle" by asking questions regarding the presence or absence of radiating pain. This new angle of questioning can make patients feel more comfortable when describing their condition.

BOX 10-2

APPROACHING SENSITIVE ISSUES

Discussing sensitive issues (e.g., alcohol use, sexual issues, suicide risk) can be uncomfortable for both the patient and the paramedic. Still, these issues must not be avoided when the information is necessary to provide good patient care. The paramedic should use these guidelines when addressing sensitive issues with patients:
- Ensure privacy.
- Be confident, direct, and firm with your questions.
- Do not apologize for asking a sensitive question.
- Do not be judgmental.
- Use terminology that is understandable, but not patronizing.
- Be patient and proceed slowly.

Defense Mechanisms

Paramedics should recognize common defense mechanisms (see Chapter 2) and if possible anticipate them. For example, a distraught parent with a seriously ill child may demonstrate regression or denial and may be unable to provide needed information at the emergency scene. Confrontation may become necessary in these and similar situations to force the parent to deal with important issues. Confrontation can clarify roles and can help others identify problems and goals. This technique should be used, however, only to obtain information critical for medical care.

> **NOTE**
>
> Confrontation must be performed in a professional way so that the patient becomes aware of inconsistencies in interfering behavior or thoughts.

Distraction

Like confrontation, distraction may be used by the paramedic to help patients identify irrational thoughts or behavior (often seen in hostile situations where patients are "acting out"). In these situations, the paramedic will need to point out unacceptable behavior and let patients know the self-defeating nature of the behavior. Often times, this distraction will prompt patients to let the paramedic "control" the situation until they can gain self-control. When dealing with a person who is angry or hostile, paramedics should:

- Not raise their voice to match that of the angry person
- Have the person identify and describe the cause of anger
- Restate the cause of the anger
- Offer a solution (if possible) or empathize and acknowledge the person's feelings

Methods to Assess Mental Status During the Interview

Observation, conversation, and exploration are methods used to assess a patient's mental status. These general methods are described in the following paragraphs. A more thorough discussion regarding assessing level of consciousness will be presented in other chapters.

Observation

The first step in assessing mental status is to observe the patient's appearance, level of consciousness, and normal or abnormal body movements. Physical characteristics, dress, and grooming can provide clues to the patient's well-being, social status, religion, culture, and self-concept. Conscious patients generally are alert and are able to converse intelligently. Body movements such as gestures and facial expressions should be appropriate to the situation. Abnormal body movements (e.g., unusual posture or gait, clenched fists) may indicate a potentially volatile situation.

Conversation

Conversation with the patient should demonstrate a patient who is oriented to person, place, and time. Verbal communications should be expressed at a usual speed or pace with even flow. Long pauses and rapid shifts in conversation are not to be expected (varies by geographical location). During normal conversation, the patient should be able to demonstrate clear thinking, a normal attention span, and the ability to concentrate on and comprehend the discussion.

> **NOTE**
>
> Identifying that the patient is oriented to person, place, and time demonstrates that remote, recent, and intermediate memory probably is intact.

A patient's responses to the environment (affect) should be appropriate to the situation. Normal reactions to stress may include autonomic responses such as sweating and trembling and unusual facial movements (e.g., muscle twitching around the mouth, nose, and eyes). Reactive movements, such as not maintaining eye contact during conversation with the paramedic, should be noted. Other behavior that may be observed during conversation and that may indicate a patient is uncomfortable or anx-ious includes grooming movements such as fixing hair and straightening clothes.

Exploration

Exploration offers a method to review the patient's internal (emotional) experiences. For example, observing the patient's mood as anxious, excited, or depressed, and noting the patient's energy level can help determine the patient's mental status. Exploration can be performed by simply interacting with the patient to observe the appropriateness of behavior and ideas.

> **NOTE**
>
> An objective assessment must consider the patient's cultural and educational background, values, beliefs, and previous experiences.

> **? CRITICAL THINKING**
>
> *Why is the mental status examination especially important both medically and legally?*

Special Interview Situations

At times, paramedics may have to use special communications techniques to interact successfully with a patient. The following discussion provides brief descriptions of situations that may require individualized approaches.

Patients Unmotivated to Talk

Although most patients are more than willing to talk, some will require more time and varying techniques for a successful interview. Difficult interviews generally stem from four sources[4]:

1. The patient's condition may affect the ability to speak.
2. The patient may fear talking because of psychological disorders, cultural differences, or age.
3. A cognitive impairment may be present.
4. The patient may intentionally want to deceive the paramedic.

Techniques to Use

The following techniques may be useful for communicating with a patient who is unmotivated to talk:

- Start the interview in the normal way. If the patient does not talk, review the nature of the call as received from the dispatch center. Take time to develop a rapport with the patient.
- Use open-ended questions to obtain a response. If unsuccessful, try direct questions.
- Provide positive feedback to any responses by the patient.
- Make sure the patient understands the questions. Consider language barriers and hearing difficulties.
- Continue asking questions regarding the critical information needed to progress with treatment. (Nonessential information may be difficult to obtain.)
- Question family members or others at the scene. If the patient has been uncommunicative for a long period, attempt to rule out pathology.
- Use summary and interpretation of events or conditions, and ask the patient if your summary and interpretation are correct.
- Ask the patient questions about your care, equipment, or profession in an attempt to create conversation. Answer all questions fully (not with one-word answers).
- Realize that all needed information may not be obtained.
- Observe patient affect and record information to establish a mental status baseline for later evaluations.
- Consider asking questions for which answers are known to establish the patient's credibility.

> **NOTE**
>
> Patients who are unconscious or unresponsive may be able to receive stimuli. Hearing is thought to be the last sensation lost with unconsciousness and the first to be regained with consciousness.[4] The paramedic must be careful not to say anything near an unconscious patient that would not be said if the patient were fully conscious.

Interviewing a Hostile Patient

As part of ensuring personal safety, the paramedic should be aware of signs of a potentially violent situation (e.g., clenched fists, rising voice level, facial expression, past history of violence toward others). If a violent situation exists or is anticipated, the EMS crew should retreat from the scene and request law enforcement personnel. If safe retreat is not an option, the paramedic should stay far enough away from the patient for personal safety (see Chapter 38). The following is a list of guidelines for interviewing a hostile patient:

- Attempt to use normal interviewing techniques.
- Never leave the patient alone without adequate assistance.
- Set limits and establish boundaries with the patient.
- Explain the advantages of cooperation to the patient.
- Follow local protocol for dealing with hostile patients, including the use of physical and chemical restraints.

Developmental Considerations When Interviewing Patients

Communicating with children and older adults usually is not difficult provided that developmental characteristics are considered. Some general guidelines for these patient groups are provided in the following paragraphs.

Communicating with Children

When communicating with children, rapport often must be established with two persons—the child and the parent. With children aged 1 to 6 years old, most conversation should be first directed toward the parent. (Offering a child a toy may provide distraction while the parent is interviewed.) The paramedic should be aware that information obtained from the parent will be from the parent's point of view and might put the parent on the defensive. The paramedic should not be judgmental if the parents have not provided proper care or safety for the child

> **NOTE**
>
> Paramedics should be aware of their nonverbal communications when interviewing children because they are especially responsive to these messages.

before EMS arrival. (The paramedic should be observant, but not confrontational.) Gradually, the paramedic should begin to make contact with the child during the parent interview by speaking at eye level and by using a quiet, calm voice. Box 10-3 lists special considerations for communicating with various age groups of children. (Dealing with pediatric patients will be further discussed in Chapter 42.)

Communicating with the Older Adult

Many older adults are dealing with age-related disease and the inevitability of their death. Interviewing older adults may take longer than interviewing younger persons. Patients in this age group may fatigue easily and may have physical disabilities that distort speech and language. Touch is generally important to most older adults. (Assessing the older adult will be further addressed in Chapter 43.)

> **NOTE**
>
> Paramedics should always address older adults using the patient's last name preceded with Mr., Mrs., or Ms. (unless the patient requests otherwise).

Hearing-impaired Patients

When dealing with a hearing-impaired patient, the paramedic should ascertain their preferred method of communications (e.g., lip reading, signing, or writing). As a rule, writing often is the best out-of-hospital method for communicating with a deaf patient. If lip

> **BOX 10-3**
>
> ### COMMUNICATIONS "TIPS" FOR VARIOUS AGE GROUPS OF CHILDREN
>
> Infants respond best to firm, gentle handling and a quiet calm voice. Older infants may have "stranger anxiety." If possible, the parent should remain in view of the child.
>
> Preschoolers see the world only from their perspective and base everything on past experience. The paramedic should use short sentences with concrete explanations.
>
> Adolescents want to be adults. They should not be communicated with as "children."

reading is preferred, the paramedic should face the patient squarely, ensure adequate lighting, speak slowly with short words and phrases, and enunciate clearly.

> **NOTE**
>
> Because many deaf patients lip read, paramedics must speak clearly in full view of deaf patients.

> **NOTE**
>
> Some deaf patients may nod "yes" even if they do not understand what is asked.
>
> If the patient is suspected of being hearing-impaired or deaf, the paramedic should try to gain the patient's attention by gentle touch, slowly waving hands in front of the patient, by speaking a little louder, or if necessary, by speaking directly into the patient's ear if no hearing aid is present. If a hearing-impaired patient needs to be transported to a medical facility, advise the emergency department staff as soon as possible so that arrangements can be made for personnel to aid in communications.

> **NOTE**
>
> Finger spelling and simple sign language are easily learned and can facilitate communications with deaf patients in the prehospital setting.

Blind Patients

When communicating with a blind patient, the paramedic should ascertain if the patient has a hearing impairment as well (although it is unusual for sightless people to also be deaf). Identification should be made in a normal voice, and all questions regarding the emergency scene and surroundings should be answered. All examination and treatment procedures should be explained in detail before touching these patients.

> **NOTE**
>
> Most patients who have disabilities are very independent and may resent unsolicited assistance.

If a sightless person has a guide dog and the situation permits, they should not be separated. If the dog has been injured during the emergency event, the paramedic should immediately advise the dispatch center to make special arrangements to care for the dog.

Patients Under the Influence of Street Drugs or Alcohol

If street drugs or alcohol are involved in an emergency situation, the paramedic should ensure personal safety and be prepared for unpredictable patient behavior. (Law enforcement assistance may be required to ensure scene safety.) During the patient interview, the paramedic should ask simple or direct questions and should avoid any action that the patient might consider threatening or confrontational (see Chapters 34 and 52).

Sexually Aggressive Patients

Paramedics should confront male or female patients who make inappropriate sexual advances to ensure that they understand the professional position of the EMS caregiver. The paramedic should document any unusual occurrences and the observations of any witnesses to any of the actions or incidents. When a

NOTE

Some EMS services use tape recorders during transport to record all interactions with sexually aggressive patients. The patient's legal consent may be required before using tape recorders.

BOX 10-4

PITFALLS TO AVOID WHEN COMMUNICATING WITH TRANSCULTURAL PATIENTS

Ethnocentrism: Viewing one's own life as the most desirable, acceptable or best; to act in a superior manner to another culture's way of life.
Cultural imposition: Imposing one's beliefs, values, and patterns of behavior on people from another culture.

patient is sexually aggressive, considering "same sex" caregivers or arranging to have a chaperon present during care and transportation is recommended.

Transcultural Considerations

When communicating with a patient from another culture, the paramedic should make a personal introduction and ask the patient to do the same. The paramedic must be aware that he or she may be viewed as a cultural stereotype to the patient and family. Therefore the role of everyone involved in providing care (paramedic, patient, family members) must be clearly understood. Box 10-4 outlines pitfalls to avoid when caring for these patients.

Personal Space

As previously mentioned, "personal space" is culturally defined and varies by individual. Table 10-1 provides general guidelines for personal space, which should be considered when communicating with patients from a different culture. Other considerations for communicating with these patients include the following:

- Some cultures expect health care workers to have all the answers to their illness.
- Different cultures accept illness or injury in different ways.
- Nonverbal communications (e.g., handshaking and touching) may be perceived differently in different cultures.
- Asian, Native Americans, Indochinese, and Arabs may consider direct eye contact impolite or aggressive; they may avert their eyes during an interview.
- The paramedic should refrain from using touch as nonverbal communications between members of different culture groups because of the ease of unintended miscommunications.
- Language barriers may present communications difficulties.

? CRITICAL THINKING

Do you know anyone whose personal space requirements are much more or much less than those listed here? How would this affect your interview with them?

TABLE 10-1	GENERAL GUIDELINES FOR PERSONAL SPACE

Intimate zone	**Social distance**
0 to 1.5 feet	4 to 12 feet
Visual distortion occurs	Used for impersonal business transactions
Best for assessing breath and other body odors	Perceptual information much less detailed
	Much of the patient interview occurs at this distance
Personal distance	
1.5 to 4 feet	**Public distance**
Perceived as extension of self	12 or more feet
Voice is moderate	Interaction with others is impersonal
Body odors are not apparent	Speaker's voice must be projected
Much of the physical assessment occurs at this distance	Subtle facial expressions are imperceptible

NOTE: These are only "general" guidelines. Some cultures are more comfortable at a variety of spaces when communicating.

S U M M A R Y

- Therapeutic communications is a planned, deliberate, professional act that uses information for desired patient-care goals.

- Communications is a dynamic process. The elements of this process include the source, encoding, the message, decoding, the receiver, and feedback.

- To effectively communicate with patients, paramedics must genuinely like people, must be able to empathize with others, and must have the ability to listen.

- Effective communications requires a suitable physical environment. Issues such as privacy, interruption, eye contact, and personal dress are external factors that can be controlled by the paramedic to enhance communications during the paramedic-patient encounter.

- The patient interview often determines the direction of the physical examination. Good emergency care involves viewing each patient as a total individual and attending to patient needs in a caring, concerned, and receptive manner.

- Open-ended and closed (direct) questions are used to obtain information from the patient. These techniques include resistance, shifting focus, recognizing defense mechanisms, and distraction.

- The first step with any patient is to assess mental status by observing the patient's appearance, level of consciousness, and normal or abnormal body movements. During normal conversation, the patient should be able to demonstrate clear thinking, a normal attention span, and the ability to concentrate on and comprehend the discussion. A patient's responses to the environment (affect) should be appropriate to the situation.

- Difficult interviews generally stem from four sources: (1) the patient's condition may impact his or her ability to speak; (2) the patient may fear talking because of psychological disorders, cultural differences, or age; (3) a cognitive impairment may be present; and (4) the patient may intentionally want to deceive the paramedic.

REFERENCES

1. Satir V: *The new peoplemaking*, Palo Alto, Calif, 1988, Science and Behavior Books.
2. Potter P and Perry A: *Fundamentals of nursing: concepts, process & practice*, ed 3, St Louis, 1993, Mosby.
3. Rathus S: *Psychology*, ed 3, New York, 1987, Holt, Rinehart & Winston.
4. *EMT–Paramedic national standard curriculum*, US Department of Transportation National Highway Traffic Safety Administration, Washington, DC, 1998, The Department.

Division Two →

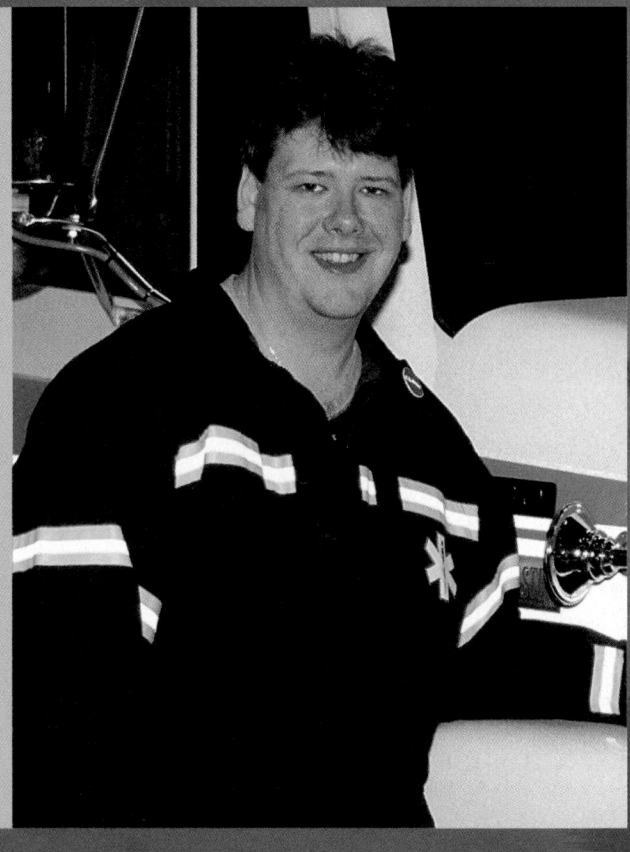

Robert McGraw,
AS-EMT-P
Program Coordinator,
Fire Science/EMS
Seminole Community
College
Sanford, Florida

"I remember a wife and her husband out on their fiftieth wedding anniversary. The man had collapsed and the wife found him and called us. As we were taking her husband away in the ambulance, the wife pulled on my arm and asked, 'He'll be home for our anniversary dinner, right?' You don't just treat the one person; you have to treat the whole family."

Airway Management and Ventilation

11 Airway Management and Ventilation

OBJECTIVES

Upon completion of this chapter, the paramedic student will be able to:

1. Distinguish between respiration, pulmonary ventilation, and external and internal respiration.
2. Explain the mechanics of respiration.
3. Relate the partial pressures of gases in the blood and lungs to atmospheric gas pressures.
4. Describe pulmonary circulation.
5. Explain the process of exchange and transport of gases in the body.
6. Describe voluntary, chemical, and nervous regulation of respiration.
7. Discuss the assessment and management of medical or traumatic obstruction of the airway.
8. Outline the causes and effects of and preventive measures for pulmonary aspiration.
9. Outline essential parameters for evaluating the effectiveness of the airway and breathing.
10. Describe the indications, contraindications, and techniques for delivery of supplemental oxygen.
11. Discuss methods of patient ventilation based on the indications, contraindications, potential complications, and use of each method.
12. Describe the use of manual airway maneuvers and mechanical airway adjuncts based on the indications, contraindications, potential complications, and techniques for each.
13. Describe assessment techniques and devices used to ensure adequate oxygenation, correct placement of the endotracheal tube, and elimination of carbon dioxide.
14. Explain variations in assessment and management of airway and ventilation problems in pediatric patients.
15. Given a patient scenario, identify possible alterations in oxygenation and ventilation based on a knowledge of gas exchange and the mechanics of breathing.

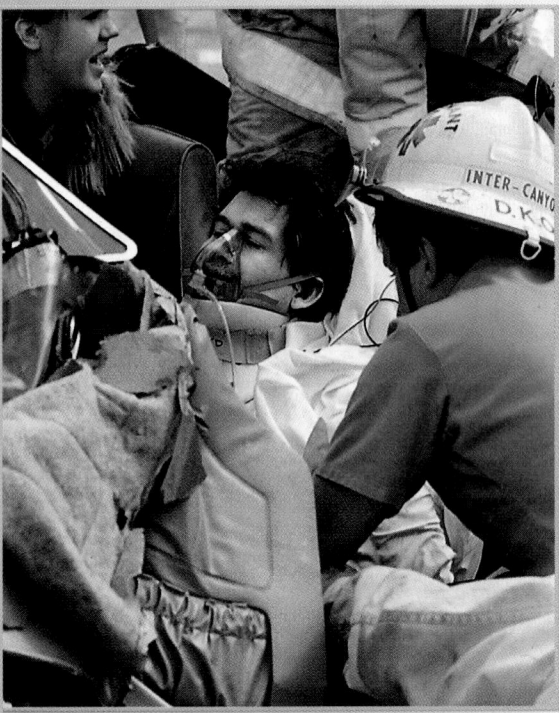

The absence of an adequate airway and ineffective ventilation are major causes of preventable death and cardiopulmonary complications in both medical and trauma patients. A thorough understanding of the respiratory system and mastery of airway management and ventilation are important aspects of prehospital emergency care.

KEY TERMS

anatomical dead space: The volume of the conducting airways from the external environment down to the terminal bronchioles.

atelectasis: An abnormal condition characterized by the collapse of lung tissue, which prevents the respiratory exchange of oxygen and carbon dioxide.

compliance: A measure of the distensibility of lung volume produced by a unit pressure change.

gag reflex: A normal neural response triggered by touching the soft palate or posterior pharynx.

hypocarbia: Diminished carbon dioxide in the blood; also known as hypocapnia.

intrapulmonic pressure: The pressure of the gas within the alveoli.

intrathoracic pressure: The pressure in the pleural space; also known as intrapleural pressure.

minute volume: The tidal volume times the respiratory rate; the amount of gas inhaled or exhaled in 1 minute.

physiological dead space: The sum of the anatomical dead space plus the volume of any nonfunctional alveoli.

pulmonary ventilation: The movement of air in and out of the lungs, which brings oxygen into the lungs and removes carbon dioxide.

respiration: The process of the molecular change of oxygen and carbon dioxide within the body's tissues.

tidal volume: The volume of air inspired or expired in a single, resting breath.

SECTION ONE
ANATOMY AND PHYSIOLOGY OF THE RESPIRATORY SYSTEM

NOTE

The reader should refer to Chapter 6 to review the anatomy of the respiratory system.

Mechanics of Respiration

Respiration is the exchange of oxygen and carbon dioxide between an organism and the environment. For this gas exchange to occur, air must move freely in and out of the lungs, bringing oxygen to the lungs and removing carbon dioxide, a process known as **pulmonary ventilation.** The two phases of respiration are:

- External respiration, or the transfer of oxygen and carbon dioxide between the inspired air and pulmonary capillaries.
- Internal respiration, or the transfer of oxygen and carbon dioxide between the capillary red blood cells and the tissue cells.

? CRITICAL THINKING

Think of two medical conditions that could impair (1) external respiration and (2) internal respiration.

Pressure Changes and Ventilation

Gas flows from an area of higher pressure or concentration to an area of lower pressure or concentration. For gas to flow into the lungs, a pressure gradient is required. This pressure gradient is produced by differences between atmospheric pressure, **intrapulmonic pressure,** and intrapleural pressure, or **intrathoracic pressure.**

Atmospheric pressure is the pressure of the gas around us. It varies with differences in altitude, but at sea level it is 760 mm Hg. Intrapulmonic pressure is the pressure of the gas within the alveoli. Depending on the size of the thorax, this pressure varies slightly above and below 760 mm Hg, depending on whether it is measured during inspiration or expiration. Intrathoracic pressure is the pressure in the pleural space. It normally is less than atmospheric pressure (usually 751 to 754 mm Hg), but it may exceed atmospheric pressure during coughing and the straining associated with bowel movements.

During inspiration the chest wall expands, which increases the size of the thoracic cavity and expands the lungs. The expansion results from muscle movement and negative pressure in the pleural space. As the thorax expands, the lung space increases, causing a drop in intrapulmonic pressure of about 1 mm Hg below atmospheric pressure. The pressure gradient results in gas flow into the lungs. At end inspiration the thorax stops expanding, the alveoli stop expanding, intrapulmonic pressure becomes equal to atmospheric pressure, and gas no longer moves into the lungs.

As the chest wall relaxes during expiration, the respiratory muscles essentially are at rest, and the process of inspiration reverses. Elastic recoil causes the thorax and lung space to decrease in size, which increases intrapulmonic pressure. The pressure gradient created in the thoracic cavity produces a decrease in alveolar volume and increases intrapulmonic pressure about 1 mm Hg over atmospheric pressure. The pressure gradient results in gas flow out of the lungs. At end expiration the opposing forces and pressures equilibrate, and thoracic volume no longer decreases. Intrapulmonic pressure becomes equal to atmospheric pressure, and gas movement out of the lungs ceases (Fig. 11-1).

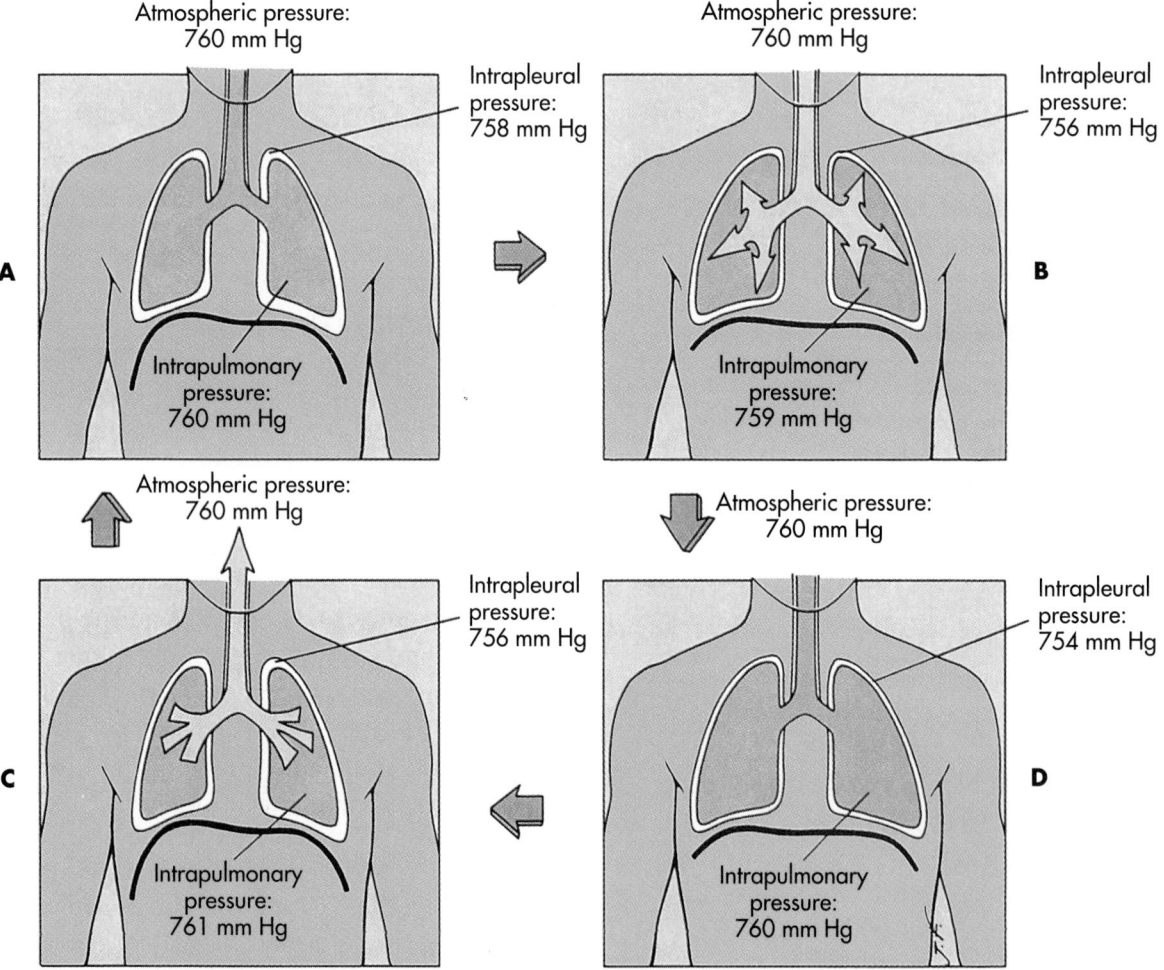

Fig. 11-1 Pressure changes during inspiration and expiration. **A,** At the end of expiration, intrapulmonary pressure equals atmospheric pressure, and no movement of air occurs. **B,** During inspiration, the volume of the pleural space increases, causing the pressure in the intrapulmonary spaces (alveoli) to decrease. Air then flows from the outside of the body, where the pressure is greater (760 mm Hg), into the alveoli, where it is lower (759 mm Hg). **C,** At the end of inspiration, intrapulmonary pressure again equals atmospheric pressure, and no movement of air occurs. **D,** During expiration, the volume of the pleural spaces decreases, causing the intrapulmonary pressure to increase. Because the intrapulmonary pressure exceeds the atmospheric pressure, air flows out of the body.

Muscles of Respiration

The expansion of the lungs and thorax is made possible by the movement of the diaphragm and the internal and external intercostal muscles (Fig. 11-2). During inspiration, the diaphragm contracts and the dome of the diaphragm flattens. This increases the superior-inferior dimension of the chest cavity. The internal and external intercostal muscles also contract, raising the ribs and increasing the anterior-posterior and side-to-side dimensions of the chest cavity.

> **? CRITICAL THINKING**
>
> *How will interruption of the chest wall from a stab wound change the mechanics of breathing?*

During expiration (a passive motion), relaxation of the diaphragm and intercostal muscles allows the elastic recoil properties of the lungs to decrease the size (or volume) of the thoracic cavity. The ease with which the lungs and thorax expand during pressure changes is referred to as **compliance.** The greater the compliance, the easier the expansion. Diseases that decrease compliance (e.g., asthma, emphysema, bronchitis, pulmonary edema) increase the energy required for breathing.

Work of Breathing

The energy required for normal, quiet breathing is about 3% of the total body expenditure in healthy people. Factors that increase the amount of energy needed for ventilation include loss of pulmonary surfactant, an increase in airway resistance, or a decrease in pulmonary compliance. These factors can increase the energy requirement to as much as one third of the total body expenditure.

The pulmonary alveoli have a natural tendency to collapse. This is the result of recoil caused by the elastic fibers in the alveolar walls and of surface tension, which is produced by the attractive forces between the water molecules in the alveolar membrane. Pulmonary surfactant lowers the surface tension by interspersing with the water molecules to reduce the cohesive force, which helps prevent collapse of the alveolus at the end of expiration.

Surfactant is continuously replenished by certain alveolar cells, and its production is thought to be stimulated by normal ventilation. If surfactant production decreases, as in pneumonia, extremely high pressures may be required to maintain lung expansion.

The elastic forces of the lung oppose lung expansion, but viscous and frictional forces often play the dominant role in impeding airflow into and out of the lungs. Much of the resistance to airflow is provided by the upper airways of the respiratory tract. The nasal passages cause about 50% of the total airway resistance during nose breathing. The mouth, pharynx, larynx, and trachea account for approximately 20% to 30% of airway resistance during quiet mouth breathing; this may increase to about 50% during periods of increased ventilation (e.g., strenuous exercise).

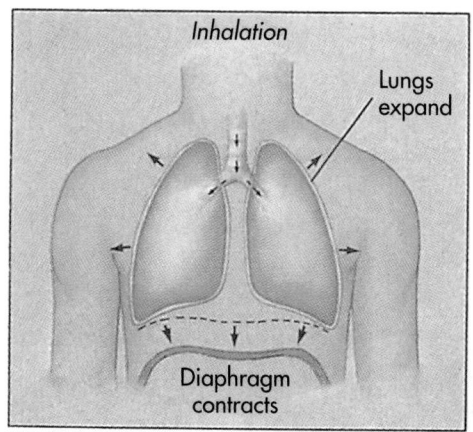 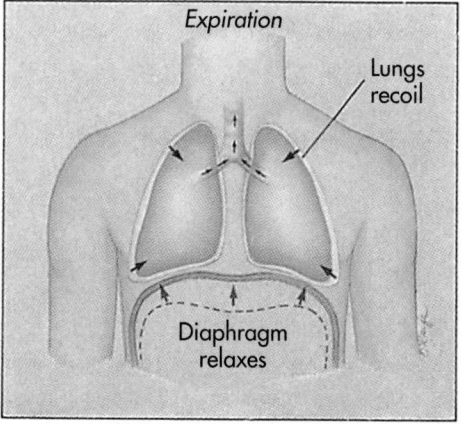

Fig. 11-2 Mechanics of breathing. During inhalation, the diaphragm contracts, increasing the volume of the thoracic cavity. The increase in volume results in a decrease in pressure, which causes air to rush into the lungs. During expiration, the diaphragm returns to an upward position, reducing the volume in the thoracic cavity. Air pressure increases and forces air out of the lungs. (From Thibodeau GA: *Structure and function of the body,* ed 9, St Louis, 1992, Mosby.)

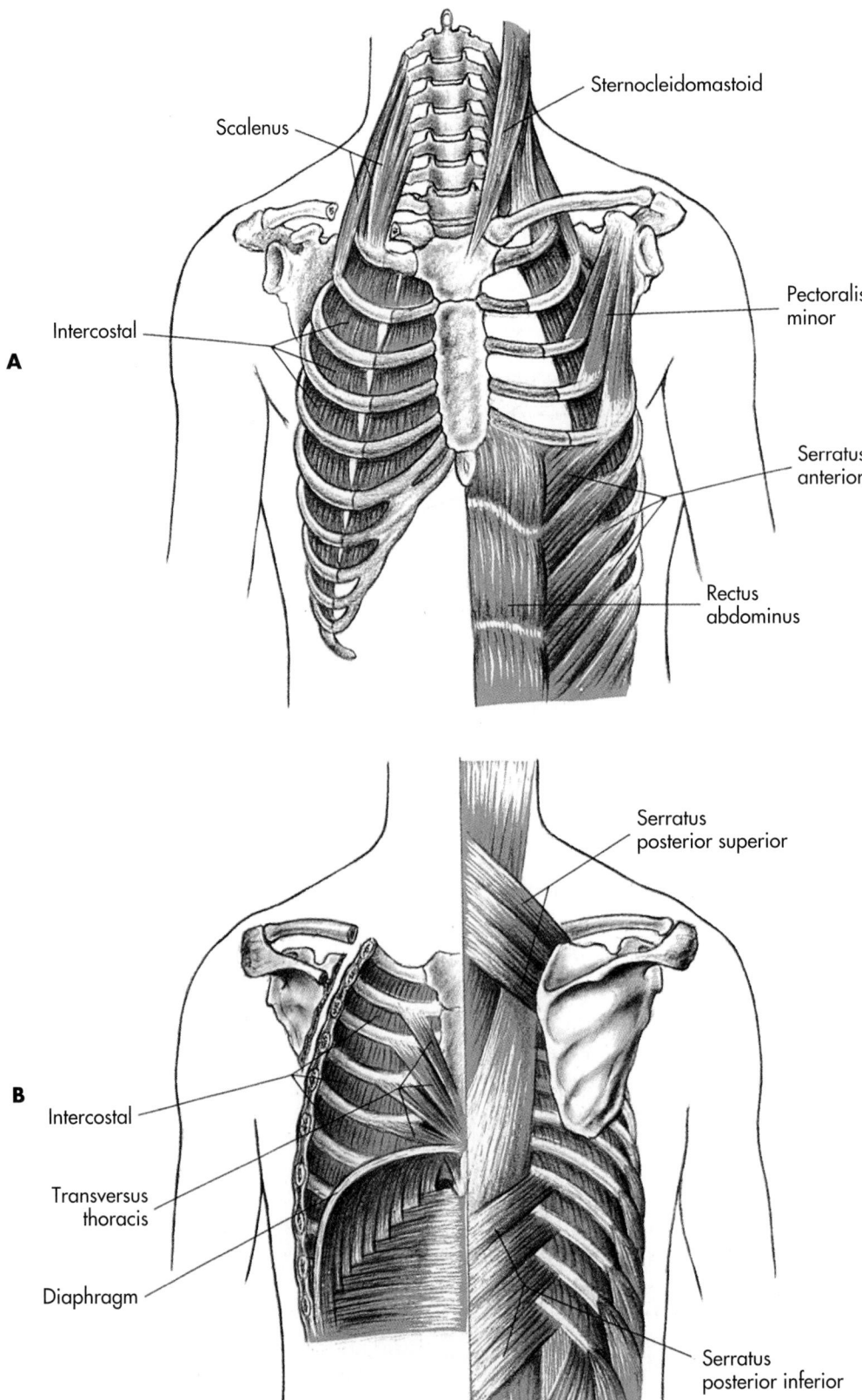

Fig. 11-3 Muscles of ventilation. **A,** Anterior view. **B,** Posterior view. (From Seidel H: *Mosby's guide to physical examination,* ed 2, St Louis, 1991, Mosby.)

Airway resistance falls dramatically as the bronchial tree continues to branch toward the alveoli because of the large increase in the total cross-sectional diameter of the airways. However, the presence of airway secretions or bronchiolar constriction can lead to increased airway resistance. These factors may occur separately but more commonly occur together (e.g., as in asthma). When resistance to airflow increases, the usual pressure gradient required for ventilation does not suffice, and muscular effort is required to create a larger pressure gradient.

Structural changes in the lung or thorax resulting from trauma or disease also may increase the amount of work required for effective ventilation. This increased work of ventilation usually is evident from the use of accessory muscles during labored breathing. These accessory muscles include the scalenes and sternocleidomastoid (deep muscles of the neck and thorax), posterior neck and back muscles, and the abdominal muscles (Fig. 11-3).

Lung Volumes and Capacities

At rest, the average adult male breathes about 12 to 24 times per minute. One fifth of this inspired air fills the upper respiratory tract and lower nonrespiratory bronchioles, never reaching the alveoli for gas exchange. This area is referred to as **anatomical dead space. Physiological dead space** refers to the anatomical dead space plus the volume of any nonfunctional alveoli. Normally the anatomical and physiological dead spaces are nearly identical. However, in patients with respiratory diseases such as emphysema, the alveolar walls begin to degenerate. The destruction of alveolar walls can increase the size of the physiological dead space up to 10 times that of anatomical dead space (Fig. 11-4).

The lungs can hold about eight times the amount of air contained in a normal resting inhalation. From the first breath of life, the lungs are never completely emptied. Even after forced expiration, a "residual volume" of air is present in the alveoli.

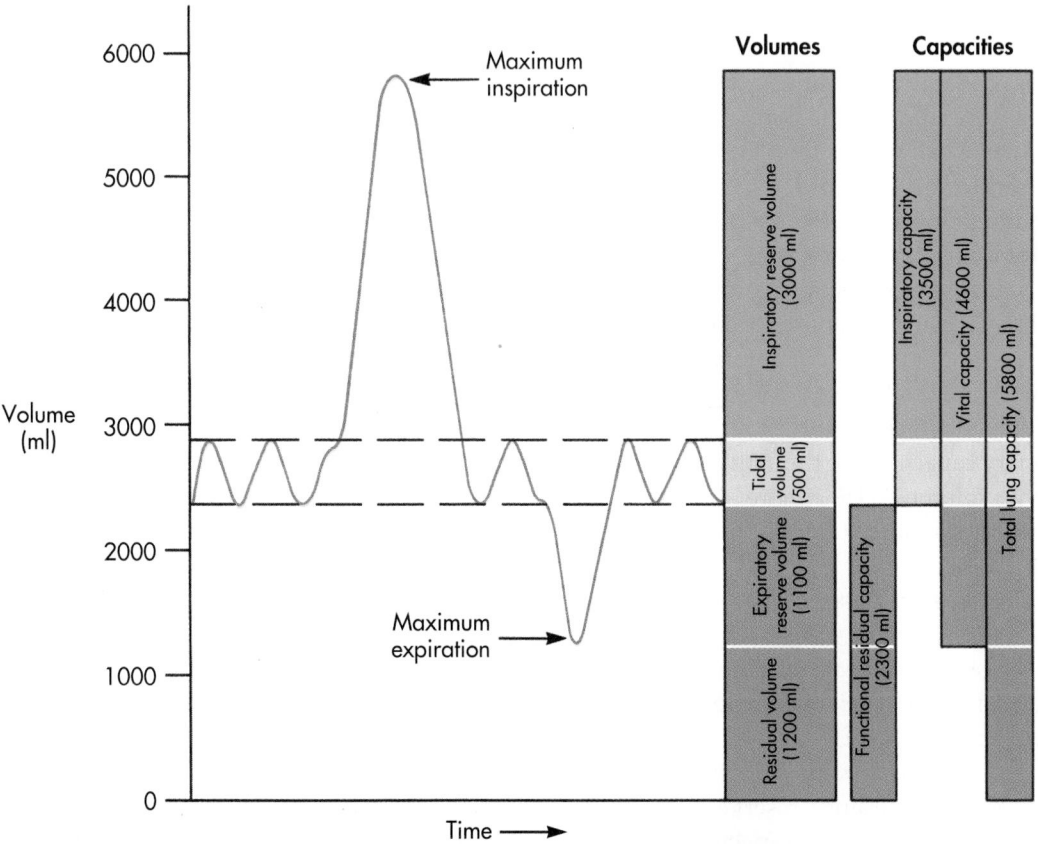

Fig. 11-4 Lung volumes and capacities. Tidal volume during resting conditions. (From Seely R: *Anatomy and physiology,* ed 2, St Louis, 1992, Mosby.)

This residual volume is replenished slowly. At least 16 breaths and sometimes more are required to renew the residual volume of air in the lungs.

Tidal volume is the volume of gas inhaled or exhaled during a normal breath. The tidal volume of the average adult male is about 500 to 600 mL. Of this, 150 mL remains in the anatomical dead space (the bronchi, bronchioles, and other prealveolar structures) until it is exhaled during the following respiratory cycle. Thus 150 mL of the atmospheric gas entering the respiratory system during each inspiration never reaches the alveoli but is merely moved in and out of the airways.

> **NOTE**
>
> A paramedic observing the rise and fall of a patient's chest is indirectly observing tidal volume.

The inspiratory reserve volume is the amount of gas that can be forcefully inspired after inspiration of the normal tidal volume. This amount is usually 2000 to 3000 mL.

The expiratory reserve volume is the amount of gas that can be forcefully expired after expiration of the normal tidal volume. The normal expiratory reserve volume usually is less than the inspiratory reserve volume (about 1200 mL).

The residual volume is the gas that remains in the respiratory system after forced expiration. The normal residual volume usually is 1000 to 1200 mL. The combined measurements of tidal volume, inspiratory reserve volume, expiratory reserve volume, and residual volume all constitute the maximum volume to which the lungs can be expanded.

Pulmonary capacities are the sum of two or more pulmonary volumes. The more common pulmonary capacities follow (Fig. 11-5):

- *Inspiratory capacity:* Inspiratory capacity is the tidal volume plus the inspiratory reserve volume. This capacity reflects the amount of gas that a person can inspire maximally after a normal expiration (about 3500 mL).
- *Functional residual capacity:* Functional residual capacity is the expiratory reserve volume plus the residual volume. This capacity reflects the amount of gas remaining in the lungs at the end of a normal expiration (about 2300 mL).

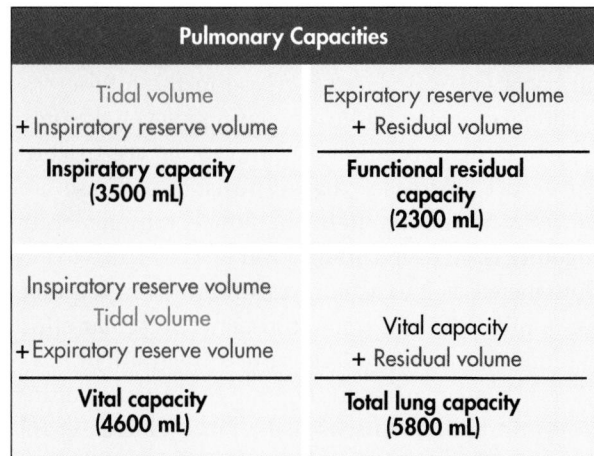

Fig. 11-5 Pulmonary capacities.

- *Vital capacity:* Vital capacity is the volume of gas that can move on deepest inspiration and expiration or the sum of the inspiratory reserve volume, the tidal volume, and the expiratory reserve volume. This capacity is about 4600 mL.
- *Total lung capacity:* Total lung capacity is the sum of the vital capacity and the residual volume (about 5800 mL).

Minute Volume and Minute Alveolar Ventilation

Minute volume is the tidal volume multiplied by the respiratory rate, or the amount of gas inhaled or exhaled in 1 minute. If, for example, the patient's respiratory rate is 10 per minute and the resting tidal volume is 500 mL, the average minute volume is 5 L per minute.

> **? CRITICAL THINKING**
>
> *Which respiratory volumes will be affected by a severe burn that encircles the chest?*

Because much of the gas inspired during respiration fills the anatomical dead space before reaching the alveoli, that amount of air is unavailable for gas exchange. The amount of inspired gas that is available for gas exchange during 1 minute is referred to as the *minute alveolar ventilation.* The minute alveolar ventilation is calculated by subtracting the

TABLE 11-1	CONCENTRATION OF GASES

GAS	CONCENTRATIONS
Gases in the Atmosphere	
Nitrogen	597 torr (78.62%)
Oxygen	159 torr (20.84%)
Carbon dioxide	0.3 torr (0.50%)
Water (vapor)	3.7 torr (6.2%)
Alveolar Gases	
Nitrogen	569 torr (74.9%)
Oxygen	104 torr (13.7%)
Carbon dioxide	40 torr (5.2%)
Water (vapor)	47 torr (6.2%)

amount of dead space from the tidal volume and then multiplying this figure by the respiratory rate:

$$\text{Minute alveolar ventilation} =$$
$$(\text{Tidal volume} - \text{Dead space}) \times \text{Respiratory rate}$$

If the tidal volume, the respiratory rate, or both increase, the minute volume also increases. Conversely, the minute volume decreases if the tidal volume, respiratory rate, or both decrease. The paramedic must note the depth of respiration (tidal volume) and the rate of ventilation to determine if the patient's respiratory status is adequate.

Measurement of Gases

The mixture of gases that make up the atmosphere exerts a combined partial pressure (described in Chapter 7) of 100%, or 760 mm Hg at sea level. Nitrogen makes up about 78.62% of the volume of dry atmospheric gas at sea level. The partial pressure resulting from nitrogen is calculated by multiplying 78.62% by 760 mm Hg, which equals 597 mm Hg, or a P_{N_2} of 597 torr. Oxygen accounts for 20.84% of the volume of atmospheric gas. The partial pressure resulting from oxygen is 20.84% multiplied by 760 mm Hg, or 159 mm Hg (a P_{O_2} of 159 torr).

Another partial pressure can be measured when gas comes into contact with water. The water molecules convert into a gas, evaporate, and exert a par-

tial pressure known as *water vapor pressure* (P_{H_2O}) (Table 11-1).

> **NOTE**
>
> Partial pressure is measured in millimeters of mercury, or torr. One torr equals 1 mm Hg.

> **NOTE**
>
> The amount of oxygen that makes up atmospheric gas commonly is rounded to 21%, carbon dioxide to less than 1% and nitrogen to 78%.

The compositions of alveolar gas and dry atmospheric gas are not the same.

This is a result of several factors: the air entering the respiratory system being humidified by the body, the exchange of oxygen and carbon dioxide between the alveoli and the blood, and the incomplete emptying of the alveoli with expiration.

Pulmonary Circulation

The process of gas exchange in the lungs is the opposite of that which occurs in the tissues throughout the rest of the body. As inspired gas enters the lungs, the respiratory system brings oxygen to the blood and removes carbon dioxide. Blood that is low in oxygen converges on the heart from all parts of the body. Passing through the right side of the heart, the blood flows into either lung through the pulmonary artery. From there it flows into the smaller pulmonary arterioles and then into capillaries that surround each of the hundreds of millions of alveoli inside the lungs (Fig. 11-6).

The alveoli, now filled with a high concentration of oxygen molecules and a low concentration of carbon dioxide from inhaled air, have the pressure gradient required for gas exchange. Oxygen molecules move into the surrounding capillaries at the same time that carbon dioxide molecules move into the alveoli to be exhaled. The blood, now rich in oxygen, flows through the pulmonary venules into the pulmonary veins, then into the left atrium, then the left ventricle, and back out through the aorta to the body's tissues. To supply enough oxygen to the body tissues, an alveolus fills and empties more than 15,000 times in a day of normal breathing.

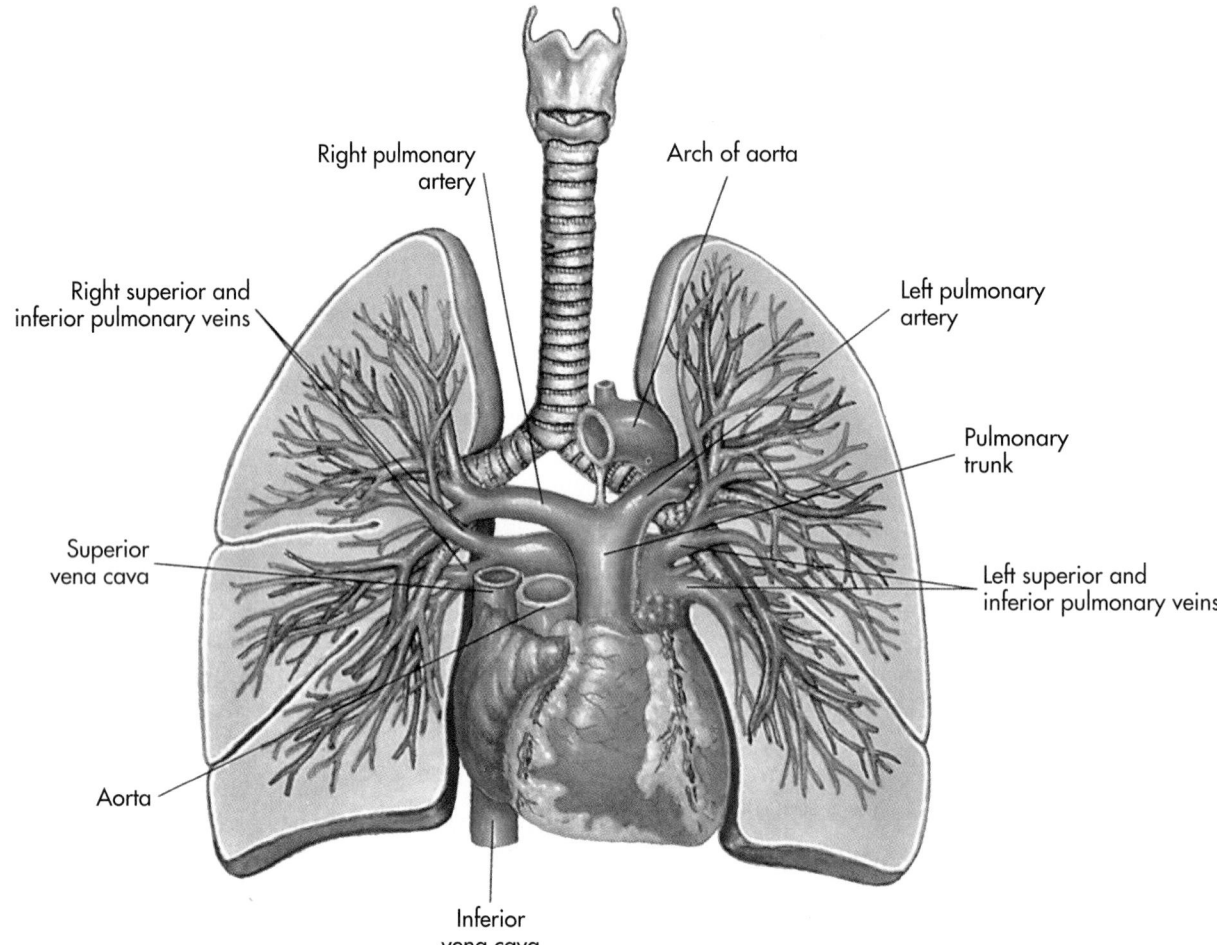

Fig. 11-6 Pulmonary circulation. (From Wilson S: *Respiratory disorders,* St Louis, 1990, Mosby.)

Exchange and Transport of Gases in the Body

The volume of oxygen taken up in the lungs may be calculated from the difference in the amount of oxygen in inspired and expired air. The volume of carbon dioxide that is eliminated may be determined in a similar fashion.

As described in Chapter 6, metabolism is the total of all the chemical changes that occur in the body. In a healthy body with a constant metabolism, the relationship between tissue carbon dioxide production and oxygen consumption is fixed. Ordinarily, the amount of oxygen taken up by the capillary blood is greater than the amount of carbon dioxide released by the blood to the alveolar gas. Therefore the expired volume is slightly less than the inspired volume.

At rest, the combined consumption of all of the body cells is about 200 mL of oxygen per minute, with about the same amount of carbon dioxide being produced. Because about 20% of atmospheric gas is oxygen, the total oxygen inspired is 20% multiplied by 5 L, or about 1 L of oxygen per minute. Of this, 200 mL crosses the alveoli into the pulmonary capillaries, and the remaining 800 mL is exhaled. The 200 mL of oxygen is added to the quantity of oxygen already in the pulmonary capillaries and is then transported to the body tissues by the circulatory system. After the body cells use the necessary oxygen, the oxygen remaining in the blood returns to the heart and lungs. This exchange of oxygen and carbon dioxide is accomplished by the passive process of diffusion, which is the tendency for molecules in solution to move from an area of higher concentration to an area of lower concentration (see Chapter 7).

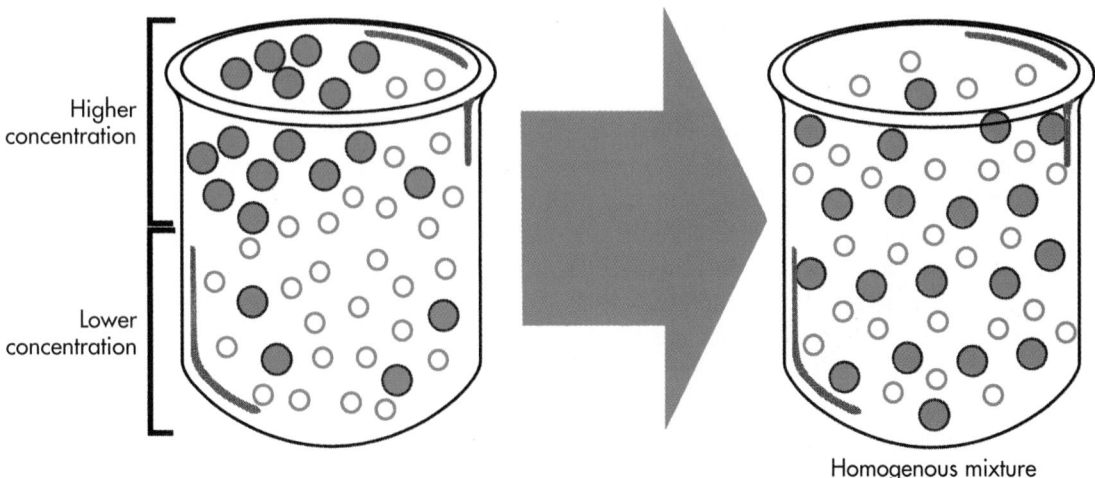

Fig. 11-7 Random movement of gas is from a higher concentration to a lower concentration until a homogenous mixture of gases is achieved.

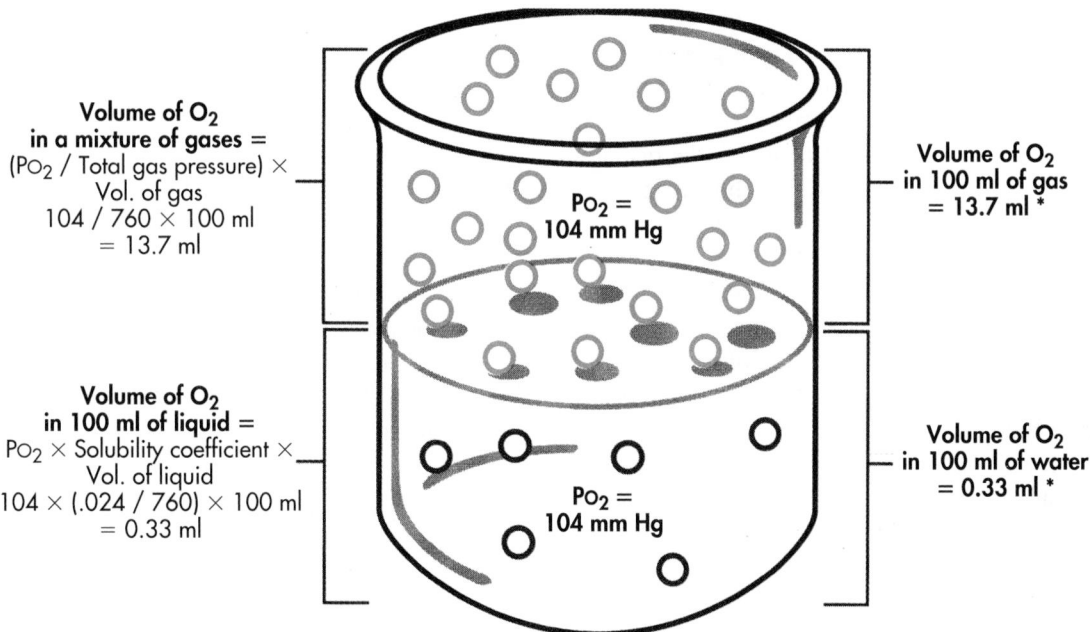

Volume of O$_2$ in a mixture of gases = (PO$_2$ / Total gas pressure) × Vol. of gas
104 / 760 × 100 ml
= 13.7 ml

PO$_2$ = 104 mm Hg

Volume of O$_2$ in 100 ml of gas = 13.7 ml *

Volume of O$_2$ in 100 ml of liquid = PO$_2$ × Solubility coefficient × Vol. of liquid
104 × (.024 / 760) × 100 ml
= 0.33 ml

PO$_2$ = 104 mm Hg

Volume of O$_2$ in 100 ml of water = 0.33 ml *

Fig. 11-8 At equilibrium, the concentration of a gas in liquid is determined by its partial pressure in the gas and by its solubility in the liquid. *At atmospheric pressure (760 mm Hg) and 37° C.

Diffusion

Molecules of gases are in constant, random motion, which is fueled by collisions with other molecules. If the blood is divided by a permeable barrier, such as a capillary wall or cell membrane, many gas molecules come into contact with and cross the barrier. The likelihood is much greater that highly concentrated molecules will strike and cross the membrane than less concentrated molecules. Thus the concen-

tration of molecules across a permeable membrane tends to equilibrate (Fig. 11-7).

The diffusion of gases through liquid is determined by the pressure of the gases and the solubility of the gases in liquid (Fig. 11-8). When a free gas comes into contact with liquid, the number of gas molecules that dissolve in the liquid is directly proportional to the pressure of the gas. When the free gas pressure is higher than the pressure of the gas in the liquid, enough molecules dissolve in the liquid for the free gas pressure to equal the dissolved gas pressure.

Conversely, if a liquid containing a dissolved gas at a high pressure is exposed to a free gas at a lower pressure, gas molecules leave the liquid and enter the free gas until the pressures become equal (the general gas law). This is the underlying theme of the exchange of gases between the cells and the capillary blood throughout the body. The free gas (PO_2) in the lungs is greater than that in the bloodstream, therefore oxygen diffuses from the lungs to the blood. The partial pressure of oxygen in the blood is higher than that in the peripheral tissues, therefore oxygen diffuses from the blood into the tissues.

In addition to the pressure of gases, the solubility of the gases in a liquid affects the behavior of the gases. The ease with which gases dissolve determines the absolute number of gas molecules that diffuse through the liquid at a given pressure. For example, if a liquid is exposed to two different gases at the same pressure, the number of molecules of each gas that will diffuse may not be identical because of the differing solubilities of the two gases.

Blood entering the pulmonary capillaries is systemic venous blood that has been circulated to the lungs via the pulmonary arteries. The partial pressure of carbon dioxide (PCO_2) is relatively high in this blood, and the partial pressure of oxygen (PO_2) is low. Because the alveoli contain a greater concentration of oxygen than the blood entering the pulmonary capillaries, oxygen molecules diffuse from the alveoli into the blood. Carbon dioxide moves from the blood, where it is more concentrated, to the alveoli, where it is less concentrated (Fig. 11-9).

The blood flowing through the pulmonary capillaries is separated from the alveolar air by a thin layer of tissue known as the *respiratory membrane.* This membrane is composed of the alveolar wall (surfactant, epithelial cells, and basement membrane), interstitial fluid, and the wall of the pulmonary capillary (basement membrane and endothelial cells). The differences in the partial pressures of oxygen and carbon dioxide on the two sides of the respiratory membrane result in the diffusion of oxygen into the blood and of carbon dioxide into the alveoli. With this diffusion, the capillary blood PO_2 rises and the PCO_2 falls. Diffusion of these gases stops when alveolar and capillary partial pressures equalize. In healthy individuals this process of gas exchange is so rapid that the blood leaving the lungs to be pumped through the arteries has nearly the same PO_2 (80 to 100 mm Hg) and PCO_2 (35 to 40 mm Hg) as alveolar air.

The diffusion of gases at the capillary-alveolar level can be affected in several ways. Some respiratory diseases (e.g., emphysema) cause destruction and collapse of the alveolar walls, a condition known as **atelectasis,** with the formation of fewer but larger alveoli. This degeneration results in a reduction of the total area available for diffusion. In some disease states the alveolar capillary membrane also may become thickened or less permeable, forcing gas molecules to travel farther and thereby decreasing the rate of diffusion. An example is pulmonary edema, in which fluid accumulates in the alveoli and pulmonary interstitial space, forcing gases to diffuse through a thicker than normal layer of fluid and tissue.

Oxygen Content of Blood

Oxygen is present in the blood in two forms: (1) physically dissolved in the blood and (2) chemically bound to hemoglobin (Hb) molecules. Compared with carbon dioxide and nitrogen, oxygen is relatively insoluble in water. Only 3 mL of oxygen can be dissolved in 1 L of blood at the normal alveolar and arterial PO_2 of 100 mm Hg. In contrast, 197 mL of oxygen (about 98%) is carried in red blood cells, where it is chemically bound to hemoglobin (oxyhemoglobin).

Hemoglobin can unload carbon dioxide and absorb oxygen 60 times faster than blood plasma.

When completely converted to oxyhemoglobin (HbO_2), each hemoglobin molecule can carry four molecules of oxygen and is said to be *fully saturated.* Hemoglobin nears full saturation at a PO_2 of 80 to 100 mm Hg.

The extent to which hemoglobin combines with oxygen increases rapidly when the PO_2 is 10 to 60 mm Hg. (About 90% of total hemoglobin is combined with oxygen when the PO_2 is 60 mm Hg.) Further increases in PO_2 produce only small increases in the binding of oxygen to hemoglobin. If PO_2 falls moderately, the amount of oxyhemoglobin decreases only slightly, still providing adequate oxygenation to tissues.

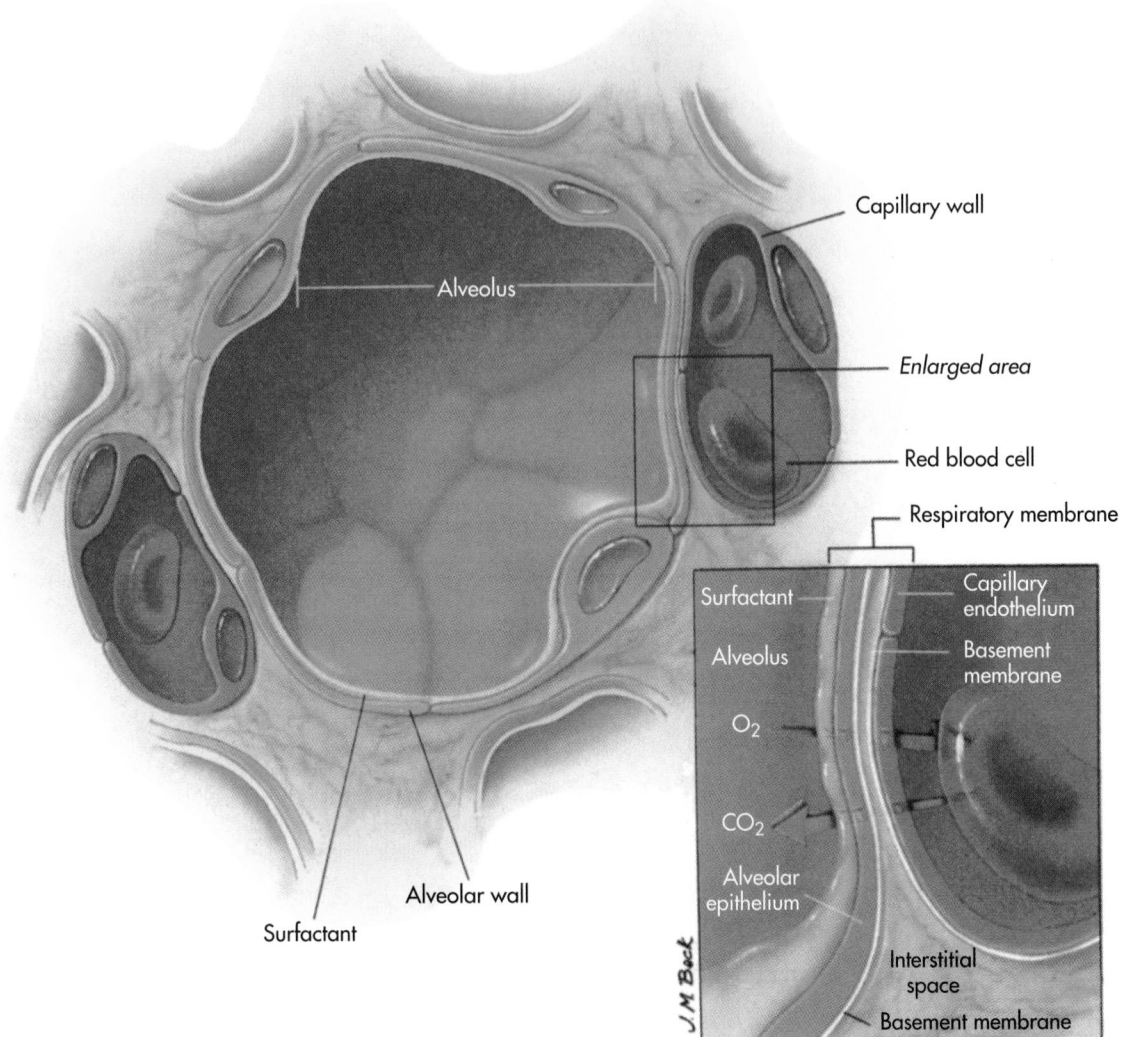

Fig. 11-9 Gas exchange structure of the lung. (From Thibodeau GA: *Structure and function of the body,* ed 9, St Louis, 1992, Mosby.)

NOTE

Understanding this adaptive plateau at higher P_{O_2} values is important when dealing with patient situations involving high altitudes, excessive exercise, and cardiac and pulmonary disease.

The partial pressure of oxygen in the blood plasma is the most important factor in determining the extent to which oxygen combines with hemoglobin. Oxyhemoglobin, however, does not contribute to the P_{O_2} of the blood. Only the physically dissolved oxygen molecules can create gas pressure. This oxygen uptake by hemoglobin molecules removes dissolved oxygen from blood plasma and maintains a low P_{O_2}, allowing diffusion to continue (Fig. 11-10).

Venous blood entering the lungs has a P_{O_2} of 40 mm Hg and a hemoglobin saturation of 75%. Oxygen diffuses from the alveoli (because of its higher P_{O_2} of 100 mm Hg) into the plasma. This diffusion raises plasma P_{O_2}, producing an increase in the uptake of oxygen by the hemoglobin molecules. In the tissue capillaries, this process is reversed. As the blood enters the capillaries, plasma P_{O_2} is greater than the P_{O_2} in the fluid surrounding the capillaries, causing diffusion across the capillary membranes to the cells of the tissues.

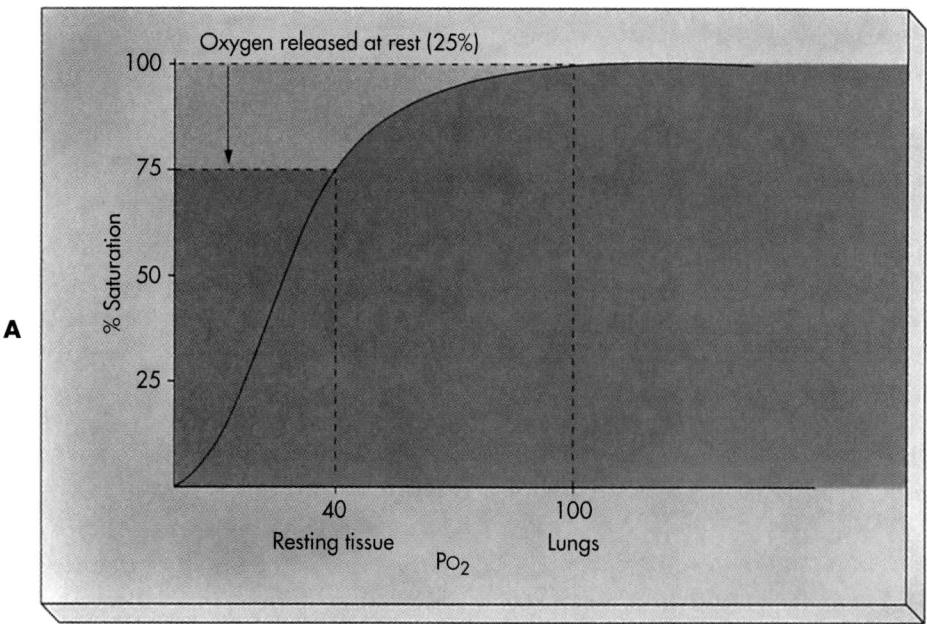

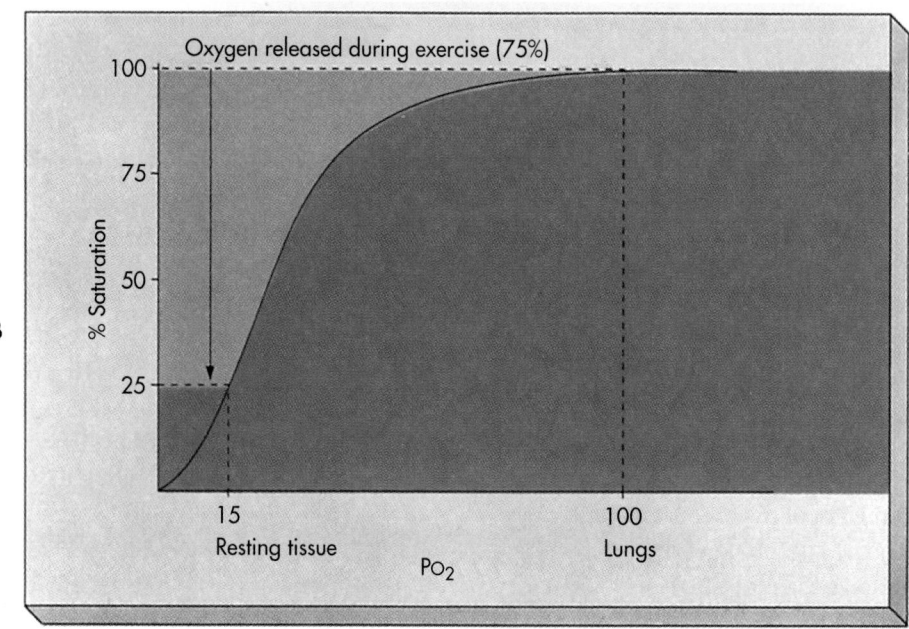

Fig. 11-10 Oxygen-hemoglobin dissociation curves. The graphs indicate the percentage of the hemoglobin saturated with oxygen as the partial pressure of oxygen increases. **A,** At the partial pressure of oxygen (P_{O_2}) in the lungs, hemoglobin is 100% saturated. At the P_{O_2} of resting tissues, hemoglobin is 75% saturated. Consequently, 25% of the oxygen picked up in the lungs is released to the tissues. **B,** In exercising tissues, the percentage saturation of hemoglobin can decrease to 25%, resulting in the release of 75% of the transported oxygen. (From Seely R: *Anatomy and physiology,* ed 2, St Louis, 1992, Mosby.)

Carbon Dioxide Content of Blood

The amount of carbon dioxide produced by the body is relatively constant and is determined by the body's rate and type of metabolism. If the metabolic rate increases (e.g., during exercise), more carbon dioxide is produced. Conversely, as the metabolic rate decreases (e.g., during sleep), so does the production of carbon dioxide. Certain types of metabolic processes also re-

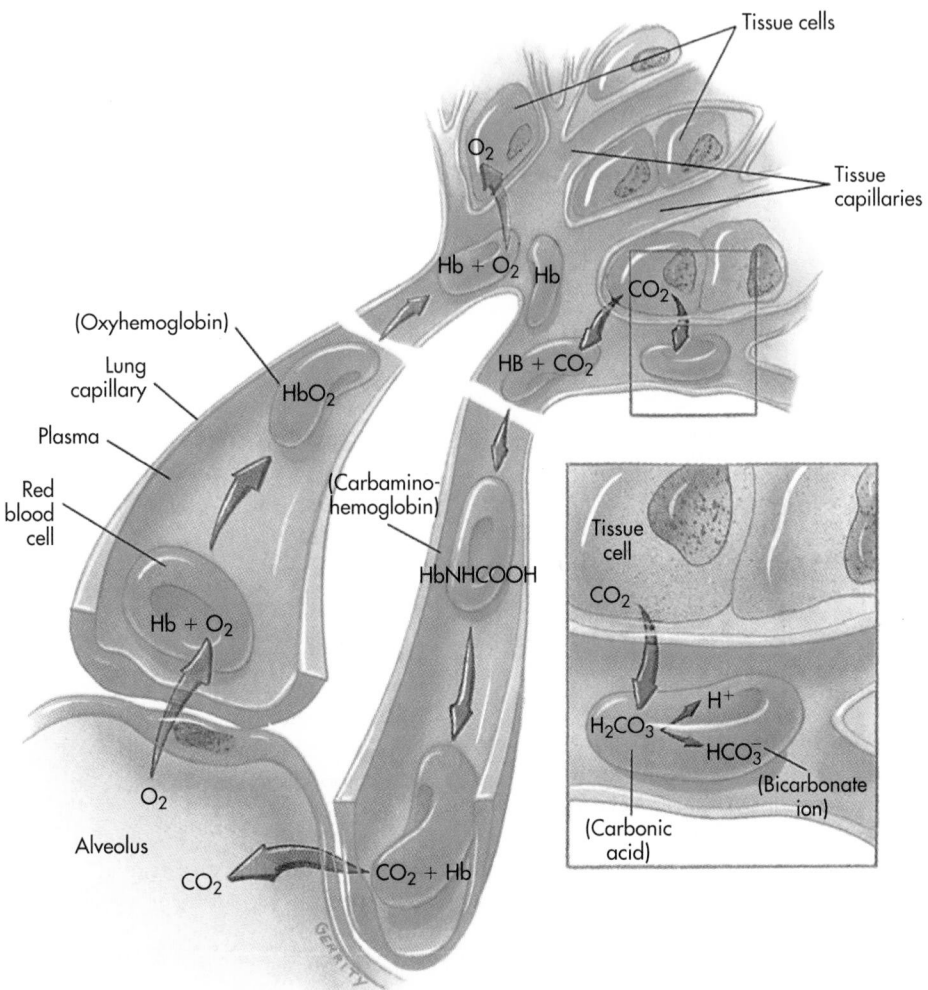

Fig. 11-11 Exchange of gases in lung and tissue capillaries. The diagram shows oxygen diffusing from alveolar air into blood and associating with hemoglobin in lung capillaries to form oxyhemoglobin. In tissue capillaries, oxyhemoglobin dissociated releasing oxygen, which diffuses from the red blood cells and then crosses the capillary wall to reach the tissue cells. At the same time, carbon dioxide diffuses in the opposite direction (into red blood cells) and associates with hemoglobin to form carbaminohemoglobin. As shown in the inset, some carbon dioxide combines with water to form carbonic acid, which dissociates to form hydrogen and bicarbonate ions. Back in lung capillaries, carbon dioxide diffuses from blood into alveolar air. (From Thibodeau GA: *Structure and function of the body*, ed 9, St Louis, 1992, Mosby.)

sult in increased carbon dioxide production. Examples include metabolism that occurs in the absence of oxygen (anaerobic metabolism) and the body's production of ketoacids in the absence of insulin.

Carbon dioxide is transported in the blood in three major forms: plasma, blood proteins, and bicarbonate ions. As with oxygen, the solubility of carbon dioxide in water is quite minimal, accounting for 8% of the carbon dioxide carried in plasma. Approximately 20% of the carbon dioxide is present in blood proteins (including hemoglobin), and about 72% is in the form of bicarbonate ions. When arterial blood flows through tissue capillaries, oxyhemoglobin gives up oxygen to the tissues and carbon dioxide diffuses from the tissues into the blood.

As a result, a small amount of the carbon dioxide dissolves in the plasma.

Oxygen-free hemoglobin binds more readily to carbon dioxide than does hemoglobin bound with oxygen. Therefore some of the carbon dioxide that diffuses into red blood cells binds to hemoglobin to form carbaminohemoglobin (HbNHCOOH). The remainder of the carbon dioxide reacts with water to form carbonic acid. Bicarbonate, in contrast to carbon dioxide, is extremely soluble in water. Venous blood rich in carbon dioxide is returned to the lungs. Because the blood P_{CO_2} is greater than that in the alveoli, carbon dioxide from the blood diffuses into the alveoli. From there it is expired and eliminated from the body (Fig. 11-11).

BOX 11-1

ABNORMAL CONDITIONS THAT CAN AFFECT BLOOD OXYGENATION

Depressed Respiratory Drive
Head injury
Central nervous system depressants (anesthetics, narcotics, sedatives)

Paralysis of Respiratory Muscles
Spinal injury
Inhalation injury
Neuromuscular diseases

**Increased Resistance
in the Respiratory Airways**
Asthma
Bronchitis
Emphysema
Congestion

**Decreased Compliance of the Lungs
and Thoracic Wall**
Interstitial lung disease as a result of inhalation of toxic substances
Infection (pneumonia, tuberculosis)
Lung cancer
Connective tissue diseases
Chronic pulmonary hypertension

Chest Wall Abnormalities
Chest wall injury (flail chest)
Scoliosis
Eschar (full-thickness burn contractions)

Decreased Surface Area for Gas Exchange
Emphysema
Tuberculosis
Pneumonia
Pulmonary edema
Atelectasis

Increased Thickness of Respiratory Membrane
Pulmonary edema (caused by heart failure, pneumonia, infections)
Interstitial fibrosis

Ventilation and Perfusion Mismatching*
Asthma
Pneumonia
Pulmonary embolus
Pulmonary edema
Myocardial infarction
Respiratory distress syndrome
Shock

**Reduced Capacity of the Blood to Transport
Oxygen**
Anemias
Hemoglobin alterations
Carbon monoxide poisoning
Methemoglobinemia

*Ventilated alveoli that are not perfused or perfused alveoli that are not ventilated.

Factors That Influence Blood Oxygenation

In healthy people, the breathing process allows blood to become fully oxygenated at the alveolar-capillary level and carbon dioxide to be eliminated. Box 11-1 presents some abnormal conditions of inadequate blood oxygenation.

Regulation of Respiration

Respiration is controlled at any instant by several factors. When evaluating any patient, it is important to consider the various mechanisms responsible for rhythmic ventilation in addition to the rate and depth of breathing.

Voluntary Control of Respiration

Breathing is primarily an involuntary process, but within limits the pattern of respiration can be consciously altered. For example, voluntary hyperventilation can lead to a decrease in blood P_{CO_2}, vasodilation of the peripheral blood vessels, a decrease in blood pressure, or a combination of these effects. Hyperventilation causes excessive loss of exhaled carbon dioxide, which produces **hypocarbia,** resulting in cerebral vascular constriction, reduced cerebral perfusion, paresthesia, dizziness, or even feelings of euphoria.

Breathing also can be affected by voluntary apnea, such as when children hold their breath. When this occurs, the arterial blood P_{CO_2} increases whereas the P_{O_2} decreases. As the apneic period continues, the abnormal levels of P_{CO_2} and P_{O_2} trigger the respiratory centers and override the individual's conscious influence. If loss of consciousness occurs, the respiratory center resumes normal function.

? CRITICAL THINKING

If a prolonged, deep breath is held what other vagal effects might the patient experience?

Nervous Control of Respiration

The inspiratory muscles (the diaphragm and intercostal muscles) are composed of skeletal muscle and cannot contract unless they are stimulated by nerve impulses. The two phrenic nerves responsible for moving the diaphragm originate from the third, fourth, and fifth cervical spinal nerves. The 11 pairs of intercostal nerves are formed from the first through the eleventh thoracic spinal nerves. The nerve impulses responsible for controlling these respiratory muscles originate within neurons of the medulla. This respiratory center is bilateral, with each lateral area composed of two groups of neurons (the inspiratory and expiratory centers) that are responsible for the basic rhythm of respiration (Fig. 11-12).

The inspiratory center neurons are spontaneously active and exhibit a pattern of activity followed by fatigue and then spontaneous activity again. When active they send impulses along the spinal cord to the phrenic and intercostal nerves, stimulating the muscles of inspiration.

The expiratory center is inactive during quiet respiration. The exact neural mechanisms that control the activity of this center are unknown. However, the expiratory center appears to be stimulated when the activity of the inspiratory center increases (e.g., heavy or labored breathing). When activated, the expiratory center reciprocates with the inspiratory center, alternating forceful inspiration with forceful expiration.

Two distinct neural mechanisms are responsible for the basic respiratory rhythm established by the inspiratory and expiratory centers: the vagal reflex (Hering-Breuer reflex) and the pneumotaxic center. The vagus nerve conveys sensory information from the thoracic and abdominal organs. Some of the vagus nerve fibers end in stretch or inflation receptors in the walls of the bronchi, bronchioles, and lungs. When the stretch receptors are stimulated by expansion of the lungs, information is conveyed by the vagus nerve to the medulla. This in turn discharges inhibitory impulses, causing inspiration to stop. The cessation of breathing is followed by deflation of the lungs. As this expiration continues, the stretch receptors are no longer stimulated, allowing the inspiratory center to become active again. Therefore the Hering-Breuer reflex limits inspiration and prevents overinflation of the lungs.

The pneumotaxic center, located in the pons superior to the respiratory center of the medulla, has an inhibitory effect on the inspiratory center. When the activity of the inspiratory center stops, inhibitory impulses no longer flow from the pneumotaxic center and the inspiratory center discharges impulses to initiate inspiration. The pneumotaxic center appears to be active only in labored breathing. In quiet breathing the stretch receptors are the primary control mechanisms for rhythmic breathing.

The apneustic center is located in the lower portion of the pons. Nerve impulses from this area stimulate the inspiratory center. The apneustic center neurons are constantly active at a baseline rate but are overridden by the pneumotaxic center when it is stimulated by demand for increased ventilation.

? CRITICAL THINKING

What alteration in breathing would you anticipate in the patient who has an injury affecting the pons?

Chemical Control of Respiration

The activities of the respiratory centers are determined by changes in oxygen and carbon dioxide concentrations and by the hydrogen ion concentration (pH) of body fluids (e.g., cerebrospinal fluid). The partial pressure of carbon dioxide is the major determinant in controlling respiration.

The chemoreceptive area in the medulla contains neurons that are sensitive to changes in carbon dioxide and pH. An increase or decrease in plasma P_{CO_2} is accompanied by changes in pH. An increase in P_{CO_2} and the resulting decrease in pH adversely affect cellular metabolism. Excess carbon dioxide must be

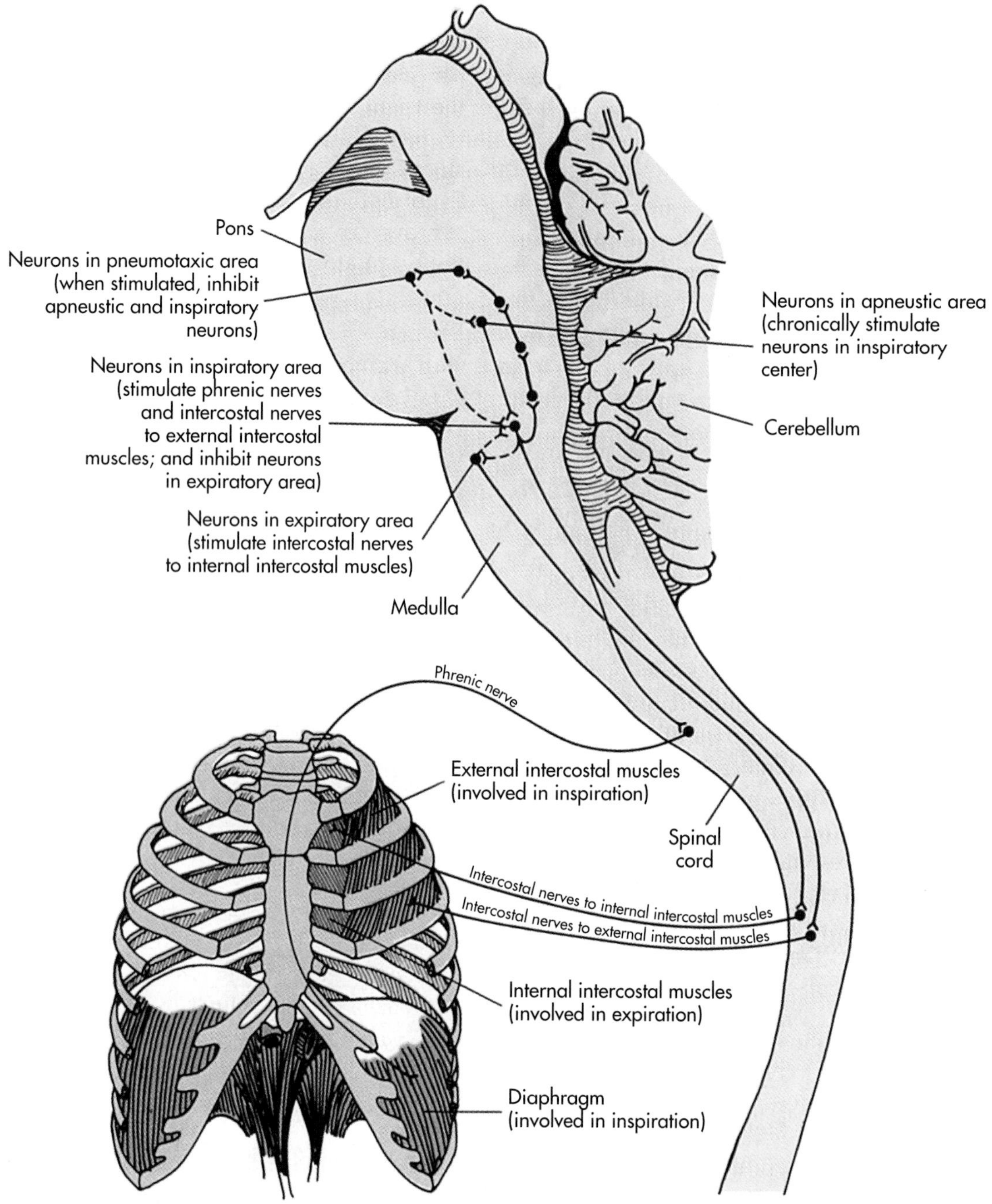

Fig. 11-12. Respiratory center and its control in the regulation of respiration.

eliminated to return the pH to normal. For example, the body responds to an increase in PCO_2 of 5 mm Hg with an increase in ventilation of 100%. Conversely, a decrease in PCO_2 inhibits ventilation, allowing the carbon dioxide produced by normal metabolism to accumulate and return the PCO_2 to normal. Through these adaptive mechanisms, the PCO_2 is maintained within a normal range of 35 to 45 mm Hg.

Compared with the body's sensitivity to pH and carbon dioxide levels, oxygen plays a relatively small part in regulating respiration. However, if the PO_2 levels in the arterial blood fall and the pH and PCO_2 are held constant, ventilation increases.

Chemoreceptors monitor arterial PO_2. They are located in the medulla and peripherally in the bifurcation of the common carotid arteries and in the arch of the aorta. These peripheral receptors are known as the *carotid* and *aortic bodies.* The carotid and aortic bodies are in intimate contact with the arterial blood of the great vessels. Therefore their blood supply is greater than their use of oxygen, and the Po_2 of their tissues is very close to that of arterial blood. The nerve fibers from these bodies enter the brain stem, where they synapse with the neurons of the medulla and initiate a respiratory response.

Although carbon dioxide and hydrogen ion concentrations are the most important regulators of respiration, reduced Po_2 in the arterial blood also may play an important stimulatory role. In conditions of shock in which the patient is hypotensive, for example, the Po_2 in the arterial blood may fall to levels low enough to stimulate the sensory receptors of the carotid and aortic bodies, leading to an increased rate and depth of ventilation. This can occur without a significant change in the blood Pco_2, although it usually is accompanied by metabolic acidosis that occurs secondary to anaerobic metabolism (see Chapter 7).

A situation in which Po_2 clearly plays a role in respiratory regulation occurs at high altitudes, where the barometric pressure is low. The low barometric pressure causes the Po_2 in the arterial blood to fall low enough to stimulate the carotid and aortic bodies. Even though the arterial Po_2 is reduced, the body's ability to eliminate carbon dioxide is not greatly affected by lowered barometric pressure. The blood carbon dioxide levels become lower than normal because of the increase in ventilation initiated in response to the lowered arterial Po_2.

Patients with severe emphysema or chronic bronchitis have chronically elevated Pco_2 and may rely on the low Po_2 as the main drive for ventilation (hypoxic drive). In diseases with chronic elevation of Pco_2, the chemoreceptors become less sensitive to a high carbon dioxide level and fail to be stimulated by it. Over time, hypoxia becomes the only remaining respiratory drive.

Control of Respiration by Other Factors

Several other factors may contribute to the control of respiration, including body temperature, drugs and medications, pain, emotion, and sleep.

An increase in body temperature caused by febrile illness or physical activity can affect the respiratory center neurons, causing an increase in ventilation. Conversely, significant decreases in body temperature can lower the ventilation rate. An extreme example of this phenomenon can occur during severe hypothermia, in which patients can appear almost apneic.

Some medications, such as *epinephrine* (Adrenalin), stimulate respiration by unknown mechanisms. The release of epinephrine increases ventilation by promoting cellular metabolism during stressful events and strenuous exercise. *Diazepam* (Valium) and *morphine* may decrease respirations. Individuals who take an overdose of narcotics or barbiturates can become apneic.

Painful stimulation anywhere in the body may produce a reflex stimulation of ventilation. Examples include performing a sternal rub and stepping into a cold shower.

An increase in the movement of air into and out of the lungs is required during expression of emotions such as laughing or crying. Stimulation of ventilation (rapid breathing) also occurs in situations involving fear and anger.

As the body's metabolism slows, so do the impulses for stimulation of the respiratory centers. Therefore during periods of decreased activity, ventilation decreases.

Modified Forms of Respiration

The cough reflex and the sneeze reflex are protective mechanisms with the function of dislodging foreign matter or irritants from the respiratory passages. Coughing generally is preceded by an inspiration of greater amplitude than normal (about 2.5 L of gas). The glottis then closes and the muscles of the thorax contract forcibly, causing an increase in intrapulmonic pressure. The pressure change in the lungs increases to about 100 mm Hg. When this pressure is reached, the vocal cords part and air escapes from the lungs at high velocity, carrying foreign materials and mucus particles.

Sneezing is a violent expulsion of gas that is forced or directed through the nasal cavity. It may occur as a result of nasal irritants, stimulation of the fifth cranial nerve (trigeminal nerve) in the nose, or exposure to bright lights. During the sneeze reflex, the uvula and the soft palate are depressed to direct air through both the nasal passages and the oral cavity.

Other forms of modified respiration include the sigh and the hiccough (in rare cases these are chronic disorders). Sighing is a slow, deep inspiration followed by a prolonged expiration. This modified respiratory effort is thought to be a protective reflex to hyperinflate the lungs and to reexpand alveoli that might have been collapsed (atelectasis).

The hiccough results from a spasmodic contraction of the diaphragm with the sudden inspiration cut short by the closure of the glottis. Hiccoughs serve no known useful physiological purpose and usually pass with time. However, they may indicate a pathological condition.

Special Considerations for Older Patients

Respiratory disorders pose special problems for the older patient, whose respiratory function may be compromised as a result of the aging process. Pulmonary changes that occur as a result of aging decrease vital capacity and increase physiological dead space. Ventilation-perfusion mismatching also tends to increase, which leads to a gradually lowered PO_2. The changes in pulmonary physiology include the following:

- Alterations in lung and chest wall compliance
  Increased thoracic rigidity
  Decreased elastic recoil (total lung capacity remains unchanged because of opposing loss of chest wall compliance and weakened respiratory muscles)
- Enlarged alveolar ducts and sacs
  Fewer alveoli
  Less alveolar surface for gas exchange

The aging process also changes the body's ventilatory control mechanisms. As an individual grows older, for example, the body's arterial PO_2 falls, although no significant change in arterial PCO_2 occurs. Several methods have been developed to calculate the expected PO_2 in older individuals. One method is to remember that a person who is 70 years old is expected to have a PO_2 of 70 mm Hg. Using this value as a baseline, one should expect a 1 mm Hg decrease in PO_2 for every year over 70 or a 1 mm Hg increase in PO_2 for every year under 70. An individual who is 65 years old, for example, would be expected to have a PO_2 of 75 mm Hg, and a 75-year-old would be expected to have a PO_2 of 65 mm Hg.

The functioning of the body's chemoreceptors also declines with age. This results in a diminished ventilatory response to hypoxia, hypercapnia, and

similar conditions and may predispose the older individual to respiratory failure.

NOTE

It is important that older patients with respiratory compromise from any cause receive immediate intervention, oxygenation, and ventilatory support.

SECTION TWO
PATHOPHYSIOLOGY

A common cause of inadequate ventilation is upper airway obstruction caused by particulate matter or vomited stomach contents (aspiration by inhalation). Establishing and maintaining a patent airway in any patient who has respiratory compromise from any cause is the most important lifesaving maneuver and should always be a first-order priority of patient care. Early detection, early intervention, and education of the general public in basic life support measures are major factors in preventing unnecessary deaths from airway compromise.

NOTE

Brain damage may occur 4 to 6 minutes after interruption of breathing and circulation. After 6 minutes of circulatory arrest, brain damage almost always occurs. After 10 minutes of circulatory arrest, some portions of the brain have been irreversibly damaged to the point of death.[1]

Foreign Body Airway Obstruction

About 3000 deaths each year result from foreign body obstruction of the airway.[2] Immediate removal of the obstruction might have prevented the resulting hypoxemia, unconsciousness, or cardiopulmonary arrest that caused these deaths. Management of foreign body airway obstruction by healthcare providers, as recommended by national standards, is summarized in Table 11-2.

	OBJECTIVES	ACTIONS		
		ADULT (OVER 8 YR)	**CHILD (1 TO 8 YR)**	**INFANT (UNDER 1 YR)**
Conscious victim	1. Assessment: Determine airway obstruction.	Ask, "Are you choking?" Determine if victim can cough or speak.		Observe breathing difficulty.
	2. Act to relieve obstruction.	Perform five subdiaphragmatic abdominal thrusts (Heimlich maneuver).		Give up to five back blows. Give five chest thrusts at the rate of one per second.
	3. Be persistent.	Repeat Step 2 until obstruction is relieved or victim becomes unconscious.		
Victim who becomes unconscious	4. Position victim.	Turn on back as unit, supporting head and neck, face up, arms by sides.		
	5. Check for foreign body.	Perform tongue-jaw lift and finger sweep.	Perform tongue-jaw lift. Remove foreign object only if visible.	
	6. Give rescue breaths.	Open airway with head-tilt/chin-lift. Attempt rescue breathing. If first ventilation attempt is unsuccessful, reposition head and reattempt ventilation.		
	7. Act to relieve obstruction.	Perform five subdiaphragmatic abdominal thrusts (Heimlich maneuver).		Give up to five back blows. Give five chest thrusts at the rate of one per second.
	8. Check for foreign body.	Perform tongue-jaw lift and finger sweep.	Perform tongue-jaw lift. Remove foreign object only if visible.	
	9. Attempt rescue breathing.	Open airway with head-tilt/chin-lift. Attempt rescue breathing (slow ventilations $1\frac{1}{2}$-2 sec each for adult and 1-$1\frac{1}{2}$ sec each for child or infant).		
	10. Be persistent.	Repeat Steps 6-8 until obstruction is relieved.*		
Unconscious victim	1. Assessment: Determine unresponsiveness.	Tap or gently shake shoulder. Shout, "Are you okay?"		Tap or gently shake shoulder.
	2. Position victim.	Turn on back as unit, supporting head and neck, face up, arms by sides.		
	3. Open airway.	Open airway with head-tilt/chin-lift.		Open airway with head-tilt/chin-lift without hyperextension.
	4. Assessment: Determine breathlessness.	Maintain an open airway. Place ear over mouth; observe chest. Look, listen, feel for breathing (3-5 sec).		
	5. Give rescue breaths.	Seal mouth to mouth with barrier device or bag-valve device.		Seal mouth to nose/mouth with barrier device.
		Attempt rescue breathing (slow ventilations $1\frac{1}{2}$-2 sec each for adult and 1-$1\frac{1}{2}$ sec each for child or infant). If first ventilation is unsuccessful, reposition head and reattempt ventilation.		
	6. Act to relieve obstruction.	Perform five subdiaphragmatic abdominal thrusts (Heimlich maneuver).		Give up to five back blows. Give five chest thrusts at the rate of one per second.
	7. Check for foreign body.	Perform tongue-jaw lift and finger sweep.	Perform tongue-jaw lift. Remove foreign object only if visible.	
	8. Provide rescue breathing.	Open airway with head-tilt/chin-lift. Attempt rescue breathing (slow ventilations $1\frac{1}{2}$-2 sec each for adult and 1-$1\frac{1}{2}$ sec each for child or infant).		
	9. Be persistent.	Repeat Steps 6-8 until obstruction is relieved.*		

*OR advanced procedures are available (i.e., Kelly clamp, Magill forceps, cricothyrotomy).

NOTE

Methods to relieve FBAO in an unconscious victim of any age have been simplified for lay rescuers. Lay rescuers are to begin standard CPR when an unrelieved, responsive choking victim becomes unresponsive, or an unresponsive person suspected of a FBAO is encountered, evaluated, and treated. The only difference from regular CPR is that the lay rescuer should open the airway widely whenever ventilations are attempted to look for a foreign object and remove it if seen. Blind finger sweeps are not to be used by lay rescuers for victims of any age.

Airway Obstruction in a Conscious Patient

Meat is the most common cause of foreign body airway obstruction in conscious adults (although a variety of other foods and foreign objects are also responsible for obstruction in children and in some adults). Factors associated with choking include large, poorly chewed pieces of food, an elevated blood alcohol level, and poorly fitting dentures. The patient often is middle-aged or older.

? CRITICAL THINKING

How can you relieve this type of obstruction using only your hands?

Foreign bodies may cause partial or complete airway obstruction. A patient with a partly obstructed airway usually can speak and can produce a forceful cough in an effort to expel the object. If air exchange is adequate, no rescuer intervention is recommended in these situations.[1] A patient with a partial obstruction should be closely monitored and encouraged to persist with spontaneous coughing and breathing efforts. If the obstruction persists or air exchange becomes inadequate (evidenced by a weak, ineffective cough, also wheezing, increased respiratory difficulty, decreased air movement, and cyanosis), the patient should be managed as though a complete airway obstruction exists.

Patients with complete airway obstruction cannot speak (aphonia), exchange air, or cough. They often grasp the neck between the thumb and fingers (a universal sign of choking). These individuals require immediate rescuer intervention. Complete airway obstruction causes hypoxemia and may precipitate an acute myocardial infarction in patients with concurrent atherosclerotic cardiovas-

cular disease. Airway obstruction inevitably leads to cardiac arrest in all patients if not corrected within minutes.

Airway Obstruction in an Unconscious Patient

Although upper airway obstruction may lead to unconsciousness and cardiopulmonary arrest, more often the obstruction is caused by unconsciousness and cardiopulmonary arrest.[1] The primary source of upper airway obstruction in an unconscious patient is the tongue.

The tongue is attached to the mandible by the muscles that form the floor of the mouth. The normal tone of these muscles allows for air exchange through a patent posterior pharynx. If a patient is unconscious or has neuromuscular dysfunction, laxity of these muscles may cause airway occlusion by the tongue. Some causes of airway obstruction by the tongue include the following:

- Cardiac arrest
- Trauma
- Stroke
- Intoxication with alcohol, barbiturates, or psychotropic drugs
- Paralysis caused by muscle relaxants
- Myasthenia gravis
- Fractured facial and nasal bones

Laryngeal Spasm and Edema

Spasmodic closure of the vocal cords often is caused by an aggressive intubation technique. (Endotracheal intubation is addressed later in this chapter.) It also may occur immediately upon extubation, especially if the patient is semiconscious. Laryngeal spasm is best managed with aggressive ventilation and a forceful upward pull of the jaw; it sometimes may require use of muscle relaxants.

NOTE

Maintaining steady pressure by the endotracheal tube against the cords sometimes overcomes the spasmodic closure.

Swelling of the glottic and subglottic tissues of the airway can lead to laryngeal closure. The formation of edema may result from inflammatory or mechanical causes such as epiglottitis, croup, allergic reaction, thermal injuries, strangulation, blunt trauma, or drowning. Associated swelling may partly or completely obstruct the airway, making aggressive airway management mandatory for the patient's survival.

Fractured Larynx

The most common cause of external trauma to the larynx is a motor vehicle crash. If a trauma patient has localized laryngeal pain on palpation or swallowing, stridor, hoarseness, difficulty with speech (dysphonia), or hemoptysis, a fracture of the larynx should be suspected. Laryngeal injury can result in a lack of support for the vocal cords, causing them to collapse into the tracheal-laryngeal lumen and obstruct the airway. Subcutaneous emphysema, dysphagia, and throat discomfort that increases with coughing or swallowing indicate the possibility of an impending airway obstruction. The paramedic should remain alert to the possibility of laryngeal fracture because laryngeal edema can rapidly occlude the airway.

Certain types of injury, such as clothesline injury and blunt trauma to the neck, may cause laryngeal fracture. A laryngeal fracture requires rapid intervention to obtain a patent airway before laryngeal edema and hemorrhage cause complete occlusion.

Tracheal Trauma

Trauma to the trachea is rare but serious. The most common site of tracheal injury is the area bordered by the cricoid cartilage and the third tracheal ring. This injury seldom occurs as an isolated event and often is associated with injuries to the surrounding esophagus and cervical spine. Central nervous system (CNS) injuries and abdominal and thoracic trauma also usually accompany tracheal injury. (Tracheal trauma is further described in Chapter 22.)

Aspiration by Inhalation

Aspiration is the active inhalation of food, a foreign body, or fluid (vomitus, saliva, blood, neutral liquids) into the airway. Depending on the type and degree of aspiration, the syndrome may precipitate spasm, mucus production, atelectasis, a change in pH (if the aspirant is acidic), or coughing. The primary means of preventing aspiration is controlling and maintaining the airway; preven-

tion is far superior to any known treatment. The paramedic should always be prepared for the possibility of aspiration in patients with a diminished level of consciousness.

Large food particles and other foreign bodies can occlude the airway and cause hypoventilation of distal lung segments. The size of the particle determines which airway is obstructed and to what extent.

About 80% of the approximately 3000 deaths each year from foreign body aspiration occur in children.[2] Running with food or other objects in the mouth, seizures, and forced feeding are among the risk factors in this age group. Hot dogs and peanuts are foods children commonly aspirate. In adults, obstruction may be caused by dental or nasal surgery, unconsciousness, swallowing of poorly chewed food, and alcohol intoxication.

Approximately 60% of foreign bodies are found in the right mainstem bronchus, 19% in the left, and 21% at the larynx or vocal cords.[3] (Because the left mainstem bronchus branches from the trachea at a 45- to 60-degree angle, foreign body occlusion of this bronchus is less likely than of the right mainstem bronchus, which is shorter, wider, and more vertical.) When the larynx or trachea is completely obstructed, the victim can die from asphyxiation within minutes.

The average adult stomach has a capacity of 1.4 L and manufactures an additional 1.4 L of gastric juices in each 24-hour period. Hydrochloric acid is manufactured by special cells in the gastric mucosa. With the assistance of a protein-dissolving enzyme (pepsin), this acid helps break down large pieces of food into smaller ones. Vomitus contains not only partly digested food particles but also acidic gastric fluid.

Saliva is a watery, slightly acidic fluid secreted in the mouth by the major salivary glands and the smaller salivary glands in the mucous membranes that line the mouth. Saliva contains the digestive enzyme amylase, which helps break down carbohydrates. In addition to this enzyme, saliva contains minerals such as sodium, calcium, and chloride; proteins; mucin (the principal constituent of mucus); urea; white blood cells; debris from the lining of the mouth; and bacteria.

The consequences of aspiration of neutral liquids (liquids that are neither acidic nor basic) are easier to reverse with supportive therapy than the consequences of aspiration of acids or bases. Nonetheless, aspiration of a large volume of neutral liquids also is associated with a high mortality rate.

Pathophysiology of Aspiration

The predisposing conditions associated with a high risk of aspiration are a diminished level of consciousness and mechanical disturbances of the airway and gastrointestinal (GI) tract.

A reduced level of consciousness may be caused by trauma, alcohol or other drug intoxication, a seizure disorder, cardiopulmonary arrest, a cerebrovascular accident, or a CNS dysfunction. The common element of these conditions is depression or loss of the **gag reflex,** with or without a full stomach.

> **NOTE**
>
> The gag reflex is a normal neural reflex triggered by touching the soft palate or posterior pharynx.

A common type of mechanical disturbance is iatrogenic (i.e., caused by medical procedures) and involves the use of various devices to control upper airway problems. Examples include removal of certain airway devices (risk of vomiting on removal), placement of a nasogastric tube (the artificial opening through the esophageal sphincter increases the risk of regurgitation and aspiration), and intubation, which requires an adequate seal at the tracheal orifice to prevent aspiration. These mechanical airway devices are discussed later in this chapter.

Other mechanical disturbances that may lead to a high risk of aspiration include tracheostomy and esophageal motility disorders such as hiatal hernia and esophageal reflux. Other individuals at risk include those with either an ileus or a mechanical bowel obstruction.

The potential for aspiration increases whenever vomiting occurs. Vomiting follows stimulation of the vomiting center of the medulla. This stimulation can result from irritation anywhere along the GI tract, from information passed to the medulla from the frontal lobes of the brain, or from disturbances in the balance mechanism of the inner ear. Once this center is stimulated, the following seven events occur:

1. A deep breath is taken.
2. The hyoid bone and larynx are elevated, opening the preesophageal sphincter.
3. The opening of the larynx is closed.
4. The soft palate is elevated, closing the posterior nares.
5. The diaphragm and the abdominal muscles are forcefully contracted, compressing the stomach and increasing the intragastric pressure.
6. The lower esophageal sphincter is relaxed, and stomach contents are propelled into the lower esophagus.
7. If the patient is unconscious or unable to protect the airway, pulmonary aspiration may occur.

Effects of Pulmonary Aspiration

The severity of pulmonary aspiration depends on the pH of the aspirated material, the volume of the aspirate, and if particulate matter (e.g., food) and bacterial contamination are present in the aspirate. It generally is accepted that when the pH level of an aspirate is 2.5 or less, a severe pulmonary response occurs. When the pH is below 1.5, the patient usually dies. The mortality among patients who aspirate material grossly contaminated (as occurs in bowel obstruction) approaches 100%.

The toxic effects on the lungs of gastric acid (with a pH of less than 2.5) can be equated with those of chemical burns. These are severe injuries that produce pulmonary changes such as destruction of surfactant-producing alveolar cells, alveolar collapse and destruction, and destruction of pulmonary capillaries. The permeability of the capillaries increases with massive flooding of the alveoli and bronchi with fluid. The resulting pulmonary edema creates areas of hypoventilation, shunting, and severe hypoxemia. The massive fluid shift from the intravascular compartment to the lungs also may produce hypovolemia severe enough to require volume replacement.

> **NOTE**
>
> The risk of pulmonary aspiration can be minimized by continuously monitoring the patient's mental status, properly positioning the patient to allow for drainage of secretions, limiting ventilation pressures to avoid gastric distention, and using suction devices and esophageal or endotracheal (ET) intubation. Airway protection should be provided if the risk of aspiration exists or promptly after an occurrence of aspiration.

SECTION THREE
AIRWAY EVALUATION

Essential Parameters of Airway Evaluation

Evaluation of the respiratory system is presented in depth in Chapter 14. This discussion is limited to essential parameters of airway evaluation that are used to note immediate and life-threatening airway compromise.

Essential Parameters

Essential parameters of airway evaluation include rate, regularity, and effort, in addition to recognition of airway problems that might indicate respiratory distress.

✓ TRICKS OF THE TRADE

Shortness of breath is subjective. You can't make patients prove to you how short of breath they are—take them at their word.

Rate, Regularity, and Effort

The normal respiratory rate in a resting adult is 12 to 24 breaths per minute. Regularity is defined as a steady inspiratory and expiratory pattern. Breathing at rest should be effortless and marked by only subtle changes in rate or regularity.

NOTE

Irregular respiratory patterns are significant until proven otherwise.

Patients in respiratory distress often compensate for their inability to breathe easily by sitting upright with the head tilted back (upright sniffing position), by leaning forward on the arms (tripod position), or by lying down with the head and thorax slightly elevated (semi-Fowler's position). These patients frequently avoid lying supine.

? CRITICAL THINKING

Why would lying in the supine position likely worsen respiratory distress?

Recognition of Airway Problems

Respiratory distress may be caused by upper or lower airway obstruction, inadequate ventilation, impairment of the respiratory muscles, ventilation-perfusion mismatching, diffusion abnormalities, or impairment of the nervous system. Dyspnea often is associated with hypoxia (Box 11-2).

NOTE

Recognition and management of respiratory failure is crucial to the patient's survival. The paramedic must remember that the brain can survive only a few minutes of anoxia and that all therapies will fail if the airway is not adequate.

Observation techniques. Visual techniques for recognizing airway problems include noting the patient's preferred position to facilitate breathing and assessing the rise and fall of the patient's chest. Other visual clues of respiratory distress include the following:
- Gasping for air
- Cyanosis
- Nasal flaring
- Pursed-lip breathing
- Retraction of the intercostal or subcostal muscles, suprasternal notch, and supraclavicular fossa during respirations

Auscultation and palpation techniques. Air movement can be evaluated by listening to respirations without using a stethoscope and by using a stethoscope to assess bilateral lung fields. Palpation of the chest wall helps determine the presence or absence of paradoxical motion and any retraction of accessory muscles.

BOX 11-2

DEFINITIONS

Hypoxia: inadequate oxygen at the cellular level
Hypoxemia: deficiency of oxygen in arterial blood
Anoxia: lack of oxygen

Other signs of respiratory distress. Other signs that indicate possible causes of respiratory distress include resistance or changing compliance when assisting or delivering respirations with a bag-valve mask (seen in asthma, chronic obstructive pulmonary disease [COPD], and tension pneumothorax), and the presence of pulsus paradoxus. Pulsus paradoxus refers to a drop of 10 mm Hg or more in systolic blood pressure on inspiration. (A change in the quality of the pulse may also be noted.) This condition is sometimes seen in patients with asthma or COPD and in those with pericardial tamponade.

NOTE

Pulsus paradoxus is difficult to measure in any setting. The more obvious signs and symptoms of respiratory distress should take precedence over this measurement.

NOTE

Pericardial tamponade results from compression of the heart caused by the accumulation of blood or fluid in the pericardial sac. It often results from blunt or penetrating chest trauma.

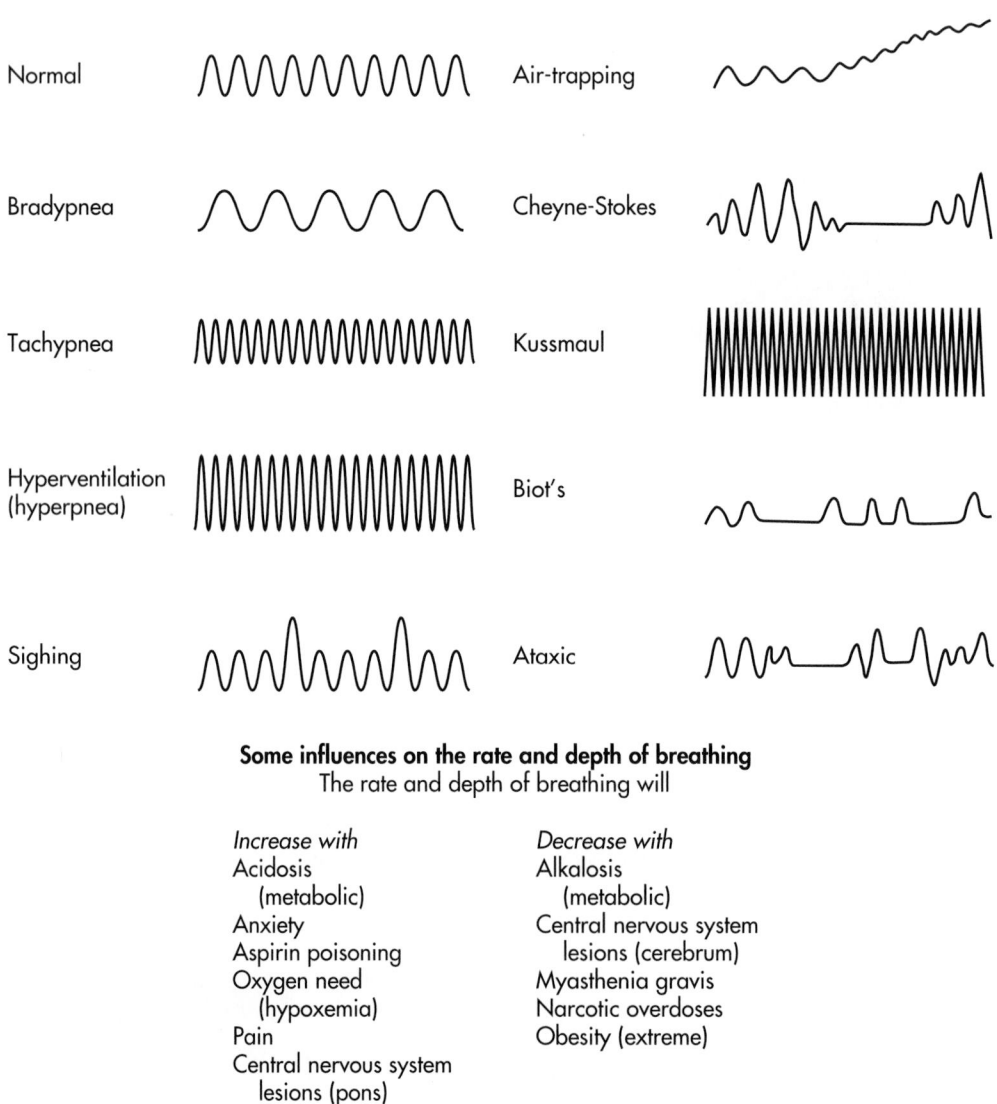

Some influences on the rate and depth of breathing
The rate and depth of breathing will

Increase with	*Decrease with*
Acidosis (metabolic)	Alkalosis (metabolic)
Anxiety	Central nervous system lesions (cerebrum)
Aspirin poisoning	Myasthenia gravis
Oxygen need (hypoxemia)	Narcotic overdoses
Pain	Obesity (extreme)
Central nervous system lesions (pons)	

Fig. 11-13 Patterns of respiration. Horizontal axis indicates relative rate; vertical swings indicate relative depth.

History. Obtaining a history to determine the evolution and duration of the dyspneic event also helps guide the direction of patient care. For example, the paramedic should ascertain if the event was sudden in onset or if it occurred gradually over time (and if so, what period of time) and if any known causes or "triggers" initiated the difficulty breathing. The paramedic also must know if the respiratory distress is constant or recurrent. Other questions that should be asked when obtaining a patient's history include the following:

- What makes it better?
- What makes it worse?
- Are there any associated symptoms (e.g., cough, chest pain, fever)?
- Has any intervention through drugs been attempted?
- Has the patient taken all medications and treatments as prescribed?

> **NOTE**
>
> It also is important to determine if the patient has been previously evaluated or hospitalized for this condition and if the patient has ever been intubated because of respiratory problems.

Changes in Respiratory Pattern

As previously stated, the breathing process should be comfortable, regular, and initiated without distress. Several abnormal respiratory patterns are seen in some ill or injured patients (Fig. 11-13 and Box 11-3). Recognizing these breathing patterns may help determine the appropriate intervention.

Inadequate Ventilation

Inadequate ventilation is said to occur when the body cannot compensate for increased oxygen demand or

---

BOX 11-3

ABNORMAL RESPIRATORY PATTERNS

Agonal respiration: A type of breathing that usually follows a pattern of gasping succeeded by apnea. It generally indicates the onset of respiratory arrest or the breathing pattern of a dying person.

Ataxic: A type of cluster or irregular breathing pattern characterized by a series of inspirations and expirations. Ataxic respiration is usually associated with a structural or compressive lesion in the medullary respiratory centers.

Biot's: A respiratory pattern involving irregular respirations varying in depth and interrupted by intervals of apnea (absence of breathing). Although similar to Cheyne-Stokes, this pattern lacks the repetitiveness and is often irregular. Biot's respiration is usually seen in patients with head injuries who have increased intracranial pressure. Unlike Cheyne-Stokes, Biot's ataxic pattern frequently produces ventilatory failure and may lead to apnea.

Bradypnea: A persistent respiratory rate slower than 12 breaths per minute. This abnormal rate may be a result of the patient "guarding" against respiratory discomfort caused by chest wall injury, respiratory failure, cerebral vascular accident (CVA), pulmonary infection, or narcotic poisoning. However, bradypnea is more commonly caused by respiratory drive depression that occurs secondary to neurological disturbances.

Central neurogenic hyperventilation: A pattern of breathing marked by rapid and regular ventilations at a rate of about 25 per minute. Increasing regularity, rather than rate, is an important diagnostic sign because it indicates an increasing depth of coma.

Cheyne-Stokes: A regular, periodic pattern of breathing with equal intervals of apnea followed by a crescendo-descrescendo sequence of respirations. Cheyne-Stokes respirations are thought to represent a level of cortical dysfunction of the brain. Although some children and older adults breathe in this pattern during sleep, it is usually seen in patients who are seriously ill or injured.

Eupnea: Normal breathing.

Hyperventilation: A persistent, rapid, and deep respiration that often results in hyperpnea. Compared with tachypnea, hyperpnea is usually slower and much deeper. Its causes include exercise, anxiety, metabolic disturbances (e.g., diabetic ketoacidosis), and CNS illness.

Kussmaul: An abnormally deep, very rapid sighing respiratory pattern characteristic of diabetic ketoacidosis or other metabolic acidosis.

Tachypnea: A persistent respiratory rate that exceeds 20 breaths per minute. It may be common in patients who are in pain, frightened, or anxious. The many other causes of tachypnea include fractured ribs, pneumonia, pneumothorax, pulmonary embolus, and pleurisy.

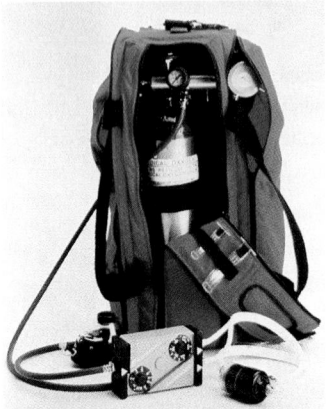

Fig. 11-14 Oxygen cylinders.

> **NOTE**
>
> Some medical experts distinguish between inadequate ventilation caused by a problem in the mechanics of breathing (usually defined by P_{CO_2}) and inadequate oxygenation but normal ventilation, as seen in pulmonary embolus and often pneumonia.

cannot maintain a normal range of oxygen/carbon dioxide balance. Numerous factors can cause inadequate ventilation, including infection, trauma, brain stem insult, and noxious or hypoxic atmosphere. A patient who has inadequate ventilation may have a number of symptoms and various respiratory rates and breathing patterns.

Supplemental Oxygen Therapy

The rationale for providing supplemental oxygen therapy is twofold: (1) enriched oxygen in the atmosphere increases the oxygen content in pulmonary capillary blood, and (2) increasing the available oxygen allows the patient to compensate without increasing the work of breathing.

Oxygen Sources

The most common form of oxygen used in the prehospital setting is pure oxygen gas, delivered in liters per minute (LPM). This gas is stored under pressure in stainless steel or lightweight alloy cylinders (Fig. 11-14). These cylinders have been color coded by the *U.S. Pharmacopeia* to distinguish various com-

> **BOX 11-4**
>
> ### CALCULATING TANK LIFE
>
> One method used to estimate the amount of oxygen available in an oxygen cylinder is to first subtract the safe residual pressure (200 psi) from the tank pressure and then multiply this number by the tank's factor (cylinder constant) to obtain the volume of gas. This volume is divided by the liters per minute (LPM) delivery to determine the tank life in minutes.
> Example:
> Tank pressure in an E cylinder is 650 psi. You are delivering 6 L/min of oxygen to the patient.
> Step 1. Subtract the safe residual pressure from the tank's psi:
> $650 - 200 = 450$
> Step 2. Multiply this number by the E cylinder factor to obtain the volume:
> $450 \times 0.28 = 126$
> Step 3. Divide the volume by the LPM delivery to determine the tank life in minutes:
> $126 \div 6 = 21$ minutes

pressed gases. Steel green and white cylinders have been assigned to all grades of oxygen. Stainless steel and aluminum cylinders are not painted. Common sizes (and their factors) that are used in emergency care include the following (Box 11-4):

D cylinder (400 L of oxygen)	Factor: 0.16
E cylinder (625 L of oxygen)	Factor: 0.28
M cylinder (3450 L of oxygen)	Factor: 1.56

> **NOTE**
>
> Oxygen cylinders are filled under a pressure of 2000 to 2200 psi, therefore safety is of prime importance when handling this equipment. The paramedic should ensure that the correct regulator is firmly attached before moving oxygen cylinders and should never handle a cylinder by the neck assembly alone.

> **NOTE**
>
> Most oxygen cylinders are considered "empty" at 200 psi (the safe residual pressure). As a rule, tanks with less than 500 psi are too low to keep in service.

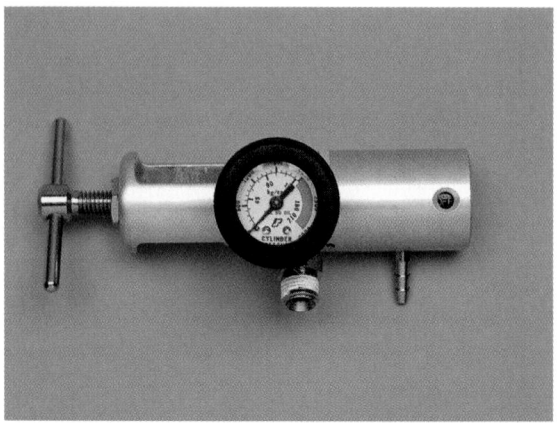

Fig. 11-15 Pressure regulator.

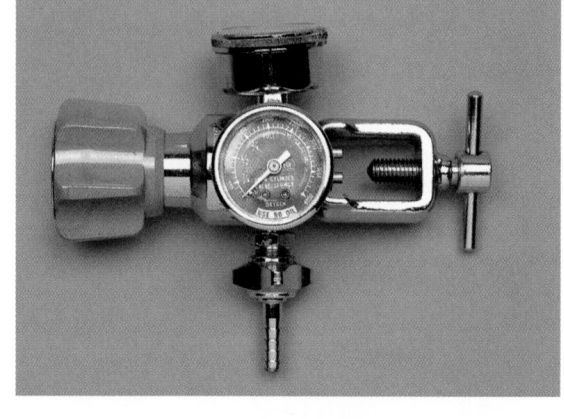

Fig. 11-16 Flowmeter.

TRICKS OF THE TRADE

Always change the oxygen bottle when the regulator reads 200 psi (the safe residual pressure). It's really embarrassing to run out of one of the most abundant resources on the planet.

Liquid Oxygen

Liquid oxygen (LOX) has been cooled to its aqueous state but converts to a gaseous state when warmed. This form of oxygen is used by some aeromedical services and by other emergency medical service (EMS) agencies when the weight and space that an oxygen system occupies must be considered. The main advantage of liquid oxygen is that a much larger volume of gaseous oxygen can be stored in an aqueous state. The disadvantages of liquid oxygen are the cost (LOX is more expensive than pressurized oxygen), the fact that the units generally require upright storage, and the special requirements for large volume storage and cylinder transfer.

Regulators

High-pressure regulators are used to transfer cylinder gas from tank to tank. They are attached to cylinder stems and allow cylinder gas to be delivered under high pressure.

Therapy regulators are used to deliver a safe pressure of oxygen to patients (Fig. 11-15). They are attached to the cylinder stem and work through a regulator mechanism whereby 50 psi escape pressure is reduced ("stepped down") to 30 psi for safe delivery to the patient.

NOTE

Therapy regulators are attached to smaller oxygen cylinders by a yoke assembly with a pin index safety system. This system prevents the paramedic from using a regulator with the wrong type of gas. It requires that the yoke pins match the corresponding holes in the valve assembly for oxygen to be delivered. Larger oxygen cylinders have valve assemblies with a threaded outlet specific to medical oxygen.

Flowmeters

Flowmeters control the amount of oxygen delivered to the patient (Fig. 11-16). These devices are connected to the pressure regulator and adjusted to deliver oxygen at a certain number of liters per minute. Some EMS agencies attach disposable humidifiers to the flowmeter to provide moisture to the dry oxygen coming from the supply cylinder. Humidified oxygen is desirable for long-term oxygen administration and for patients with croup, epiglottitis, or bronchiolitis (see Chapter 27).

Oxygen Delivery Devices

Several oxygen delivery devices can be used to provide supplemental oxygen to prehospital patients who have spontaneous respirations. They are the nasal cannula, simple face mask, partial rebreather mask, nonrebreather mask, and Venturi mask (Table 11-3).

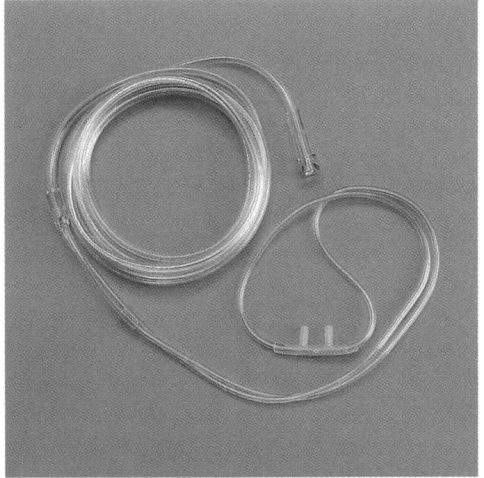

Fig. 11-17 Nasal cannula.

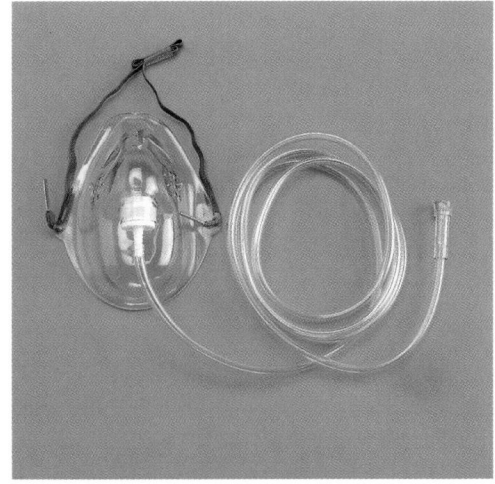

Fig. 11-18 Simple face mask.

TABLE 11-3	OXYGEN DELIVERY DEVICES	
DEVICE	**FLOW RATE**	**O₂% DELIVERED**
Nasal cannula	1-6 L/min	24%-44%
Simple face mask	6-10 L/min	35%-60%
Partial rebreather	6-10 L/min	35%-60%
Nonrebreather	10-15 L/min	80%-95%
Venturi mask	4-8 L/min	24%-50%

L/min, Liters per minute.

The nasal cannula (Fig. 11-17) delivers low-concentration oxygen to patients by way of two small plastic prongs placed into the nostrils. Nasal cannulas are contraindicated for patients with poor respiratory effort, severe hypoxia, and apnea and for those who breathe primarily through the mouth. As a rule, the nasal cannula is well tolerated, but it does not deliver high-volume/high-concentration oxygen. The relationship of approximate oxygen concentrations to liter per minute flow is listed in Table 11-4.

The simple face mask (Fig. 11-18) is a soft, clear plastic mask that conforms to the patient's face. Small perforations in the mask allow atmospheric gas to be mixed with oxygen during inhalation and

> **NOTE**
>
> The maximum oxygen flow rate for a nasal cannula is 6 L/min.

> **NOTE**
>
> It is difficult to obtain oxygen concentrations greater than 30% to 35% via nasal cannula. This is a result of the mouth breathing that occurs during oxygen administration, which decreases the concentration of inspired oxygen. The nasal cannula, therefore, is limited to patients who would benefit from low-concentration oxygen delivery (e.g., some patients with chest pain and patients who have chronic pulmonary disease). The device also is ineffective if the patient's nares are occluded by blood or mucus.

permit the patient's exhaled air to escape. Oxygen concentrations of 35% to 60% can be delivered through this device with a flow rate of 6 to 10 L/min. Because a flow rate of less than 6 L/min can produce an accumulation of carbon dioxide in the mask, oxygen delivery through *any* face mask should always exceed this minimum. Flow rates beyond 10 L/min do not enhance oxygen concentration.

> **NOTE**
>
> All masks must be well fitted to the patient's face for optimal benefit. Any leaks will decrease the oxygen concentration.

The partial rebreather mask (Fig. 11-19) has an attached oxygen reservoir bag that should be filled before the patient uses the mask. This device has vent ports covered by one-way disks that allow a portion of the patient's exhaled gas to enter the reservoir bag and be reused. The remainder of the

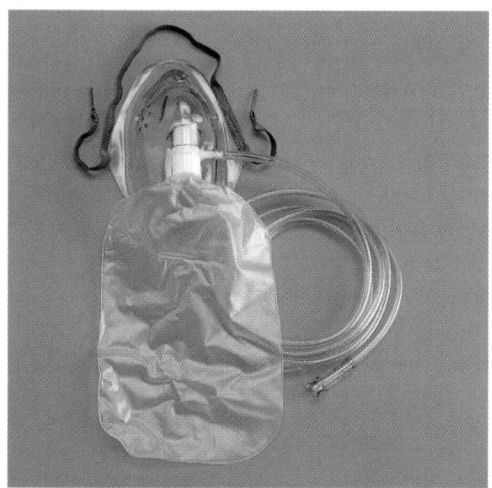

Fig. 11-19 Partial rebreather.

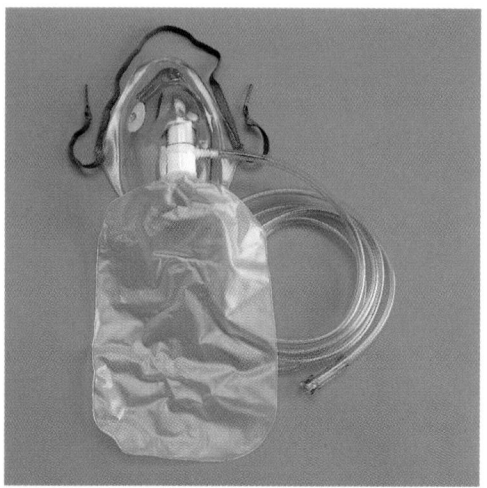

Fig. 11-20 Nonrebreather mask.

carbon dioxide–loaded gas escapes to the atmosphere. Oxygen concentrations of 35% to 60% can be delivered with a flow rate that prevents the reservoir bag from collapsing completely on inspiration. Partial rebreather masks are contraindicated for patients with apnea or poor respiratory effort. As with the simple face mask, delivery of volumes above 10 L/min through this device does not enhance oxygen concentration.

The nonrebreather mask (Fig. 11-20) is similar in design to the partial nonrebreather. However, a flutter valve assembly in the mask piece prevents the patient's exhaled air from returning to the reservoir bag. This device delivers oxygen concentrations ranging above 95% with an adequate flow rate that keeps the reservoir bag partly inflated during inspiration. The paramedic should ensure that the mask is seated firmly over the patient's mouth and nose and that the reservoir bag is never less than two thirds full. This device most commonly is used in patients who require high-concentration oxygen delivery (10 to 15 L/min). Like other masks, it is contraindicated for patients with apnea or poor respiratory effort.

? CRITICAL THINKING

What could happen if the oxygen source is disconnected from a nonrebreather mask?

NOTE

Patients with severe respiratory distress may require up to 20 L/min to maintain inflation of the reservoir bag.

TABLE 11-4	APPROXIMATE OXYGEN CONCENTRATION TO LITER PER MINUTE FLOW	
LITERS PER MINUTE		**OXYGEN CONCENTRATION**
1		24%
2		28%
3		32%
4		36%
5		40%
6		44%

The Venturi mask (Fig. 11-21) is a high-airflow oxygen entrainment delivery device that delivers a precise fraction of inspired oxygen (FiO_2) at typically low concentrations. The device was originally designed to deliver 30% to 40% concentrations but has since been adapted to deliver higher oxygen percentages. The Venturi mask uses "jet mixing" of atmospheric gas and oxygen to achieve the desired mixture.

Various sized color-coded adapters are attached to the mask to control the oxygen flow rate. (Standard size adapters are 3-, 4-, and 6-L/min.) The color codes and adapters state the exact liter flow to use to obtain the precise FiO_2. Choosing a different liter flow drastically alters the FiO_2 delivered. The various Venturi masks deliver 24% to 50% oxygen and are recommended for patients who rely on a hypoxic respiratory drive (e.g., those with chronic obstructive pulmonary disease). The main benefit of the Venturi mask is that it allows precise regulation

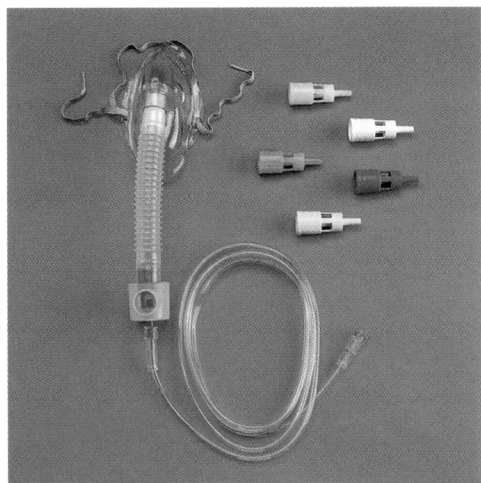

Fig. 11-21 Venturi mask.

of FiO₂. In addition, its use permits the paramedic to titrate oxygen for the patient with COPD so as not to exceed the patient's hypoxic drive while allowing enrichment of supplemental oxygen.

> **NOTE**
>
> Care must be taken to match the appropriate FiO₂ to the correct flow rate or the Venturi mask will not deliver the indicated FiO₂.

Ventilation

Patient ventilation can be provided by several methods in the prehospital setting, including rescue breathing (mouth to mouth, mouth to nose, mouth to stoma), mouth to mask breathing, bag-valve devices, and automatic transport ventilators.

Rescue Breathing

As previously discussed, inspired air has an oxygen concentration of about 21%. Of this 21% approximately 4% is used by the body, and the remaining 17% is exhaled. Ventilation by rescue breathing can accordingly provide adequate oxygenation to a patient with respiratory insufficiency.

The advantages of rescue breathing are that it requires no equipment and it is immediately available. The disadvantages are the limitation of the vital capacity of the rescuer (about 700 to 1000 mL are needed to effectively ventilate an adult patient) and the low concentration of oxygen in expired air compared with other methods of ventilation with sup-

plemental oxygen delivery. It also may be difficult for the rescuer to force air past obstructions in the airway. A risk exists of disease transmission through direct body fluid contact and of unknown communicable disease at the time of the event. Complications common to all rescue breathing techniques include the following:

- Hyperinflation of the patient's lungs
- Gastric distention
- Blood/body fluid contact concerns
- Rescuer hyperventilation

> **? CRITICAL THINKING**
>
> **What are two harmful effects of gastric distention during artificial ventilation?**

Mouth-to-Mouth Method

The following guidelines should be observed when delivering ventilations mouth to mouth:

1. If no spinal injury is suspected, position the patient with optimal head-tilt and chin-lift. (If spinal injury is suspected, maintain in-line stabilization and maintain an open airway through the jaw-thrust without head-tilt technique, described later in this chapter.) If necessary, clear the airway of vomitus, body fluids, and foreign objects.
2. Pinch the patient's nostrils closed.
3. Inhale a deep breath.
4. Seal your mouth over the patient's mouth, which should be slightly open.
5. Exhale into the patient's mouth until the chest rises and resistance is produced by the patient's lung expansion.

> **NOTE**
>
> Mouth-to-mouth breathing will likely result in the exchange of saliva between the victim and the rescuer. Transmission of the hepatitis B virus (HBV) and the human immunodeficiency virus (HIV) during rescue breathing has not been documented. However, rare instances of herpes transmission during cardiopulmonary resuscitation (CPR) have been reported.[1] When possible, personal barrier protection devices should be used.

6. Break contact with the patient's mouth to allow for passive exhalation.

7. Repeat the process, providing a full ventilation of 700 to 1000 mL (more than 2 seconds in duration) every 5 to 6 seconds as needed.

Mouth-to-Nose Method

Mouth-to-nose ventilation is very similar to the technique described for mouth-to-mouth rescue breathing. The differences in the mouth-to-nose method are as follows:

- If no spinal injury is suspected, one hand must be kept on the patient's forehead to maintain an open airway while the rescuer's other hand is used to close the patient's mouth. (If a spinal injury is suspected, the jaw-thrust without head-tilt technique should be used, and the rescuer's cheek is used to seal the patient's mouth.)
- The patient's nose is left open.
- The rescuer's mouth is placed over the patient's nose with as tight a seal as possible.
- During passive exhalation by the patient, the rescuer's mouth is removed from the patient's nose and the patient's mouth is opened for exhalation. The head-tilt or jaw-thrust position must be maintained to ensure an open airway.
- Mouth-to-nose ventilation may be appropriate for patients who have injuries to the mouth and lower jaw and for patients with missing teeth or dentures (which makes a tight seal around the mouth difficult). It also may overcome psychological barriers in having mouth-to-mouth contact with a patient.

Ventilation of infants and children. To provide ventilations to infants and children, the paramedic should use the mouth-to-mouth-and-nose technique as described below:

1. Position the patient with a *slight* head-tilt and chin-lift sufficient to open the airway. Hyperextension of a pediatric patient's neck may occlude the airway. (Use spinal precautions as needed.)
2. When ventilating, the rescuer's mouth should cover both the mouth and the nose of the infant or small child up to 1 year of age.
3. Use smaller breaths than for an adult patient, but the breaths should be large enough to make the chest rise.
4. When allowing for passive exhalation, break contact with the patient's mouth and nose.

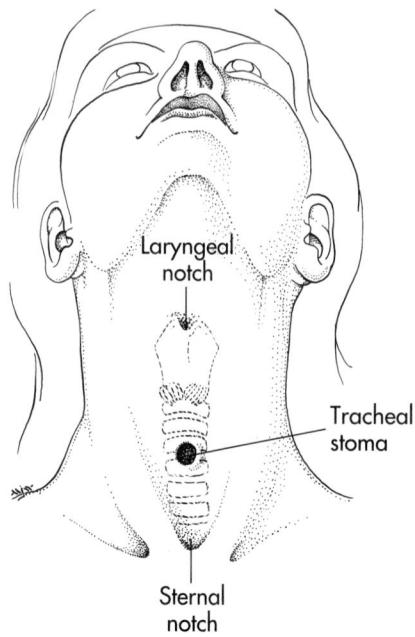

Fig. 11-22 Stoma.

5. Provide slow ventilations (1 to 1½ seconds in duration) every 3 seconds.

Mouth-to-Stoma Method

A stoma is a temporary or permanent surgical opening in the neck of a patient who has had a laryngectomy or tracheostomy (Fig. 11-22). The airway of such a patient has been surgically interrupted, and the larynx is no longer connected to the trachea (Box 11-5).

The stoma created by a laryngectomy is large and round, and the edge of the tracheal lining can be seen attached to the skin. The stoma in tracheostomy patients is usually no more than several millimeters in diameter and contains one or two concentric tubes made of plastic or metal. The method of ventilating these patients is the same, regardless of the type of stoma.

> **NOTE**
>
> Stomas and breathing tubes may become clogged with secretions, encrusted mucus, and foreign matter, leading to inadequate ventilation.

If cleaning is necessary, wipe the neck opening with gauze. If the breathing tubes are clogged, they can be removed or suctioned. The tracheostomy

BOX 11-5

SPECIAL CONSIDERATIONS FOR PATIENTS WHO HAVE HAD A LARYNGECTOMY

When providing care for patients with laryngectomies, it may sometimes be necessary to suction the tracheostomy tube or to remove, clean, and replace a tube that has become obstructed by mucus. (Patients with laryngectomies have a less effective cough, and mucus plugs commonly obstruct breathing tubes.) The steps for suctioning a breathing tube are as follows:

1. Preoxygenate the patient.
2. Inject 3 mL of sterile saline down the trachea.
3. Step 2 usually results in coughing; if it does not, instruct the patient to exhale.
4. Insert the suction catheter until resistance is met (without negative pressure).
5. Step 4 usually results in coughing; if it does not, instruct the patient to cough or exhale.
6. Suction while withdrawing the catheter.

If the breathing tube cannot be cleared and requires replacement, follow these steps:

1. Lubricate a same-size tracheostomy tube or ET tube (5.0 or larger).
2. Instruct the patient to exhale.
3. Gently insert the tube 1 to 2 cm beyond the balloon cuff.
4. Inflate the cuff.
5. Confirm the patient's comfort and verify the patency and proper placement of the tube.

NOTE

Stenosis (spontaneous narrowing of a stoma) may be life threatening, and it makes replacing a tracheostomy tube difficult or impossible. In such situations an endotracheal tube must be placed before total obstruction occurs.

---

tube or stoma is suctioned by passing a sterile suction catheter through the external opening into the trachea. *Do not insert the catheter more than 3 to 5 inches (7 to 12 cm) into the trachea.* Once the airway is partly open, begin ventilations by the mouth-to-stoma method (mouth-to-stoma ventilation is bacteriologically cleaner than the mouth-to-mouth method) by using a pediatric-size pocket mask over the top of the stoma or by securing the airway with an ET tube placed through the stoma.

The technique for stoma ventilation is basically the same as that for other methods of artificial ventilation. However, the patient's head should be kept straight (rather than tilted back), with the patient's shoulders slightly elevated. This position permits more effective ventilation. If the patient's chest does not rise or if air is heard to escape through the patient's upper airway, the patient may be a "partial neck breather." These patients are able to inhale and exhale some air through their nose and mouth. Should this occur, the patient's nostrils must be pinched closed and the mouth sealed with the palm of one hand during ventilation.

Mouth-to-Mask Devices

Mouth-to-mask devices have become popular as an alternative to mouth-to-mouth methods of ventilation. These masks are of a clear, flexible construction and are available with one-way valves, bacterial filters, and ports for supplemental oxygen delivery (Fig. 11-23). They are produced by a number of manufacturers and are available in a variety of sizes. The mouth-to-mask technique offers several advantages:

- It eliminates direct contact with the patient's mouth and nose.
- Supplemental oxygen delivery is possible.
- The one-way valve eliminates exposure to exhaled gases and sputum.
- It is easy to apply.
- It provides more effective ventilation than the mouth-to-mouth method or a bag-valve-mask device.
- It is aesthetically more acceptable than mouth-to-mouth ventilation.

NOTE

Mouth-to-mask ventilation is indicated for apnea from any mechanism. It is useful, however, only when it is readily available.

Technique

The mask device can be used in patients with or without spontaneous respirations. If immediately

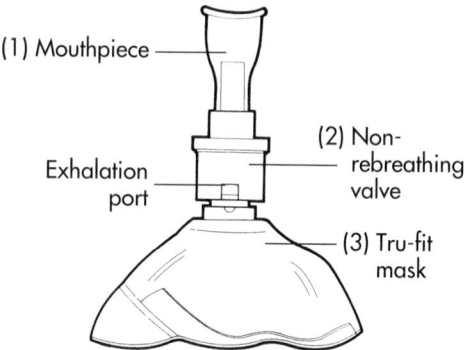

Fig. 11-23 Mouth-to-mask device.

(1) Mouthpiece

(2) Non-rebreathing valve

Exhalation port

(3) Tru-fit mask

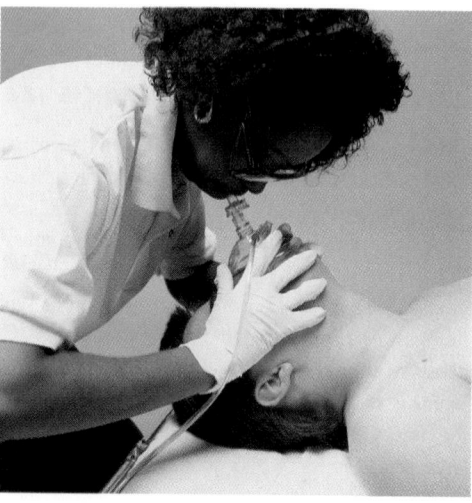

Fig. 11-24 Mouth-to-mask ventilation technique (cephalic technique).

available, mouth-to-mask is the preferred method of initial ventilation (Fig. 11-24). To apply the mask, follow these steps:

1. If no spinal injury is suspected, position the patient with optimal head-tilt and chin-lift. The use of an oropharyngeal or nasopharyngeal airway is indicated in an unconscious patient. (If a spinal injury is suspected, spinal precautions should be used.)
2. Connect the one-way valve to the mask. Oxygen tubing should be connected to the inlet port with an oxygen flow rate of 15 L/min. Using supplemental oxygen provides a higher concentration of oxygen in the inspired air. An oxygen flow rate of 10 L/min, combined with rescuer ventilations, can supply an oxygen concentration of 50%. An oxygen flow rate of 15 L/min provides an inspired oxygen concentration of about 80%.
3. Position yourself at the patient's head (cephalic technique) or side (lateral technique). If necessary, clear the airway of secretions, vomitus, and foreign objects. Place the mask on the patient's face, creating an airtight seal. Use the thumb side of the palm with both hands, and apply pressure to the sides of the mask. If using the cephalic technique, apply upward pressure to the mandible just in front of the ear lobes, using the index, middle, and ring fingers of both hands while maintaining head-tilt. If using the lateral technique, seal the mask by placing the index finger and thumb of the hand closer to the top of the patient's head along the border of the mask and place the thumb of the other hand along the lower margin of the mask. Place the remaining fingers of the hand closer to the patient's feet and lift the jaw while performing a head-tilt-chin-lift.

4. Blow into the opening of the mask, observing chest rise and fall. If available, a second rescuer should apply cricoid pressure (Sellick's maneuver) to help prevent gastric inflation during positive pressure ventilation and to reduce the possibility of regurgitation and aspiration (Box 11-6).
5. Remove the mask from the patient's face to allow for passive exhalation.

If oxygen is not available, tidal volumes and inspiratory times for mouth-to-mask ventilation should be the same as for mouth-to-mouth breathing (10 mL/kg or 700 to 1000 mL more than 2 seconds). If supplemental oxygen (minimum flow rate of 10 L/min) is used with the face mask, provide lower tidal volumes of 6 to 7 mL/kg (400 to 600 mL) over 1 to 2 seconds until the chest rises.[4]

Bag-Valve Devices

Bag-valve devices consist of a self-inflating bag and a nonrebreathing valve (Fig. 11-25). They can be used with a mask, an ET tube, or another invasive airway device. An adequate bag-valve unit should have (1) a self-refilling bag that is disposable or easily cleaned or sterilized, (2) a nonjam valve system that allows a minimum oxygen inlet flow of 15 L/min, (3) a non-pop-off valve, (4) standard 15- and 22-mm fittings, (5) a system for delivering high-concentration oxygen through an inlet port at the back of the bag or by an oxygen reservoir, and (6) a nonrebreathing valve.[5]

BOX 11-6

CRICOID PRESSURE (SELLICK'S MANEUVER)

Pressure applied to the solid ring of the cricoid cartilage can occlude the esophagus, reducing the risk of regurgitation and possible aspiration. It can also help minimize gastric distention during bag-valve-mask (BVM) ventilation. Cricoid pressure is indicated if vomiting is likely or if the patient is unconscious while intubation or artificial ventilation is performed. Cricoid pressure should be used with caution if cervical spine injury is suspected because it may further compromise the injury. Complications include laryngeal trauma with excessive force and esophageal rupture from unrelieved high gastric pressures.

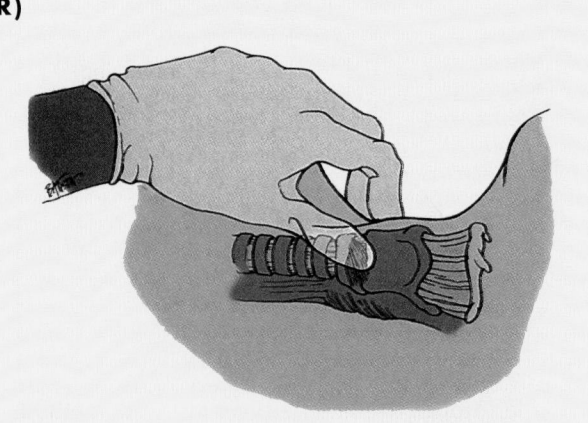

The device also should perform under all common environmental conditions and extremes of temperature and should be available in both adult and pediatric sizes.

> **NOTE**
>
> All paramedics should be proficient in delivering effective oxygenation and ventilation with a bag-valve device to adults, children, and infants. It is the preferred method of ventilatory support, particularly if the transport time is short.[6]

When the bag-valve device is compressed, air is delivered to the patient through a one-way valve. The air inlet to the bag is closed during delivery. When the bag is released, the patient's expired gas passes through an exhalation valve into the atmosphere, preventing the patient's gas from reentering the bag-valve device. As the patient exhales, atmospheric air and supplemental oxygen from the reservoir refill the bag.

Use of the bag-valve device with a mask is difficult because of the problem of creating an effective mask seal on the patient's face while maintaining an open airway. For this reason, it has been recommended that two rescuers use the device, one holding the mask and maintaining the airway while the second compresses the bag with two hands. If three rescuers are available, one rescuer can be solely responsible for maintaining the mask seal while providing spinal precautions as indicated.

When properly used, the bag-valve device has many benefits. The rescuer can provide a wide range of inspiratory pressures and volumes to adequately ventilate patients of varying sizes and underlying pathological conditions. It can be used to assist patients with shallow respirations, it performs adequately in extremes of environmental temperatures, and oxygen concentrations ranging from 21% (room air concentration) to nearly 100% (using supplemental oxygen and a reservoir) can be achieved. In addition, manual compression of the bag can give the rescuer a sense of the patient's lung compliance, which is an advantage over mechanical methods of ventilation.

Technique

Ventilation with the bag-valve device is best accomplished when the patient has been intubated. If the patient has not been intubated, the bag-valve device may be used with a mask. The following technique is recommended for use with the bag-valve-mask (BVM) device:

1. The rescuer is positioned at the top of the patient's head.
2. If no spinal injury is suspected, the patient should be in the optimal head-tilt chin-lift position, and the patient's head should be elevated in extension. If a spinal injury is suspected, spinal precautions should be used.
3. If necessary, the airway should be cleared of secretions, vomitus, and foreign objects. If the patient is

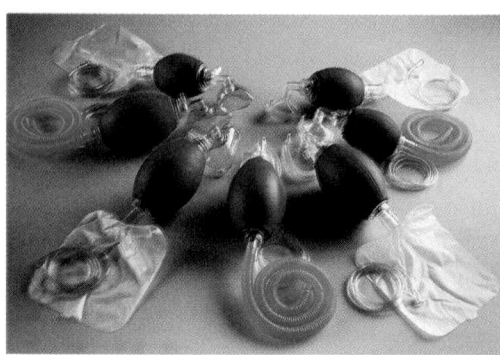

Fig. 11-25 Disposable and reusable adult and pediatric bag-valve devices.

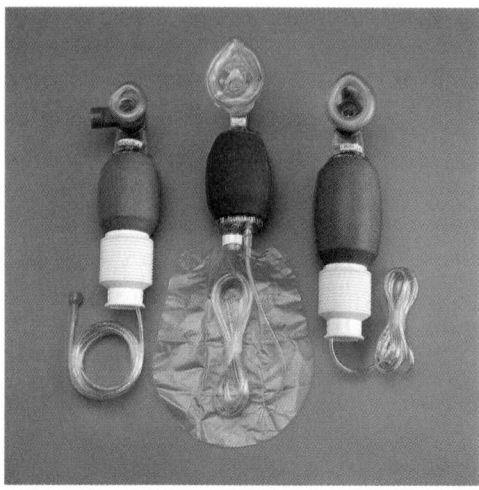

Fig. 11-26 Pediatric bag-valve-mask device.

unconscious, an oropharyngeal or nasopharyngeal airway should be inserted. The patient's mouth should remain open under the mask.

4. An oxygen source is connected, and the reservoir is flushed with high-concentration oxygen.
5. The mask is placed on the patient's face, making a tight seal. This can be accomplished by placing the thumb on the nose area, placing an index finger on the chin, and spreading the remaining fingers along the mandible. The anterior displacement of the mandible must be maintained. To compress the bag, the rescuer's other hand presses the bag against his or her body (e.g., the thigh), or another rescuer compresses the bag with two hands as recommended by the American Heart Association (AHA). The bag should be compressed smoothly, delivering 6 to 7 mL/kg of air (approximately 500 mL for the average adult) over 2 seconds. (A third rescuer may provide cricoid pressure.)

Pediatric Considerations

Smaller bag-valve devices are needed for infants and children to reduce the chances of overinflation and subsequent barotrauma. Bag-valve devices are used primarily to provide ventilatory support in pediatric patients who are in respiratory arrest. BVM devices equipped with a fish-mouth- or leaf-flap-operated outlet valve should not be used to provide supplemental oxygen to a spontaneously breathing infant or child, because if the valve fails to open during inspiration, the child receives only the exhaled

gases contained within the mask itself. For this reason, bag-valve devices for ventilation of full-term neonates, infants, and children should have a minimum volume of 450 to 500 mL.[7] At least 10 to 15 L/min of oxygen flow are required to maintain an adequate oxygen volume in the reservoir of a pediatric bag (Fig. 11-26).

> **NOTE**
>
> A child's flat nasal bridge makes achieving a mask seal difficult, and compressing the mask against the face may result in obstruction. The mask seal is best achieved with jaw displacement using two rescuers to provide BVM ventilation.

Technique. The following procedure is used to artificially ventilate a pediatric patient with a bag-valve-mask device:

1. Ensure a proper mask fit by using a length-based resuscitation tape or by measuring from the bridge of the nose to the cleft of the chin.
2. Ensure a proper mask position and seal. Place the mask over the mouth and nose (avoid compressing the eyes). With one hand, place a thumb on the mask at the apex and place the index finger on the mouth at the chin (like a C clamp). With gentle pressure, push down on the mask to establish an adequate seal. Maintain the airway

by lifting the bony prominence on the chin, with the remaining fingers placed on the mandible, forming an E. Avoid putting pressure on the soft area under the chin.

3. Provide ventilations at a rate of one breath every 3 seconds.
4. Obtain chest rise with each ventilation. Saying "squeeze" with each ventilation should provide adequate volume to initiate chest rise. *Do not overinflate.*
5. Allow adequate time for exhalation by releasing the bag and saying, "release, release."
6. Continue with ventilations using the "squeeze, release, release" method.
7. Assess BVM ventilation by observing adequate rise and fall of the chest, by listening for lung sounds at the third intercostal space and midaxillary line, and by assessing for improvement in skin color or heart rate, or both.

? CRITICAL THINKING

What should you do if you find that it is suddenly more difficult to ventilate a non-intubated patient?

Automatic Transport Ventilators

Several time-cycled, gas-powered, automatic transport ventilators (ATVs) are available for field use or intrahospital transport when caring for patients who require ventilatory support (Fig. 11-27). Most of these ventilators consist of a plastic control module connected by tubing to any 50-psi gas source (e.g., air or different concentrations of oxygen, including 100% oxygen). The exit valve of the control module is connected by one or two tubes (based on

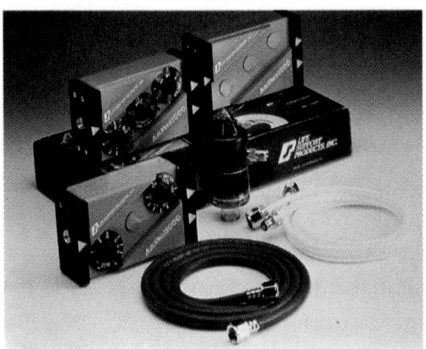

Fig. 11-27 Autovent 1000, 2000, and 3000.

the model) to the patient valve assembly to deliver selected tidal volumes (400 to 1200 mL for adults, 200 to 600 mL for children). Another control selects respiratory rates from 8 to 22 breaths per minute for adults and 8 to 30 breaths per minute for children. (Most ATVs are not to be used in children under 5 years of age.) Most units provide a 40 L/min flow of oxygen, which remains constant regardless of changes in the patient's airway or lung compliance.

NOTE

ATVs should have a default rate of 10 breaths per minute for adults and 20 breaths per minute for children, with the ability to adjust the rate once the patient is intubated with a tracheal tube or alternative airway.[8]

The volume of gas delivered by the automatic ventilator is determined by the length of time the manual trigger is depressed or by the inspiratory effort of the spontaneously breathing patient. Most units are designed to limit the inspiratory pressure to 60 to 80 cm of water. When this pressure is reached, an audible alarm sounds, and excess gas flow is vented off, preventing possible lung damage. ATVs allow the paramedic to use both hands to obtain a tight mask seal on a patient who has not been intubated and to perform other tasks when the ventilator is used with ET intubation. Cricoid pressure also can be applied with one hand while the other hand seals the mask on the face. Most ATVs are contraindicated for patients who are awake,

BOX 11-7

PERSONAL PROTECTIVE EQUIPMENT

The Centers for Disease Control and Prevention (CDC) recommend that healthcare workers, in addition to taking the normal precautions for personal protection from communicable diseases, use masks, eyewear (e.g., safety glasses and face shields), and gowns when splashes of blood or other body fluids are likely. Because of the possibility during airway management procedures of patient reactions such as vomiting and coughing and the potential for exposure to blood and other body fluids, the paramedic should take barrier precautions.

who have obstructed airways, and or who have increased airway resistance (e.g., pneumothorax, asthma, pulmonary edema).

Airway Management

Science and technology have produced numerous adjuncts for providing airway management. However, the paramedic must not neglect basic airway management in favor of a procedure that is technically more difficult than necessary to secure a safe and functional airway. Airway management should progress rapidly from the least to the most invasive modality. Box 11-7 presents recommendations on personal protective equipment.

> **NOTE**
>
> Because unconscious patients lack the muscular tone and control to maintain a patent airway, *the airways of all unconscious patients must be established and maintained in the initial assessment.* The paramedic also should remember that any injury severe enough to cause loss of consciousness is severe enough to cause spinal injury. *Spinal precautions should be considered in all trauma patients who need airway management or ventilatory support until an x-ray film of the spine has been made.*

Manual Techniques for Airway Management

Manual techniques for airway management have been described by the AHA and the American Red Cross (ARC). These include the head-tilt chin-lift method, the jaw-thrust, and the jaw-thrust without head-tilt.

> **NOTE**
>
> Manual maneuvers to open a patient's airway are contraindicated in patients who are responsive and when resistance is met when attempting to open the mouth. All manual maneuvers are hazardous in the presence of spinal injury, and none protect against aspiration.

The head-tilt chin-lift method (Fig. 11-28) is preferred for opening the airway when a spinal injury is not suspected. The head-tilt is accomplished by placing one hand on the victim's forehead and applying firm backward pressure with the palm to tilt the head back. The fingers of the other hand then are placed under the bony part of the lower jaw (near the chin) and lifted to bring the chin forward, supporting the jaw and helping to maintain the head-tilt position.

If no spinal injury is suspected, the jaw-thrust maneuver (Fig. 11-29) may be used to gain additional forward displacement of the mandible. This is accomplished by grasping the angles of the patient's lower jaw and lifting with both hands, one on each side, displacing the mandible forward while tilting the head back.

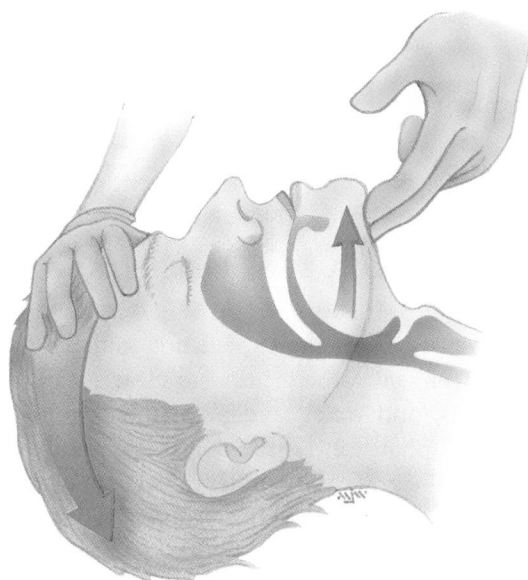

Fig. 11-28 Head-tilt chin-lift maneuver.

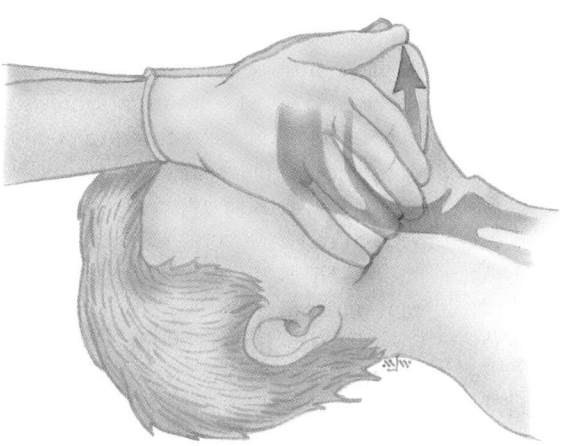

Fig. 11-29 Jaw-thrust maneuver.

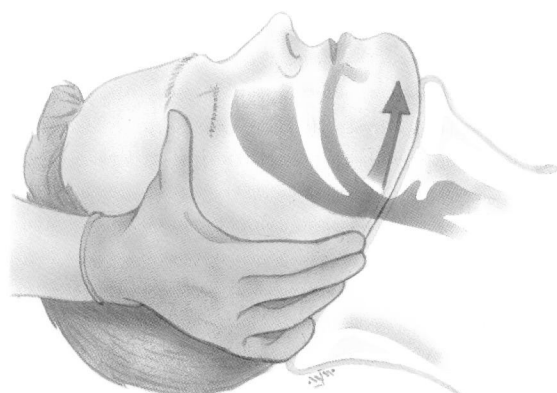

Fig. 11-30 Jaw-thrust without head-tilt maneuver.

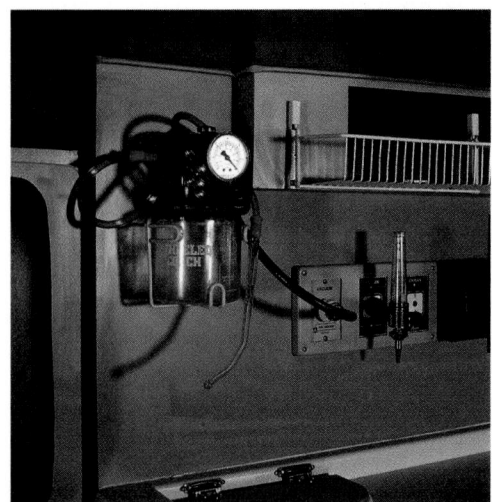

Fig. 11-31 Fixed suction unit.

If a spinal injury is suspected, the jaw-thrust without head-tilt maneuver (Fig. 11-30) should be used to open the airway. During this maneuver, the patient's head should be stabilized and the cervical spine immobilized with neutral, in-line stabilization. The jaw-thrust maneuver should then proceed without extending the neck.

Suction

Suction can be used to remove vomitus, saliva, blood, food, and other foreign objects that might occlude the airway or increase the likelihood of pulmonary aspiration by inhalation. Because many factors can predispose an individual to aspiration, every patient should be regarded as a possible aspiration victim.

Suction Devices

Fixed and portable mechanical suction devices are available through a number of manufacturers. Fixed suction devices (Fig. 11-31) are mounted in patient care areas of hospitals and nursing homes and in many emergency vehicles. These systems are electrically operated by vacuum pumps or powered by the vacuum produced by a vehicle engine manifold. Fixed suction devices furnish an air intake of at least 40 L/min and provide a vacuum of more than 300 mm Hg when the tube is clamped.

Portable suction devices (Fig. 11-32) may be oxygen or air powered, electrically powered, or manually powered. These devices should furnish an air intake of no less than 20 L/min to operate effectively.

Suction Catheters

Suction catheters are used to clear the oral cavity and airway passages of secretions and debris. The two broad classifications of catheters are the whistle-tip suction catheter and the tonsil-tip suction catheter.

The whistle-tip catheter is a narrow, flexible tube used primarily for tracheobronchial suctioning to clear secretions through either an ET tube or the nasopharynx (Fig. 11-33). This catheter is designed with molded ends and side holes to produce minimal trauma to the mucosa. A side opening in the proximal end is covered with the thumb to produce suction. Using sterile technique, the catheter is advanced to the desired location, and suction is applied intermittently as the catheter is withdrawn.

> **NOTE**
>
> Soft-tip catheters should be lubricated before insertion.

The tonsil-tip (Yankauer) suction catheter is a rigid pharyngeal catheter used to clear secretions, blood clots, and other foreign material from the mouth and pharynx (Fig. 11-34). It is carefully inserted into the oral cavity under direct visualization and slowly withdrawn while suction is activated.

Before any suctioning procedure is initiated, all equipment should be checked and the suction set between 80 and 120 mm Hg. (Higher suction is needed for tracheobronchial suctioning.) The pa-

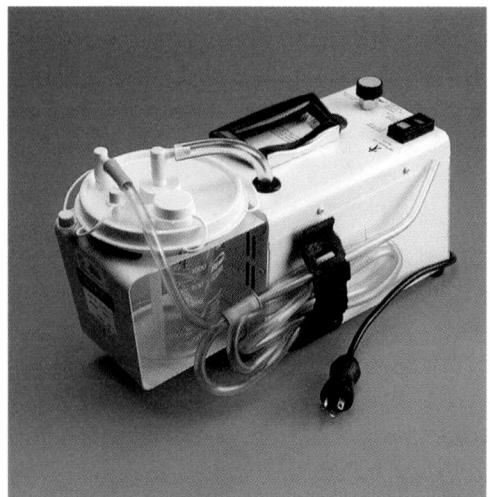

Fig. 11-32 Portable suction unit.

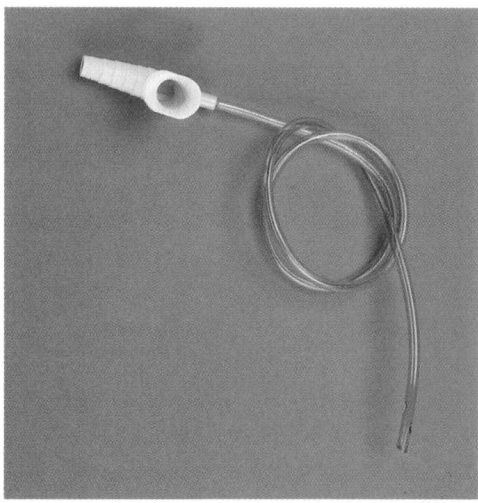

Fig. 11-33 Soft (whistle-tip) suction catheter.

tient's lungs should be oxygenated with 100% oxygen for at least 2 minutes before suction is initiated, if possible. *Suction should never be applied for longer than 10 to 15 seconds in adult patients or longer than 5 seconds in pediatric patients.* If additional suctioning is needed, the patient's lungs should be reoxygenated before the procedure is repeated. Possible complications from suctioning include the following:

- Sudden hypoxemia that occurs secondary to decreased lung volume during the suction application
- Severe hypoxemia that may lead to cardiac rhythm disturbances and cardiac arrest
- Airway stimulation that may increase arterial pressure and cardiac rhythm disturbances
- Coughing that may result in increased intracranial pressure with reduced blood flow to the brain and increased risk of herniation in patients with head injury
- Soft tissue damage to the respiratory tract

Tracheobronchial Suctioning

Before tracheobronchial suctioning is performed through an ET tube, the patient must be oxygenated with 100% oxygen for 5 minutes.[7] Using sterile technique, the catheter is advanced to the desired location (about at the level of the carina). Suction is applied intermittently by closing the side opening as the catheter is withdrawn in a rotating motion. The patient's cardiac rhythm should be monitored throughout the procedure. If dysrhythmias or

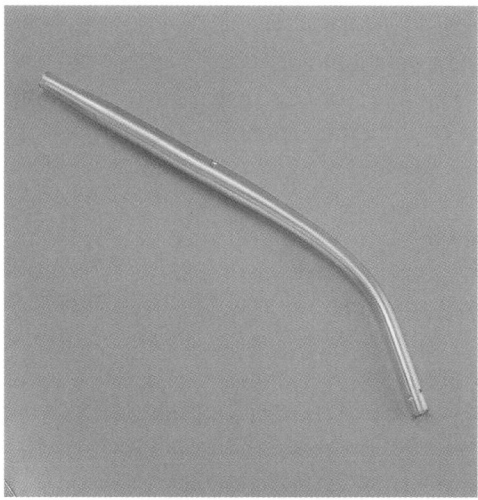

Fig. 11-34 Rigid (tonsil-tip [Yankauer]) suction catheter.

bradycardia develop, suction should be discontinued and the patient manually ventilated and oxygenated. Before the suction procedure is repeated, the patient should be ventilated with 100% oxygen for about 30 seconds.

> **NOTE**
>
> For tracheal suction, a Y-Piece or T-Piece or a lateral opening should lie between the suction tube and the source of the on-off suction control.

NOTE

It may be necessary to inject 3 to 5 mL of sterile saline down the ET tube to loosen secretions.

Gastric Distention

Gastric distention results from air being trapped in the stomach. As the stomach diameter increases from the trapped air, it pushes against the diaphragm and interferes with lung expansion. The abdomen becomes increasingly distended (especially in small children), and resistance may be felt to BVM ventilation.

Management. Management of gastric distention begins by slightly increasing the BVM ventilation inspiratory time. (Large-volume suction should be readily available.) If possible, the patient should be placed in a left lateral recumbent position, and manual pressure should be slowly applied to the epigastric region. Gastric distention that cannot be managed with these noninvasive techniques may require insertion of a gastric tube (Fig. 11-35).

Gastric Tubes

Gastric decompression for gastric distention or emesis control can be accomplished through naso-

NOTE

Gastric distention is very common when ventilating patients who have not been intubated.

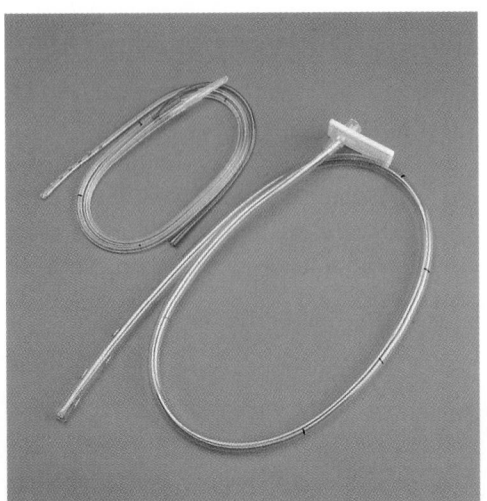

Fig. 11-35 Top: nasogastric/orogastric tube. Bottom: oral gastric lavage tube.

gastric (NG) or orogastric decompression. The steps for each procedure are listed below:

NOTE

Gastric decompression is performed with extreme caution in patients who have esophageal trauma or esophageal disease. It is contraindicated if an esophageal obstruction is present. NG decompression should not be attempted in a patient with facial trauma or esophageal varices.

Nasogastric decompression
1. Prepare the patient.
   a. Place the head in a neutral position.
   b. Preoxygenate.
   c. Instill a topical anesthetic or intravenous (IV) *lidocaine* (per medical direction or protocol).
   d. Locate the larger naris.
2. Lubricate the NG tube with viscous lidocaine (Xylocaine) per protocol.
3. Advance the tube gently along the nasal floor and into the stomach. (Having the patient swallow during insertion may help advance the tube into the esophagus and prevent tracheal insertion.)
4. Confirm placement.
   a. Auscultate the epigastric region while injecting 30 to 50 mL of air.
   b. Note gastric contents in the NG tube.
   c. Ensure that no reflux appears around the NG tube.
5. Secure the NG tube in place.

Orogastric decompression
1. Prepare the patient and tube as described above for NG insertion.
2. Introduce the orogastric tube down the midline of the oropharynx and into the stomach.
3. Ensure placement and secure the orogastric tube as described above for NG insertion.

Complications of gastric decompression. Regardless of the method chosen, gastric decompression is uncomfortable for the patient and may induce nausea and vomiting even when the gag reflex is suppressed. Gastric tubes also interfere with mask seals and with visualization of airway structures during intubation. Complications of the procedures include nasal, esophageal, or gastric trauma, tracheal placement, supragastric placement, and gastric tube obstruction.

Mechanical Adjuncts in Airway Management

Use of mechanical devices in airway management should never delay the opening of a compromised airway. These devices should be used only after efforts have been made to open the airway manually.

Nasopharyngeal Airway (Nasal Airway)

The nasal airway is used to maintain an airway in a semiconscious or an unconscious patient (Fig. 11-36). Insertion of a nasal airway may also be a useful temporizing maneuver to control the airway in patients with seizures or possible cervical spine injury and also before nasotracheal intubation (described later in this chapter). In addition, this adjunct may serve as a guide for insertion of a nasogastric tube.

> **? CRITICAL THINKING**
>
> *Think about two or three specific patient conditions that would warrant the use of a nasal airway.*

> **NOTE**
>
> In very young patients, airway secretions and debris may obstruct small nasal airways, making them unreliable.

Description

The nasal airway is soft and pliable. It has a gentle curve, and the outer end is flared. Nasal airways are available in a variety of sizes to accommodate infants and adults. They vary from 17 to 20 cm long and sizes 12 to 36 French. (As with most other catheters, the French Scale System is used to indicate internal diameter. Each unit of the scale equals about $\frac{1}{3}$ mm. A 21-French catheter, for example, is 7 mm in diameter.)

To determine the correct size, the paramedic should choose an airway that has a tube length equal to the distance between the tip of the patient's nose and the tragus of the ear, which is the cartilaginous area anterior to the external auditory canal (Fig. 11-37). The following are the recommended sizes of nasopharyngeal airways:

- Large adult: 8-9 mm internal diameter (24-27 French)
- Medium adult: 7-8 mm internal diameter (21-24 French)
- Small adult: 6-7 mm internal diameter (18-21 French)

Insertion

The nasal airway should be lubricated with a water-soluble lubricant to minimize resistance in the nasal cavity. The device is placed in the nostril with the beveled tip (designed to protect nasal structures) directed toward the nasal septum. The airway is gently passed close to the midline, along the floor of the nostril, following the natural curvature of the nasal

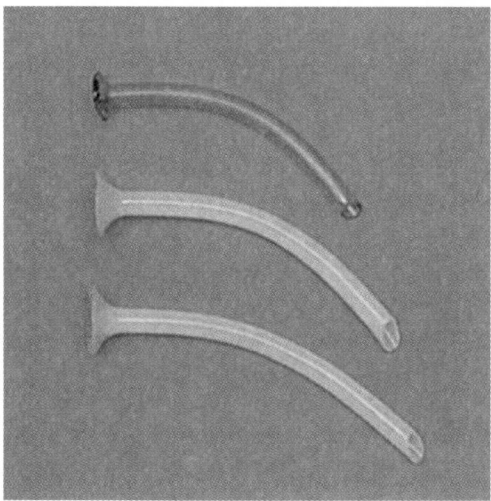

Fig. 11-36 Nasal airways.

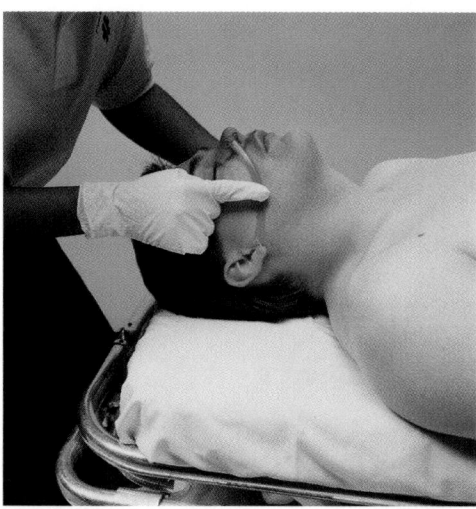

Fig. 11-37 Measuring a nasal airway.

passage. The insertion should be made perpendicular to the coronal plane of the face. The airway should not be forced. If resistance is encountered, rotating the tube slightly may help, or insertion can be attempted through the other nostril (Fig. 11-38).

After insertion, the nasal airway rests in the posterior pharynx behind the tongue. If the patient begins to gag after insertion of the airway, the tube may be stimulating the posterior pharynx. Removal of the airway or withdrawing it 0.5 to 1 cm and rein-

> **NOTE**
>
> Nasal airways (and NG tubes) are contraindicated in patients who have fractures of the basal skull or facial bones because inadvertent intracranial placement is a potential complication.

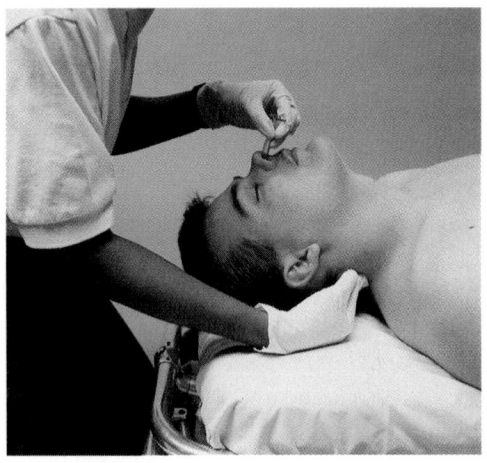

Fig. 11-38 Insertion of a nasal airway.

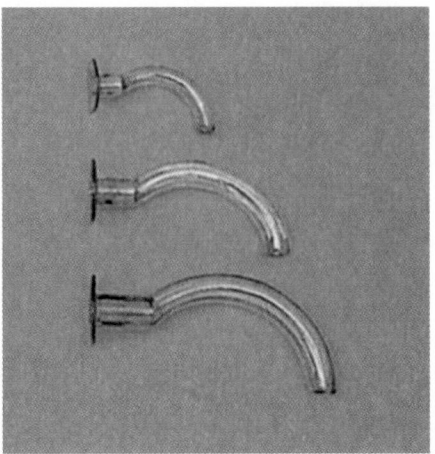

Fig. 11-39 Oral airways.

serting it may be indicated. The paramedic should remember to maintain displacement of the mandible by head-tilt chin-lift or by jaw-thrust without head-tilt when using this airway.

Advantages

- A nasal airway is well tolerated by conscious and semiconscious patients with an intact gag reflex.
- Insertion is a quick procedure.
- A nasal airway may be used when insertion of an oropharyngeal airway is contraindicated or difficult because of oral trauma or soft tissue injury.

Possible Complications

- Long nasal airways may enter the esophagus.
- The airway may precipitate laryngospasm and vomiting in patients with a gag reflex.
- It may injure nasal mucosa, causing bleeding and possibly airway obstruction.
- Small-diameter airways may become obstructed by mucus, blood, vomitus, and the soft tissues of the pharynx.
- A nasal airway does not protect the lower airway from aspiration.
- It is difficult to suction through.

Oropharyngeal Airway (Oral Airway)

Oral airways are designed to prevent the tongue from obstructing the glottis. They are indicated in unconscious or semiconscious patients who have no gag reflex and who are not intubated.

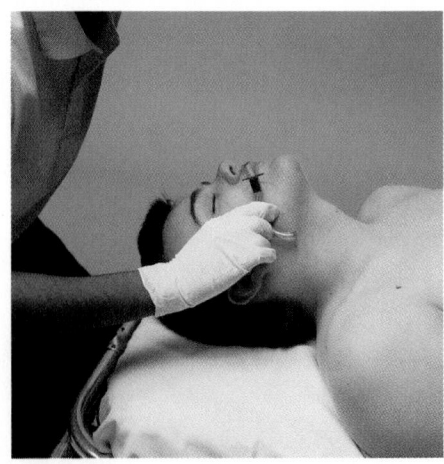

Fig. 11-40 Measuring an oral airway.

Description

The oral airway is a semicircular device designed to hold the tongue away from the posterior wall of the pharynx. Most oropharyngeal airways are made of disposable plastic. The two types of airways most frequently used are the Guedel, distinguished by its tubular design, and the Berman, distinguished by airway channels along each side (Fig. 11-39).

> **NOTE**
>
> The cuffed oropharyngeal airway (COPA) is a modified oral airway with a distal inflatable cuff and proximal standard 15-mm connector to allow for attachment of a bag-valve device. The COPA may be a useful adjunct in airway management during resuscitation.

Like nasopharyngeal airways, oral airways are available in a variety of sizes, from infant to adult. The size is based on the distance in millimeters from the flange to the distal tip. The proper size for the patient may be determined by placing the airway next to the face so that the flange is at the level of the patient's central incisors and the bite block segment is parallel to the patient's hard palate. The airway should extend from the corner of the mouth to the tip of the ear lobe or the angle of the jaw (Fig. 11-40). The following sizes are recommended[7]:

- Large adult: 100 mm (Guedel size 5)
- Medium adult: 90 mm (Guedel size 4)
- Small adult: 80 mm (Guedel size 3)

Insertion

Before any oral airway is inserted, the mouth and pharynx should be cleared of all secretions, blood, or vomitus. In an adult or older child, the oral airway may be inserted upside down or at a 90-degree angle to avoid catching the tongue during insertion (Fig. 11-41, A). As the oral airway passes the crest of the tongue, it is rotated into the proper position so that it is situated against the posterior wall of the oropharynx. Another method of insertion, recommended for pediatric patients and usable in adult patients, is to use a tongue blade to displace the tongue inferiorly and anteriorly. The airway is then inserted and moved posteriorly toward the back of the oropharynx, following the normal curvature of the oral cavity (Fig. 11-41, B). Regardless of the method of insertion, trauma to the face and oral cavity should be avoided. In addition, the paramedic should be sure that the patient's lips and tongue are not caught between the teeth and the airway.

> **? CRITICAL THINKING**
>
> *Why is this method of oral airway insertion used for infants and young children?*

Proper placement of the airway is confirmed by observable chest wall expansion and good breath sounds on auscultation of the lungs during ventilation. The paramedic should remember that even with an oral airway in place, the patient's head must be kept in proper position to help ensure a patent airway.

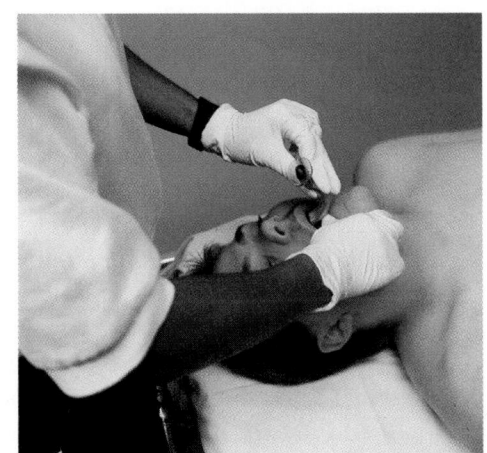 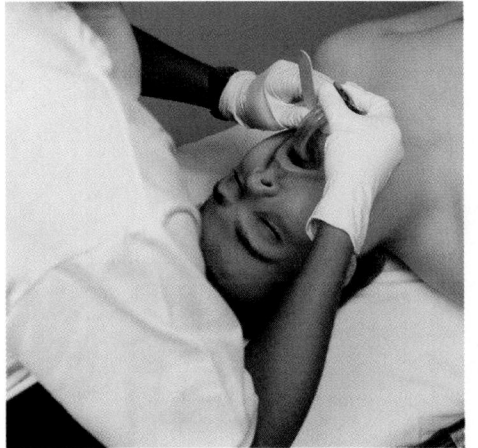

Fig. 11-41 A, Inserting an airway upside down. **B,** Alternative method of inserting an oral airway.

Advantages

- An oral airway secures the tongue forward and down, away from the posterior pharynx.
- It provides easy access for airway suction.
- It serves as a bite block to protect an ET tube and the airway in the event of convulsions.

Possible Complications

- Oral airways that are too small may fall back into the oral cavity, occluding the airway.
- Long airways may press the epiglottis against the entrance of the trachea, producing a complete airway obstruction.
- The airway may stimulate vomiting and laryngospasm in a patient with a gag reflex.
- It does not protect the lower airway from aspiration.
- It may push the tongue back and obstruct the airway if improperly inserted.

Advanced Airway Procedures

Advanced airway procedures described in this text include endotracheal intubation, digital or blind intubation, nasotracheal intubation, the laryngeal mask airway (LMA), and multilumen airways. All of these advanced airway procedures require special training. Before initiating any advanced procedure, paramedics should have direct authorization from medical direction or be operating under protocols that have been developed and approved by medical direction and the EMS agency. The para-

medic also should be aware that long-term complications may result from advanced airway procedures, even when the procedures are properly performed. These complications include aspiration, tracheal stenosis, transient dysphagia, and voice changes.

Endotracheal Intubation

Tracheal intubation is the preferred technique for airway control in patients who are unable to maintain a patent airway. Indications for tracheal intubation include the following situations:

- When the rescuer is unable to ventilate an unconscious patient with conventional methods (mouth-to-mask method, BVM)
- When the patient cannot protect his or her own airway (coma, respiratory and cardiac arrest)
- When prolonged artificial ventilation is needed

In addition, tracheal intubation provides the following advantages:

- Isolates the airway, preventing aspiration of material into the lower airway
- Facilitates ventilation and oxygenation
- Facilitates suctioning of the trachea and bronchi
- Prevents wasted ventilation and gastric insufflation during positive-pressure ventilation
- Provides a route for the administration of some medications: *lidocaine* (Xylocaine), *epinephrine* (Adrenalin), *atropine*, and *naloxone* (Narcan)

Description

The common ET tube is a flexible tube that is open at both ends (Fig. 11-42). The proximal end has a standard 15-mm adapter that connects to various oxygen delivery devices for positive-pressure ventilation. The distal end of the tube is beveled to facilitate placement between the vocal cords, and the adult tube (5 or larger) has a balloon cuff that occludes the remainder of the tracheal lumen. This cuff prevents aspiration around the tube and minimizes air leaks during ventilation. The cuff is attached by the inflating tube to a one-way inflating valve with an inlet port designed to accept a syringe for inflation. A properly positioned ET tube with its cuff inflated permits administration of high concentrations of oxygen at controlled pressures. In addition to the common ET tube,

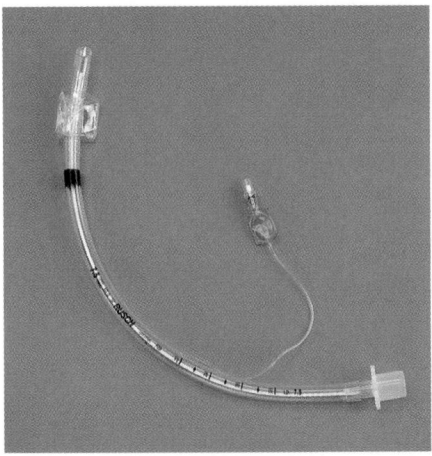

Fig. 11-42 ET tube.

specialized variations are available. They include the following:

- Armored or anode tubes that have an inner spiral of flat metal to prevent kinking or compression
- "Trigger" tubes that have a thin cord running down the anterior wall of the tube, to which a ring is attached proximally. (Pulling on the ring with a finger or thumb increases the curvature. This ring may help maneuver the tube anteriorly without a stylet.)
- Some ET tubes have medication ports for ET drug administration.

Endotracheal Tube Sizes

The markings on the ET tube indicate the internal diameter of the tube in millimeters. (The tubes are available in graduated sizes from 2.5 to 10 mm.) The length of the tube from the distal end is indicated in centimeters at several levels. Recommended ET tube sizes are 7.0 to 8.0 mm internal diameter for men and 7.0 mm internal diameter for women.[9]

Infant and pediatric ET tubes are available with and without balloon cuffs. Cuffed ET tubes are indicated only for children over the age of 8 to 10 years. Children under 8 to 10 years of age have a circular narrowing at the level of the cricoid cartilages. This narrowing serves as a functional cuff, allowing minimal air leakage at the cricoid ring. Accordingly, uncuffed ET tubes are recommended for this age group.

> **NOTE**
>
> Cuffed tracheal tubes for young children may be appropriate under circumstances where high ventilatory pressures are indicated. Examples include status asthmaticus and acute respiratory distress syndrome (ARDS). (See Chapter 27.)

Various methods may be used to determine the correct ET tube size for infants and children. An estimate of tracheal tube size for children older than 1 year may be made by use of one of the following equations[9]:

Uncuffed Tube

Tracheal tube size (mm) = (age in years/4) + 4

Cuffed Tube

Tracheal tube size (mm) = (age in years/4) + 3

An alternative method to select an appropriately sized ET tube is to use length-based resuscitation tapes (for children up to 35 kg). (See Chapter 42.) Suggested sizes for ET tubes and suction catheters for adult and pediatric patients are listed in Table 11-5.[9]

TABLE 11-5	PEDIATRIC AND ADULT TRACHEAL TUBE AND SUCTION CATHETER SIZES*	
APPROXIMATE AGE/SIZE (WEIGHT)	**INTERNAL DIAMETER OF TRACHEAL TUBE, mm**	**SUCTION CATHETER SIZE, F**
Premature infant (<1 kg)	2.5	5
Premature infant (1 to 2 kg)	3.0	5 or 6
Premature infant (2 to 3 kg)	3.0 to 3.5	6 or 8
0 month to 1 year/ infant (3 to 10 kg)	3.5 to 4.0	8
1 year/small child (10 to 13 kg)	4.0	8
3 years/child (14 to 16 kg)	4.5	8 or 10
5 years/child (16 to 20 kg)	5.0	10
6 years/child (18 to 25 kg)	5.5	10
8 years/child to small adult (24 to 32 kg)	6.0 cuffed	10 or 12
12 years/adolescent (32 to 54 kg)	6.5 cuffed	12
16 years/adult (50+ kg)	7.0 cuffed	12
Adult female	7.0 cuffed	12 or 14
Adult male	7.0 to 8.0 cuffed	14

*These are approximations and should be adjusted on the basis of clinical experience. Tracheal tube selection for a child should be based on the child's size or age. One size larger and one size smaller should be allowed for individual variation. Color-coding based on length or size of the child may facilitate approximation of correct tracheal tube size.

Necessary Equipment

A laryngoscope is required for visualizing the glottis during tracheal intubation. Although various makes are available, all have several features in common. The standard laryngoscope includes a handle made of plastic or stainless steel. The handle contains the batteries for the light source and attaches to a plastic or stainless steel blade with a bulb placed in the distal third. The electrical contact between the blade and the handle is made at a connection point called the *fitting*. The indentation of the blade is attached to the bar of the handle. When the blade is elevated to a right angle with the laryngoscope handle, the blade snaps into place and the bulb lights (Fig. 11-43). (Failure of the bulb to light may be the result of a loose connection between the bulb and the bulb socket, a damaged bulb, or faulty batteries.) Other necessary equipment includes a 10-mL syringe for cuff inflation, water-soluble lubricant, and suction equipment.

Two types of blades (available in various sizes) are used with the laryngoscope: a straight blade, such as the Miller, Wisconsin, or Flagg blade (Fig. 11-44), and a curved blade, such as a MacIntosh blade (Fig. 11-45). The tip of a straight blade is applied directly to the epiglottis to expose the vocal cords. Advocates of the straight blade claim it provides more exposure of the glottis and less need for a stylet. A straight blade usually is recommended for infant intubation because it provides greater displacement of the tongue into the floor of the mouth and better visualization of the glottic structures.

> **? CRITICAL THINKING**
>
> *Ask several paramedics and anesthesiologists which laryngoscope blade they prefer, and why.*

The curved blade design is intended to displace the tongue to the left and to elevate the epiglottis without touching it. Advocates of the curved blade claim it reduces the chance of dental trauma and provides more room for passage of the ET tube. The choice of blade is a matter of personal preference and the patient's anatomy. Paramedics should acquire expertise in using both curved and straight blades because some patients can be intubated more easily with one type than the other. Occasions also may arise when only one type of blade is available. Versatility with both curved and straight blades may enhance patient survival.

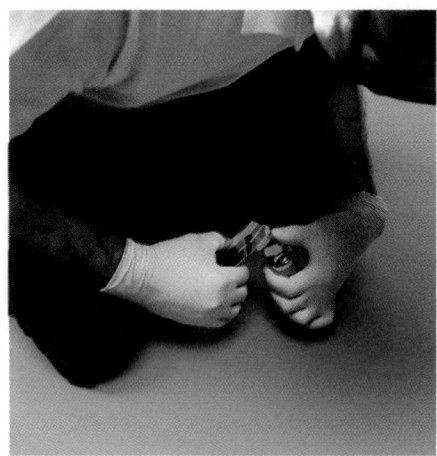

Fig. 11-43 Attaching blade to laryngoscope handle.

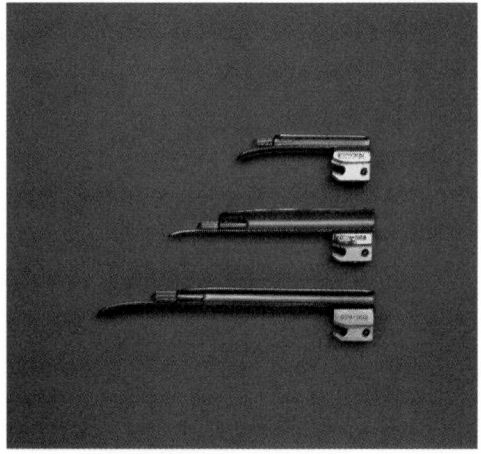

Fig. 11-44 Straight blades.

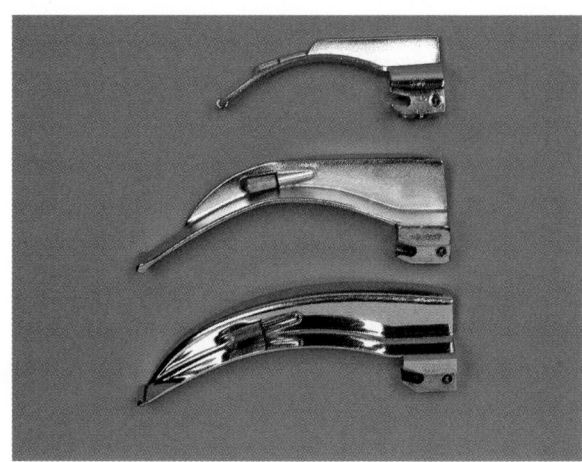

Fig. 11-45 Curved blades.

A malleable stylet (preferably plastic coated) may be inserted through the ET tube before intubation (Fig. 11-46). The stylet will conform to any desired configuration and may facilitate proper placement of the ET tube. If used, the stylet must be recessed at least 1 to 2 cm from the distal end of the ET tube to prevent injury to the patient. Recession of the stylet tip is maintained by bending the proximal end of the stylet over the

> **NOTE**
>
> A gum elastic bougie can be used to assist with ET tube placement. This large flexible device is placed in the trachea, after which the tracheal tube is passed over the bougie and into position in the trachea.

> **NOTE**
>
> Patient ventilation should be established by other means before intubation (e.g., mouth-to-mask method, BVM). The adequacy of ventilation should be assessed by observing the chest rise and fall during ventilation, by auscultating for breath sounds, and by noting the patient's skin color. When preparing for intubation, the paramedic should remember that the patient's lungs should be first hyperventilated with 100% oxygen for 1 to 2 minutes. In addition, the time required for intubation (i.e., the time lapse without ventilating the patient's lungs) should not exceed 30 seconds. If intubation is not completed within this time, the procedure should be stopped and the patient's lungs well ventilated and oxygenated for 15 to 30 seconds by other means before attempting intubation again. If the patient has a perfusing rhythm, pulse oximetry and ECG monitoring should be continuous during intubation attempts.

proximal rim of the adapter so that it does not advance through the lumen with manipulation of the ET tube. If the stylet is allowed to extend beyond the distal end of the tube, the mucosal surface of the larynx or trachea or the vocal cords may be damaged.

Some physicians also authorize the use of Magill forceps, a scissor-style clamp that has circular tips (Fig. 11-47), to help direct the tip of the ET tube into the larynx during intubation and to remove some foreign bodies. Use of this device requires special training and authorization from medical direction.

Preparing for Intubation

Before intubation, all equipment should be examined and tested for defects. The cuff of the ET tube should be checked for integrity by inflating the balloon with 5 to 8 mL of air and checking for leaks in the cuff or inlet port. The blade of the laryngoscope should be snapped into place to examine the light bulb. The bulb should be secured in its socket and checked for brightness ("light, bright, and tight").

Anatomical Considerations

The ET tube may be passed into the trachea through the mouth (orotracheal method) or through the nose (nasotracheal method). The orotracheal method is used most commonly and is performed under direct visualization of the glottic opening. The nasotracheal route essentially is a "blind" technique. The following anatomical structures are important landmarks during intubation:

- The trachea is in the midline of the neck and has its superior entry at the level of the glottic opening. In

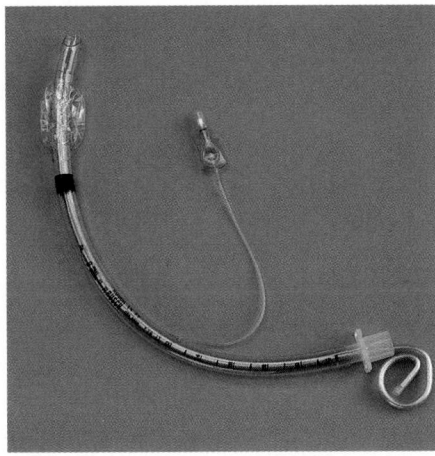

Fig. 11-46 ET tube with malleable stylet.

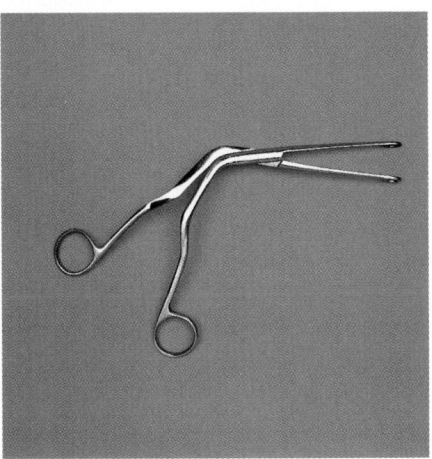

Fig. 11-47 Magill forceps.

REMOVAL OF FOREIGN BODIES BY DIRECT LARYNGOSCOPY

Direct laryngoscopy and use of Magill forceps to remove foreign bodies should be attempted only after manual techniques of clearing the airway have been unsuccessful. The steps in removing a foreign body from the airway by direct laryngoscopy are as follows:

1. Assemble the necessary laryngoscopic equipment. (Have suction ready for immediate use in case of vomiting.)
2. Place the supine patient in the sniffing position (Fig. 11-48) with the head extended.
3. Hyperventilate the patient with supplemental oxygen, if possible.
4. Insert the laryngoscope, visualizing the glottic opening and surrounding structures.
5. If foreign matter is visualized, grasp the foreign matter with Magill forceps or a Kelly clamp and remove it from the airway.

NOTE: Forceps removal of foreign matter should only be attempted with direct visualization of the obstruction. Even then, caution must be exercised to avoid soft tissue damage from the teeth of the forceps.

6. If spontaneous respirations resume within 5 seconds, remove the laryngoscope blade and monitor the patient.
7. If spontaneous respirations do not resume, insert an ET tube, administer 100% oxygen, and assess the patient's circulatory status.

If complete foreign body obstruction of the upper airway cannot be relieved, needle cricothyrotomy or transtracheal jet insufflation may be warranted (described later in this section). These advanced airway procedures provide oxygenation until tracheal intubation or tracheostomy can be performed in a controlled setting.

orotracheal intubation, the vocal cords should be visualized while passing the tube to ensure passage into the trachea.

- The uvula is suspended from the midline of the soft palate and is used as a guide in placing the laryngoscope properly.
- The epiglottis is attached to the base of the tongue and should be visualized and elevated to expose the glottis and vocal cords. Pressure on the solid ring of the cricoid (Sellick's maneuver) can occlude the esophagus, reducing the risk of

regurgitation during the intubation attempt. It also may help to better visualize the entrance of the trachea by pushing it slightly posteriorly.

- The trachea extends to the level of the second intercostal space anteriorly, at which point it bifurcates into left and right mainstem bronchi. The right main bronchus branches off at a very slight angle to the trachea, whereas the left branches at a 45- to 60-degree angle.

NOTE

Because of this anatomical configuration, it is more common for an ET tube that has been advanced too far to enter the right main bronchus, bypassing and occluding the origin of the left main bronchus. If this occurs, atelectasis and pulmonary insufficiency of the left lung may result. It therefore is important for the paramedic to evaluate ET tube placement by auscultating both lungs. With proper ET tube placement, breath sounds should be of almost equal intensity over both lung fields. Certain pathological conditions (e.g., pneumothorax, hemothorax, surgical removal of a lung) may result in unequal breath sounds even when an ET tube is in the proper position.

Orotracheal Intubation

In preparation for orotracheal intubation, the non-trauma patient should be placed in the sniffing position (see Fig. 11-48) so that the neck is flexed at the fifth and sixth cervical vertebrae and the head is extended at the first and second cervical vertebrae. This allows the three axes of the mouth, pharynx, and trachea (oropharyngeolaryngeal axis) to be aligned for direct visualization of the larynx. (If trauma is not a factor, it may be helpful to place several layers of towels under the patient's head for elevation.)

The tube should be lubricated, and a stethoscope, stylet, and suction equipment (with large-bore catheters) should be readily available. As in all advanced airway procedures, the patient's lungs should be hyperventilated with 100% oxygen for 1 to 2 minutes before intubation. The orotracheal intubation procedure is as follows (Fig. 11-49):

1. Position yourself at the patient's head.
2. Inspect the oral cavity for secretions and foreign material. Suction the mouth and pharynx if needed.

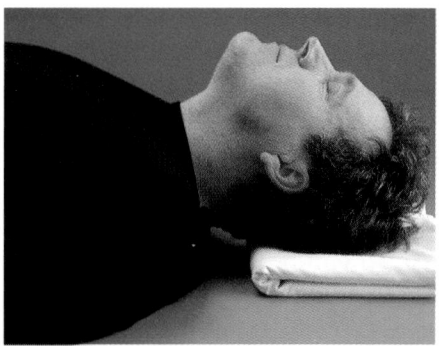

Fig. 11-48 Sniffing position.

3. Open the patient's mouth with the fingers of the right hand. Retract the patient's lips on the teeth or gums to avoid pinching them in the blade. The "crossed-finger technique" also may be useful in opening the patient's mouth. To perform this procedure, cross the right thumb and index finger to form an X. Place the thumb on the patient's lower incisors and the index finger on the patient's upper incisors, and apply crossed-finger pressure to open the patient's mouth.

A

B

C

D

E

F

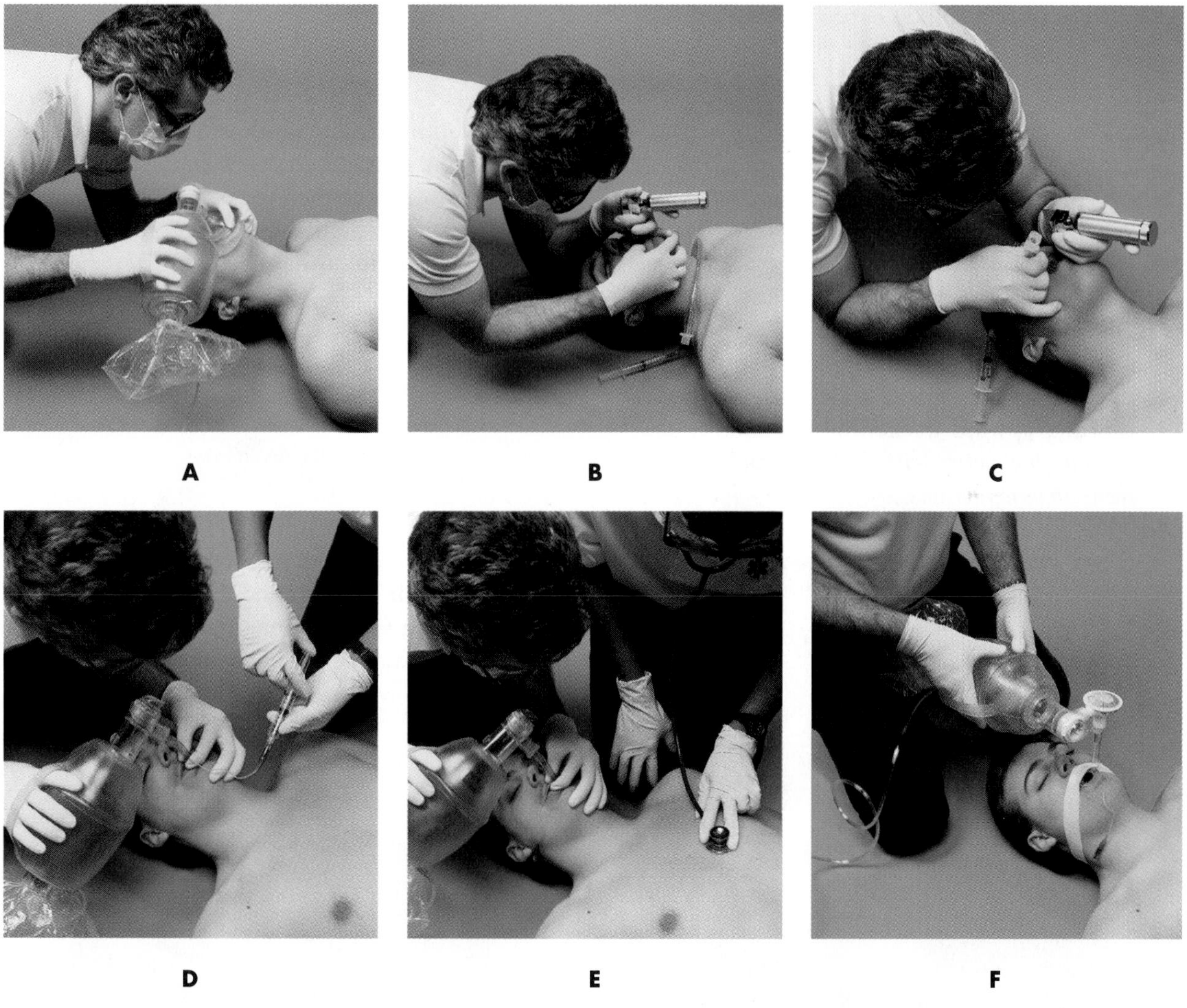

Fig. 11-49 A, Before intubation, hyperventilate the patient's lungs with 100% oxygen for at least 1 to 2 minutes. **B,** With the laryngoscope held in the left hand, insert the blade into the right side of the mouth, displacing the tongue to the left. **C,** Advance the ET tube through the right corner of the mouth and, under direct vision, through the vocal cords. **D,** Inflate the cuff with about 10 mL of air and ventilate the patient's lungs with a mechanical airway device. **E,** Confirm ET placement by primary and secondary confirmation methods. **F,** Secure the ET tube to the patient's head and face and provide ventilatory support with supplemental oxygen.

4. Grasp the lower jaw with the right hand and draw it forward and upward. Remove any dentures.

5. Holding the laryngoscope in the left hand, insert the blade in the right side of the mouth, displacing the tongue to the left. Move the blade toward the midline and the base of the tongue and identify the uvula. Gentleness and avoiding pressure on the lips and teeth are essential.

> **NOTE**
>
> Whenever possible, a second rescuer should apply cricoid pressure during tracheal intubation in adults to protect against regurgitation of gastric contents and to help facilitate tube placement. The second rescuer should apply backward, upright, rightward pressure (BURP) to help bring the vocal cords into the field of vision of the paramedic who is performing the intubation.

6. When using a curved blade, advance the tip of the blade into the vallecula, the space between the base of the tongue and the pharyngeal surface of the epiglottis (Fig. 11-50). When using a straight blade, insert the tip under the epiglottis (Fig. 11-51). The glottic opening is exposed by exerting upward traction on the handle. *Never use a prying motion with the handle and do not use the teeth as a fulcrum.*

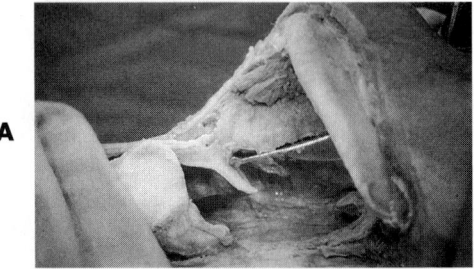

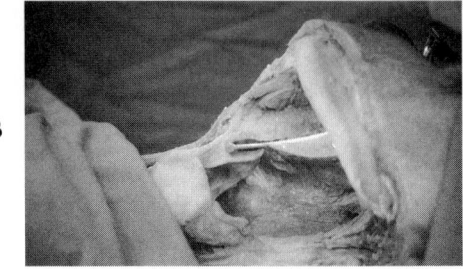

Fig. 11-50 A, The tip of the blade is inserted into the vallecula. **B,** Pressure is directed caudally and anteriorly, lifting to expose the vocal cords.

7. Advance the ET tube through the right corner of the mouth and, under direct vision, through the vocal cords (Fig. 11-52). If a stylet has been used, it should be removed from the tube after the tube passes through the cords into the trachea.

8. After viewing the vocal cords, ensure that the proximal end of the cuffed tube has advanced past the cords about 1 to 2.5 cm (½ to 1 inch) (Fig. 11-53). The tip of the tube should then be halfway between the vocal cords and the carina. This position allows some displacement of the tube tip during flexion or extension of the patient's neck without extubation or movement of the tip into the mainstem bronchus. (In the average adult, the distance from teeth to carina is 27 cm. The paramedic should observe the depth markings on the ET tube during intubation. In the average adult, the tube is properly positioned when the patient's teeth are between the 19- and 23-cm marks on the tube, placing the tip of the tube 2 to 3 cm above the carina.)

> **NOTE**
>
> The average tube depth in men is 22 cm ("teeth and tube at 22"). The average tube depth in women is 21 cm.

9. Inflate the cuff with about 10 mL of air to prevent any air leaks around the tracheal cuff seal.[5]

10. Attach the tube to a mechanical airway device and ventilate the patient's lungs.

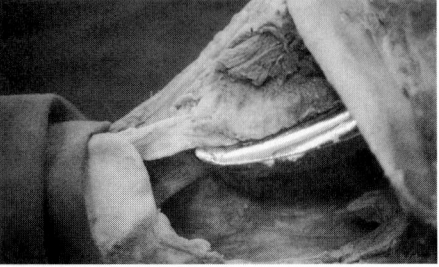

Fig. 11-51 The blade is used to lift the epiglottis, directly exposing the vocal cords.

11. During ventilation, confirm accurate tube placement with primary and secondary confirmation methods[10]:

a. Primary confirmation methods
   Initially confirm proper tube placement by auscultating over the epigastrium, the mid-axillary, and anterior chest line on the right and left sides of the chest. If stomach gurgling is present or chest expansion is absent, immediately remove the tracheal tube and reattempt intubation after oxygenating the patient's lungs with 100% oxygen for 15 to 30 seconds. When appropriate tube placement has been confirmed, reconfirm and note the tube mark at the front of the patient's teeth, secure the tube to the patient's head and face with tape or a commercially available device, and reevaluate lung sounds to ensure that the tube was not inadvertently repositioned. Finally, an oral airway or bite block should be inserted to prevent the patient from biting down and occluding the airway.

NOTE

If breath sounds are decreased or absent in the left lung, the tube may have passed into the right mainstem bronchus, effectively bypassing the origin of the left main bronchus. If this is the case, the cuff should be deflated and the tube withdrawn 1 to 2 cm; the cuff should be reinflated and tube placement should be verified as above.

NOTE

Securing the tube is as critical as the intubation itself. Adjuncts include securing the maxilla rather than the mandible, using tincture of benzoin to facilitate tape adhesion, and use of commercial devices designed to quickly secure the ET tube with or without tape.

b. Secondary confirmation methods
   Secondary confirmation is obtained with mechanical devices. These devices include end-tidal carbon dioxide detectors, esophageal detectors, and pulse oximetry for patients who have a perfusing rhythm. These devices are described later in this chapter.

Transillumination technique (lighted stylet). Malleable fiberoptic stylets, or "light wands" (Fig. 11-54), have a high-intensity light at the distal end that is powered by a small battery housing at the operator end. This method has the advantage of not requiring manipulation of the patient's head and neck because visualization of the vocal cords is not required or

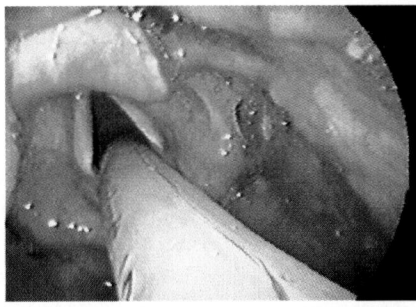

Fig. 11-53 ET tube passing through the vocal cords.

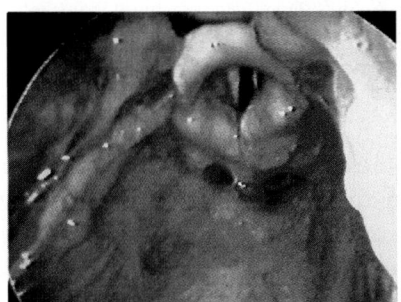

Fig. 11-52 View of the vocal cords.

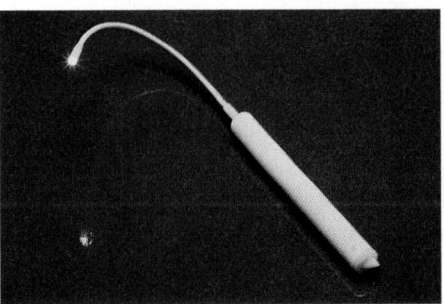

Fig. 11-54 Light wand for fiberoptic intubation.

attempted. Placement of the ET tube is facilitated by observation of the light from the end of the ET tube passing through the soft tissues of the neck. These stylets are 6 mm in diameter and are therefore too large for pediatric use. The procedure for fiberoptic intubation is as follows:

1. Position yourself at the side of the patient's head. If a spinal injury is suspected, have a second rescuer maintain in-line spinal immobilization.
2. Ensure hyperventilation with 100% oxygen for 1 to 2 minutes before intubation.
3. Lift the patient's tongue and mandible anteriorly by hand to position the epiglottis.
4. Advance the ET tube in combination with the lighted stylet through the oropharynx and the glottis. Transillumination of the skin of the neck will cause the airway structures to become more distinct. When the thyroid and cricoid cartilages are illuminated by a bright circle of light, the stylet should be held stationary and the ET tube advanced 1 to 2 cm.
5. Inflate the cuff and remove the stylet. Verify proper tube placement using primary and secondary methods.
6. Secure the tube as previously described.

If the illumination produces a dim, indistinct light, the esophagus has probably been intubated. If this occurs, the ET tube should be removed and the patient's lungs should be hyperventilated with 100% oxygen before reattempting the intubation. A disadvantage to this method is that ambient light may make it difficult to see illumination produced by the stylet. This problem can be minimized by darkening the work area during intubation or by placing several layers of dark blankets around the patient's neck during the procedure.

Lighted stylets can also be used to help verify placement after intubation by other methods. Once the cuff has been inflated and lung sounds auscultated, the stylet is advanced through the ET tube. A bright light inferior to the thyroid cartilage indicates proper placement. In addition, the list of indicators of proper ET positioning should be applied to evaluate correct placement.

Digital or blind intubation. Before the advent of laryngoscopes, intubation was performed by inserting the intubator's fingers into the patient's mouth to guide the ET tube into the trachea. Although this is not a common prehospital procedure, digital intubation may be necessary in cases of patient entrapment, in patients whose airway is blocked from view by large amounts of blood or other secretions, or if equipment fails. Digital intubation also may be applied in certain disaster situations in which victims are widespread and equipment is in short supply. The procedure for digital intubation is as follows:

1. Position yourself at the patient's left side. If a spinal injury is suspected, have a second rescuer maintain in-line spinal immobilization.
2. Ensure hyperventilation with 100% oxygen for 1 to 2 minutes before intubation.
3. Use a bite-stick or other device to hold the patient's mouth open to protect the rescuer's fingers.
4. Bend the tube and stylet combination into a J or hockey stick configuration.
5. Insert the gloved left middle and index fingers into the patient's mouth. Alternating fingers, "walk" down the patient's tongue, pulling the tongue and epiglottis away from the glottic opening.
6. When a flap of cartilage covered by mucous membrane is felt with the middle finger, the epiglottis has been located (Fig. 11-55, *A*). Maintain contact and advance the ET tube with the right hand, using the index finger of the left hand as a guide (Fig. 11-55, *B*). The index finger maintains the tube position against the middle finger, leading the tip of the tube into the glottic opening. It may be helpful for a second rescuer to perform Sellick's maneuver to occlude the esophagus and help prevent aspiration.

> **NOTE**
>
> Correct ET tube placement should be reverified often. At a minimum, verification should be made each time a patient is moved or has a sudden change in condition.

7. Once the cuff of the ET tube passes the tips of the paramedic's fingers, inflate the cuff, remove the stylet, and verify placement in the usual manner.
8. Secure the tube as previously described.

Potential Complications from Intubation Procedures
Trauma may occur during intubation, including the following:

- Lacerated lips or tongue
- Dental trauma from the laryngoscope
- Lacerated pharyngeal or tracheal mucosa
- Tracheal rupture
- Avulsion of an arytenoid cartilage
- Vocal cord injury
- Vomiting and aspiration of stomach contents
- Intubation may produce significant releases of epinephrine and norepinephrine, leading to hypertension, tachycardia, or cardiac rhythm disturbances.
- Intubation may lead to vagal stimulation (particularly in infants and children), resulting in bradycardia and hypotension.
- Intubation may increase intracranial pressure in patients with a head injury.
- The esophagus may be accidentally intubated.
- A bronchus may be accidentally intubated.
- Rupture of the cuff, inflation port malfunction, or severance or kinking of the inflation tube may cause cuff malfunction and air leakage.

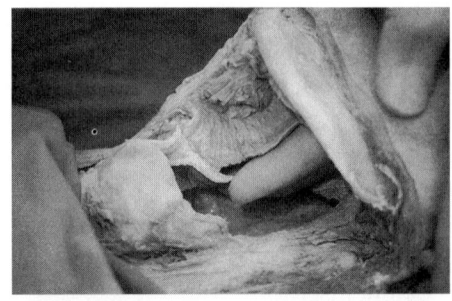

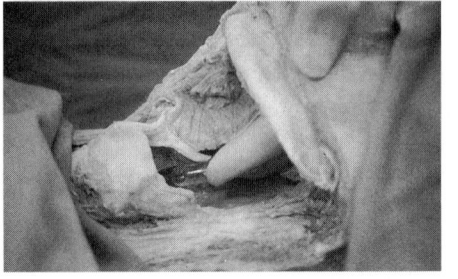

Fig. 11-55 A, Locate the epiglottis with the tips of the fingers of one hand. **B,** Using the palpated epiglottis as a landmark, guide an ET tube into the larynx.

Nasotracheal Intubation

Nasotracheal intubation may be the airway procedure of choice in patients who have spontaneous respirations when laryngoscopy is difficult or the motion of the cervical spine must be limited. Examples of such conditions include the following:

- Medication overdose
- Asthma or anaphylaxis
- Chronic obstructive pulmonary disease (COPD)
- Stroke
- Seizure (status epilepticus with constant seizure activity)
- Altered mental status

These and other situations may make it difficult to align the oropharyngeolaryngeal axis, precluding successful orotracheal intubation. It should be recognized that nasotracheal intubation is a "blind" procedure and carries a significant risk of improper tube placement because the paramedic cannot directly visualize the vocal cords.

Generally, conscious patients tolerate a nasotracheal tube better than an orotracheal tube. In addition, a nasotracheal tube usually causes less recurrent trauma to the tracheal mucosa because less intratracheal tube movement occurs with head motion than with an orotracheal tube. When time permits, the patient should be prepared by use of a vasoconstrictor spray (e.g., phenylephrine) and topical anesthetic (e.g., lidocaine [Xylocaine] jelly). These measures make the patient more comfortable and less susceptible to nasal hemorrhage that occurs secondary to the procedure. If time permits, placement of a soft nasopharyngeal airway before the procedure may indicate which nostril is more passable and may compress the mucosa to allow a less traumatic placement.

> **NOTE**
>
> Nasotracheal intubation is contraindicated in patients who are apneic, who have midfacial fractures, or are suspected of having basal skull fractures (described in Chapter 22), who have bleeding disorders, or who are taking Coumadin or are likely to receive **heparin** or fibrinolytics. Other contraindications include severe nasal trauma, pharyngeal hemorrhage, acute epiglottitis, suspected laryngeal fracture, and suspected increased intracranial pressure.

Insertion

1. Choose a cuffed ET that is 1 mm smaller than optimal for oral intubation. (Most ET tubes are designed for both orotracheal and nasotracheal

intubation procedures.) Prepare and check all necessary equipment (balloon cuff, syringe, suction, stethoscope). Stylets are not used in nasotracheal intubation because the stylet reduces the flexibility and increases the risk of injury during blind insertion.

2. Ensure that the patient's lungs have been well oxygenated and hyperventilated for 1 to 2 minutes before insertion.

3. Lubricate the ET tube with a water-soluble or lidocaine jelly.

4. Insert the tube with the flange facing the nasal septum and advance the tube along the nasal floor of the nostril that is clearer and more direct. If both nares appear open, advance through the largest nostril first. If the chosen nostril is impassable, try the other nostril before selecting an ET tube that is 0.5 mm smaller in diameter.

5. Stand beside the patient with one hand on the tube and the thumb and index finger of the other hand palpating the larynx. The curve of the tube should follow the natural curvature of the airway. Gently advance the tube while rotating it medially 15 to 30 degrees until maximal airflow is heard through the tube. Gently and swiftly advance the tube during early inspiration. Voluntary tongue extrusion in cooperative patients is helpful, or the tongue can be wrapped with gauze and pulled forward. Flexion of the neck (if no spinal instability is suspected) and posterior pressure on the thyroid cartilage may help position the larynx.

6. Externally observe the advancement of the tube toward the carina. "Misting" or condensation on the tube should be evident as the tube approaches tracheal placement. This phenomenon occurs because the patient's exhaled breath has a high concentration of water vapor, which promptly condenses on exposure to cooler room air.

NOTE

Tube misting is not always a reliable indicator of proper tube position.

7. On completion of intubation, verify proper tube placement as previously described. Inflate the cuff with about 10 mL of air and secure the tube in place. Ventilations may then be assisted with supplemental oxygen, or the patient's lungs can be ventilated by mechanical means.

8. If intubation fails, withdraw the tube and redirect it after ventilation and oxygenation of the patient. It may be possible to recognize tube misplacement by inspecting and palpating the neck for bulges.

Possible Complications

- Epistaxis
- Vagal stimulation
- Injury to the nasal septum or turbinates
- Retropharyngeal laceration
- Vocal cord injury
- Avulsion of an arytenoid cartilage
- Esophageal intubation
- Intracranial tube placement if the patient has a basilar skull fracture

Intubation with Spinal Precautions

Nasal or oral intubation may be performed in patients with suspected spinal injury.

1. Auscultate for bilateral breath sounds while manual or mechanical ventilations are in progress. This provides a baseline.

2. A second person should apply manual in-line stabilization from the patient's side. The second individual places his or her hands over the patient's ears. The little fingers should be under the occipital skull and the thumbs on the face over the maxillary sinuses. Stabilization (without distraction) should be maintained in a neutral position throughout the procedure. Thin padding under the patient's head may be necessary to maintain neutral, in-line positioning.

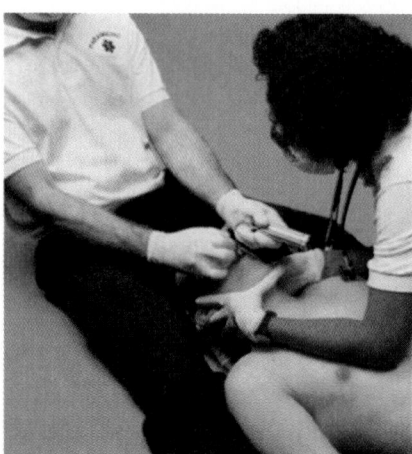

Fig. 11-56 Intubation in a sitting position.

3. In one method of intubation, the paramedic is positioned at the patient's head. The legs straddle the patient's shoulders and arms, and the patient's head is secured between the paramedic's thighs. The grip of both rescuers keeps the head from moving during the intubation. In this position, it may be necessary for the paramedic to lean back to visualize the vocal cords (Fig. 11-56). Another method is for the paramedic to lie prone at the patient's head. When using this technique, the second rescuer maintains the in-line position alone (Fig. 11-57).

Extubation

Removal of the ET tube is not usually indicated in the prehospital setting. However, if the patient develops intolerance to the tube (and cannot be sedated to improve tolerance), medical direction may recommend extubation. If time permits, the patient's lungs should be hyperventilated with 100% oxygen before the procedure. To remove the ET tube, the paramedic should tilt the patient or backboard to one side and proceed as follows:

1. Have suction available. (The oral cavity and the area above the cuff should be suctioned before extubation.)
2. Deflate the cuff completely.
3. Swiftly withdraw the tube on cough or expiration.
4. Assess respiratory status.
5. Provide high-concentration oxygen and assist ventilations as needed.

Advantages of ET Intubation

- It provides complete airway control.
- It helps prevent aspiration.
- Positive-pressure ventilation can be delivered.
- Tracheal suctioning is possible.
- It prevents gastric distention.
- High concentrations of oxygen and large volumes of ventilation can be delivered.
- It may provide a route for some medications.

Special Considerations for Pediatric Intubations

In addition to the differences in airway and ventilation procedures for pediatric patients, the anatomical differences of the pediatric airway must be considered.[6] These anatomical differences are listed below:

1. The infant's upper airway is relatively small, and the tongue is disproportionately large. Therefore posterior displacement of the tongue easily obstructs the airway. In addition, the larger tongue of the pediatric patient tends to make laryngoscopy more difficult.
2. The epiglottis is omega shaped and is narrower and longer in children than in the adult. Because of this, the epiglottis is more difficult to control with a laryngoscopic blade. The larynx lies more anteriorly in relation to the base of the tongue than in the adult, and it is also elevated under the base of the tongue, making visualization more difficult. The glottic opening is at the third cervical vertebra in premature neonates, the third to

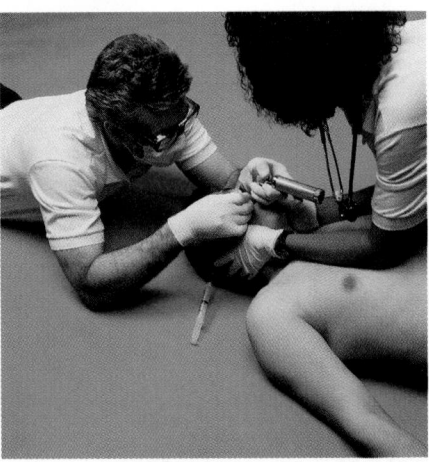

Fig. 11-57 Intubation in a prone position.

fourth cervical vertebra in term neonates, and the fourth to fifth cervical vertebra in adults.

3. During the first few months of life, the vocal cords of the infant slope from back to front, frequently causing the ET tube to "hang up" in the angle formed by the cords. This problem can be minimized by rotating the ET tube or by having a second rescuer perform Sellick's maneuver during intubation.

4. The cricoid cartilage is the narrowest part of the airway in the infant and young child. As the child reaches 8 to 10 years of age, the vocal cords become the narrowest part, and this position is maintained into adulthood.

5. The distance from the vocal cords to the carina varies and can be correlated with the patient's height. This distance is about 4 to 5 cm at birth and 6 to 7 cm at age 6. During placement of the ET tube, it is recommended that the tube be advanced until breath sounds are lost unilaterally (usually on the left side). It should then be slowly withdrawn until breath sounds return, indicating that the tube tip is at the carina. After the return of breath sounds, the tube should be withdrawn 2 to 3 cm farther, placing it at a safe distance above the carina and below the cords. The tube should then be secured with tape or a commercial device.

6. Children use their diaphragm as the major muscle for ventilation and require full diaphragmatic excursion to breathe. Gastric distention caused by swallowing air or artificial ventilation can inhibit the child's respiratory efforts. Infants are nose breathers until 3 to 5 months of age.

7. Deciduous teeth begin to develop at about 6 months and are lost between 6 and 8 years. They may become dislodged during airway procedures such as intubation and oral airway insertion and by the child biting on the airway.

During any airway procedure, the paramedic should remember that the airway structures of the pediatric patient are very fragile and easily damaged. Therefore great caution must be exercised so as not to injure these patients.

Adjuncts to Aid in Confirming ET Tube Placement

Several adjuncts often can aid in determining correct ET tube placement. These include end-tidal carbon dioxide detectors, bulb- or syringe-type esophageal detection devices, and pulse oximeters.

End-Tidal Carbon Dioxide Detectors

End-tidal carbon dioxide detectors are designed to help verify ET placement and to recognize inadvertent esophageal intubation. They also can provide a noninvasive estimate of alveolar ventilation, carbon dioxide production, and arterial carbon dioxide content. Their use as an adjunct to assessment of ET tube placement is strongly encouraged.[7]

> **NOTE**
>
> The correct depth of insertion in centimeters for children over age 2 can be approximated by adding one half the patient's age to 12.
>
> $$\frac{\text{Age (y)}}{2} + 12$$
>
> As an alternative, the depth of insertion in centimeters also can be estimated by multiplying the internal diameter of the tube by 3.[7]
>
> Depth of insertion = internal diameter $\times$ 3

> **NOTE**
>
> Color indicators of colorimetric CO_2 detectors can be affected by the presence of vomitus and by a patient's recent consumption of carbonated beverages (if the ET tube is placed in the esophagus).

The two types of carbon dioxide detectors are disposable colorimetric devices and the electronic monitor. Colorimetric devices are made of a white plastic and contain a chemical indicator in the upper part that is sensitive to carbon dioxide gas. When the de-

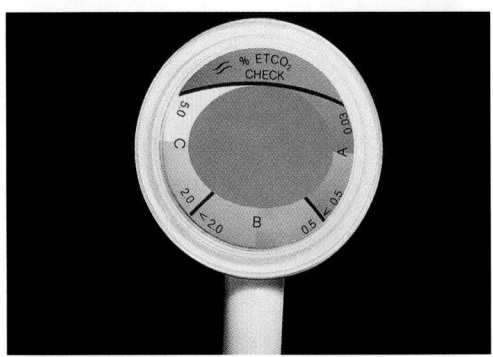

Fig. 11-58 Colorimetric end-tidal CO_2 detector.

tector is attached to an ET tube, the color of the indicator changes with elevated carbon dioxide concentrations, such as would be expected in the tracheal but not esophageal environment (Fig. 11-58). Any color change indicates tracheal placement; no color change indicates esophageal intubation.

✓ TRICKS OF THE TRADE

A memory aid for colorimetric devices is: yellow (yes, the tube is correctly placed); tan (think about it; the tube may not be properly placed); and purple (problem; the tube is not in the trachea).

Electronic devices can confirm successful tracheal tube placement within seconds of an intubation attempt, and subsequent tracheal dislodgement.[10] They use an infrared analyzer to measure the percentage of carbon dioxide gas at each phase of respiration (Fig. 11-59). The information is displayed in a digital waveform on the monitor or printout. Both devices may be useful as an indicator of circulation during some cardiac arrest situations because an increase in end-tidal carbon dioxide concentrations seems to be related to effective perfusion during external chest compression.[12]

? CRITICAL THINKING

Your patient is in full arrest so your ETCO₂ detector is inconclusive and you can't get the oxygen saturation monitor to work. You are not sure if you hear breath sounds clearly. What should you do?

NOTE

With very low cardiac output during cardiopulmonary resuscitation, the carbon dioxide detector may show no color change even when the ET tube is in the trachea. A second method (e.g., an esophageal detector) to confirm tube placement should be used.

Bulb- and Syringe-Type Esophageal Detectors

Esophageal detection devices (e.g., the Toomey syringe), are attached to the end of the ET tube (Fig. 11-60). They operate on the principle that the esophagus is a collapsible tube. As such, a vac-

uum will be created in the bulb device (after it is compressed) or when negative pressure is applied to the syringe device if the ET tube is in the esophagus. If the ET tube has been correctly placed in the trachea, the bulb device easily refills with air or the syringe device is easily aspirated after negative pressure is applied. Esophageal detection devices also can be used to verify correct placement of multilumen airways (described later in this chapter).

Pulse Oximetry

Pulse oximeters (Fig. 11-61) help in determining effective patient oxygenation by measuring the transmission of red and near-infrared light through arterial beds. Hemoglobin absorbs red and infrared light waves differently when it is bound with oxygen (oxyhemoglobin) than when it is not (reduced hemoglobin). Oxyhemoglobin absorbs more infrared than red light, and reduced hemoglobin absorbs more red than infrared light. Pulse oximetry reveals arterial saturation by measuring this difference.

The oximeter probe is placed on a thin tissue, such as a finger, toe, or ear lobe. One side of the probe emits wavelengths of light into the arterial bed. The other side detects the presence of red or infrared light. Using this balance of red and infrared colors, the oximeter calculates the oxygen saturation of the blood and displays it on the monitor screen.

The percentage of hemoglobin saturated with oxygen is denoted as Sa_{O_2} and depends on a number of factors, including P_{CO_2}, pH, temperature, and whether the hemoglobin is normal or altered. The lower range of normal for Sa_{O_2} is 93% to 95%. The

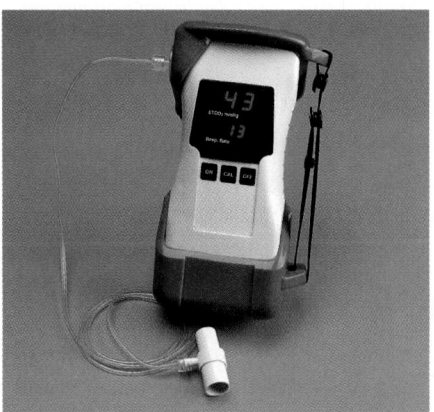

Fig. 11-59 Digital (or electronic) end-tidal CO_2 detector.

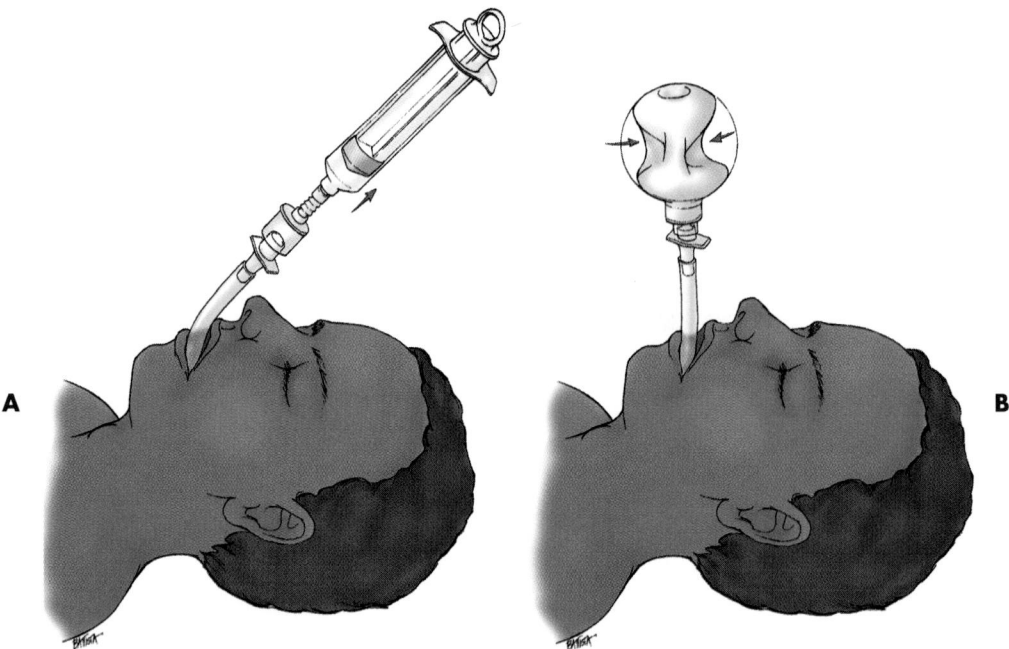

Fig. 11-60 Esophageal intubation detector. **A,** Syringe. **B,** Bulb. (From Shade B: *Mosby's EMT-Intermediate textbook,* St Louis, 1997, Mosby.)

upper range is 99% to 100%. Once the SaO_2 falls below 90% (corresponding to a PO_2 of 60 mm Hg), further decreases are associated with a marked decline in oxygen content (Box 11-8).

Because difficulties and inaccuracies may result from the use of pulse oximeters, paramedics should consider them as only another tool to assist in patient monitoring. Circumstances that may produce false readings include the following[13]:

- Dyshemoglobinemia (hemoglobin saturated with compounds other than oxygen [e.g., carbon monoxide, methemoglobinemia])
- Excessive ambient light (sunlight, fluorescent lights) on the oximeter's sensor probe
- Patient movement
- Hypotension
- Hypothermia/vasoconstriction
- Patient use of vasoconstrictive drugs
- Patient use of nail polish
- Jaundice

Laryngeal Mask Airway

The laryngeal mask airway (LMA) is an advanced airway control device that may be used in the prehospital setting when conventional ET intubation is unsuccessful, when access to the patient is limited, there is a possibility of unstable neck injury, or ap-

propriate positioning of the patient for tracheal intubation is impossible.[14] The LMA also allows ET intubation through the device, which allows easier placement of the ET tube.

> **NOTE**
>
> The LMA does not provide absolute protection against aspiration, however aspiration using this device is uncommon. A small portion of patients cannot be adequately ventilated with the LMA. The device is contraindicated in conscious patients and in those with an intact gag reflex.

Description and Method of Insertion

The LMA is available in several sizes (size 1 for neonates to size 5 for adults.) It consists of a proximal tube with standard adapters for connecting ventilatory devices. The tube is connected to a distal mask that is inflated by means of a pilot tube and balloon.

The LMA is inserted through the mouth into the pharynx. It is advanced until resistance is felt as the distal portion of the tube locates in the hypopharynx. When the device is properly inserted, the black line marked on the LMA rests midline against the patient's upper lip. Inflating the cuff seals the larynx and leaves distal opening of the tube just above

COMPARISON OF OXYGEN SATURATION AND PARTIAL PRESSURE (Po_2)

With 90% saturation, Po_2 drops to 60 mm Hg
With 75% saturation, Po_2 drops to 40 mm Hg
With 50% saturation, Po_2 drops to 27 mm Hg

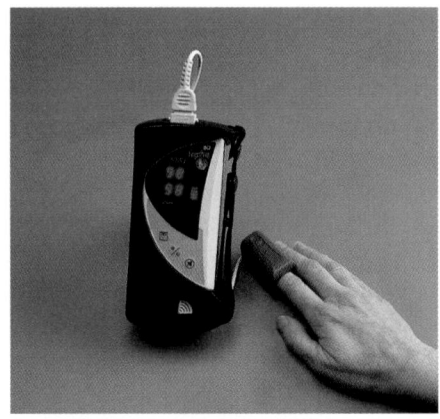

Fig. 11-61 Pulse oximeter.

the glottis, providing a clear and secure airway. After the pilot cuff is inflated, proper placement is confirmed by observing equal rise and fall of the chest, by ensuring bilateral breath sounds, and with end-tidal CO_2 detectors, esophageal detectors, and pulse oximetry monitoring (in a patient who has a perfusing rhythm). Use of the LMA requires special training and authorization from medical direction.

NOTE

The LMA may be difficult to maintain during patient movement, making it problematic to use during patient transport.

Necessary Equipment
- Water-soluble lubricant
- Syringes
- Bag-valve device
- Oxygen source and connecting tubing
- Suction equipment
- Stethoscope

Common Advantages
- Less skilled training or maintenance is required than for ET intubation
- Does not require laryngoscopy or visualization of the vocal cords
- Minimal spinal movement is required for insertion
- Allows for ET intubation through the LMA

Common Disadvantages
- The patient must be unresponsive without a gag reflex
- Not all patients can be adequately ventilated with the LMA
- The airway must be removed when the patient becomes responsive or agitated

- The airway should be replaced with an ET tube as soon as possible

Common Contraindications
- Presence of a gag reflex
- Caustic ingestion
- Esophageal trauma or disease

Multilumen Airways

Multilumen airways (e.g., the Esophageal Tracheal Combitube [ETC] and the pharyngeal tracheal lumen [PtL]), allow for either esophageal or tracheal insertion. They use a plastic tube with twin lumens that are separated by a partition wall. One tube resembles an ET tube and has an open distal end. The second tube is blocked by an obturator at the distal end. Both tubes use low-pressure balloons that provide a seal for either the trachea or esophagus, depending on placement. When inflated, the large pharyngeal balloon fills the space between the base of the tongue and the soft palate, anchoring the tube in position. The multilumen airway most commonly finds its way into the esophagus because of the stiffness and curve of the tube and the shape and the structure of the pharynx.

NOTE

Multimen airways should be considered an alternative method of airway control when conventional tracheal intubation is indicated but is unsuccessful or unavailable. The LMA and ETC (preferred over the PtL) provide superior ventilation compared with face masks in cardiac arrest.[14]

Insertion

Multilumen airways are inserted by gently guiding the device into the esophagus or trachea. (This insertion is accomplished without hyperextension or flexion of the patient's head and without visualization of the glottic opening.) The pharyngeal and distal balloons are then inflated, isolating the oropharynx above the upper balloon and the esophagus (or trachea) below the lower balloon. Ventilation is initially provided through the esophageal lumen (because of the high probability of esophageal placement after blind insertion). In this position, air passes into the pharynx and beyond the glottis into the trachea. Placement is confirmed by primary and secondary confirmation methods previously described. Figure 11-62 illustrates placement of the ETC airway.

If breath sounds and chest movement are absent with ventilation through the esophageal lumen, ventilation should be performed through the tracheal lumen without changing the position of the airway. Air passes through this lumen directly into the trachea. Placement is confirmed in the usual manner.

> **NOTE**
>
> Multilumen airways reduce but do not eliminate the risk of aspiration.

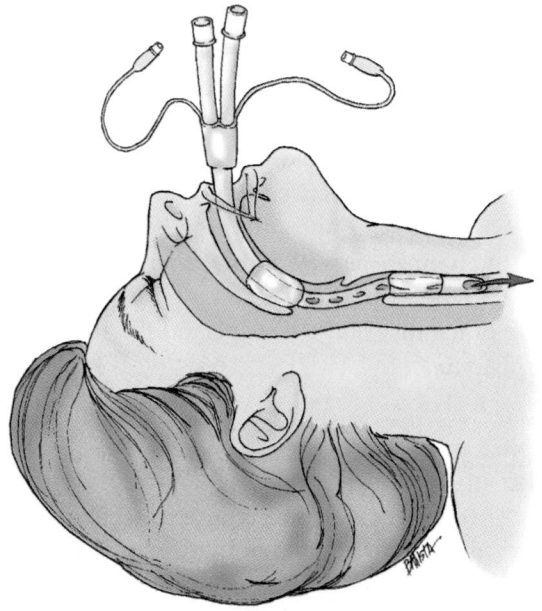

Fig. 11-62 Placement of the ETC airway. (From Shade B: *Mosby's EMT-Intermediate textbook,* St Louis, 1997, Mosby.)

Necessary Equipment

- Water-soluble lubricant
- Syringes
- BVM
- Oxygen source and connecting tubing
- Suction equipment
- Stethoscope

The various kinds of balloon system devices available share advantages, disadvantages, and contraindications. These common elements are described next:

Common Advantages

- Airways cannot be improperly placed.
- Less skilled training or maintenance is required than for endotracheal intubation.
- Minimal spinal movement is required for insertion.
- Suctioning is easily accomplished.

Common Disadvantages

- The patient must be unresponsive and without a gag reflex.
- The airway must be removed when the patient becomes responsive or agitated.
- Proper identification of tube location may be difficult, leading to ventilations through the wrong lumen.
- The trachea cannot be suctioned when the tube is in the esophagus.
- The airway should be replaced with an ET tube as soon as possible.

Common Contraindications

- Patients under 5 feet tall or younger than 14 years of age
- Caustic ingestion
- Esophageal trauma or disease
- Presence of a gag reflex

Pharmacological Adjuncts to Airway Management and Ventilation

Sedation is sometimes used in airway management and ventilation to reduce anxiety, induce amnesia, and decrease the gag reflex. Possible indications for use include combative patients, patients who require aggressive airway management but who are too alert to tolerate intubation, and agitated trauma patients. Classes of drugs that commonly are used for sedation in these situations include tranquilizers, barbiturates, benzodiazepines, and narcotics.

> **NOTE**
>
> Sedating a patient with a tenuous airway is dangerous because the patient may experience respiratory arrest. The paramedic should always consult with medical direction.

Paralytic Agents in Emergency Intubation

Paralysis for the purpose of emergency intubation involves the use of neuromuscular blocking drugs. They are indicated for use with combative patients (e.g., patients with head injury) who need to be intubated. These drugs are contraindicated in the following situations:

- Patients who will be difficult to ventilate (e.g., facial hair)
- Patients who will be difficult to intubate (e.g., short necks, obstructions)

> **NOTE**
>
> Neuromuscular blockers do not inhibit pain or seizure activity.

Pharmacology

As described in Chapter 8, neuromuscular blockers produce skeletal muscle paralysis by binding to the nicotinic receptor for acetylcholine (ACh) at the neuromuscular junction. To review, the neuromuscular junction is the point of contact between the nerve ending and the muscle fiber (see Chapter 6). When nerve impulses pass through this junction, ACh and other chemicals are released, causing the muscle to contract. The two types of neuromuscular blocking drugs are depolarizing agents and nondepolarizing agents.

Depolarizing agents substitute themselves into the neuromuscular junction and bind to the receptors for ACh. Because these drugs produce depolarization of the muscular membrane, they often lead to fasciculations (uncontrollable muscle twitching) and some muscular contractions. An example of a depolarizing agent is *succinylcholine* (Anectine).

Nondepolarizing agents bind to the receptors for ACh and block the uptake of ACh at the neuromuscular junction without initiating depolarization of the muscle membrane. Examples of nondepolarizing drugs include *vecuronium* (Norcuron) and *pancuronium* (Pavulon). These drugs have a longer onset and duration than depolarizing agents.

> **NOTE**
>
> **Succinylcholine** (Anectine) has a rapid onset of action and the briefest duration of action of all neuromuscular blocking drugs, making it the drug of choice for emergency endotracheal intubation.

> **NOTE**
>
> Because these blocking agents produce complete paralysis, ventilatory support must be provided and the efficacy of ventilation and oxygenation closely monitored. If the patient is conscious, explain the effects of the medication before administering it. Premedication with **atropine** should be strongly considered, particularly in the pediatric age group. Premedication with **lidocaine** (Xylocaine) may blunt any increase in intracranial pressure associated with intubation. Finally, **diazepam** (Valium), **etomidate** (Amidate), **midazolam** (Versed), or another sedative approved by medical direction should be used in any conscious patient undergoing neuromuscular blockade.

Rapid Sequence Intubation (RSI)

Rapid sequence intubation is a technique that involves the virtually simultaneous administration of a potent sedative agent and a neuromuscular blocking agent, usually *succinylcholine* (Anectine), for the purpose of ET intubation. RSI provides optimal intubation conditions while minimizing the risk of aspiration of gastric contents. RSI is indicated in the following situations[15]:

- Emergency intubation is warranted.
- The patient has a "full" stomach.
- Intubation is predicted to be successful (see the box on p. 423).
- If intubation fails, ventilation is predicted to be successful.

RSI is not indicated for patients in cardiac arrest or deeply comatose patients when immediate intubation is required. Relative contraindications include concern that intubation or mask ventilation

NOTE

The purpose of RSI is to avoid positive-pressure ventilation (in a patient who needs intubation and who is at risk of aspiration) until the ET tube is correctly placed in the trachea with the cuff inflated.

would be unsuccessful; significant facial or laryngeal edema, trauma, or distortion; or a spontaneously breathing patient who requires upper airway muscle tone and positioning (e.g., upper airway obstruction, epiglottitis).[16]

The central concept of RSI is to take the patient from the starting point (e.g., conscious, breathing) to a state of unconsciousness with complete neuromuscular paralysis and then to achieve intubation *without* interposed mechanical ventilation. The six steps of RSI (the six "Ps") are preparation, preoxygenation, pretreatment, paralysis (with sedation), placement of the tube, and postintubation management (Box 11-9). Each step is described below:

1. Preparation
   a. Assess the patient for difficulty of intubation (e.g., using the Mallampati score on p. 423).
   b. Prepare all drugs and equipment.
   c. Ensure one or more patent IV lines.
   d. Explain the procedure to the patient.
2. Preoxygenation (to be done simultaneously with preparation)

NOTE

RSI requires special training and authorization from medical direction. The effectiveness of RSI performed in the field should be monitored through a quality improvement process.

   a. Preoxygenate the patient with 100% oxygen for 5 minutes (an essential step of the "no-bagging" approach of RSI).
   b. Consider the use of a pulse oximeter.
3. Pretreatment (to be done 3 minutes before intubation)
   a. Consider *lidocaine* (Xylocaine) to blunt a rise in intracranial pressure and to prevent laryngospasm.
   b. Consider beta blockers or opioids to reduce sympathoadrenal response to intubation.
4. Paralysis (with sedation)
   a. Administer a sedative (per protocol) to produce unconsciousness, immediately followed by a rapid push of the neuromuscular blocker.

? CRITICAL THINKING

How will you determine if a patient needs more sedation after a paralytic has been administered?

   b. Perform Sellick's maneuver as the patient loses consciousness to prevent regurgitation. (Once neuromuscular blockade has been established, active vomiting cannot occur.)
   c. Do not initiate ventilations unless the patient's oxygenation saturation falls below 90%.
   d. Within 45 seconds of administration of *succinylcholine* (Anectine), the patient will be relaxed enough for intubation.
5. Placement
   a. Perform orotracheal intubation and confirm placement.
6. Postintubation management
   a. Secure the tube in place.
   b. Initiate mechanical ventilation.
   c. Monitor the patient continuously.

Translaryngeal Cannula Ventilation

Translaryngeal cannula ventilation (also known as *percutaneous transtracheal ventilation* and *needle cricothyrotomy*) may be valuable in the initial stabilization of a patient whose airway cannot be managed by manual measures and in patients who cannot be intubated by oral or nasal means. It is a temporary procedure to provide oxygenation when the airway is obstructed as a result of edema of the

SIGNS OF A POTENTIALLY DIFFICULT INTUBATION[9]

The potential difficulty of an intubation can be judged by the accessibility of the oropharynx. Visibility of the oropharynx ranges from complete visualization, including the tonsillar pillars (indicating an easy intubation) to no visualization at all, with the uvula pressed against the tongue (indicating a difficult intubation).

Other situations that indicate a potentially difficult intubation include the following:

- An immobilized trauma patient
- Children
- A short neck that makes visualization of the cords more difficult
- Prominent upper incisors that limit working space
- Receding mandible that may limit line of vision
- Limited jaw opening
- Limited cervical mobility
- Upper airway conditions (e.g., burns, neck injury, epiglottitis)
- Facial trauma
- Laryngeal trauma

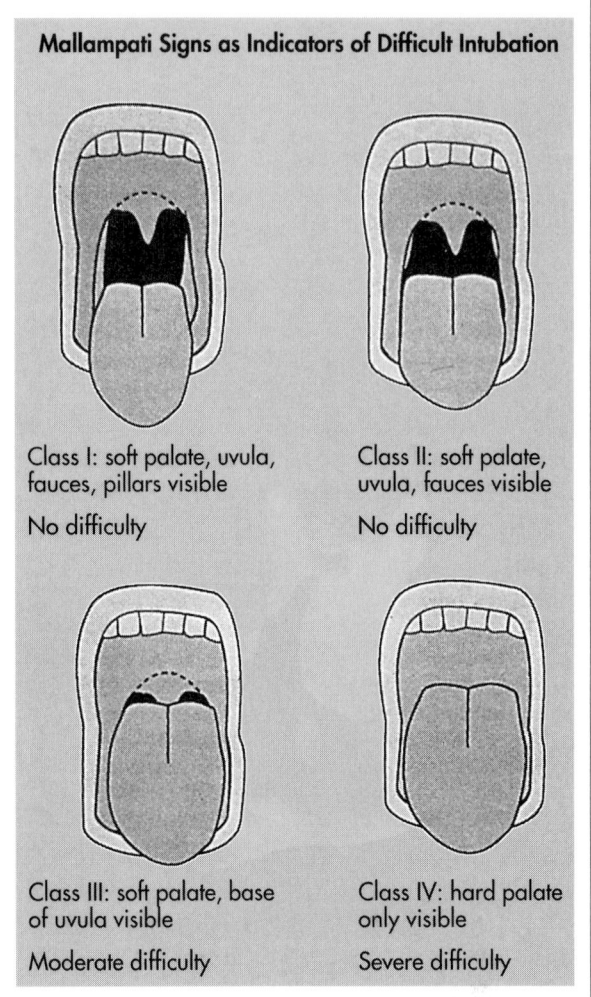

Mallampati Signs as Indicators of Difficult Intubation

Class I: soft palate, uvula, fauces, pillars visible
No difficulty

Class II: soft palate, uvula, fauces visible
No difficulty

Class III: soft palate, base of uvula visible
Moderate difficulty

Class IV: hard palate only visible
Severe difficulty

glottis, fracture of the larynx, or severe oropharyngeal hemorrhage. Translaryngeal cannula ventilation requires special training and authorization from medical direction.

Description

Translaryngeal cannula ventilation provides high-volume/high-pressure oxygenation of the lungs through cannulation of the trachea below the glottis. The procedure delivers a large volume of oxygen through a small port at high pressure to the lungs compared to other methods (50 psi versus 1 psi through a therapy regulator).

Necessary Equipment

- A 12- or 14-gauge over-the-needle catheter with a 5- or 10-mL syringe
- Alcohol or povidone-iodine swabs
- Adhesive tape or appropriate ties
- Pressure-regulating valve and pressure gauge attached to a high-pressure (30 to 60 psi) oxygen supply (Most oxygen tanks and regulators can provide 50 psi at 15 L/min or when opened to flush.)
- High-pressure tubing connecting the high-pressure regulating valve to a hand-operated release valve (5-foot tubing is recommended)

- A release valve connected by tubing to the catheter (this may be provided through a Y or T connector, through a three-way stopcock directly attached to the high-pressure tubing, or by cutting a hole in the oxygen line to provide a "whistle-stop" effect).

Technique

The following steps should be taken for translaryngeal cannula ventilation (Fig. 11-63):

1. Ensure that the patient is supine and the cricothyroid membrane has been identified. (If a spinal injury is suspected, in-line stabilization may be provided as for nasal and tracheal intubation.)

2. Stabilize the larynx using the thumb and middle finger of one hand. With the other hand, palpate the small depression below the thyroid cartilage (the "Adam's apple"), sliding the index finger down to locate the cricothyroid membrane.

? CRITICAL THINKING

What conditions could make the anatomic landmarks for translaryngeal cannulation or cricothyrotomy difficult to locate?

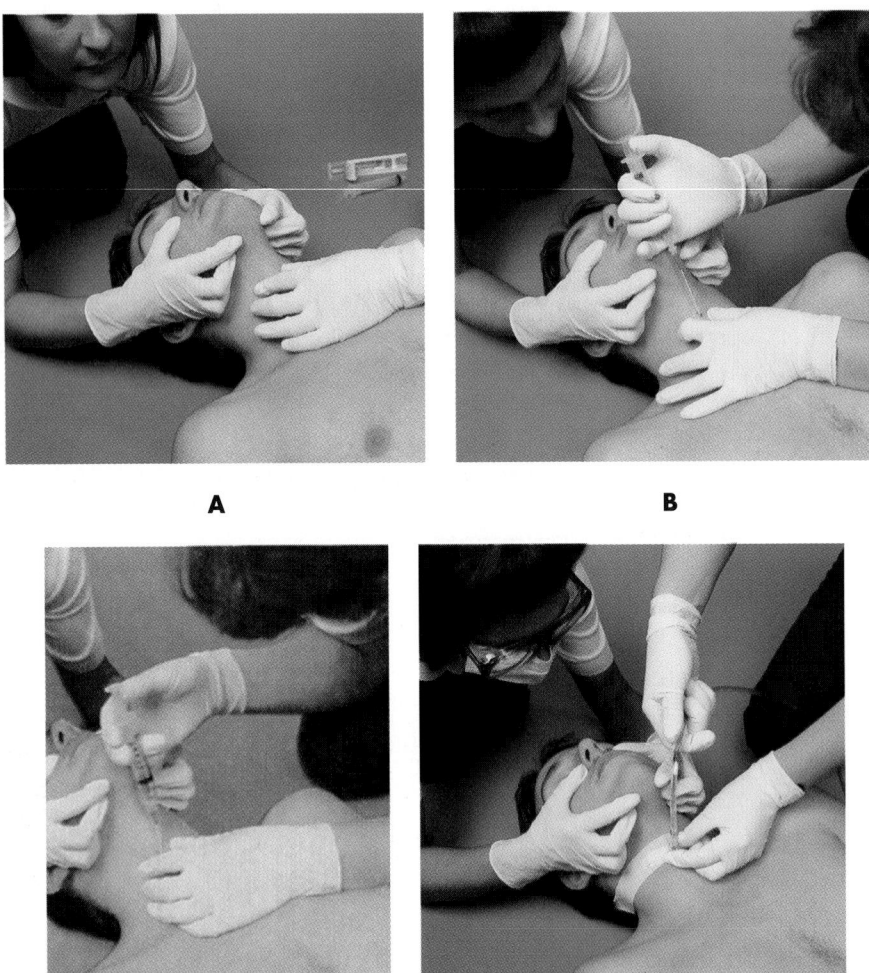

A

B

C

D

Fig. 11-63 A, Stabilize the larynx and identify the cricothyroid membrane. **B,** Insert the needle of the syringe downward through the midline of the membrane toward the carina. **C,** During insertion, apply negative pressure to the syringe. The entrance of air into the syringe indicates that the needle is in the trachea. **D,** After removing the needle and syringe, stabilize the catheter and connect the end of the oxygen tubing from the hub of the cannula to the oxygen regulator. Provide for a release valve.

3. Insert the needle of the syringe downward through the midline of the membrane at a 45- to 60-degree angle toward the patient's carina, applying negative pressure to the syringe during insertion (Fig. 11-64, *A*). The entrance of air into the syringe indicates that the needle is in the trachea.

4. Advance the catheter over the needle toward the carina and remove the needle and syringe (Fig. 11-64, *B*). Care must be taken not to kink the catheter when removing the needle and syringe.

5. Hold the hub of the catheter to prevent accidental dislodgment during the time required to provide ventilation. Connect the end of the oxygen tubing from the hub of the cannula to the oxygen regulator. Provide for a release valve as previously described.

When the release valve is closed, oxygen under pressure is introduced into the trachea. The pressure is adjusted to a level that allows adequate lung expansion. The patient's chest must be observed carefully and the release valve opened to allow for exhalation. The correct ratio of inflation to deflation varies, depending on whether upper airway obstruction is present. For an open upper airway, an inspiratory-to-expiratory ratio of 1 to 4 seconds is adequate. Ratios of approximately 1 to 8 seconds are needed to prevent barotrauma (injuries caused by excessive pressures [e.g., pneumothorax]) when the upper airway is obstructed.[17]

> **NOTE**
>
> Should the chest remain inflated during the period of exhalation, a proximal complete airway obstruction may be present and a longer expiratory time should be used. If this does not produce adequate deflation, a second large-bore catheter may be inserted through the cricothyroid membrane next to the first one. If the chest continues to remain distended, a cricothyrotomy should be performed.

Advantages

- Translaryngeal cannula ventilation is simple, inexpensive, and effective when properly performed.
- It requires minimal spinal manipulation.
- It is the least invasive of surgical procedures.
- It can be initiated quickly.

Disadvantages

- It is an invasive procedure.
- It requires constant monitoring.
- It requires "jet ventilation."
- It does not protect the airway.
- It does not allow for efficient elimination of carbon dioxide.
- It may adequately ventilate the patient's lungs for only 30 to 45 minutes.

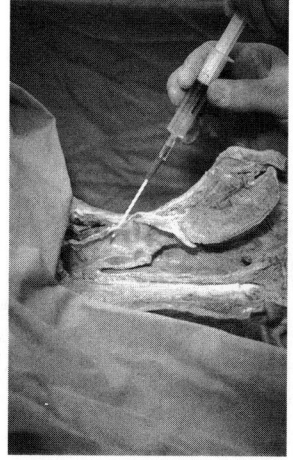 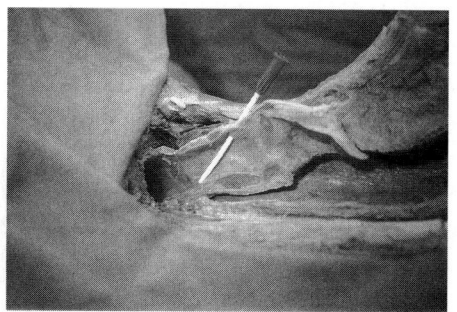

Fig. 11-64 Needle cricothyrotomy. **A,** Insert a large-bore catheter through the cricothyroid membrane, directing it caudally. Aspirate on the syringe as it is passed; when air is aspirated, the airway has been entered. **B,** Slide the catheter off the stylet into the larynx.

Possible Complications

- High pressure during ventilation and air entrapment may cause pneumothorax.
- Hemorrhage might occur at the insertion site, and the thyroid and esophagus might be perforated if the needle is advanced too far.
- It does not allow direct suctioning of secretions.
- Subcutaneous emphysema may occur.

Method of Removal

Because translaryngeal cannula ventilation is a temporary emergency procedure to allow time for other airway management techniques, removal should only follow successful orotracheal or nasotracheal intubation or commencement of a more definitive surgical airway, such as cricothyrotomy or tracheostomy. Removal entails withdrawing the catheter and dressing the wound.

Cricothyrotomy

Cricothyrotomy is a surgical procedure that allows rapid entrance to the airway through the cricothyroid membrane. The procedure can be performed quickly, is much faster and technically easier than a tracheostomy, and does not manipulate the cervical spine.

Description

Cricothyrotomy can provide ventilation and oxygenation for patients in whom airway control is not possible by other means. It should not be performed on patients who can be orally or nasally intubated. Although few situations require this surgical procedure, relative indications for cricothyrotomy include severe facial or nasal injuries that preclude oral or nasal intubation, massive midfacial trauma, possible spinal trauma preventing adequate ventilation, anaphylaxis, and chemical inhalation injuries. Like translaryngeal cannula ventilation, cricothyrotomy requires special training and authorization from medical direction.

Necessary Equipment

Commercially prepared cricothyrotomy kits are available through a number of manufacturers. If such a kit is not available, the following equipment is required:

- Scalpel blade
- 6 (preferred) or 7 ET tube or tracheostomy tube
- Antiseptic solution
- Oxygen source
- Suction device
- Bag-valve device

Technique

In patients suspected of having a spinal injury, in-line stabilization should be maintained throughout the procedure. If possible, the neck should be cleaned with alcohol or another antiseptic solution. The technique for performing the surgical procedure follows (Fig. 11-65):

1. Locate the anatomical landmarks of the neck and identify the cricothyroid membrane.
2. Make a 2-cm horizontal incision with the scalpel at the level of the cricothyroid membrane. (Some physicians may recommend a vertical skin incision rather than a horizontal one.)
3. Open the incision of the cricothyroid membrane by inserting the scalpel handle. Rotate it 90 degrees to allow placement of a 6 or 7 ET tube or tracheostomy tube that does not damage the larynx. The cuff should be inflated and the tube securely tied.

> **NOTE**
>
> Use of a smaller diameter ET tube may facilitate successful placement. The paramedic should be careful not to advance the tube beyond a few centimeters once in the airway to avoid mainstem intubation.

4. Provide ventilation by a bag-valve device with the highest available oxygen concentration.
5. Determine adequacy of ventilation through bilateral auscultation and observation of rise and fall of the chest.

Possible Complications

- Prolonged execution time
- Hemorrhage

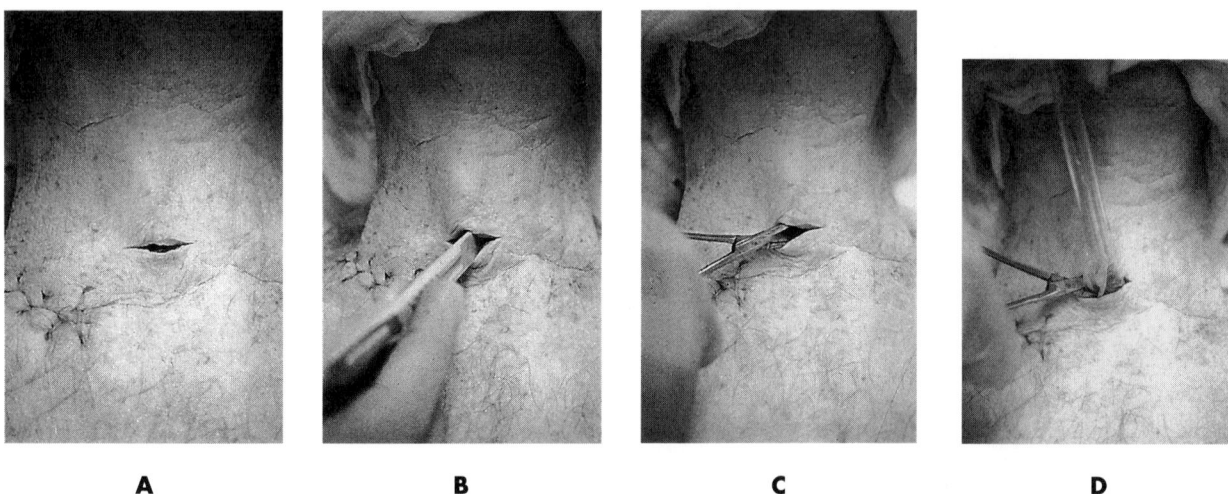

A   B   C   D

Fig. 11-65 A, Make an incision through the cricothyroid membrane. **B,** Open the hole by twisting the handle of a scalpel in it or **C,** by opening it with a clamp. **D,** Insert the ET tube.

- Aspiration
- Possible misplacement
- False passage
- Perforation of the esophagus
- Injury to the vocal cords and carotid and jugular vessels lateral to the incision (the patient must be immobilized)
- Subcutaneous emphysema

Contraindications

- Inability to identify anatomical landmarks
- Underlying anatomical abnormality (e.g., tumor, subglottic stenosis)

- Tracheal transsection
- Acute laryngeal disease caused by trauma or infection
- Small child under 10 years of age (In these patients, inserting a 12- to 14-gauge catheter over the needle may be safer than a cricothyrotomy.)

Method of Removal

The removal of adjuncts used during an emergency cricothyrotomy should not be attempted in the prehospital setting.

S U M M A R Y

- A thorough understanding of the respiratory system and mastery of airway management and ventilation are important aspects of emergency care.

- The two phases of respiration are (1) external respiration, or the transfer of oxygen and carbon dioxide between the inspired air and pulmonary capillaries, and (2) internal respiration, or the transfer of oxygen and carbon dioxide between the peripheral blood capillaries and the tissue cells.

- The mixture of gases that compose the atmosphere exerts a combined partial pressure of 100%, or 760 mm Hg at sea level. The amount of oxygen that composes atmospheric gas is 21%; carbon dioxide 0.03 %; and nitrogen 78%.

- As inspired gas enters the lungs, the respiratory system brings oxygen to the blood and removes carbon dioxide.

- The 200 mL of oxygen that crosses the alveoli each minute is added to the quantity of oxygen already in the pulmonary capillaries and then transported to the body tissues by the circulatory system. After the body cells use the necessary oxygen, the oxygen remaining in the blood returns to the heart and lungs. This exchange of oxygen and carbon dioxide is accomplished by the passive process of diffusion.

- Respiration is controlled at any instant by several factors. Breathing is primarily an involuntary process, but within limits the pattern of respiration can be consciously altered. The inspiratory muscles are composed of skeletal muscle and cannot contract unless they are stimulated by nerve impulses. The activities of the respiratory centers are determined by changes in oxygen and carbon dioxide concentrations and by the pH of the body fluids.

- The elderly cannot compensate effectively for alterations in airway and ventilation. Pulmonary changes that occur as a result of aging decrease vital capacity and increase physiological dead space. PO_2 also tends to be gradually lower as age increases.

- Causes of inadequate ventilation include upper airway obstruction and aspiration by inhalation. Establishing and maintaining a patent airway in any patient who has respiratory compromise from any cause is the most important lifesaving maneuver and should always be a first-order priority of patient care.

- Essential parameters of airway evaluation include rate, regularity, and effort and recognition of airway problems that might indicate respiratory distress.

- The most common form of oxygen used in the prehospital setting is pure oxygen gas, delivered in liters per minute (LPM). Therapy regulators are used to deliver a safe pressure of oxygen to patients. Flowmeters control the amount of oxygen delivered to the patient. Several oxygen delivery devices can be used to provide supplemental oxygen to prehospital patients who have spontaneous respirations. They are the nasal cannula, simple face mask, partial rebreather mask, nonrebreather mask, and Venturi mask.

- There are several methods by which patient ventilation can be provided in the prehospital setting. These methods include rescue breathing (mouth-to-mouth, mouth-to-nose, mouth-to-stoma), mouth-to-mask breathing, use of bag-valve devices, and automatic transport ventilators.

- Emergency airway management should progress rapidly from the least to the most invasive modality. Manual techniques for airway management include the head-tilt chin-lift method, the jaw-thrust, and the jaw-thrust without head-tilt.

- Suction catheters are used to clear the air passages of secretions and debris.

- Gastric decompression for gastric distention or emesis control can be accomplished through nasogastric or orogastric decompression.

- Mechanical devices for airway management include the nasal airway, oral airway, endotracheal intubation, digital intubation, nasotracheal intubation, laryngeal mask airway, multilumen airways, translaryngeal cannula ventilation, and cricothyrotomy.

- Rapid sequence intubation (RSI) is a technique that involves the virtually simultaneous administration of a potent sedative agent and a neuromuscular blocking agent for the purpose of ET intubation.

- Anatomical differences in the pediatric airway must be considered when managing a child's airway. Specifically, the child's upper airway structures have significantly different proportions and orientation to each other relative to the adult airway. Smaller bag-valve devices are needed for infants and children to reduce the chances of overinflation and subsequent barotrauma.

- Three adjuncts can often aid in determining correct ET placement. These are end-tidal carbon dioxide detectors, pulse oximeters, and esophageal detector devices.

■ REFERENCES

1. American Heart Association: *Basic life support for healthcare providers*, Dallas, 1997, The Association.
2. National Safety Council, *Injury facts*, Chicago, 1999, The Council.
3. Tintinalli J et al: *Emergency medicine: a comprehensive study guide*, ed 2, New York, 1988, McGraw-Hill.
4. American Heart Association: Guidelines 2000 for cardiopulmonary resuscitation and emergency cardiovascular care, International Consensus on Science, *Circulation* 102(8):37, 2000.
5. American Heart Association: *Advanced cardiac life support*, Dallas, 1997, The Association.
6. American Heart Association: Guidelines 2000 for cardiopulmonary resuscitation and emergency cardiovascular care, International Consensus on Science, *Circulation* 102(8):267, 2000.
7. American Heart Association: *Pediatric advanced life support*, Dallas, 1997, American Heart Association.
8. American Heart Association: Guidelines 2000 for cardiopulmonary resuscitation and emergency cardiovascular care, International Consensus on Science, *Circulation* 102(8):96, 2000.
9. American Heart Association: Guidelines 2000 for cardiopulmonary resuscitation and emergency cardiovascular care, International Consensus on Science, *Circulation* 102(8):300, 2000.
10. American Heart Association: Guidelines 2000 for cardiopulmonary resuscitation and emergency cardiovascular care, International Consensus on Science, *Circulation* 102(8):101, 2000.
11. American College of Surgeons: *Upper airway management: advanced trauma life support*, Chicago, 1985, The College.
12. Garnet R et al: End-tidal carbon dioxide monitoring during cardiopulmonary resuscitation, *JAMA* 257(4):1379, 1987.
13. Mackreth B: Assessing pulse oximetry in the field, *JEMS* 15(6):56, 1990.
14. American Heart Association: Guidelines 2000 for cardiopulmonary resuscitation and emergency cardiovascular care, International Consensus on Science, *Circulation* 102(8):98, 2000.
15. Rosen P, Barkin R: *Emergency medicine: concepts and clinical practice*, ed 4, St Louis, 1998, Mosby.
16. American Heart Association: Guidelines 2000 for cardiopulmonary resuscitation and emergency cardiovascular care, International Consensus on Science, *Circulation* 102(8):302, 2000.
17. Stothert J et al: High pressure transtracheal ventilation: the use of large-gauge intravenous-type catheters in the totally obstructed airway, *Am J Emerg Med* 8:184, 1990.

Division Three ⟶

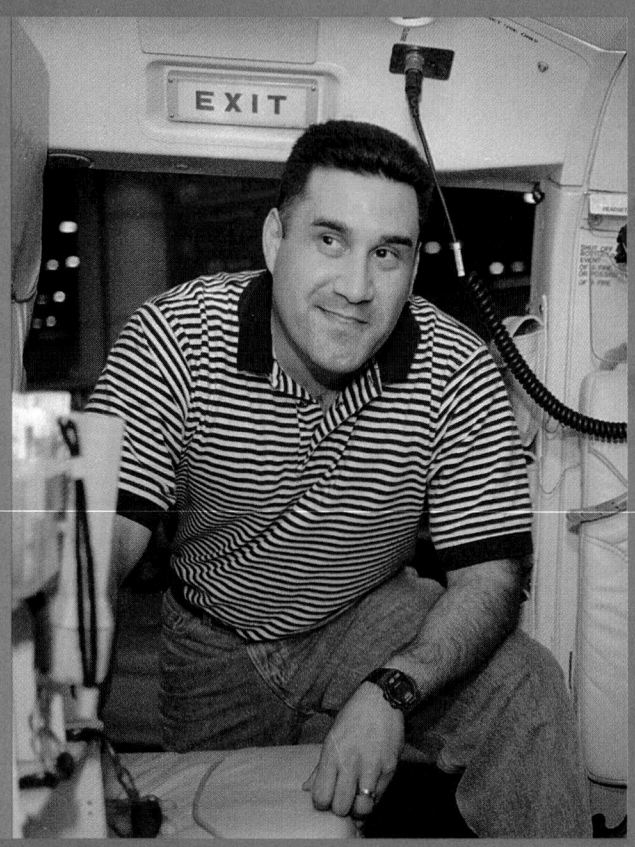

Alberto Vazquez, EMT-P
Moore County EMS
Fayetteville,
North Carolina

"One time a whole platoon of guys got hit by lightning. We had to do all the triage and assess the scene. Later, I stopped and thought how that wasn't a 'normal' situation—but at the time you don't realize what is normal and what's not. You just do your job."

Patient Assessment

IN THIS DIVISION

12 History Taking

OBJECTIVES

Upon completion of this chapter, the paramedic student will be able to:

1. **Describe the purpose of effective history taking in prehospital patient care.**

2. **List components of the patient history as defined by the Department of Transportation.**

3. **Outline effective patient interviewing techniques to facilitate history taking.**

4. **Identify strategies to manage special challenges in obtaining a patient history.**

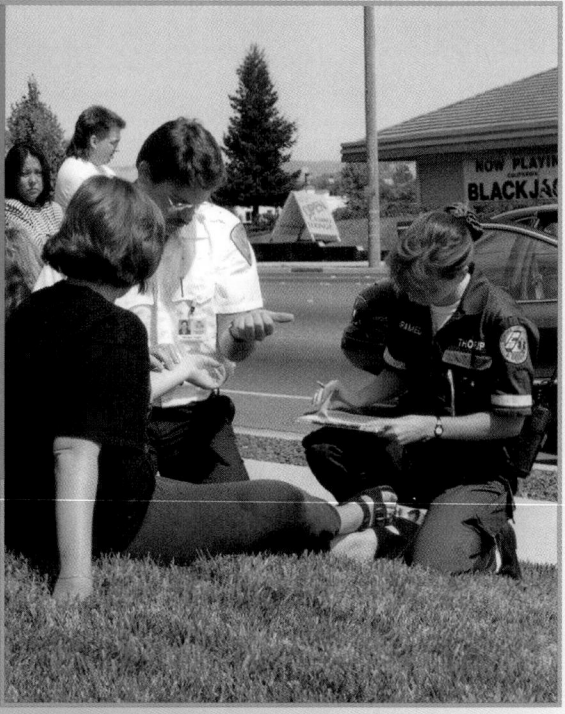

History taking *refers to information gathered during an interview with a patient. It provides an account of medical and social occurrences in a patient's life and environmental factors that may have a bearing on the patient's condition. Obtaining a patient history provides structure to patient assessment and often is essential to establish priorities in patient care.*

KEY TERMS

chief complaint: A patient's primary complaint.

current health status: Focuses on the patient's current state of health, environmental conditions, and personal habits.

family history: Illness or disease in a patient's family or family's background that may be relevant to the patient complaint.

history taking: Information gathered during the patient interview.

present illness: Identifies the chief complaint and provides a full, clear, chronological account of the symptoms.

significant past medical history: A patient's medical background that may offer insight into the patient's current problem.

Content of the Patient History

The patient history is composed of several components—each of which has a specific purpose. These components provide a "snapshot" of patients and their condition. Box 12-1 lists the components of the patient history as defined by the Department of Transportation's EMT-Paramedic National Standard Curriculum.[1]

> **NOTE**
>
> This chapter provides an overview of history taking. Other methods that can be used to obtain a comprehensive patient history are presented throughout this text by subject matter.

Techniques of History Taking

As emphasized in Chapter 10, the paramedic should "set the stage" for a good paramedic-patient encounter by establishing a favorable first impression and by making the environment conducive to free-flow communication. The paramedic should do the following:

- Establish a professional demeanor with the patient.
- Ensure patient comfort and provide a safe environment.

BOX 12-1

CONTENT OF THE PATIENT HISTORY

Date and Time
Identifying Data
    Age
    Sex
    Race
    Birthplace
    Occupation
Source of Referral
    Patient referral
    Referral by others
Source of History
    Patient
    Family
    Friends
    Police
    Others
Reliability
    Variable (memory, trust, motivation)
    Determined at the end of the evaluation
Chief Complaint
    Main part of history
    The one or more symptoms for which the patient
        is seeking medical care
Present Illness
    Identifies the chief complaint
    Provides a chronological account of the patient's
        symptoms
Past History
Current Health Status
Review of Body Systems

- Greet the patient by name or surname and avoid demeaning terms (e.g., "Granny" or "Hon").
- Avoid entering the patient's personal space.
- Inquire about the patient's feelings.
- Be sensitive to the patient's feelings and experiences.
- Watch for signs of uneasiness.
- Use language that is appropriate and easily understood.

- Ask open-ended questions and direct questions (if needed).
- Use therapeutic communications techniques.

Opening questions may incorporate facilitation, reflection, clarification, empathetic responses, confrontation, interpretation, and asking patients about their feelings (Box 12-2). These methods should use the techniques of therapeutic communications described in Chapter 10.

Chief Complaint

The **chief complaint** is the patient's primary complaint. It is the main part of the patient's health history and usually is the reason for the EMS response. The complaint may be verbal (e.g., complaint of chest pain) or nonverbal (e.g., pain or distress expressed by a facial grimace). Most chief complaints are characterized by pain, abnormal function, a change in the patient's normal state, or an unusual observation made by the patient (e.g., heart palpitations). The paramedic should be aware that a chief complaint may be misleading or that a problem may be more serious than the patient's chief complaint may present. For example, the patient who has fallen down a flight of steps may complain of an injured ankle, but physical examination may reveal suspected internal injuries. After determining the chief complaint (and stabilizing any life-threatening situations), the paramedic should obtain a history of the present illness and any significant medical history.

? CRITICAL THINKING

What illnesses or injuries could cause a chief complaint of confusion?

History of Present Illness

The **present illness** identifies the chief complaint and provides a full, clear, and chronological account of the symptoms. Obtaining a thorough history of the present illness requires skill both in asking appropriate questions related to the chief complaint and in interpreting the patient's response to those questions. For example, a patient's complaints of low back pain suggest a muscle strain. During direct questioning in the interview, however, he reveals history of a burning sensation with urination and a low-grade fever for the past several days, suggesting a urinary tract infection or renal stones. Thus, the history of the present illness may be more important than the obvious chief complaint. The mnemonic *OPQRST* helps define the patient's complaint by focusing on essential elements of assessment (Box 12-3). Using this memory device will

BOX 12-2

TECHNIQUES FOR OPENING QUESTIONS

Facilitation

Your posture, actions, or words should encourage the patient to say more.

Maintain eye contact.

Use phrases, such as "go on," "I'm listening," to encourage the patient to continue talking.

Reflection

Repeating, or "echoing," the patient's words to encourage additional responses usually will not bias the patient's story or interrupt the patient's train of thought.

Clarification

Ask questions to better understand ambiguous statements or words.

Empathetic Responses

Use therapeutic communications techniques to interpret the patient's feelings.

Confrontation

Some issues or responses may require confronting patients about their feelings.

Interpretation

You may need to make an inference from the patient's responses. (Interpretation goes beyond confrontation.)

Ask About the Patient's Feelings

Use therapeutic communications techniques to encourage patients to explain how they feel.

NOTE

The paramedic should take notes while obtaining the health history. Most patients realize that it is difficult to remember all details and are comfortable with note taking.

help lead the paramedic through a thorough sequence of questions to better understand the chief complaint.

Significant Past Medical History

After gaining a clear understanding of the patient's chief complaint, the paramedic should gather other **significant past medical history** (e.g., diabetes, cardiac, or respiratory disorders) that may offer additional insight into the patient's current problem. Important past medical history information may include the following:

- General state of health
- Medications and allergies
- Childhood illnesses
- Adult illnesses
- Psychiatric illnesses
- Accidents and injuries
- Surgeries
- Hospitalizations

TRICKS OF THE TRADE

Body piercing has become increasingly popular. When assessing your patient, be alert for pierced tongues, which can cause airway and speech problems.

A variety of mnemonics or memory devices are used to remember relevant questions for gathering medical history. One example is the *SAMPLE Sur-*

vey (Box 12-4). Although the depth and focus of the patient interview are based on the particular episode, the paramedic should gather as much information as possible at the scene and during transport to the hospital.

NOTE

Using the results of questions to think about associated problems and body system changes related to the patient's complaint is known as *clinical reasoning*.

Current Health Status

Current health status focuses on the patient's current state of health, environmental conditions, and personal habits (Box 12-5). Information regarding allergies, medications, last oral intake, and family history are especially important to the patient's current health status. Patients with abdominal pain also should be questioned regarding their last menstrual period (in female patients who are of childbearing age) and last bowel movement. Finally, events that occurred before the emergency also should be identified.

Allergies

Although few emergency medications produce an allergic reaction, information regarding allergies is important and useful to others involved in the patient's care. For example, the patient may be sensitive to tetanus prophylaxis, antibiotics, radiographic contrast medium, and other drugs administered during treatment. Allergies to food and other substances may

---

BOX 12-3

OPQRST MNEMONIC

O (Onset/Origin):	What were you doing when the pain started? Do you have a history of this problem?
P (Provokes):	What provokes the symptoms? What makes the symptoms better? What makes it worse?
Q (Quality):	What does the pain feel like? Is it sharp, dull, burning, or tearing?
R (Region):	Where is the symptom? Where does it go? Is it in one or more areas?
S (Severity):	On a scale of 1 to 10, with 1 being the least and 10 being the worst, what number would you assign your pain or discomfort?
T (Time):	How long have you had this symptom? When did it start? When did it end? How long did it last?

BOX 12-4

ELEMENTS OF THE SAMPLE SURVEY

S:	Signs and symptoms
A:	Allergies
M:	Medications
P:	Past medical history
L:	Last meal or oral intake
E:	Events before the emergency

BOX 12-5

PERSONAL HABITS AND ENVIRONMENTAL CONDITIONS

Personal Habits

Tobacco use
Alcohol, other drugs and related substances
Diet
Screening tests
Immunizations
Sleep patterns
Exercise and leisure activities
Use of safety measures
Home situation, spouse, or significant other person
Physical abuse or violence
Sexual history
Daily life
Important experiences
Religious beliefs
Patient outlook

Environmental

Home conditions: housing; cleanliness; temperature; economic condition; pets and their health
Occupation: description of past and present work; exposure to heat, cold, and industrial toxins
Travel: exposure to contagious diseases; residence in tropics; water and milk supply; and other possible sources of infection
Military record: geographical areas; exposure to chemicals

---

also offer valuable information about the patient's condition. If the patient is unconscious or unable to converse, the paramedic should look for medical alert information and question family members or friends about the patient's allergies.

NOTE

Many persons have a life-threatening allergy to latex—a common substance found in many EMS emergency care equipment.

? CRITICAL THINKING

What would you do if you couldn't recognize the names or indications for the patient's home medicines?

Medications

The paramedic should ask if the patient takes any medications on a regular basis and, if so, for what reasons. The patient's compliance with a medication regimen also should be ascertained if possible. The medication history may provide clues to the chief complaint. For example, a diabetic patient

---

✓ TRICKS OF THE TRADE

When obtaining a medication history, don't forget to ask about herbs and other over-the-counter medications. Just because they are available, over-the-counter doesn't mean that they are safe. Some medications may have interactions with the patient's regular prescribed medications.

---

may have taken her insulin but eaten irregularly. Other examples include a patient with chest pain who takes various cardiac drugs, an irrational patient who takes prescribed sedatives, and a trauma patient who takes blood-thinning drugs. Although the patient's medication history may not always be relevant to the present problem, it can indicate potential problems that may be encountered during the patient care episode.

Last Oral Intake

The time of the last meal or fluid consumption is important when considering potential airway problems in a patient who loses consciousness or begins to deteriorate. Determining the patient's last oral intake also may help rule out problems such as food poisoning and food allergies. For example, symptoms of certain types of food poisoning do not usually appear for several hours after ingestion. In contrast, patients who are sensitive to certain food substances, such as peanut oil or shellfish, would develop an allergic reaction immediately after eating.

> **NOTE**
>
> The time of the patient's last oral intake helps determine the appropriateness of surgery. Surgery for a patient who has consumed food or drink within the previous 6 to 8 hours generally is delayed if possible because stomach contents may be aspirated during induction of anesthesia. If immediate surgery is indicated after recent oral intake, a nasogastric tube is inserted to evacuate the stomach.

Family History

Family history of illness or disease may be relevant to the patient complaint. The paramedic should establish whether there is a family history of heart disease, high blood pressure, cancer, tuberculosis, stroke, diabetes, kidney disease, current contagious illness, or other ailments. The presence or absence of hereditary diseases such as hemophilia or sickle cell anemia also should be established during the patient interview.

> **NOTE**
>
> Through experience, the paramedic will develop a "personal line" of questioning to further analyze a patient's particular symptom.

Last Menstrual Period

The paramedic should obtain a menstrual history when interviewing female patients between the ages of 12 and 55 years who have abdominal pain. This line of questioning may prompt the patient to discuss other significant symptoms such as vaginal discharge, bleeding, and pregnancy history. The patient's response should determine the need to pursue additional questions regarding contraceptive use, venereal disease, urinary tract infections, and ectopic pregnancy (see Chapter 39).

Last Bowel Movement

The paramedic should question a patient regarding bowel habits to determine if they have been normal or abnormal. If a patient with abdominal pain describes a recent history of diarrhea, constipation, or bloody bowel movements, this information will be important to the receiving physician as the patient is assessed for bowel obstruction, dehydration, or lower gastrointestinal bleeding. During this time, the paramedic also should ask the patient about any symptoms of abnormal urinary function, such as blood in the urine, urethral discharge, pain or burning with urination, frequent urination, or the inability to void.

Events Before the Emergency

The patient and/or bystanders should be questioned about events or actions that may have occurred before the emergency. For example, was a fainting episode preceded by exertion or straining? Did a loss of consciousness occur before or after a fall? The paramedic should attempt to correlate any event with the progression of an illness or injury.

Getting More Information

With experience, paramedics will develop communication skills that will allow them to get more complete information about a patient's illness or injury. By obtaining more information about a patient's symptom or complaint, paramedics will be able to use clinical reasoning to evaluate associated problems and possible effects on body systems. Defining the attributes of a symptom (Box 12-6) generally requires the paramedic to ask direct questions and may involve obtaining a history regarding sensitive topics such as alcohol or other drug use, physical abuse or violence, and sexual issues.

Special Challenges

History taking often presents special challenges. Each patient is unique, and each patient encounter will be slightly different from all others. The paramedic must be able to quickly adapt to the special requirements of each encounter so that the necessary information can be obtained quickly. Some challenges that commonly affect history taking are listed in the following paragraphs.

BOX 12-6

ATTRIBUTES OF A SYMPTOM

Location
    Where is it?
    Does it radiate?
Its Quality
    What is it like?
    Can you describe it to me?
Its Quantity or Severity
    How bad is it?
    Quantify the pain on a 1 to 10 scale.
Its Timing
    When did it start?
    How long does it last?
The Setting in which It Occurs
    Emotional response
    Environmental factors
    Factors that make it better or worse
    Associated manifestations

Silence

Silence is often uncomfortable and has many meanings and uses. For example, patients may use silence to collect thoughts, remember details, or decide whether they trust the paramedic. Silence also can effectively diffuse an emotionally tense event. The paramedic should stay alert for nonverbal clues of distress or anxiety (e.g., worried expression, loss of eye contact), which often precede a silent period during the patient encounter. As a rule, when patients are ready to talk again, they will express feelings more clearly.

NOTE

A patient's silence also may be secondary to a paramedic's lack of sensitivity, understanding, or compassion. An appropriate and caring "bedside manner" is essential to good patient care.

Overly Talkative Patients

Interviewing overly talkative patients can be frustrating when there is a limited amount of time to obtain a health history. Although there are no per-

fect solutions in these situations, the following techniques may be helpful:

- Accept a less comprehensive history.
- Give the patient "free rein" for the first several minutes.
- Ask questions that invite brief "yes" or "no" answers when appropriate.
- Summarize the patient's comments frequently.
- Refocus the discussion as needed.

? CRITICAL THINKING

What single question would you ask a patient to identify the priority chief complaint when they have given you a list of multiple problems?

Patients with Multiple Symptoms

Some patients (especially older patients) have a longer medical history because of age, chronic illness, and medication use. In addition, many older patients are likely to suffer from concurrent illnesses. The paramedic should anticipate a longer interview and use the techniques presented in Chapter 10 to help patients with multiple symptoms "focus" on the most relevant aspects of the chief complaint.

Anxious Patients

It is normal for the patient, family members, and bystanders to be anxious in an emergency situation. The paramedic should be sensitive to nonverbal clues of anxiety and should be supportive in a calm and confident approach. The professional and car-

✓ TRICKS OF THE TRADE

When assessing a patient, don't forget to think about what is on the patient's mind. In a car crash, for example, the patient may be worried about insurance, whose fault the crash was, where the car will be towed, getting a rental car, and how this event will affect the rest of his or her life. "Everything is going to be okay" is never an appropriate response.

ing attitude of the paramedic often will help reduce the patient's anxiety.

False Reassurance

Providing false reassurance (e.g., "it's all right" or "everything's going to be okay") may be tempting for the paramedic as a way to comfort an ill or injured patient. Early reassurance or "over-reassurance" also should be avoided until it can be provided with confidence. False reassurances may block open communications between the paramedic and the patient. Appropriate verbal reassurances in most patient-care situations include the following:

- There is hope (when appropriate).
- The paramedic is listening.
- Care is available.
- The patient will be treated with dignity and respect.
- The patient's medical condition is understood.

Anger and Hostility

Like anxious behavior, anger and hostility are natural responses in some emergency situations. The paramedic should expect these reactions at times to be displaced toward the EMS crew. Although personal and scene safety must always be ensured, anger and hostility toward the patient is never appropriate. Maintaining a calm manner, demonstrating confidence, setting limits on acceptable behavior, and attempting to calm the patient is the most effective approach.

Intoxication

Patients who are intoxicated with alcohol or other drugs should be managed with caution because their behavior may be unpredictable. Intoxicated patients should not be challenged or aggravated. As in managing patients who are angry or hostile, the

> **NOTE**
>
> A patient who appears intoxicated may be suffering from medical illness or an injury that mimics an inebriated or drug-induced state.

paramedic must ensure personal and scene safety and establish limits for acceptable behavior. To ensure scene safety, assistance from law enforcement personnel should be requested when necessary.

Crying

Crying can reduce tension and may help reestablish the patient's emotional stability during an emergency. If crying is excessive or uncontrollable, the paramedic should hold the patient's hand (if appropriate) and use direct eye contact to help control the crying. Reducing exhaustive crying conserves energy and promotes comfort.

> **NOTE**
>
> The paramedic should show compassion for a crying patient. Many patients use crying as a way to express very strong emotions. Impatience often will worsen the crying episode.

Depression

Communicating with a depressed patient can be difficult. There are many types and causes of depression (see Chapter 38). The depression seen in an emergency event often is the result of a moderate-to-high level of anxiety and may be enhanced by alcohol or substance use. The paramedic should use the communication techniques previously described for anxious patients. If possible, the seriousness of the patient's depressed state should be identified. A physician's evaluation is encouraged.

Sexually Attractive or Seductive Patients

Paramedics and patients may be sexually attracted to each other. The paramedic should recognize these feelings as normal, but they should not affect professional behavior. If a patient becomes seductive or makes sexual advances, the paramedic should firmly set limits of acceptable behavior and make it clear that the patient relationship is professional. As discussed in Chapter 10, providing same-sex care often is the best practice. If this is not possible, an additional caregiver (or other chaperone) should remain with the patient.

Confusing Behavior or Histories

Because emergencies are often emotionally charged events, the paramedic should be prepared to encounter relatively confusing historical information or inappropriate or abnormal behavior. Factors that may contribute to these situations include mental illness, delirium, dementia, drug use, illness, and injury. Although identifying a pattern of patient behavior is difficult, the paramedic should try to identify one (e.g., signs and symptoms consistent with a particular disorder) and attempt to lead the patient in an appropriate line of questioning.

Developmental Disabilities

The paramedic should not overlook the aptitude of patients with developmental disabilities to provide adequate information. These patients should be interviewed just like other patients, using easily understood words and phrases. Obvious omissions in the patient's answers indicate the need for additional questioning posed in a rephrased or clarified format. If the patient has severe mental retardation, the paramedic should attempt to obtain information from family or friends (see Chapter 45).

Communication Barriers

As discussed in Chapter 10, barriers to communication may result from social or cultural differences and from sight, speech, or hearing impairments. The paramedic should find assistance if possible. Family members, translators, and those with special training in communicating with the blind or the deaf may be helpful in these situations.

Talking with Family and Friends

Because friends and family are often at the scene of an emergency, they should be considered a reliable source of information when the patient cannot provide all necessary information because of illness or injury. If family or friends are unavailable and addi-

tional patient information is needed, the paramedic should try to locate a third party (e.g., a neighbor) who can help supply the missing data.

✓ TRICKS OF THE TRADE

Expect older adults to be slower in answering questions. They tend to put more emphasis on words and will choose them carefully.

There is an old saying in medicine: "You can't find a fever if you don't take a temperature." This means that you have to investigate your patient's complaint. This is "Columbo" medicine.

Ask only one question at a time. The "right question" will yield valuable results. As a rule, your patient is your best historian.

The reason you were dispatched to the scene may not be the "real" reason you were called. Listen carefully to what the patient tells you. For example, did the patient with a broken arm fall over the pet or did she fall because she couldn't see the pet? If you ignore the real reason you were called, the patient may suffer consequences in the days to come.

There's an old saying in medicine: "When you hear the sound of galloping hoofs, think horses, not zebras." This means that you should look for the obvious, not the obscure.

If you think the patient may be a member of a gang and the emergency is gang-related, it is in your best interest not to cut their clothing (their "colors") in public because this is a sign of disrespect. If possible, move the patient to the ambulance or explain why you need to the cut the clothing; generally, the patient and his friends will agree.

Sometimes it isn't the patient who needs your care as much as the family needs respite from whatever they are facing. Caring for a bed-ridden family member who can't feed herself, who soils herself, or can't remember loved ones can take a toll. Leaving the patient in this environment could lead to potential abuse.

Treat the patient—not the wound. Investigate each situation.

When dealing with patients from other cultures, be very careful about using hand signals. For example, a "thumbs up" may be a positive gesture in some cultures but an offensive gesture in others.

SUMMARY

- Obtaining a patient history provides structure to patient assessment and often establishes priorities in patient care.

- Content of the patient history includes date and time, identifying data, source of referral, history, reliability, chief complaint, present illness, past history, and review of body systems.

- The paramedic should ensure patient comfort, avoid entering the patient's personal space, be sensitive to the patient's feelings, watch for signs of uneasiness, use appropriate language, ask open-ended and direct questions, and use therapeutic communications techniques.

- Challenges that can affect history taking include silence, overly talkative patients, patients with multiple symptoms, anxious patients, false reassurance, anger and hostility, intoxication, crying, depression, sexually attractive or seductive patients, confusing behavior or histories, developmental disabilities, communication barriers, and talking with family and friends.

REFERENCE

1. *EMT–Paramedic national standard curriculum*, U.S. Department of Transportation National Highway Traffic Safety Administration, 1998, Washington, DC, The Department.

13 Techniques of Physical Examination

OBJECTIVES

Upon completion of this chapter, the paramedic student will be able to:

1. **Describe physical examination techniques commonly used in the prehospital setting.**
2. **Describe the examination equipment commonly used in the prehospital setting.**
3. **Describe the general approach to physical examination.**
4. **Outline the steps of a comprehensive physical examination.**
5. **Detail the components of the mental status examination.**
6. **Distinguish between normal and abnormal findings in the mental status examination.**
7. **Outline the steps in the general patient survey.**
8. **Distinguish between normal and abnormal findings in the general patient survey.**
9. **Describe physical examination techniques used for assessment of specific body regions.**
10. **Distinguish between normal and abnormal findings when assessing specific body regions.**
11. **State modifications to the physical examination that are necessary when assessing children.**
12. **State modifications to the physical examination that are necessary when assessing the older adult.**

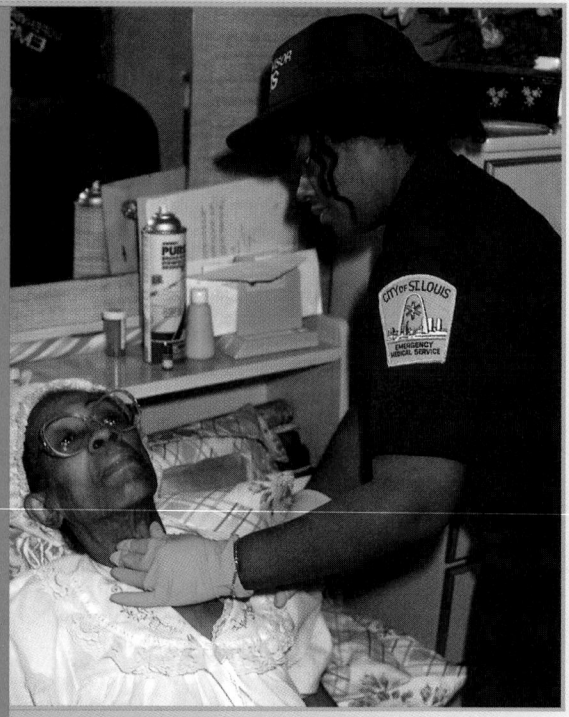

The paramedic must have a wide range of knowledge and skills to perform a comprehensive **physical examination** and to make effective clinical patient care decisions. This chapter presents the techniques of a general physical examination and discusses the relevant pathophysiological significance of the physical findings. Some of the examination techniques presented in this chapter will not routinely be used when assessing patients in the prehospital setting. Although some techniques will have application to examinations performed in the field, others will more likely be performed in the expanded scope of practice activities.

KEY TERMS

auscultation: A technique that requires the use of a stethoscope and is used to assess body sounds produced by the movement of various fluids or gases in organs or tissues.

inspection: A visual assessment of the patient and surroundings.

palpation: A technique in which an examiner uses the hands and fingers to gather information from a patient by touch.

percussion: A technique used to evaluate the presence of air or fluid in body tissues.

physical examination: An assessment of a patient that includes examination techniques, measurement of vital signs, an assessment of height and weight, and the skillful use of examination equipment.

Physical Examination: Approach and Overview

The physical examination consists of examination techniques, measurement of vital signs, an assessment of height and weight, and the skillful use of examination equipment (Box 13-1).

Examination Techniques

The examination techniques commonly used in the physical examination are **inspection**, **palpation**, **percussion**, and **auscultation**. These terms are referred to frequently throughout this text as they relate to the evaluation of specific body systems. Depending on the situation, these examination techniques may be the sole method available for patient evaluation (e.g., assessment of an unconscious

trauma patient) or may be integrated with history taking and other patient care procedures. If time permits, the paramedic should explain each examination technique that requires touch to the patient before initiating it.

Inspection

Inspection is the visual assessment of the patient and surroundings. This examination technique can alert the paramedic to the patient's mental status and possible injury or underlying illness. Patient hygiene, clothing, eye gaze, body language, body position, skin color, and odor are significant inspection findings. If the emergency response was to the patient's home, the paramedic should make a visual inspection for cleanliness, prescription medicines, illegal drug paraphernalia, weapons, and signs of alcohol use. These and other observations can play an important role in determining patient care activities.

BOX 13-1

COMPONENTS OF THE PHYSICAL EXAMINATION

Examination techniques
  Inspection
  Palpation
  Percussion
  Auscultation
Measurement of vital signs
  Pulse
  Respirations
  Blood pressure
  Temperature (especially in children)
Assessment of height and weight
Equipment
  Stethoscope
  Ophthalmoscope
  Otoscope
  Blood pressure cuff

? CRITICAL THINKING

What will you look for during your initial patient inspection when you arrive at the scene of a motor vehicle crash?

443

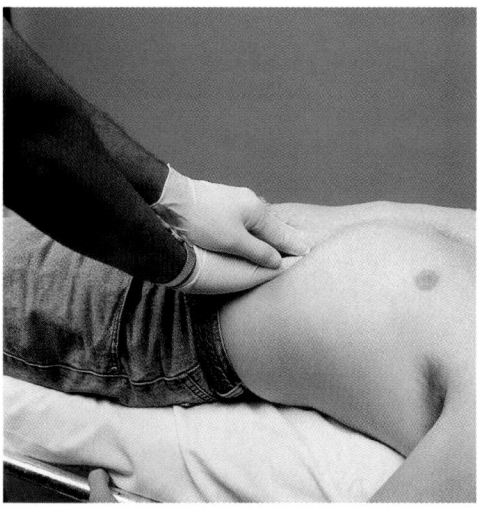

Fig. 13-1 Deep bimanual palpation.

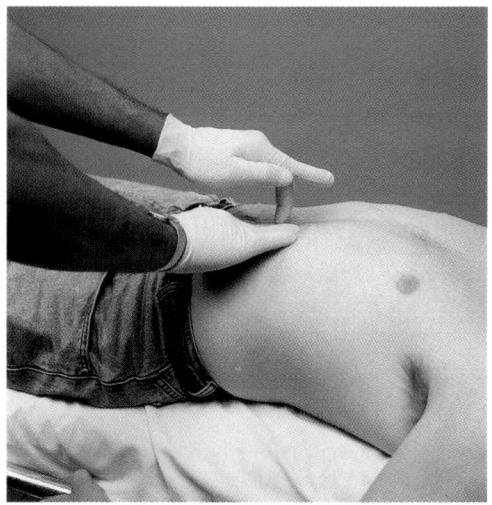

Fig. 13-2 Percussion technique.

BOX 13-2

PERCUSSION TONES AND EXAMPLES

PERCUSSION TONE	EXAMPLE
Tympany (the loudest)	Gastric bubble
Hyperresonance	Air-filled lungs (e.g., COPD, pneumothorax)
Resonance	Healthy lungs
Dullness	Liver
Flat (the quietest)	Muscle

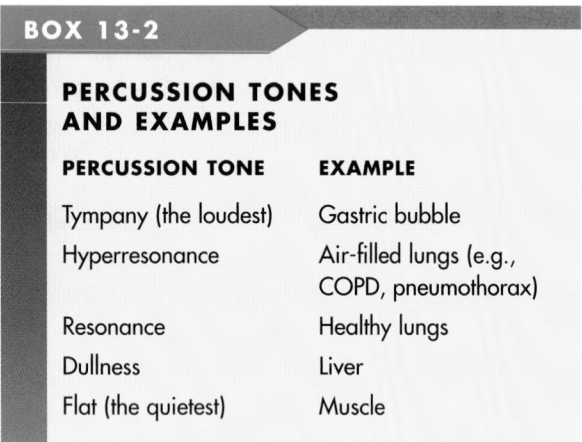

Palpation

Palpation is a technique in which the paramedic uses the hands and fingers to gather information by touch. Generally, the palmar surface of the fingers and the finger pads are used to palpate for texture, masses, fluid, and crepitus, and to assess skin temperature (Fig. 13-1). Palpation may be either superficial or deep; the applications for each are addressed throughout this chapter. Examining a patient by palpation is a form of invasion of the patient's body, so the approach should be gentle and initiated with respect.

Percussion

Percussion is used to evaluate the presence of air or fluid in body tissues. The technique is performed by the paramedic's striking one finger against another to produce vibrations and sound waves of underlying tissue. Sound waves are heard as percussion tones (resonance) and are determined by the density of the tissue being examined. The denser the body area, the lower the pitch of the percussion tone. To percuss, the paramedic places the first joint of the middle finger of the nondominant hand on the patient, keeping the rest of the hand poised above the skin. The fingers of the other hand should be flexed and the wrist action loose. The wrist of the dominant hand is then snapped downward with the tip of the middle finger tapping the joint of the finger that is on the body surface. The tap should be sharp and rigid, percussing the same area several times to interpret the tone (Fig. 13-2). Percussion tones and examples of each are described in Box 13-2.

> **NOTE**
>
> As with any other examination technique, percussion requires practice to obtain the skill needed for the physical examination.

Auscultation

Auscultation requires the use of a stethoscope and is used to assess body sounds produced by the movement of various fluids or gases in the patient's organs or tissues. Auscultation is best performed in a relatively quiet environment where attention can be focused on each body sound being assessed. The paramedic should isolate a particular area to note characteristics of intensity, pitch, duration, and quality. In the prehospital

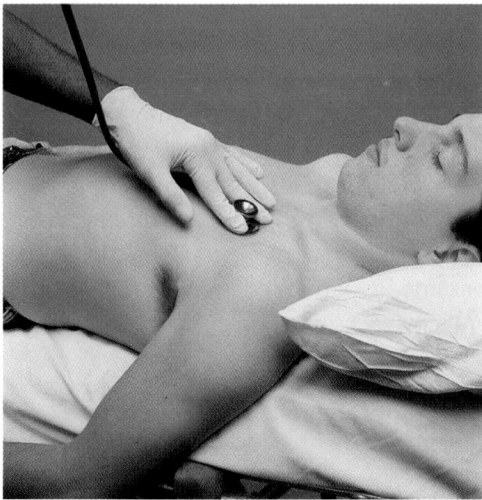

Fig. 13-3 Position of the stethoscope between the index and middle fingers.

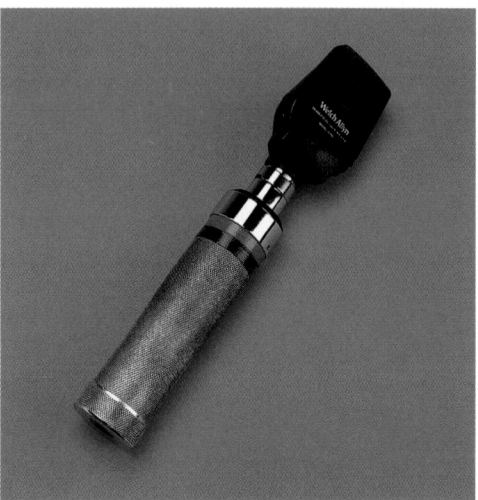

Fig. 13-4 Ophthalmoscope.

setting, auscultation is most often used to assess blood pressure and to evaluate breath sounds, heart sounds, and bowel sounds. To auscultate, the diaphragm of the stethoscope should be placed firmly against the patient's skin for stabilization (Fig. 13-3). If a bell endpiece is used, it should be positioned lightly on the body surface to prevent the damping of vibrations.

> **NOTE**
>
> The bell and diaphragm endpieces of a stethoscope selectively emphasize sounds of different frequencies. The bell is central for listening to low-pitched sounds (e.g., certain heart sounds). In contrast, the diaphragm filters out low-pitched sounds and therefore emphasizes high-pitched ones. Examples of high-pitched sounds include breath sounds and bowel sounds.

Examination Equipment

Equipment used during the comprehensive physical examination includes the stethoscope, ophthalmoscope, otoscope, and blood pressure cuff. The ophthalmoscope and otoscope are "nontraditional" EMS tools that are being introduced to the paramedic with expanded scope of practice. These devices will not routinely be used when assessing patients in the prehospital setting.

Stethoscope

The stethoscope is used to evaluate sounds created by the cardiovascular, respiratory, and gastrointesti-

nal systems. There are three major types of stethoscopes: acoustic stethoscopes, magnetic stethoscopes, and electronic stethoscopes.

Acoustic stethoscopes transmit sound waves from the source to the paramedic's ears. Most have a rigid diaphragm that transmits high-pitched sounds and a bell endpiece that transmits low-pitched sounds.

Magnetic stethoscopes have a single diaphragm endpiece that contains an iron disc and a permanent magnet. The air column of the diaphragm is activated as magnetic attraction is established between the iron disc and the magnet. A frequency dial adjusts for high-, low-, and full-frequency sounds.

Electronic stethoscopes convert sound vibrations into electrical impulses. These impulses are amplified and transmitted to a speaker where they are converted to sound. These devices may be advantageous for use in the prehospital setting to compensate for environmental noise.

Ophthalmoscope

The ophthalmoscope is used to inspect structures of the eye, including the retina, choroid, optic nerve disc, macula (an oval, yellow spot at the center of the retina), and retinal vessels (see Chapter 6). The device has a battery light source, two dials, and a viewer (Fig. 13-4). The dial at the top of the battery changes the light image. The dial at the top of the viewer allows for the selection of lenses. (Five lenses are available, but the large white light generally is used.)

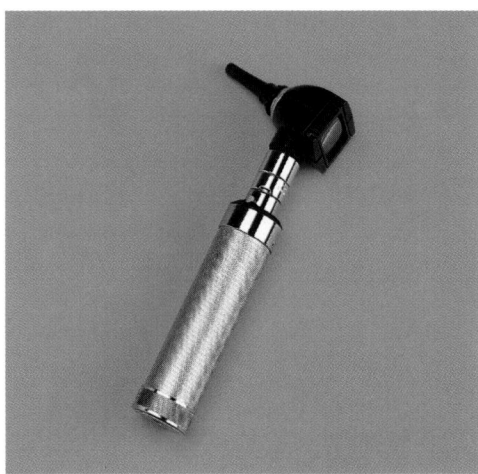

Fig. 13-5 Otoscope.

Otoscope

The otoscope is used to examine deep structures of the external and middle ear. The device is essentially an ophthalmoscope with a special ear speculum attached to the battery tube (Fig. 13-5). Ear speculums come in a number of sizes to conform to various ear canals. (The paramedic should choose the largest speculum that fits comfortably in the patient's ear.) The light from the otoscope allows for visualization of the tympanic membrane.

Blood Pressure Cuff

The blood pressure cuff (sphygmomanometer) most commonly is used (along with the stethoscope) to measure systolic and diastolic blood pressure. The common blood pressure cuff used in the prehospital setting consists of a pressure gauge that registers millimeter calibrations, a synthetic plastic cuff with velcro closures that encloses an inflatable rubber bladder, and a pressure bulb with a release valve. Blood pressure cuffs are available in a number of sizes. Adult widths should be one third to one half the circumference of the limb. For children, the width should cover about two thirds of the upper arm or thigh. (Blood pressure cuffs that are too large will give a falsely low reading; cuffs that are too small will give a falsely high reading.)

> **NOTE**
>
> Electronic vital-sign devices are available and are used by hospitals and some EMS agencies to monitor the patient's blood pressure, pulse rate, body temperature, and oxygen saturation at regular intervals.

General Approach to the Physical Examination

The physical examination is performed systematically, with special emphasis placed on the patient's present illness and chief complaint. The paramedic should remember that most patients view a physical exam with some apprehension and anxiety. Often, they will initially feel vulnerable and exposed. Establishing a professional trust early in the paramedic-patient encounter and ensuring the patient's privacy when possible are very important.

Overview of a Comprehensive Physical Examination

The physical examination is a systematic assessment of the body that includes the following components:

- Mental status
- General survey
- Vital signs
- Skin
- Head, eyes, ears, nose, and throat (HEENT)
- Chest
- Abdomen
- Posterior body
- Extremities (peripheral vascular and musculoskeletal)
- Neurological exam

> **NOTE**
>
> The Centers for Disease Control and Prevention and the Occupational Safety and Health Administration have recommended that health care workers wear gloves "when handling blood-soiled items, body fluids, excretions and secretions, as well as surfaces, materials, and objects exposed to them."[1] This textbook assumes that all paramedics are gloved during appropriate patient care activities. Personal protective measures are listed on the inside cover of this book and are further addressed in Chapter 37.

Mental Status

The first step in any patient-care encounter is to note the patient's appearance and behavior and to assess for level of consciousness. A healthy patient is expected to be alert and responsive to touch, verbal instruction, and painful stimuli.

Appearance and Behavior

As previously mentioned, a visual assessment of the patient can provide important information. Abnormal findings may include drowsiness, obtundation, stupor, or coma. A patient who is obtunded is insensitive to unpleasant or painful stimuli from a reduced level of consciousness, usually produced by anesthetic or analgesics. Stupor is a state of lethargy and unresponsiveness. Stuporous patients usually are unaware of their surroundings. Coma is a state of profound unconsciousness. A patient in coma has no spontaneous eye movements, does not respond to verbal or painful stimuli, and cannot be aroused.

> **NOTE**
>
> Some medical direction agencies discourage the use of these terms to describe a patient's mental status, since they are vague and open to interpretation. Describing the patient's reactions and verbal and motor responses with indices such as the *AVPU scale* or *Glasgow coma scale* (described in Chapters 14 and 22) often is considered better patient information.

Posture, Gait, and Motor Activity

The paramedic should observe the patient's posture, gait, and motor activity by assessing pace, range, character, and appropriateness of movement. For example, most patients without physical disabilities can walk with good balance and without a limp, discomfort, or fear of falling. Abnormal findings may include ataxia (uncoordinated movement), paralysis, restlessness, agitation, bizarre body posture, immobility, and involuntary movements.

Dress, Grooming, Personal Hygiene, and Breath or Body Odors

Dress, grooming, and personal hygiene should be appropriate for the patient's age, lifestyle, occupation, and socioeconomic group. Dress should be appropriate for environmental temperature and weather conditions. (Older adults and children who are improperly dressed for environmental temperatures or who have poor physical hygiene may be victims of neglect by a caregiver.) Medical jewelry (e.g., copper bracelets for arthritis, medical identification insignias) should be noted. Hair, fingernails, and cosmetics may reflect the patient's lifestyle, mood, and personality. These findings can indicate a decreased interest in appearance (e.g., grown-out hair or faded nail polish) that may help estimate the length of an illness.

Breath or body odors can indicate underlying conditions or illness. Examples of breath odors include alcohol, acetone (seen with some diabetic conditions), feces (seen with bowel obstruction), and halitosis from throat infections and poor dental and oral hygiene. Renal and liver disease and poor physical hygiene also may result in body odor.

Facial Expression

Facial expressions may reveal anxiety, depression, elation, anger, or withdrawal. The paramedic should be alert to changes in facial expression while the patient is at rest, during conversation, during the examination, and when questions are asked. Facial expressions should be appropriate to the situation.

Mood, Affect, and Relation to Person and Things

Like facial expression, the patient's mood and affect should be appropriate to the situation. Mood and affect are expressed verbally and nonverbally. Examples of abnormal findings include an unusual happiness in the presence of major illness, indifference, responses to imaginary people or objects, and unpredictable mood swings.

> **NOTE**
>
> *Affect* refers to the person's feelings as they appear to others or an outward manifestation of a person's feelings or emotions.

> **? CRITICAL THINKING**
>
> **What physical clues do you look for in your friends or your partner that tell you about their mood?**

Speech and Language

Normal speech is understandable and moderately paced. The paramedic should assess the quantity, rate, loudness, and fluency of the patient's speech patterns. Abnormal findings include aphasia (loss of speech), dysphonia (abnormal speaking voice), dysarthria (poorly articulated speech), and speech and language that changes with mood.

Thought and Perceptions

A healthy person's thoughts and perceptions are logical, relevant, organized, and coherent. Patients should have an insight into their illness or injury and should be able to demonstrate a level of judgment in making decisions or plans about their situation and their care. Although accurately assessing a person's thoughts and perceptions is difficult, the following usually are considered abnormal findings:

- Abnormal thought processes
  Flight of ideas
  Incoherence
  Confabulation
- Abnormal thought content
  Obsessions
  Compulsions
  Delusions
  Feelings of unreality
- Abnormal perceptions
  Illusions
  Hallucinations

Memory and Attention

Healthy persons normally are oriented to person, place, and time ("oriented times 3"). There are several other methods that can be used to assess a patient's memory and attention. These include asking the patient to count from 1 to 10 using only even or odd numbers (digit span), multiplying by sevens (serial sevens), and spelling simple words backward. The paramedic also should assess the patient's remote memory (e.g., birthdays), recent memory (e.g., events of the day), and the patient's new learning ability. New learning ability can be evaluated by giving the patient new information (e.g., the year and model of the ambulance) and then later asking the patient to recall that information.

General Survey

After the patient's level of consciousness and mental status have been assessed, a general survey of the patient should be performed. In addition to the assessments described above, the patient should be evaluated for signs of distress, apparent state of health, skin color and obvious lesions,

height and build, sexual development, and weight. Vital signs also should be assessed during the general survey.

Signs of Distress

Obvious signs of distress include those that result from cardiorespiratory insufficiency, pain, and anxiety. Examples of these signs and symptoms are as follows:

- Cardiorespiratory insufficiency
  Labored breathing
  Wheezing
  Cough
- Pain
  Wincing
  Sweating
  Protectiveness of a painful body part or area
- Anxiety
  Restlessness
  Anxious expression
  Fidgety movement
  Cold, moist palms

> **? CRITICAL THINKING**
>
> *Combine one symptom from each of the categories of distress, and visualize how a patient with these symptoms might look and act.*

Apparent State of Health

A patient's apparent state of health can be assessed by observation. The paramedic should note the patient's general appearance as being acutely or chronically ill, frail, feeble, robust, or vigorous.

Skin Color and Obvious Lesions

Skin color can vary by body part and from person to person. A patient's normal skin color is of course dependent on race and can range in tone from pink or ivory to deep brown, yellow, or olive. Skin color is best assessed by evaluating skin that usually is not exposed to the sun (e.g., the palms) or skin that has less pigmentation (e.g., lips and nail beds). Abnormal skin colors and their possible causes are described in Box 13-3. Obvious skin lesions that can indicate illness or injury include rashes, bruises, scars, and discoloration.

Height and Build

Patients generally can be described as average, tall, or short, with a slender, lanky, muscular, or stocky build. All of these factors can reflect overall health. For example, a patient can be excessively thin (as seen with some eating disorders) or trim and muscular.

Sexual Development

The paramedic should ascertain if sexual characteristics are appropriate for the patient's age and sex. Normal changes associated with puberty include facial hair and deepening of the voice in men, increased breast size in women, and hair growth in the axillary and groin areas in both sexes.

Weight

Ideally, a patient's body weight should be proportionate to height (Fig. 13-6). Weight conditions

---

BOX 13-3

ABNORMAL SKIN COLOR AND POSSIBLE CAUSES

COLOR	POSSIBLE CAUSES
Pallor (decrease in color)	Shock, dehydration, fright
Cyanosis (bluish color)	Cardiorespiratory insufficiency, cold environment
Jaundice (yellow-orange color)	Liver disease, RBC destruction
Red	Fever, inflammation, carbon monoxide poisoning

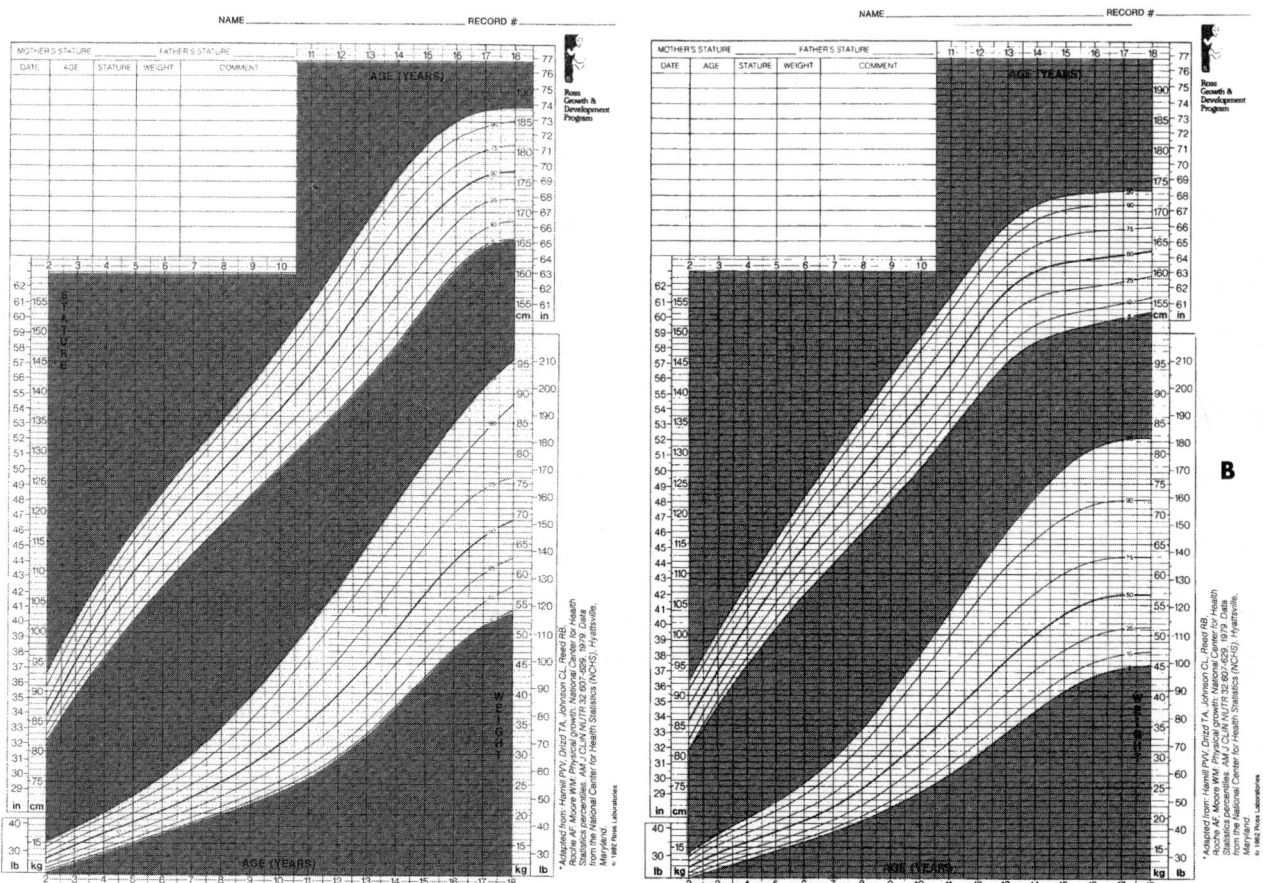

Fig. 13-6 Physical growth curves and NCHS percentiles for children, age 2 through 18 years, for height and weight. **A**, Boys. **B**, Girls.

that easily are observed in the general survey include patients who are emaciated (excessively lean from lack of nutrition), plump, or obese. A recent gain or loss of weight is an important finding and may be clinically significant. Like body height and build, body weight can reflect the patient's level of health, age, and lifestyle.

? CRITICAL THINKING

Think about three medical conditions that might result in significant weight loss and then three that might cause a significant weight gain.

NOTE

Medical obesity can be defined as body weight that is 20% above desirable body weight for a person's age, sex, height, and body build.

Vital Signs

Vital signs generally are considered to include pulse, blood pressure, respirations, skin condition, and pupil size and reactivity.

Pulse. A normal resting pulse rate for an adult is usually between 60 and 100 beats per minute; it may be affected by the patient's age and physical condition. A child's pulse rate may be 80 to 100 beats per minute, for example, and a well-trained athlete's pulse rate may be 50 to 60 beats per minute. Factors such as pregnancy, anxiety, and fear also may produce a higher-than-normal pulse rate in healthy individuals.

Pulse rates may be obtained at the carotid artery in the neck or at any pulse site where the artery lies close to the skin surface. To evaluate the radial pulse, the pads of the paramedic's index and middle fingers are placed at the distal end of the patient's wrist, just medial to the radial styloid. If pulsations are regular, they should be counted for 15 seconds and multiplied by four to determine the number of beats per minute. In addition to the number of times the heart beats per minute, the regularity and strength of the pulse should be assessed. For example, the pulse can be characterized as regular or irregular, weak or strong. Application of an ECG monitor also may be useful in evaluating cardiovascular status after initial assessment of the pulse.

Blood pressure. The systolic blood pressure is the reading that identifies the amount of pressure exerted against the arterial walls when the heart contracts. Diastolic blood pressure is the amount of pressure exerted against the arterial walls during relaxation of the heart. For all age groups, normal systolic blood pressure is considered to be less than 140 mm Hg; normal diastolic pressure should be less than 90 mm Hg.

Blood pressure is best measured by auscultation. The blood pressure cuff is placed on the patient's arm with the lower end of the cuff positioned 1 to 2 inches (2 to 5 cm) above the antecubital space. The cuff is inflated to a point approximately 30 mm Hg above where the brachial pulse can no longer be palpated. The stethoscope is placed over the brachial artery, and the cuff is slowly deflated at a rate of 2 to 3 mm Hg per second. As the pressure falls, the paramedic should observe the gauge and note where the first sound or pulsation is heard. This is the patient's systolic pressure. The point at which the sounds change in quality or become muffled is noted as the patient's diastolic pressure.

NOTE

Determining accurate diastolic pressure sometimes is difficult. The difference between the point of muffled tones and the complete disappearance of pulsations varies by individual. In some persons the difference is a few mm Hg; at the opposite end of the range are people whose pulsations never totally disappear. The ability to measure accurate diastolic pressures develops from experience and requires careful listening in a quiet environment.

Blood pressure may be estimated by palpation when vascular sounds are difficult to hear with a stethoscope because of environmental noise, but this method is less accurate than auscultation and can only estimate systolic pressure. To estimate blood pressure by palpation, the paramedic should locate the brachial or radial pulse and apply the blood pressure cuff as previously described. Finger contact is maintained at the pulse location as the cuff slowly deflates. When the pulse becomes palpable, the gauge reading denotes the systolic pressure. Like pulse rates, a patient's blood pressure may be unusually high because of fear or anxiety. Other factors, such as a patient's age and normal level of physical activity, may be responsible for unusual blood pressure readings.

Respirations. The normal respiratory rate for adults is between 12 and 24 breaths per minute (Table 13-1). The respiratory rate is obtained by watching the patient breathe, by feeling for chest movement, or by auscultating the patient's lungs. The paramedic should count the patient's respirations for 30 seconds and multiply by two to determine breaths per minute. Rhythm and depth of respirations are assessed by visualization and auscultation of the thorax. Abnormal findings include shallow, rapid, noisy, or deep breathing; asymmetrical chest wall movement; accessory respiratory muscle involvement; or congested, unequal, or diminished breath sounds.

Skin. Skin color, temperature, and moisture provide additional information about the patient's status. As previously discussed, a patient's skin color and the presence of bruises, lesions, or rashes may indicate serious illness or injury.

Skin temperature may be normal (warm), hot, or cold. Skin that is hot to the touch indicates a possible fever or heat-related illness or injury. Cold skin may indicate decreased tissue perfusion and cold-related illness or injury. The dorsal surface of the hand is more sensitive than the palmar surface and should be used to estimate body temperature. Body temperature can be measured more accurately by applying plastic heat-sensitive tape to the patient's skin or by using standard mercury clinical thermometers, electronic thermometers, or tympanic membrane thermometers. Evaluations of body temperature may have specific applications in emergencies, such as febrile seizures and hyperthermic and hypothermic emergencies.

Many EMS services use tympanic membrane thermometers or electronic thermometers that obtain readings within seconds. With a standard thermometer, temperature readings are obtained by placing the thermometer under the conscious patient's tongue for 4 to 6 minutes, under the patient's armpit for 10 minutes, or in the patient's rectum for 5 to 8 minutes. (Rectal readings provide the most accurate assessment but may be impractical for prehospital use.) Normal body temperature is 37° C (98.6° F). Standard clinical thermometers record body temperatures from 34.4° C (94° F) to 40° C (106° F).

Skin moisture usually is classified as dry (normal) or wet (clammy or diaphoretic). Diaphoretic skin may indicate a hemodynamic deficit, such as hypovolemia, or another illness or injury that results in decreased tissue perfusion or increased sweat gland activity. Examples are cardiovascular and heat-related emergencies, respectively.

Pupils. Examining the pupils for response to light may yield information on the neurological status of some patients. Normally, the pupils are equal and constrict when exposed to light. (The acronym *PERRL* indicates that the pupils are equal, round, and react to light.) When testing the pupils for light response, the paramedic shines a penlight directly into one eye. The normal reaction is for the pupil exposed to the light to constrict with a consensual constriction of the opposite eye. Abnormal pupillary reactions and possible causes are provided in Table 13-2.

TABLE 13-1		AVERAGE VITAL SIGNS BY AGE	
AGE	**PULSE**	**RESPIRATIONS**	**BLOOD PRESSURE**
Newborn	120-160	40-60	80/40
1 year	80-140	30-40	82/44
3 years	80-120	25-30	86/50
5 years	70-115	20-25	90/52
7 years	70-115	20-25	94/54
10 years	70-115	15-20	100/60
15 years	70-90	15-20	110/64
Adult	60-80	12-20	120/80

TABLE 13-2	ABNORMAL PUPIL REACTIONS
PUPIL SIZE	**POSSIBLE CAUSES**
Equal	
Dilated or unreponsive	Cardiac arrest, CNS injury, hypoxia or anoxia, drug use (LSD, atropine, amphetamines)
Constricted or unresponsive	CNS injury or disease, narcotic drug use (heroin, morphine), eye medications
Unequal	
One dilated or unresponsive	Cerebrovascular accident (CVA), head injury, direct trauma to the eye, eye medications

Anatomical Regions

The remainder of this chapter will discuss physical examination techniques as they pertain to anatomical regions of the body. The paramedic should always be aware that anatomical and physiological components of the human body are age-related and vary by individual.

Skin

In addition to the general assessment of the skin that has been previously described, the comprehensive physical examination should include an evaluation of the skin's texture and turgor, hair, and fingernails and toenails (all of which are a part of the integumentary system).

BOX 13-4

ABNORMAL NAIL FINDINGS

Clubbing: A change in the angle between the nail and nail base that approaches or exceeds 180 degrees; associated with flattening and often enlargement of the fingertips; may indicate chronic cardiac or respiratory disease.

Paronychia: Inflammation of the skin at the base of the nail; may result from local infection or trauma.

Onycholysis: The separation of a nail from its bed; associated with psoriasis, dermatitis, fungal infection, and other conditions.

Terry's nails: The presence of transverse white bands that cover the nail except for a narrow zone at the distal tip; associated with cirrhosis.

White spots: The presence of white spots that appear in the nail plate; usually result from minor injury or cuticle manipulation.

Transverse white lines: Longitudinal white streaks in the nail plate; may indicate a systemic disorder.

Psoriasis: Pitting, discoloration, and subungual thickening of the nail plate; may lead to splinter hemorrhages.

Splinter hemorrhages: Red or brown linear streaks in the nail bed; associated with minor nail trauma, bacterial endocarditis, and trichinosis.

Beau's lines: Transverse depressions in the nail that inhibit nail growth; associated with systemic illness, severe infection, and nail injury.

Skin Texture and Turgor

The texture of the skin normally is smooth, soft, and flexible. In older adults, however, the skin may be wrinkled and leathery from decreases in collagen, subcutaneous fat, and sweat glands. Abnormal skin texture may result from lesions, rashes, tumors, and localized trauma.

Turgor refers to the skin's elasticity (which normally decreases with age). To test skin turgor, the paramedic should pinch ("tent") a fold of skin and assess the ease and speed at which the skin returns to its normal position. (Skin on the back of the patient's hand or over the sternum are good areas to test for turgor.) Tented skin that does not quickly return to its normal position may indicate dehydration.

Hair

As part of the examination, the paramedic should inspect and palpate the patient's hair, noting quantity, distribution, and texture. Important findings include a recent change in the growth or loss of hair, which may result from chemotherapy or hormone and endocrine disorders (e.g., menopause, diabetes). Thinning hair is common in both older men and women.

Fingernails and Toenails

Color, shape, and the presence or absence of lesions should be noted when the paramedic is assessing the patient's fingernails and toenails. Uncolored nails usually are transparent, and healthy nails are smooth and firm on palpation. Abnormal findings in the nails are described in Box 13-4. With age, nails often develop longitudinal striations and may have a yellow tint because of insufficient calcium.

Head, Ears, Eyes, Nose, and Throat

An examination of the structures of the head and neck involves inspection, palpation, and auscultation.

Head and Face

To examine the head, the paramedic should inspect the skull for shape and symmetry, keeping in mind that hair can hide abnormalities. The hair should be parted in several places to assess for scaliness, lumps, or other lesions. The assessment should employ a systematic palpation, moving from front to back, noting any swelling, tenderness, indentations, or depressions. The scalp should move freely over the skull, and the patient should not complain of pain or discomfort during the examination.

The face should be inspected for symmetry, expression, and contour. Any asymmetry, involuntary movements, masses, or edema should be noted. Facial skin should be evaluated for color, pigmentation, texture, thickness, hair distribution, and any lesions.

Eyes

The paramedic should verify that both eyes can see by soliciting the patient's history regarding visual disturbances or by asking the patient to demonstrate visual acuity. Visual acuity can be assessed by asking the patient to read printed material, count fingers at a distance, demonstrate the ability to distinguish light from dark, and through the use of various eye charts (e.g., a *Snellen chart*) (Fig. 13-7).

Both eyes should move equally well in all four directions (up, down, right, left). To evaluate visual fields, the paramedic should ask the patient to look at his or her nose. The paramedic then extends his or her arms with elbows at right angles and wiggles both index fingers at the same time to test peripheral vision. By asking the patient to identify finger movement and to visually track a moving object (e.g., a pencil, finger, or penlight), the paramedic can determine if visual fields are grossly normal. This assessment should be performed in all four quadrants. The eyes also should be surveyed for normal position and alignment.

> **? CRITICAL THINKING**
>
> *When you perform an examination of the eyes, you are evaluating components of at least four body systems. What are they?*

The orbital area should be inspected for edema and puffiness, and the eyebrows should be free of scaliness. Inspection of the eyelids consists of noting the width of palpebral fissures (the elliptical opening between the upper and lower lids), edema, color, lesions, condition and direction of the eyelashes, adequacy of lid closure, and drainage. The paramedic also should briefly inspect the regions of the lacrimal gland and lacrimal sac for

swelling, noting excessive tearing or dryness of the eye.

The conjunctiva and sclera are examined by asking the patient to look up while both lower lids are depressed with the thumbs. The sclera should be white; the cornea and the iris should be clearly visible; and the pupils should be of equal size, round, and reactive to light (Fig. 13-8). The paramedic should palpate the lower orbital rim to determine structural integrity.

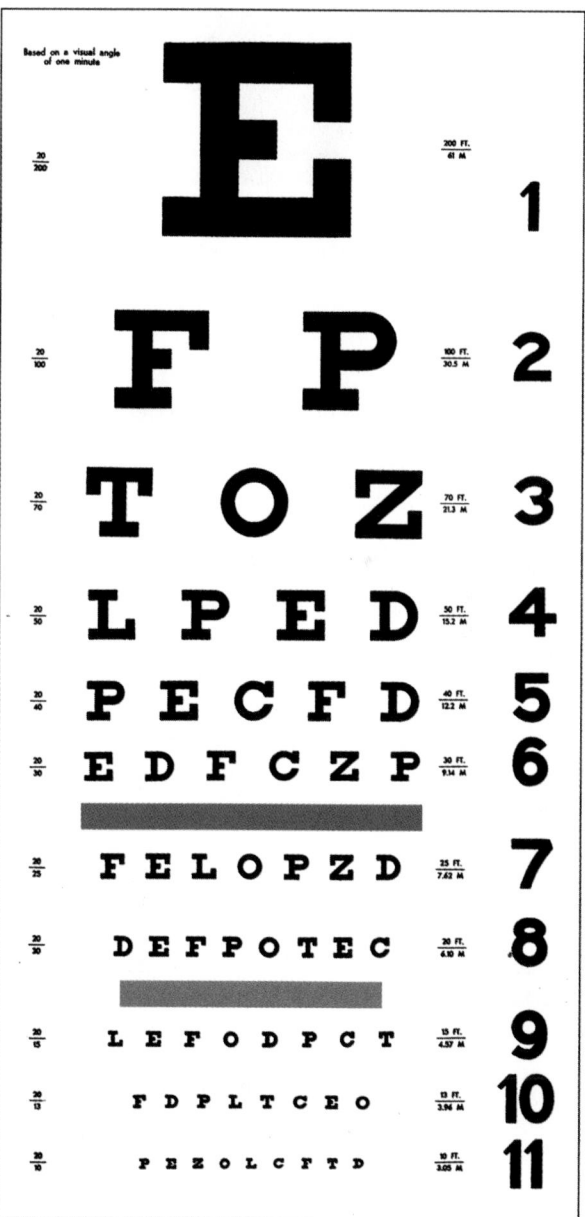

Fig. 13-7 Snellen chart. (From Seidel HM et al: *Mosby's guide to physical examination*, ed 2, St Louis, 1991, Mosby.)

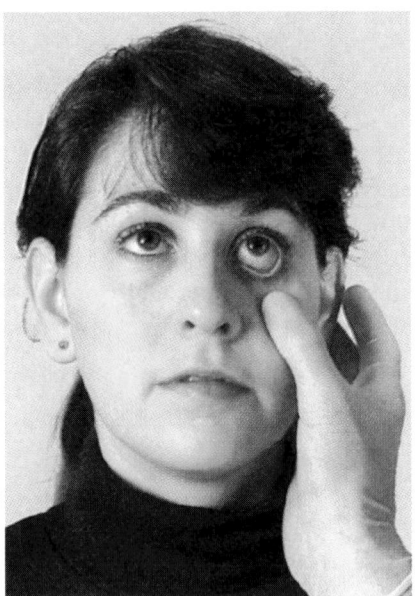

Fig. 13-8 Cornea and sclera. (From Seidel HM et al: *Mosby's guide to physical examination,* ed 2, St Louis, 1991, Mosby.)

> **NOTE**
>
> The paramedic should be alert to the presence of contact lenses and ocular prostheses when examining a patient's eyes.

Ophthalmoscope Examination

The ophthalmoscope is used to evaluate the cornea for foreign bodies, lacerations, abrasions, and infection; the anterior chamber for hyphema (accumulation of blood) or hypopyon (accumulation of pus); the fundus to assess retinal vessels, the optic nerve, and retina; the vitreous; and to assess for foreign bodies under the eyelid (Fig. 13-9).

> **NOTE**
>
> Ophthalmoscopic examinations should be performed in a darkened room so that the pupils are somewhat dilated. Contacts do not need to be removed.

To perform an examination with an ophthalmoscope, the paramedic should follow these steps for each eye:

1. Ask the patient to fixate on a distant object.
2. Sit facing the patient at same seat height.
3. Turn on the ophthalmoscope light and select the 0 lens setting.

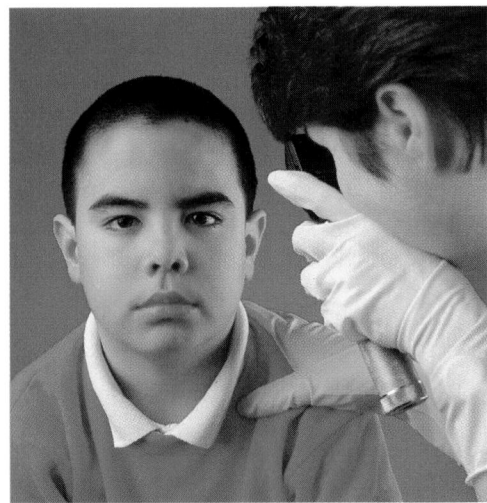

Fig. 13-9 Paramedic using an ophthalmoscope.

4. Use the right hand and eye to examine the patient's right eye and the left hand and eye to examine the patient's left eye.
5. Direct the patient to look over your shoulder, keeping both eyes open.
6. Hold the scope against your face and shine the light on the patient's pupil at a distance of about 10 inches from the face. A bright orange glow in the pupil ("red reflex") can normally be seen.
7. Move the light slowly toward the pupil to see the structures of the fundus. Rotate the lens to improve focus as needed.
8. Inspect the size, color, and clarity of the disc and integrity of vessels; assess for retinal lesions and appearance of the macula. A normal examination will reveal the following (Fig. 13-10)[2]:
   - A clear, yellow optic nerve disc
   - Reddish-pink (European-American) or darkened (African-American) retina
   - Light red arteries and dark red veins
   - A 3:2 vein-to-artery ratio in size proportion
   - The avascular macula

Ears

The external ear and surrounding tissues should be inspected for signs of bruising, deformity, or discoloration. There should be no discharge from either ear canal. Pulling gently on the ear lobes (lobules) should not produce pain or discomfort. The paramedic should palpate the skull and facial bones surrounding the ear and inspect the mastoid area for tenderness or discoloration. An alert, hearing patient who

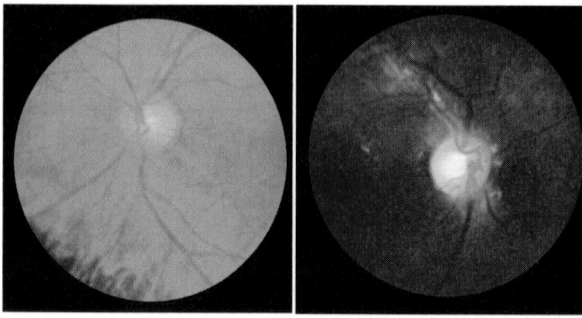

Fig. 13-10 Normal fundus examination. (From Potter PA, Perry AG: *Fundamentals of nursing: concepts, process, and practice,* ed 3, St Louis, 1993, Mosby.)

speaks the same language as the paramedic should be able to respond to questions without excessive requests for repetition. Hearing-aid devices should be noted. An assessment of gross auditory acuity can be made by covering one ear at a time and asking the patient to repeat short test words spoken by the paramedic in soft and loud tones.

Otoscopic Examination

An otoscope is used to evaluate the inner ear for discharge and foreign bodies and to assess the eardrum (see Chapter 6). The paramedic performs an otoscopic exam using the following steps for each ear (Fig. 13-11):

1. Select the appropriate size speculum.
2. Check the ear for foreign bodies before inserting the speculum.
3. Instruct the patient not to move during the examination to avoid injury to the canal and tympanic membrane. (Infants and young children may need to be restrained.)
4. Turn on the otoscope and insert the speculum into the ear canal, slightly down and forward. To ease insertion, pull the auricle up and backward in adults; back and downward in infants.
5. Identify cerumen and look for foreign bodies, lesions, or discharge.
6. Visualize and inspect the tympanic membrane for tears or breaks. A normal examination will reveal the following:
   - Cerumen will be dry (tan or light yellow) or moist (dark yellow or brown).
   - The ear canal should not be inflamed (a sign of infection).
   - The tympanic membrane should be translucent or pearly gray (pink or red indicates inflammation).

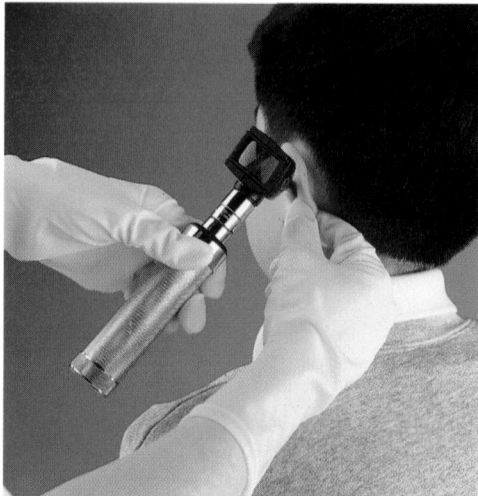

Fig. 13-11 Paramedic performing an otoscopic exam.

Nose

The nose should be inspected for shape, size, color, and stability. The column of the nose should be midline with the face, and the nares should be symmetrically positioned. (Slight asymmetry of nares is considered normal.) The paramedic should palpate the column of the nose and surrounding soft tissues for pain, tenderness, or deformity. The frontal and maxillary sinuses may be inspected for the presence of swelling and palpated for tenderness along the bony brow on each side of the nose and the zygomatic processes.

Discharge from the nose can have a number of causes. For example, cerebrospinal fluid may be present as a result of head trauma; a bloody discharge (epistaxis) may result from trauma or from mucosal erosions involving blood vessels, hypertension, or bleeding disorders; and a mucus discharge commonly results from allergy, upper respiratory tract infection, sinusitis, or cold exposure.

Mouth and Pharynx

The lips should be inspected for symmetry, color, edema, and skin surface irregularities. The lips should be pink. Pallor of the lips is associated with anemia; cyanosis is associated with cardiorespiratory insufficiency; red lips occasionally are a late finding in carbon monoxide poisoning. There should be no swelling, deformity, or pain on palpation.

Healthy gums in the oral cavity are pink and free of lesions and swelling. Patchy areas of pigmentation in the mouths of African-Americans are not

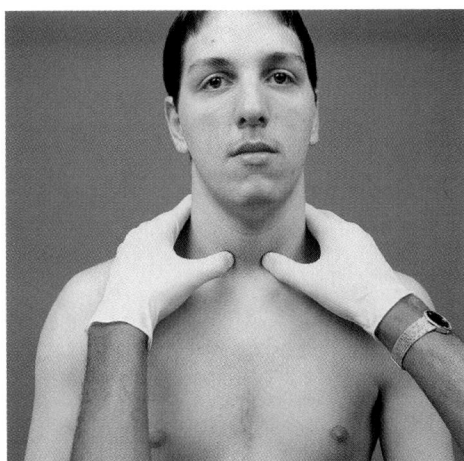

Fig. 13-12 Position of the thumbs to evaluate the midline position of the trachea.

uncommon. Enlarged gums may indicate pregnancy, leukemia, poor oral hygiene, puberty, or use of some medications (e.g., *phenytoin* [Dilantin]). The mouth should be free of loose or broken teeth. Dental appliances may be present.

The tongue should be inspected for size and color. It should be positioned in the midline of the oral cavity and appear nonswollen, dull red, moist, and glistening. To inspect the oropharynx, a tongue blade can be used to depress the tongue. The normal palate is white or pink. If the oral cavity is inflamed or covered with exudate, an infection may be present. (Specific breath odors may indicate alcohol or other drug consumption or illness.) The tonsils normally are pink and smooth without edema, ulceration, or inflammation.

> **NOTE**
>
> A patient with a typical "sore throat" often will have a reddened and edematous uvula and tonsillar pillars. A yellow exudate will sometimes be present.

Neck

The neck should be inspected in the patient's normal anatomical position. If trauma is suspected, use spinal precautions. The trachea should be midline, and there should be no use of accessory muscles or tracheal tugging during respiration. To palpate the neck, the paramedic places both thumbs along the sides of the distal trachea and systematically moves the hands toward the head (Fig. 13-12). Care should be taken not to apply bilateral pressure to the carotid arteries because syncope or bradycardia may result.

The lymph nodes should be nontender. (Tender or swollen lymph nodes usually are the result of inflammation.) The thyroid and cricoid cartilages should be pain-free and move when the patient swallows. Bubbling or crackling sensations that can be palpated in the soft tissues of the neck may indicate the presence of subcutaneous emphysema. Distended neck veins or prominent carotid arteries should be noted (see Chapter 28).

Head and Cervical Spine

The temporomandibular joint (TMJ) connects the mandible of the jaw to the temporal bone of the skull and can sometimes become painful or dislocated. Normally the patient should be able to open and close the mouth without pain or limitation in movement. TMJ dysfunction is a relatively common complaint.

For the patient who has not undergone trauma, the cervical spine should be inspected and palpated for tenderness or deformities. Range of motion can be tested in the following manner:

- Flexion: Touching the chin to the chest
- Rotation: Touching the chin to each shoulder
- Lateral bending: Touching each ear to each shoulder
- Extension: Tilting the head backward

> **NOTE**
>
> Any movement of the neck of a trauma patient for performing a general or neurological examination must be accompanied by continuous manual protection and stabilization of the spine (see Chapter 23).

Chest

A thorough knowledge of the structure of the thoracic cage is required to perform an adequate respiratory and cardiac assessment. In addition to protecting the vital organs within the thorax, the ribs provide support for respiratory movements of the diaphragm and intercostal muscles (see Chapter 6). A loss of thoracic structural integrity (e.g., a flail segment) prevents or limits respiratory function.

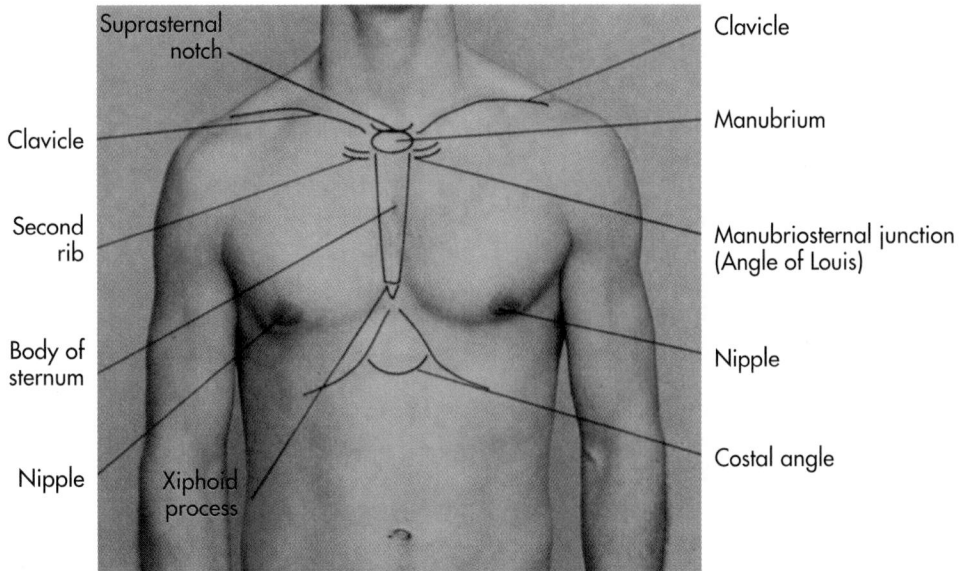

Fig. 13-13 Topographical landmarks of the chest. (From Seidel H: *Mosby's guide to physical examination,* ed 2, St Louis, 1991, Mosby.)

The ribs of the thorax also are used as anatomical landmarks in locating specific areas for examination. Fig. 13-13 shows the topographical landmarks of the chest. The thorax can be evaluated by using imaginary lines to document physical examination findings (Fig. 13-14).

TRICKS OF THE TRADE

Remember that bullet holes and stab wounds like to hide in armpits. Don't overlook these areas!

Inspection

The chest wall should be inspected for symmetry on both the anterior and posterior surfaces. Although the thorax is not completely symmetrical, a visual inspection of one side should offer a reasonable comparison to the other. Chest wall diameter often is increased in patients with obstructive pulmonary disease, resulting in a barrel-shaped appearance of the thorax. Other chest wall deformities or asymmetry are described in Box 13-5. The paramedic should inspect the skin and nipples for cyanosis and pallor and should be alert to the presence of suture lines from chest wall surgery and skin pockets enclosing implanted pacemaker devices or implanted central venous lines. The patient's respira-

BOX 13-5

CHEST WALL ABNORMALITIES

Funnel chest: An indentation of the lower sternum above the xiphoid process.
   Pigeon chest: A prominent sternal protrusion.
   Thoracic kyphosis: A posterior deviation of the spine that results in increased convexity of the chest.
   Scoliosis: A lateral deviation of the spine that results in an abnormal curvature.

tory status should be evaluated by inspection, palpation, percussion, and auscultation. The pattern or rhythm of respirations and any use of accessory respiratory muscles (e.g., intercostal or supraclavicular retractions, or both) should be noted.

? CRITICAL THINKING

Evaluate breathing in a supine patient or friend while standing to the person's side, then at the head, and finally at the feet. Which position provides the best view of the symmetry of the thorax?

Palpation

The thorax should be palpated for pulsations, tenderness, bulges, depressions, crepitus, subcuta-

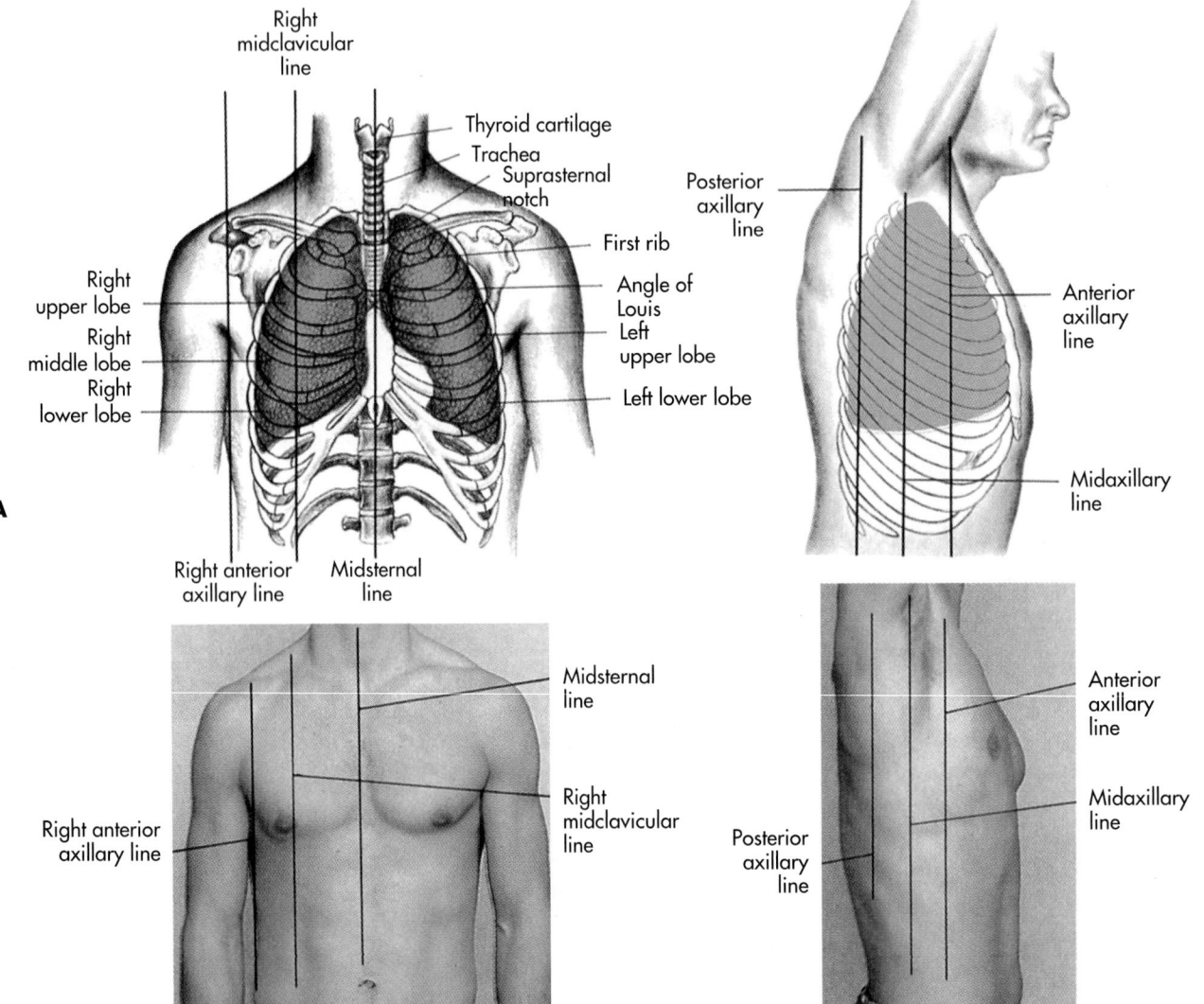

Fig. 13-14 Thoracic landmarks. **A,** Anterior thorax. **B,** Right lateral thorax. (From Seidel H: *Mosby's guide to physical examination,* ed 2, St Louis, 1991, Mosby.)

neous emphysema, and unusual movement and position. The examination begins with the paramedic noting the position of the trachea, which should be midline and directly above the sternal notch. Starting with the patient's clavicles, the paramedic firmly palpates both sides of the patient's chest wall simultaneously, front to back and right side to left side. The examination should proceed systematically, without pain or discomfort.

To evaluate the anterior chest wall for equal expansion during inspiration, the paramedic places both thumbs along the patient's costal margin and the xiphoid process, with palms lying flat on the chest wall. Equal movement should be noted as the

patient inhales and exhales. The posterior chest wall is evaluated for symmetrical respiratory movement by placing the thumbs along the spinous processes at the level of the tenth rib (Fig. 13-15).

Percussion

Percussion should be performed in symmetrical locations from side to side to compare the percussion note (Fig. 13-16). Resonance usually is heard over all areas of healthy lungs. Hyperresonance is associated with hyperinflation and may indicate pulmonary disease, pneumothorax, or asthma. Dullness or flatness suggests the presence of fluid and/or pulmonary congestion. The level and move-

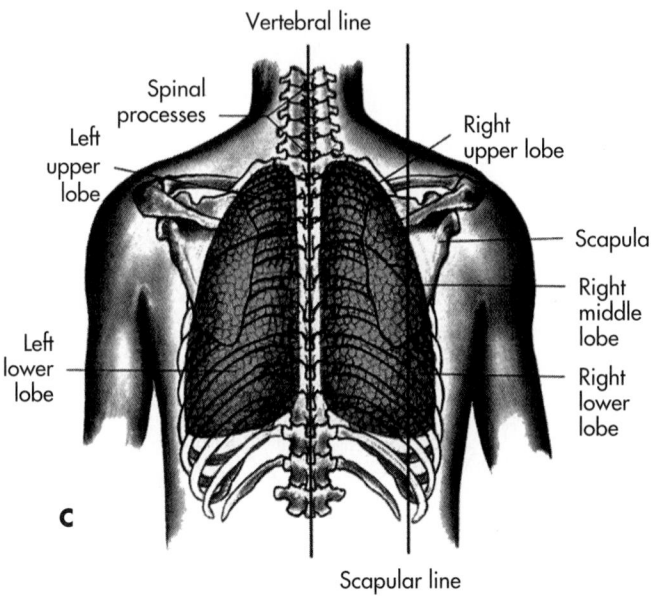

C

Scapular line

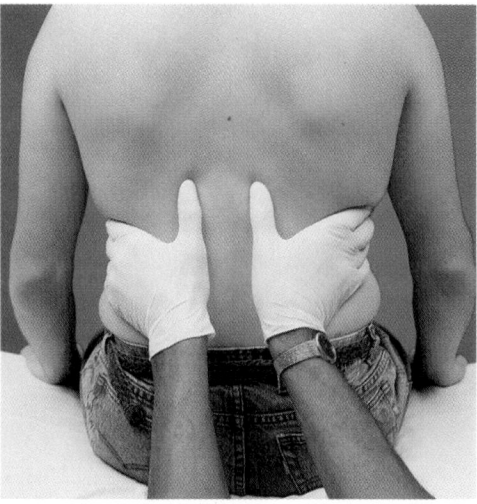

Fig. 13-15 Palpating the thoracic expansion. The thumbs are at the level of the tenth ribs.

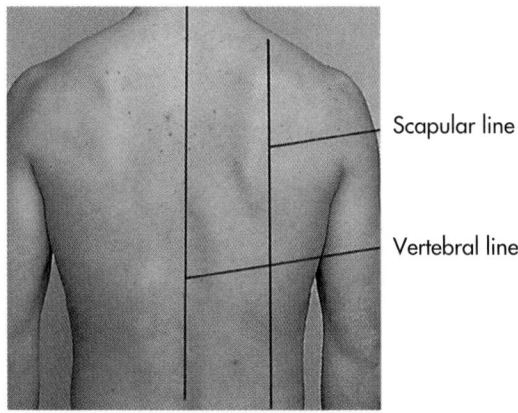

Fig. 13-14 cont'd   C, Posterior thorax.

ment of the diaphragm during breathing (diaphragmatic excursion) may be limited by disease (e.g., emphysema, tumor) or pain (e.g., rib fracture).

Auscultation

The thorax is best auscultated with the patient sitting upright (if possible) and breathing deeply and slowly through an open mouth during the examination. The paramedic should be alert to the possibility of resulting hyperventilation and fatigue, which may occur in ill and older patients.

The paramedic uses the diaphragm of the stethoscope to auscultate the high-pitched sounds of the patient's lungs by holding the stethoscope firmly on the patient's skin and listening carefully as the patient inhales and exhales. The chest auscultation should be systematic as well as thorough, allowing evaluation of both the anterior and the posterior lung fields (Fig. 13-17).

Breath Sounds

Air movement creates turbulence as it passes through the respiratory tree and produces breath sounds during inhalation and exhalation. During inhalation, air moves first into the trachea and major bronchi and then into progressively smaller airways to its final destination, the alveoli. During exhalation, the air flows from small airways to larger ones, which creates less turbulence. Therefore normal breath sounds generally are louder during inspiration.

Normal Breath Sounds

Normal breath sounds are classified as *vesicular*, *bronchovesicular*, and *bronchial*. Vesicular breath sounds are heard over most of the lung fields and are the major normal breath sound. Lungs considered "clear" make normal vesicular breath sounds. These sounds are low pitched and soft and have a long inspiratory phase and a shorter expiratory phase (Fig. 13-18).

Vesicular breath sounds are further classified as *harsh* or *diminished*. Harsh vesicular sounds may result from vigorous exercise in which ventilations are rapid and deep. They also occur in children who

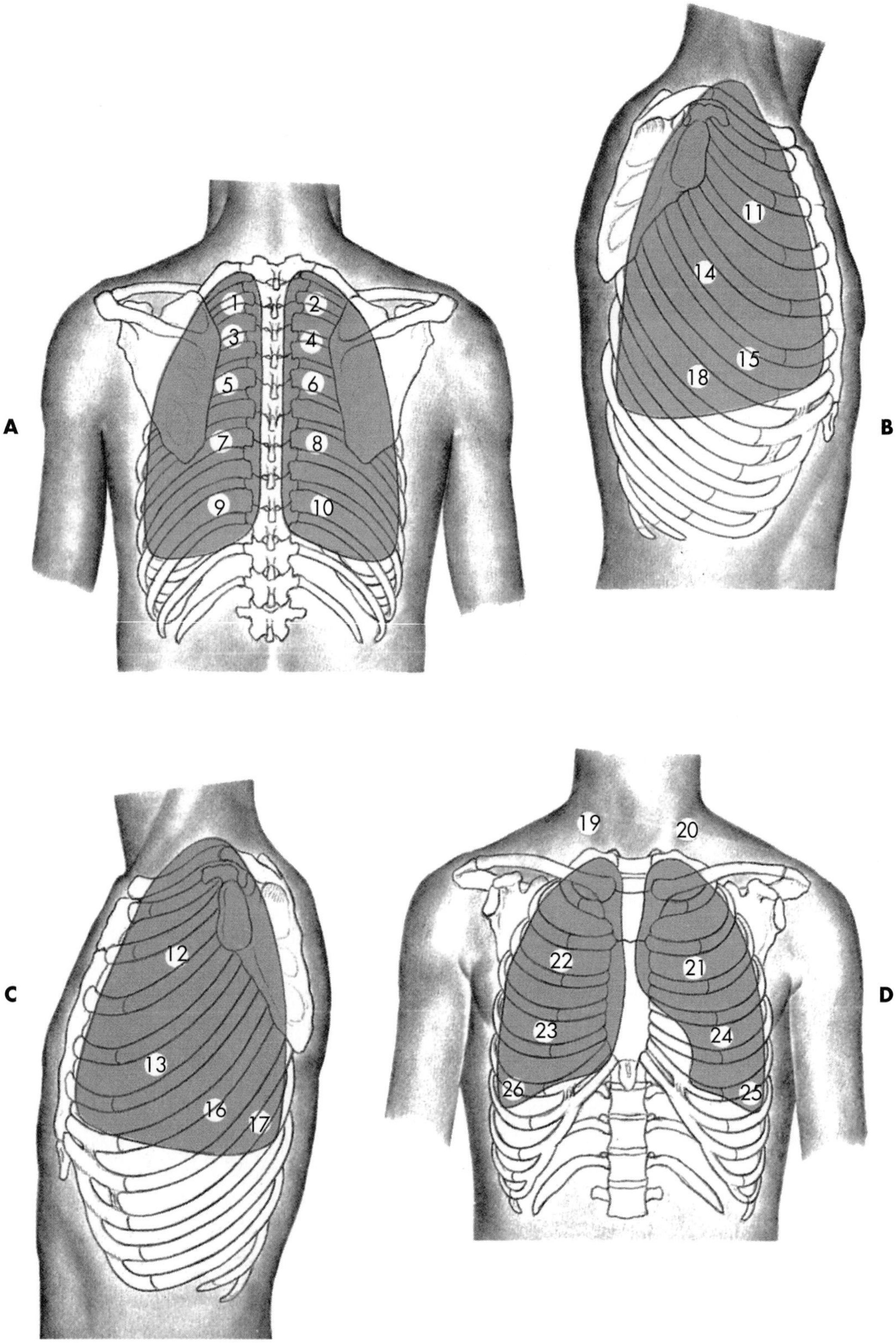

Fig. 13-16 Suggested sequence for systematic percussion and auscultation of the thorax. **A,** Posterior thorax. **B,** Right lateral thorax. **C,** Left lateral thorax. **D,** Anterior thorax. (From Seidel H: *Mosby's guide to physical examination,* ed 2, St Louis, 1991, Mosby.)

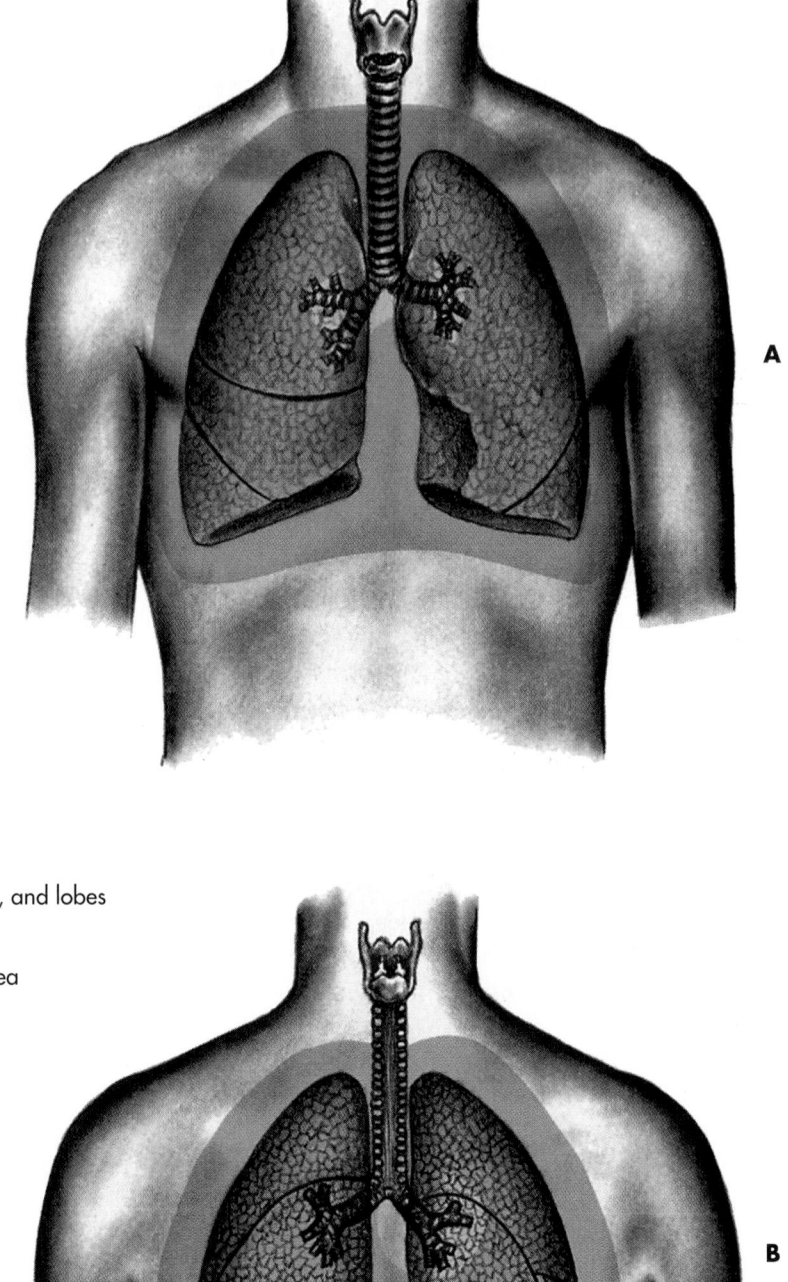

KEY:

Bronchovesicular
over main bronchi

Vesicular over lesser
bronchi, bronchioles, and lobes

Bronchial over trachea

Fig. 13-17 Normal auscultatory sounds on the anterior **(A)** and posterior **(B)** chest wall. (From Seidel H: *Mosby's guide to physical examination,* ed 2, St Louis, 1991, Mosby.)

Ill   *Well*

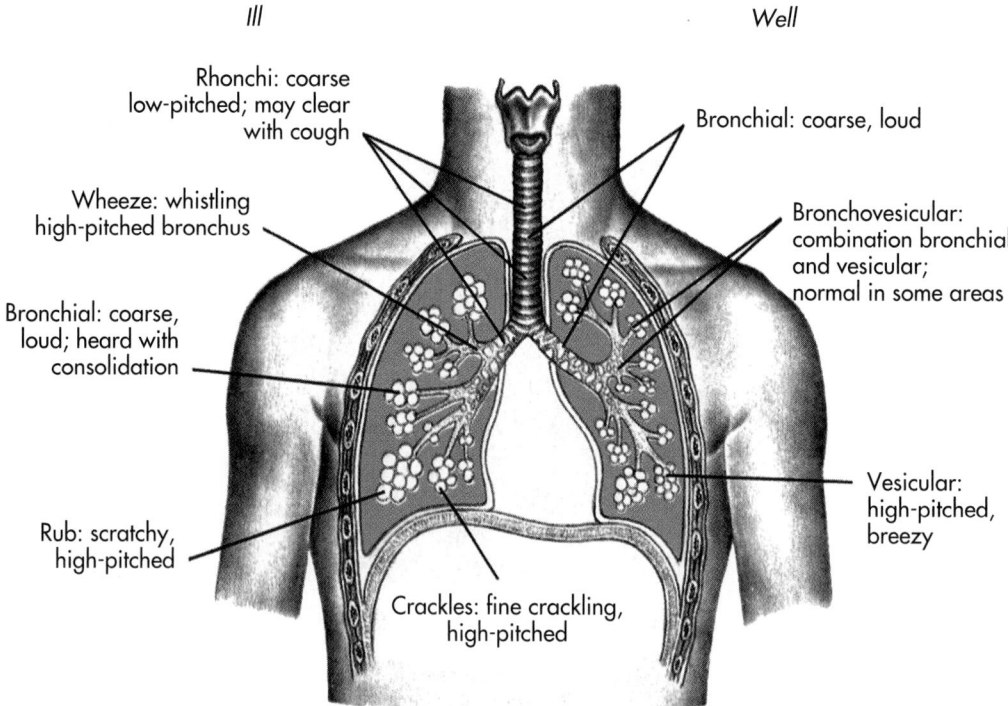

Rhonchi: coarse low-pitched; may clear with cough

Bronchial: coarse, loud

Wheeze: whistling high-pitched bronchus

Bronchovesicular: combination bronchial and vesicular; normal in some areas

Bronchial: coarse, loud; heard with consolidation

Vesicular: high-pitched, breezy

Rub: scratchy, high-pitched

Crackles: fine crackling, high-pitched

Fig. 13-18 Schema of breath sounds in ill and well patients. (From Seidel H: *Mosby's guide to physical examination,* ed 2, St Louis, 1991, Mosby.)

have thin and elastic chest walls in which breath sounds are more easily audible. Vesicular breath sounds may be diminished in older people, who have less ventilation volume, and in obese or very muscular persons, whose additional overlying tissue muffles the sound.

Bronchovesicular breath sounds are heard over the major bronchi and over the upper right posterior lung field. They are louder and harsher than vesicular breath sounds and are considered to be of medium pitch. Bronchovesicular breath sounds have equal inspiration and expiration phases and are heard throughout respiration.

Bronchial breath sounds are heard only over the trachea and are the highest in pitch. They are coarse, harsh, loud sounds with a short inspiratory phase and a long expiration. A bronchial sound heard anywhere but over the trachea is considered an abnormal breath sound.

Abnormal Breath Sounds

Abnormal breath sounds are classified as *absent, diminished,* and *incorrectly located bronchial sounds* and *adventitious breath sounds.* Absent breath sounds may indicate total cessation of the breath-

ing process (e.g., complete airway obstruction), or they may be absent only in a specific area. Causes of localized absent breath sounds include endotracheal tube misplacement, pneumothorax, and hemothorax.

Diminished breath sounds may result from any condition that lessens the airflow. Examples include endotracheal tube misplacement, pneumothorax, partial airway obstruction, and pulmonary disease. Although some airflow is present, diminished breath sounds usually indicate that some portion of the alveolar tissue is not being ventilated.

Bronchial breath sounds auscultated in the peripheral lung field indicate the presence of fluid or exudate in the alveoli, either of which may block airflow. Diseases that contribute to this condition are tumors, pneumonia, and pulmonary edema.

Adventitious Breath Sounds

Adventitious breath sounds are abnormal sounds that are heard in addition to normal breath sounds. They may be divided into two categories: *discontinuous* and *continuous.* Adventitious breath sounds result from obstruction of either the large or small airways and are most commonly heard during inspiration. Adventitious breath sounds are classified as *crackles* (formerly known as *rales*), wheezes, and rhonchi (Fig. 13-19).

Discontinuous breath sounds. Crackles are the high-pitched, discontinuous sounds (similar to the sound of hair being rubbed between the fingers) that usually are heard during the end of inspiration. They indicate disease of the small airways or alveoli, or both, and may be heard anywhere in the peripheral lung field. There is some debate about the etiology of crackles. Some experts believe that the alveoli become filled with fluid, mucus, or pus and tend to close on expiration. With inspiration, the air forces the alveoli open again, producing a "popping" sound. Others contend that the popping sound is produced by air movement through the fluid.

The most typical causes of crackles are pulmonary edema and pneumonia in its early stages. Because gravity draws fluid downward, they often start in the bases of the lungs. Crackles may be further classified as *coarse crackles* (wet, low-pitched sounds) and *fine crackles* (dry, high-pitched sounds). Crackles are discrete and sometimes difficult to hear and may be overridden by louder respiratory sounds. If the paramedic suspects crackles when auscultating the chest, he or she should ask the patient to cough. A cough may clear secretions and make crackles more easily audible.

Continuous breath sounds. Wheezes (also known as *sibilant wheezes*) are high-pitched, "musical" noises that are usually louder during expiration. They are caused by high-velocity air traveling through narrowed airways and may occur because of asthma and other constrictive diseases as well as congestive heart failure. When wheezing occurs in a localized area, a foreign body obstruction, tumor, or mucus plug should be suspected. Wheezes are classified as *mild*, *moderate*, and *severe* and should be described as occurring on inspiration or expiration, or both.

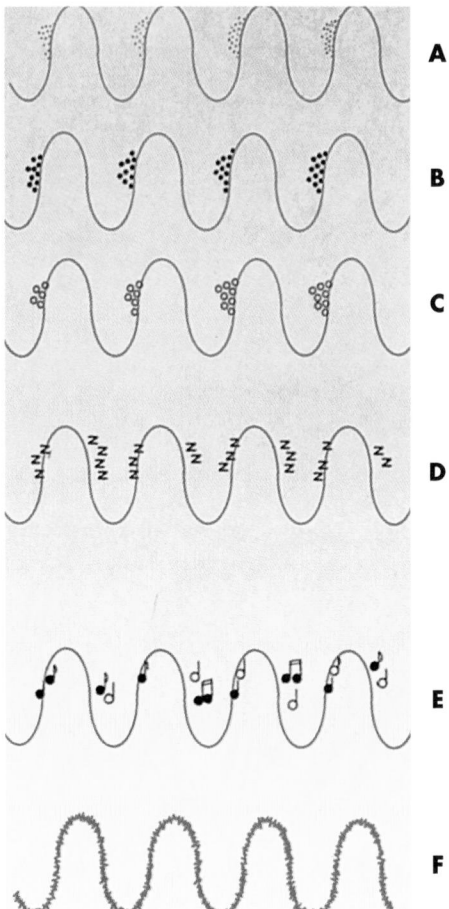

Fig. 13-19 Adventitious breath sounds. **A,** Fine crackles. **B,** Medium crackles. **C,** Coarse crackles. **D,** Rhonchi. **E,** Wheeze. **F,** Pleural friction rub. (From Seidel H: *Mosby's guide to physical examination*, ed 2, St Louis, 1991, Mosby.)

Rhonchi (also known as *sonorous wheezes*) are continuous, low-pitched, rumbling sounds usually heard on expiration. Although rhonchi sound similar to wheezes, they do not involve the small airways. They are less discrete than crackles and are easily auscultated. Rhonchi are caused by the passage of air through an airway obstructed by thick secretions, muscular spasm, new tissue growth, or external pressure collapsing the airway lumen. They may result from any condition that increases secretions. Examples are pneumonia, drug overdose, and long-term postoperative recovery.

Stridor usually is an inspiratory, crowing-type sound that can be heard without the aid of a stethoscope. It indicates significant narrowing or obstruction of the larynx or trachea and may be caused by epiglottitis, viral croup, foreign body aspiration, or

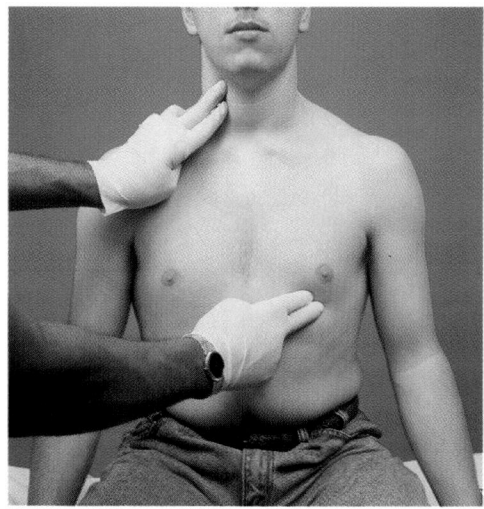

Fig. 13-20 Simultaneous palpation of the carotid artery and apical impulse.

a combination of these factors. Stridor is heard best over the site of origin, usually the larynx or trachea. Stridor often indicates a life-threatening problem, especially in children, and its presence requires careful observation for ventilatory failure and hypoxia.

Pleural friction rub. Although it occurs outside the respiratory tree, a pleural friction rub also may be considered an adventitious breath sound. It is a low-pitched, dry, rubbing, or grating sound caused by the movement of inflamed pleural surfaces as they slide on one another during breathing. The friction rub may be auscultated on both inspiration and expiration and usually is loudest over the lower lateral anterior surface of the chest wall. Presence of a pleural friction rub may indicate pleurisy, viral infection, tuberculosis, or pulmonary embolism.

Heart

In the prehospital setting, the heart must be examined indirectly. However, information about the size and effectiveness of pumping action is obtained through a skilled assessment that includes palpation and auscultation.

Palpation

The apical impulse is the visible and palpable force produced by the contraction of the left ventricle. Palpating this impulse may be useful to compare the relationship of other pulses with the ventricular

cycle. The hearts of some patients with cardiac irregularities, for example, do not always produce a peripheral pulse with every ventricular contraction. By palpating or auscultating the apical impulse and the carotid pulse simultaneously, the paramedic can note these pulse deficits (Fig. 13-20). Factors such as obesity, large breasts, and muscularity may make this landmark difficult to see or palpate.

Auscultation

Heart sounds may be auscultated for frequency (pitch), intensity (loudness), duration, and timing in the cardiac cycle. A thorough evaluation of heart sounds requires a high level of skill and experience, a quiet environment, and sufficient time to listen closely. Two basic heart sounds, however, may be assessed relatively quickly and improve understanding of the patient's condition. These are the basic heart sounds, S1 and S2, which are normal heart sounds that occur when the myocardium contracts. They are best heard toward the apex of the heart at the fifth intercostal space. For evaluation of heart sounds, the patient should be sitting up and leaning slightly forward (Fig. 13-21, *A*), supine (Fig. 13-21, *B*), or in a left lateral recumbent position (Fig. 13-21, *C*). These positions bring the heart closer to the left anterior chest wall. To listen for S1, the paramedic should instruct the patient to breathe normally and hold the breath in expiration. To listen for S2, the patient should breathe normally again and hold the breath in inspiration.

Heart sounds may be muffled or diminished by obesity or obstructive lung disease and by the presence of fluid in the pericardial sac surrounding the heart muscle. This usually is the result of penetrating or severe blunt chest trauma, cardiac tamponade, or cardiac rupture and is considered a true emergency. Other causes of muffled or diminished heart sounds include infectious uremic pericarditis and malignancy. (See Chapters 24 and 28 for further discussion of abnormal heart sounds.)

Inflammation of the pericardial sac may produce a rubbing sound audible with a stethoscope. This is a pericardial friction rub, which may result from infectious pericarditis, myocardial infarction, uremia, trauma, and autoimmune pericarditis. These rubs have a scratching, grating, or squeaking quality and tend to be louder on inspiration. They can be differentiated from pleural friction rubs by their continued presence when the patient holds the breath.

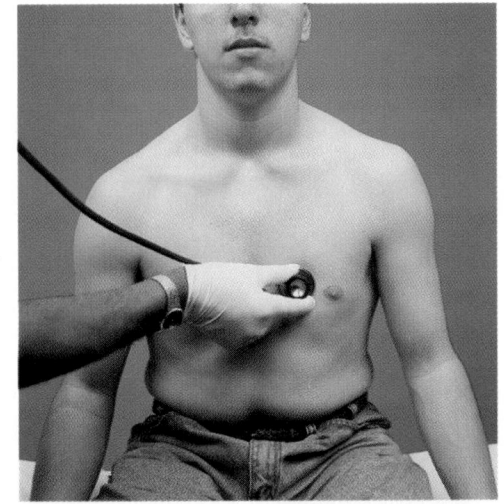

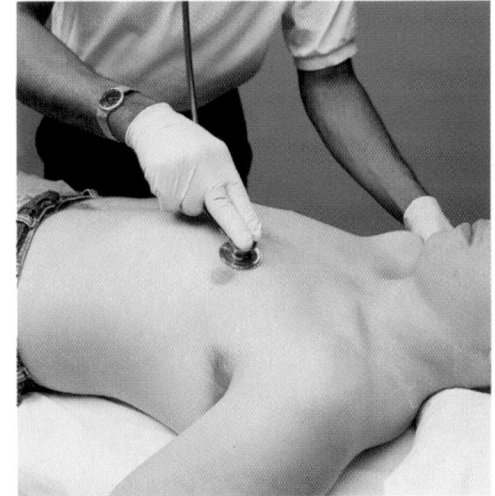

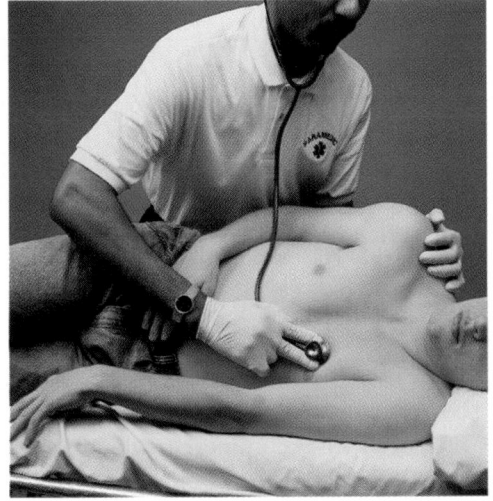

Fig. 13-21 Patient positions for auscultation. **A,** Sitting up, leaning slightly forward. **B,** Supine. **C,** Left lateral recumbent.

Extra Sounds

Extra sounds that can sometimes be heard during auscultation or felt by palpation include heart murmurs, bruits, and thrills. Heart murmurs are prolonged extra sounds that are caused by a disruption in the flow of blood into, through, or out of the heart. Most murmurs are caused by valvular defects. Some heart murmurs are very serious, while others (e.g., some that occur in children and adolescents) are benign and have no apparent cause. Heart murmurs can be detected during auscultation of the heart.

A bruit is an abnormal sound or murmur that may be heard while the carotid artery or another organ or gland is being auscultated, and may indicate local obstruction. Bruits usually are low pitched and relatively hard to hear. To assess blood flow in the carotid artery, the paramedic should place the bell of the stethoscope over the carotid artery at the medial end of the clavicle, and ask the patient to hold his or her breath (Fig. 13-22).

Thrills are similar to bruits, but are described as fine vibrations or tremors that may indicate blood flow obstruction. They may be palpable over the site of an aneurysm or on the precordium. Like murmurs and bruits, thrills may be serious or benign.

Abdomen

The abdomen is divided by two imaginary lines that separate the abdominal region into four quadrants: upper right, lower right, upper left, and lower left (Fig. 13-23). These quadrants and their contents

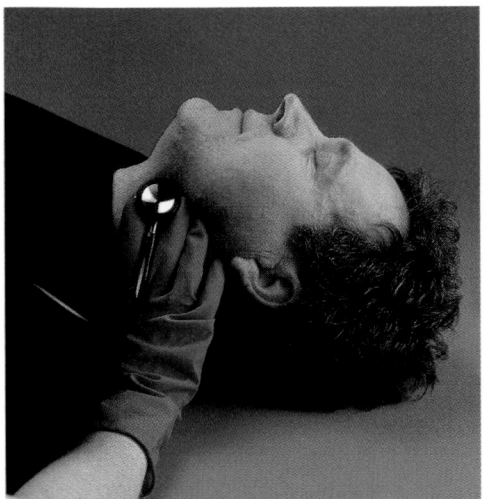

Fig. 13-22 Evaluation of carotid bruit.

(Chapter 6) provide the basis for inspection, auscultation, percussion, and palpation (Box 13-6).

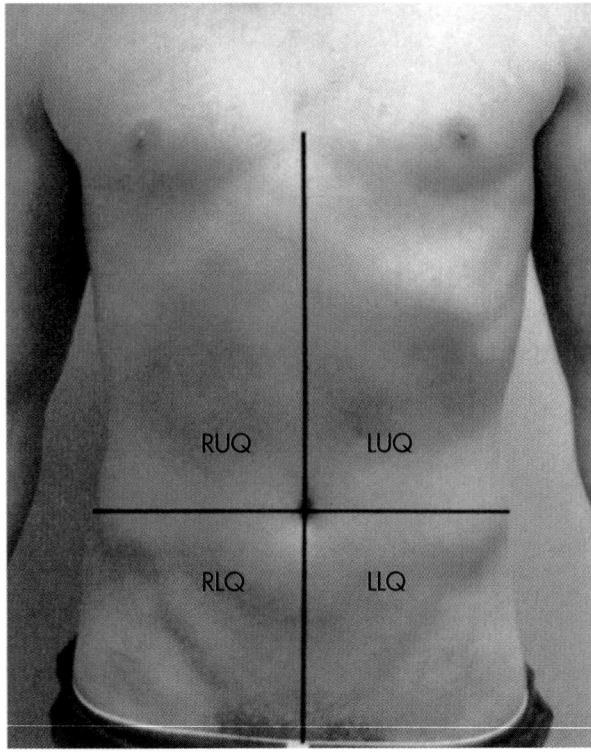

Fig. 13-23 Four quadrants of the abdomen. (From Seidel H: *Mosby's guide to physical examination,* ed 2, St Louis, 1991, Mosby.)

NOTE

When examining a patient's abdomen, the paramedic should make sure that the patient is comfortable (with an empty bladder, if possible) and in a supine position. The paramedic's hands and stethoscope should be warm. The patient should be approached slowly and respectfully, and any painful area should be examined last.

TRICKS OF THE TRADE

Discoloration found in the flank, called *Grey-Turner's sign,* may indicate possible kidney injury.

Inspection

The paramedic should visually inspect the abdomen for signs of cyanosis, pallor, jaundice, bruising, discoloration, swelling (ascites), masses, and aortic pulsations. Surgical scars and implanted devices such as automatic implanted cardioverter defibrillators (AICDs) also should be noted. The abdomen should be evenly round and symmetrical. Symmetrical distention of the abdomen may result from obesity, enlarged organs, fluid, or gas. Asymmetrical distention may result from hernias, tumor, bowel obstruction, or enlarged abdominal organs. A flat abdomen is common in athletic adults, and convex abdomens are common in children and in adults with poor exercise habits. The umbilicus should be free of swelling, bulges, and signs of inflammation. The normal umbilicus usually is inverted, or it may protrude slightly.

TRICKS OF THE TRADE

Discoloration around the umbilicus, called *Cullen's sign,* may indicate peritoneal bleeding.

Abdominal movement during respiration should be smooth and even. As a rule, males have more abdominal involvement than females during respiration, so limited abdominal movement in the symptomatic male may indicate an abdominal pathological condition. Visible pulsations in the upper abdomen may be normal in thin adults, but marked pulsations may indicate an abdominal aortic aneurysm.

BOX 13-6

ABDOMINAL QUADRANTS

Right Upper Quadrant
Liver and gallbladder
Pylorus
Duodenum
Head of pancreas
Right adrenal gland
Portion of right kidney
Hepatic flexure of colon
Portions of ascending and transverse colon

Left Upper Quadrant
Left lobe of liver
Spleen
Stomach
Body of pancreas
Left adrenal gland
Portion of left kidney
Splenic flexure of colon
Portions of transverse and descending colon

Right Lower Quadrant
Lower pole of right kidney
Cecum and appendix
Portion of ascending colon
Appendix
Bladder (if distended)
Ovary and salpinx
Uterus (if enlarged)
Right ureter

Left Lower Quadrant
Lower pole of left kidney
Sigmoid colon
Portion of descending colon
Bladder (if distended)
Ovary and salpinx
Uterus (if enlarged)
Left ureter

Auscultation

Noting the presence or absence of bowel sounds to assess motility and to discover vascular sounds has limited value in the prehospital setting because it does not affect or determine the approach to patient care. In addition, the time required for thorough bowel sound assessment (about 5 minutes per quadrant) far exceeds the justifiable scene time for most patients. If auscultation is to be performed, however, it should always precede palpation, since the latter maneuvers may alter the intensity of bowel sounds.

To auscultate bowel sounds, the paramedic holds the diaphragm of the stethoscope on the abdomen with light pressure. If bowel sounds are present, they usually are heard as rumblings or gurgles that occur irregularly, ranging in frequency from 5 to 35 per minute. Auscultation should be done in all four quadrants, and a minimum of 5 minutes per quadrant is required to determine that normal bowel sounds are absent. Increased bowel sounds may indicate gastroenteritis or intestinal obstruction. Decreased or absent bowel sounds may indicate peritonitis (inflammation of the lining of the abdominal cavity) or ileus (inactive peristaltic activity resulting from one of several causes).

Percussion and Palpation

Percussion and palpation of the abdomen may be useful to detect the presence of fluid, air, and solid masses. The paramedic should use a systematic approach, moving either from side to side or in a clockwise direction, noting any rigidity, tenderness, or abnormal skin temperature or color. The patient's face should be observed for signs of pain or discomfort. If the patient is complaining of abdominal pain, the painful quadrant should be examined last so that the patient will not unnecessarily tighten or "guard" the abdominal area. The abdominal assessment should begin with a light palpation, using an even pressing motion. As previously stated, the paramedic's hands should be warm, and sharp and quick jabs should be avoided. Palpation may be done simultaneously with percussion.

Percussion should begin by evaluating all four quadrants of the abdomen for a general assessment of tympany and dullness. (Tympany is the major sound that should be noted during percussion because of the normal presence of air in the stomach and intestines. Dullness should be heard over organs and solid masses.) When one is percussing the abdomen, it is best to proceed from an area of tympany to an area of dullness, because the change in sound is easier to detect. Individual assessments of the liver and spleen (described in the following paragraphs) may be done when the abdomen is examined if indicated by patient complaint or mechanism of injury.

> **NOTE**
>
> Patients who may require surgery for abdominal illness or injury will be best served by rapid assessment, stabilization, and transport to an appropriate medical facility.

Percussion and Palpation of the Liver

The liver is percussed by beginning just above the umbilicus in the right midclavicular line in an area of tympany. Percussion should continue in an upward direction until the change from tympany to dullness occurs. This change usually occurs slightly below the costal margin and indicates the lower border of the liver. To determine the upper border of the liver, the percussion should begin in the same midclavicular line at the midsternal level, proceeding downward until the tympany from the lung area changes to dullness (usually between the fifth and seventh intercostal spaces). Liver size is related to age and sex. It will usually be proportionately larger in adults than in children and larger in males than in females.

For palpation of the liver, the patient should be supine, comfortable, and have a relaxed abdomen. The examination should be performed from the patient's right side and begins by placing the left hand

under the patient in the area of the eleventh and twelfth ribs (Fig. 13-24). The right hand should be placed on the abdomen, with the fingers pointing toward the patient's head and extended, resting just below the edge of the costal margin. The conscious patient should be instructed to breathe deeply through the mouth. During exhalation, the hand under the patient is pressed upward, and the right hand is gently pushed in and up. If the liver is felt, it should be firm and nontender. (A healthy liver usually cannot be palpated unless the patient is thin.)

Percussion and Palpation of the Spleen

For percussion of the spleen, the patient must be lying supine or in a right lateral recumbent position. Percussion should begin at the area of lung tympany, just posterior to the midaxillary line on the left side. When one is percussing downward, a change from tympany to dullness should be heard between the sixth and tenth ribs. Large areas of dullness suggest an enlarged spleen. Stomach contents and air-filled or feces-filled intestines make splenic assessment by percussion difficult since these and other factors may affect percussion tones of dullness and tympany.

Palpation is a more useful assessment technique for evaluating the spleen. The patient should be lying supine with the paramedic positioned at the patient's left side. The left hand is placed under the patient, supporting the lower left rib cage. The right hand is placed just below the patient's lower left costal margin (Fig. 13-25). The area should be

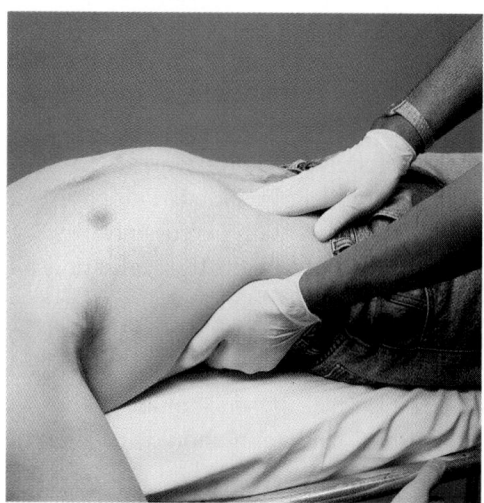

Fig. 13-24 Palpation of the liver.

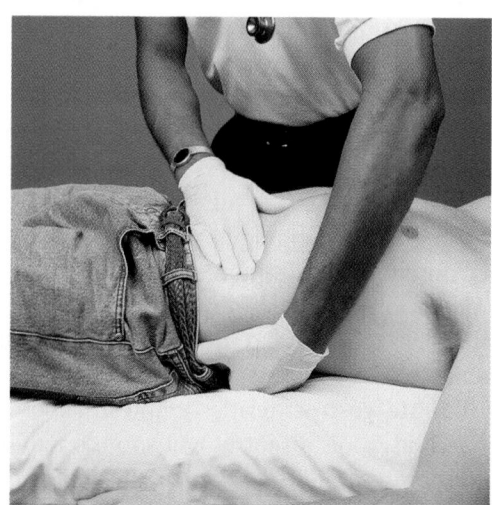

Fig. 13-25 Palpation of the spleen.

gently palpated by lifting up the left hand, and pressing down with the right. (A normal spleen usually cannot be palpated in an adult. A palpable spleen is probably enlarged three times its normal size.)

> **NOTE**
>
> Palpation of the spleen can produce rupture of the organ. It should be performed with caution.

> ✓ **TRICKS OF THE TRADE**
>
> Assume any female of childbearing age to be pregnant until proven otherwise.

Female Genitalia

An examination of the genitalia of either sex can be awkward and uncomfortable for the patient and the paramedic. When possible, same-sex paramedics should perform these examinations. In the absence of same-sex caregivers, a chaperone should be present during the examination.

The external genitalia should be visually inspected to note any swelling, redness, discharge, bleeding, or evidence of trauma. Discoloration or tenderness may be the result of traumatic bruising. Ulcers, vesicles, and discharges (with or without pain) indicate sexually transmitted disease. If touching the anal area is necessary, gloves should be changed to prevent bacteria from being introduced into the vaginal area.

> **?** CRITICAL THINKING
>
> *Why is it advisable to examine a patient's genitalia in the presence of another prehospital care provider?*

Male Genitalia

When examining the male genitalia, the paramedic should visually inspect the area for bleeding and signs of trauma. The shaft of the penis should be nontender and flaccid. Patients with leukemia, sickle cell disease, or spinal injury may have a persistent painful erection (priapism, a rare condition).

The urethral opening should be free of blood (a possible result of pelvic trauma) or discharge (a sign of sexually transmitted disease). The scrotum should be nontender and slightly asymmetrical. A swollen or painful scrotum may result from infection, herniation, testicular torsion, or trauma.

> ✓ **TRICKS OF THE TRADE**
>
> Discoloration of the genitals, called *Coopernail's sign*, may indicate peritoneal bleeding.

Anus

Examination of the anus is indicated in the presence of rectal bleeding or trauma to the area. It can be accomplished with the patient in one of several positions; however, most patients will find the side-lying position to be most comfortable. (The patient's privacy should be protected with appropriate drapes.) Inspection of the sacrococcygeal and perineal areas should consider abnormal findings such as lumps, ulcers, inflammation, rashes, and excoriations (surface injury caused by scratching or abrasions). Inflamed external hemorrhoids are common in adults and pregnant women.

Method of Testing for Occult Blood

A sample of feces can be tested for occult (microscopic) blood with Hemoccult test supplies (Fig. 13-26). To test for occult blood, the paramedic should follow these steps:

1. Explain the procedure to the patient. If possible, ask the patient to produce a stool specimen that

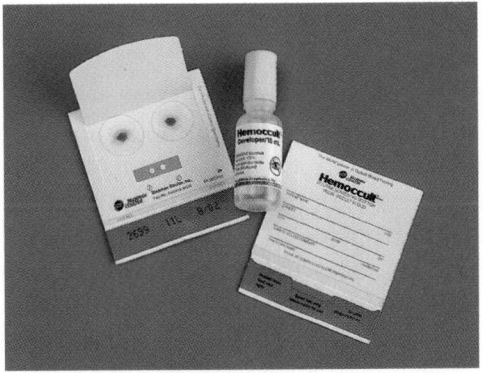

Fig. 13-26 Hemoccult kit.

is not mixed with urine or water. If necessary, a sample specimen can be collected by inserting a gloved finger into the rectum.

2. Use clean disposable gloves and a wooden applicator to collect a small sample of fecal material.
3. Apply a thin smear of stool to each of the specimen papers in the test card. Close the slide cover.
4. Turn the test card over and open the flap. Apply two drops of Hemoccult developing solution on each paper sample and control strip in the test card.
5. Test results are visible in 30 to 60 seconds. Blue indicates occult blood. No change in color indicates negative results.
6. Properly dispose of all materials.

Extremities

When examining the upper and lower extremities, paramedics should pay attention to function as well as structure (see Chapter 6). The patient's general appearance, body proportions, and ease of movement are important observations. In particular, the paramedic should note any limitation in the range of motion or an unusual increase in the mobility of a joint. Abnormal findings include the following:

- Signs of inflammation
  Swelling
  Tenderness
  Increased heat
  Redness
  Decreased function
- Asymmetry
- Crepitus
- Deformities
- Decreased muscular strength
- Atrophy

Examining Upper and Lower Extremities

A systematic assessment of the upper and lower extremities includes an evaluation of the skin and tissue overlying the muscles, cartilage, and bones; and joints for soft tissue injury, discoloration, swelling, and masses. The upper and lower extremities should be reasonably symmetrical in both structure and muscularity. The circulatory status of each extremity should be assessed during the examination by determining skin color, temperature, sensation,

and the presence of distal pulses. Bones, joints, and surrounding tissues of the extremities should be assessed for structural integrity and continuity. Muscle tone should be firm and nontender. Joints are assessed for function by moving each joint through its full range of motion (see Chapter 6). A normal range of motion occurs without pain, deformity, limitation, or instability.

Hands and Wrists

The paramedic should inspect both hands and wrists for contour and positional alignment. Palpate the wrists, hands, and joints of each finger for tenderness, swelling, or deformity. To determine range of motion, request the patient to flex and extend the wrists, make a fist, and touch the thumb to each fingertip. All movements should be performed without pain or discomfort.

Elbows

The paramedic should inspect and palpate the elbows in both the flexed and extended positions. To determine the elbow's range of motion, the paramedic should ask the patient to rotate the hands from palm up to palm down. The grooves between the epicondyle and olecranon should be inspected by palpation. Pain and tenderness should not be present when the examiner presses on the lateral and medial epicondyle.

Shoulders and Related Structures

The shoulders should be inspected and palpated for symmetry and integrity of the clavicles, scapulae, and humeri. Pain, tenderness, or asymmetric contour may indicate a fracture or dislocation. The patient should be able to shrug shoulders and raise and extend both arms without pain or discomfort. The following regions should be palpated, noting any tenderness or swelling (Fig. 13-27):

- Sternoclavicular joint
- Acromioclavicular joint
- Subacromial area
- Bicipital groove

Ankles and Feet

The patient's feet and ankles should be inspected for contour, position, and size. Tenderness, swelling, and deformity are abnormal findings on palpation. The toes should be straight and aligned with each

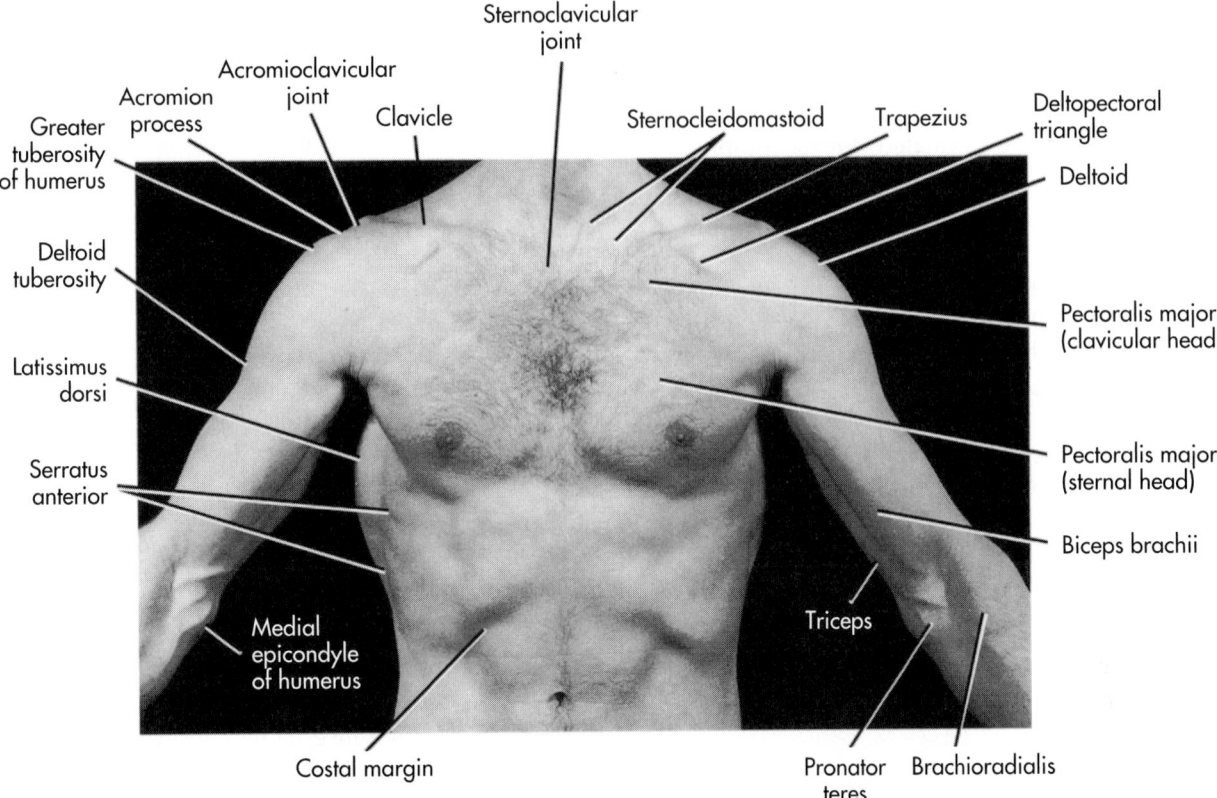

Fig. 13-27 Evaluation of shoulder and related structures. (From Snell RS, Smith MS: *Clinical anatomy for emergency medicine,* St Louis, 1993, Mosby.)

other. Range of motion can be determined by requesting the patient to bend the toes, point the toes, and rotate the feet both inward and outward from the ankle. These movements should be possible without pain or discomfort. All surfaces of the ankles and feet should be inspected for deformities, nodules, swelling, calluses, corns, and skin integrity.

Pelvis, Hips, and Knees

The structural integrity of the pelvis should be verified. To palpate the iliac crest and the symphysis pubis, the paramedic places both hands on each anterior iliac crest, pressing downward and outward (Fig. 13-28). To determine stability, the paramedic places the heel of the hand on the symphysis pubis and presses downward. Deformity and point tenderness of the pelvis may be signs of fracture, masking major structural and vascular injury.

The hips should be inspected and palpated for instability, tenderness, and crepitus. The supine or unconscious patient can be examined by assessing the structural integrity of the iliac crest. A mobile patient should be able to walk without discomfort.

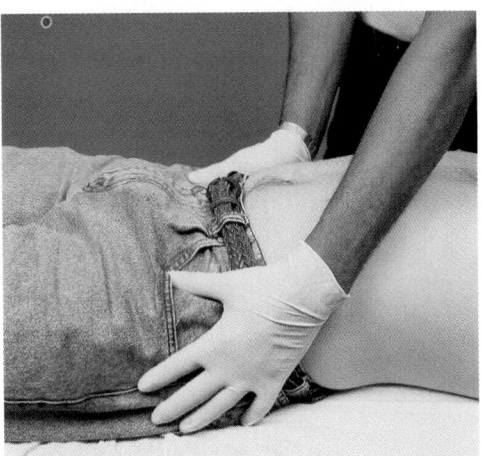

Fig. 13-28 Palpating the pelvis for stability.

A supine patient should be able to raise the legs and knees and rotate the legs inward and outward.

The knees should be inspected and palpated for swelling and tenderness. The patella should be smooth, firm, nontender, and midline in position. The patient should be able to bend and straighten each knee without pain.

Peripheral Vascular System

The peripheral vascular system includes arteries, veins, the lymphatic system and lymph nodes, and the fluids exchanged in the capillary bed. These components can be evaluated during the physical examination of the upper and lower extremities.

Arms

While evaluating the arms, the paramedic should inspect from fingertips to shoulders, noting size, symmetry, swelling, venous pattern, color of the skin and nail beds, and texture of the skin. If arterial insufficiency is noted because of a weak radial pulse, the brachial pulse should be palpated. Epitrochlear nodes and brachial nodes should be nonswollen and nontender (Fig. 13-29).

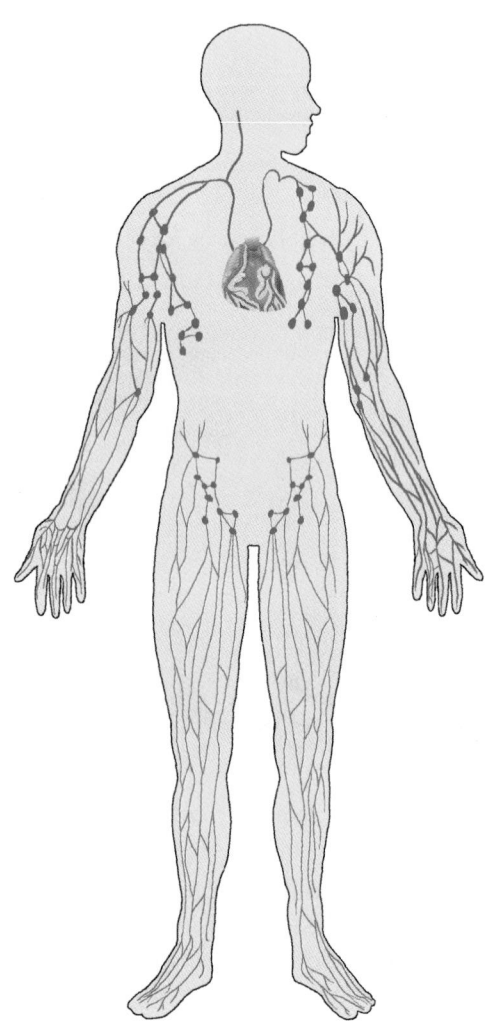

Fig. 13-29 Nodes of upper and lower extremities.

> **NOTE**
>
> A fine venous network on upper and lower extremities often is visible. The paramedic should be alert for enlargement of superficial veins during the examination.

Legs

During examination of the lower extremities, the patient should be supine and appropriately draped. (Shoes, socks, and hosiery should be removed for a thorough examination.) The paramedic should visually inspect from the groin and buttocks to the feet, noting the following:

- Size and symmetry
- Swelling
- Venous pattern and venous enlargement
- Pigmentation
- Rashes, scars, or ulcers
- Color and texture of the skin
- Presence or absence of hair growth (indicating compromised arterial circulation)

The superficial inguinal nodes in the groin should be palpated to assess for swelling and tenderness. All lower extremity pulse sites should be assessed to evaluate circulation, strength, and regularity. These include the femoral pulse, the popliteal pulse, the dorsalis pedis pulse, and the posterior tibial pulse (see Chapter 6). The temperature of the feet and legs should be warm, indicating adequate circulation. The presence of pitting edema can be evaluated over the dorsum of each foot, behind each medial malleolus, and over the shins by pressing firmly on the skin with the thumb for at least 5 seconds. Edema is said to be pitting when depression of the tissue remains after removal of finger pressure.

Abnormal Findings

Findings that are considered abnormal during a peripheral vascular assessment include the following:

- Swollen or asymmetrical extremities
- Pale or cyanotic skin
- Weak or diminished pulses
- Skin that is cold to the touch
- Absence of hair growth
- Pitting edema

Spine

A comprehensive physical examination includes an assessment of the spine, beginning with a visual assessment of the cervical, thoracic, and lumbar curves. From the patient's side, the paramedic should note any curvature of the spine, including that associated with abnormal lordosis, kyphosis, and scoliosis. In addition, the paramedic should look for any differences in the height of the shoulders or iliac crest that may result from abnormal spinal curvature.

? CRITICAL THINKING

If there is no deformity of the spine found during the examination, can spine fracture or dislocation be ruled out?

Cervical Spine

The patient's neck should be in a midline position. If the patient is alert and denies neck pain, the paramedic should palpate the posterior aspect for point tenderness and swelling. (The only palpable landmark should be the spinous process of the seventh cervical vertebra at the base of the neck.) In the absence of suspected injury, the paramedic tests range of motion by directing the patient to bend the head forward, backward, and from side to side. These movements should not cause pain or discomfort.

NOTE

To test range of motion, the paramedic should never attempt to move the neck of an individual who is unconscious or who is unable or unwilling to do so on his or her own. Spontaneous cervical muscle spasm frequently is associated with significant cervical spine injury in the trauma victim.

Thoracic and Lumbar Spine

The paramedic should inspect the thoracic and lumbar areas for signs of injury, swelling, and discoloration. Palpation should begin at the first thoracic vertebrae and move downward to the sacrum. Under normal conditions, the spine is nontender to palpation. Range of motion can be evaluated by requesting the patient to bend at the waist forward and backward and to each side, and also to rotate the upper trunk from side to side in a circular motion.

Nervous System

Detail of an appropriate neurological examination varies greatly and depends on the origin of the patient's complaint (e.g., peripheral nervous system vs. central nervous system problems). The examination may be performed separately, but more often the evaluation is completed during other assessments. A neurological examination may be organized into five categories:

- Mental status and speech
- Cranial nerves
- Motor system
- Sensory system
- Reflexes

Mental Status and Speech

As previously discussed, a healthy patient should be oriented to person, time, and place. Patients should also be able to organize thoughts and converse freely (provided there are no hearing or speech impediments). Abnormal findings include unconsciousness, confusion, slurred speech, aphasia, dysphonia, and dysarthria.

Cranial Nerves

The 12 cranial nerves can be categorized as sensory, somatomotor and proprioceptive, and parasympathetic (see Chapter 6). The following methods can be used to assess each of the cranial nerves:

Cranial Nerve I Olfactory: Test sense of smell with spirits of ammonia.

Cranial Nerve II Optic: Test for visual acuity (previously described).

Cranial Nerve II and III Optic and Oculomotor: Inspect the size and shape of the pupils; test the pupil response to light.

Cranial Nerve III, IV, VI Oculomotor, Trochlear, Abducens: Test extraocular movements by asking the patient to look up and down, to the left and right, and diagonally up and down to the left and right (the six cardinal directions of gaze).

Cranial Nerve V Trigeminal: Test motor movement by asking the patient to clench the teeth while you palpate the temporal and masseter muscles. Test sensation by touching the fore-head, cheeks, and jaw on each side.

Cranial Nerve VII   Facial: Inspect the face at rest and during conversation, noting symmetry, tics, or abnormal movements. Ask the patient to raise the eyebrows, frown, show both upper and lower teeth, smile, and puff out both cheeks. Strength of the facial muscles can be assessed by asking the patient to close eyes tightly so they cannot be opened, and gently attempt to raise the eyelids. Observe for weakness or asymmetry.

Cranial Nerve VIII   Acoustic: Assess hearing acuity (previously described).

Cranial Nerve IX and X   Glossopharyngeal and Vagus: Assess the patient's ability to swallow with ease; to produce saliva; and to produce normal voice sounds. Instruct the patient to hold the breath, and assess for normal slowing of the heart rate. Testing for the gag reflex also will test the cranial nerves.

Cranial Nerve XI   Spinal Accessory: Ask the patient to raise and lower the shoulders, and to turn the head.

Cranial Nerve XII   Hypoglossal: Ask the patient to stick out the tongue and to move it in several directions.

Motor System

An evaluation of a patient's motor system includes observing the patient during movement and while at rest. Abnormal involuntary movements should be evaluated for quality, rate, rhythm, and amplitude. Other body movement assessments include posture, level of activity, fatigue, and emotion.

Muscle Strength

Muscle strength should be bilaterally symmetrical, and the patient should be able to provide reasonable resistance to opposition. One method to evaluate muscle strength in the upper extremities is to instruct the patient to extend the elbow and to pull it toward the chest while using opposing resistance (Fig. 13-30, *A*). Muscle strength in the lower extremities is evaluated by requesting the patient to push the soles of the feet against the paramedic's palms. Next, the patient is directed to pull the toes toward the head while the paramedic provides opposing resistance (Fig. 13-30, *B*). Both of these actions should be easily performed by the patient without evident fatigue. Other methods that can be used to evaluate muscle strength and agility (illustrated in Chapter 6) include testing for flexion, extension, and abduction of the upper and lower extremities.

Coordination

To evaluate a patient's coordination, the paramedic should assess the patient's ability to perform rapid alternating movements. These include point-to-point movements, gait, and stance.

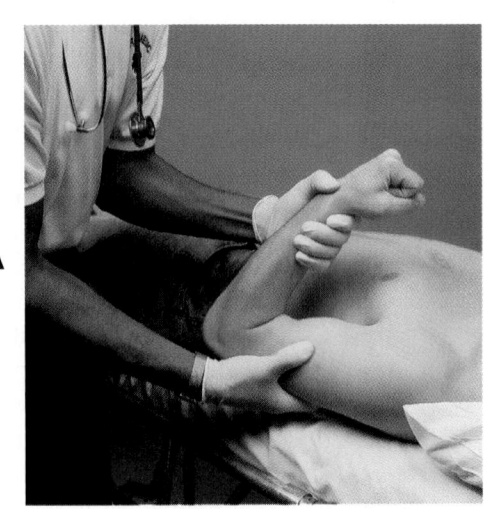
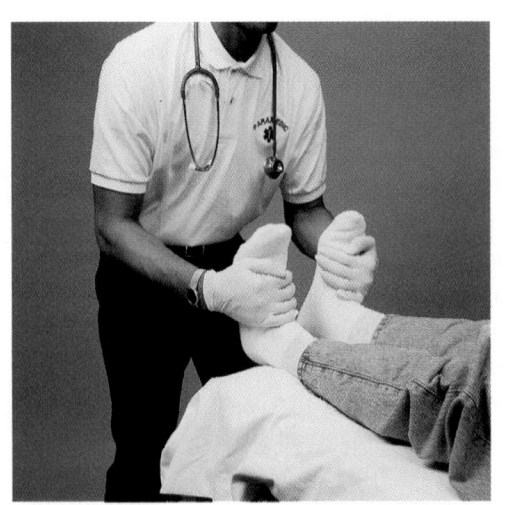

Fig. 13-30 Evaluating muscle strength of the upper **(A)** and lower **(B)** extremities.

One point-to-point movement that the patient can easily perform is to touch the finger to the nose, alternating hands. Another test is to instruct the patient to touch each heel to the opposite shin. Both movements should be performed numerous times and quickly to assess coordination, which should be smooth, rapid, and accurate.

Gait can be evaluated in several ways. A healthy patient should be able to perform each of the following tasks without discomfort or losing balance:

- Walk heel to toe
- Walk on the toes
- Walk on the heels
- Hop in place
- Do a shallow knee bend
- Rise from a sitting position without assistance

> **NOTE**
>
> The paramedic should take into consideration the patient's age and physical condition in determining the appropriateness of these examinations.

Stance and balance can be evaluated by using the Romberg test and the Pronator Drift test. To perform the Romberg test, ask the patient to stand erect with the feet together and arms at the sides. The eyes should initially be open and then closed. Although slight swaying is normal, a loss of balance is abnormal (a positive Romberg sign). A patient also should be able to stand in this position with one foot raised for 5 seconds without losing balance.

> **NOTE**
>
> The paramedic should stay close to the patient being tested for stance and balance so that injury from a fall or loss of balance can be avoided.

The Pronator Drift test (also known as an *arm drift test*) is performed by having the patient close the eyes and hold both arms out from the body. A normal test will reveal that both arms move the same or both arms do not move at all. Abnormal findings include one arm that does not move in concert with the other or one arm that drifts down compared with the other.

Sensory System

The sensory pathways of the nervous system conduct sensations of pain, temperature, position, vibration, and touch. A healthy patient is expected to be responsive to each of these stimuli. Common assessments of the sensory system include evaluating the patient's response to pain and light touch. Each of the responses should be considered in relation to dermatomes (see Chapter 6).

In conscious patients, a sensory examination should be performed with light touch on each hand and each foot. If the patient cannot feel light touch or is unconscious, sensation may be evaluated by gently pricking the hands and soles of the feet with a sharp object that will not penetrate the skin (e.g., a paper clip or cotton swab). The sensory examination should proceed from head to toe, comparing symmetrical areas on each side of the body as well as distal and proximal areas of the body. A lack of sensory response may indicate spinal cord damage (see Chapter 23).

Physical Examination of Infants and Children

Examining the ill or injured child requires special assessment skills. Children differ physiologically, psychologically, and anatomically from adults, so pediatric patient assessment must take age and development into account.

Approaching the Pediatric Patient

The assessment and management objectives in caring for critically ill or injured children are similar to those for any other patient encounter. The approach to the pediatric patient must differ, however. The initial encounter with the sick or injured child sets the tone for the entire patient care episode, so the paramedic must consider the patient's age and be sensitive to how the child perceives the emergency environment. The following six guidelines should be considered when approaching the pediatric patient[3]:

1. Remain calm and confident. The parent's anxiety is infectious. Stay under control and take charge of the situation in a gentle but firm manner.

2. Do not separate the child from the parent unless absolutely necessary. In fact, once parents are reassured, encourage them to touch, hold, or cuddle the child when such actions are practical. This comforts the parents as well as the child.

3. Establish rapport with the parents as well as the child. Much of a child's fear and anxiety reflects the parent's behavior. When the family is calm, the child is reassured and is less fearful.

4. Be honest with both child and parent. In simple, direct, nonmedical language, explain to both the parent and the child what is happening as it occurs. When a procedure is going to hurt, inform the child. Never lie. Do not give the impression that there are options when none exist. For example, do not say, "Would you like to go for a ride in the ambulance?" The child may answer "No."

5. Whenever possible, assign one emergency caregiver to stay with the child. This person should obtain the history and be the primary person to initiate therapy. Even in a few moments, one person who remains on the child's level can establish a trusting relationship.

6. Observe the patient before the physical examination. When possible, the paramedic should initially assess the alert child without touching the patient. After the physical examination begins, the child's behavior may drastically change, making it difficult to assess whether the behavior is a reaction to a physical state or to the perceived intrusion. The patient's general appearance, skin signs, level of consciousness, respiratory rate, and behavior usually can be assessed easily before approaching the patient. During this observation, also note any particular area of the body that appears painful. Avoid manipulating this area until the end of the examination and inform the child that you will give warning before you touch the area.

? CRITICAL THINKING

The next time you are in a room with an infant or small child, try this "across the room" assessment technique. What can you tell about the level of distress and cardiopulmonary function by doing this?

General Appearance

A child's general appearance is best assessed from a distance. While the patient is in safe, familiar surroundings (e.g., a parent's arms), the paramedic should visually assess the child's level of consciousness, spontaneous movement, respiratory effort, and skin color. The child's body position also can provide helpful information; for example, the child may be lying limp or sitting upright to facilitate breathing. Other clues (e.g., crying, eye contact, concentration, distractibility) may help determine the child's willingness to cooperate during the physical examination.

A visual inspection of the child's general appearance is a fairly reliable indicator of the patient's need for emergency care. Children who are seriously ill or injured usually do not attempt to disguise or hide their condition and generally exhibit behavior that reflects the severity of the situation. Therefore the patient's general appearance is a valuable assessment tool for the paramedic. Table 13-3 provides the important components of general appearance in initial assessment of the pediatric patient.

Physical Examination

A hands-on examination is best conducted through an age-related evaluation. The following guidelines will vary according to the child's development but may be used as a reference for examination procedures. Parents and family members also may be a source of information during the examination. Questions regarding "normal" behavior and activity levels may be directed to the parents.

Birth to 6 Months

Children under 6 months of age typically are not frightened by the approach of a stranger, and the physical examination is relatively easy. During the examination, special consideration should be given to maintaining the child's body temperature.

Healthy and alert infants usually are in constant motion and may have a lusty cry. If the patient is under 3 months of age, poor head control is normal. Infants are "abdominal breathers," which causes the stomach to protrude and the infant's chest wall to retract during inspiration. This diaphragmatic involvement may give the impression of labored breathing. Skin color, nasal flaring, and intercostal

TABLE 13-3	COMPONENTS OF GENERAL APPEARANCE FOR ASSESSING PEDIATRIC PATIENTS
ASSESSMENT FINDING	**EVALUATION CONSIDERATIONS**
Alertness	How perceptive is the child, and how responsive is he or she to the presence of a stranger or to other aspects of the environment?
Distractibility	How readily does a person, object, or sound draw the child's attention? For example, drawing a child's attention to a toy when the child initially appeared disinterested in the surroundings is a positive sign.
Consolability	Can a distressed child be comforted? For example, stopping a child from crying by speaking softly or offering a pacifier or a toy is an encouraging sign.
Speech or cry	Is the speech or cry strong and spontaneous? Weak and muffled? Hoarse? Absent unless stimulated? Absent altogether?
Spontaneous activity	Does the child appear flaccid? Do the extremities move only in response to stimuli, or are there spontaneous movements?
Color	Is there pallor, a flushed appearance, cyanosis, or mottling? Does the skin coloring of the trunk differ from that of the extremities?
Respiratory efforts	Are there intercostal, supraclavicular, or suprasternal retractions in the resting state? Nasal flaring also indicates respiratory difficulty.
Eye contact	Does the child appear to gaze aimlessly, or does he or she maintain eye contact with objects or people? Even very small infants, when well, preferentially fix their gaze on a face rather than other objects.

muscle retraction are the best indicators of respiratory insufficiency.

In the infant, assessing the fontanelles is particularly important. These sutures between the flat bones of the skull are fairly wide to allow a "give" in the skull during the birth process. (The anterior fontanelle, known as the *soft spot*, usually is present up to the age of 18 months.) The anterior fontanelle should be level with the skull or slightly depressed and soft. It usually bulges during crying and may feel firm if the child is lying down. In the absence of injury, the fontanelle is best examined with the child in an upright position. A sunken fontanelle may indicate dehydration, and a bulging fontanelle in the noncrying upright infant may indicate an increase in intracranial pressure.

7 Months to 3 Years

Patients from 7 months to 3 years of age often are difficult to evaluate. They have little capacity to understand the emergency event and are likely to experience emotional problems as a result of illness, injury, or hospitalization. Children of this age fear strangers and may show separation anxiety. If possible, parents should be present and be allowed to hold the child during the examination. The paramedic should approach the child with a quiet, reassuring voice, and if time permits, allow the patient to become accustomed to the examination environment.

During the physical assessment, each activity should be explained in short, simple sentences, even though it may not improve cooperation. It is best to be gentle and firm and to complete the examination as quickly as possible. If physical restraint is necessary and if patient care activities will not be hindered, the child should be restrained with hands rather than mechanical devices (e.g., backboards).

4 to 10 Years

Children in the 4- to 10-year age group are developing a capacity for rational thought and may be very cooperative during the physical examination. Depending on the child's age and the emergency scenario, he or she may be able to provide a limited history of the event. These children also may experience separation anxiety and may view their illness or injury as punishment. Therefore the paramedic should approach the child slowly and speak in quiet and reassuring tones. Questions should be simple and direct.

During the examination, the child should be allowed to participate by holding the stethoscope, penlight, or other pieces of equipment. This "helping" activity may lessen the child's fear and improve the paramedic-patient relationship. Children of this age group have a limited understanding of their bodies and are reluctant to allow the paramedic to see or touch their "private parts" (seldom necessary in the prehospital setting). All examination procedures should be explained simply and completely, and the child should be advised of any expected pain or discomfort.

Adolescents (11 to 18 Years of Age)

Adolescents generally understand what is happening and usually are calm, mature, and helpful. These patients are more adult than child and should be treated as such. Adolescents are preoccupied with their bodies and usually are very concerned about modesty, disfigurement, pain, disability, and death. If appropriate, reassurance should be provided about these concerns during the examination.

During the patient interview, the patient's need for privacy should be respected. Some adolescents may be hesitant to reveal pertinent history in the presence of family and friends. If the adolescent gives incomplete answers or appears uncomfortable during the interview, the parents and patient should be interviewed privately. The possibility of alcohol or other drug use should be considered, as well as the possibility of pregnancy.

Physical Examination of Older Adults

As in pediatric patients, age-related physiological and psychological variations in older adults may create special challenges in patient assessment. However, the paramedic should not assume that all older adults are victims of age-related disorders. Individual differences in knowledge, mental reasoning, experience, and personality influence how these patients respond to examination.

Communicating with the Older Adult

Some older adults have sensory losses that make communications more difficult. Hearing and visual impairments, for example, are not uncommon. In addition, some older adults experience some memory loss and may become easily confused. Extra time may be needed to communicate effectively with these patients.

TRICKS OF THE TRADE

When interviewing a patient (especially an older adult), make your questions specific. If you ask, "What's wrong?" you open an entire Pandora's box of complaints about the head, back, belly, bowels, and legs.

The paramedic should remain close to the patient during the interview. The older adult generally perceives a reassuring voice and gentle touch as comforting. Short and simple questions are best. Speaking more loudly than usual may be necessary, and questions may have to be repeated. The paramedic must be patient and careful not to patronize or offend patients by assuming that they have a hearing impairment or cannot understand a particular line of questioning.

Patient History

Older patients often have multiple health problems present simultaneously. Patients may be vague and nonspecific when describing their chief complaint, making it difficult to isolate a nonapparent injury or illness. In addition, normal signs and symptoms of illness or injury may be absent because of decreased sensory function in some older adult patients.

Older adult patients with multiple health problems often take several medications, which increases the risk of illness from medication use and misuse. The paramedic should attempt to gather a complete medication history and must be alert to the relationship among drug interactions, disease, and the aging process.

As part of the history, the patient's functional abilities and any recent changes in daily activities should be assessed. Many older adults attribute these changes to age and will not mention them unless asked. This information may help indicate patient conditions that are not readily observable and may reveal the need for other pertinent lines of questioning. Examples of functional activities to be discussed with the patient include the following:

- Walking
- Getting out of bed
- Dressing
- Driving a car
- Using public transportation
- Preparing meals
- Taking medications
- Sleeping habits
- Bathroom habits

Physical Examination

During examination, the older adult patient's comfort should be ensured. The paramedic should clearly explain examination procedures and sensi-tively answer all questions. Many older patients with chronic illness may have lived with pain or discomfort for quite some time. Therefore their perception of what is painful may be quite different from that of other patients. Signs such as grimacing or wincing during the physical examination should be observed and may indicate pain or a possible injury site. If the situation permits, the examination should be performed slowly and gently with consideration of the patient's feelings and needs.

Many older adults believe they will die in a hospital, so if transportation is necessary, patients may become fearful and anxious. The paramedic should be sensitive to these concerns and if appropriate, reassure patients that their condition is not serious. The paramedic should attempt to calm these patients and advise them that they will be well cared for in the hospital. All examination findings should be carefully recorded (see Chapter 17).

S U M M A R Y

- The examination techniques commonly used in the physical examination are inspection, palpation, percussion, and auscultation.

- Equipment used during the comprehensive physical examination includes the stethoscope, ophthalmoscope, otoscope, and blood pressure cuff.

- The physical examination is performed systematically, with special emphasis placed on the patient's present illness and chief complaint.

- The physical examination is a systematic assessment of the body that includes mental status, general survey, vital signs, skin, head, eyes, ears, nose and throat, chest, abdomen, posterior body, extremities, and neurological examination.

- The first step in any patient care encounter is to note the patient's appearance and behavior and to assess for level of consciousness. This may include assessment of: posture, gait and motor activity; dress, grooming, hygiene, and breath or body odors; facial expression; mood, affect, and relation to person and things; speech and language; thought and perceptions; and memory and attention.

- During the general survey, the patient should be evaluated for signs of distress, apparent state of health, skin color and obvious lesions, height and build, sexual development, and weight. Vital signs also should be assessed.

- The comprehensive physical examination should include an evaluation of the skin's texture and turgor, hair, and fingernails and toenails.

- Examination of the structures of the head and neck involves inspection, palpation, and auscultation.

- A thorough knowledge of the structure of the thoracic cage is required to perform an adequate respiratory and cardiac assessment. Air movement creates turbulence as it passes through the respiratory tree and produces breath sounds during inhalation and exhalation. In the prehospital setting, the heart must be examined indirectly. However, information about the size and effectiveness of pumping action is obtained through a skilled assessment that includes palpation and auscultation.

- The four quadrants of the abdomen and their contents provide the basis for inspection, auscultation, percussion, and palpation of this body region.

- An examination of the genitalia of either sex can be awkward and uncomfortable for the patient and the paramedic. The genitalia should be inspected for bleeding and signs of trauma (if indicated).

- Examination of the anus is indicated in the presence of rectal bleeding or trauma to the area.

- When examining the upper and lower extremities, the paramedic should direct his or her attention to function as well as structure.

- Assessment of the spine begins with a visual assessment of the cervical, thoracic, and lumbar curves and continues with a region-by-region examination for pain, swelling, and range of motion.

- A neurological examination may be organized into five categories: mental status and speech, cranial nerves, motor system, sensory system, and reflexes.

- When approaching the pediatric patient, remain calm and confident, avoid separation of child and parent, establish a rapport with parents and child, be honest, assign one caregiver to the child, and observe the child before beginning the physical examination.

- The paramedic should not assume that all older adults are victims of age-related disorders. Individual differences in knowledge, mental reasoning, experience, and personality will influence how these patients respond to examination.

REFERENCES

1. Centers for Disease Control and Prevention: *Curriculum guide for public-safety and emergency-response workers: prevention of transmission of human immunodeficiency virus and hepatitis B virus,* Atlanta, 1989, US Government Printing Office.

2. Potter P, Perry A: *Fundamentals of nursing: concepts, process, and practice,* ed 3, St Louis, 1993, Mosby.

3. Seidel J, Henderson D, editors: *Prehospital care of pediatric patients,* California EMSC Project, Los Angeles, 1987, American Academy of Pediatrics.

14 Patient Assessment

OBJECTIVES

Upon completion of this chapter, the paramedic student will be able to:

1. Identify the components of the scene size-up.
2. Identify the priorities in each component of patient assessment.
3. Outline the critical steps in initial patient assessment.
4. Describe findings in the initial assessment that may indicate a life-threatening condition.
5. Discuss interventions for life-threatening conditions that are identified in the initial assessment.
6. Identify the components of the focused history and physical examination for medical patients.
7. Identify the components of the focused history and physical examination for trauma patients.
8. List the components of the detailed physical examination.
9. Describe the on-going assessment.
10. Distinguish priorities in the care of the medical versus trauma patient.

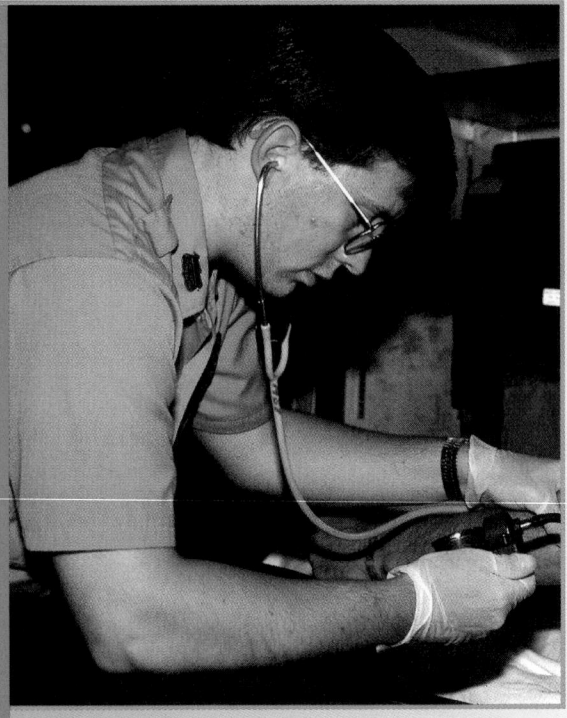

The prehospital environment usually lacks on-scene emergency physicians and diagnostic services. Therefore priorities of care must be established based on patient assessment. These priorities include scene safety, recognition and stabilization of life-threatening conditions, and identification of patients who require rapid stabilization and transport for definitive care.

KEY TERMS

focused history: A component of patient assessment to ascertain the patient's chief complaint, history of present illness, past medical history, and current health status.

general impression: An immediate assessment of the environment and the patient's chief complaint used to determine if the patient is ill or injured and the nature of the illness or the mechanism of injury.

initial assessment: A component of the patient assessment to recognize and manage all immediate life-threatening conditions.

ongoing assessment: A repeat of the initial assessment that is performed throughout the paramedic-patient encounter.

priority patients: Patients who need immediate care and transport.

scene size-up: An assessment of the scene to ensure scene safety for the paramedic crew, patient(s), and bystanders; a quick assessment to determine the resources needed to adequately manage the scene.

Scene Size-Up and Assessment

Scene size-up and assessment are the initial steps taken during every EMS response to ensure scene safety for the paramedic crew, patient(s), and bystanders. The assessment of the scene and surroundings will provide valuable information to the paramedic. The priorities in scene size-up and assessment include the following:

- Determine the nature of the incident.
- Determine the maximum potential number of people already ill or injured and requiring care.
- Assess for hazards at the scene.
- Initiate a mass casualty plan if indicated (see Chapter 49).
- Notify the dispatch center to request additional resources (e.g., law enforcement, fire, rescue, utility companies) and to alert area hospitals (as needed).
- Determine the best access routes and staging areas for responders.
- Secure the area as rapidly as possible, clearing unnecessary people from the scene.
- Begin triage (if needed).

Even scenes that appear safe may be dangerous. Paramedics should never enter a potentially unsafe scene until they know it is safe to approach the patient. Examples of unsafe scenes include crash and rescue scenes, toxic substances and low-oxygen areas, crime scenes where there is a potential for violence, and scenes that have unstable surfaces (e.g., slope, ice, water).

TRICKS OF THE TRADE

Remember the saying "Dead heroes don't save lives."

? CRITICAL THINKING

Do you know a paramedic who has been injured on a scene? What caused the injury? Could it have been prevented?

NOTE

Personal safety is the paramedic's first priority.

Protective Clothing

The National Fire Protection Association[1] (NFPA) and Occupational Safety and Health Administration (OSHA)[2,3] standards for protective clothing and personal protective equipment have been adopted by many emergency response agencies. At a minimum, paramedics should have access to the following personal protective equipment:

- Impact-resistant protective helmet with ear protection and chin-strap
- Safety goggles with vents to prevent fogging
- Lightweight, puncture-resistant "turn-out coat"
- Slip-resistant waterproof gloves
- Boots with steel insoles and steel toe protection
- Self-contained breathing apparatus

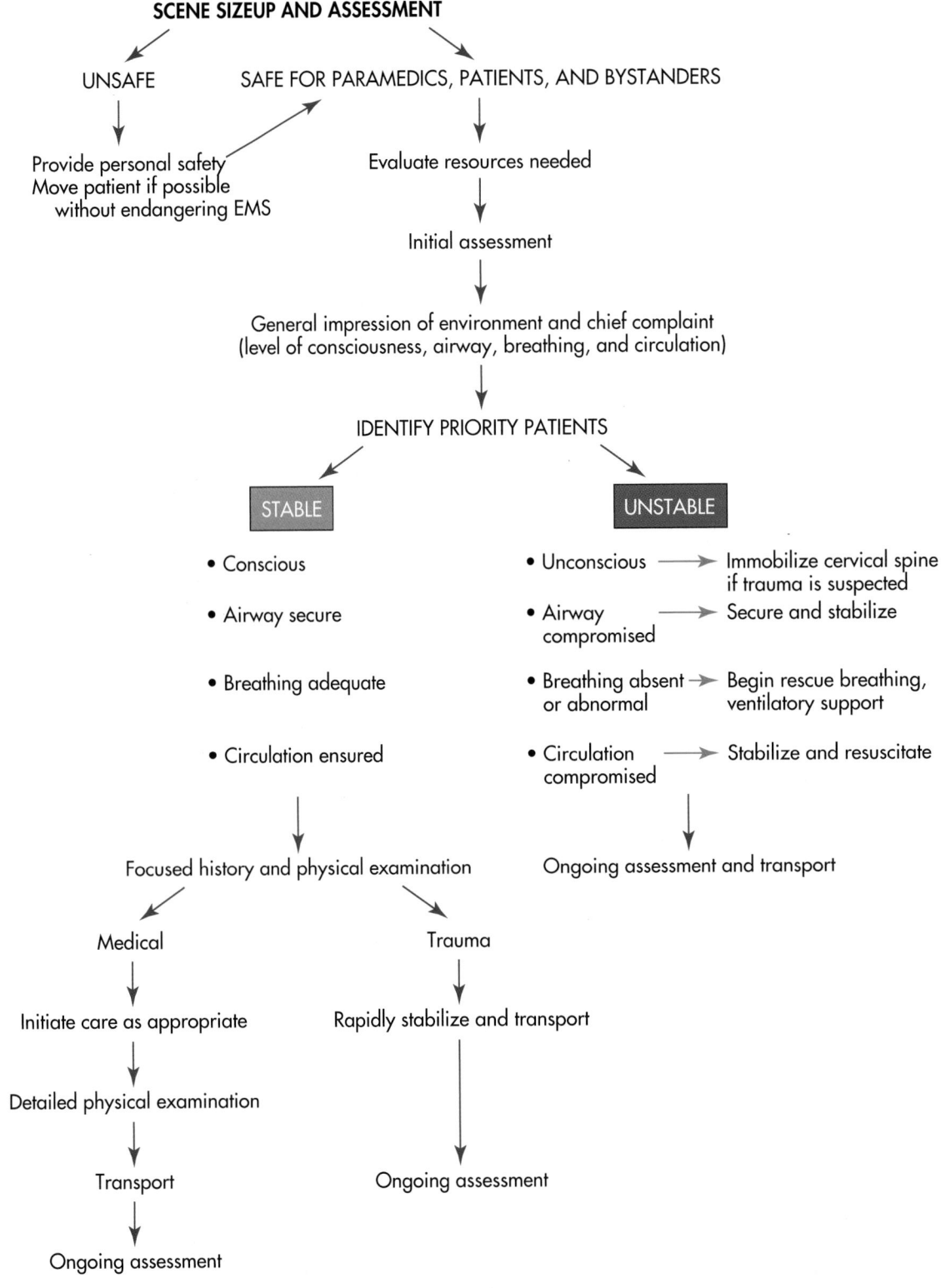

Fig. 14-1 Components of patient assessment.

Personal Protection from Bloodborne Pathogens

OSHA's bloodborne pathogen standard (described in Chapter 9 and summarized on the inside cover of this textbook) established criteria for workplace protection from bloodborne diseases. These measures should be observed when there is a potential for contact with human blood or body fluids. In these situations, the paramedic should wear eye protection, gloves, gown, and mask, if necessary.

Patient Assessment Priorities

After determining that the scene is safe and that necessary resources are available or have been requested, the emergency team can begin patient assessment (Fig. 14-1). Patient assessment entails the following four priorities[4]:

1. *Initial assessment*: to recognize and manage all immediate life-threatening conditions. Resuscitation may be necessary for critical patients (Box 14-1).
2. *Focused history and physical examination*: to obtain vital signs, reassess changes in the patient's condition, and perform appropriate physical examination for trauma and medical patients.
3. *Detailed physical examination*: to gather additional patient information.
4. *Ongoing assessment*: to continue monitoring the patient's status en route to the hospital and to provide treatment as necessary.

Initial Assessment

An **initial assessment** is performed on all patients to establish priorities of care. It is composed of the paramedic's general impression of the patient, the assessment for life-threatening conditions, and the identification of **priority patients** who need immediate care and transport.

General Impression of the Patient

The **general impression** is the paramedic's immediate assessment of the environment and the patient's chief complaint. It is used to determine if the patient is ill or injured and the nature of the illness or the mechanism of injury. As part of the general impression, the paramedic should identify the patient's approximate age, sex, and race.

BOX 14-1

RESUSCITATION

Resuscitation may be indicated during the initial assessment. The paramedic begins resuscitative measures such as airway maintenance, ventilatory assistance, and CPR immediately after recognizing the life-threatening condition that necessitates each respective maneuver. Several emergency care procedures generally are initiated in situations involving seriously ill or injured patients. Nearly all medical and trauma patients, for example, need some form of supplemental oxygen. Other resuscitation procedures for medical and trauma patients are listed below:

Resuscitation Procedures for Medical Patients
- Oxygen and airway control
- Inserting an intravenous line to administer drugs or volume-expanding fluid
- Administering resuscitation medications
- Applying a pneumatic antishock garment (PASG) if appropriate
- Administering electrical therapy (defibrillation, cardioversion, external pacing)

Resuscitation Procedures for Trauma Patients
- Oxygen and airway control
- Cervical spine immobilization
- Inserting intravenous lines for volume-expanding fluid
- Administering resuscitation medications
- Applying a PASG, if appropriate

Assessment for Life-Threatening Conditions

To assess for life-threatening conditions, the paramedic should conduct a systematic evaluation of the patient's level of consciousness, airway, breathing, and circulation.

Level of Consciousness

The first priority with any patient is to assess the level of consciousness. This usually can be accomplished by a cordial exchange with the patient (e.g., "I'm a paramedic, how can I help you?"). If the patient appears unconscious, gentle tactile stimulation (e.g., rubbing the patient's shoulder), along with questions such as "Are you okay?" and "Can you hear me?" may elicit a response. If the patient is unconscious or if spinal injury is suspected, the patient's cervical spine should be immobilized (see Chapter 23). The patient's level of consciousness can be quickly assessed by using the mnemonic evaluation *AVPU* (Box 14-2).

✓ **TRICKS OF THE TRADE**

Unconscious patients cannot maintain their airway. Open it, keep it open, and maintain it with an adjunctive airway device.

? CRITICAL THINKING

What does the level of consciousness tell you about the patient's oxygenation and circulation?

Airway

The airway should be assessed for patency by determining if the patient can speak, noting signs of airway obstruction or respiratory insufficiency (stridor, gurgling), and by inspecting the oral cavity for foreign objects. Any condition that compromises the delivery of oxygen to body tissues is potentially life threatening and must be managed immediately. Factors that may compromise the airway include the following:

- Tongue obstructing the airway in an unconscious patient
- Loose teeth or foreign objects in the patient's airway
- Epiglottitis
- Upper airway obstruction from any cause
- Facial and oral bleeding
- Vomitus
- Soft-tissue trauma to the patient's face and neck
- Facial fractures

A compromised airway must be secured manually or with adjunct equipment (e.g., using modified jaw thrust, chin lift, oral or nasal airways, suction, or endotracheal [ET] or esophageal intubation with multilumen airways). When performing an airway procedure for patients who may have cervical spine injury, manipulation of the cervical spine should be minimal, and the head and neck should be stabilized in a neutral position. All patients must have an airway established and maintained during the initial assessment.

NOTE

Securing a patent airway should always receive priority above spinal immobilization. However, both are important tasks in the initial assessment.

The patient whose airway is obstructed by a foreign object should be managed using the guidelines currently recommended by the American Heart Association and the American Red Cross. If these maneuvers fail, medical direction may recommend direct laryngoscopy or cricothyrotomy (see Chapter 11).

Breathing

Breathing is assessed by evaluating the rate, depth, and symmetry of chest movement. The chest wall should be exposed and palpated for structural integrity, tenderness, and crepitus, observing for accessory respiratory use of the muscles of the neck, chest, and abdomen. The paramedic should auscultate for the presence of bilateral breath sounds and listen to the patient's speech. A patient who has difficulty speaking without pain or who cannot talk without gasping for air may need ventilatory support. Respiratory abnormalities discovered during the physical examination that may indicate a potentially life-threatening condition include the following:

- Cyanosis
- Respiratory distress with dyspnea or hypoxia
- Asymmetrical chest wall movement
- Chest injury (e.g., tension pneumothorax, flail segment, open chest wound)
- Tracheal deviation
- Distended neck veins

BOX 14-2

AVPU SCALE OF LEVEL OF CONSCIOUSNESS

A—Alert
V—Responds to verbal stimulus
P—Responds to painful stimulus
U—Unresponsive

Ill or injured patients with ineffective respirations need ventilatory support supplemented with high-concentration oxygen. If the respiratory rate of a critically ill or injured patient is less than 10 or more than 28 per minute, ventilatory assistance may be necessary. Assisted ventilation may be synchronized with the patient's respiratory efforts or interspersed as needed to maintain adequate oxygenation. Depending on the patient's condition, ET intubation may be indicated.

> **? CRITICAL THINKING**
>
> *Are there any situations when a patient's respirations are between 10 and 28 that would require assisted ventilation?*

If respirations are absent, rescue breathing via a pocket mask should be initiated followed by positive-pressure ventilation via a bag-valve device or demand valve and ET intubation. Spinal precautions and barrier protection should be considered during all airway procedures.

Circulation

The patient's circulatory status is evaluated after assessing airway and breathing. For trauma patients, this evaluation includes a quick head-to-toe visual survey to identify and control severe bleeding. The paramedic should quickly assess the patient's skin color, moisture, and temperature and evaluate the pulse for quality, rate, and regularity.

Pulse. A quick evaluation of the patient's pulse may reveal a normal heart rate, tachycardia, bradycardia, asystole, or an irregular heart rate. The location of an obtainable pulse also may provide a rough estimate of the patient's systolic blood pressure. If the carotid pulse is present but the radial pulse is not palpable, for example, the systolic blood pressure is generally between 60 and 80 mm Hg (Table 14-1).

Capillary Refill. Capillary filling time (the capillary refill test) may provide information regarding the patient's cardiovascular status. This test is performed by blanching the patient's nail bed or the fleshy eminence at the base of the thumb and observing the time it takes for normal color to return. A filling time of more than 2 seconds, caused by shunting and capillary closure to peripheral capillary beds,

indicates inadequate circulation and impaired cardiovascular function. Because factors such as the patient's age, gender, and environment may affect the filling time, this test should only be used as a possible indicator of circulatory status. Other signs and symptoms of inadequate circulation and impaired cardiovascular function include:

- Altered or decreased level of consciousness
- Distended neck veins
- Increased respiratory rate
- Pale, cool, diaphoretic skin
- Distant heart sounds
- Restlessness
- Thirst

> **? CRITICAL THINKING**
>
> *How do age, gender, and the environment affect capillary refill?*

> **NOTE**
>
> The capillary refill test is considered most reliable in children younger than 12 years of age.

When an unconscious person lacks a carotid pulse, chest compressions and cardiac arrest protocols should be implemented. In cases of severe external hemorrhage, bleeding should be controlled using direct pressure, elevation, and pressure points (see Chapter 20). In most cases, these procedures will stabilize the patient during transportation. Regardless of the cause, all patients with circulatory compromise need rapid stabilization, which may include intravenous fluids, other medications, and transportation to an appropriate medical facility.

TABLE 14-1	PULSE SITE AND BLOOD PRESSURE ESTIMATES	
	PULSE SITE	**ESTIMATED MINIMAL SYSTOLIC BLOOD PRESSURE**
	Radial	80 mm Hg
	Femoral	70 mm Hg
	Cartoid	60 mm Hg

Identify Priority Patients

Using the findings from the initial assessment, the paramedic should identify priority patients who need stabilization and rapid transport. A sampling of priority patients includes those who have:

- Poor general impression
- Decreased level of consciousness (depressed or absent gag or cough reflex)
- No response to commands (unresponsiveness)
- Difficulty breathing
- Shock (hypoperfusion)
- Complicated childbirth
- Chest pain with a systolic pressure less than 100 mm Hg
- Uncontrolled bleeding
- Severe pain anywhere
- Multiple injuries

Focused History and Physical Examination—Medical Patients

The **focused history** and physical examination for medical patients is dictated by the patient's overall condition and level of consciousness. If the patient is responsive, the paramedic should assess the patient's history by identifying the chief complaint, history of present illness, past medical history, and current health status. An appropriate physical examination is then performed using the techniques presented in Chapter 13. A baseline set of vital signs (including an assessment for orthostatic hypotension, further described in Chapter 19) should be obtained, and emergency care provided based on signs and symptoms in consultation with medical direction.

If the patient is unconscious, a rapid head-to-toe assessment should be performed to identify any life-threatening conditions. Particular attention should be given to the airway of any patient with a decreased level of consciousness. Baseline vital signs should be assessed, and if possible, a patient history should be obtained from family, friends, bystanders, and/or medical identification devices.

Focused History and Physical Examination—Trauma Patients

A focused history for a trauma patient is performed to identify and permit reconstruction of the mechanism of injury. Significant mechanisms of injury that identify priority patients include:

- Ejection from a vehicle
- Death in same passenger compartment
- Falls from greater than 20 feet
- Vehicle rollover
- High-speed vehicle collision
- Vehicle–pedestrian collision
- Motorcycle crash
- Injuries that cause unresponsive or altered mental status
- Penetration of the head, chest, or abdomen
- Hidden injuries (e.g., those caused by seat belts and air bags) (Box 14-3)

BOX 14-3

HIDDEN INJURIES

Personal restraint devices (lap and shoulder belts) can cause injury, even when properly used. Examples of hidden injuries (injuries that are not visible) that can result from personal restraint devices include chest injury, pelvic injury, and internal organ injury.

Air bags also can be a source of hidden injury during a motor vehicle crash. These devices may be ineffective in preventing injury if the driver or passenger is not wearing a seat belt. The paramedic should inspect the steering wheel for deformity by "lifting and looking" under the bag after the patient is removed from the car. Any visible deformation of the steering wheel should be regarded as an indicator of potentially serious internal injury. Improper placement of child safety seats also may cause injury to children during air bag deployment.

? CRITICAL THINKING

If a patient has a mechanism of injury other than those listed here, does that mean the patient has no life-threatening injuries?

Mechanisms of injury considered significant with infants and children include falls greater than 10 feet, bicycle collision, and medium-speed vehicle collision.

Rapid Trauma Physical Examination

A rapid trauma examination should be performed to identify life-threatening conditions on all patients with a significant mechanism of injury. In responsive patients, symptoms should be sought before and during the trauma assessment. The rapid trauma physical examination is composed of the following:

- Continued spinal immobilization
- Mental status assessment
- Inspection and palpation of the head, neck, chest, abdomen, pelvis, and extremities for injuries or signs of injuries
- Inspection of the posterior surfaces of the body
- Baseline vital signs
- Patient history (chief complaint, history of present illness, past medical history, current health status)

A patient without any significant mechanism of injury (e.g., a cut finger) should receive an appropriate assessment focused on the injury site. Baseline vital signs and a patient history also should be obtained.

Detailed Physical Examination

The detailed physical examination should be patient- and injury-specific. A patient with a minor injury (e.g., a sprained ankle) should not require a complete physical examination. Conversely, an older patient with difficulty breathing should receive a detailed physical examination. A comprehensive and detailed physical examination (described in Chapter 13) includes the following:

- Mental status assessment
  Appearance and behavior
  Posture and motor activity
  Speech and language
  Mood
  Thought and perceptions
  Insight and judgment

  Memory and attention
- General survey
  Level of consciousness
  Signs of distress
  Apparent state of health
  Skin color and obvious lesions
  Height and build
  Sexual development
  Weight
  Posture, gait, and motor activity
  Dress, grooming, and personal hygiene
  Odors of breath or body
  Facial expression
- Examination of:
  Skin
  Head
  Eyes
  Ears
  Nose and sinuses
  Mouth and pharynx
  Neck
  Thorax and lungs
  Cardiovascular system
  Abdomen
  Genitalia
  Anus and rectum
  Peripheral vascular system
  Musculoskeletal system
  Nervous system
- Baseline vital signs

Ongoing Assessment

The **ongoing assessment** is a repeat of the initial assessment. As the name implies, this assessment should be performed throughout the paramedic-patient encounter. For stable patients (nonpriority patients), the ongoing assessment should be repeated and recorded every 15 minutes. If the patient is unstable (a priority patient), the ongoing assessment should be performed every 5 minutes (at a minimum). The purpose of the ongoing assessment is to:

- Reassess mental status
- Reassess airway
- Monitor breathing for rate and quality
- Reassess circulation
- Reestablish patient priorities

? CRITICAL THINKING

The ongoing assessment can identify "trends" in the patient's condition. What does that mean?

NOTE

The paramedic should observe for changes (that occur over time) in the patient's condition, which may indicate the need for a change in care or treatment.

During the on-going assessment, the paramedic should also reassess and record vital signs, further investigate the patient complaint or injury, and assess the effectiveness of any interventions. This entails assessing the patient's response to patient-care activities and determining the need to maintain or modify the management plan.

NOTE

A continuous assessment of the patient and thorough documentation of assessment findings may help the paramedic recognize a "trend" in the assessment components. For example, a patient may have been cyanotic, hypotensive, and disoriented at the scene. After administering intravenous fluid therapy and high-concentration oxygen, this patient may have improved color and blood pressure and may appear to be more alert during transport. The documenting and reporting of trends in assessment components will be valuable to other health care professionals who will assume care of the patient upon arrival at the emergency department.

Care of Medical versus Trauma Patients

Much of the definitive care for medical patients can often be initiated in the prehospital setting. For some cardiac patients and patients with respiratory difficulties and other medical emergencies, appropriate care can be instituted by paramedic crews. With these medical patients, the scene time may be slightly longer.

In contrast, most trauma patients can receive definitive care only when rapidly stabilized and transported to an appropriate medical facility. Patients with internal bleeding, major fractures, head injury, and multiple-system trauma need life-saving care that can only be provided by specially trained physicians and support staff. Minimal time should be spent at the scene with these patients. Most trauma life-support training programs (e.g., *Basic Trauma Life Support* [BTLS], *Prehospital Trauma Life Support* [PHTLS], and *Advanced Trauma Life Support* [ATLS]) recommend that patients requiring immediate transport be stabilized and prepared for transport ("packaged") within 10 minutes after EMS arrival. Field management should be limited to airway control and ventilatory support, spinal immobilization, and major fracture stabilization. If initiated, intravenous fluid therapy should be done en route to the hospital. (Trauma management is further addressed in Division Four: Trauma.)

S U M M A R Y

- Scene size-up consists of the initial steps performed on every EMS response to ensure scene safety and to provide valuable information to the paramedic.

- Patient assessment comprises five priorities: initial assessment, resuscitation, focused history and physical examination, detailed physical examination, and ongoing assessment.

- The initial assessment includes the paramedic's general impression of the patient, the assessment for life-threatening conditions, and the identification of priority patients requiring immediate care and transport.

- Assessing for life-threatening conditions entails a systematic evaluation of the patient's level of consciousness, airway, breathing, and circulation.

- The paramedic begins resuscitative measures such as airway maintenance, ventilatory assistance, and cardiopulmonary resuscitation (CPR) immediately after recognizing the life-threatening condition that necessitates each respective maneuver.

- The focused history and physical examination for medical patients is dictated by the patient's overall condition and level of consciousness.

- A focused history for a trauma patient is performed to reconsider the mechanism of injury. A rapid trauma examination should be performed on all patients with a significant mechanism of injury to identify life-threatening conditions.

- The detailed physical examination should be patient- and injury-specific and should include an assessment of mental status, general survey, a head-to-toe examination, and baseline vital signs.

- The ongoing assessment is a repeat of the initial assessment.

REFERENCES

1. *Standards on protective clothing for structural fire fighting; NFPA 1999* (1971, 1976, 1981 rev. 1997), National Fire Protection Association, Quincy, Mass, The Association.
2. *Fire brigade regulation*, 29 CFR 1910.156, Occupational Safety and Health Administration, Washington, DC, 1980, The Administration.
3. *Hazardous waste operations and emergency response (HAZWOPER)*, standard 1910.120, Occupational Safety and Health Administration, Washington, DC, 1990, The Administration.
4. *EMT–Paramedic national standard curriculum*, US Department of Transportation National Highway Traffic Safety Administration, Washington, DC, 1998, US Government Printing Office.

15 Clinical Decision Making

OBJECTIVES

Upon completion of this chapter, the paramedic student will be able to:

1. List the key elements of paramedic practice.
2. Discuss the limitations of protocols, standing orders, and patient-care algorithms.
3. Outline the key components of the critical thinking process for paramedics.
4. Identify elements necessary for an effective critical thinking process.
5. Describe situations that may necessitate the use of the critical thinking process while delivering prehospital patient care.
6. Describe the six elements required for effective clinical decision making in the prehospital setting.

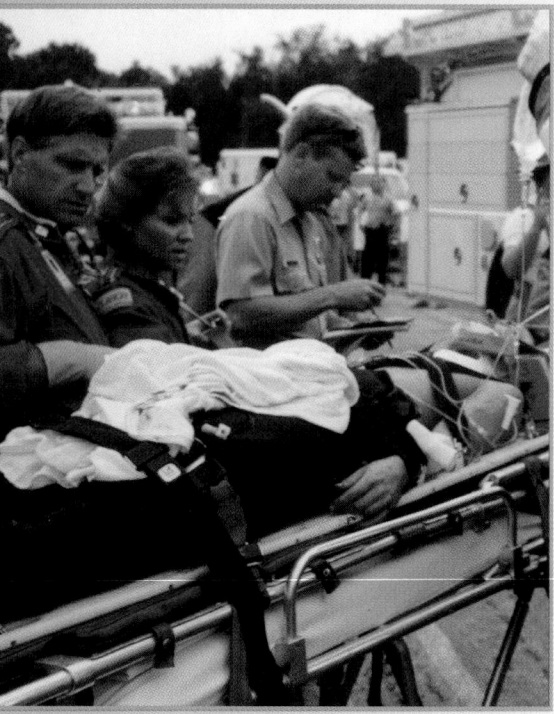

Unique to the EMS profession is the uncertainty of the prehospital environment, which is heavily influenced by factors that do not exist in other medical settings. The paramedic must be able to do the following: gather, evaluate, and synthesize information; develop and implement appropriate patient management plans; apply judgment and exercise independent decision making; and think and work effectively under pressure. These are the cornerstones of effective paramedic practice.

application of principle: A component of critical thinking during which patient care decisions are made based on the examiner's conceptual understanding of the situation and the interpretation of data gathered from the patient.

concept formation: A component of critical thinking that refers to all elements that are gathered to form a general impression of the patient.

data interpretation: A component of critical thinking whereby the examiner gathers the necessary data to form a field impression and working diagnosis.

evaluation: A component of critical thinking whereby an assessment is made of the patient's response to care.

reflection on action: A component of critical thinking (usually performed after the event) whereby a patient-care episode is evaluated for possible improvement in future responses of a similar nature.

The Spectrum of Prehospital Care

As described in Chapter 13 and Chapter 14, the paramedic must have a wide spectrum of knowledge and skills to make effective patient care determinations in the prehospital setting. On any given workday, the paramedic may be exposed to obvious critical life-threats, potential life-threats, and non–life-threatening situations (Box 15-1). And on each call, the EMS provider will be expected to provide appropriate care and treatment.

Protocols, standing orders, and patient-care algorithms help promote a standardized approach to patient care for "classic" patient presentations by clearly defining and outlining performance parameters. However, these standards have several limitations: (1) they may not apply to nonspecific patient complaints that do not fit the "model"; (2) they

do not speak to multiple disease etiologies or multiple treatment modalities; and (3) they promote linear thinking ("cookbook medicine"). The paramedic must develop critical thinking skills to assist in unique patient care situations.

Critical Thinking Process for Paramedics

There are specific components, stages, and sequences associated with the critical thinking process.[1] These include **concept formation**, **data interpretation**, **application of principle**, **evaluation**, and **reflection on action** (Fig. 15-1).

Concept Formation

Concept formation refers to all elements gathered to form a general impression of the patient (the "what" of the patient story). These are described in Chapter 13 and include the following:

- Scene assessment (mechanism of injury, social setting)
- Chief complaint

BOX 15-1

SPECTRUM OF PREHOSPITAL CARE

Obvious Critical Life-threats
Major multisystem trauma
Devastating single-system trauma
End-stage disease presentations
Acute presentations of chronic conditions

Potential Life-threats
Serious multisystem trauma
Multiple disease etiologies

Non–life-threatening Presentations
Minor illness or injury
EMS system misuse

TRICKS OF THE TRADE

Just when you think "you've seen it all," a patient presentation will take you by surprise. *Always expect the unexpected.*

493

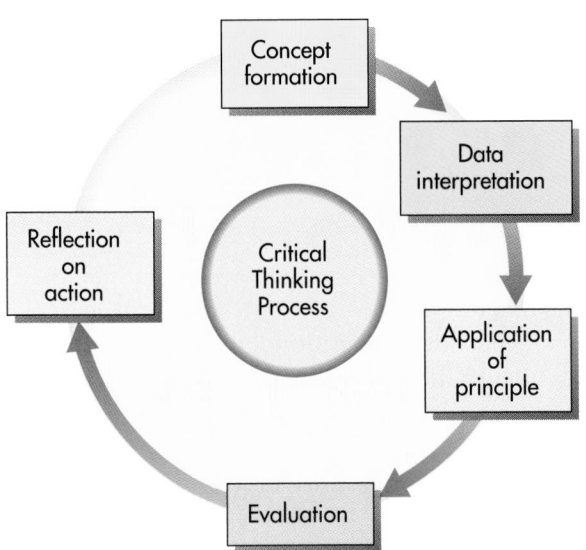

Fig. 15-1 Critical thinking process.

- Patient history
- Patient affect
- Initial assessment and physical examination
- Diagnostic tests

Data Interpretation

Following concept formation, the paramedic must gather the necessary data (the "working phase" of patient care) to form a field impression and working diagnosis. The quality of data interpretation depends on the paramedic's knowledge of anatomy and physiology, pathophysiology, and previous experience in providing patient care. During data interpretation, the paramedic attempts to obtain a complete "picture" of the patient's situation. The success of this component of critical thinking can be greatly affected by the paramedic's attitude and the way in which the paramedic-patient interaction proceeds (see Chapter 10).

Application of Principle

The next step in the critical thinking process is the application of principles of appropriate patient care, based on the paramedic's conceptual understanding of the situation and the interpretation of data gathered from the patient. Once the field impression and working diagnosis are established, treatment and intervention are initiated (often through protocols and standing orders) or direct/on-line medical direction.

Evaluation

The patient's response to the care rendered by the paramedic must be continuously evaluated. Evaluation includes the following:

- Reassessment of the patient (ongoing assessment)
- Reflection of action (effectiveness of the intervention)
- Revision of field impression (a change in the working diagnosis)
- Review of the appropriateness of the protocol, standing orders, or direct orders for the patient
- Revision of the treatment or intervention as needed

Reflection on Action

Reflection on action occurs "after the event." It usually is performed through a run critique whereby the patient-care episode is evaluated for possible improvement in similar future emergency responses. Reflection on action provides paramedics with an avenue to add to or modify their experience base.

Fundamental Elements of Critical Thinking for Paramedics

For an effective critical thinking process, several fundamental elements must be present. These include adequate knowledge and the ability to do the following:

- Focus on specific and multiple elements of data simultaneously
- Gather and organize data and form concepts
- Identify and deal with medical ambiguity (patients who don't fit the "model")
- Differentiate between relevant and irrelevant data
- Analyze and compare similar situations from past experience
- Recall situations where the working diagnosis was incorrect
- Articulate decision-making reasoning and construct arguments to support or discount the decision

Field Application of Assessment-Based Patient Management

Assessment-based patient management places tremendous responsibility on the paramedic. The paramedic must have a systematic means of: analyzing a patient's problems, determining how to solve them, carrying out a plan of action, and evaluating its effectiveness. The success of assessment-based patient management in the prehospital setting depends on an integration of interpersonal skills, scientific knowledge, and physical activities (skills).

The Patient Acuity Spectrum

EMS is activated on a daily basis for countless reasons, and few prehospital calls constitute true life-threatening emergencies. Minor medical and trauma events require little critical thinking and result in relatively easy decision making for the paramedic. Likewise, patients with obvious life-threats pose limited critical thinking challenges because they often fit the "model" for standardized treatment modalities (e.g., cardiac arrest). Patients who fall on the acuity spectrum between minor and life-threatening events pose the greatest critical think-

ing challenges for the paramedic. Examples include patients with mild-to-moderate respiratory distress and patients with diffuse abdominal pain.

Thinking Under Pressure

Hormonal influences from the "fight or flight" response (described in Chapter 2) can have both positive and negative impacts on critical decision making. The response provides for enhanced visual and auditory acuity and improved reflexes and muscle strength. These can be positive when critical decisions must be made and activities must be performed. The negative aspects of the response may include diminished critical thinking skills that can result from a decrease in concentration and assessment ability. Mental conditioning that results in "instinctive performance" and "automatic responses" for technical procedures is the key to effective performance under pressure.

Mental Checklist for Thinking Under Pressure

Mental conditioning takes practice. A "checklist" for thinking under pressure may help facilitate behavior that will improve the paramedic's ability to concentrate during stressful events. The mental checklist the paramedic should use is as follows:

- Stop and think
- Scan the situation
- Decide and act
- Maintain clear and concise control
- Regularly and continually reevaluate the patient

> **? CRITICAL THINKING**
>
> *Do you think you can improve your performance under pressure by practicing imaginary critical situations in your head? Why or why not?*

Practicing this mental checklist when working under pressure will result in facilitating behaviors that improve clinical decision making. These positive behaviors include staying calm (not panicking), assuming a plan for the worst situation (erring on the side of the patient), and maintaining a systematic assessment pattern. In addition, the paramedic can learn to balance the various styles of situation analysis, data processing, and decision-making (Box 15-2).

STYLES OF SITUATION ANALYSIS, DATA PROCESSING, AND DECISION MAKING

1. Situational Analysis Styles: Reflective versus Impulsive

Health care professionals should avoid "closing off" data pursuit and the list of differential diagnoses too quickly.

Examples:

Reflective: When performing endotracheal intubation, consider pros and cons of each blade type for intubating a difficult airway.

Impulsive: Immediately grabbing the straight blade because it is the blade the paramedic "always uses."

2. Data-processing Styles: Divergent versus Convergent

Health care professionals should avoid the tendency to collect partial data that may lead them down the incorrect diagnostic or therapeutic path. This is a corollary of number 1.

Examples:

Divergent: Consulting with drug references and medical direction for suggestions on new drugs carried on an EMS vehicle.

Convergent: "The package insert says to do this . . ."

3. Decision-making Styles: Anticipatory versus Reactive

Anticipatory decision making is the process most used by health care professionals and is based on continuing data collection and evolution of the patient's condition.

Examples:

Anticipatory: Treat the patient's early signs and symptoms of an anaphylactic reaction with oxygen, **epinephrine** (Adrenalin), and **diphenhydramine** (Benadryl). Be prepared to intubate.

Reactive: Wait until the patient has respiratory difficulty before initiating treatment.

Putting It All Together— "The Six Rs"

To put all components required for effective clinical decision making into action, the paramedic can think in terms of "the six Rs" listed next (Fig. 15-2):

1. *Read the patient.* The paramedic should observe the patient's level of consciousness and skin color. Position of the patient should be noted along with any obvious deformity or asymmetry. Talking to the patient will determine the chief complaint and identify the presence of a worsening or preexisting condition. Skin temperature and moisture should be evaluated, and the pulse should be assessed for rate, strength, and regularity. Auscultating the lungs will reveal upper or lower airway problems. The paramedic should identify all life-threats and obtain an accurate set of vital signs.

NOTE

Vital signs can be used as a triage tool to estimate severity and can assist the paramedic in identifying the majority of life-threatening conditions. The paramedic should remember that vital signs can be affected by the patient's age, physical and medical conditions, and the use of current medications.

✓ TRICKS OF THE TRADE

Although vital sign assessment is important, you should never rely solely on the patient's "numbers." Treating numbers instead of what the patient is telling you is a bad practice that will get you (and the patient) into trouble.

2. *Read the scene.* As part of the scene size-up, the paramedic should assess general environmental conditions, evaluate the immediate surroundings, and attempt to identify any mechanism of injury.

3. *React.* All life-threats should be managed in the order in which they are found. The paramedic should determine the most common and probable cause of the life-threat that fits the patient's initial presentation. If a clearly defined and recognizable presentation of medical illness cannot be identified in a priority patient, treatment should be based on presenting signs and symptoms.

4. *Reevaluate.* Reevaluation includes a focused and detailed assessment to analyze the pa-

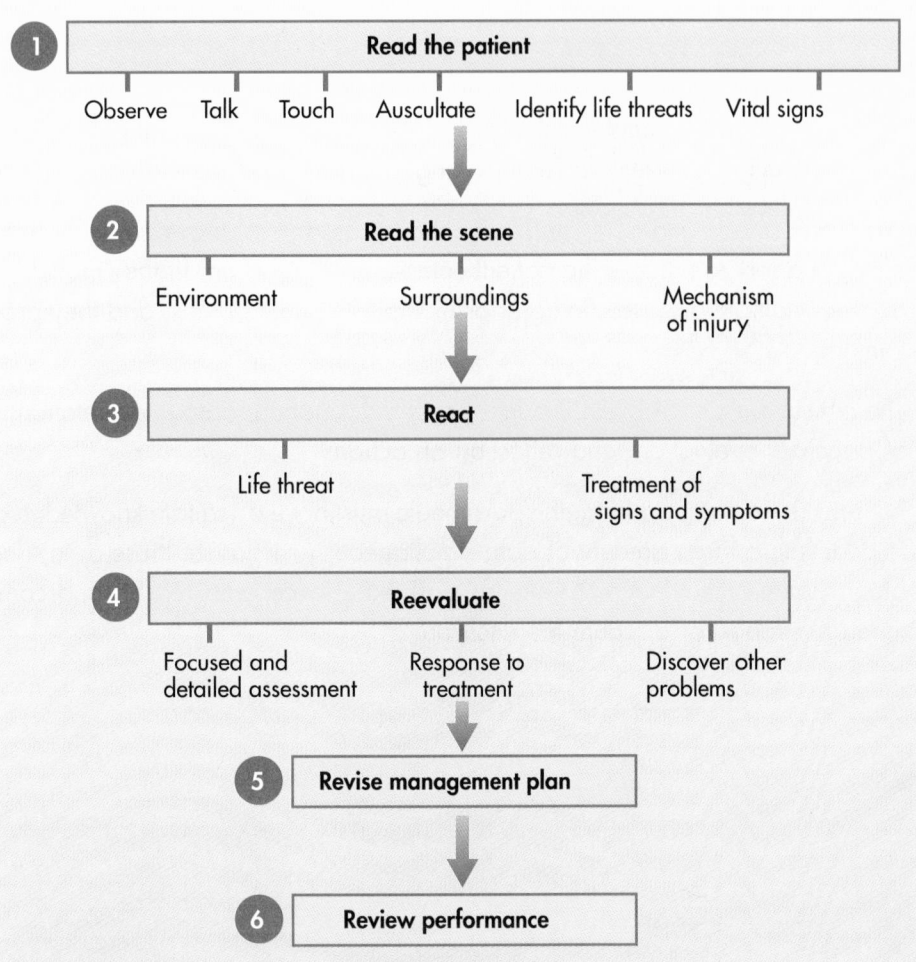

Fig. 15-2 The six Rs.

tient's response to management and interventions. Reevaluation also may lead the paramedic to discover other problems that were not evident during the initial assessment.

5. *Revise management plan.* Findings obtained during reevaluation may require that the management plan be revised to more clearly address the needs of the patient. The facts that patient conditions change and that patients do not respond uniformly to identical treatment intervention highlight the importance of ongoing assessment.

6. *Review performance at run critique.* Reviewing the specifics of the call through a run critique allows for the identification of areas that can

be improved on similar calls in the future. The interest and investment of paramedics in the outcome of their personal cases often is the strongest stimulus to favorably change their practice patterns. This process also enhances the paramedic's experience base, which leads to improvement of data interpretation skills.

? CRITICAL THINKING

How do you think a very negative or punitive run critique would influence your ability to perform under a similar circumstance in the future?

SUMMARY

- The paramedic must be able to do the following: gather, evaluate, and synthesize information; develop and implement appropriate patient management plans; apply judgment and exercise independent decision making; and think and work effectively under pressure.

- Protocols, standing orders, and patient-care algorithms have several limitations: they may not apply to nonspecific patient complaints that do not fit the "model," they do not address multiple disease etiologies or multiple treatment plans, and they promote linear thinking.

- The critical thinking process includes concept formation, data interpretation, application of principle, evaluation, and reflection on action.

- For effective critical thinking, the paramedic must have adequate knowledge and be able to deal with a large amount of data simultaneously, organize those data, deal with ambiguity, relate the situation to similar past experience, and reason and construct arguments to support or discount the decision.

- When using assessment-based patient management, the paramedic must analyze a patient's problems, determine how to solve them, carry out a plan of action, and evaluate its effectiveness.

- Effective clinical decision making requires the paramedic to read the patient, read the scene, react, reevaluate, revise the management plan, and review performance at a run critique.

REFERENCE

1. *EMT-Paramedic national standard curriculum*, US Department of Transportation National Highway Traffic Safety Administration, Washington, DC, 1998, The Department.

16 Communications

Upon completion of this chapter, the paramedic student will be able to:

1. *Outline the chain of EMS communications.*
2. *Describe the role of communications in EMS.*
3. *Define common EMS communications terms.*
4. *Describe the primary modes of EMS communications.*
5. *Describe how EMS communications are regulated.*
6. *Describe the role of dispatching as it applies to prehospital emergency medical care.*
7. *Outline techniques for relaying EMS communications clearly and effectively.*

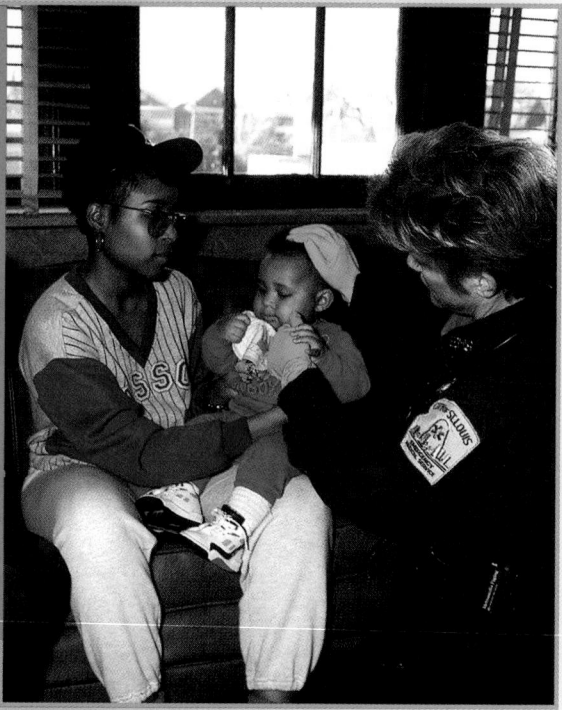

EMS communications *refers to the delivery of patient and scene information (either in person, in writing, or through communications technology) to other members of the emergency response team. These members include telecommunicators, EMS providers, emergency response workers, EMS system control and administration staff, and medical direction. This chapter addresses the complexities of communications that are vital components of the EMS system.*

duplex mode: A communications mode with the ability to transmit and receive traffic simultaneously through two different frequencies, one to transmit and one to receive.

EMS communications: The delivery of patient and scene information (either in person, in writing, or through communications technology) to other members of the emergency response team.

Federal Communications Commission: A federal agency with jurisdiction over interstate and international telephone and telegraph services and satellite communications.

multiplex mode: A communications mode with the ability to simultaneously transmit two or more different types of information, in either or both directions, over the same frequency.

simplex mode: A communications mode with the ability to transmit or receive in one direction at a time. Simultaneous transmission cannot occur.

SOAP format: A memory aid used to organize written and verbal patient reports; it includes subjective data, objective data, assessment data, and plan of patient management.

telemedicine: Refers to technological communications that allow for the transmission of photographs, video, and other information to be sent directly from the scene to a hospital for physician evaluation and consultation.

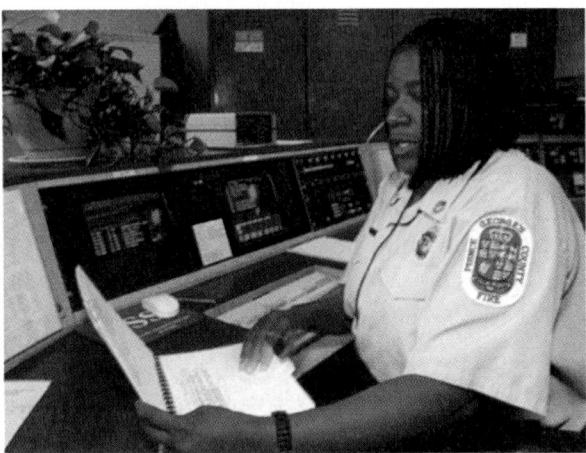

Fig. 16-1 Communication console (dispatch).

Phases of Communications During a Typical EMS Event

Five phases of communications occur during a typical EMS event.[1] These are (1) occurrence of the event; (2) detection of the need for emergency services; (3) notification and emergency response; (4) EMS arrival, treatment (including consultation with medical direction), and preparation for transport; and (5) preparation of EMS for the next emergency response.

In many urban areas, the public requests assistance via telephone to a communications center or public safety answering point (PSAP). Communications specialists receive the information, and in the most modern systems, digitalized information about the origin of the call and history of the response to that location is automatically displayed on a console (Fig. 16-1). The call taker then passes the information via digital technology to the telecommunicator, who sends a response unit to the scene. (Prearrival instructions also may be provided to the caller by the telecommunicator in some PSAP systems.)

> **NOTE**
>
> As described in Chapter 1, a telecommunicator is a person trained in public safety telecommunications. The term applies to call takers, dispatchers, radio operators, data terminal operators, or any combination of such functions in a PSAP located in a fire, police, or EMS communications center.

After the EMS unit has been dispatched to the scene, the paramedic crew advises the communications center of response and arrival status via radio or cellular phone and contacts medical direction for consultation and to give status reports. Care is rendered at the emergency scene; the patient is packaged for transport and delivered to the receiving facility.

Following the completion of paperwork, the EMS vehicle is made ready for the next emergency call.

The Role of Communications in EMS

Verbal, written, and electronic communications allow the delivery of information between the party requesting help and the telecommunicator; between the telecommunicator and paramedic; between the paramedic, patient, hospital, and direct/on-line medical direction; and between the paramedic and hospital personnel who receive the patient on emergency department arrival (Fig. 16-2). Effective delivery of communications can occur only when certain elements are in place. These elements comprise the basic model of communications.

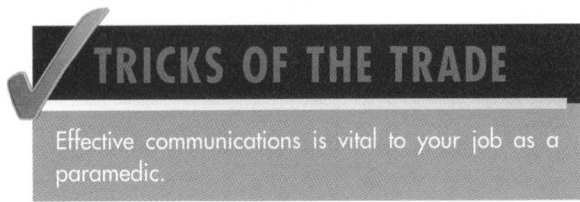

TRICKS OF THE TRADE

Effective communications is vital to your job as a paramedic.

The Basic Model of Communications

Communications, whether verbal, nonverbal, or written, serve a vital information function for decision making. It is the process by which one individual or group transmits meaning to others. The basic model of communications describes the relationships between an idea, encoding, a sender, a medium or channel, a receiver, decoding, and feedback (Fig. 16-3).

The idea is the intended meaning of the communications. Conveying the idea requires the sender to organize or manipulate the intended meaning (encoding) through a medium or channel (e.g., written or oral communications, facial or body expression, voice modulation), and interpretation (decoding) by the receiver who can then provide feedback to the initial idea that was communicated. If communications are completely successful, there will be an overlap between the idea being communicated by the sender and the feedback provided by the receiver (i.e., the receiver would interpret the decoding of the idea in a way identical to that intended by the sender). Four common barriers to successful communications are listed as follows[2]:

1. Attributes of the receiver. Different people react in different ways to the same message or idea for a variety of personal reasons (e.g., cultural differences, language barriers) that may affect their interpretations of the message. An example is a patient from one culture who may find personal touch to be comforting, whereas a patient from another culture may be offended by it.

? CRITICAL THINKING

What tends to happen to you when you are involved in a conversation with someone who continually interrupts you?

2. Selective perception. People have a tendency to listen to only part of an idea or message and "block out" other information for a variety of reasons (e.g., values, mood, and motives of the sender) or when new information conflicts with established values, beliefs, or expectations. Example: the input of a recently licensed paramedic is not welcomed or respected by a paramedic supervisor.

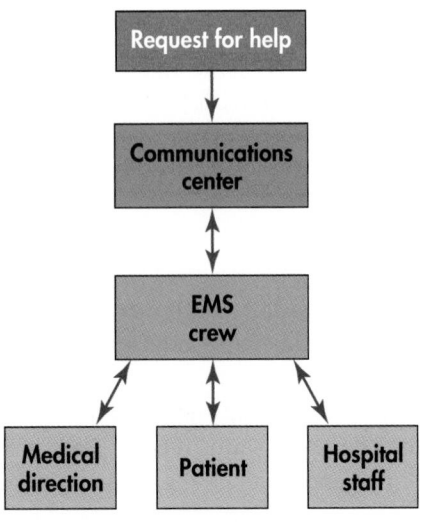

Fig. 16-2 EMS communications.

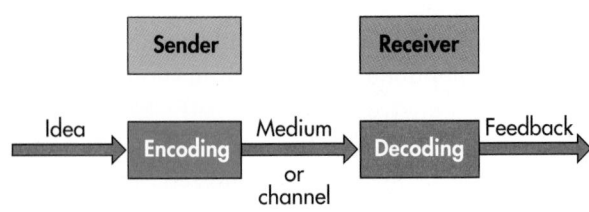

Fig. 16-3 Basic model of communications.

3. Semantic problems. Words commonly used in communications may carry different meanings for different people. Two common semantic problems are the use of vague or abstract words or phases that invite varying interpretation and the use of medical terminology and technical language ("lingo") that the receiver cannot understand. Example: a paramedic refers to a patient as "comatose" during a radio report to the hospital, and medical direction asks for further clarification using the AVPU scale.

4. Time pressures. Time pressures can lead to distortions in communications. A major temptation when pressed for time is to "short-circuit" channels. In these cases the immediate demands of the situation are met, but a number of unintended consequences can result. Example: medications administered in the field during a cardiac arrest were not documented, causing confusion about the next appropriate drug and billing problems after the event.

The paramedic should consider this basic communications model and the common barriers to successful communications when conveying information to or receiving information from telecommunicators, co-workers, patient(s), bystanders, medical direction, and hospital personnel.

Proper Verbal Communications During an EMS Event

The role of proper verbal communications during an EMS event is to exchange system information and patient information with other members of the emergency response team.

Terminology used in EMS communications should be unambiguous and conveyed in short-narrative form. Technical or semantic jargon that cannot be clearly understood by all parties should be avoided. Although some EMS services use a code to shorten radio transmissions, the English language usually is preferred for written and verbal communications.

> **NOTE**
>
> The paramedic should remember that many radio and phone communications are recorded and may be replayed for patient-care audits, media broadcasts, disciplinary hearings, and during legal proceedings. Professionalism in all communications is very important.

> **NOTE**
>
> The use of "scanners" by the general public to monitor emergency services is prevalent in many communities. The paramedic should be aware of this and preserve patient confidentiality by not speaking the name of the patient or providing descriptive phrases over unsecured airwaves.

Proper Written Communications During an EMS Event

Written documentation during an EMS event serves several important functions. It provides a written and legal record of the incident, conveys important clinical information from one component of the medical chain (EMS) to the next (ED), and is expected as part of professional work. Written documentation of patient care activities also becomes part of the patient's medical record (see Chapter 17). Other important ways in which written data can be used within the EMS system include the following:

1. Medical audit
2. Quality improvement/quality management
3. Billing
4. Data collection
5. Research

In addition to the patient care report (PCR), other types of documentation that may be required by an EMS agency include the following:

- Personnel records documenting training and work assignments
- Call records that list or log dates, times, and other specifics of a call
- Vehicle maintenance records documenting vehicle service at regular intervals
- Vehicle and equipment cleaning records documenting procedures used to disinfect vehicle and emergency equipment
- Drug and equipment inventory records verifying daily checks of drug and fluid expiration, security measures of controlled substances as required by state and federal drug enforcement agencies, and monitor-defibrillator, radio, and telemetry checks
- Incident reports that document problem calls or unusual circumstances
- Records of significant exposures to communicable disease

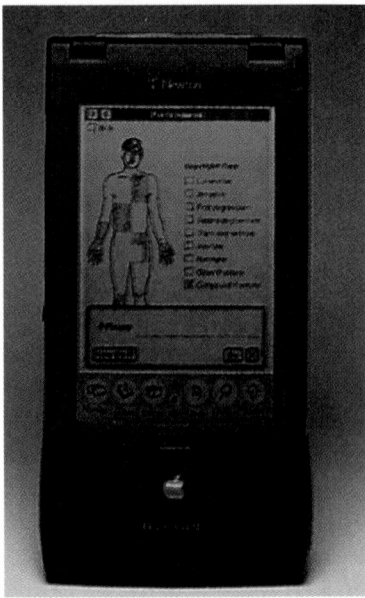

Fig. 16-4 Pen-based computer. (From Shade B: *Mosby's EMT-Intermediate textbook,* St Louis, 1997, Mosby.)

Technological Advances in the Collection and Exchange of Information

Technology continues to change the way EMS collects and exchanges information and reduces dependence on traditional means of verbal and written communications. Examples include portable wireless voice and data devices, satellite terminals, global positioning systems for tracking emergency vehicles, diagnostic devices, and hand-held, pen-based computers (Fig. 16-4). These and other devices sometimes allow for "real-time capture" of EMS events and information. They also may affect the role of medical direction in delivering patient care by providing advanced notification, thereby reducing time to in-hospital diagnosis and therapy.

Communications Systems

Emergency communications technology has industry-specific terminology (Box 16-1). An overview of simple and complex communications systems is provided here.

Simple Systems

The minimum radio communications equipment requirements for an ambulance service include a self-contained desktop transceiver with a speaker, microphone, antenna, and mobile unit, and a two-way radio with multiple-frequency capability in the vehicle. Most EMS services also use hand-held portable radios (often called *portables*) capable of communications contact with the base station and data-recording apparatus for all communications. The portable radio protects the crew and facilitates optimal patient care by permitting continued contact with the communications center and medical direction. The recording apparatus provides medical

BOX 16-1

COMMUNICATIONS TERMINOLOGY

911: A three-digit telephone number to facilitate the reporting of an emergency requiring response by a public safety agency

911 Service area: The geographical area that has been granted authority by a state or local governmental body to provide 911 service

Abandoned call: A call placed to 911 in which the caller disconnects before the call can be answered by the Public Safety Answering Point (PSAP) attendant

Advanced mobile phone service (AMPS): The analog radio interface used in cellular telephone systems

Alternate PSAP: A PSAP designated to receive calls when the primary PSAP is unable to do so

Alternate routing: The capability of routing 911 calls to a designated alternate location(s) if all 911 trunks to a primary PSAP are busy or out of service. May be activated upon request or automatically, if detectable, when 911 equipment fails or the PSAP itself is disabled.

Amplitude modulated: The encoding of a carrier wave by variation of its amplitude in accordance with an input signal

Attendant position: The customer premises equipment (CPE) at which calls are answered and responded to by the telecommunicator

Automatic alarm and automatic alerting device: Any automated device that will access the 911 system for emergency services upon activation and does not provide for two-way communication. Many states prohibit the dialing of 911 by an automated device.

Automatic call distributor: Equipment that automatically distributes incoming calls to available PSAP attendants in the order the calls are received or queues calls until an attendant becomes available

Automatic location identification (ALI): The automatic display at the PSAP of the caller's telephone number, the address or location of the telephone, and supplementary emergency services information

Automatic number identification (ANI): Telephone number associated with the access line from which a call originates

Backup public safety answering point (PSAP): Typically a disaster recovery answering point that serves as a backup to the primary PSAP and is not co-located with the primary PSAP

Basic 911: An emergency telephone system that automatically connects 911 callers to a designated answering point. Call routing is determined by originating central office only. Basic 911 may or may not support ANI and/or ALI.

Call relay: Forwarding of pertinent information by a PSAP attendant to the appropriate response agency. Not to be confused with telephone relay service.

Calling party hold: The capability of the PSAP to maintain control of a 911 caller's access line, even if the caller hangs up

Calling party's number (CPN): The call-back number associated with a wireless telephone. Similar to ANI for wireline telephones. (Ref. NENA 03-002.)

Cell: The wireless telecomunications (cellular or PCS) antenna serving a specific geographical area

Circuit route: The physical path between two terminal locations

Computer-aided dispatch (CAD): A computer-based system that aids PSAP attendants by automating selected dispatching and record-keeping activities

Consolidated PSAP: A facility where one or more Public Safety Agencies choose to operate as a single 911 entity

Dedicated trunk: A telephone circuit used for a single purpose; such as transmission of 911 calls

Direct dispatch: The performance of 911 call answering and dispatching by personnel at the primary PSAP

Diverse routing: The practice of routing circuits along different physical paths to prevent total loss of 911 service in the event of a facility failure

Emergency call: A telephone request for public safety agency emergency services that requires immediate action to save a life, report a fire, or stop a crime. May include other situations as determined locally.

Emergency ring back: The capability of a PSAP attendant to ring the telephone on a held circuit. Requires calling party hold. Also known as *re-ring*. A basic 911 feature.

Emergency service (ES) trunks: Message trunks capable of providing ANI, connecting the serving central office of the 911 calling party and the designated E911 Control Office

Enhanced 911 (E911): An emergency telephone system that includes network switching, database and CPE elements capable of providing selective routing, selective transfer, fixed transfer, ANI, and ALI

Forced disconnect: The capability of a PSAP attendant to disconnect a 911 call even if the calling party remains off-hook. Used to prevent overloading of 911 trunks.

Global positioning system (GPS): A satellite-based location determination technology (LDT)

Highway call box: A telephone enclosed in a box and placed along a highway that allows a motorist to summon emergency and nonemergency assistance.

BOX 16-1

COMMUNICATIONS TERMINOLOGY—cont'd

Management information dystem (MIS): A program that collects, stores, and collates data into reports enabling interpretation and evaluation of performance, trends, traffic capacities, and so on

Master street address guide (MSAG): A database of street names and house number ranges within their associated communities defining emergency service zones (ESZs) and their associated emergency service numbers (ESNs) to enable proper routing of 911 calls.

National Emergency Number Association (NENA): A not-for-profit corporation established in 1982 to further the goal of "One Nation – One Number." NENA is a networking source and promotes research, planning, and training. NENA strives to educate, set standards, and provide certification programs, legislative representation, and technical assistance for implementing and managing 911 systems.

Primary public safety answering point (PSAP): A PSAP to which 911 calls are routed directly from the 911 Control Office (see **PSAP**)

Public safety answering point (PSAP): A facility equipped and staffed to receive 911 calls. A Primary PSAP receives the calls directly. If the call is relayed or transferred, the next receiving PSAP is designated a Secondary PSAP.

Selective routing (SR): The routing of a 911 call to the proper PSAP based on the location of the caller. Selective routing is controlled by the ESN, which is derived from the customer location.

Telecommunicator: As used in 911, a person who is trained and employed in public safety telecommunications. The term applies to call takers, dispatchers, radio operators, data terminal operators, or any combination of such functions in a PSAP.

Trunk: Typically, a communication path between central office switches or between the 911 Control Office and the PSAP.

From National Emergency Number Association (NENA) Technical Committee and PSAP Operational Standards Committee: *NENA Master Glossary of 911 Terminology,* March 1998, National Emergency Number Association.

---

and legal protection for the service and can verify the communications transmissions when contact is disrupted.

TRICKS OF THE TRADE

Always ensure that at least one member of your crew is able to contact the communications center at a moment's notice. A safe scene can quickly become unsafe.

Complex Systems

More sophisticated communications systems can include remote consoles, high-power transmitters, repeaters, satellite receivers, and high-power multifrequency vehicle radios. Some services also use mobile transmitter steering, vehicular repeaters, mobile encode-decode capabilities, mobile data terminals, microwave links, and other sophisticated communications devices.

Base Stations

Base stations usually are located on a high spot such as a hill, mountain, or tall building for optimal transmission and reception. Base stations generally are connected via telephone lines to dispatch centers, where all elements of the EMS response are coordinated. Depending on locale, one dispatch center may be responsible for all fire, police, and EMS communications activities. Base station transmitters usually are equipped with an antenna to boost their signal.

Mobile Transceivers

Vehicle-mounted transmitters usually operate at lower outputs than base stations. They provide a range of 10 to 15 miles over average terrain. Transmission over flat land or water increases this range, and transmission over mountainous terrain, dense foliage, or urban areas with tall buildings decreases the range. Transmitters with higher outputs are available and may provide greater ranges for transmission. Multichannel units are preferred over single-channel radios because of the many channels used in an EMS system.

Portable Transceivers

Portable transceivers are handheld or hand-carried devices used when working away from the emergency vehicle. These devices typically have a limited range; many systems boost the signal of these portable radios through a mobile or vehicular repeater. Portable transceivers may be single-channel or multichannel units.

Repeaters

Repeaters act as a special type of long-range transceiver. They receive transmissions from a low-power portable or mobile radio on one frequency and simultaneously retransmit it at a higher power on another frequency. Repeaters may be fixed or vehicle mounted; EMS systems commonly use both. Repeaters are necessary for effective radio communications over large geographical areas and are used to increase coverage from portable/mobile-to-portable/mobile. They allow low-power units to hear other radio messages and allow two or more low-power units to communicate with one another when distances or obstructions would normally hinder communications.

Remote Console

Most EMS systems use dispatch services located away from base stations. These remote centers control all base-station functions and are connected via dedicated telephone lines, microwave, or other radio means. Hospitals also are often equipped with a terminal that receives and displays telemetry transmissions as well as providing communications with field paramedic crews. Consoles for these systems include an amplifier, a speaker, a telemetry oscilloscope, a microphone, receiving capabilities, and remote control circuits.

Satellite Receivers and Terminals

Depending on the geographical area and terrain, satellite receivers sometimes are used to ensure that low-power units are always within communications coverage. The satellite receivers are strategically located and are connected to the base station or repeater by dedicated phone lines, radio, or microwave relay. "Voting systems" (also used in other types of communications systems) automatically select the strongest or best audio signal among multiple satellite receivers and the main base station receiver.

Portable satellite terminals may provide a means of transmitting important data when other communications systems are not available (e.g., during major disasters). Commonly available satellite terminals incorporate ground stations and transportable stations and provide voice, data, and video communications.

Encoders and Decoders

Selective call encoders are devices that resemble a telephone dial or the buttons of a push-button telephone. When activated, the encoder transmits tone pulses or pairs of tones over the air. Receivers with decoders are programmed to recognize specific codes that open the audio circuits of the receivers. Two-tone sequential paging signals by means of two pairs of specific frequency tones to selectively address pagers and alert monitors. A selective-address system normally incorporates a code for calling all units within radio range (all-call).

> **NOTE**
>
> Hospitals in certain regions throughout the United States are tied together by radio systems known as *Hospital Emergency Administrative Radio/HEAR* (Motorola) or *Emergency Administrative Communications/EACOM* (General Electric). These radios use 1500-Hz rotary pulse dialing, which transmits specific groups of rotary tone pulses to selectively address hospital-based receivers. Most ambulance services have access to this system.

Cellular Telephones

Many EMS services use cellular telephones (both analog and digital) as an alternative to dedicated EMS communications systems. In addition to having more channels, a cellular telephone provides a moderately secure communications link between EMS personnel and area hospitals. It also allows the on-line physician to speak directly with the patient. Disadvantages of cellular telephone use for emergency services include network usage that might limit channel access or produce problems in maintaining continuous communications in some areas, lack of priority access, and the inability of calls to be monitored by other members of an emergency response team. Therefore many EMS agencies using cellular telephones have backup radio communications capabilities (see the box below).

Digital

Digital modes of communications include digital phones, telemetry, fax transmissions, and digital signals used in some wireless phone, paging and alerting systems. Telemetry and facsimiles are transmitted using electronic signals that are converted into audio tones. These tones are converted back into electronic signals by the receiver's decoder so they can be displayed or printed. An example of telemetry is the transmission of a patient's ECG.

Computer

Computer technology (e.g., that used with AEDs and other devices) has the potential to "save" every step of data entry. Computers allow for (1) documentation in near "real time"; (2) sorting information in many categories; (3) creation of multiple reporting formats; and (4) quick on-line and retrieval system data. Computer terminals also are used by some communications centers to automatically dispatch units for emergency calls. As with most technologies, computer devices are subject to human error and machine limitations and therefore require regular upgrades and user education.

CELLULAR PHONE TECHNOLOGY

An analog cell phone is really a radio that allows two people to communicate on one frequency. The analog signal fluctuates with the rise and fall of the caller's voice, producing a wildly oscillating electrical wave (a "copy" of speech) that can be heard at the receiver's end. Digital cell phones use the same radio technology but different frequencies and compress the caller's voice into digital 1s and 0s that remain stable for the length of their travel. The digital information is then converted back to voice at the receiver's end. The digital signal is generally considered to provide better sound quality and a more secure method of transmission than using analog technology. Finally, digital technology provides a platform for future wireless services, such as data transmission and interactive computers.

Operation Modes Used for EMS Communications

The operation modes commonly used in EMS communications include simplex, multiplex, duplex, and trunked.

Simplex Mode

The **simplex mode** (Fig. 16-5) requires both a transmitter and receiver at each end of the communications path. Both elements operate on the same fre-

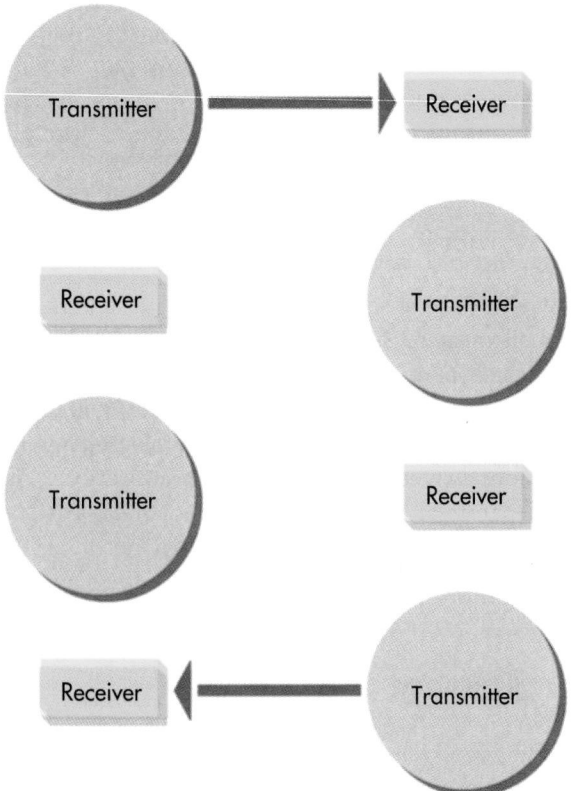

Fig. 16-5 Required equipment for simplex mode includes a transmitter and a receiver at each end of the communications path, both operating on the same frequency. In the simplex mode, only one end may operate at a time.

quency, but only one end may operate at a time. This mode allows speakers to send a message without interruption; however, it slows the communications process and takes away the ability to "discuss" a case.

Duplex Mode

The **duplex mode** (Fig. 16-6) uses two frequencies that allow both ends to communicate simultaneously. The advantage of this mode is that either

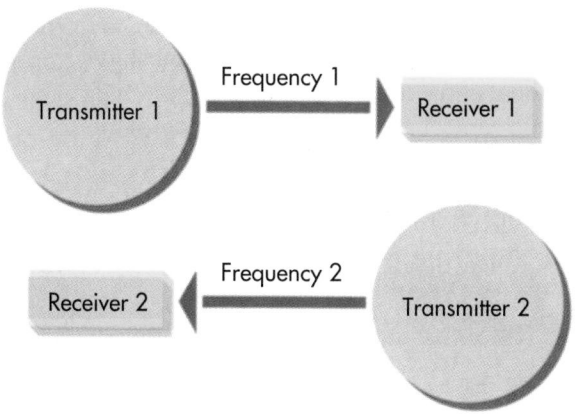

Fig. 16-6 Duplex mode requires two frequencies so both ends can communicate simultaneously.

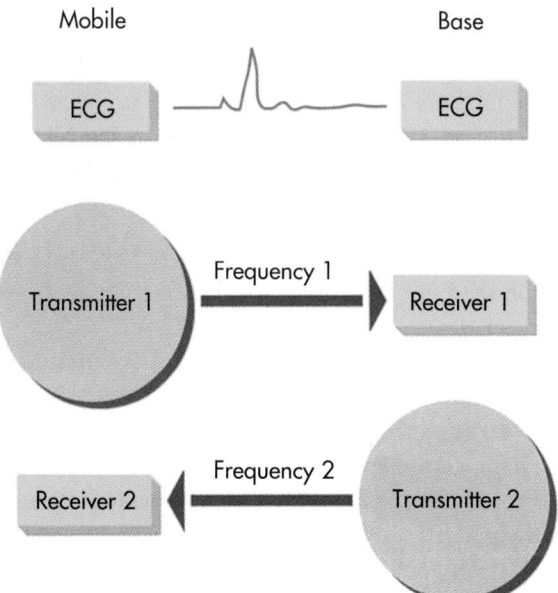

Fig. 16-7 Multiplex mode operates similar to duplex mode with added capabilities, such as simultaneous ECG and voice transmission.

party can interrupt the other to facilitate discussion. There is a tendency, however, for each end to interrupt the other.

Multiplex Mode

The **multiplex mode** (Fig. 16-7) has the advantage of transmitting telemetry and voice simultaneously from a field unit. With this mode, either party can interrupt as necessary, thereby facilitating discussion. As with the duplex mode, each party has a tendency to interrupt the other. In addition, voice transmission may interfere with the transmission of data. This is the most common mode in use today with most EMS services.

Trunked System

Trunking refers to systems that have five or more repeaters, each on a different channel, that work as a group. The trunking system may belong to a single user (e.g., a specific EMS agency or police department) or it may be shared by a number of different public service agencies. When radio transmissions are originated, computerized scanning automatically finds an available repeater in the system and then switches that transmission to the selected repeater. As one fleet captures an open channel, it locks out all other users who share the system, preventing interference from other agencies. The trunked system is of particular advantage in major metropolitan operations where radio frequencies are heavily used.

Components and Functions of Dispatch Communications Systems

The dispatch communications system is the public safety answering point (see the box on p. 510). Some functions of an effective EMS dispatch communications system include the following[3]:

- Receive and process calls for EMS assistance. The dispatcher receives and records calls for EMS assistance and selects an appropriate course of action for each call. This function involves obtaining as much information as possible about the emergency event, including name, call back number, and address, and it may include dealing with distraught callers.

911, ENHANCED 911, AND COMPUTER-AIDED DISPATCH SYSTEMS

As described in Chapter 1, 911 was designated in 1988 as the universal emergency telephone number by the American Telephone and Telegraph Company to provide the public with a toll-free number to reach a public safety answering point (PSAP). (This service is still not available universally.) Since then, enhanced 911 (E911) has been developed and is used in many areas of the country. This advanced system allows for automatic caller location and identification and displays the caller's phone number and address on a terminal at the communications center.

The most sophisticated communications centers use a computer-aided dispatch (CAD) system that monitors available resources and makes an assignment decision based on access and routes for the ambulance closest to the map grid displayed on the terminal. Global positioning systems tell the telecommunicator or system status controller which unit is closest to the origin of the call by air miles. That unit is then dispatched to the emergency scene. The telecommunicator monitors the call from beginning to end and records status changes by digital audio tape.

systems, computer-aided dispatching may be used. This advanced technology allows one or more of the following capabilities or functions:

Automatic entry of 911
Automatic call notification/request for assistance
Automatic interface to automatic vehicle location with or without map display
Automatic interface to mobile data terminal
Computer messaging among multiple radio operators, call takers, or both
Dispatch note taking, reminder aid, or both
Emergency medical dispatch review
Manual or automatic updates of unit status
Manual entry of call information
Radio control and display of channel status
Standard operating procedure review
Telephone control and display of circuit status

✓ TRICKS OF THE TRADE

The communications center can be your "lifeline" that helps ensure personal safety.

- Dispatch and coordinate EMS resources. The dispatcher directs the appropriate emergency vehicle(s) to the correct address. In addition, the dispatcher coordinates the movements of emergency vehicles while en route to the scene, to the medical facility, and back to the operations base.
- Relay medical information. The dispatcher may provide a telecommunications channel among appropriate medical facilities and EMS personnel, fire, police, rescue workers, and private citizens. The channel may consist of telephone, radio, or biomedical telemetry.
- Coordinate with public safety agencies. The dispatcher provides for communications between public safety units (fire, law enforcement, rescue) and elements of the EMS system to facilitate coordination of services such as traffic control, escort, fire suppression, and extrication. To ensure that all these events take place in an integrated, well-coordinated system, the dispatcher must know the location and status of all EMS vehicles and the availability of support services. In larger

Dispatcher Training

Many EMS and public service agencies require specialized medical training for their dispatch personnel. This training may include the *Association of Public Communications Officials (APCO) and Emergency Medical Dispatch (EMD) Program* (based on the NHTSA National Standard Curriculum for EMD). EMDs are trained to do the following[4]:

- Use locally approved EMD guidecards (customized to local protocols and EMS response priorities)
- Quickly and properly determine the nature of the call
- Determine the priority of the call
- Dispatch the appropriate response
- Provide the caller with instructions to help treat the patient until the responding EMS unit arrives

A base of training in EMS helps the telecommunicator understand functions of the EMS system, personnel capabilities, and equipment limitations. It also provides the dispatcher with appropriate protocols to give prearrival instructions that might mitigate the event before the arrival of an EMS unit. A variety of dispatching systems and procedures are in place throughout the United States. These systems range from very simple "call received–ambulance dispatched" types of programs to the more sophisticated call prioritization–prearrival instructions systems.

Call Prioritization–Prearrival Instructions Systems

In the call screening–prearrival instructions system an EMD, paramedic, or nurse determines what type of assistance is required for a particular emergency call. This may include referring the caller to other services, choosing BLS or ALS response, selecting private or public EMS service, and determining use of audible and visual lights warning devices. While dispatching the appropriate unit to respond, dispatchers provide the caller with prearrival instructions. Prearrival instructions are important for the following reasons:

- They provide immediate assistance to the caller.
- They complement the call prioritization process.
- They allow the telecommunicator to provide updated information to responding units.
- They may be lifesaving in critical incidents.
- They provide emotional support for the caller, bystander, or victim.

? CRITICAL THINKING

What are some potential consequences of a dispatching error?

Regulation

Radio communications in the United States are regulated by the **Federal Communications Commission** (FCC). This commission develops rules and regulations for the use of all radio equipment and frequencies. In addition to the FCC, state and local governments may have rules and regulations for radio operations. The paramedic must be knowledgeable about these agencies and follow their guidelines. The primary functions of the FCC include the following:

- Licensing and frequency allocation
- Establishing technical standards for radio equipment

- Establishing and enforcing rules and regulations for equipment operation, including monitoring frequencies for appropriate usage and spot-checking for appropriate licenses and records

? CRITICAL THINKING

Why are these rules and regulations necessary for effective EMS communications?

Procedures for EMS Communications

Most EMS systems use a standard radio communications protocol that includes the desired format for message transmission and key words and phrases. Following this format aids in professional and efficient radio communications within the system. General guidelines for radio communications include the following:

- Think before you speak (formulate the message) to ensure that communications will be effective.
- Speak at close range (2 to 3 inches) when talking into a microphone.
- Speak slowly and clearly. Enunciate each word distinctly and avoid words that are difficult to hear.
- Speak in a normal pitch without emotion.
- Be brief and concise. Break up long messages into shorter ones.
- Avoid codes unless they are systems-approved. Avoid dialect or slang.
- Advise the receiving party when the transmission has been completed.
- Confirm the receiving party has received the message.

? CRITICAL THINKING

Provide three reasons why a concise EMS radio report is essential.

Relaying Patient Information

A standard format of transmission may be developed as a protocol for some EMS services. This allows efficient use of medical communications systems by limiting radio air time. In addition, physicians can quickly receive information regarding the patient's condition, and the potential for omitting any significant information is lessened.

Patient information can be reported to the hospital or dispatcher by radio or telephone. Although the order of information delivery may vary by EMS system and scenario, the radio report should be brief and concise and contain the following[1]:

- Unit and provider identification
- Description of the scene or incident
- Patient's age, sex, and approximate weight (for drug orders)
- Patient's chief complaint
- Associated symptoms
- Brief, pertinent history of present illness or injury
- Pertinent past medical history, medications, and allergies
- Pertinent physical examination findings
  Level of consciousness
  Vital signs
  Neurological examination
  General appearance and degree of distress
  ECG results (if applicable)
  Trauma Index or Glasgow Coma Scale (if applicable)
  Other pertinent observations and significant findings
- Any treatment given
- Estimated time of arrival (ETA)
- Request for orders from or further questions for medical direction physician

NOTE

The use of telemetry to transmit a patient's ECG usually is reserved for the patient who requires 12-lead diagnosis before the administration of some drugs. Telemetry transmission uses excessive air time. If warranted, 15 to 30 seconds of telemetry transmission usually are adequate.

The SOAP Format

The **SOAP format** (or a similar method) is used by many paramedics as a memory aid to organize written and verbal patient reports. *SOAP* is an acronym for the following:

- **S**ubjective data: All patient symptoms including chief complaint, associated symptoms, past history, current medications and allergies, and information provided by bystanders and family
- **O**bjective data: Pertinent physical examination information including vital signs, level of consciousness, physical examination findings, ECG, pulse oximetry readings, and blood glucose determinations, and so on
- **A**ssessment data: The paramedic's clinical impression of the patient based on subjective and objective data
- **P**lan of patient management: Treatment that has been provided and any requests for additional treatment

General Procedures for the Exchange of Information

When communicating with medical direction, the paramedic should repeat all orders received from the physician and confirm any orders that are unclear or seem inappropriate. The receiving hospital also should be informed of any significant changes in the patient's status before and during transport. General procedures of the exchange of information include the following:

- Protect the patient's privacy.
- Use proper unit numbers, hospital numbers, names, and titles.
- Avoid slang or profanity.
- Use the "echo" procedure (repeating what was heard) when receiving directions from the dispatcher or physician.
- Obtain confirmation that the message was received.

SUMMARY

- EMS communications refers to the delivery of patient and scene information to other members of the emergency response team.

- Verbal, written, and electronic communications allow the delivery of information between the party requesting help and the dispatcher, between the dispatcher and paramedic, and between the paramedic, hospital, and direct/on-line medical direction.

- Communications technology has industry-specific terminology.

- The primary modes of EMS communications include simplex mode, duplex mode, multiplex mode, trunking system, digital, and computer.

- Radio communications in the United States are regulated by the FCC. The paramedic must be knowledgeable about regulatory agencies and follow their guidelines.

- The functions of an effective dispatch communications system include receiving and processing calls for EMS assistance, dispatching and coordinating EMS resources, relaying medical information, and coordinating with public safety agencies.

- A standard format of transmission of patient information allows efficient use of medical communications systems, allows physicians to quickly receive information, and lessens the potential for omitting any significant information.

REFERENCES

1. Department of Transportation National Highway Traffic Safety Administration: *Paramedic national standard curriculum*, Washington, DC, 1998, The Department.
2. Szilagyi A, Wallace M: *Organizational behavior and performance*, ed 5, Glenview, Ill, 1990, Addison-Wesley.
3. US Department of Transportation National Highway Traffic Safety Administration: *Emergency medical dispatch: national standard curriculum*, Washington, DC, 1996, US Government Printing Office.
4. APCO Institute: *Emergency medical dispatch services*, South Daytona, Fla, 1998, The Institute. www.apcointl.org/institute/pages/emd/htm.

17 Documentation

OBJECTIVES

Upon completion of this chapter, the paramedic student will be able to:

1. Identify the purpose of the patient care report.
2. Describe the uses of the patient care report.
3. Outline the components of an accurate, thorough patient care report.
4. Describe the elements of a properly written EMS document.
5. Describe an effective system for documentation of prehospital patient care.
6. Identify differences necessary when documenting special situations.
7. Describe the appropriate method to make revisions or corrections to the patient care report.
8. Recognize consequences that may result from inappropriate documentation.

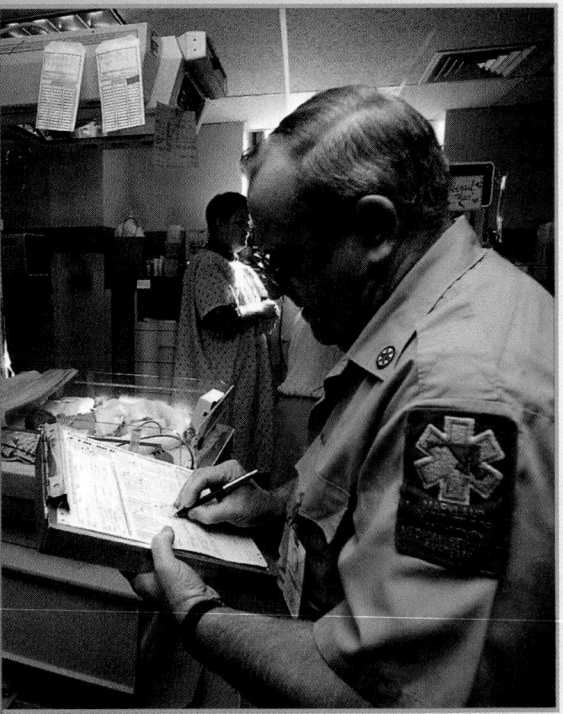

The patient care report (PCR) is used to effectively document the essential elements of patient assessment, care, and transport.[1] It is a legal document that, next to providing good patient care, is the paramedic's best protection from liability action.

KEY TERMS

narrative: The portion of the patient care report that allows for a chronological description of the call.

pertinent negative findings: Findings that warrant no medical care or intervention but that, by seeking them, show evidence of the thoroughness of the examination and history of the event.

NOTE

Record-keeping requirements vary throughout the United States. As a safety measure to guard against statute-of-limitation issues, most EMS records (including PCRs) are maintained a minimum of 10 years (see Chapter 4). *Accurate documentation leads to accurate recall if litigation occurs.*

Importance of Documentation

There are many reasons for thorough, written documentation. It provides a written and legal record of the incident and often is used by physicians and nurses to better understand the patient's initial condition and the type of care given before hospital treatment. The EMS agency and medical direction also may use the report to monitor care in the field, evaluate individual performance, conduct review conferences and other educational forums, and identify system issues regarding quality improvement. Examples of quality improvement issues that may be identified through the PCR and may result in policy changes to improve patient care include the following:

- Minimizing time spent on the scene for critical trauma patients
- Adding new medications to better manage some medical emergencies
- Changing the placement of emergency vehicles during peak response times in certain demographic areas

The PCR also provides the paramedic with a means of documenting unique scene situations that

---

BOX 17-1

IMPORTANCE OF DOCUMENTATION

Written documentation provides for the following:
- A written record of the incident
- A legal record of the incident
- Professionalism
- Medical audit
- Quality improvement
- Billing and administration
- Data collection

---

may have affected patient care (e.g., a long response time because of traffic congestion; an entrapment of the patient that required prolonged extrication), and tracking particular patient care skills (e.g., intravenous lines, intubations, defibrillations) that may be required for relicensure or recertification. The PCR data also are a primary source for administrative and billing information (pertinent administrative information) necessary for the economic survival of many EMS agencies (Box 17-1).

NOTE

Accurate billing leads to increased revenue for EMS systems.

NOTE

The PCR may be the only way for a paramedic to accurately recall events of an emergency call during testimony that occurs years after the incident. The paramedic must include as much detail as possible in the PCR for present and future use.

General Considerations

The PCR (Box 17-2) should be carefully detailed and legible. Because it is viewed as a legal document and

BOX 17-2

PREHOSPITAL CARE REPORT DATA

- Dates
- Response times
- Difficulties en route
- Communication difficulties
- Scene observations
- Reasons for extended on-scene time
- Previous care provided
- Time of extrication
- Time of patient transport
- Reason for hospital selection (trauma center designation, patient choice, or other concerns)

BOX 17-3

COMPONENTS OF THE NARRATIVE PORTION OF THE PATIENT CARE REPORT

- Initial contact
- All patient care activities (including medications and treatments)
- Initial assessment and vital signs
- Chief complaint
- Pertinent significant medical history
- Clock time of hospital contact
- Time of physician orders and advice (name of physician)
- Pertinent negative findings
- Pertinent oral statements
- Changes in patient status
- Patient response to treatment
- Vital sign reassessment
- ECG interpretation
- Use of support services
- Time and condition of patient on delivery
- Name of receiving health care worker

part of the patient's medical record, the use of slang terminology or medical abbreviations that are not universally accepted should be avoided (Table 17-1).

NOTE

Many EMS systems develop agency-approved medical abbreviations.

The report should include all dates and response times and describe any difficulties encountered en route and during patient treatment, extrication, or transport. The report also should include observations at the scene, any previous medical care provided (and by whom), and time of patient extrication, if appropriate. The times of all significant occurrences and interventions are useful to the receiving physician and should be recorded. In particular, the PCR provides a legal and accurate recording of the following incident times:

- Time of call
- Time of dispatch
- Time of arrival at the scene
- Time at patient's side
- Time of vital sign assessments
- Time(s) of medication administration and certain medical procedures as defined by local protocol
- Time of departure from the scene
- Time of arrival at the medical facility (when transporting a patient)
- Time back in service

? CRITICAL THINKING

How can documentation of specific "times" on the patient care report be useful?

The Narrative

The **narrative** portion of the PCR allows for a chronological description of the call. It should be documented concisely and clearly, using simple words and avoiding uncommon abbreviations, unnecessary terms, and duplication of information. A standard format should be established by medical direction and followed by the paramedic. This helps ensure completeness and facilitates quality-improvement reviews (Box 17-3).

NOTE

Documentation should never be used by the paramedic to creatively construct patient care. If the paramedic didn't document it—it wasn't done. Conversely, if it wasn't done—don't document it.

TABLE 17-1 COMMON ABBREVIATIONS

NOTE: Abbreviations in common use can vary widely from place to place. Each institution's list of acceptable abbreviations is the best authority for its records.

°C	degrees Centigrade	CO_2	carbon dioxide
°F	degrees Farenheit	COPD	chronic obstructive pulmonary disease
μg	microgram	CPK	creatine phosphokinase
μm	micrometer	CPR	cardiopulmonary resuscitation
℥	dram	CSF	cerebrospinal fluid
@	at	CT	computed tomography
aa	of each	CVA	cerebrovascular accident, costovertebral angle
ABG	arterial blood gas		
ac	before meals	CVP	central venous pressure
ad lib	freely as desired	D&C	dilation and curettage
ADL	activities of daily living	D5W	5% dextrose in water
Ag	silver, antigen	db, dB	decibels
AIDS	acquired immunodeficiency syndrome	dc	discontinue
ALS	amyotrophic lateral sclerosis	DIC	disseminated intravascular coagulation
AM	morning	diff	differential blood count
a.m.a.	against medical advice	dil	dilute
AMI	acute myocardial infarction	DJD	degenerative joint disease
amp	ampule	dl	deciliter
ARC	AIDS-related complex	DM	diastolic murmur
ARDS	acute respiratory distress syndrome	DNR	do not resuscitate
AS	aortic stenosis	DOE	dyspnea on exertion
ASD	atrial septal defect	dx, DX	diagnosis
Ba	barium	EBV	Epstein-Barr virus
BE	barium enema	ECF	extracellular fluid
bid	two times a day	ECG	electrocardiogram
BM, bm	bowel movement	ECT	electroconvulsive therapy
BMR	basal metabolic rate	EDC	estimated date of confinement
BP	blood pressure	EDD	estimated date of delivery
BPH	benign prostatic hypertrophy	EEG	electroencephalogram
BRP	bathroom privileges	EKG	electrocardiogram
BSA	body surface area	elix	elixir
BUN	blood urea nitrogen	EMG	electromyogram
c̄	with	ENG	electronystagmography
c/o	complains of	ER	emergency room
Ca	calcium, cancer, carcinoma	ERG	electroretinogram
CAD	coronary artery disease	ESR	erythrocyte sedimentation rate
cap	capsule	ESRD	end-stage renal disease
CAT	computed axial tomography	EST	electroshock therapy
cath.	catheter, catheterize	f℥	fluid ounce
CBC	complete blood count	FANA	fluorescent antinuclear antibody test
CBR	complete bed rest	Fe	iron
CC	chief complaint	FEV	forced expiratory volume
cc	cubic centimeter	FHR	fetal heart rate
CCU	coronary care unit, critical care unit	FRC	functional residual capacity
CDC	Centers for Disease Control	FUO	fever of unknown origin
CEA	carcinoembryonic antigen	Fx, fx	fracture, fractional urine test
CFT	complement-fixation test	g, gm, Gm	gram
cg	centigram		
CHF	congestive heart failure	Gc, GC	gonococcus
CHO	carbohydrate	GI	gastrointestinal
Cl	chlorine	gr	grain
cm	centimeter	grav I, II, III, etc	pregnancy one, two, three, etc
cm^3	cubic centimeter		
CNS	central nervous system	gt, gtt	drop, drops
CO	carbon monoxide	GTT	glucose tolerance test

From Potter PA, Perry AG: *Fundamentals of nursing: concepts, process, and practice,* ed 4, St Louis, 1997, Mosby.

TABLE 17-1   COMMON ABBREVIATIONS—cont'd

GU	genitourinary	mcg	microgram
GYN, Gyn	gynecological	MCH	mean corpuscular hemoglobin
		MCHC	mean corpuscular hemoglobin concentration
H_2O	water		
h	hour	MCV	mean cell volume, mean corpuscular volume
H^+	hydrogen ion		
h/o	history of	mg	milligram
H&P	history and physical examination	Mg	magnesium
HAV	hepatitis A virus	MG	myasthenia gravis
Hb	hemoglobin	MI	myocardial infarction
HBAg	hepatitis B antigen	MICU	medical intensive care unit
HBV	hepatitis B virus	mL	milliliter
Hct, HCT	hematocrit	mm	millimeter
Hg	mercury	mm^3	cubic millimeter
Hgb	hemoglobin	mm Hg	millimeters of mercury
HIV	human immunodeficiency (AIDS) virus	MRI	magnetic resonance imaging
HLA	human lymphocyte antigen	MS	multiple sclerosis
hs	at bedtime	MW	molecular weight
HSV	herpes simplex virus	N	nitrogen
I&O	intake and output	Na	sodium
IC	inspiratory capacity	NICU	neonatal intensive care unit
ICP	intracranial pressure	NIH	National Institutes of Health
ICU	intensive care unit	nm	nanometer
IDDM	insulin-dependent diabetes mellitus	NMR	nuclear magnetic resonance
IE	immunoelectrophoresis	NPO	nothing by mouth
Ig	immunoglobulin	NS	normal saline
IgA, etc	immunoglobulin A, etc	O_2	oxygen
IM	intramuscular	OD	right eye; optical density; overdose
IOP	intraocular pressure	OL	left eye
IPPB	intermittent positive pressure breathing	OOB	out of bed
IV	intravenous	ORIF	open reduction and internal fixation
IVP	intravenous push; intravenous pyelogram	OS	left eye
IVU	intravenous urogram	OT	occupational therapy
JRA	juvenile rheumatoid arthritis	OTC	over-the-counter
K	potassium	oz, ℥	ounce
kg	kilogram	P&A	percussion and auscultation
KUB	kidney, ureters, and bladder (radiograph)	$PaCO_2$	partial pressure of carbon dioxide (arterial blood)
KVO	keep vein open		
L	liter	PaO_2	partial pressure of oxygen (arterial blood)
L&A	light and accommodation		
LBBB	left bundle branch block	para I, II, etc	unipara, bipara, etc
LE	lupus erythematosus		
LGV	lymphogranuloma venereum	PAT	paroxysmal atrial tachycardia
LLL	left lower lobe	pc	after meals
LLQ	left lower quadrant	PCG	phonocardiogram
LMP	last menstrual period	PCO_2	partial pressure of carbon dioxide
LNMP	last normal menstrual period	PCP	pulmonary capillary pressure, phencyclidine
LP	lumbar puncture		
LUL	left upper lobe	PCV	packed cell volume
LUQ	left upper quadrant	PCWP	pulmonary capillary wedge pressure
LVH	left ventricular hypertrophy	PD	interpupillary distance; postural drainage
m	meter		
m, min, ♏	minim	PE	pulmonary embolism, physical examination
		PEEP	positive end expiratory pressure
		PEG	pneumoencephalography
MAP	mean arterial pressure	per	through, by way of

From Potter PA, Perry AG: *Fundamentals of nursing: concepts, process, and practice,* ed 4, St Louis, 1997, Mosby.

TABLE 17-1 ▶ COMMON ABBREVIATIONS—cont'd

PERRLA	pupils equal, round, and reactive to light and accommodation	SICU	surgical intensive care unit
PET	positron emission tomography	SIDS	sudden infant death syndrome
PG	prostaglandin	Sig	write on label
pH	hydrogen ion concentration (acidity and alkalinity)	SLE	systemic lupus erythematosus
		sol	solution, dissolved
PID	pelvic inflammatory disease	sos	if necessary
PKU	phenylketonuria	sp. gr., SG, sg	specific gravity
PM	postmortem		
PM	evening	SQ, subq	subcutaneous
PMS	premenstrual syndrome	SR	sedimentation rate
PND	paroxysmal nocturnal dyspnea, post-nasal drip	ss	half
		SSS	sick sinus syndrome, specific soluble substance, short-stay surgery
PO_2	partial pressure of oxygen		
PO, po	orally	STAT	immediately
PPD	purified protein derivative	STD	sexually transmitted disease
ppm	parts per million	STS	serologic test for syphilis
p.r.n.	when required, as often as necessary	susp	suspension
PT	physical therapy; prothrombin time	T_3	triiodothyronine
PTT	partial thromboplastin time	T_4	tetraiodothyronine
PUO	pyrexia of unknown origin	T&A	tonsillectomy and adenoidectomy
PVC	premature ventricular contraction	TAB	typhoid and paratyphoid A and B
q	every	TAH	total abdominal hysterectomy
q2h	every 2 hours	TAT	tetanus antitoxin; thematic apperception test
q3h	every 3 hours		
q4h	every 4 hours	TB, TBC	tuberculosis
qd	every day	TBG	thyroxin-binding globulin
qh	every hour	TG	triglyceride
qid	four times a day	TIA	transient ischemic attack
qn	every night	TIBC	total iron-binding capacity
qod	every other day	tid	three times a day
qns	quantity not sufficient	TKO	to keep open
R/O	rule out	TLC	total lung capacity; thin layer chromatography
RA	rheumatoid arthritis		
RBBB	right bundle branch block	TPN	total parenteral nutrition
RDA	recommended daily (dietary) allowance	TPR	temperature, pulse, and respirations
RDS	respiratory distress syndrome	tr, tinct	tincture
Rh+	positive Rh factor	TST	triple sugar iron test
Rh−	negative Rh factor	UIBC	unsaturated iron-binding capacity
RHD	rheumatic heart disease	URI	upper respiratory infection
RLL	right lower lobe	UTI	urinary tract infection
RLQ	right lower quadrant	V&T	volume and tension
RML	right middle lobe	VC	vital capacity
ROM	range of motion	VD	venereal disease
ROS	review of systems	VDA	visual discriminatory acuity
RS	Reiter's syndrome	VDH	valvular disease of the heart
RSV	Rous sarcoma virus	VDRL	Venereal Disease Research Laboratory (test for syphilis)
RUL	right upper lobe		
RUQ	right upper quadrant	VS	vital signs
Rx	take; treatment	VSD	ventricular septal defect
$\bar{s}$	without	V_T	tidal volume
SB	sternal border	W/V	weight/volume
SC	subcutaneous	WBC	white blood cell, white blood count
sib.	sibling	WNL	within normal limits
		WR	Wasserman reaction

Pertinent negative findings may help determine the course of treatment and should be recorded. Pertinent negative findings (e.g., the absence of diminished breath sounds) are findings that warrant no medical care or intervention but that, by seeking them, show evidence of the thoroughness of the paramedic's examination and history of the event. Pertinent oral statements made by the patient and other on-scene persons also should be recorded. Statements that may have an impact on subsequent patient care or resolution of the situation include the following:

- Mechanism of injury
- Patient's behavior
- First-aid interventions before EMS arrival
- Safety-related information (including disposition of weapons)
- Information of interest to crime scene investigators
- Disposal of valuable personal property (e.g., jewelry, wallets)

? CRITICAL THINKING

Why should you note the previous care given by bystanders in your report?

NOTE

The paramedic should put into quotation marks any statements directly made by patients or others that relate to possible criminal activity or admission of suicidal intention.

NOTE

Failed skills (e.g., an unsuccessful IV or ET intubation attempt) also should be documented on the PCR.

The narrative also should include the use of support services (e.g., helicopter, coroner, rescue/extrication) and mutual aid assistance. Finally, the PCR should be signed by the paramedic, listing everyone who participated in patient care before emergency department delivery. Because a copy of the report is placed in the patient's hospital medical record, leaving a finished copy with the patient at the receiving hospital may be necessary. This requires developing a systematic approach to completing the report in a timely fashion so the EMS crew can be available for service.

NOTE

The PCR is valuable in providing the attending physician and ED staff the advantage of understanding the events and the care rendered in the prehospital setting. If possible, the report should be left with the patient at the hospital.

Elements of a Properly Written EMS Document

A properly written EMS document is accurate, legible, timely, unaltered, and free of nonprofessional or extraneous information. A brief description of each of these elements is listed as follows:

1. *Accurate and complete.* For accurate documentation, all pertinent information must be provided in both the narrative and check-box sections of the report. Completing all areas of the report (even if a section was unused) demonstrates a precise and comprehensive document. The paramedic should ensure that medical terms, abbreviations, and acronyms are properly used and correctly spelled.
2. *Legible.* Legibility means that handwriting, especially in the narrative portion of the report, can be read by others without difficulty. Check-box markings should be clear and consistent from the top page of the report to all underlying pages.
3. *Timely.* Ideally, documentation should be completed immediately after the patient interaction. Delays in recording can result in serious omissions and may be interpreted as negligence.
4. *Unaltered.* If errors are made while writing the report, the paramedic should draw a single line through the error, and date and initial it (Fig. 17-1). Any alterations to a completed report should be accompanied by an appropriate "revision/correction" supplement with the date and time of revision.
5. *Free of nonprofessional/extraneous information.* The PCR must be free of jargon, slang, personal bias, libelous or slanderous remarks, and irrelevant opinion or impression.

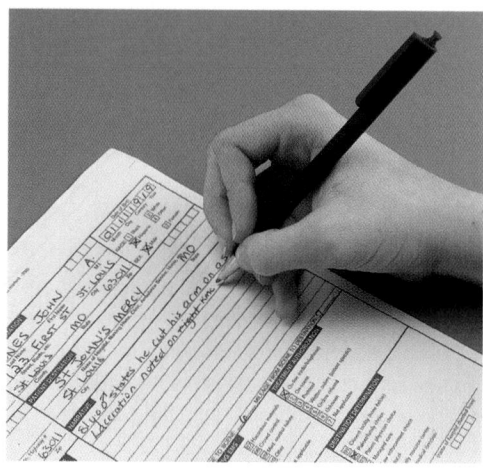

Fig. 17-1 Correcting a PCR.

Systems of Narrative Writing

As with all other aspects of emergency care, the paramedic should develop a systematic approach for writing the narrative portion of the patient care report. Many approaches for writing the narrative can be used; however, the paramedic should adopt only *one* approach and use it consistently to avoid omissions in report writing. Examples of systems that are used to write the narrative include the SOAP method; SAMPLE history; a physical approach from head to toe; a review of primary body systems; a chronological, call incident approach; a patient management approach; and others. Regardless of the system used to organize the narrative, the paramedic must ensure that objective (versus subjective) elements of documentation comprise the report.

? CRITICAL THINKING

How many meanings can you think of for the word lethargic? Look it up in the dictionary. Should you use this word to document a patient's mental status? Why?

Special Considerations of Documentation

Several considerations of documentation deserve special mention. Three of these include a patient's refusal of care and/or transport, situations and events where transportation is not needed, and situations involving mass casualties. Other situations that require careful documentation (e.g., caring for intoxicated patients, cases of abuse and neglect) are described in Chapter 4 and Chapter 44, respectively.

Patient Refusal of Care and/or Transport

As described in Chapter 4, a patient's refusal of care and/or transport is a major area of potential liability for paramedics and EMS agencies. Thorough documentation of these situations is crucial and should include the following:

- The paramedic's advice to the patient regarding the benefits of treatment and the risks associated with refusing care
- The advice rendered by medical direction via telephone or radio

- Clinical information (e.g., the patient's level of consciousness) that suggests competency
- The signatures of any witnesses(es) to the event, according to local protocol
- A complete narrative, including quotations or statements made by others

> **NOTE**
>
> If the patient refuses care and/or transport, the paramedic should carefully document the incident and make it clear that the patient may call again for help, despite the initial refusal. When possible, friends or family should be encouraged to stay with the patient.

When Care and Transportation is Not Needed

There will be occasions when care and transportation of a patient will not be warranted, either as a result of the patient's condition or a canceled request for help. After evaluation of the patient or scene, if the paramedic determines that circumstances do not warrant EMS transport (e.g., a car crash without injuries or a patient who has left the scene), the dispatch center should be advised, and the event should be documented. If the EMS unit is canceled en route to the scene, the paramedic should make note of the canceling authority (e.g., dispatch center, EMS supervisor) and time of the cancellation. Like refusal of care, thorough documentation of these events can protect the paramedic from potential liability.

Situations Involving Mass Casualties

During a major incident where there are a large number of patients, comprehensive documentation may have to be postponed until patients are triaged and transported for definitive care (see Chapter 49). These are difficult and unusual situations. In these circumstances, the paramedic should know and follow local documentation procedures.

Document Revision/Correction

As previously stated, revising or correcting a patient care report may sometimes be necessary. Most EMS agencies provide separate report forms for this purpose. If a separate report is needed, the paramedic should do the following:

- Note the purpose of the revision or correction and why the information did not appear on the original document
- Note the date and time the revision or correction was made
- Ensure that the revision or correction was made by the original author of the document
- Make the revision or correction as soon as the need for it is realized

Acceptable methods for making corrections or adding supplemental information to a document vary by agency. Some methods include making the revision on the original form with initials, date, and time; writing corrections in the narrative; or attaching a new report to the original. Supplemental narratives can be written on a separate form and attached to the original. The paramedic should follow the policies established by the EMS agency and medical direction for revising and/or correcting reports.

> **? CRITICAL THINKING**
>
> *What would you do if you were asked by your supervisor to change your documentation so the insurance company would pay for the transport?*

Consequences of Inappropriate Documentation

Inappropriate documentation may have medical and legal implications. An incomplete, inaccurate, or

> **BOX 17-4**
>
> ### THE PARAMEDIC'S RESPONSIBILITY FOR DOCUMENTATION
>
> As part of professional responsibility, the paramedic should do the following:
> - View the task of documentation as one of utmost importance
> - Assume responsibility for self-assessment of all documentation
> - Appreciate the importance of good documentation among peers
> - Strive to set a good example to others regarding the completion of the documentation task
> - Respect the confidential nature of an EMS report

illegible PCR may cause subsequent caregivers to provide inappropriate care to a patient. For example, if the paramedic failed to mention a patient with chest pain had an allergy to *lidocaine* (Xylocaine), and that patient later became unconscious in the emergency department as a result of a ventricular rhythm disturbance, a lethal medication for that patient could inadvertently be administered. A PCR that is thoroughly completed in a professional manner may greatly influence the decision of an attorney who is considering the merits of an impending lawsuit for negligence or malpractice. (The converse also is true if documentation is not thorough and professional.)

NOTE

Thorough documentation is an important means for paramedics to represent themselves as professionals.

Finally, documentation should never become routine or superficial to the paramedic (Box 17-4). Good and appropriate documentation should be completed in a timely manner and with careful attention to detail. This will ensure that the PCR is medically and legally sound.

SUMMARY

- The patient care report is used to effectively document the essential elements of patient assessment, care, and transport.

- The reasons for written documentation include its use by the medical community involved in the patient's care, as a legal record, and for data collection.

- The patient care report should include dates and response times, difficulties encountered, observations at the scene, previous medical care provided, a chronological description of the call, and significant times.

- A properly written EMS document is accurate, legible, timely, unaltered, and free of non-professional or extraneous information.

- Many approaches for writing the narrative can be used; however, the paramedic should adopt only one approach and use it consistently to avoid omissions in report writing.

- Special documentation will be necessary when a patient refuses care and/or transport, care or transportation is not needed, or mass casualty incidents occur.

- Most EMS agencies provide separate forms for revisions or corrections of the patient care report.

- Inappropriate documentation may have medical and legal implications.

REFERENCE

1. US Department of Transportation National Highway Traffic Safety Administration: *EMT-Paramedic national standard curriculum*, Washington, DC, 1998, The Department.

Division Four →

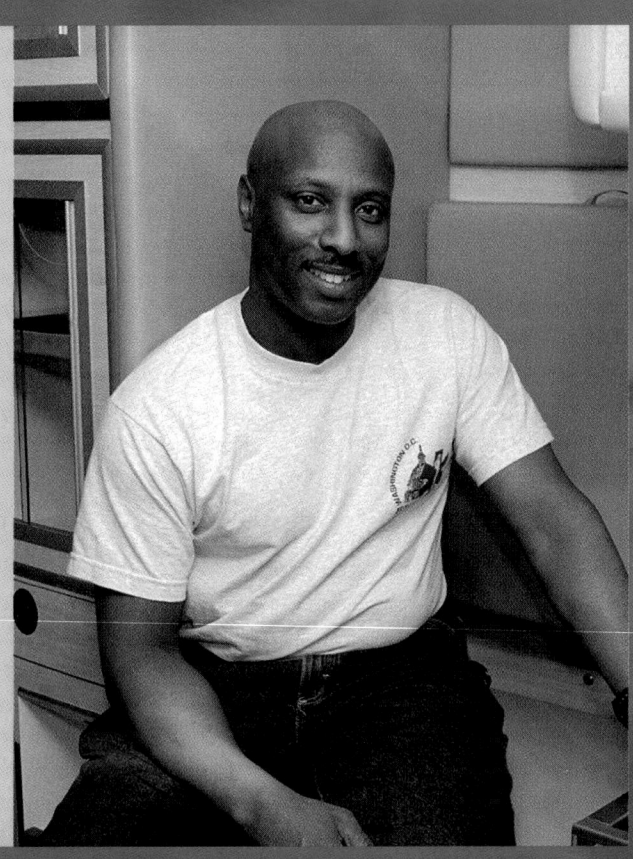

Calvin Haupt, EMT-P
District of Columbia
Fire and Emergency
Medical Services
Washington, D.C.

"One of my most memorable rescues involved a car that had rolled over in a creek. We were the first ones on the job. The water was about 40 degrees and it was rising inside the car. We had to turn the car over to get to the lady who was trapped inside. Luckily, I was small enough to climb inside the car and help her out."

Trauma

IN THIS DIVISION

18 Trauma Systems and Mechanism of Injury

OBJECTIVES

Upon completion of this chapter, the paramedic student will be able to:

1. Describe the incidence and scope of traumatic injuries and deaths.
2. Identify the role of each component of the trauma system.
3. Predict injury patterns based on a knowledge of the laws of physics related to forces involved in trauma.
4. Describe injury patterns that should be suspected when injury occurs related to a specific type of blunt trauma.
5. Describe the role of restraints in injury prevention and injury patterns.
6. Discuss how organ motion can contribute to injury in each body region depending on the forces applied.
7. Identify selected injury patterns associated with motorcycle and all-terrain vehicle (ATV) collisions.
8. Describe injury patterns associated with pedestrian collisions.
9. Identify injury patterns associated with sports injuries, blast injuries, and vertical falls.
10. Describe factors that influence tissue damage related to penetrating injury.

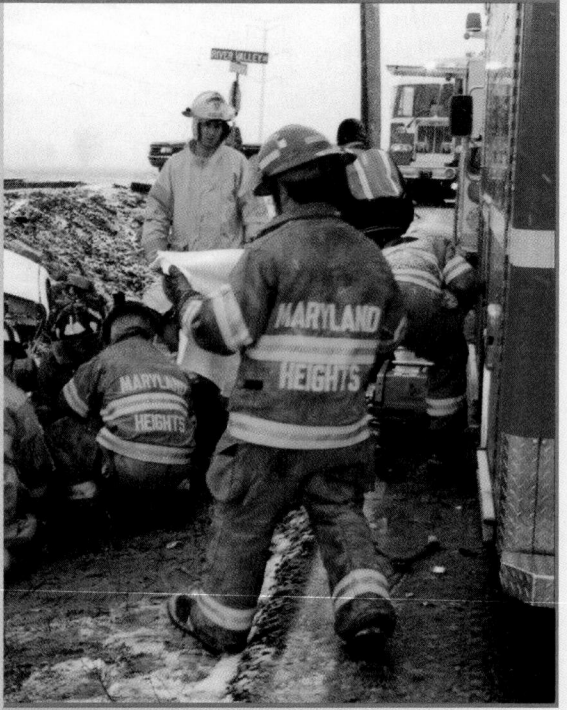

Trauma is a major cause of morbidity and mortality. The paramedic must have an appreciation of trauma systems and be able to recognize mechanisms of injury to enhance patient assessment and emergency care.

blunt trauma: An injury produced by the wounding forces of compression and change of speed, both of which can disrupt tissue.

cavitation: A temporary or permanent opening produced by a force that pushes body tissues laterally away from the tract of a projectile.

kinematics: The process of predicting injury patterns that can result from the forces and motions of energy.

penetrating trauma: An injury produced by crushing and stretching forces of a penetrating object that results in some form of tissue disruption.

Epidemiology of Trauma

Unintentional injury is a devastating medical and social problem. It is the leading cause of death among persons 1 to 36 years of age and the fifth leading cause of death among all Americans.[1] Trauma deaths in 1998 were exceeded only by HIV infection for persons 34 to 37 years of age and by cardiovascular disease and cancer among all other age groups. In 1998, there were about 92,000 accidental deaths in the United States. The National Safety Council estimates that the total number of unintentional injuries in the United States approaches 61 million annually. Of these, 9 million are disabling, 350,000 result in permanent impairment, and 8.4 million result in permanent disabilities. The economic effect of unintentional injuries in the United States exceeds $480 billion each year.

> **NOTE**
>
> In any given 10-minute period in the United States, two persons are killed and about 370 suffer a disabling injury. Costs amount to more than 9 million dollars.

Trends in Trauma Deaths

Deaths from unintentional injury are increasing yearly. Since most deaths by trauma are preventable, this increase emphasizes the need for increased safety and health efforts to reverse the trend. Motor vehicle crashes, falls, poisoning by solids and liquids, fire and burns, and drowning have been the top five causes of trauma deaths since 1970[1] (Fig. 18-1).

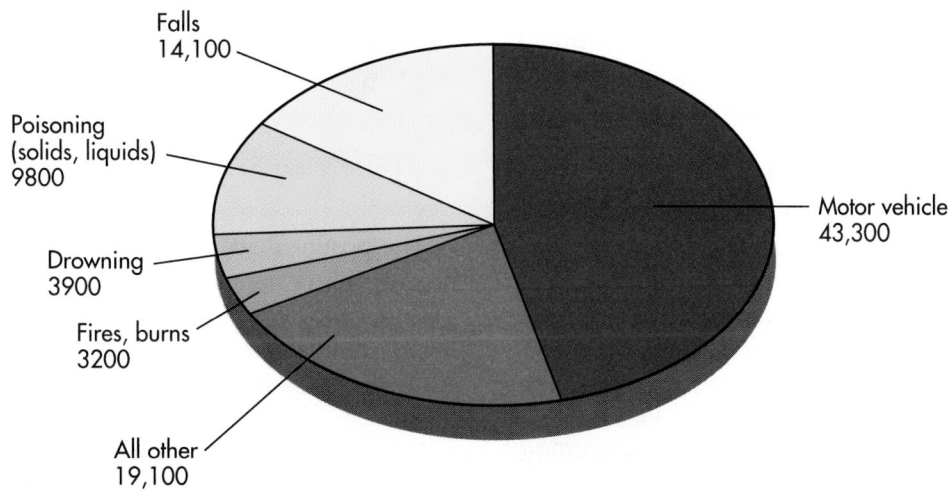

Falls
14,100

Poisoning
(solids, liquids)
9800

Drowning
3900

Fires, burns
3200

All other
19,100

Motor vehicle
43,300

Fig. 18-1 Deaths from unintentional injury by event, United States, 1996. (From *National Safety Council Accident Facts,* 1997 edition, p. v, National Safety Council.)

PREVENTION OF TRAUMA DEATHS

Deaths from trauma occur in three periods: immediate, early, and late. Each period presents its own unique problems.[4]

Immediate

Immediate death occurs within seconds or minutes of the injury. Lacerations of the brain, brain stem, upper spinal cord, heart, aorta, or other large vessels usually cause these deaths. Few if any patients in this category can be saved. Effective injury prevention programs are the only way to reduce the number of these deaths.

Early

The second peak of death occurs within the first 2 to 3 hours after injury. The causes of these deaths usually are major head injury, hemopneumothorax, ruptured spleen, lacerated liver, pelvic fracture, or multiple injuries associated with significant blood loss. Most of these injuries are treatable with available techniques, but the time lapse between injury and definitive care is critical.

Late

The third peak of death occurs days or weeks after the injury. These deaths most often result from sepsis, infection, or multiple organ failure. Prehospital emergency care focused on early recognition and management of life-threatening injury can play an important role in preventing these late deaths from trauma.

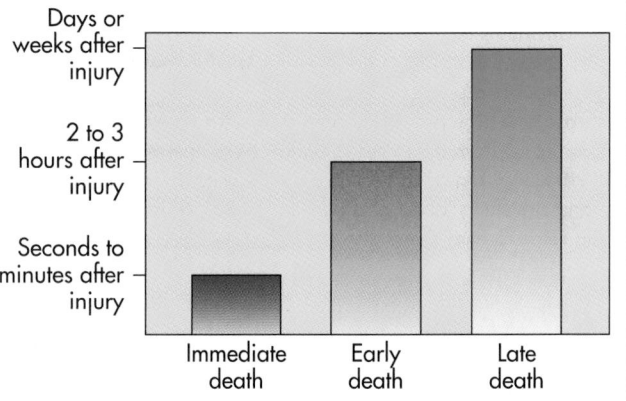

NOTE

Fatalities caused by motor vehicle crashes are decreasing, but the number of deaths from firearms and other causes is increasing. The death rate resulting from firearms is 289 per 100,000 population among those 15 to 24 years of age.[2]

? CRITICAL THINKING

What other measures will you take, while on duty as a paramedic, to decrease the risk of traumatic injury to you or your co-workers?

Phases of Trauma Care

Trauma care is divided into three phases: preincident, incident, and postincident.[3] The preincident phase refers to prevention of intentional and unintentional trauma deaths. Paramedics and other health care professionals play an important role in this phase through public education (for example, use of personal restraint systems and motorcycle helmets and appropriate use of 911) and by promoting legislation that supports injury prevention programs. (See the injury prevention information in Appendix C.)

The incident phase is the trauma event. Since the paramedic can prevent many of these events through education and by practicing personal safety, his or her role in this phase is to "practice what you preach" and to teach by example. The paramedic can accomplish this by driving safely and using personal restraint systems while on and off duty.

NOTE

During the incident phase, the application of active (for example, seat belts) and passive (for example, air bags) systems can significantly alter the outcome of a trauma event.

The postincident phase is when the paramedic employs his or her expertise and skills (the delivery of emergency care to injured patients). Important responsibilities for the paramedic in this phase include the following:

- Performing lifesaving maneuvers
- Properly preparing the patient for transportation to an appropriate medical facility
- Promptly transporting the patient to the appropriate medical facility (Box 18-1)

THE GOLDEN HOUR

The first hour after severe injury is known as the *golden hour*. It is a critical period in which surgical intervention for the trauma patient can enhance survival and reduce complications. The paramedic must recognize patients in this category and ensure that prehospital care activities do not unnecessarily delay patient transportation. The paramedic can best serve these patients through rapid assessment, stabilization of life-threatening injuries, and rapid transportation to an appropriate medical facility for definitive care.

NOTE

The factor most critical to any severely injured patient's survival is the length of time that elapses between the incident and definitive care[3] (see the box on p. 528).

Trauma Systems

The eight components of a sophisticated trauma system are as follows[5]:

1. Injury prevention
2. Prehospital care, including management, transportation, and trauma triage guidelines
3. Emergency department care
4. Interfacility transportation if needed
5. Definitive care
6. Trauma critical care
7. Rehabilitation
8. Data collection and trauma registry

? CRITICAL THINKING

How can you learn more about the components of the trauma system during your career as a paramedic?

The paramedic plays an important role in the trauma system by being involved in injury prevention programs, by entering appropriate patients into the trauma care system, and by participating in data collection and research that can influence health care improvements in caring for injured patients (Box 18-2).

TRAUMA REGISTRIES

Trauma registries allow for the collection of injury data by individual hospitals or groups of hospitals on a local, regional, or state level. The American College of Surgeons (ACS) funded these registries (for example, the *National Trauma Data Bank*) and software programs (for example, *NATIONAL TRACS*) to provide for online data management and a national reciprocity of injury data for a variety of commercial registry programs. Trauma registries generate periodic standard reports that provide statistical data to allow facilities to compare trends and other important information regarding trauma care.

Trauma Centers

As described in Chapter 1, the U.S. Department of Health and Human Services (USDHHS) released the *Position Paper on Trauma Center Designation* in 1980. Since then, states have developed comprehensive trauma systems. More than 800 hospitals now have a designated specialty in trauma.[6]

Trauma Center Classification

The American Medical Association (AMA) recommended categorization of hospital emergency services in the early 1970s.[7] In 1990 the Task Force of the American College of Surgeons (ACS) Committee on Trauma published *Resources for Optimal Care of the Injured Patient*. It described three levels (since revised to include four levels) of trauma centers based on resources (essential and desired), admissions, staff, research, and education involvement.

A level I trauma center can provide total care for every aspect of injury and is qualified to care for the most severely injured patient, especially in the surgical critical care setting; it is followed by level II, III, and IV facilities. Categorization of hospital resources identifies hospitals capable of handling trauma patients and enables EMS providers to rapidly transport patients to the most appropriate medical facilities. Based on ACS guidelines, some government agencies have designated certain institutions as trauma centers. Other specialized care facilities, such as pediatric trauma centers, burn centers, hyperbaric centers, and poison treatment centers, provide care for critically ill or injured patients with special needs.

in Chapter 48.) Air transportation should be considered in the following situations:

- The time needed to transport a patient by ground to an appropriate facility poses a threat to the patient's survival and recovery.
- Weather, road, or traffic conditions would seriously delay the patient's access to definitive care.
- Critical care personnel and equipment are needed to adequately care for the patient during transportation.

NOTE

The ACS Committee on Trauma also established guidelines for field triage, interhospital triage to specialized care facilities, and mass casualty triage. These criteria are based on the patient's condition, mechanism of injury, injury severity indices, and available patient care resources.

? CRITICAL THINKING

Where can you find the trauma triage criteria for your area?

Transportation Considerations

Determination of the appropriate level of care and hospital destination is based on the patient's needs and condition and the advice of medical direction. Once the paramedic determines the level of care needed and the destination facility, he or she can make decisions regarding the mode of transportation (ground or air ambulance).

Ground Transportation

As a rule, the paramedic should use ground transportation by ambulance if the appropriate facility can be reached within a "reasonable time." Reasonable time is defined by national standards (for example, definitive care within 60 minutes after the injury for severe trauma) and local protocol. Factors that affect the decision to use ground or air transportation include geographical location, topographical area, population, weather, availability of resources, traffic conditions, and time of day.

Aeromedical Transportation

The availability and use of aeromedical services varies throughout the United States. Aeromedical services can provide rapid response time, high-quality medical care, and rapid transportation to appropriate care facilities. Helicopters also can provide aerial surveillance and transportation of additional personnel and equipment to the emergency scene. Paramedic crews should consult with medical direction and follow local protocol regarding use of aeromedical services. (Use of aeromedical services is further addressed

SECTION ONE

KINEMATICS

Energy

A transfer of energy from an external source to the human body causes injuries. The extent of injury is determined by the type and amount of energy applied, how quickly it is applied, and to what part of the body it is applied.

Physical Laws

Knowledge of four basic laws of physics is required to understand the wounding forces of trauma:

1. *Newton's first law of motion.* An object, whether at rest or in motion, remains in that state unless acted upon by an outside force.
2. *Conservation of energy law.* Energy cannot be created nor destroyed; it can only change form. Energy can take mechanical, thermal, electrical, chemical, and nuclear forms.
3. *Newton's second law of motion:* Force (F) equals mass (M) multiplied by acceleration (a) or deceleration (d).

$$F = M \times a \ or \ F = M \times d$$

4. *Kinetic energy:* Kinetic energy (KE) equals half the mass (M) multiplied by the velocity squared (V^2).

$$KE = \frac{1}{2}m \times V^2$$

As the kinetic energy formula indicates, velocity is much more important than mass in determining total kinetic energy. For example, an automobile and its unrestrained 150-pound driver are traveling 60 miles per hour. According to Newton's first law of motion, the automobile remains in motion until acted upon by an outside force. If the driver gradually applies the brakes, the friction of the brakes slowly converts the mechanical energy of the automobile to thermal energy (conservation of energy law); the energy transfer occurs gradually through the slow deceleration. If the automobile strikes a tree, however, and is instantaneously stopped, the tree absorbs the mechanical energy, the automobile, and the driver. When the front of the car has stopped, the rear of the car continues forward until all of the energy of its motion is absorbed. The driver is traveling in the same direction and at the same speed as the automobile before impact, so like the rear of the car, the driver continues forward. The driver suffers injuries in anatomical areas that strike the vehicle.

In this sequence the motion of the front of the car is stopped by the tree, the steering column continues forward and stops against the dashboard, the driver's sternum stops against the steering column, and the driver's chest cavity and its contents hit the sternum and are crushed from behind by the posterior thorax, deforming the entire chest. The kinetic energy in this example is calculated as follows:

KE = - of the mass times the velocity squared, or

$$KE = \frac{1}{2}m \times V^2$$

$$KE = \frac{150}{2} \times 60^2$$

$$KE = 270,000 \text{ units of energy}$$

As shown in this calculation, the 150-pound driver traveling 60 miles per hour must change 270,000 units of kinetic energy (known as *foot pounds*, calculated as pounds multiplied by miles per hour) into another form of energy when he or she stops. In addition, since force equals mass multiplied by acceleration (Newton's second law of motion), the 150-pound driver is moving forward in the vehicle with about 9000 foot-pounds of force when stopped by the steering column. The energy of the body's motion causes tissue destruction as this energy is absorbed into the body cells when the body stops. This example illustrates the principle, but the actual total force also is determined by the true rate of deceleration, or "g" force, and several other factors.

? CRITICAL THINKING

Can you apply these same four laws of physics to another traumatic situation, such as a fall onto concrete? What force is applied? What factors influence the kinetic energy?

NOTE

Lap and shoulder restraints and air bags increase the distance over which the body stops its movement. This can decrease the deceleration force considerably.

Kinematics

Kinematics is the process of predicting injury patterns. Specific types and patterns of injuries are associated with certain mechanisms. In addition to individual factors, such as age, and protective factors, such as restraint systems, helmets, and air bags, the paramedic should consider the following when evaluating the trauma patient:

- Mechanism of injury
- Force of energy applied
- Anatomy
- Energy (for example, mass; velocity; distance; thermal, electrical, chemical forms)

SECTION TWO
BLUNT TRAUMA

Blunt Trauma

Blunt trauma is an injury produced by the wounding forces of compression and change of speed (usually deceleration), which can disrupt tissue. Direct compression, or pressure on a structure, is the most common type of force applied in blunt trauma. The amount of injury depends on the length of time of compression, the force of compression, and the area compressed. For example, compression of the thorax can lead to rib fracture or pneumothorax. Other compression injuries include contusions and lacerations of solid organs and rupture of hollow (air-filled) organs.

Acceleration is an increase and deceleration is a decrease in the velocity of a moving object; both can produce significant injury. For example, when a vehicle stops abruptly, the occupant's body continues its constant velocity after the impact until it decelerates as a result of striking the steering wheel, restraint system, or dashboard. The external aspect of the body is forcibly stopped, but the contents of the cranial, thoracic, and peritoneal cavities remain in motion because of inertia. Tissues can be stretched, crushed, ruptured, lacerated, or sheared from their points of attachment as a result. Examples of change-of-speed injuries include concussion, cardiac or pulmonary contusion, organ laceration, and aortic tear.

Motor Vehicle Collision

The various injuries produced by blunt trauma are best illustrated through examination of motor vehicle collisions, although forces that cause blunt trauma can result from a variety of impacts. As described in the previous example, a motor vehicle collision involves three separate impacts as the energy is transferred: (1) the vehicle strikes an object, (2) the occupant collides with the inside of the car, and (3) the internal organs collide inside the body. The injuries that result from automobile crashes depend on the type of collision, the position of the occupant inside the vehicle, and the use or nonuse of active or passive restraint systems.

Motor vehicle collision is classified by type of impact, including head-on, lateral, rear-end, rotational, and roll-over. The forces of compression and change of speed produce predictable injury patterns in each type of collision.

Head-On (Frontal) Impact

Head-on collisions result when forward motion stops abruptly (for example, when one automobile collides with another traveling in the opposite direction). The first collision occurs when the automobile hits the second vehicle, resulting in damage to the front of the car. As the vehicle abruptly stops, the occupant continues to move at the speed of the automobile before impact. The front seat occupant continues forward into the restraint system, steering column, or dashboard, resulting in the second collision. The occupant who is not restrained usually travels in one of two pathways in relationship to the dashboard: down-and-under or up-and-over. The precise course of this pathway determines how the organs collide inside the body and the extent of tissue damaged.

In the down-and-under pathway, the occupant travels downward into the vehicle seat and forward into the dashboard or steering column (Fig. 18-2). The knees become the leading part of the body, striking the dashboard, with the upper legs absorbing most of the impact. Predictable injuries include knee dislocation, patellar fracture, femur fracture, fracture or posterior dislocation of the hip, fracture of the acetabulum, vascular injury, and hemorrhage. After the initial impact of the knees into the dashboard, the body rotates forward. As the chest wall hits the steering column or dashboard, the

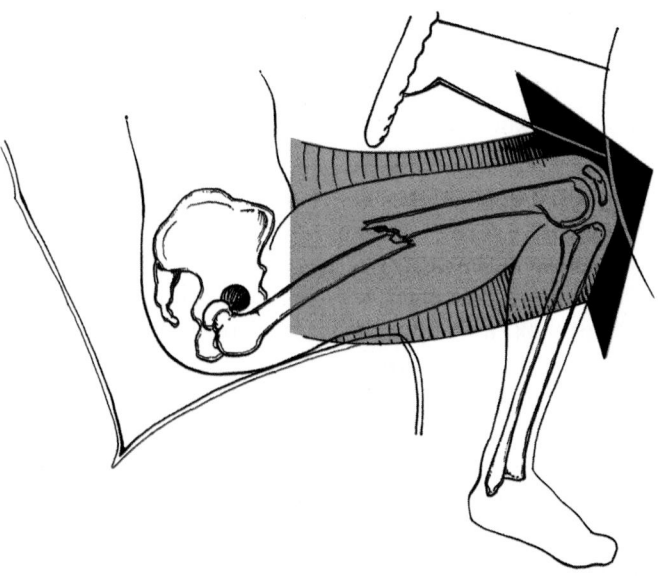

Fig. 18-2 Down-and-under pathway.

head and torso absorb energy as indicated in the description of the up-and-over pathway.

? CRITICAL THINKING

How does the use of lap and shoulder restraints influence the patterns of injury described here?

In the up-and-over pathway, as the body in forward motion strikes the steering wheel, the ribs and underlying structures absorb the momentum of the thorax (Fig. 18-3). Predictable injuries from this transfer of energy include rib fracture, ruptured diaphragm, hemopneumothorax, pulmonary contusion, cardiac contusion, myocardial rupture, and vascular disruption (most notably, aortic rupture).

If the abdomen is the point of impact, compression injuries can occur to the hollow abdominal organs, solid organs, and lumbar vertebrae. The kidneys, liver, and spleen are subject to vascular tears from supporting tissue, including the disruption of renal vessels from their points of attachment to the inferior vena cava and descending aorta. Predictable injuries include liver laceration, spleen rupture, internal hemorrhage, and abdominal organ incursion into the thorax (ruptured diaphragm).

If the occupant's head is the leading point of impact, the cervical vertebrae absorb the continued momentum of the body. Cervical flexion, axial loading, and/or hyperextension (further described in

Chapter 23) can result in fracture or dislocation of the cervical vertebrae. In addition, severe angulation of the cervical vertebrae can damage the soft tissues of the neck and cause spinal cord injury and spinal instability, even without fracture. Other predictable injuries include trauma to the brain (for example, concussion, contusion, shearing injury, edema) and intracranial vascular disruption, resulting in subdural or epidural hematoma.

Lateral Impact

Lateral impact occurs when a vehicle is struck from the side. Injury patterns depend on whether the damaged automobile remains in place or moves away from the point of impact. The external shell of an automobile that remains in place after impact usually intrudes into the passenger compartment, directing force at the lateral aspect of the occupant's body. Predictable injuries result from compression to the torso, pelvis, and extremities. Examples of these injuries include fractured ribs, pulmonary contusion, ruptured liver or spleen (depending on the side involved), fractured clavicle, fractured pelvis, and head and neck injury.

> **NOTE**
>
> Some automobiles are equipped with side-impact air bags that can guard against injury in some lateral impacts.

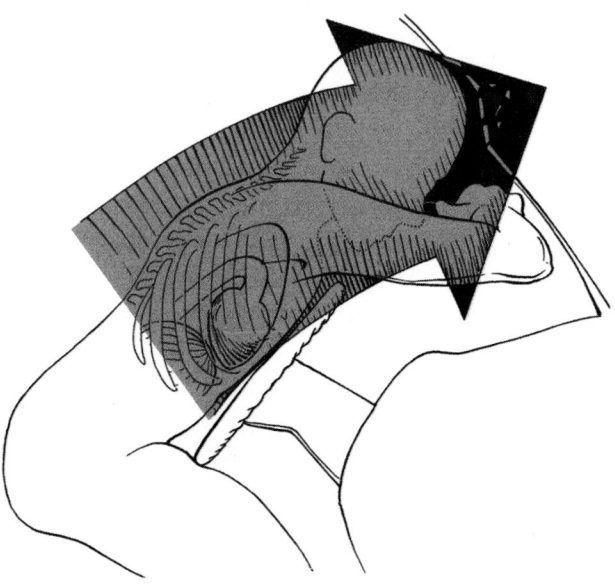

Fig. 18-3 Up-and-over pathway.

If the damaged vehicle moves away from the point of impact, the occupant accelerates away from the point of impact, moving laterally with the car. The effects of inertia on the head, neck, and thorax produce lateral flexion and rotation of the cervical spine. This movement can result in neurological injury and tears or strains of the lateral ligaments and supporting structures of the neck. Injuries also can occur on the side of the passenger opposite the impact as the occupant is propelled toward the other side of the car. If other occupants are in the automobile, secondary collision with other passengers is likely.

Rear-End Impact

A vehicle struck from behind rapidly accelerates, causing the vehicle to move forward under the occupant. The greater the difference in the forward speed of the two vehicles, the greater the force and damaging energy of the initial impact. For example, if a vehicle traveling 50 mph strikes a stationary vehicle, the damaging energy is greater than when a vehicle traveling 50 mph strikes a vehicle traveling 30 mph. Thus in forward collisions, the sum of both vehicles' speeds is the velocity that produces damage. In rear-end collisions, the difference between the two speeds is the damaging velocity.

Predictable injuries in rear-end collisions include back and neck injuries and cervical strain or fracture caused by hyperextension. The cervical portion of the spine is particularly susceptible to secondary hyperextension, which is caused by the rapid forward acceleration of the vehicle and subsequent relative rearward forces on the occupant. If the automobile undergoes a second collision by striking an object in front of it, the paramedic should suspect injuries associated with frontal impact.

Rotational Impact

Rotational impacts occur when an off-center portion of the automobile (usually the front quarter) strikes an immovable object or one that is moving more slowly or in the opposite direction. The part of the vehicle striking the object stops during impact. The remainder of the vehicle continues in forward motion until the energy is completely transformed. The occupant moves inside the vehicle with the forward motion and usually is struck by the side of the car as the vehicle rotates around the point of impact. A rotational impact results in injuries common to both head-on and lateral collisions.

Roll-Over Accidents

In roll-over crashes or collisions the occupant tumbles inside the automobile and is injured wherever the body strikes the vehicle. The various impacts occur at many different angles, which can cause multiple-system injuries. Predictable injuries sustained in roll-over collisions are difficult to categorize. These crashes can produce any of the injury patterns associated with other types of collisions.

Restraints

Public awareness programs in personal safety and various state laws regarding seat belt protection have increased automobile occupant use of personal restraints in recent years. According to the National Safety Council, among passenger vehicle occupants over 4 years of age, seat belts saved an estimated 10,750 lives in 1997; an additional 9600 could have been saved if *all* passengers over 4 years of age had worn seat belts.[1]

> **NOTE**
>
> As of December 1999, 49 states and the District of Columbia have laws in effect requiring the use of seat belts; the only exception is New Hampshire.

A significant hazard to unrestrained occupants is ejection from the vehicle after impact. Among crashes in which a fatality occurred in 1995, only 2% of restrained passenger-car occupants were ejected, compared with 25% of those who were unrestrained.[1,7] In addition, 1 of every 13 ejection victims suffers a spinal fracture, and ejected victims are killed 6 times more often than those who are not ejected.[3] The high mortality rate among ejected victims results in part from the occupant being subjected to a second impact as the body strikes the ground or another object outside the vehicle.

> **? CRITICAL THINKING**
>
> *How can you apply this knowledge about ejection statistics to your practice in each of the phases of trauma care (preincident, incident, and postincident)?*

The four restraining systems available in the United States are lap belts, diagonal shoulder straps, air bags, and child safety seats, all of which significantly reduce injuries. If they are inappropriately worn, however, these protective devices also can produce injuries.

Lap Belts

The lap belt, used alone or in combination with a diagonal shoulder strap, is the most commonly used active restraint system. When properly applied, the occupant should direct the lap belt at a 45-degree angle to the floor between the anterior-superior iliac spine and the femur. A lap belt worn tightly enough to remain in this position absorbs energy forces and protects the abdominal cavity by transferring energy to the strong, bony pelvis.

If the lap belt is incorrectly worn above the anterior-iliac spine, the forward motion of the body during impact is absorbed by vertebrae T12, L1, and L2. As the thorax is propelled forward, the abdominal organs are compressed between the vertebral column and the lap belt, which can cause injury to the liver, spleen, duodenum, and pancreas. An indicator of these abdominal injuries is the presence of abrasions or a lap belt imprint over the abdomen.

Significant injury can result even when the occupant uses a lap belt correctly. These injuries occur from angulation of the lumbar spine, pelvis, thorax, and head around the restraint system and from failure of the restraint system to sufficiently decrease the impact forces. Injuries that can occur during high-speed impacts include sternal fractures, chest wall injuries, lumbar vertebral fractures, head injuries, and maxillofacial trauma.

Diagonal Shoulder Straps

Use of a diagonal shoulder strap helps absorb the forward motion of the thorax after impact. When the occupant wears the shoulder strap with the lap belt, the shoulder strap prevents the thorax, face, and head from striking the dashboard, windshield, or steering column. Clavicular fracture can result from the position of the shoulder strap. Organ collision inside the body with resultant internal organ injury, cervical fracture, and spinal cord injury can still occur during high-speed impacts, even when personal restraint systems are used.

Air Bags

Although some automobiles are equipped with side-impact air bags to protect against lateral impacts, the more common air bag is a frontal air bag that inflates from the center of the steering wheel and dashboard during frontal impact. These devices cushion the forward motion of the occupant when used with a lap and shoulder belt. Frontal air bags deflate rapidly and are effective only with an initial frontal collision. They are ineffective in lateral or roll-over impacts. These systems do not prevent movement in the down-and-under pathway. Thus the occupant's

AIR BAG CONSIDERATIONS

Most air bag injuries are minor cuts, bruises, or abrasions and are far less serious than the skull fractures and brain injuries that air bags prevent. However, 87 people have been killed by air bags as of November 1, 1997. These deaths are tragic but rare events. The one fact that is common to all who died is that they were too close to the air bag when it started to deploy. For some, this occurred because they were sitting too close to the air bag. More often this occurred because they were not restrained by seat belts or child safety seats and were thrown forward during pre-crash braking.

The vast majority of people can avoid being too close and can minimize the risk of serious air bag injury by making simple changes in behavior. Shorter drivers can adjust their seating position. Front seat adult passengers can sit a safe distance from their air bag. Infants and children 12 and under should sit in the back seat. And everyone can buckle up. The limited number of people who may not be able to make these changes may benefit from having the opportunity to turn off their air bags when necessary. Consumers can choose to have an on-off switch installed for the air bags in their vehicle if they are, or a user of their vehicle is, in a risk group listed below:

- People who *must* transport infants riding in rear-facing infant seats in the front passenger seat.
- People who *must* transport children ages 1 to 12 in the front passenger seat.
- Drivers who *cannot* change their customary driving position and keep 10 inches between the center of the steering wheel and the center of their breastbone.
- People whose doctors say that, due to their medical condition, the air bag poses a special risk that *outweighs* the risk of hitting their head, neck, or chest in a crash if the air bag is turned off.

knees may still be the point of impact, resulting in leg, pelvis, and abdominal injuries.

An air bag can produce significant injury if it is deployed in close proximity (10 inches or closer) to the occupant. Deployment in these situations can produce spinal fractures, hand and eye injury, and facial and forearm abrasions. The following groups are at higher risk of injury from air bag deployment[8]:

- Infants and children less than 12 years of age
- Adults of short stature (less than 5' 2")
- Older adults
- Persons with special medical conditions

> **NOTE**
>
> Children less than 12 years of age should ride in the rear seat. Infants in rear-facing safety seats should not ride in the front seat of a vehicle with a passenger side air bag.

> **NOTE**
>
> Although the benefits of air bags far outweigh the risks, 74 children and 58 adults (though April 1, 1999) were killed by air bags that deployed in otherwise survivable crashes.[1] This must be compared with the estimated 3000 lives saved by air bags in otherwise lethal crashes.

Child Safety Seats

The leading cause of death in children under 4 years of age is injuries sustained in motor vehicle crashes. For each of these deaths, the U.S. Department of Health, Education, and Welfare estimates that thousands more suffer debilitating injury. The National Safety Council reports that an estimated 2894 lives have been saved by child restraints from 1975 through 1997, with 312 in 1997 alone.

All 50 states and the District of Columbia now require child safety seats for select age groups of children. The seats are available in several shapes and sizes to accommodate the different stages of physical development, including infant carriers, booster seats, and toddler seats. Child safety seats use a combination of lap belts, shoulder belts, full-body harnesses, and harness-and-shield apparatus to protect the child during vehicle collision. Predictable injuries likely to occur even with the appropriate use of child safety seats include blunt abdominal

trauma, change-of-speed injuries from deceleration forces, and neck and spinal injury.

> **NOTE**
>
> A significant amount of misuse of child safety seats (for example, location, installation, and strapping) occurs. Public education in their correct use is an important prevention measure.

Organ Collision Injuries

Organ motions and their injuries are a result of deceleration and compression forces. Recognition of these injuries requires a high degree of suspicion using the principles of kinematics.

Deceleration Injuries

When body organs are put into motion after an impact, they continue to move in opposition to the structures that attach them to the body. Therefore there is a risk of separation of body organs from their attachments. Injury to the vascular pedicle or mesenteric attachment can lead to brisk or exsanguinating hemorrhage.

Head Injuries

When the head strikes a stationary object, the cranium comes to an abrupt stop, but brain tissue inside the cranium continues to move until it is compressed against the skull (Fig. 18-4). This movement can cause brain tissue to be bruised, crushed, or lacerated and blood vessels attached to the brain and skull to be torn, producing intracranial hemorrhage. Other

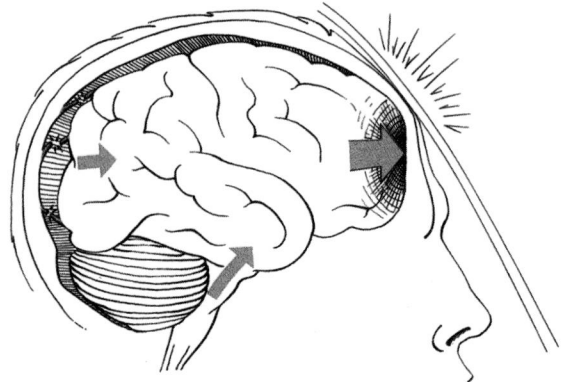

Fig. 18-4 After cessation of forward motion of the skull, the brain continues its motion, resulting in possible contusion and intracerebral hemorrhage.

injuries associated with deceleration of the head include CNS injury, caused by stretching of the spinal cord and its attachments, and cervical fracture.

Thoracic Injuries

The aorta frequently is injured by severe, lethal deceleration forces. It is affixed at several points, most proximally by the aortic valve in the descending portion, just below the arch by the ligamentum arteriosum, and along the descending aorta by its attachment to the thoracic spine. As the thorax strikes a stationary object, the heart and aorta continue in motion in opposition to their attachment at the lower end of the aortic arch. The aorta usually is sheared at the level of its ligamentum arteriosum attachment (Fig. 18-5). Frank rupture of the aorta leads to rapid exsanguination, but transection and dissection through the internal lining (intima and media) can tamponade, allowing patients to arrive at an emergency department and survive the injury.

Abdominal Injuries

When deceleration forces are applied to the abdomen, intraabdominal organs and retroperitoneal structures (most commonly the kidneys) are affected. The forward motion of the kidneys can shear them away from their vascular pedicle (Fig. 18-6), and the forward motion of the small and large intestines can result in mesenteric tears. The downward and forward motion of the liver can cause separation at its midpoint from its vascular and hepatic duct pedicle, and the forward motion of the spleen, which is restrained by the diaphragm and abdominal wall attachments, can result in tear of the splenic capsule.

Compression Injuries

Compressive forces can injure any portion of the body. This discussion is limited to injuries of the head, thorax, and abdomen.

Head Injuries

Compression injuries to the head can result in open fractures, closed fractures, and bone fragment penetration (depressed skull fracture). Associated injuries include brain contusion and lacerations of brain tissue. Compression forces to the skull also can produce hemorrhage from fractured bone, meningeal vessels, or the brain itself. If facial structures are involved in the injury, soft tissue trauma and facial bone fractures can occur (see Chapter 22). The paramedic should also consider CNS injury and assume cervical fracture when evaluating injuries to the head. Compression injury to the vertebral bodies can result in compression fracture, hyperextension, and hyperflexion injury.

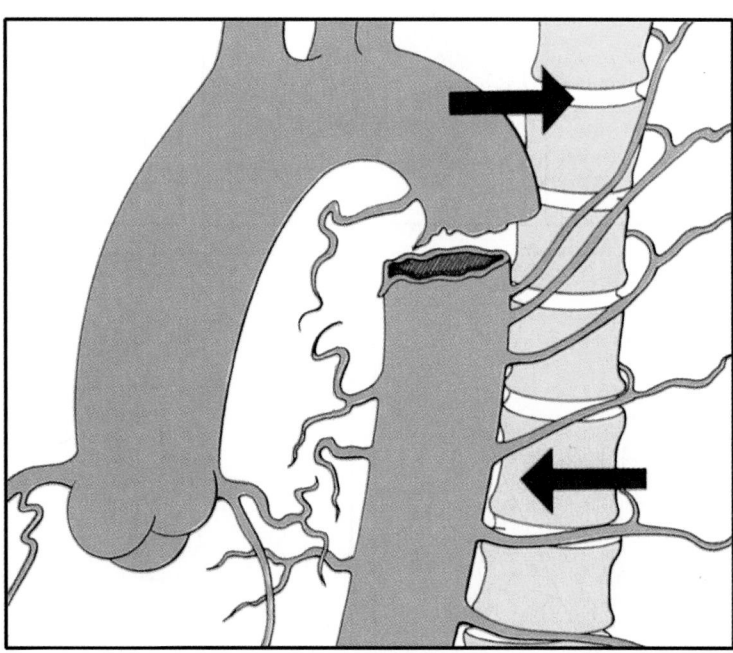

Fig. 18-5 Shearing forces along the descending aorta move in opposition to the attachments at the lower end of the aortic arch. (From Moylan J: *Principles of trauma surgery*, ed 2, New York, 1992, Gower Medical Publishing.)

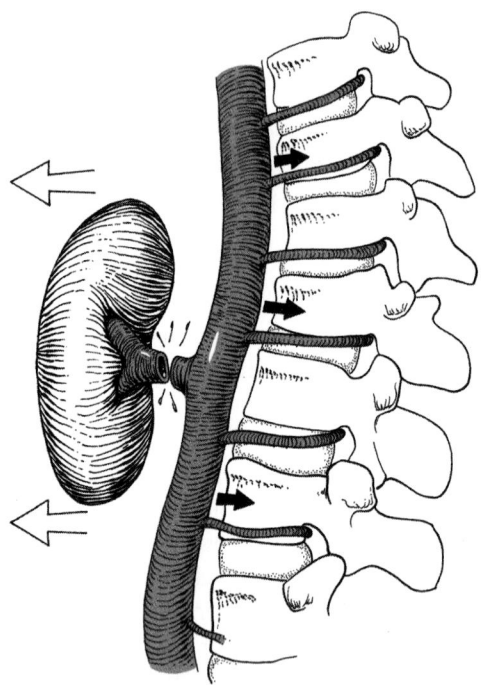

Fig. 18-6 Forward motion of the kidney can cause separation at its midpoint from its vascular pedicle.

Thoracic Injuries

Compression injury to the thorax frequently involves the lungs and heart. Associated injuries to external structures include fractured ribs and sternum, which can lead to an unstable chest wall, open pneumothorax, or both.

A serious lung injury that can occur from compression forces results from a "paper-bag effect." This injury occurs when increased intrathoracic pressure causes rupture of the lungs. For example, when an automobile driver is threatened by an approaching vehicle, he or she notes the potential collision and instinctively takes a deep breath and holds it. This protective inhalation fills the lungs (paper bag) with air against the closed glottis and creates a closed container (Fig. 18-7). As the thorax strikes the steering column, the inward motion of the chest wall causes an increase in lung pressure, resulting in alveolar rupture (as when a hand strikes the paper bag). This phenomenon is thought to be responsible for most pneumothoraces after automobile trauma.[9] Penetration of a fractured rib through the pleura and laceration of the lung also

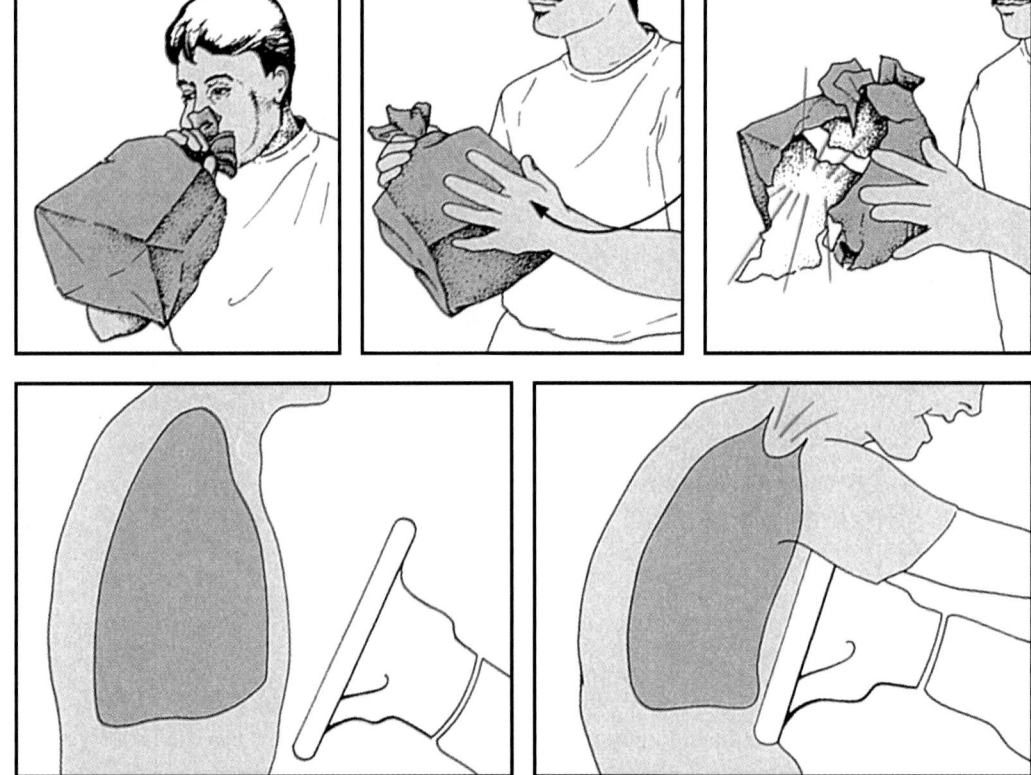

Fig. 18-7 In a crash or collision, the lungs are similar to an air-filled paper bag held tightly at the neck and compressed with the other hand. Thoracic compression against the closed glottis causes the lungs to pop. (From Moylan J: *Principles of trauma surgery*, ed 2, New York, 1992, Gower Medical Publishing.)

contribute to pneumothorax after blunt trauma to the chest.

During compression injury to the thorax, the heart can become trapped between the sternum and the thoracic spine. Depending on the force of energy applied, increased intraabdominal compression and retrograde hydrostatic pressure on the aorta can rupture the aortic valve. Compression of the patient's heart between the sternum and the vertebral column can cause cardiac dysrhythmias, myocardial contusion, or atrial or ventricular rupture.

Abdominal Injuries

Compression injuries to the abdominal cavity can have serious effects, such as solid organ rupture, vascular organ hemorrhage, and hollow organ perforation into the peritoneal cavity. Common injuries include rupture of the bladder, especially if it is full, and lacerations to the spleen, liver, and kidneys.

Just as the paper-bag effect produces a pneumothorax in thoracic injury, compression of the abdominal cavity can cause increases in intraabdominal pressure that exceed the tensile strength (resistance to length-wise stretch) of the walls of hollow organs or the diaphragm. Predictable injuries include rupture or herniation of the diaphragm and rupture of hollow organs such as the gallbladder, urinary bladder, duodenum, colon, stomach, and small bowel.

Other Motorized Vehicular Collisions

Injuries from other motorized vehicular collisions include those involving motorcycles, all-terrain vehicles (ATVs), snowmobiles, motor boats, water bikes, jet skis, and farm machinery. This text discusses only motorcycles and ATVs because of their common recreational use and popularity.

> **NOTE**
>
> According to the National Highway Traffic Safety Administration (NHTSA), about 55,000 motorcycle riders and passengers are injured each year, and more than 2000 die from their injuries.

Small motorized vehicles are considered to be more dangerous than other motor vehicles because they offer minimal protection to the rider from the transfer of energy associated with collisions. The injuries sustained in small motor vehicle crashes usually are more severe than those received from automobile crashes. As with other types of motor vehicle collision, predictable injuries depend on the type of collision that occurs.

Motorcycle Collision

Common motorcycle collisions result from head-on impact and angular impact and from laying the motorcycle down.

Head-On Impact

A motorcycle's center of gravity is above the front axle, forward of the rider's seat. When the motorcycle strikes an object that stops its forward motion, the rest of the bike and the rider continue forward until acted on by an outside force. Typically, the motorcycle tips forward and the rider is propelled over the handlebars. Secondary impacts with the handlebars or other objects stop the forward motion of the rider. Predictable injuries caused by these secondary impacts include head and neck trauma and compression injuries to the chest and abdomen. If the feet remain on the foot rests during impact, the midshaft of the femur absorbs the rider's forward motion, which can result in bilateral fractures to the femur and lower leg. Severe perineal injuries can result if the rider's groin strikes the tank or handlebars of the motorcycle.

Angular Impact

When a motorcycle strikes an object at an angle, the rider often is caught between the cycle and the second object. Predictable injuries include crushing-type injuries to the patient's affected side, such as open fractures to the femur, tibia, and fibula and fracture and dislocation of the malleolus.

Laying the Motorcycle Down

Professional racers and recreational riders often use the strategy of laying the motorcycle down before striking an object. This protective maneuver separates the rider from the motorcycle and the object by allowing the rider to slide away from the bike. Predictable injuries include massive abrasions ("road rash") and fractures to the affected side as the rider slides on the ground or pavement. Although these injuries can be severe, they usually are less serious than those that occur from other types of impacts.

ATVs

Injuries from crashes involving ATVs are different from those seen in motorcycle collisions. ATVs have a higher center of gravity than motorcycles and a large, flat front tire that makes them difficult to steer. A specific balance different than that required for riding motorcycles or bicycles is necessary to keep the ATV from overturning.

The natural tendency of the rider to put a foot down to support the ATV when stopping can lead to the rear tire running over the rider's foot, catching the leg, and throwing the rider forward off the vehicle and onto his or her shoulder or crushing the rider. Predictable injuries from ATV collisions include extremity injury and fracture, clavicular fracture, and serious head and neck injuries.

Personal Protective Equipment

Protective equipment for riders of small motor vehicles includes boots, leather clothing, eye protection, and helmets. Helmets are structured to absorb the energy of an impact, thereby reducing injuries to the face, skull, and brain, and are estimated to be 29% effective in preventing fatal injuries.[1] Nonuse of helmets increases head injuries by more than 300%.[3]

Pedestrian Injuries

In 1998, 145,000 people were injured in auto-pedestrian collisions in the United States. Of those injuries, 5900 were fatal.[1] All auto-pedestrian collisions can produce serious injuries and require a high degree of suspicion for multiple-system trauma.

Three primary mechanisms of injury (multiple impacts) exist in auto-pedestrian collisions. The first impact occurs when the bumper of the vehicle strikes the body, the second occurs as the pedestrian strikes the hood of the vehicle, and the third occurs when the pedestrian strikes the ground or another object.

Predictable injuries depend on whether the pedestrian is an adult or a child. Variations in the height of the pedestrian in relation to the bumper and hood of the car affect the injury pattern. The velocity of the vehicle also is a major factor. However, even low speeds can result in serious trauma because of the mass of the vehicle and the transfer of energy. Another consideration in evaluating an auto-pedestrian

incident is the possibility of the patient suffering a second collision from another vehicle.

Adult Pedestrian

Most adult pedestrians threatened by an approaching vehicle attempt to protect themselves by turning away from the oncoming automobile. Therefore injuries often are a result of lateral or posterior impacts. During the initial impact, the adult usually is struck by the vehicle bumper in the lower legs, producing lower-extremity fractures.

The second impact occurs as the pedestrian falls toward the hood of the vehicle. This impact can result in fractures to the femur, pelvis, thorax, and spine and produce intraabdominal or intrathoracic injury. The head and spine also can be injured if the victim strikes the hood or windshield.

The third impact occurs as the victim strikes the ground or is thrown against another object. This can result in significant damage to the hip and shoulder of the affected side as the body makes contact with the landing surface. Sudden deceleration and compression forces associated with this impact can cause fractures, internal hemorrhage, and head and spinal injury.

Child Pedestrian

Unlike adults, who try to protect themselves from auto-pedestrian injury, children tend to face the oncoming vehicle. Therefore their injuries often are the result of a frontal impact. Because children are smaller than most adults, the initial impact of the automobile occurs higher on the body, usually above the knees or pelvis. Predictable injuries from the initial impact include fractures to the femur and pelvic girdle as well as internal hemorrhage.

The second impact occurs as the front of the vehicle's hood continues forward, making contact with the victim's thorax. The victim immediately is thrown backward, forcing the head and neck to flex forward. Depending on the position of the patient in relation to the automobile, the child's head and neck may contact the vehicle's hood. Predictable injuries include abdominopelvic and thoracic trauma, facial trauma, and head and neck injury.

The third impact occurs as the child is thrown downward to a landing surface. Because of the child's smaller size and weight, he or she can fall under the vehicle and be dragged for some distance or fall to the side of the vehicle and be run over by the front or rear wheels. Predictable injuries consist of those previously described and may include traumatic amputation.

Other Causes of Blunt Trauma

Other common causes of blunt trauma include sports injuries, blast injuries, and vertical falls.

Sports Injuries

Sports are practiced by participants of all ages. Common sports associated with frequent injuries include contact sports, such as football, basketball, hockey, and wrestling; high-velocity activity sports, such as downhill skiing, water skiing, bicycling, roller blading, and skateboarding; racquet sports; and water sports, such as swimming and diving. Although sporting activities provide a variety of health benefits, they also can produce severe injury. Sports-related injuries account for 15% of all spinal cord injuries in the United States each year.[2]

Sports-related injuries are caused by forces of acceleration and deceleration, compression, twisting, hyperextension, and hyperflexion. The paramedic can use the general principles of kinematics to predict injuries by ascertaining the following:

- What energy forces were transferred to the patient?
- To what part of the patient's body was the energy transferred?
- What associated injuries should be considered as a result of the energy transfer?
- How sudden was the acceleration or deceleration?
- Was compression, twisting, hyperextension, or hyperflexion involved in the injury?

? CRITICAL THINKING

Sports-related injuries often occur out-of-doors. What other considerations will you have for patient care based on the environment?

If the patient used protective equipment, the paramedic should evaluate it to help determine the mechanism of injury. For example, the condition

and structural stability of a helmet can provide clues as to the amount of energy transferred to the patient during the injury. Other examples include broken skis, broken hockey sticks, and structural deformities of bicycles.

Blast Injuries

Blast injury is damage to a patient exposed to a pressure field that is produced by an explosion of volatile substances. Explosions of this nature primarily have been a wartime concern. However, in recent years the number of blast injuries from homemade bombs used in social protests and terrorist activities has increased. Other causes include exploding automobile batteries, industrial use of volatile substances, chemical reactions in clandestine drug laboratories, explosions in mining, and transportation incidents or crashes involving hazardous materials.

? CRITICAL THINKING

In all incidents related to blast injury, what is your first consideration on the scene?

Blasts release large amounts of energy in the form of pressure and heat. If this release of energy is confined in a casing (for example, a bomb), the pressure ruptures the casing and ejects fragments of the housing at a high velocity. The remaining energy is transmitted to the surrounding environment and can severely injure bystanders. Blast injuries are classified as *primary, secondary, tertiary,* and *miscellaneous.*

Primary Blast Injuries

Primary blast injuries result from sudden changes in environmental pressure. These injuries usually occur in gas-containing organs and suffer the most severe damage when poorly supported tissue is displaced beyond its elastic limit. The organs and tissues most vulnerable to primary blast injury are the ears, lungs, CNS, and gastrointestinal tract. Predictable damage to these areas includes hearing loss, pulmonary hemorrhage, cerebral air embolism, abdominal hemorrhage, and bowel perforation. Thermal burns also can result from the release of energy in the form of heat. These injuries are likely to occur on unprotected areas that are close to the source of explosion (for example, the face and hands) (see Chapter 21). In closed spaces, because of blast reflection, victims farther from the explosion may be as severely injured as those close to the explosion.

Secondary Blast Injuries

Secondary blast injuries usually result when bystanders are struck by flying debris (for example, glass, metal, or falling mortar). In addition to the obvious injuries such as lacerations and fractures, flying debris can cause high-velocity missile-type injuries if nails, screws, or casing fragments are part of the debris.

Tertiary Blast Injuries

Tertiary blast injuries occur when victims are propelled through space by an explosion and strike a stationary object. These injuries are similar to those sustained in vertical falls and ejections from automobiles or small motor vehicles. In most cases, the sudden deceleration from the impact causes more damage than the acceleration through space because the deceleration is more sudden. Injuries from these forces include damage to the abdominal viscera, CNS, and musculoskeletal system.

Miscellaneous Blast Injuries

Miscellaneous blast injuries result from radiation exposure and inhalation of dust and toxic gases (further described in Chapter 51). Predictable injuries include those to the eyes, lungs, and soft tissues.

Vertical Falls

Falls accounted for 16,000 deaths in 1998 and were the second leading cause of accidental death in the United States.[1] In predicting injuries associated with falls, the paramedic should evaluate the distance fallen, body position of the patient on impact, and type of landing surface struck. Injuries associated with vertical falls are a result of deceleration and compression.

NOTE

More than half of all falls occur in homes; nearly four out of five involve a person 65 years of age or older.

Although falls from some levels are rarely associated with fatal injury, falls from distances greater than three times the height of an individual (15 to 20 feet) are more likely to be associated with severe injuries. As a point of reference for these distances,

the roof of a one-story house is about 15 feet from the ground, and the roof of a two-story house is about 30 feet from the ground.

? CRITICAL THINKING

What patients may be susceptible to serious injury from low-level falls?

Adults who have fallen more than 15 feet usually land on their feet. A predictable injury from this vertical fall is bilateral calcaneus fractures. As the energy dissipates from the initial impact, the head, torso, and pelvis push downward, and the body is forced into flexion. When this occurs, hip dislocations and compression fractures of the spinal column in the thoracic and lumbar areas are seen. About 10% of patients with calcaneal fracture have associated spinal fractures. If the patient leans forward or attempts to break the fall with outstretched hands, bilateral Colles' fractures to the wrists (clinically evident by the so-called "silver fork deformity") are likely.

If the distance fallen is less than 15 feet, most adults land in the position in which they fell. For example, an adult who falls head first strikes the landing surface with the head, arms, or both. Predictable injuries depend on the body part that strikes the landing surface and the route of transfer of energy through the body. The paramedic should suspect internal injuries if the trunk of the body is the initial impact area.

NOTE

Older adult patients sustain a high number of low-distance falls, often resulting in hip fracture.

Children tend to fall head first, regardless of distance fallen or body position during the fall, because their heads are proportionally larger and heavier. For this reason, children who experience a vertical fall usually are victims of head injury.

NOTE

The ability of the landing surface to absorb energy influences the severity of injury. For example, less damage is expected from a fall on a soft, grassy surface than from a fall on asphalt or concrete.

SECTION THREE
PENETRATING TRAUMA

Penetrating Trauma

All penetrating objects, regardless of velocity, cause tissue disruption (**penetrating trauma**). This damage occurs as a result of two types of forces: crushing and stretching. The character of the penetrating object, its speed of penetration, and the type of body tissue that it passes through or into determine which of the two mechanisms of injury predominates.

Cavitation

Cavitation is an opening produced by a force that pushes body tissues laterally away from the tract of a projectile. The amount of cavitation produced by the transfer of energy is directly related to the density

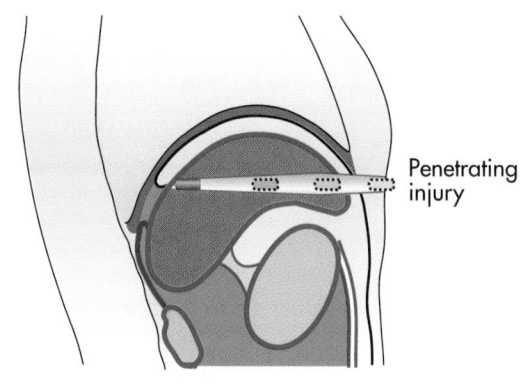

Penetrating injury

Permanent cavitation

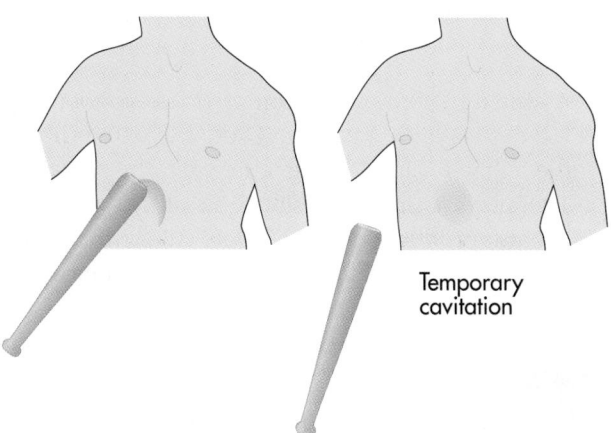

Temporary cavitation

Fig. 18-8 Permanent and temporary cavitation.

(number of particles) of tissue in a given body area and the ability of the body tissue to return to its original shape and position. For example, a person who receives a high-velocity blow to the abdomen experiences abdominal cavitation at the moment of impact. However, because of the lower density of the abdominal musculature, the cavitation is temporary (lasting only a few microseconds) even in the presence of severe intraabdominal injury (Fig. 18-8).

Permanent cavities are produced by penetrating injuries in which the transfer of energy exceeds the tensile strength of the tissue. Tissues with high water density (for example, liver, spleen, and muscle) or solid density (for example, bone) are more prone to permanent cavitation. Certain injuries (for example, a stab wound to the abdomen) can produce cavitations as tissues are displaced in frontal and lateral directions.

Ballistics

The energy created and dissipated by the object into surrounding tissues determines the effect of a projectile on the body. The paramedic should consider the principles of kinematics when dealing with injuries from penetrating trauma. To review, kinetic energy equals half the mass of an object multiplied by the square of its velocity. With reference to ballistic trauma, doubling the mass doubles the energy, but doubling the velocity quadruples the energy. Therefore a small-caliber bullet traveling at a high speed can produce more serious injury than a wide-caliber bullet traveling at a lower speed, as long as the wide-caliber bullet does not strike a major vessel or organ.

Damage and Energy Levels of Projectiles

Injuries caused by penetrating trauma result from three energy levels: low, medium, and high. This discussion considers hand-driven weapons as low-energy projectiles and bullets as medium- and high-energy projectiles.

Low-energy projectiles such as knives, needles, and ice picks cause tissue damage by their sharp, cutting edges (Fig. 18-9). The amount of tissue crushed in these injuries usually is minimal because the amount of force applied in the wounding process is small. The more blunt the penetrating object, the more force that must be applied to cause penetration. The more force needed to cause penetration, the more tissue crushed. The damage of tissue from low-energy injuries usually is limited to the pathway of the projectile.

When evaluating a patient with a stab wound, the paramedic should attempt to identify the type of wounding object and consider the possibility of multiple wounds, embedded penetrating objects, extensive internal damage to organs of the thorax and abdomen, and penetration of multiple body cavities. A high degree of suspicion also is indicated for stab wounds to areas of the back and flank, since these may be associated with penetrating hollow visceral injuries and injuries to retroperitoneal organs. Penetrating injuries of the thorax can involve the abdomen, just as abdominal injuries can involve the thorax.

> ### ? CRITICAL THINKING
>
> **Your patient has a stab wound in the midaxillary line, lateral to the left nipple. What organs may be affected by this mechanism? What else would you like to know about this injury?**

Firearms that have a muzzle velocity of less than 1500 feet per second are usually the cause of medium-energy injuries. All handguns and some rifles are medium-energy weapons. The injury tract produced by medium-energy weapons usually is two to three times the diameter of the projectile.

Firearms with a muzzle velocity of more than 1500 feet per second are usually the cause of high-energy injuries. Examples of high-energy weapons include military rifles, AR-15s, M-16s, AK 47/74s, and some deer rifles. As with medium-energy injuries, the injury tract produced by high-energy weapons usually is two to three times the diameter of the projectile.

Implications of soft body armor. Some EMS agencies have adopted soft body armor policies as additional protection for paramedics against blunt and penetrating trauma. Most agencies follow U.S. Department of Justice guidelines to determine the type of body armor protection for the types of weapons most commonly found in their community. There are seven levels of body armor protection. Authorities generally recommend a type III or higher protection level for EMS providers. These soft vests protect against low- and some medium- and high-velocity weapons (see Chapter 52).

Wounding Forces of Medium- and High-Energy Projectiles
A firearm cartridge is composed of a bullet made of metal, gunpowder to propel the bullet, a primer to explode and ignite the gunpowder, and a cartridge case that surrounds these components. When the trigger is pulled, the metal hammer strikes the firing pin, which ignites the primer. The gunpowder ignites and forces the bullet to exit the cartridge case.

> **NOTE**
>
> There were 900 unintentional firearm deaths in the United States in 1998.[1]

The mechanism of injury from firearms is related to the energy created and dissipated by the bullet into the surrounding tissues. When a firearm is discharged, several events affect this dissipation of energy and ultimately the wounding forces of the missile:

1. As the missile travels through air, it experiences wind resistance, or drag. The greater the drag, the greater the slowing effect on the missile. Therefore a firearm discharged at close range usually produces a more severe injury than the same firearm discharged at a greater distance.

> **NOTE**
>
> In civilian shooting incidents, the average distance from gun to victim is 7 yards (a very short range).

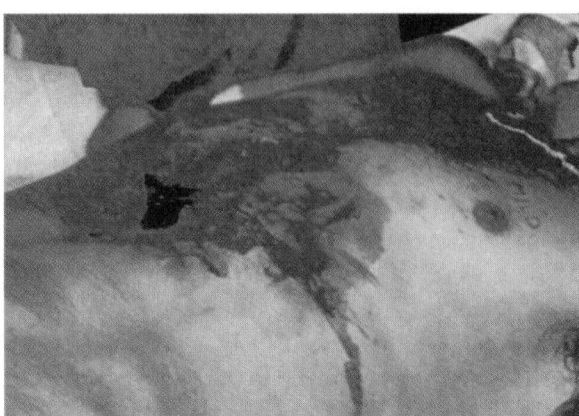

Fig. 18-9 Stab wound in which a knife has pierced the liver and pancreas and entered the splenic vein.

2. As the missile travels through air, a sonic pressure wave spreads out behind the missile. Because the speed of sound in tissue is about four times the speed of sound in air, the sonic pressure wave jumps ahead and precedes the missile through the tissue. This pressure wave displaces tissue and sometimes stretches it dramatically.

3. The localized crush of tissue in the missile's path and the momentary stretch of the surrounding tissue cause tissue disruption.

When a projectile strikes a body, tissue stretches at the point of impact to allow entry of the penetrating object (temporary cavitation). Because the projectile's energy exceeds the tensile strength of the tissue, tissue crush occurs, impelling surrounding tissues outward from the path of the projectile (permanent cavitation). The differences in wounds caused by projectiles vary with the amount and location of crushed and stretched tissue (Fig. 18-10). The wounding forces of a missile depend on the projectile mass, deformation, fragmentation, type of tissue struck, striking velocity, and range.[8]

Projectile mass. Tissue crush is limited by the physical size or profile of the projectile. If the missile strikes point first, the crushed area is no larger than the diameter of the bullet. If the missile is tilted as it strikes the body, the amount of crushed tissue is no larger than the length and longitudinal cross section of the bullet.

Deformation. Some firearm missiles deform when striking tissue (for example, expanding hollow- or soft-point hunting bullets). The points of these projectiles typically flatten on impact. The diameter of the bullet expands, creating a larger area of crushed tissue. Military use of these bullets in war is forbidden. Military bullets now are not intended to kill, but to produce injury.

Fragmentation. Each piece of missile crushes its own path through tissue, causing extensive tissue damage. These fragments produce a larger frontal area than a single, solid bullet and disperse energy into the surrounding tissues rapidly. Tissues weaken from the multiple fragment tracts and increase the subsequent stretch of the temporary cavity. The higher the velocity, the more likely the bullet is to fragment. If a bullet fragments, there may be no exit wound.

Type of tissue struck. Tissue disruption varies greatly with tissue type. For example, elastic tissues such as the bowel wall, lung, and muscle tolerate stretch much better than nonelastic organs such as the liver.

Striking velocity. The velocity of a missile determines the extent of cavitation and tissue deformation. Low-velocity missiles localize injury to a small radius from the center of the injury tract and have little disruptive effect, pushing the tissue aside. High-velocity missiles produce more serious injuries

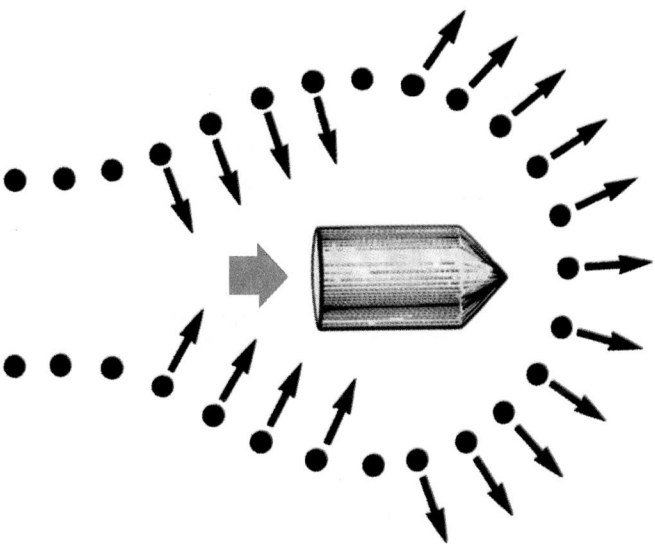

Fig. 18-10 Bullet passing through tissue. Outward stretching of the permanent cavity as the tissue particles move away from the penetrating missile cause the temporary cavity. (From Moylan J: *Principles of trauma surgery*, ed 2, New York, 1992, Gower Medical Publishing.)

because they lose more energy to the tissues and produce more cavitation.

Bullet yaw, or "tumble," in tissue also contributes to cavitation and tissue damage. A wedge-shaped bullet's center of gravity is nearer to the base than to the nose. As the missile strikes body tissue, it slows rapidly. Momentum carries the base of the bullet forward, and the center of gravity becomes the leading part of the missile. This forward rotation around the center of mass causes an end-over-end motion, producing more energy exchange and more tissue damage.

Range. The distance of the weapon from the target is a significant factor in the severity of ballistic trauma. Air resistance (drag) slows the missile significantly; therefore increasing the distance of the projectile from the target decreases the velocity at the time of impact.

If the firearm is discharged at close range (within 3 feet), cavitation can occur from the combustion of powder and the forceful expansion of gases. The gas and powder can enter the body cavity and cause internal explosion of tissue. This is common with shotgun wounds but less common with handguns because the latter produce a small amount of gas and create a small entrance wound. The expansion of only gas can cause extensive tissue destruction, especially in an enclosed area (for example, the skull).

Shotgun Wounds

Shotguns are short-range, low-velocity weapons that fire multiple lead pellets, which are encased in a larger shell. Each pellet (there may be 9 to 400 or more, depending on pellet size and gauge of gun) is considered a missile capable of producing tissue damage. Each shell contains pellets, gunpowder, and a plastic or paper wad that separates the pellets from the gunpowder. This wad of unsterile material increases the potential for infection in shotgun wounds.

The energy transferred to body tissue and the resultant tissue damage depends on the gauge of the gun, size of the pellets, powder charge, and dis-

> **NOTE**
>
> The explosion of gas explains how "blanks" (ammunition without projectiles) can cause injury or death when fired at short range.

tance from the victim. For example, a 12-gauge, full-choke shotgun with number 6 shot (275 pellets) concentrates 95% of the pellets into a 7-inch circle at 10 yards. At close range a shotgun injury can create extensive tissue damage similar to that from a high-velocity missile weapon.

Entrance and Exit Wounds

The presence of entrance and exit wounds is affected by several factors, including range, barrel length, caliber, powder, and weapon (Fig. 18-11). In general, an entrance wound over soft tissue is round or oval and may be surrounded by an abrasion rim or collar. If the firearm is discharged at intermediate or close range, powder burns (tattooing) may be present (see the box on p. 548).

Exit wounds, if present, are generally larger than entrance wounds because of the cavitational wave that occurs as the bullet passes through the tissues. As the bullet exits the body, the skin can "explode," resulting in ragged and torn tissue. This splitting and tearing often produces a star-burst or stellate wound.

> **? CRITICAL THINKING**
>
> ***You locate an entrance wound but no exit wound on a patient who was shot. Does this mean that the injury is not serious?***

If the muzzle is in direct contact with the skin at the time of firearm discharge, expanding gases can enter the tissue and produce crepitus. These burning gases also can produce thermal injury at the entrance site and along the injury tract.

> **NOTE**
>
> The paramedic should describe and document the appearance of all wounds but refrain from commenting or speculating on which is the entry or exit wound. Identifying a wound as an entry or exit wound can result in the paramedic being served a subpoena to testify in court in an area that is beyond the scope of paramedic practice.

Special Considerations for Specific Injuries

Identification of ballistic injuries requires a thorough examination and a high degree of suspicion because penetrating trauma from high- and medium-velocity missiles is unpredictable.

Head injuries. Gunshot wounds to the head typically are devastating because of direct destruction of brain tissue and subsequent swelling. In addition, patients with head wounds frequently sustain severe face and neck injuries, resulting in significant blood loss, difficulty in maintaining airway control, and spinal instability.

As a medium-energy projectile penetrates the skull, the energy is absorbed within the closed space of the cranium. The resulting force of the injury compresses brain tissue against the cranial cavity, often fracturing orbital plates and separating the dura from the bone. Depending on the characteristics of the missile, the bullet may not have sufficient force to exit the skull after penetration, as occurs with 0.22- and 0.25-caliber handguns. In these injuries the bullet follows the curvature of the skull's interior, producing significant damage.

High-velocity wounds to the skull produce massive destruction because pieces of the skull and brain typically are destroyed. At close range, this results in part from the large quantities of gas produced by combustion of the propellant. If the weapon is held in contact with the head, the gas follows the bullet into the cranial cavity, producing an explosive effect.

Thoracic injuries. Gunshot wounds to the thorax can result in severe injury to the pulmonary and vascular systems. If the lungs are penetrated by a missile, the pleura and pulmonary parenchyma (the tissue of an organ, as distinguished from supporting and connective tissue) are likely to be disrupted, producing a pneumothorax. On occasion, the pulmonary defect allows air that cannot be expelled to continue to flow into the thoracic cavity. The subsequent increase in pressure can eventually cause collapse of the lung and a shift in the mediastinum to the unaffected side (tension pneumothorax).

Vascular trauma from penetrating injuries can result in massive internal and external hemorrhage. For example, if the pulmonary artery or vein, venae

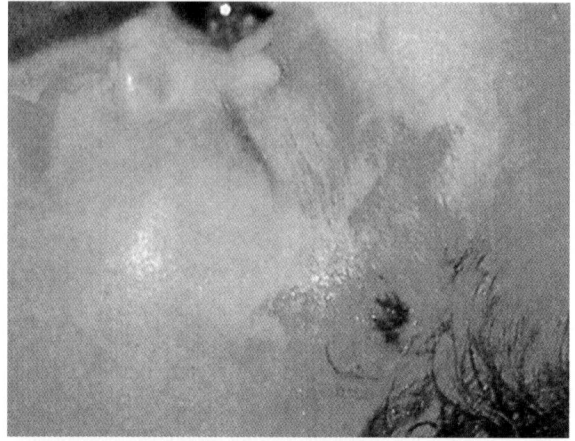

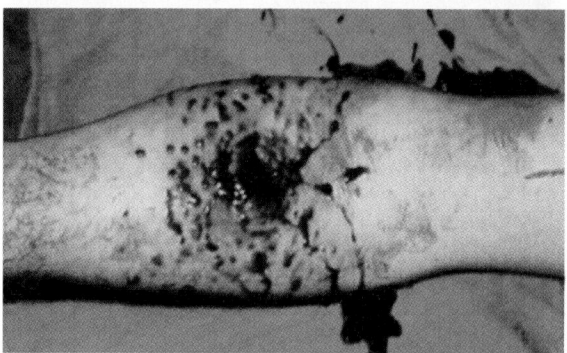

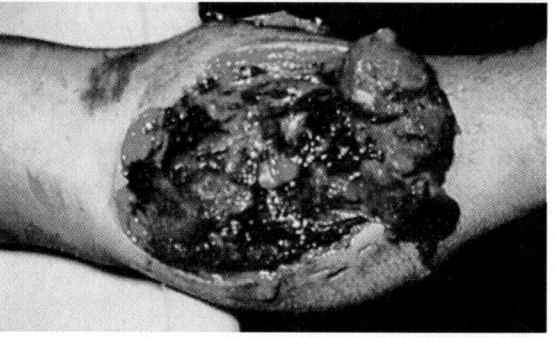

Fig. 18-11 A, The powder marks show that this 0.22-caliber bullet wound was inflicted at close range. **B,** A short-range shotgun wound to the forearm. **C,** Exit wound caused by a powerful shotgun fired at close range. (From London PS: *A color atlas of diagnosis after recent injury,* Ipswich, England, 1990, Wolfe Medical Publications.)

cavae, or aorta is destroyed, exsanguination can occur within minutes. Other vascular injuries from penetrating trauma to the thorax can result in hemothorax and, if the heart is involved, myocardial rupture or pericardial tamponade.

Penetrating injury can cause thoracic trauma in the absence of visible chest wounds. For example, a bullet can enter the abdomen and travel upward through the diaphragm and into the thorax. The

FORENSIC CONSIDERATIONS IN MANAGING GUNSHOT WOUNDS

Lifesaving procedures always take precedence over forensic considerations. However, the paramedic should not touch or move weapons or other environmental clues unless it is absolutely necessary for patient care procedures. Other forensic considerations follow:

- Document the exact condition of the patient and wound appearance on arrival at the scene, including environment of the patient and body position in relation to objects and doorways.
- Disturb the scene as little as possible.
- If possible, cut or tear clothing along a seam to avoid altering tears made by a penetrating object.
- Avoid cutting through a bullet hole in the clothing.
- Do not shake clothing.
- Keep all clothing in a paper bag rather than a plastic bag that may alter evidence and do not give it to the victim's family members.
- Save any avulsed tissue for forensic pathology.
- If the bullet is retrieved, place it in a padded container to prevent marring and secure the evidence until is delivered to the authorities (obtain a receipt).

paramedic should evaluate all victims of abdominal gunshot wounds for thoracic injury and victims of thoracic gunshot wounds for abdominal injury.

Abdominal injuries. Gunshot wounds to the abdomen usually require surgery to determine the extent of injury. Penetrating trauma can affect multiple organ systems, causing damage to air-filled and solid organs, vascular injury, trauma to the vertebral column, and spinal cord injury. The paramedic should assume a serious injury when managing victims of penetrating abdominal trauma, even if they appear to be stable.

Extremity injuries. Gunshot wounds to the extremities occasionally are life threatening and can result in lifelong disability. Special considerations with these injuries include vascular injury with bleeding into soft tissues and damage to nerves, muscles, and bones. The paramedic should evaluate any extremity that has sustained penetrating trauma for bone injury, motor and sensory integrity, and the presence of adequate blood flow (for example, pulses and capillary refill).

Vessels can be injured by being struck by the bullet or by temporary cavitation. Either mechanism can damage the lining of the blood vessel, producing hemorrhage or thrombosis. Penetrating trauma can damage muscle tissue by stretching it as the muscle expands away from the path of the missile. Stretching that exceeds the tensile strength of the muscle produces hemorrhage.

Bone struck by a penetrating object can be deformed and fragmented. If this occurs, the transfer of energy causes pieces of bone to act as secondary missiles, crushing their way through surrounding tissue. This can result in extensive damage and additional tissue disruption.

SUMMARY

- Trauma is the leading cause of death among persons 1 to 36 years of age and the fifth leading cause of death among all Americans.

- Trauma care is divided into three phases: preincident, incident, and postincident.

- Components of the trauma system include injury prevention, prehospital care, emergency department care, interfacility transportation (if needed), definitive care, trauma critical care, rehabilitation, data collection, and trauma registry.

- Injuries are caused by a transfer of energy from some external source to the human body. The extent of injury is determined by the type of energy applied, how quickly it is applied, and to what part of the body it is applied.

- Blunt trauma is an injury produced by the wounding forces of compression and change of speed, which can disrupt tissues.

- The three restraining systems available in the United States are lap belts, diagonal shoulder straps, and air bags, all of which significantly reduce injuries. However, if they are inappropriately worn, these protective devices also can produce injuries.

- Organ motions and their injuries are a result of deceleration and compression forces. Recognition of these injuries requires a high degree of suspicion using the principles of kinematics.

- Small motorized vehicles, such as motorcycles, all-terrain vehicles (ATVs), snowmobiles, motor boats, water bikes, and farm machinery, are considered to be more dangerous than other motor vehicles because they offer minimal protection to the rider from the transfer of energy associated with collisions.

- All auto-pedestrian collisions can produce serious injuries and require a high degree of suspicion for multiple-system trauma.

- Although sporting activities provide a variety of health benefits, they also can produce severe injury. Sports-related injuries account for 15% of all spinal cord injuries in the United States each year.

- Blast injury is damage to a patient exposed to a pressure field that is produced by an explosion of volatile substances. Blasts release large amounts of energy in the form of pressure and heat.

- Falls from greater than three times the height of an individual (15 to 20 feet) are associated with an increased incidence of severe injuries. In predicting injuries associated with falls, the paramedic should evaluate the distance fallen, body position of the patient on impact, and type of landing surface struck.

- All penetrating objects, regardless of velocity, cause tissue disruption. The character of the penetrating object, its speed of penetration, and the type of body tissue it passes through or into determine whether crushing or stretching forces will cause injury.

REFERENCES

1. National Safety Council: *Injury facts*, Chicago, 1999, The Council.
2. Rosen P, Barkin R: *Emergency medicine: concepts and clinical practice*, ed 3, St Louis, 1998, Mosby.
3. National Association of Emergency Medical Technicians: *PHTLS: basic and advanced prehospital life support*, ed 4, St Louis, 1999, Mosby.
4. Baker C et al: Epidemiology of trauma deaths, *Am J Surg* 140:144, 1980.
5. US Department of Transportation, National Highway Traffic Safety Administration: *Paramedic national standard curriculum*, Washington, DC, 1998, US Government Printing Office.
6. American Hospital Association: *Hospital statistics 1994-1995*, Chicago, 1995, The Association.
7. Kuehl A, editor: *EMS medical director's handbook*, St Louis, 1989, Mosby.
8. American Heart Association: *Currents in emergency cardiac care*, vol 9, no 2, Dallas, 1998, The Association.
9. McSwain N, Kerstein M: *Evaluation and management of trauma*, Norwalk, Conn, 1987, Appleton-Century-Crofts.

19 Hemorrhage and Shock

Upon completion of this chapter, the paramedic student will be able to:

1. Describe how to recognize signs and symptoms of internal or external hemorrhage.

2. Define shock.

3. Outline the factors necessary to achieve adequate tissue oxygenation.

4. Describe how the diameter of resistance vessels influences preload.

5. Describe the function of the components of blood.

6. Outline the changes in the microcirculation during the progression of shock.

7. List the causes of hypovolemic, cardiogenic, neurogenic, anaphylactic, and septic shock.

8. Describe pathophysiology as a basis for signs and symptoms associated with the progression through the stages of shock.

9. Describe key assessment findings to distinguish the etiology of the shock state.

10. Outline the prehospital management of the patient in shock based on knowledge of the pathophysiology associated with each type of shock.

11. Discuss how to integrate the assessment and management of the patient in shock.

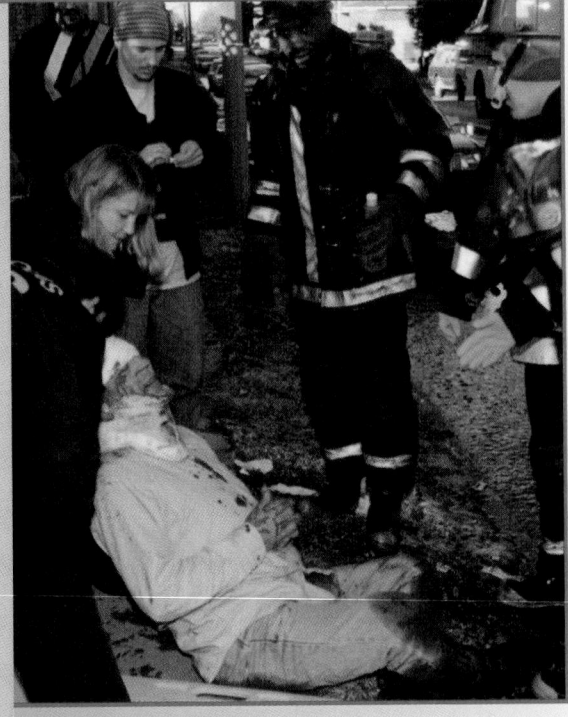

Severe medical illnesses and traumatic events threaten the human body's internal environment. During these events the protective systems of the body attempt to compensate in an effort to maintain cellular oxygenation. The paramedic must be able to integrate pathophysiological principles and assessment findings to formulate a field impression and to implement a treatment plan for the patient with hemorrhage or shock.

disseminated intravascular coagulation: A grave coagulopathy that results from the overstimulation of the body's clotting and anticlotting processes in response to disease or injury.

Fick principle: The principle used to determine cardiac output; assumes that the quantity of oxygen delivered to an organ is equal to the amount of oxygen consumed by that organ plus the amount of oxygen carried away from that organ.

hemostasis: The termination of bleeding by mechanical or chemical means or by substances that arrest the blood flow.

pulse pressure: The difference between systemic and pulmonic pressure.

Hemorrhage

Hemorrhage occurs when there is a disruption, or "leak," in the vascular system. Sources of hemorrhage can be external or internal.

External Hemorrhage

External hemorrhage results from soft tissue injury (described in Chapter 20) and accounts for nearly 10 million emergency department visits in the United States each year.[1] Most soft tissue trauma is accompanied by mild hemorrhage and is not life threatening, but it can carry significant risks of morbidity and disfigurement. The seriousness of the injury depends on the anatomical source of the hemorrhage

NOTE

Education and prevention "before the event" are the best ways to avoid significant trauma. Strategies include community education (for example, use of seat belts), enforcement (for example, helmet laws), and environment and engineering (for example, installing "walk signals" at a busy intersection). These and other prevention strategies can help reduce the occurrence of significant injury (see Appendix C).

(arterial, venous, capillary), the degree of vascular disruption, and the amount of blood loss that can be tolerated by the patient.

Internal Hemorrhage

Internal hemorrhage can result from blunt or penetrating trauma and acute or chronic medical illnesses. Internal bleeding that can cause hemodynamic instability usually occurs in one of four body cavities: the chest, abdomen, pelvis, or retroperitoneum. Intracranial hemorrhage also can cause grave hemodynamic instability. Internal hemorrhage is associated with higher morbidity and mortality rates than external hemorrhage. Signs and symptoms that can indicate significant internal hemorrhage include the following:

- Bright red blood from mouth, rectum, or other orifice
- Coffee-ground appearance of vomitus
- Melena (black, tarry stools)
- Hematochezia (passage of red blood through the rectum)
- Dizziness or syncope on sitting or standing
- Orthostatic hypotension (described later in this chapter)

? CRITICAL THINKING

Why do you think internal hemorrhage is associated with an increase in morbidity and mortality rates?

Physiological Response to Hemorrhage

The termination of bleeding by chemical means (**hemostasis**) is the body's initial response to hemorrhage. This vascular reaction (further described in Chapter 20) involves local vasoconstriction, formation of a platelet plug, coagulation, and the growth of fibrous tissue into the blood clot that permanently closes and seals the injured vessel. If hemorrhage is severe, these mechanisms can fail, resulting in shock (hypoperfusion).

Defining Shock

Shock was defined by Gross in 1850 as a "rude unhinging of the machinery of life"[2] and has since been redefined by many others. Robert M. Hardaway, professor of surgery at Texas Tech University School of Medicine in El Paso, Texas, defines shock this way[3]:

I believe that the best definition of shock is inadequate capillary perfusion. As a corollary of this broad definition, almost anyone who dies, except one who is instantly destroyed, must go through a stage of shock—a momentary pause in the act of death.

Shock is not a single entity with a specific cause and treatment but rather a complex group of physiological abnormalities that can result from a variety of disease states and injuries. Because of the many complexities involved in shock, it is not adequately defined by pulse rate, blood pressure, or cardiac function, and it cannot be reduced to hypovolemia or loss of systemic vascular resistance. Shock may affect an entire organism, or it may occur at a tissue or cellular level, even with normal hemodynamics. An understanding of cellular physiology is necessary to recognize subtle aspects of shock and to properly assess the severity of various stages of shock.

Tissue Oxygenation

To achieve adequate oxygenation of tissue cells (perfusion), three distinct components of the cardiovascular system must function properly: the heart, vasculature, and lungs. When any one of these malfunctions, a decrease in cellular oxygenation can occur.

> **NOTE**
>
> Chapter 6 provides a review of the anatomy of the respiratory and cardiovascular systems.

Heart

The pumping action of the heart produces pressure changes that circulate blood throughout the body. This repetitive pumping action is referred to as the *cardiac cycle.*

Cardiac output (described in Chapter 7) is a crucial determinant of organ perfusion and depends on several factors, including strength of contraction, rate of contraction, and amount of venous return available to the ventricle (preload). The formula to determine cardiac output is as follows:

$$\text{Cardiac output (CO)} = \text{Heart rate (HR)} \times \text{Stroke volume (SV)}$$

In 1870, Adolph Fick developed the first method for measuring cardiac output in healthy animals and people. The method, called the **Fick principle,** assumes that the quantity of oxygen delivered to an organ is equal to the amount of oxygen consumed by that organ plus the amount of oxygen carried away from that organ. The Fick principle frequently is used to estimate perfusion either to an organ or to the whole body when oxygen content of both the arterial and venous blood is known and oxygen consumption is assumed to remain fixed (Box 19-1).

Vasculature

The entire vascular system is lined with smooth, low-friction endothelial cells. All vessels larger than capillaries have layers of tissue surrounding the endothelium. These layers of tissue, or tunicae, provide supporting connective tissue to counter the pressure of blood contained in the vascular system, elastic properties to dampen pressure pulsations and minimize flow variations throughout the cardiac cycle, and muscle fibers to control the vessel diameter. The vascular system maintains blood flow by changes in pressure and peripheral vascular resistance.

Fluid flows through a tube in response to pressure gradients between the two ends of the tube. The difference in pressure between the two ends determines flow, not the absolute pressure in the tube. In many animals, including humans, the two ends are the aorta and the vena cavae.

Systemic pressure (left-sided pressure) and pulmonic pressure (right-sided pressure) are measurements of pressure in the vascular system. Systemic pressure, like pulmonic pressure, has two phases: systolic and diastolic. The difference between these two pressures is the **pulse pressure**. Pressure is greatest at its origin (the heart) and least at its terminating point (the venae cavae). This pressure gradient changes significantly at the arteriole as a result of peripheral vascular resistance.

NOTE

Pulse pressure reflects the tone of the arterial system and is more sensitive to changes in perfusion than the systolic or diastolic pressures alone.

The peripheral vascular resistance (afterload) is the total resistance against which blood must be pumped. It is a measure of friction between the vessel walls and fluid and between the molecules of the fluid themselves (viscosity), both of which oppose flow. When the resistance to flow increases, blood pressure must increase for the flow to remain constant. Resistance to blood flow increases with increased fluid viscosity or vessel length and decreased vessel diameter.

Viscosity is the physical property of a liquid characterized by the degree of friction between its component molecules (for example, between the blood cells and between the plasma proteins). Viscosity normally plays a minor role in blood flow regulation because it remains fairly constant in healthy individuals. Vessel length in the human body also remains fairly constant. Vessel diameter is the primary factor affecting the resistance to blood flow.

? CRITICAL THINKING

How do firefighters use these principles of viscosity and vessel diameter when fighting a fire?

Major arteries are large and offer little resistance to flow unless they have an abnormal narrowing (stenosis). Arterioles have a much smaller diameter than arteries and offer the major resistance to blood flow. The smooth muscle in the arteriole walls can relax or contract, changing the diameter of the inside of the arteriole as much as fivefold. Thus the vasoconstriction or vasodilation

BOX 19-1

THE FICK PRINCIPLE

1. An adequate amount of oxygen must be available to red blood cells through the alveolar membrane in the lungs to ensure hemoglobin saturation with oxygen. This requires adequate ventilation of the lungs through the patient's airway, a high partial pressure of oxygen in inspired air (FiO_2), and minimal obstruction to the diffusion of oxygen across the alveolar capillary membrane.
2. The red blood cells must be circulated to the tissue cells. This requires adequate cardiac function, an adequate volume of blood flow, and proper routing of blood through the vascular channels.
3. The red blood cells must be able to adequately load oxygen in the pulmonary capillaries and unload the oxygen at the site of peripheral tissue cells. This requires normal hemoglobin levels, circulation of the oxygenated red blood cells to the tissues in need, close approximation of the tissue cells to the capillaries to allow for diffusion of oxygen, and ideal conditions of pH, temperature, and other factors. Fick principle (Tissue oxygenation) = (Arterial oxygen content − Venous oxygen content) × Perfusion

of these vessels primarily regulate arterial blood pressure.

Microcirculation

The body's microcirculation is divided into pulmonary microcirculation and peripheral microcirculation. Separate pumps, the right and left heart, respectively, produce pressure in each of these divisions.

At any given moment, about 5% of the total circulating blood is flowing through the capillaries. This 5% is exchanging nutrients and metabolic end products. The muscular arterioles, which are the major resistance vessels, regulate regional blood flow to the capillary beds. The venules and veins serve as collecting channels and storage (capacitance) vessels, normally containing 70% of the blood volume. The mechanisms that control blood flow to the tissues are described in Chapter 7 and include the following:

- Local control of blood flow by the tissues
- Nervous control of blood flow
  - Baroreceptor reflexes
  - Chemoreceptor reflexes
  - CNS ischemia response
  - Hormonal mechanisms
    - Adrenal-medullary mechanism
    - Renin-angiotensin-aldosterone mechanism
    - Vasopressin mechanism
  - Reabsorption of tissue fluid

Lungs

Adequate oxygenation of tissue cells requires that adequate oxygen be made available to the red blood cells at the capillary membrane in the lungs (the first component of the Fick principle). The high partial pressure of oxygen in inspired air, adequate depth and rate of ventilation, and matching of pulmonary ventilation (described in Chapter 11) and perfusion make adequate oxygenation possible.

> **? CRITICAL THINKING**
>
> *Think of something that could impair each of these components of adequate oxygenation.*

Body as a Container

The healthy body is a smooth-flowing fluid delivery system inside a container. The container must be filled to achieve adequate preload and tissue oxygenation. Although the external size of the container of any human body is relatively constant, the volume of the vascular component in the container is directly related to the diameter of the resistance vessels, which can change rapidly. Any change in the diameter of the vessels changes the volume of fluid that the container holds, thereby affecting preload.

An example of this principle is a 5-L container, the normal container size for a 70-kg adult male (Fig. 19-1). If the fluid volume is 5 liters, preload is adequate. With a strong myocardium, cardiac output and perfusion also are adequate. If 2 liters of this fluid have been lost, either externally or internally, the remaining 3 liters are inadequate to sup-

ply an effective preload. Since cardiac output depends on preload, a decrease in preload significantly decreases cardiac output.

If the patient is hypovolemic and the 5-liter container has remained the same size despite the 3-liter volume, the patient becomes hypotensive because of decreased cardiac output. However, if the container is reduced to 3 liters by compensatory mechanisms (for example, vasoconstriction), the 3-liter container can provide adequate preload to the heart with the 3 liters of available fluid. This is at the expense of certain tissues that are not perfused in this constricted state.

If fluid is adequate for a 5-liter container but the container size has been enlarged to 7 liters by illness or injury that results in vasodilation, the 5 liters of fluid do not provide adequate preload for the container (relative hypovolemia). Factors that occasionally are responsible for vasodilation include cardiac

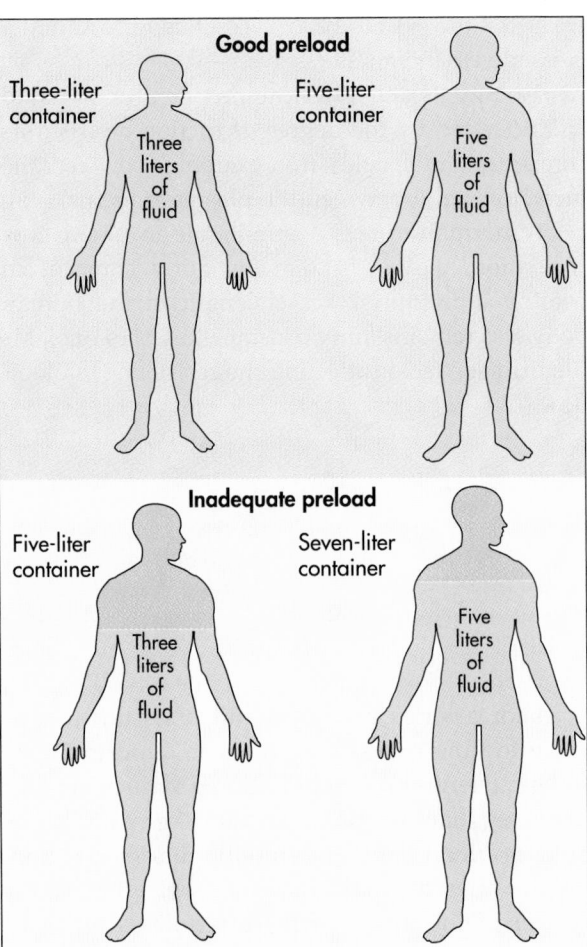

Fig. 19-1 Fluid versus container volume.

and blood pressure medications, allergic reaction, heat- and cold-related injuries, and alcohol or other drug use.

Blood and Its Components

The average adult male has a blood volume of 7% of total body weight, and the blood volume of the average adult female is 6.5% of total body weight (70 mL multiplied by kg body weight). Normal adult blood volume is 4.5 to 5 liters. This amount remains fairly constant in the healthy body. (Blood and its components are further described in Chapter 6.)

Plasma is about 92% water and is the blood's solvent (the liquid portion of blood). Salts, minerals, sugars, fats, and proteins are circulated in the body through plasma. Plasma contains three major proteins: albumin, globulin, and fibrinogen. Albumin is the most plentiful plasma protein. It is similar in consistency to egg white and gives blood its gummy texture. This large protein helps keep the water concentration of blood low enough to allow water to diffuse readily from tissues into blood. Globulins (alpha, beta, and gamma) serve two main functions: alpha and beta globulins transport other proteins, and gamma globulins provide immunity to disease. Fibrinogen aids in blood clotting by forming a web of protein fibers that binds blood cells together.

In addition to helping the body maintain its blood supply, plasma proteins serve several purposes. Should blood acidity change, the proteins can act together as an acid or base to correct it. If the body runs short of food, plasma protein also can temporarily meet the nutritional needs of the body.

Although oxygen dissolves in plasma, the plasma can only carry about 1% of the oxygen that the body demands. Red blood cells (erythrocytes) transport the other 99%. Red blood cells make up about 45% of the blood and are the most abundant cells in the body. Red blood cells provide oxygen to tissues and remove carbon dioxide. Each red blood cell contains approximately 270 million hemoglobin molecules. These molecules allow erythrocytes to pick up oxygen in the lungs and release it to body tissues.

White blood cells (leukocytes) defend the body against various pathogens (bacteria, viruses, fungi, and parasites). The bone marrow and lymph glands constantly produce and maintain a reserve of white blood cells, but not many are present in a healthy bloodstream (white cells are outnumbered by red cells 600 to 1). When a pathogen invades the body, the leukocyte reserves are released.

Another part of the body's defense mechanism is platelets, which prevent blood from escaping. Platelets are formed in the red bone marrow and work by swelling and adhering together to form sticky plugs, thereby initiating the clotting phenomenon (see Chapter 20).

Capillary-Cellular Relationship in Shock

The progression of shock in the microcirculation follows a sequence of stages related to changes in capillary perfusion and cellular necrosis (Fig. 19-2).[2]

Stage 1: Vasoconstriction

Vasoconstriction begins as minimal perfusion to the capillaries continues. Oxygen and substrate delivery to the cells supplied by these capillaries decreases; anaerobic metabolism replaces aerobic metabolism, and production of lactate and hydrogen ions increases. Shortly thereafter, the lining of the capillaries can begin to lose its ability to retain large molecular structures within its walls, permitting protein-containing fluid to leak into the interstitial spaces. This is known as the *leaky capillary syndrome*.

> **? CRITICAL THINKING**
>
> *If this "leak" persists, what effect will it have on preload and cardiac output?*

Arteriovenous (AV) shunts open, particularly in the skin, kidneys, and gastrointestinal tract, causing less flow to the arterioles and therefore less flow through the capillaries. Sympathetic stimulation produces pale, sweaty skin; a rapid, thready pulse (caused by hypovolemia and vasoconstriction); and an elevation in blood glucose level. The release of epinephrine dilates coronary, cerebral, and skeletal muscle arterioles and constricts other arterioles. As a result, blood is shunted to the heart, brain, and skeletal muscle, and capillary flow to the kidneys and abdominal viscera decreases. If the vasoconstriction

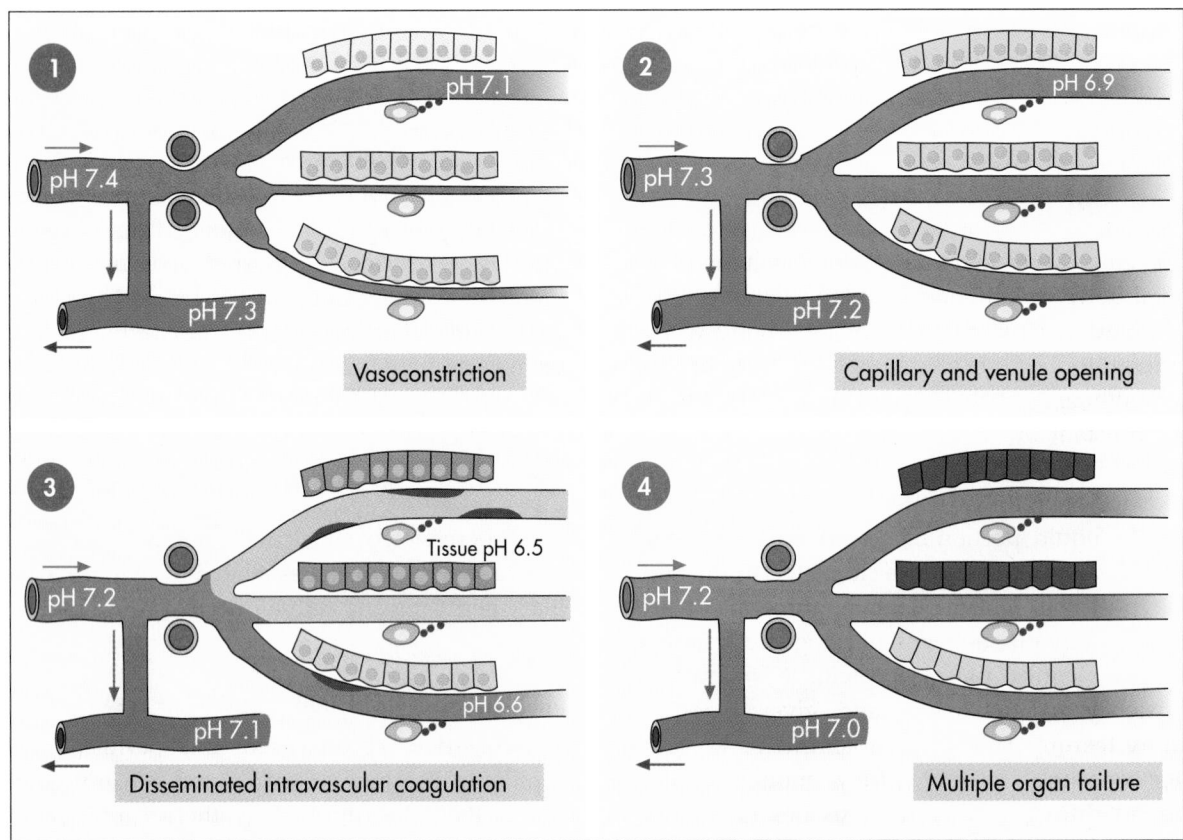

Fig. 19-2 Diagram of the microcirculation in shock, progressing from (1) vasoconstriction, (2) capillary and venule opening, (3) DIC, and (4) multiple organ failure. (Adapted from Hardaway R, editor: *Shock: the reversible stage of dying,* Littleton, Mass, 1988, PSG Publishing.)

stage of shock is not treated by prompt restoration of circulatory volume, shock progresses to the next stage.

> **NOTE**
>
> Stage one of shock occurs when intravascular blood volume is decreased by about 15%. Blood pressure and heart rate usually are normal at this stage of compensation. This stage is reversible if the hemorrhage is controlled.

Stage 2: Capillary and Venule Opening

As the progression of shock continues, the precapillary sphincter relaxes, with some resultant expansion of the vascular space. Because postcapillary sphincters resist local effects, they remain closed, causing blood to pool or stagnate in the capillary system and producing capillary engorgement. Arte-

rial hypotension, secondary arteriolar vasoconstriction, and opening of AV shunts result in less blood flow through arterioles and contribute to the stagnation of blood flow in the capillaries.

The vascular space expands greatly as increasing hypoxemia and acidosis lead to the opening of additional venules and capillaries. When this occurs, even normal blood volume may be inadequate to fill the container. The capillary and venule capacity can become great enough to reduce the volume of available blood for the great veins and venae cavae, resulting in decreased venous return and a fall in cardiac output. In addition, the viscera (lungs, liver, kidneys, and gastrointestinal mucosa) can become

> **? CRITICAL THINKING**
>
> *What happens to the function of the heart as acidosis increases?*

congested. The low arterial blood pressure, extremely constricted arterioles, presence of AV shunts, and many open capillaries result in stagnant capillary flow.

Sluggish blood flow and the reduced delivery of oxygen result in increased anaerobic metabolism and the production of lactic acid. The respiratory system attempts to compensate for the acidosis by increasing ventilation to release carbon dioxide, producing a partially compensated metabolic acidosis. As the acidosis increases and pH falls, the red blood cells may cluster together (Rouleaux formation). This halts perfusion in the vital visceral capillaries, affecting nutritional flow and preventing the removal of cellular metabolites. Clotting mechanisms also are affected, leading to hypercoagulability. This stage of shock often progresses to the third stage if fluid resuscitation is inadequate or delayed, or if the shock state is complicated by trauma or sepsis.

> **NOTE**
>
> Stage two of shock occurs with a 15% to 25% decrease in intravascular blood volume. Heart rate, respiratory rate, and capillary refill are increased and pulse pressure is decreased at this stage. Blood pressure may still be normal.

Stage 3: Disseminated Intravascular Coagulation

Stage 3 of shock is resistant to treatment (refractory shock) but is still reversible. Blood begins to coagulate in the microcirculation, clogging capillaries. This is referred to as **disseminated intravascular coagulation** (DIC). Clumps of red blood cells may occlude the capillaries. This occlusion decreases capillary perfusion, prevents delivery of oxygenated substrates such as glucose, and prevents removal of metabolites. As a result, distal tissue cells switch to anaerobic metabolism, and lactic acid production increases.

As stage 3 of shock continues, lactic acid accumulates around the cell. The cell no longer has the energy needed to maintain homeostasis. Water and sodium leak into the cell through the cellular membrane, potassium leaks out, and the cells swell and die (also known as the *wash out* phase). Microinfarcts develop in the viscera. Microthrombi produce capillary congestion, fluid leaks, rupture, and hemorrhage. The pulmonary capillaries become perme-

able, leading to pulmonary edema, which decreases the absorption of oxygen and results in possible alterations in carbon dioxide elimination. This can lead to acute respiratory failure or adult respiratory distress syndrome (further described in Chapter 27). If shock and DIC continue, the patient progresses to multiple organ failure.

> **NOTE**
>
> Stage three of shock occurs with a 25% to 35% decrease in intravascular blood volume. At this stage, hypotension occurs. This stage of shock usually requires blood replacement.

> **NOTE**
>
> Blood pressure in the shock patient is classified as *normotensive* (normal), *hypotensive* (a systolic pressure of 70 to 100 mm Hg with signs and symptoms of shock), or *profoundly hypotensive* (a systolic pressure less than 70 mm Hg).[4]

Stage 4: Multiple Organ Failure

The amount of cellular necrosis required to produce organ failure varies with each organ and depends on the underlying condition of the organ. Usually hepatic failure occurs first, followed by renal failure and heart failure. However, if any given area of capillary occlusion persists for more than 1 to 2 hours, the cells nourished by that capillary undergo changes that rapidly become irreversible. In this stage of shock, blood pressure falls dramatically (to levels of 60 mm Hg or less). Even if blood pressure is returned to normal after a couple of hours, the cell's ability to obtain energy from oxygen through anaerobic metabolism fails and the cell dies from inadequate capillary perfusion (described in the beginning of this discussion). Inadequate tissue perfusion and cell death are the results of irreversible shock.

If cellular necrosis damages a critical amount of the vital organ, the organ soon fails. Failure of the liver and kidneys is common and often presents early in this stage. Capillary blockage can cause heart failure. Gastrointestinal bleeding and sepsis can result from gastrointestinal mucosal necrosis; pancreatic necrosis can lead to further clotting disorders and severe pancreatitis. Pulmonary thrombosis can produce hemorrhage and fluid loss into the alveoli, leading to death from respiratory failure.

> **NOTE**
>
> Stage four of shock occurs when intravascular blood volume is decreased by 35% to 40%.

Classifications of Shock

More than 100 types of shock have been discussed in the medical literature. A common classification of shock for use in emergency care is to describe the syndrome based on the initiating cause (for example, hypovolemia) (see Chapter 7). Although these classifications are separate and distinct, two or more types often are combined. For example, hypovolemia may occur in septic shock, or elements of cardiogenic shock may occur in hypovolemic shock. Regardless of the classification, the underlying defect is inadequate tissue perfusion.

Hypovolemic Shock

In the United States, hypovolemic shock most frequently is caused by hemorrhage but also can be secondary to dehydration (commonly seen with severe diarrhea and vomiting). In either case, there is a loss of circulating volume. Scenarios that can lead to hypovolemic shock include hemorrhage, burns, severe or prolonged diarrhea, vomiting, endocrine disorders, and internal third space loss, as in peritonitis. In addition to loss of circulating volume, tissue injury resulting from trauma can exacerbate shock by causing microemboli and further activating the inflammatory and coagulation systems.

> **NOTE**
>
> Since most patients with shock have hypovolemia, shock is assumed to be hypovolemic in origin until proven otherwise. The paramedic should initially manage the patient with shock with a fluid bolus unless the lungs are wet (identified by crackles). Crackles on physical examination indicate cardiogenic shock instead.

Cardiogenic Shock

Cardiogenic shock results when the cardiac pump cannot deliver adequate circulating blood volume for tissue perfusion. This can be due to inadequate filling of the heart, poor contractility, or outflow obstruction. The patient in cardiogenic shock usually suffers from an acute myocardial infarction, a serious cardiac rhythm disturbance, cardiac tamponade, tension pneumothorax, cardiac contusion, severe valvular heart disease, cardiomyopathy, pulmonary embolism, or dissecting aortic aneurysm. Cardiogenic shock occurs in 5% to 10% of patients hospitalized for myocardial infarction. The associated mortality rate in these patients approaches 80%.

> **? CRITICAL THINKING**
>
> *Why does cardiogenic shock develop in a patient who has had a severe myocardial infarction?*

> **NOTE**
>
> Shock that develops from cardiac tamponade, tension pneumothorax, or pulmonary embolism also is known as *obstructive shock* because the common pathophysiology in these conditions is obstruction to blood flow.

Neurogenic Shock

Neurogenic shock (also known as *spinal cord, distributive,* or *vasogenic shock*) results from vasomotor paralysis below the level of injury. Normal vasomotor tone through sympathetic nervous system control is lost, and there is a resultant decrease in peripheral vascular resistance. The loss of sympathetic impulses and resultant vasodilation increases the size of the container (so to speak), so even normal intravascular volume is insufficient to fill the vascular compartment and perfuse the tissues. Because of the nature of the injuries responsible for this syndrome, respiratory insufficiency, head injury, or both also may be present.

> **NOTE**
>
> Fainting may be due to mild, readily reversible vasogenic shock that can occur in the absence of injury. It also may be secondary to decreased cardiac output secondary to bradycardia.

Anaphylactic Shock

Anaphylactic shock occurs when the body is exposed to a substance that produces a severe allergic reaction. Common causes include antibiotic agents (especially penicillins), venoms, and insect stings. Physiological responses result from the release of histamine and other mediators, which act on receptors in both the systemic and pulmonary microcirculation and on bronchial smooth muscle. Histamine causes arterioles and capillaries to dilate and increases capillary membrane permeability. Intravascular fluid leaks into the interstitial space, resulting in a decrease in intravascular volume. In addition, many of the mediators released cause constriction of both the upper and lower airways with the potential for complete airway obstruction (see Chapter 31).

Septic Shock

Septic shock most often results from a serious systemic bacterial infection. It is thought to be mediated through toxins that are either a part of the microorganism (endotoxin—gram-negative sepsis) or are released by the organism (exotoxin—gram-positive shock). These toxins stimulate the release of complex vasoactive agents that affect arterioles, capillaries, and venules, altering microcirculatory pressure and capillary permeability. Septic shock can result from staphylococcal and streptococcal infections, pneumonia, postoperative infections, and infections resulting from indwelling urinary catheters. Between 40,000 and 100,000 people develop septic shock each year. It most often is seen in older adults (particularly nursing home residents), alcoholics, neonates, and patients who are immunosuppressed (for example, patients with cancer, human immunodeficiency virus [HIV] infection, or sickle cell disease).

Stages of Shock

Hypoperfusion and its associated anaerobic metabolism are categorized by stages of the body's response to the shock syndrome. The three stages are (1) compensated shock, (2) uncompensated (or decompensated) shock, and (3) irreversible shock.[5] Table 19-1 lists the stages of shock and the signs and symptoms of each.

Compensated Shock

Compensated shock (Fig. 19-3) is associated with some decreased tissue perfusion, but the body's compensatory responses are sufficient to overcome the decrease in available fluid. An increase in catecholamine production maintains cardiac output and a normal systolic blood pressure.

The decrease in perfusion and subsequent increase in acidosis lead to a chemoreceptor response that increases the rate and depth of ventilation (to compensate for acidosis by decreasing PCO_2). Sympathetic stimulation increases heart rate and contractility, causes bronchodilation, leads to increases in peripheral vascular resistance, and decreases capillary flow in some capillary beds, such as the gastrointestinal tract. The patient may exhibit delayed capillary refill and cool skin as the blood is shunted to the vital organs. In spite of maintaining normal blood pressure and urinary output, some patients may exhibit signs of decreased CNS perfusion (lethargy, confusion, combativeness), even at this stage. If the underlying cause of shock is untreated, the compensatory mechanisms collapse.

TABLE 19-1	STAGES OF SHOCK		
SIGNS AND SYMPTOMS	**COMPENSATED SHOCK**	**UNCOMPENSATED SHOCK**	**IRREVERSIBLE SHOCK**
Heart rate	Mild tachycardia	Moderate tachycardia	Bradycardia, severe dysrhythmias
Level of consciousness	Lethargy, confusion, combativeness	Confusion, unconsciousness	Coma
Skin	Delayed capillary refill, cool skin	Delayed capillary refill, cold extremities, cyanosis	Pale, cold, clammy skin
Blood pressure	Normal or slightly elevated measurement	Decreased systolic and diastolic pressure	Frank hypotension

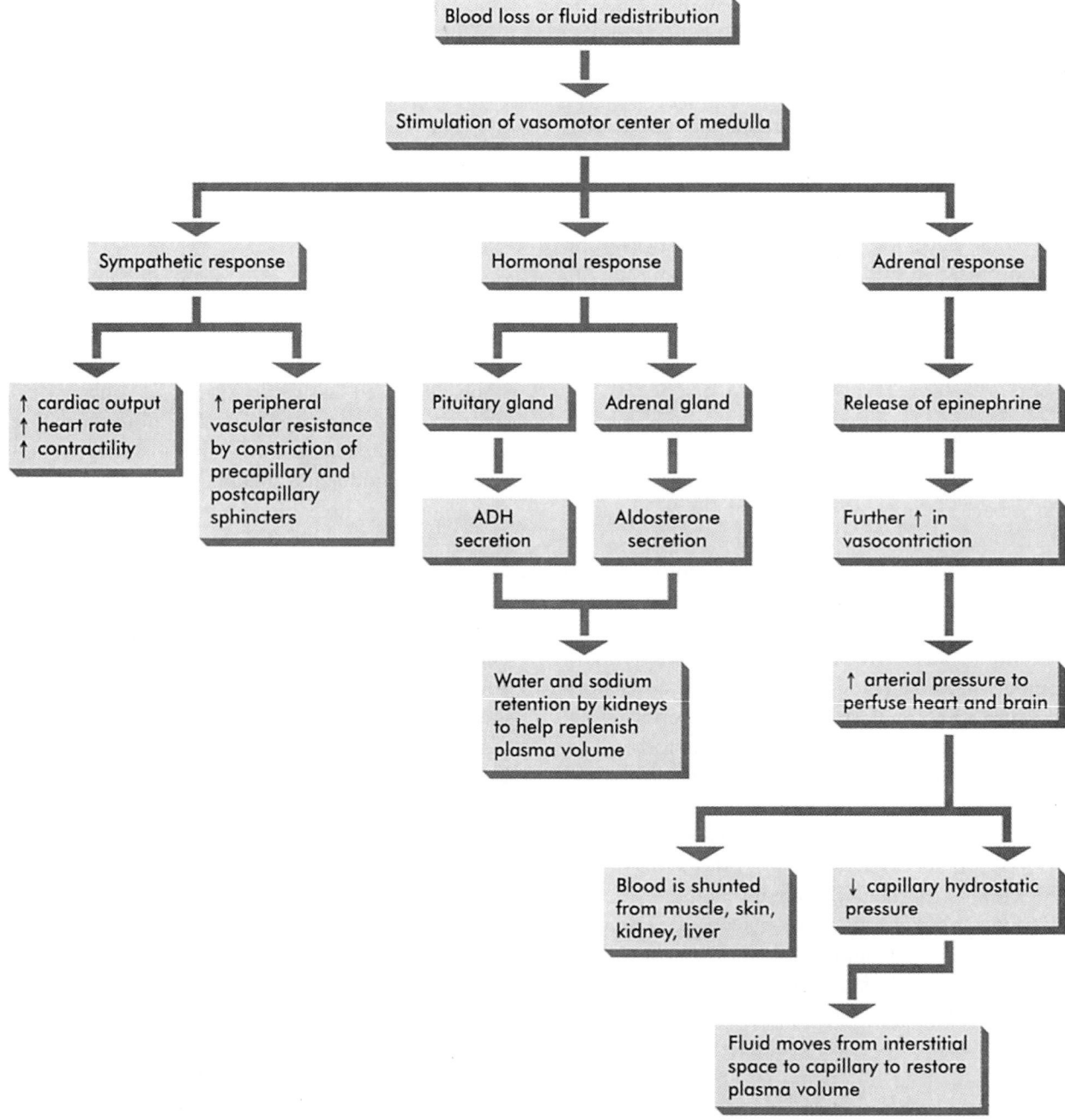

Fig. 19-3 Compensated shock. This stage of shock is reversible.

Uncompensated Shock

Uncompensated shock (Fig. 19-4) occurs when the body is no longer able to maintain systemic blood pressure. The systolic pressure usually drops before the diastolic pressure since it is more dependent on blood volume. Diastolic pressure may rise initially because of vasoconstriction. The decrease in systolic pressure, along with maintained or increased diastolic pressure, can lead to a very narrow pulse pressure. The pulse pressure can be narrowed to such an extent that it is not detectable with a blood pressure cuff.

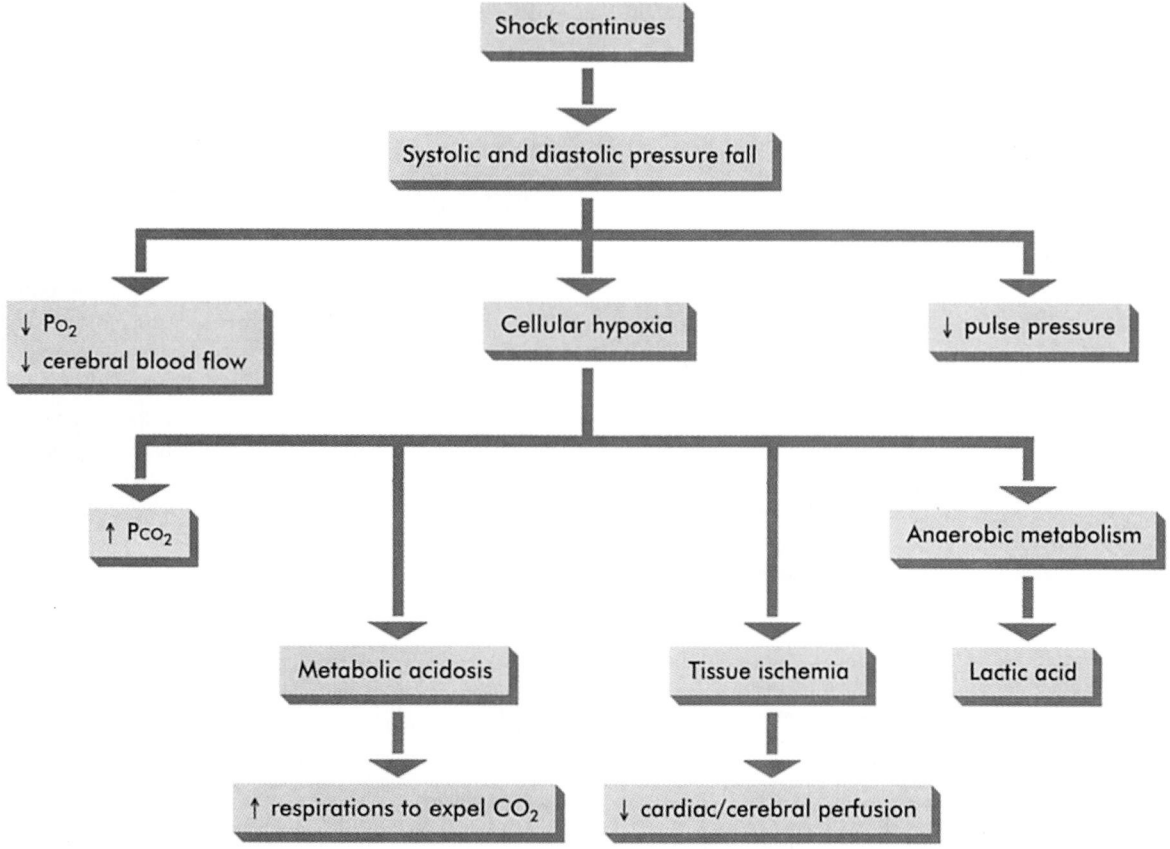

Fig. 19-4 Uncompensated shock. This stage of shock is reversible.

As the body's compensatory mechanisms begin to fail, both systolic and diastolic pressure drop and cerebral blood flow decreases. Po_2 may drop, but Pco_2 usually remains normal or low unless the patient has a head or chest injury that leads to hypoventilation. The clinical signs of uncompensated shock include hypotension, tachycardia, tachypnea, delayed capillary refill, and decreased urinary output (5 to 15 mL/hour). Shunting of blood and tissue hypoxia may cause the patient to have cold extremities and cyanosis. Effects on the cardiovascular system include a decreased preload and an increased rate of contraction secondary to catecholamine stimulation. Although myocardial contractions initially can be stronger as a result of catecholamine release, in the latter phases of uncompensated shock, myocardial strength may decrease as a result of the following factors:

1. Ischemia can result from a reduction of circulating red blood cells, a lower oxygen saturation (Po_2), and decreased coronary perfusion secondary to hypotension (especially diastolic hypotension).

2. Cardiodepressant substances (for example, myocardial toxin released from the ischemic pancreas) can depress heart function in late shock.

3. Necrosis of myocardium (essentially simulating myocardial infarction) can result from associated ischemia.

4. Decreased preload can lead to decreased contractility.

5. Acidosis can lead to decreased contractility.

6. Cardiac rhythm disturbances can result from hypoxia.

Irreversible Shock

The progression of cellular ischemia and necrosis and subsequent organ death, even with the restoration of oxygenation and perfusion, indicate the third stage of shock (Fig. 19-5). Despite a return to normal perfusion, patients with irreversible shock as a result of massive cellular damage do not survive. Cells and the vital organs begin to die from the lack of energy. The membrane pumps fail, and the various organelles in the cells sequentially break down, so necrosis is inevitable even if cell perfusion is restored.

Decompensation may occur suddenly, or it may be delayed from 1 day to 3 weeks after the onset of shock. The clinical signs of irreversible shock in-clude bradycardia; serious dysrhythmias; frank hy-potension; evidence of multiple organ failure; and pale, cold, and clammy skin. Cardiopulmonary col-lapse usually is imminent in these patients.

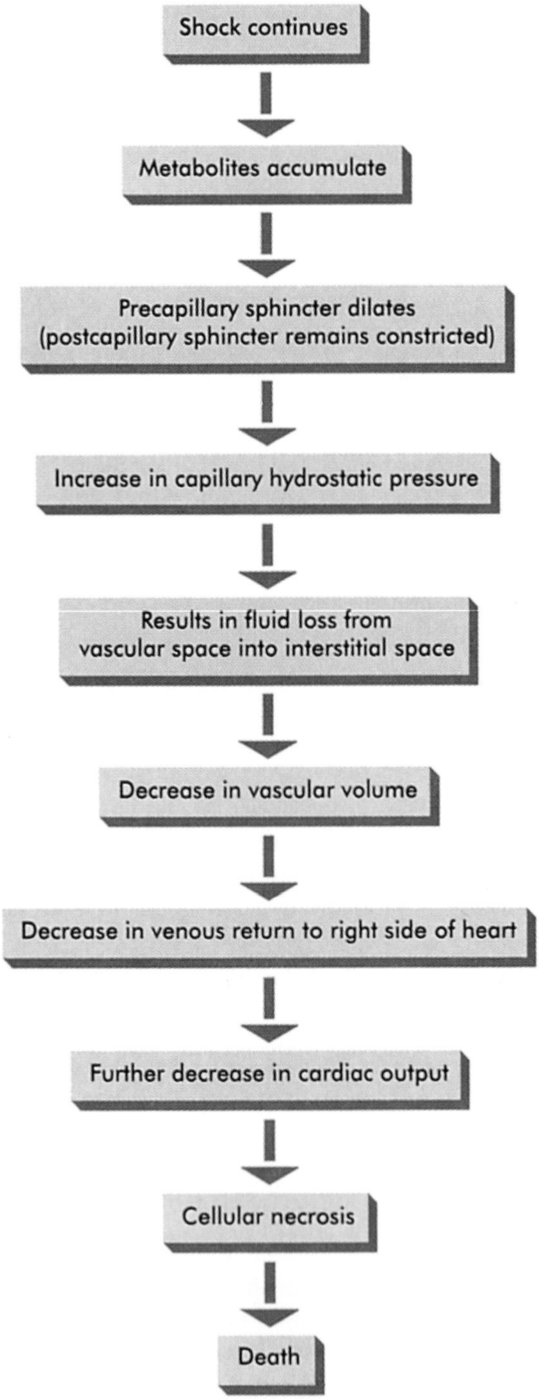

> **NOTE**
>
> During the prehospital management of shock, it is im-possible to distinguish between uncompensated and ir-reversible shock. Prehospital management of the shock victim should always focus on resuscitation, especially since irreversible shock is more a function of time than degree. Rapid resuscitation and transportation to an appropriate medical facility can abort the irreversible stage of shock.

> **NOTE**
>
> The use of large volumes of crystalloid in the field is con-troversial, especially in patients with ongoing hemor-rhage.[6,7] Several recent animal studies and controlled human trials suggest that minimal fluid resuscitation may be advantageous in patients with ongoing hemor-rhage. In these studies, the rapid control of hemorrhage and use of blood or blood products for volume expan-sion were associated with improved survival over those given fluid resuscitation. Medical direction and estab-lished protocol should guide fluid resuscitation for pa-tients in shock who are normotensive, hypotensive, or profoundly hypotensive.

Variations in Physiological Response to Shock

Many variations in physiological response occur among patients in shock. Determining factors in-clude the following:

- Age and relative health
  - Older adults, who are less able to compensate
  - Children, who compensate longer and deterio-rate faster
  - General physical condition
  - Preexisting disease

Fig. 19-5 Irreversible shock. Regardless of fluid replace-ment and an initial favorable response in blood pressure, death will ensue within 1 day to 3 weeks.

The flowchart depicts:

Shock continues → Metabolites accumulate → Precapillary sphincter dilates (postcapillary sphincter remains constricted) → Increase in capillary hydrostatic pressure → Results in fluid loss from vascular space into interstitial space → Decrease in vascular volume → Decrease in venous return to right side of heart → Further decrease in cardiac output → Cellular necrosis → Death

> **? CRITICAL THINKING**
>
> *What diseases can influence a patient's response to shock?*

- Ability to activate compensatory mechanisms
  - Medications, some of which can interfere with compensatory mechanisms
- Specific organ system affected

Management and Treatment Plan for the Shock Patient

The management and treatment plan for the patient in shock focuses on the assessment of oxygenation and perfusion of the body organs. The goals of the treatment plan are to ensure a patent airway, to provide adequate oxygenation and ventilation, and to restore perfusion.

Initial Assessment

The initial assessment can help identify the adequacy of cellular perfusion. The following five-step description of the initial assessment focuses on evaluating the shock victim, but the paramedic should be aware of common objectives in evaluating any patient with other types of serious illness or injury:

1. *Airway.* The airway must be opened and patency must be maintained to ensure adequate air movement.
2. *Breathing.* The respiratory pattern often reflects the adequacy of ventilation and can offer clues to the presence of shock. For example, if the patient is acidotic, the rate and depth of ventilation increase in an attempt to reduce carbon dioxide content of the blood and compensate for the metabolic acidosis.

? CRITICAL THINKING

Should you administer oxygen to a patient with early signs and symptoms of shock if the SaO$_2$ reading is normal?

---

3. *Circulation.* Evaluation of the patient's circulatory status should begin by assessing the patient for any uncontrolled arterial bleeding. In cases of external hemorrhage, control can almost always be obtained by applying direct pressure. (See Chapter 20 for methods to control external bleeding.) This usually suffices until the patient can be trans-

ported to the emergency department for definitive care. Pressure dressings (for example, bandages, a pneumatic antishock garment [PASG]) can be applied to control hemorrhage. If the paramedic suspects internal bleeding, rapid transportation to an appropriate medical facility is the highest priority after securing an airway and ensuring adequate ventilation. The paramedic should suspect internal bleeding in any trauma patient with signs of shock, especially those without evidence of external blood loss. It may become even more obvious on observation or palpation of the abdomen or pelvis.

NOTE

Treatment for internal hemorrhage must be directed at definitive care to stop the bleeding. Thus rapid transportation of the patient to an appropriate medical facility is of utmost importance. Studies suggest that application of the PASG is not indicated in the prehospital setting with the possible exception of pelvic fracture with hemodynamic instability or when prolonged transportation is anticipated.[1] As previously discussed, the use of crystalloid in the field in patients with acute hemorrhage is controversial. Most EMS systems are still initiating intravenous (IV) fluid therapy in the field with normal saline or lactated Ringer's solution, which should be performed en route to avoid a delay of definitive care.

The rate, character, and location of the patient's pulse should be evaluated as part of the circulatory assessment. Pulse rates increase fairly early in shock to help maintain an adequate cardiac output. The strength of contraction also may increase, but this often is negated by the decrease in preload. Tachycardia normally will not occur until the patient has suffered a 10% to 15% volume depletion (relative to container size) as a result of blood loss or an increase in container size. The character of the pulse can be strong or weak, which permits estimation of the effectiveness of the filling volume of the artery being palpated and an indirect measurement of systolic pressure. The paramedic also can use the location of the palpable pulse (described in Chapter 14) as an indirect measure of systolic pressure.

Tissue perfusion sometimes can be estimated by evaluating the skin's color, moisture, and temperature. These guidelines can be unreliable in patients exposed to extremes of temperature and in those suffering from septicemia and shock caused by neurological injury. Evaluation of the fingers and toes (the most distal points of circulation) is important, since these areas can be the first to indicate inadequate tissue perfusion. If ambient temperatures are moderate and tissue perfusion is adequate, these areas will be pink, warm, and dry.

The capillary refill test (described in Chapter 14) can offer useful information on the pediatric patient's tissue perfusion. These measurements should be used only as a guide because the accuracy of this test can be affected by environmental conditions and by the patient's general health, age, and gender.

4. *Disability*. Evaluation of the patient's level of consciousness is important in assessing cerebral oxygenation. The patient can become restless, agitated, and confused as cerebral ischemia develops. In addition to shock, cerebral edema and intracranial hemorrhage from head injury can compromise cerebral perfusion. Any significant alteration in the patient's sensorium should be considered an indicator of a critical perfusion deficit, whether it be from shock or from an increase in intracranial pressure. The patient's level of consciousness can be measured with the AVPU Scale or other evaluation methods (see Chapter 22).

NOTE

Some authorities contend that assessment of cerebral function is the best way to determine appropriate blood pressure for the trauma patient because the brain is the most sensitive organ to changes in physiological state. The goals of this patient-focused method of shock management are to ensure that systolic pressure is at least 90 mm Hg and that the patient has positive peripheral pulses and is awake or responsive to stimuli.[8]

---

5. *Exposure of the body surfaces*. The paramedic should expose the body surfaces in the initial assessment as indicated by scenario or mechanism of injury. Visual inspection can reveal life-threatening conditions hidden by clothing.

Differential Shock Assessment Findings

Although shock is assumed to be hypovolemic until proven otherwise, assessment findings that can help the paramedic differentiate between hypovolemic shock and other causes of shock include the following:

1. *Cardiogenic shock*. The patient often has a chief complaint of chest pain, dyspnea, or extreme heart rates (tachycardia, bradycardia, other dysrhythmias). Some patients also show signs of congestive heart failure such as jugular vein distention (described in Chapters 24 and 28).
2. *Distributive shock* (neurogenic shock, anaphylactic shock, septic shock). The patient's history or scene assessment may reveal a mechanism that suggests vasodilation. Signs and symptoms of distributive shock that are unusual in the presence of hypovolemic shock include warm flushed skin (especially in dependent areas), and those of neurogenic shock include a normal pulse rate (relative bradycardia).
3. *Obstructive shock (caused by obstruction to blood flow)*. These patients often are the victim of major chest injury (usually penetrating) or reveal a history that is consistent with pulmonary embolism (for example, recent surgery or long-bone fracture). Patients with cardiac tamponade or tension pneumothorax often have jugular vein distention. Patients with tension pneumothorax also almost always have decreased breath sounds on the affected side.

Detailed Physical Examination

After the initial assessment and management of any life-threatening conditions, the paramedic should evaluate the patient further. A systematic approach provides the means to evaluate potentially life-threatening conditions and to further assess the patient's perfusion status. This assessment should begin with baseline measurements of the patient's vital signs and evaluation of the patient's electrocardiogram.

? CRITICAL THINKING

Can blood donation cause a fluid deficit large enough to cause shock? If so, how is that fluid deficit managed?

The paramedic should expect the pulse rate to increase above normal limits after a fluid deficit of 10% to 15%. Some patients, however, continue to have normal pulse rates even though a volume deficit of this magnitude exists. Therefore the patient's pulse rate should only be considered one factor in evaluating the patient's level of perfusion.

Bradycardia, which can result from hypoxemia, concomitant neurological injury, increased vagal tone, preexisting illness, or prior medication use, also can indicate severe myocardial ischemia, a primary cause of cardiogenic shock. Bradycardic rhythms frequently occur just before cardiac arrest. Immediately after the paramedic notes a bradycardic rhythm, he or she should optimize oxygenation by increasing FiO_2 and assisting ventilations if necessary.

The diastolic pressure initially rises as peripheral vascular resistance increases with increased vascular tone. This decreases the container size and selectively shunts blood away from certain portions of the body. When the heart can no longer pump blood to keep the container full on the arterial side, the diastolic pressure begins to drop. The paramedic should expect this when the deficit in ratio of fluid to container size is greater than 20% to 25%.

The systolic pressure falls when the heart can no longer pump enough blood to fill the container at the end of cardiac contraction. Systolic pressure usually is more sensitive to volume depletion than is diastolic pressure and therefore drops first. However, as the fluid deficit approaches 25%, systolic and diastolic pressure both begin to drop.

The paramedic should consider evaluation of orthostatic vital signs in conscious patients suspected of being volume depleted, provided that he or she does not suspect spinal injury or another condition precluding this assessment. A rise from a recumbent position to a sitting or standing position associated with a fall in systolic pressure (after 1 minute) of 10 to 15 mm Hg and/or a concurrent rise in pulse rate (after 1 minute) of 10 to 15 beats per minute indicates a significant (at least 10%) volume depletion (postural hypotension) and a decrease in perfusion status.

A fluid deficit can still exist after the systolic pressure returns to normal after fluid replacement. Therefore fluid replacement initiated in the prehospital setting should continue until indicators of adequate tissue perfusion are present (for example, improved skin color, capillary refill of less than 2 seconds in pediatric patients, normal pulse oximetry readings).

Resuscitation

Resuscitation of the shock victim is aimed at restoring adequate peripheral tissue oxygenation as quickly as possible. As previously stated, the paramedic accomplishes this by ensuring adequate oxygenation, maintaining an effective ratio of volume to container size, and rapidly transporting the victim to an appropriate medical facility.

> **NOTE**
>
> Overresuscitation of trauma patients can occur. It is particularly important in patients with closed head injury or pulmonary or cardiac contusion to avoid "fluid overload." As previously stated, medical direction and established protocol should guide fluid resuscitation for the shock patient.

Red Blood Cell Oxygenation

Adequate oxygenation of red blood cells is a primary requirement for adequate tissue oxygenation. For red blood cell oxygenation to be adequate, the patient must have a patent airway and ventilation must be supported with a high FiO_2. If necessary, ventilation should be assisted with positive pressure. In addition, any abnormality that interferes with adequate ventilation (for example, obstructed airway, pneumothorax, hemothorax, open chest wound, unstable chest wall) should be corrected (see Chapter 24).

Ratio of Volume to Container Size

The second component needed to maintain adequate oxygen-carrying capacity requires that the container be full of fluid. The paramedic can accomplish this by decreasing the size of the container, especially in shock states not associated with hemorrhage. In addition, in some cases of distributive shock, vasoactive medications can be used to manage the shock when reduction of container size is the primary concern. Volume replacement also can be necessary in these patients.

> **NOTE**
>
> Vasoactive agents generally are not recommended to treat patients in hypovolemic shock until fluid volume replacement is complete, which rarely occurs in the prehospital setting.

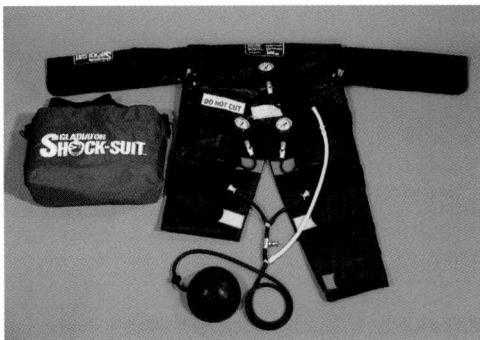

Fig. 19-6 JOBST Gladiator Shock Suit. (Courtesy Jobst Institute, Inc., Toledo, Ohio.)

Pneumatic Antishock Garment

The PASG (Fig. 19-6) is thought by some to be effective in managing shock through the following mechanisms[9]:

- The PASG reduces vessel diameter and artificially increases peripheral resistance in the tissues beneath the PASG, which maintains perfusion pressure to the patient's other vital organs.
- The PASG can arrest hemorrhage by tamponading any bleeding vessels in the abdomen, pelvis, or lower extremities.
- The PASG can help stabilize pelvic and lower-extremity fractures when inflated, thus decreasing movement and subsequent blood loss.

Although decisions on the use of the PASG are left to local protocol and medical direction, pulmonary edema, cardiogenic shock, ruptured diaphragm, and hemorrhage within the chest cavity generally are considered contraindications for the PASG.[2,9] Some medical direction authorities feel that use of a PASG also is contraindicated in the following situations:

- Impaled objects in the abdomen (precluding inflation of the abdominal section of the garment)
- Advanced pregnancy (third trimester pregnancy precludes inflation of the abdominal compartment)
- Evisceration (no inflation of the abdominal compartment)

> **NOTE**
>
> The benefits of a PASG have been questioned by the scientific community. The paramedic should follow the recommendations of medical direction regarding the use of this device.

General PASG guidelines. The paramedic should apply the PASG when indicated after the lower extremities and abdomen have been inspected for major wounds. He or she must always position the garment below the level of the patient's lowest rib, and the patient's blood pressure and lung sounds should be monitored before, during, and after inflation. The paramedic should stop inflation when an adequate blood pressure has been obtained. He or she must inflate the leg compartments before or with the abdominal compartment. *The paramedic should never inflate the abdominal compartment before the leg compartments.* Doing so can cause the abdominal compartment to act as a constrictive band that reduces venous return from the legs.

> **? CRITICAL THINKING**
>
> *What effect can inflation of the abdominal compartment of the PASG before the leg segments have on cardiac output?*

After PASG inflation, the garment should seldom if ever be deflated in the prehospital setting and only with a physician's direction. The abdominal compartment is deflated before the leg compartments. The patient should be closely monitored during the deflation process because removal of the garment before fluid replacement commonly results in a rapid fall of blood pressure and cardiac output, which can lead to cardiac arrest.

Changes in environmental temperature and atmospheric pressure can cause a significant fluctuation in the pressure within the PASG. The paramedic should constantly monitor the patient when moved from a cold environment to a warm one or when transported by air. The relationship among temperature, atmospheric pressure, and pressure within the PASG is as follows:

- A rise in temperature raises the pressure within the PASG, and a fall in temperature decreases the pressure.
- A fall in atmospheric pressure causes an increase in PASG pressure, and a rise in atmospheric pressure produces a decrease in garment pressure.

The PASG is not without complications even with appropriate use. Sustained inflation of the garment for more than 1 to 2 hours can lead to decreased tissue perfusion, ischemia of the underlying tissues (including the development of compartment syndrome[10]), and loss of the limb, even without underlying fracture.

Fluid Resuscitation in Shock

Almost every shock victim, with the exception of patients in cardiogenic shock, requires volume expanders as part of resuscitation. The selection of IV fluids for initial volume replacement varies according to medical direction. In prehospital care, the most common emergency requiring fluid replacement is volume depletion secondary to hemorrhage or dehydration. The type of fluid replacement needed depends on the nature and extent of the volume loss (Box 19-2). The two main categories of fluids used in resuscitation are crystalloids and colloids.

> **NOTE**
>
> As previously stated, recent studies have questioned the practice of aggressive fluid resuscitation in uncontrolled hemorrhage associated with major trauma. These findings suggest that aggressive crystalloid fluid resuscitation can worsen hemorrhage by diluting clotting factors and increasing blood pressure. The paramedic should follow the recommendations for fluid resuscitation provided by medical direction.

Crystalloids. Crystalloid solutions are created by dissolving crystals such as salts and sugars in water. These solutions do not have as much osmotic pressure as colloid solutions and can be expected to equilibrate more quickly between the vascular and extravascular spaces. Two thirds of the infused crystalloid fluid leaves the vascular space within 1 hour, so 3 mL of a crystalloid solution is needed to replace 1 mL of blood. Examples of crystalloid solutions are lactated Ringer's solution, normal saline, and glucose solutions in water.

Hypertonic solutions have higher osmotic pressure than that of body cells and include 5% dextrose in 0.9% sodium chloride, 7.5% saline, and 5% dextrose in 0.45% sodium chloride. Hypotonic solutions have a lower osmotic pressure than that of body cells (for example, distilled water and 0.45% sodium chloride [0.45% NaCl]).

Lactated Ringer's solution is the fluid of choice for resuscitating patients in shock. It is a well-balanced solution containing many of the chemicals

> **BOX 19-2**
>
> ## FLUID RESUSCITATION IN SHOCK
>
> ### Crystalloids
> - Hypertonic sodium chloride
> - Hypotonic sodium chloride
> - Balanced salt solutions (isotonic)
>   - Lactated Ringer's solution
>   - Normal saline
>
> ### Colloids
> - Blood
>   - Typed and crossmatched
>   - Type-specific
>   - Packed red blood cells
> - Plasma
> - Plasma substitutes
>   - Dextran
>   - Hetastarch (Hespan)
>   - Plasma protein fraction (Plasmonate)

> **NOTE**
>
> Strong consideration is being given to the use of small 250-mL boluses of hypertonic saline solutions instead of large volumes of isotonic crystalloids in resuscitating patients in shock. The increased osmolar state found in the hypertonic solution draws fluid into the vessels from the interstitial spaces and requires only small amounts to improve blood pressure. Another advantage to hypertonic solutions is packaging; the bags are significantly smaller and lighter.

found in human blood. Lactated Ringer's solution contains sodium chloride, small amounts of potassium and calcium, and 28 mEq of lactate, which can act as a buffer to neutralize acidity when metabolized by the liver. One third of the infused solution remains in the vascular space after 1 hour.

Normal saline contains 154 mEq/L of sodium and has no buffering capabilities. Although preferred by some physicians, the higher chloride content of normal saline is less desirable than the more balanced lactated Ringer's solution. As in lactated Ringer's solution, nearly one third of the infused normal saline remains in the vascular space after 1 hour, making it an equally effective volume expander. Studies have not shown superiority of one option over the other.

Glucose-containing solutions (for example, D5W) have immediate volume expansion effects, but the glucose leaves the intravascular compartment rapidly with a resultant free water increase. The volume-replacement benefits of glucose solutions only last 5 to 10 minutes while the glucose is metabolized, so its use as a replacement fluid in volume deficits is inappropriate. Glucose solutions are most often used to maintain vascular access for administration of IV medications.

> **NOTE**
>
> D5W is an isotonic solution. When administered, however, the dextrose molecules leave the circulation so rapidly that its effect is that of a hypotonic solution.

Colloids. Colloid solutions contain molecules (usually protein) that are too large to pass through the capillary membrane. These solutions exhibit osmotic pressure and remain within the vascular compartment for a considerable time. Examples of colloid solutions are whole blood, plasma, packed red blood cells, and plasma substitutes. Whole blood, packed red blood cells, and plasma generally are reserved for in-hospital use.

Whole blood replacement is sometimes indicated after initial fluid resuscitation with a crystalloid solution in patients who have had a major loss of blood. Whole blood replacement rarely is given. Rather, packed red cells are transfused, and other blood components are transfused as necessary. Whole blood is drawn in a citrate solution to prevent clotting and is refrigerated until needed. According to blood bank regulations, the blood can be stored up to 3 weeks in refrigeration, but clotting factors and platelets deplete progressively. A type and crossmatch should be obtained when possible before a patient is given blood to determine the patient's ABO group and Rh type (described in Chapter 7) and to determine if other antibodies are present that can cause a transfusion reaction.

Centrifugation separates packed red blood cells from the plasma component of blood. Like whole blood, packed red cells must be typed and crossmatched and can be refrigerated for up to 3 weeks. The advantage of packed red blood cells over whole blood is that the volume of hemoglobin per unit is almost twice that of whole blood. In addition, because there is no plasma, circulatory overload is less likely, transfusion reactions are less frequent, and transfusion hepatitis is less common.

> **NOTE**
>
> Several types of blood transfusion reactions can occur during or up to 96 hours after infusion. Symptoms range from mild fever to life-threatening shock. If a reaction is suspected (for example, during an interhospital transfer), the paramedic should stop the transfusion and contact medical direction.

Blood plasma is procured by separating the blood cells from the whole citrated blood. Blood plasma, which can be given without concern for ABO compatibility, contains fibrinogen, albumin, gamma globulins, hemoagglutinins (an agglutinin that clumps red blood corpuscles), prothrombin (a chemical that is part of the clotting cascade, the precursor of thrombin), other clotting factors, sugars, and salts. Blood plasma sometimes is used to restore effective blood volume in patients with circulatory failure associated with burns, traumatic shock, and hemorrhage. It more commonly is used to correct clotting deficiencies.

Although plasma substitutes do not increase oxygen-carrying capacity by replacing red blood cells nor improve clotting by the addition of plasma protein, they sometimes are used to restore circulating blood volume as an emergency treatment for hypovolemia caused by blood loss. Plasma substitutes such as dextran, plasma protein fraction, and hetastarch have osmotic properties similar to those of plasma. They therefore stay in the intravascular space longer than crystalloid solution. Plasma substitutes do not carry the HIV or hepatitis viruses, do not require typing and crossmatching before admin-

> **NOTE**
>
> Studies of experimental solutions for volume replacement associated with severe hemorrhage are underway. These blood substitutes contain hemoglobin from red blood cells (treated to destroy viruses). The solutions do not have toxic effects associated with free hemoglobin, do not require typing or crossmatching, can be stored up to several months, and can have future application in the prehospital setting.

istration, and are readily available. Their use is appealing, particularly in mass casualty situations when blood products are scarce because susceptible patients can be allergic to some plasma substitutes. However, they do have adverse effects, including increased bleeding tendencies and immune suppression. Emergency vehicles can carry plasma substitutes, but expense and storage problems make them impractical for general use in the prehospital setting.

Theory of fluid flow. The flow of fluid through a catheter is directly related to its diameter (to the fourth power) and inversely related to its length. Therefore a catheter with a large diameter has a much greater flow than a catheter with a small diameter; short catheters provide somewhat faster flow rates than longer catheters of equal diameter. Other factors that affect the flow of fluid include the diameter and length of the tubing, the size of the vein, and the viscosity and temperature of the IV fluid. (Viscosity is affected by temperature; warm fluids generally flow better than cold ones.) Pressure bags are available that pressurize the IV system to 300 mm Hg to maximize the rate of fluid administration. Table 19-2 lists the maximum rate of fluid flow for various gauges of 2-inch Medicut catheters without pressure on the bag at a height of 1 meter above the patient.[11] When aggressive fluid resuscitation is indicated, the paramedic should do the following:

- Use short, large-diameter catheters.
- Use warm fluids of low viscosity (if possible).
- Keep the tubing short, and pressurize the IV system.

? CRITICAL THINKING

Aside from flow, what other advantages do warmed fluids offer for the patient in shock who requires a large-volume fluid bolus?

Key Principles in Managing Shock

The paramedic should follow these key principles as part of the plan for managing shock:

1. Establish and maintain an open airway.
2. Administer high-concentration oxygen, and assist ventilation as needed.
3. Control external bleeding (if present).

TABLE 19-2	NEEDLE GAUGES AND MAXIMUM FLUID FLOW

NEEDLE GAUGE (I.D.)	MAXIMUM FLUID FLOW
18 gauge	4.81 L/hr or 80 mL/min
16 gauge	7.45 L/hr or 124 mL/min
14 gauge	9.67 L/hr or 161 mL/min

4. By order of medical direction or per protocol, initiate IV fluid replacement if appropriate. Two large-bore IV lines of a volume-expanding fluid commonly are established in cases of hypovolemia. *The administration of IV fluids in the prehospital setting should not delay patient transportation because crystalloid solutions cannot restore the oxygen-carrying capacity of blood.* Generally, the patient is best served by rapid assessment, airway stabilization, immobilization, and rapid transportation to an appropriate medical facility. Many EMS authorities recommend that IV therapy for shock resuscitation be initiated en route to the hospital.
5. Consider use of a PASG (per protocol), especially if transportation time is long, pelvic fractures are suspected, or a patient is deteriorating despite IV therapy.
6. Maintain the patient's normal body temperature. Patients in shock often are unable to conserve body heat and easily become hypothermic.
7. In the absence of spinal or head injury and if hypovolemia is suspected and ventilation is adequate, consider positioning the patient in the modified Trendelenburg position (legs elevated 15 to 18 inches).
8. Monitor cardiac rhythm and oxygen saturation.
9. Frequently reassess vital signs en route to the emergency department.

Management of Specific Forms of Shock

In addition to the general management appropriate to all victims of shock, certain management guidelines are specific to each etiological classification.

Hypovolemic shock. The management of hypovolemic shock is not considered complete until the circulatory deficit and its cause or causes are corrected. This includes crystalloid fluid replacement in cases of simple dehydration or volume replacement resulting from hemorrhage, definitive surgery, critical care support, and postoperative rehabilitation.

Cardiogenic shock. The management of cardiogenic shock focuses on improving the pumping action of the heart and managing cardiac rhythm irregularities. The paramedic should initiate fluid resuscitation in the adult with 100 to 200 mL of a volume-expanding fluid, as long as the patient has no crackles in the lung fields, which would indicate pulmonary edema. If the patient improves, fluid therapy should continue cautiously until the blood pressure stabilizes and the pulse rate decreases. The paramedic should assess lung sounds frequently. If the patient shows signs of increased lung congestion, the paramedic should adjust the rate of infusion to keep the vein open.

Drug therapy for cardiogenic shock varies according to cause and can include vasopressors, vasodilators, inotropic drugs, and antidysrhythmics (usually after fluid infusion) (see Chapter 28). Patients with cardiogenic shock secondary to myocardial ischemia or infarction require reperfusion strategies and possible circulatory support (for example, intraaortic balloon pump). The paramedic must manage obstructive causes of cardiogenic shock immediately, including tension pneumothorax and cardiac tamponade (see Chapter 24).

Neurogenic shock. The management of neurogenic shock is similar to the management for hypovolemia. However, the paramedic must take care during fluid therapy to avoid circulatory overload. Throughout the resuscitation phase, the paramedic should closely monitor the patient's lung sounds for signs of pulmonary congestion. In addition, patients in neurogenic shock may respond to the administration of vasopressors (for example, *dopamine* [Intropin]).

Anaphylactic shock. Subcutaneous administration of *epinephrine* (Adrenalin) is the treatment of choice in acute anaphylactic reactions. Depending on the severity of reaction, other treatment modalities can include oral, IV, or intramuscular administration of antihistamines such as *diphenhydramine* (Benadryl). The paramedic can initiate bronchodilators to treat bronchospasm and steroids to reduce the inflammatory response.

Crystalloid volume replacement also is indicated to compensate for the increased container size caused by vasodilation that results from histamine release during an anaphylactic reaction. Paramedics should anticipate the need for aggressive airway management in any allergic reaction (see Chapter 31).

Septic shock. The management of septic shock in the prehospital setting can include the management of hypovolemia (if present) and the correction of metabolic acid-base imbalance. Depending on the patient's response to the infection, prehospital care may involve fluid resuscitation, respiratory support, and the administration of vasopressors to improve cardiac output. If possible, the paramedic should obtain a thorough patient history to help identify the septic focus. There is an increased risk of septic shock in any immunocompromised group, such as those with HIV infection, some cancer patients receiving chemotherapy, and patients with indwelling urinary or vascular catheters.

Integration of Patient Assessment and the Treatment Plan

The goals of prehospital care for the patient with severe hemorrhage or shock include rapid recognition of the event, initiation of treatment, prevention of additional injury, rapid transport to an appropriate medical facility by ground or air ambulance, and advanced notification of the receiving facility. The paramedic should follow guidelines established by local protocol and medical direction in determining the appropriate prehospital level of care for patients and in identifying the appropriate medical facility for patient transport.

S U M M A R Y

- The seriousness of external hemorrhage depends on the anatomical source of the hemorrhage, the degree of vascular disruption, and the amount of blood loss that can be tolerated by the patient. Internal bleeding that can cause instability usually occurs in one of three body cavities: the chest, abdomen, or retroperitoneum.

- Shock is not a single entity with a specific cause and treatment but rather a complex group of physiological abnormalities that can result from a variety of disease states and injuries.

- To achieve adequate oxygenation of tissue cells (perfusion), three distinct components of the cardiovascular system must function properly: the heart, vasculature, and lungs.

- The healthy body is a smooth-flowing fluid delivery system inside a container. The volume of the container is directly related to the diameter of the resistance vessels, which can change rapidly.

- Normal adult blood volume is 4.5 to 5 liters.

- The progression of shock in the microcirculation follows a sequence of stages related to changes in capillary perfusion and cellular necrosis. These stages include vasoconstriction, capillary and venule opening, disseminated intravascular coagulation (DIC), and multiple organ failure.

- A common classification of shock for use in emergency care is to describe the syndrome based on the initiating cause (hypovolemic, cardiogenic, neurogenic, anaphylactic, or septic).

- Hypoperfusion and its associated anaerobic metabolism can be categorized by stages of the body's response to the shock syndrome. The three component stages are compensated shock, uncompensated (or decompensated) shock, and irreversible shock.

- Variations in physiological response to shock can occur based on the patient's age and relative health, his or her ability to activate compensatory mechanisms, and the specific organ affected.

- The management and treatment plan for the patient in shock focuses on the assessment of oxygenation and perfusion of the body organs. The goals of the treatment plan are to ensure a patent airway, to provide adequate oxygenation and ventilation, and to restore perfusion. The initial survey can help identify the adequacy of cellular perfusion.

◼ REFERENCES

1. Rosen P, Barkin R: *Emergency medicine: concepts and clinical practice*, ed 4, St Louis, 1999, Mosby.
2. Mann FC: Systems of surgery, *Bull John Hopkins Hospital* 25:205, 1914.
3. Hardaway R, editor: *Shock: the reversible stage of dying*, Littleton, Mass, 1988, PSG Publishing.
4. American Heart Association: *Advanced cardiac life support*, Dallas, 1997, The Association.
5. US Department of Transportation, National Highway Traffic Safety Administration: *EMT-Paramedic national standard curriculum*, Washington, DC, 1998, The Department.
6. Owens T et al: Limiting initial resuscitation of uncontrolled hemorrhage reduced internal bleeding and subsequent volume requirements, *J Trauma* 39(2):209, 1995.
7. Dalton A: Prehospital intravenous fluid replacement in trauma: an outmoded concept? *J R Soc Med* 88(4): 213P, 1995.
8. Criss E: Trauma management in the new millennium, *JEMS* 24(12):34, 1999.
9. National Association of Emergency Medical Technicians: *PHTLS: basic and advanced prehospital trauma life support*, ed 4, St Louis, 1999, Mosby.
10. Chisholm C, Clark D: Effect of the pneumatic antishock garment on intramuscular pressure, *Ann Emerg Med* 13(8):581, 1984.
11. Haynes B et al: Catheter introducers for rapid fluid resuscitation, *Ann Emerg Med* 12(10):606, 1983.

20 Soft Tissue Trauma

OBJECTIVES

Upon completion of this chapter, the paramedic student will be able to:

1. *Describe the normal structure and function of the skin.*

2. *Describe the pathophysiologic responses to soft tissue injury.*

3. *Discuss pathophysiology as a basis for key signs and symptoms, and describe the mechanism of injury and signs and symptoms of specific soft tissue injuries.*

4. *Outline management principles for prehospital care of soft tissue injuries.*

5. *Describe, in the correct sequence, patient management techniques for control of hemorrhage.*

6. *Identify the characteristics of general categories of dressings and bandages.*

7. *Describe prehospital management of specific soft tissue injuries not requiring closure.*

8. *Discuss factors that increase the potential for wound infection.*

9. *Describe the prehospital management of selected soft tissue injuries.*

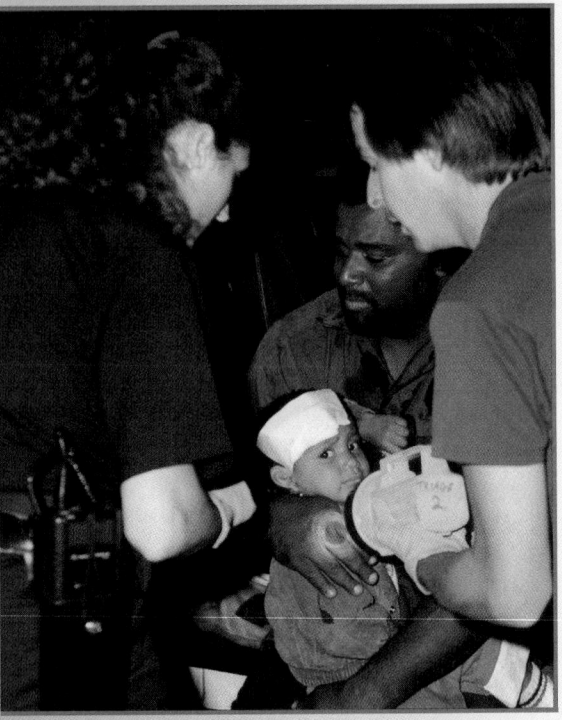

The skin and its accessory organs are the primary cosmetic structures of the body and perform many functions that are critical to survival. The paramedic must thoroughly understand soft tissue trauma to quickly assess life-threatening injury and to intervene to promote normal healing and function.

KEY TERMS

abrasion: A partial-thickness injury caused by scraping or rubbing away of a layer or layers of skin.

amputation: A complete or partial loss of a limb secondary to mechanical force.

avulsion: A full-thickness skin loss in which the wound edges cannot be approximated.

compartment syndrome: The result of a crush injury, usually caused by compressive forces or blunt trauma to muscle groups confined in tight fibrous sheaths with minimal ability to stretch.

crush injury: Injury from exposure of tissue to a compressive force sufficient to interfere with the normal structure and metabolic function of the involved cells and tissues.

crush syndrome: A life-threatening and sometimes preventable complication of prolonged immobilization; a pathologic process that causes destruction, alteration, or both, of muscle tissue.

hematoma: A closed injury characterized by blood vessel disruption and swelling beneath the epidermis.

puncture wound: An open injury that results from contact with a penetrating object.

rhabdomyolysis: An acute, sometimes fatal, disease characterized by destruction of skeletal muscle.

NOTE

Each year about 35 million people in the United States seek care in emergency departments for soft tissue injuries that result from falls, motor vehicle crashes, blunt and penetrating trauma, and burns. Although most soft tissue injuries are not life threatening, more than 63,000 people died as a result of these injuries in 1998[1] (see the Injury Prevention section in Appendix C).

Anatomy and Physiology

The skin is a tough, supple membrane that covers the entire body. It constitutes the largest and most dynamic organ of the body, covering more than 20 square feet and comprising 16% of total body weight. The skin comprises two distinct layers of tissue: the outer layer (epidermis) and the inner layer (dermis) (Fig. 20-1).

Epidermis

The epidermis is a thin, avascular epithelial tissue that derives its nourishment from the capillaries of the dermis. Although it is only as thick as a page of this text, the epidermis is composed of five layers: stratum basale, the innermost layer; stratum spinosum; stratum granulosum; stratum lucidum; and stratum corneum, the most superficial layer of the epidermis. The stratum corneum is composed of about 20 layers of dead skin cells that are filled with the waterproofing protein keratin.

Dermis

The dermis lies beneath the epidermis and contains connective tissue, elastic fibers, blood vessels, lymph vessels, and motor and sensory fibers. The dermis also houses other structures of the integumentary system, including hair, nails, and sebaceous and sweat glands. This layer of skin provides protection against bacterial invasion and helps maintain fluid balance.

Connective tissue and elastic fibers in the dermis give skin its strength and elasticity. Blood vessels in the dermis nourish all skin cells and aid in body temperature regulation through vasoconstriction or vasodilation. Nerves in the dermis generate impulses to dermal muscles and glands. These nerves also are responsible for carrying impulses away from sensory receptors in the skin in response to pain, touch, heat, and cold.

? CRITICAL THINKING

Predict the consequences of destruction of a large segment of skin, including the dermis, based on your knowledge of its functions.

573

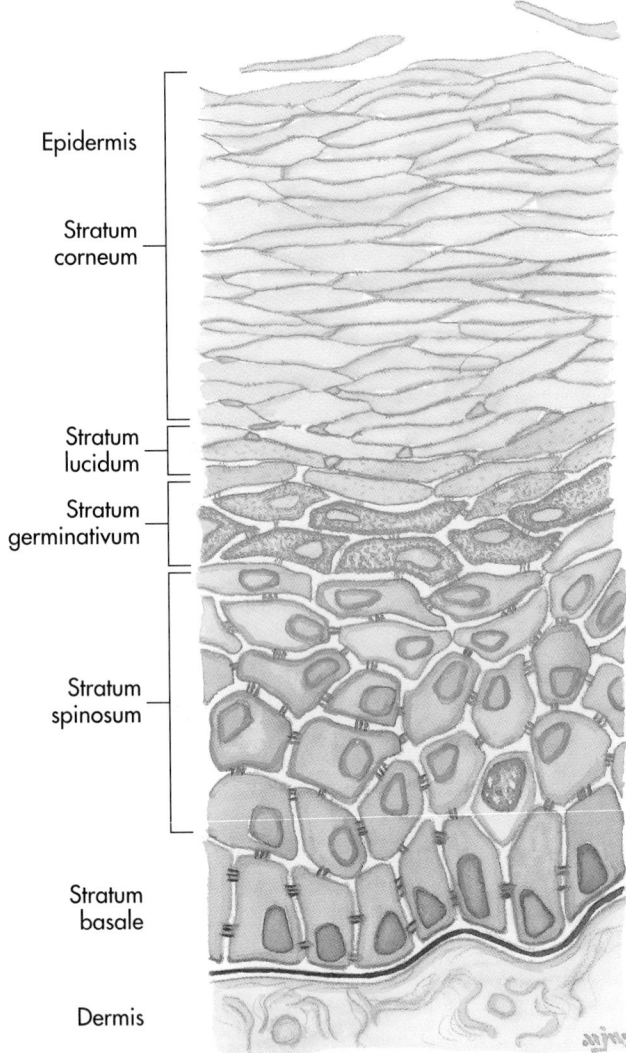

Epidermis

Stratum
corneum

Stratum
lucidum

Stratum
germinativum

Stratum
spinosum

Stratum
basale

Dermis

Fig. 20-1 Tissue layers of the skin.

> **NOTE**
>
> The dermis has a reservoir of defensive and regenerative elements that combat infection and repair deep wounds by use of specialized white blood cells, lymphatics, and other cellular components.

The dense layer of fibrous tissue (deep fascia) beneath the dermis provides for insulation, cushioning, caloric reserve, and body substance and shape. The primary function of this tissue is to support and protect underlying structures.

Pathophysiology

Surface trauma can interfere with the normal preservation of body fluids and electrolytes and with the maintenance of body temperature. The two physiologic responses to surface trauma are vascular and inflammatory reactions that can lead to healing, scar formation, or both. The extent and success of these responses are influenced by the amount of tissue disruption.

Hemostasis of Wound Healing

As described in Chapter 19, hemostasis is the initial physiologic response to wounding. This vascular reaction involves vasoconstriction, formation of a platelet plug, coagulation, and the growth of fibrous tissue into the blood clot that permanently closes and seals the injured vessel.

Vasoconstriction secondary to injury is rapid but temporary. In response to injury, severed blood vessels constrict and retract with the aid of the surrounding subcutaneous tissues. This vessel spasm slows blood loss immediately and may completely close the ends of the injured vessels. The vasoconstriction response typically is sustained for as long as 10 minutes, during which time blood coagulation mechanisms are activated to produce a blood clot.

Platelets adhere to injured blood vessels and to collagen in the connective tissue that surrounds the injured vessel. As platelets contact collagen, they swell, become sticky, and secrete chemicals that activate other surrounding platelets. This process causes the platelets to adhere to one another and creates a "platelet plug" in the injured vessel. If the opening in the vessel wall is small, the plug may be sufficient to stop blood loss completely. For larger wounds, however, a blood clot is necessary to arrest the flow of blood (Fig. 20-2).

Blood coagulation occurs as a result of a chemical process that begins within seconds of a severe vessel injury and within 1 to 2 minutes of a minor wound. Coagulation progresses rapidly; within 3 to 6 minutes after the rupture of a vessel, the entire end of the vessel is filled with a clot. Within 30 minutes the clot retracts and the vessel is further sealed. The blood-clotting mechanism is a complex biologic process that includes the following three mechanisms:

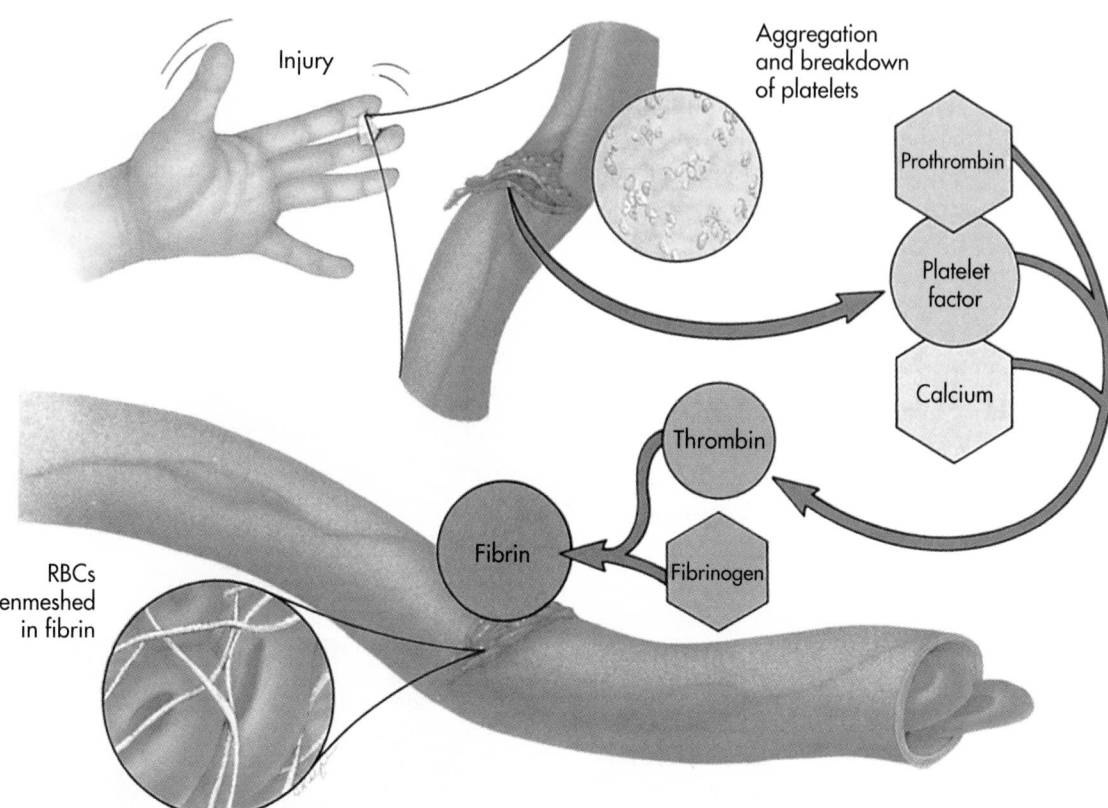

Fig. 20-2 The complex clotting mechanism can be distilled into three basic steps: release of platelet factors at the injury site, formation of thrombin, and trapping of red blood cells in fibrin to form a clot. (From Thibodeau GA, Patton KT: *Structure and function of the body,* ed 9, St Louis, 1992, Mosby.)

1. Prothrombin activator is formed in response to rupture or damage of the blood vessel.
2. Prothrombin activator stimulates the conversion of prothrombin to thrombin.
3. Thrombin acts as an enzyme to convert fibrinogen into fibrin threads that entrap platelets, blood cells, and plasma to form the clot.

? CRITICAL THINKING

List some drugs that may impair the normal clotting functions.

NOTE

The process of hemostasis usually is protective and is necessary for survival. In some instances, however, hemostasis can result in responses that threaten life and function. For example, blood clots that form in atherosclerotic vessels can lead to myocardial infarction or stroke.

Certain diseases or genetic factors that interrupt the clotting cascade can impair hemostasis, thereby retarding the process of clot formation. Examples include hemophilia, thrombocytopenia (low platelet count), and liver disease, which affects the production of clotting factors. Various medications also can impair coagulation. *Aspirin* decreases platelet activity, and warfarin (Coumadin) suppresses the liver's ability to make certain clotting factors. In any patient with impaired hemostasis, even minor trauma can result in uncontrollable and life-threatening hemorrhage.

Inflammatory Response

The release of chemicals from the injured vessel and various blood components (platelets, white blood cells) causes localized vasodilation of arterioles, precapillary sphincters, and venules, increasing the permeability of the affected capillaries and vessels. Plasma, plasma proteins, electrolytes, and chemical substances from the leaking venules accumulate in the extracellular space for about 72 hours after the injury. Blood flow increases to the area of injury to supply the metabolic demands of the tissues during healing and results in the redness, swelling, and pain associated with inflammation.

The transportation of granulocytes, lymphocytes, and macrophages to the injured area also increases local blood flow. These specialized cells prepare the wound for eventual healing by clearing foreign bodies and dead tissue, and they trigger neovascularization (new vessel formation). Within 12 hours of the injury, new epithelial cells are regenerated (the epithelialization phase) and begin the process of healing through reestablishment of skin layers.

Collagen is the principal structural protein of most body tissues. The normal repair of tissues depends on collagen synthesis and deposition. In the healthy body, fibroblasts synthesize and deposit collagen within 48 hours after injury. Collagen increases the tensile strength of the tissue, but most injured tissue will not regain its full strength and function until at least 4 months later.[2]

Alterations of Wound Healing

Many factors can affect or alter wound healing, including anatomic factors, concurrent drug use, medical condition and disease, and high-risk wounds.

Anatomic Factors

Some tissues of the body heal better and faster than others because of body region and skin tension lines. The elasticity of the skin and various forces (lines of tension) vary in different areas of the body and are affected by muscular contraction and movements of flexion and extension, thereby affecting wound healing and scar formation. For example, a soft tissue injury to the forearm generally will heal better and faster than one located over a joint. Other anatomic factors that may adversely affect wound healing and scar formation include oily skin and pigmentation.

Concurrent Drug Use, Existing Medical Conditions, and Disease

A patient's concurrent drug use and existing medical conditions or disease can delay or interfere with the normal wound-healing process through various mechanisms. Common drugs that can alter wound healing include corticosteroids, nonsteroidal antiinflammatory drugs (NSAIDs; *aspirin*), penicillin, colchicine, anticoagulants, and antineoplastic agents. Medical conditions and diseases that can result in delayed healing include the following:

- Advanced age
- Severe alcoholism
- Acute uremia
- Diabetes
- Hypoxia
- Peripheral vascular disease (PVD)
- Malnutrition
- Advanced cancer
- Hepatic failure
- Cardiovascular disease

✓ TRICKS OF THE TRADE

Patients who have diabetes, especially elderly patients, are particularly susceptible to poor wound healing. Always ask these patients about wounds and skin sores that are slow to heal.

High-Risk Wounds

High-risk wounds have an increased potential for infection because of the location of the wound or the nature of the wounding force. Examples of high-risk wounds include those located on or near the hands, feet, and perineal areas. Wound forces that are associated with a high risk for infection include those produced by human and animal bites, foreign bodies, and injection (for example, high-pressure grease guns). Other high-risk wounds are those contaminated with organic material or that have significant devitalized tissue; crush wounds; and any wounds in patients who are immunocompromised or who have poor peripheral circulation.

✓ TRICKS OF THE TRADE

High-pressure grease gun injuries often look minor but are very serious wounds. These injuries need to be evaluated by a physician.

Abnormal Scar Formation

Abnormal scar formation can result in a keloid or hypertrophic scar. A keloid is the excessive accumulation of scar tissue that extends beyond the original wound borders. This abnormal scar is more common in darkly pigmented patients and in those who have injuries to the ears, upper extremities, lower abdomen, or sternum. A hypertrophic scar has an excess accumulation of scar tissue confined within the original wound borders. It is more common in areas of high tissue stress, such as the flexion creases across joints.

Wounds Requiring Closure

Although all serious wounds should be evaluated by a physician, the paramedic should expect the following types of wounds to require closure:

- Wounds to cosmetic regions (face, lips, eyebrows, etc.)
- Gaping wounds
- Wounds over tension areas (for example, joints)
- Degloving injuries (described later in this chapter)
- Ring finger injuries
- Skin tearing

> ## ✓ TRICKS OF THE TRADE
>
> If you are working in the emergency department and are asked to "prep" a patient with a lacerated eyebrow for wound closure, *never shave the eyebrow.* Doing so destroys the landmarks necessary for an accurate closure.

There are many techniques that are used to close a wound, including suture, tape, staples, and tissue adhesives.

> **NOTE**
>
> The American Red Cross and the U.S. Army are evaluating dry fibrin-glue sealant bandages that contain freeze-dried fibrinogen, thrombin, and calcium as a method to stop hemorrhage.[3] After these bandages are applied to a wound, contact with the wound's plasma reconstitutes and activates the fibrinogen, thrombin, and calcium and initiates a "super-clotting" cascade to arrest hemorrhage. These and similar bandages may have future application for prehospital care of wounds.

Pathophysiology and Assessment of Soft Tissue Injuries

Soft tissue injuries are classified as closed or open, depending on the absence or presence of a break in the continuity of the epidermis. Although soft tissue wounds often are the most evident injury, they generally are considered low-priority injuries unless life-threatening hemorrhage or associated airway compromise is present.

Closed Wounds

Closed soft tissue injuries usually are associated with minimal blood loss, although some can cause significant hemorrhage in the cavities of the thorax, abdomen, pelvis, or soft tissues of the legs. This text classifies closed wounds as contusion, hematoma, and crush injury.

Contusions and Hematomas

Blunt trauma causes contusions and hematomas. A contusion is characterized by blood vessel disruption beneath the epidermis, resulting in swelling, pain, and ecchymosis that can occur 24 to 48 hours after the injury. A **hematoma** is a collection of blood beneath the skin. It may occur with a contusion but represents a larger amount of tissue damage and the disruption of larger vessels (Fig. 20-3). These wounds usually are superficial but are sometimes associated with underlying fractures, vascular involvement, and significant hemorrhage.

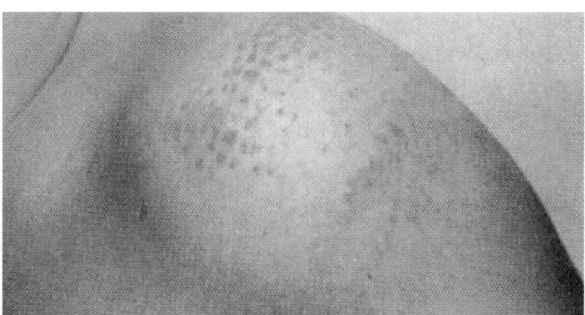

Fig. 20-3 Spotty bruising on a well-padded part of the shoulder. (From London PS: *A colour atlas of diagnosis after recent injury,* Ipswich, England, 1990, Wolfe Medical Publications.)

Crush Injury

Crush injury can occur when a crushing force is applied to a body area (Fig. 20-4). These injuries can be severe and are sometimes associated with internal organ rupture, major fractures, and hemorrhagic shock. Overlying skin may remain intact with crush injury, even in the presence of severe injury and shock. Crush injuries are further described later in this chapter.

? CRITICAL THINKING

What are some mechanisms of crush injury?

Open Wounds

Open soft tissue injuries are classified as abrasion, laceration, puncture, avulsion, amputation, and bites. (NOTE: Burns that include open and closed injury are addressed in Chapter 21.)

Abrasion

An **abrasion** is a partial-thickness injury caused by the scraping or rubbing away of a layer or layers of skin (Fig. 20-5). The wound usually results from friction with a hard object or surface (for example, in sports injuries and motorcycle crashes). Although these wounds often are superficial, they are painful and are at high risk for infection from contamination.

Laceration

A laceration results from a tear, a split, or an incision of the skin (Fig. 20-6). Blunt forces that typically produce a jagged injury or a knife or other sharp object cause lacerations, resulting in a linear wound, or incision. The sizes and depths of lacerations vary greatly, depending on the injury sites and wounding mechanism, and lacerations can be sources of significant bleeding.

Puncture

Contact with a sharp, pointed object such as a wooden splinter, needle, staple, glass, or nail commonly causes a **puncture wound** (Fig. 20-7). Although the entrance wound generally is small, these injuries are often associated with deep penetration

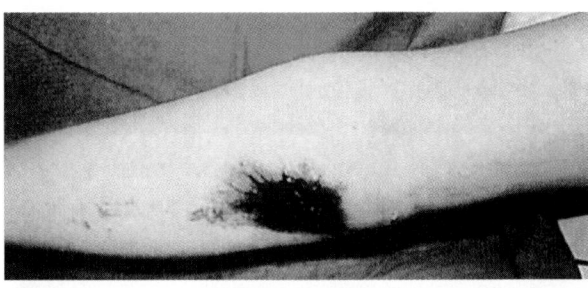

Fig. 20-5 Deep abrasion caused by a fall from a bicycle. (From London PS: *A colour atlas of diagnosis after recent injury*, Ipswich, England, 1990, Wolfe Medical Publications.)

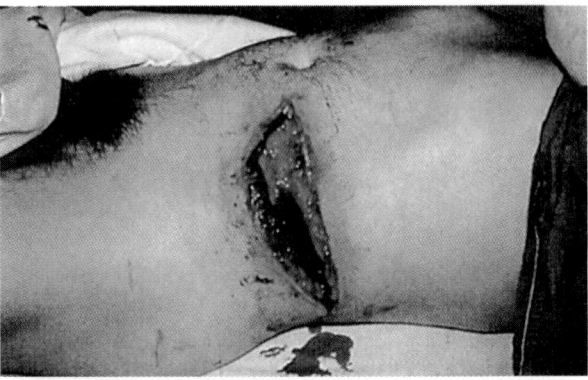

Fig. 20-6 Large wound caused by a broken power saw. (From London PS: *A colour atlas of diagnosis after recent injury*, Ipswich, England, 1990, Wolfe Medical Publications.)

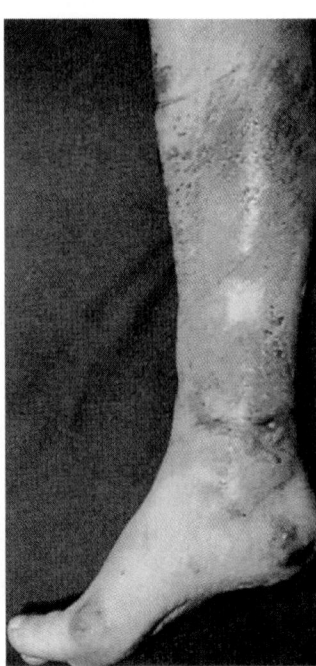

Fig. 20-4 Appearance of a woman's leg after it had been run over by the wheel of a milk van. (From London PS: *A colour atlas of diagnosis after recent injury*, Ipswich, England, 1990, Wolfe Medical Publications.)

and injury to underlying tissues. Punctures can be difficult to assess in the prehospital setting; an injury that appears to be minor can conceal a considerable amount of internal damage.

In some penetrating injuries, the wounding object remains embedded or impaled in the wound (Fig. 20-8). If this occurs to the chest or abdomen, severe bleeding and major underlying damage to internal organs can occur. Examples include the following:

- Chest injury
  - Pneumothorax (simple, open, tension)
  - Hemothorax
  - Pericardial tamponade
  - Penetrating heart wound
  - Rupture of the esophagus, aorta, diaphragm, mainstem bronchus
- Abdominal injury
  - Hollow and solid organ damage
  - Peritonitis (bacterial, chemical)
  - Evisceration

? CRITICAL THINKING

Why should a person always seek medical care to have a penetrating object removed?

Injection injury. Injection of a substance into the body under high pressure (for example, grease, paint, turpentine, dry-cleaning fluids, and molten plastics) can also cause a puncture wound (Fig. 20-9).

These injuries often have life- or limb-threatening potential and require rapid surgical decompression and debridement. These injuries usually are associated with minimal bleeding and may not appear serious. Numbness and blanching of the involved area frequently occur because of increased tissue pressure of the injected substance. Most patients with injection injuries are surgical emergencies and are at high risk for development of compartment syndrome. Definitive care for injection injuries generally requires hospitalization and surgical intervention to prevent infection. Amputation may be necessary if treatment is delayed.

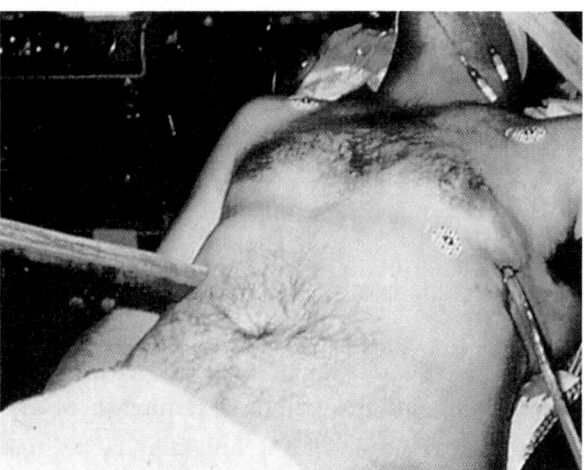

Fig. 20-8 Piece of wood impaled in the right chest, piercing the diaphragm and lacerating the spleen, stomach, and liver. (From London PS: *A colour atlas of diagnosis after recent injury*, Ipswich, England, 1990, Wolfe Medical Publications.)

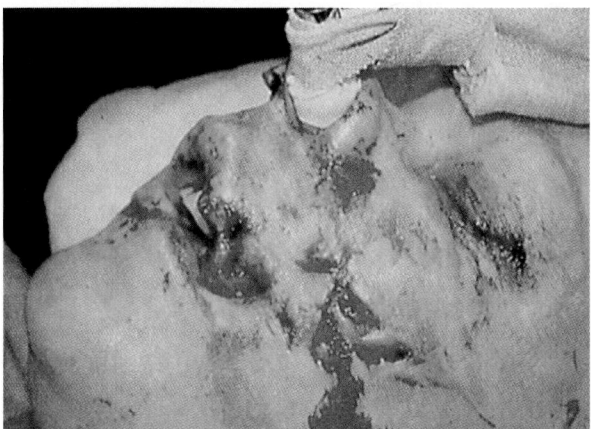

Fig. 20-7 Puncture wounds caused by broken glass from a shattered windshield. (From London PS: *A colour atlas of diagnosis after recent injury*, Ipswich, England, 1990, Wolfe Medical Publications.)

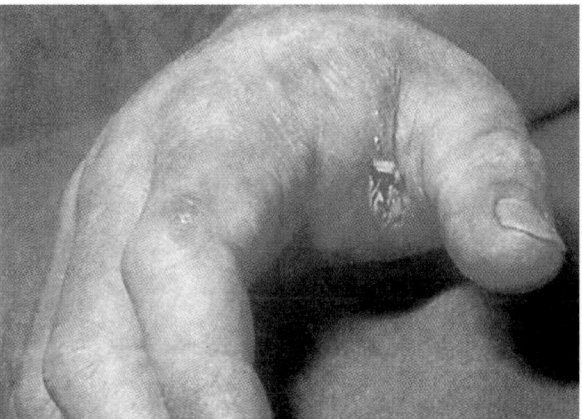

Fig. 20-9 Injection of paraffin into the hand resulted in amputation of the index finger. (From London PS: *A colour atlas of diagnosis after recent injury*, Ipswich, England, 1990, Wolfe Medical Publications.)

Avulsion

An **avulsion** is a full-thickness skin loss (Fig. 20-10) in which the wound edges cannot be approximated. Frequently involved body areas are the ear lobes, nose tip, and fingertips. Common causes of avulsion injury are industrial equipment, such as meat slicers or sawing devices, and domestic violence, such as human bites.

A degloving injury is a type of avulsion in which shearing forces separate the skin from the underlying tissues (Fig. 20-11). Common causes of degloving injury are industrial machinery that entangles an extremity, producing circumferential tearing; finger jewelry caught on a stationary object, producing a shearing of the soft tissue and possibly of the bone of the digit; and machinery that entraps hair, resulting in scalp avulsion. Degloving injuries are sometimes associated with underlying skeletal damage and massive loss of tissue in the affected area. Bleeding can be significant.

Amputation

Traumatic **amputation** involves a complete or partial loss of a limb secondary to mechanical force (Fig. 20-12). The digits, lower leg, hand and forearm, and the distal portion of the foot are most frequently injured in this fashion. Bleeding is a potentially fatal complication of amputation injury. In situations in which a complete amputation has occurred, injured arteries often retract, and hemorrhage may be less severe than in partial amputation injuries.

Bites

An animal or human bite wound frequently is a combination of puncture, laceration, avulsion, and crush injury (Fig. 20-13). The great pressure of the injuring jaw, which can be as great as 400 psi, can involve deep structures such as tendons, muscles, and bones. Complications from bite wounds, particularly human bites, include abscesses, lymphangitis, cellulitis, osteomyelitis, tenosynovitis, tuberculosis, hepatitis B, and tetanus. Other less common com-

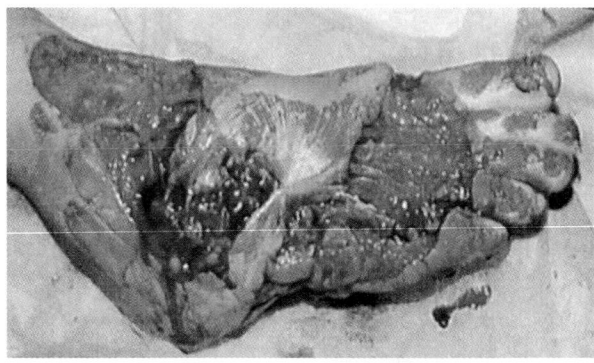

Fig. 20-11 Degloving injury of the foot. (From London PS: *A colour atlas of diagnosis after recent injury*, Ipswich, England, 1990, Wolfe Medical Publications.)

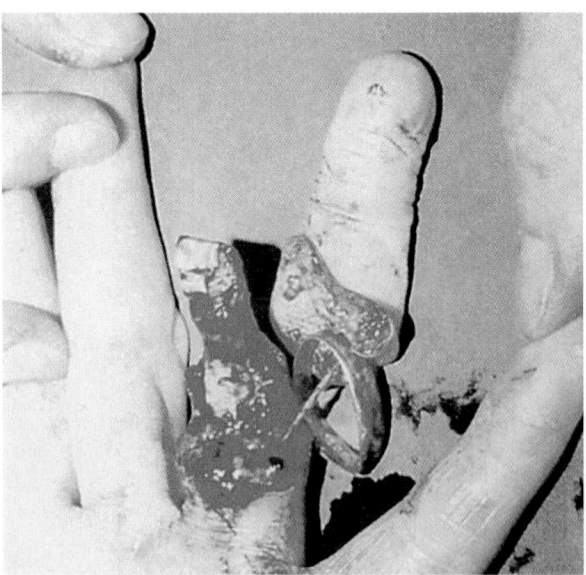

Fig. 20-10 Ring avulsion injury. (From London PS: *A colour atlas of diagnosis after recent injury*, Ipswich, England, 1990, Wolfe Medical Publications.)

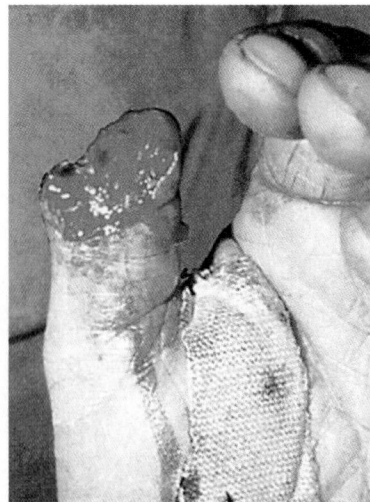

Fig. 20-12 Amputation of the fingertip. (From London PS: *A colour atlas of diagnosis after recent injury*, Ipswich, England, 1990, Wolfe Medical Publications.)

plications of mammalian bites include the transmission of diseases such as actinomycosis, syphilis, and rarely, rabies. All patients who have been bitten should seek physician evaluation.

NOTE

Although it is theoretically possible for a human bite to transmit HIV, the Centers for Disease Control and Prevention (CDC) suggest that the potential for salivary transmission of the virus is remote.[4]

Crush Injury

Crush injury is one of the three injuries that occur when tissue is exposed to a compressive force sufficient to interfere with the normal structure and metabolic function of the involved cells and tissues. The degree of injury produced by the crushing force depends on the amount of pressure applied to the body, the amount of time the pressure remains in contact with the body, and the specific body region in which the injury occurs. A massive crush injury to vital organs can cause immediate death.

NOTE

Compression injuries include crush injury, compartment syndrome, and crush syndrome.

Crush injury usually involves the upper or lower extremities, torso, or pelvis. It can result from entrapment under a heavy object, as in a foundation collapse, or from some other massive compressive force. Examples of situations that can cause crush injury include the following:

- Collapse of masonry or steel structures
- Collapse of earth (for example, mud slides and earthquakes)

- Motor vehicle crashes
- Warfare injuries
- Industrial accidents

NOTE

Prolonged application of a PASG and improperly applied casts can also cause crush injury.

Compartment Syndrome

Compartment syndrome is a result of crush injury and is a surgical emergency (Fig. 20-14). It usually results from compressive forces or blunt trauma to muscle groups confined in tight fibrous sheaths with minimal ability to stretch (below the knee, above the elbow). Other less common causes of compartment syndrome include the following:

- Extreme exertional exercise
- Low-level repetitive injury
- Electrical injury

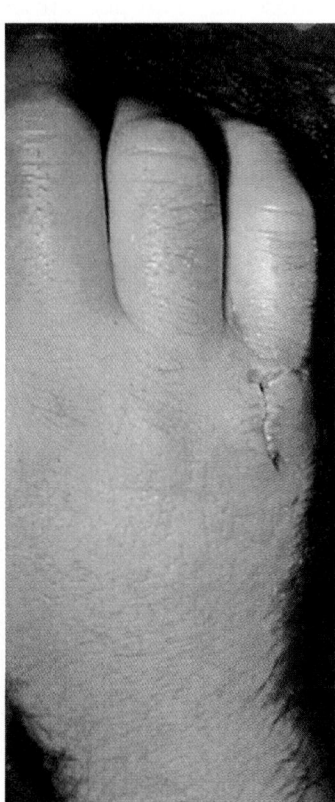

Fig. 20-13 Human bite to the hand. (From London PS: *A colour atlas of diagnosis after recent injury,* Ipswich, England, 1990, Wolfe Medical Publications.)

- Hemorrhage into a compartment (for example, coagulopathy among hemophiliacs)
- Circumferential deep burns and electrical burns
- Vascular occlusion
- High-pressure injection injuries
- Immobilization with pressure necrosis (for example, among alcoholics, drug addicts, and victims of stroke)

> **? CRITICAL THINKING**
>
> **Why would alcoholics, drug addicts, and stroke victims be at risk for compartment syndrome?**

Compartment syndrome develops as associated hemorrhage and edema increase pressure in the closed fascial space (compartment). This results in ischemia to the muscle, which causes further muscle cell swelling. As the intracompartmental pressure continues to rise, circulation is compromised, and irreversible ischemic damage to tissue develops within several hours to several days after injury. In addition to muscular damage, any nerves that travel through the compartment can undergo necrosis if the condition remains untreated. Signs and symptoms of compartment syndrome in an extremity include those of vascular insufficiency (the "five Ps") (Box 20-1). Other signs and symptoms that can indicate the presence of compartment syndrome include the following:

- Pain seemingly out of proportion to injury
- Swelling (tautness of the compartment)
- Tenderness to palpation

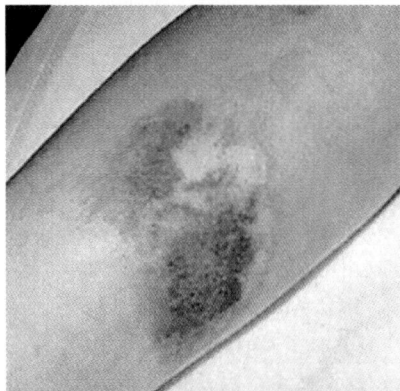

Fig. 20-14 Appearance that can follow prolonged crushing, as when an unconscious person lies on a body part for several hours.

- Weakness of the involved muscle groups
- Pain on passive stretch (earliest finding)

Recognition of compartment syndrome requires a high degree of suspicion based on patient history and mechanism of injury. Although most frequently associated with tibial fracture of the lower leg, compartment syndrome also can occur with crush injury or fracture of the femur, forearm, or upper arm. Delayed treatment can result in nerve death, muscle necrosis, and crush syndrome.

Crush Syndrome

Crush syndrome is a life-threatening and sometimes preventable complication of prolonged immobilization or compression. It is a pathologic process that causes destruction or alteration of muscle tissue. Crush syndrome is relatively rare and is most likely to occur in catastrophic events in which patient rescue and extrication are delayed beyond 4 to 6 hours (for example, earthquake or building collapse). Prehospital management of crush syndrome often determines patient outcome.

The exact mechanism of crush syndrome is unknown. It is believed that the compressive forces of entrapment produce a pathologic process that disrupts vascular integrity and causes loss of cellular architecture and structure of the membrane system. Patients with crush syndrome may appear stable for hours or days, as long as the compressive forces remain in place. However, when the patient is released from the entrapment, three detrimental processes occur simultaneously that can ultimately lead to death:

1. Oxygen-rich blood returns to the ischemic extremity, producing a pooling of intravascular volume into crushed tissue. This reperfusion

> **BOX 20-1**
>
> **FIVE Ps OF VASCULAR INSUFFICIENCY**
>
> 1. Pain
> 2. Paresis (late finding)
> 3. Paresthesia
> 4. Pallor (variable)
> 5. Pulselessness (late finding)

phenomenon reduces total circulating volume, often leading to clinical shock.

2. With the return of oxygen-rich blood, various toxic substances and waste products of anaerobic metabolism are released into the systemic circulation, causing metabolic acidosis. High levels of intracellular solutes and water are released from damaged cells, resulting in hyperkalemia, hyperuricemia, hypocalcemia, and hyperphosphatemia.

3. Myoglobin is released from the damaged muscle cells of the injured extremity and filtered through the kidneys (**rhabdomyolysis**), resulting in acute renal failure.

Blast Injuries

As described in Chapter 18, severe injuries can result from an initial air blast, from flying debris, and from secondary contact with another object as the victim is thrown by the blast. Examples of situations that can result in blast injury include natural gas or gasoline explosions, fireworks explosions, explosions in grain elevators, and terrorist bombs. Scene and personal safety is of paramount importance. Paramedics

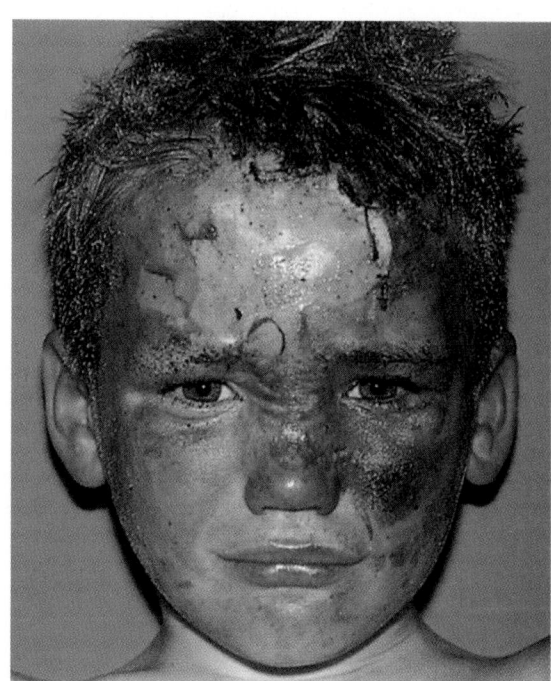

Fig. 20-15 Blast injury to the face. His eardrums were normal. He was admitted because of the risk of swelling to his face and airway with potential airway obstruction. (From Beattie T et al: *Pediatric emergencies,* London, 1997, Mosby-Wolfe.)

should not enter the scene where a blast injury occurred until it has been made safe by appropriate authorities (for example, law enforcement, fire service, specialized rescue teams, HAZMAT teams, and other public service agencies).

Injuries from blasts can be superficial or deep, injuring internal organs (Fig. 20-15). Patients who suffer blast injury require rapid stabilization (airway and ventilatory support with spinal precautions; circulatory support) and rapid transportation for physician evaluation. Blast injuries and associated trauma can be difficult to identify in the prehospital setting; these patients will need extensive evaluation in a trauma center. Compression injuries that occur to air-filled organs include rupture of the following:

- Eardrum
- Sinuses
- Lungs
- Stomach
- Intestines

? CRITICAL THINKING

What injury do you suspect if a patient who has suffered a blast injury has a sudden onset of hearing loss?

NOTE

Barotrauma is a physical injury sustained as a result of exposure to changes in atmospheric pressure. Barotrauma, a common affliction of scuba divers, can result from air blasts or excessive pressures with use of mechanical airway devices (see Chapter 36).

Management Principles for Soft Tissue Injuries

Personal and scene safety is always the priority in any emergency response. If indicated, law enforcement and rescue personnel should assure the paramedic that the scene is safe for entry and that any perpetrators have been apprehended. Assistance from other public service agencies also may be needed if other types of dangers exist, such as hazardous materials and bombs.

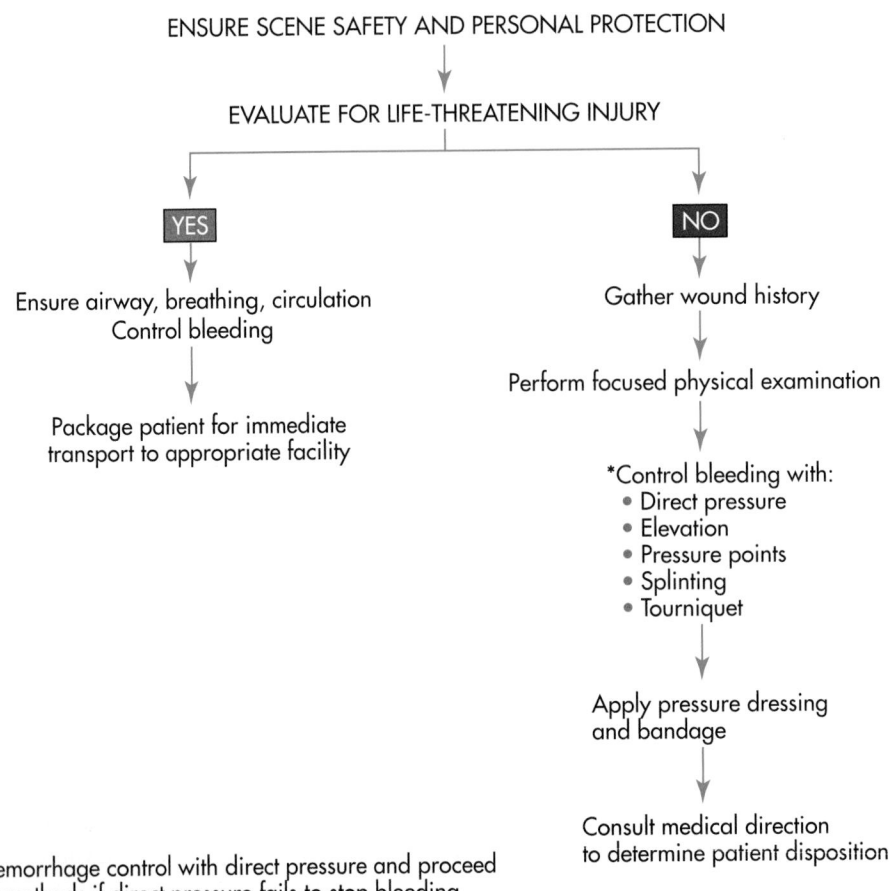

ENSURE SCENE SAFETY AND PERSONAL PROTECTION

EVALUATE FOR LIFE-THREATENING INJURY

YES

Ensure airway, breathing, circulation
Control bleeding

Package patient for immediate
transport to appropriate facility

NO

Gather wound history

Perform focused physical examination

*Control bleeding with:
• Direct pressure
• Elevation
• Pressure points
• Splinting
• Tourniquet

Apply pressure dressing
and bandage

Consult medical direction
to determine patient disposition

*Begin hemorrhage control with direct pressure and proceed
to other methods if direct pressure fails to stop bleeding.

Fig. 20-16 Treatment plan for a patient with soft tissue injury.

Treatment Priorities

Assessment of life-threatening injuries and resuscitation precedes evaluation and intervention of non–life-threatening soft tissue injuries. The paramedic evaluates wounds that do not pose a threat to life later in the physical examination. General wound assessment should include a history of the wounding event and careful examination of the injury. Fig. 20-16 illustrates a treatment plan based on assessment findings for a patient with soft tissue injury.

Wound History

A wound history should include the following:

- Time of injury
- Environment where the injury occurred (risk of infection is greater in unclean environments)
- Mechanism of injury and likelihood of concurrent or associated injuries
- Volume of blood loss
- Severity of pain

- Medical history, including use of medications that may impair hemostasis
- Tetanus immunization

Physical Examination

Physical examination of a wound should include the following:

- Inspection of the wound for bleeding, size, depth, presence of foreign bodies, amount of tissue lost, edema, and deformity
- Inspection of the area surrounding the wound for damage to underlying structures, arteries, nerves, tendons, or muscle

> **? CRITICAL THINKING**
>
> *Will you perform this physical examination on every wound in the prehospital setting?*

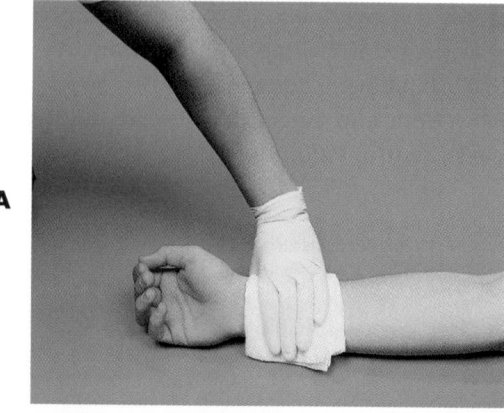

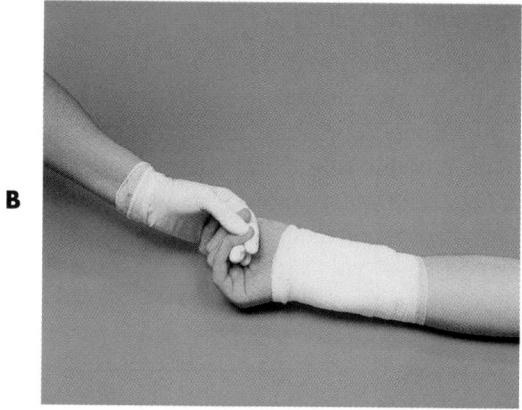

Fig. 20-17 **A**, Application of direct pressure to control hemorrhage. **B**, Pressure dressing.

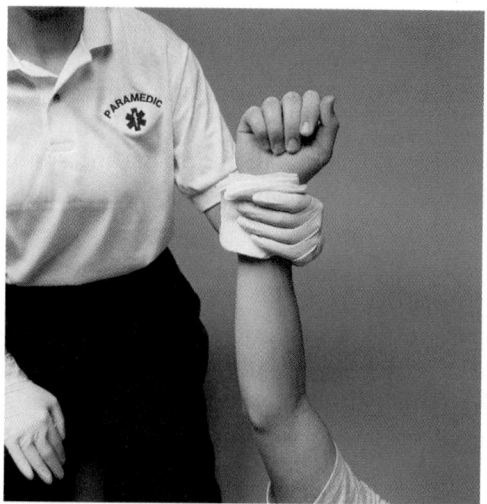

Fig. 20-18 Elevation to control hemorrhage.

- Assessment of sensory or motor function of the extremity
- Evaluation of the perfusion status of the wound and tissue distal to the wound
- Palpation of the injury and associated structures to evaluate capillary refill, distal pulses, tenderness, temperature, edema, and crepitus (if underlying bony injury is suspected)

Hemorrhage and Control of Bleeding

Blood loss frequently is associated with soft tissue injury and may be the result of damage to arteries, veins, capillaries, or a combination thereof. Generally, arterial bleeding is characterized as bright red and spurting, venous bleeding as dark reddish-blue and flowing, and capillary bleeding as bright red and oozing. However, it often is difficult to differentiate among the types of vessel hemorrhage. In the prehospital setting, the primary concern in hemorrhage, regardless of origin, is to control the bleeding process.

Methods of hemorrhage control include direct pressure, elevation, pressure point, immobilization by splinting, pneumatic pressure devices (air splints, PASG), and rarely the use of tourniquets.

> **NOTE**
>
> As in any patient encounter in which contact with body fluids is likely, the paramedic must take personal protective measures.

Direct Pressure

The paramedic can control external hemorrhage by applying direct pressure over the injury site (Fig. 20-17). Direct pressure controls most types of hemorrhage within 4 to 6 minutes. To maintain control, a pressure dressing can be applied over the site and held in place with a self-adherent roller bandage. The paramedic must continue direct pressure, even with a pressure dressing. Once the paramedic has applied the dressing, he or she should not remove it because removal can disrupt the fresh blood clot. If bleeding resumes and the dressing becomes soaked with blood, the paramedic should apply another dressing on top of the first one and hold it in place with direct pressure until the bleeding is controlled.

Elevation

The paramedic can control or reduce venous bleeding in an extremity by elevating the extremity above the level of the heart (Fig. 20-18). Elevation alone usually does not control hemorrhage and should be considered a supplement to direct pressure.

Pressure Point

The paramedic should attempt pressure-point control if direct pressure and elevation have not controlled hemorrhage. The chosen artery must be proximal to the injury site and must overlie a bony structure against which it can be compressed. Examples of pressure-point sites include the temporal artery to control bleeding from the scalp, the brachial artery to control bleeding from the forearm, and the femoral artery to control bleeding from the leg (Fig. 20-19). The paramedic should maintain pressure-point control (Fig. 20-20) for at least

10 minutes and may need to continue compression during patient transportation. The paramedic may need to complement combinations of direct pressure, elevation, and proximal pressure-point compression to control vigorous hemorrhage.

? **CRITICAL THINKING**

Why should the pressure point chosen to control hemorrhage be proximal to the injury?

Immobilization by Splinting

Patient movement promotes blood flow and can disrupt the clot or increase vascular injury. Therefore the paramedic should immobilize the patient whenever possible (Fig. 20-21). The paramedic can immobilize extremity injuries with appropriate splinting devices, or the patient can be fully immo-

Fig. 20-19 Arterial pressure points. (From doCarmo P: *Basic EMT skills and equipment,* St Louis, 1988, Mosby.)

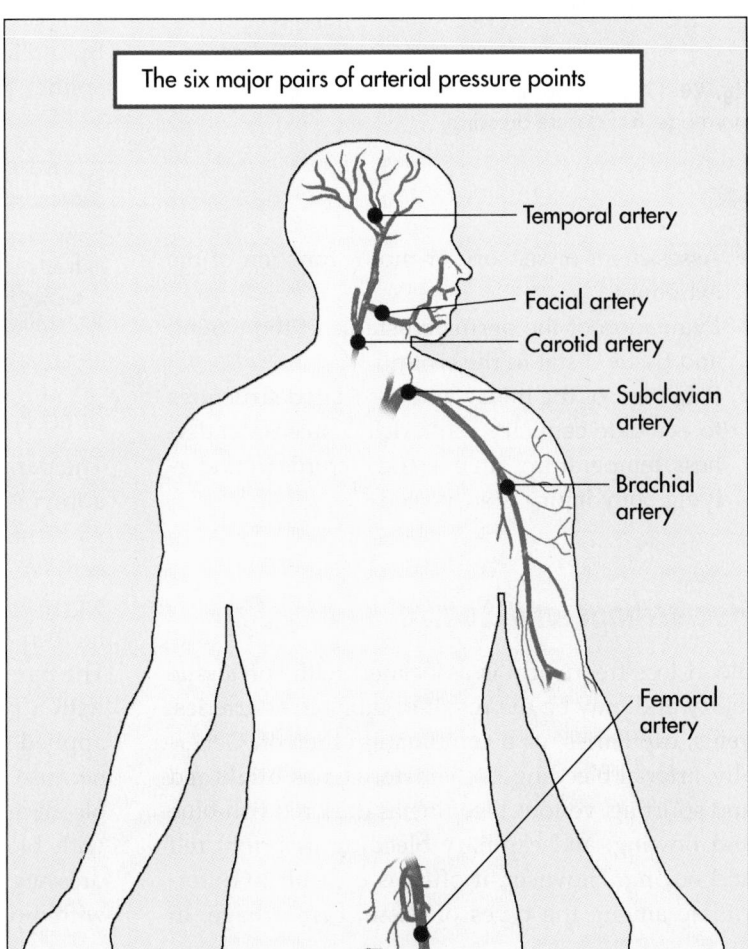

The six major pairs of arterial pressure points

Temporal artery

Facial artery

Carotid artery

Subclavian artery

Brachial artery

Femoral artery

bilized with a long spine board. Immobilization is not effective alone as a method to control bleeding and should be used as an adjunct.

Pneumatic Pressure Devices

Pneumatic pressure devices, such as inflatable air splints applied to an extremity or the use of the PASG, can provide uniform direct pressure to an immobilized injury site. The paramedic should apply these devices over a dressed wound only after other methods have controlled the bleeding (Fig. 20-22).

Tourniquet

Tourniquet use has little or no indication in the emergency management of hemorrhage (Fig. 20-23). Use of a tourniquet is associated with damage to nerves and blood vessels and eventual loss of the extremity. An inadequately applied tourniquet can produce venous occlusion, only restricting the outflow but not the inflow of blood and producing an increase in blood loss. Therefore the paramedic should only consider a tourniquet as a last resort when all other methods have failed and when its use is essential to save the patient's life. An example of such an extreme circumstance is a partial or complete traumatic amputation of a limb. Even in these cases, other methods of hemorrhage control often are effective. Guidelines for application of a tourniquet are as follows:

1. Consult with medical direction.

2. Select a site for the tourniquet. The site should be about 2 inches proximal to the wound and over the supplying brachial or femoral artery. A blood pressure cuff applied over the brachial artery also can act as a tourniquet. If a blood pressure cuff is used, note the time of application on the cuff itself.

3. Place the tourniquet (commercially prepared or wide, flat material) within 2 inches of the wound and over the artery to be compressed. Never use thin material such as rope or twine because it may damage underlying tissue. If a blood pressure cuff is used as a tourniquet, inflate the cuff until the cuff pressure exceeds the arterial pressure or to the point at which the hemorrhage stops.

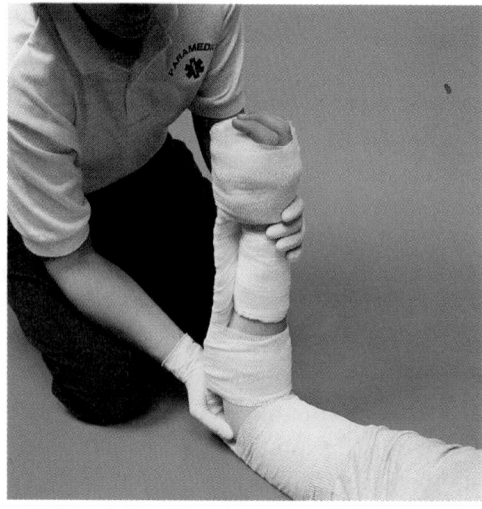

Fig. 20-21 Immobilization by splinting to control hemorrhage.

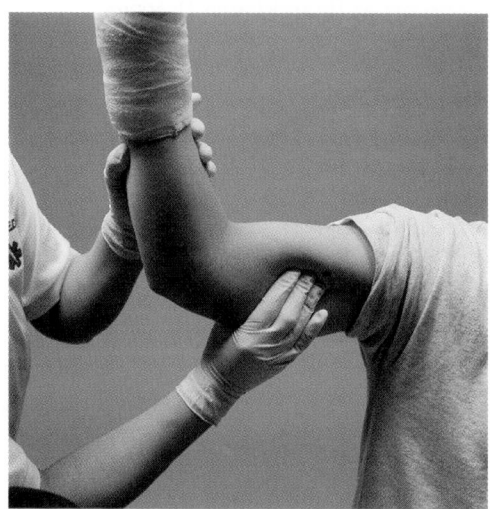

Fig. 20-20 Pressure-point control.

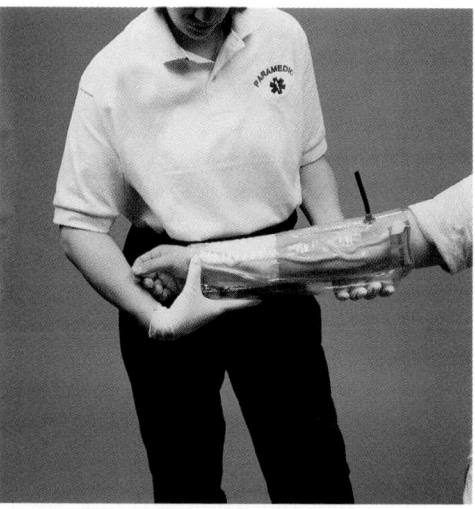

Fig. 20-22 Application of pneumatic pressure device to control hemorrhage.

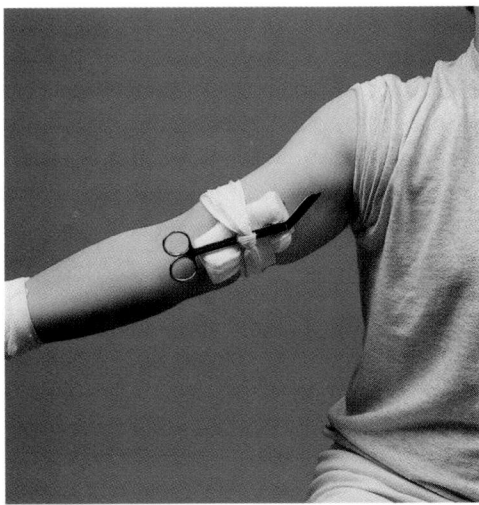

Fig. 20-23 Application of a tourniquet to control hemorrhage.

4. Place the pad (a roll of gauze or thick folded dressings) over the artery to be compressed.
5. Encircle the tourniquet twice around the extremity and pad, and tie it in a half knot over the pad.
6. Place a windlass (stick, pen, or similar object) on the half knot, and secure it in place with a square knot.
7. Tighten the windlass by twisting *only* until hemorrhage stops. Secure the windlass in that position. Never loosen the tourniquet once it is tightened.
8. Note the time of tourniquet application and secure it to the patient, or clearly mark "TK" on the patient's forehead. Document the tourniquet procedure on the patient care report.

Dressing Materials Used with Soft Tissue Trauma

There is a variety of bandages and dressings used in trauma care. The six general categories of dressings are as follows:

1. *Sterile dressings* are processed to eliminate bacteria. They should be used whenever infection of the wound is a concern.
2. *Nonsterile dressings* are not sterilized and can be used when infection is not a prime concern.
3. *Occlusive dressings* do not allow the passage of air through the material. These dressings are useful in treating wounds of the thorax and major vessels where negative pressure can cause air to enter the body, resulting in a pneumothorax or air embolism, respectively (see Chapter 24).
4. *Nonocclusive dressings* allow air to pass through the material and are indicated for managing most soft tissue injuries.
5. *Adherent dressings* attach to the wound surface by incorporating wound exudate into the dressing mesh. Use of these dressings can sometimes assist in controlling acute bleeding.
6. *Nonadherent dressings* allow the passage of wound exudate and do not adhere to the wound surface. These dressings do not damage the wound when removed and often are used after wound closure.

Bandages hold dressings in place. Bandages are classified as absorbent, nonabsorbent, adherent, and nonadherent. Like dressings, bandages are sterile or nonsterile.

Complications of Improperly Applied Dressings and Bandages

Improperly applied dressings and bandages can harm the patient and cause discomfort. For example, dressings that are applied too loosely often do not stop bleeding. Bandages that are applied too tightly can cause tissue ischemia and structural damage to vessels, nerves, tendons, muscles, and skin.

Basic Concepts of Open Wound Dressing

The basic concepts of open wound dressing include the following steps:

1. Assess the wound for size, depth, location, and contamination.
2. Properly prepare the wound for dressing. Prehospital care usually is limited to cleaning the injured surface of gross contaminants by irrigation of the wound with sterile water or normal saline. Do not attempt extensive debridement in the prehospital setting. Apply antibacterial ointment if the patient is not allergic (per protocol).
3. Apply the appropriate dressing.

4. Secure the dressing in place with bandages or gauze wrappings.
5. Tape the loose ends of the bandage.

Management of Specific Soft Tissue Injuries Not Requiring Closure

The paramedic encounters many minor open wounds that do not require closure or physician evaluation. In these situations, the paramedic provides "basic first-aid" and instructions for self-care to the patient.

Dressings and Bandages

Depending on the nature and location of the patient's injury, dressings, bandages, and immobilization may be indicated to properly care for the wound. (Fig. 20-24, *A* to *J* illustrates basic dressing and bandaging procedures for various wounds.) Open wounds that always require physician evaluation include those with the following:

- Neural, muscular, or vascular compromise
- Tendon or ligament compromise
- Heavy contamination
- Cosmetic complications
- Foreign bodies

> **NOTE**
>
> Patients with soft tissue injuries that pose a threat to life or limb require rapid assessment, stabilization, and rapid transportation for physician evaluation.

Evaluation

Local protocol may permit the paramedic to manage and release the patient with minor soft tissue injury to his or her own care or manage and refer the patient to his or her private physician for follow-up care. Some EMS systems allow paramedics to provide tetanus vaccine and written and verbal instructions to these patients who will not be transported by ambulance for physician evaluation.

Tetanus Vaccine

Tetanus is a serious and sometimes fatal disease of the central nervous system (CNS), caused by infection of

> **NOTE**
>
> About half a million cases of tetanus occur worldwide each year; in the United States only about 100 cases are reported annually. All cases occur in nonimmunized people, mostly in those over 50 years of age.

> ✓ **TRICKS OF THE TRADE**
>
> Soft tissue wounds (scrapes and abrasions) are common injuries for rescue personnel and other emergency care providers. Your tetanus immunization needs to be up to date.

a wound with spores of the bacterium *Clostridium tetani*. The patient can be protected against tetanus by periodic immunization with a tetanus vaccine.

Adults receive a combined immunization against diphtheria and tetanus (DT), and children receive vaccinations against diphtheria, pertussis (whooping cough), and tetanus (DPT) routinely in the United States. After initial immunization during childhood, children receive "booster" vaccines every 5 to 10 years. Patients who have not previously been immunized against tetanus receive tetanus immune globulin (TIG) because it confers immediate immunity. During wound care, the paramedic should ascertain the patient's last tetanus immunization and any prior allergic reactions to tetanus preparations. Normal side effects from the vaccine include slight fever, sore injection site, or minor rash. The tetanus vaccine is contraindicated in infants less than 6 weeks of age, in pregnant patients, and in those who are hypersensitive to the vaccine.

> ? **CRITICAL THINKING**
>
> *Why is it important for you to be knowledgeable about and to ask the patient about tetanus vaccination if it is not carried on your ambulance?*

Patient Instructions

Verbal and written instructions (for example, a "patient instruction sheet") regarding wound care

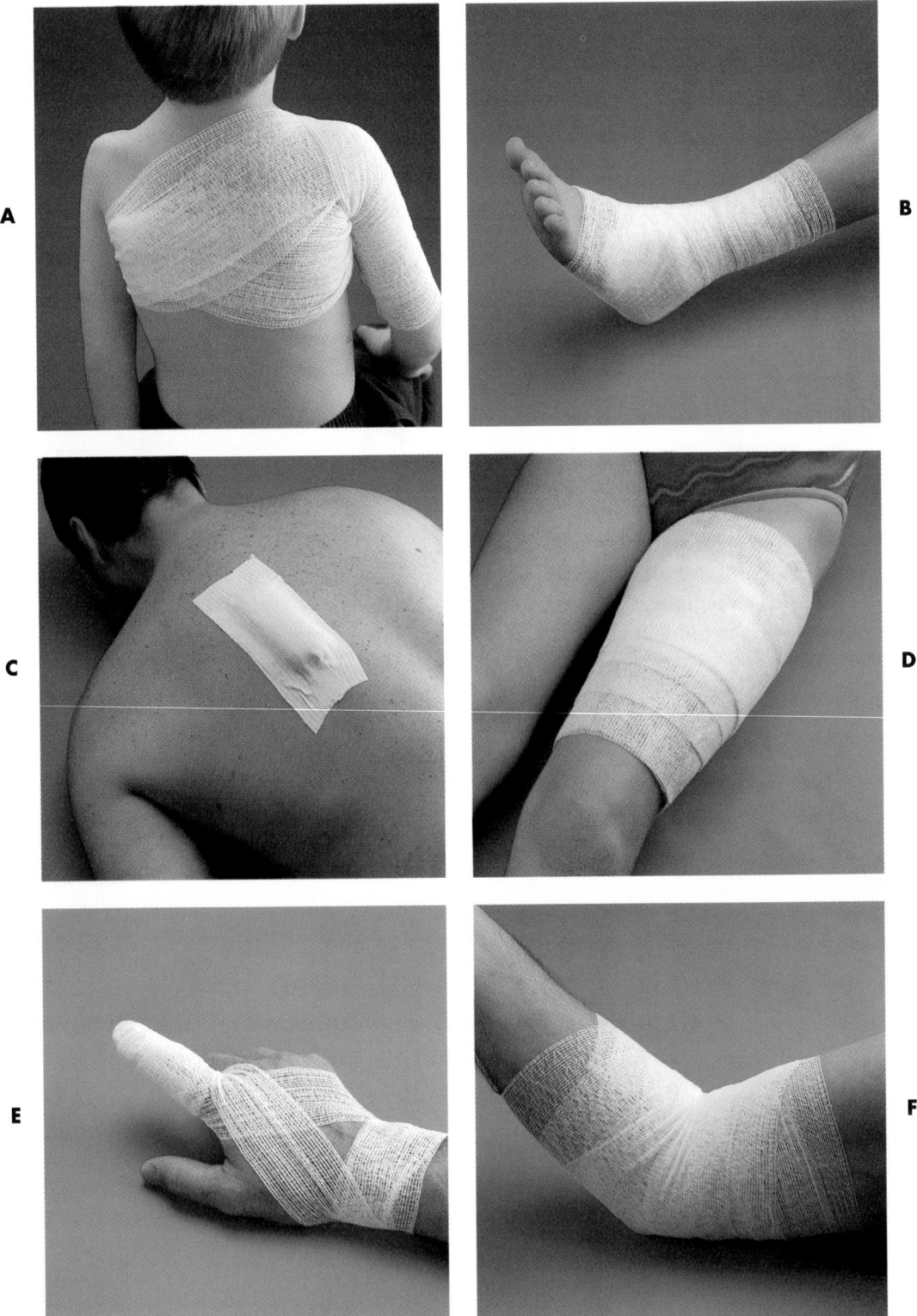

Fig. 20-24 Various dressings. **A,** Shoulder dressing. **B,** Ankle dressing. **C,** Torso dressing. **D,** Thigh dressing. **E,** Finger dressing. **F,** Elbow dressing.

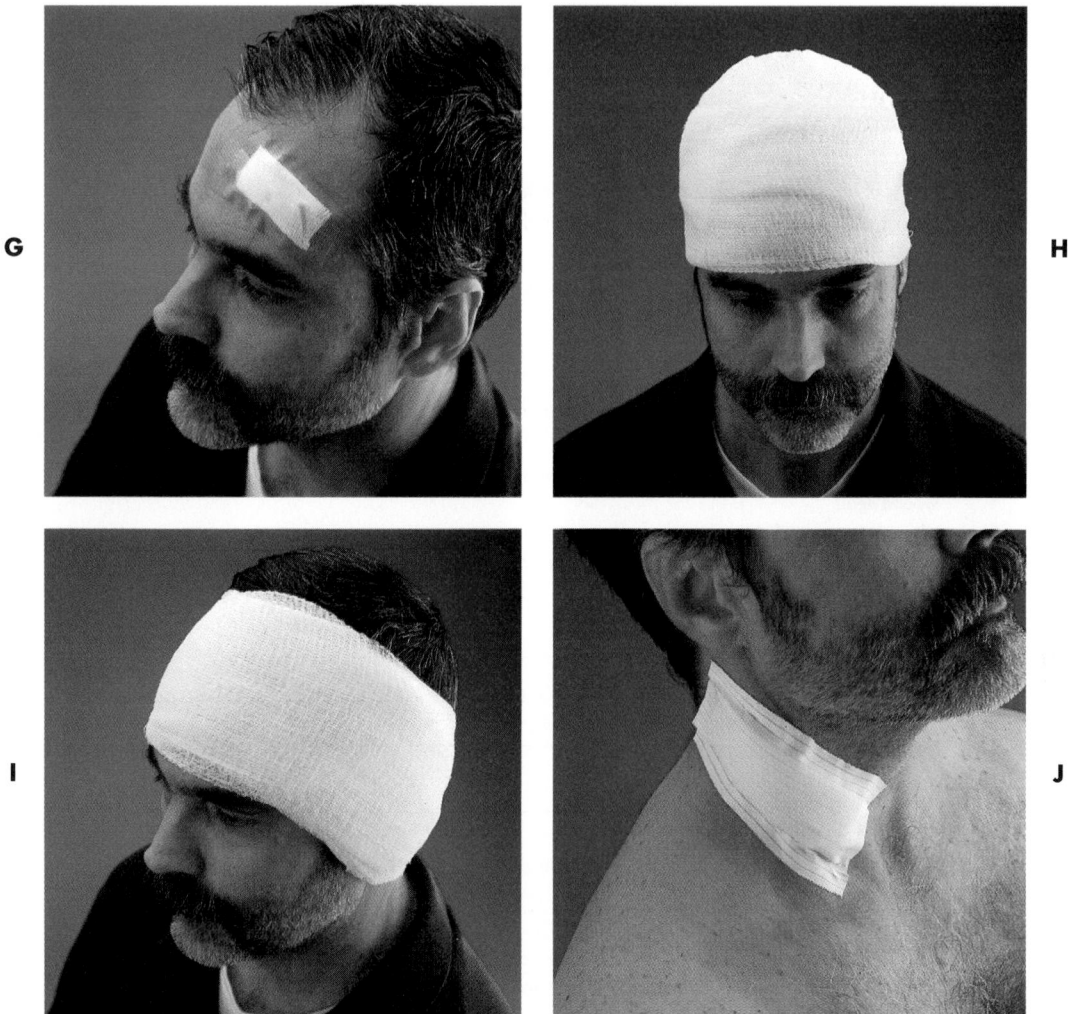

Fig. 20-24 cont'd G, Forehead dressing. **H**, Scalp dressing. **I**, Ear/mastoid dressing. **J**, Neck dressing.

(Fig. 20-25) should be provided to all patients who are not transported for physician evaluation. These instructions should include the following:

- Protection and care of wounded area
- Dressing change and follow-up
- Wound cleansing recommendations
- Signs of wound infection

Wound Infection

Infection is a common complication of soft tissue injury that results from a break in the continuity of the skin and subsequent exposure to the nonsterile external environment. Most infections are minor, but some can be quite serious. The goals of wound care are to prevent infection and protect from infection. Factors that influence the likelihood of infection include unclean wounds and wound mechanisms (for example, wounds contaminated by soil, dirt, or grease) and a patient's poor state of health. These factors can have both local and systemic complications and can affect the patient's general recovery.

Causal Factors of Wound Infection

There are many causal factors of wound infection. Nine of the most common are as follows[1]:

1. *Time.* The risk of infection can be greatly reduced if the wound is cleaned and repaired within 8 to 12 hours after injury. Bacterial proliferation to a

---

WOUND CARE INSTRUCTION SHEET

Patient name: _____

1. Call your physician. He/she may have further instructions to offer for your care.
2. Keep the wound and dressing as dry as reasonably possible, since water aids bacterial growth.
3. Remove the dressing applied after 2 days.
4. Check for signs of infection:
    a. Swelling
    b. Excessive redness
    c. Pain
    d. Heat—either locally or systemically as reflected by a fever
    e. Excessive drainage from wounds
5. Reapply a sterile gauze dressing, taping it down at the edges. Repeat this every 2 days until the wound heals.
6. Wounds in areas of high mobility, such as around joints, are subject to excessive tension. Appropriate precautions should be taken to decrease the motion of the affected joint to assist in healing.

Other instructions: _____

_____

_____

Treatment rendered: _____

Tetanus: Yes / No   Type: _____

I hereby acknowledge that I have read the instructions above, that they have been explained to me, that I understand them, and that I have received a copy of them.

I understand that I have had emergency treatment only and that I may be released before all of my medical problems are known and treated. I will arrange for the follow-up care as instructed.

_____   _____
Responsible Party's Signature   Relationship

_____   _____
Witness   Title

Original to Patient Care Report   _____
Copy to Patient   Date/Time

Fig. 20-25 Sample instruction sheet for wound care.

level that can result in infection can occur as early as 3 hours after injury.

2. *Mechanism.* Lacerations caused by fine cutting forces resist infection better than crush injuries. High-velocity missile injuries can produce internal damage that may not be apparent for several days.

3. *Location.* Injuries of the foot, lower extremity, hand, and perineum have a higher-than-normal risk for infection.

4. *Severity.* The more tissue damage produced by the injury, the higher the risk for infection.

5. *Contamination.* The presence of foreign matter in a wound decreases resistance to infection. Of

particular concern are wounds contaminated by soil, saliva, and feces.

6. *Preparation*. Body, facial, and head hair removed by clipping versus shaving is less likely to result in wound infection. Shaving can cause additional injury by abrading the skin and potentially moving skin flora into the larger wound.
7. *Cleansing*. Wound cleansing should be performed with normal saline and a high-pressure syringe.
8. *Technique of repair*. Wounds at high risk for infection (for example, animal bites) may need to be cleaned, debrided, and left open for 4 to 5 days, and then closed through traditional techniques.
9. *General patient condition*. Elderly patients and patients with concurrent illness or preexisting disease (for example, diabetes) often are less able to ward off infection.

Assessment of Wound Healing

A paramedic can assess a wound for proper healing by doing the following:

- Examine dressings for excess drainage. Change saturated dressings to prevent contamination of the wound.
- Examine wounds for early signs of infection or delayed healing. Inflammation, edema, and bloody drainage are normal during the first 3 days but should gradually subside as the wound heals.

Signs of wound infection include increasing inflammation or edema, purulent drainage, foul odor, persistent pain, delayed healing, and fever. If any of these is present, the paramedic should consult with medical direction for proper patient disposition (for example, patient transportation to the emergency department or patient referral to a private physician for follow-up care).

Special Considerations for Soft Tissue Injuries

As previously stated, assessment of life-threatening injuries and resuscitation precede evaluation of and intervention for non–life-threatening soft tissue injuries. After ensuring adequate airway, breathing, and circulatory status (with spinal precautions if indicated); controlling severe hemorrhage; and main-

taining normal body temperature, wound care can proceed. Special considerations for specific wounds are described in the following sections.

Penetrating Chest or Abdominal Injury

The paramedic must appropriately cover an open wound to the chest or abdomen with sterile and occlusive dressings. Open chest wounds can involve severe pulmonary injuries, including pneumothorax and tension pneumothorax (described in Chapter 24). Major complications of penetrating abdominal injury include hemorrhage from a major vessel or solid organ and perforation of a segment of bowel (see Chapter 25). The paramedic should observe the following guidelines in managing a penetrating wound to the chest or abdomen in which an impaled object is present:

1. Do not remove the impaled object; severe hemorrhage or damage to underlying structures can occur.
2. Do not manipulate the impaled object unless it is necessary to shorten the object for extrication or for patient transportation.
3. Control bleeding with direct pressure applied around the impaled object.
4. Stabilize the object in place with bulky dressings, and immobilize the patient to prevent movement.

Avulsion

Prehospital management of avulsed tissue varies by protocol, but two guidelines generally apply:

1. If the tissue is still attached to the body:
    a. Clean the wound surface of gross contaminants with sterile saline.
    b. Gently fold the skin back to its normal position.
    c. Control bleeding, dress the wound with bulky pressure dressings, and maintain direct pressure.

> **NOTE**
>
> The paramedic should not delay patient transportation to find avulsed tissue or amputated body parts if they are not readily available. The paramedic should advise law enforcement officers or other health care providers at the scene of the ambulance destination so that the avulsed tissue or amputated body part can be transported at a later time, if found.

2. If the tissue is completely separated from the body:
   a. Control the bleeding with application of direct pressure.
   b. Retrieve the avulsed tissue if possible.

? **CRITICAL THINKING**

Why should you use normal saline or lactated Ringer's solution versus sterile water to wrap or clean avulsed tissue?

---

c. Wrap the tissue in gauze, either dry or moistened with lactated Ringer's or saline solution (per protocol).
d. Seal the tissue in a plastic bag.
e. Place the sealed bag on crushed ice.

NOTE

To prevent additional tissue damage, the paramedic should not place the tissue directly on ice.

Amputations

As with other open wounds, the paramedic should attempt hemorrhage control for amputation with direct pressure and elevation. The wound may require use of a tourniquet, but the paramedic should avoid it if possible because the resultant damage can interfere with reimplantation attempts. The paramedic should retrieve and manage the amputated limb in the same manner as avulsed tissue.

Crush Syndrome

Crush syndrome is complex and difficult to diagnose and treat because of the many variables involved, such as the extent of tissue damage, duration and force of compression, patient's general health, and associated injuries. Management of crush syndrome is controversial, and a medical direction physician familiar with this pathologic process must supervise prehospital care.

Paramedics should consider the potential for crush syndrome when prolonged immobilization or compression occurs. He or she must coordinate emergency care with rescue efforts so that the timing of the release from entrapment follows medical treatment to prevent the development of hypovolemic shock and crush syndrome. The steps in patient care management are as follows[5]:

1. Provide airway and ventilatory support, including high-concentration oxygen administration.
2. Maintain body temperature.
3. Aggressively hydrate the patient to manage hypovolemia and to maintain urine output. Consider an initial bolus of 1 to 1.5 liters (up to 12 liters may be needed within the first 24 hours). The ideal fluid for crush syndrome is D5½NS.
4. Alkalinize the urine with sodium bicarbonate (beginning at 1 amp/L) to maintain a urine pH greater than 6.5. This controls hyperkalemia and acidosis and can prevent acute myoglobinuric renal failure and sudden cardiac dysrhythmias. Manage severe hyperkalemia with *insulin* and *dextrose* (25 mL $D_{50}W$, followed by 10 units regular *insulin* IV) if necessary. *Calcium chloride* generally is not indicated unless there is a danger of hyperkalemia dysrhythmia.
5. Maintain urine output with a diuresis goal of at least 300 mL/hr. Consider *mannitol* (Osmitrol), 10 g or 20% solution added to each liter of IV fluid. Do not administer loop diuretics (for example, *furosemide* [Lasix]) because they can acidify the urine.
6. It can be beneficial to use arterial tourniquets before the release of a crushed limb. If intracompartmental pressure is greater than 40 mm Hg, fasciotomy may be indicated to preserve the limb and cutaneous sensation. Performing a field fasciotomy requires special training and authorization from medical direction.
7. A physican may need to perform surgical amputation when extrication is impossible.

NOTE

Field fasciotomy or amputation carries an increased risk for infection and sepsis.

---

8. After extrication, care may include transporting the patient for hyperbaric oxygen treatment to restore tissue perfusion and to decrease tissue necrosis and muscle edema. (Hyperbaric therapy is further described in Chapter 36.)

SUMMARY

- The skin and its accessory organs are the primary cosmetic structures of the body and perform many functions that are critical to survival. The skin is composed of two distinct layers of tissue: the outer layer (epidermis) and the inner layer (dermis).

- Surface trauma can interfere with the normal preservation of body fluids and electrolytes and with the maintenance of body temperature. The two physiologic responses to surface trauma are vascular and inflammatory reactions that can lead to healing, scar formation, or both. Many factors can affect or alter wound healing.

- Soft tissue injuries are classified as closed or open as determined by the absence or presence of a break in the continuity of the epidermis. Closed wounds include contusions, hematomas, and crush injury. Open wounds are classified as abrasion, laceration, puncture, avulsion, amputation, and bite.

- Assessment of life-threatening injuries and resuscitation precedes evaluation and intervention of non–life-threatening soft tissue injuries. General wound assessment should include a history of the wounding event and careful examination of the injury.

- Methods of hemorrhage control include direct pressure, elevation, pressure point, immobilization by splinting, and pneumatic pressure devices.

- The general categories of dressings used in trauma care are sterile dressings, nonsterile dressings, occlusive dressings, nonocclusive dressings, adherent dressings, and nonadherent dressings. The general categories of bandages are absorbent, nonabsorbent, adherent, and nonadherent.

- Depending on the nature and location of the patient's injury, dressings, bandages, and immobilization may be indicated to properly care for a wound.

- The goals of wound care are to prevent infection and protect from infection. Factors that influence the likelihood of infection include unclean wounds and wound mechanisms and a patient's poor state of health.

- Special considerations for specific wounds include penetrating chest or abdominal injury, avulsion, amputations, and crush syndrome.

REFERENCES

1. National Safety Council: *Injury facts*, Itasca, Ill, 1999, The Council.
2. Rosen P, Barkin R: *Emergency medicine: concepts and clinical practice*, ed 4, St Louis, 1999, Mosby.
3. American Red Cross: *Fibrin sealant bandage chosen as "best of new" by Popular Science*, 1998. Available at www.redcross.org.
4. Centers for Disease Control and Prevention, US Department of Health and Human Services, Public Health Service: *Guidelines for prevention and transmission of human immunodeficiency virus and hepatitis B virus to health-care and public safety workers*, Atlanta, 1989, The Department.
5. US Department of Transportation, National Highway Traffic Safety Administration: *EMT-Paramedic national standard curriculum*, Washington, DC, 1998, US Government Printing Office.

21 *Burns*

OBJECTIVES

Upon completion of this chapter, the paramedic student will be able to:

1. Describe the incidence, patterns, and sources of burn injury.

2. Describe the pathophysiology of local and systemic responses to burn injury.

3. Classify burn injury according to depth, extent, and severity based on established standards.

4. Discuss the pathophysiology of burn shock as a basis for key signs and symptoms.

5. Outline the physical examination of the burned patient.

6. Describe the prehospital management of the patient who has sustained a burn injury.

7. Discuss pathophysiology as a basis for key signs, symptoms, and management of the patient with an inhalation injury.

8. Outline the general assessment and management of the patient who has a chemical injury.

9. Describe specific complications and management techniques for selected chemical injuries.

10. Describe the physiological effect of electrical injury as they relate to each body system based on an understanding of key principles of electricity.

11. Outline assessment and management of the patient with electrical injury.

12. Describe the distinguishing features of radiation injury and considerations in the prehospital management of these patients.

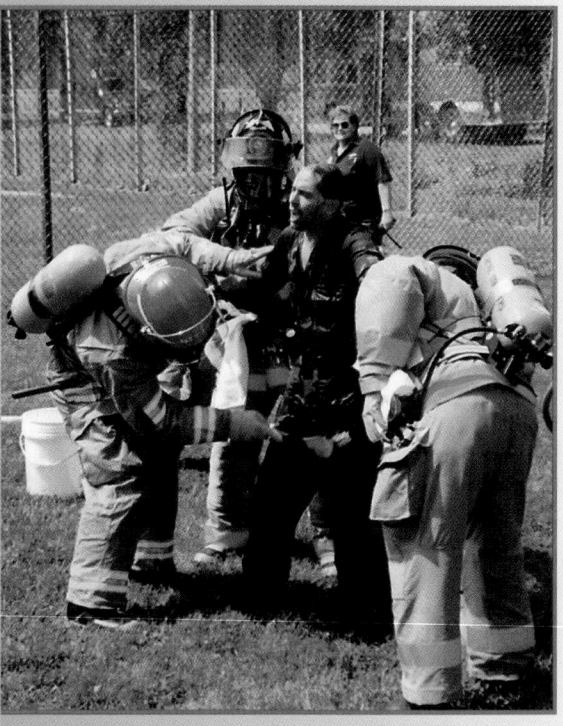

Management of burns often poses a challenge for the paramedic. Understanding the consequences of burn injury and appropriate prehospital management can reduce morbidity and mortality in this complex patient group.

KEY TERMS

eschar: A scab or dry crust resulting from a thermal or chemical burn.

first-degree burn: A burn injury where only a superficial layer of epidermal cells is destroyed.

fourth-degree burn: A full-thickness burn injury that penetrates the subcutaneous tissue, muscle, fascia, periosteum, or bone.

inhalation injury: An upper and/or lower airway injury that results from thermal and/or chemical exposure.

Lund and Browder chart: A method to estimate burn injury that assigns specific numbers to each body part; accounts for developmental changes in percentages of body surface area.

rule of nines: A method to estimate burn injury that divides the total body surface area (TBSA) into segments that are multiples of 9%.

second-degree burn: A burn injury that extends through the epidermis to the dermis (superficial partial-thickness); considered a deep partial-thickness injury if it extends to the basal layers of the skin.

third-degree burn: A burn injury where the entire thickness of the epidermis and dermis is destroyed.

Incidence and Patterns of Burn Injury

Burns are a devastating form of trauma associated with high mortality rates, lengthy rehabilitation, cosmetic disfigurement, and permanent physical disabilities. Each year, more than 2 million Americans seek medical attention for burns. Of these, 70,000 are hospitalized and up to 10,000 die as a result of thermal injury or burn-related infection.[1] Physiological and systemic complications that contribute to thermal injury deaths are listed in Box 21-1.

> **NOTE**
>
> Fires and burns were the fifth leading cause of unintentional injury deaths in 1998.[2]

Morbidity and mortality rates from burn injury follow significant patterns with regard to gender, age, and socioeconomic status. For example, two thirds of all fire fatalities are men; the death rate from thermal injury is highest among children and older adults; and three fourths of all fire deaths occur in the home, with the highest incidence in lower-income households.[2] A key component of the professional role of the paramedic is community education to stress prevention as the most effective management of these injuries. (See Appendix C.)

Major Sources of Burns

A burn injury is caused by an interaction between energy (thermal, chemical, electrical, or radiation) and biological matter. The majority of burns are thermal and commonly result from flames, scalds, or contact with hot substances. (*Frostbite*, also considered a thermal injury, is addressed in Chapter 36.)

Chemical burns are caused by substances capable of producing chemical changes in the skin, with or without heat production. Although heat may be generated during the burning process, the chemical changes in the skin, not the heat, produce the greatest injury. Chemical burns differ from thermal burns in that the topical agent generally adheres to the skin for prolonged periods, producing continuous tissue destruction. The severity of the chemical injury is related to the type of agent, its concentration and volume, and the duration of contact. Chemical agents that frequently cause burn injury include acids and alkalis, which are found in many household cleaning products and organic compounds. Chemical burns are associated with high morbidity, especially when they involve the eyes.

> **NOTE**
>
> **Inhalation injury** may result from thermal and/or chemical exposure. Inhalation burns are described later in this chapter.

PHYSIOLOGICAL AND SYSTEMIC COMPLICATIONS OF THERMAL INJURIES

Depending on the severity of thermal injury, physiological and systemic complications may include the following:

- Fluid loss
- Electrolyte loss
- Acidosis
- Renal failure
- Liver failure
- Heart failure
- Hypoxia
- Anoxia
- Dysrhythmias
- Hypothermia
- Hypovolemia
- Infection

Electrical injuries (including lightning injuries) result from direct contact with an electric current or arcing of electricity between two contact points near the skin. In direct contact injury, the current itself is not considered to have any thermal properties, but the potential energy of the current is transformed into thermal energy when it meets the electrical resistance of biological tissue interposed between the entrance and exit sites. Arc injuries are localized at the termination of current flow and are caused by the intense heat or flash that occurs when the current "jumps," making contact with the skin. Flame burn also may occur as a result of arcing if the heat generated ignites clothing or other fuel source near the patient.

? CRITICAL THINKING

If electrical energy is transformed to heat causing tissue damage in a human, why doesn't an electrical cord feel hot when you touch it?

Radiation injury is caused by *ionizing* and *nonionizing* radiation (described later in this chapter). Burns may result from a high level of radiation exposure to a specific body area, but radiation injuries make up a very small percentage of burn injuries.

Pathophysiology of Thermal Burn Injury

NOTE

Anatomy and physiology of the skin is presented in Chapter 6 and Chapter 20. The reader should refer to those chapters for review.

Studies have shown that surface temperatures of 44° C (111° F) do not produce burns unless exposure time exceeds 6 hours.[3] At temperatures between 44° C and 51° C (111° F and 124° F), the rate of epidermal necrosis approximately doubles with each degree of temperature rise. At 70° C (185° F) or greater, the exposure time required to cause transepidermal necrosis is less than 1 second. The degree of tissue destruction depends on the temperature and duration of exposure. Factors that influence the body's ability to resist burn injury include the water content of the skin tissue; thickness and pigmentation of the skin; presence or absence of insulating substances such as skin oils or hair; and peripheral circulation of the skin, which affects dissipation of heat.

? CRITICAL THINKING

Based on these facts and your knowledge of life span development, who would you predict would have a deeper burn from the same energy source: an 18-year-old or a 75-year-old? Why?

Local Response to Burn Injury

Burn injury immediately destroys cells or so completely disrupts their metabolic functions that cellular death ensues. Cellular damage is distributed over a spectrum of injury. Some cells are destroyed instantly, others are irreversibly injured, and some injured cells may survive if rapid and appropriate intervention is provided in the prehospital setting and in-hospital care.

Major burns have three distinct zones of injury (*Jackson's Thermal Wound Theory*), which usually appear in a "bull's eye" pattern (Fig. 21-1). The central area of the burn wound, which has sustained the most intense contact with the thermal source, is the *zone of coagulation*. In this area, coagulation necrosis

Burn zones

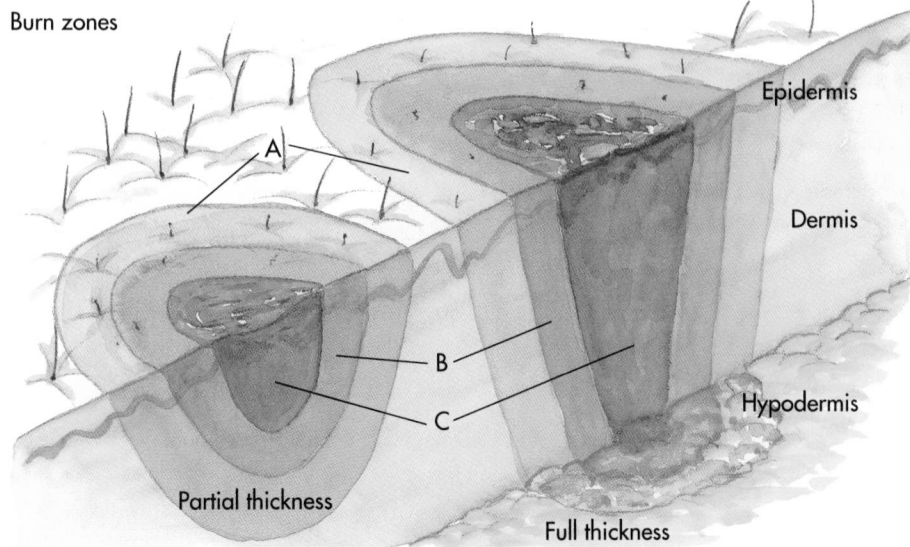

Epidermis

Dermis

Hypodermis

Partial thickness

Full thickness

Fig. 21-1 Three zones of intensity: (*A*) zone of hyperemia (peripheral); (*B*) zone of stasis (intermediate); and (*C*) zone of coagulation (central).

of the cells has occurred, and the tissue is nonviable. The *zone of stasis* surrounds the critically injured area and consists of potentially viable tissue despite the serious thermal injury. In this zone, cells are ischemic because of clotting and vasoconstriction. The cells die within 24 to 48 hours after injury if no supportive measures are undertaken. At the periphery of the zone of stasis is the *zone of hyperemia*. This zone has increased blood flow as a result of the normal inflammatory response. The tissues in this area recover in 7 to 10 days if infection or profound shock does not develop.

Tissue damage from burns depends on the degree of heat and duration of exposure to the thermal source. As a rule, the burn wound swells rapidly because of the release of chemical mediators, which cause an increase in capillary permeability and a fluid shift from the intravascular space into the injured tissues. The increased permeability is accentuated by injury to the sodium pump in the cell walls. As sodium moves into the injured cells, it causes an increase in osmotic pressure that increases the inflow of vascular fluid into the wound. Finally, the normal process of evaporative loss of water to the environment is dramatically accelerated (5 to 15 times that of normal skin) through the burned tissue. In a small wound, these physiological alterations produce a classic local inflammatory response (pain, redness, swelling) without major systemic effects. If the wound covers a large body surface area, however, these local tissue responses can produce major systemic effects and life-threatening hypovolemia.

Systemic Response to Burn Injury

As local events occur at the injury site, other organ systems become involved in a general response to the stress caused by the burn. One of the earliest manifestations of the systemic effects of a large thermal injury is hypovolemic shock with a decrease in venous return, decreased cardiac output, and increased vascular resistance (except in the hyperemic zone). This hypovolemic state, when combined with hemolysis (the breakdown of red blood cells), rhabdomyolysis, and subsequent hemoglobinuria and myoglobinuria (myoglobin in the urine) seen with major burns and electrical injury, can lead to renal failure. Other systemic responses to major burn injury are listed in Box 21-2.

Classifications of Burn Injury

Burns (body surface area involvement and depth) must be assessed and classified as accurately as possible in the field to ensure proper treatment and transport to an appropriate medical facility and to monitor progression of tissue damage. However, this typically is not possible in the prehospital setting because of the progressive nature of the injury. The amount of tissue damage may not be evident for hours or sometimes days after a burn injury.

SYSTEMIC RESPONSES TO MAJOR BURN INJURY

- Pulmonary response
  Hyperventilation to meet increased metabolic needs
- Gastrointestinal response
  Decrease in splanchnic perfusion that may lead to mucosal hemorrhage and transient adynamic ileus
  Vomiting and aspiration
  Stress ulcers
- Musculoskeletal response
  Decreased range of motion from immobility and edema
  Possible osteoporosis and demineralization (late)
- Neuroendocrine response
  Increased amounts of circulating epinephrine and norepinephrine and transient elevation of aldosterone levels
- Metabolic response
  Elevated metabolic rate, particularly with infection or surgical stress
- Immune response
  Altered immunity, resulting in increased susceptibility to infection
  Depressed inflammatory response
- Emotional response
  Physical pain
  Isolation from loved ones and familiar surroundings
  Fear of disfigurement, deformities, and disability
  Altered self-image
  Depression

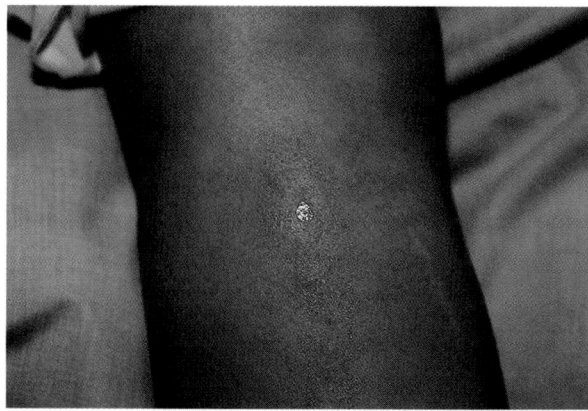

Fig. 21-2 First-degree burn.

First-degree Burns

First-degree burns characteristically are painful, red, and dry, and blanch with pressure (Fig. 21-2). They typically occur secondary to prolonged exposure to low-intensity heat or a short-duration flash exposure to a heat source. In first-degree burns, only a superficial layer of epidermal cells is destroyed, and they slough (peel away from healthy tissue underneath the wound) without residual scarring. These injuries usually heal within 2 to 3 days. An example of a first-degree burn is *sunburn*.

Second-degree Burns

Second-degree burns may be divided into two groups: superficial partial-thickness and deep partial-thickness wounds. The superficial partial-thickness injury is characterized by blisters and commonly is caused by skin contact with hot but not boiling water or other hot liquids, explosions producing flashburns, hot grease, and flame.

In superficial partial-thickness second-degree burns (Fig. 21-3), injury extends through the epidermis to the dermis, but the basal layers of the skin are not destroyed, and the skin regenerates within a few days to a week. Edematous fluid infiltrates the dermal-epidermal junction, creating the blisters characteristic of this depth of wound. Intact blisters provide a seal that protects the wound from infection and excessive fluid loss. (For this reason, blisters should not be broken in the prehospital setting.) The injured area usually is red, wet, and painful and may blanch when the tissue around the injury is compressed. In the absence of infection, these wounds heal without scarring, usually within 14 days.

Depth of Burn Injury

Burns are classified in terms of depth as first, second, and third degree. First- and second-degree burns are superficial, and partial-thickness burns usually heal without surgery if uncomplicated by infection or shock. Third-degree burns are full-thickness burns that usually require skin grafts.

NOTE

Other depth classifications may be preferred by medical direction.

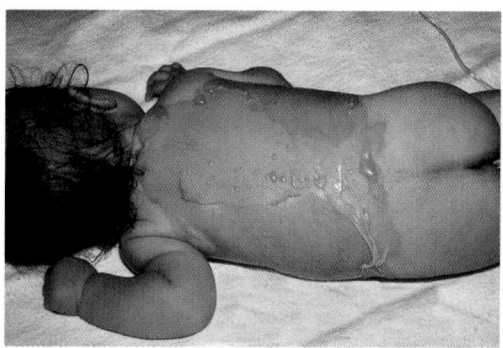

Fig. 21-3 Superficial partial-thickness second-degree burn. (Courtesy St John's Mercy Medical Center, St Louis, Mo.)

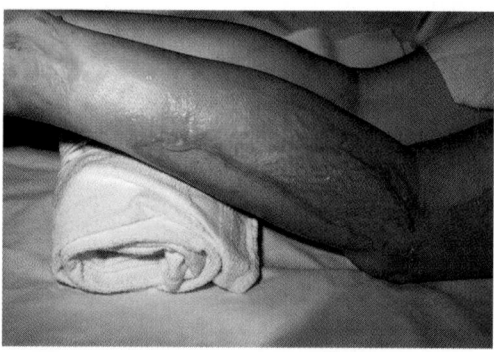

Fig. 21-4 Deep partial-thickness burn. (Courtesy St John's Mercy Medical Center, St Louis, Mo.)

If the depth of the second-degree burn involves the basal layer of the dermis, it is considered a deep partial-thickness burn (Fig. 21-4). As in superficial partial-thickness burns, edema forms at the epidermal-dermal junction. Sensation in and around the wound may be diminished because of the destruction of basal-layer nerve endings. The injury may appear red and wet or white and dry, depending on the degree of vascular injury. Wound infection and subsequent sepsis and fluid loss are major complications of these injuries. If uncomplicated, deep partial-thickness burns generally heal within 3 to 4 weeks. Skin grafting may be necessary to promote timely healing and minimize thick scar tissue formation, which may severely restrict joint movements and cause persistent pain and disfigurement.

Third-degree Burns

In **third-degree burns,** the entire thickness of the epidermis and dermis is destroyed; thus skin grafts are necessary for timely and proper healing (Fig. 21-5). The wound is characterized by coagulation necrosis of the cells and appears pearly white, charred, or leathery. A definitive sign of third-degree burn is a translucent surface in the depths of which thrombosed veins are visible. **Eschar,** a tough, nonelastic coagulated collagen of the dermis, is present in these injuries.

Sensation and capillary refill are absent in third-degree burns because small blood vessels and nerve endings are destroyed. This often results in large plasma volume loss, infection, and sepsis. Natural wound healing may produce contracture deformity

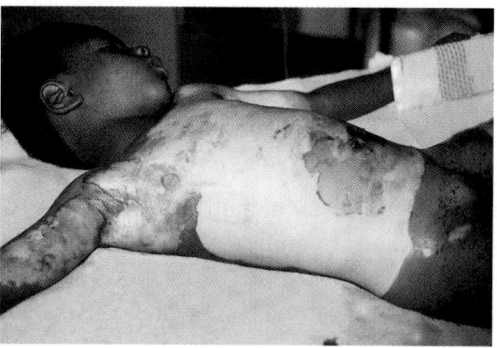

Fig. 21-5 Third-degree burn. (Courtesy St John's Mercy Medical Center, St Louis, Mo.)

and severe scarring. Therefore surgical intervention with skin grafting is necessary to close full-thickness wounds, minimize complications, and allow restoration of maximal function.

Some burn classifications also include a **fourth-degree burn** to describe a full-thickness injury that penetrates the subcutaneous tissue, muscle, fascia, periosteum, or bone. These burns usually result from incineration-type exposure and electrical burns in which heat is sufficient to destroy tissues below the skin.

Extent and Severity of Burn Injury

There are several methods to evaluate the extent of burn injury. Two common methods include the **rule of nines** and the **Lund and Browder chart.** In addition, the American Burn Association has devised a categorization of burns to determine severity. The paramedic should use a method for determining the extent of burn injury approved by medical direction.

? CRITICAL THINKING

Why is the calculation of body surface area different for children less than 10 years of age?

Rule of Nines

The rule of nines commonly is used in the prehospital setting. The measurement divides the total body surface area (TBSA) into segments that are multiples of 9%. This method provides a rough estimate of burn injury size and is most accurate for adults and children older than 10 years of age. Fig. 21-6 explains the rule of nines.

If the burn is irregularly shaped or has a scattered distribution throughout the body, the rule of nines is difficult to apply. In these situations, burn size can be estimated by visualizing the patient's palm as an indicator of percentage (the "rule of

palms"). The surface of the patient's palm equals about 1% of the total body surface area.

NOTE

Only second- and third-degree burns are included when calculating TBSA. For large burns, TBSA may more easily be calculated by subtracting the percentage of unburned area from 100.

Lund and Browder Chart

The Lund and Browder chart (Fig. 21-7) is a more accurate method of determining the area of burn injury because it assigns specific numbers to each body part. It is used to measure burns in infants and young children because it allows for developmental

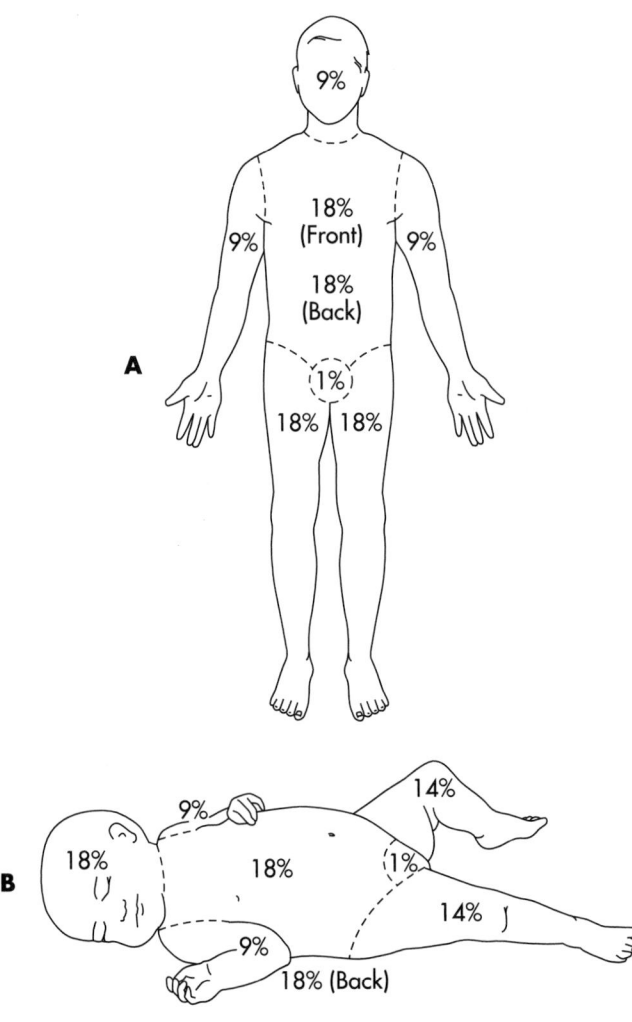

Fig. 21-6 The rule of nines. **A,** Adult. **B,** Infant. (From Rosen P, Barkin R: *Emergency medicine: concepts and clinical practice,* ed 4, St Louis, 1998, Mosby.)

BOX 21-3

AMERICAN BURN ASSOCIATION CATEGORIZATION

Major Burn
 25% of the body surface or greater
 Functionally significant involvement of hands, face, feet, or perineum
 Electrical or inhalation injury
 Concomitant injury
 Severe preexisting medical problems

Moderate Burn
 15% to 25% body surface area
 No complications or involvement of hands, face, feet, or perineum
 No electrical injury, inhalation injury, concomitant injury, or severe preexisting medical problem

Minor Burn
 15% or less body surface area
 No involvement of face, hands, feet, or perineum
 No electrical burns, inhalation injury, severe preexisting medical problems, or complications

changes in percentages of body surface area. For example, the adult head is 9% of TBSA, but the newborn head is 18% TBSA.

American Burn Association Categorization

Using the criteria established by the American Burn Association, burn injuries are categorized as *major,* *moderate,* and *minor* (Box 21-3).

In determining severity, factors such as the patient's age, the presence of concurrent medical or surgical problems, and the complications that accom-

pany certain types of burns, such as those of the face and neck, hands and feet, and genitalia, also must be considered. For example, burns of the face and neck may cause respiratory compromise or interfere with the ability to eat or drink. Burns of the hands and feet may interfere with ambulation and activities of daily living. Perineal burns present a high risk of infection because of the contaminants in this region and may disrupt the normal patterns of elimination.

Burn Center Referral Criteria

Many EMS services use the categorizations previously described or other criteria as the basis for determining which patients need transport to specialized burn centers. According to the Committee on Trauma of the American College of Surgeons and the American Burn Association, burn injuries usually

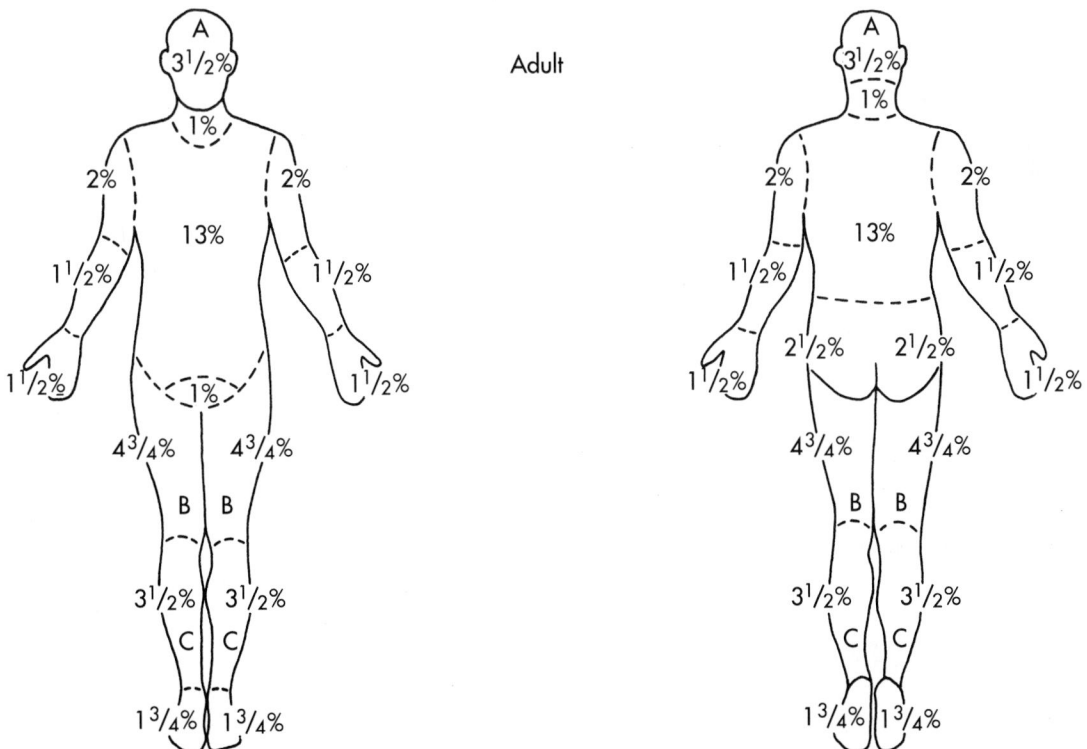

Age	0-1	1-4	5-9	10-14	15
A—1/2 of head	9 1/2%	8 1/2%	6 1/2%	5 1/2%	4 1/2%
B—1/2 of one thigh	2 3/4%	3 1/4%	4%	4 1/4%	4 1/2%
C—1/2 of one leg	2 1/2%	2 1/2%	2 3/4%	3%	3 1/4%

Fig. 21-7 Lund and Browder chart. (From Lee G: *Flight nursing: principles and practice,* St Louis, 1991, Mosby.)

requiring referral to a burn center include the following 11 guidelines[4]:

1. Second- and third-degree burns that in combination cover more than 10% of the body surface area in patients under 10 or over 50 years of age
2. Second- and third-degree burns that in combination cover more than 20% of the body surface area of patients in the other age groups
3. Second- and third-degree burns that involve the face, hands, feet, genitalia, or perineum or those that involve skin overlying major joints
4. Third-degree burns over more than 5% body surface area in any age group
5. Significant electrical burns, including lightning injury
6. Significant chemical burns
7. Inhalation injury
8. Burn injury in patients with preexisting illnesses that could complicate management, prolong recovery, or affect mortality
9. Burns in any patient in whom concomitant trauma poses an increased risk of morbidity or mortality and who may be initially treated in a trauma center until stable before transfer to a burn center
10. Burns in children seen in hospitals without qualified personnel or equipment for their care (they should be transferred to a burn center with these capabilities)
11. Burn injuries in patients who require special social and emotional or long-term rehabilitative support, including cases involving suspected child abuse and neglect

Pathophysiology of Burn Shock

Shock can occur from large BSA burns. Shock results from local and systemic responses to thermal trauma that lead to edema and accumulation of vascular fluid in the tissues in the area of injury. Locally there is a brief initial decrease in blood flow to the area (the *emergent phase*) followed by a marked increase in arteriolar vasodilation. A concurrent release of vasoactive substances from the burned tissue causes increased capillary permeability, producing intravascular fluid loss and wound edema (the *fluid shift phase*). The fluid loss into the injured tissues and the marked increase in evaporative fluid loss secondary to the break in the epithelial barrier contribute to produce hypovolemia.

? CRITICAL THINKING

What life- or limb-threatening problems can develop from this swelling?

The greatest loss of intravascular fluid occurs in the first 8 to 12 hours, followed by a continued, moderate loss over the next 12 to 16 hours. At some point within 24 hours, the extravasation of fluid greatly diminishes (the *resolution phase*), and equilibrium between the intravascular space and the interstitial space is reached. Shock and organ failure (most commonly acute renal failure) can occur as a consequence of hypovolemia (see Chapter 7 and Chapter 19). In response to hypovolemia, the body attempts to compensate for diminished circulating blood volume with a reduction in cardiac output and an elevation in peripheral vascular resistance. With volume replacement, cardiac output can increase to levels above normal (the *hypermetabolic phase* of thermal injury) (Fig. 21-8).

Fluid Replacement

Within minutes of a major burn injury, all capillaries in the circulatory system (not just those in the area of the burn) lose their capillary seal. This increase in capillary permeability prevents the creation of an osmotic gradient between the intravascular and extravascular space, allowing colloid solutions to quickly equilibrate across the capillary barrier and into the interstitium. The process of burn shock continues for about 24 hours, at which time the capillary seal is restored.[5] Therefore therapy for burn shock is aimed at supporting the patient through the period of hypovolemic shock. Crystalloid solution (e.g., lactated Ringer's solution) usually is considered the fluid of choice in initial resuscitation.

> **NOTE**
>
> Fluid resuscitation in burns is controversial. Medical direction may recommend that fluid resuscitation not be initiated in the prehospital setting if transport to a hospital can be accomplished within 30 minutes.[6] Transport should not be delayed to initiate IV therapy.

Assessment of the Burn Patient

Emergency care for a burn patient, like any other trauma patient, begins with the initial assessment to recognize and treat life-threatening injuries. In burn patients, however, the dramatic appearance of burns, the patient's intense pain, and the characteristic odor of burnt flesh may easily distract the paramedic from life-threatening problems. It is important that the EMS provider should confidently assess and direct efforts away from the burn wound and toward the patient as a whole.

> ✓ **TRICKS OF THE TRADE**
>
> If the wound is so grotesque that it distracts you—cover it up, and go on!

> **NOTE**
>
> As with all other emergency responses, personal and scene safety is the number one priority.

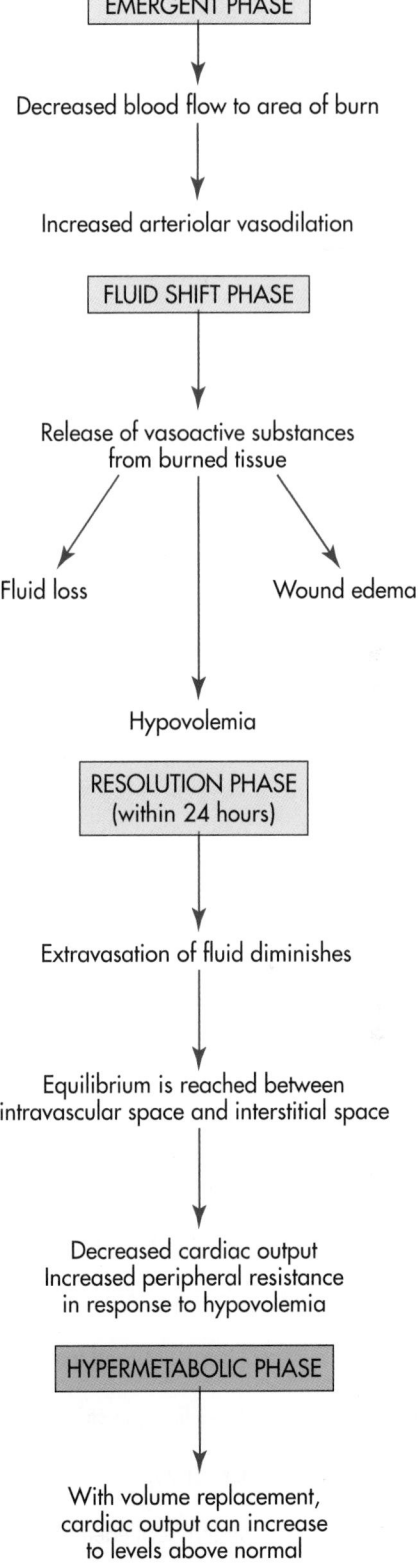

Fig. 21-8 Phases of burn shock.

Initial Assessment

Evaluation of the patient's airway is a major concern in the initial assessment, particularly for the patient with an inhalation injury (described later in this chapter). The paramedic should observe for stridor (an ominous sign that indicates the patient's upper airway is at least 80% narrowed), facial burns, soot in the nose or mouth, singed facial or nasal hair, edema of lips and the oral cavity, coughing, inability to swallow secretions in the pharynx, hoarse voice, and circumferential neck burns. Airway management should be aggressive with these patients (Fig. 21-9).

> **? CRITICAL THINKING**
>
> *Why should you perform frequent reassessment of the airway of a patient who has a large burn when your initial assessment reveals that the airway is patent?*

Breathing should be evaluated for rate, depth, and the presence of wheezes, crackles, or rhonchi. The patient's circulatory status should be evaluated by assessing the presence, rate, character, and rhythm of pulses; capillary refill; skin color and temperature; pulse oximetry, which may be inaccurate in the presence of carbon monoxide; and obvious arterial bleeding.

The patient's neurological status should be determined by using the AVPU scale or a similar method. Deviations from normal should be carefully evaluated for underlying cause. Abnormalities include hypoxia, decreased cerebral perfusion from hypovolemia, and cerebral injury resulting from head trauma. After the initial assessment is completed, a history of the event should be obtained while the physical examination is performed.

An accurate history from the patient or bystanders can help the paramedic determine the potential for inhalation injury, concomitant trauma, or preexisting conditions that may influence the physical examination or patient outcome. When obtaining the patient history, the following information should be ascertained:

1. What is the patient's chief complaint (e.g., pain, dyspnea)?
2. What were the circumstances of the injury?
   - Did it occur in an enclosed space?
   - Were explosive forces involved?
   - Were hazardous chemicals involved?
   - Is there related trauma?

- Burns around nose or mouth

- Soot in mouth or nose: singed nasal hairs

- Intraoral burns: burned tongue

- Intraoral swelling (no stridor)

- Hoarseness of voice

- Visible pharyngeal edema

- Inspiratory stridor

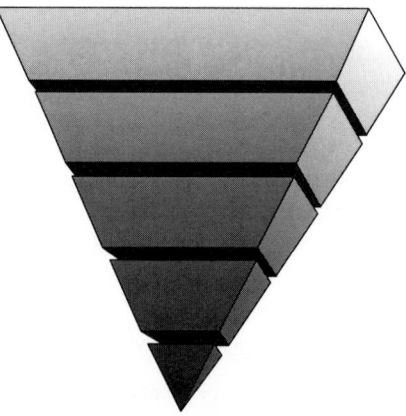

Fig. 21-9 Probability of upper airway obstruction.

3. What was the source of the burning agent (e.g., flame, metal, liquid, chemical)?
4. Does the patient have any significant medical history?
5. What medications does the patient take (including recent ingestion of illegal drugs or alcohol)?
6. Did the patient lose consciousness at any time? (Suspect inhalation injury.)
7. What is the status of tetanus immunization?

Physical Examination

At the beginning of the physical exam, a complete set of vital signs should be assessed. The blood pressure should be obtained in an unburned extremity, if available. If all extremities are burned, sterile gauze may be placed under the blood pressure cuff and an attempt made to auscultate a blood pressure. Patients with severe burns or pre-existing cardiac or medical illness should be monitored by ECG. Lead placement may need to be modified to avoid placing electrodes over burned areas (see Chapter 28). Field care and hospital destination are determined by the depth, size, location, and extent of burned tissue and the presence of associated illness or injury.

General Principles in Burn Management

Goals for prehospital management of the severely burned patient include preventing further tissue injury, maintaining the airway, administering oxygen and ventilatory support, providing fluid resuscitation (per protocol), providing rapid transport to an appropriate medical facility, using clean technique to minimize the patient's exposure to infectious agents, and providing psychological and emotional support. Patients with burns also should be evaluated for other types of life-threatening trauma; some will have additional injuries associated with the burn event. Examples include blunt or penetrating trauma sustained in automobile crashes, blast injury, and skeletal or spinal injury from attempts to escape the thermal source or contact with electrical current.

Stopping the Burning Process

The first step in managing any burn is to stop the burning process. This step must be accomplished with the safety of the emergency crew in mind because it often occurs in close proximity to the source that caused the burn. With minor first-degree burns, the burning process can be terminated by cooling the local area with cold water (but not ice-cold water). Ice, snow, or ointments should not be applied to the burn because these agents may increase the depth and severity of thermal injury. In addition, ointments may impair or delay assessment of the injury when the patient arrives in the emergency department.

> ### ✓ TRICKS OF THE TRADE
>
> Many people still believe that putting butter on a burn is an appropriate intervention. Help put this harmful remedy to rest.

In cases of severe burns, the patient should be rapidly and safely moved from the burning source to an area of safety if possible. A person whose clothing is in flames or smoldering should be placed on the floor or ground and rolled in a blanket to smother the flames and/or doused with large quantities of the cleanest available water. (Cold water to rapidly decrease skin temperature is preferred.) Contaminated water sources, such as a lake or river, should be avoided. These patients should never be allowed to run or remain standing. Running may fan the flame, and an upright position may increase the likelihood of the patient's hair being ignited.

> ### NOTE
>
> The National Fire Protection Association (NFPA) developed a training program called *Stop, Drop, and Roll.* The program was designed to teach children and adults that in the event their clothing catches fire, they should: *stop* (do not run); *drop* (cover your face with your hands and drop to the ground in a prone position); and *roll* (to smother the fire until the flames are extinguished).

The patient's clothing should be completely removed while cooling the burn so that heat is not trapped under the smoldering cloth. If pieces of smoldering cloth have adhered to the skin, they should be cut, not pulled, away. Melted synthetic fabrics that cannot be removed should be soaked in cold water to stop the burning process. After the burn is cooled, the patient with a large body surface area injury should be covered with a clean, preferably sterile sheet, over which blankets are placed when ambient temperatures are low.

> **NOTE**
>
> The duration of cooling is controversial; it should continue at least until pain is relieved and probably for a total duration of 15 to 30 minutes.[7]

Airway, Oxygen, and Ventilation

The adequacy of airway and ventilatory efforts should be evaluated in all burn patients. High-concentration humidified oxygen should be administered if available to any patient with severe burns, and ventilation should be assisted as needed. If inhalation injury is suspected, the patient should be closely observed for signs of impending airway obstruction. Life-threatening laryngeal edema may be progressive and may make tracheal intubation difficult if not impossible. The decision to intubate these patients should not be delayed.

> **NOTE**
>
> Every attempt should be made to intubate the patient's lungs with a normal (not smaller) size ET tube. These patients often are difficult to ventilate, even with an appropriately sized tube.

Circulation

The need for fluid resuscitation is based on the severity of the injury, the patient's vital signs, and transport time to the receiving hospital. Some authorities contend that prompt intervention of IV therapy in the critically burned patient is essential to prevent long-term complications such as burn shock and renal failure. (The paramedic should consult with medical direction and follow local protocol regarding fluid replacement.)

If IV therapy is to be performed, it should be initiated with a large-bore catheter in a peripheral vein in an unburned extremity. (The arm is the preferred site.) If an unburned site is not available, the catheter may be inserted through burned tissue, although the risk of subsequent infection is greater. Care should be taken to secure the catheter with a dressing; tape may not adhere to the injured area as it begins to leak fluid.

> **NOTE**
>
> The administration of pain medication is an early intervention. Medical direction may recommend that patients with large burns be given IV *morphine* or *meperidine* (Demerol). Other pharmacological therapy that may be given after arrival in the emergency department includes topical applications (e.g., silver sulfadiazine, special synthetic dressings), oral analgesics, and tetanus immunization.

If transport of the burn patient is delayed or a lengthy interfacility transport is anticipated, other patient care procedures may be required. These include the placement of a nasogastric tube to prevent gastric distention or vomiting and placement of an indwelling urinary catheter to measure urine output and to maintain patency of the urethra in patients with burns to the genitalia (see Chapter 46).

> **? CRITICAL THINKING**
>
> *How should you administer pain medicine to a patient with a large burn? Why did you choose this route?*

Special Considerations

Although all burn injuries warrant good patient assessment and care, burns of specific body regions require special consideration. These include burns to the face and extremities and circumferential burns.

Burns of the face swell rapidly and may be associated with airway compromise. The head of the ambulance stretcher should be elevated at least 30 degrees if not contraindicated by spinal trauma to minimize the edema. If the patient's ears are burned, the use of a pillow should be avoided to minimize additional injury to the area.

If burns involve the extremities or large areas of the body, all rings, watches, and other jewelry should be removed as soon as possible to prevent vascular compromise with increased wound edema. Peripheral pulses should be reassessed frequently, and the burned limb should be elevated above the patient's heart if possible.

✓ **TRICKS OF THE TRADE**

To prevent any "misunderstanding," a patient's jewelry or other personal belongings removed during emergency care should be inventoried, documented on the PCR, and placed in a bag marked with the patient's name. The name of the person (family member, ED personnel) who received the items also should be recorded.

Burn injuries that encircle a body region can pose a threat to the patient's life or limbs. Circumferential burns that occur to an extremity may produce a tourniquet-like effect, which may quickly compromise circulation and cause irreversible damage to the limb. Circumferential burns of the chest can severely restrict movement of the thorax and may significantly impair chest wall compliance. If this occurs, the depth of respirations is reduced, tidal volume is decreased, and the patient's lungs may become difficult to ventilate, even by mechanical means. Definitive treatment for circumferential burns involves an in-hospital surgical procedure known as *escharotomy*, whereby incisions are made through deep burns to reduce compartment pressure and allow adequate blood volume to flow to and from the affected limb or thorax.

Inhalation Burn Injury

Smoke inhalation injury is present in about 20% to 35% of all patients admitted to burn centers[8]; more than 50% of the 12,000 fire deaths each year are directly related to smoke inhalation or inhalation injury.[1] Prehospital considerations in caring for patients with inhalation injury include recognition of the dangers inherent in the fire environment, pathophysiology of inhalation injury, and early detection and treatment of impending airway or respiratory problems.

NOTE

The reader should refer to Chapter 6 and Chapter 11 to review airway anatomy.

Smoke inhalation most commonly occurs in a closed environment such as a building, an automobile, or an airplane and is caused by the accumulation of toxic byproducts of combustion. Inhalation injury also can occur in an open space; therefore all burn victims should be evaluated for this injury. Dangers that contribute to inhalation injury in a fire environment are as follows:

- Heat
- Consumption of oxygen by the fire
- Production of carbon monoxide
- Production of other toxic gases

NOTE

Inhalation injury also may occur in the absence of significant thermal injury from exposure to toxic gases (e.g., carbon monoxide).

Pathophysiology

Smoke inhalation and inhalation injury compose a broad group of consequences secondary to combustion. For this text, these consequences are classified as carbon monoxide poisoning, inhalation injury above the glottis (*supraglottic*), and inhalation injury below the glottis (*infraglottic*).

Carbon Monoxide Poisoning

Carbon monoxide is a colorless, odorless, tasteless gas produced by incomplete combustion of carbon-containing fuels. Carbon monoxide does not physically harm lung tissue, but it causes a reversible displacement of oxygen on the hemoglobin molecule, forming carboxyhemoglobin (COHb). The result is low circulating volumes of oxygen despite normal partial pressures. In addition, the presence of COHb requires that tissues be very hypoxic before oxygen is released from the hemoglobin to fuel the cells.

Carbon monoxide has about 250 times the affinity for hemoglobin that oxygen has. Therefore small concentrations of carbon monoxide in inspired air can result in severe physiological impairments, including tissue hypoxia, inadequate cellular oxygenation, inadequate cellular and organ function, and eventually death. The physical effects of carbon monoxide poisoning are related to the level of COHb in the blood (see the box below).

Treatment of the patient with carbon monoxide poisoning includes ensuring a patent airway, providing adequate ventilation, administering high-concentration oxygen, and possible pharmacological therapy (sodium thiosulfate, 12.5 g) for severely poisoned patients. The half-life of carbon monoxide at room air is about 4 hours. This can be reduced to 30 to 40 minutes if 100% oxygen and adequate ventilation are provided. The use of hyperbaric oxygen therapy to promote increased oxygen uptake on parts of the hemoglobin molecule not yet bound by carbon monoxide is controversial in treating carbon monoxide poisoning. The paramedic should follow local protocol.

> **NOTE**
>
> As discussed in Chapter 11, the pulse oximeter is unreliable in determining effective patient oxygenation in carbon monoxide poisoning.

PHYSICAL EFFECTS OF CARBON MONOXIDE BLOOD LEVELS

Carbon monoxide levels less than 10% usually do not cause symptoms; they are common in smokers, traffic police, truck drivers, and others who are chronically exposed to carbon monoxide. At levels of 20%, a healthy patient may complain of headache, nausea, vomiting, and loss of manual dexterity. At 30% the patient may become confused and lethargic, and ECG abnormalities may be present. At levels between 40% and 60%, coma may develop. Levels above 60% often are fatal. Tachypnea and cyanosis usually are not present in these patients because arterial oxygen tension is normal. Patients with high COHb levels may have a skin appearance that is bright red, but more commonly the patient has normal or pale skin and lip coloration.

In addition to carbon monoxide, other volatile byproducts (e.g., cyanide, hydrogen sulfide) may be released when some materials are burned. Inhalation of these toxins can result in inhalation poisoning (e.g., *thiocyanate intoxication*) and may require pharmacological therapy (e.g., Pasadena cyanide antidote kit, formerly the *Lily Cyanide Poison Kit*), further described in Chapter 34.

? CRITICAL THINKING

Can carbon monoxide poisoning be ruled out if the patient does not have these signs or symptoms?

Inhalation Injury Above the Glottis

The structure and function of the airway superior to the glottis make it particularly susceptible to injury if exposed to high temperatures. The upper airway is very vascular and has a large surface area, which allows it to normalize temperatures of inspired air. Because of this design, actual thermal injury to the lower airway is rare because the upper airway sustains the impact of injury when environmental air is superheated.

Thermal injury to the airway can result in immediate edema of the pharynx and larynx (above the level of the true vocal cords), which can rapidly progress to complete airway obstruction (Fig. 21-10). Signs and symptoms of upper airway inhalation injury include the following:

- Facial burns
- Singed nasal or facial hairs
- Carbonaceous sputum

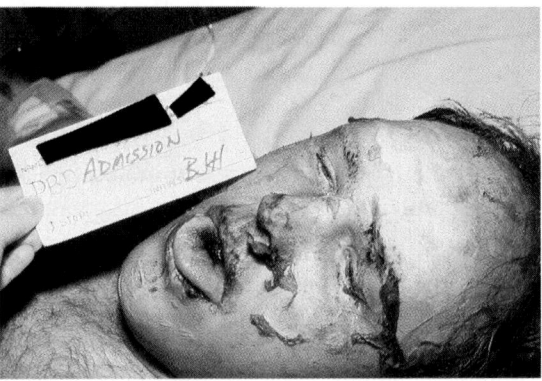

Fig. 21-10 Inhalation injury.

- Edema of the face, oropharyngeal cavity, or both
- Signs of hypoxemia
- Hoarse voice
- Stridor
- Brassy cough
- Grunting respirations

Prompt recognition and protection of the airway are critical in these patients. If impending airway obstruction is suspected, early nasotracheal or orotracheal intubation may be warranted because progressive edema can make emergency intubation extremely hazardous if not impossible.

Inhalation Injury Below the Glottis

The two primary mechanisms of direct injury to the lung parenchyma are heat and toxic material inhalation. Thermal injury to the lower airway is rare; causes include inhalation of superheated steam, which has 4000 times the heat-carrying capacity of dry air; aspiration of scalding liquids; and explosions, which occur as the patient is breathing high concentrations of oxygen under pressure.

Most fire-related lower-airway injuries result from the inhalation of toxic chemicals such as the gaseous byproducts of burning materials. Signs and symptoms of lower-airway injury may be immediate but more frequently are delayed, beginning several hours after the exposure. These include the following:

- Wheezes
- Crackles or rhonchi
- Productive cough
- Signs of hypoxemia
- Spasm of bronchi and bronchioles

Prehospital care should be directed at ensuring a patent airway and providing high-concentration oxygen and ventilatory support. Specific airway and ventilatory management, which may include nasal or oral tracheal intubation and pharmacological therapy with bronchodilators, should be coordinated with on-line/direct medical direction.

Chemical Burn Injury

Caustic chemicals frequently are present in the home and workplace, and unintentional exposure is common. Three types of caustic agents frequently are associated with burn injuries: alkalis, acids, and organic compounds. Alkalis (strong bases with a high pH), occur in hydroxides and carbonates of sodium, potassium, ammonium, lithium, barium, and calcium. These compounds commonly are found in oven cleaners, household drain cleaners, fertilizers, heavy industrial cleaners, and the structural bonds of cement and concrete. Strong acids are in many household cleaners, such as rust removers, bathroom cleaners, and swimming pool acidifiers (Fig. 21-11).

Organic compounds are chemicals that contain carbon. Most organic compounds, such as wood and coal, are harmless chemicals. However, several organic compounds produce caustic injury to human tissue. These include phenols and creosote and petroleum products such as gasoline. In addition to their role in producing chemical burns, organic compounds may be absorbed by the skin, causing serious systemic effects. The severity of chemical injury is related to the chemical agent, concentration and volume of the chemical, and duration of contact.

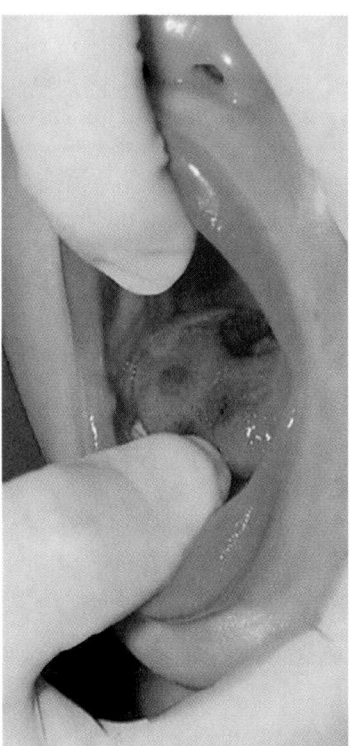

Fig. 21-11 Intraoral chemical burns sustained by a boy who has ingested bleach. (From Beattie TF, Hendry GM, Duguid KP: *Pediatric emergencies*, London, 1997, Mosby-Wolfe.)

Assessment

Exposure factors often can be assessed during the patient history. When dealing with a chemical exposure, the paramedic should ascertain the following:

- Type of chemical substance. If the container is available and can be safely transported, it should be taken to the medical facility.
- Concentration of chemical substance
- Volume of chemical substance
- Mechanism of injury (local immersion of a body part, injection, splash)
- Time of contamination
- First aid administered before EMS arrival
- Appearance (chemical burns vary in color)
- Pain

Management

As with all burn injuries, the safety of the rescuers must be the first consideration in managing the victim of chemical injury. (Law enforcement, fire service, and special rescue personnel may be needed to secure the scene before entry.) The paramedic must consider the use of protective gear before approaching the scene. Depending on the scene and the chemical agent(s) involved, personal protection may include gloves, eye shields, protective garments, and appropriate breathing apparatus. The treatment of chemical injuries varies little from that of thermal burns during the initial assessment. Treatment is directed at stopping the burning process. This can best be accomplished by the following:

1. Remove all clothing, including shoes, which can trap concentrated chemicals.
2. Brush off powdered chemicals.
3. Irrigate the affected area with copious amounts of water.
   a. In otherwise stable patients, irrigation takes priority over transportation unless irrigation can be continued en route to the emergency department.

> **NOTE**
>
> A response to a hazardous materials incident requires special safety considerations and trained rescue personnel (see Chapter 51).

   b. If a large body surface area is involved, a shower should be used for irrigation, if readily available.

Chemical Burn Injury to the Eyes

Chemical exposure to the eyes (e.g., from mace, pepper spray, other irritants) may cause damage ranging from superficial inflammation (*chemical conjunctivitis*) to severe burns. Patients with these conditions have local pain, visual disturbance, lacrimation (tearing), edema, and redness of surrounding tissues. Management guidelines include flushing the eyes with water by using a mild flow from a hose, intravenous tubing, or water from a container. (The affected eye should be irrigated from the medial to the lateral aspect to avoid flushing the chemical into the unaffected eye.) Irrigation should be continued during transport. If contact lenses are present, they should be removed.

> **NOTE**
>
> When retracting the lids to irrigate the eyes, the paramedic should take care to apply pressure only to the bony structures surrounding the eye, avoiding pressure on the globe.

Some EMS services use nasal cannulas to irrigate both eyes simultaneously. The cannula is placed over the bridge of the nose, with the nasal prongs pointing down toward the eyes. The cannula is attached to an intravenous administration set using either normal saline or lactated Ringer's solution and run continually into both eyes (Fig. 21-12). Irrigation lenses (e.g., *Morgan Therapeutic Lens*) may be useful for prolonged eye irrigation in adults, provided that edema is absent and there are no lacerations or penetrating wounds of the globe or eyelids. The use of these devices in the prehospital setting is controversial and requires special training and authorization from medical direction.

> **NOTE**
>
> A chemical burn to the eye can be frightening for the patient who fears loss of sight from the injury. The paramedic should attempt to calm the patient and explain the importance of thorough eye irrigation, which may be uncomfortable. This often will improve the patient's cooperation.

Use of Antidotes or Neutralizing Agents

According to the American Burn Association, no agent has been found to be superior to water for treating most chemical burns.[9] Consequently the use of antidotes or neutralizing agents should be avoided in initial prehospital management of most burn injuries. Many neutralizing agents produce heat and may increase injury when applied to the wound.

In special circumstances, such as when an industrial complex within a response area is known to use a chemical agent with a specific antidote, medical direction may elect to have the EMS stock the neutralizer. In this situation, paramedics should receive special training on the indications, contraindications, use, and side effects of these agents.

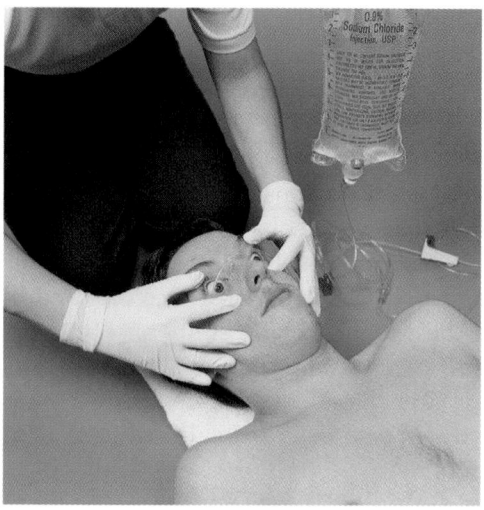

Fig. 21-12 Use of nasal cannula for eye irrigation.

Specific Chemical Injuries

Although the primary treatment for most chemical burns is copious irrigation with water, several specific chemical injuries warrant further discussion. These include petroleum, hydrofluoric acid, phenols, ammonia, and alkali metals.

Petroleum

In the absence of flame, products such as gasoline and diesel fuel can cause significant chemical burns if prolonged contact occurs (e.g., entrapment in a motor vehicle crash surrounded by spilled gasoline). Initially the injury appears to be only a first- or second-degree burn when in fact it may be a full-thickness injury. Systemic effects such as central nervous system depression, organ failure, and death may result from the absorption of various hydrocarbons. In addition, lead toxicity can occur if the exposure was from gasoline containing tetraethyl lead.

Hydrofluoric Acid

Hydrofluoric acid, one of the most corrosive materials known, is used in industry for cleaning fabrics and metals, for glass etching, and in the manufacture of silicone chips for electronic equipment. Both the hydrogen ion and fluoride ion are damaging to tissue. Fluoride inhibits several chemical reactions essential to cell survival, and it continues to penetrate and kill cells when it is neutralized by binding to calcium or magnesium. Thus endogenous or exogenous hydrofluoric acid has the potential to produce very deep, painful, and severe injuries. If large body surface areas are involved or there has been exposure to high concentrations of the acid, the patient may experience severe hypocalcemia and even death. Even the most minor-appearing wounds that involve hydrofluoric acid should be evaluated at an appropriate medical facility.

Irrigation of the exposed area with copious amounts of water should be initiated in the prehospital setting. On arrival in the emergency department, patient treatment may include subcutaneous administration of a 10% **calcium gluconate** solution directly into the burn site.

Phenol

Phenol (*carbolic acid*) is an aromatic hydrocarbon derived from coal tar. It is widely used in industry as a disinfectant in cleaning agents and in the manufacture of plastics, dyes, fertilizers, and explosives. Skin contact with phenol can result in local tissue coagulation and systemic toxicity if the agent is absorbed. A soft tissue injury from phenol exposure may be painless because of the agent's anesthetic properties. Minor exposures may cause central nervous system depression and dysrhythmias. Patients with significant exposures (10% to 15% TBSA) may require systemic support and should be carefully observed for signs of respiratory failure.

Wounds should be copiously irrigated with large volumes of water. After irrigation, medical direction may recommend that the wound be swabbed with a suitable solvent such as glycerol, vegetable oil, or soap and water to bind phenol and prevent its systemic absorption.

Ammonia

Ammonia is a noxious, irritating gas and strong alkali that is very soluble in water. It is an extremely hazardous solution if introduced into the eye and may result in tissue necrosis and blindness. The patient with an ammonia "burn" to the eye will probably have swelling or spasm of the eyelids. These patient injuries must be irrigated with water or a balanced salt solution for up to 24 hours.

Respiratory injury from ammonia vapors depends on the concentration and duration of exposure. For example, short-term, high-concentration exposure usually results in upper-airway edema, whereas long-term low-concentration exposure may damage the lower respiratory tract. Initial care for patients with respiratory injury includes high-concentration oxygen administration, ventilatory support as needed, and rapid transport to an appropriate medical facility.

Alkali Metals

Sodium and potassium are highly reactive metals that can ignite spontaneously. Water is generally

---

PRINCIPLES OF ELECTRICITY

Tissue damage produced by electric current is a function of six factors: *amperage, voltage, resistance, type of current, current pathway,* and *duration of current flow.*

1. Amperage. Amperage is a measure of the current flow (intensity) per unit of time. One ampere (amp) is a passage of 1 coulomb of charge per second past any point in the circuit. Thus a 10-amp flow means that 10 coulombs of electricity are passing a point per second.

2. Voltage. Voltage is a continuous force (tension) applied to any electric circuit that produces a flow of electricity. Volts are the potential driving force for electrical current. One volt is the force needed to drive 1 amp of current in a circuit with 1 ohm of resistance. High-voltage electrical injuries result from contact with a source of 1000 volts or greater. High-tension accidents commonly range from 7200 to 19,000 volts but may involve current with as high as 100,000 to 1 million volts.

3. Ohm. An ohm is a measure of the resistance of an electrical conductor. Electrical resistance is composed of four factors: (1) resistivity, the capacity of a material to resist current flow; (2) the size of the object pathway; (3) the length of the object pathway; and (4) temperature. Resistance to the flow of electricity varies greatly within the body because various tissues have different resistance to current flow. Tissue resistance to electrical flow in the body is highest in bone, decreasing progressively through the fat, skin, muscle, blood, and nerve tissue.

4. Type of current. Two basic forms of electric current are in common usage: direct current (DC) and alternating current (AC). The type of current can in-

fluence patterns and severity of injury. DC flows in one direction only. It frequently is used in industry and is the type of current produced by batteries. DC commonly is used in electrosurgical devices and defibrillators and is characterized by high amperage and low voltage.

AC reverses the direction of flow at regular intervals (60-cycle current has 60 reversals per second). These alterations in current direction can cause tetanic muscle contractions, which may "freeze" the victim to the source until the current is terminated. Household current in the United States generally is AC and either 120 or 220 volts. AC is a more common cause of electrical injury.

5. Current pathway. Electricity normally flows along a continuous pathway known as an *electric circuit.* Although the current pathway can be somewhat unpredictable, as a rule, low-voltage current (less than 1000 volts) follows the path of least resistance and high-voltage current follows the shortest path. In either case, the greater the current flow, the greater the heat generated.

The pathway of the current through the body is important because it gives a clue as to what anatomical structures are damaged. For example, if the current travels from one hand to the other, it may flow across the heart and provoke ventricular fibrillation or other dysrhythmias.

6. Duration of flow. Tissue injury results from the conversion of electrical energy into heat. The amount of heat produced is directly proportional to the square of the current strength multiplied by the resistance of the tissue multiplied by the duration of the current flow (Joule's law). Therefore injury is directly proportional to the duration of contact with the electrical source.

contraindicated when these metals are imbedded in the skin because they react with water and produce large amounts of heat. Physically removing the metal or covering it with oil minimizes the thermal injury.

Electrical Burn Injuries

Electrical injuries account for 4% to 6.5% of admissions to burn centers and are responsible for about 500 deaths each year.[2] An understanding of the principles of current and the path of destruction it may produce in the body is essential for good patient care and personal safety at the scene of an electrocution (see the box on p. 614).

Types of Electrical Injury

Three basic types of injury may occur as a result of contact with electric current: *direct contact burns, arc injuries,* and *flash burns.* Direct contact burns occur when electric current directly penetrates the resistance of the skin and underlying tissues. The hand and wrist are common entrance sites, and the foot is a common exit site (Fig. 21-13). Although the skin may initially resist current flow, continued contact with the source lessens resistance and permits increased current flow. The greatest tissue damage occurs directly under and adjacent to the contact points and may include fat, fascia, muscle, and bone. Tissue destruction may be massive at the entrance and exit sites; however, it is the area between these wounds that poses the greatest threat to the patient's life.

Arc injuries occur when a person is close enough to a high-voltage source that the current between two contact points near the skin overcomes the resistance in the air, passing the current flow through the air to the bystander. Temperatures generated by these sources can be as high as 2000° C to 4000° C (3632° F to 7232° F), and the arc may jump as far as 10 feet.

Flame and flash burn injuries can occur when the heat of electric current ignites a nearby combustible source. Common injury sites include the face and eyes (*Welder's flash*). Flash burns also may ignite a person's clothing or cause fire in the surrounding environment. No electrical current passes through the body in this type of burn.

Effects of Electrical Injury

Electrical injuries often are unpredictable and vary according to the parameters described. However, certain physiological effects should be anticipated by the paramedic crew.

The skin is almost always the first point of contact with electrical current. Direct contact and passage of current through tissue may produce extensive areas of coagulation necrosis. The entrance site is often a characteristic "bull's-eye" wound and may appear dry, leathery, charred, or depressed. The exit wound may be ulcerated and may have an "exploded" appearance where areas of tissue are missing.

TRICKS OF THE TRADE

The entrance site of an electrical injury can "hide" and may be difficult to find, particularly in a patient with an altered level of consciousness. Look for the wound in the "not-so-common" places such as between the fingers and toes and in the patient's hairline.

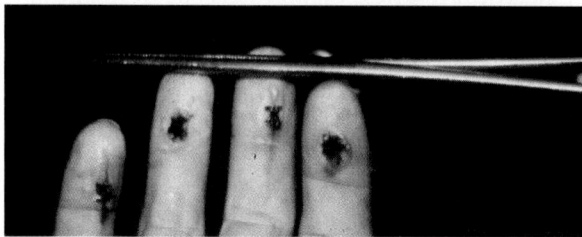

A

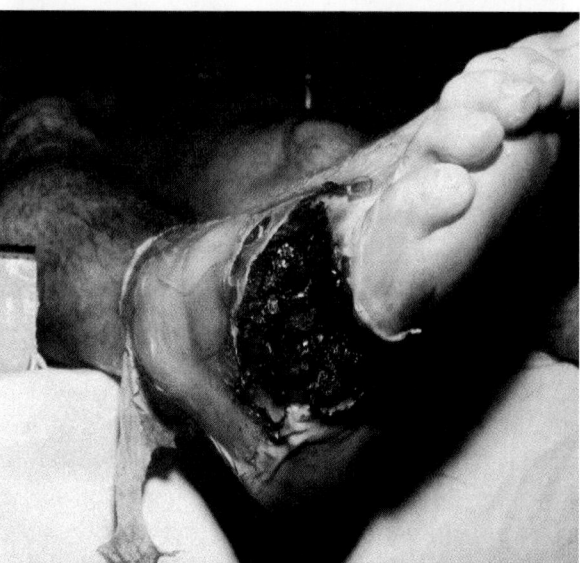

B

Fig. 21-13 Direct contact burn. **A,** Entry wound (hand). **B,** Exit wound (foot).

Oral burns frequently are seen in children under 2 years of age. These wounds typically are caused by chewing or sucking on a low-tension electrical cord. Oral burns may be associated with injury to the tongue, palate, and face.

Hypertension and tachycardia associated with a large release of catecholamines is a common finding in electrical injury. Electrical current also may cause significant dysrhythmias (including ventricular fibrillation and asystole) and damage to the myocardium as it passes through the body. If the patient has suffered cardiac arrest and early rescue and resuscitation can be initiated by the paramedic, success rates are high.

> **NOTE**
>
> As little as 100 milliamperes can cause ventricular fibrillation.

Nerve tissue is an excellent conductor of electrical current and may therefore be commonly affected in electrical injuries. Central nervous system damage may result in seizures or coma with or without focal neurological findings; peripheral nerve injury may lead to motor or sensory deficits, which may be permanent. If the current passes through the brain stem, respiratory arrest or depression, cerebral edema, or hemorrhage may rapidly lead to death.

Electrical injury can cause extensive necrosis of blood vessels. These injuries, although they may not be evident on EMS arrival, can cause immediate or delayed internal hemorrhage or arterial or venous thrombosis and embolism with subsequent complications.

Damage within the extremities after an electrical burn is similar to crush injury (described in Chapter 20) in that severe muscle necrosis releases myoglobin, and hemolysis releases hemoglobin, which can precipitate in the renal tubules, producing acute renal failure. (Some patients may require amputation of the affected extremity as a result of decreased circulation and compartment syndrome.) In the electrocuted patient, severe muscle spasms can produce bony fractures and dislocations, even of major joints. In addition, a patient may fall after the electrical shock and sustain significant skeletal trauma, including damage to the cervical spine.

Acute renal failure is a serious complication that affects about 10% of significant direct-contact electrical injuries. It may result from a combination of myoglobin or hemoglobin sludging in the renal tubules, disseminated intravascular coagulation secondary to tissue damage, hypovolemic shock, and DC damage. Although acute renal failure is not of immediate consequence in the prehospital environment, prompt fluid resuscitation and management of shock may have a positive impact on a significant number of these patients.

Ventilation may be impaired when electrical burns produce central nervous system injury or chest wall dysfunction. If the respiratory center is disrupted, hypoventilation can lead to immediate patient death. Contact with any AC sources has also been documented to produce respiratory arrest and death from tetany of the muscles of respiration.

Conjunctival and corneal burns and ruptured tympanic membranes are common in some electrical injuries. Cataracts and hearing loss also may appear as late as 1 year after the event.

Numerous other internal structures may be damaged secondary to electrical injury, including the abdominal organs and urinary bladder. Submucosal hemorrhage may occur in the bowel, and various forms of ulceration are possible. Each patient requires a thorough physical assessment and a high degree of suspicion for associated trauma.

Assessment and Management

Patient assessment should begin by ensuring that no hazards exist for the rescuers or bystanders. If the patient is still in contact with the electrical source, the electric company, fire department, or other specially trained personnel should be summoned before approaching the patient. Once the scene is safe, patient intervention may begin.

> **? CRITICAL THINKING**
>
> *What will you do if you respond to a scene and there is a child still in contact with electrical current having tetanic movements, with a large crowd gathered around screaming at you to help? The fire department is 3 minutes away. How will you feel?*

Initial Assessment

The initial assessment should proceed as for all other trauma patients, with particular care taken to immobilize the cervical spine. If the patient is not breathing, assisted ventilation should proceed immediately. Intubation should be performed as soon as possible because apnea may persist for lengthy periods. A patient who is breathing should have a patent airway maintained and respirations supported with supplemental high-concentration oxygen. If the patient is in cardiac arrest, resuscitation efforts should be implemented according to protocol. If possible, a history should be obtained, including the following:

- Patient's chief complaint (e.g., injury, disorientation)
- Source, voltage, and amperage of the electrical injury
- Duration of contact
- Level of consciousness before and after the injury
- Past significant medical history

> **NOTE**
>
> The source, voltage, and type of current (AC versus DC) is essential information for the attending physician to estimate internal damage from external wounds.

Physical Examination

The physical exam should be particularly thorough to search for entrance and exit wounds or any associated trauma caused by tetany or a fall. The paramedic should remember that there may have been multiple pathways of current and therefore multiple wounds. All of the patient's clothing and jewelry should be removed and the areas between the patient's fingers and toes should be examined for sites of entry or exit. Distal pulses, motor function, and sensation should be carefully assessed in all extremities and well documented to monitor for possible development of compartment syndrome. Entrance and exit wounds should be covered with sterile dressings, and any associated trauma should be managed appropriately.

Internal damage from electrical current may be much more significant than external wounds, and frequent reassessment is necessary because of the progressive nature of electrical injury. In addition, ECG monitoring should be implemented at the scene and continued during patient transport. As previously discussed, electrical injury may cause a variety of dysrhythmias, some of which can be lethal.

Management

Early fluid resuscitation is critical in managing patients with severe electrical injury to prevent hypovolemia and subsequent renal failure. If possible, two large-bore intravenous lines should be established in an extremity without entry or exit wounds. The fluid of choice generally is lactated Ringer's solution or normal saline without glucose, and the flow rate should be determined by the patient's clinical status.

In the emergency department or during interhospital transfer, the patient's intravenous fluid rates will be regulated to maintain a urine output of 75 to 100 mL/hr, which decreases the potential for renal damage caused by myoglobin. In addition, emergency department management may include administration of **sodium bicarbonate** to maintain an alkaline urine, which increases the solubility of hemoglobin and myoglobin and thus minimizes the incidence of renal failure.

Lightning Injury

Lightning strikes the earth about 7.4 million times each year and accounts for about 90 deaths each year.[2] It comprises DC of up to 200,000 amps at a potential of 100 million or more volts, with temperatures that vary between 16,000° F and 60,000° F (8871° C and 33,315° C). Lightning injuries can occur from a direct strike or by a side flash (splash) between a victim and a nearby object that has been struck by lightning. About 30% of those struck by lightning die.

> **NOTE**
>
> Lightning strikes are most common in Florida, Texas, and North Carolina.

Lightning strikes produce tissue injuries that differ from other types of electrical injury because the pathway of tissue damage often is *over* rather than *through* the skin (Fig. 21-14). Because the duration of the lightning is short (1/100 to 1/1000 second), skin burns are less severe than those seen with other high-voltage current, and third-degree burns are rare. Common lightning burns are linear, feathery, and punctate (pinpoint) in appearance. In addition, depending on the severity of the strike, the patient may suffer cardiac and respiratory arrest, which are the most common causes of death in lightning injuries.

Lightning injuries may be classified as minor, moderate, or severe. Patients with minor lightning injuries usually are conscious and frequently are confused and amnestic. Burns or other signs of injury are rare, and vital signs usually are stable.

Patients with moderate injury may be combative or comatose and may have associated injuries from the impact of the lightning strike. First- and second-degree burns are common, as is tympanic membrane rupture. These patients may have serious internal organ damage and should be carefully observed for signs and symptoms of cardiorespiratory dysfunction.

Severe lightning injuries include those that cause immediate brain damage, seizures, respiratory paralysis, and cardiac arrest. Prehospital care is directed at basic and advanced life support measures and rapid transport to an appropriate medical facility.

Assessment and Management

Like all other emergency responses, scene safety is the first priority. If the electrical storm is still in progress, all patient care activities should take place in a sheltered area. To prevent injury from subsequent lightning strikes, the paramedic crew should stay away from objects that project from the ground, including trees, fences, and high buildings, and avoid areas of open water. If rescue attempts in an open area are necessary, the paramedic should stay low to the ground.

Prehospital management of lightning injuries is the same as for other severe electrical injuries. Initial patient care is directed at airway and ventilatory support; basic and advanced life support; patient immobilization; fluid resuscitation to prevent hypovolemia and renal failure; pharmacological therapy (per protocol) to manage seizures (if present) and promote excretion of myoglobin and to treat dysrhythmias; wound care; and rapid transport to an appropriate medical facility.

NOTE

Cardiopulmonary resuscitation should be initiated immediately for patients who appear "dead" because resuscitation is possible after lightning injury.

Radiation Exposure

The most common radiation accidents involve sealed radioactive sources used in industrial radiography and nondestructive testing. Victims of these types of accidents rarely require emergency care. However, EMS personnel may be summoned to building fires and transportation crashes potentially involving radioactive materials, so an understanding of the hazards of radiation exposure is important.

NOTE

Safety issues regarding radiation have been excellent overall throughout the world. However, hazards associated with radiation became well known as a result of the disastrous accident at the Chernobyl Nuclear Power Station in the Soviet Union in 1986 and the serious potential for disaster that occurred at Three Mile Island in Pennsylvania in 1979.

? CRITICAL THINKING

What industries in your area use radioactive materials? Is there a preplan for accidents at that site?

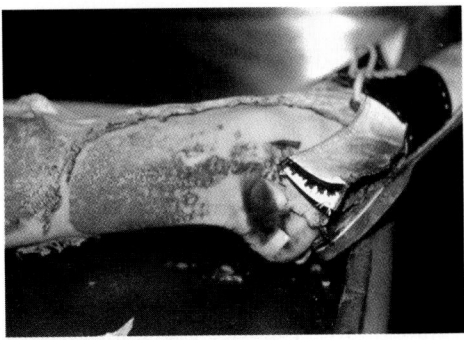

Fig. 21-14 Lightning injury. (Courtesy Michael Graham, MD.)

Characteristics of Radioactive Particles

Radioactive particles generally are classified into three types: *alpha, beta,* and *gamma.* Alpha particles are large, travel only a few millimeters, and have minimal penetrating ability. They may be stopped by paper, clothing, or skin and are considered the least dangerous external radiation source. However, if alpha particles enter the body through inhalation, ingestion, or absorption, they can damage internal organs and interfere with the body's chemical functions. Internal exposure to alpha radiation is considered the most dangerous form of internal radiation exposure.

Beta particles are one-seven thousandth the size of alpha particles but have considerably more energy and penetrating power. Beta particles can penetrate subcutaneous tissue and usually enter the body through damaged skin, ingestion, or inhalation. Protection from alpha and beta radiation requires full protective clothing, including a positive-pressure SCBA.

Gamma rays and x-rays are the most dangerous forms of penetrating radiation, requiring lead shields for protection. Gamma rays have 10,000 times the penetrating power of alpha particles and 100 times the penetrating power of beta particles. Protective clothing does not stop gamma rays. Gamma rays possess both internal and external hazards and may produce localized skin burns and extensive internal damage.

Harmful Effects from Radiation Exposure

Nonionizing radiation includes radio waves and microwaves and usually is not considered dangerous. Ionizing radiation is produced by nuclear weapons, reactors, radioactive material, and x-ray machines. Although it is rare, the exposure to ionizing radiation poses a threat to victims and rescue personnel.

> **NOTE**
>
> Radiation is a hazardous material. The paramedic crew should not enter the scene until the scene has been made safe by appropriate authorities.

The amount of emitted radiation is expressed in *roentgens* and indicates the ionization produced in the air by gamma or x-radiation. Other units used to measure radiation are the *rad* (radiation absorbed dose), and the *rem* (roentgen equivalent man). A rad is a measure of both the amount of ionized radiation being emitted and the amount that has been absorbed and is active within the body tissues. A rem is used to assess the biological effects of the different types of radiation. For emergency purposes, rescue personnel should assume that 1 roentgen = 1 rad = 1 rem.

Doses of less than 100 rem usually do not cause significant acute problems. Doses from 100 to 200 rem may cause symptoms but are not life threatening. When an exposure of 200 rem is approached, nausea, vomiting, and diarrhea begin within 2 to 4 hours. After an exposure of 450 rems, 50% mortality can be expected within 30 days if no medical care is given. Victims of radiation accidents rarely show immediate signs or symptoms of exposure. Therefore all victims of possible exposure should be presumed to have a radiation injury until proved otherwise. (See the box on p. 620.)

> **NOTE**
>
> An object or a person who has been exposed to radiation is not "radioactive." It is only the *presence* of radioactive residue that poses a threat to rescuers.

Emergency Response to Radiation Accidents

If the EMS crew has been advised that radioactive materials are present at an emergency scene, they should approach the site with caution and not enter the scene until it has been secured by proper authorities (see Chapter 51). Rescue personnel, emergency vehicles, and the command post should be positioned 200 to 300 feet upwind of the site. Emergency workers should not eat, drink, or smoke at the accident site or in any rescue vehicle. The appropriate local authorities should be contacted (state radiological health office, local specialists), and medical direction should be notified. Protective clothing suitable for other hazardous material releases should be worn by all emergency workers, and dose meters should be available for all rescue personnel. SCBAs should be used if fire, smoke, or gas is present.

TYPES OF RADIATION INJURY

The harmful effects from radiation may be classified as *external irradiation, contamination by radioactive materials, incorporation of radioactive materials,* and *combined radiation injury.*

External irradiation occurs when all or part of the body is exposed to penetrating radiation from an external source. An example of external irradiation is a medical x-ray. The degree of radiation injury depends on the intensity of radiation, which in turn depends on the duration of exposure and the distance from the source. A patient who has been exposed to large amounts of radiation may have nausea, vomiting, and diarrhea. In severe cases, additional symptoms may include weight loss, hair loss, fever, bleeding, mouth and throat sores, skin burns, lowered body resistance, vesiculation, and ulceration. The effects from this type of radiation are not contagious, and providing emergency care poses no risks to the rescuer.

Contamination occurs when radioactive materials in the form of gases, liquids, or solids are released into the environment, contaminating people internally, externally, or both. When radioactive material remains on the patient's clothing or skin or in open wounds, a potential hazard is present for both the rescuer and the patient. Patients who have been contaminated should be considered medical emergencies and may pose significant risk to emergency providers.

Incorporation refers to the uptake of radioactive materials by body cells, tissues, and target organs such as bone, liver, thyroid, or kidney. Incorporation is impossible unless contamination has occurred.

A combination radiation injury involves external irradiation, contamination, incorporation, or some combination of these. This type of exposure usually is the result of a major incident and may be complicated by a patient's physical injury.

After exposure to radiation, individuals may be at risk for delayed complications, which include cell and chromosomal changes, subsequent reproductive genetic aberrations, cell death, and sterility. In addition, diseases such as anemia and various forms of cancer may develop.

Personal Protection from Radiation

The Federal Emergency Management Agency (FEMA) recommends that basic radiation protection for both the rescuer and the patient include the following four factors[10]:

1. Time: The less time spent in a radiation field, the less radiation exposure. If adequate personnel are available, a rotating team approach can be used to keep individual radiation exposure to a minimum.
2. Distance: The farther a person is from the source of radiation, the lower the radiation dose. Even moving several feet away from a radioactive source greatly reduces the level of exposure.
3. Shielding: The general principle of shielding is that the denser the material, the greater its ability to stop the passage of radiation. Lead shields provide the best protection from exposure. However, vehicles, mounds of dirt, and pieces of heavy equipment placed between the radiation source and the rescuer and victim also can diminish exposure levels. Protective clothing and SCBAs may provide adequate protection from all alpha and some beta radiation, but protective clothing does not prevent penetration of gamma rays. If adequate shielding is not readily available, rescuers should use the time and distance factors to reduce radiation exposure.
4. Quantity: Limiting the amount of radioactive material in a specific area lessens the radiation exposure. Examples include removing contaminated clothing, bagging all contaminated items, and moving containers of radioactive material from the area.

Emergency Care for Victims of Radiation Accidents

Patients who have been irradiated are not radioactive. However, when external contamination occurs and radioactive material remains on the patient's clothing and skin or in open wounds, the rescuer should consult with medical direction and follow agency protocol. The effects of radiation exposure may be immediate (e.g., burns) or delayed.

With the exception of dealing with contaminants and containing their spread, there are no emergency care procedures specific to radiation injury. All external bleeding should be controlled, the spine immobilized, open wounds covered, and fractures stabilized in normal fashion. The EMS crew should move the patient away from the radiation source as soon as possible. Lifesaving care should not be delayed for patient transfer or decontamination procedures. Intravenous fluid replacement should be initiated if indicated, using strict aseptic technique. If an IV line is not needed for specific therapy, its use should be avoided to prevent introducing contaminants into the body.

Radiation Decontamination Procedures

Radiation emergencies involving patients may be defined as either *clean*, meaning that the patient was exposed but not contaminated, or *dirty*, meaning that the patient was contaminated. Only properly trained personnel (e.g., Hazmat teams and qualified county, state, or federal health department personnel) should attempt to decontaminate radiation victims at the scene. A patient who is to be transported to a hospital for decontamination should be isolated from the environment (described in Chapter 51), and all patient effects should be transported with the patient.

S U M M A R Y

- Each year more than 2 million Americans seek medical attention for burns. Morbidity and mortality rates from burn injury follow significant patterns with regard to gender, age, and socioeconomic status. A burn injury is caused by an interaction between thermal, chemical, electrical, or radiation energy and biological matter.

- Tissue damage from burns depends on the degree of heat and duration of exposure to the thermal source. As local events occur at the injury site, other organ systems become involved in a general response to the stress caused by the burn.

- Burns are classified in terms of depth as first, second, and third degree. The rule of nines provides a rough estimate of burn injury size (extent) and is most accurate for adults and for children older than age ten. The Lund and Browder chart is a more accurate method of determining the area of burn injury. Severity of burn injury and burn center referral guidelines are based on standards that take into account the depth, extent, and severity of the burn wound; the source of injury; patient age; presence of concurrent medical or surgical problems; and the body region that is burned.

- Shock after thermal injury results from edema and accumulation of vascular fluid in the tissues in the area of injury and systemic hypovolemia if the burn is large.

- Emergency care for a burn patient begins with the initial assessment to recognize and treat life-threatening injuries.

- Goals for prehospital management of the severely burned patient include preventing further tissue injury, maintaining the airway, administering oxygen and ventilatory support, providing fluid resuscitation, providing rapid transport to an appropriate medical facility, using aseptic (clean) technique to minimize the patient's exposure to infectious agents, managing pain, and providing psychological and emotional support.

- Prehospital considerations in caring for patients with inhalation injury include recognition of the dangers inherent in the fire environment, pathophysiology of inhalation injury, and early detection and treatment of impending airway or respiratory problems.

- The severity of chemical injury is related to the chemical agent, concentration and volume of the chemical, and duration of contact. Treatment is directed as stopping the burning process by using copious irrigation.

- Three types of injury may occur as a result of contact with electric current: direct contact burns, arc injuries, and flash burns. Once the scene is safe, patient intervention may begin. Internal damage from electrical current may be much more significant than external wounds.

- Persons injured by radiation rarely require emergency care. Radioactive particles are classified into three types: alpha, beta, and gamma. The Federal Emergency Management Agency recommends that basic radiation protection for both the rescuer and the patient include four factors: minimize time in the radiation field; maintain a safe distance from the source; place shielding between the rescuers and the source; and limit the amount of radioactive material in a specific area.

REFERENCES

1. National Institute of General Medical Sciences, National Institutes of Health: *Trauma, burn, shock and injury: facts and figures*, Bethesda, Md, 1999, The Institute.
2. National Safety Council: *Injury facts*, Itasca, Ill, 1999, The Council.
3. Achauer B: *Management of the burned patient*, Norwalk, Conn, 1987, Appleton & Lange.
4. Committee on Trauma American College of Surgeons: *Resources for optimal care of the injured patient*, Chicago, 1999, The Committee.
5. Faldmo L et al: Management of acute burns and shock resuscitation, *Clin Iss Crit Care Nurs* 4(2):351, 1993.
6. Rosen P, Barkin R: *Emergency medicine: concepts and clinical practice*, ed 4, St Louis, 1998, Mosby.
7. American Heart Association: Guidelines 2000 for cardiopulmonary resuscitation and emergency cardiovascular care, International Consensus on Science, *Circulation* 102 (8):79, 2000.
8. US Department of Transportation National Highway Traffic Safety Administration: *EMT-Paramedic national standard curriculum*, Washington, DC, 1998, The Department.
9. Nebraska Burn Institute: *Advanced burn life support provider's manual*, Lincoln, 1990, The Institute.
10. Federal Emergency Management Agency: *Radiological emergency management*, http://www.fema.gov.

22 Head and Facial Trauma

OBJECTIVES

Upon completion of this chapter, the paramedic student will be able to:

1. **Describe the mechanisms of injury, assessment, and management of maxillofacial injuries.**

2. **Describe the mechanisms of injury, assessment, and management of ear, eye, and dental injuries.**

3. **Describe the mechanisms of injury, assessment, and management of anterior neck trauma.**

4. **Describe the mechanisms of injury, assessment, and management of injuries to the scalp, cranial vault, or cranial nerves.**

5. **Distinguish between types of traumatic brain injury based upon an understanding of pathophysiology and assessment findings.**

6. **Outline the prehospital management of the patient with cerebral injury.**

7. **Calculate a Glasgow coma scale, trauma score, revised trauma score, and pediatric trauma score when given appropriate patient information.**

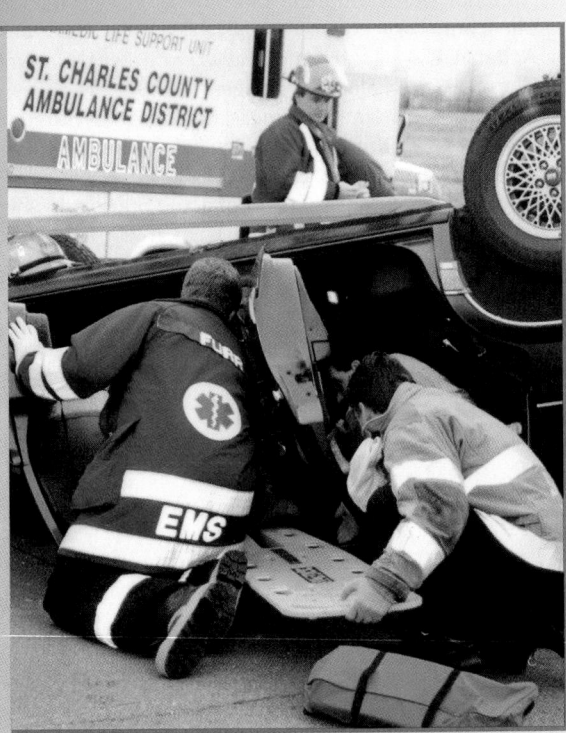

Head injuries affect nearly 4 million people each year in the United States, and about 50,000 patients with severe head trauma die each year before reaching the emergency department.[1] The categories of head trauma discussed in this chapter include maxillofacial trauma; ear, eye, and dental trauma; anterior neck trauma; and trauma to the skull and brain.

KEY TERMS

antegrade amnesia: The loss of memory for events that occurred immediately after recovery of consciousness.

Battle's sign: Ecchymosis over the mastoid process caused by a fracture of the temporal bone.

cerebral perfusion pressure: A measure of the amount of blood flow to the brain calculated by subtracting the intracranial pressure from the mean systemic arterial blood pressure.

Cushing's triad: Increased systolic pressure, widened pulse pressure, and decrease in the pulse and respiratory rate, which result from increased intracranial pressure.

decerebrate posturing: A position in which a comatose patient's arms are extended and internally rotated and the legs are extended with the feet in forced plantar flexion; usually observed in patients who have compression of the brainstem.

decorticate posturing: A position in which the comatose patient's upper extremities are rigidly flexed at the elbows and at the wrists; usually observed in patients who have a lesion in the mesencephalic region of the brain.

intracerebral hematoma: An accumulation of blood or fluid within the tissue of the brain.

LeFort fracture: A fracture pattern that can be produced in the midface region.

mean arterial pressure: The arithmetic mean of the blood pressure in the arterial portion of the circulation.

raccoon's eyes: Ecchymosis of one or both orbits caused by fracture of the base of the sphenoid sinus.

retrograde amnesia: The loss of memory for events that occurred before the event that precipitated the amnesia.

subarachnoid hematoma: A collection of blood or fluid in the subarachnoid space.

> **NOTE**
>
> The reader should refer to Chapter 6 to review anatomy of the head, neck, and face.

> **NOTE**
>
> The reader should refer to the Injury Prevention section located in Appendix C.

Maxillofacial Injury

In descending order of frequency, major causes of maxillofacial trauma are motor vehicle crashes, home accidents, athletic injuries, animal bites, intentional violent acts, and industrial injuries. Maxillofacial trauma may be classified as soft tissue injuries and facial fractures.

Soft Tissue Injuries

The face receives its blood supply from the branches of the internal and external carotid arteries. Because of this rich vascular supply, soft tissue injuries to the face often appear to be quite serious (Fig. 22-1). With the exception of a compromised upper airway and the potential for significant bleeding, however, damage to the tissues of the maxillofacial area is seldom life threatening. Depending on the mechanism of injury, facial trauma may range from minor cuts and abrasions to more serious injuries involving extensive soft tissue lacerations and avulsions. If possible, the paramedic should obtain a thorough history from the patient, including mechanism of injury; events leading up to the injury; time of injury; associated medical problems; and allergies, medications, and last oral intake.

> **?** CRITICAL THINKING
>
> *Why might it be difficult to obtain a history from a patient with this type of injury?*

> **NOTE**
>
> Soft tissue injuries to the nose and mouth are common with facial injuries. Special care should be taken with these patients to ensure a clear and open airway.

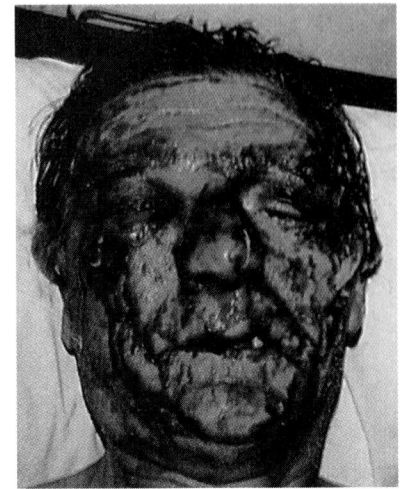 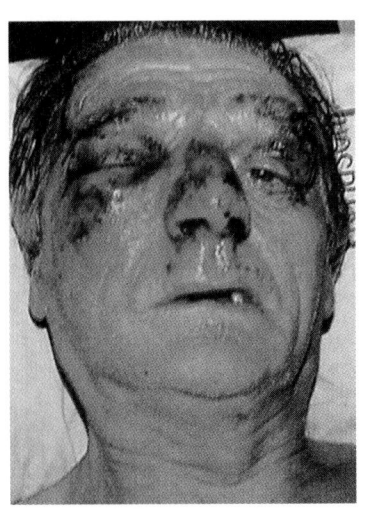

Fig. 22-1 A, Appearance of a patient after being attacked. **B,** Appearance of same man after cleansing. (From London PS: *A colour atlas of diagnosis after recent injury,* Ipswich, England, 1990, Wolfe Medical Publications, Ltd.)

6. Control bleeding through direct pressure and pressure bandages.

Facial Fractures

Although facial bones can withstand tremendous forces from energy impact, facial fractures are common after blunt trauma. The anatomical structure of the facial bones allows "stepwise" fracture to absorb the impact of blunt trauma. Blunt trauma injuries may be classified anatomically as fractures to the mandible, midface, zygoma, orbit, and nose. Signs and symptoms of facial fractures include:

- Pain
- Swelling
- Ecchymosis
- Lacerations and bleeding
- Numbness
- Dental malocclusion
- Limitation of mandibular excursion
- Visual disturbances
- Limited ocular movements
- Asymmetry of cheekbone prominences
- Discontinuity of the orbital rim
- Crepitus
- Displacement of the nasal septum

Fractures of the Mandible

The mandible is the single facial bone in the lower third of the face. Because of its prominence, fractures to this bone rank second in frequency after nasal fractures. The mandible is a hemicircle of bone and may break in multiple locations, often distant from the point of impact. Signs and symptoms spe-

Fig. 22-2 Fracture of the middle third of the face. (From London PS: *A colour atlas of diagnosis after recent injury,* Ipswich, England, 1990, Wolfe Medical Publications, Ltd.)

Management

1. Use spinal precautions (described in Chapter 23).
2. Assess the airway for obstruction caused by blood, vomitus, bone fragments, broken teeth, dentures, and damage to the anterior neck.
3. Apply suction as needed.
4. Secure and maintain the airway through oral or nasal adjuncts, tracheal intubation, or cricothyrotomy as indicated.
5. Ensure adequate ventilation and oxygenation.

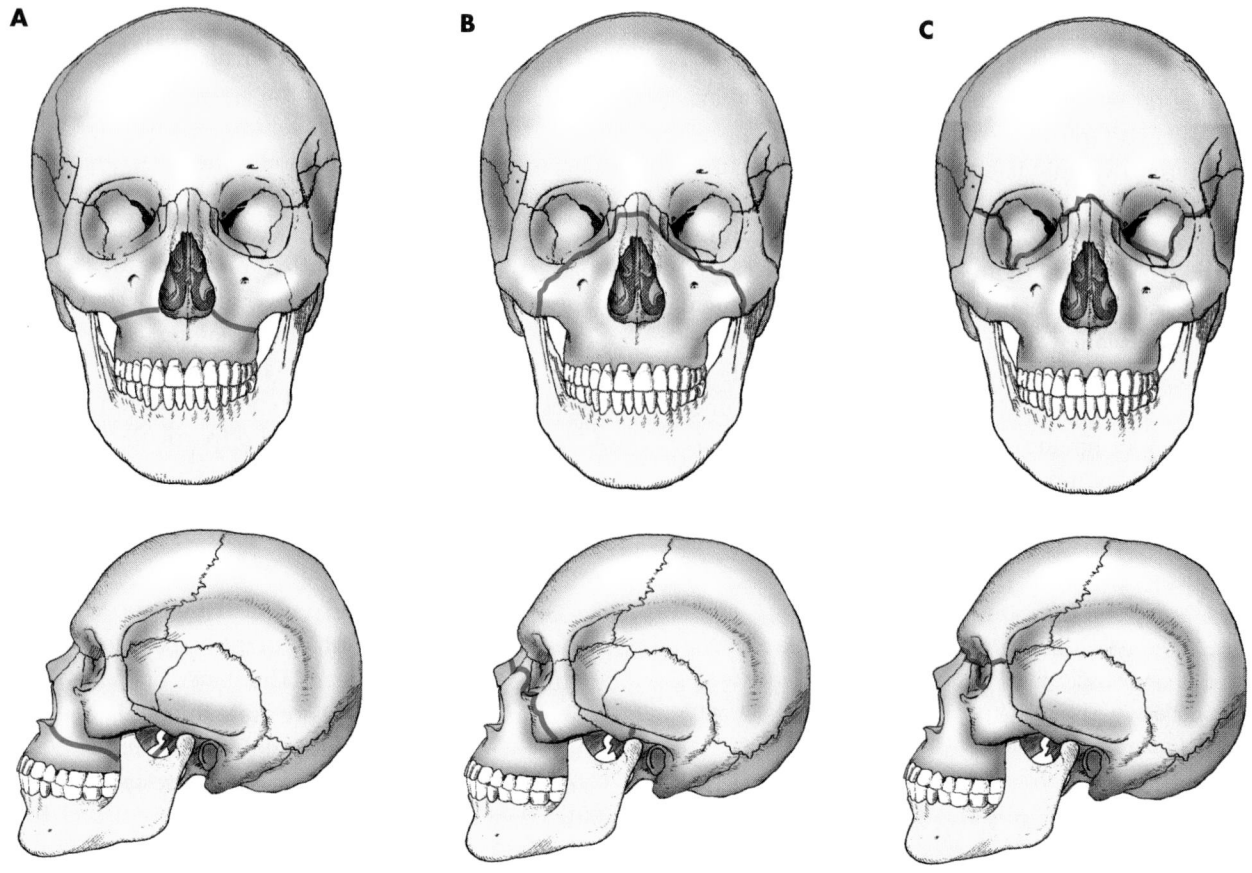

Fig. 22-3 **A,** LeFort I facial fractures (lateral and frontal views). **B,** LeFort II fractures (lateral and frontal views). **C,** LeFort III fractures (lateral and frontal views). (From Sheehy S: *Emergency nursing,* ed 3, St. Louis, 1992, Mosby.)

cific to mandibular fractures include malocclusion (patients may complain that their teeth do not "feel right" when their mouths are closed), numbness in the chin, and inability to open the mouth. The patient also may have difficulty swallowing and excessive salivation. Most patients with mandibular fractures require hospitalization.

Anterior dislocation of the mandible in the absence of fracture also may occur as a result of blunt trauma to the face (rare), an abnormally wide yawn, and dental treatment requiring that the jaws remain open for long periods. In these movements, the condylar head advances forward beyond the articular eminence of the temporal bone. The jaw-closing muscles spasm, and the mouth becomes locked in a wide-open position. The patient usually experiences severe pain from the muscle spasm and anxiety and discomfort that perpetuate the spasm. Mandibular dislocations are manually reduced in the emergency department with the aid of a muscle relaxant or sedative, or in the operating room with a general anesthetic.

? CRITICAL THINKING

What will be your patient care priority with these patients?

Fractures of the Midface

The middle third of the face includes the maxilla, zygoma, floor of the orbit, and nose. Fractures to this region result from direct or transmitted force (e.g., blunt trauma to the mandible transmitted to produce fractures to the maxilla). They often are associated with central nervous system injury and spinal trauma (Fig. 22-2).

LeFort fractures. In 1901, a cadaver study done by LeFort described three patterns of injuries **(LeFort fracture)** that can be produced in the midface region (Fig. 22-3). The LeFort I fracture involves the maxilla up to the level of the nasal fossa. The LeFort II involves the nasal bones and medial orbits and generally is shaped like a pyramid. The LeFort III entails craniofacial dislocation involving all of the bones of the face. Depending on the severity of injury, different combinations of LeFort fractures may be present.

Signs and symptoms specific to midface fractures include midfacial edema, unstable maxilla, lengthening of the face ("donkey face"), epistaxis, numb upper teeth, nasal flattening, and cerebrospinal fluid rhinorrhea (CSF leakage caused by ethmoid cribriform plate fracture). Patients with midface fractures usually are hospitalized. These patients (particularly those with LeFort II and III fractures) are at risk of having a seriously compromised airway and of having nasogastric or even nasotracheal tubes placed intracranially.

> **NOTE**
>
> As described in Chapter 11, nasal airways, nasogastric tubes, and nasotracheal intubation are contraindicated in patients who have fractures of the basal skull or facial bones.

> **NOTE**
>
> CSF leakage from the ear or nose should be allowed to drain freely. The paramedic should make no attempts to control CSF leakage with direct pressure.

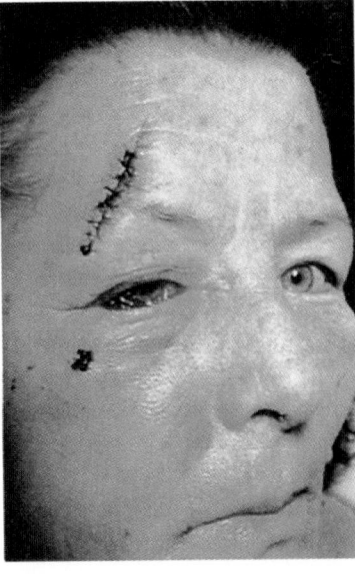

Fig. 22-4 Fracture of the zygomatic bone. (From London PS: *A colour atlas of diagnosis after recent injury*, Ipswich, England, 1990, Wolfe Medical Publications, Ltd.)

Fractures of the Zygoma

The zygoma (malar eminence) articulates with the frontal, maxillary, and temporal bones. It commonly is called the *cheekbone* and seldom is fractured because of its sturdy construction. When fractures occur, they usually are a result of physical assaults and motor vehicle crashes. Zygomatic fractures frequently are associated with orbital fractures and manifest similar clinical signs (Fig. 22-4). They are differentiated with radiological imaging. Signs and symptoms specific to zygomatic fractures include flatness of a usually rounded cheek area; numbness of the cheek, nose, and upper lip (particularly if an orbital fracture is involved); epistaxis; and altered vision.

Fractures of the Orbit

The orbital contents are protected by a bony ring that resembles a pyramid, with the apex pointed toward the back of the head. The bones of the walls, floor, and roof of the orbit are quite thin and are easily fractured by direct blows and transmitted forces. In addition, many orbital fractures are associated with other facial injuries, such as LeFort II and III fractures.

A blowout fracture to the orbit can occur when an object of greater diameter than that of the bony orbital rim strikes the globe of the eye and surrounding soft tissue (Fig. 22-5). This impact pushes the globe into the orbit, compressing the orbital contents. The sudden increase in intraocular pressure is transmitted to the orbital floor, the weakest part of the orbital structure. If the orbital floor fractures, the orbital contents may herniate into the maxillary sinus, where soft tissue and extraocular muscles may be entrapped in the defect. Signs and symptoms of blowout fractures include periorbital edema, subconjunctival ecchymosis, diplopia (double vision), enophthalmos (recessed globe), epistaxis, anesthesia in the region of the infraorbital nerve (anterior cheek), and impaired extraocular movements.

> **? CRITICAL THINKING**
>
> *How do you assess for extraocular movements?*

Orbital fractures often are associated with other fractures, such as LeFort II and III injuries and those of the zygomatic complex. In addition, injury to the orbital contents is common and should be suspected with any facial fracture.

Fractures of the Nose

Of all the facial bones, the nasal bones have the least structural strength and are fractured most frequently. The external portion of the nose, formed mostly of hyaline cartilage, is supported mainly by the nasal bones and the frontal processes of the maxillary bones. Injuries to the nose may depress the dorsum of the nose, displace it to one side, or result only in epistaxis and swelling without apparent skeletal deformity. Fractures to the orbit also may be present. In children, minimal displacement of nasal bones can result in growth changes and ultimate deformity.

Management of Facial Fractures

1. Assume that the spine has been injured and use spinal precautions (facial fractures are associated with a high percentage of concomitant cervical spine fractures).
2. Assess the airway for obstruction caused by blood, vomitus, bone fragments, broken teeth, dentures, and damage to the anterior neck.
3. Apply suction as needed.
4. Secure and maintain the airway through oral adjuncts, nasal adjuncts (in the absence of suspected midface or basal skull fracture), tracheal intubation, or cricothyrotomy as indicated.
5. Ensure adequate ventilation and oxygenation.
6. Control bleeding through direct pressure and pressure bandages.
7. Control epistaxis (which may be severe) by external direct pressure (compression of the anterior nares).

? CRITICAL THINKING

Why wouldn't you want the blood to drain posteriorly?

NOTE

To prevent blood from draining down the throat, mild epistaxis is best controlled in the conscious patient by instructing the patient to sit upright or to lean forward (if spinal precautions are not indicated) while compressing the nares. An unconscious patient should be positioned on the side (if not contraindicated by injury). If bleeding is severe, the patient should be evaluated for hemorrhagic shock.

Nasal and Ear Foreign Bodies

The insertion of foreign bodies (e.g., beans and crayons) in the nose or ear is not uncommon in children and may cause infection if the foreign bodies are not detected and removed. These patients may need to be transported for physician evaluation. A foreign body in the ear should be removed if it can be easily retrieved. As a rule, a foreign body in the nose

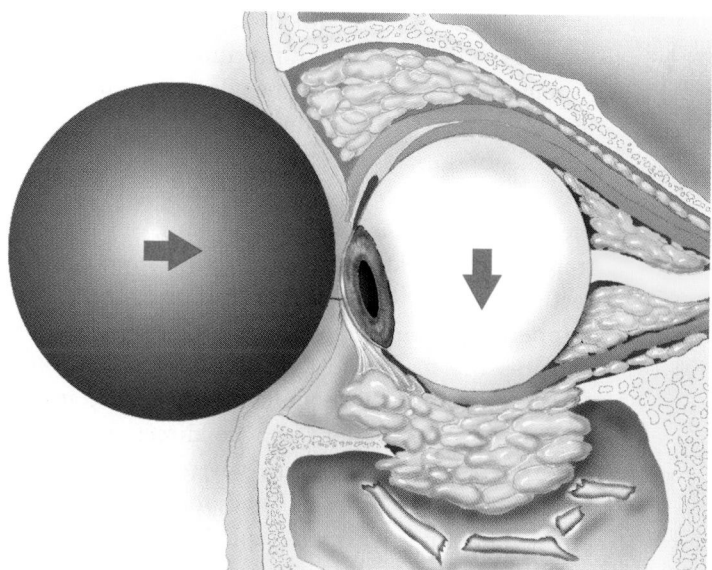

Fig. 22-5 Artist's impression of a blowout fracture caused by the impact of a ball. (From Ragge N: *Immediate eye care*, London, 1990, Wolfe Medical Publications, Ltd.)

should not be removed in the prehospital setting unless it is contributing to airway compromise or unless it can be easily removed without equipment.

Ear, Eye, and Dental Trauma

The ears, eyes, or teeth may be injured separately or in association with other forms of head trauma. Injury to these regions may be minor or may result in permanent sensory function loss and disfigurement. Regardless of the severity, ear, eye, and dental trauma should be evaluated and treated only after life-threatening problems have been addressed.

Ear Trauma

Trauma to the ear may include lacerations and contusions, thermal injuries, chemical injuries, traumatic perforations, and barotitis.

Lacerations and Contusions

Lacerations and contusions usually result from blunt trauma and are particularly common in victims of domestic violence (Fig. 22-6). These injuries are treated by direct pressure to control bleeding and the application of ice or cold compresses to decrease soft tissue swelling. If a portion of the outer ear (pinna) has been avulsed, the avulsed tissue should be retrieved if possible, wrapped in moist gauze, sealed in plastic, placed on ice, and transported with the patient for surgical repair.

> **NOTE**
> Cartilage tears often heal poorly and are easily infected.

Thermal Injuries

Thermal injuries may occur from prolonged exposure to extreme cold or in exposure of lesser duration to extreme heat. Contact with hot liquids or electrical currents also can lead to thermal injury. Prehospital management usually is limited to soft tissue dressings to prevent contamination and patient transportation for physician evaluation.

Chemical Injuries

Strong acids or alkali produce burns on contact. Emergency care consists of copious irrigation. After irrigation, the ear and ear canal should be bathed with saline or sterile water, allowing the irrigation liquid to remain in the ear canal for 2 to 3 minutes. This procedure should be repeated 3 to 4 times, after which the ear should be dried and covered to prevent contamination. The patient should be transported for physician evaluation.

Traumatic Perforations

The tympanic membrane can be perforated by penetrating objects such as a cotton-tipped applicator or from great pressure differentials resulting from explosions (blast injuries) or scuba diving (barotrauma). These injuries usually heal spontaneously without treatment, but evaluation by a physician is recommended.

If the injury is caused by a penetrating object, it should be stabilized in place, and the ear should be covered to prevent further contamination. If the inner or middle ear canal has been contaminated (e.g., by swimming water or a foreign object), antibiotic therapy usually is prescribed. Serious complications that may result from perforations include facial nerve palsy frequently accompanied by temporal bone fractures, hearing loss, and vertigo.

Barotitis

Barotitis occurs when an individual is exposed to changes in barometric pressure great enough to produce inflammation and injury to the middle ear. Barotitis can result, for example, from flying at high altitudes and from scuba diving.

Gas pressure in the air-filled spaces of the middle ear normally is in equilibrium with the environment. Boyle's law (further described in Chapter 36) states that at constant temperature, the volume of gas is inversely proportional to the pressure. On ascent, gas expands, and on descent, it contracts. Therefore, when gases become trapped or partially trapped, they expand in direct proportion to the decrease in pressure. When trapped gas cannot reach equilibrium with ambient pressure, pain and the sensation of a blocked ear may develop. To equalize the pressure in the middle ear, the patient can be directed to bear down (Valsalva maneuver), yawn, swallow, and move the lower jaw. These methods may cause the eustachian tube to open, equalizing pressure in the middle ear cavity.

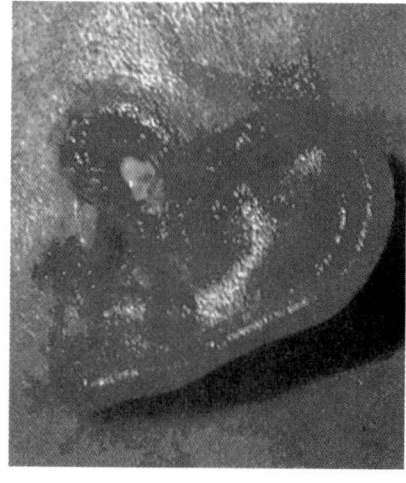 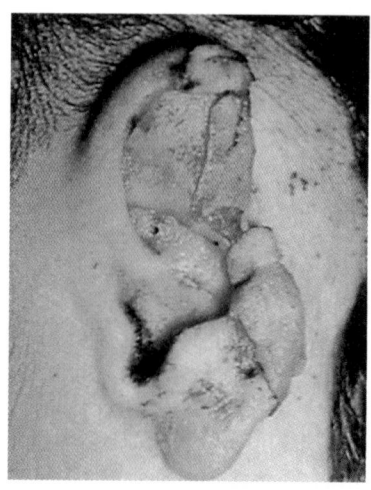

Fig. 22-6 A, Partially detached pinna. **B,** Loss of rim. (From London PS: *A colour atlas of diagnosis after recent injury,* Ipswich, England, 1990, Wolfe Medical Publications, Ltd.)

Eye Trauma

More than 2000 eye and orbital injuries are estimated to occur each day in the United States.[2] Common causes of eye injury are blunt and penetrating trauma from motor vehicle crashes, sport and recreational activities, and violent altercations; chemical exposure from household and industrial accidents; foreign bodies; and animal bites and scratches.

Evaluation

Acute eye injuries may be difficult to identify because a patient with normal vision may have a serious underlying injury. Symptoms requiring a high degree of suspicion include:

- Obvious trauma with eye injury
- Visual loss or blurred vision that does not improve with blinking, indicating possible damage to the globe, ocular contents, or optic nerve
- Loss of a portion of the visual field, indicating possible detachment of the retina, hemorrhage into the eye, or optic nerve injury

Evaluation of eye injury should include a thorough history and measurement of visual acuity, pupillary reaction, and extraocular movements.

> **NOTE**
>
> The prehospital assessment of a patient's vision will be a rough estimation at best. Vision will be reevaluated in the emergency department under controlled circumstances.

> **? CRITICAL THINKING**
>
> *Aside from trauma, what are some other causes of visual disturbances?*

History. A thorough history should include the following information:

- Exact mode of injury
- Previous ocular, medical, and drug history, including cataracts, glaucoma, and presence of hepatitis or HIV
- Use of eye medications
- Use of corrective glasses or contact lenses
- Presence of ocular prostheses
- Duration of symptoms and treatment interventions that may have been attempted before EMS arrival

Visual acuity. Measurement of visual acuity is usually the first step in any examination of the patient's eyes. (The exception is a chemical burn to the eye; in this case, irrigation should precede visual acuity measurement.) To measure visual acuity, the paramedic should use a hand-held visual acuity chart (e.g., Snellen chart) or any printed material with small, medium, and large point sizes (e.g., an IV fluid bag). The distance that the printed matter was held from the patient's face should be recorded.

The vision of each eye should be measured separately while covering the untested eye with material that will occlude vision without applying pressure. The injured eye should be tested first for acuity comparison to the uninjured eye. If corrective lenses are worn, acuity should be measured with lenses first and then without lenses. Illiteracy or foreign language limitations may require alternative methods of evaluation, such as finger-counting, hand motion, and presence or absence of light perception. Abnormal responses to any of these methods indicate significant loss of vision.

? CRITICAL THINKING

What factors in the prehospital setting may make assessment of visual acuity difficult on some calls?

NOTE

The two types of vision are central and peripheral. Central vision is vision that results from images falling on the macula of the retina. Peripheral vision is the capacity to see objects that reflect light waves falling on areas of the retina distant from the macula.

Pupillary Reaction

Pupils should be black, round, and equal in size and should react to light in concert; both eyes should constrict in response to light and dilate in response to dark. Abnormal pupillary responses after blunt trauma to the eye are common. They may be caused by tearing but more commonly are caused by direct trauma to the pupillary sphincter. They also may suggest a more serious injury involving the optic nerve or globe. Causes of pupil abnormalities in the absence of recent injury include drug use, cataracts, previous surgical procedures, ocular prosthesis, anisocoria (normal or congenital unequal pupil size), CNS disease, strokes, and previous injury. All of the patient's pupil abnormalities should be documented.

Extraocular movements.
Extraocular muscles are responsible for movements of the globe. Voluntary muscles, which are innervated by cranial nerves III, IV, and VI, are attached to the outside of the eyeball and bones of the orbit and move the globe in any desired direction. Involuntary eye muscles, which are innervated by sympathetic nerves, are located within the eye. Examples of involuntary eye muscles are the iris and the ciliary muscle, which dilate

and constrict the pupil and change the shape of the lens, respectively.

To evaluate the eyes' extraocular movement, the paramedic should instruct the patient to visually track the movement of an object (e.g., finger, pencil, penlight) up, down, to the right, and to the left. Abnormalities in movement may indicate orbital content edema, cranial nerve injury, contusions or lacerations of extraocular muscles, or muscle entrapment in a fracture. Patients with limited or abnormal extraocular movements frequently complain of double vision in one or more directions of gaze. All findings should be documented.

Evaluation and Management of Specific Eye Injuries

Although few eye injuries are truly urgent, all victims of ocular trauma should be evaluated by a physician. Some patients require specialized care by an ophthalmologist. If a serious injury that may require specialized care is suspected, medical direction should be advised as soon as possible so that services will be available when the patient arrives in the emergency department (Fig. 22-7).

Foreign bodies in the cornea, conjunctiva, or eyelid usually are evidenced by a patient complaint of foreign body sensation (especially when opening and closing the eyelids) and by profuse tearing. If a foreign body is suspected, the inner surface of the upper and lower lid and conjunctiva should be inspected and the foreign body removed by gentle, copious irrigation with clear fluid (e.g., tap water, normal saline, or sterile water).

NOTE

Medical direction may recommend that an ophthalmic anesthetic, such as **tetracaine** (Pontocaine), be applied for patient comfort.

Corneal abrasion occurs when the outer layers of the cornea are rubbed away. The injury often results from a foreign body scratching the cornea, and it also is common in those who wear contact lenses. Patients with a corneal abrasion usually complain of pain and foreign body sensation under the upper eyelid, photophobia (abnormal light sensitivity), excessive tearing, and sometimes a decrease in visual acuity. Often these signs and symptoms are delayed. Prehospital management of corneal abrasion is gentle irrigation

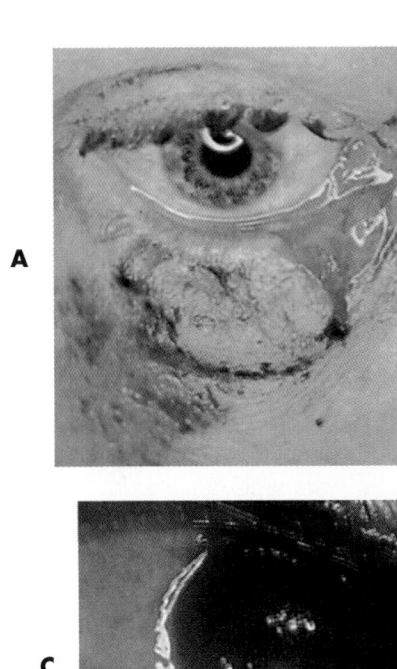

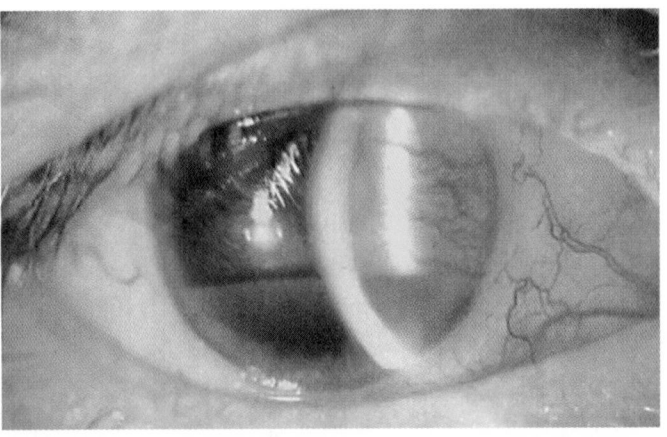

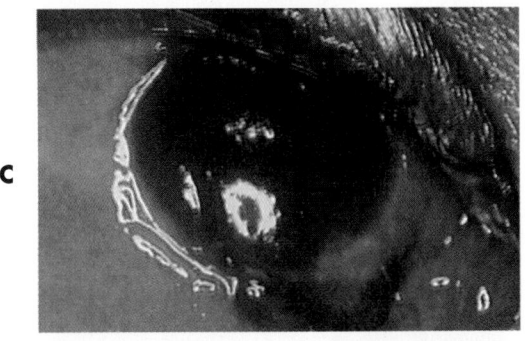

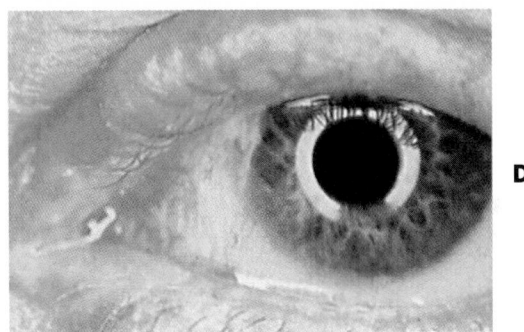

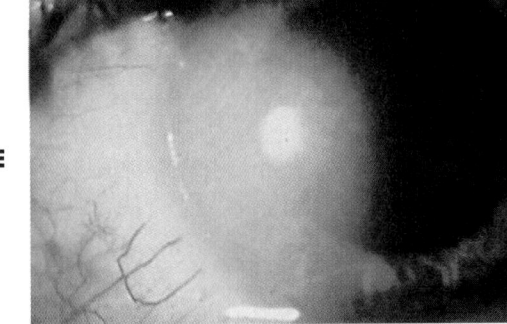

Fig. 22-7 A, Avulsion of lid. **B,** Hyphema.
C, Ruptured globe. **D,** Acid burn. **E,** Alkali burn.
(From Ragge N: *Immediate eye care,* London,
1990, Wolfe Medical Publications, Ltd.)

with clear fluid and the application of a double patch to both eyes to prevent consensual eye movement and resultant aggravation (Fig. 22-8). Corneal abrasions generally heal within 24 to 48 hours.

> **? CRITICAL THINKING**
>
> *Will the patient with a suspected corneal abrasion need physician evaluation?*

> **NOTE**
>
> The paramedic should follow local protocol regarding the use of wet versus dry dressings for eye injury.

Blunt trauma to the eye or its adjacent structures may result in a contusion injury, traumatic hyphema (bleeding into the anterior chamber), or globe or scleral rupture. Signs and symptoms of these injuries are:

Contusion injury
- Traumatic dilation or constriction of the pupil
- Pain
- Photophobia
- Blurred vision
- Tears of the iris (tear-shaped pupil)

Traumatic hyphema
- Traumatic dilation or, less commonly, constriction of the pupil

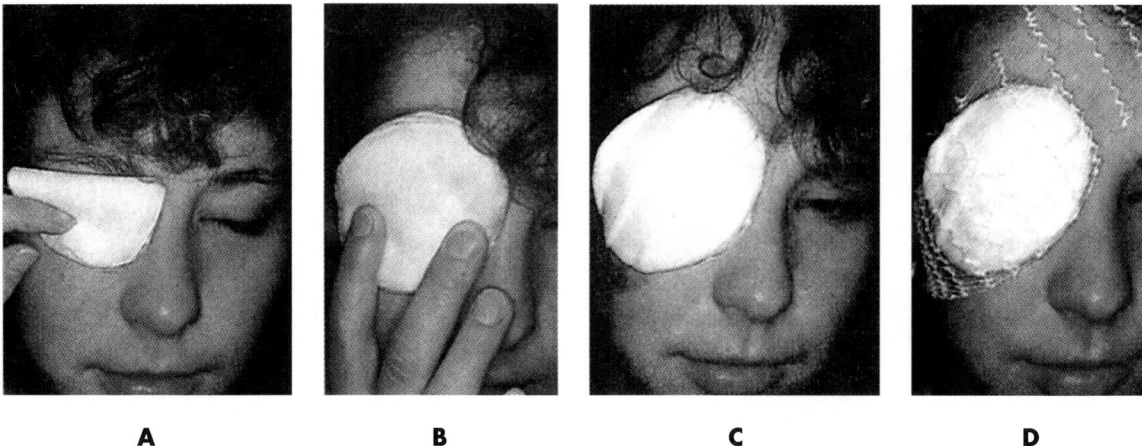

A   **B**   **C**   **D**

Fig. 22-8 A, A folded pad is placed over the closed eye. **B,** A second unfolded pad is placed over the top of the first pad. **C,** Tape is applied along the length of the pad. **D,** The pads are secured firmly in place. (From Ragge N: *Immediate eye care,* London, 1990, Wolfe Medical Publications, Ltd.)

- Decrease in visual acuity
- Blood in the anterior chamber (may be visible with penlight)

Globe or scleral rupture

- Decrease in visual acuity to hand movements or light perception
- Lowered intraocular pressure (soft eye)
- Pupil irregularity
- Hyphema

Blunt injury to the eye may be associated with other serious injuries, such as orbital fracture, vitreous hemorrhage, and dislocation of the lens. Prehospital care should be limited to control of any bleeding with gentle, direct pressure; protection of the affected eye with a metal shield or cardboard cup; and rapid transportation for physician evaluation. If traumatic hyphema or globe or scleral rupture is suspected, the paramedic should immobilize the patient's head and spine, elevate the head of spine board 40 degrees to decrease intraocular pressure, and instruct the patient to avoid any activity that might increase intraocular pressure (e.g., straining, coughing).

Penetrating injury to the eye may be associated with embedded foreign bodies, lid avulsions, and lacerations to the lids, sclera, or cornea. Penetrat-

ing globe injuries can damage retinal structures and cause a loss of vitreous humor and subsequent blindness. Any bleeding should be controlled by gentle, direct pressure, and the globe should be protected from dehydration or contamination from foreign bodies by covering the orbital area with plastic or damp, sterile dressings and an eye shield.

Protruding intraocular foreign bodies should be stabilized and covered with a cardboard cup secured with tape, and the unaffected eye should be covered to prevent consensual movement. No attempt should be made to remove the object. If necessary, the penetrating object may be shortened judiciously to facilitate transport (consult with medical direction). Oxygen and IV fluids also may be recommended in these situations.

Chemical injury to the eye (described in Chapter 21) may be associated with loss of corneal epithelial tissue, globe perforation, and scarring and deformation of eyelids and conjunctiva. These injuries are true emergencies and require immediate intervention. A chemical exposure generally mandates extensive, continuous irrigation of both eyes with a neutral fluid for 20 minutes before patient transport (if effective irrigation can be performed) and while en route to the emergency department.

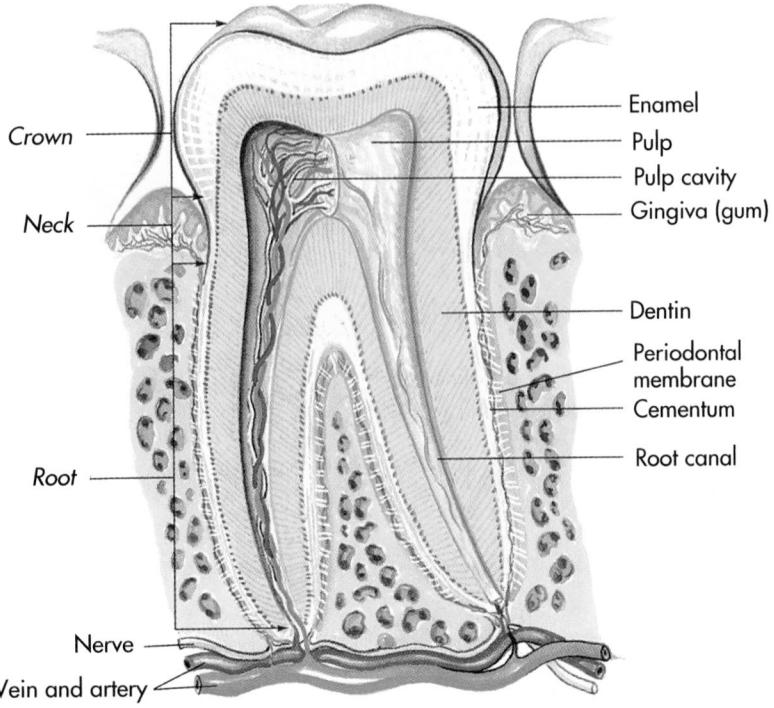

Fig. 22-9 Longitudinal section of a tooth. (From Thibodeau GA, Patton KT: *Structure and function of the body*, ed 9, St. Louis, 1992, Mosby.)

? CRITICAL THINKING

Should you wait until medical direction is contacted before you begin irrigation of the eye?

Contact Lenses

Contact lenses are of three general types: hard, soft hydrophilic, and rigid gas-permeable. Hard lenses are microlenses that are sometimes prescribed for astigmatism. (These lenses rarely are used today.) Soft hydrophilic lenses usually are large in diameter (extending onto the conjunctiva) and retain 25% to 85% hydration. Soft lenses may be designed for daily or extended wear. Rigid gas-permeable lenses are similar in size to microlenses and have a low water content and high oxygen permeability. Gas-permeable lenses generally are removed at the end of each day but may be designed for intermediate wear (up to 7 days) or permanent wear (up to 3 months).

As a rule, paramedics should not attempt to remove contact lenses in patients with eye injuries.

To do so may cause additional damage and aggravate the injury. If management of an eye injury is complicated by the presence of contact lenses (e.g., chemical burns to the eyes), medical direction may recommend that the lenses be removed. If the patient is unable to remove the lenses, the paramedic may be instructed to do so (see the box on the next page).

Dental Trauma

The normal adult mouth has 32 teeth. Each tooth consists of two sections: the crown, which projects above the gingiva (the portion of the oral mucosa surrounding the tooth), and the root, which fits into the bony socket (alveolus) of the maxilla or mandible. Three layers make up the hard tissues of the teeth: the enamel, the dentin (ivory), and the cementum. The soft tissues of the teeth include the pulp and the periodontal membrane (Fig. 22-9).

The teeth and associated alveolar process may be injured alone or in combination with fractures of the jaw or facial bones. The two most common

REMOVAL OF CONTACT LENSES

Removal of Hard and Rigid Gas-Permeable Lenses

1. With gloved hands, separate the eyelids so that the margins of the lids are beyond the top and bottom edges of the lens.
2. Gently pass the eyelids down and forward to the edges of the lens.
3. Move the eyelids toward each other, forcing the lens to slide out between them.
4. Store the lens in a container with water or saline and label the container with the patient's name. If a contact lens container is not available, store each lens in a separate container and label as left or right.
5. If lens removal is difficult, the lens should be gently moved downward from the cornea to the conjunctiva overlying the sclera until arrival in the emergency department.

NOTE: Special suction cups are also available for the removal of hard and rigid contact lenses. This device should be moistened with saline or sterile water before contacting the lens.

Removal of Soft Lenses

1. With gloved hands, pull down the lower eyelid.
2. Gently slide the soft lens down onto the conjunctiva.
3. Using a pinching motion, compress the lens between the thumb and index finger.
4. Remove the lens from the eye.
5. Store the lens in a container (marked right or left) with water or saline and label the container with the patient's name.

types of dental trauma involve fractures and avulsions of the anterior teeth. If a tooth is fractured, the oral cavity should be carefully searched for tooth fragments. Removal of fragments reduces the risk of aspiration and obstruction of the airway.

NOTE

Lacerations and avulsions to the tongue and surrounding mucous membranes commonly occur with dental trauma. These injuries often are painful, may bleed profusely, and may compromise the patient's airway.

Tooth avulsions are common, and many teeth can be saved with proper emergency treatment.[3] Permanent teeth that have been avulsed have a good survival rate if reimplanted and stabilized within 1 hour. (Deciduous teeth, or "milk teeth," are not generally reimplanted because they may become fused to the bone, delaying formation and eruption of the permanent tooth.) If the avulsed tooth has been extraoral for less than 15 minutes, medical direction may recommend reimplanting the tooth into the original socket. The paramedic should take care not to reimplant the tooth backwards and be alert for possible aspiration. If reimplantation is impossible, the paramedic should follow the guidelines established by the American Dental Association and the American Association of Endodontists:

1. Never place an avulsed tooth in anything that can dry or crush the outside of the tooth.
2. Do not handle the tooth roughly. Do not rinse it off or rub, scrape, or disinfect the outside of the tooth in any way. (Any adherent membrane or fibrous tissue should be left in place to avoid stripping off the periodontal membrane and ligament, which are critical to the survival of a reimplanted tooth.)
3. Place the tooth in a nurturing, break-resistant storage device (e.g., Emergency Tooth Preserving System) with a tightly fitted top and soft inner walls.
4. Store the tooth in a pH-balanced, isotonic, glucose-, calcium-, and magnesium-enriched cell-preserving fluid (e.g., Hank's solution). Use refrigerated fresh whole milk as the best alternative storage medium (powdered milk is not suitable). For very short periods (1 hour or less), use sterile saline. Do not use tap water because it damages the periodontal ligament.
5. Advise medical direction of avulsed teeth so that appropriate services will be available when the patient arrives in the emergency department.

Anterior Neck Trauma

Anterior neck injuries are caused by blunt and penetrating trauma (Fig. 22-10). These injuries may result in damage to the skeletal structures, vascular structures, nerves, muscles, and glands of the neck.

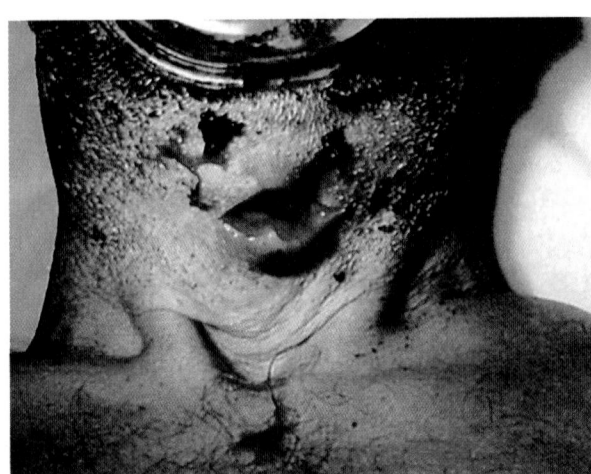

Fig. 22-10 A self-inflicted stab wound that had entered the pharynx. (From London PS: *A colour atlas of diagnosis after recent injury,* Ipswich, England, 1990, Wolfe Medical Publications, Ltd.)

Common mechanisms of injury to the anterior neck are:

- Motor vehicle crashes
- Neck striking dashboard or steering column
- Hyperextension and hyperflexion injuries
- Sport and recreational activities
- Contact sports (boxing, karate, basketball, football, hockey)
- ATVs and other small motor vehicles ("clothesline" injuries to the neck from running into wires, ropes, fences)
- Water sports (jet skiing, water skiing)
- Snow skiing
- Horseback riding
- Industrial accidents
- "Strangulation" injuries from clothing, jewelry, or personal equipment getting caught in machinery
- Violent altercations
- Stab wounds (knives, screwdrivers, ice picks)
- Missile injury from firearms
- Blows to the neck
- Hangings

> **NOTE**
>
> With both blunt and penetrating neck injuries, cervical spine injury must be assumed until ruled out by clinical examination and cervical radiography. Radiographic examination alone does not rule out cervical spine injury (see Chapter 23).

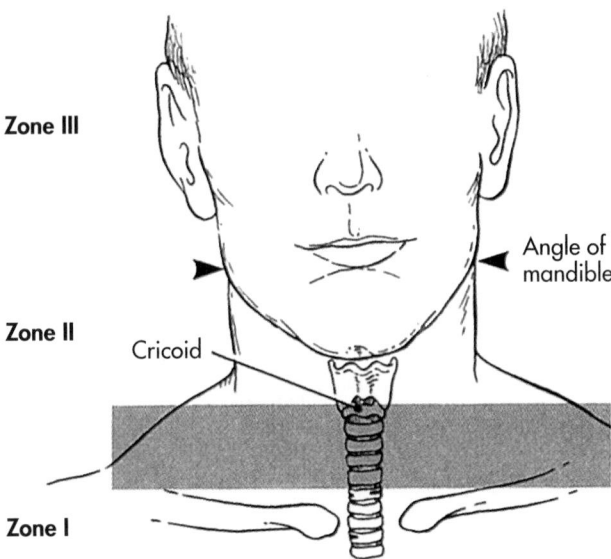

Fig. 22-11 Zones of the neck. The junction of zone 1 and zone 2 is variously described as the cricoid cartilage or top of the clavicles. (From Moore EE: *Early care of the injured patient,* ed 4, Philadelphia, 1990, Decker.)

Evaluation

For purposes of evaluating the trauma patient, the neck can be divided into three zones defined by horizontal planes (Fig. 22-11).[1] Zone I represents the base of the neck, extending from the sternal notch to the top of the clavicles or the cricoid cartilage. Injuries to this zone carry the highest mortality rate because of the risk of injury to major vascular and thoracic structures (subclavian vessels and jugular veins, lungs, esophagus, trachea, cervical spine, cervical nerve roots).

Zone II extends from the clavicles or cricoid cartilage cephalad to the angle of the mandible. The carotid artery, jugular vein, trachea, larynx, esophagus, and cervical spine are the vital structures in this zone. Because of its relative size, zone II injuries are the most common but have a lower mortality rate than zone I injuries.

Zone III is the part of the neck above the angle of the mandible. The risk of injury to the distal carotid artery, salivary glands, and pharynx is greatest in this zone.

Soft Tissue Injuries

Soft tissue injuries to the neck from blunt trauma often produce hematomas and associated edema or direct laryngeal or tracheal injury, both of which can result in airway compromise. Penetrating trauma may produce lacerations and puncture wounds with resultant vascular, laryngeal-tracheal, or esophageal injury. Uncommonly, blunt trauma also may cause vascular injuries. As with all other scenarios of trauma, initial evaluation and resuscitation must begin with rapid assessment, control of the airway, and consideration for spinal injury.

? CRITICAL THINKING

Is prehospital airway control always possible in patients with anterior neck injuries?

Hematomas and Edema

Edema of the pharynx, larynx, trachea, epiglottis, and vocal cords may produce enough pressure in the neck tissues to completely obstruct the airway. If the airway is compromised (evidenced by dyspnea, inspiratory stridor, cyanosis, or changes in voice quality), oral or nasal intubation with spinal precautions should be considered. Intubation stabilizes damaged areas of the neck, protects the airway, and provides a means for ventilatory support. (A slightly smaller endotracheal tube may be needed to ensure passage through the airway.)

NOTE

Fractured or transected airways may be totally or partially obstructed or occluded by attempts at oral or nasal intubation. In these cases (if the patient is moving air), rapid transportation with high-concentration oxygen is perhaps the most prudent course.

If blood or vomitus that cannot be cleared with suction obstructs the airway or if progressive edema makes direct intubation impossible, cricothyrotomy or translaryngeal cannula ventilation (described in Chapter 11) may be indicated. Other measures that may prove helpful in treating edematous airways include the administration of cool, humidified oxygen and slight elevation of the patient's head (if not contraindicated by the injury).

Lacerations and Puncture Wounds

Lacerations and puncture wounds may be superficial or deep. Superficial injuries usually can be managed by covering the wound to prevent further contamination. Deep, penetrating wounds are associated with more serious injuries to underlying structures. These injuries may require aggressive airway therapy and ventilatory support, suction, hemorrhage control by direct pressure, and fluid replacement. Signs and symptoms of significant penetrating neck trauma include:

- Shock
- Active bleeding
- Tenderness to palpation
- Mobility and crepitus
- Large or expanding hematoma
- Pulse deficit
- Neurological deficit (stroke, brachial plexus injury, spinal cord injury)
- Dyspnea
- Hoarseness
- Stridor
- Subcutaneous emphysema
- Hemoptysis
- Dysphagia
- Hematemesis

? CRITICAL THINKING

Why is rapid transportation especially important when caring for a patient with anterior neck injuries?

Vascular Injury

Blood vessels are the most commonly injured structures in the neck; they may be injured by blunt or penetrating trauma. Vessels at risk of injury include the carotid, vertebral, subclavian, innominate, and internal mammary arteries and the jugular and subclavian veins. Laceration of these major vessels can result in rapid exsanguination if bleeding is not controlled.

After securing the airway with spinal precautions and providing adequate ventilatory support, prehospital management of vascular injury to the anterior neck should be directed at controlling hemorrhage by constant, direct pressure. The paramedic should apply pressure only to the affected vessels so blood flow to the brain is not obstructed. If bleeding cannot be controlled in this manner, medical direction may advise tamponading the vessels with direct, gloved finger pressure.

If a venous injury is suspected, the patient should be kept supine or in a slight Trendelenburg position to prevent air embolism (a rare but lethal complication). If an air embolism is suspected (previously described in Chapter 9), the immobilized patient should be turned on the left side, head lower than feet, to attempt to trap the air embolus in the right ventricle.

Fluid replacement for hypovolemia should be guided by medical direction and may include using large-bore catheters and isotonic crystalloid (lactated Ringer's solution or normal saline). If penetrating injury to the base of the neck (zone I) has occurred, placement of at least one IV line in a lower extremity should be considered in the event that upper-extremity venous drainage has been compromised by the laceration. Medical direction may recommend that a second IV line be placed in the upper extremity on the side opposite the injury.

? CRITICAL THINKING

Why might application of PASG be harmful with this type of injury?

Laryngeal or Tracheal Injury

Injury secondary to blunt or penetrating trauma to the anterior neck may cause fracture or dislocation of the laryngeal and tracheal cartilages, hemorrhage, or swelling of the air passages, all of which can significantly compromise the airway and cause respiratory distress. Because airway injury can lead to death in head and neck trauma patients, rapid and judicious control of the airway and prevention of aspiration are crucial. In addition, a high degree

of suspicion for associated vascular disruption and esophageal, chest, and intraabdominal injury is an important aspect of preventing death. Injuries that may be associated with laryngeal and tracheal trauma include:

- Fracture of the hyoid bone resulting in laceration and distortion of the epiglottis
- Separation of the hyoid and thyroid cartilages resulting in epiglottis dislocation, aspiration, and subcutaneous emphysema
- Fractures of the thyroid cartilage resulting in epiglottis and vocal cord avulsion, arytenoid dislocation, and aspiration of blood and bone fragments
- Dislocation or fracture of the cricothyroid resulting in long-term laryngeal stenosis, laryngeal nerve paralysis, and laryngotracheal avulsion
- Fracture to the trachea resulting in tracheal avulsion, complete airway obstruction, and subcutaneous emphysema

Emergency airway management of laryngeal and tracheal trauma is controversial. Some medical direction agencies recommend oral or nasal intubation; others may feel that intubation attempts may contribute to the potential for anoxic injury and further damage the airway structures. Alternative methods of airway management include use of bag-valve-mask ventilation, cricothyrotomy, and translaryngeal cannula ventilation.

If penetrating trauma causes complete disruption of the laryngotracheal complex, medical direction may recommend dissection through the wound so that the exposed distal trachea can be directly cannulated with a cuffed endotracheal tube.

Regardless of the method chosen, emergency care is directed at securing the airway with spinal precautions, providing adequate ventilatory support, controlling hemorrhage, treating for shock, and providing rapid transport to an appropriate medical facility for definitive surgical care.

Esophageal Injury

Esophageal injuries should be suspected in patients with trauma to the neck or chest. Specific injuries that require a high degree of suspicion for associated esophageal injury include tracheal fractures, penetrating trauma from stab or gunshot wounds, and ingestion of caustic substances.

> **NOTE**
>
> Esophageal perforation is associated with a high mortality rate from mediastinitis, caused by the release of gastric contents into the thoracic cavity. If not contraindicated by mechanism of injury, the patient with a suspected esophageal tear should be placed in a semi-Fowler's position (an inclined position with the upper half of the body raised by elevating the head or stretcher about 30 degrees) to prevent reflux of gastric contents.

Esophageal injury is difficult to diagnose and may be overlooked as the paramedic focuses on more obvious life-threatening injuries. Signs and symptoms may include subcutaneous emphysema, neck hematoma, and oropharyngeal or nasogastric blood (indicating esophageal perforation).

> **?** CRITICAL THINKING
>
> *Are these signs and symptoms so unique that you will be able to distinguish esophageal injury as the cause versus other kinds of traumatic conditions?*

Head Trauma

The anatomical components of the skull are the scalp, followed by the cranial vault, under which are the dural membrane, the arachnoid membrane, the pia, and the brain substance. Injuries to the skull may be classified as soft tissue injuries to the scalp and skull fractures.

> **NOTE**
>
> All patients with head or neck trauma must be assumed to have a spinal injury until ruled out by clinical examination and radiography in the emergency department. (Spinal precautions [including helmet issues] will be presented in Chapter 23.) This text assumes that spinal precautions will be employed for *all* patients with a significant mechanism of injury.

Soft Tissue Injuries to the Scalp

The most common scalp injury is an irregular linear laceration. Like the face, the scalp is very vascular. Therefore scalp lacerations may give rise to profuse bleeding and resultant hypovolemia, particularly in infants and children. Other, less frequent scalp injuries include stellate wounds, avulsions, and subgaleal hematomas (Fig. 22-12).

Management of soft tissue injuries to the scalp includes efforts to prevent contamination of open wounds, use of direct pressure or pressure dressings to decrease blood loss, and fluid replacement if needed. The paramedic also should consider the potential for underlying skull fracture and brain and spinal trauma as indicated by the mechanism of injury. Aside from the possibility of excessive blood loss, scalp lacerations that occur as a single entity rarely produce life-threatening complications.

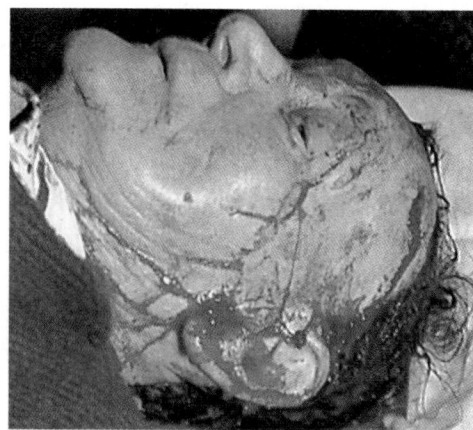

Fig. 22-12 Even small wounds from the scalp can bleed profusely. (From London PS: *A colour atlas of diagnosis after recent injury*, Ipswich, England, 1990, Wolfe Medical Publications, Ltd.)

If not contraindicated by injury, all patients with head or facial trauma should be positioned on a stretcher or spine board with the head elevated 30 degrees (semi-Fowler's position).

Skull Fractures

Skull fractures may be classified as *linear fractures, basilar fractures, depressed fractures,* and *open vault fractures* (Fig. 22-13). Complications associated with these injuries are cranial nerve injury, vascular involvement (e.g., meningeal artery, dural sinuses),

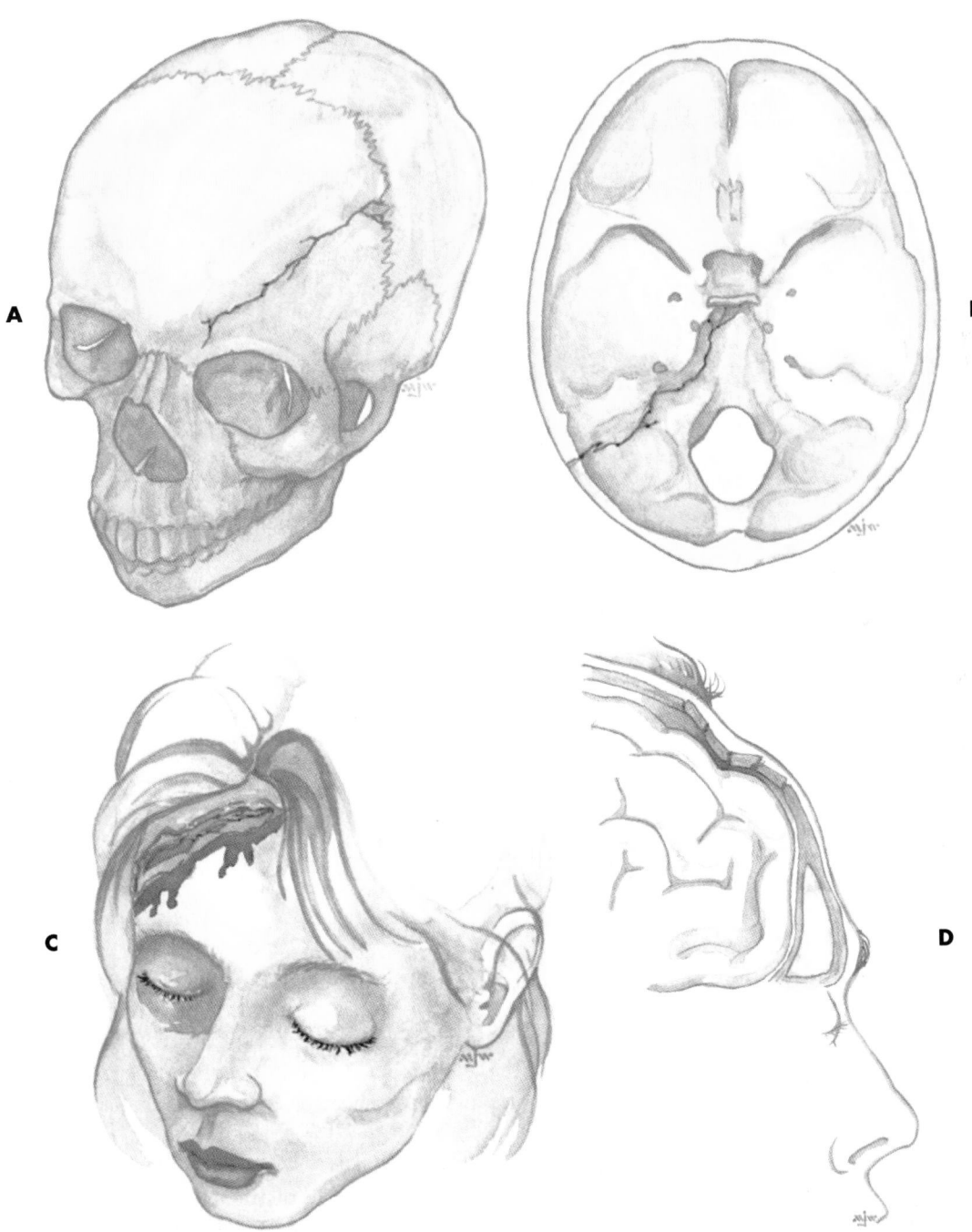

Fig. 22-13 Skull fractures. **A,** Linear skull fracture. **B,** Basilar skull fracture. **C,** Open vault fracture. **D,** Depressed skull fracture.

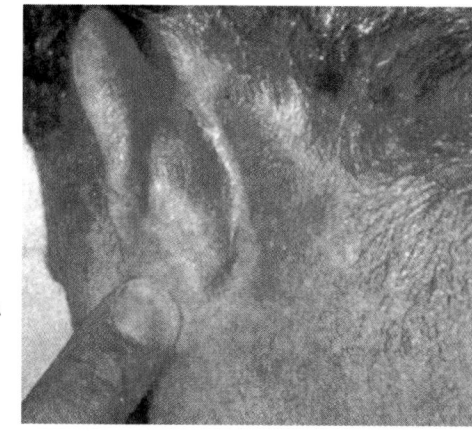

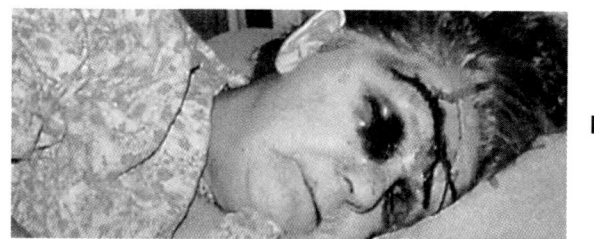

Fig. 22-14 A, Battle's sign. **B,** Raccoon's eyes. (From London PS: *A colour atlas of diagnosis after recent injury,* Ipswich, England, 1990, Wolfe Medical Publications, Ltd.)

infection, underlying brain injury, and dural defects caused by depressed bone fragments. With all injuries to the head, the paramedic should consider the potential for spinal injury and take appropriate spinal precautions.

Linear Fractures

Linear fractures (seen as straight lines on x-ray film) account for 80% of all fractures to the skull.[4] They usually are not depressed and often occur without an overlying scalp laceration. As an isolated injury, these fractures generally have a low rate of complication. However, if the fracture is associated with scalp laceration, infection is possible. In addition, linear fractures that cross the meningeal groove in the temporal-parietal area, midline, or occipital area may lead to epidural bleeding from the middle cerebral artery.

? CRITICAL THINKING

Will you be able to detect linear skull fractures on examination in the prehospital setting?

Basilar skull fractures. Basilar skull fractures usually are associated with major impact trauma. These injuries may occur when the mandibular condyles perforate into the base of the skull, but more commonly result from an extension of a linear fracture into the floor of the anterior and middle fossae. Basilar skull fractures can be difficult to see on x-ray

films and usually are diagnosed clinically by the following signs and symptoms:

- Ecchymosis over the mastoid process resulting from fracture to the temporal bone (**Battle's sign**) (Fig. 22-14, *A*)
- Ecchymosis of one or both orbits caused by fracture of the base of the sphenoid sinus (**raccoon's eyes**) (Fig. 22-14, *B*)
- Blood behind the tympanic membrane caused by fractures of the temporal bone (hemotympanum)
- Cerebrospinal fluid leakage, which can result in bacterial meningitis

NOTE

Battle's sign and racoon's eyes usually do not occur until some time after the injury. If they are present on EMS arrival, the ecchymosis is probably the result of a previous injury.

Other complications associated with basilar skull fractures include cranial nerve injuries and massive hemorrhage from vascular involvement of the carotid artery. Treatment for basilar skull fractures includes bed rest, in-hospital observation, and evaluation for hearing loss due to acoustic nerve injury.

Depressed Skull Fractures

Depressed skull fractures usually result from a relatively small object striking the head at high speed and therefore commonly are associated with scalp lacerations. The frontal and parietal bones are most

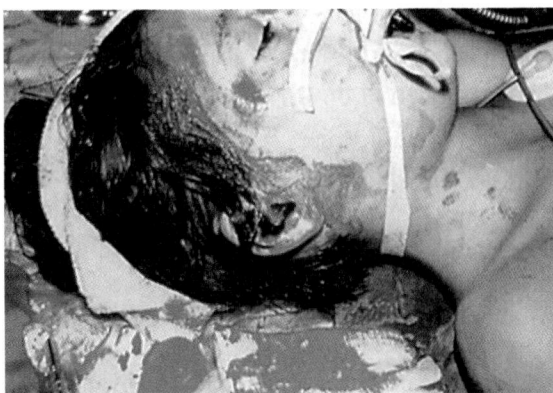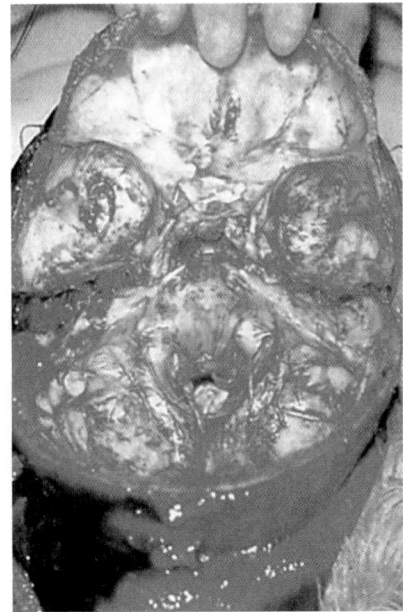

Fig. 22-15 Severe fracture of the base of the skull. (From London PS: *A colour atlas of diagnosis after recent injury,* Ipswich, England, 1990, Wolfe Medical Publications, Ltd.)

often affected by these fractures. It is estimated that 30% of patients with depressed skull fractures have associated hematomas and cerebral contusions.[4] If the depression is greater than the thickness of the skull, dural laceration also is likely. Patients with depressed skull fractures frequently require surgical removal of the bone fragments (craniectomy).

Open-Vault Fractures

Open-vault fractures result when there is direct communication between a scalp laceration and cerebral substance (Fig. 22-15). Because of the nature of these injuries and the force required to produce them, they often are associated with multiple-system trauma and a high mortality rate. Communication between the intracranial contents and the external environment may lead to infection (meningitis). Open-vault fractures require surgical repair. Prehospital management usually is limited to spinal immobilization, ventilatory support, efforts to prevent contamination, and rapid transportation to an appropriate medical facility.

Cranial Nerve Injuries

Twelve pairs of cranial nerves leave the brain and pass through openings in the skull called *foramina*. Injury to cranial nerves usually is associated with

skull fractures. Signs and symptoms of common cranial nerve injuries are:

- Cranial nerve I (olfactory nerve)
  - Loss of smell
  - Impairment of taste (dependent on food aroma)
  - Hallmark of basilar skull fracture
- Cranial nerve II (optic nerve)
  - Blindness in one or both eyes
  - Visual field defects
- Cranial nerve III (oculomotor nerve)
  - Ipsilateral (same side), dilated, fixed pupil
  - Especially compression by the temporal lobe
  - Mimicking of direct ocular trauma
- Cranial nerve VII (facial nerve)
  - Immediate or delayed facial paralysis
  - Basilar skull fracture
- Cranial nerve VIII (auditory nerve)
  - Deafness
  - Basilar skull fracture

Brain Trauma

A *brain injury* is defined by the National Head Injury Foundation as "a traumatic insult to the brain capable of producing physical, intellectual, emotional, social, and vocational change."[4] Categories of brain injury include mild and moderate diffuse injury, diffuse axonal injury, and focal injury.[5]

Mild Diffuse Injury (Concussion)

Concussion is a fully reversible brain injury that does not result in structural damage to the brain. It is caused by mild-to-moderate impact to the skull, movement within the cranial vault, or both. It occurs when the function of the brainstem (particularly the reticular activating system) or both cerebral cortices is temporarily disturbed, resulting in a brief altered level of consciousness, usually less than 5 minutes.

> **NOTE**
>
> If the patient has been unconscious for more than 5 minutes, the paramedic should suspect a more serious injury caused by contusion or hemorrhage.

The loss of consciousness usually is followed by periods of drowsiness, restlessness, and confusion, with a fairly rapid return to normal behavior. The patient may have no recall of the events before the injury (**retrograde amnesia**) or immediately after recovery of consciousness (**antegrade amnesia**). This short-term memory loss may produce anxiety, and the patient frequently asks repetitive questions (e.g., "Where am I? What happened?"). Other signs and symptoms of concussion are vomiting; combativeness; transient visual disturbances (e.g., light flashes, wavy lines); defects in equilibrium and coordination; and changes in blood pressure, pulse rate, and respiration (rare). After physician evaluation, treatment generally consists of in-hospital or home observation by a reliable observer for 24 to 48 hours.

> **? CRITICAL THINKING**
>
> *Why should the patient with a new onset of retrograde or antegrade amnesia not be considered a reliable historian?*

A concussion injury affects the patient most severely at the time of impact and is followed by improvement. It is the most common and least serious type of brain injury. *Any patient whose condition wors-* *ens over time or whose level of consciousness deteriorates rather than improves must be suspected of having a more serious injury.* Therefore it is important to document baseline measurements of level of consciousness, memory status, and neurological function (e.g., Glasgow coma scale, AVPU scale) in any victim of head injury.

Moderate Diffuse Injury

Moderate injuries are those that result in minute petechial bruising of brain tissue. Involvement of the brainstem and reticular activating system lead to unconsciousness. These injuries account for 20% of all severe head injuries and 45% of all cases of diffuse injury.[4] Often these patients will have basilar skull fracture. Most will survive their injury, but permanent neurological impairment is common.

A patient with moderate diffuse injury initially will be unconscious, followed by persistent confusion, disorientation, and amnesia of the event. During recovery, these patients often experience an inability to concentrate, frequent periods of anxiety, uncharacteristic mood swings, and sensorimotor deficits (e.g., an altered sense of smell). Patients with moderate diffuse injury are managed like those with concussion; frequently reassess the level of consciousness and ensure an adequate airway and tidal volume.

> **NOTE**
>
> If possible, patients with head injury should be moved to a quiet, calm area. Exposure to bright lights should be avoided (patients often are photophobic), and constant reorientation may be necessary.

Diffuse Axonal Injury

Diffuse axonal injury (DAI) is the severest form of brain injury. It results from brain movement within the skull secondary to acceleration or deceleration forces. These forces cause shearing, stretching, or tearing of nerve fibers with subsequent axonal (nerve cell) damage. DAI may be classified as mild, moderate, or severe. Mild DAI is associated with coma of 6 to 24 hours and has a mortality rate of 16%.[4] Moderate DAI is more common and is distinguished by coma lasting more than 24 hours and abnormal posturing. The associated mortality rate of moderate DAI approaches 24%.[6]

> **? CRITICAL THINKING**
>
> *Is it possible for a patient with a diffuse axonal injury to die as a result of that condition?*

Severe DAI (formerly known as *brainstem injury*) involves severe mechanical shearing of many axons in both cerebral hemispheres extending to the brainstem. Severe DAI occurs in 16% of all severe head injuries and in 36% of all cases of DAI.[4] These patients often are unconscious for prolonged periods and may exhibit abnormal posturing and other signs of increased intracranial pressure (ICP). Prehospital care for these patients is focused on ensuring an adequate airway and tidal volume.

> **NOTE**
>
> Hypoxia must be prevented (to avoid secondary injury to brain tissue) in all patients with head injury.

Focal Injury

Focal injuries are specific, grossly observable brain lesions. Included in this category are lesions that result from skull fracture (previously described), contusion, edema with associated increased ICP, ischemia, and hemorrhage.

> **NOTE**
>
> The brain occupies 80% of intracranial space. It is divided into four areas: the brainstem (consisting of the medulla, pons, and midbrain), the diencephalon (including the thalamus and hypothalamus), the cerebrum, and the cerebellum. The intracranial contents consist of brain water (58%), brain solids (25%), cerebrospinal fluid (7%), and intracranial blood (10%).

Cerebral Contusion

A cerebral contusion is bruising of the brain in the area of the cortex or deeper within the frontal (most common), temporal, or occipital lobes. This bruis-

ing produces a structural change in the brain tissue and results in greater neurological deficits and abnormalities than are seen with concussions. These abnormalities may include seizures, hemiparesis, aphasia, and personality changes. If the brainstem also is contused, the patient may lose consciousness. In some cases, the comatose state may be prolonged, lasting hours to days or longer. Of the patients who die from head injury, 75% have cerebral contusions at autopsy.[4]

If applied force is sufficient to cause the brain to be displaced against the irregular surfaces of the skull, tiny blood vessels in the pia mater may rupture. The brain substance may be damaged locally at the site of impact (coup) or on the contralateral side (contrecoup) opposite the site of impact. Contrecoup injuries commonly are caused by deceleration of the head, as in a fall or motor vehicle crash.

As a rule, cerebral contusions usually heal without intervention. Like patients with concussion, these patients usually improve, although the time to heal and level of improvement differ in these two conditions. The most important complication associated with cerebral contusion is increased ICP manifested by headache, nausea, vomiting, seizures, and a declining level of consciousness. These signs usually are delayed responses that are not seen in the prehospital emergency setting.

Edema

Significant injuries to the brain often result in swelling of the brain tissue with or without associated hemorrhage. The swelling, which results from humoral and metabolic responses to injury, leads to marked increases in ICP. This can in turn lead to decreased cerebral perfusion (described below) or herniation.

Ischemia

Ischemia can result from vascular injuries, secondary vascular spasm, or increased intracranial pressure. In any case, focal or more global infarcts can result.

Hemorrhage

The same forces that result in concussion and contusion also may cause serious vascular damage with resultant hemorrhage into or around brain tissue. These injuries may cause epidural or subdural hematomas, which compress the underlying brain tissue, or intraparenchymal hemorrhage (bleeding directly into the brain tissue). Hemorrhage often is associated with cerebral contusions and skull fractures.

Cerebral blood flow. Although the brain accounts for only 2% of adult weight, 20% of total body oxygen use and 25% of total body glucose use are devoted to brain metabolism.[4] Oxygen and glucose delivery are controlled by cerebral blood flow.

Cerebral blood flow is a function of **cerebral perfusion pressure** (CPP) and resistance of the cerebral vascular bed. CPP is determined by the **mean arterial pressure** (MAP) (the diastolic pressure plus one-third pulse pressure) minus intracranial pressure. As ICP approaches MAP, the gradient for flow decreases and cerebral blood flow is restricted. Therefore, when intracranial pressure increases, CPP decreases. As CPP decreases, cerebral vasodilation occurs, which results in increased cerebral blood volume (increasing ICP) and further cerebral vasodilation.

? CRITICAL THINKING

What happens to the flow of oxygen to the brain, and CO_2 from the brain to the capillaries, when ICP is increasing and CPP is decreasing?

NOTE

CPP can be maintained with a systolic pressure of at least 70 mm Hg.[4]

Vascular tone in the normal brain is regulated by carbon dioxide pressure (P_{CO_2}), oxygen pressure (P_{O_2}), and autonomic and neurohumoral control;

P_{CO_2} has the greatest effect on intracerebral vascular diameter and subsequent resistance. For example, if P_{CO_2} is increased from 40 to 80 torr, cerebral blood flow is doubled, resulting in increased brain blood volume and intracranial pressure.

Intracranial pressure. The normal range of intracranial pressure is 0 to 15 torr. When intracranial pressure rises above this level because of an expanding mass or diffuse swelling, the body's ability to maintain CPP is compromised, and cerebral blood flow is diminished. As the cranial vault continues to fill (because of brain edema or expanding hematoma), the body attempts to compensate for the decline in CPP by a rise in MAP (Cushing reflex). However, this increase in cerebral blood flow further elevates the intracranial pressure. As it continues to rise, cerebrospinal fluid is displaced to compensate for the expansion. If unresolved, the brain substance may herniate over the edge of the tentorium (one of three extensions of the dura mater that separates the cerebellum from the occipital lobe of the cerebrum) or through the foramen magnum (Fig. 22-16).

Early signs and symptoms of increased ICP include headache, nausea and vomiting, and altered level of consciousness (Box 22-1). These eventually are followed by increased systolic pressure, widened pulse pressure, and a decrease in the pulse and irregular respiratory pattern (**Cushing's triad**). As the volume continues to expand in the cranial vault, herniation of the temporal lobe through the tentorium causes compression of cranial nerve III, producing a dilated pupil and loss of the light reflex on the side of compression. The patient rapidly becomes unresponsive to verbal and painful stimuli and may exhibit the ominous signs of **decorticate posturing** (characterized by extension of the legs and flexion of the arms at the elbows) or **decere-**

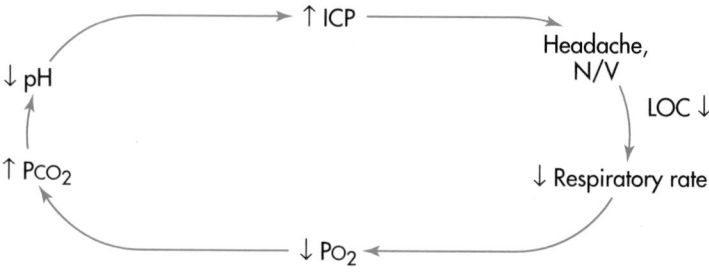

Fig. 22-16 Effects of increased intracranial pressure.

brate posturing (characterized by extension of all four extremities) (Fig. 22- 17).

❓ CRITICAL THINKING

Why is cranial nerve III affected by this shift in brain tissue?

Respiratory patterns. As intracranial pressure continues to rise, abnormal respiratory patterns (described in Chapter 11) may develop. Respiratory abnormalities associated with increased intracranial pressure and significant brainstem injury include hypoventilation, Cheyne-Stokes breathing (which may accompany decorticate posturing), central neurogenic hyperventilation (which may accompany decerebrate posturing), and ataxic breathing. The clinical significance of decorticate (flexion) and decerebrate (extension) posturing and respiratory patterns are not of major clinical importance other than to identify the need for intervention and treatment (intubation and consideration of immediate neurosurgical intervention).

NOTE

Some motion of the limbs, albeit abnormal, is better than no motion of the limbs (which indicates a worse level of neurological function).

Types of Brain Hemorrhage

Traditionally, brain hemorrhages are classified according to their location as epidural, subdural, subarachnoid, or cerebral (intraparenchymal) (Fig. 22-18).

Epidural hematoma. An epidural hematoma (accounting for 0.5% to 1% of all head injuries[4]) is a collection of blood between the cranium and the dura in the epidural space. It usually is a rapidly developing

BOX 22-1

LEVELS OF INCREASING ICP

Cerebral cortex and upper brainstem
Blood pressure rises, pulse rate slows
Pupils remain reactive
Cheyne-Stokes respirations may be present
Patient will initially try to localize and remove painful stimuli (eventually withdraws and flexion occurs)
All effects are reversible at this stage

Middle brainstem
Wide pulse pressure and bradycardia
Pupils become nonreactive or sluggish
Central neurogenic hyperventilation develops
Abnormal posturing (extension)
Few patients function normally with injury at this level

Lower portion of brainstem/medulla
Pupil "blown" (fixed and dilated) on same side of injury
Respirations become ataxic
Patient will be flaccid
Irregular pulse rate
QRS, S-T, and T-wave changes will be present
Blood pressure will fluctuate
These patients generally do not survive

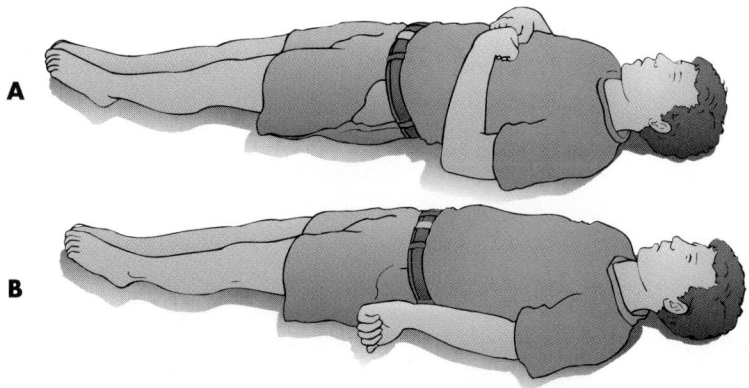

Fig. 22-17 A, Abnormal flexion (decorticate posturing). **B,** Abnormal extension (decerebrate posturing). (From Sheehy S: *Emergency nursing*, ed 3, St. Louis, 1992, Mosby.)

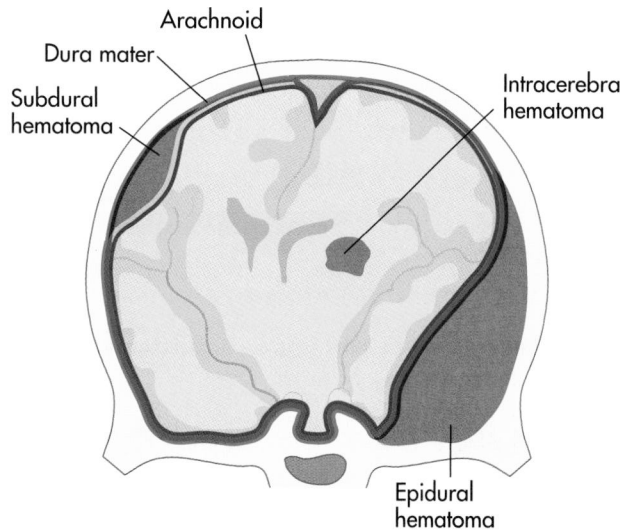

Arachnoid
Dura mater
Subdural hematoma
Intracerebral hematoma
Epidural hematoma

Fig. 22-18 Varieties of intracranial hemorrhage.

lesion associated with a laceration or tear of the middle meningeal artery. This hemorrhage frequently occurs as a result of a linear or depressed skull fracture in the temporal bone, although bleeding from other sites also can produce epidural hemorrhage. If the source of hemorrhage is predominantly venous, deterioration usually is not as rapid because low-pressure vessels bleed more slowly.

Fifty percent of patients with epidural hematoma have a transient loss of consciousness, followed by a lucid interval in which neurological status returns to normal.[4] (The remaining 50% of patients with acute epidural hematoma never recover consciousness.) The lucid interval usually lasts between 6 and 18 hours, during which time the hematoma enlarges. As ICP rises, the patient develops a headache with lethargy, decreasing level of consciousness, and contralateral hemiparesis. In the early stages of an epidural hematoma, the patient's complaints may be only headache and drowsiness. Immediate recognition and rapid transportation to an appropriate medical facility for surgical intervention are the cornerstones of definitive therapy. Common causes of epidural hematoma include low-velocity blows to the head, violent altercations, and deceleration injuries. About 15% to 20% of these patients die.[4]

Subdural hematoma. A subdural hematoma is a collection of blood between the dura and the surface of the brain in the subdural space. This injury usually results from bleeding of the veins that bridge the subdural space. Associated contusion or laceration of the brain frequently is present. It often is the result of blunt head trauma and commonly is associated with skull fracture. Subdural hematomas are classified as *acute* (50% to 80% mortality rate), *subacute* (25% mortality rate), and *chronic* (20% mortality rate),[4] depending on the time lapse between the injury and development of symptoms. As a general rule, if symptoms occur within 24 hours, the hematoma is considered acute; between 2 and 10 days, subacute; and after 2 weeks, chronic. Subdural hematomas are more common than epidural hematomas.

Signs and symptoms of subdural hematoma are similar to those of epidural hematoma and include headache, nausea and vomiting, decreasing level of consciousness, coma, abnormal posturing, paralysis, and, in infants, bulging fontanelles. These findings may be quite subtle because of the slow evolution of the hematoma in the subacute and chronic phases. Definitive care consists of surgical evacuation of the hematoma. Individuals at increased risk of developing subdural hematoma include older adults and patients with clotting deficiencies (e.g., alcoholics, hemophiliacs, persons who take anticoagulants) and patients with cortical atrophy (older adults, alcoholics).

Subarachnoid hemorrhage. A **subarachnoid hemorrhage** refers to intracranial bleeding into the CSF, resulting in bloody CSF and meningeal irritation. Bleeding that results from trauma, rupture of an aneurysm, or arteriovenous anomaly may extend into the brain if the force of the bleeding from the broken vessel is sudden and severe. Patients with this injury often complain of a sudden and severe headache that initially is localized and then spreads (from meningeal irritation), becoming dull and throbbing. Other characteristics of a subarachnoid hemorrhage include dizziness, neck stiffness, unequal pupils, vomiting,

? CRITICAL THINKING

What could account for delays in surgical treatment, causing subsequent death, in patients who have an epidural hematoma?

? CRITICAL THINKING

What causes the vomiting, seizures, and loss of consciousness in a patient with subarachnoid hemorrhage?

seizures, and loss of consciousness. Severe hemorrhage may result in coma and death. Permanent brain damage is common in those who survive.

Cerebral hematoma. An **intracerebral hematoma** may be defined as a collection of more than 5 mL of blood somewhere within the substance of the brain, most commonly in the frontal or temporal lobe.[4] This injury usually results from multiple lacerations produced by penetrating head trauma or a high-velocity deceleration injury in which vessels are torn as the brain moves across rough surfaces of the skull. It also may occur as the brain is compressed and distorted from increased intracranial pressure. Cerebral hematoma often is associated with subdural hemorrhage and skull fracture. Signs and symptoms may be immediate or delayed, depending on the size and location of the hemorrhage. Once symptomatology presents, the patient usually deteriorates rapidly. The mortality rate after surgical evacuation of the hematoma (if possible) is more than 40%.[4]

Penetrating Injury

Penetrating injuries to the brain usually are caused by missiles fired from handguns and stab wounds caused by sharp instruments such as knives, scissors, screwdrivers, and nails. Less frequently, penetrating trauma may result from falls and high-velocity motor vehicle crashes. Associated injuries include skull fracture; damage to cerebral arteries, veins, or venous sinuses; and intracranial hemorrhage. Complications include infection and post-traumatic epilepsy. Definitive care for these injuries requires neurosurgical intervention.

Assessment and Neurological Evaluation

Prehospital management of the patient with a head injury is determined by a number of factors, including the mechanism and severity of injury and the patient's level of consciousness. Associated injuries affect priorities of emergency care.

Airway and ventilation. Initial steps in treating all patients with head trauma are to ensure an open airway with spinal precautions and provide adequate ventilatory support with high-concentration oxygen. Airway management may include oral or nasal adjuncts, multilumen devices, or nasal or tracheal intubation to maintain and protect the airway. Tracheal intubation and ventilatory support usually are recommended in all patients with head injuries who have a Glasgow coma scale (GCS) score of 8 or less[4] (described later in the chapter).

> **? CRITICAL THINKING**
>
> *Imagine what a patient with a GCS of 8 or lower would look like. Why should these patients be intubated? What if their GCS improves rapidly?*

> **NOTE**
>
> Nasal intubation may increase ICP and should be avoided, if possible.

> **NOTE**
>
> Patients with signs and symptoms of increasing ICP should be ventilated at a rate *not to exceed 30 breaths/minute.*[4]

Patients with head injuries are likely to vomit. If the patient has a decreased level of consciousness after the airway is secured, a nasogastric tube should be inserted to decompress the stomach. In the presence of facial fractures, rhinorrhea (CSF discharge from the nose), or otorrhea (CSF discharge from the ear), an orogastric tube rather than a nasogastric tube should be inserted to avoid possible intubation of the cranial cavity through the fracture site. In addition, the patient should be well stabilized on a long spine board for safe repositioning, and suction equipment with large-bore suction catheters should be available. Ventilatory support should be focused on maintaining adequate oxygenation and optimizing cerebral perfusion. An elevated PO_2 can help buy time against the ill effects of intracranial hemorrhage and elevated ICP.

Circulation. After the airway has been secured while maintaining spinal protection, support of the patient's cardiovascular function becomes the next priority. Major external bleeding should be controlled, and the patient's vital signs should be assessed to establish a baseline for future evaluations. A cardiac monitor will detect changes in rhythm (particularly bradycardia and tachycardia) that can occur with increasing ICP and brainstem injury.

Persistent hypotension that results from an isolated head injury is a rare and terminal event, with the exception of head injury in infants and small children. *Closed head injury in the adult does not produce hypovolemic shock.* Therefore a patient with head injuries who also is hypotensive should be evaluated for other sources of hemorrhage and the possibility of neurogenic shock from spinal cord trauma.

> **NOTE**
>
> It is important to adequately resuscitate the head-injured patient so that cerebral perfusion pressure can be maintained.

The blood pressure of every patient should be maintained at normal levels with fluid replacement (per medical direction). Rapid infusion of isotonic fluids may be indicated for hemorrhagic shock but probably should be used cautiously in patients with evidence of hypotension secondary to neurogenic shock. In the latter patient group, vasopressors also may be helpful in maintaining blood pressure. Neurogenic shock may be distinguished from hemorrhagic shock by the following:

- A relatively bradycardic response (e.g., a pulse of 80 with a blood pressure of 80 mm Hg)
- Skin that often is warm and dry (not cool and clammy)
- No evidence of significant blood loss or hypovolemia
- Paralysis and loss of spinal reflexes

Neurological examination. Conscious patients should be interviewed to determine their memory status before and after the injury and to learn of significant medical history (e.g., heart disease, hypertension, diabetes, epilepsy, medication use, alcohol or other drug use, allergies). The history also should include the mechanism of injury and the events leading up to the injury (e.g., loss of consciousness before or after the accident).

The motor skills of conscious patients should be evaluated to determine their ability to follow commands and to note any paralysis. (Hemiparesis or hemiplegia, especially with a sensory deficit on the same side, indicates brain damage rather than spinal trauma.) If the patient is unconscious on EMS arrival, bystanders should be interviewed about the history of the event and the length of time the patient has been unconscious. The most important indicator of increasing ICP is deterioration in the patient's sensorium. Therefore level of consciousness should be evaluated by use of the AVPU Scale or by the GCS and reevaluated several times during the encounter with the patient.

> **? CRITICAL THINKING**
>
> *How reliable will the patient be regarding the duration of their loss of consciousness?*

The patient's pupils should be assessed for position, size, and reactivity to light. Abnormal pupillary responses may indicate an increase in ICP and cranial nerve involvement. However, alcohol and some other drugs can cause abnormal pupillary reactions, but they commonly are bilateral (except for certain eye drops, if placed in one eye). If the patient is conscious, extraocular movement also should be evaluated.

Fluid therapy. In the absence of hypotension, fluid therapy normally should be restricted in a patient with head injury to minimize cerebral edema.[4] If the patient is hemodynamically stable, an IV line of crystalloid fluid should be established to keep the vein open. If significant hypovolemia is present from another injury, the patient should be managed with aggressive fluid therapy (guided by medical direction) and rapid transportation to an appropriate medical facility. In this circumstance, the injury causing hypovolemia usually is more immediately life threatening than the head injury. As a rule, hypotension in the presence of head injury initially should be managed with fluid boluses to maintain a systolic blood pressure of 90 to 100 mm Hg in the adult male less than 40 years of age.[4]

Drug therapy. Drug therapy in the prehospital setting for head injury is controversial. Pharmacological agents that may be prescribed by medical direction to decrease cerebral edema or circulating blood volume include *mannitol* (Osmotrol), *furosemide*

(Lasix), and other diuretics. If used, medical direction may require the insertion of an indwelling urinary catheter to carefully monitor urine output before administration of these agents. Hypotension leading to hypoperfusion may occur as a complication of diuretic use in patients with head injuries.

> **NOTE**
>
> The administration of glucose (***dextrose 50%***) is contraindicated in patients with head injuries unless hypoglycemia is confirmed. Concentrated glucose may exacerbate cerebral damage.

Anticonvulsant agents such as ***phenytoin*** (Dilantin) and ***diazepam*** (Valium), generally are reserved for head-injured patients who develop seizure activity. As a rule, these drugs are not used in the initial management of head injuries because of their sedating effects. Some medical direction agencies may prescribe anticonvulsant agents as a prophylactic measure to prevent a rise in ICP that often accompanies sudden seizure activity. Intravenous ***lidocaine*** (Xylocaine) has been shown to blunt increases in ICP that normally occur during endotracheal intubation.[4]

In addition, the use of sedatives and paralytics for some patients with head injuries may be indicated for airway management and to facilitate transport of combative patients (particularly during aeromedical transport). The paramedic should follow local protocol and consult with medical direction regarding the use of these drugs.

Injury Rating Systems

Several injury rating systems (also known as *indices* or *scales*) are used to triage, guide patient care, predict patient outcome, identify changes in patient status, and evaluate trauma care in epidemiological studies and quality-assurance reviews. These indices are especially important to prehospital personnel in determining patient care needs with reference to hospital resources. Rating systems commonly used in emergency care include the Glasgow coma scale, Trauma Score, Revised Trauma Score, and Pediatric Trauma Score.

Glasgow Coma Scale

The Glasgow coma scale (GCS) evaluates eye opening, verbal and motor responses, and brainstem reflex function. The scale is considered one of the best indicators of eventual clinical outcome[4] and should be part of any neurological examination for patients with head injury (Table 22-1). A GCS of 13 to 15 is associated with mild head injury; 8 to 12, moderate injury; and less than 8, severe head injury.

> **NOTE**
>
> Intubation is recommended by the American College of Surgeons for patients with GCS score of 8 or less.[1]

Trauma Score

The Trauma Score (TS) was developed in 1980 to predict outcome for patients with blunt or penetrating injuries. It was based on the trauma index, an earlier measurement that used a numerical injury rating system based on a patient's injured body region; type of injury; and cardiovascular, central nervous system, and respiratory status. The TS modified the trauma index to include systolic blood pressure, capillary refill, respiratory rate, and the GCS (Table 22-2). The TS has limited use in the prehospital setting and does not adequately predict mortality for isolated, severe head injury.

TABLE 22-1	GLASGOW COMA SCALE		
Eye Opening		**Motor Response**	
Spontaneous	4	Obeys command	6
To voice	3	Localizes pain	5
To pain	2	Withdrawn (pain)	4
None	1	Flexion (pain)	3
		Extension (pain)	2
		None	1
Verbal Response		**Total GCS Points**	
Oriented	5	14-15 = 5	
Confused	4	11-13 = 4	
Inappropriate words	3	8-10 = 3	
Incomprehensible words	2	5-7 = 2	
None	1	3-4 = 1	

TABLE 22-2	CALCULATION OF TRAUMA SCORE USING THE GLASGOW COMA SCALE

Glasgow Coma Scale

Eye-opening response	Spontaneous	4
	To voice	3
	To pain	2
	None	1
Best verbal response	Oriented	5
	Confused	4
	Inappropriate words	3
	Incomprehensible sounds	2
	None	1
Best motor response	Obeys command	6
	Localizes pain	5
	Withdraws (pain)	4
	Flexion (pain)	3
	Extension (pain)	2
	None	1
TOTAL	Apply this score to GCS portion of TS below:	3-15

Trauma Score

GCS (total points from above)	14-15	5
	1-13	4
	8-10	3
	5-7	2
	3-4	1
Respiratory rate	10-24/min	4
	25-35/min	3
	36/min or greater	2
	1-9/min	1
	None	0
Respiratory expansion	Normal	1
	Retractive/none	0
Systolic blood pressure	90 mm Hg or greater	4
	70-89 mm Hg	3
	50-69 mm Hg	2
	0-49 mm Hg	1
	No pulse	0
Capillary refill	Normal	2
	Delayed	1
	None	0
TOTAL TRAUMA SCORE		1-16

Trauma score	16	15	14	13	12	11	10	9	8	7	6	5	4	3	2	1
Percentage survival	99	98	96	93	87	76	60	42	26	15	8	4	2	1	0	0

From Moore EE, editor: *Early care of the injured patient,* ed 4, Philadelphia, 1990, BC Decker.

Revised Trauma Score

The Revised Trauma Score (RTS) uses the GCS with measurements for systolic blood pressure and respiratory rate that are divided into five intervals (Table 22-3). (The RTS essentially is the same as the TS, except for the consideration of capillary refill.) A range of values for these physiological measurements is assigned a number between 0 and 4. These numbers are then added to give a total between 0 and 12. The American College of Surgeons recommends that patients who have a revised trauma score of 11 or less be transferred to level I trauma centers.[7]

Pediatric Trauma Score

The Pediatric Trauma Score (PTS) grades six characteristics commonly seen in pediatric trauma patients: size (weight), airway, central nervous system, systolic blood pressure, open wound, and skeletal injury (Table 22-4). The American College of Surgeons recommends that any pediatric trauma patient with a PTS of less than 8 be transported to a level I trauma center.[7] Although specifically designed for pediatric patients, the PTS has demonstrated no advantages over the RTS.

In addition to these assessment protocols, the paramedic may use other methods to categorize patients and to determine the need for immediate transport. One method of patient status coding is the *CUPS system*, which assigns patients to one of four categories (Box 22-2). Regardless of the method chosen, the paramedic must remember that assessment is a dynamic process in which patients' conditions frequently change. Constant monitoring of the patient is crucial, and changes in patient status may alter the course of a treatment plan.

TABLE 22-3 REVISED TRAUMA SCORE

GCS	SPB	RR	CODED VALUES
13-15	>89	10-29	4
9-12	76-89	>29	3
6-8	50-75	6-9	2
4-5	1-49	1-5	1
3	0	0	0

SPB, Systolic blood pressure, *RR*, respiratory rate.
From Moore EE, editor: *Early care of the injured patient*, ed 4, Philadelphia, 1990, BC Decker.

BOX 22-2 CUPS SYSTEM OF PATIENT CATEGORIZATION

CPR: The patient is in respiratory or cardiac arrest.
Unstable: The patient is in shock, with or without accompanying respiratory distress.
Potentially unstable: The patient has marginal vital signs and requires close monitoring. The victim's survivability may well be affected by transport or treatment delay.
Stable: The patient is in no distress. Vital signs are within normal limits, and there are no respiratory problems.

TABLE 22-4 COMPONENTS OF THE PEDIATRIC TRAUMA SCORE

COMPONENT	+2	+1	−1
Size	≥20 kg	10-20 kg	≤10 kg
Airway	Normal	Maintainable	Unmaintainable
CNS	Awake	Obtunded	Coma
SBP	≥90 mm Hg	50-90 mm Hg	≤50 mm Hg
Open wound	None	Minor	Major
Skeletal injuries	None	Closed fracture	Open or multiple fractures

CNS, Central nervous system; *SPB*, systolic blood pressure.
From Moore EE, editor: *Early care of the injured patient*, ed 4, Philadelphia, 1990, BC Decker.

SUMMARY

- Major causes of maxillofacial trauma are motor vehicle crashes, home accidents, athletic injuries, animal bites, intentional violent acts, and industrial injuries.

- With the exception of compromised airway and the potential for significant bleeding, damage to the tissues of the maxillofacial area is seldom life threatening. Blunt trauma injuries may be classified as fractures to the mandible, midface, zygoma, orbit, and nose.

- Injury to the ears, eyes, or teeth may be minor or may result in permanent sensory function loss and disfigurement. Trauma to the ear may include lacerations and contusions, thermal injuries, chemical injuries, traumatic perforation, and barotitis. Evaluation of the eye should include a thorough history and measurement of visual acuity, pupillary reaction, and extraocular movements.

- Anterior neck injuries may result in damage to the skeletal structures, vascular structures, nerves, muscles, and glands of the neck.

- Injuries to the skull may be classified as soft tissue injuries to the scalp and skull fractures. Skull fractures may be classified as linear fractures, basilar fractures, depressed fractures, and open vault fractures.

- Categories of brain injury include diffuse axonal injury (DAI) and focal injury. DAI may be mild (concussion), moderate, or severe. Focal injuries are specific, grossly observable brain lesions. Included in this category are lesions that result from skull fracture, contusion, edema with associated increased ICP, ischemia, and hemorrhage.

- Prehospital management of the patient with head injuries is determined by a number of factors, including the mechanism and severity of injury and the patient's level of consciousness; associated injuries affect the priorities of care.

- Several injury rating systems are used to triage, guide patient care, predict patient outcome, identify changes in patient status, and evaluate trauma care. Rating systems commonly used in emergency care include the Glasgow coma scale, Trauma Score, Revised Trauma Score, and Pediatric Trauma Score.

REFERENCES

1. Rosen P, Barkin R: *Emergency medicine: concepts and clinical practice,* ed 4, St. Louis, 1998, Mosby.
2. National Safety Council: *Injury facts,* Itasca, Ill., 1999, The Council.
3. American Association of Endodontists: *Treating the avulsed permanent tooth,* Chicago, 1998, The Association. *http://www.aae.org*
4. U.S. Department of Transportation National Highway Traffic Safety Administration: *EMT-Paramedic national standard curriculum,* Washington, DC, 1998, The Department.
5. Hickey J: *The clinical practice of neurological and neurosurgical nursing,* ed 4, Philadelphia, 1997, Lippincott.
6. *Trauma nursing from resuscitation through rehabilitation,* ed 2, Philadelphia, 1994, WB Saunders.
7. American College of Surgeons, Committee on Trauma: *Resources for optimal care of the injured patient: 1999,* 1999, The College.

23 Spinal Trauma

OBJECTIVES

Upon completion of this chapter, the paramedic student will be able to:

1. Describe the incidence, morbidity, and mortality related to spinal injury.
2. Predict mechanisms of injury that are likely to cause spinal injury.
3. Describe the anatomy and physiology of the spine and spinal cord.
4. Outline the general assessment of a patient with suspected spinal injury.
5. Distinguish between types of spinal injury.
6. Describe prehospital evaluation and assessment of spinal cord injury.
7. Identify prehospital management of the patient with spinal injuries.
8. Distinguish between spinal shock, neurogenic shock, and autonomic hyperreflexia syndrome.
9. Describe selected nontraumatic spinal conditions and the prehospital assessment and treatment of them.

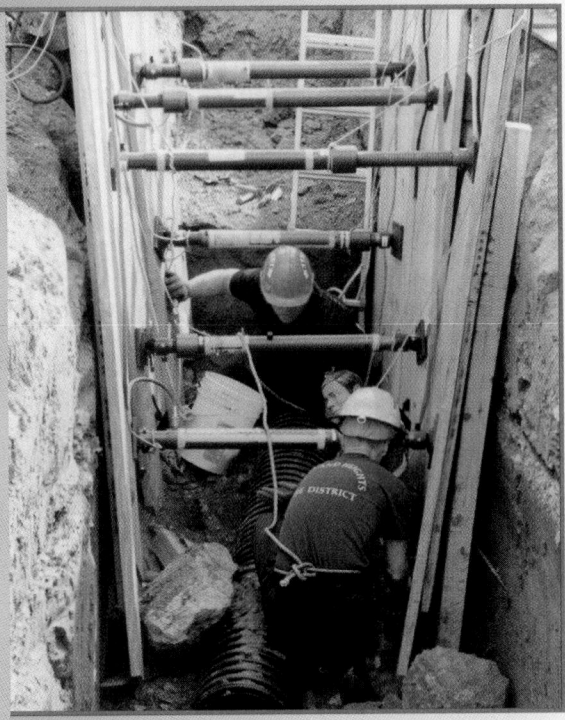

More than 200,000 victims of spinal injury are currently living in the United States, and more than 10,000 new spinal cord injuries (SCI) will occur this year.[1] Of these patients, an estimated 4200 will die before admission to a hospital. Education in injury prevention, prehospital assessment, and proper handling and transportation of these patients can decrease morbidity and mortality.

KEY TERMS

anterior cord syndrome: A spinal cord injury usually seen in flexion injuries; caused by pressure on the anterior aspect of the spinal cord by a ruptured intervertebral disk or fragments of the vertebral body extruded posteriorly into the spinal canal.

axial loading: Vertical compression of the spine that results when direct forces are transmitted along the length of the spinal column.

Brown-Sequard syndrome: A hemitransection of the spinal cord. In the classic presentation, pressure on half of the spinal cord results in weakness of the upper and lower extremities on the ipsilateral (same) side and loss of pain and temperature on the contralateral (opposite) side.

central cord syndrome: A spinal cord injury commonly seen with hyperextension or flexion cervical injuries; characterized by greater motor impairment of the upper than lower extremities.

distraction: A spinal injury that occurs if the cervical spine is suddenly stopped while the weight and momentum of the body pull away from it.

neurogenic hypotension: Hypotension secondary to spinal shock; caused by a loss of sympathetic tone to the vessels.

spinal shock: Refers to a temporary loss of all types of spinal cord function distal to a cord injury.

subluxation: A partial dislocation.

transection: A complete or incomplete lesion to the spinal cord.

Incidence, Morbidity, and Mortality

Most spinal cord injuries result from motor vehicle crashes (48%), followed by falls (21%), penetrating injuries from acts of violence (15%), and sport injuries (14%). The median age of spinal injury victims is 25 years, with men outnumbering women four to one.[1] The incidence of spinal cord injury is highest in men between ages 16 and 30 years.

Forty percent of trauma patients with neurological deficit will have a temporary or permanent spinal cord injury. In addition to the devastating emotional and psychological impact on victims and their families, the annual cost to society exceeds $5 billion. The cost of lifelong care for a 25-year-old victim with permanent SCI is estimated at $1.7 million.[2]

NOTE

The reader should refer to Appendix C for a discussion of injury prevention strategies.

Traditional Spinal Assessment Criteria

Traditional spinal assessment criteria have focused on mechanism of injury (MOI) with spinal immobilization considerations for two specific patient groups: (1) unconscious injury victims, and (2) any patient with a "motion" injury. This mechanism-of-injury criterion covers all patients with a potential for spinal injury, but it is not always practical in the prehospital setting. Prehospital assessment can be enhanced by applying clear, clinical guidelines (clinical criteria) for evaluating spinal cord injury, which includes the following signs and symptoms (in the absence of other injuries, altered mental status, or use of intoxicants):

- Pain
- Distribution of tenderness
- Painful movement
- Deformity
- Cuts/bruises over spinal area
- Paralysis
- Paresthesias
- Weakness or neurological deficit

Mechanism of Injury/Nature of Injury

When determining mechanism of injury in a patient who may have spinal trauma, the paramedic

CLINICAL CRITERIA VS. MECHANISM OF INJURY

- Initial management is based solely on MOI
- Positive MOI requires spinal immobilization
- Negative MOI (without signs and symptoms) requires no spine immobilization
- Uncertain MOI requires further clinical assessment and evaluation to determine need for spinal immobilization

can classify the MOI as *positive, negative,* or *uncertain.*[3] This classification, combined with the clinical criteria for spinal injury listed previously, can help identify situations in which spinal immobilization is appropriate.

? CRITICAL THINKING

What are the disadvantages of immobilizing patients on long spine boards?

Positive MOI

In a positive MOI, the forces exerted on the patient are highly suggestive of spinal cord injury. A positive MOI always requires full spinal immobilization. Examples of positive MOIs include:

- High-speed motor vehicle crashes
- Falls from greater than three times the patient's height
- Violent situations occurring near the patient's spine (e.g., blunt and penetrating injuries)
- Sports injuries
- Other high-impact situations

In the absence of signs and symptoms of SCI, some medical-direction agencies may recommend

✓ TRICKS OF THE TRADE

When assessing a patient with a suspected spinal injury, especially one with a positive MOI, it is more important than ever to ask open-ended questions. People tend to respond to "yes" and "no" questions by nodding or shaking their heads.

that a patient with a positive MOI *not* be immobilized.[3] These recommendations will be based on the paramedic's assessment when patient history is reliable and there are no distracting injuries (described later in this chapter).

Negative MOI

A negative MOI includes events where force or impact does not suggest a potential for spinal injury. In the absence of SCI signs and symptoms, negative MOI injuries do not require spinal immobilization. Examples of negative MOIs include:

- Dropping an object on the foot
- Twisting an ankle while running
- Isolated soft tissue injury

Uncertain MOI

When the impact or force involved in the injury is unknown or uncertain, clinical criteria must be the basis used to determine the need for spinal immobilization (Box 23-1). Examples of uncertain MOIs include:

- Tripping or falling to the ground and hitting the head
- Falls from 2 to 4 feet
- Low-speed motor vehicle crashes ("fender benders")

Assessment of uncertain MOIs. When evaluating the need for spinal immobilization in which there is an uncertain MOI, the paramedic must ensure that the patient is "reliable." A reliable patient is one who is calm, cooperative, sober, alert, and oriented. Examples of patients who would be considered "unreliable" are those who:

- Have acute stress reactions from sudden stress of any type
- Have brain injury
- Are intoxicated
- Have abnormal mental status
- Have distracting injuries
- Have problems communicating

? CRITICAL THINKING

Why isn't patient "reliability" always easy to assess quickly in the prehospital setting?

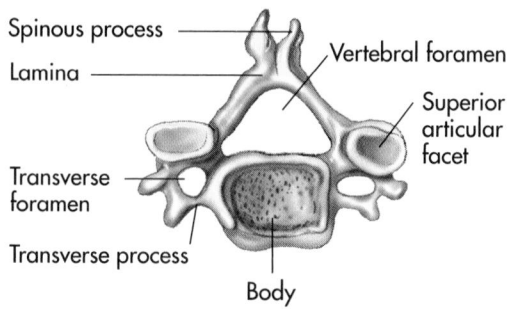

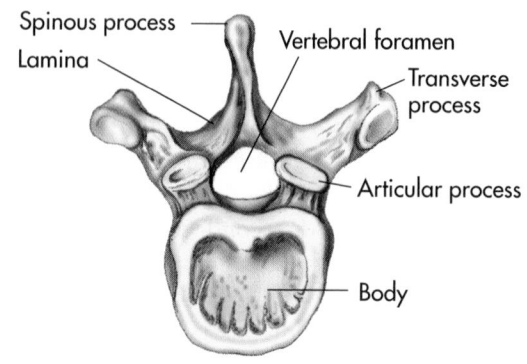

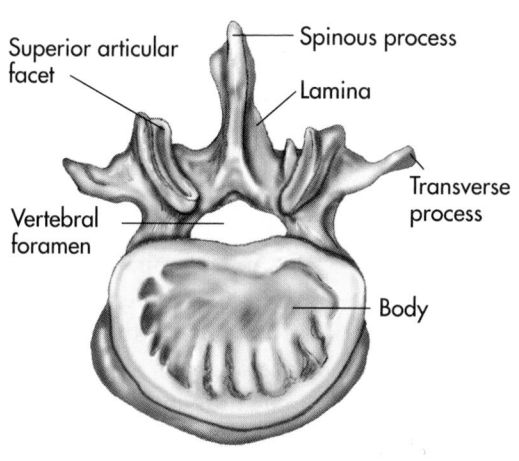

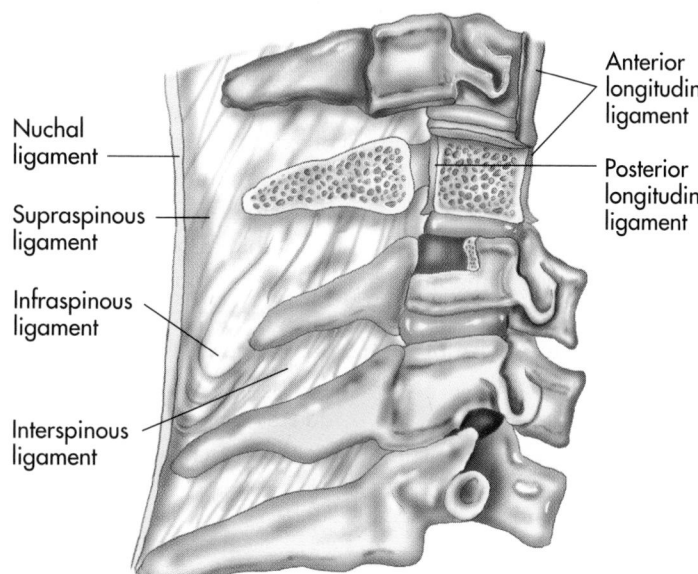

Fig. 23-1 Vertebral bodies and elements of the spine. (From Rosen P, Barkin R: *Emergency medicine: concepts and clinical practice,* ed 4, St Louis, 1998, Mosby.)

> **NOTE**
>
> When in doubt as to the mechanism or nature of injury, the paramedic should employ full spinal immobilization.

Review of Spinal Anatomy and Physiology

As described in Chapter 6, the spinal column is composed of 33 bones (vertebrae) divided into five sections: 7 cervical, 12 thoracic, 5 lumbar, 5 sacrum (fused), and 4 coccyx (fused). The anterior elements of the spine include vertebral bodies, intervertebral disks, and anterior and posterior longitudinal ligaments that connect the vertebral bodies anteriorly and inside the canal (Fig. 23-1).

Each vertebra consists of a solid body (bearing most of the weight of the vertebral column), a posterior and anterior arch, a posterior spinous process, and, in some vertebrae, a transverse process. Ligaments between the spinous processes provide support for the movements of flexion and extension, whereas those between the lamina provide support during lateral flexion. The spinal cord lies in the spinal canal, with the spinal nerve roots passing out through the vertebral foramen.

> **NOTE**
>
> The reader should refer to Chapter 6 to review spinal anatomy and related structures.

General Assessment of Spinal Injury

Spinal injury most commonly results from the spine being forced beyond its physiological limits of motion (Fig. 23-2). The adult skull, which weighs about 16 to 22 lb, sits on top of the first cervical vertebrae (C1), or the atlas. The second cervical vertebrae (C2), or the axis and its odontoid process, allow the head to move with about a 180 degree range of motion. Because of the weight and position of the head in relation to the thin neck and cervical vertebrae, the cervical spine is particularly susceptible to injury (27% to 33% of all cervical spine injuries occur in the C1 to C2 region).[3] Other spinal components that affect physiological limits of motion are the posterior neck muscles, which permit up to 60 degrees of flexion and 70 degrees of extension without stretching of the spinal cord, and the sacrum, which is joined to the pelvis by immovable joints.

The specific mechanisms of injury that frequently cause spinal trauma are axial loading; extremes of flexion, hyperextension, or hyperrotation; excessive lateral bending; and distraction. These energy forces may result in stable and unstable injuries, based on the extent of disruption to spinal structures and the relative strength of the structures remaining intact.

Axial Loading

Axial loading (vertical compression) of the spine results when direct forces are transmitted along the length of the spinal column. Examples include striking the head against a windshield of an automobile, shallow diving injuries, vertical falls, and being struck on the head or a helmet with a heavy object. These forces may produce compression fracture or a crushed vertebral body without SCI, and most commonly occur from T12 to L2.[3]

Flexion, Hyperextension, and Hyperrotation

Extremes in flexion, hyperextension, or hyperrotation may result in fracture, ligamentous injury, or muscle injury. Spinal cord injury is caused by impingement into the spinal canal by **subluxation** (dislocation) of one or more cervical vertebrae. Examples of these motion extremes include rapid acceleration or deceleration forces from motor vehicle crashes, hangings, and midfacial skeletal or soft tissue trauma. Serious injuries often result from a combination of loading *and* rotational forces, producing displacement or fracture of one or more vertebrae.

Lateral Bending

Excessive lateral bending may result in dislocations and bony fractures to the cervical and thoracic spine. The injury occurs as a sudden lateral impact moves the torso sideways. Initially, the head tends to remain in place until pulled along by the cervical attachments. Examples of lateral bending include side or angular collisions from motor vehicle crashes and injuries from contact sports. The mechanism of this lateral force requires less movement before injury than flexion or extension caused by frontal or rear impacts.

Distraction

Distraction may occur if the cervical spine is suddenly stopped while the weight and momentum of the body pull away from it. This force or stretching may result in tearing and laceration of the spinal cord. Examples of distraction include intentional or accidental hangings (e.g., suicide, schoolyard or playground accidents).

Other Mechanisms

Other less common mechanisms of spinal injury include blunt and penetrating trauma and electrical injury. The spinal cord, like the brain, may become concussed, contused, and lacerated and may develop hematomas and edema in response to blunt trauma. Examples include spinal injuries that result from direct blows, as from falling tree limbs or other heavy objects.

Penetrating trauma to the spine may be caused by missile-type injuries or stab wounds to the neck, chest, or abdomen. These forces may result in laceration of the spinal cord or nerve roots over a wide area and occasionally may produce a complete **transection** (lesion). In addition, areas of edema or contusion adjacent to the laceration may disrupt cord tissue.

Spinal trauma may occur from direct electrical injury or by the violent muscle spasms that accompany electrical shock (described in Chapter 21).

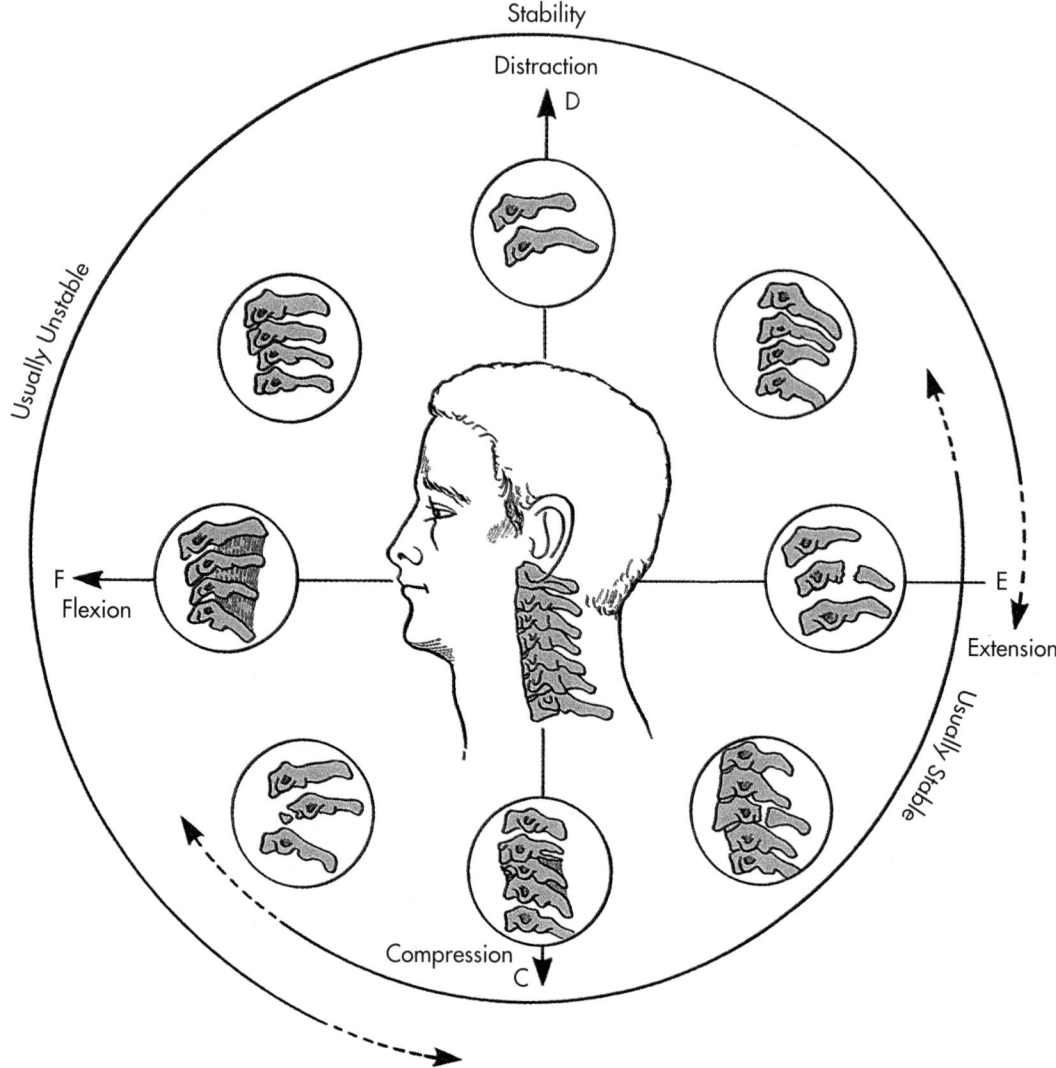

Fig. 23-2 Mechanisms of cervical spine injury and fracture or dislocation. The mechanism of cervical injury (flexion versus extension) determines the type of cervical spine fracture or dislocation. (From Moore EE, editor: *Early care of the injured patient*, ed 4, Philadelphia, 1990, BC Decker.)

Classifications of Spinal Injury

Spinal injuries may be classified as sprains and strains, fractures and dislocations, sacral and coccygeal fractures, and cord injuries. Regardless of the specific injury, all patients with suspected spinal trauma and signs and symptoms of SCI should be immobilized, and unnecessary movement should be avoided until injury to the spine or spinal cord can be excluded by clinical examination and radiography. An unstable spine can only be ruled out by radiography or lack of any potential mechanism for the injury. As a guideline, the presence of spine injury and an unstable spine should be assumed with the following[3]:

- Significant trauma and use of intoxicating substances
- Seizure activity
- Complaints of pain in the neck or arms (or paresthesia in the arms)

> **NOTE**
>
> Spinal injury (bony injury) can occur with or without spinal cord injury. Likewise, a patient may have spinal cord injury without bony injury. *Spinal cord injury without radiological abnormality* (SCIWORA) is a more common finding in children.

- Neck tenderness on examination
- Unconsciousness as a result of head injury
- Significant injury above the clavicle
- A fall more than three times the patient's height
- A fall and fracture of both heels (associated with lumbar fractures)
- Injury from a high-speed motor vehicle crash

> **NOTE**
>
> Most bony and ligamentous injuries are associated with prompt, severe, and persistent cervical muscle spasm.

The damage produced by the injury forces can be further complicated by the patient's age (calcification from the aging process), preexisting bone diseases (osteoporosis, spondylosis, rheumatoid arthritis, Paget's disease), and congenital spinal cord anomalies (e.g., fusion, narrow spinal canal). Spinal cord neurons do not regenerate to any great extent. Therefore any injury to the central nervous system that produces cellular death often results in irreparable damage and permanent loss of function. The role of the paramedic in protecting this critical area cannot be overemphasized.

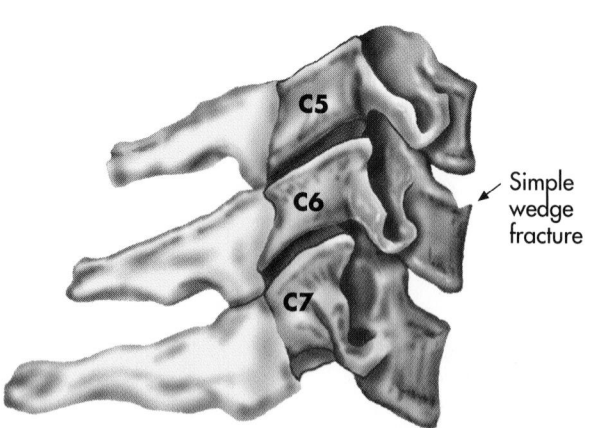

Fig. 23-3 Lateral view of simple wedge fracture. (From Rosen P, Barkin R: *Emergency medicine: concepts and clinical practice,* ed 4, St Louis, 1998, Mosby.)

Sprains and Strains

Sprains and strains usually result from hyperflexion and hyperextension forces. A hyperflexion sprain occurs when the posterior ligamentous complex tears at least partially. This sprain can also result in tears of the joint capsules and may allow partial dislocation (subluxation) of the intervertebral joints. Hyperextension strains are common in low-velocity, rear-end automobile collisions and are commonly known as *whiplash*. Injury occurs as the occiput is thrown backward against the posterior thorax during impact, damaging anterior soft tissues of the neck.

> **?** **CRITICAL THINKING**
>
> *How can the paramedic distinguish between sprain/strain and spinal fracture in the prehospital setting?*

> **NOTE**
>
> Whiplash injuries have decreased in recent years due to the introduction of head-rests and high-back seats by automobile manufacturers. (This is an example of an engineering control method of injury prevention.)

With both sprains and strains, local pain may be produced by spasms of the neck muscles and injury to the vertebrae, intervertebral disks, and ligamentous structures. The pain usually is described as a nonradiating, aching soreness of the neck or back muscles. Discomfort often varies in intensity with changes in posture.

On examination, a deformity of the spine may be palpable if subluxation has occurred, and the patient may complain of associated point tenderness and swelling. Until the diagnosis is excluded by radiography, these patients should be treated as if they have an unstable cervical spine injury with a potential for spinal cord damage. After the diagnosis is confirmed, treatment of cervical sprain or strain usually is symptomatic and occasionally may include a cervical collar to decrease neck movement, heat application, and analgesics.

Fractures and Dislocations

The most frequently injured spinal regions in descending order are C5 to C7, C1 to C2, and T12 to L2.[3] Of these injuries, the most common are wedge-shaped compression fractures and "teardrop" fractures or dislocations. Neurological deficits associated with these fractures and dislocations vary with the location and extent of injury. Although the spine and spinal cord are anatomically closely related, the spine can be fractured without spinal cord injury and vice versa. In addition, multiple-level spinal injuries are common.

Wedge-shaped fractures (Fig. 23-3) are hyperflexion injuries that usually result from compressive force applied to the anterior portion of the vertebral body with stretching of the posterior ligament complex (commonly seen in industrial accidents and falls). These fractures usually occur in the mid or lower cervical segments or at T12 and L1. They generally are considered stable because the posterior ligamentous complex is rarely totally disrupted.

Teardrop fractures and dislocations (Fig. 23-4) are extremely unstable injuries that result from a combination of severe hyperflexion and compression forces commonly seen in motor vehicle crashes. During impact, the vertebral body is fractured, the anterior-inferior corner of the vertebral body being displaced anteriorly. Unlike simple wedge fractures, these fractures may be associated with neurological abnormalities. These are among the most unstable injuries of the spine. A number of other spinal injuries are associated with the mechanisms of flexion, extension, rotation, and axial loading. Most of these are unstable and require careful immobilization.

Sacral and Coccygeal Fractures

The majority of serious spinal injuries occur in the cervical, thoracic, and lumbar regions. This is partly because of the location of the spinal cord and its ter-

mination in the adult spine at about L2 and because of the protection provided by the ring structure of the pelvis and the musculature of the buttocks and lower back. However, fractures through the foramina of S1 and S2 are fairly common and may compromise several sacral nerve elements. Such fractures may result in loss of perianal sensory motor function and in bladder and sphincter disturbances.

The sacrococcygeal joint also may be injured as a result of direct blows and falls. Patients frequently complain that they have "broken their tailbone" and experience moderate pain from the mobile coccyx. Diagnosis usually is confirmed by a physician through a rectal examination.

Cord Injuries

Spinal cord injury may be further classified as *primary* and *secondary* injuries. Primary injuries occur at the time of impact. Secondary injury occurs after the initial injury and can include swelling, ischemia, and movement of bony fragments. Like other tissues, the spinal cord can be concussed, contused, compressed, and lacerated, all of which can cause temporary or permanent loss of cord-mediated functions distal to the injury from compression or ischemia. Bleeding from damaged blood vessels also can occur in the cord's tissue, causing an obstruction

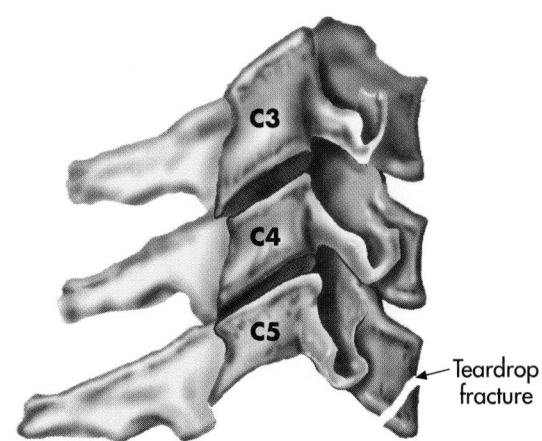

Fig. 23-4 Lateral view of teardrop fracture. (From Rosen P, Barkin R: *Emergency medicine: concepts and clinical practice*, ed 4, St Louis, 1998, Mosby.)

to spinal blood supply. The severity of these injuries depends on the amount and type of force that produced them and the duration of the injury.

Cord Lesions

Lesions (transections) to the spinal cord are classified as *complete* or *incomplete*. Complete lesions usually are associated with spinal fracture or dislocation. Patients have total absence of pain, pressure, and joint sensation and complete motor paralysis below the level of injury. Autonomic dysfunction may be associated with complete cord lesions depending on the level of cord involvement. Manifestations of autonomic dysfunction include:

- Bradycardia caused by loss of sympathetic autonomic activity
- Hypotension caused by loss of vasomotor control and peripheral vascular resistance
- Priapism
- Loss of sweating and shivering
- Poikilothermy (body temperature varying with ambient temperature)
- Loss of bowel and bladder control

> **? CRITICAL THINKING**
>
> *Why should you immobilize a patient already demonstrating signs and symptoms that indicate a complete cord lesion?*

The paramedic should be familiar with several incomplete spinal cord syndromes. Knowledge of these rare syndromes helps the EMS provider understand the mechanism of injury and the potential for further injury. The three syndromes indicating incomplete lesions of the spinal cord are:

1. **Central cord syndrome**: Central cord syndrome, commonly seen with hyperextension or flexion cervical injuries, is characterized by greater motor impairment of the upper than lower extremities. Signs and symptoms of central cord syndrome are:
   a. Paralysis of the arms
   b. *Sacral sparing* (the preservation of sensory or voluntary motor function of the perineum, buttocks, scrotum, or anus)

> **? CRITICAL THINKING**
>
> *How will the prehospital care differ for a patient who has signs or symptoms of one of these syndromes?*

2. **Anterior cord syndrome**: Anterior cord syndrome, usually seen in flexion injuries, is caused by pressure on the anterior aspect of the spinal cord by a ruptured intervertebral disk or fragments of the vertebral body extruded posteriorly into the spinal canal. Signs and symptoms include:
   a. Decreased sensation of pain and temperature below the level of the lesion (including lesions of the sacral region)
   b. Intact light touch and position sensation
   c. Paralysis
3. **Brown-Sequard syndrome**: Brown-Sequard syndrome is a hemitransection of the spinal cord. It may result from a ruptured intervertebral disk or encroachment on the spinal cord by a fragment of vertebral body, often after knife or missile injuries. In the classic presentation, pressure on half of the spinal cord results in weakness of the upper and lower extremities on the ipsilateral (same) side and loss of pain and temperature on the contralateral (opposite) side.

Pharmacological therapy for incomplete cord injury. The benefits of pharmacological agents (glucocorticoids, *naloxone* [Narcan], calcium-channel blockers, GM-1 Ganglioside [Sygen], and others) in the management of incomplete cord injury are controversial. These drugs are hypothesized to provide some type of "damage control" following some spinal cord injuries. Some are thought to work by reducing the toxicity of "excitatory" amino acids that cause cells to die; others, by encouraging the growth of new neurons or by reducing inflammation of the injured spinal cord and the bursting open of damaged cells.[2] Many drugs (and combinations of drugs) are currently being tested in both animal and clinical trials.

Methylprednisolone (Solu-Medrol), a synthetic steroid that reduces posttraumatic spinal cord edema and inflammation, routinely is used in victims of spinal cord injury. Studies have found that patients treated with this drug (30 mg/kg IV bolus followed by an infusion of 5.4 mg/kg/hr for 23 hours) within 8 hours of injury show significant neurological improvement at 6 weeks when compared with patients who were treated with a placebo.[4] Paramedics should consult with medical direction and follow local protocol regarding the use of these pharmacological agents in the prehospital setting.

Evaluation and Assessment of Spinal Cord Injury

Spinal cord trauma should be evaluated only after all life-threatening injuries have been assessed and treated. As with any scenario of serious illness or injury, the paramedic's first priority must be scene survey (including ensuring personal safety) and assessment of the patient's airway, breathing, and circulation. The second priority is to preserve spinal cord function and avoid secondary injury to the spinal cord.

The primary injury to the spine occurs at impact. Therefore the critical role of paramedics is to prevent secondary injury that could result from unnecessary movement of an unstable spinal column, hypoxemia, edema, or shock (which may reduce perfusion of the injured cord). These goals are best met by maintaining a high degree of suspicion for the presence of spinal trauma (based on scene survey, kinematics, and history of the event), providing early spinal immobilization, and rapidly correcting any volume deficit through fluid replacement, PASG application (per protocol), and oxygen administration.

After any life-threatening problems encountered in the initial assessment are treated, a neurological examination should be performed. This examination may be done in the field or en route to the receiving hospital if the patient's condition requires rapid transportation. Thorough documentation of the paramedic's findings provides an important baseline for further assessment and evaluation after the patient is delivered to the emergency department. The components of the neurological examination include evaluation of motor and sensory findings and reflex responses.

Motor Findings

Conscious patients should be questioned about pain in the neck or back with and without palpation and ability to move arms and legs. If possible, the strength and motion of all four extremities should be tested by asking the patient to flex the elbows (biceps, C6), extend the elbows (triceps, C7), and abduct/adduct the fingers (C8, T1). In unconscious patients, painful stimuli in the hands and lower extremities may initiate an involuntary muscle reflex unless the patient is in profound coma.

Upper Extremity Neurological Function Assessment

To test interosseous muscle function (controlled by T1 nerve roots), the paramedic should instruct the patient to spread the fingers of both hands and to keep them apart while the paramedic squeezes the second and fourth fingers. Normal resistance should be "spring-like" and equal on both sides.

To test the extensors of the hands and fingers (controlled by C7 nerve roots), the paramedic should instruct the patient to hold wrists or fingers straight out and to keep them out with the paramedic pressing down on the fingers. (The arm should be supported at the wrist to avoid testing arm function and other nerve roots.) Moderate resistance should be felt to moderate pressure. Both sides should be evaluated if not contraindicated by injury.

Lower Extremity Neurological Function Assessment

To test plantar flexors of the foot (controlled by S1,2 nerve roots), the paramedic should place his or her hands at the sole of each foot and instruct the patient to push against the hands. Both sides should feel equal and strong.

To test dorsal flexors of the foot and great toe (controlled by L5 nerve roots), the paramedic should hold the patient's foot (with fingers on toes) and instruct the patient to pull them back or toward the nose. Both sides should feel equal and strong.

> **NOTE**
>
> Any movement of the patient for performing a general or neurological examination must be accompanied by continuous, manual protection and in-line stabilization of the spine. Once stabilized, the entire spine should be palpated. Any report of pain on palpation indicates the need to immobilize the spine.

Sensory Findings

In conscious patients, sensory examination should be performed with light touch on each hand and each foot (while the patient's eyes are closed) to evaluate the ability to feel this type of stimuli. (Light touch is carried by more than one nerve tract.) Sensation should be equal on both sides. The patient also should be questioned about weakness, numbness, paresthesia, or radicular pain ("shooting pain" that travels along a nerve).

If the patient cannot feel light touch or is unconscious, sensation may be evaluated by gently pricking the hands and soles of the feet with a sharp object that will not penetrate the skin (e.g., the end of a pen or broken Q-tip). One method of examination proceeds from head to toe; recording the level at which sensation stops or the unconscious patient ceases to respond to a painful stimulus by marking that location on the patient's skin with ink or a marker. Another method is to begin the sensory assessment by moving from an area of no sensation to an area where sensation begins, and then marking that location with ink or marker. (These marks make it possible to accurately compare sensory level after repeated examinations.) Lack of response to stimulation in the upper extremities indicates cord damage in the cervical region; failure of only the lower extremities to respond indicates cord injury in the thoracic region, lumbar regions, or both.

? CRITICAL THINKING

How will you respond to the patient who fearfully asks you, "Why can't I move or feel my arms or legs?"

Dermatomes (described in Chapter 6) correspond to spinal nerves (Box 23-2), so the following four landmarks may be useful for a quick sensory evaluation in the prehospital setting[3]:

1. C2 to C4 dermatomes provide a collar of sensation around the neck and over the anterior chest to below the clavicles.
2. T4 dermatome provides sensation to the nipple line.
3. T10 dermatome provides sensation to the umbilicus.
4. S1 dermatome provides sensation to the soles of the feet.

Reflex Responses

Reflex responses seldom are evaluated in the prehospital setting. Some abnormal responses are easily observed, however, and may indicate autonomic injury. These responses include loss of temperature control, hypotension, bradycardia, and priapism. Another pathological reflex includes the presence of Babinski's sign (the plantar reflex), which is a reflex movement in which the great toe bends upward

---

BOX 23-2

COMMON NERVE ROOT AND MOTOR/SENSORY CORRELATION

NERVE ROOT	MOTOR	SENSORY
C3,4	Trapezius (shoulder shrug)	Top of shoulder
C3,4,5	Diaphragm	Top of shoulder
C5,6	Biceps (elbow flexion)	Thumb
C7	Triceps (elbow extension) Wrist/finger extension	Middle finger
C8, T1	Finger abduction/adduction	Little finger
T4	Nipple	
T10	Umbilicus	
L1,2	Hip flexion	Inguinal crease
L3,4	Quadriceps	Medial thigh/calf
L5	Great toe/foot dorsiflexion	Lateral calf
S1	Knee flexion	Lateral foot
S1,2	Foot plantar flexion	
S2,3,4	Anal sphincter tone	Perianal

✓ TRICKS OF THE TRADE

To check for priapism in male patients with suspected spinal injury, gently sweep the pubic area with the back of your hand.

when the outer edge of the sole of the foot is scratched (Fig. 23-5).

Other Methods of Evaluation

Visual inspection also may indicate the presence of injury and its level. For example, transection of the cord above C3 often results in respiratory arrest. Lesions that occur at C4 may result in paralysis of the diaphragm, whereas transections that occur at C5 to C6 usually spare the diaphragm, permitting diaphragmatic breathing. This is because the intercostal muscles are sequentially innervated between C4 to C5 and T12. Accordingly, intercostal muscle groups may be paralyzed with cervical or thoracic lesions below the level where diaphragmatic innovation takes place. (The higher the lesion, the greater the loss of intercostal muscle function.)

The patient's body position also may provide clues about neurological injury. For example, a patient with a spinal cord injury at C6 may lie with the arms flexed at the elbows and wrists ("hold-up" position).

General Management of Spinal Injuries

The absence of neurological deficits does not rule out significant spinal injury. More than 50% of patients with cervical spinal injuries have normal responses to motor, sensory, and reflex examinations.[1] Therefore, if the paramedic suspects a spinal injury for any reason, the patient's spine must be protected. In addition, the patient's ability to walk should not be a factor in determining the need for spinal precautions. As previously stated, an unstable spine can be ruled out only by clinical examination, radiography, and the lack of any potential mechanism for spinal injury. General principles of spinal immobilization include:

1. The primary goal is to prevent further injury.
2. The spine should be treated as a long bone with a joint at either end (the head and pelvis).

3. Always use "complete" spinal immobilization. (It is impossible to splint and isolate a specific injury site. It also is common to have spine fractures in more than one location.)
4. Spinal immobilization begins in the initial assessment and must be maintained until the spine is completely immobilized on a long spine board.
5. The patient's head and neck must be placed in a neutral, in-line position unless contraindicated by condition or mechanism of injury. (Neutral positioning allows for the most space for the spinal cord, thereby reducing cord hypoxia and excess pressure.)

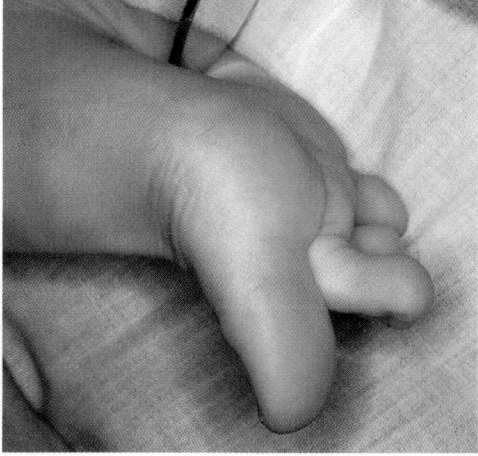

Fig. 23-5 Babinski's sign: dorsiflexion of the great toe with or without fanning of the toes. (Courtesy Gary Quick, M.D.)

Spinal Stabilization/Immobilization Techniques

Immediately on recognizing a possible or potential spine injury, the patient's head and neck should be manually protected. The basic principle to follow is that the head and neck must be maintained in line with the long axis of the body. If other injuries require treatment, the patient's head and neck position must be maintained without interruption.

A number of commercial immobilization devices are designed for prehospital use. When properly applied to patients who are sitting, standing, or lying, these devices can provide adequate spinal protection. However, no mechanical device should be considered for application until the head and neck have been stabilized with manual in-line immobilization.

> **NOTE**
>
> All spinal immobilization techniques discussed in this text follow the guidelines recommended by the Prehospital Trauma Life Support Committee of the National Association of Emergency Medical Technicians in cooperation with the Committee on Trauma of the American College of Surgeons.[4]

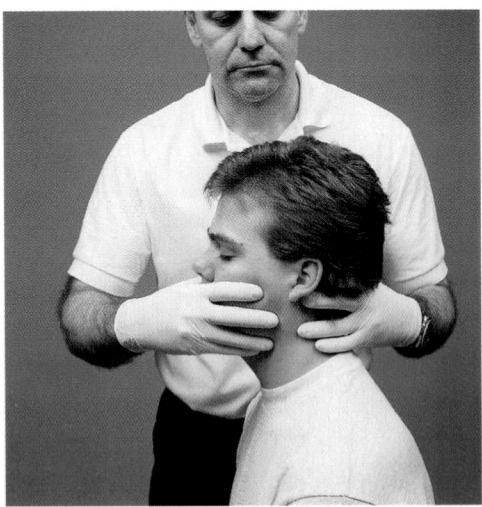

Fig. 23-6 Manual in-line immobilization from the side.

Manual In-Line Immobilization

Manual in-line immobilization should be applied without traction, applying only enough tension to relieve the weight of the head from the cervical spine. After manual immobilization has been initiated, it must be continued without interruption until the head and spine are immobilized to an appropriate mechanical device (short spine board or vest, long spine board).

> **NOTE**
>
> Manual in-line immobilization can be accomplished from almost any patient position.

Contraindications for moving the patient's head to an in-line position are listed below. If any of these contraindications occur, all manual movement of the patient's head should stop, and the head and neck should be stabilized in the position found. Contraindications include:

- Resistance to movement
- Neck muscle spasm
- Increased pain
- The presence or increase in neurological deficits during movement (e.g., numbness, tingling, loss of motor function)
- Compromise of the airway or ventilation
- Severe misalignment of the head away from the midline of the shoulders and body axis (rare)

Manual immobilization from the sitting or standing patient's side.
1. Stand alongside the patient, holding the back of the head with one hand. Place the thumb and first finger of the other hand on each cheek, just below the zygomatic arch (Fig. 23-6).
2. Tighten the position of both hands without moving the head or neck.
3. Move the head to an in-line position if needed. Maintain this position by bracing the elbows against your torso for support.

Manual in-line immobilization from the front of the sitting or standing patient.
1. Stand in front of the patient and place the thumb of each hand on the patient's cheeks, just below the zygomatic arch.

2. Place the little fingers of each hand on the posterior aspect of the patient's skull.
3. Spread the remaining fingers of each hand on the lateral planes of the head and increase the strength of the grip (Fig. 23-7).
4. Move the head to an in-line position if needed. Maintain this position by bracing the elbows against your torso for support.

Manual in-line immobilization with a supine patient.

1. Kneel or lie at the patient's head and place the thumbs of each hand just below the zygomatic arch of each cheek (Fig. 23-8).
2. Place the little fingers of each hand on the posterior aspect of the patient's skull.
3. Spread the remaining fingers of each hand on the lateral planes of the head and increase the strength of the grip.
4. Move the head to an in-line position if needed. Maintain this position by bracing the elbows against your torso or ground surface for support.

> ## ✓ TRICKS OF THE TRADE
>
> What exactly do you do with the hands of a patient who has been immobilized on a long spine board? A quick and simple solution is to gently tie the hands with a cravat in a figure-eight until the patient is in the ambulance. This keeps patients from flailing the arms while you carry them.

Log-roll with spinal precautions. Log-rolling methods are used when it is necessary to move patients with possible spinal injury. Examples include moving patients onto a mechanical immobilization device and turning patients from a prone to a supine position. Log-rolling maneuvers require a minimum of four rescuers to provide adequate spinal protection.

> ## NOTE
>
> The position of the patient's arms during log-rolling maneuvers may affect thoracic-lumbar motion and further compromise spinal stability. One method that may minimize lateral motion and help to maintain neutral alignment of the pelvis and legs is to position the patient with arms extended at the side, palms on lateral thighs.

Log-roll of the supine patient.

1. Rescuer 1 should be positioned at the patient's head, providing in-line manual stabilization (Fig. 23-9). A rigid cervical collar should be applied and a long spine board placed at the patient's side. (If there is an obvious spinal injury with paralysis or if shock is suspected, the PASG should be prepared on the spine board per protocol.)
2. Rescuers 2 and 3 should be positioned at the patient's midthorax and knees. The patient's arms should be extended at the sides, palms on lateral thighs. The legs should be brought together for neutral alignment.

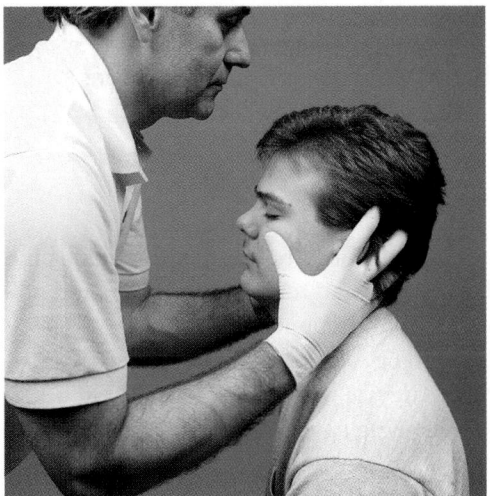

Fig. 23-7 Manual in-line immobilization from the front.

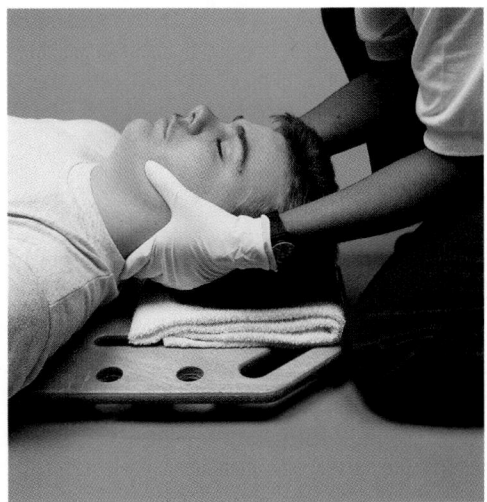

Fig. 23-8 Manual in-line immobilization with a supine patient.

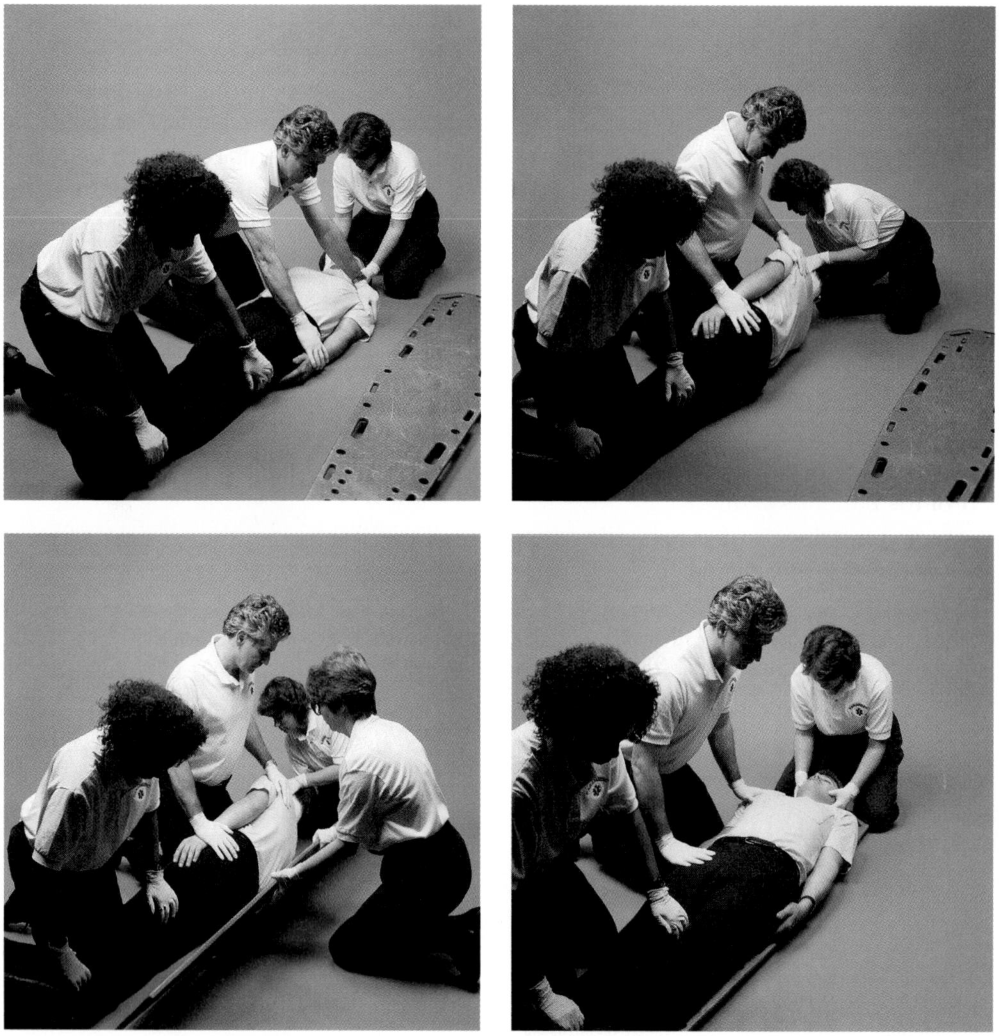

Fig. 23-9 A, To log-roll a supine patient, rescuer 1 is positioned at the patient's head, providing in-line manual stabilization. Rescuers 2 and 3 are positioned at the patient's midthorax and knees. **B,** While maintaining immobilization, the rescuers slowly log-roll the patient onto his or her side perpendicular to the ground in one organized move. **C,** Rescuer 4 positions the long spine board by placing the device flat on the ground or at a 30- to 40-degree angle against the patient's back. **D,** In one organized move, the rescuers slowly log-roll and center the patient onto long spine board.

3. Rescuer 2 grasps the far side of the patient at the shoulder and wrist. Rescuer 3 grasps the hips (just distal of the wrists) and both lower extremities at the ankles.
4. In one organized move, the rescuers slowly log-roll the patient onto his or her side and slide the spine board under the patient. In-line support of the patient's head must be maintained by rotating it exactly with the torso to avoid flexion or hyperextension. In addition, the ankles must be slightly elevated to maintain lateral and anterior-posterior alignment.
5. Rescuer 4 positions the long spine board by placing the device flat on the ground or at a 30- to 40-degree angle against the patient's back.
6. In one organized move, the rescuers slowly log-roll and center the patient on the long spine board.

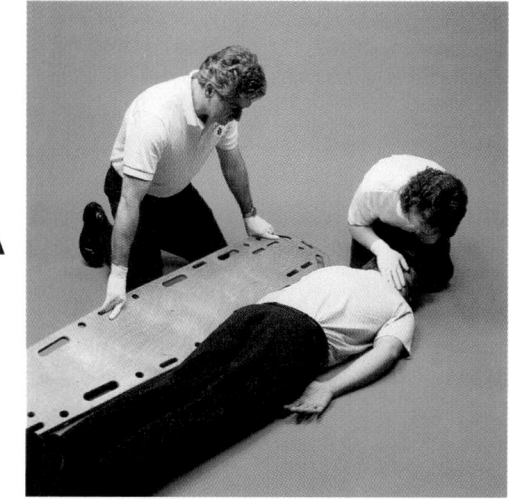

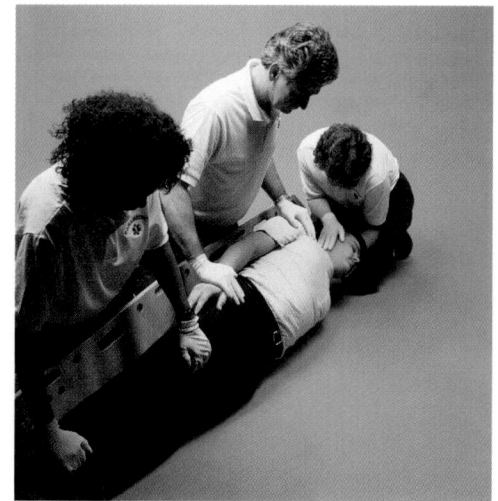

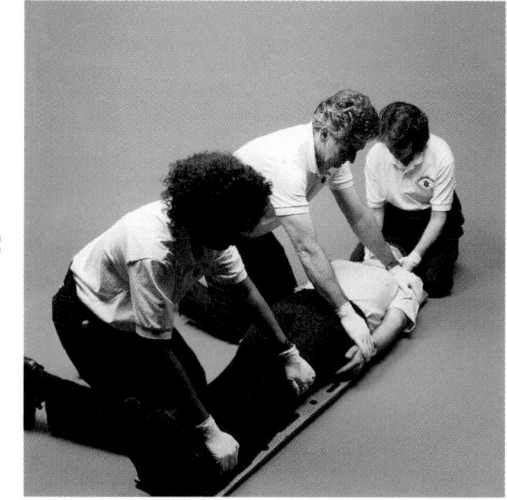

Fig. 23-10 A, Rescuer 1 places his or her hands in a position that provides in-line stabilization and that accommodates the rotation of the patient with the torso. Rescuer 2 positions the long spine board. **B,** In one organized move, the patient is rotated away from the direction of his or her initial prone position. **C,** In one organized move, the rescuers slowly log-roll and center the patient onto the long spine board. A rigid cervical collar is then applied.

Log-roll of the prone patient. The general principles used in log-rolling supine patients can be applied to a patient who is in a prone or semiprone position. The procedure incorporates the same initial alignment of the patient's arms and legs and the same rescuer responsibilities for maintaining alignment. The two major differences in this log-roll maneuver are rescuer 1's hand position during the log-roll and the application of the rigid cervical collar, which can be applied only after the patient is in a supine position (Fig. 23-10).

1. Rescuer 1 places his or her hands in a position that provides in-line stabilization and that accommodates rotation of the patient with the torso.

2. In one organized move, the patient is rotated away from the direction of the initial prone position.
3. The long spine board is placed on a flat surface or positioned between the patient's back and the rescuers at the patient's side.
4. In one organized move, the rescuers slowly log-roll and center the patient on the long spine board.
5. A rigid cervical collar is applied.

Mechanical Devices

Spinal immobilization equipment covered includes rigid cervical collars, short spine boards, and long spine boards. For this text, only *general* principles of spinal immobilization by mechanical devices are

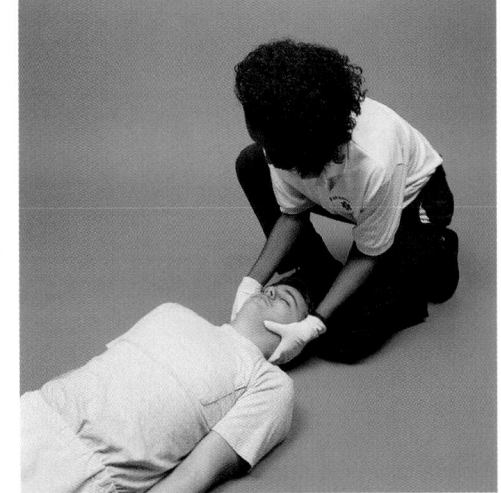

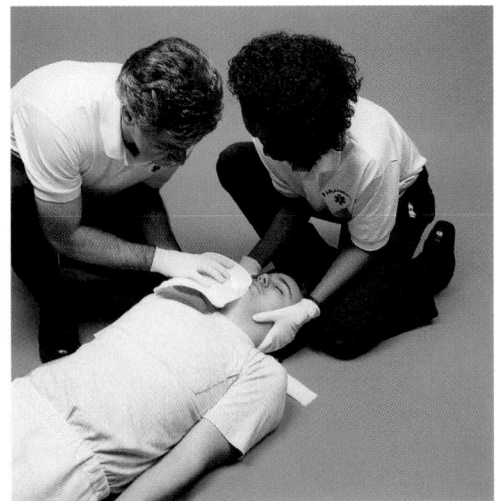

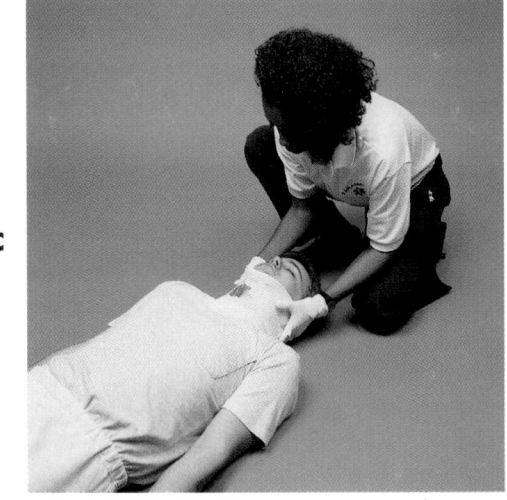

Fig. 23-11 A, Rescuer 1 applies manual in-line immobilization and maintains this position throughout the procedure. **B,** Rescuer 2 positions the collar and secures it with Velcro straps. **C,** Rescuer 1 spreads fingers and maintains support until the patient is secured to a short or long spine board.

presented. The specific methods of application vary by device. Paramedics should familiarize themselves with the equipment used in their locale and follow the application guidelines of the equipment manufacturer.

Rigid cervical collars. Rigid cervical collars are designed to protect the cervical spine from compression. Although these devices may reduce movement and some range of motion of the head, they do not by themselves provide adequate immobilization of the spine. These mechanical devices must always be used in conjunction with manual in-line stabilization or mechanical immobilization by a suitable device (e.g., vest, short spine board, long spine board). To apply a rigid cervical collar, the

paramedic should follow these general steps, which demonstrate the application of the Stifneck Collar (Fig. 23-11):

1. Rescuer 1 applies manual in-line immobilization from behind the patient and maintains this position throughout the procedure.
2. Rescuer 2 properly angles the collar for placement.
3. Rescuer 2 positions the collar bottom.
4. Rescuer 2 sets the collar in place around the patient's neck.
5. Rescuer 2 secures the collar with the Velcro straps.
6. Rescuer 1 spreads his or her fingers and maintains support until the patient is secured to a short or long spine board.

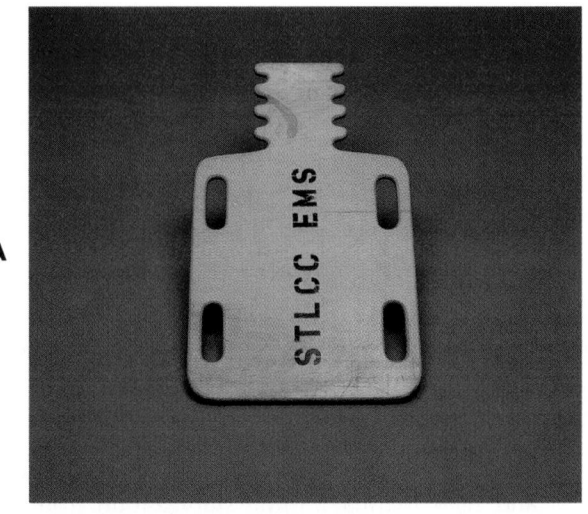
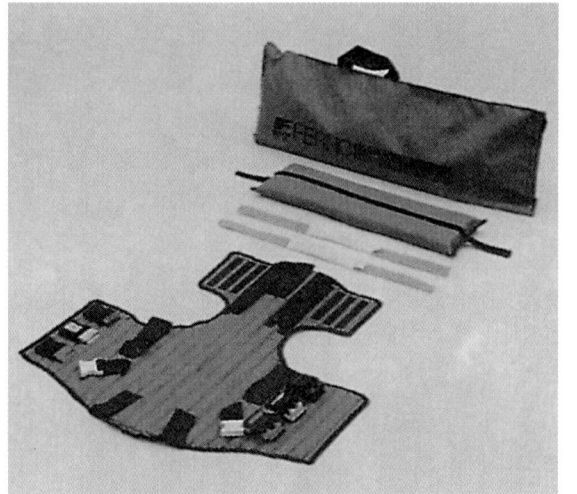

Fig. 23-12 A, Wooden short spine board. **B,** Kendrick's Extrication Device (KED). (**B,** Courtesy Ferno Washington, Wilmington, Ohio.)

Rigid cervical collars are available in a number of sizes (or are adjustable) to accommodate the various physical characteristics of patients. Choosing the appropriate size reduces flexion or hyperextension that may occur during patient extrication and packaging and as a result of acceleration and deceleration forces that normally occur during patient transportation in emergency vehicles. The following guidelines apply to the use of rigid cervical collars:

- Rigid cervical collars must not inhibit the patient's ability to open his or her mouth or to clear his or her airway in case vomiting occurs.
- Rigid cervical collars must not obstruct airway passages or ventilations.
- Rigid cervical collars should be applied only after the head has been brought into a neutral in-line position.

Short spine boards. Short spine boards or other short spine extrication devices are used to splint the cervical and thoracic spine. These mechanical devices vary in design and are available from a number of equipment manufacturers (Fig. 23-12). Short spine boards generally are used to provide spinal immobilization in situations in which the patient is in a sitting position or a confined space. After short spine board immobilization, the patient is transferred to a long spine board device for complete spinal immobilization. Examples of short spine boards include the plastic or synthetic half backboard, the Kendrick's Extrication Device (KED), the Oregon Spine Splint II, and the Hare Extrication Device. General principles of short spine board application, demonstrated with the KED, are (Fig. 23-13):

? CRITICAL THINKING

Think of some situations where spinal column immobilization is needed when the use of the short board would NOT be indicated?

1. After manual in-line immobilization and the application of a rigid cervical collar, the short spine board device is placed behind the patient. It should be positioned snugly beneath the patient's axillae to prevent it from moving up the torso.

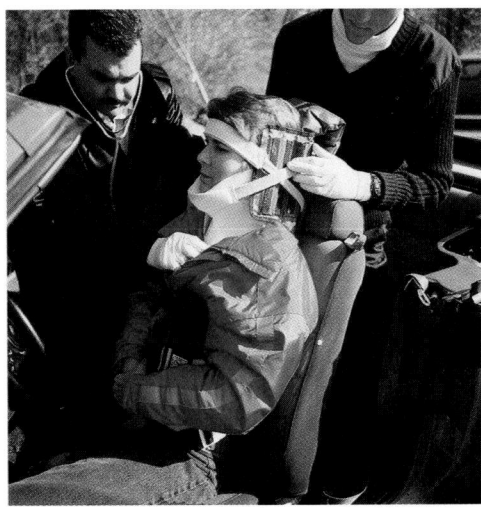

Fig. 23-13 KED application.

2. Immobilize the upper and middle torso by fastening the upper, middle, and lower chest straps. The upper strap can be relatively tight without impairing chest excursion. The middle and lower straps should be snug so that fingers cannot be slipped beneath the straps. Readjust as needed.

3. Position and fasten each groin strap separately, forming a loop. These straps prevent the KED from moving up and the lower end from moving laterally.

4. Pad as needed and secure the head to the short spine board.

5. Carefully move the patient as a unit to a long spine board by rotating the patient and KED onto the board. The legs are held proximal to the knees and are lifted during the transition.

NOTE

Short spine board application should be considered only if the patient's condition allows. If the patient is unstable because of life-threatening injury, the need for immediate resuscitation, or if the time required to apply the device would jeopardize the patient's life (e.g., a patient with a carotid pulse, but absent radial pulse), the patient's head and neck should be stabilized with manual, in-line support, and the patient should be moved as a unit to a long spine board.

---

6. Center the patient on the long spine board, release the leg straps, and slowly lower the patient's legs to an in-line position.

7. Secure the patient and KED to the long spine board, maintaining a neutral in-line position with the long axis of the body. Then slightly loosen the KED chest straps.

The steps required for rapid extrication may vary depending on the size and make of the vehicle and the patient's location inside the vehicle. A general description of the steps required for rapid extrication are listed below:

1. Rescuer 1 supports the patient's head and neck and uses manual in-line stabilization from behind the patient or from the patient's side (Fig. 23-14). This stabilization is maintained by rescuer 1 throughout the extrication procedure.

2. After a rapid initial assessment, a rigid cervical collar is applied, and a long spine board is positioned near the vehicle.

3. Rescuer 2 helps support the patient's midthorax as rescuer 3 frees the patient's lower extremities for extrication.

4. On rescuer 2's command, the patient is rotated so that his or her back faces the open doorway. The patient's feet are positioned on the passenger seat by rescuer 3. Each movement during the rotation of the patient should be coordinated, stopping so that the rescuers and the patient can be repositioned as needed to limit unwanted patient movement.

5. The long spine board should be inserted on the car seat at the patient's buttocks, and the patient should carefully be lowered onto the backboard.

6. The patient is centered on the long spine board and secured as described below.

Long spine board with supine patient. Like short spine boards, long spine boards are available in a variety of configurations. These include plastic and synthetic spine boards, metal alloy spine boards, vacuum mattress splints, and split litters (scoop stretchers) that must be used in conjunction with a long spine board. The following description of securing patients on a long spine board may be applied to any long spinal immobilization device.

Immobilizing the torso to a long spine board must always precede immobilization of the head to

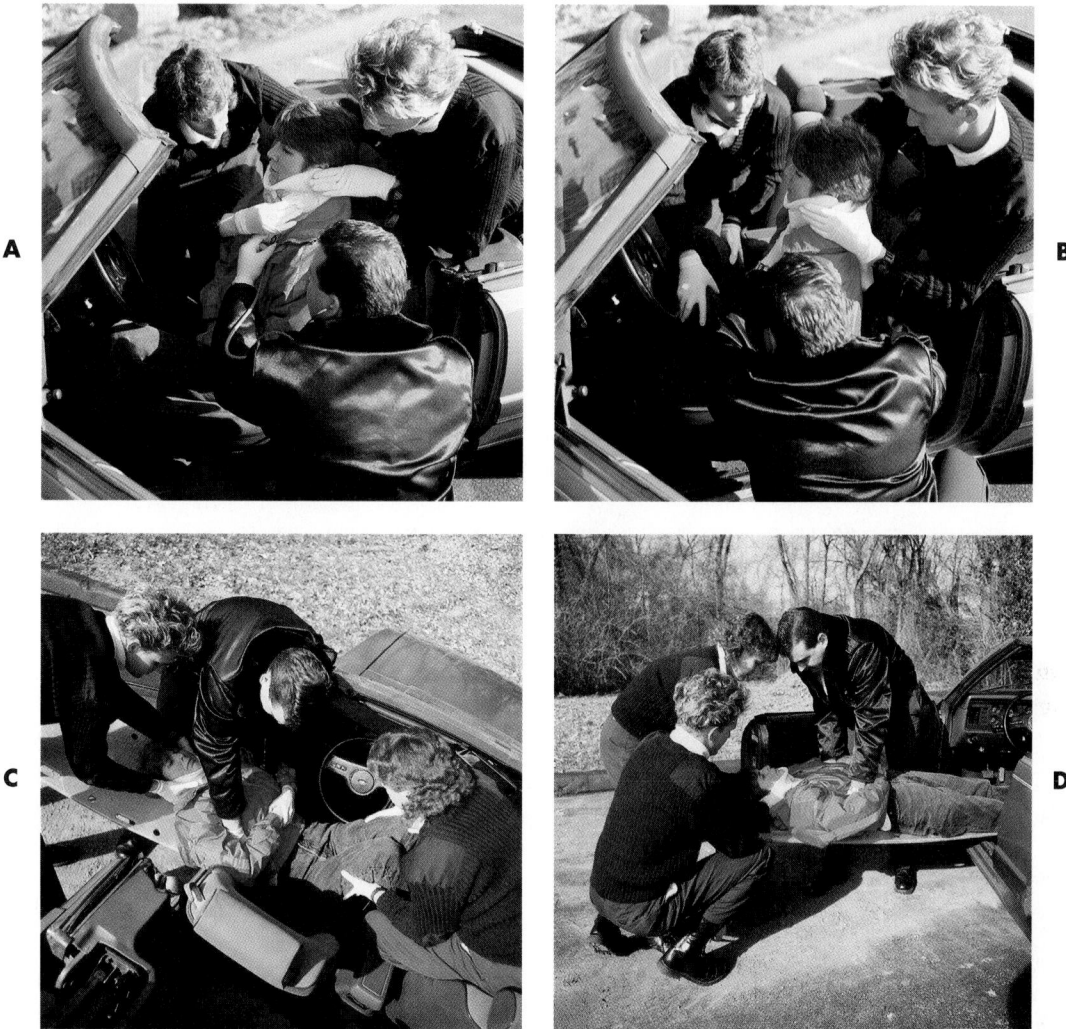

Fig. 23-14 A, Rescuer 1 supports the patient's head and neck and uses manual in-line stabilization throughout the procedure. **B,** After a rapid primary assessment, rescuer 2 helps support the patient's midthorax as rescuer 3 frees the patient's lower extremities for extrication. **C,** The patient is carefully lowered onto the long spine board. **D,** The patient is centered and secured on the long spine board.

prevent angulation of the cervical spine. The torso must not be allowed to move up, down, or to either side. Straps should be placed at the shoulders or chest to avoid compression and lateral movement of the thorax, around the midtorso, and across the iliac crest to prevent movement of the lower torso. Care should be taken not to tighten the straps to the point that chest excursion is inhibited.

After immobilization of the torso, the head and neck should be immobilized in a neutral, in-line position. When most adults are placed on a long or short spinal device, a significant space is produced

between the back of the head and the spine board. Therefore noncompressible padding (e.g., commercial padding, folded towels) should be added (body shims) before securing the head (Fig. 23-15, *A*). The amount of padding required for in-line immobilization varies by patient and must be evaluated on an individual basis. Too little padding may cause hyperextension of the head, and too much padding may cause flexion; both may increase spinal cord damage. Children have proportionally larger heads than adults and may require padding under the torso to allow the head to lie in a neutral position on

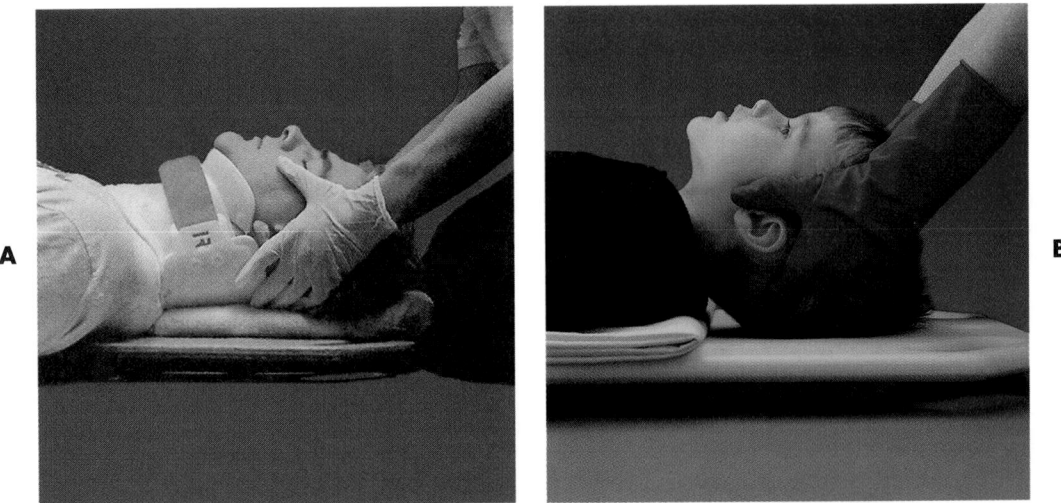

Fig. 23-15 Padding requirements for adult **(A)** and pediatric **(B)** patients.

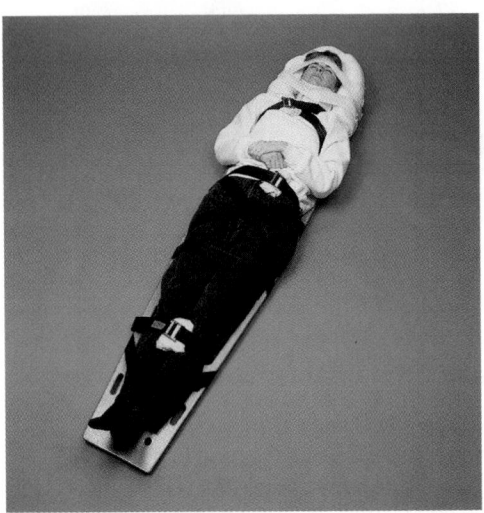

Fig. 23-16 Long spine board immobilization (supine patient).

the board (Fig. 23-15, *B*). The padding (if needed) should be firm and extend the full length and width of the torso from the buttocks to the top of the shoulders to prevent movement and misalignment of the spine.

The head is secured to the spinal device by placing commercial pads or rolled blankets on both sides of the head and securing them with the included straps, 2- to 3-inch tape strips, or a self-adhering firm wrap such as Colban, Medi-Rip, or Elastoplast. (Elastic or gauze bandages do not provide adequate fixation.) The upper forehead should be secured across the supraorbital ridge. The lower

portion of the head should be secured across the anterior portion of the rigid cervical collar. Chin straps, sandbags, and intravenous bags are considered less optimal in immobilizing the head to a spinal device.

The patient's legs should be secured to the long spine board, with two or more straps applied above and below the knees. Towels, blankets, or suitable padding may be placed on both sides of the patient's lower legs to minimize movement and help maintain the patient's central position on the spinal device (Fig. 23-16).

Before moving the patient, the patient's arms should be secured to the spinal device for safety. This is best accomplished by placing the patient's arms at his or her side (palms in) and securing them with a separate strap placed across the forearms and torso.

Long spine board with standing patient. Patients who are standing may also be secured to a long spine board using the following technique (Fig. 23-17):

1. Rescuer 1 applies manual, in-line immobilization from behind the patient and maintains this position throughout the procedure. A rigid cervical collar is applied.
2. Rescuer 2 slides the long spine board behind the patient from the side, and the patient's upper and lower torso are secured to the spine board.

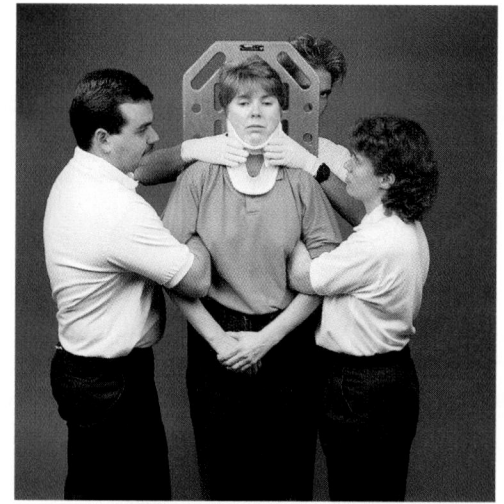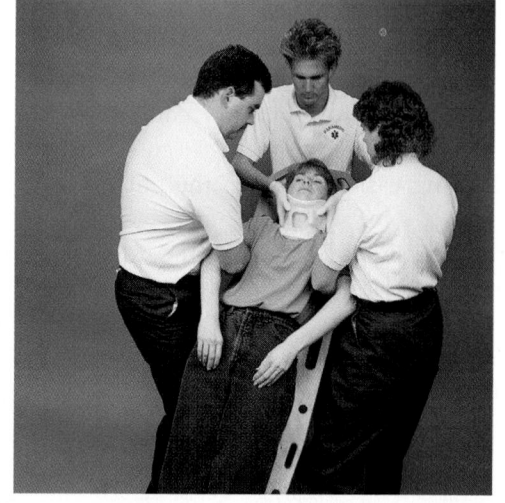

Fig. 23-17 A, While rescuer 1 maintains manual in-line stabilization, the patient is supported by rescuers 2 and 3. **B,** In one organized move, the patient is lowered to the ground on the long spine board for further immobilization.

3. Padding (if needed) is placed behind the patient's head, and the head is secured to the spine board.
4. After immobilization of the patient's torso, neck, and head, the patient is lowered halfway to the ground by rescuers 1 and 2. Rescuer 3 stabilizes the foot end of the spinal device. As the spine board is lowered about halfway, movement of the board stops to reposition hand-holds on the board.
5. The patient is lowered to the ground and secured to the board as described.

Fig. 23-18 Infant and pediatric immobilization board. (Courtesy Life Support Products Inc., Irvine, Calif.)

> **NOTE**
>
> If the patient becomes unstable during backboard procedures, manual in-line stabilization should be maintained, and the patient should be supported by rescuers 2 and 3 as he or she is lowered to the ground on the long spine board for further immobilization.

Immobilizing Pediatric Patients

As with adult patients, prehospital care of a pediatric patient with suspected spine trauma should be managed with manual in-line immobilization, a rigid cervical collar, and a long spinal immobilization device. A variety of pediatric immobilization devices are available from various equipment man-ufacturers (Fig. 23-18). If special pediatric immobilization devices are not available, children may be secured on an adult long spine board. (A great deal of padding, however, will be needed to fill voids and prevent movement.)

Helmet Issues

The purpose of helmets is to protect the head and brain, not the neck (which leaves the cervical spine vulnerable to injury). The various types of helmets include full-face or open-face designs (used in motorcycling, bicycling, roller blading, and other activities), and helmets designed for sports such as football and motor-cross. Factors that the paramedic should consider when determining the need to remove a helmet from an injured patient who requires airway management and spinal immobilization include:

- Athletic trainers may have special equipment (and training) to remove facepieces from sports helmets, allowing easier access to the patient's airway
- Sports garb (e.g., shoulder pads) could further compromise the cervical spine if only the helmet were removed
- The firm fit of a helmet may provide firm support for the patient's head

> **NOTE**
>
> Airway management and cervical spine immobilization must be done for all patients with a significant injury whether or not a helmet is present.

Helmet Removal

Removing a helmet from an injured patient in the prehospital setting (vs. in-hospital removal) is controversial and should be guided by medical direction. If the patient's airway cannot be adequately

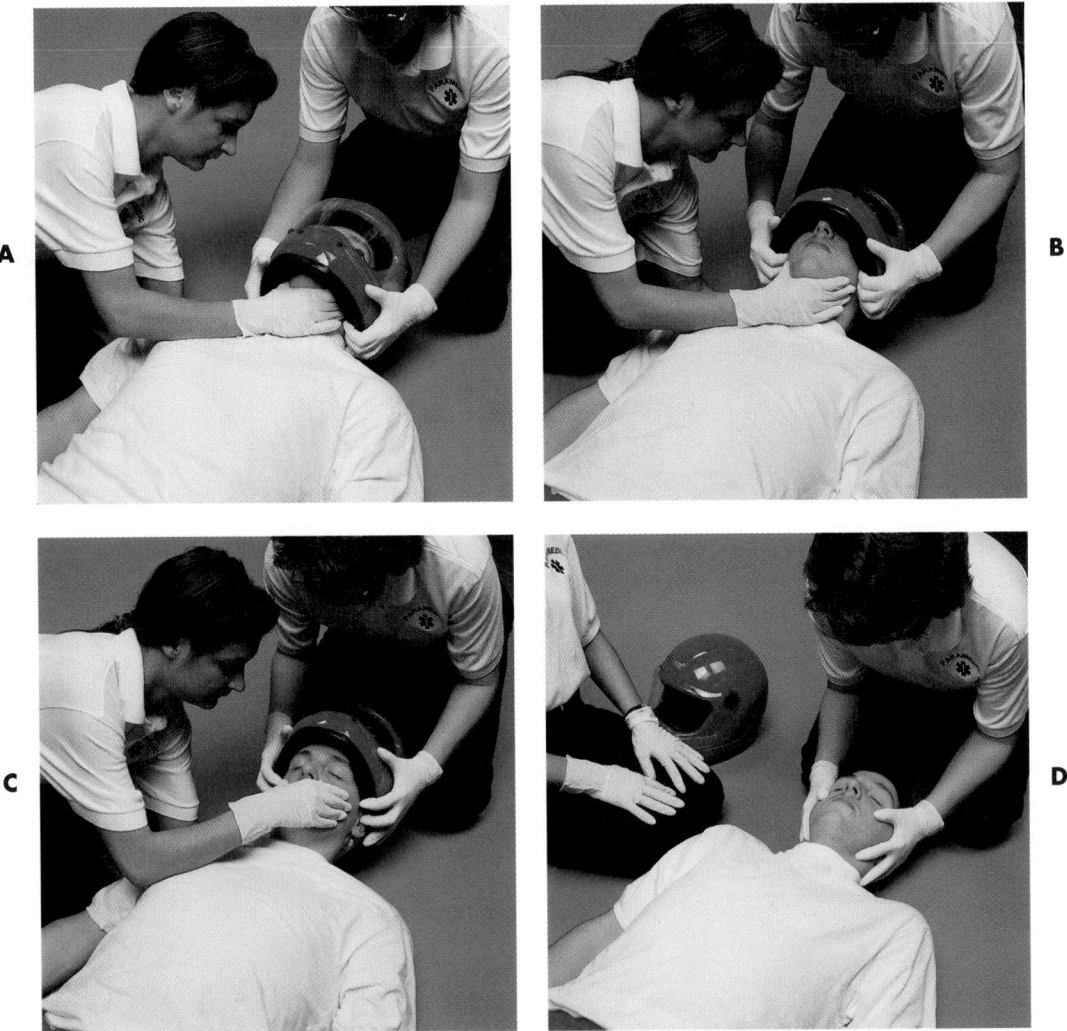

Fig. 23-19 A, Rescuer 1 immobilizes the helmet and head in an in-line position. Rescuer 2 grasps the patient's mandible by placing the thumb at the angle of the mandible on one side and two fingers at the angle on the other side. Rescuer 2's other hand is placed under the neck at the base of the skull, producing in-line immobilization of the patient's head. **B,** Rescuer 1 carefully spreads the sides of the helmet away from the patient's head and ears. **C,** The helmet is then rotated toward the rescuer to clear the nose and removed from the patient's head in a straight line. **D,** After the removal of the helmet, rescuer 1 applies in-line immobilization. A rigid cervical collar is applied.

accessed or secured, or if the helmet hinders emergency care procedures (e.g., spinal immobilization), the helmet should be removed in the field. The following steps in full-face helmet removal are recommended by the American College of Surgeons Committee on Trauma[4]:

1. Rescuer 1 immobilizes the helmet and head in an in-line position (Fig. 23-19). This is accomplished by the rescuer pressing his or her palms on each side of the helmet with the fingertips curled over its lower margin.
2. Rescuer 2 removes the face shield and chin strap, assessing the patient airway and ventilatory status.
3. Rescuer 2 grasps the patient's mandible by placing the thumb at the angle of the mandible on one side and two fingers at the angle on the other side. Rescuer 2's other hand is placed under the neck at the base of the skull, taking over in-line immobilization of the patient's head.
4. Rescuer 1 carefully spreads the sides of the helmet away from the patient's head and ears. The helmet is then rotated toward the rescuer to clear the patient's nose and removed from the patient's head in a straight line. Just before removing the helmet from under the patient's head, rescuer 1 assumes in-line immobilization by squeezing the sides of the helmet against the patient's head.

> **NOTE**
>
> The paramedic should consult with medical direction if the patient complains of increased pain during removal of the helmet or if the helmet is difficult to remove in the field.

5. Rescuer 2 repositions his or her hands to support the head and to prevent it from dropping as the helmet is completely removed. This is accomplished by the rescuer placing a hand further up on the occipital area of the head and by grasping the maxilla with the thumb and first fingers of the other hand on each side of the nose. After this position is secured, rescuer 2 takes over in-line immobilization.
6. Rescuer 1 rotates the helmet about 30 degrees, following the curvature of the patient's head. The helmet is completely removed by carefully pulling it in a straight line.

7. After removal of the helmet, rescuer 1 applies in-line immobilization, and a rigid cervical collar is applied.

> **NOTE**
>
> A key point to remember during helmet removal is that in-line immobilization must be maintained throughout the procedure. Therefore the rescuers should never remove their hands at the same time. In addition, the helmet must be rotated in one direction to clear the nose and in the opposite direction to clear the back of the patient's head.

Spinal Immobilization in Diving Accidents

Most diving accidents involve injury to the patient's head, neck, and spine. If the patient is still in the water when EMS arrives, the patient should be managed as follows:

1. Ensure scene and personal safety. Only rescuers trained in water rescue should enter the water (Fig. 23-20).
2. A supine patient should be floated to a shallow area without unnecessary movement of the spine.
3. A prone patient should be approached from the top of the head. One arm of the rescuer should be positioned under the patient so that the head, neck, and torso are supported. The rescuer's other arm should be placed across the patient's head and back, splinting the head and neck between the rescuer's arms. The patient should be carefully turned to a supine position, and airway and breathing should be quickly assessed by the paramedic. (Rescue breathing may be initiated in the water.)
4. A second rescuer slides a long spine board or other rigid device under the patient's body while the first rescuer continues to support the patient's head and neck without flexion or extension. A rigid cervical collar should be applied. Manual in-line immobilization must be maintained throughout the rescue.
5. The spinal immobilization device should be floated to the edge of the water and lifted out.
6. The patient should be completely immobilized on the long spine board as previously described.

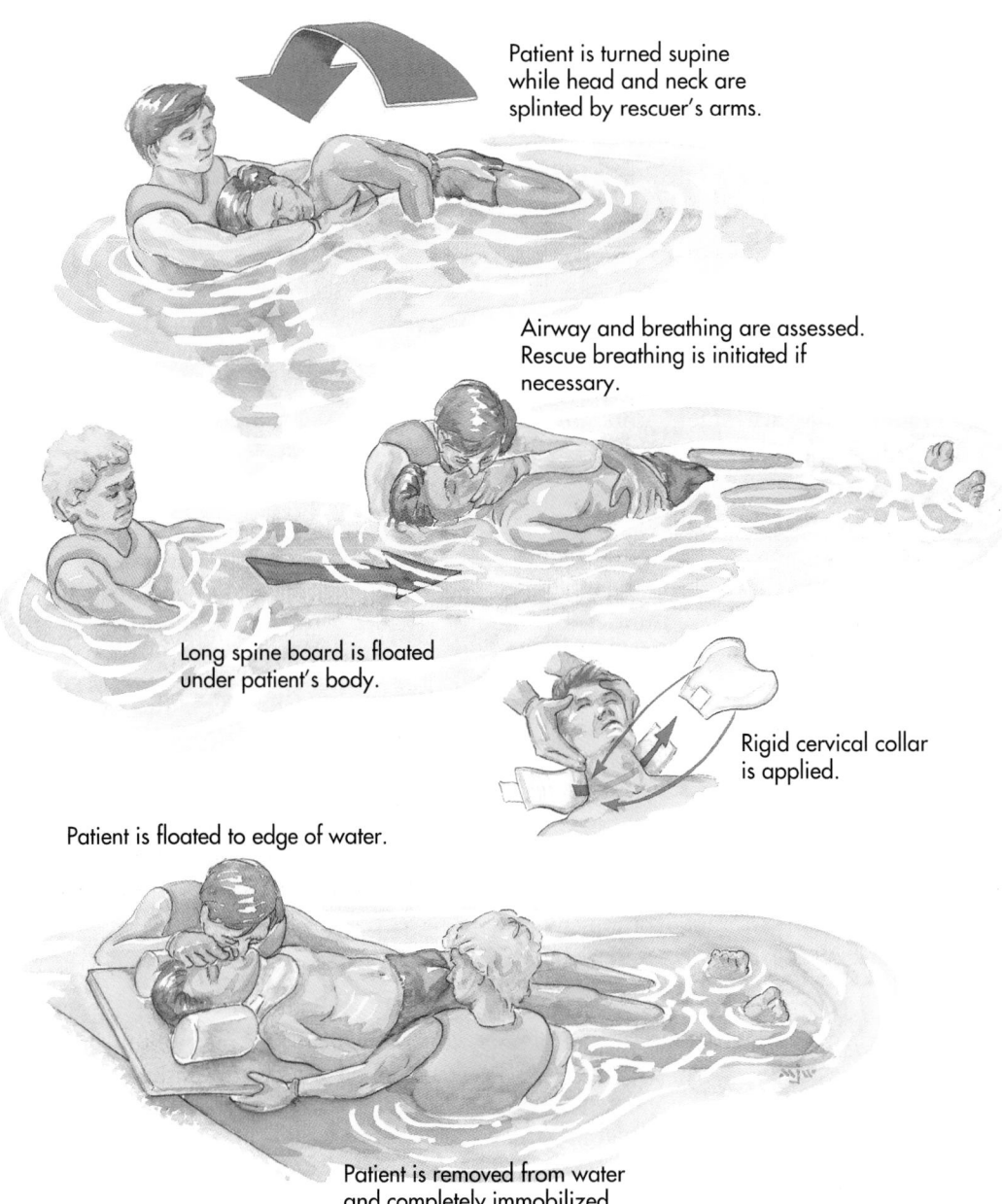

Patient is turned supine while head and neck are splinted by rescuer's arms.

Airway and breathing are assessed. Rescue breathing is initiated if necessary.

Long spine board is floated under patient's body.

Rigid cervical collar is applied.

Patient is floated to edge of water.

Patient is removed from water and completely immobilized.

Fig. 23-20 Extrication of a diving accident victim. Rescue breathing with barrier protection can begin in the water.

Cord Injury Presentations

Three cord injury presentations deserve special mention. These include spinal shock, neurogenic hypotension, and autonomic hyperreflexia syndrome.

Spinal Shock

Spinal shock refers to a temporary loss of all types of spinal cord function distal to the injury. Signs and symptoms of spinal shock include flaccid paralysis distal to the injury site and loss of autonomic function, which may be demonstrated by hypotension, vasodilation, loss of bowel and bladder control, priapism, and loss of thermoregulation. Spinal shock does not always involve permanent, primary injury. The autonomic dysfunction usually resolves within 24 hours, but rarely, may last a few days to a few weeks. Careful handling of these patients to avoid secondary injury is crucial. Initial management includes full spinal immobilization, high-concentration oxygen administration, positioning the secured patient in a Trendelenburg position (elevating the foot-end of the long spine board) providing it does not impair ventilation, and administering IV crystalloids (per protocol).

> **NOTE**
>
> Spinal shock refers to the appearance of complete spinal cord injury, for which vascular function is later regained. Neurogenic hypotension results from vasodilation that causes hypoperfusion.

Neurogenic Hypotension

Neurogenic hypotension (neurogenic shock) secondary to spinal shock results from the blockade of vasoregulatory fibers, motor fibers, and sensory fibers. This "block" produces a loss of sympathetic tone to the vessels or vasodilation. These patients often present with relative hypotension (a systolic blood pressure of 80 to 100 mm Hg); warm, dry, and pink skin (from cutaneous vasodilation); and relative bradycardia.

> **NOTE**
>
> Neurogenic hypotension should always be a "diagnosis of exclusion" in a trauma patient.

Neurogenic hypotension is rare and initially should not be considered as a cause of hypovolemia in the spine-injured patient. The paramedic should consider other causes of hypotension, including internal hemorrhage, cardiac tamponade, and tension pneumothorax. If hypotension is severe, shock management should be initiated (per protocol).

Autonomic Hyperreflexia Syndrome

Autonomic hyperreflexia syndrome may occur after resolution of spinal shock, and is associated with chronic SCI patients who have injuries at T6 or above.[3] (The syndrome often is precipitated by a distended bladder or rectum.) The effects of this syndrome result from a massive, uncompensated cardiovascular response that stimulates the sympathetic nervous system. The stimulation of sensory receptors below the level of cord injury causes the intact autonomic nervous system to respond with arteriolar spasm that increases blood pressure. The cerebral, carotid, and aortic baroreceptors sense the rise in blood pressure and respond by stimulating the parasympathetic nervous system to decrease heart rate and dilate the peripheral and visceral vessels. Because of the cord injury, however, vasodilation is not possible, and blood pressure skyrockets to dangerous and life-threatening levels. The characteristics of this syndrome include:

- Paroxysmal hypertension (up to 300 mm Hg)
- Pounding headache
- Blurred vision
- Sweating (above the level of injury) with flushing of the skin
- Increased nasal congestion
- Nausea
- Bradycardia (30 to 40 bpm)
- Distended bladder or rectum

Emptying of the bladder or bowel often relieves the syndrome. Blood pressure may need to be controlled with antihypertensive agents. These patients are best managed in the hospital setting under close physician supervision.

Nontraumatic Spinal Conditions

The nontraumatic spinal conditions to be discussed in this chapter include low back pain (LBP), degenerative disk disease, spondylosis, herniated intervertebral disk, and spinal cord tumors.

Low Back Pain

It is estimated that between 60% and 90% of the U.S. population experience some form of low back pain (LBP).[5] Low back pain usually affects the area between the lower rib cage and the gluteal muscles,

> **? CRITICAL THINKING**
>
> *What are some other medical conditions that may cause the patient to present with a chief complaint of low back pain?*

and often radiates into the thighs. About 1% of those with low back pain have sciatica (pain in the lumbar nerve root accompanied by neurosensory and motor deficits in the thigh and leg). Most LBP is idiopathic, making a precise diagnosis difficult. Causes of this condition include:

- Tension from tumors
- Disk prolapse
- Bursitis
- Synovitis
- Degenerative joint disease
- Abnormal bone pressure
- Inflammation caused by infection (e.g., osteomyelitis)
- Fractures
- Ligament strains

Risk factors associated with low back pain include occupations that require repetitive lifting, exposure to vibrations from vehicles or industrial machinery, and osteoporosis (elderly women report more symptoms than men).

Low back pain must come from innervated structures, but deep pain and the way it is referred to other parts of the body varies by individual. Although the disk has no specific innervation, irritation of surrounding membranes that have pain receptors often occurs (especially in the presence of disk prolapse). The source of most low back pain occurs at L3,4,5 and S1. Other areas of abundant pain receptors are found in anterior and posterior longitudinal ligaments which are vulnerable to strains and sprains.

Degenerative Disk Disease

Degenerative disk disease is a common finding in persons over 50 years of age. Causes of this condition include biochemical and biomechanical alterations in the tissue of the intervertebral disk that occur with aging. The associated narrowing of the disk results in variable segmental instability and occasional low back pain.

Spondylosis

Spondylosis is a structural defect of the spine that involves the lamina or vertebral arch. It usually occurs in the lumbar spine between superior and inferior articulating facets. (Rotational "stress" fractures

are common at the affected site.) Heredity appears to be a significant factor for this condition.

Herniated Intervertebral Disk

Herniated intervertebral disk (herniated nucleus pulposus) refers to a tear in the posterior rim of the capsule that encloses the gelatinous center of the disk. Rupture of the disk usually is caused by trauma, degenerative disk disease, and improper lifting (most common). Men between the ages of 30 and 50 are more prone to develop this condition. Disks that most commonly are affected are L5-S1, and L4-L5. (It also will occasionally be seen in the cervical area at C5-C6 and C6-C7.) These injuries may have an immediate onset, or may develop over months to years.

Spinal Cord Tumors

Tumors in the spinal cord may develop from cord compression, degenerative changes in bones and joints, or from an interruption in the cord's blood supply. These tumors are classified by cell type, growth rate, and structure of origin. Clinical manifestations are dependent on tumor type and location and may include bilateral or asymmetric motor dysfunction, paresis, spasticity, pain, temperature dysfunction, sensory changes, and other abnormalities.

Assessment and Management of Nontraumatic Spinal Conditions

As previously stated, nontraumatic spinal conditions such as low back pain are difficult to diagnose. Assessment and management are based on the patient's chief complaint, the physical examination, and through the evaluation of associated risk factors. Signs and symptoms that commonly are seen with nontraumatic spinal conditions include:

- Discomfort
- Difficulty in standing erect
- Pain with straining (e.g., coughing, sneezing)
- Limited range of motion
- Alterations in sensation, pain, and temperature
- Upper extremity pain or paresthesia that increases with motion
- Motor weakness

Management

Management of patients with back pain in the pre-hospital setting primarily is supportive to decrease pain and discomfort. Some patients are best managed with immobilization on a full spine board or vacuum-type stretcher to prevent movement. Full spinal immobilization is not required unless the condition is a result of trauma. In-hospital evaluation may include various testing such as computerized tomography (CT scan), electromyelography, and magnetic resonance imaging (MRI).

S U M M A R Y

- Most spinal cord injuries result from motor vehicle crashes, followed by falls, penetrating injuries from acts of human violence, and sport injuries.

- The paramedic can classify the mechanism of injury (MOI) as positive, negative, or uncertain. This, combined with the clinical guidelines for evaluating spinal cord injury, includes the following signs and symptoms: pain; tenderness; painful movement; deformity; cuts/bruises over spinal area; paralysis; paresthesias; and weakness. This classification system can help identify situations in which spinal immobilization is appropriate.

- The spinal column is composed of 33 vertebrae divided into five sections: 7 cervical, 12 thoracic, 5 lumbar, 5 sacrum (fused), and 4 coccyx (fused).

- The specific mechanisms of injury that frequently cause spinal trauma are axial loading; extremes of flexion, hyperextension, or hyperrotation; excessive lateral bending; and distraction.

- Spinal injuries may be classified as sprains and strains, fractures and dislocations, sacral and coccygeal fractures, and cord injuries. The spinal cord may sustain primary or secondary injury. Lesions (transections) of the spinal cord are classified as complete or incomplete.

- After evaluation and management of the life threats, the second priority is to preserve spinal cord function and avoid secondary injury to the spinal cord. These goals are best met by maintaining a high degree of suspicion for the presence of spinal trauma, by providing early spinal immobilization, rapidly correcting any volume deficit, and oxygen administration.

- General principles of spinal immobilization include: prevention of further injury; treating the spine as a long bone with a joint at either end (the head and pelvis); always using "complete" spine immobilization; beginning spinal immobilization in the initial assessment and maintaining it until the spine is completely immobilized on the long spine board; and, placing the patient's head in a neutral, in-line position, unless contraindicated.

- Spinal shock refers to a temporary loss of all types of spinal cord function distal to the injury.

- Neurogenic hypotension secondary to spinal shock produces a loss of sympathetic tone to the vessels causing relative hypotension; warm, dry, and pink skin; and relative bradycardia.

- Autonomic hyperreflexia syndrome results from a massive, uncompensated cardiovascular response that stimulates the sympathetic nervous system causing an increase in blood pressure and other symptoms.

- Some nontraumatic spinal conditions include low back pain, degenerative disk disease, spondylolysis, herniated intervertebral disk, and spinal cord tumors. Management of patients with non-traumatic back pain in the prehospital setting is primarily supportive to decrease pain and discomfort.

REFERENCES

1. Rosen P, Barkin R: *Emergency medicine: concepts and clinical practice,* ed 4, St Louis, 1998, Mosby.
2. Foundation for Spinal Cord Injury Prevention: *Spinal cord injury facts,* National Spinal Cord Injury Statistical Center, Detroit, 1999, www.fscip.org/facts.
3. U.S. Department of Transportation National Highway Traffic Safety Administration: *EMT-Paramedic national standard curriculum,* Washington, DC, 1998, The Department.
4. National Association of Emergency Medical Technicians: *PHTLS: basic and advanced prehospital life support,* ed 4, St Louis, 1999, Mosby.
5. McCance K, Huether S: *Pathophysiology: the biological basis for disease in adults and children,* ed 2, St Louis, 1994, Mosby.

24 Thoracic Trauma

OBJECTIVES

Upon completion of this chapter, the paramedic student will be able to:

1. Discuss the epidemiology and mechanism of injury associated with thoracic trauma.
2. Describe the mechanism of injury, signs and symptoms, and management of skeletal injuries to the chest.
3. Describe the mechanism of injury, signs and symptoms, and prehospital management of pulmonary trauma.
4. Describe the mechanism of injury, signs and symptoms, and prehospital management of injuries to the heart and great vessels.
5. Outline the mechanism of injury, signs and symptoms, and prehospital care of the patient with esophageal and tracheobronchial injury and diaphragmatic rupture.

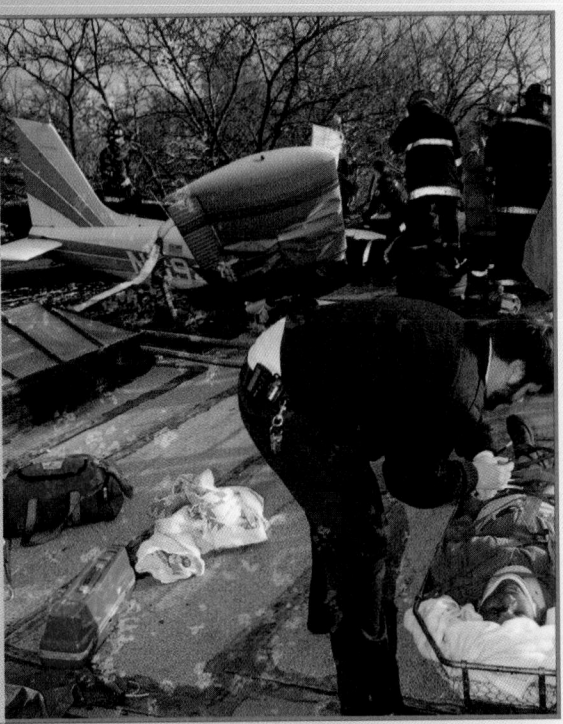

Chest injuries are directly responsible for more than 20% of all traumatic deaths (regardless of mechanism) and account for about 16,000 deaths per year in the United States.[1] Chest injuries are caused by blunt trauma, penetrating trauma, or both, and frequently result from motor vehicle crashes, falls from heights, blast injuries, blows to the chest, chest compression, gunshot wounds, and stab wounds. Thoracic trauma may be classified as skeletal injury, pulmonary injury, heart and great vessel injury, and diaphragmatic injury. (Anterior neck trauma is discussed in Chapter 22.)

> **NOTE**
>
> Education is the best strategy to prevent chest injuries. Examples include community educational programs in gun safety, sports training, and use of personal restraint systems. (See Appendix C.)

Skeletal Injury

Skeletal injuries may be caused by blunt or penetrating trauma. Specific injuries discussed in this chapter are clavicular fractures, rib fractures, flail chest, and sternal fractures.

> **NOTE**
>
> The reader should refer to Chapter 6 for a review of the structures that make up the thoracic cavity.

Clavicular Fractures

The clavicle is the most commonly fractured bone, and an isolated clavicular fracture is seldom a significant injury (Fig. 24-1). It is common in children who fall on their shoulders or outstretched arms and in athletes involved in contact sports. Management usually is accomplished with a sling and swathe that immobilizes the affected shoulder and arm or a clavicle strap (described in Chapter 26). These injuries usually heal well within 4 to 6 weeks.

Signs and symptoms of clavicular fractures include pain, point tenderness, and evident deformity. A rare complication that may be associated with clavicular fracture is injury to the subclavian vein or artery from bony fragment penetration, producing a hematoma or venous thrombosis.

Rib Fractures

Rib fractures most commonly occur on the lateral aspect of ribs 3 through 8, where they are least protected by musculature (Fig. 24-2). Fractures are more likely in adults than in children because younger patients have more resilient cartilage. Morbidity or mortality from rib fractures is dependent on the patient's age and the number and location of the fractures.

> **? CRITICAL THINKING**
>
> *Why would you expect greater underlying pulmonary injury in a child versus an adult with rib fractures?*

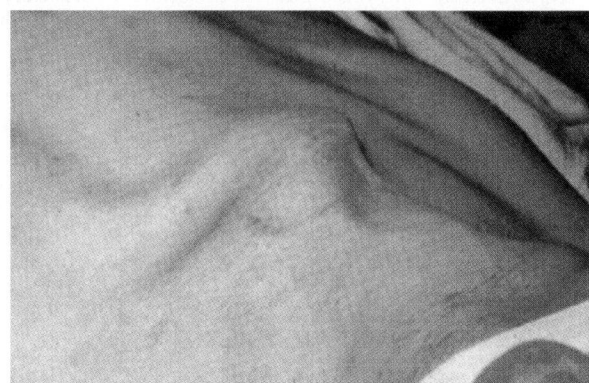

Fig. 24-1 Fracture of the left clavicle seen from above the left shoulder. (From London PS: *A colour atlas of diagnosis after recent injury,* Ipswich, England, 1990, Wolfe Medical Publications, Ltd.)

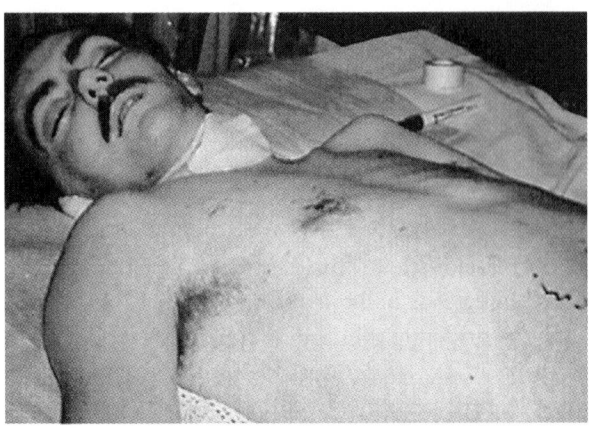

Fig. 24-2 Chest wall asymmetry caused by rib fractures. (From London PS: *A colour atlas of diagnosis after recent injury,* Ipswich, England, 1990, Wolfe Medical Publications.)

Simple rib fractures usually are very painful but rarely life threatening. Most patients can localize the fracture by pointing to the area (confirmed by palpation). Occasionally movement or crepitance can be felt. Complications of rib fracture include splinting, which leads to atelectasis, and ventilation-perfusion mismatch (ventilated alveoli that are not perfused or perfused alveoli that are not ventilated). Management is aimed at relieving pain. The paramedic should encourage the patient to cough and to breathe deeply. Pain may be relieved by splinting the patient's arm against the chest wall with a sling and swathe (avoiding circumferential splinting) and by administering analgesics per protocol. Based on the mechanism of injury, the paramedic should consider the possibility of more serious trauma such as closed pneumothorax and internal bleeding. Fractures to the lower ribs, 8 through 12, may be associated with spleen, kidney, or liver injuries.

Great force is required to fracture the first and second ribs because of their shape and the protected location provided by the scapulae, clavicles, and upper chest musculature. Fractures to these ribs may be associated with myocardial contusion, bronchial tears, and vascular injury.

Flail Chest

A flail chest may occur when two or more adjacent ribs are fractured in two or more places (Fig. 24-3).

This injury usually is not detected in the prehospital setting because of the muscle spasm that accompanies the injury. Within 2 hours after the injury, however, the muscle spasm subsides and the injured segment of the chest wall may begin to move in a paradoxical (contrary) fashion with inspiration and expiration.

NOTE

Paradoxical breathing describes a condition in which part of the lung deflates during inspiration and inflates during expiration. It commonly is associated with chest trauma such as an open chest wound or rib cage injury.

NOTE

Causes of flail chest include vehicle crashes, falls, industrial accidents, assault, and birth trauma. Mortality rates are 20% to 40% because of associated injuries.[2] Mortality rates increase with advanced age, seven or more rib fractures, three or more associated injuries, shock, and head injury.

During inspiration the diaphragm descends, lowering the intrapleural pressure. The unstable chest wall is pushed ("sucked") inward by the negative intrathoracic pressure as the rest of the chest wall expands. During expiration, the diaphragm rises and the intrapleural pressure exceeds atmospheric pressure, causing the unstable chest wall to move outward. Patients with flail chest often develop hypoxia because of the underlying pulmonary contusion usually associated with this injury. The contusion, which results from interstitial and alveolar hemorrhage, is associated with decreased vital capacity and vascular shunting of deoxygenated blood. Signs and symptoms of flail chest include tenderness and bony crepitus on palpation and paradoxical motion (a late sign).

Prehospital management of patients with flail chest includes assisting ventilation with positive pressure via a bag-valve-mask, use of high-concentration supplemental oxygen, and fluid replacement as needed. Field stabilization of the flail segment is controversial. In one method, the paramedic attempts to splint the flail segment in the in-

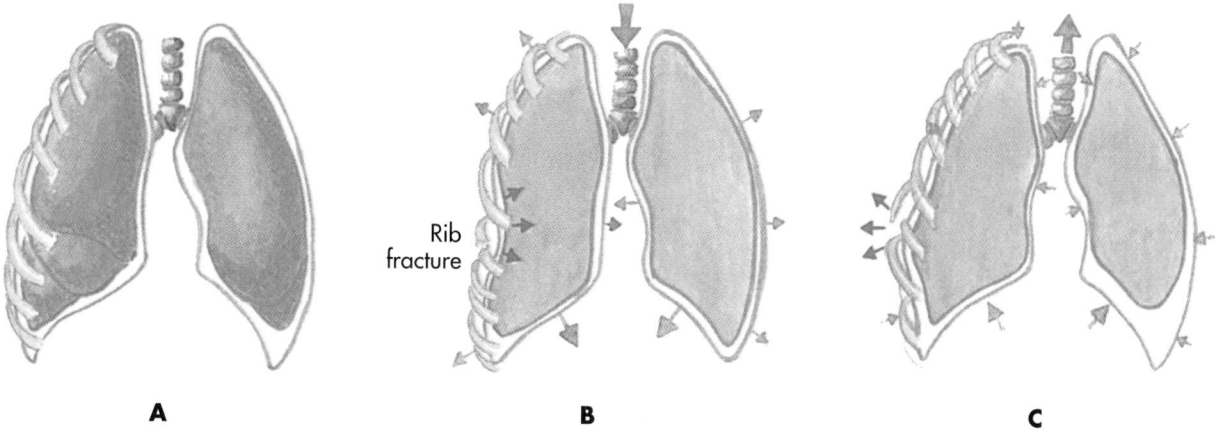

Fig. 24-3 Flail chest. **A,** Normal lungs. **B,** Flail chest during inspiration. **C,** Flail chest during expiration.

ward position with simple hand pressure or bulky dressings or towels taped to the chest wall. Although this splinting can reduce vital capacity, it may increase the efficiency of ventilation. Many authorities recommend intubation and positive-pressure ventilation (internal splinting) in patients with respiratory distress and a flail chest. Intubation also may be indicated if the chest injury is associated with shock, other severe injuries, head injury, or pulmonary disease, or if it occurs in patients over age 65. A large percentage of patients with significant chest injury progress to respiratory failure, requiring long-term ventilatory support and hospitalization.

? CRITICAL THINKING

Why is positive-pressure ventilation the management of choice for this injury?

NOTE

Prehospital use of positive end-expiratory pressure (PEEP) to keep alveoli open at the end of exhalation may be recommended by some medical direction agencies. This procedure requires special equipment and training (see Chapter 27).

Sternal Fractures

Sternal fractures are uncommon, but serious. They usually result from a direct blow to the chest, as when it strikes a steering column or dashboard, or from a massive crush injury (Fig. 24-4). Sternal fractures usually are very painful and may be associated with an unstable chest wall, myocardial injury, or cardiac tamponade. Signs and symptoms include a history of significant anterior chest trauma, tenderness, and abnormal motion or crepitation over the sternum. Prehospital management includes maintaining a high degree of suspicion for associated injuries, airway maintenance, ventilatory support, ECG monitoring, and rapid transport to an appropriate medical facility. Associated injuries that often contribute to morbidity and mortality include:

- Pulmonary and myocardial contusion
- Flail chest
- Vascular disruption of thoracic vessels (rare)
- Intraabdominal injuries
- Head injury

NOTE

Sternal fractures occur in only 5% to 8% of patients with blunt chest trauma but carry a 25% to 45% mortality rate.[2]

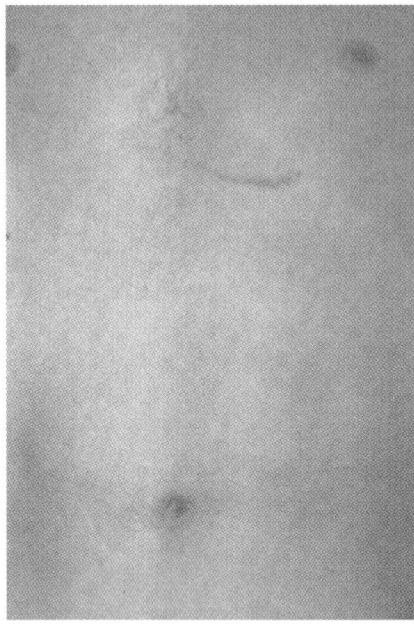

Fig. 24-4 Well-marked band of spotty bruising caused by a steering wheel impact. (From London PS: *A colour atlas of diagnosis after recent injury,* Ipswich, England, 1990, Wolfe Medical Publications.)

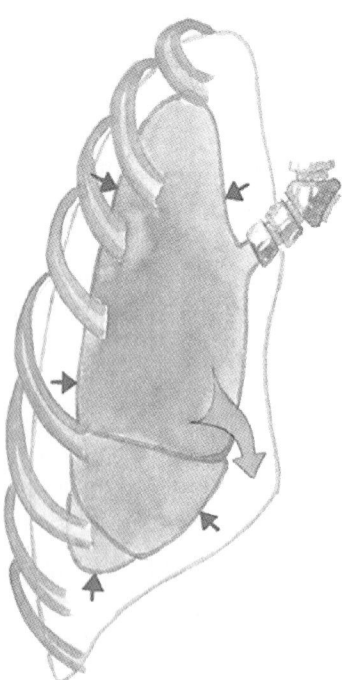

Fig. 24-5 Simple pneumothorax.

Pulmonary Injury

Pulmonary injuries may be classified as closed pneumothorax, tension pneumothorax, open pneumothorax, hemothorax, pulmonary contusion, and **traumatic asphyxia.** Any of these injuries can result in respiratory insufficiency. Prehospital management must be directed at ensuring an open airway, providing ventilatory support, correcting immediately life-threatening ventilatory problems (e.g., tension pneumothorax), and rapid transport for definitive care.

Closed Pneumothorax

A closed pneumothorax (simple pneumothorax) is caused by the presence of air in the pleural space and a partially or totally collapsed lung (Fig. 24-5). A common cause of pneumothorax is a fractured rib that penetrates the underlying lung. Pneumothoraces also may occur in the absence of rib fractures from excessive pressure on the chest wall against a closed glottis (paper-bag effect described in Chapter 18), and from a rupture or tear of the lung parenchyma and visceral pleura with no demonstrable cause (spontaneous pneumothorax).

> **NOTE**
>
> Closed pneumothorax occurs in 10% to 30% of patients with blunt chest trauma and in almost 100% of patients with penetrating chest trauma.[2]

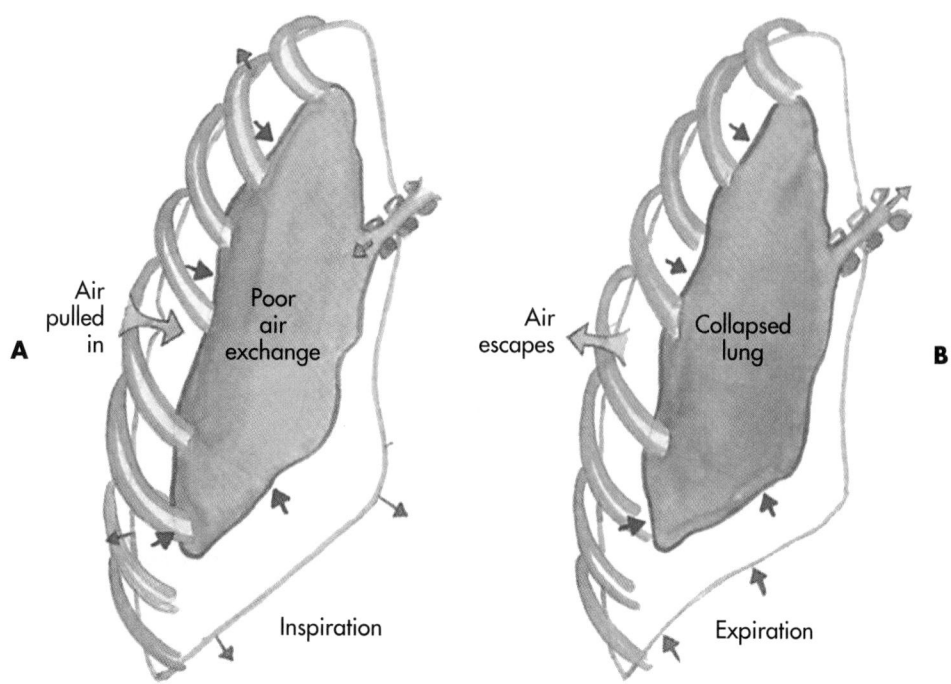

Fig. 24-6 Open pneumothorax. **A,** Air enters the pleural cavity during inspiration. **B,** Air exits the pleural cavity during expiration.

Signs and symptoms of a closed pneumothorax include chest pain, dyspnea, and tachypnea. Auscultation may disclose decreased or absent breath sounds on the affected side. Prehospital management is directed at ventilatory support with high-concentration oxygen and careful monitoring for signs of a tension pneumothorax. The patient should be transported in a semisitting position of comfort unless contraindicated by the mechanism of injury. If the patient's respirations are fewer than 12 or more than 28 breaths per minute, ventilatory assistance with a bag-valve-mask may be indicated.

NOTE

If the patient is standing, air will accumulate in the apices. If the patient is supine, air will accumulate in the anterior chest.

Most healthy patients have large circulatory and ventilatory reserve capacities. Therefore closed pneumothoraces usually are not life threatening. Life-threatening consequences may develop, however, if the pneumothorax is a tension pneumothorax, if it occupies more than 40% of the hemithorax, or if it occurs in a patient with shock or preexisting pulmonary or cardiovascular diseases.

✓ TRICKS OF THE TRADE

If your patient suffers an open pneumothorax, consider intubation before decompression. If the patient is intubated, an occlusive dressing will probably not be necessary as long as the wound is no larger than four-fifths the size of the trachea.

Open Pneumothorax

An open pneumothorax develops when the injury to the chest allows the pleural space to be exposed to atmospheric pressure (Fig. 24-6). The severity of the injury is directly proportional to the size of the wound. When a chest wound is larger than the normal pathway for air through the nose and mouth, atmospheric pressure forces the air through the open wound and into the thoracic cavity during inspiration. As the air accumulates in the pleural space, the lung on the injured side collapses and begins to shift toward the uninjured side. Very little air enters the tracheobronchial tree to be exchanged with intrapulmonary air on the affected side, which results in decreased alveolar ventilation and decreased perfusion. The normal side also is adversely affected because expired air may enter the lung on the collapsed side, only to be rebreathed into the functioning lung with the next ventilation. This may result in severe ventilatory dysfunction, hypoxemia, and death unless the situation is rapidly recognized and corrected.

> **NOTE**
>
> Small open chest wounds may act like a ball-valve—allowing air in, but not out. The accumulation of air may result in a shift in the patient's mediastinum, decreasing the patient's preload.

Signs and symptoms of open pneumothorax include shortness of breath, pain, and a sucking or gurgling sound as air moves in and out of the pleural space through the open chest wound (giving rise to the term *sucking chest wound*). Prehospital management of an open pneumothorax entails (Fig. 24-7):

1. Closing the chest wound. This can be accomplished through applying an occlusive petrolatum gauze dressing (covered with sterile dressings) and securing it with tape. Medical direction may recommend that only three sides of the dressing be taped to provide for a "venting" mechanism (or one-way valve) that allows spontaneous decompression of a developing tension pneumothorax.

> **NOTE**
>
> The paramedic should be particularly alert for the development of a tension pneumothorax in patients who have a dressing that does not provide a venting mechanism.

2. Providing ventilatory support with high-concentration oxygen. Airway management includes assisting ventilations with a bag-valve-device and intubation.
3. Managing for shock through the administration of crystalloid (per protocol).
4. Rapidly transporting the patient to an appropriate medical facility.

Tension Pneumothorax

When air within the thoracic cavity cannot exit the pleural space, a tension pneumothorax may develop (Fig. 24-8). This is a true emergency that results in profound hypoventilation and death if it is not immediately recognized and managed.

When air is allowed to leak into the pleural space during inspiration and becomes trapped during expiration, an increase in pleural pressure results. The increase in pressure produces a shift in the mediastinum and further compresses the lung on the uninjured side. In addition, venous return to the heart is decreased by compression of the vena cava, resulting in decreased cardiac output. Signs and symptoms of a tension pneumothorax include:

- Anxiety
- Cyanosis

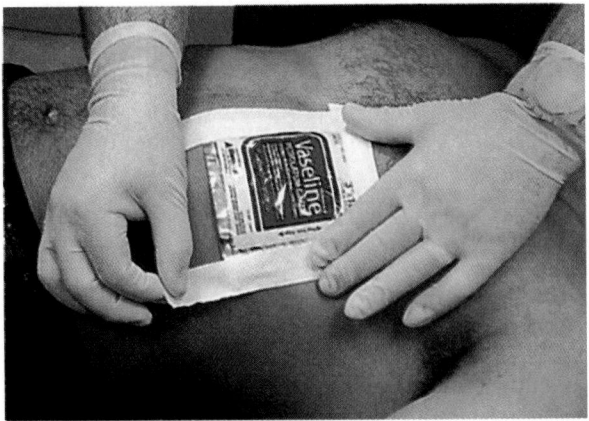

Fig. 24-7 Sealing a chest wound.

- Increasing dyspnea
- Tracheal deviation (a late sign)
- Tachycardia
- Hypotension
- Diminished or absent breath sounds on the injured side
- Distended neck veins (unless the patient is hypovolemic)
- Unequal expansion of the chest (tension does not fall with respiration)
- Subcutaneous emphysema

? CRITICAL THINKING

Why may the neck veins be distended in a patient with a tension pneumothorax?

Tension pneumothorax may be confirmed by radiography in the hospital setting, although waiting for x-ray confirmation is considered less-than-optimal management. In the prehospital setting, a suspected tension pneumothorax, evidenced by increasing dyspnea, compromised ventilation, tachycardia, tachypnea, and unilateral decreased or absent breath sounds, should be managed aggressively. Emergency care is directed at reducing the pressure in the pleural space (returning the intrapleural pressure to atmospheric or subatmospheric levels).

Tension Pneumothorax Associated with Penetrating Trauma

An open pneumothorax that has been sealed with an occlusive dressing may result in a tension pneumothorax. In such cases, increased pleural pressure can be relieved by momentarily removing the dressing. When the dressing has been lifted from the wound, there should be an audible release of air from the thoracic cavity. If this does not occur and the patient's condition remains unchanged, the paramedic should gently spread the chest wound

NOTE

The maneuver of removing the dressing to relieve pleural pressure may need to be done periodically during transport. If the tension is not relieved with this procedure, thoracic decompression (needle thoracentesis) should be performed.

open to allow the trapped air to escape. After the pressure has been released, the wound should again be sealed.

Tension Pneumothorax Associated with Closed Trauma

A tension pneumothorax that develops in a patient with closed chest trauma must be relieved through thoracic decompression with either a large-bore needle or a commercially available thoracic decompression kit. The paramedic should consult with medical direction before initiating this procedure.

Needle decompression is accomplished by inserting a 2-inch, 12- or 14-gauge hollow needle or catheter into the affected pleural space, usually in

NOTE

If the tension is not relieved with initial decompression, insertion of a second or third needle may be indicated.[2]

? CRITICAL THINKING

Put your finger on the correct location on your chest to place a needle for decompression of a tension pneumothorax.

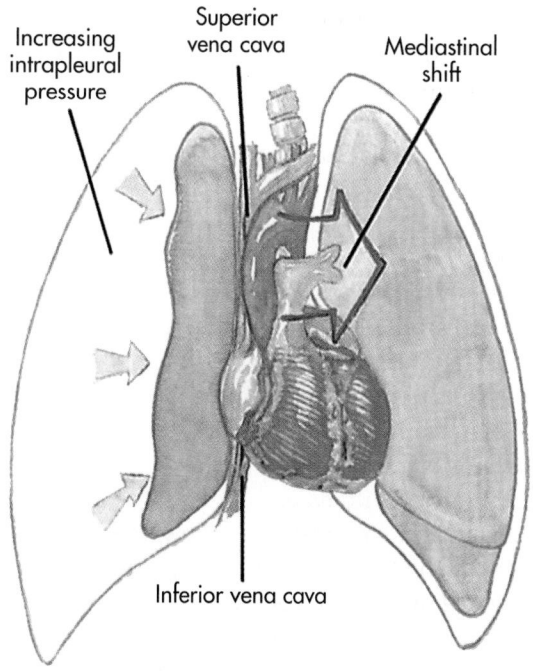

Fig. 24-8 Tension pneumothorax.

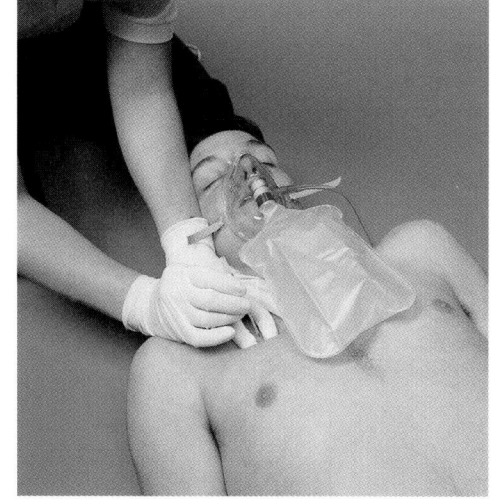

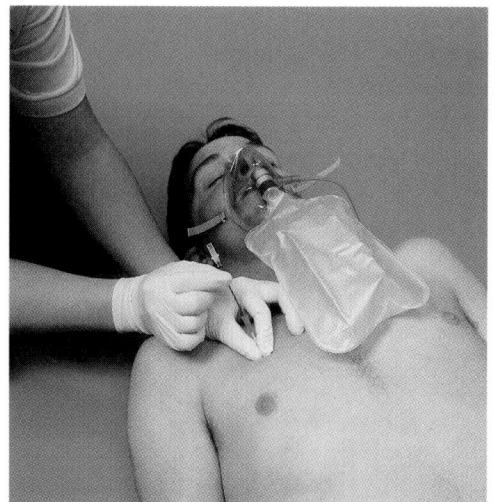

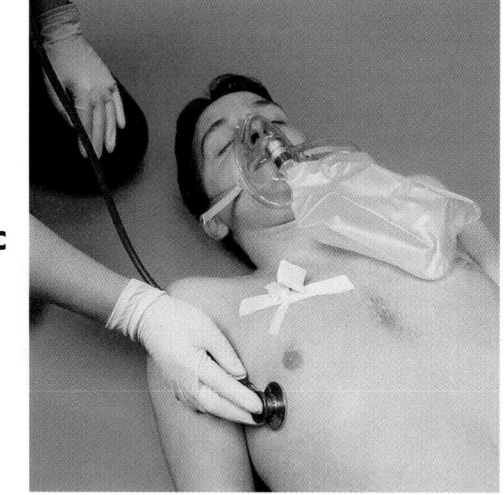

Fig. 24-9 A, Insert a 2-inch, 14- or 16-gauge hollow needle or catheter into the affected pleural space, usually in the second intercostal space in the midclavicular line. **B,** After needle insertion, there should be an audible rush of air as pressure escapes from the pleural space. **C,** Secure the catheter in place with tape, and prevent the reentry of air into the pleural space. Carefully monitor the patient's respiratory status.

the second intercostal space in the midclavicular line (Fig. 24-9). The needle should be inserted just above the third rib to avoid the nerve, artery, and vein that lie just beneath each rib. After insertion of the needle, there should be an audible rush of air as pressure escapes from the pleural space (confirming the tension pneumothorax), and the patient should show signs of improvement (i.e., the patient will be easier to ventilate or will demonstrate less labored breathing). The needle or catheter should be secured in place with tape.

If time and circumstances allow, the hub of the needle can be occluded during inspiration by a one-way valve to prevent reentry of air into the pleural space. This can be accomplished by cutting a finger from a sterile glove (rinsed with sterile water) and creating a small hole at the fingertip. The finger is slipped over the hub of the needle and secured with a rubber band. An alternative method is to attach special tubing and a flutter valve (per protocol) to the hub of the needle instead of a finger from a sterile glove. Both methods permit air to escape from but not enter the pleural space.

Hemothorax

A hemothorax is the accumulation of blood in the pleural space caused by bleeding from the lung parenchyma or damaged vessels (Fig. 24-10). If this condition is associated with a pneumothorax, it is called a *hemopneumothorax*. Blood loss may be massive in these patients; each side of the thorax can hold 30% to 40% (2000 to 3000 mL) of the patient's blood volume.[2] (A severed intercostal artery can easily bleed 50 mL per minute.) Therefore patients with a hemothorax frequently have hypovolemia and hypoxemia.

As blood continues to fill the pleural space, the lung on the affected side may collapse, and rarely, the mediastinum may even shift away from the hemothorax, compressing the unaffected lung. The resultant respiratory and circulatory compromise are responsible for the following signs and symptoms:

- Tachypnea
- Dyspnea
- Cyanosis (often not evident in hemorrhagic shock)
- Diminished or decreased breath sounds (dullness on percussion)
- Hypovolemic shock
- Narrowed pulse pressure
- Tracheal deviation to the unaffected side (rare)

Prehospital care for patients with a hemothorax is directed at correcting ventilatory and circulatory compromise. This entails administering high-concentration oxygen; ventilatory support with bag-valve-mask, intubation, or both; administration of volume-expanding fluids to correct the hypovolemia; and rapid transport to an appropriate medical facility.

? CRITICAL THINKING

> *Why is hemothorax associated with a higher mortality rate than simple, closed pneumothorax?*

NOTE

A hemothorax that is associated with great vessel or cardiac injury carries a high mortality rate: 50% of these patients will die immediately; 25% will live for 5 to 10 minutes; 25% may live longer than 30 minutes.[2]

Pulmonary Contusion

Pulmonary contusion most commonly is caused by rapid deceleration forces that cause the lung to contact the chest wall (e.g., motor vehicle crashes, injuries producing a flail chest). These forces result in rupture of the alveoli with hemorrhage and interstitial edema. (Pulmonary contusion less frequently results from penetrating trauma and high-energy shock waves from an explosion in air or water.) Over 50% of patients with blunt chest trauma have pulmonary contusion.[2]

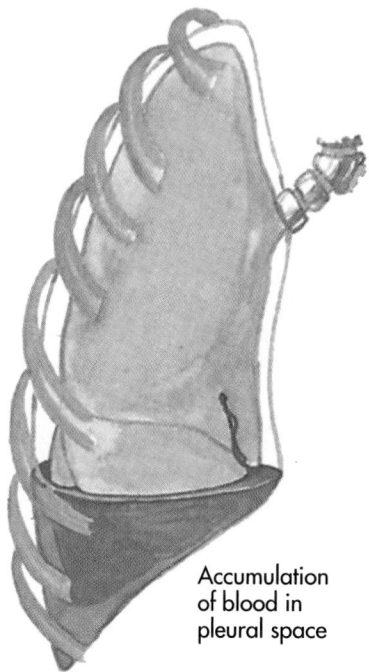

Accumulation of blood in pleural space

Fig. 24-10 Hemothorax.

During the sudden inertial deceleration and direct impact, fixed and mobile parts of the lung parenchyma move at different speeds, resulting in stretching and shearing of alveoli and intravascular structures (inertial effect). This kinetic wave of energy is partially reflected at the alveolar membrane surface, with the remainder causing a localized release of energy (spalding effect). Overexpansion of air in the lungs occurs, after the primary energy wave has passed (implosion effect), from low-pressure rebound shock waves that produce overstretching and damage to lung tissue. The combination of these physical mechanisms result in alveolar and capillary damage with interstitial and intraalveolar extravasation of blood. Because the contused area of the lung is not able to function properly after injury, profound hypoxemia may develop. The degree of respiratory complication is directly related to the size of the contused area.

Signs and symptoms of pulmonary contusion initially are subtle and should be suspected based on the kinematics of the event and the presence of associated injuries. Common signs and symptoms include:

- Tachypnea
- Tachycardia

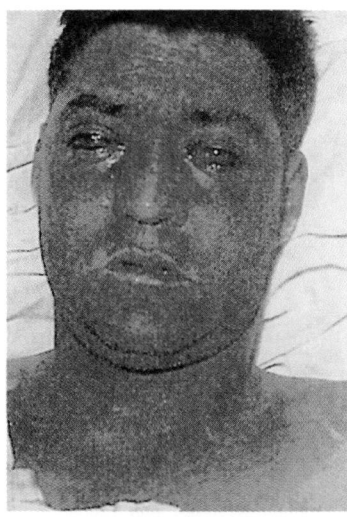

Fig. 24-11 Discoloration of traumatic asphyxia, which results from forcible compression of the chest. (From London PS: *A colour atlas of diagnosis after recent injury,* Ipswich, England, 1990, Wolfe Medical Publications.)

- Cough
- Hemoptysis
- Apprehension
- Respiratory distress
- Dyspnea
- Evidence of blunt chest trauma
- Cyanosis

? CRITICAL THINKING

Will you always be able to distinguish between simple pneumothorax and pulmonary contusion in the prehospital setting? Why?

Emergency care for pulmonary contusion includes ventilatory support and high-concentration oxygen administration. Patients with associated injuries or preexisting pulmonary or cardiovascular disease should be closely monitored for the need to assist ventilations with a bag-valve device, intubation, or both. Although pulmonary contusions may be associated with major thoracic injury, they generally heal spontaneously over several weeks.

Traumatic Asphyxia

Traumatic asphyxia is a term used to describe a severe crushing injury to the chest and abdomen (Fig. 24-11). It results from an increase in intrathoracic

pressure that forces blood from the right side of the heart into the veins of the upper thorax, neck, and face. Although the forces involved in this phenomenon may produce lethal injury, traumatic asphyxia alone is not life threatening[1] (although brain hemorrhages, seizures, coma, and death have been documented as occasional sequela).

Signs and symptoms of traumatic asphyxia include reddish purple discoloration of the face and neck (skin below the area remains pink), jugular vein distention, and swelling or hemorrhage of the conjunctiva (subconjunctival petechiae may appear). Emergency care for the patient is directed at ensuring an open airway, providing adequate ventilation, and caring for associated injuries. The paramedic should be prepared to manage hypovolemia and shock when the compressive force is released.

Heart and Great Vessel Injury

Trauma to the heart and great vessels may result from blunt or penetrating injury and associated forces. The injuries discussed in this section are myocardial contusion, pericardial tamponade, myocardial rupture, and traumatic aortic rupture.

Myocardial Contusion

The clinical findings in myocardial contusion are often subtle and frequently overlooked for the following reasons: (1) multiple injuries direct attention elsewhere, (2) there often is little evidence of thoracic injury, and (3) signs of cardiac injury may not be present on initial examination. Contusions to the myocardium usually result from motor vehicle collision as the chest wall strikes the dashboard or steering column. (Sternal and multiple rib fractures

NOTE

Blunt myocardial injury occurs in 16% to 76% of patients who suffer blunt trauma to the chest.[2]

? CRITICAL THINKING

How would you manage a cardiac rhythm disturbance resulting from a myocardial contusion?

are common.) Therefore a deformed dashboard or steering column should alert the paramedic to the possibility of a cardiac injury.

The extent of injury may vary from a localized bruise to a full-thickness injury to the wall of the heart with hemorrhage and edema. The accumulation of blood in the pericardium (**hemopericardium**) may occur from a lacerated epicardium or endocardium, resulting in cardiac rupture or a traumatic myocardial infarction. The fibrinous reaction at the contusion site may lead to delayed rupture or ventricular aneurysm.

Patients with a myocardial contusion may have no symptoms or may complain of chest pain similar to that of a myocardial infarction. Other signs and symptoms include ECG abnormalities, new cardiac murmur, pericardial friction rub (late), persistent tachycardia, and palpitations. Emergency care for these patients is similar to that for myocardial infarction: oxygen administration, ECG monitoring, and pharmacological therapy for dysrhythmias and hypotension. Any intervention that increases myocardial oxygen consumption should be avoided.

Pericardial Tamponade

Penetrating trauma (and rarely blunt trauma) may cause tears in the heart chamber walls, allowing blood to leak from the heart. If the pericardium has been torn sufficiently, this blood leaks into the thoracic cavity and the patient rapidly exsanguinates. However, the pericardium often remains intact, in which case the blood enters the pericardial space, causing increased pericardial pressure. The increase

> **NOTE**
>
> Pericardial tamponade occurs in less than 2% of patients who suffer chest trauma.[2]

> **NOTE**
>
> Penetrating injuries such as those from some knife and gunshot wounds may result in exsanguination rather than tamponade because the pericardium has too large a wound to maintain the blood in the pericardial space. Gunshot wounds carry a higher mortality than stab wounds.[2]

in pericardial pressure does not allow the heart to expand and refill with blood, resulting in a decrease in stroke volume and cardiac output. Myocardial perfusion decreases because of pressure effects on the walls of the heart and decreased diastolic pressures. Associated ischemic dysfunction may result in myocardial infarction.

Most patients with pericardial tamponade initially demonstrate peripheral vasoconstriction (which tends to raise the diastolic blood pressure more than the systolic blood pressure, causing a decrease in pulse pressure) and an increase in heart rate to compensate for the decrease in cardiac output. Up to this point, pericardial tamponade and hemorrhagic shock have similar manifestations. However, one very important clinical finding often allows differentiation of the two forms of shock. This clinical finding first was described by Beck in 1935 and, with two other clinical clues, makes up what is known as **Beck's triad** (seen only in 30% of patients with pericardial tamponade).[2]

Beck's triad consists of elevated central venous pressure (evidenced by jugular vein distention), muffled heart sounds, and hypotension. A pulsus paradoxus, which is difficult to measure in the prehospital setting, also may occur in pericardial tamponade. This is evidenced by a systolic blood pressure that drops more than 10 to 15 mm Hg during inspiration compared with expiration. The first element of Beck's triad, elevated central venous pressure, is the single best way to distinguish pericardial tamponade from hemorrhagic shock.[1] Other signs and symptoms of pericardial tamponade include:

- Tachycardia
- Respiratory distress
- Narrow pulse pressure
- Cyanosis of the head, neck, and upper extremities
- ECG changes

> **NOTE**
>
> It is important to stress that entities other than pericardial tamponade can present with hypotension and elevated central venous pressure. These are most notably tension pneumothorax in the trauma victim and cardiogenic shock. It also is true that patients with tamponade and hemorrhage may not initially demonstrate elevated venous pressure.

Pericardial tamponade is a true emergency. These patients must have pericardial blood removed and the source of the bleeding stopped to survive the injury. Prehospital management includes careful monitoring, oxygen administration, fluid replacement, and rapid transport to an appropriate medical facility where needle pericardiocentesis can be performed to aspirate blood from the pericardial sac. Removal of as little as 20 mL may drastically improve cardiac output.[2]

Myocardial Rupture

Myocardial rupture occurs when blood-filled chambers of the ventricles are compressed with sufficient force to rupture the chamber wall, septum, or valve. The injury is nearly always immediately fatal, but death may be delayed for 2 to 3 weeks (after blunt trauma).[2] Motor vehicle crashes are responsible for most cases of myocardial rupture, accounting for 15% of fatal thoracic injuries.[1] Other proposed mechanisms include:

- Deceleration or shearing forces that disrupt the inferior and superior venae cavae
- Upward displacement of blood (causing an increase in intracardiac pressure) after abdominal trauma
- Direct compression of the heart between the sternum and vertebrae
- Laceration from a rib or sternal fracture
- Complications of myocardial contusion

These patients often present with a significant mechanism of injury and with signs and symptoms of congestive heart failure and cardiac tamponade. Prehospital care for these patients is primarily supportive and includes airway and ventilatory support and rapid transport for definitive care. The possibility of a tension pneumothorax should be considered with these patients, since signs and symptoms of it mimic myocardial rupture with tamponade.

Traumatic Aortic Rupture

Traumatic aortic rupture is thought to be a result of shearing forces that develop between tissues that decelerate at different rates (Fig. 24-12). Common mechanisms of injury include rapid deceleration in high-speed motor vehicle crashes, falls from great heights, and crushing injuries. It has been estimated that one out of every six people who die in motor vehicle crashes sustains a rupture of the aorta.[1] Of these patients, 80% to 90% die at the scene as a result of massive hemorrhage. About 10% to 20% survive the first hour because the bleeding is tamponaded by the surrounding adventitia of the aorta and intact visceral pleura. Of these, however, 30% have ruptures within 6 hours—thus the need for a rapid and pertinent evaluation and transport to an appropriate medical facility.

> **NOTE**
>
> Aortic rupture is responsible for 15% of all blunt trauma deaths.[2]

The usual site of damage to the aorta is in the distal arch just beyond the takeoff of the left subclavian artery and proximal to the ligamentum arteriosum. The ligamentum arteriosum and descending tho-

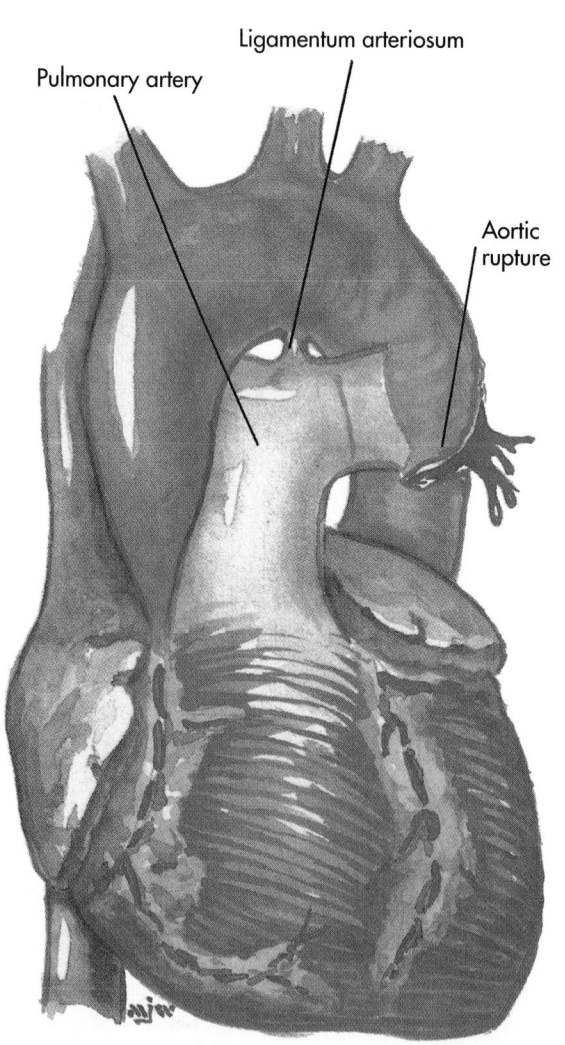

Pulmonary artery

Ligamentum arteriosum

Aortic rupture

Fig. 24-12 Aortic rupture.

racic arch are relatively fixed, whereas the transverse portion of the arch is relatively mobile. If shearing forces exceed the tensile strength of the arch, the junction of the mobile and fixed points of attachment may partially be torn. If the outer layer of tissue surrounding the aorta remains intact, the patient may survive long enough for surgical repair.

Because aortic rupture is a severe injury (with an 80% to 90% fatality rate within the first hour), the paramedic should always consider the possibility of this injury in any trauma patient who has unexplained shock and an appropriate mechanism of injury (rapid deceleration). Upper-extremity hypertension with absent or decreased amplitude of femoral pulses can occur in patients with aortic rupture (thought to result from compression of the aorta by the expanding hematoma). Other patients have generalized hypertension secondary to increased sympathetic discharge. About 25% of these patients have a harsh systolic murmur over the pericardium or interscapular region. Rarely, paraplegia is seen with a normal cervical and thoracic spine. This is secondary to decreased blood flow through the anterior spinal artery, which is in the thoracic region and is composed of branches from the posterior intercostal arteries, which in turn are branches from the thoracic aorta.

Prehospital management of these patients includes advising medical direction of the suspected rupture, high-concentration oxygen administration, ventilatory support with spinal precautions, judicious fluid replacement (avoiding overhydration), and rapid transport for surgical repair.

> **NOTE**
>
> Patients who are normotensive should have limited replacement fluids to prevent an increase in pressure in the remaining aortic wall tissue.

Penetrating Wounds of the Great Vessels

Penetrating wounds of the great vessels (aorta, pulmonary arteries and veins, superior and inferior venae cavae) usually involve injury to the chest, abdomen, or neck. These wounds often are accompanied by massive hemothorax, hypovolemic shock, cardiac tamponade, and enlarging hematomas that may cause compression of the vena cava, trachea, esophagus, great vessels, and heart. Prehospital care for patients with penetrating injury to the great vessels is directed at providing airway and ventilatory support, managing hypovolemia with judicious fluid therapy (guided by medical direction), and rapid transport for definitive care.

Other Thoracic Injuries

Other injures that may be associated with blunt or penetrating trauma to the thorax include esophageal and tracheobronchial injuries (described in Chapter 22) and diaphragmatic rupture.

Esophageal and Tracheobronchial Injuries

Esophageal injuries most frequently are caused by penetrating trauma (e.g., missile and knife wounds). They also can result from spontaneous perforation caused by cancer and anatomic distortions produced by diverticulae or gastric reflux, both of which can lead to violent emesis.[2] Assessment findings may include pain, fever, hoarseness, dysphagia, respiratory distress, and shock. If esophageal perforation occurs in the cervical region, local tenderness, subcutaneous emphysema, and resistance to neck movement may be noted. Esophageal perforation that occurs lower in the thoracic region may result in mediastinal and subcutaneous emphysema, mediastinitis, and splinting of the chest wall.

Tracheobronchial injuries are rare (occurring in less than 3% of victims of blunt or penetrating chest trauma) but carry a mortality rate greater than 30%.[2] Most injuries occur within 3 cm of the carina, but they can occur anywhere along the tracheobronchial tree. Signs and symptoms of tracheobronchial injury include:

- Severe hypoxia
- Tachypnea
- Tachycardia
- Massive subcutaneous emphysema
- Dyspnea
- Respiratory distress
- Hemoptysis

> **NOTE**
>
> A tension pneumothorax that does not respond to needle decompression or the continuous flow of air from the needle following decompression should alert the paramedic to the possibility of a tracheobronchial injury.

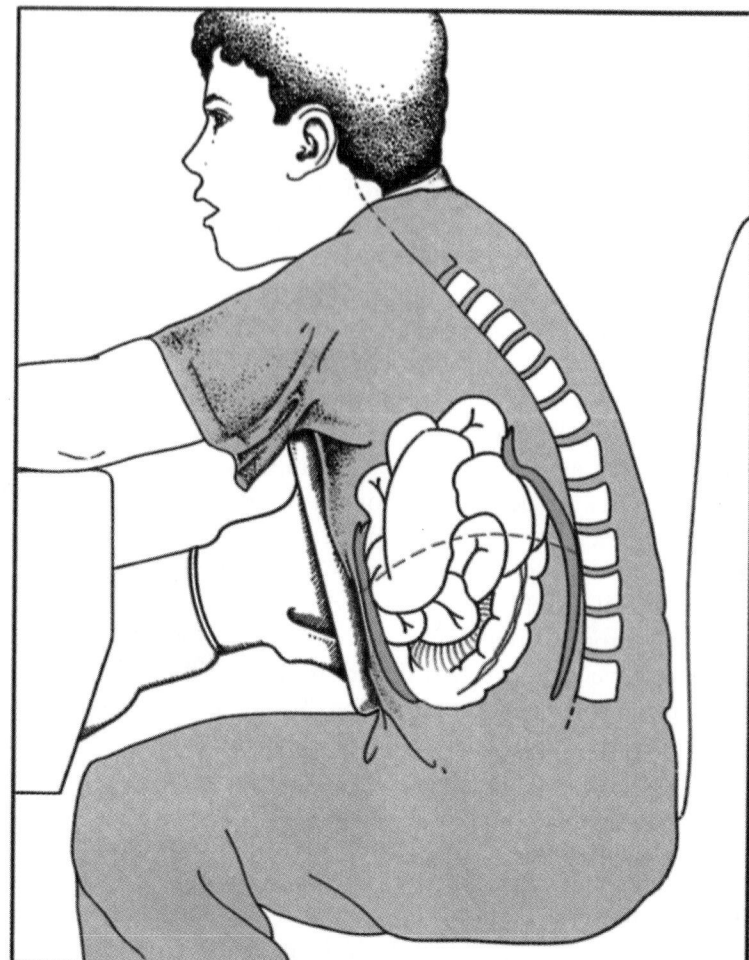

Fig. 24-13 Diaphragmatic rupture. A rapid compression of the abdomen may increase intraabdominal pressure, causing the abdominal contents to rupture through the thin diaphragmatic wall and enter the chest cavity. (From Moylan EE: *Principles of trauma surgery,* ed 2, New York, 1992, Gower Medical Publishing.)

Emergency care for patients with esophageal or tracheobronchial injury is directed at providing airway, ventilatory, and circulatory support, and rapid transport for definitive care at an appropriate medical facility.

Diaphragmatic Rupture

As described in Chapter 6, the diaphragm is a sheet of voluntary muscle that separates the abdominal cavity from the thoracic cavity. When rapid compression of the abdomen results in a sharp increase in intraabdominal pressure (e.g., blunt trauma to the trunk), the pressure differences may cause abdominal contents to rupture through the thin diaphragmatic wall and enter the chest cavity (Fig. 24-13). Diaphragmatic rupture is detected more on the left side than on the right. Ruptures on either side, however, may allow intraabdominal organs to enter the thoracic cavity, where they may cause compression of the lung with a reduction in ventilation, a decrease in venous return, a decrease in cardiac out-

put, and shock. Multiple injuries often are present in patients with diaphragmatic rupture because of the mechanical forces involved.

Signs and symptoms of a ruptured diaphragm include abdominal pain, shortness of breath, and decreased breath sounds. If a majority of the abdominal contents are displaced into the chest, the abdomen may have a hollow or empty appearance and bowel sounds may be present in the affected hemithorax. Prehospital management includes oxygen administration, ventilatory support as needed (positive pressure may worsen the injury), volume-expanding fluids, and rapid transport in a supine position to an appropriate medical facility for surgical repair. Some medical direction agencies also may recommend that a nasogastric tube be placed to decompress the stomach.

? CRITICAL THINKING

What is the advantage of placing a nasogastric tube in a patient who has a diaphragmatic rupture?

S U M M A R Y

- Thoracic trauma is caused by blunt or penetrating trauma resulting from motor vehicle crashes, falls from heights, blast injuries, blows to the chest, chest compression, gunshot wounds, and stab wounds.

- Fractures of the clavicle, ribs, or sternum, and flail chest may be caused by blunt or penetrating trauma. Complications of skeletal trauma of the chest may include cardiac, vascular, or pulmonary injuries.

- Closed pneumothorax may be life threatening if it is a tension pneumothorax, occupies more than 40% of the hemithorax, or occurs in a patient with shock or preexisting pulmonary or cardiovascular disease. Open pneumothorax may result in severe ventilatory dysfunction, hypoxemia, and death unless it is rapidly recognized and corrected. Tension pneumothorax is a true emergency that results in profound hypoventilation and death if it is not immediately recognized and managed. Hemothorax may result in massive blood loss. These patients often have hypovolemia and hypoxemia. Pulmonary contusion results when trauma to the lung causes alveolar and capillary damage. Severe hypoxemia may develop and is directly related to the size of the contused area. Traumatic asphyxia results from forces that cause an increase in intrathoracic pressure. When it occurs alone, it is often not lethal, but brain hemorrhages, seizures, coma, and death have been reported following these injuries.

- The extent of injury from myocardial contusion may vary from a localized bruise to a full-thickness injury to the wall of the heart, resulting in cardiac rupture, ventricular aneurysm, or a traumatic myocardial infarction. Pericardial tamponade occurs if 150 to 200 mL of blood enters the pericardial space acutely, resulting in a decrease in stroke volume and cardiac output. Myocardial rupture refers to an acute traumatic perforation of the ventricles or atria. It is nearly always immediately fatal, but death may be delayed for several weeks after blunt trauma. Aortic rupture is a severe injury with an 80% to 90% mortality in the first hour. The paramedic should consider aortic rupture in any trauma patient who has unexplained shock after rapid deceleration injury.

- Esophageal injuries most frequently are caused by penetrating trauma (e.g., missile and knife wounds). Tracheobronchial injuries are rare (occurring in less than 3% of victims of blunt or penetrating chest trauma) but carry a mortality rate greater than 30%. A tension pneumothorax that does not respond to needle decompression or the continuous flow of air from the needle following decompression should alert the paramedic to the possibility of a tracheobronchial injury.

- Diaphragmatic ruptures may allow intraabdominal organs to enter the thoracic cavity, where they may cause compression of the lung with a reduction of ventilation, a decrease in venous return, a decrease in cardiac output, and shock.

REFERENCES

1. Rosen P, Barkin R: *Emergency medicine: concepts and clinical practice,* ed 4, St Louis, 1998, Mosby.

2. US Department of Transportation, National Highway Traffic Safety Administration: *EMT-Paramedic national standard curriculum,* Washington, DC, 1998, The Department.

25 Abdominal Trauma

OBJECTIVES

Upon completion of this chapter, the paramedic student will be able to:

1. Identify mechanisms of injury associated with abdominal trauma.
2. Describe mechanisms of injury, signs and symptoms, and complications associated with abdominal solid organ, hollow organ, retroperitoneal organ, and pelvic organ injuries.
3. Outline the significance of injury to intra-abdominal vascular structures.
4. Describe the prehospital assessment priorities for the patient suspected to have abdominal injury.
5. Outline the prehospital care of the patient with abdominal trauma.

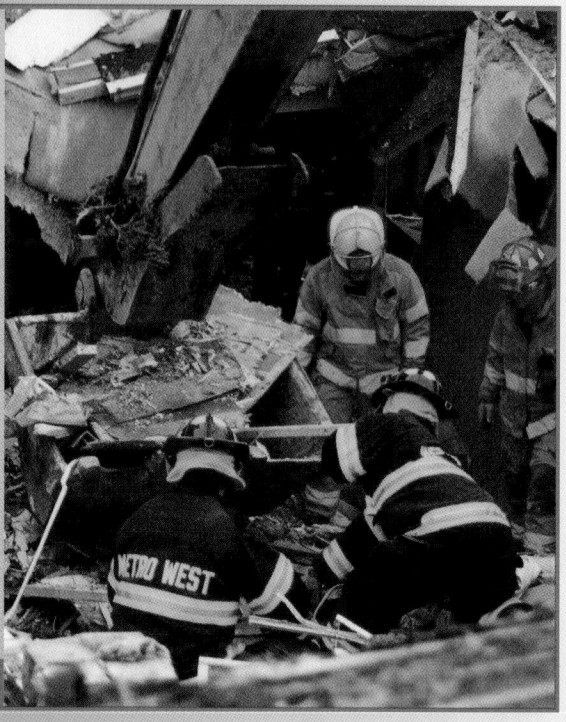

Abdominal trauma may be difficult to evaluate in the prehospital setting. This is due to the wide spectrum of potential injuries to multiple organs; physical findings that sometimes are lacking or exaggerated; and altered levels of pain perception that occur as a result of preexisting conditions, shock, alcohol or other drug use, head injury, or other factors. Therefore the paramedic must exercise a high degree of suspicion based on the mechanism of injury and kinematics. Death from abdominal trauma usually is a result of continuing hemorrhage and delay of surgical repair.

hematuria: The abnormal presence of blood in the urine.
hemoperitoneum: The presence of extravasated blood in the peritoneal cavity.
Kehr's sign: Pain in the left shoulder thought to be caused by referred pain secondary to irritation of the adjacent diaphragm.

NOTE

Like most other types of trauma, many abdominal injuries can be prevented. Participating in community programs (e.g., promoting gun safety legislation) and emphasizing the need for using personal restraints are excellent prevention strategies. (See Appendix C.)

Mechanisms of Abdominal Injury

Abdominal injury may result from blunt or penetrating trauma. Regardless of the organ injury, prehospital management usually is limited to securing the airway with spinal precautions, providing ventilatory support, providing wound management, managing shock with fluid replacement and application of a pneumatic antishock garment (PASG) (per protocol), and rapidly transporting the patient for definitive care (Box 25-1).

BOX 25-1

PREHOSPITAL CARE FOR ABDOMINAL INJURY

1. Secure the airway with spinal precautions.
2. Provide ventilatory support.
3. Provide wound management.
4. Manage shock with fluid replacement and PASG (per protocol).
5. Rapidly transport the patient for definitive care.

Blunt Trauma

Blunt trauma to abdominal organs usually results from compression or shearing forces (see Chapter 18). Compression forces may cause the abdominal viscera to be crushed between solid objects (e.g., the steering column and spinal vertebrae). Shearing forces may produce a tear or rupture of the solid organs or blood vessels as they become stretched at their points of attachment (stabilizing ligaments or blood vessels). The degree of injury usually is related to the quantity and duration of force applied and the type of abdominal structure injured (fluid filled, gas filled, solid, hollow). Blunt abdominal trauma may be a result of motor vehicle and motorcycle collisions (including injuries that result from use of personal restraints), pedestrian injuries, falls, assaults, and blast injuries (Fig. 25-1).

? CRITICAL THINKING

Why are young children more susceptible to abdominal organ injury than adults?

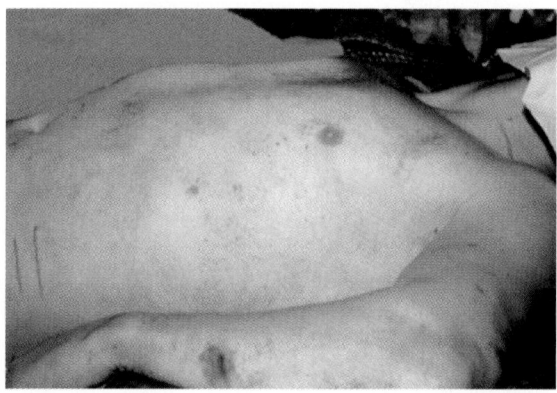

Fig. 25-1 Marks of impact sustained by the front-seat passenger in a car crash. The victim suffered rupture of the diaphragm and spleen.

Penetrating Trauma

Penetrating injury may result from stab wounds, gunshot wounds, or impaled objects. Major complications of penetrating trauma are hemorrhage from a major vessel or solid organ and perforation of a segment of bowel. As a rule, injuries from penetrating trauma do not have as high a mortality rate as those that result from blunt trauma.[2]

Specific Abdominal Injuries

Abdominal injury may be classified as solid organ, hollow organ, retroperitoneal organ, pelvic organ, or vascular injury (Fig. 25-2).

Solid Organ Injury

Injury to solid organs usually results in rapid and significant blood loss. The two solid organs most

? CRITICAL THINKING

When will shock associated with injury to the liver or spleen develop?

commonly injured are the liver and spleen; both are primary sources of exsanguination.

Liver

The liver is the largest organ in the abdominal cavity. Because of its location, it is commonly injured from trauma to the eighth through twelfth ribs on the right side of the body and from trauma to the upper central part of the abdomen. Injury to the liver should be suspected in any patient with a steering wheel injury, lap belt injury, or history of epigastric trauma. After injury, blood and bile escape into the peritoneal cavity, producing signs and symptoms of shock and peritoneal irritation, respectively.

Spleen

The spleen lies in the upper left quadrant of the abdomen and is slightly protected by the organs surrounding it medially and anteriorly and by the lower portion of the rib cage. Injury to this organ commonly is associated with other intraabdominal injuries. Splenic injury should be suspected in motor vehicle crashes and in falls or sport injuries in which there was an impact to the lower left chest, flank, or upper left abdomen. Although about 40% of patients with splenic injures have no symptoms, the patient may complain of pain in the left shoulder (**Kehr's sign**), thought to be caused by referred pain secondary to irritation of the adjacent diaphragm from splenic hematoma or **hemoperitoneum.**

Hollow Organ Injury

Injuries to the hollow abdominal organs may result in sepsis, wound infection, and abscess formation, particularly if trauma to the intestine remains undiagnosed for an extended period. In contrast to solid organ injury, in which hemorrhage is the major

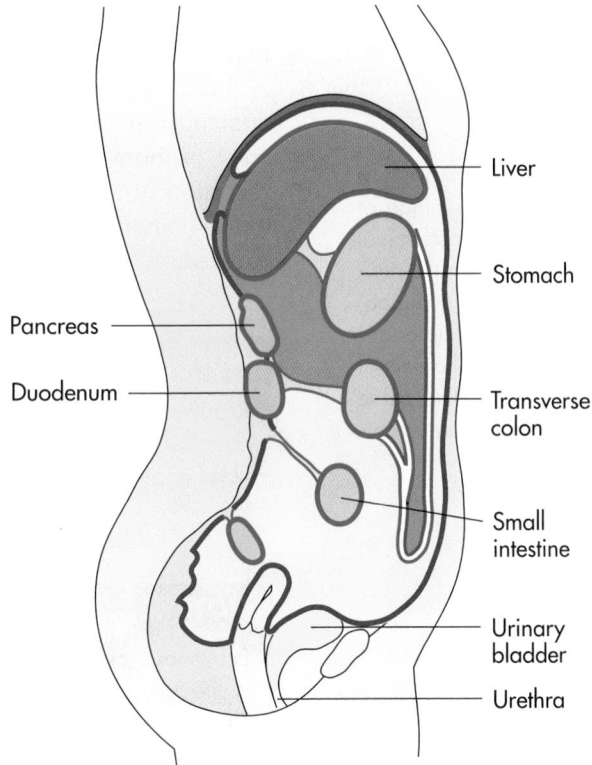

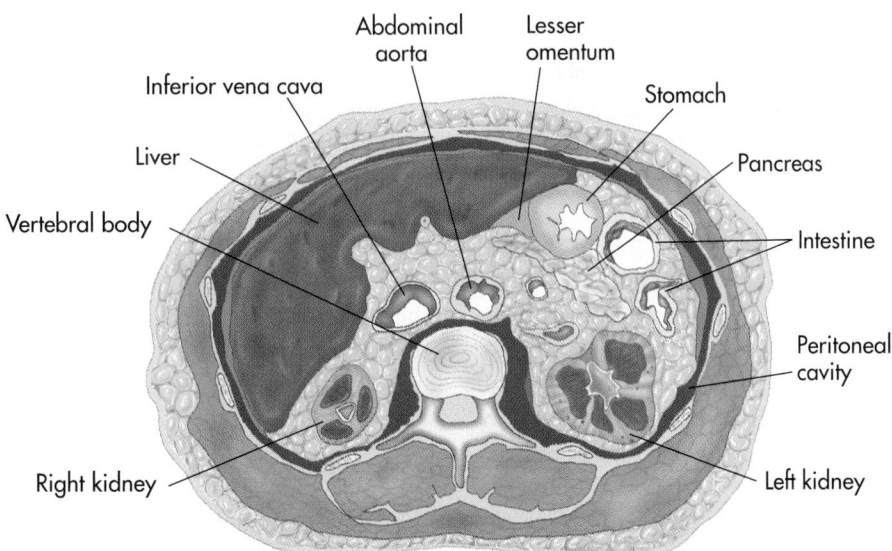

Fig. 25-2 Hollow, solid, retroperitoneal, and pelvic organs.

cause of symptoms, injury to the hollow organs results in symptoms from spillage of their contents (resulting in peritonitis) (Box 25-2).

Stomach

The stomach is not commonly injured after blunt trauma because of its protected location in the abdomen. Penetrating trauma, however, may cause gastric transection or laceration. Patients with this condition may exhibit signs of peritonitis rather rapidly from leakage of acidic gastric contents. Diagnosis of injury to the stomach usually is confirmed during surgery unless nasogastric drainage returns blood.

BOX 25-2

PERITONEAL IRRITATION

Peritonitis usually is acute and quite painful and may be delayed for hours or days following a hollow-viscus injury. It results from the spillage of enzymes, acids, and bacteria into the abdominal cavity that produces a chemical irritation to the peritoneum, the membrane that lines the wall of the abdomen and covers the abdominal organs. (Blood is not a chemical irritant to the abdomen.) The pain of peritonitis usually is localized (via somatic nerve fibers) but also may be diffuse. Signs and symptoms of peritonitis include:

1. Pain
2. Tenderness on percussion or palpation
3. Guarding, rigidity
4. Fever (if untreated)
5. Distention (a late finding)

   NOTE: The adult abdomen can accommodate 1.5 L of fluid with no abdominal distention.

NOTE

The stomach is damaged in about 1% of cases of blunt abdominal trauma and in about 19% of cases of penetrating trauma.[1]

Colon and Small Intestine

The colon and small intestine are similar to the stomach and duodenum in that injury to these organs is probably a result of penetrating trauma (e.g., a gunshot wound to the abdomen or buttocks) rather than blunt trauma. However, the large and small bowel also may be injured by compression forces in high-speed motor vehicle crashes and in deceleration injuries associated with wearing personal restraints. Because of the amount of force required to injure the colon and small intestine, other injuries usually are present. Peritoneal contamination with bacteria is a common problem.

NOTE

The colon is damaged in about 6% of cases of blunt abdominal trauma, and the small intestine in about 7% of cases; in penetrating trauma to the abdomen, the colon is damaged in about 16% of cases, and the small intestine in about 26% of cases.[1]

Retroperitoneal Organ Injury

Retroperitoneal organ injury may occur as a result of blunt or penetrating trauma to the anterior abdomen, posterior abdomen (particularly the flank area), or thoracic spine. Hemorrhage within the retroperitoneal area may be massive. Most retroperitoneal hemorrhages result from pelvic and/or lumbar fractures.

NOTE

Retroperitoneal structures are damaged in about 9% of cases of blunt abdominal injuries and in about 11% of cases of penetrating trauma.[1]

NOTE

Ecchymosis of the flanks (Turner's sign) or umbilicus (Cullen's sign) indicates retroperitoneal hemorrhage. These signs, however, usually are delayed 12 hours to several days.

Kidneys

The kidneys are solid organs that lie in the retroperitoneal space but that may be injured with abdominal trauma as well. Injuries may involve contusion fractures and lacerations, resulting in hemorrhage, urine extravasation, or both. Contusions usually are self-limiting and heal with bed rest and forced fluids. Fractures and lacerations are more severe and may require surgical repair, depending on which part of the kidney is damaged.

Ureters

The ureters are hollow organs rarely injured by blunt trauma because of their flexible structure. When injury occurs, it usually results from penetrating abdominal or flank wounds (e.g., stab wounds, firearm injuries).

? CRITICAL THINKING

What functions of the pancreas may be disrupted after injury? What might be the effects of spillage of pancreatic juices into the abdominal cavity?

Pancreas

The pancreas is a solid organ that lies within the retroperitoneal space. Injury, although rare, usually is caused by compressive or penetrating forces applied to the upper left quadrant, as in steering wheel and bicycle handlebar impalement. The pancreas more commonly is injured in penetrating trauma (particularly with firearms) than in blunt trauma.

Duodenum

The duodenum lies across the lumbar spine and seldom is injured, because of its location in the retroperitoneal area, near the pancreas. When great force from blunt trauma or penetrating injury occurs, the duodenum may be crushed or lacerated. Injury to this organ usually is associated with concurrent pancreatic trauma; it is confirmed through surgery.

Pelvic Organ Injury

Injury to pelvic organs usually results from motor vehicle crashes that produce pelvic fractures. Other, less frequent causes of pelvic organ injury are penetrating trauma, straddle-type injuries from falls, pedestrian accidents, and some sexual acts. Because the pelvis provides support and protection for multiple organ systems, there is great potential for associated injury. The most common associated injuries are those to the urinary bladder and urethra.

> **NOTE**
>
> Fractures of the pelvis often are associated with severe retroperitoneal hemorrhage and carry a mortality rate that ranges from 6.4% to 19%.[1] Pelvic fractures are further described in Chapter 26.

> **NOTE**
>
> The urinary bladder and surrounding structures are damaged in about 6% of cases of abdominal trauma.[1]

Urinary Bladder

The urinary bladder is a hollow organ that may be ruptured by blunt trauma, penetrating trauma, or pelvic fracture. Rupture is more likely if the bladder is distended at the time of injury. With rupture, the integrity of the peritoneum may be broken, and urine may extravasate into the peritoneal cavity. Bladder injury should be suspected in inebriated patients subjected to lower abdominal trauma. Gross **hematuria** (blood in the urine) may be present, or the patient may complain that he or she is unable to void.

Urethra

Urethral disruption occurs more frequently in men and usually is secondary to blunt trauma associated with pelvic fracture. The patient may complain of an inability to urinate and abdominal pain. Blood at the meatus indicates urethral injury.

> **NOTE**
>
> Passage of an indwelling urinary catheter is contraindicated in these patients.

Vascular Structure Injury

Intraabdominal arterial and venous injuries may be life threatening because of their potential for massive hemorrhage. These injuries usually occur from penetrating trauma but may also arise from compression or deceleration forces applied to the abdomen. As in solid organ injury, vascular injury usually presents as hypovolemia and occasionally is associated with a palpable abdominal mass. The major vessels most frequently injured are the aorta; the inferior vena cava; and the renal, mesenteric, and iliac arteries and veins (see Chapter 6). Vascular structure injury carries a high mortality rate if it is not surgically repaired soon after the traumatic event.

> **? CRITICAL THINKING**
>
> *How can you attempt to manage profound shock from massive vascular injury associated with a severe pelvic fracture?*

Assessment

The most significant indicator of severe abdominal trauma is the presence of unexplained shock. In addition to the mechanism of injury and classic presentation of hypovolemia, other signs and symptoms that should alert the paramedic to the possibility of severe abdominal trauma are abdominal wall injuries (e.g., bruising and discoloration to the abdomen, abrasions) and:

- Obvious bleeding
- Pain, abdominal tenderness or guarding
- Abdominal rigidity, distention

> **NOTE**
>
> Most abdominal distention in trauma patients is a result of swallowed air. Adults and especially children frequently swallow air when under stress. In addition, mask-assisted ventilation may force air down the esophagus. A patient who has abdominal distention from hemorrhage probably is in hemorrhagic shock.

- Evisceration (Box 25-3)
- Rib fractures
- Pelvic fractures

> **BOX 25-3**
>
> ### EVISCERATION
>
> An evisceration is the protrusion of an internal organ or peritoneal contents through a wound or surgical incision, especially in the abdominal wall. The presence of an evisceration from abdominal trauma generally is associated with major intraperitoneal injury. The wound is managed in the prehospital setting by covering the eviscerated contents with a moist, sterile gauze or trauma dressing to prevent further contamination and drying. No attempt should be made to replace eviscerated organs into the peritoneal cavity; to do so would increase the risk of infection and complicate surgical evaluation of the injury.

> **NOTE**
>
> The absence of these signs and symptoms does not preclude the presence of abdominal injury. The paramedic must maintain a high degree of suspicion based on the nature of the injury.

Management

Emergency care of patients with abdominal trauma usually is limited to stabilizing the patient and rapid transport to an appropriate medical facility for surgical intervention. The most important components of on-scene care are:

- A thorough scene survey to identify forces involved in abdominal trauma
- Rapid evaluation of the patient and mechanism of injury
- Airway maintenance with spinal precautions
- High-concentration oxygen administration
- Ventilatory support as needed
- Reduction of continued hemorrhage by pressure application
- Fluid replacement with volume expanders and PASG (per protocol)
- Cardiac monitoring

While en route to the hospital, a comprehensive physical examination and ongoing assessment can be performed. This includes obtaining a focused history; vital sign assessment (and reassessment); and inspection, percussion, and palpation of the abdomen. Auscultation of the abdomen for the presence of bowel sounds can establish a baseline measurement for hospital personnel. This assessment, however, should never delay patient transport.

SUMMARY

- Blunt trauma to abdominal organs usually results from compression or shearing forces.

- Penetrating injury may result from stab wounds, gunshot wounds, or impaled objects.

- The two solid organs most commonly injured are the liver and spleen; both are primary sources of exsanguination. Injuries to the hollow abdominal organs may result in sepsis, wound infection, and abscess formation.

- Injury to the retroperitoneal organs (kidneys, ureters, pancreas, duodenum) may cause massive hemorrhage.

- Injury to the pelvic organs (bladder, urethra) usually results from motor vehicle crashes that produce pelvic fractures.

- Abdominal vascular structure injuries may be life threatening because of their potential for massive hemorrhage.

- The most significant indicator of severe abdominal trauma is the presence of unexplained shock.

- Emergency care of patients with abdominal trauma involves stabilizing the patient and rapid transport to an appropriate medical facility for surgical intervention.

REFERENCES

1. Rosen P, Barkin R: *Emergency medicine: concepts and clinical practice*, ed 4, St Louis, 1998, Mosby.

2. US Department of Transportation, National Highway Traffic Safety Administration: *EMT-Paramedic national standard curriculum*, 1998, Washington, DC, The Department.

26 Musculoskeletal Trauma

OBJECTIVES

Upon completion of this chapter, the paramedic student will be able to:

1. Describe the features of each classification of musculoskeletal injury.

2. Describe the features of bursitis, tendonitis, and arthritis.

3. Given a specific patient scenario, outline the prehospital assessment of the musculoskeletal system.

4. Outline general principles of splinting.

5. Describe the significance and prehospital management principles for selected upper-extremity injuries.

6. Describe the significance and prehospital management principles for selected lower-extremity injuries.

7. Identify prehospital management priorities for open fractures.

8. Describe principles for realignment of angular fractures and dislocations.

9. Outline the process for referral of patients with minor musculoskeletal injury.

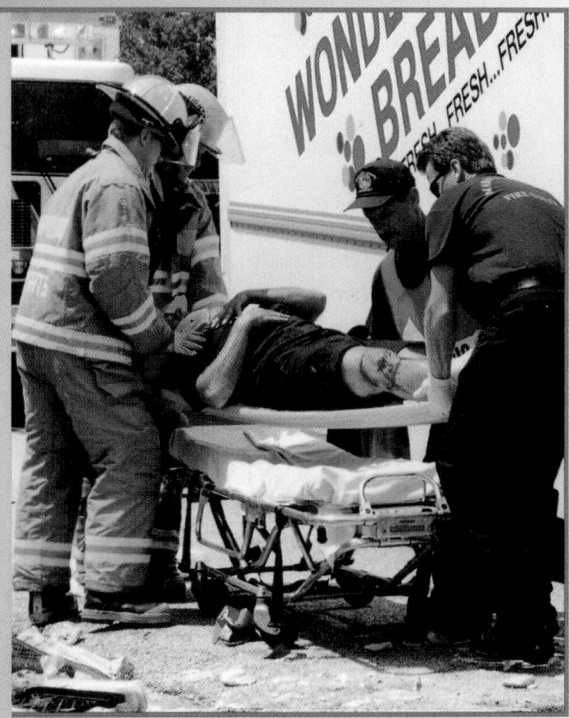

Musculoskeletal trauma occurs in 70% to 80% of patients who experience traumatic injury (occurring as an isolated injury or with other injuries).[1] Although extremity trauma is seldom life threatening, early recognition and management may prevent long-term, debilitating complications.

KEY TERMS

DCAP-BTLS: An acronym for wound assessment that includes deformity, contusions, abrasions, penetrations or punctures, burns, tenderness, lacerations, and swelling.

false movement: An unnatural movement of an extremity, usually associated with fracture.

fracture: A break in the continuity of bone or cartilage.

joint dislocation: An injury that occurs when the normal articulating ends of two or more bones are displaced.

sprain: A partial tearing of a ligament caused by a sudden twisting or stretching of a joint beyond its normal range of motion.

strain: An injury to the muscle or its tendon from overexertion or overextension.

NOTE

Extremity trauma usually results from motor vehicle crashes, falls, acts of violence, and contact sports.[2] Prevention strategies include proper sports training (interfacing with athletic trainers regarding the use of protective equipment), use of personal restraints, gun safety and education, and fall prevention (e.g., high-rise window guards). (See Appendix C.)

NOTE

The reader should refer to Chapter 6 to review the anatomy of the musculoskeletal system.

Classifications of Musculoskeletal Injuries

The musculoskeletal system and associated neurovascular structures are made up of bones, nerves, vessels, muscles, tendons, ligaments, and joints. Injuries that result from application of traumatic forces to these tissues include fractures, sprains, strains, and joint dislocations. The paramedic should not attempt to differentiate these injuries in the prehospital setting. Patients with suspected extremity trauma should be managed as though a fracture exists. Problems associated with musculoskeletal injuries include:

- Hemorrhage
- Instability
- Loss of tissue
- Simple laceration and contamination
- Interruption of blood supply
- Nerve damage
- Long-term disability

? CRITICAL THINKING

How could long-term disability result from a musculoskeletal injury?

Musculoskeletal injuries can result from direct trauma (e.g., blunt force applied to an extremity), indirect trauma (e.g., a vertical fall that produces a spinal fracture distant from the site of impact), or pathological conditions (e.g., some forms of arthritis; malignancy). The paramedic should carefully evaluate the scene and consider kinematics when caring for a patient with musculoskeletal injury (see Chapter 18).

Fractures

A **fracture** is any break in the continuity of bone or cartilage (Fig. 26-1). It may be complete or incomplete, depending on the line of fracture through the bone. Fractures also are classified as *open* or *closed*,

---

NOTE

As described in Chapter 6, the head of long bones in children is separated from the shaft of the bone by the epiphyseal plate until the bone stops growing. Fractures that involve the epiphyseal plate (epiphyseal fractures) are serious injuries that may result in separation or fragmentation of the plate and in permanent angulation or deformity of an extremity.

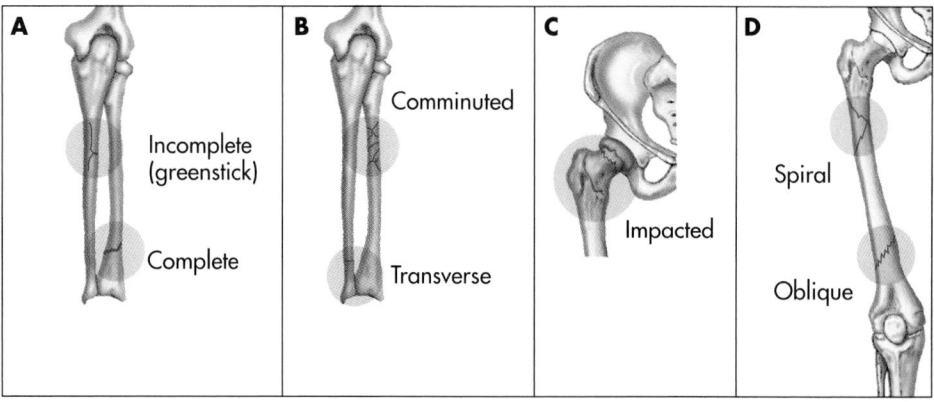

Fig. 26-1 Bone fractures. **A,** Complete and incomplete. **B,** Comminuted and transverse. **C,** Impacted. **D,** Oblique and spiral. (Illustrator David J. Mascaro and Associates.)

depending on the integrity of the skin near the fracture site (Box 26-1). Fractures of long bones may result in moderate to severe hemorrhage within the first 2 hours, releasing as much as 550 mL of blood in the lower leg from a tibial or fibular fracture, 1000 mL of blood in the thigh from a femoral fracture, and 2000 mL of blood from a pelvic fracture.[1]

Sprains

A **sprain** is partial tearing of a ligament caused by a sudden twisting or stretching of a joint beyond its normal range of motion. Two common areas for sprains are the knee and ankle. Sprains are graded by severity (Table 26-1). A first-degree sprain has no joint instability because only a few ligamentous fibers are torn. Swelling and hemorrhage are minimal. (Repeated first-degree sprains can result in ligamentous stretching.) A second-degree sprain causes more disruption than first-degree injuries. The joint usually is still intact, but there is increased swelling and ecchymosis. In third-degree sprains the ligaments are totally disrupted. If third-degree sprains are accompanied by a dislocation, nerve or vascular compromise to the extremity is possible.

> **NOTE**
>
> Some second-degree sprains and most third-degree sprains often present in the same manner as a fracture.

Strains

A **strain** is an injury to the muscle or its tendon from overexertion or overextension. Strains commonly occur in the back and arms and may be accompanied by a significant loss of function. Severe strains may cause an avulsion of bone from the attachment site.

Joint Dislocations

A **joint dislocation** occurs when the normal articulating ends of two or more bones are displaced. Joints

TABLE 26-1	GRADING OF SPRAINS BY SEVERITY		
	FIRST-DEGREE SPRAIN	**SECOND-DEGREE SPRAIN**	**THIRD-DEGREE SPRAIN**
	No joint instability	Joint usually remains intact	Total disruption of ligaments
	Minimal swelling/ hemorrhage	Increased swelling/ ecchymosis	Nerve or vascular compromise is possible

that frequently are dislocated are those of the shoulders, elbows, fingers, hips, knees, and ankles. The injury should be suspected when a joint is deformed or does not move with normal range of motion. A complete dislocation is called a *luxation;* an incomplete dislocation is called a *subluxation.* All dislocations can result in great damage and instability.

? CRITICAL THINKING

Why are dislocation injuries associated with a high incidence of vascular or nerve damage?

Inflammatory and Degenerative Conditions

Several inflammatory and degenerative conditions may present or be complicated by extremity injury (Box 26-2). These include bursitis, tendonitis, and arthritis.

Bursitis

Bursitis is inflammation of a bursa (a small, fluid-filled sac that acts as a cushion at a pressure point near joints). The most important bursae are around the knee, elbow, and shoulder. The condition usually is a result of pressure (e.g., prolonged kneeling on a hard surface), friction, or slight injury to the membranes surrounding the joint. Management generally consists of rest, ice, and analgesics, after which the condition usually subsides. In rare cases, bursectomy may be performed.

BOX 26-2

AGE-ASSOCIATED CHANGES IN BONES

As a person ages, morphological changes in bones occur, some of which may increase the likelihood of injury or complicate the healing process. These changes include:

1. A decrease in the water content of intervertebral disks (increasing the risk of herniation)
2. Loss of $\frac{1}{2}$ to $\frac{3}{4}$ inch in stature, causing a shortened trunk and the formation of an arc-shaped vertebral column that is prone to injury
3. Thoracic rigidity caused by ossification of costal cartilage (may lead to shallow breathing)
4. Porous and brittle bones that are prone to fracture
5. Bone disorders (e.g., osteoporosis) that increase the risk of fracture

NOTE

The application of ice to an injury during the first 24 hours generally reduces pain and swelling, after which heat (e.g., warm soaks) often is prescribed to increase circulation.

Tendonitis

Tendonitis is inflammation of a tendon, often caused by injury. Symptoms include pain, tenderness, and, occasionally, restricted movement of the muscle attached to the affected tendon (e.g., pain in the shoulder when the arm is raised above a certain angle). Management usually includes nonsteroidal antiinflammatory drugs (NSAIDs) and sometimes corticosteroid drugs that are injected around the tendon.

Arthritis

Arthritis (further described in Chapter 43) is inflammation of a joint that is characterized by pain, swelling, stiffness, and redness. The condition is not a single disease, but rather refers to joint disease (involving one or many joints) that can occur from a number of causes. Arthritis varies in severity from a mild ache and stiffness to severe pain and, later, to joint deformity.

Osteoarthritis (degenerative arthritis) is the most common. It results from wear and tear on the joints and evolves in middle age. The pain from this condition generally is managed with antiinflammatory agents.

Rheumatoid arthritis is the most severe type of inflammatory joint disease. It is an autoimmune disorder in which the body's immune system acts against and damages joints and surrounding soft tissues. Many joints, most commonly those in the hands, feet, and arms, become extremely painful, stiff, and deformed. Drugs used to treat this condition include NSAIDs to decrease pain and antirheumatic drugs and immunosuppressant agents to arrest or slow the progress of the disease.

Gouty arthritis is a form of joint disease in which uric acid accumulates in joints in the form of crystals, causing inflammation. The first attack of this form of arthritis usually involves only one joint (e.g., the base of the big toe) and lasts a few days. Subsequent attacks may be more severe and may affect more joints (e.g., knee, ankle, wrist, foot, and small joints of the hand). Pain and inflammation from gouty arthritis is controlled with large doses of NSAIDs or corticosteroid injections. Other management may include drugs to inhibit the formation of or increase the excretion of uric acid, and diet modifications.

Signs and Symptoms of Extremity Trauma

Signs and symptoms of extremity trauma may range from subtle complaints of discomfort to obvious deformity or open fracture. Field evaluation should be rapid, assuming significant injury. Common signs and symptoms of extremity trauma include:

- Pain on palpation or movement
- Swelling, deformity
- Crepitus
- Decreased range of motion
- **False movement** (unnatural movement of an extremity)
- Decreased or absent sensory perception or circulation distal to the injury (evidenced by alterations in skin color and temperature, distal pulses, and capillary refill)

? CRITICAL THINKING

How can a paramedic distinguish between a serious sprain and a fracture in the prehospital setting?

NOTE

This text presents immobilization strategies for fractures and dislocations as they pertain to isolated extremity injuries. Again, extremity trauma is seldom life threatening, so patients with multiple-system traumatic injury should first be managed for conditions that compromise the airway, breathing, circulation (including internal and external hemorrhage in the extremities), and spinal stability. If rapid transport is indicated by the patient's condition or mechanism of injury, injured extremities can be stabilized by fully immobilizing the patient on a long spine board.

Assessment

Musculoskeletal assessment can be divided into four classes of patients:

1. Patients with life- or limb-threatening injuries or conditions, including life- or limb-threatening musculoskeletal trauma
2. Patients with other life- or limb-threatening injuries and only simple musculoskeletal trauma
3. Patients with no other life- or limb-threatening injuries but with life- or limb-threatening musculoskeletal trauma
4. Patients with only isolated, non–life or limb-threatening injuries

---

BOX 26-3

THE SIX *Ps* OF MUSCULOSKELETAL ASSESSMENT

Pain or tenderness
Pallor (pale skin or poor capillary refill)
Paresthesia (pins-and-needles sensation)
Pulses (diminished or absent)
Paralysis (inability to move)
Pressure

The paramedic should conduct an initial assessment to determine if there are any life-threatening conditions. He or she should care for those conditions first; never overlook musculoskeletal trauma; and never allow a horrible-looking, but noncritical, musculoskeletal injury to distract from the priorities of care. Evaluation of an injured extremity should always include an assessment for the "six *P*'s of musculoskeletal assessment": pain, pallor, paresthesia, pulses, paralysis, and pressure (Box 26-3). The paramedic also should evaluate an extremity's neurovascular status by assessing the distal pulse, motor function, and sensation (before and after movement or splinting), and should inspect and palpate the injured area for **DCAP-BTLS**:

- Deformity
- Contusions
- Abrasions
- Penetrations or punctures
- Burns
- Tenderness
- Lacerations
- Swelling

The assessment should include a comparison with the opposite, uninjured extremity. If extremity trauma is suspected, the injury should be immobilized by splinting.

TRICKS OF THE TRADE

Use a pen to mark the location of a distal pulse on the patient's skin. It helps others who care for the patient to check the pulse and to identify where you found it.

General Principles of Splinting

The goal of splinting is immobilization of the injured body part. Immobilization by splinting helps alleviate pain; decreases tissue injury, bleeding, and contamination in an open wound; and simplifies and facilitates transport of the patient. The general principles of splinting are listed in Box 26-4.

Types of Splints

A wide variety of splints and splinting materials are available through a number of equipment manufacturers. These splints can be broadly categorized as rigid, soft or formable, and traction splints.

Rigid splints cannot be changed in shape and require that the body part be positioned to fit the splint's design. Examples of rigid splints include board splints, contoured metal and plastic splints, and some cardboard splints (Fig. 26-2). Rigid splints

---

BOX 26-4

GENERAL PRINCIPLES OF SPLINTING

1. Splint joints and bone ends above and below.
2. Immobilize open and closed fractures in the same manner.
3. Cover open fractures to minimize contamination.
4. Check pulses, sensation, and motor function before and after splinting.
5. Stabilize the extremity with gentle, in-line traction to a position of normal alignment.
6. Immobilize a long bone extremity in a straight position that can easily be splinted.
7. Immobilize dislocations in a position of comfort; ensure good vascular supply.
8. Immobilize joints as found; joint injuries are only aligned if there is no distal pulse.
9. Apply cold to reduce swelling and pain.
10. Apply compression to reduce swelling.
11. Elevate the extremity if possible.

NOTE: Immobilization requires a minimum of two rescuers.

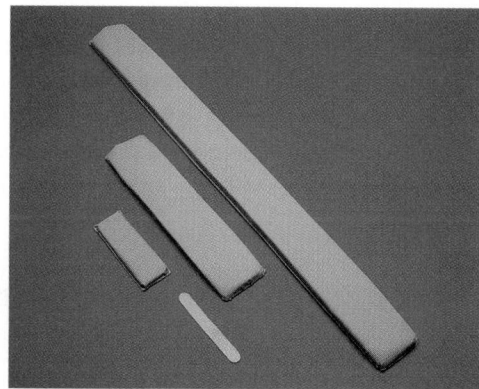

Fig. 26-2 Rigid splints.

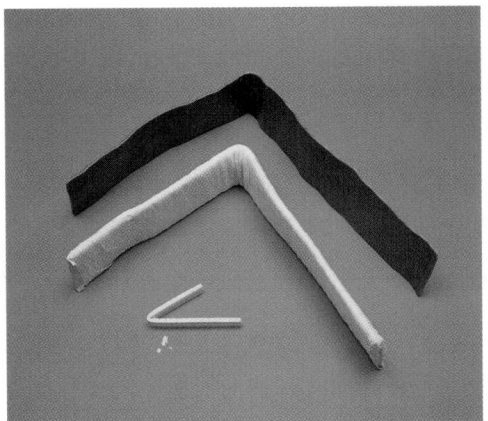

Fig. 26-3 Formable splints.

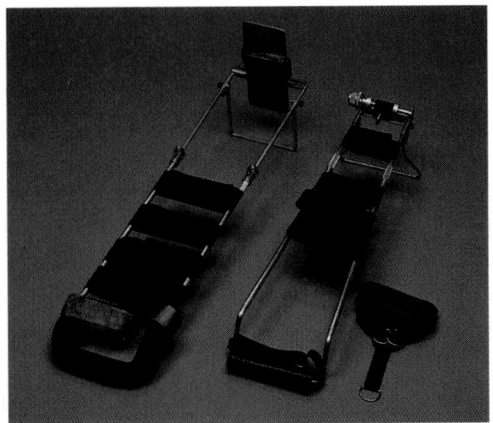

Fig. 26-4 Traction splints.

should be padded before use to accommodate for anatomical shape and patient comfort.

Soft or formable splints can be molded into various shapes and configurations to accommodate the injured body part. Examples of soft or formable splints include pillows, blankets, slings and swathes, vacuum splints, some cardboard splints, wire ladder splints, and padded, flexible aluminum splints (Fig. 26-3). Inflatable air splints also are considered to be soft or formable splints, but they are not designed to be used for injuries proximal to the knee or elbow.

✓ TRICKS OF THE TRADE

It's important to communicate with your partners during splinting. Coordination in splinting can reduce pain and decreases the risk of making a closed fracture into an open one.

Traction splints are specifically designed for midshaft femoral fractures. These splints do not apply or maintain sufficient traction to reduce a femoral fracture but provide enough traction to stabilize and align it. Examples include Thomas half-ring, Hare traction, and Sager traction splints (Fig. 26-4).

✓ TRICKS OF THE TRADE

If you misplace the ankle hitch to your Hare traction splint, one can easily be improvised using a cravat.

Upper-Extremity Injuries

Upper-extremity injuries can be classified as fractures or dislocations to the shoulder, humerus, elbow, radius and ulna, wrist, hand, and finger (Fig. 26-5). Clavicular injury was discussed in Chapter 24. Most upper-extremity injuries can be adequately immobilized by application of a sling and swathe.

Shoulder Injury

Shoulder injuries are common in the older adult because of weaker bone structure and frequently result from a fall on an outstretched arm. Patients with anterior fracture or dislocation (accounting for 90% of cases) often will be positioned with the affected arm/shoulder close to the chest (with the lateral aspect of the shoulder appearing flat instead of rounded) and a deep depression between the head of the humerus and the acromion laterally ("hollow shoulder"). Patients with posterior fracture or dislocation may be positioned with the arm above the head. Management includes:

1. Assessment of neurovascular status
2. Application of a sling and swathe (Fig. 26-6)
3. Application of ice

NOTE

Ice should be placed in a plastic bag and applied for 20-minute periods to the injury site. Refreezable packs of gelled solution are inefficient and should not be used.

Based on the position of the affected arm/shoulder, splinting may need to be improvised to hold

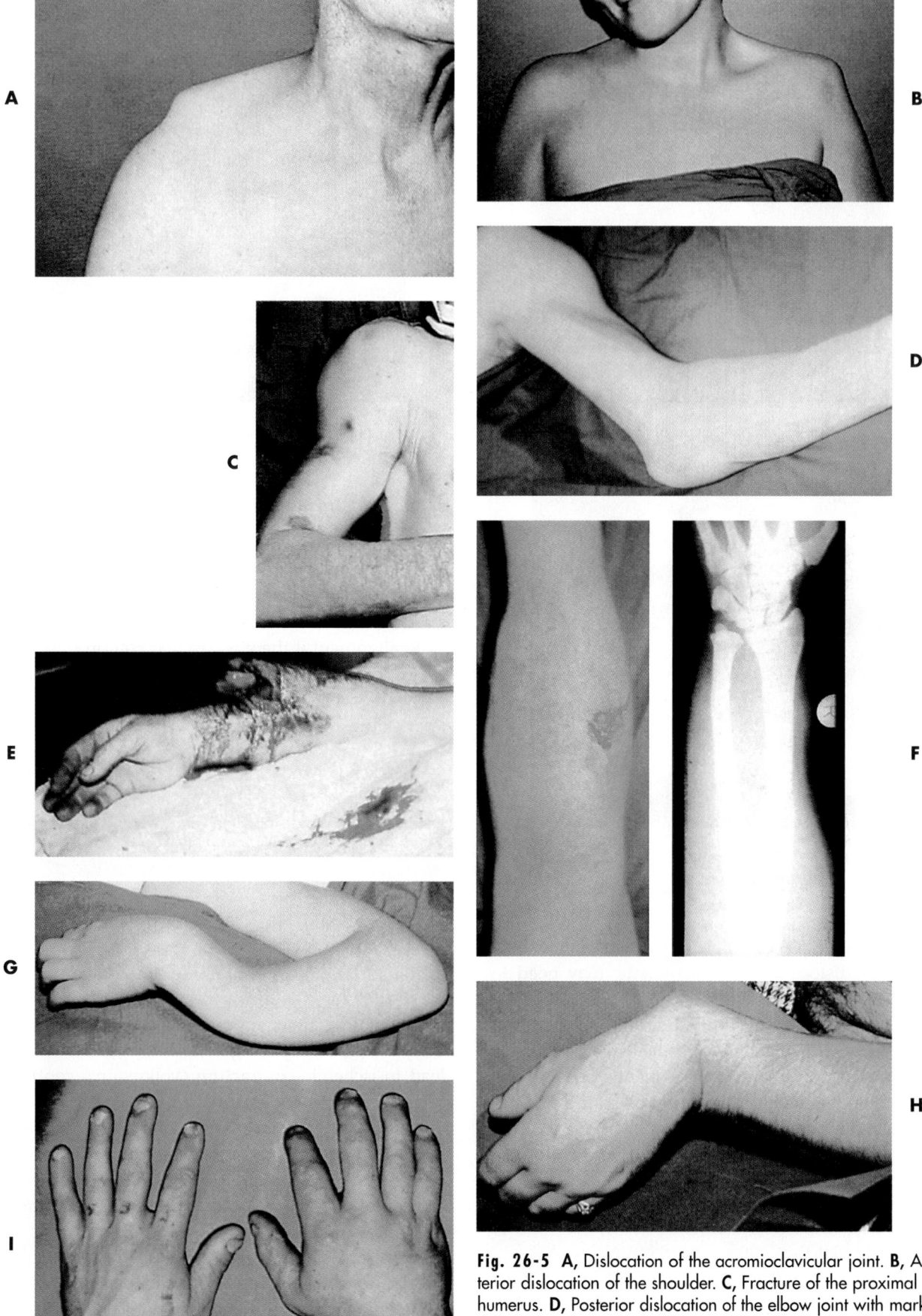

Fig. 26-5 **A,** Dislocation of the acromioclavicular joint. **B,** Anterior dislocation of the shoulder. **C,** Fracture of the proximal humerus. **D,** Posterior dislocation of the elbow joint with marked deformity. **E,** Severe open fracture of the forearm. **F,** Penetration of the forearm caused by a nail gun. **G,** Greenstick fracture with marked deformity. **H,** Fracture of the distal radius. **I,** Hand injury from a motorcycle crash. (From London PS: *A colour atlas of diagnosis after recent injury,* Ipswich, England, 1990, Wolfe Medical Publications, Ltd.)

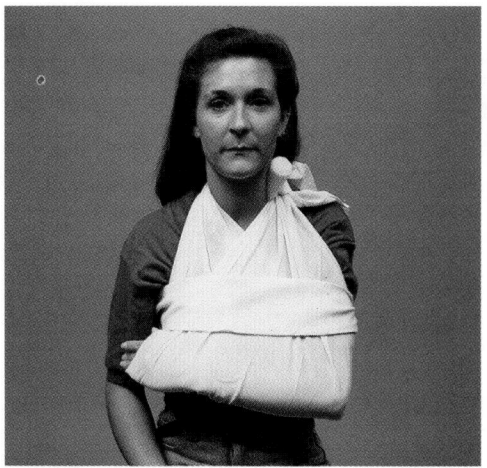

Fig. 26-6 Immobilization of the shoulder.

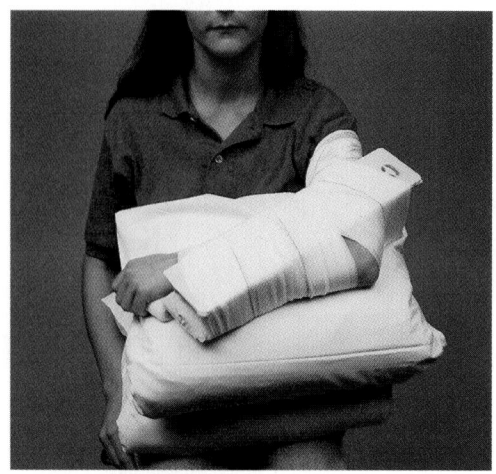

Fig. 26-8 Immobilization of the elbow.

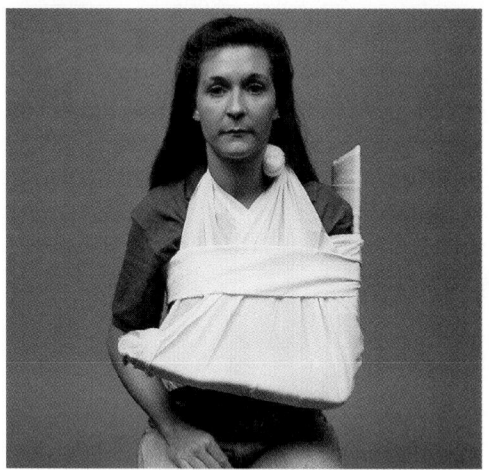

Fig. 26-7 Immobilization of the humerus.

shaft, and a fracture of the humeral neck may cause axillary nerve damage. Internal hemorrhage into the joint also may be a complication. Management includes:

1. Assessment of neurovascular status
2. Realignment if there is vascular compromise
3. Application of a rigid splint and sling and swathe (Fig. 26-7), or splinting the extremity with the arm extended

> **NOTE**
>
> If the patient has a possible cervical spine injury, the sling should not be tied around the patient's neck.

4. Application of ice

Elbow Injury

Elbow injuries are common in children and athletes. They are especially dangerous in children and may lead to ischemic contracture (Volkmann's contracture) with serious deformity to the forearm and a clawlike hand. The mechanism of injury usually involves falling on an outstretched arm or flexed elbow. Associated complications include laceration of the brachial artery and radial nerve damage. Management includes:

1. Assessment of neurovascular status
2. Splinting in the position found with a pillow, blanket, rigid splint, or sling and swathe (Fig. 26-8)
3. Application of ice

the injury in place. For example, with some fractures or dislocations, the paramedic may need to use a rolled blanket with a cravat through the center, position the blanket roll under the elevated arm and secure it like a sling, and then swathe the arm to prevent movement. If the patient's arm is positioned above the head, it should be splinted in position. Alternatively, traction can be applied on the long axis of the arm to obtain a better position for immobilization.

Humeral Injury

Upper-arm fractures are common in older adults and children and often are difficult to stabilize. Radial nerve damage may be present if a fracture occurs in the middle or distal portion of the humeral

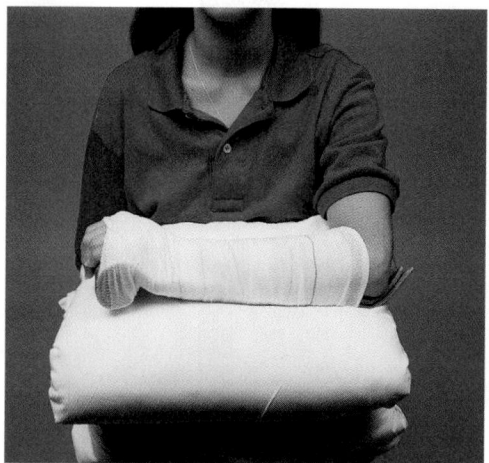

Fig. 26-9 Immobilization of the forearm.

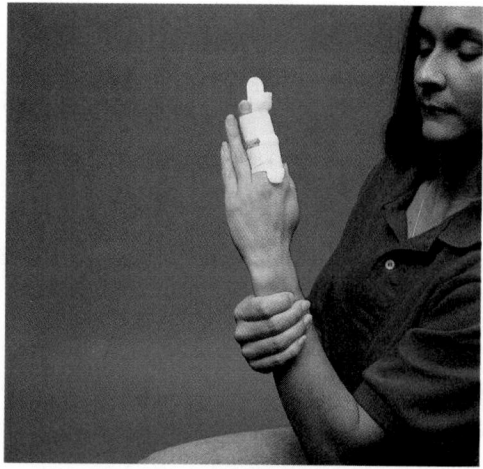

Fig. 26-10 Immobilization of the finger.

Radial, Ulnar, or Wrist Injury

Like most other upper-extremity injuries, injuries to the radius, ulna, and wrist usually are a result of a fall on an outstretched arm. Wrist injuries may involve the distal radius, ulna, or any of the eight carpal bones. The most common wrist injury involves a fracture with "silver-fork" deformity of the distal radius with dorsal angulation (Colles' fracture). Forearm injury is common in both children and adults. Management includes:

1. Assessment of neurovascular status
2. Splinting in the position found with rigid or formable splints or a sling and swathe (Fig. 26-9)
3. Application of ice and elevation

? CRITICAL THINKING

What effect does application of a cold pack have on musculoskeletal injuries?

Hand (Metacarpal) Injury

Injury to the hand frequently results from contact sports, violence (fighting), and work-related crushing injuries. A common metacarpal injury is boxer's fracture, which results from direct trauma to a closed fist, fracturing the fifth metacarpal bone. These injuries also may be associated with hematomas and open wounds. Although the boxer's fracture is the most common metacarpal fracture, any of the metacarpals can be fractured, depending on the

mechanism of injury. Hand injuries should be splinted in the position of function (as with a hand grasping a football) with rigid or formable splints (previously described for a radial, ulnar, or wrist injury). Management includes:

1. Assessment of neurovascular status
2. Splinting with a rigid or formable splint (pillow, blanket) in the position of function
3. Application of ice and elevation

Finger (Phalangeal) Injury

Injured fingers may be immobilized with foam-filled aluminum splints or tongue depressors or by simply taping the injured finger to an adjacent one ("buddy splinting"). Although finger injuries are common, they should not be considered trivial. Serious injuries include thumb metacarpal fractures and any open or markedly comminuted metacarpal or proximal phalangeal fracture. Management includes:

1. Assessment of neurovascular status
2. Splinting as previously described (Fig. 26-10)
3. Application of ice and elevation

Lower-Extremity Injuries

Lower-extremity injuries include fractures to the pelvis and fractures or dislocations to the hip, femur, knee and patella, tibia and fibula, ankle and foot, and phalanx (Fig. 26-11).

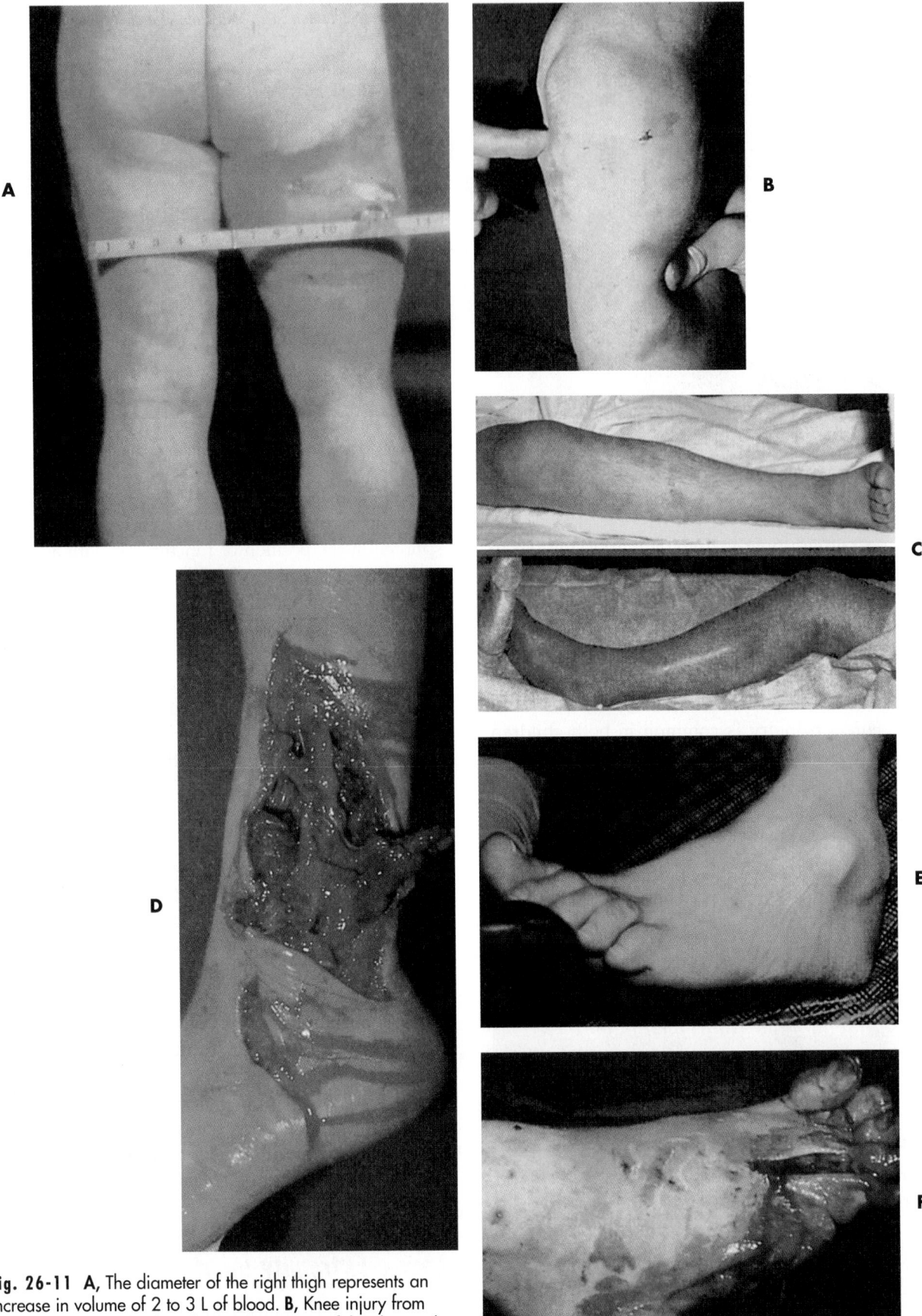

Fig. 26-11 **A,** The diameter of the right thigh represents an increase in volume of 2 to 3 L of blood. **B,** Knee injury from a pedestrian-automobile collision. **C,** Fracture of the tibia and fibula. **D,** Open fracture to the lower leg. **E,** Subtalar dislocation. **F,** Foot that was run over by the wheel of a railway coach. (From London PS: *A colour atlas of diagnosis after recent injury,* Ipswich, England, 1990, Wolfe Medical Publications, Ltd.)

Compared with upper-extremity injuries, lower-extremity injuries are associated with greater wounding forces and more significant blood loss. They also are more difficult to manage in the patient with multiple injuries and may be life threatening (e.g., femoral and pelvic fractures).

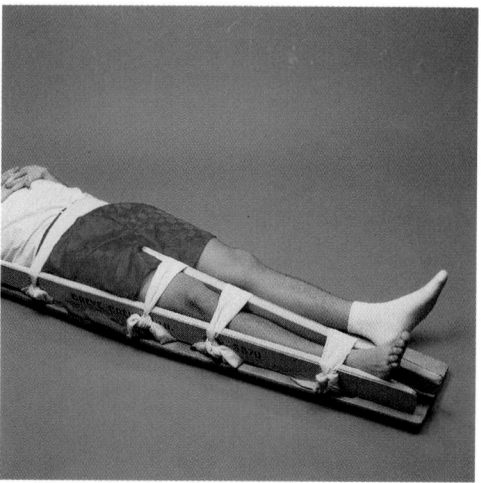

Fig. 26-12 Immobilization of the hip.

Pelvic Fracture

As described in Chapter 25, blunt or penetrating injury to the pelvis may result in fracture, severe hemorrhage, and associated injury to the urinary bladder and urethra. Since the pelvis is surrounded by heavy muscles and other soft tissues, deformity may be difficult to see. Injury to the pelvis should be suspected based on the mechanism of injury or the presence of tenderness on palpation of the iliac crests (described in Chapter 14). Management includes:

1. High-concentration oxygen administration
2. Management for shock (pneumatic antishock garment [PASG] per protocol)
3. Full-body immobilization on a long spine board (adequately padded for comfort)
4. Regular monitoring of vital signs
5. Rapid transport (essential)

Trauma to the abdomen and pelvic area may be complicated by pregnancy (further described in Chapter 40).

✓ **TRICKS OF THE TRADE**

Discoloration of the genitals (Coopernail's sign) can indicate pelvic fracture with internal bleeding.

As described in Chapter 19, the PASG may be useful in arresting hemorrhage by tamponading bleeding vessels in the pelvis or lower extremities, and in stabilizing pelvic and lower-extremity fractures. Decisions on the use of PASG are left to local protocol and medical direction.

Hip Injury

Hip injuries commonly occur in older adults as a result of a fall, and in younger patients as a result of major trauma. If the hip is fractured at the femoral head and neck, the affected leg usually is shortened and externally rotated. By comparison, dislocations of the hip usually are evidenced by a shortened and internally rotated leg. Management includes:

1. Assessment of neurovascular status
2. Splinting with a long spine board (Fig. 26-12) and generously padding the patient for comfort during transport (slight flexion of the knee or padding beneath the knee may improve comfort).
3. Frequent monitoring of vital signs

Femoral Injury

Injury to the femur usually results from major trauma, as in motor vehicle crashes and pedestrian accidents. It also is a fairly common result of child abuse.

Fractures to the femur usually are evident from the powerful thigh muscles producing overriding of the bone fragments. The patient generally has a shortened leg that is externally rotated and midthigh swelling from hemorrhage, which can be life threatening. These fractures should be immobilized in the field with a traction splint. Management includes:

1. High-concentration oxygen administration
2. Management for shock

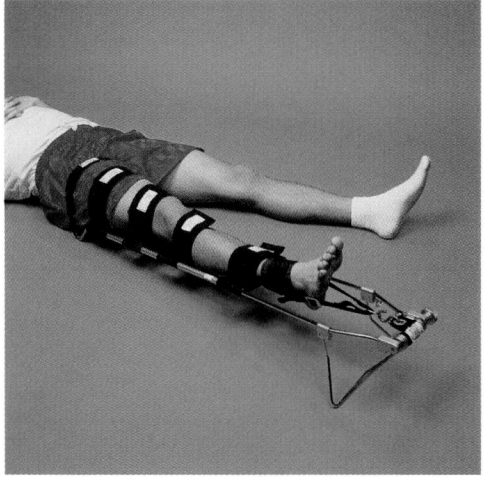

Fig. 26-13 Application of traction splint.

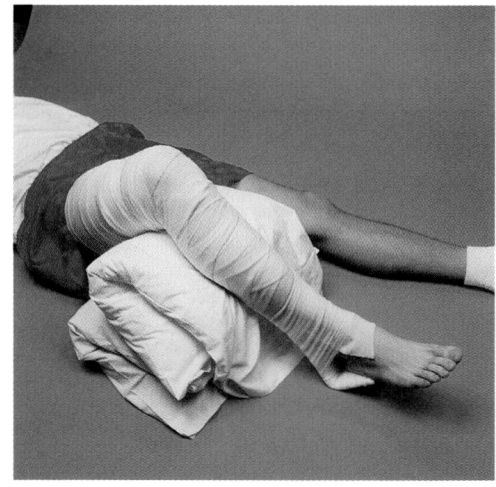

Fig. 26-14 Immobilization of the knee.

3. Assessment of neurovascular status
4. Application of a traction splint (Fig. 26-13)
5. Regular monitoring of vital signs

> **NOTE**
>
> Traction splints are only to be used to immobilize mid-shaft femoral fractures. They are contraindicated for fractures to the lower third of the leg, pelvic fractures, hip injury, knee injury, and avulsion or amputation of the ankle and foot. It is recommended that the patient be positioned on a long spine board before traction splint application.

> **NOTE**
>
> Fractures of the proximal femur may present similar to an anterior hip dislocation, with a shortened and internally rotated leg.

If concurrent injuries are contributing to the development of shock and if local protocol advocates the use of PASG in conjunction with a traction splint, the traction splint should be applied *over* the PASG only after it has been inflated. Any traction device placed under the PASG may promote continued hemorrhage, tissue damage, and compromised circulation to the injured extremity.

Knee and Patellar Injury

Fractures to the knee (supracondylar fracture of the femur, intraarticular fracture of the femur or tibia) and fractures and dislocations of the patella commonly result from motor vehicle crashes, pedestrian accidents, contact sports, and falls on a flexed knee. The relationship of the popliteal artery to the knee joint is important and may give rise to vascular injury (particularly with posterior dislocations). Management includes:

1. Assessment of neurovascular status
2. Splinting in the position found with a rigid or formable splint (Fig. 26-14) that effectively immobilizes the hip and ankle

> **NOTE**
>
> Traction splints are not to be used to immobilize a knee or patellar injury.

3. Application of ice and elevation, if possible

Tibial and Fibular Injury

Injuries to the tibia and fibula may result from direct or indirect trauma or twisting injury. If the injury is associated with the knee, popliteal vascular

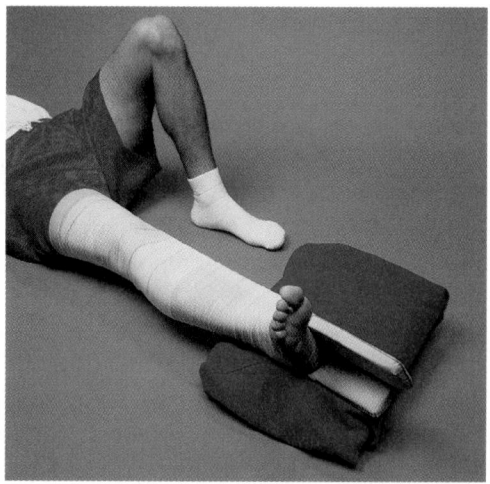

Fig. 26-15 Immobilization of the lower leg.

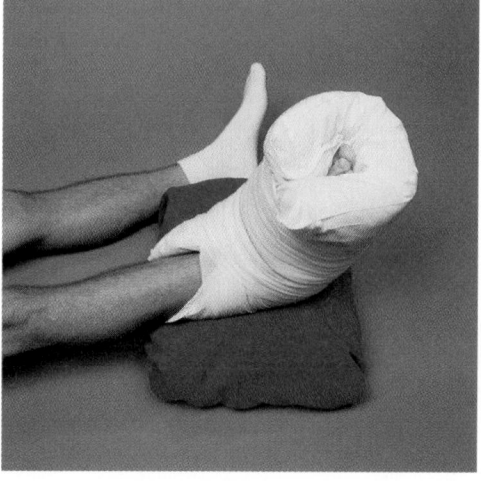

Fig. 26-16 Immobilization of the foot and ankle.

injury should be suspected. Management includes:

1. Assessment of neurovascular status
2. Splinting with a rigid or formable splint (Fig. 26-15)
3. Application of ice and elevation

Foot and Ankle Injury

Fractures and dislocations of the foot and ankle may result from a crush injury, a fall from a height, or a violent rotary force. The patient usually complains of point tenderness and is hesitant to bear weight on the extremity. Management includes:

1. Assessment of neurovascular status
2. Application of a formable splint, such as a pillow, blanket, or air splint (Fig. 26-16)
3. Application of ice
4. Elevation

Phalangeal Injury

Toe injuries often are caused by "stubbing" the toe on an immovable object. These injuries usually are managed by buddy taping the toe to an adjacent toe for support and immobilization. Management includes:

1. Assessment of neurovascular status
2. Buddy splinting

3. Application of ice
4. Elevation

Open Fractures

Patients with open fractures require special care and evaluation by the paramedic. Fractures may be open in two ways: *from within,* as when a bone fragment pierces the skin, or *from without* (e.g., after a gunshot wound). An open fracture also may have made contact with the skin some distance from the fracture site. Although most open fractures are obvious because of associated hemorrhage, a small puncture wound may not be immediately apparent and bleeding may be minimal. Therefore the paramedic must consider any soft tissue wound in the area of a suspected fracture to be evidence of an open fracture.

Open fractures are considered a true surgical emergency because of the potential for infection. Most authorities agree that open wounds associated with fractures should be covered with sterile, dry dressings. They should not be irrigated in the field or soaked with any type of antiseptic solution. Hemorrhage should be controlled with direct pressure and pressure dressings.

If a bone end or bone fragment is visible, it should be covered with a dry, sterile dressing and splinted. Bone ends that slip back into the wound during immobilization should be noted and reported to the receiving hospital so that surgical debridement can take place.

Straightening Angular Fractures and Reducing Dislocations

Angular fractures and dislocations may pose significant problems regarding splinting and, in some situations, patient extrication and transport. If the paramedic thinks it is necessary to attempt manipulation of a fracture or dislocation to facilitate transport or to improve circulation to the injured extremity, he or she should consult with medical direction.

✓ TRICKS OF THE TRADE

Always measure a splint against the uninjured extremity, especially if the fracture is angulated. Muscle spasm may cause the affected limb to shorten.

NOTE

Limb-threatening injuries include knee dislocation, fracture or dislocation of the ankle, and subcondylar fractures of the elbow.[1] These serious injuries require rapid transport for physician evaluation.

? CRITICAL THINKING

Aside from narcotic analgesics, what other drugs may be indicated to relieve muscle spasm, provide anesthesia, and relax the patient while reducing a dislocation or fracture?

As a rule, fractures and dislocated joints should be immobilized in the position of injury, and the patient transported to the emergency department for realignment (reduction). However, if transport is delayed or prolonged, an attempt to reposition a grossly deformed fracture or dislocated joint should be made if circulation is impaired. With the exception of the elbow, which should never be manipulated in the prehospital setting, a grossly deformed fracture or dislocation often can be realigned if necessary without causing additional damage or extreme discomfort to the patient. The injury should be handled carefully, and gentle, firm traction should be applied in the direction of the long axis of the extremity. If there is obvious resistance to alignment, the extremity should be splinted without repositioning.

Specific Techniques for Specific Joints

A brief description of specific techniques for realigning extremity injuries is provided in the following discussion.[1] Only *one* attempt at realignment should be made in the prehospital setting, *only if* there is severe neurovascular compromise (e.g., extremely weak or absent distal pulses), and *only* after consulting with medical direction. Manipulation (if indicated) should be performed as soon as possible after the injury and should be avoided in the presence of other severe injuries. If not contraindicated by other injuries, the use of analgesics (e.g., *midazolam* [Versed]) for the realignment procedure should be considered.

NOTE

The paramedic should always assess and document pulse, sensation, and motor function before and after manipulating any injured extremity or joint.

Finger Realignment

- Apply in-line traction along the shaft of the finger.
- Continue with slow and steady traction until the finger is realigned and the patient feels relief from pain.
- Immobilize the finger with a splint device or by buddy splinting.

Shoulder Realignment

- Attempt only in the absence of severe back injury.
- Check circulatory and sensory status.
- Apply slow, gentle longitudinal traction with countertraction exerted on the axilla.
- Slowly (and without force) bring the extremity to the midline and realign in the anatomical position while maintaining traction.
- Immobilize with a sling and swathe.

Hip Realignment

- Apply in-line traction along the shaft of the femur with the hip and knee flexed at 90 degrees.
- Continue with slow and steady traction to relax the muscle spasm. Successful realignment will be noted by a "pop" into the joint, a sudden relief of pain, and easy manipulation of the leg to full extension.
- Immobilize the leg in full extension with the patient positioned on a long spine board; reevaluate pulses and neurovascular status.
- If full extension is not achieved, immobilize the leg at a flexion not to exceed 90 degrees with pillows or blankets; place the patient supine.

Knee Realignment

- Apply gentle and steady traction while moving the injured joint into normal position.
- Successful realignment will be noted by a "pop" into the joint, loss of deformity, relief of pain, and increased mobility.

NOTE

A knee dislocation should not be confused with a patellar dislocation (a non–limb-threatening injury). An attempt to reposition a dislocation of the knee into anatomical position should be made if transport time is delayed or prolonged more than 2 hours, even if distal circulation is normal. Realignment should not be attempted if the dislocation is associated with other severe injuries.[1]

- Immobilize the leg in full extension (or slight flexion for comfort); position the patient supine on a long spine board.

Ankle Realignment

- Apply in-line traction on the talus while stabilizing the tibia.
- Successful realignment will be noted by a sudden rotation to a normal position.
- Immobilize the ankle in the same manner as for a fracture.

Referral of Patients with Minor Musculoskeletal Injury

Some patients with minor musculoskeletal injury (e.g., a minor sprain) will not require EMS transport. To make this determination, the paramedic should:

- Evaluate the need for immobilization.
- Evaluate the need for radiography based on the patient's condition and mechanism of injury.
- Evaluate the need for private physician assessment versus emergency department assessment based on the patient's condition and mechanism of injury.
- Consult with medical direction.

? CRITICAL THINKING

What should be documented on these calls?

Patients who are not transported to the hospital should receive advice on how to care for their injury (e.g., through an instruction sheet that explains the application of immobilization, elevation, cold, heat, rest, use of analgesics, and indications for physician follow-up). If there is any doubt about the seriousness of the patient's injury, he or she should be transported to the emergency department for physician evaluation.

✓ TRICKS OF THE TRADE

Part of the transport decision should include an assessment of the patient's current level of function compared with that person's normal level of function.

S U M M A R Y

- Injuries that can result from application of traumatic forces to the musculoskeletal system include fractures, sprains, strains, and joint dislocations. Problems associated with musculoskeletal injuries include hemorrhage, instability, loss of tissue, simple laceration and contamination, interruption of blood supply, and long-term disability.

- Several inflammatory and degenerative conditions may present or be complicated by extremity injury. These include bursitis, tendonitis, and arthritis.

- Common signs and symptoms of extremity trauma include pain on palpation or movement, swelling or deformity, crepitus, decreased range of motion, false movement, and decreased or absent sensory perception or circulation distal to the injury.

- Once the paramedic has assessed for life-threatening conditions, the extremity injury should be examined for pain, pallor, paresthesia, pulses, paralysis, and pressure. In addition, DCAP-BTLS should be evaluated for the injured extremity.

- Immobilization by splinting helps alleviate pain; decreases tissue injury, bleeding, and contamination in an open wound; and simplifies and facilitates transport of the patient. Splints can be categorized as rigid, soft or formable, and traction splints.

- Upper-extremity injuries can be classified as fractures or dislocations to the shoulder, humerus, elbow, radius and ulna, wrist, hand, and finger. Most upper-extremity injuries can be adequately immobilized by application of a sling and swathe.

- Lower-extremity injuries include fractures to the pelvis and fractures or dislocations to the hip, femur, knee and patella, tibia and fibula, ankle and foot, and phalanx.

- Although most open fractures are obvious because of associated hemorrhage, a small puncture wound may not be immediately apparent, and bleeding may be minimal. Therefore the paramedic must consider any soft tissue wound in the area of a suspected fracture to be evidence of an open fracture. Open fractures are considered a true surgical emergency because of the potential for infection.

- Only *one* attempt at realignment should be made in the prehospital setting, *only* if there is severe neurovascular compromise (e.g., extremely weak or absent distal pulses), and *only* after consulting with medical direction.

- The paramedic should evaluate the need for private physician assessment versus emergency department assessment based on the patient's condition and mechanism of injury.

REFERENCES

1. US Department of Transportation, National Highway Traffic Safety Administration: *EMT-Paramedic national standard curriculum*, Washington, DC, 1998, The Department.
2. Rosen P, Barkin R: *Emergency medicine: concepts and clinical practice*, ed 4, St Louis, 1998, Mosby.

Division Five ⟶

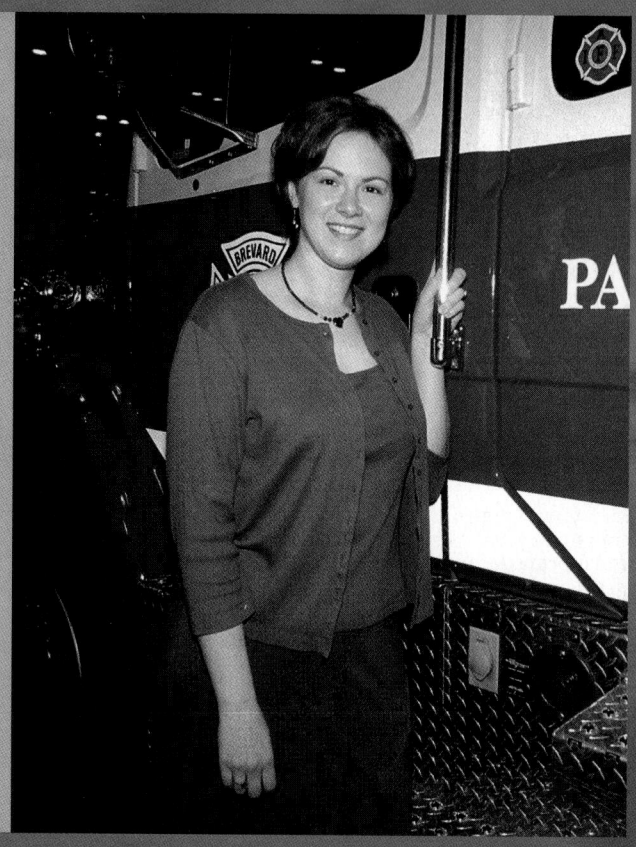

**Kimberly Davanzo,
EMT-PIC,
Flight Paramedic
Midwest Medflight
Ypsilanti, Michigan**

"The first cardiac arrest I experienced—it was on my first shift as a medic. We got a call for a GI bleed, but then the person went into full arrest. I started CPR, scared to death that I didn't know what I was doing. Suddenly, the patient reached up and grabbed my arm; we had brought him back. I'll always remember that as a one in a million call."

Medical

IN THIS DIVISION

27 Pulmonary

OBJECTIVES

Upon completion of this chapter, the paramedic student will be able to:

1. *Distinguish pathophysiology of respiratory emergencies related to ventilation, diffusion, and perfusion.*

2. *Describe causes, complications, signs and symptoms, and prehospital management of patients with a diagnosis of obstructive airway disease, pneumonia, adult respiratory distress syndrome, pulmonary thromboembolism, upper respiratory infection, spontaneous pneumothorax, hyperventilation syndrome, and lung cancer.*

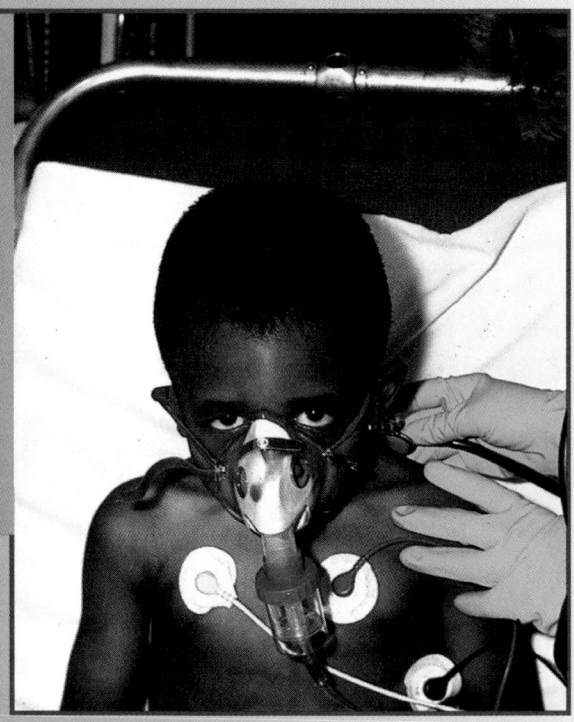

Respiratory emergencies are common in the prehospital setting, accounting for 28% of all chief complaints in all EMS calls.[1] Since more than 300,000 people die as a result of respiratory emergencies each year in the United States,[2] patients with respiratory emergencies require the highest priority of care. The paramedic must be able to quickly assess a patient with respiratory distress, identify the cause, initiate management, and provide appropriate care while en route to the hospital.

KEY TERMS

bronchiectasis: An abnormal dilation of the bronchi caused by a pus-producing infection of the bronchial wall.

hyperventilation syndrome: Abnormally deep or rapid breathing that results in excessive loss of carbon dioxide (producing respiratory alkalosis).

spontaneous pneumothorax: A condition that results when a subpleural bleb ruptures, allowing air to enter the pleural space from within the lung.

status asthmaticus: A severe, prolonged asthma exacerbation that has not been broken with repeated doses of bronchodilators.

NOTE

There are many different pulmonary diseases that act in a variety of different ways on a number of body systems. However, all respiratory problems (acute or chronic) can be categorized as impacting ventilation, diffusion, or perfusion. Management can be initiated rapidly and effectively once the problem has been identified as a ventilation, diffusion, or perfusion defect (or a combination of defects) (Table 27-1).

NOTE

Prevention strategies to avoid respiratory illness include smoking prevention/cessation programs, control of air pollution, and provision of smoke-free workplace and public locations. (See Appendix C.)

NOTE

The reader should refer to Chapters 6 and 11 to review upper and lower airway anatomy and related physiology of ventilation and respiration.

Pathophysiology

A variety of problems can impact the pulmonary system's ability to achieve gas exchange to provide for cellular needs and the excretion of wastes (see Chapters 6 and 11). Specific pathophysiologies that are responsible for respiratory emergencies include those related to ventilation, diffusion, and perfusion. Risk factors associated with the development of respiratory disease are listed in Box 27-1. The following discussion of physiology will serve as a review.

BOX 27-1

RISK FACTORS ASSOCIATED WITH THE DEVELOPMENT OF RESPIRATORY DISEASE

Intrinsic Factors

Genetic predisposition may influence the development of:

    Asthma
    Obstructive lung disease
    Cancer

Cardiac or circulatory pathologies may influence the development of:

    Pulmonary edema
    Pulmonary emboli

Stress may increase the:

    Severity of respiratory complaints
    Frequency of exacerbations of asthma and
        COPD

Extrinsic Factors

Smoking increases the:

    Prevalence of COPD and cancer
    Severity of virtually all respiratory
        disorders

Environmental pollutants increase the:

    Prevalence of COPD
    Severity of all obstructive airway
        disorders

TABLE 27-1	VENTILATION, DIFFUSION, AND PERFUSION DEFECTS

PROBLEM	EXAMPLE
Ventilation	
Upper airway obstruction	Foreign body, epiglottitis
Lower airway obstruction	Asthma, airway edema
Chest wall impairment	Trauma, muscular dystrophy
Neurogenic dysfunction	CNS depressant drugs, stroke
Diffusion	
Inadequate oxygen in ambient air	Fire environments, CO poisoning
Alveolar pathology	Lung disease, inhalation injury
Interstitial space pathology	Pulmonary edema, near-drowning
Capillary bed pathology	Severe atherosclerosis
Perfusion	
Inadequate blood volume or hemoglobin levels	Shock, anemia
Impaired circulatory blood flow	Pulmonary embolus
Capillary wall pathology	Trauma

Ventilation

Ventilation refers to the process of air movement in and out of the lungs. For ventilation to occur, the following must be intact:

- Neurological control to initiate ventilation
- Nerves between the brain stem and the muscles of respiration
- Functional diaphragm and intercostal muscles
- Patent upper airway
- Functional lower airway
- Alveoli that are functional and noncollapsed

Specific pathophysiologies associated with ventilation include upper and lower airway obstruction, chest wall impairment, and problems in neurological control. Emergency interventions for ventilation problems include ensuring that the upper and lower airways are open and unobstructed and providing assisted ventilations.

Diffusion

Diffusion refers to the process of gas exchange between the air-filled alveoli and the pulmonary capillary bed. Gas exchange is driven by simple diffusion in which gases move from areas of high concentration to areas of low concentration (until the concentrations are equal). For diffusion to occur, the following must be intact:

- Alveolar and capillary walls that are not thickened
- Interstitial space between the alveoli and capillary wall that is not enlarged or filled with fluid

Specific pathophysiologies associated with diffusion include inadequate oxygen concentration in ambient air, alveolar pathology, interstitial space pathology, and capillary bed pathology. Emergency interventions for diffusion problems include providing high-concentration oxygen and taking measures to reduce inflammation in the interstitial space.

Perfusion

Perfusion refers to the process of circulating blood through the pulmonary capillary bed. For perfusion to occur, the following must be intact:

- Adequate blood volume
- Adequate hemoglobin within the blood
- Pulmonary capillaries that are not occluded
- Properly functioning left side of the heart that provides smooth flow of blood through the pulmonary capillary bed

Specific pathophysiologies associated with perfusion include inadequate blood volume, impaired circulatory blood flow, and capillary wall pathology. Emergency interventions for perfusion problems include ensuring adequate circulating volumes and hemoglobin levels and optimizing left-sided heart function as necessary.

Assessment Findings

Pulmonary complaints may be associated with exposure to a wide variety of toxic environments that have deficient ambient oxygen. During scene size-up, it is critical to ensure a safe environment for all EMS personnel before initiating patient contact. Rescue personnel with specialized training and equipment should be utilized as necessary to ensure scene safety.

Initial Assessment

A major focus of the initial assessment is the recognition of life-threatening conditions. (A variety of pulmonary conditions offer a very real risk for patient death.) Recognition of life threats and the initiation of resuscitation take priority over detailed assessment. Signs of life-threatening respiratory distress in adults include:

- Alterations in mental status
- Severe cyanosis
- Absent breath sounds
- Audible stridor
- One- or two-word dyspnea
- Tachycardia
- Pallor and diaphoresis
- Presence of retractions and/or the use of accessory muscles to assist with breathing

Focused History and Physical Exam

The paramedic should ascertain the patient's chief complaints, which may include dyspnea, chest pain, productive or nonproductive cough, hemoptysis, wheezing, and signs of respiratory infection (e.g., fever, increased sputum production). The history should be focused on the patient's previous experiences with similar or identical symptoms. The patient's objective description of severity often is an accurate indicator of the severity of the present episode if the pathology is chronic.

> **NOTE**
>
> Asking the patient "what happened the last time you had an attack this bad?" is an extremely useful predictor of the current episode's course.

Known Pulmonary Diagnosis

If the diagnosis is not known to the paramedic, an effort should be made to learn whether it is primarily related to ventilation, diffusion, perfusion, or a combination of defects. After a history of the present illness is obtained, a medication history that includes current medications, medication allergies, cardiac medications, and pulmonary medications (e.g., inhaled, oral, or parenteral sympathomimetics; inhaled or oral corticosteroids; chromolyn sodium; methylxanthines; antibiotics) should be obtained.

> **NOTE**
>
> It is important to ask patients if intubation was ever required to manage their respiratory disease. A history of previous intubation is an accurate indicator of severe pulmonary disease and suggests that intubation may be required again.

Physical Examination

The physical examination begins with a general impression of the patient, noting the patient's position, mentation, ability to speak, respiratory effort, and skin color (see Chapter 14). Vital signs should be assessed with the following considerations[1]:

1. Pulse rate. Tachycardia is a sign of hypoxemia and may result from the use of sympathomimetic medications. Bradycardia with a pulmonary etiology is an ominous sign of severe hypoxemia and imminent cardiac arrest.
2. Blood pressure. Hypertension may result from the use of sympathomimetic medications.
3. Respiratory rate. The respiratory rate is not an accurate indicator of respiratory status unless it is very slow. Trends are essential in evaluating the patient with chronic respiratory disease. A slowing rate in the presence of an unimproved condition suggests exhaustion and impending respiratory insufficiency. Abnormal respiratory patterns (described in Chapter 11) that may be seen in patients with respiratory disease include eupnea, tachypnea, Cheyne-Stokes, central neurogenic hyperventilation, Kussmaul, ataxic, apneustic, and apnea.

The patient's face and neck should be assessed for the presence of pursed-lip breathing and use of accessory muscles. Pursed-lip breathing helps maintain pressure within the airways (even during exhalation) to support bronchial walls internally that have lost their external support as a result of disease. The use of accessory muscles can quickly result in respiratory fatigue. The patient should be questioned about sputum production. An increasing

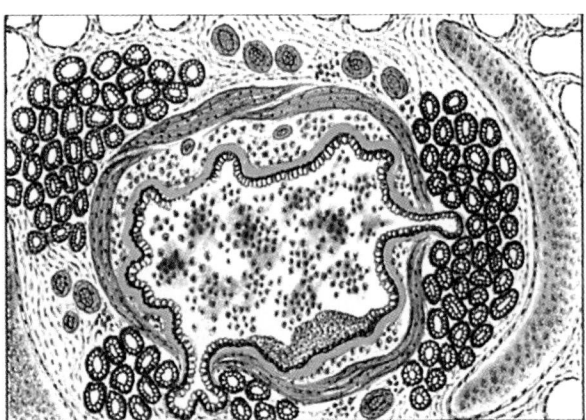

Fig. 27-1 Chronic bronchitis. Bronchi are filled with excess mucus. (From Wilson SF: *Respiratory disorders,* St Louis, 1990, Mosby.)

amount of sputum suggests infection. Thick, green, or brown sputum may indicate pneumonia; yellow or pale gray sputum may be related to allergic or inflammatory etiologies; pink, frothy sputum is associated with severe and late stages of pulmonary edema. The patient's neck should be evaluated for jugular vein distention that may accompany right-sided heart failure caused by severe pulmonary congestion.

The patient's chest should be inspected for injury and any indicators of chronic disease (such as a barrel chest from long-standing chronic obstructive pulmonary disease). Other components of the chest examination include noting accessory muscle use or retractions to facilitate breathing, evaluating chest wall symmetry, and auscultating the patient's lungs for normal and abnormal breath sounds.

The patient's extremities should be assessed for peripheral cyanosis, clubbing of the fingers, and carpopedal spasm. Peripheral cyanosis is caused by an excess of deoxygenated hemoglobin in the blood. Clubbing is an abnormal enlargement of distal phalanges that indicates long-standing chronic hypoxemia. Carpopedal spasm (spasms of the hands, thumbs, feet, or toes) often is associated with hypocapnia, resulting from long periods of rapid, deep respiration. All of these are important findings in a patient with respiratory disease and should be documented on the patient care report and communicated to medical direction.

Diagnostic Testing

Diagnostic testing that may be appropriate for some patients with respiratory disease includes the use of pulse oximetry, peak flow meters, and capnometry. Pulse oximeters measure oxygen saturation. Peak flow meters (described later in this chapter) provide a baseline assessment of airflow for patients with obstructive lung disease. Capnometry can provide an ongoing assessment of endotracheal tube position in patients who require intubation (see Chapter 11).

Obstructive Airway Disease

Obstructive airway disease is a major health problem in the United States, affecting some 17 million Americans.[2] Predisposing factors that contribute to obstructive pulmonary disease include smoking, environmental pollution, industrial exposures, and various pulmonary infectious processes. Obstructive airway disease is a triad of distinct diseases that often coexist: chronic bronchitis and emphysema (together referred to as *COPD*) and asthma. Although these diseases are presented separately in this chapter, the paramedic should remember that different degrees of each frequently are present in the same patient.

> **? CRITICAL THINKING**
>
> **Will patients with COPD always be able to "name" their disease when you ask about their history?**

Chronic Bronchitis

Chronic bronchitis is a clinical description that refers to inflammatory changes and excessive mucus production in the bronchial tree (Fig. 27-1). It affects about 20% of men in the United States and is characterized by hyperplasia and hypertrophy of mucus-producing glands that results from prolonged exposure to irritants (most commonly, cigarette smoke). The condition clinically is diagnosed by the presence of cough with sputum production occurring on most days for at least 3 months of the year and for at least 2 consecutive years.[1] The alveoli are not seriously affected, and diffusion remains relatively normal.

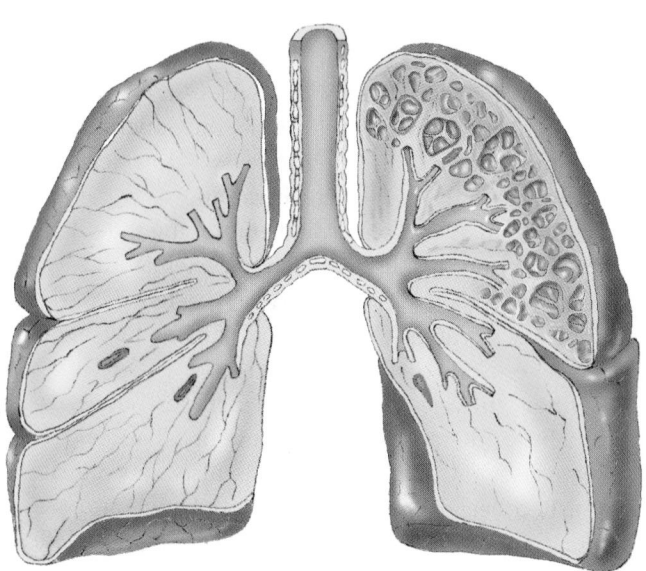

Fig. 27-2 Cystic changes of lobar emphysema resulting from destruction of alveoli. (From Wilson SF: *Respiratory disorders*, St Louis, 1990, Mosby.)

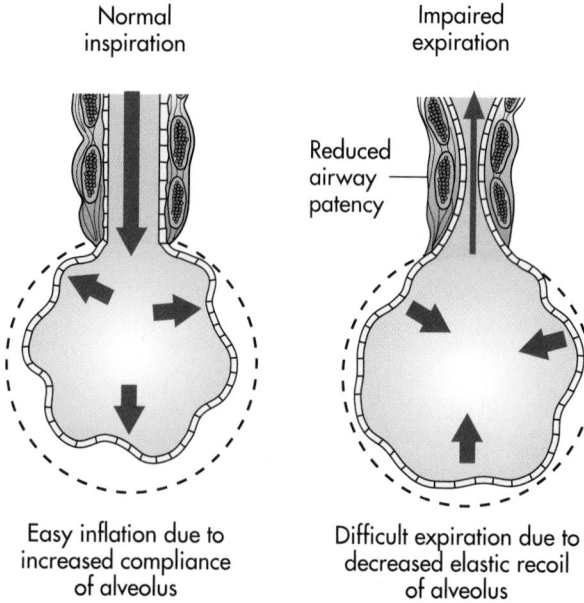

Normal inspiration

Impaired expiration

Reduced airway patency

Easy inflation due to increased compliance of alveolus

Difficult expiration due to decreased elastic recoil of alveolus

Fig. 27-3 Mechanisms of air trapping in COPD: Mucus plugs and narrowed airways cause air trapping and hyperinflation on expiration. During inspiration, the airways enlarge, allowing gas to flow past the obstruction. This mechanism of air trapping occurs in asthma and chronic bronchitis. Mechanism of air trapping in emphysema: Damaged or destroyed alveolar walls no longer support and hold open the airways, and alveoli lose their property of elastic recoil. Both of these factors contribute to collapse during expiration. (From Wilson SF: *Respiratory disorders*, St Louis, 1990, Mosby.)

Patients with severe chronic bronchitis (sometimes called *blue bloaters* when they appear cyanotic) have a low oxygen pressure (PO_2) because of altered ventilation-perfusion relationships in the lung and hypoventilation. The hypoventilation leads to hypercapnia, hypoxemia, and increases in arterial carbon dioxide pressure (PCO_2). Patients with chronic bronchitis have frequent respiratory infections that eventually result in scarring of lung tissue. In time, irreversible changes occur in the lung, which may lead to emphysema or **bronchiectasis** (an abnormal dilation of the bronchi caused by a pus-producing infection of the bronchial wall).

Emphysema

Emphysema is an anatomical description of pathological changes in the lung; it is the end stage of a process that progresses slowly for many years. The disease is characterized by permanent abnormal enlargement of the air spaces beyond the terminal bronchioles, destruction of the alveoli, and failure of the supporting structures to maintain alveolar integrity (Fig. 27-2). Besides reducing the alveolar functional surface area, it reduces elasticity, leading

to trapping of air. Thus residual volume increases while vital capacity remains relatively normal.

The associated reduction in arterial PO_2 leads to increased red blood cell production and polycythemia (an elevated hematocrit value). This elevation in hematocrit is much more common in the "blue bloater" (patient with chronic bronchitis) than in the "pink puffer" (patient with predominantly emphysema) because the former is more often chronically hypoxemic. Decreases in alveolar membrane surface area and in the number of pulmonary capillaries in the lung decrease the area for gas exchange and increase resistance to pulmonary blood flow.

Patients with emphysema have some resistance to airflow in and out of the lungs, but most of the hyperexpansion results from air trapping secondary to the loss of elastic recoil (Fig. 27-3). Patients with chronic bronchitis have increased airway resistance during inspiration and expiration, whereas patients with emphysema have increased airway resistance only on expiration. Normally an involuntary act, expiration becomes a muscular act in patients with COPD. Over time, the chest becomes rigid (barrel shaped), and the patient must use accessory muscles of the neck, chest, and abdomen to breathe. Full deflation of the lungs becomes increasingly difficult and finally impossible. Often, the patient with emphysema is thin because of poor dietary intake and the increased caloric consumption required for the work of breathing (Table 27-2).

? CRITICAL THINKING

What effect might application of a cervical collar, short spine board or vest, and immobilization supine on a long backboard have on a patient with COPD who has sustained trauma?

NOTE

Patients with emphysema often develop bullae (thin-walled cystic lesions in the lung) from the destruction of alveolar walls. When bullae collapse, they increase the diffusion defect seen with these patients and can lead to pneumothorax.

Assessment

Patients with COPD generally are aware of and have adapted to their illness. A request for emergency care indicates that a significant change has occurred in the patient's condition. The patient with COPD usually presents with an acute episode of worsening dyspnea that is manifested even at rest, an increase or change in sputum production, or an increase in the malaise that accompanies the disease. Other common complaints include inability to sleep and recurrent headaches.

On EMS arrival, the patient with COPD is likely to be in respiratory distress. Often, the patient is sitting upright and leaning forward to facilitate breathing, using pursed-lip breathing to maintain positive airway pressures, and employing the use of accessory muscles. Increases in hypoxemia and hypercarbia may be evidenced by tachypnea, diaphoresis, cyanosis, confusion, irritability, and drowsiness.

Other physical findings include wheezes, rhonchi, and crackles (described in Chapter 13). Breath sounds and heart sounds also may be diminished because of reduced air exchange and the increased diameter of the thoracic cavity. In late stages of decompensation, the patient may have peripheral cyanosis, clubbing of the fingers, and signs of right-sided heart failure. The patient's ECG may reveal cardiac dysrhythmias or signs of atrial enlargement (see Chapter 28).

Management

The primary goal of prehospital care for these patients is correction of hypoxemia through improved airflow. This can be accomplished through oxygen administration and pharmacological therapy. This therapy can produce serious side effects and complications, particularly if the patient has used medication before EMS arrival. Therefore it is important for the paramedic to obtain a thorough medical history regarding medication use, home oxygen use, and drug allergies.

All patients in respiratory distress should have an IV line established and a cardiac monitor applied. If the patient has a productive cough, cough-

TABLE 27-2	COMPARISON OF SIGNS AND SYMPTOMS OF EMPHYSEMA AND CHRONIC BRONCHITIS	
EMPHYSEMA		**CHRONIC BRONCHITIS**
Thin, barrel-chest appearance		Typically overweight
Nonproductive cough		Productive cough with sputum
Wheezing and rhonchi		Coarse rhonchi
Pink complexion		Chronic cyanosis
Extreme dyspnea or exertion		Mild, chronic dyspnea
Prolonged inspiration (purse-lip breathing)		Resistance on inspiration and expiration

ing should be encouraged. Any sputum should be collected and delivered with the patient for laboratory analysis.

Some patients with COPD rely on a hypoxic drive for their ventilatory effort; however, *the paramedic should never withhold oxygen because of fear of decreasing hypoxic drive while providing emergency care in the prehospital setting.* High-concentration oxygen should be administered via a nonrebreather mask if indicated. Pulse oximetry to measure oxygen saturation should be considered. Some of these patients will require ventilatory assistance.

Medications used in the prehospital setting to relieve bronchospasm and reduce constricted airways are beta agonists such as *metaproterenol* (Alupent) and *albuterol* (Proventil). Other drugs that may be given after physician evaluation include steroids (*methylprednisolone* [Solu-Medrol]), nebulized anticholinergics (e.g., *atropine*), and occasionally methylxanthines such as *aminophylline* (Amoline) for bronchodilation and stimulation of the respiratory drive[3] (Box 27-2). (See the Emergency Drug Index for specific drug therapy.)

TRICKS OF THE TRADE

If your patient needs to use a nebulizer and cannot follow directions or self-administer the medication, pull the reservoir mask from a nonrebreather mask and attach the nebulizer. This allows the patient to inhale the prescribed medication without having to hold onto the apparatus.

Asthma

Asthma, or reactive airway disease, is a common disorder that affects 10 to 15 million Americans (4% to 5% of the U.S. population) and is responsible for 4000 to 5000 deaths each year.[3] Asthma is most common in children and young adults but can occur in any decade of life. Exacerbating factors tend to be extrinsic in children and intrinsic in adults (Fig. 27-4). Childhood asthma often improves or resolves with age, but adult asthma usually is persistent.

Pathophysiology of an Asthma Exacerbation

Asthma generally occurs in acute episodes of variable duration, between which the patient is relatively symptom free. The exacerbation is character-

ized by reversible airflow obstruction caused by bronchial smooth muscle contraction; hypersecretion of mucus, resulting in bronchial plugging; and inflammatory changes in the bronchial walls. With increased resistance to airflow, there is alveolar hypoventilation, marked ventilation-perfusion mismatching (leading to hypoxemia), and carbon dioxide retention (stimulating hyperventilation) (Fig. 27-5). The obstruction of inspiration and marked obstruction of expiration results in positive end expiratory pressure *(auto-PEEP)* secondary to air trapping.

During an acute asthma exacerbation, the combination of increased airway resistance, increased respiratory drive, and air trapping creates excessive demand on the muscles of respiration. This leads to greater accessory muscle use and increases the potential for respiratory fatigue. If labored breathing continues, excessive positive intrathoracic pressure may decrease left ventricular preload. The result is a transient reduction in cardiac output and systolic blood pressure, with the subsequent physical findings of pulsus paradoxus. If the episode continues unabated, hypoxemia and the hemodynamic alterations may lead to death (near-fatal asthma). In the prehospital setting, cardiac arrest in patients with severe asthma has been linked to[4]:

- Severe bronchospasm and mucous plugging leading to asphyxia (the most common cause of asthma-related death)
- Cardiac dysrhythmias due to hypoxia
- Tension pneumothorax (often bilateral)

Other conditions that may be present in patients with near-fatal asthma include cardiac disease,

---

NOTE

Most asthma-related deaths occur outside the hospital.

BOX 27-2

PHARMACOLOGICAL AGENTS FOR COPD

Adrenergic stimulants
Albuterol
Metaproterenol
Atropine
Magnesium

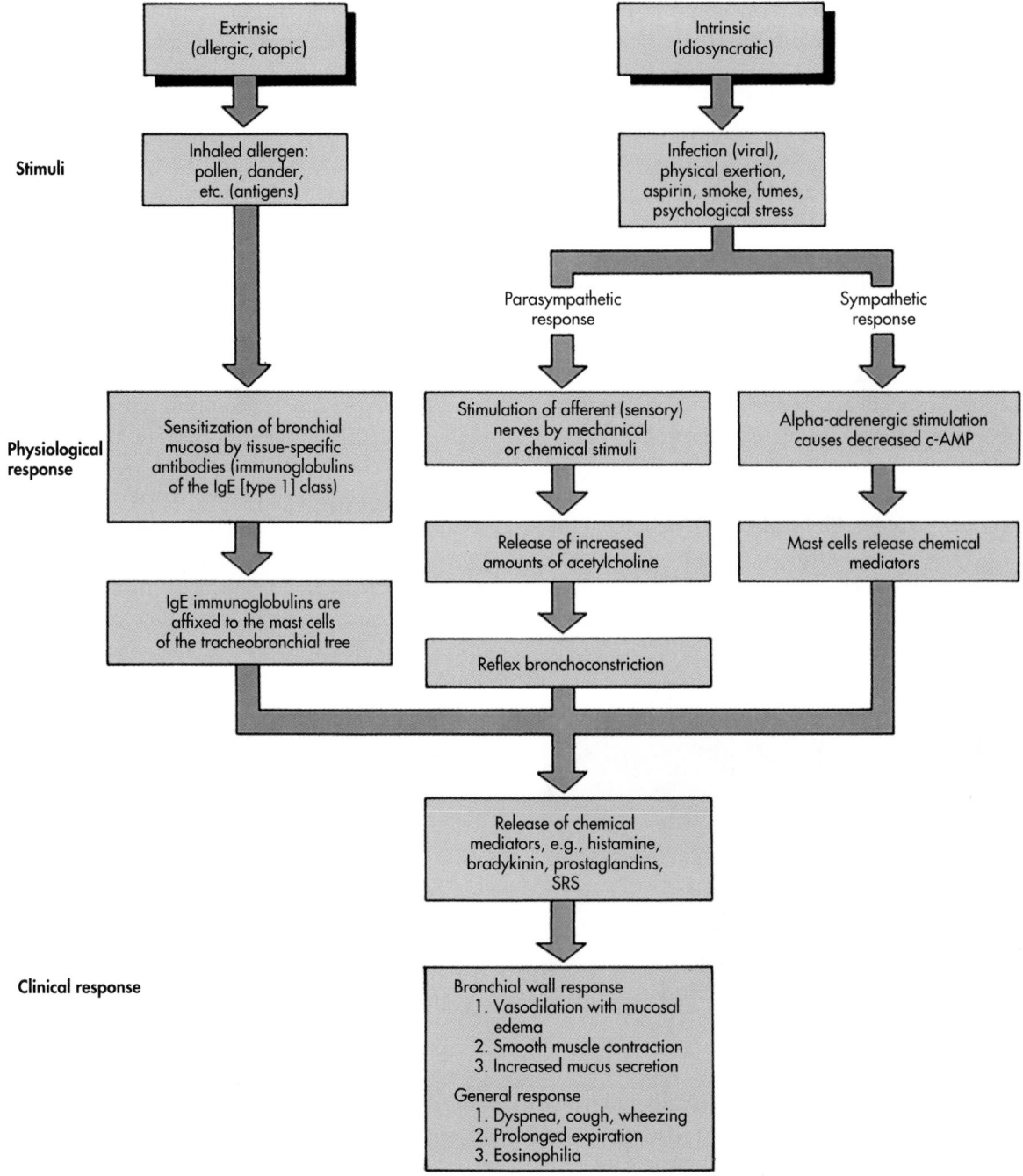

Fig. 27-4 Proposed pathogenesis of extrinsic and intrinsic bronchial asthma. (From Wilson SF: *Respiratory disorders,* St Louis, 1990, Mosby.)

pulmonary disease, acute allergic bronchospasm or anaphylaxis, drug use/misuse (beta blockers, cocaine and opiates), and recent discontinuation of long-term corticosteroids therapy (associated with adrenal insufficiency).

NOTE

Caution: Thoracic decompression in a patient with severe refractory asthma *without* pneumothorax might puncture the visceral pleura of the hyperinflated lung, producing a pneumothorax (most likely under tension).[5]

Assessment

On EMS arrival, the patient usually is sitting upright, leaning forward with hands on knees (tripod position), and using accessory muscles to facilitate breathing. The typical asthmatic is in obvious respiratory distress, with rapid and loud respirations. Audible wheezing may be present. The patient's mental status should be noted and monitored carefully. Lethargy, exhaustion, agitation, and confusion are ominous signs of impending respiratory failure. An initial history must be quickly obtained. Questions regarding the onset, relative severity, medication use, allergies, and precipitating cause of the exacerbation should be specific and to the point.

> **NOTE**
>
> It is important to ascertain if the patient previously required intubation to manage his or her asthma.

On auscultation, there may be a prolonged expiratory phase, usually with wheezing from the movement of air through the narrowed airways. Inspiratory wheezing (unlike inspiratory stridor) does not indicate upper airway occlusion but suggests that the large and midsize muscular airways are obstructed to a greater degree than if only expiratory wheezes are heard. Inspiratory wheezes also may suggest large airway secretions. A silent chest may indicate such severe obstruction that flow rates are too low to generate breath sounds. Other signs of severe asthma include:

- Findings of obtundation
- Diaphoresis and pallor
- Retractions
- Inability to speak after only one or two words
- Poor, floppy muscle tone
- Pulse rate greater than 130 beats per minute
- Respirations greater than 30 breaths per minute

> **NOTE**
>
> Asthma exacerbations are true medical emergencies. Management should be aggressive. Deterioration can be expected, rapid, and fatal, so the paramedic's observation of the patient must be vigilant. Initial patient management should be directed at ensuring an adequate airway, providing supplemental oxygen, and reversing the bronchospasm.

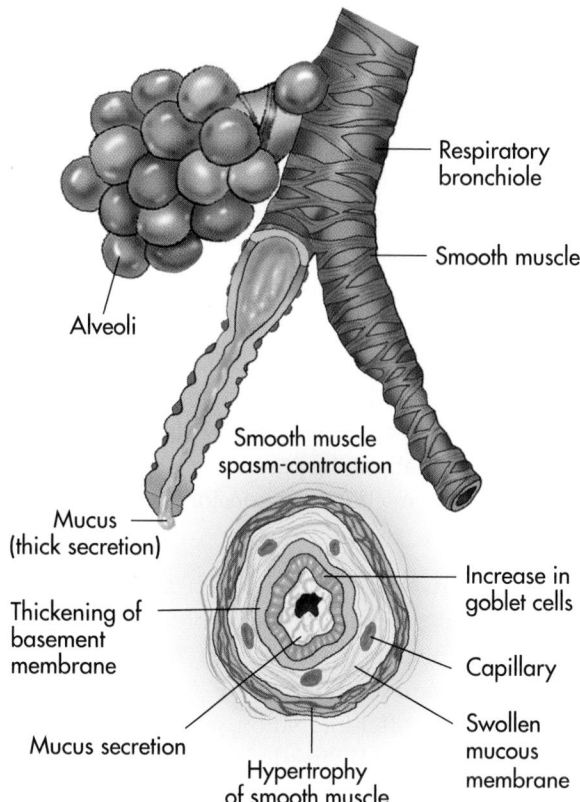

Fig. 27-5 With bronchial asthma, the bronchiole is obstructed on expiration, particularly by muscle spasm, edema of the mucosa, and thick secretions. (From Wilson SF: *Respiratory disorders,* St Louis, 1990, Mosby.)

- Pulsus paradoxus greater than 20 mm Hg
- Altered mental status or severe agitation

Management

After providing high-concentration oxygen, pharmacological therapy is based on the patient's age and medication use before EMS arrival. The initial medications prescribed by medical direction will probably be those with a short onset of action (e.g., **Albuterol** [Proventil, Ventolin]). Other medications that may be used to manage asthma are listed in Box 27-3. Medical direction also may prescribe rehydration through the administration of IV fluids. All patients with acute asthma should be transported in a position of comfort

> **? CRITICAL THINKING**
>
> *What options do you have to promote bronchodilation if the patient is unable to hold the nebulizer mouthpiece or needs to be ventilated using a bag-valve device?*

NOTE

Albuterol (Proventil, Ventolin) is the current cornerstone of asthma treatment in the United States. It stimulates beta-adrenergic receptors and thus acts as a rapid bronchodilator. Side effects include transient tachycardia and tremor.

to maximize the use of respiratory muscles and monitored for cardiac rhythm disturbances.

In some cases, endotracheal intubation will be required to manage the airway of a patient with a severe asthma exacerbation. If a conscious patient requires ET intubation, the paramedic should consult with medical direction and consider the following critical points[4]:

- Provide adequate sedation with *ketamine* (Ketalor), a benzodiazepine, or barbiturate.
- Paralyze the patient with *succinylcholine* (Anectine) or *vecuronium* (Pavulon)
- Immediately after intubation, give 2.5 to 5 mg *albuterol* (Proventil) directly into the ET tube
- Confirm ET tube placement with primary and secondary confirmation methods (described in Chapter 11)
- Ventilate at 8 to 10 breaths per minute to allow for the escape of air and to avoid sudden hypotension (especially in elderly patients with emphysema)

NOTE

Tracheal intubation only supports the patient's failing ventilatory efforts—it does not solve the problem.

BOX 27-3

ASTHMA MEDICATIONS

Nebulized Beta$_2$ Agonists
    Albuterol (Proventil, Ventolin, Salbutamol)
    Metoproterenol (Alupent)
IV Corticosteroids
    Methylprednisone (Solu-Medrol)
    Hydrocortisone
IV Aminophylline
IV **Magnesium Sulfate**
SQ or IM **Epinephrine** (Adrenalin) or Terbutaline (Brethine)
Ketamine (Ketalar)
Heliox (helium:oxygen)

NOTE

Even after tracheal intubation, the patient's lungs may continue to be difficult to ventilate. The absence of any significant obstruction to airflow immediately after tracheal intubation suggests that the diagnosis of acute asthma may have been incorrect, and the problem may be in the upper airway.[4]

Pulmonary function tests. Pulmonary function tests to measure peak expiratory flow rate (PEFR) can help determine the severity of an asthma exacerbation and evaluate the effectiveness of management in reversing airway obstruction. Peak flow meters (Fig. 27-6) can be used in the prehospital setting for this purpose. Their use requires a cooperative patient (who can make a maximal respiratory effort) and coaching by the paramedic.

To determine baseline airflow (before drug administration), the patient is instructed to fully inflate the lungs and forcefully exhale into the flow meter. The reading is then compared with standard tables based on height, sex, and race. The measurement is repeated throughout the course of management to evaluate the patient's response to drug therapy.

NOTE

Most children less than 5 years of age cannot adequately perform PEFR tests. This test also should not be performed in a patient with severe respiratory distress. Drug therapy to reverse the bronchospasm is the priority.

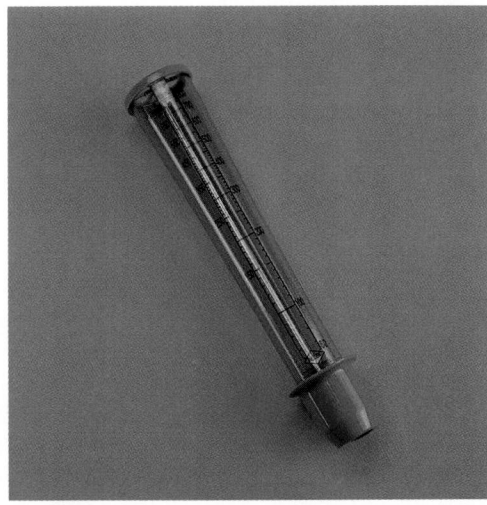

Fig. 27-6 Peak flow meter.

Status Asthmaticus

Status asthmaticus refers to a severe, prolonged asthma exacerbation that has not been broken with repeated doses of bronchodilators. It may be of sudden onset (resulting from spasm of the airways), or it may be more insidious. Frequently it is precipitated by a viral respiratory infection or prolonged exposure to allergen(s). Status asthmaticus is a true emergency that requires early recognition and immediate transport. These patients are in imminent danger of respiratory failure.

> ### ? CRITICAL THINKING
>
> *When a patient being managed for status asthmaticus is reassessed, would decreasing respiratory and heart rates indicate a good or bad outcome? Why?*

Patient management guidelines for status asthmaticus are the same as those for acute asthma exacerbations, but the urgency of rapid transport is more important. In addition, these patients usually are dehydrated and require IV fluid administration. The patient's respiratory status should be closely monitored, high-concentration oxygen should be administered, and the need for intubation and aggressive ventilatory support should be anticipated. Continuous bronchodilator therapy may be ordered by medical direction to manage these patients.

Differential Considerations

Although wheezing commonly is associated with asthma, it also may be present with other diseases that cause dyspnea (Table 27-3). For example, tachypnea, wheezing, and respiratory distress may indicate heart failure, pneumonia, pulmonary edema, pulmonary embolism, pneumothorax, toxic inhalation, foreign body aspiration, and various other pathological states. Only through gathering a complete history and performing a thorough patient assessment can appropriate emergency care decisions be made.

> **NOTE**
>
> Wheezes may be present in *all* types of obstructive lung disease.

> ✓ **TRICKS OF THE TRADE**
>
> Never take a patient suffering from asthma for granted. These patients can "crash" rapidly. Asthma is a complicated disease and should be approached with trepidation.

> **NOTE**
>
> The frequency of community-acquired pneumonia (an infection acquired from the environment, including infections acquired indirectly from the use of medications) has risen in recent years as a result of the increased percentage of the population over age 65 and the increasing number of patients taking immunosuppressive drugs for the treatment of malignancy, transplantation, or autoimmune disease.

Pneumonia

Pneumonia is a group of specific infections (not a single disease) that cause an acute inflammatory process of the respiratory bronchioles and the alveoli; it is the fifth most common cause of death from infectious disease in the United States[1] (Fig. 27-7). Pneumonia can be caused by bacterial, viral, or

TABLE 27-3	DISEASES AND SYMPTOMS ASSOCIATED WITH WHEEZING
DISEASE	**ASSOCIATED SYMPTOMS**
Asthma	Productive cough, tightness in chest
Bacterial pneumonia	Productive cough, pleuritic pain
Chronic bronchitis	Chronic, productive cough
Emphysema	Cough
Foreign body aspiration	Cough
Heart failure	Cough, orthopnea, nocturnal dyspnea
Pneumothorax	Sudden, sharp pleuritic pain
Pulmonary congestion	Tachypnea, cough
Pulmonary embolism	Sudden, sharp pleuritic pain
Toxic inhalation	Cough, pain

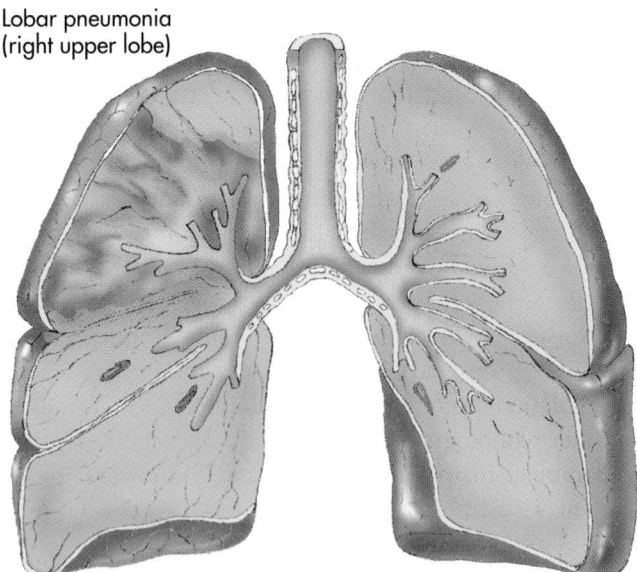

Lobar pneumonia
(right upper lobe)

Pneumococcal pneumonia

Fig. 27-7 Pneumonia is an inflammatory process of the respiratory bronchioles and alveoli that is caused by infection. (From Wilson SF: *Respiratory disorders*, St Louis, 1990, Mosby.)

fungal infection; associated risk factors include cigarette smoking, alcoholism, exposure to cold, and extremes of age (the very young and very old). These diseases may be spread by droplets or contact with infected persons or through aspiration of bacteria from one's own nasopharynx. Pneumonia may be classified as viral, bacterial, mycoplasmal, or aspiration pneumonia.

Viral Pneumonia

Influenza A is the most common type of viral pneumonia (see the box in the right column). It often occurs as epidemics in populations of small groups such as schoolchildren, army recruits, and nursing home residents. The interstitial infection caused by

NOTE

Pneumonia generally presents with classic signs and symptoms (typical pneumonia) that include a productive cough, pleuritic chest pain, and fever that produces "shaking chills." It also may present with nonspecific complaints (particularly in older adults and debilitated patients) that include a nonproductive cough, headache, fatigue, and sore throat (atypical pneumonia).

INFLUENZA

Influenza is a generalized, acute, febrile disease associated with upper and lower respiratory tract viral infection. It usually is characterized by the abrupt onset of a severe and protracted cough, fever, headache, myalgia, and mild sore throat. Of all the viruses, influenza and parainfluenza viruses are the most common causes of serious respiratory infections and have significant morbidity and mortality rates.

Influenza viruses A, B, and C (and their many mutagenic strains) are known for their potential to cause respiratory infections rapidly after exposure (usually within 24 to 48 hours). The viruses are inhaled in aerosolized mucus droplets from infected persons and are deposited on and penetrate the surface of upper respiratory tract mucosal cells. The virus-containing exudate eventually spreads to the lower respiratory tract, causing interstitial inflammation and destruction of the ciliated epithelium. The impaired mucociliary clearance often leads to a secondary bacterial infection, which may result in pneumonia or acute respiratory failure, particularly in patients with chronic lung disease.

Influenza is particularly significant because of the potential for widespread epidemics of the disease in high-risk populations (e.g., adults and children with chronic cardiorespiratory or metabolic disorders, residents of nursing homes and other institutions, health care workers). Current vaccines with minimal side effects are effective against some strains of the virus. If uncomplicated, influenza is self-limiting. Acute symptoms last 2 to 7 days and are followed by a convalescent period of about 1 week.

the virus predisposes the patient to secondary bacterial pneumonia.

Bacterial Pneumonia

The pneumococcus bacillus (*Streptococcus pneumoniae*) accounts for 90% of bacterial pneumonias. It affects 1 in 500 persons annually, with a peak incidence in winter and early spring. A vaccine now available is 80% to 90% effective against this type of pneumonia in adults. Bacterial pneumonia can result from aspiration of oropharyngeal contents. Thus patients in a coma or with seizures, suppressed cough reflex, and increased secretions are predisposed to develop the disease. Other predisposing risk factors that may contribute to the development of bacterial pneumonia include:

- Infection
    Upper respiratory infection (influenza)
    Postoperative infection
- Foreign body aspiration
- Alcohol or other drug addiction
- Cardiac failure
- Stroke
- Syncope
- Pulmonary embolism
- Chronic illness
    Chronic respiratory disease
    Diabetes mellitus
    Congestive heart failure
- Prolonged immobilization
- Compromised immune status

Mycoplasmal Pneumonia

Mycoplasmal pneumonia is caused by infection with *Mycoplasma pneumoniae.* Exposure to the organism causes mild upper respiratory infection in school-age children and young adults. Transmission is believed to be through infected respiratory secretions, so the condition spreads quickly among family members. This form of pneumonia may be treated effectively with antibiotics such as erythromycin, macrolide antibiotics (which include azithromycin [Zithromax] and clarithromycin [Biaxin]), and the newest fluoroquinolones (levofloxacin [Levaquin]).

> **NOTE**
>
> EMS personnel should consider receiving pneumonia vaccines to protect against infection.

Aspiration Pneumonia

Aspiration pneumonia is an inflammation of the lung parenchyma resulting from introduction of foreign material into the tracheobronchial tree. The syndrome is common in patients who have an altered level of consciousness (e.g., from head injury, seizure activity, use of alcohol or other drugs, anesthesia, infection, shock), intubated patients, and those who have aspirated foreign bodies. Factors common to victims of aspiration include depression of the cough or gag reflex, inability of the patient to

handle secretions or gastric contents, and alterations in physiological mechanisms to protect the airway.

Aspiration pneumonia may be nonbacterial (e.g., after aspiration of stomach contents, toxic materials, or inert substances), which typically is called *pneumonitis* to distinguish it from infectious pneumonia, or bacterial (as a secondary complication). Bacterial aspiration pneumonia has a poor prognosis, even with antibiotic therapy.

Management

The pathophysiology of pneumonia depends on the etiological agent. In viral and mycoplasmal pneumonias, the inflammatory response in the bronchi damages the ciliated epithelium, causing congestion and, in some cases, hemorrhage. Signs and symptoms include chest pain, cough, fever, dyspnea, and occasionally hemoptysis. Patients usually complain of general malaise and upper respiratory and gastrointestinal symptoms. Auscultation of the chest may reveal wheezing and fine crackles. In uncomplicated cases, symptoms usually abate in 7 to 10 days.

Bacterial pneumonia begins with infection in the alveoli that progressively fills the alveoli with fluid and purulent sputum. As the infection spreads from alveolus to alveolus, large areas of the lung, sometimes entire lobes, may become consolidated (filled with fluid and cellular debris). Consolidation reduces the available surface area of respiratory membranes and decreases the ventilation-perfusion ratio, both of which may lead to hypoxemia. Patients with bacterial pneumonia usually have acute shaking chills, tachypnea, tachycardia, cough, and sputum production. The sputum may be rust colored (classic for pneumococcus) but more commonly is yellow, green, or gray. Additional symptoms include malaise, anorexia, flank or back pain, and vomiting. If the disease is uncomplicated and treated with antibiotics, the patient begins to recover within 3 to 5 days, although antibiotics usually are continued for a total of 7 to 10 days.

The physiological effects of aspiration pneumonia are based on the volume and pH of the aspirated substances. If the pH is below 2.5, as may occur in the aspiration of stomach contents, atelectasis, pulmonary edema, hemorrhage, and cell necrosis may occur. In addition, the alveolar-capillary membrane may be damaged, leading to exudation and, in severe cases, adult respiratory distress syndrome (described later on this page). Patient presentation varies with the scenario and the severity of the insult (e.g., near-drowning, foreign body aspiration, aspiration of gastric contents). Clinical features may include dyspnea, cough, bronchospasm, wheezes, rhonchi, crackles, cyanosis, and pulmonary and cardiac insufficiency. Of these patients, 25% to 45% develop pulmonary infection.

? CRITICAL THINKING

What measures can the paramedic take to minimize the patient's risk of aspiration?

Prehospital care for patients with pneumonia includes airway support, oxygen administration, ventilatory assistance as needed, IV fluids to support blood pressure and to thin and loosen mucus, cardiac monitoring, and transport for physician evaluation. (Bronchodilator therapy also may be indicated for some patients.) In cases of aspiration, suctioning of the airway may be required. General patient management usually includes bed rest, analgesics, decongestants, expectorants, antipyretics, and antibiotic therapy. In severe cases, bronchoscopy and mechanical ventilation may be part of definitive patient care.

Adult Respiratory Distress Syndrome

Adult respiratory distress syndrome (ARDS) is a fulminant form of respiratory failure characterized by acute lung inflammation and diffuse alveolar-capillary injury.[6] All disorders that result in ARDS cause severe pulmonary edema. The syndrome develops as a complication of injury or illness such as trauma, gastric aspiration, cardiopulmonary bypass surgery, gram-negative sepsis, multiple blood transfusions, oxygen toxicity, toxic inhalation, drug overdose, pneumonia, and infections. Regardless of the specific cause, increased capillary permeability (high-permeability noncardiogenic pulmonary edema) results in a clinical condition in which the lungs are wet and heavy, congested, hemorrhagic, and stiff, with decreased perfusion capacity across alveolar membranes. As a result, there is a decrease in pulmonary compliance, requiring higher airway pressure for each breath.

NOTE

Cardiogenic pulmonary edema (high-pressure pulmonary edema) is discussed in Chapter 28.

The pulmonary edema associated with ARDS leads to severe hypoxemia, intrapulmonary shunting, reduced lung compliance, and, in some cases, irreversible parenchymal lung damage. Unique to this syndrome is that most patients who develop this condition have healthy lungs before the event that caused the disease. ARDS is more common in men than in women and has a mortality rate of over 65%. Complications include respiratory failure, cardiac dysrhythmias, disseminated intravascular coagulation, barotrauma, congestive heart failure, and renal failure.

Management

All patients with ARDS should be given high-concentration oxygen and ventilatory support. Depending on the underlying cause of ARDS, prehospital management may include fluid replacement to maintain cardiac output and peripheral perfusion, drug therapy to support mechanical ventilation, the use of pharmacological agents such as corticosteroids to stabilize pulmonary, capillary, and alveolar walls and diuretics (all of these treatments are controversial).

Patients with ARDS usually have tachypnea, labored breathing, and impaired gas exchange 12 to 72 hours after the initial injury or medical crisis. Because the syndrome often is a complication of another illness or injury, the paramedic should consider the pathophysiology of the underlying problem and provide supplemental oxygen and ventilatory support to improve arterial oxygenation (assessed by pulse oximetry). Most patients with moderate to severe respiratory distress require me-

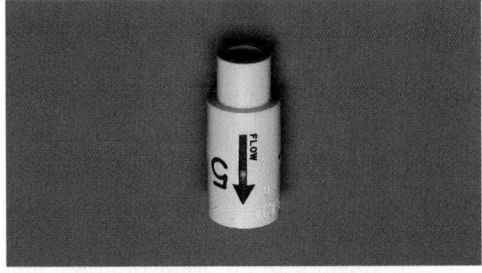

Fig. 27-8 Boehringer valve. (Courtesy Boehringer Laboratories, Inc., Norristown, Pa.)

chanical ventilatory support with positive end-expiratory pressure (PEEP) or continuous positive airway pressure (CPAP), both of which provide positive-pressure ventilation. Both PEEP and CPAP increase PO_2 by decreasing intrapulmonary shunting and ventilation-perfusion mismatch.

> **NOTE**
>
> PEEP and CPAP may produce adverse circulatory effects, including decreased venous return, decreased cardiac output, and pulmonary barotrauma. This type of ventilatory support requires special training and authorization from medical direction.

Positive End-Expiratory Pressure

PEEP maintains a degree of positive pressure at the end of exhalation to keep alveoli open and to push fluid from the alveoli back into the interstitium or capillaries. Ventilatory support with PEEP can be accomplished in the prehospital setting through intubation and the use of a Boehringer valve, a cylinder in which a metal ball is suspended (Fig. 27-8). The Boehringer valve is connected to the expiratory port of a bag-valve device and creates PEEP by forcing the patient to exhale against the weight of the metal ball (available in 5-, 10-, and 15-cm water pressures).

Continuous Positive Airway Pressure

CPAP transmits positive pressure into the airways of a spontaneously breathing patient throughout the respiratory cycle. The increase in airway pressure allows for better diffusion of gases and reexpansion of collapsed alveoli, resulting in improvement of gas exchange and a reduction in the work of breathing. CPAP can be applied invasively (via an ET tube, creating PEEP) or noninvasively via a face or nose mask. Mask CPAP is provided through a tight-fitting face mask connected to a battery-operated breathing circuit with an adjustable FiO_2 and PEEP valve that delivers 5- to 10-cm water pressure. CPAP reduces the inspiratory work of breathing and lowers mean airway pressures. In addition to managing patients with pulmonary congestion, CPAP also may benefit pa-

> **NOTE**
>
> Patients who receive CPAP require a lot of coaching and reassurance from the paramedic.

tients with acute blunt and penetrating pulmonary injury and those with obstructive airway disease.[3]

Biphasic Positive Airway Pressure

Biphasic positive airway pressure (BiPAP) conceptually combines partial ventilatory support and CPAP. BiPAP is applied by face mask or nose mask through a noninvasive ventilator device with two settings that provides a 5-cm water pressure difference between inspiratory positive airway pressure (IPAP) and expiratory positive airway pressure (EPAP). BiPAP is a leak-tolerant system (CPAP is not) that allows IPAP and EPAP settings to be titrated to reach a desired PEEP range. In selected patients with respiratory distress caused by COPD, pulmonary edema, pneumonia, and asthma, BiPAP may obviate the need for ET intubation.

Pulmonary Thromboembolism

Pulmonary thromboembolism (pulmonary embolism [PE]) refers to blockage of a pulmonary artery by a clot or other foreign material that has traveled there from another place of origin, usually the lower extremities (Fig. 27-9). It is a relatively

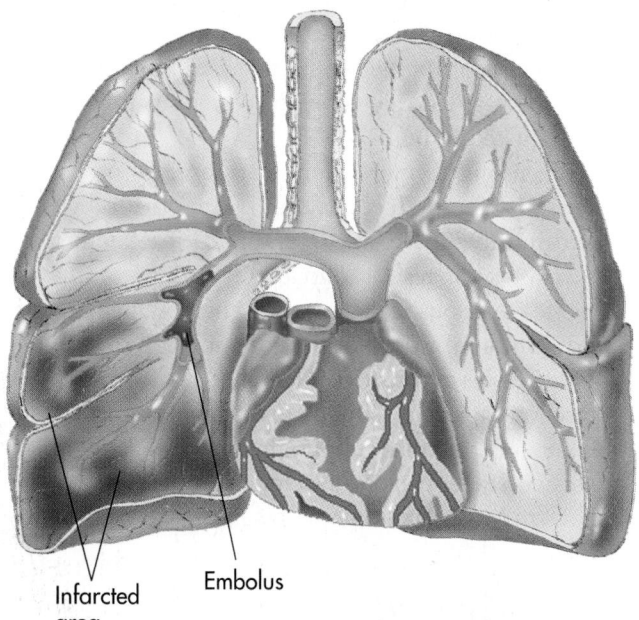

Infarcted area

Embolus

Fig. 27-9 PE is the blockage of a pulmonary artery by foreign matter, such as a thrombus, that usually arises from a peripheral vein, fat, air, or tumor tissue. The blockage obstructs blood supply to the lung tissue. (From Wilson SF: *Respiratory disorders,* St Louis, 1990, Mosby.)

NOTE

Pulmonary embolism is responsible for 5% of all sudden deaths.[1]

✓ TRICKS OF THE TRADE

A young woman who takes birth control pills and smokes cigarettes has an increased risk for venous thrombosis. If she is hyperventilating, you should suspect a pulmonary embolism until proven otherwise.

common disorder that affects about 650,000 individuals each year in the United States. Of this number, about 50,000 (less than 10%) patients die, 10% within the first hour after blockage.[3]

PE usually begins as a venous disease. It most often is caused by migration of a thrombus from the large veins of the lower extremities, but it also can occur as a result of fat, air, sheared venous catheters, amniotic fluid, or tumor tissue. The clot or embolus dislodges and travels through the venous system to the right side of the heart. From there, it migrates to the pulmonary arteries, obstructing blood supply to a section of lung. The most common sites for thrombus formation are the deep veins of the legs and pelvis. Six factors that contribute to the development of venous thrombosis are listed in Box 27-4.

When one or more pulmonary arteries occlude, the embolism produces an area of lung that is ventilated but hypoperfused. In response, a reflex bronchoconstriction results from local hypocarbia and the release of various mediators (most notably, histamine and serotonin) from the clot formation. This causes blood vessels to constrict. If the patient's vascular obstruction is severe (60% or greater blockage of the pulmonary vascular supply), hypoxemia, acute pulmonary hypertension, systemic hypotension, and shock may rapidly occur, with subsequent death.

Signs and Symptoms

An embolus may be small, moderate, or massive. Therefore the patient with PE may present very differently, with a wide variety of signs and symptoms. Signs and symptoms depend on the location and size of the clot and may include dyspnea,

cough, hemoptysis (rare), pain, anxiety, syncope, hypotension, diaphoresis, tachypnea, tachycardia, fever, and distended neck veins. In addition, chest splinting, pleuritic pain, pleural friction rub, crackles, and localized wheezing may be present. The paramedic should consider a PE in any patient who has cardiorespiratory problems that cannot be otherwise explained, particularly when risk factors are present.

? CRITICAL THINKING

What information in the patient assessment may help distinguish PE from other conditions that cause similar signs and symptoms?

BOX 27-4

CONTRIBUTING FACTORS FOR THE DEVELOPMENT OF VENOUS THROMBOSIS

1. Venostasis
   a. Extended travel
   b. Prolonged bed rest
   c. Obesity
   d. Advanced age
   e. Burns
   f. Varicose veins
2. Venous injury
   a. Surgery of the thorax, abdomen, pelvis, or legs
   b. Fractures of the pelvis or legs
3. Increased blood coagulability
   a. Malignancy
   b. Oral contraceptives
   c. Congenital or acquired coagulopathies
4. Pregnancy
5. Disease
   a. Chronic lung disease
   b. Congestive heart failure
   c. Sickle cell anemia
   d. Cancer
   e. Atrial fibrillation
   f. Myocardial infarction
   g. Previous pulmonary embolism
   h. Previous deep vein thrombosis
   i. Infection
   j. Diabetes mellitus
6. Multiple trauma
   a. Long bone fracture
   b. Pelvic fracture

Management

Prehospital care primarily is supportive. Supplemental high-concentration oxygen should be administered, a cardiac monitor applied, pulse oximetry utilized, and an IV line of normal saline or lactated Ringer's solution established. The patient should be transported in a position of comfort. Definitive care requires hospitalization and fibrinolytic or *heparin* therapy.

> **NOTE**
>
> Fibrinolytic agents rarely are used in the prehospital setting for the management of PE.

Upper Respiratory Infection

Upper respiratory infections (URIs) affect the nose, throat, sinuses, and larynx. They are among the most common of all illnesses, affecting nearly 80 million persons each year.[1] These illnesses (which include the common cold, pharyngitis, tonsillitis, sinusitis, laryngitis, and croup) rarely are life threatening. They often, however, exacerbate underlying pulmonary conditions and may lead to significant infections in patients with suppressed immune function. A variety of bacteria and viruses can cause URIs. Group A streptococci are responsible for 20% to 30% of cases; 50% of cases have no demonstrated bacterial or viral cause.[1] Signs and symptoms of upper respiratory infection include:

- Sore throat
- Fever
- Chills
- Headache
- Facial pain (sinusitis)
- Purulent nasal drainage
- Halitosis
- Cervical adenopathy
- Erthyematous pharynx

> **NOTE**
>
> Hand washing and covering the mouth during sneezing and coughing are essential in preventing the spread of respiratory infections.

> **? CRITICAL THINKING**
>
> **When can a URI become life threatening? Think of two or three examples.**

Management

Most URIs are self-limiting and require little or no prehospital intervention. Prehospital care is symptomatic and is based in part on the presence of underlying pulmonary conditions, in which oxygen administration may be appropriate. Other interventions that may be indicated for patients with associated respiratory illness include the administration of bronchodilators or corticosteroids. Throat cultures (if obtained at the scene) require family notification of results and physician follow-up. The paramedic should follow local protocol.

Spontaneous Pneumothorax

A primary **spontaneous pneumothorax** usually results when a subpleural bleb (a cystic lesion on a lobe of the lung) ruptures, allowing air to enter the pleural space from within the lung. This type of pneumothorax may occur in apparently healthy persons, usually between 20 and 40 years of age. Often, these persons are men who are tall and thin and have long, narrow chests. (In contrast, a secondary spontaneous pneumothorax may sometimes develop from an underlying disease process such as COPD.)

> **NOTE**
>
> In recent years, the number of spontaneous pneumothoraces has increased in some populations. These groups include persons with AIDS who have pneumonia and drug abusers who deeply inhale free-base cocaine, marijuana, or inhalants (such as glue or solvents).

Most primary spontaneous pneumothoraces are well tolerated by the patient if the pneumothorax does not occupy more than 20% of the hemithorax (partial pneumothorax). Signs and symptoms include shortness of breath and chest pain that often is sudden in onset, pallor, diaphoresis, and tachypnea. In severe cases where the pneumothorax occupies more than 20% of the hemithorax, the following signs and symptoms may be present:

- Altered mentation
- Cyanosis
- Tachycardia
- Decreased breath sounds on the affected side
- Local hyperresonance to percussion
- Subcutaneous emphysema

Management

Prehospital care is based on the patient's symptoms and degree of respiratory distress. High-concentration oxygen administration is indicated to help resolve the pneumothorax, and airway, ventilatory, and circulatory support may be required in severe cases. These patients should be transported in a position of comfort for physician evaluation and possible decompression of the pleural space. In some cases, surgery may be indicated to allow for lung reexpansion or to prevent recurrence.

Hyperventilation Syndrome

Hyperventilation syndrome refers to abnormally deep or rapid breathing that results in excessive loss of carbon dioxide (producing respiratory alkalosis). As a result, the syndrome produces hypocarbia that leads to cerebrovascular constriction, reduced cerebral perfusion, paresthesias, dizziness, or even feelings of euphoria. There are multiple causes of hyperventilation syndrome, some of which include:

- Anxiety
- Hypoxia
- Pulmonary disease
- Cardiovascular disorders
- Metabolic disorders
- Neurological disorders
- Drugs
- Fever
- Infection
- Pain
- Pregnancy

Signs and symptoms of hyperventilation syndrome include dyspnea with rapid breathing and high minute volume, chest pain, circumoral tingling, and carpopedal spasm. Other assessment findings vary, based on the cause of the syndrome.

Management

If the syndrome clearly is caused by anxiety (psychogenic dyspnea—a diagnosis of exclusion), prehospital care will primarily be supportive, consisting of calming measures and reassurance. If the paramedic suspects that the syndrome is a result of illness (e.g., diabetes, renal disease) or drug ingestion, emergency care also may include oxygen administration, and airway and ventilatory support. All patients who are hyperventilating should be calmed, and the paramedic should coach the patient's ventilations. If the hyperventilation is severe or complicated by illness or drug ingestion, transport for physician evaluation is indicated. The paramedic should consult with medical direction.

Lung Cancer

Lung cancer is an epidemic in the United States, with an estimated 150,000 new cases being reported each year. Most cases of lung cancer develop in persons between the ages of 55 and 65. Of the new cases reported, most will die of the disease within 1 year, 20% will have local lung involvement, 25% will have spread to the lymph system, and 55% will have distant metastatic cancer.[3] The most common cause of lung cancer is cigarette smoking. Other risk factors include passive smoking (exposure to someone else's cigarette smoke) and exposure to asbestos, radon gas, dust, coal products, ionizing radiation, and other toxins.

> **NOTE**
>
> Heavy smokers (those who smoke more than 20 cigarettes per day) have a 25 times greater chance of developing lung cancer than nonsmokers.[2]

Pathophysiology

Like other cancers, lung cancer is an expression of the uncontrolled growth of abnormal cells. (At least a dozen different cell types of tumors are associated with primary lung cancer.) The two major cell types of lung cancer are *small cell lung cancer* and *non–small cell lung cancer* (which is further divided into *squamous cell carcinoma, adenocarcinoma,* and *large cell carcinoma*). Each cell type has a different growth pattern and a different response to treatment. Most abnormal cell growth begins in the bronchi or bronchioles.

> **NOTE**
>
> The lung also is a fairly common site of metastasis of cancers with other primary sites (e.g., breast cancer).

Signs and Symptoms

Signs and symptoms of early-stage disease often are nonspecific and attributed by the person to the effects of smoking. These include coughing, sputum production, lower airway obstruction (noted by wheezing), and respiratory illness (e.g., bronchitis). As the disease progresses, signs and symptoms may include:

- Cough
- Hemoptysis (which may be severe)

> **NOTE**
>
> Patients with cancer also may call EMS for conditions related to their chemotherapy or radiation therapy, which is toxic to both normal body cells and malignant cells. Associated complaints often include nausea and vomiting, fatigue, and dehydration. Emotional and psychological support for these patients is indicated.

- Dyspnea
- Hoarseness or voice change
- Dysphagia
- Weight loss/anorexia
- Weakness

Management

Most patients with lung cancer are aware of their disease. Prehospital management includes airway, ventilatory, and circulatory support; oxygen administration (based on symptoms and pulse oximetry); and transport for physician evaluation. Depending on the severity of the patient's condition, medical direction also may recommend IV fluids to improve hydration and to thin sputum, pharmacological agents such as bronchodilators and corticosteroids to improve breathing, and analgesics to relieve pain. End-stage patients may have advance directives or DNR orders. In these cases, emotional support also will be required for family and loved ones.

> **NOTE**
>
> Some patients will have an indwelling vascular access device in place. Paramedics should consult with medical direction regarding the use of these devices as a means of vascular access (see Chapter 9).

SUMMARY

- Specific pathophysiologies that are responsible for respiratory emergencies include those related to ventilation, diffusion, and perfusion.

- Obstructive airway disease is a triad of distinct diseases that often coexist: chronic bronchitis, emphysema, and asthma. The patient with chronic obstructive pulmonary disease usually presents with an acute episode of worsening dyspnea that is manifested even at rest, an increase or change in sputum production, or an increase in the malaise that accompanies the disease. The primary goal of prehospital care for these patients is correction of hypoxemia through improved air flow.

- Asthma, or reactive airway disease, is characterized by reversible airflow obstruction caused by bronchial smooth muscle contraction, hypersecretion of mucus resulting in bronchial plugging, and inflammatory changes in the bronchial walls. The typical patient with asthma is in obvious distress, with rapid and loud respirations. Initial medications in the prehospital setting will probably be those with a short onset of action.

- Pneumonia is a group of specific infections (bacterial, viral, or fungal) that cause an acute inflammatory process of the respiratory bronchioles and the alveoli. Pneumonia usually presents with classic signs and symptoms that include a productive cough and associated fever that produces "shaking chills." Prehospital care of patients with pneumonia includes airway support, oxygen administration, ventilatory assistance as needed, IV fluids, cardiac monitoring, and transport.

- Adult respiratory distress syndrome is a fulminant form of respiratory failure characterized by acute lung inflammation and diffuse alveolar-capillary injury. It develops as a complication of illness or injury causing a condition in which the lungs are wet and heavy, congested, hemorrhagic, and stiff, with decreased perfusion capacity across alveolar membranes.

- Pulmonary thromboembolism refers to a blockage of a pulmonary artery by a clot or other foreign material. When one or more pulmonary arteries occlude, the embolism produces a section of lung that is ventilated but hypoperfused. Prehospital care primarily is supportive.

- Upper respiratory infections (URIs) affect the nose, throat, sinuses, and larynx. Signs and symptoms of URI include sore throat, fever, chills, headache, cervical adenopathy, and erythematous pharynx. Prehospital care is based on the patient's symptoms.

- A primary spontaneous pneumothorax usually results when a subpleural bleb ruptures, allowing air to enter the pleural space from within the lung. Signs and symptoms include shortness of breath and chest pain that often are sudden in onset, pallor, diaphoresis, and tachypnea. Prehospital care is based on the patient's symptoms and degree of distress.

- Hyperventilation syndrome refers to abnormally deep or rapid breathing that results in excessive loss of carbon dioxide. If the syndrome clearly is caused by anxiety, prehospital care will primarily be supportive, consisting of calming measures and reassurance. If the paramedic suspects that the syndrome is a result of illness or drug ingestion, emergency care may include oxygen administration and airway and ventilatory support.

- Lung cancer is an expression of the uncontrolled growth of abnormal cells. As the disease progresses, signs and symptoms may include cough, hemoptysis, dyspnea, hoarseness, and dysphagia. Prehospital management includes airway, ventilatory, and circulatory support.

REFERENCES

1. US Department of Transportation, National Highway Traffic Safety Administration: *EMT-Paramedic national standard curriculum,* Washington, DC, 1998, The Department.
2. American Lung Association: *Data and statistics,* http://www.lungusa.org/data/index.html.
3. Rosen P, Barkin R: *Emergency medicine: concepts and clinical practice,* ed 4, St Louis, 1998, Mosby.
4. American Heart Association: Guidelines 2000 for cardiopulmonary resuscitation and emergency cardiovascular care, International Consensus on Science, *Circulation* 102 (8):237, 2000.
5. American Heart Association: Guidelines 2000 for cardiopulmonary resuscitation and emergency cardiovascular care, International Consensus on Science, *Circulation* 102 (8):240, 2000.
6. McCance L, Huether S: *Pathophysiology: the biologic basis for disease in adults and children,* ed 3, St Louis, 1998, Mosby.

28 Cardiology

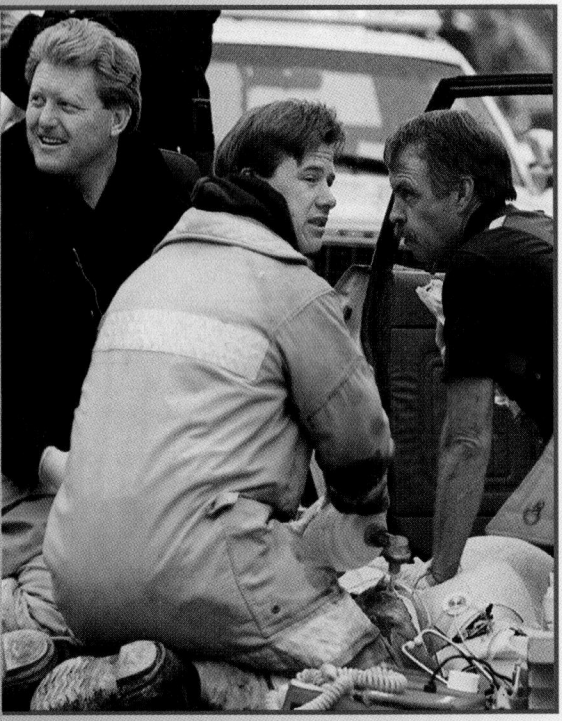

Cardiovascular disease accounts for more than 930,000 deaths in the United States each year. About two thirds of sudden death due to coronary disease takes place outside the hospital and usually occurs within 2 hours after onset of symptoms.[1] It is possible that a large number of these deaths can be prevented by rapid entry into the EMS system, prompt provision of CPR, and early defibrillation.

KEY TERMS

automaticity: A property of specialized excitable tissue that allows self-activation through spontaneous development of an action potential.

AV dissociation: A conduction disturbance in which atrial and ventricular contractions occur rhythmically but are unrelated to each other.

bundle of Kent: An accessory pathway between the atria and ventricles outside of the conduction system; a congenital anomaly that causes Wolff-Parkinson-White syndrome.

cardiac ejection fraction: The percentage of ventricular volume released during contraction.

hypertensive encephalopathy: A set of symptoms, including headache, convulsions, and coma, that result solely from elevated blood pressure.

P wave: The first complex of the electrocardiogram, representing depolarization of the atria.

paroxysmal nocturnal dyspnea (PND): An abnormal condition of the respiratory system, characterized by sudden attacks of shortness of breath, profuse sweating, tachycardia, and wheezing that awaken a person from sleep; often associated with left ventricular failure and pulmonary edema.

paroxysmal supraventricular tachycardia (PSVT): An ectopic rhythm in excess of 100 beats per minute and usually faster than 170 beats per minute that begins abruptly with a premature atrial or junctional beat and is supported by an atrioventricular nodal reentry mechanism or by an atrioventricular reentry involving an accessory pathway.

PR interval: The time elapsing between the beginning of the P wave and the beginning of the QRS complex in the electrocardiogram.

premature atrial contraction (PAC): A cardiac dysrhythmia characterized by an atrial beat occurring before the expected excitation and indicated on the electrocardiogram as an early P wave.

premature junctional contraction (PJC): A single contraction that occurs during sinus rhythm earlier than the next expected sinus beat and is caused by premature discharge of an ectopic focus in the atrioventricular junctional tissue.

premature ventricular contraction (PVC): A cardiac dysrhythmia characterized by a ventricular beat preceding the expected electrical impulse and indicated on the electrocardiogram as an early, wide QRS complex without a preceding related P wave.

proarrhythmia: A serious tachydysrhythmia or bradydysrhythmia seemingly generated by antidysrhythmic agents.

QRS complex: The principal deflection in the electrocardiogram, representing ventricular depolarization.

QT interval: The time elapsing from the beginning of the QRS complex to the end of the T wave, representing the total duration of electrical activity of the ventricles.

R-on-T phenomenon: The occurrence of a ventricular depolarization during a vulnerable period of relative refractoriness.

refractory period: The period after effective stimulation during which excitable tissue fails to respond to a stimulus of threshold intensity.

resting membrane potential (RMP): The electrical charge difference inside a cell membrane measured relative to just outside the cell membrane.

ST segment: The early part of repolarization in the electrocardiogram of the right and left ventricles.

Starling's law of the heart: A rule that the force of the heartbeat is determined by the length of the fibers making up the myocardial walls.

T wave: A deflection in the electrocardiogram after the QRS complex, representing ventricular repolarization.

threshold potential: The value of the membrane potential at which an action potential is produced as a result of depolarization in response to a stimulus.

torsades de pointes: An unusual bidirectional ventricular tachycardia.

U wave: The gradual deviation from the T wave in the electrocardiogram, thought to represent the final stage of repolarization of the ventricles.

ventricular bigeminy: A cardiac rhythm disturbance characterized by two ventricular beats in rapid succession followed by a longer interval.

ventricular tachycardia (VT): A tachycardia that usually originates in the Purkinje fibers.

ventricular trigeminy: A cardiac dysrhythmia characterized by three ventricular beats in rapid succession followed by a longer interval.

? CRITICAL THINKING

How many of your friends or family have had a heart attack or stroke? How has that illness affected their lives?

Risk Factors and Prevention Strategies

Although death rates from myocardial infarction have declined over the past several decades, coronary artery disease (CAD) and resultant sudden death is still a major cause of morbidity and mortality and is the most prominent medical emergency in the United States today.[1] This decline in death rates is due in large part to heightened public awareness, increased availability of automated external defibrillators (AEDs), improved cardiovascular diagnosis and therapy, use of cardiovascular drugs by persons at high risk, improved revascularization techniques, and improved and more aggressive risk factor modification.

Risk Factors and Risk Factor Modifications

Persons at high risk for cardiovascular disease include those with diabetes, hypertension, hypercholesterolemia, hyperlipidemia, a family history of premature cardiovascular disease, and known CAD. Their risk can be significantly increased if they have additional risk factors such as obesity, cigarette smoking, and a sedentary lifestyle (Box 28-1). Clearly, some risk factors cannot be changed. Others, however, can be changed or modified through the following:

- Cessation of smoking
- Medical management and control of blood pressure, diabetes, cholesterol, and lipid disorders
- Exercise
- Weight loss
- Diet
- Stress reduction

> **NOTE**
>
> Modification of cardiovascular risk factors can alter the rate of progression of arterial disease and reduce the incidence of acute myocardial infarction (AMI), sudden death, renal failure, and stroke.

Prevention Strategies

Prevention strategies for cardiovascular disease that can be supported and practiced by paramedics and other health care professionals include educational programs about nutrition in their communities, cessation of smoking (smoking prevention for children), early recognition and management of hypertension and cardiac symptoms, and prompt intervention (including CPR and AED). These and other prevention strategies may help reduce risk factors at a young age and may have the greatest impact on risk factor modification. (See Appendix C.)

BOX 28-1

RISK FACTORS FOR CARDIOVASCULAR DISEASE

Risk Factors
Age
Family history
Prior myocardial infarction
Diabetes
Hypertension
Hyperlipidemia
Hypercholesterolemia
Male sex
Cigarette smoking
Cocaine use
Carbohydrate intolerance

Possible Contributing Risk Factors
Poor diet
Female sex
Obesity
Oral contraceptive use
Sedentary lifestyle
Stress
Personality type
Psychosocial tensions

SECTION ONE
ANATOMY AND PHYSIOLOGY OF THE HEART

Anatomy

The anatomy of the heart is described and illustrated in Chapter 6. Readers are encouraged to refer to that chapter for a review.

The coronary arteries are the exclusive suppliers of arterial blood to the heart muscle, delivering 200 to 250 mL of blood to the myocardium each minute during rest (Fig. 28-1). The left coronary artery carries about 85% of the blood supply to the myocardium, and the right coronary artery carries the remainder. The coronary arteries originate just above the aortic valve where the aorta exits the heart. These arteries run along the epicardial sur-

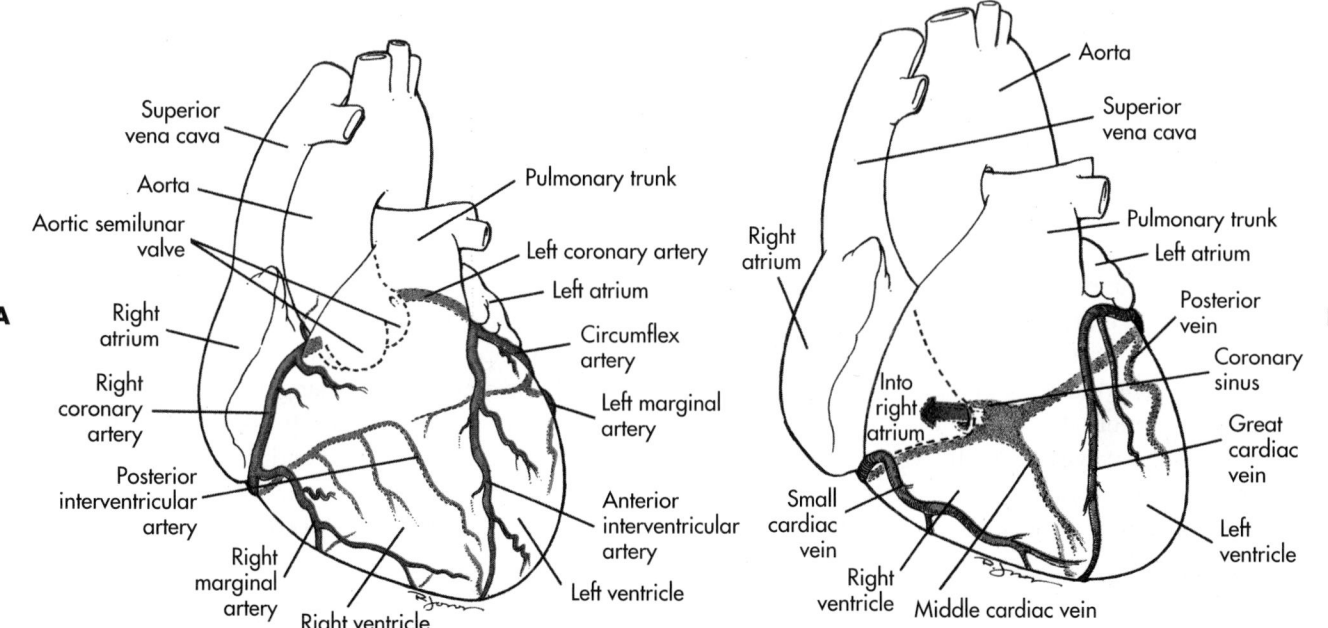

Fig. 28-1 Blood vessels providing circulation of the heart. **A,** Arteries. **B,** Veins. The anterior surface of the heart is represented. The vessels of the anterior surface are seen directly and have a darker color, whereas the vessels of the posterior surface are seen through the heart and have a lighter color. (From Sims/Illustrator: Rusty Jones.)

face and divide into smaller vessels as they penetrate the myocardium and the endocardial (inner) surface.

The left main coronary artery subdivides into the left anterior descending and circumflex arteries. The former supplies the anterior wall of the more muscular left ventricle and the interventricular septum. The latter feeds the lateral and posterior portions of the left ventricle and part of the right ventricle. The right coronary artery and the left anterior descending artery supply most of the right atrium and ventricle and the inferior aspect of the left ventricle. In addition to the blood supply provided by these arteries, many anastomoses exist between arterioles of coronary arteries that provide collateral circulation. These anastomoses play an important role in providing alternative routes of blood flow in the event of blockage in one or more of the coronary vessels.

> ? CRITICAL THINKING
>
> **Why is collateral circulation important?**

Coronary capillaries permit the exchange of nutrients and metabolic wastes. The capillaries merge to form coronary veins. These veins deliver most of the blood to the coronary sinus, which empties directly into the right atrium. The coronary sinus is the major vein draining the myocardium.

Physiology

The heart can be thought of as two pumps in one: a low-pressure pump (right atrium and right ventricle) supplying the pulmonary vasculature and a high-pressure pump (left atrium and left ventricle) supplying the systemic vasculature. The right atrium receives venous blood from the systemic circulation and from the coronary veins. Most of this deoxygenated blood in the right atrium then passes to the right ventricle as the ventricle relaxes from the previous contraction. Once the right ventricle receives about 70% of its volume, the right atrium contracts, and blood remaining in the atrium is pushed into the ventricle. Contraction of the right ventricle pushes blood against the tricuspid valve (forcing it closed) and through the pulmonic valve (forcing it open), allowing blood to enter the lungs via the pulmonary arteries. From the pulmonary arteries, the deoxygenated blood enters the pulmonary capillary bed, where gas exchange takes place.

From the lungs, the blood travels through four pulmonary veins back to the left atrium. The mitral valve opens, and blood flows to the left ventricle. Once the left ventricle receives about 70% of its volume, the left atrium contracts and the remaining blood is pushed into the ventricle. The blood passing from the left atrium to the left ventricle opens the bicuspid valve when the ventricle relaxes to complete left ventricular filling. As the left ventricle contracts, blood is pushed against the bicuspid valve (closing it) and against the aortic valve (opening it), allowing blood to enter the aorta. From the aorta, blood is distributed first to the heart itself and then throughout the systemic arterial circulation.

> **NOTE**
>
> The atria function primarily as "primer pumps." Under most conditions, the ventricles can pump sufficient amounts of blood to maintain homeostasis without the help of the atria. However, under conditions of stress, when the heart may pump 300% to 400% more blood than during rest, the priming pump action of the atria becomes important in maintaining pumping efficiency.

Cardiac Cycle

The pumping action of the heart is a product of rhythmic, alternate contraction (systole) and relaxation (diastole) of the atria and ventricles. (When *systole* and *diastole* are used without reference to specific chambers, they mean *ventricular systole* or *diastole*.) These heartbeats occur about 70 times per minute in resting adults. Pressure changes produced within the heart chambers by contraction are responsible for blood movement, as blood moves from areas of high pressure to areas of low pressure (Fig. 28-2).

Ventricular Systole and Diastole

As the ventricular myocardium begins to contract during ventricular systole, ventricular pressure exceeds atrial pressure, causing the atrioventricular (AV) valves to close. As the contraction proceeds, ventricular pressure continues to rise until it exceeds that in the pulmonary artery on the right side of the heart and in the aorta on the left side. At that time, the pulmonary and aortic valves open and blood flows from the ventricles into those arteries (ejection).

After ventricular contraction, ventricular relaxation begins and ventricular pressure falls rapidly. When the pressure falls below the pressure in the aorta or the pulmonary trunk, blood is forced back toward the ventricles, closing the pulmonic and aortic valves. As ventricular pressure drops below atrial pressure, the tricuspid and mitral valves open, and blood flows from the atria into the ventricles. Atrial systole occurs during ventricular diastole.

> **? CRITICAL THINKING**
>
> *What would happen if the valves were scarred and became stiff?*

Stroke Volume

The stroke volume (SV) is the amount of blood ejected from each ventricle with one contraction. SV depends on preload (the volume of blood returning to the heart), afterload, and myocardial contractility.

Preload

During diastole, blood flows from the atria into the ventricles. The volume of blood returning to each ventricle (end-diastolic volume) normally reaches 120 to 130 mL. As the ventricles empty during systole, their volume decreases to 50 to 60 mL (end-systolic volume). Therefore the amount of blood ejected during each cardiac cycle (SV) is about 70 mL.

In a patient with a healthy heart, the capacity to increase stroke volume is great. The strong contraction of a heart during exercise, for example, can reduce the volume returning to each ventricle to as little as 10 to 30 mL. If large amounts of blood flow into the ventricles during diastole, their end-diastolic volume can be as much as 200 to 250 mL. In this way, SV can be increased to more than double that of normal. The heart's ability to pump more strongly when it has a larger preload is explained by a concept known as ***Starling's law of the heart.***

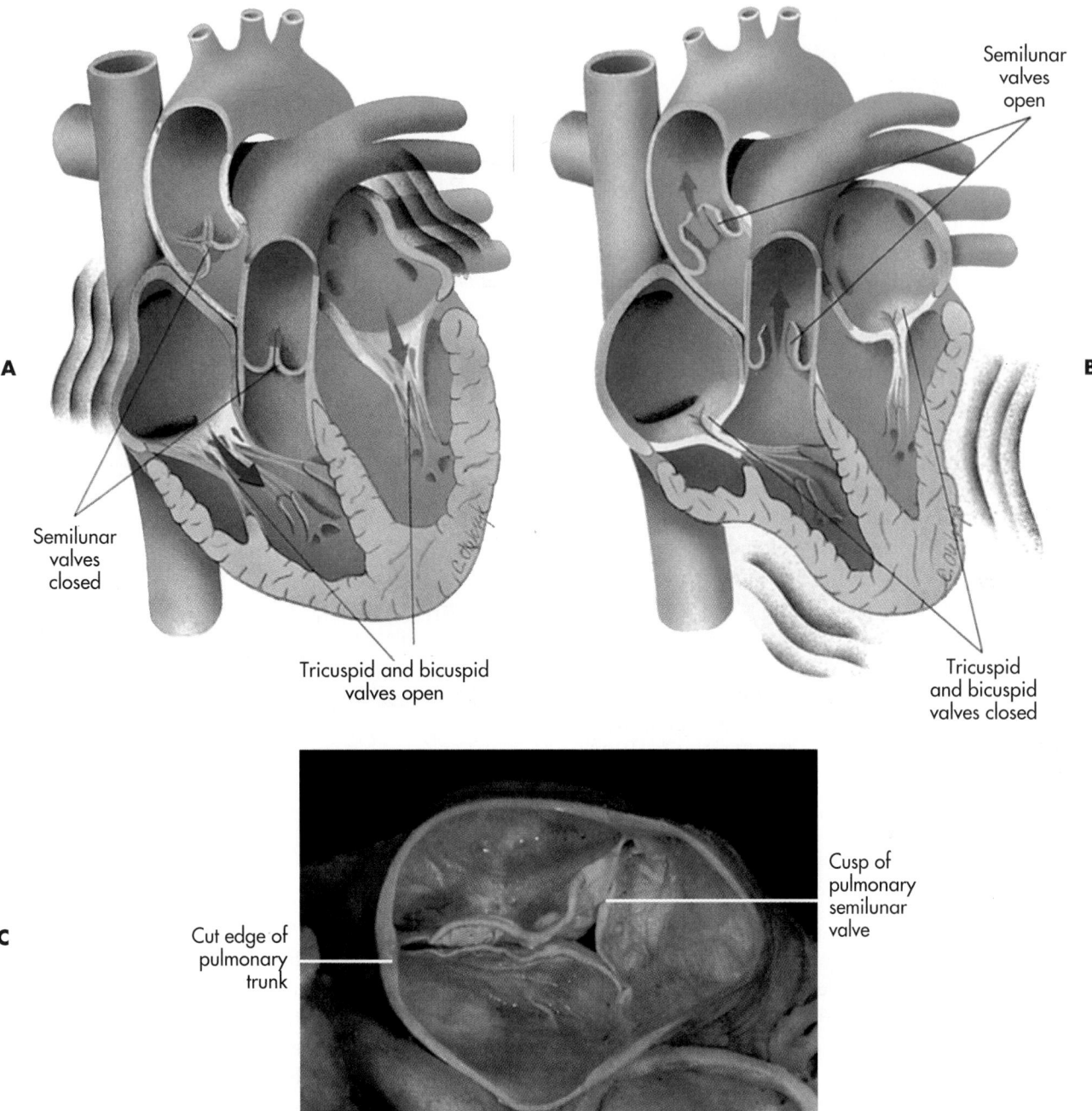

A

Semilunar
valves
closed

Tricuspid and bicuspid
valves open

B

Semilunar
valves
open

Tricuspid
and bicuspid
valves closed

C

Cut edge of
pulmonary
trunk

Cusp of
pulmonary
semilunar
valve

Fig. 28-2 Heart action. **A,** During atrial systole (contraction), cardiac muscle in the atrial wall contracts, forcing blood through the atrioventricular valves and into the ventricles. **B,** During the ventricular systole that follows, the atrioventricular valves close, and blood is forced out of the ventricles through the semilunar valves into the arteries. **C,** The pulmonary semilunar valves as seen from above (superior). (From Thibodeau GA: *Structure and function of the body,* ed 9, St Louis, 1992, Mosby.)

Starling's law of the heart. According to Starling's law (Fig. 28-3), myocardial fibers contract more forcefully when stretched. (This ability of stretched muscle to contract with increased force is characteristic of all striated muscle, not just cardiac muscle.) The primary mechanism by which Starling's law affects SV and ultimately cardiac output is as follows: When the ventricles are filled with larger-than-normal volumes of blood (increased preload), they contract with greater-than-normal force to deliver their entire contents to the systemic circulation.

The most important feature of the heart's ability to adapt itself to changing volumes in venous return is that, within reasonable limits, changes in arterial pressure have minimal effect on cardiac output. In other words, the heart can pump either a small amount of blood or a large amount, depending on the amount of venous return. The heart automatically adapts as long as the total quantity of blood does not exceed the physiological limit that the heart can pump. Venous return is the most important factor in SV, with arterial pressure causing a lesser effect in the form of afterload.

Afterload

Afterload is a result of peripheral vascular resistance—the total resistance against which blood must be pumped. An increase in peripheral vascular resistance decreases SV because of the increased pressure in the aorta that the ventricular muscle must overcome to open the aortic valve and push blood through. Conversely, a decrease in peripheral vascular resistance increases SV if there is sufficient volume of fluid in the system.

Myocardial Contractility

The intrinsic state of the myocardium, along with the activity of the autonomic nervous system, plays a major role in the function of the heart. Ischemia or various drugs can decrease myocardial contractility by decreasing the number of functional myocardial cells (as occurs in myocardial infarction) or by decreasing the ability of the individual myocardial cells to contract (e.g., as a result of hypoxia or the administration of beta blockers).

Cardiac Output

Cardiac output is the amount of blood pumped by the ventricles per minute. Cardiac output can increase by increasing the heart rate, SV, or both, and is calculated as follows:

$$\text{Cardiac output} = \text{SV} \times \text{Heart rate}$$

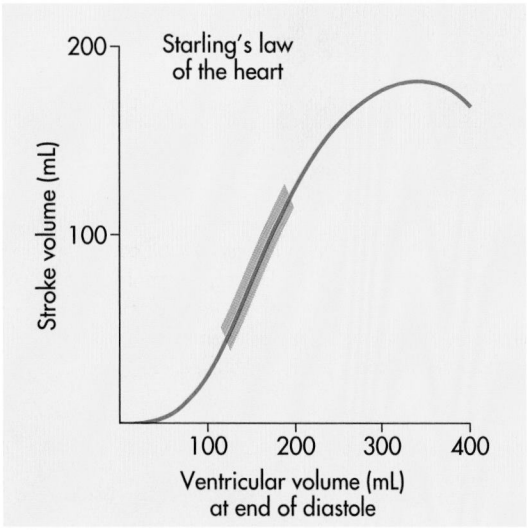

Fig. 28-3 Starling's law of the heart. (From Thibodeau GA: *Anatomy and physiology handbook,* St Louis, 1993, Mosby.)

Peripheral vascular resistance modifies cardiac output through its effect on SV. Vasodilation of the arteries, for example, decreases peripheral vascular resistance and arterial pressure (afterload), thereby producing an increase in cardiac output. In contrast, vasoconstriction of arteries and the smaller arterioles increases peripheral vascular resistance and tends to decrease cardiac output. However, constriction of the venous circulation by increasing filling of the heart, and through Starling's law, enables the heart to contract more forcefully and maintains or increases cardiac output.

Nervous System Control of the Heart

In addition to the body's intrinsic control in regulating the heart, extrinsic control by the parasympathetic and sympathetic nerves of the autonomic nervous system is a major factor influencing the heart rate, conductivity, and contractility. Control is achieved by a group of nerves, the cardiac plexus, that innervate the atria and ventricles. The atria are well supplied with large numbers of sympathetic and parasympathetic nerve fibers, but the ventricles mainly are supplied by sympathetic nerves.

The parasympathetic nervous system primarily is concerned with vegetative functions, whereas the sympathetic nervous system helps prepare the body to respond to stress. These sympathetic and parasympathetic control systems work in a "check and balance" manner, stimulating the heart to increase or decrease cardiac output according to the body's metabolic demands.

> **? CRITICAL THINKING**
>
> *How is the behavior of the autonomic nervous system similar to how you regulate the hot and cold taps in your shower?*

Parasympathetic Control

Parasympathetic innervation of the heart is through the vagus nerve. Innervation by these fibers has a continuous inhibitory influence on the heart, primarily by decreasing the heart rate and, to a lesser extent, contractility. The vagus nerve may be stimulated in several ways. Examples include the Valsalva maneuver, carotid sinus massage (described later in this chapter), pain, and distention of the uri-

nary bladder. Acetylcholine is the chemical mediator of the parasympathetic nervous system.

Although strong parasympathetic stimulation can decrease the heart rate to 20 or 30 beats per minute, it generally has little effect on SV. In fact, SV may increase with a decreased heart rate because the longer time interval between heartbeats allows the heart to fill with a volume of blood and thus contract more forcefully (Starling's law).

Sympathetic Control

Sympathetic nerve fibers originate in the thoracic region of the spinal cord and form the thoracic and cervical sympathetic ganglia. Their postganglionic fibers release the chemical mediator norepinephrine, which stimulates an increase in the heart rate (positive chronotropic effect) and an increase in the force of muscle contraction (positive inotropic effect). Sympathetic stimulation of the heart causes dilation of coronary blood vessels. Along with the constriction of peripheral vessels, this ensures that increased oxygen demands of the heart are met by an increase in blood and oxygen supply. The cardiac effects of norepinephrine result from stimulation of cell surface alpha- and beta-adrenergic receptors.

> **NOTE**
>
> As described in Chapter 8, *inotropic* refers to the force of energy of muscular contractions; *chronotropic* refers to the regularity and rate of the heartbeat; and *dromotropic* refers to conduction velocity. Effects are classified as positive or negative. For example, positive inotropism is a process that increases the strength of contraction; negative dromotropism is a process that decreases conduction velocity.

Strong sympathetic stimulation of the heart may increase the heart rate significantly. When rates are markedly accelerated (greater than 150 beats per minute), the time available for diastolic filling decreases, and ventricular filling is markedly reduced. This produces a decrease in SV.

Hormonal Regulation of the Heart

Sympathetic impulses are transmitted to the adrenal medulla at the same time that they are transmitted to all blood vessels. These impulses cause the adrenal medulla to secrete the hormones epinephrine and norepinephrine into the circulating blood. These hormones are secreted in response to increased physical activity, emotional excitement, or stress.

Epinephrine has essentially the same effect on cardiac muscles as norepinephrine and therefore increases the rate and force of contraction. In addition, epinephrine causes blood vessels to constrict in the skin, kidneys, GI tract, and other viscera and causes dilation of skeletal and coronary vessels. Epinephrine takes longer to act on the beta-adrenergic receptors of the heart than direct sympathetic innervation does, but the effect lasts longer. Norepinephrine causes constriction of peripheral blood vessels in most areas of the body and stimulates cardiac muscle.

Role of Electrolytes

Myocardial cells, like all other cells of the human body, are bathed in an electrolyte solution. The major electrolytes that influence cardiac function are calcium, potassium, and sodium. Magnesium, a major intracellular cation, plays an important role as well.

? CRITICAL THINKING

What drugs can alter the normal balance of electrolytes in the body?

SECTION TWO
ELECTROPHYSIOLOGY OF THE HEART

Much of coronary care is based on an understanding and manipulation of the electrical and mechanical properties of cardiac function. It is important for the paramedic to understand the concepts of an inadequate electrical conduction system and the effect that myocardial ischemia has on cardiac rhythms. The two basic groups of cells within the myocardium that are important for cardiac function are the specialized cells of the electrical con-

duction system responsible for the formation and conduction of electrical current, and the working myocardial cells that possess the property of contractility.

Electrical Activity of Cardiac Cells and Membrane Potentials

As described in Chapter 7, ions are charged particles that are electrically positive or negative, depending on their ability to accept or donate electrons. In solutions containing electrolytes, the electrostatic attraction of particles with unlike (opposite) charges and the repulsion between particles with like charges result in a tendency to produce ion pairs, which maintain electrical neutrality throughout the solution.

Electrically charged particles may be thought of as small magnets. They require energy to push them apart if they have opposite charges and to push them together if they have like electrical charges. Thus separated particles with opposite charges have an electrical magnetic-like force of attraction that gives them potential energy (Fig. 28-4). The effect of this is to establish a membrane potential between the inside and the outside of the cell. The electrical charge (potential difference) between the inside and outside of cells is expressed in millivolts (mV) (1 mV = 0.001 volt). This potential energy is released when the cell membrane separating the negatively charged ions inside the cell and the positively charged ions outside the cell becomes permeable to them.

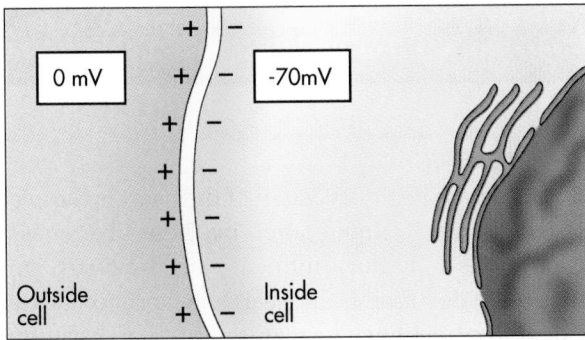

Fig. 28-4 Electrical activity of cardiac cells and membrane potentials.

Resting Membrane Potential

When the cell is in its "resting" state, the electrical charge difference is referred to as a **resting membrane potential (RMP).** The term *potential* is used in the electrical sense as a synonym for *voltage.* Because the inside of the cell is negative compared with the outside of the cell membrane and the RMP is recorded from the inside of the cell, it is reported as a negative number (about −70 to −90 mV).

The RMP is a result of the equilibrium between two opposing forces: the concentration gradient of ions (primarily potassium) across a permeable cell membrane and the electrical forces produced by the separation of positively charged ions from their negative ion pair. The RMP primarily is established by the difference between the intracellular potassium ion level and the extracellular potassium ion level. The ratio of 148:5 produces a large chemical gradient for potassium ions to leave the cell, but the negative intracellular charge relative to the extracellular charge tends to keep potassium ions in the cell (Fig. 28-5).

Sodium ions, positively charged ions on the outside of the cell, have a chemical and electrical gradient, which would tend to cause them to move intracellularly. Depolarization (electrical conduction) takes place when sodium ions rush into the cell, making the cell more positive on the inside compared with the outside.

Diffusion Through Ion Channels

The cell membrane is relatively permeable to potassium, somewhat less permeable to calcium chloride, and minimally permeable to sodium. The cell membrane appears to have individual protein-lined channels that allow passage of a specific ion or group of ions. These permeability characteristics are influenced by their electrical charge, their size, and the proteins that open and close the channels (gating proteins).

The potassium ion channels are smaller than the sodium ion channels and thus prevent sodium from passing. Potassium ions are small enough to pass through sodium ion channels, but the concentration gradient and strong electrical gradient for sodium ions from the outside to the inside of the cell favor the influx of sodium ions through the sodium ion channels over the egress of potassium ions during rapid depolarization (the rapid entry of sodium

ions into cells). Rapid depolarization creates a local area of current known as the *action potential.* After one patch of membrane is depolarized, the electrical charge spreads along the cell surface, opening more channels (Fig. 28-6).

The contribution of unpaired ions to the RMP depends on two factors: (1) the diffusion of ions through the membrane by way of the ion channels, which creates an imbalance of charges, and (2) the active transport of ions through the membrane by way of the sodium-potassium exchange pump, which also creates an imbalance of charges.

? CRITICAL THINKING

Which of these processes of electrolyte transfer requires energy to occur?

Sodium-Potassium Exchange Pump

The specialized sodium-potassium exchange pump actively pumps sodium ions out of the cell and

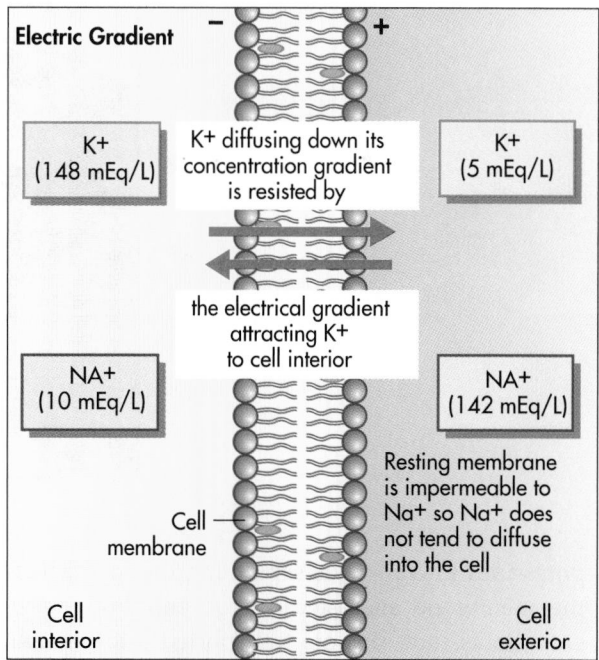

Fig. 28-5 At equilibrium (resting conditions), the tendency for potassium ions to diffuse out of the cell is opposed by the potential difference (electrical gradient) across the cell membrane. Because the resting membrane is not permeable to sodium ions, sodium ions do not tend to diffuse into the cell. (From Sims/Illustrator: Rusty Jones.)

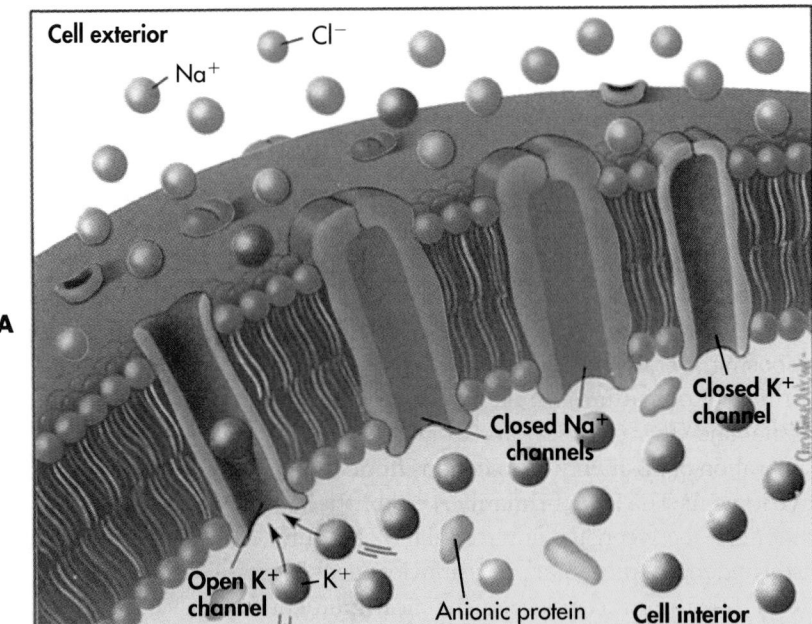

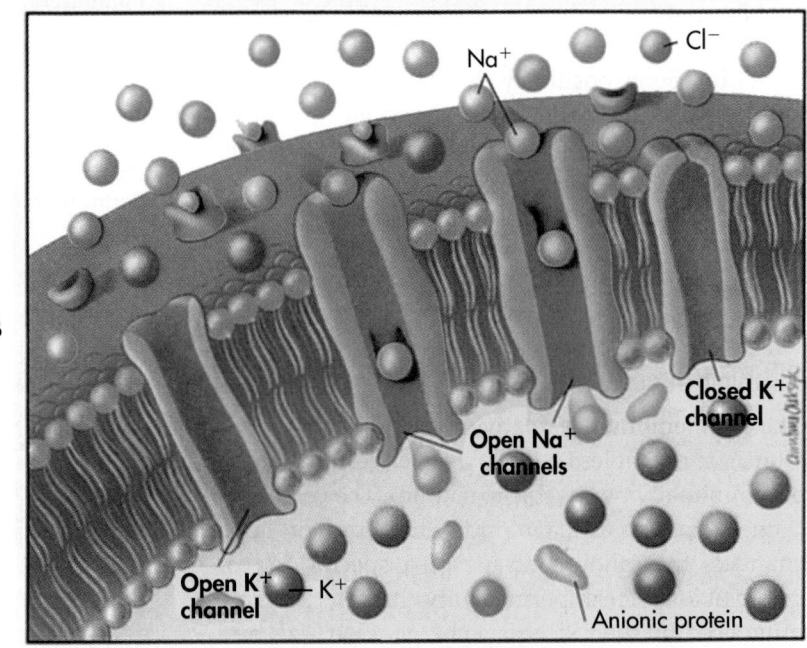

Fig. 28-6 Effect of a stimulus that causes a voltage change across the cell membrane on the permeability of the cell membrane. **A,** Sodium channels remain closed in a resting or un-stimulated cell membrane. **B,** Depolarization of the cell membrane causes sodium channels to open. Sodium ions then diffuse down their concentration gradient into the cell, causing depolarization of the cell membrane.

potassium ions in, thus separating the ions across the membrane against their concentration gradients. Potassium ions are transported into the cell, increasing their concentration in the cell; sodium ions are transported out of the cell, increasing their concentration outside (Fig. 28-7).

The sodium-potassium exchange pump normally transports three sodium ions out for every two potassium ions taken in. Therefore more positively charged ions are transferred outward than inward,

returning the cell to its resting state, where the number of negative charges inside the cell is equal to the number of positive charges outside the cell.

Pharmacological Actions

In cardiac muscle, sodium and calcium ions can enter the cell through two separate channel systems in the cell membrane: fast channels and slow channels. Fast channels are sensitive to small changes in membrane potential. As the cell drifts toward

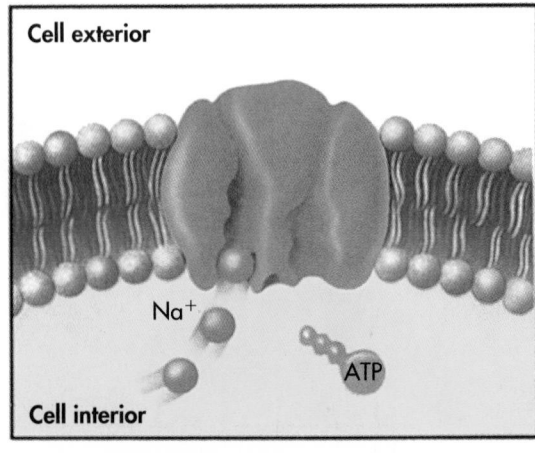
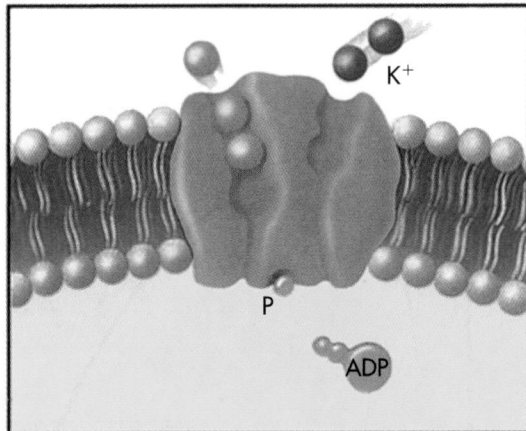
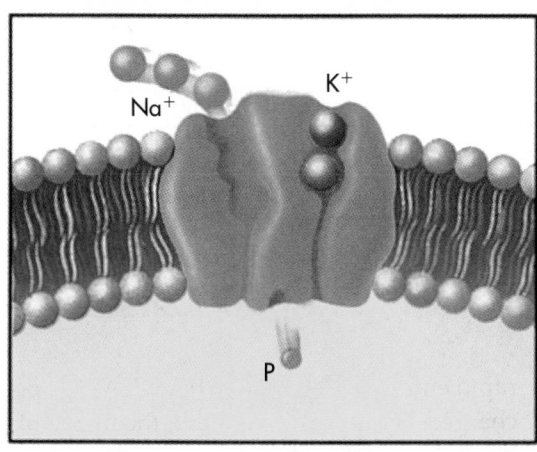
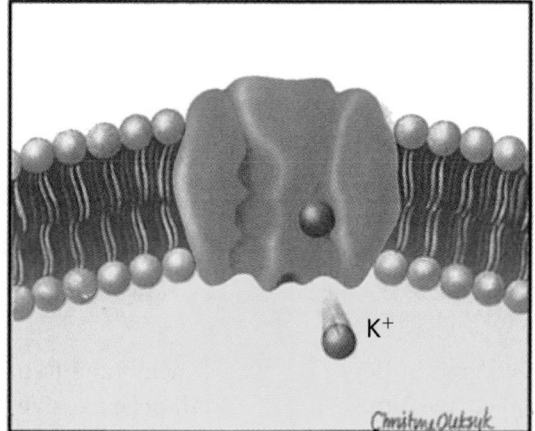

Fig. 28-7 The sodium-potassium exchange pump actively transports sodium ions out of the cell across the cell membrane and potassium ions into the cell across the cell membrane. Adenosine triphosphate is used as the energy source, and the pump can transport up to three sodium ions for every two potassium ions transported. (Illustrator Christine Oleksyk.)

threshold level (the point at which a cell depolarizes), fast sodium channels open, resulting in a rush of sodium ions intracellularly and in very rapid depolarization. The slow channel has selective permeability to calcium and to a lesser extent to sodium.

> **NOTE**
>
> Calcium plays both an electrical role by contributing to the number of positive charges in the cell and a contractile role in that it is the ion necessary for cardiac muscle contraction to occur.

An understanding of ion channels helps the paramedic understand how the heart rate and contractility can be manipulated pharmacologically. For example, calcium channel blockers (which se-

lectively block the slow channel), such as ***verapamil*** (Isoptin) and ***diltiazem*** (Cardizem), limit the movement of calcium ions into the cell without altering its voltage dependence. Other examples, such as ***procainamide*** (Pronestyl, a type I antidysrhythmic) owe much of their antidysrhythmic effects to their ability to block the fast inward sodium channel.

Cell Excitability

Nerve and muscle cells are capable of producing action potentials, a property known as *excitability*. When these cells are stimulated, a series of changes in the RMP normally causes depolarization of a small region of the cell membrane. If the stimulus is

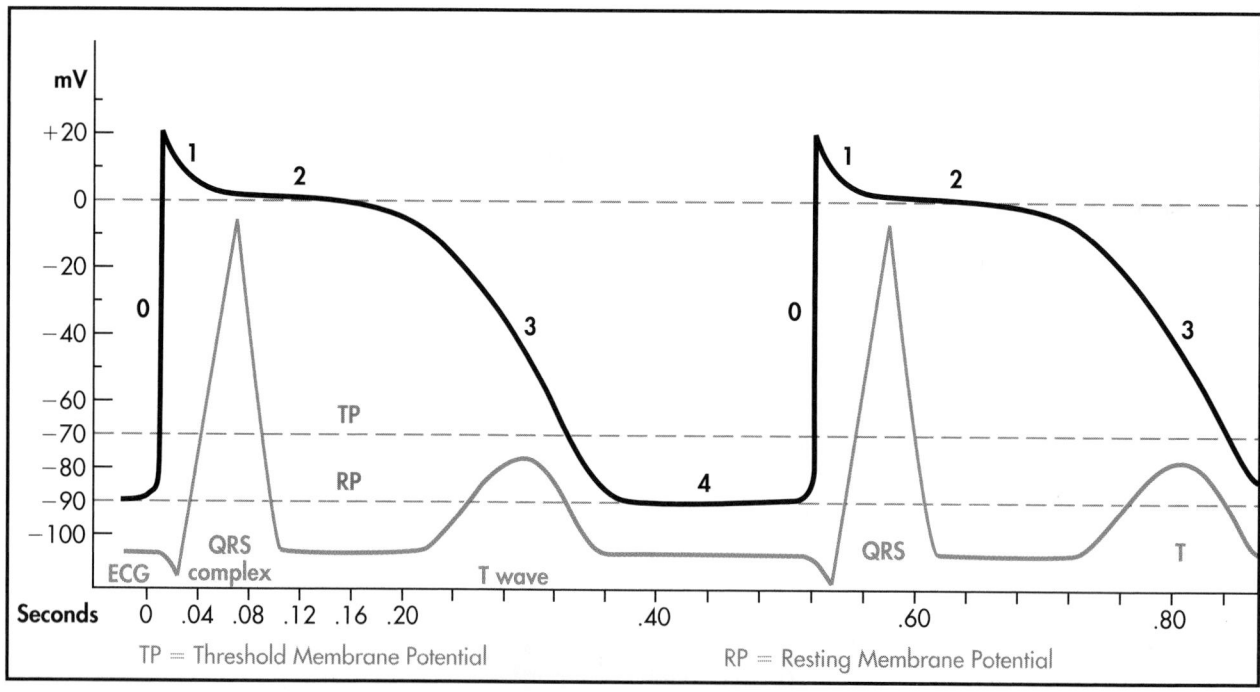

Fig. 28-8 Cardiac action potential of myocardial cells.

strong enough to depolarize a cell membrane to a level called the **threshold potential,** an explosive series of permeability changes takes place to produce an action potential that spreads over the entire cell membrane.

Propagation of Action Potential

An action potential at any point on the cell membrane acts as a stimulus to adjacent regions of the cell membrane. Therefore the excitation process, once started, is propagated (or spread) along the length of the cell and onto the next cell, and so on. A stimulus that is strong enough to cause a cell to reach threshold and depolarize (action potential) starts a cascade of depolarization from one cell to another (the all-or-none principle). The cardiac action potential can be divided into five phases (phases 0 through 4) (Fig. 28-8).

Phase 0

Phase 0 (the rapid depolarization phase) represents the very rapid upstroke of the action potential, which occurs when the cell membrane reaches threshold potential. During this phase, the fast sodium channels open momentarily, permitting

rapid entry of sodium into the cell. As the positively charged ions flow into the cell, the inside of the cell becomes positive compared with the outside, leading to muscular contraction.

Phase 1

During phase 1 (the early rapid depolarization phase), the fast sodium channels close, the flow of sodium into the cell stops, and potassium continues to be lost from the cell. This results in a decrease in the number of positive electrical charges inside the cell and a drop in the membrane potential, returning the cell membrane to its resting permeability state.

Phase 2

Phase 2 (the plateau phase) is the prolonged phase of repolarization of the action potential. During this phase, calcium enters the myocardial cells, triggering a large secondary release of calcium from intracellular storage sites and initiating contraction. Calcium slowly enters the cell through the slow calcium channels as potassium continues to leave the cell. The inward calcium current maintains the cell in a prolonged depolarization state (allowing time for completion of one muscle contraction before another depolarization begins), stimulates the release of intracellular stores of calcium, and aids in the contraction process.

Phase 3

Phase 3 (the terminal phase of rapid repolarization) results in the inside of the cell becoming markedly negative and the membrane potential returning to its resting state. This phase is initiated by closing of the slow calcium channels and by an increase in permeability with an outflow of potassium. Repolarization is completed by the end of this phase.

Phase 4

Phase 4 represents the period between action potentials, when the membrane has returned to its RMP. During this phase, the inside of the cell is negative with respect to the outside, but there is still an excess of sodium in the cell and potassium outside the cell. This activates the sodium-potassium exchange pump, and the excess sodium is transported out of the cell and the potassium back in. During phase 4, pacemaker cells have a slow depolarization from their most negative membrane potential to a level at which threshold is reached and phase 0 begins all over again.

Refractory Period of Cardiac Muscle

Cardiac muscle, like all excitable tissue, has a **refractory period** associated with the action potential. During the absolute refractory period, the cardiac muscle cell is completely insensitive to further stimulation. Because the depolarization phase of cardiac muscle is prolonged, the refractory period also is prolonged (Fig. 28-9).

The refractory period ensures that the cardiac muscle is completely relaxed before another action potential can be initiated. The refractory period of the ventricles is of about the same duration as that of the action potential. The refractory period of the atrial muscle is much shorter than that of the ventricles, allowing the rate of atrial contraction to be much faster than that of the ventricles. There also is

> **? CRITICAL THINKING**
>
> *How are the relative and absolute refractory periods of the heart similar to the flushing mechanism of your toilet?*

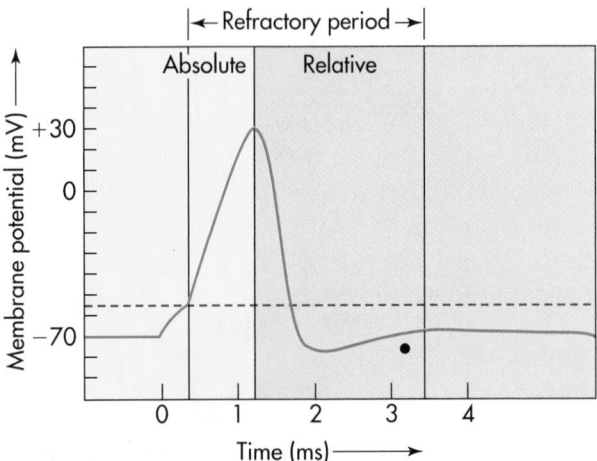

Fig. 28-9 Refractory period. (From Thibodeau GA, Patton KT: *Anatomy and physiology,* ed 2, St Louis, 1993, Mosby.)

a relative refractory period during which the muscle cell is more difficult than normal to excite but nonetheless can still be stimulated.

Electrical Conduction System of the Heart

The conduction system of the heart is composed of two nodes and a conducting bundle (Fig. 28-10). The two nodes are contained within the walls of the right atrium and are named according to their location. The sinoatrial (SA) node is medial to the opening of the superior vena cava, and the atrioventricular (AV) node is medial to the right AV valve. The AV node and the bundle of His form the AV junction, which serves as the only electrical link between the atria and ventricles in a normal heart. The bundle of His passes through a small opening in the fibrous skeleton to reach the interventricular septum, where it divides into right and left bundle branches. The left bundle branch then subdivides into the anterior-superior and posterior-inferior fascicles, which provide pathways for impulse conduction. A third fascicle of the left bundle branch that innervates the interventricular septum and the base of the heart also has been identified.

The right and left bundle branches extend beneath the endocardium on either side of the septum to the apical portions of the right and left ventricles, respectively. The bundle branches subdivide into smaller branches and become Purkinje fibers. The

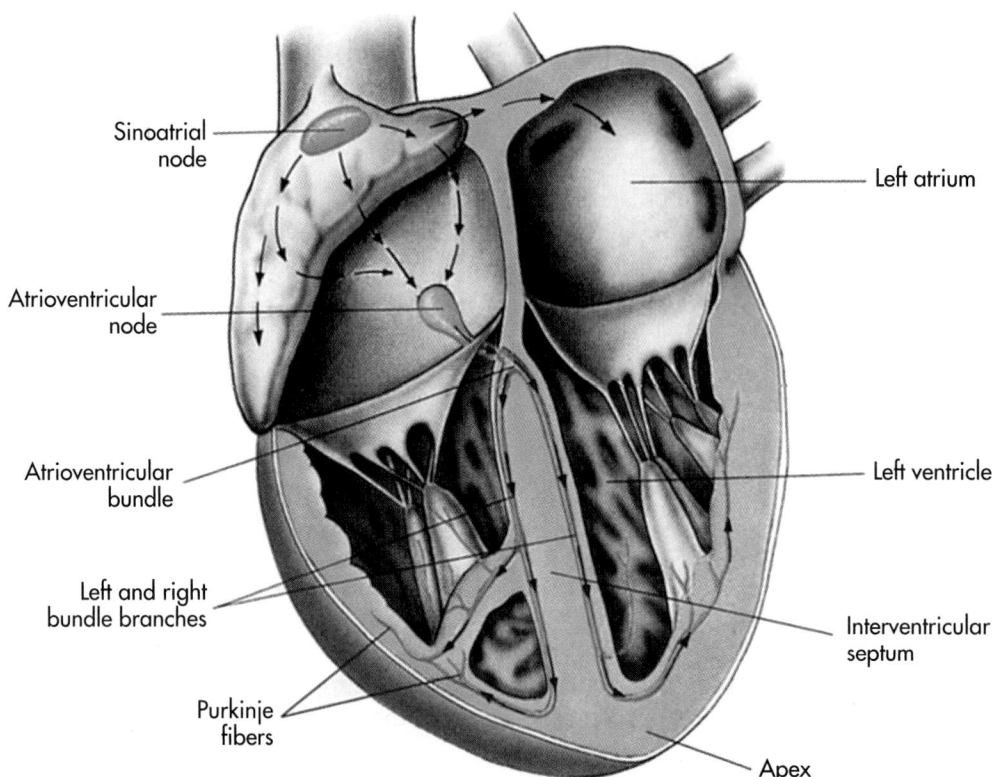

Fig. 28-10 Conduction system of the heart. Impulses *(arrows)* travel across the wall of the right atrium from the SA node to the AV node. The AV bundle extends from the AV node through the fibrous skeleton and into the interventricular septum, where it divides into right and left bundle branches. The bundle branches descend to the apex of the ventricle and then branch repeatedly for distribution throughout the ventricular walls. (Illustrator Barbara Cousins.)

terminal Purkinje fibers contact myocardial fibers through which electrical impulses spread from cell to cell in the remaining myocardium (resulting in contraction). The rapid conduction along these fibers causes depolarization of all right and left ventricular cells more or less simultaneously, ensuring a single coordinated contraction.

Pacemaker Activity

In skeletal and most smooth muscle, the individual cells contract only in response to impulses arising from hormonal stimulation or neurotransmitters from the efferent branch of the central nervous system. However, unlike most other muscle cells, cardiac fibers have specialized cells (pacemaker cells) capable of generating electrical impulses spontaneously (a property known as **automaticity**). Pacemaker cells depolarize in a repetitive manner. This rhythmic activity occurs because these tissues do not have a stable RMP. Instead, the RMP gradually

decreases with time from its maximum repolarization potential until it reaches a critical threshold, at which time depolarization results. If the heart's normal pacemaker cells of the SA node fail to generate an electrical impulse, other pacemaker cells take over. These pacemaker cells also are capable of spontaneous depolarization and subsequent spread of an action potential, although it occurs usually at a slower intrinsic rate.

Sequence of Excitation in Cardiac Muscle

Under normal circumstances, the dominant pacemaker function of the heart is supplied by the SA node. This is because the SA node reaches its threshold for depolarization at a faster rate than other specialized tissues. The rapid rate of the SA node normally prevents the discharge of slower pacemakers from becoming dominant. If impulses from the SA node do not develop normally, however, the next specialized tissue to reach its threshold level would assume the pacemaker duties.

Cardiac cells, with their characteristic automaticity, serve as a "fail-safe" mechanism for initiating electrical impulses. The "backup" cells (intrinsic pacemakers) are arranged in cascade fashion; the farther from the SA node, the slower the intrinsic firing rate. In order, the location of cells with pacemaker capabilities and rates of spontaneous discharge are the SA node (60 to 100 discharges per minute); AV junctional tissue (40 to 60 discharges per minute); and the ventricles, including the bundle branches and Purkinje fibers (20 to 40 discharges per minute) (Fig. 28-11).

From the SA node, the excitation spreads throughout the right atrium. Through internodal tracts, impulses travel directly from the right to the left atrium and to the base of the right atrium, resulting in virtually simultaneous contraction of both atria. About 0.04 second is required for the impulse of the SA node to spread to the AV node. From there, propagation of the action potentials within the AV node is slow compared with the rate in the remainder of the conducting system. As a result, there is a delay of 0.11 second from the time the action potentials reach the AV node until they pass to the AV bundle. The total delay of 0.15 second allows atrial contraction to be completed before ventricular contraction begins.

After leaving the AV node, the impulse picks up speed and travels rapidly through the bundle of His and the left and right bundle branches. The action potential passes quickly through the individual Purkinje fibers, ending in near-simultaneous stimulation and contraction of the left and right ventricles. Ventricular contraction begins at the apex. Once stimulated, the special arrangement of muscle layers in the wall of the heart produce a wringing action that proceeds toward the base of the heart.

Autonomic Nervous System Effects on Pacemaker Cells

The effects of autonomic nervous system stimulation on the heart rate are mediated through the chemical neurotransmitters acetylcholine and norepinephrine. Acetylcholine causes the cell membrane of the SA node to become more permeable to potassium ions, resulting in hyperpolarization. This delays the pacemaker reaching threshold and therefore decreases the heart rate. Parasympathetic ef-

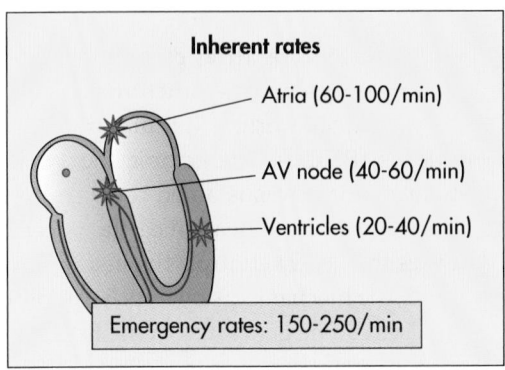

Fig. 28-11 Intrinsic pacemakers in the atria, AV node, and ventricles can discharge at their own inherent rate when normal pacemaking fails. (Redrawn from Dubin D: *Rapid interpretation of EKGs,* ed 3, Tampa, Fla., 1983, Cover Publishing.)

fects also may result from stimulation of the cardiac branch of the vagus nerve to the heart, as occurs in vigorous carotid sinus massage, which may abolish the threshold potential altogether.

> **NOTE**
>
> Excessive vagal stimulation may result in asystole (the absence of electrical and mechanical activity in the heart), hence the reason why asystole sometimes is referred to as the "ultimate bradycardia."

> **? CRITICAL THINKING**
>
> *What else can cause unintentional vagal stimulation?*

Norepinephrine increases the heart rate by increasing the rate of depolarization. The result is an increase in pacemaker discharge rate in the SA node. Norepinephrine increases the flow of potassium and calcium ions into the cell during depolarization of the action potential. As a result, sympathetic stimulation leads to an increase in the heart rate and the force of cardiac contraction.

Mechanisms of Ectopic Electrical Impulse Formation

An ectopic beat results when the pacemaker function is assumed for one beat by cells other than those in the SA node. These isolated events sometimes are referred to as *premature beats* because they occur early in diastole before the SA node normally is scheduled to discharge. The new pacemaker is called an *ectopic focus.* Depending on the location of the ectopic focus, the premature beats may be of atrial origin **(premature atrial complexes [PACs]),** junctional origin, **(premature junctional complexes [PJCs]),** or ventricular origin **(premature ventricular complexes [PVCs]).** The ectopic focus may be intermittent or may be sustained and assume the pacemaker duties of the heart (i.e., the pacemaker site that fires the fastest controls the heart).

The two basic mechanisms by which ectopic electrical impulses can be generated in the heart are enhanced automaticity and reentry.

Enhanced Automaticity

Enhanced automaticity is caused by an acceleration in depolarization that commonly results from an abnormally high leakage of sodium ions into the cells, causing the cells to reach threshold prematurely. As a result, the rate of electrical impulse formation in potential pacemakers increases beyond their inherent rate.

Enhanced automaticity is responsible for dysrhythmias in Purkinje fibers and other myocardial cells. This condition may occur secondary to excess catecholamines (i.e., norepinephrine, epinephrine), digitalis toxicity, hypoxia, hypercapnia, myocardial ischemia or infarction, increased venous return (preload), hypokalemia or other electrolyte abnormalities, or *atropine* administration.

Reentry

Reentry is the reactivation of myocardial tissue for the second or subsequent time by the same impulse (Fig. 28-12). It occurs when the progression of an electrical impulse is delayed, blocked, or both, in one or more segments of the heart's electrical conduction system. A delayed or blocked impulse that enters cardiac cells that have just become repolarized may produce single or repetitive ectopic beats. Reentry dysrhythmias can occur in the SA node, atria, AV junction, bundle branches, or Purkinje fibers. Reentry is the most common mechanism in producing ectopic beats, including cases of PVCs, **ventricular tachycardia (VT), ventricular fibrillation (VF), atrial fibrillation, atrial flutter,** and **paroxysmal supraventricular tachycardia (PSVT).**

The reentry mechanism requires that, at some point, conduction through the heart takes parallel pathways, each having a different conduction speed and different refractory characteristics. A premature impulse, for example, may find one branch of a conducting pathway still refractory from the passage of the last normal impulse. If the impulse passes (somewhat slowly) along a parallel conducting pathway, by the time the impulse reaches the previously blocked pathway, it may have had time to recover its ability to conduct. If the two parallel paths connect at an area of excitable myocardial tissue, the depolarization process from the slower path may enter the now repolarized tissue and give rise to a new impulse spawned from the original impulse. Common causes of delayed or blocked electrical impulses include myocardial ischemia, certain drugs, and hyperkalemia.

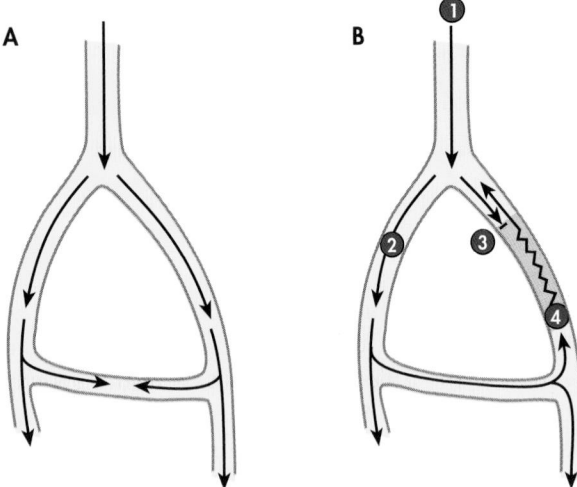

Fig. 28-12 Reentry within terminal Purkinje fibers. **A,** Conduction through normal Purkinje fibers. The conduction velocity is uniform. **B,** Conduction through a severely depressed segment of terminal Purkinje fibers. The impulse *(1)* travels normally through normal tissue *(2)* and is blocked at the severely depressed tissue *(3)*, but returns, with delay, through this tissue from the opposite direction. (From Marriott H: *Advanced concepts in arrhythmias,* ed 2, St Louis, 1989, Mosby.)

SECTION THREE
ASSESSMENT OF THE CARDIAC PATIENT

Assessment

A focused evaluation of any patient should identify a chief complaint, cover the history of the event and significant past medical history, and include a physical examination. These elements are important in determining the cause of the emergency event, directing initial patient care, and anticipating potential problems during patient transport to a medical facility. The following discussion of patient assessment serves as a framework for approaching a patient with a cardiovascular problem.

Chief Complaint

Cardiovascular disease may present with a variety of symptoms. It is the paramedic's responsibility to obtain an appropriate history of each symptom and apply the information to form a diagnostic impression in any patient with a possible coronary event. Common chief complaints include chest pain or discomfort, including shoulder, arm, neck, or jaw pain or discomfort; dyspnea; syncope; and abnormal heartbeat or palpitations.

NOTE

In some patients (particularly older adults), cardiovascular problems commonly present with atypical symptoms such as mental status changes, abdominal or gastrointestinal symptoms, and vague complaints of being ill.

Chest Pain or Discomfort

Chest pain or discomfort is the most common chief complaint of patients with myocardial infarction. However, many causes of chest pain are unrelated to cardiac disease (e.g., pulmonary embolus, pleurisy, and reflux esophagitis). Therefore a history of chest pain is important. The OPQRST method (or a similar method) should be used to obtain the following information when possible:

O: Onset/Origin? What does the pain feel like? What were you doing when the pain began? Do you have a past history of similar pain?

P: Provokes? What makes the pain better? What makes the pain worse? (e.g., relief with rest or *nitroglycerin;* worsening with exercise or eating fried foods)

Q: Quality? Is the pain sharp or tearing, burning, heavy, or squeezing?

R: Region? Where does it hurt? (Try to localize it.) Does it radiate? Where to?

S: Severity? How badly does it hurt? Have you ever had pain like this before? How would you rate your pain on a scale of 1 to 10?

T: Time? How long have you had the pain? Is the pain constant or does it come and go?

NOTE

Cocaine-induced chest pain is one of the most common complaints of cocaine users. Cocaine use can cause serious cardiac toxicity from the drug's effect on the heart coupled with central nervous system stimulatory effects on the cardiovascular system. Although rare, AMI can occur in these patients, even in the absence of risk factors for ischemic heart disease.[1]

Dyspnea

Dyspnea often is associated with myocardial infarction and is a primary symptom of pulmonary congestion caused by heart failure. Other common causes of dyspnea that may be unrelated to heart disease include chronic obstructive pulmonary disease, respiratory infection, pulmonary embolus, and asthma. Historical factors important in differentiating breathing difficulties include the following:

- Duration and circumstances of onset of dyspnea
- Anything that aggravates or relieves the dyspnea, including medications
- Previous episodes
- Associated symptoms
- Orthopnea
- Prior cardiac problems

Syncope

Syncope is caused by a sudden decrease in cerebral perfusion. Cardiac causes of syncope result from events that decrease cardiac output. The most common cardiac disorders associated with syncope are dysrhythmias. Other causes of syncope in the medical patient include stroke, drug or alcohol intoxication, aortic stenosis, pulmonary embolism, and hypoglycemia. In the older patient, syncope may be the only symptom of a cardiac problem. Young, otherwise healthy people may have a syncopal episode resulting from increased vagal tone (vasovagal syncope) that produces hypotension and bradycardia. The history of a syncopal event should include:

- Presyncope aura (nausea, weakness, lightheadedness)
- Circumstances of occurrence (e.g., patient's position before the event, severe pain, emotional stress)

? CRITICAL THINKING

Syncopal events often occur in public places, such as a church. How can you decrease the feelings of embarrassment that the patient may have during this situation?

- Duration of syncopal episode
- Symptoms before syncopal episode (palpitation, seizure, incontinence)
- Other associated symptoms
- Previous episodes of syncope

Abnormal Heartbeat and Palpitations

Many patients are aware of their own heartbeat, particularly if it is irregular ("skipping beats") or rapid ("fluttering"). Palpitations sometimes are a normal occurrence but also may indicate a serious dysrhythmia. Important information to obtain from these patients includes:

- Pulse rate
- Regular versus irregular rhythm
- Circumstances of occurrence
- Duration
- Associated symptoms (chest pain, diaphoresis, syncope, confusion, dyspnea)
- Previous episodes, frequency
- Medication (drug stimulant) or alcohol use

Significant Past Medical History

Past medical history is an important aspect of any patient assessment. If possible, the paramedic should determine the following six points:

1. Is the patient taking prescription medications, particularly cardiac medications? Common medications that should alert the paramedic to a possible coronary event include:
   a. *Nitroglycerin*
   b. Beta blockers (e.g., *propranolol* [Inderal], *atenolol* [Apo-Atenol])
   c. Calcium channel blockers
   d. Antihyperlipidemics
   e. Digitalis
   f. Diuretics
   g. Antihypertensives
   h. Other antidysrhythmics
2. Is the patient being treated for any other illness?
3. Has the patient ever had any of the following?
   a. Myocardial infarction or episodes of angina pectoris
   b. Coronary artery bypass procedure or angioplasty
   c. Heart failure
   d. Hypertension
   e. Diabetes
   f. Chronic lung disease
4. Does the patient have any allergies?
5. Are there any other associated risk factors for a cardiac event?
   a. Patient age
   b. Smoking
   c. Diabetes
   d. Family history
   e. Obesity
   f. Hypercholesterolemia (increased serum cholesterol level)
   g. Routine medications that may cause cardiac symptoms
   h. Cardiac effects from illicit drug use (e.g., cocaine, methamphetamine)
6. Does the patient have an implanted pacemaker or ICD?

Physical Examination

The "classical presentation" of myocardial infarction is pain or discomfort beneath the sternum (often described as *crushing, pressure, squeezing,* or *burning*) that often lasts more than 30 minutes. Associated signs and symptoms may include apprehension, diaphoresis, dyspnea, nausea and vomiting, and a sense of impending doom (e.g., patients feel that they are going to die). Unfortunately, at times the presentation is atypical. The paramedic's skill in gathering a pertinent medical history and performing a focused physical examination directs patient care and may greatly influence patient outcome.

When caring for a patient with chest pain caused by a coronary event, the paramedic should remember that the patient is experiencing a devastating episode with the potential for life-threatening consequences. These patients should be calmed and reassured to decrease their anxiety.

Initial Assessment

In most medical emergencies involving conscious patients, the primary elements of the initial assessment (airway, breathing, and circulation) can be evaluated during the initial paramedic-patient encounter. Vital sign assessment and a quick neurological examination evaluate the following:

- Level of consciousness (Alterations in the patient's level of consciousness may indicate decreased cerebral perfusion caused by poor cardiac output. If possible, determine the normal level of function for this patient.)
- Respirations
- Pulse (rate, regularity)
- Blood pressure

Physical Examination

The physical examination of the cardiac patient should be systematic and complete, using a "look-listen-feel" approach.

Look

Skin color, capillary refill, skin moisture
    Indications of adequate hemoglobin oxygenation
        (pulse oximetry)

Indications of cardiac function (peripheral perfusion)
Jugular vein distention (JVD)
    An increase in central venous pressure can produce engorgement of internal jugular veins. JVD should be evaluated with the patient's head elevated at 45 degrees. (Normal venous pressure is 1 to 2 cm.)
    JVD may be difficult to assess in obese patients.
Peripheral and presacral edema
    Edema may be caused by chronic back-pressure in systemic venous circulation.
    Edema is most obvious in dependent areas (ankles and sacral region in bedridden patients).
    Edema may be nonpitting (with minimal or no depression of tissue after removal of finger pressure) or pitting (when depression of tissue remains after removal of finger pressure).
Additional indicators of cardiac disease
    Nitroglycerin patch
    Midsternal scar from coronary surgery
    Implanted pacemaker or automatic ICD (left upper chest; abdominal wall)
    Medical alert information

Listen

Lung sounds
    Assess for equality.
    Assess for adventitious sounds that may indicate pulmonary congestion or edema.
Heart sounds (Box 28-2)
    Carotid artery bruit: assessed if contemplating carotid sinus massage

Feel

Peripheral or presacral edema
    Pulse
    Rate
    Regularity
    Equality
    Pulse deficit
Skin
    Diaphoretic pale skin is an indicator of peripheral vasoconstriction and sympathetic stimulation.
    Cyanosis is an indicator of poor oxygenation.
    Fever usually is an indicator of infection.

NOTE

The apical pulse (described in Chapter 13) can best be evaluated at the **point of maximum impulse (PMI).** The PMI is the location at which the apical impulse is most readily seen or palpated—often in the fifth intercostal space, just medial to the left midclavicular line. The PMI can be used to assess for pulse deficit and can help locate the left ventricle's apex. It also identifies the location of the mitral valve for assessing heart sounds.

BOX 28-2

HEART SOUNDS

Heart sounds can typically be auscultated with a stethoscope during ventricular systole and diastole. When the ventricles contract, both AV valves close nearly simultaneously. This closure causes a vibration of the valves and surrounding fluid and results in a low-pitched sound (often described as a "lubb" sound). Closing of the aortic and pulmonary semilunar valves at the end of ventricular systole produces a higher-pitched sound (described as "dubb"). These normal heart sounds are referred to as S_1 and S_2, respectively.

Rarely, a third heart sound can be heard near the end of the first third of diastole (S_3). The third heart sound (caused by turbulent flow of blood into the ventricles) may be normal but may be an indicator of congestive heart failure. A fourth heart sound (S_4) may be heard during the end of diastole. It is thought to result from turbulence and chamber stretching from the atrial contraction during this part of the cardiac cycle and is often a sign of congestive heart failure in adults.

NOTE: Both the S_3 and S_4 contribute to "gallop" rhythms, which are useful clinical indicators of congestive heart failure. Heart sounds are difficult to distinguish in the field. The evaluation of heart sounds should never delay emergency care or transport; they do not alter prehospital patient management.

S_1: First heart sound occurs with closure of AV valves during ventricular systole.

S_2: Second heart sound occurs with closure of aortic and pulmonic valves and signifies the beginning of ventricular diastole.

S_3: Extra heart sound is heard after S_2 and is compatible with heart failure but not always present.

S_4: Extra heart sound is heard in late diastole (just before S_1); it is associated with atrial contractions and often heard in patients with congestive heart failure.

The electrocardiogram (ECG) is a graphic representation of the heart's electrical activity generated by depolarization and repolarization of the atria and ventricles. It is a valuable diagnostic tool for identifying a number of cardiac abnormalities, including abnormal heart rates and rhythms, abnormal conduction pathways, hypertrophy or atrophy of portions of the heart, and the approximate location of ischemic or infarcted cardiac muscle.

Evaluation of the ECG requires a systematic approach that includes descriptive analysis (assessing the ECG tracing) and clinical impression (applying ECG analysis in assessing the patient). The ECG tracing is only a reflection of the heart's electrical activity. It does not provide information on mechanical events such as force of contraction or blood pressure.

? CRITICAL THINKING

Aside from blood pressure, how will you evaluate the mechanical activity of the heart?

Basic Concepts of ECG Monitoring

The summation of all the action potentials transmitted through the heart during the cardiac cycle can be measured on the surface of the body. This measurement is obtained by applying electrodes on the body's surface that are connected to an ECG machine. The voltage changes are fed to the machine, amplified, and displayed visually on the oscilloscope, graphically on ECG paper, or both. Voltage may be positive (seen as an upward deflection on the ECG tracing); negative (seen as a downward deflection on the ECG tracing); or isoelectric, when no electrical current is detected (seen as a straight baseline on the ECG tracing).

ECG Leads

ECG machines can provide many views of the heart's electrical activity by monitoring voltage changes between any number of electrodes applied

TABLE 28-1		COMPARISON OF VARIOUS LEADS
I, II, III	Limb lead	Bipolar
aV_R, aV_L, aV_F	Limb lead	Unipolar
V_1-V_6	Chest lead	Unipolar

From Phalen T: *The 12-lead ECG in acute myocardial infarction,* St Louis, 1996, Mosby.

in various places on the body. Each pair of electrodes is referred to as a *lead*. A standard ECG performed in the hospital is recorded by viewing the heart's electrical activity from 12 leads. Many EMS services in the United States have equipment that provides 12-lead monitoring.

An ECG lead consists of two surface electrodes of opposite polarity (one positive and the other negative) or one positive surface electrode and one reference point. A lead composed of two electrodes of opposite polarity is called a *bipolar lead*. A lead composed of a single positive electrode and a reference point is a unipolar lead. Bipolar leads constitute the standard limb leads (I through III). Unipolar leads make up the augmented limb leads (aV_R, aV_L, and aV_F) and the precordial leads (V_1 through V_6) (Table 28-1).

Each lead assesses the electrical activity of the heart from a slightly different angle. The various leads produce different ECG tracings. If the depolarization moves toward a positive electrode, the ECG tracing for that particular lead shows an upward deflection. If the wave moves away from a positive electrode, a negative deflection appears on the ECG tracing (Fig. 28-13).

Standard Limb Leads

Standard limb leads record the difference in electrical potential between the left arm, the right arm, and the left leg electrodes, which represent the axes (the average direction of the heart's electrical activity) of the standard limb leads. If these axes are moved so that they cross a common midpoint without changing their orientation, they form a triaxial reference system (three intersecting lines of reference). Lead I is a lateral (leftward) lead that assesses the heart's electrical activity from a vantage point defined as 0 degrees on a circle divided into an upper negative 180 degrees and a lower positive 180 degrees. Leads II and III are inferior leads that assess the heart's

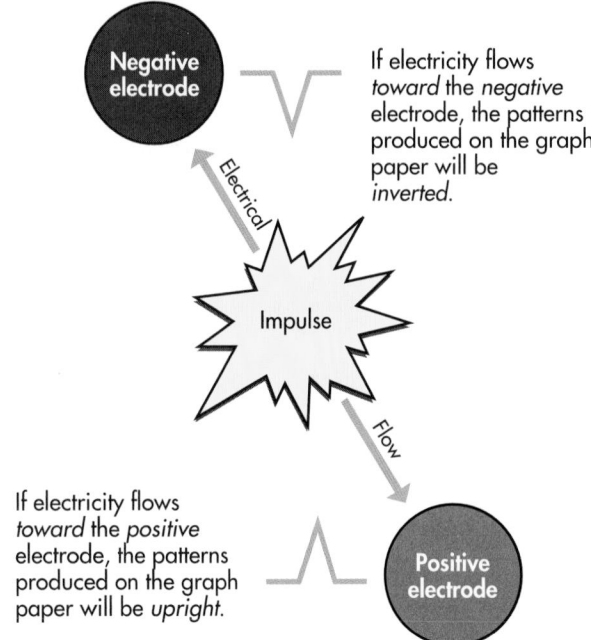

Negative electrode

If electricity flows *toward* the *negative* electrode, the patterns produced on the graph paper will be *inverted.*

Impulse

If electricity flows *toward* the *positive* electrode, the patterns produced on the graph paper will be *upright.*

Positive electrode

Fig. 28-13 Rule of electrical flow. (From Walraven G: *Basic arrhythmias,* ed 3, Englewood Cliffs, N.J., 1992, Prentice Hall.)

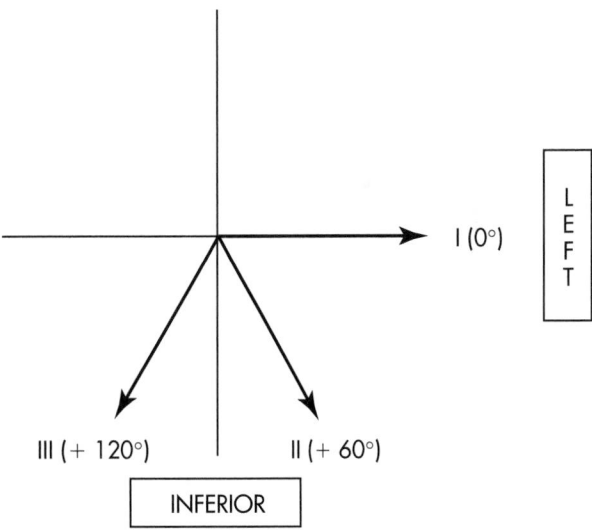

I (0°)

L E F T

III (+ 120°)   II (+ 60°)

INFERIOR

Fig. 28-14 Electrical vantage points of the three standard limb leads. (From Grauer K: *Practical guide to ECG interpretation,* St Louis, 1992, Mosby.)

electrical activity from vantage points of +60 degrees and +120 degrees, respectively (Fig. 28-14). The electrodes of the three bipolar leads are placed on the following areas of the body:

Lead	Positive electrode	Negative electrode
I	Left arm	Right arm
II	Left leg	Right arm
III	Left leg	Left arm

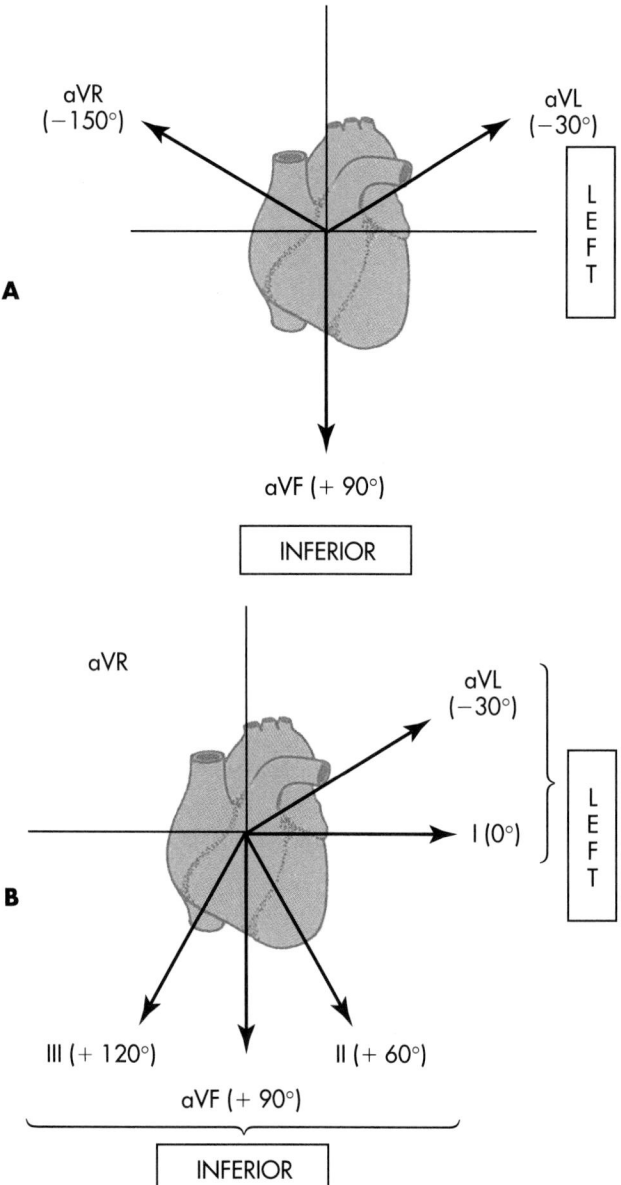

Fig. 28-15 A, Electrical vantage points of the three augmented limb leads. **B,** Combined electrical vantage points. Leads II, III, and aV_F are considered inferior leads; leads I and aV_L are considered lateral leads. (From Grauer K: *Practical guide to ECG interpretation,* St Louis, 1992, Mosby.)

Augmented Limb Leads

Augmented limb leads record the difference in electrical potential between the respective extremity lead sites and a reference point with zero electrical potential at the center of the electrical field of the heart. As a result, the axis of each lead is formed by the line from the electrode site (on the right arm, left arm, or left leg) to the center of the heart. The aV_R, aV_L, and aV_F leads intersect at dif-

ferent angles than the standard limb leads and produce three other intersecting lines of reference, which together with the standard limb leads make up the hexaxial reference system. Augmented limb leads use the same set of electrodes as the standard limb leads. They measure an axis between the two bipolar leads by electronically combining the negative electrodes.

> **NOTE**
>
> Augmented limb leads "augment" the voltage of the positive lead to increase the size of the ECG complexes.

Lead aV_L acts as a lateral (leftward) lead that records the heart's electrical activity from a vantage point that looks down from the left shoulder (−30 degrees). Lead aV_F acts as an inferior lead, recording the heart's electrical activity from a vantage point that looks up from the left lower extremity (+90 degrees). Lead aV_R is a distant recording electrode that looks down at the heart from the right shoulder. Based on these lead descriptions, the lateral, or left-sided, leads are I and aV_L, and the inferior leads are II, III, and aV_F (Fig. 28-15).

> **? CRITICAL THINKING**
>
> *Why is aV_R seldom used in ECG analysis? What "view" of the heart does it provide?*

Modified Lead Recording

Placement of the limb leads can be altered to mimic the precordial leads (V_1 through V_6) and can help evaluate conduction in specific areas of the heart. These leads are referred to as *modified chest leads* and become MCL_1 through MCL_6. Modified chest leads that are particularly useful for monitoring cardiac activity in the prehospital setting are MCL_1 and MCL_6. These leads may help distinguish between supraventricular tachycardia with aberration and ventricular tachycardia and can help diagnose conduction blocks in the bundle branches (described later in this chapter).

> **NOTE**
>
> Modified chest leads have the same "look" as V leads.

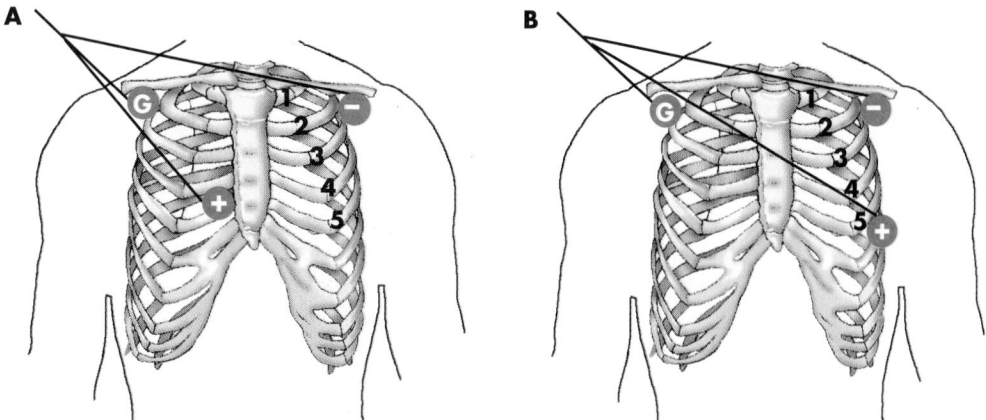

Fig. 28-16 Monitor lead placement for MCL₁ **(A)** and MCL₆ **(B).** (From Goldberger A: *Treatment of cardiac emergencies,* ed 5, St Louis, 1990, Mosby.)

When MCL₁ is viewed, the positive electrode is placed in the V₁ position (in the fourth intercostal space, just to the right of the patient's sternum) and the negative electrode is placed anteriorly, just below the lateral end of the left clavicle. Electrical activity in MCL₆ is observed by placing the positive electrode on the left midaxillary line at the level of the fifth intercostal space (as for lead V₆). The negative electrode is placed anteriorly, just below the left shoulder (Fig. 28-16).

Routine ECG Monitoring

Routine monitoring of cardiac rhythm in the prehospital setting, emergency department, or coronary care unit usually is obtained in lead II or MCL₁; these are the best leads to monitor for dysrhythmias because of their ability to visualize P waves. Considerable information can be gathered from a single monitoring lead, and in many situations, cardiac monitoring by a single lead is sufficient. For example, a paramedic can determine how fast the heart is beating, how regular the heartbeat is, and how long conduction lasts in different parts of the heart. Single-lead monitoring has limitations, however; it may fail to reveal various abnormalities (particularly ST-segment changes that signal myocardial injury or infarction) in the ECG tracing.

12-Lead ECG Monitoring

A 12-lead ECG is obtained through 10 electrodes: four limb leads (right arm, right leg, left arm, left leg) and six chest leads (V₁ through V₆). The four

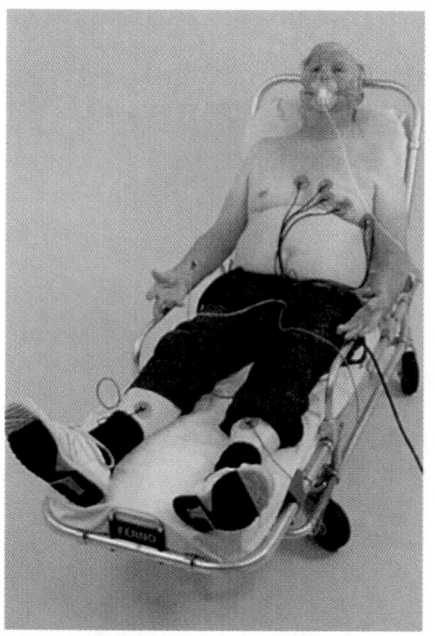

Fig. 28-17 To obtain a 12-lead ECG when using a 12-lead monitor or machine, simply attach the cables to the electrodes, ask the patient to be still, and push the record button. Acquisition requires only 10 seconds. (From American College of Emergency Physicians: *Paramedic field care: a complaint-based approach,* St Louis, 1997, Mosby.)

limb leads provide readings of leads I, II, and III, and aV_F, aV_L, and aV_R. Each lead of the 12-lead ECG views the left ventricle from the position of its positive electrode. Monitoring 12 leads is performed with a 12-lead monitor that obtains the leads simultaneously and provides a readout in conventional three- or four-column format (Fig. 28-17). As

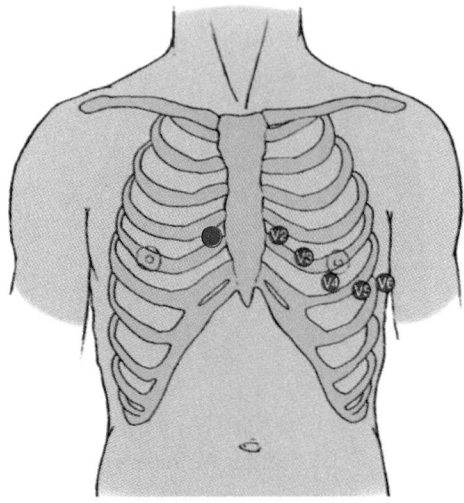

Fig. 28-18 Proper chest lead placement. (From Phalen T: *The 12-lead ECG in acute myocardial infarction*, St Louis, 1996, Mosby.)

NOTE: 15-lead ECGs are not routinely performed in the prehospital setting.

described later in this chapter, 12-lead ECG monitoring can be used to help:

- Identify ST-segment and T-wave changes relative to myocardial ischemia, injury, and infarction.
- Identify VT in wide-complex tachycardia.
- Determine the electrical axis and the presence of fascicular blocks.
- Determine the presence and location of bundle branch blocks.

Precordial Leads

The six precordial leads used in 12-lead (and 9-lead) ECG monitoring are projected through the anterior chest wall toward the patient's back (the negative end of each chest lead) (Fig. 28-18). These positive leads are placed on the chest in reference to the thoracic landmarks and record the heart's electrical activity in the transverse or horizontal plane. Leads V_1 and V_2 are septal leads, V_2 through V_4 are anterior leads, and V_4 through V_6 are lateral precordial leads (see the box in the right column).

Proper placement of the chest leads at specific intercostal spaces is essential for an accurate reading. One method (Fig. 28-19) to locate the appropriate intercostal spaces is to[2]:

1. Locate the jugular notch and move downward until the sternal angle is found.

2. Follow the articulation to the right sternal border to locate the second rib. Just below the second rib is the second intercostal space.
3. Move down two intercostal spaces and position the V_1 electrode in the fourth intercostal space, just to the right of the patient's sternum.
4. Move across the sternum to the corresponding intercostal space and position V_2 to the left of the patient's sternum.
5. From V_2, palpate down one intercostal space and follow the fifth intercostal space to the midclavicular line to place the V_4 electrode.
6. Place lead V_3 midway between V_2 and V_4.
7. Place V_5 in the anterior axillary line in a straight line with V_4 (where the arm joins the chest).
8. Place V_6 in the midaxillary line, level with V_4 and V_5. (It may be more convenient to place V_6 first, and then V_5.)

9-Lead ECG Monitoring

In the absence of a 12-lead machine, a standard 3-lead monitor can be used to obtain a multi-lead (9-lead) ECG reading. (The 9-lead ECG does not include aV_R, aV_L, or aV_F but still provides valuable information about the lateral, anterior, and inferior wall.) To obtain a 9-lead reading from a standard 3-lead monitor, the paramedic should enable the

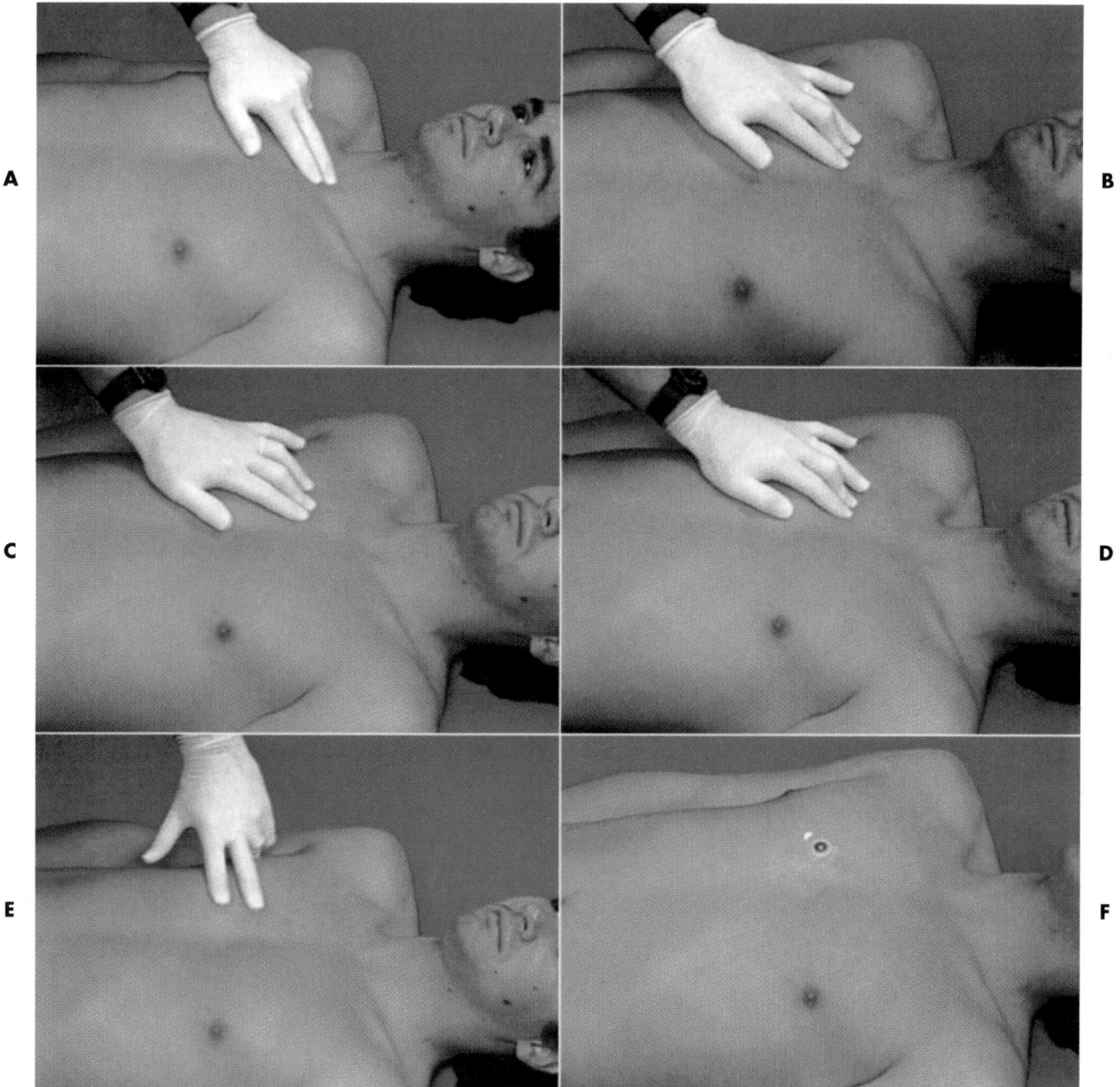

Fig. 28-19 A, Locate the jugular notch. **B,** Palpate for the angle of Louis. **C,** Follow the angle of Louis to the patient's right until it articulates with the second rib. **D,** Locate the second intercostal space (immediately below the second rib). **E,** From the second intercostal space the third and fourth intercostal spaces can be found. **F,** V_1 is positioned in the fourth intercostal space just to the right of the sternum.   *continued*

machine's diagnostic setting (if available) and follow these steps:

1. Run leads I, II, and III first. Obtain a representative sample of each lead and label it.
2. Leave the monitor in lead III (the negative electrode at the left shoulder) and move the left leg cable (the red lead wire) to each of the MCL positions (from V_1 to V_6) to obtain a readout. Label each sample.
3. Arrange the readouts in a standard 9-lead order: I, II, and III in the first column; MCL_1, MCL_2, and MCL_3 in the middle column; and MCL_4, MCL_5, and MCL_6 in the last column (Fig. 28-20).

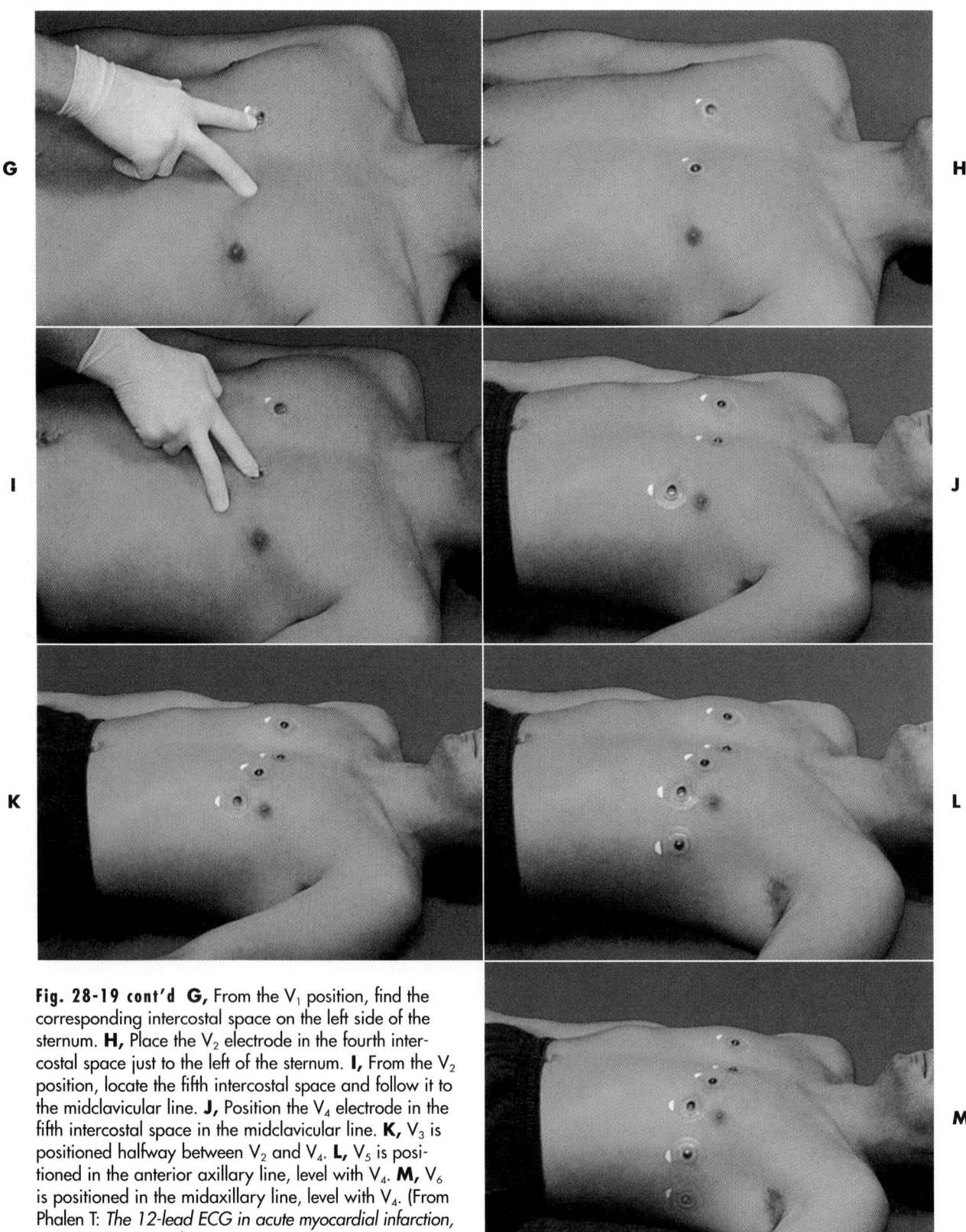

Fig. 28-19 cont'd G, From the V₁ position, find the corresponding intercostal space on the left side of the sternum. **H,** Place the V₂ electrode in the fourth intercostal space just to the left of the sternum. **I,** From the V₂ position, locate the fifth intercostal space and follow it to the midclavicular line. **J,** Position the V₄ electrode in the fifth intercostal space in the midclavicular line. **K,** V₃ is positioned halfway between V₂ and V₄. **L,** V₅ is positioned in the anterior axillary line, level with V₄. **M,** V₆ is positioned in the midaxillary line, level with V₄. (From Phalen T: *The 12-lead ECG in acute myocardial infarction,* St Louis, 1996, Mosby.)

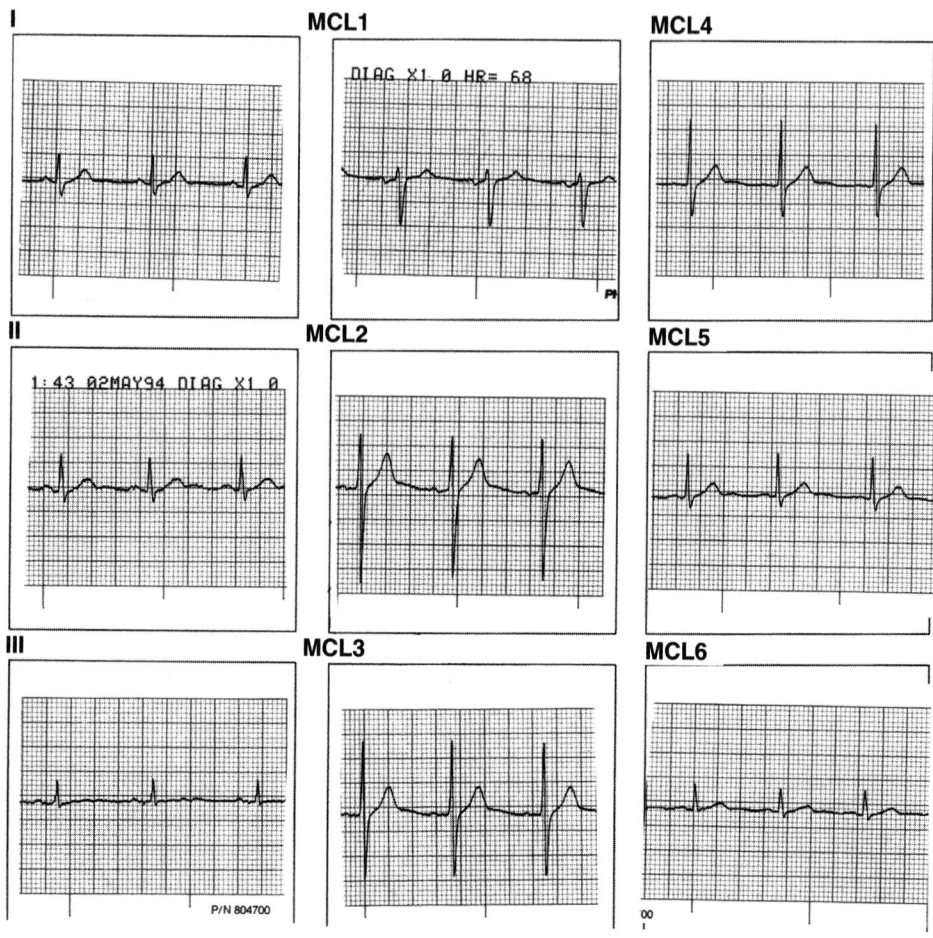

Fig. 28-20 Nine-lead ECG readout.

Application of Monitoring Electrodes

The most commonly used electrodes for continuous ECG monitoring are pregelled, stick-on disks that easily can be applied to the chest wall. The following guidelines should be observed to minimize artifacts in the signal and to make effective contact between the electrode and the skin:

1. Choose an appropriate area of skin, avoiding large muscle masses and large quantities of hair, which may prevent the electrode from lying flat against the skin.

2. Cleanse the area with alcohol to remove dirt and body oil. When attaching electrodes to the ex-

tremities, use the inner surfaces of the arms and legs. If necessary, trim excess body hair before placing the electrodes. If the patient is extremely diaphoretic, use tincture of benzoin to aid in securing application or use diaphoretic electrodes.

3. Attach the electrodes to the prepared site.
4. Attach the ECG cables to electrodes. Most ECG cables are marked for right arm, left arm, and left leg application.
5. Turn on the ECG monitor and obtain a baseline tracing.

If the signal is poor, the cable connections should be rechecked along with the effectiveness of the patient's skin contact with the electrodes. Other common causes of a poor signal include excessive body hair, dried conductive gel, poor electrode placement, and diaphoresis.

ECG Graph Paper

The paper used in recording ECGs is standardized to allow comparative analysis of an ECG wave. The graph paper is divided into squares 1 mm in height and width. The paper is further divided by darker lines every fifth square, both vertically and horizontally. Each large square is 5 mm high and 5 mm wide (Fig. 28-21).

As the graph paper moves past the stylus of the ECG machine, it measures time and amplitude. Time is measured on the horizontal plane (side to side). When the ECG is recorded at the standard pa-

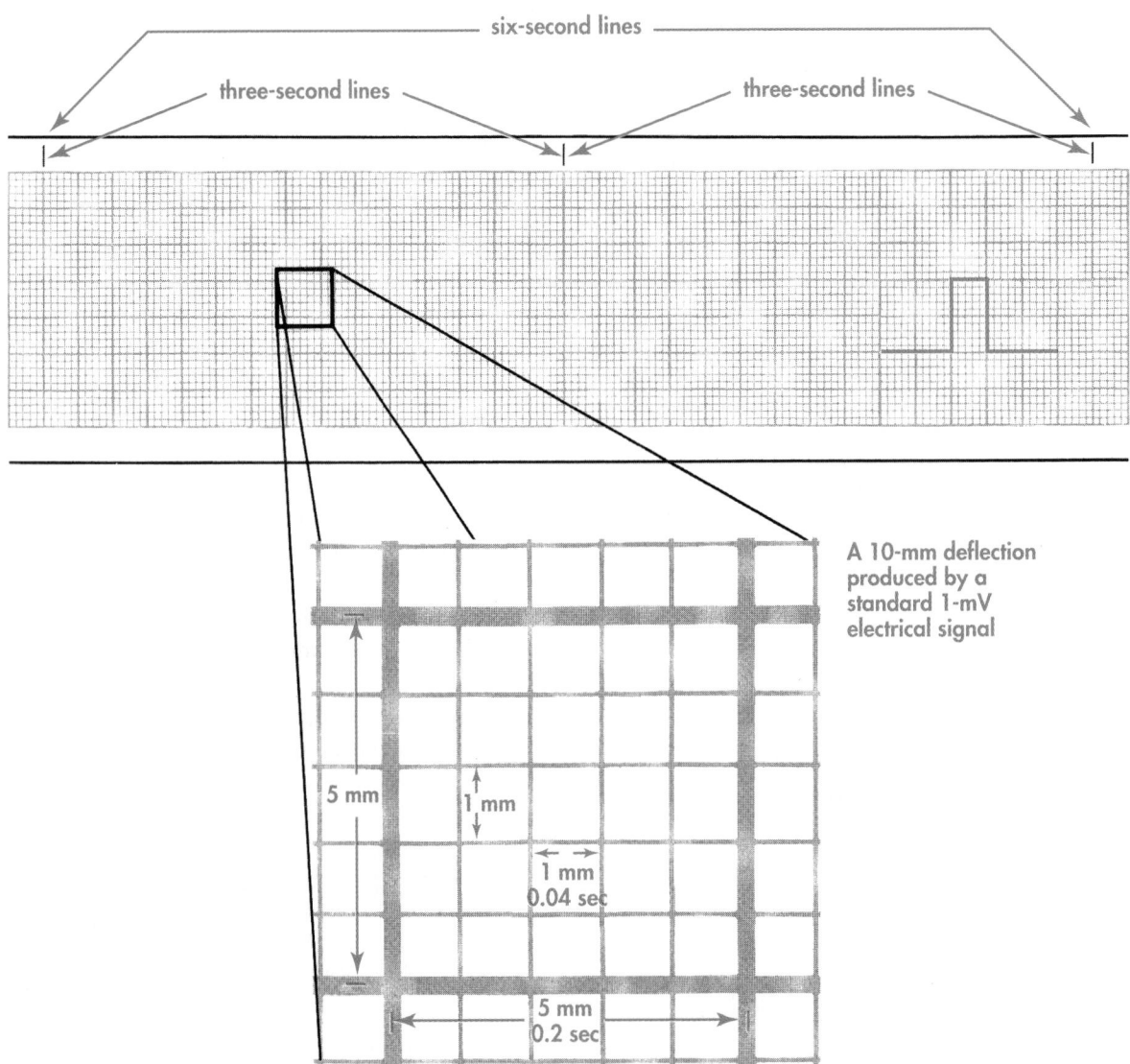

Fig. 28-21 ECG graph paper. (From Huszar R: *Basic dysrhythmias*, ed 2, St Louis, 1994, Mosby.)

per speed of 25 mm per second, each small square is equal to 1 mm (0.04 second) and each large square (the dark vertical lines) is equal to 5 mm (0.20 second). These squares measure the length of time it takes an electrical impulse to pass through a specific part of the heart.

Amplitude is measured on the vertical axis (top to bottom) of the graph paper. Each small square of the graph paper is equal to 0.1 mV, and each large square (five small squares) is equal to 0.5 mV. The sensitivity of the 12-lead ECG machine is standardized. When properly calibrated, a 1-mV electrical signal produces a 10-mm deflection (two large squares) on the ECG tracing. ECG machines equipped with calibration buttons should have a calibration curve placed at the beginning of the first ECG tracing (generally a 1-mV burst, represented by a 10-mm "block" wave).

Time-interval markings are denoted by short vertical lines and usually are located on the top of the ECG graph paper. When the ECG is recorded at the standard paper speed, the distance between each short vertical line is 75 mm (3 seconds). Each 3-second interval contains 15 large squares (0.2 second multiplied by 15 squares equals 3 seconds). These markings are used as a method of heart rate calculation (i.e., counting the number of QRS complexes in 6 seconds and multiplying by 10).

Relationship of the ECG to Electrical Activity

Each waveform seen on the oscilloscope or recorded on the ECG graph paper represents the conduction of an electrical impulse through a specific part of the heart. All waveforms begin and end at the isoelectric line, which represents the absence of electrical activity in cardiac tissue. A deflection above the baseline is positive and indicates an electrical flow toward the positive electrode. A deflection below the baseline is negative and indicates an electrical flow away from the positive electrode.

The normal ECG consists of a **P wave, QRS complex,** and **T wave.** Occasionally, a **U wave** also can be seen after the T wave. If present, it usually is a positive deflection and may be associated with electrolyte abnormalities. Other key components of the ECG that should be evaluated include the **PR interval, ST segment,** and **QT interval.** The combination of these waves represents a single heartbeat, or one complete cardiac cycle (Fig. 28-22). The electrical events of the cardiac cycle are followed by their mechanical counterparts. The descriptions of ECG waveform components refer to those that would be seen in lead II monitoring.

P Wave

The P wave is the first positive (upward) deflection on the ECG, representing atrial depolarization. It usually is rounded and precedes the QRS complex. The P wave begins with the first positive deflection from the baseline and ends at the point where the wave returns to the baseline. The duration of the P wave normally is 0.10 second or less, and its amplitude is 0.5 to 2.5 mm. The P wave usually is followed by a QRS complex. However, if conduction disturbances are present, a QRS complex does not always follow each P wave.

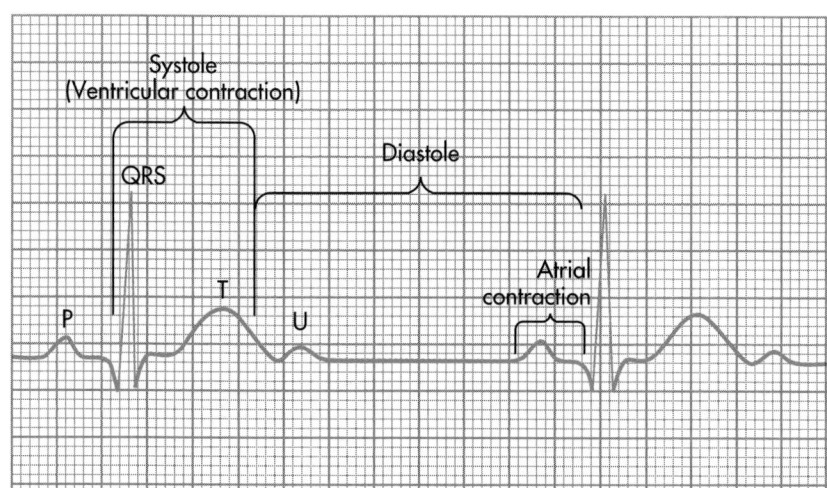

Fig. 28-22 Summary of the electrical basis of the ECG. (From Grauer K: *Practical guide to ECG interpretation,* St Louis, 1992, Mosby.)

Fig. 28-23 QRS complexes with more than one positive or negative deflection. (From Grauer K: *Practical guide to ECG interpretation,* St Louis, 1992, Mosby.)

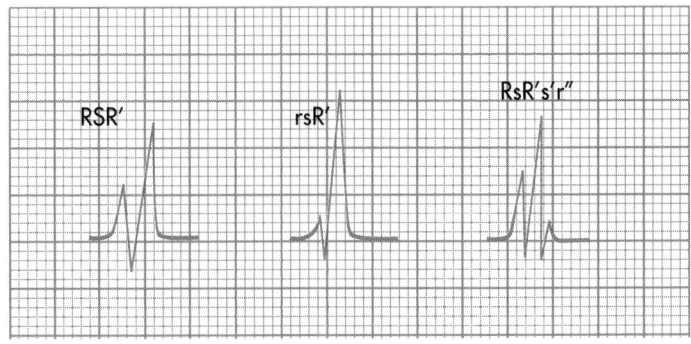

PR Interval

The PR interval is the time it takes for an electrical impulse to be conducted through the atria and the AV node up to the instant of ventricular depolarization. The PR interval is measured from the beginning of the P wave to the beginning of the next deflection on the baseline (the onset of the QRS complex). The normal PR interval is 0.12 to 0.20 second (three to five small squares on the graph paper) and depends on the heart rate and the conduction characteristics of the AV node. When the heart rate is fast, the PR interval normally is of shorter duration than when the heart rate is slow. A normal PR interval indicates that the electrical impulse has been conducted through the atria, AV node, and bundle of His normally and without delay.

QRS Complex

The QRS complex generally is composed of three individual waves: the Q, R, and S waves. The QRS complex begins at the point where the first wave of the complex deviates from the baseline and ends where the last wave of the complex begins to flatten at, above, or below the baseline. The direction of the QRS complex may be predominantly positive (upright), predominantly negative (inverted), or biphasic (partly positive, partly negative). The shape of the normal QRS complex is narrow and sharply pointed (when conduction is normal). Its duration generally is 0.08 to 0.10 second (2 to 2½ small squares on the graph paper) or less, and its amplitude normally varies from less than 5 mm to more than 15 mm.

The Q wave is the first negative (downward) deflection of the QRS complex on the ECG, although it may not be present in all leads, and represents depolarization of the interventricular septum. The R wave is the first positive deflection after the P wave. Sub-sequent positive deflections in the QRS complex that extend above the baseline and that are taller than the first R wave are called *R prime (R′), R double prime (R″)*, and so on. The S wave is the negative deflection that follows the R wave. Subsequent negative deflections are called *S prime (S′), S double prime (S″)*, and so on. Although there may be only one Q wave, there can be more than one R wave and one S wave in the QRS complex. The R and S waves represent the sum of electrical forces resulting from depolarization of the right and left ventricles (Fig. 28-23).

? CRITICAL THINKING

What is the significance of a QRS duration of >0.10 seconds?

The QRS complex follows the P wave and marks the approximate beginning of mechanical systole of the ventricles, which continues through the onset of the T wave. The QRS complex represents ventricular depolarization, or the conduction of an electrical impulse from the AV node through the bundle of His, Purkinje fibers, and the right and left bundle branches that results in ventricular depolarization.

ST Segment

The ST segment represents the early phase of repolarization of the right and left ventricles. It immediately follows the QRS complex and ends with the onset of the T wave. The point at which it "takes off" from the QRS complex is called the *J point*. In a normal ECG, the ST segment begins at baseline and has a very slight upward slope.

The position of the ST segment commonly is judged as normal or abnormal using the baseline of the PR or TP interval as a reference. Deviations

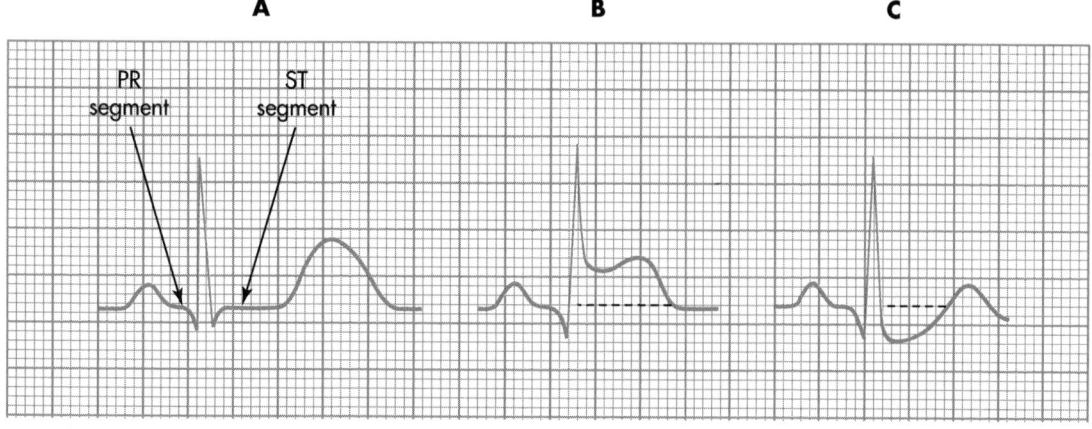

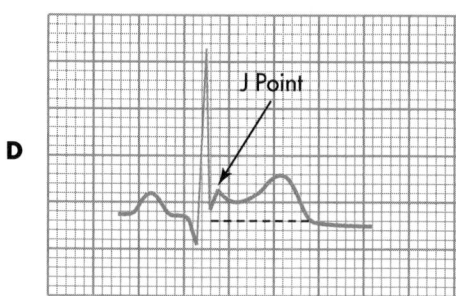

Fig. 28-24 ST-segment deviations. **A,** Use of the PR segment as a baseline. **B,** The ST segment is elevated with respect to the PR-segment baseline. **C,** The ST segment is depressed with respect to the PR-segment baseline. **D,** J point (ST-segment elevation). A prominent notch marks the takeoff of the ST segment. (From Grauer K: *Practical guide to ECG interpretation,* St Louis, 1992, Mosby.)

above this baseline are referred to as *ST-segment elevation,* and those below it are referred to as *ST-segment depression* (Fig. 28-24). Certain conditions can cause depression or elevation of the PR interval, thus affecting the reference for ST-segment abnormalities. Usually the baseline from the end of the T wave to the beginning of the P wave maintains its isoelectric position and can be used as a reference. Abnormal ST segments may be seen in infarction, ischemia, and pericarditis; after digitalis administration; and in other disease states.

T Wave

The T wave represents repolarization of the ventricular myocardial cells and occurs during the last part of ventricular systole. The T wave is identified as the first deviation from the ST segment and ends where the wave returns to the baseline. This wave may be above or below the isoelectric line and usually is slightly rounded and slightly asymmetrical. Deep and symmetrically inverted T waves may be indicative of cardiac ischemia. A T wave elevated more than half the height of the QRS complex (peaked T wave) may indicate new onset of ischemia of the myocardium or hyperkalemia.

QT Interval

The QT interval is the period from the beginning of ventricular depolarization (onset of the QRS complex) until the end of ventricular repolarization, or the end of the T wave (Fig. 28-25). During the initial portion of this interval, the heart is completely refractory to all premature stimuli (the absolute refractory period). During the latter portion of this interval (from the peak of the T wave onward), the conduction system is in a relative refractory period in which premature impulses may depolarize the heart while it is vulnerable. Commonly prescribed medications that may prolong the QT interval include quinidine, *procainamide* (Pronestyl), and disopyramide (type IA antidysrhythmics). These antidysrhythmics, by virtue of their effect on the QT interval, may lead to potentially lethal dysrhythmias, including VT, VF, and an unusual bidirectional ventricular dysrhythmia called **torsades de pointes.**

> **NOTE**
>
> If the heart rate is under 100 beats per minute, the QT interval probably is prolonged if it is greater than half of the R-R interval.[3]

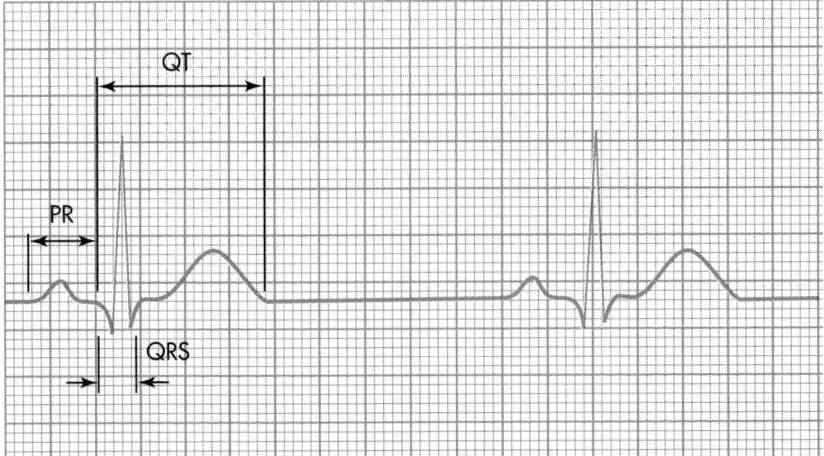

Fig. 28-25 PR, QT, and QRS intervals. (From Grauer K: *Practical guide to ECG interpretation*, St Louis, 1992, Mosby.)

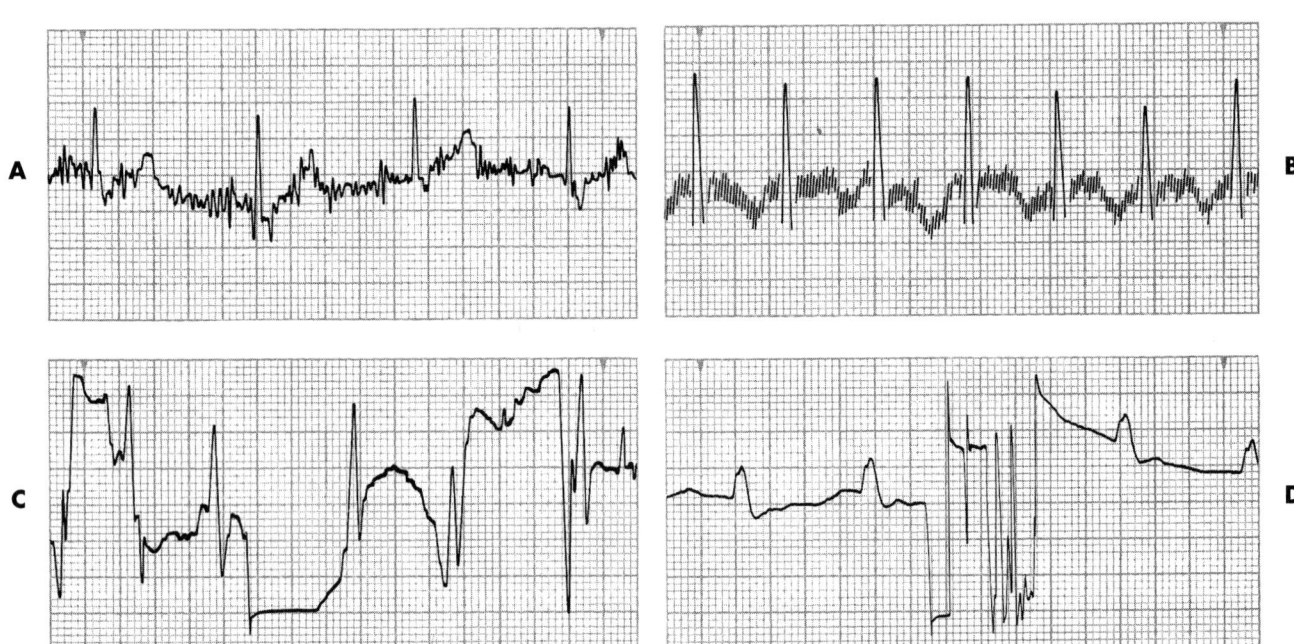

Fig. 28-26 Artifacts. **A,** Muscle tremors. **B,** AC (60-cycle) interference. **C,** Loose electrodes. **D,** Biotelemetry. (From Huszar R: *Basic dysrhythmias*, ed 2, St Louis, 1994, Mosby.)

Artifacts

Artifacts are deflections on the ECG display or tracing produced by factors other than the heart's electrical activity (Fig. 28-26). Common causes of artifacts are improper grounding of the ECG machine, patient movement, loss of electrode contact with the patient's skin, patient shivering or tremors, and external chest compression. Two types of artifacts that deserve special mention are alternating current interference (60-cycle interference) and biotelemetry-related interference.

Alternating-current (AC) interference may occur in a poorly grounded AC-operated ECG machine or when an ECG is obtained near high-tension wires or transformers. This results in a thick baseline composed of 60-cycle waves. The P waves may not be discernible because of the interference, but the QRS complex usually is visible. AC interference also may be caused by the patient or the lead cable touching a metal object such as a bed rail. Placing a blanket between the metal object and the patient may correct the interference.

Biotelemetry-related interference may occur when biotelemetry ECG signals are poorly received. This may result from weak batteries or from ECG transmission in areas with poor signaling conditions or at great distances from a base station receiver. Biotelemetry-related interference may produce sharp spikes and waves that have a jagged appearance.

Steps in Rhythm Analysis

Evaluation of an ECG requires a systematic approach to analyzing a given rhythm. There are numerous methods that can be used for rhythm interpretation. This text employs a method that first looks at the QRS complex (the most important observation in life-threatening dysrhythmias); followed by P waves and the relationship between the P waves and the QRS; rate; rhythm; and, finally, the PR interval. Regardless of the method chosen to analyze a given rhythm, a consistent format should be used. This section of the text will discuss rhythm interpretation as it pertains to standard 3-lead ECG monitoring. Evaluation of 12-lead ECG monitoring will be presented later in this chapter.

? CRITICAL THINKING

> **What does the ECG tell you about perfusion?**

NOTE

Five questions that must be asked in any rhythm analysis to determine the presence or potential for life-threatening rhythm disturbances are:
1. Is the patient sick?
2. What is the heart rate?
3. Are there normal-looking QRS complexes?
4. Are there normal-looking P waves?
5. What is the relationship between the P waves and the QRS complexes?

Step 1: Analyze the QRS Complex

The QRS complex should be analyzed for regularity and width. QRS complexes less than or equal to 0.10 second wide (less than three small squares) are supraventricular in origin and normal. Complexes that are equal to or greater than 0.12 second wide indicate either a conduction abnormality in the ventricles or that the focus originates in the ventricles and is abnormal (Fig. 28-27). When an abnormal QRS width is being evaluated, the lead with the widest QRS complex should be identified because a portion of the QRS complex may be blended with the baseline in some leads.

Step 2: Analyze the P Waves

The normal P wave in lead II is positive and smoothly rounded and usually precedes each QRS complex, indicating that the pacemaker originates in the SA node (Fig. 28-28). Therefore the following five components should be observed when evaluating P waves:

1. Are P waves present?
2. Are the P waves regular (can they be mapped out similar to R-R intervals)?
3. Is there one P wave for each QRS complex, and is there a QRS complex following each P wave?
4. Are they upright or inverted?
5. Do they all look alike? (P waves that look alike and are regular are likely from the same focus.)

Step 3: Analyze the Rate

Analyzing the heart rate may be done in a number of ways. The methods for calculating the heart rate presented in this text are heart rate calculator rulers, the triplicate method, the R-R method, and the 6-second count method.

The heart rate is determined by analyzing the ventricular rate (the QRS complex), as it is ultimately depolarization and contraction of the ventricles that produce cardiac output. However, if the atrial and ventricular rates are different (as may occur in certain dysrhythmias), they should be calculated separately. The normal adult heart rate is between 60 and 99 beats per minute. If the ventricular rate is below 60 beats per minute, it is considered a bradycardia; if the rate is equal to or greater than 100 beats per minute, it is considered a tachycardia.

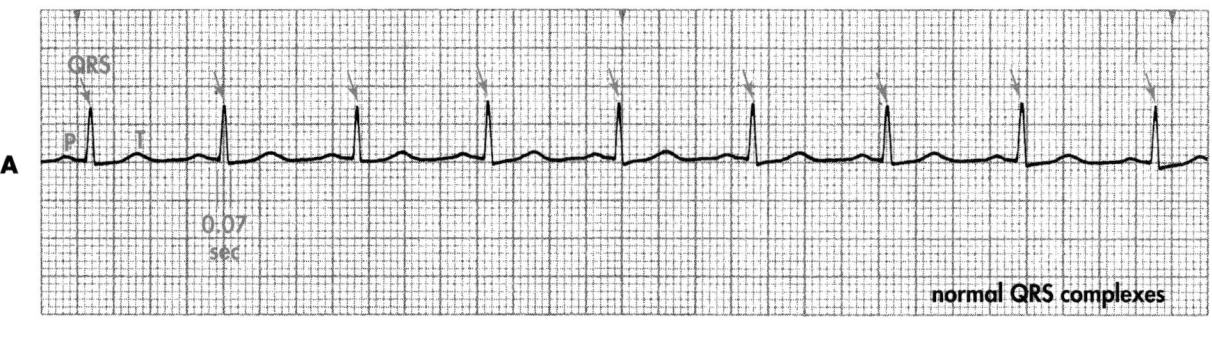

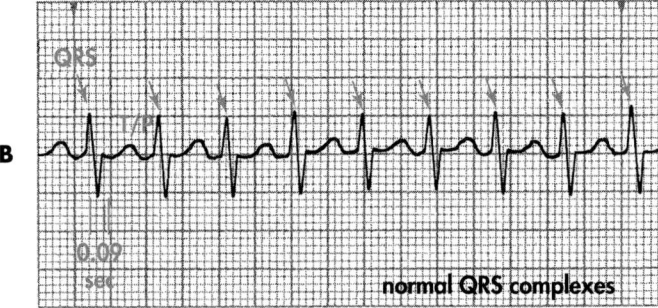

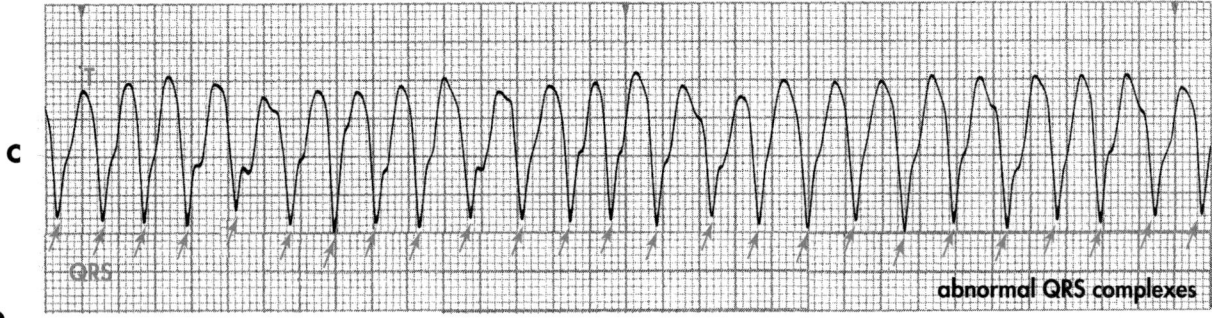

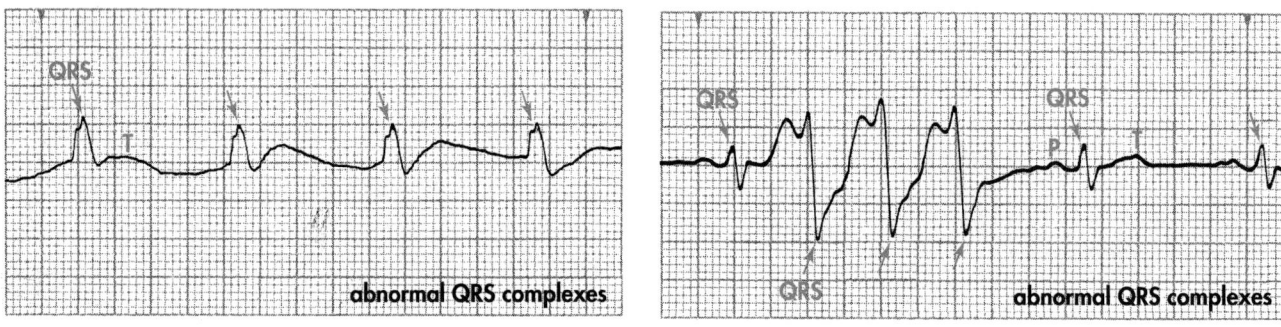

Fig. 28-27 A and **B,** Normal QRS complexes. **C** through **E,** Abnormal QRS complexes. (From Huszar R: *Basic dysrhythmias,* ed 2, St Louis, 1994, Mosby.)

Heart Rate Calculator Rulers

Heart rate calculator rulers (Fig. 28-29) are available from a number of manufacturers, and the directions for use supplied with them should be followed. Heart rate calculator rulers are reasonably accurate if the rhythm is regular. However, a mechanical device

or tool should not be solely relied on to determine the heart rate, since one may not be readily available.

Triplicate Method

The triplicate method of determining the heart rate (Fig. 28-30) is accurate only if the rhythm is

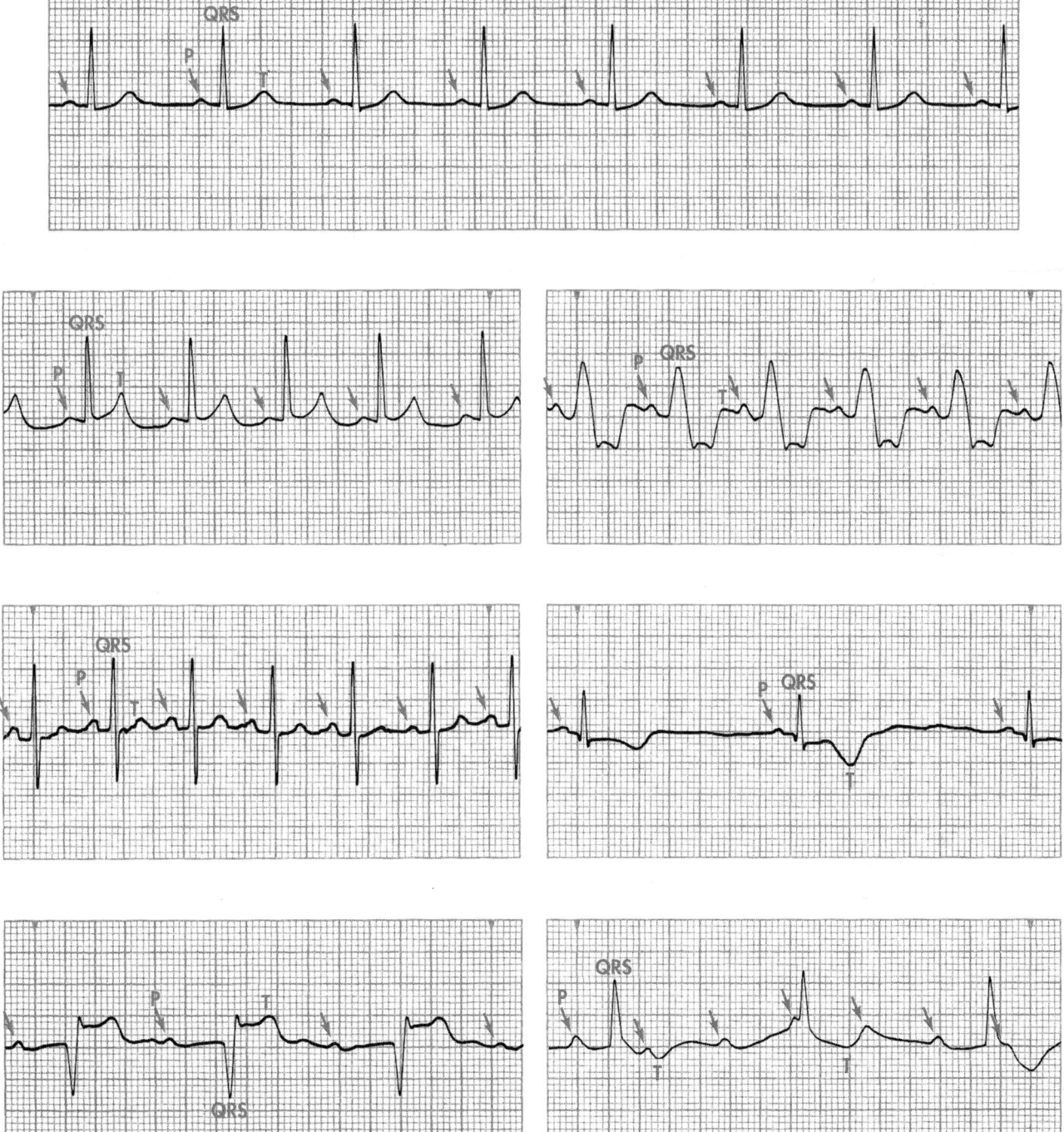

Fig. 28-28 Normal P waves. (From Huszar R: *Basic dysrhythmias,* ed 2, St Louis, 1994, Mosby.)

regular and greater than 50 beats per minute. The method requires memorizing two sets of numbers: 300-150-100 and 75-60-50. These numbers are derived from the distance between the heavy black lines (each representing $1/300$ minute). Therefore

two $1/300$-minute units are equal to $2/300$ minute, which is equal to $1/150$ minute, or a heart rate of 150 beats per minute; three $1/300$-minute units are equal to $3/300$ minute, which is equal to $1/100$ minute, or a heart rate of 100 beats per minute. Using these

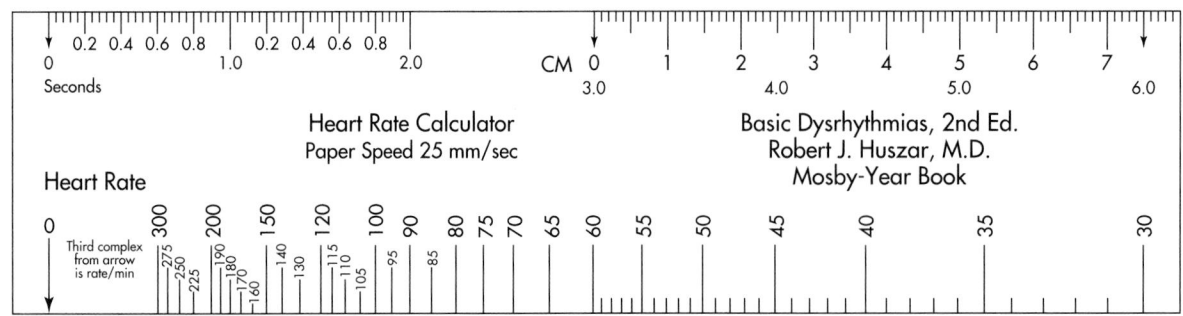

Fig. 28-29 Heart rate calculator ruler. (From Huszar R: *Basic dysrhythmias,* ed 2, St Louis, 1994, Mosby.)

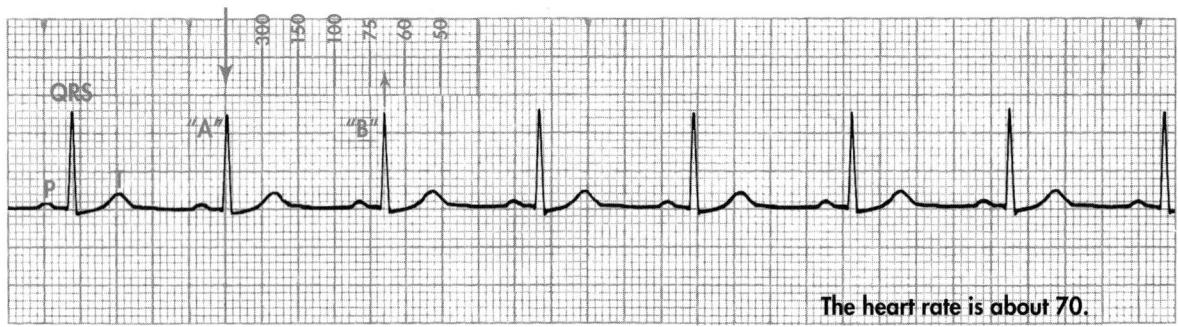

Fig. 28-30 Triplicate method. (From Huszar R: *Basic dysrhythmias,* ed 2, St Louis, 1994, Mosby.)

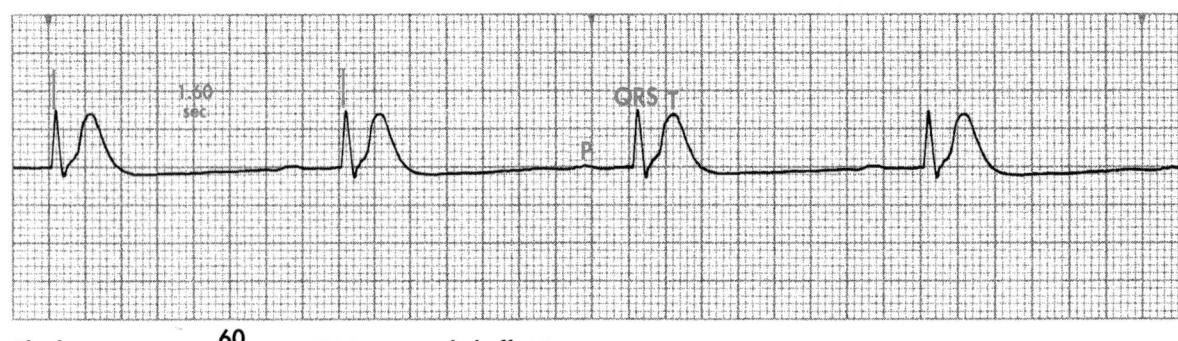

The heart rate = $\dfrac{60}{1.60 \text{ sec}}$ = 37.5 or, rounded off, 38.

Fig. 28-31 R-R interval method 1. (From Huszar R: *Basic dysrhythmias,* ed 2, St Louis, 1994, Mosby.)

triplicates, the heart rate can be calculated as follows:

1. Select an R wave that lines up with a dark vertical line.
2. Number the next six dark vertical lines consecutively from left to right as 300-150-100 and 75-60-50.
3. Identify where the next R wave falls with reference to the six dark vertical lines. If the R wave

falls on 75, the heart rate is 75 beats per minute. If the R wave falls halfway between 100 and 150, the heart rate is about 125 beats per minute.

R-R Method

The R-R method may be used several different ways to calculate the heart rate. Like the triplicate method, the rhythm must be regular to obtain an accurate reading. However, the R-R method works equally well for slow rates.

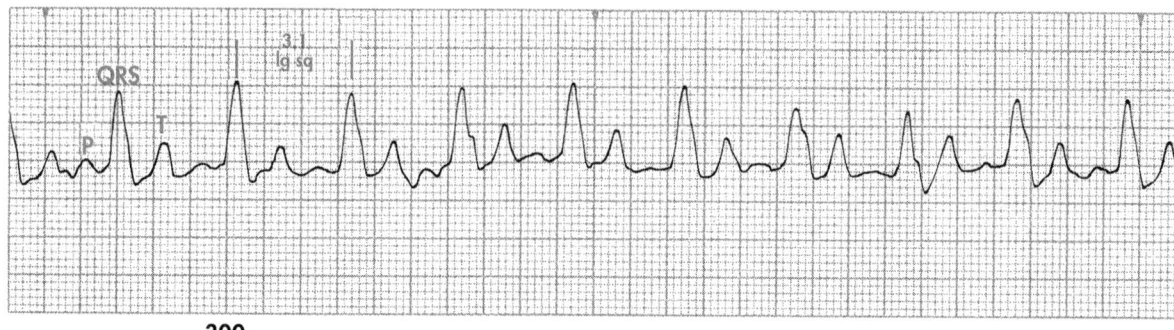

The heart rate = $\dfrac{300}{3.1 \text{ lg sq}}$ = 97.

Fig. 28-32 R-R interval method 2. (From Huszar R: *Basic dysrhythmias*, ed 2, St Louis, 1994, Mosby.)

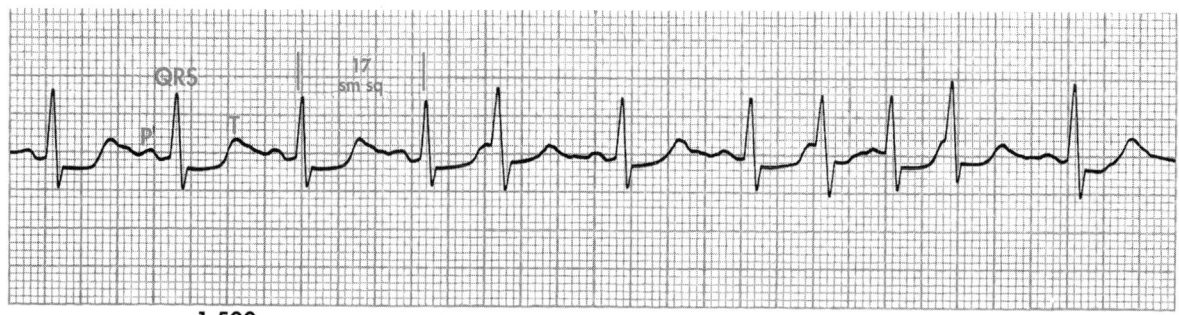

The heart rate = $\dfrac{1,500}{\text{---}}$ = 88.

Fig. 28-33 R-R interval method 3. (From Huszar R: *Basic dysrhythmias*, ed 2, St Louis, 1994, Mosby.)

Method 1. Measure the distance in seconds between the peaks of two consecutive R waves and then divide this number into 60 to obtain the heart rate (Fig. 28-31).

Method 2. Count the large squares between the peaks of two consecutive R waves and divide this number into 300 to obtain the heart rate (Fig. 28-32).

Method 3. Count the small squares between the peaks of two consecutive R waves and divide this number into 1500 to obtain the heart rate (Fig. 28-33).

Six-Second Count Method

The 6-second count method (Fig. 28-34) is the least accurate method of determining the heart rate. It may be used, however, to quickly obtain an approximate rate in regular and irregular rhythms.

? CRITICAL THINKING

Which of these rate calculation methods is fastest? Which is most accurate?

As previously stated, the short vertical lines at the top of most ECG graph papers are divided into 3-second intervals when run at a standard speed of 25 mm per second. Two of these intervals are equal to 6 seconds. The heart rate is calculated by counting the number of QRS complexes in a 6-second interval and multiplying this number by 10.

Step 4: Analyze the Rhythm

To analyze the ventricular rhythm, the paramedic should compare the R-R intervals on the ECG tracing in a systematic way from left to right. This measurement may be taken using ECG calipers or pen and paper. If calipers are used, one tip of the caliper is placed on the peak of one R wave and the other tip is adjusted so that it rests on the peak of the adjacent R wave. The caliper is then used to map the distance of the R-R interval to evaluate evenness and regularity.

In the absence of calipers, a similar method of evaluating the R-R interval may be employed using pen and paper. The straight edge of the paper is

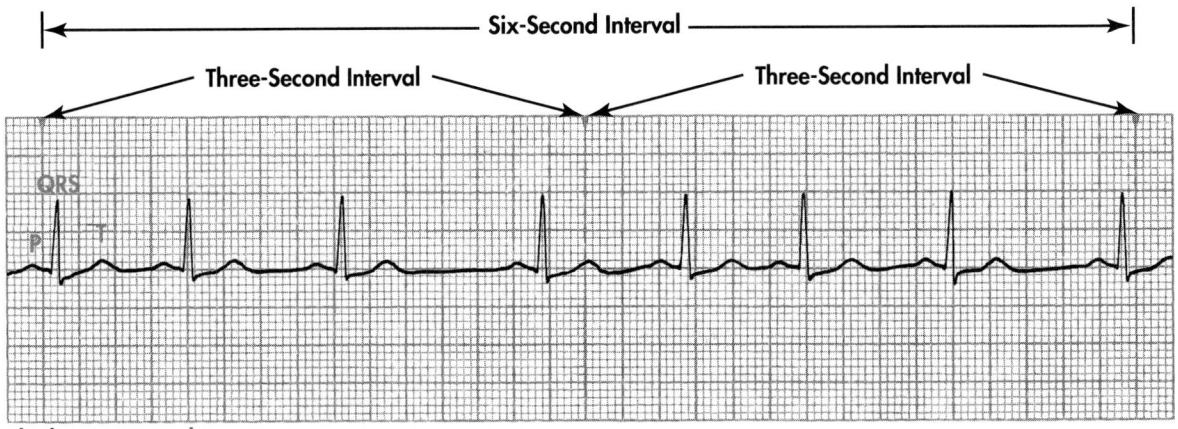

Fig. 28-34 Six-second count method. (From Huszar R: *Basic dysrhythmias,* ed 2, St Louis, 1994, Mosby.)

The distances between the R waves are determined:

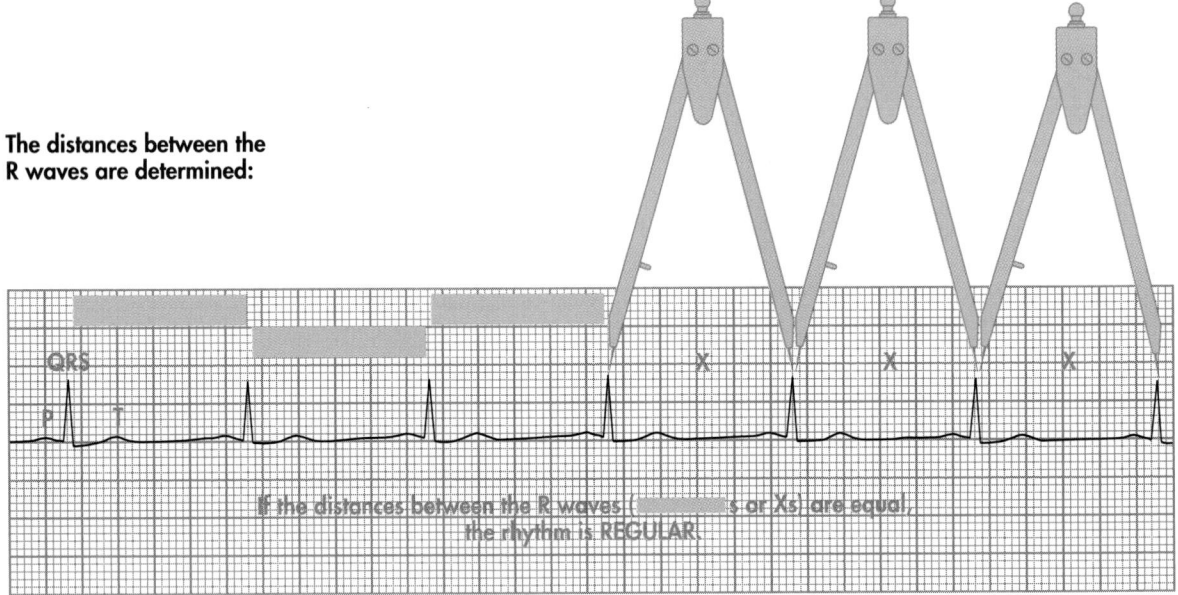

If the distances between the R waves (lines or Xs) are equal, the rhythm is REGULAR.

1. by estimating the R-R intervals,

2. by measuring the R-R intervals with ECG calipers,* or

| 14.5 | 9.5 | 8.0 | 8.0 | 14.0 | 14.5 | 14.5 | 9.0 | 8.0 | 14.0 | 15.0 | 15.0 | 9.5 |

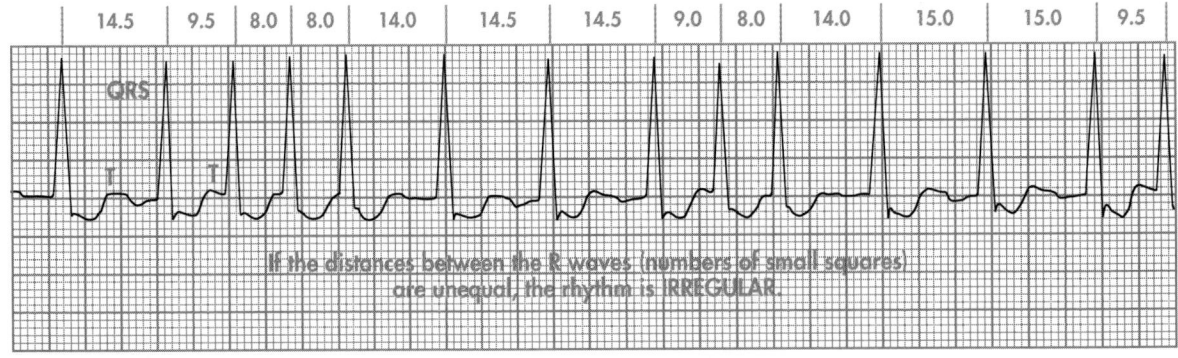

If the distances between the R waves (numbers of small squares) are unequal, the rhythm is IRREGULAR.

3. by counting the small squares between the R waves.

* If calipers are not available, mark off the distance between two R waves on a piece of paper and compare this distance with the other R-R intervals.

Fig. 28-35 Determining the rhythm. (From Huszar R: *Basic dysrhythmias,* ed 2, St Louis, 1994, Mosby.)

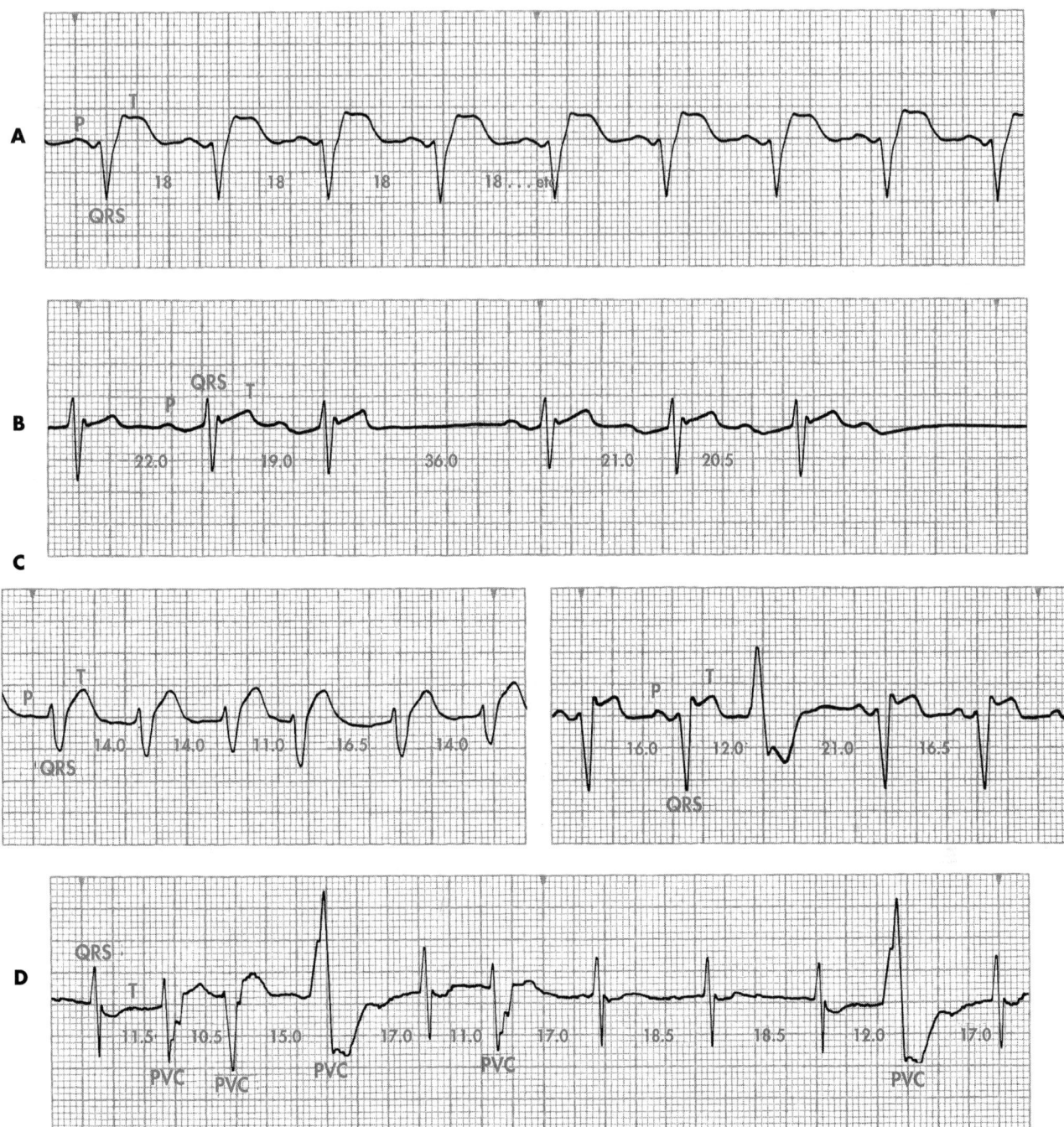

Fig. 28-36 A, Regular rhythm. **B,** Regularly irregular rhythm. **C,** Occasionally irregular rhythm.
D, Irregularly irregular rhythm. (From Huszar R: *Basic dysrhythmias,* ed 2, St Louis, 1994, Mosby.)

placed near the peaks of the R waves, and the distance between the two other consecutive R waves is marked off. This R-R interval is then compared with the other R-R intervals in the ECG tracing (Fig. 28-35).

If the distances between the R waves are equal or vary by less than 0.16 second (four small squares), the rhythm is "regular." If the shortest and longest R-R intervals vary by more than 0.16 second, the rhythm is "irregular." Irregular rhythms may be further classified as *regularly irregular* (patterned irregularity or "group beating"), *occasionally irregular* (only one or two R-R intervals being unequal), or *irregularly irregular* (totally irregular rhythm in which there is no relationship between the R-R intervals) (Fig. 28-36).

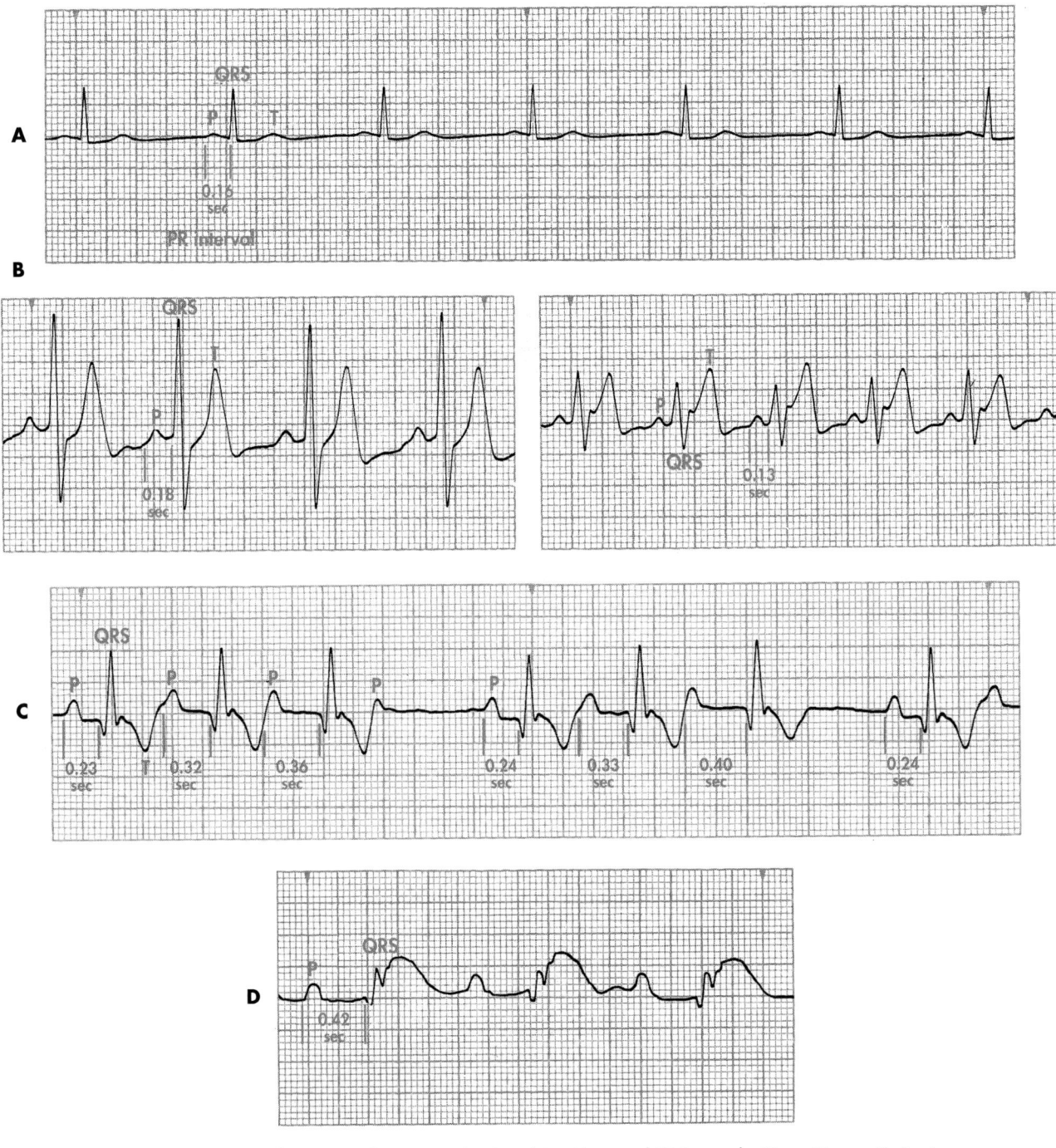

Fig. 28-37 A and **B,** Normal PR intervals. **C** and **D,** Abnormal PR intervals. (From Huszar R: *Basic dysrhythmias,* ed 2, St Louis, 1994, Mosby.)

Step 5: Analyze the PR Interval

The PR interval indicates the time it takes for an electrical impulse to be conducted through the atria and AV node. It should be constant across the ECG tracing. A prolonged PR interval (greater than 0.20 second) indicates a delay in the conduction of the impulse through the AV node or bundle of His and is called an *AV block.* A short PR interval (less than 0.12 second) indicates that the impulse progressed from the atria to the ventricles through pathways other than the AV node (Fig. 28-37). This is known as an *accessory pathway syndrome,* the most common of which is Wolff-Parkinson-White syndrome (described later in this chapter).

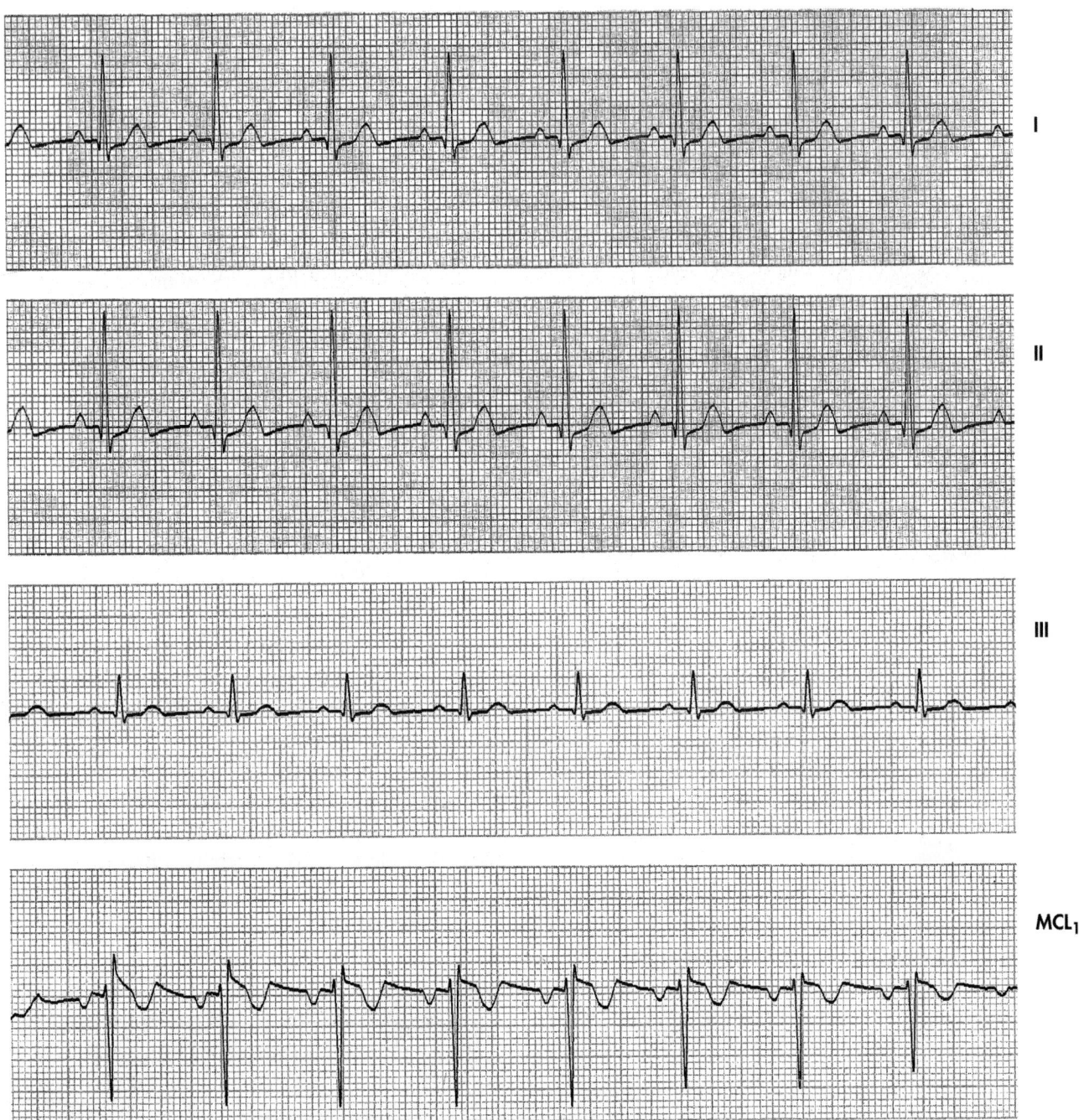

Fig. 28-38 Normal sinus rhythm.

Analyzing a Rhythm Using the Five Steps

To review, the normal sequence of atrial and ventricular activation as it relates to the ECG tracing is as follows: Each P wave (atrial depolarization) is followed by a normal QRS complex (ventricular depolarization) and T wave (ventricular repolarization). All QRS complexes are preceded by P waves; the PR interval is within normal limits, and the R-R interval is regular. The five steps in ECG rhythm interpretation can be applied to the rhythm in Fig. 28-38.

SECTION SIX

INTRODUCTION TO DYSRHYTHMIAS

Cardiac dysrhythmias can result from a number of physiological, pharmacological, and disease processes, including:

- Myocardial ischemia or necrosis
- Autonomic nervous system imbalance
- Distention of heart chambers
- Acid-base abnormalities
- Hypoxemia
- Electrolyte imbalance
- Drug effects or toxicity
- Electrical injury
- Hypothermia
- Central nervous system injury

In addition to these potential causes of dysrhythmias, some cardiac rhythm disturbances are normal, even in patients who have healthy hearts (e.g., sinus tachycardia from stress or anxiety). *Regardless of the etiology or type of dysrhythmia, management should focus on the patient and the underlying cause and not merely the dysrhythmia.*

> **NOTE**
>
> Special considerations regarding cardiac rhythm disturbances and resuscitation for infant and pediatric patients are addressed in Chapters 41 and 42.

Classifications

The classification of dysrhythmias can be based on a number of factors, including changes in automaticity versus disturbances in conduction, cardiac arrest (lethal) rhythms and non–cardiac arrest (nonlethal) rhythms, and site of origin. For learning purposes, this text classifies rhythms by rate and pacemaker site (e.g., ventricular tachycardia and sinus bradycardia) and includes the following five groups:

1. Dysrhythmias originating in the SA node
   a. Sinus bradycardia
   b. Sinus tachycardia
   c. Sinus dysrhythmia
   d. Sinus arrest
2. Dysrhythmias originating in the atria
   a. Wandering pacemaker
   b. Premature atrial complex (PAC)
   c. Paroxysmal supraventricular tachycardia (PSVT)
   d. Atrial flutter
   e. Atrial fibrillation
3. Dysrhythmias originating in the AV node and surrounding tissues
   a. Premature junctional complex (PJC)
   b. Junctional escape complexes or rhythms
   c. Accelerated junctional rhythm
4. Dysrhythmias originating in the ventricles
   a. Ventricular escape complexes or rhythms
   b. Premature ventricular complex (PVC)
   c. Ventricular tachycardia (VT)
   d. Ventricular fibrillation (VF)
   e. Asystole
   f. Artificial pacemaker rhythms
5. Dysrhythmias that are disorders of conduction
   a. AV blocks
      (1) First-degree AV block
      (2) Second-degree AV block Type I (or Wenckebach)
      (3) Second-degree AV block Type II
      (4) Third-degree AV block
   b. Disturbances of ventricular conduction
   c. Pulseless electrical activity (PEA)
   d. Preexcitation syndrome: Wolff-Parkinson-White syndrome

> **NOTE**
>
> Broadly speaking, there are only four cardiac arrest rhythms: VF, VT, asystole, and assorted PEA rhythms. The two non–cardiac arrest rhythms that are important to consider in prehospital care are those that are too slow (less than 60 beats per minute) and those that are too fast (more than 120 beats per minute).[1]

The text presents each dysrhythmia as it would appear in lead II monitoring. For comparison, the same dysrhythmia also is shown as it would appear in leads I, III, and MCL$_1$. We discuss the interpretation and emergency management, if required, of each dysrhythmia.

All management modalities presented in this chapter follow the recommendations of the American Heart Association (AHA) and are referenced to the appropriate management algorithm.

Algorithms are illustrative methods used to summarize information, and some contain prehospital and in-hospital management recommendations. The following nine guidelines apply to all management algorithms[1]:

CLASSES OF RECOMMENDATIONS 2000

Class I
Definitely recommended
Interventions always acceptable, safe, and effective
Considered standard of care
Interventions supported by *excellent* research-based evidence

Class IIa
Acceptable and useful
Interventions acceptable, safe, and useful
Considered intervention of choice
Interventions supported by *good* research-based evidence

Class IIb
Acceptable and useful
Interventions acceptable, safe, and useful
Considered as an optional or alternative intervention
Interventions supported by *fair* research-based evidence

Indeterminate
Interventions in early stages of research and documentation or lack sufficient quantity or quality of research
No recommendation until further research is available

Class III
Unacceptable, not useful; may be harmful
Intervention with no evidence of benefit; may be harmful to patient
Evidence of benefit is completely lacking or research suggests or confirms harm

From American Heart Association: *Guidelines 2000 for cardiopulmonary and emergency cardiovascular care,* International Consensus on Science, Dallas, 2000, The Association.

1. First, manage the patient, not the monitor.
2. Algorithms for cardiac arrest presume that the condition under discussion continually persists, that the patient remains in cardiac arrest, and that CPR is always performed.
3. Apply different interventions whenever appropriate indications exist.
4. The algorithms are designed to outline the most common assessments and actions performed for the majority of patients, but they are not designed to be either all-inclusive or restrictive.[4] The flow diagrams present treatments mostly in sequential order of priority. Indicated next to a treatment or pharmacological agent may be a class recommendation (See box for a description of the classes of recommendations). The algorithm's footnotes contain additional important information related to assessment, treatment, and evaluation.
5. Adequate airway, ventilation, oxygenation, chest compression, and defibrillation are more important than administration of medications and take precedence over initiating an IV line or injecting pharmacological agents.
6. Several medications (*epinephrine* [Adrenalin], *lidocaine* [Xylocaine], and *atropine*) can be administered via an endotracheal tube, but the endotracheal dose is 2 to 2½ times the IV dose for adults.
7. With a few exceptions, IV medications should always be administered rapidly in bolus method.
8. After each IV medication, give a 20- to 30-mL bolus of IV fluid and immediately elevate the extremity. This enhances delivery of drugs to the central circulation, which may take 1 to 2 minutes.
9. Last, manage the patient, not the monitor.

Dysrhythmias Originating in the SA Node

Most sinus dysrhythmias result from increases or decreases in vagal tone. The SA node generally receives sufficient inhibitory parasympathetic impulses from the vagus nerve to keep the heart rate well below the intrinsic discharge rate of the pacemaker cells. However, if vagal discharge increases, the heart rate becomes bradycardic; if vagal discharge decreases, sympathetic stimulation results in sinus tachycardia. Dysrhythmias that originate in the SA node include sinus bradycardia, sinus tachycardia, sinus dys-rhythmia, and sinus arrest. ECG features common to all SA node dysrhythmias include:

- Normal duration of QRS complex (in the absence of bundle branch block)
- Upright P waves in lead II
- Similar appearance of all P waves

- Normal duration of PR interval (in the absence of AV block)

Sinus Bradycardia
Description
Sinus bradycardia (Fig. 28-39) results from slowing of the pacemaker rate of the SA node.

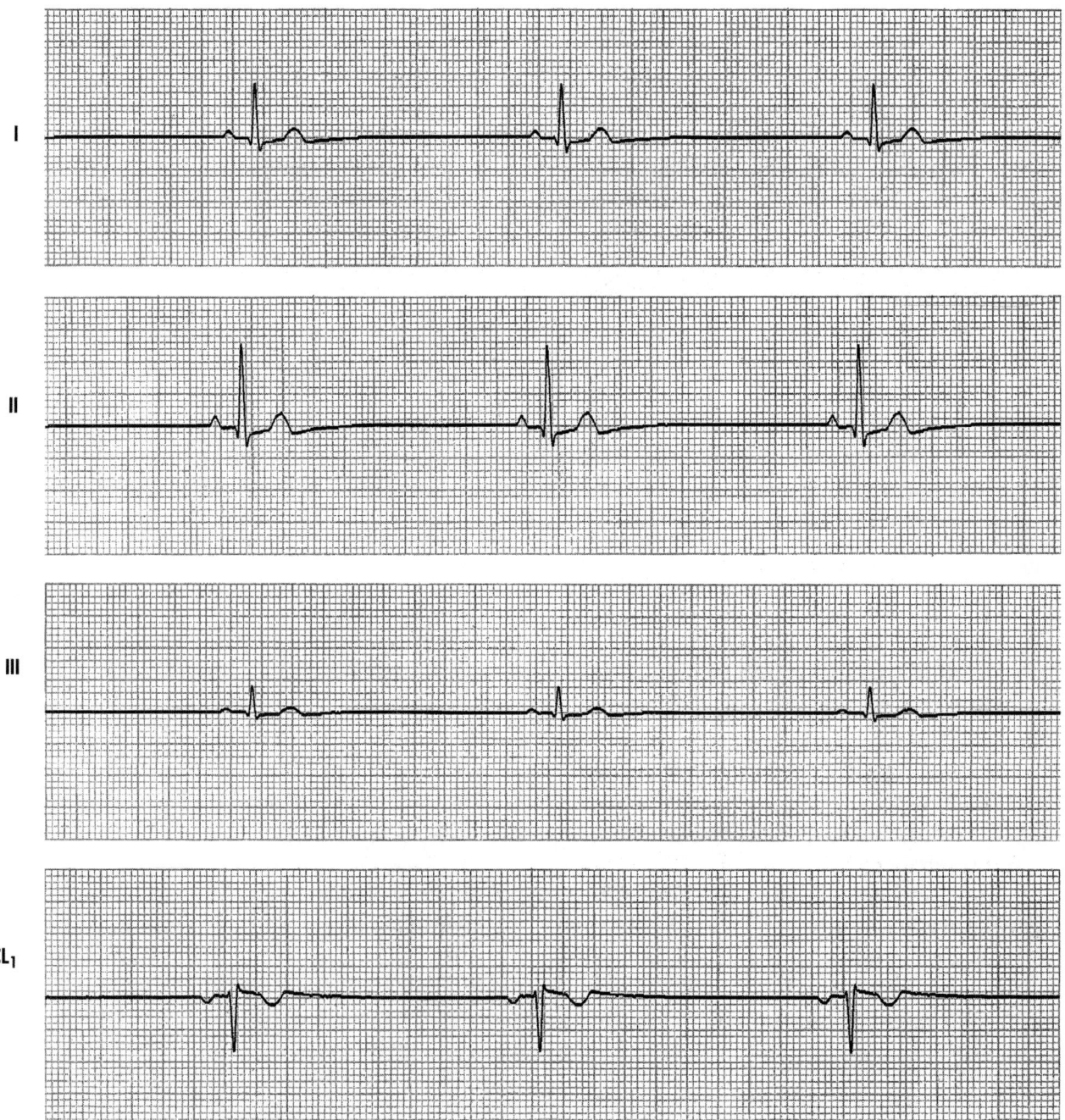

Fig. 28-39 Sinus bradycardia.

Etiology

- Intrinsic sinus node disease
- Increased parasympathetic vagal tone
- Hypothermia
- Hypoxia
- Drug effects (e.g., digitalis, beta blockers, calcium channel blockers)
- Myocardial infarction

Rules for Interpretation (Lead II monitoring)

QRS complex: Less than 0.12 second, provided there is no ventricular conduction disturbance.

P waves: Normal and upright; one P wave before each QRS complex.

Rate: Less than 60 beats per minute.

Rhythm: Regular.

PR interval: 0.12 to 0.20 second and constant (normal), provided no AV block is present.

Clinical Significance

Decreased rate may compromise cardiac output, resulting in hypotension, angina pectoris, or central nervous system symptoms (e.g., lightheadedness, vertigo, syncope). Sinus bradycardia may be associated with nausea and vomiting and is associated with vasovagal syncope. Conversely, sinus bradycardia may be beneficial by reducing myocardial oxygen consumption in the setting of myocardial infarction, provided the patient is well perfused. Sinus bradycardia also may follow the application of carotid sinus pressure (carotid sinus massage). This dysrhythmia is common during sleep and in well-conditioned athletes.

> ### ? CRITICAL THINKING
>
> *Take a poll of your classmates. How many have a resting heart rate <60 beats per minute?*

Management (Fig. 28-40)

Prehospital intervention usually is unnecessary unless hypotension, altered mental status due to inadequate perfusion, or ventricular irritability is present (these are more common with rates below 50 beats per minute). Management for symptomatic bradycardia is aimed at increasing the heart rate to improve cardiac output. Inotropic support may also be required. Treatment options for symptomatic bradycardia include oxygen, transcutaneous pacing, *atropine*, a *dopamine* infusion, an *epinephrine* infusion, and an *isoproterenol* infusion. Transcutaneous pacing is considered a Class I intervention for all symptomatic bradycardias. If the patient fails to respond to *atropine* or is critically unstable, begin transcutaneous pacing immediately. Transcutaneous pacing is indicated for symptomatic bradycardias that are related to a conduction delay or block at or below the His-Purkinje level (infranodal). Consider sedation for the patient to decrease discomfort caused by the transcutaneous pacer stimuli.

For mild symptoms related to the bradycardia, *atropine* may be administered intravenously 0.5–1 mg and may be repeated every 3 to 5 minutes. Maximum dosage for *atropine* is 0.03–0.04 mg/kg. Frequency of *atropine* administration is based on the patient's condition. *Atropine* should be administered at shorter intervals, every 3 minutes, for severely unstable patients.

Atropine should be used with caution in the setting of acute myocardial infarction due to the increased myocardial oxygen demand, and increased heart rates may worsen ischemia or increase the zone of infarction. *Atropine* may be beneficial when used for treatment of nodal behavior blocks and asystole; however, it is contraindicated for infranodal behavior blocks such as second degree type II and complete heart block with a wide QRS complex (greater than or equal to 120 ms). In the presence of infranodal behavior atrioventricular blocks, *atropine* rarely increases the heart rate and may actually worsen the rhythm.

If hypotension persists after atropine administration, add a *dopamine* infusion at 2–20 mcg/kg/min. Also, if the patient remains hypotensive and severely distressed with transcutaneous pacing and good mechanical capture, a *dopamine* infusion may be initiated.

An *epinephrine* infusion is indicated for symptomatic bradycardia after *atropine* and transcutaneous pacing fail. However, an *epinephrine* infusion (2–10 mcg/min) may be administered earlier if the patient displays acute symptoms and is deteriorating quickly.

In the treatment of symptomatic bradycardia, *isoproterenol* should only be used as an immediate and temporary measure to improve hemodynamic status. *Isoproterenol* is a pure beta agonist producing positive chronotropic and inotropic properties. The potent

Symptomatic Bradycardia

Basic Life Support

Perform Primary ABCD Survey
(Correct critical problems IMMEDIATELY as they are identified)
- Assess responsiveness, **A**irway, **B**reathing, **C**irculation, ensure availability of monitor/**D**efibrillator

Advanced Life Support

Perform Secondary ABCD Survey
Administer oxygen, establish IV access, attach cardiac monitor
Administer fluids as needed (O_2, IV, monitor, fluids)
BREATHING
Assess vital signs, attach pulse oximeter, and monitor blood pressure
Obtain and review 12-lead ECG, portable chest x-ray
Perform a focused history and physical exam

Identify the patient's cardiac rhythm
Is the patient experiencing serious signs and symptoms due to the bradycardia?

SIGNS	SYMPTOMS
Low blood pressure, shock, pulmonary congestion, congestive heart failure, angina, acute MI, ventricular ectopy	Chest pain, weakness, fatigue, dizziness, lightheadedness, shortness of breath, exercise intolerance, decreased level of responsiveness

- If no serious signs and symptoms, observe
- If serious signs and symptoms are present, further intervention depends on the cardiac rhythm identified.

Is the QRS narrow or wide?

NARROW-QRS BRADYCARDIA	WIDE-QRS BRADYCARDIA
- **Sinus bradycardia** - **Junctional rhythm** - **Second-degree AV block type I** - **Third-degree (complete) AV block** - Atropine 0.5 to 1.0 mg IV. May repeat every 3 to 5 minutes to a total dose of 2.5 mg (0.03 to 0.04 mg/kg). Total cumulative dose should not exceed 2.5 mg over 2.5 hours*. - Transcutaneous pacemaker (TCP). Pacing should not be delayed while waiting for IV access or for atropine to take effect. - Dopamine infusion 5 to 20 mcg/kg/min - Epinephrine infusion 2 to 10 mcg/min - Isoproterenol infusion 2 to 10 mcg/min (low doses)	- **Second-degree AV block type II** - **Third-degree (complete) AV block** - **Ventricular escape (idioventricular) rhythm** - Transcutaneous pacemaker as an interim device until transvenous pacing can be accomplished - Dopamine infusion 5 to 20 mcg/kg/min - Epinephrine infusion 2 to 10 mcg/min - Isoproterenol infusion 2 to 10 mcg/min (low doses)

*Ryan TJ et al: ACC/AHA guidelines for the management of patients with acute myocardial infarction: 1999 update: a report of the American College of Cardiology/American Heart Association Task Force on Practice Guidelines (Committee on Management of Acute Myocardial Infarction). Available at http://www.acc.org/clinical guidelines and http://www.americanheart.org. Accessed on 1/31/01.

Fig. 28-40 Bradycardia algorithm. (From Aehlert B: *ACLS quick review study guide*, ed 2, St Louis, 2002, Mosby.)

SEQUENCE OF CARE FOR SYMPTOMATIC BRADYCARDIA

Atropine
TCP (if available)
Dopamine (Intropin)
Epinephrine (Adrenalin) infusion
Isoproterenol (Isuprel) infusion

DOPAMINE INFUSION

- Low-dose dopamine: 1 to 5 mcg/kg/min. A low dose of dopamine produces a dopaminergic effect that increases renal, mesenteric, and cerebrovascular vessel dilation.
- Moderate-dose dopamine: 5 to 10 mcg/kg/min. At moderate doses, dopamine improves contractility, cardiac output, and blood pressure through alpha- and beta-1 receptor stimulation.
- High-dose dopamine: 10 to 20 mcg/kg/min. Higher doses of dopamine have an alpha-adrenergic effect producing peripheral arterial and venous vasoconstriction.

EPINEPHRINE INFUSION

- Epinephrine infusions are generally reserved for critically unstable patients with bradycardia close to a pulseless state or asystole. An epinephrine infusion may be prepared by mixing 1 mg of epinephrine 1:1000 into 500 mL of D_5W or 0.9 NS. The concentration is 2 mcg/mL. The recommended rate of infusion is 2 to 10 mcg/min.

CRITICAL POINTS TO REMEMBER

1. Manage the patient, not the monitor.
2. Bradycardia may be "normal" for some individuals.
3. A slow rate doesn't always make the patient ill and in some instances is beneficial.

effects of isoproterenol may increase myocardial oxygen consumption, exacerbate ischemia, and induce dysrhythmias. **Isoproterenol** is not the treatment of choice for symptomatic bradycardia, and if used, administer only in low doses.

Sinus Tachycardia

Description
Sinus tachycardia (Fig. 28-41) results from an increase in the rate of sinus node discharge.

? CRITICAL THINKING

What effect will the arrival of your ambulance likely have on the heart rate and blood pressure of a conscious, alert patient?

Etiology
This dysrhythmia is common and may result from multiple factors, including:

- Exercise
- Fever
- Anxiety
- Ingestion of caffeine or alcohol
- Smoking
- Hypovolemia
- Hyperthyroidism
- Anemia
- Congestive heart failure
- Administration of **atropine** or any vagolytic or sympathomimetic drug (e.g., cocaine, phencyclidine, **epinephrine** [Adrenalin] **isoproterenol** [Isuprel])

Rules for Interpretation (Lead II Monitoring)
QRS complex: Less than 0.12 second, provided there is no ventricular conduction disturbance.
P waves: Normal and upright; one before each QRS complex.
Rate: Equal to or greater than 100 beats per minute.
Rhythm: Regular.
PR interval: 0.12 to 0.20 second (normal), provided no AV conduction block is present.

Clinical Significance
Sinus tachycardia in healthy individuals generally is a benign dysrhythmia. If it is associated with

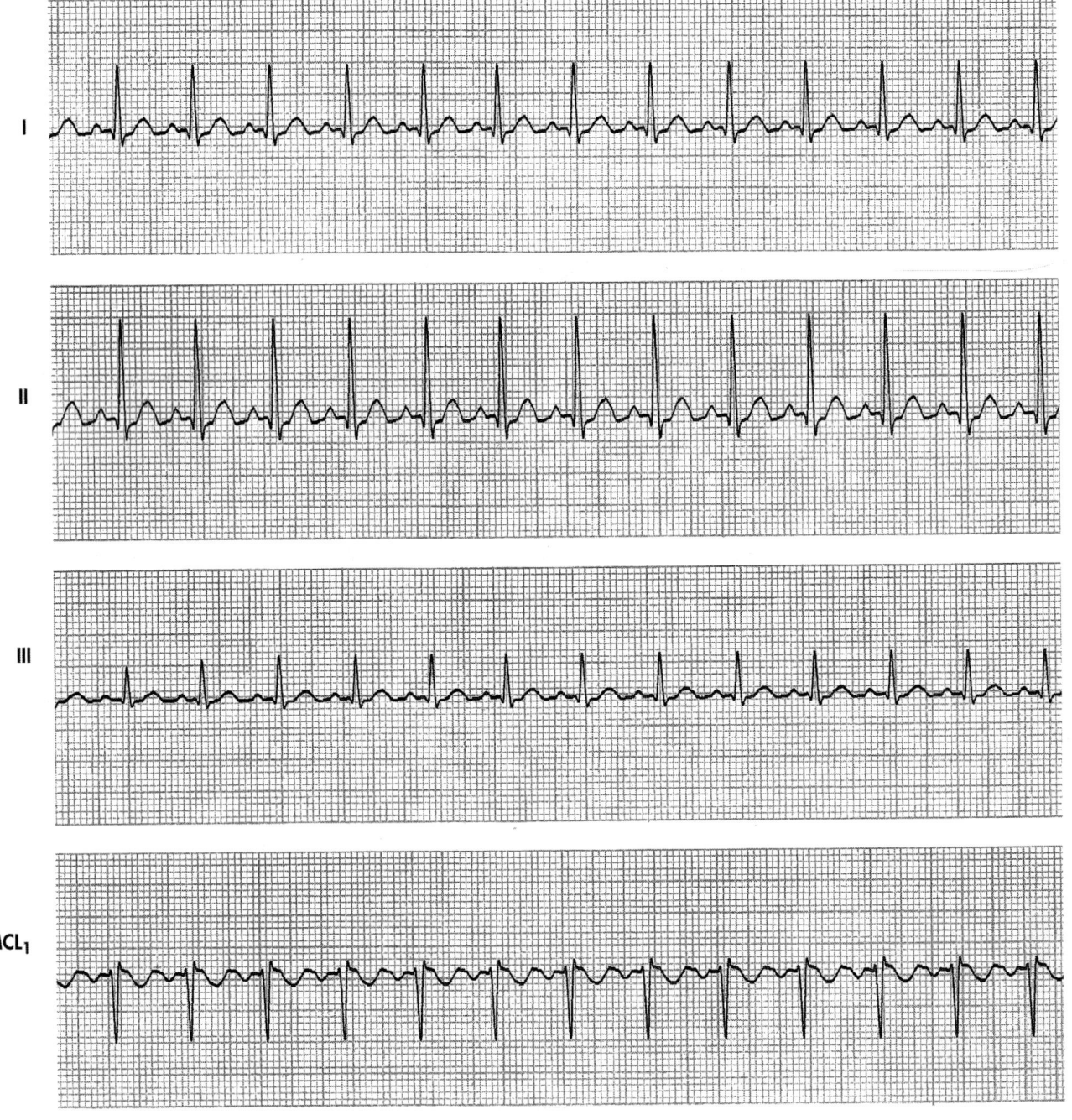

Fig. 28-41 Sinus tachycardia.

myocardial infarction, however, the tachycardia may increase the oxygen requirements of the heart, increase myocardial ischemia, and predispose the patient to more serious rhythm disturbances.

Management

Sinus tachycardia usually does not require management. When the underlying cause is removed, the tachycardia usually resolves gradually and spontaneously.

Sinus Dysrhythmia

Description

Sinus dysrhythmia (Fig. 28-42) is present when the difference between the longest and shortest R-R intervals is greater than 0.16 second.

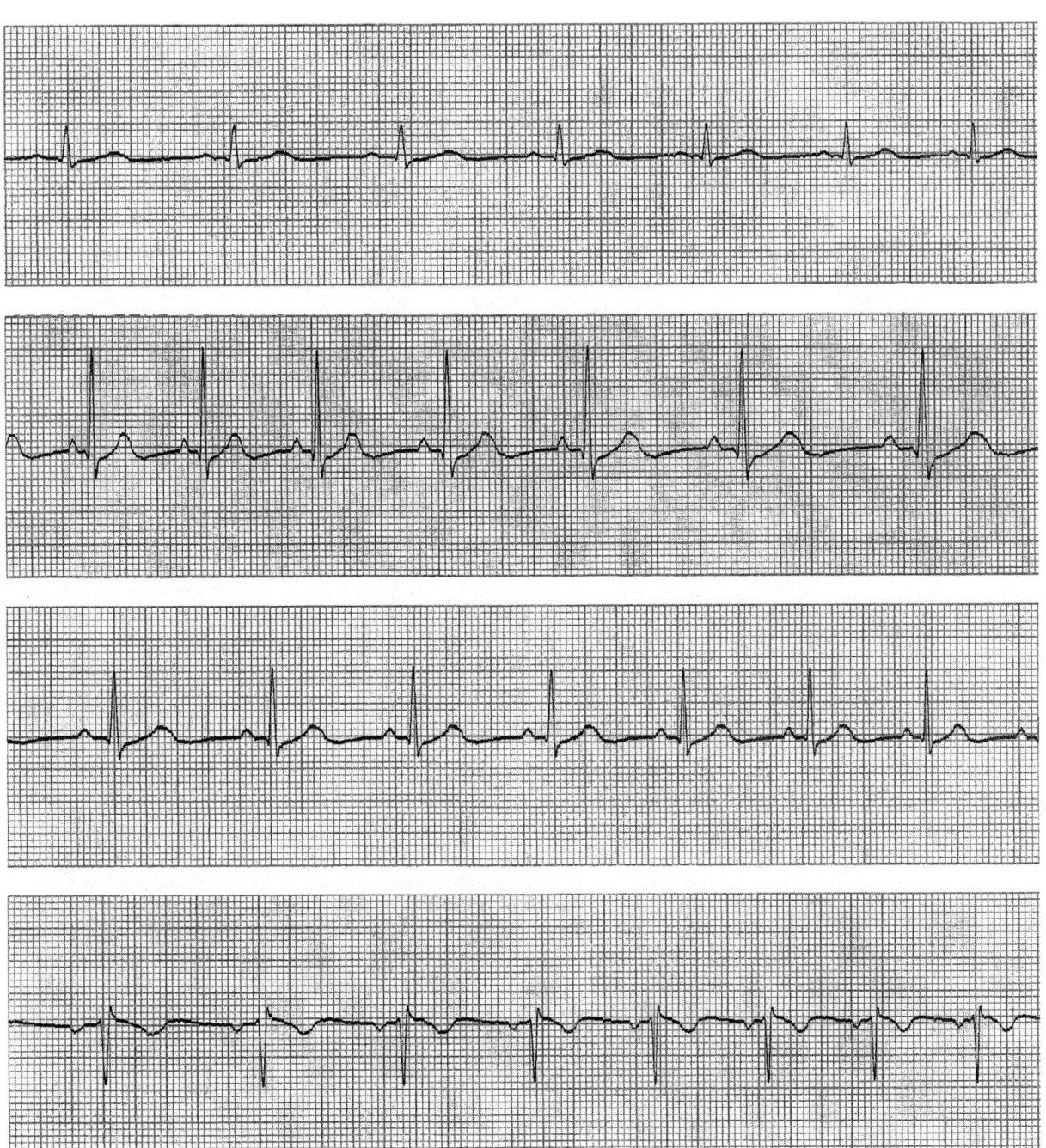

Fig. 28-42 Sinus dysrhythmia.

Etiology

Sinus dysrhythmia usually is normal. It commonly is related to the respiratory cycle and to changes in intrathoracic pressure, which cause the heart rate to increase during inspiration and decrease during expiration. Although sinus dysrhythmia sometimes occurs normally in healthy individuals, it is more common in patients with heart disease or myocardial infarction and in patients receiving certain drugs such as digitalis and *morphine.*

Rules for Interpretation (Lead II Monitoring)

QRS complex: Less than 0.12 second, provided no ventricular conduction disturbance is present.

P waves: Normal and upright; one P wave before each QRS complex.

Rate: Usually 60 to 99 beats per minute (varies with respiration).

Rhythm: Irregular (changes occur in cycles and usually follow the patient's respiratory pattern).

PR interval: 0.12 to 0.20 second and constant (normal).

Clinical Significance

This dysrhythmia is common in children, young adults, and older adults and may be associated with palpitations, dizziness, and syncope (rare).

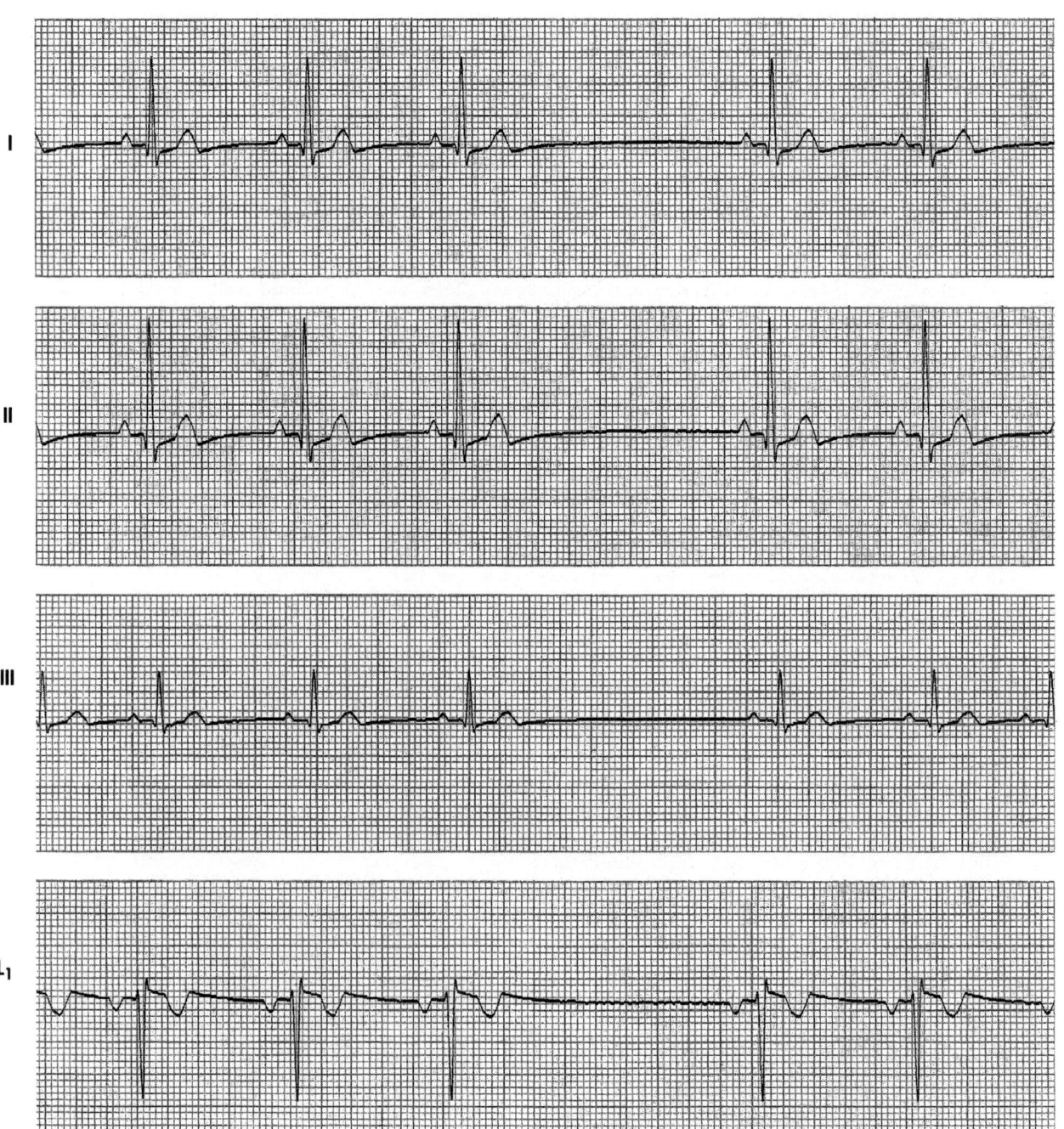

I

II

III

MCL₁

Fig. 28-43 Sinus arrest.

Management

Sinus dysrhythmia usually is of no clinical significance and requires no management.

Sinus Arrest

Description

Sinus arrest (Fig. 28-43) results from a marked depression in SA node automaticity. The failure of the sinus node causes short periods of cardiac standstill until lower-level pacemakers discharge (escape beats) or the sinus node resumes its normal function.

Etiology

Sinus arrest may be precipitated by an increase in parasympathetic tone on the SA node, hypoxia or ischemia, excessive administration of digitalis or *propranolol* (Inderal), hyperkalemia, or damage to the SA node (AMI, degenerative fibrotic disease).

Rules for Interpretation (Lead II Monitoring)

QRS complex: Less than 0.12 second, provided there is no bundle branch conduction disturbance.

P waves: Normal and upright. If the electrical impulse is not generated by the SA node or blocked from entering the atria, atrial depolarization does not occur and the P wave is dropped.

Rate: Normal to slow, depending on the frequency and duration of sinus arrest.

Rhythm: Irregular when sinus arrest is present.

PR interval: PR intervals (when the P wave is present) of the underlying rhythm are normal (0.12 to 0.20 second) in the absence of AV block. Junctional escape beats may occur with no P waves.

Clinical Significance

Frequent or prolonged episodes of sinus arrest may compromise cardiac output by decreasing the heart rate and abolishing the atrial contribution to ventricular filling. If an escape pacemaker does not take over, ventricular asystole may result, causing lightheadedness followed by syncope. With this dysrhythmia, there is danger that sinus node activity will completely cease and that an escape pacemaker may not take over pacing (resulting in asystole).

Management

If the patient is asymptomatic, close observation is all that is required. In symptomatic patients with marked bradycardia, management may include the administration of *atropine* or TCP (see Fig. 28-40).

Dysrhythmias Originating in the Atria

Atrial dysrhythmias may originate in the tissues of the atria or in the internodal pathways. Common causes of atrial dysrhythmias are ischemia, hypoxia, and atrial dilation caused by congestive heart failure, mitral valve abnormalities, or increased pulmonary artery pressures. Atrial dysrhythmias include wandering pacemaker, PACs, PSVT, atrial flutter, and atrial fibrillation. ECG features common to all atrial dysrhythmias (provided there is no ventricular conduction disturbance) include:

- Normal QRS complexes
- P waves (if present) that differ in appearance from sinus P waves
- Abnormal, shortened, or prolonged PR intervals

Wandering Pacemaker

Description

Wandering pacemaker (Fig. 28-44) (or wandering atrial pacemaker) is the passive transfer of pacemaker sites from the sinus node to other latent pacemaker sites in the atria and AV junction. The shift in the site usually is transient—back and forth along the SA node, atria, and AV junction.

Etiology

Wandering pacemaker is a variant of sinus dysrhythmia. It may be nonpathological in the very young, older adults, and well-conditioned athletes. The dysrhythmia generally is caused by the inhibitory vagal effect of respiration on the SA node and AV junction. Other causes include associated underlying heart disease and the administration of digitalis. A variant of wandering atrial pacemaker is multifocal atrial tachycardia (MAT). This rhythm disturbance resembles wandering pacemaker, but it is associated with rates frequently in the 120- to 150-per-minute range and is always considered pathological. Multifocal atrial tachycardia most often is found in patients with severe chronic obstructive pulmonary disease and may respond to management of this underlying disorder.

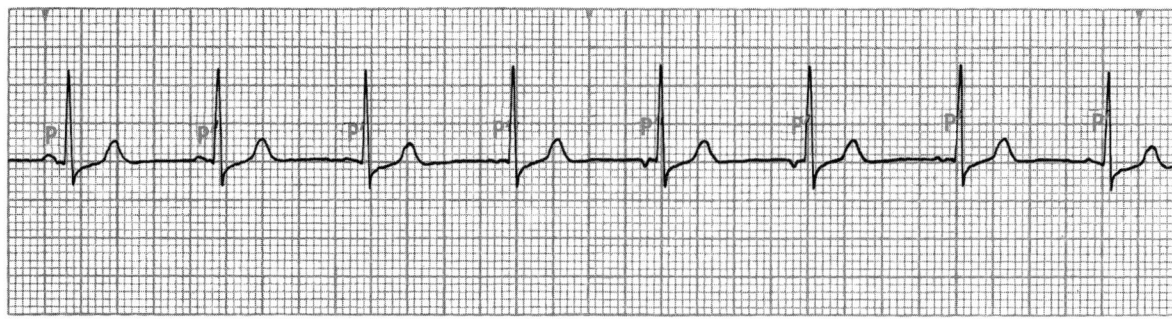

Fig. 28-44 Wandering atrial pacemaker. (From Huszar R: *Basic dysrhythmias,* ed 2, St Louis, 1994, Mosby.)

NOTE

MAT frequently is misdiagnosed as atrial fibrillation with rapid ventricular response.

Rules for Interpretation (Lead II Monitoring)

QRS complex: Usually less than 0.12 second, provided no conduction block occurs in the bundle branches.

P waves: Change in P-wave morphology from beat to beat. In lead II, the P waves may be upright, rounded, notched, inverted, biphasic, or buried in the QRS complex.

Rate: Usually 60 to 99 beats per minute. The rate may gradually slow when the pacemaker site shifts from the SA node to the atria or AV junction and increase when the pacemaker site shifts back to the SA node.

Rhythm: Irregular.

PR interval: Varies.

Clinical Significance

A wandering pacemaker usually is not clinically significant and causes no detrimental effects. Other atrial dysrhythmias (such as atrial fibrillation) occasionally are associated with this dysrhythmia.

Management

A wandering pacemaker occasionally is a benign rhythm and no management is required. MAT, however, may be precipitated by acute exacerbation of emphysema, congestive heart failure, or acute mitral valve regurgitation. Management is aimed at the underlying cause.

Premature Atrial Complex

Description

A premature atrial complex (PAC) (Fig. 28-45) is a single electrical impulse originating in the atria, outside the sinus node. The impulse creates a PAC (P wave) and, if conducted through the AV node, also causes a QRS complex before the next expected sinus beat. Since the PAC usually depolarizes the SA node prematurely, the timing of the SA node is reset. The next expected P wave of the underlying rhythm appears earlier than it would have if the SA node had not been disturbed (noncompensatory pause). PACs may originate from a single ectopic pacemaker site or from multiple sites in the atria. The electrophysiological mechanism responsible for PACs probably is enhanced automaticity or a reentry mechanism.

? CRITICAL THINKING

What will you feel when you palpate the pulse of a patient with PACs?

Etiology

PACs may result from the following:

- Increase in catecholamines and sympathetic tone
- Use of caffeine, tobacco, or alcohol
- Use of sympathomimetic drugs (*epinephrine* [Adrenalin], *isoproterenol* [Isuprel], *norepinephrine* [Levophed])
- Electrolyte imbalance
- Hypoxia
- Digitalis toxicity
- Cardiovascular disease
- In some cases, no apparent cause

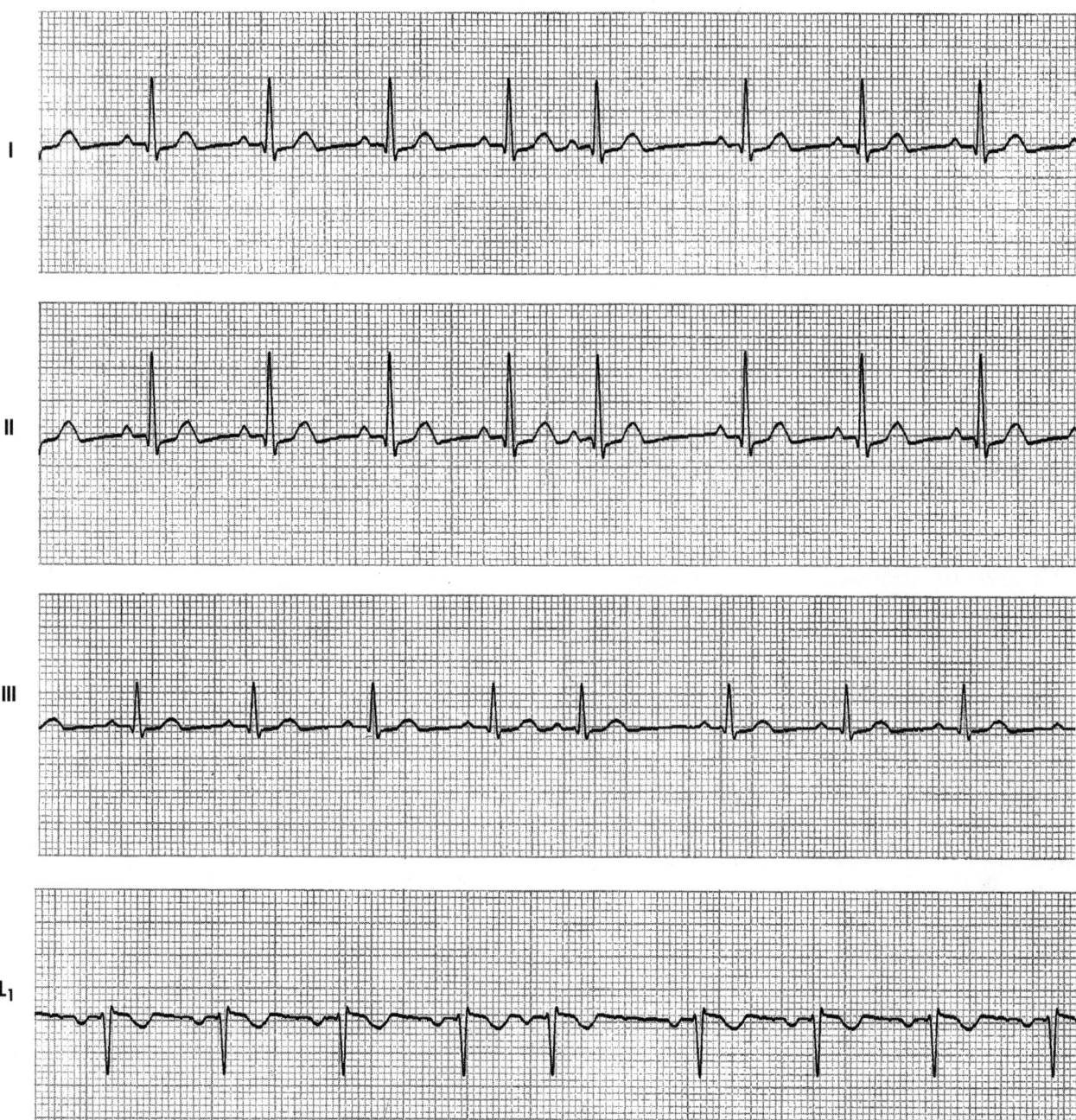

Fig. 28-45 PAC.

Rules for Interpretation (Lead II Monitoring)

QRS complex: Usually less than 0.12 second. The QRS complex may be greater than 0.12 second and appear bizarre if the PAC is abnormally conducted. It may be absent as a result of a temporary complete AV block (nonconducted PAC) that occurs during the refractory period of the AV node or ventricles.

> **NOTE**
>
> PACs with aberrancy may resemble PVCs. It is important to distinguish between these two types of dysrhythmias so that the patient is managed appropriately.

P waves: The P wave of a PAC differs in shape from a sinus P wave. It occurs earlier than the next

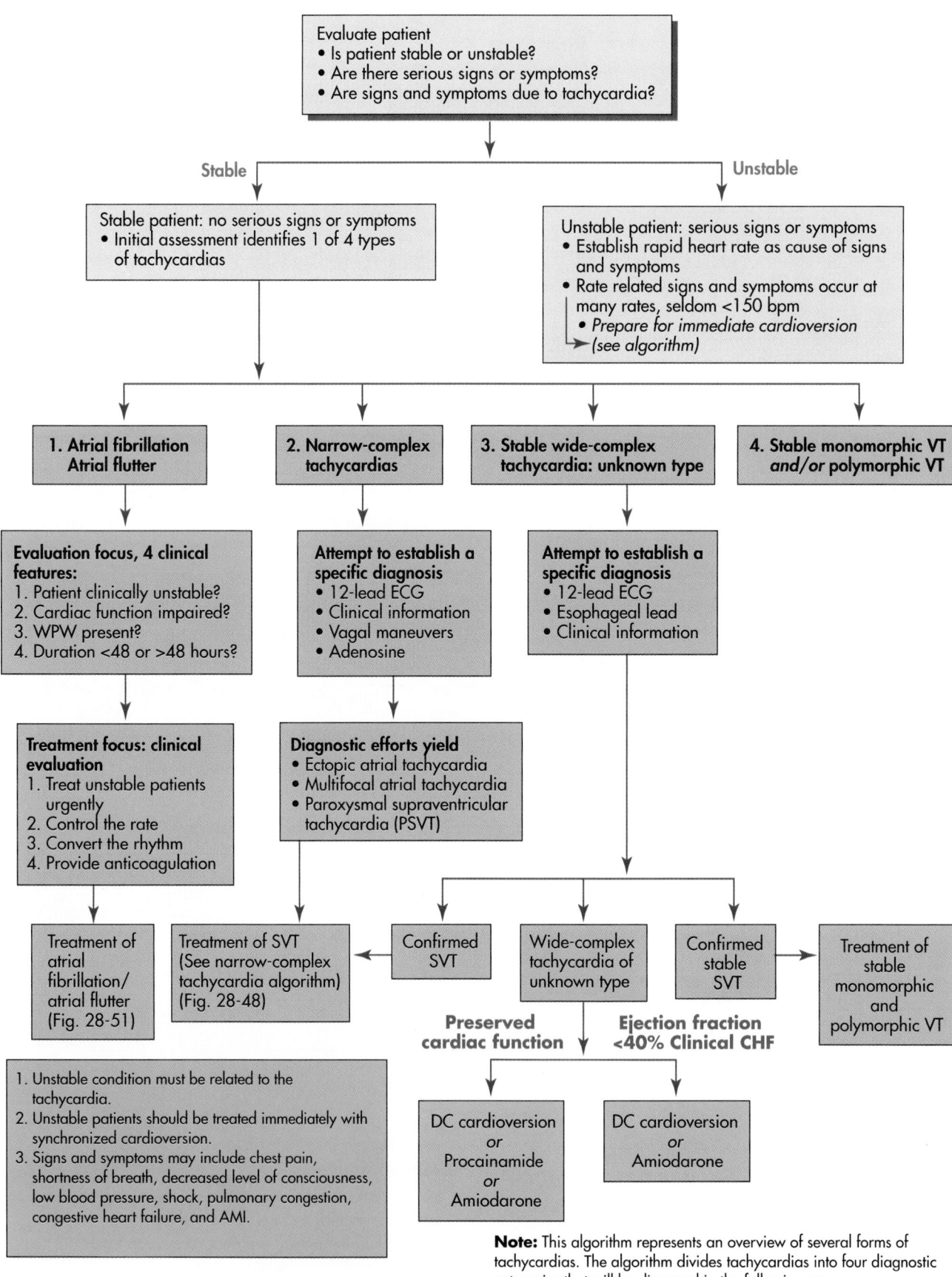

Fig. 28-46 The tachycardia overview algorithm.

expected sinus P wave and may be so early that it is superimposed or hidden in the preceding T wave. The preceding T wave should be evaluated to see if its morphology is altered by the presence of a P wave.

Rate: Depends on the underlying rhythm.

Rhythm: Usually the underlying rhythm is sinus and regular with irregular premature beats when the PACs occur.

PR interval: Usually in the normal range but differs from those of the underlying rhythm. The PR interval of a PAC varies from 0.20 second when the pacemaker site is near the SA node to 0.12 second when the pacemaker is near the AV junction.

Clinical Significance

Isolated PACs in patients with healthy hearts are not significant. Frequent PACs that occur in patients with heart disease may predispose the patient to serious supraventricular dysrhythmias such as MAT, atrial tachycardia, atrial flutter, atrial fibrillation, or PSVT.

Management

Prehospital care of asymptomatic patients usually only requires observation. If nonconducted PACs are frequent and the patient becomes symptomatic from bradycardia, TCP or *atropine* may be indicated (see Fig. 28-40).

Supraventricular Tachycardia and Paroxysmal Supraventricular Tachycardia

Description

Supraventricular tachycardias (SVTs) include paroxysmal supraventricular tachycardia (PSVT), nonparoxysmal atrial tachycardia, multifocal atrial tachycardia, junctional tachycardia, atrial flutter, and atrial fibrillation (Fig. 28-46). This section of the text will present PSVT, an SVT that begins abruptly.

PSVT (Fig. 28-47) can originate in the atria (paroxysmal atrial tachycardia [PAT]) or AV junction (paroxysmal junctional tachycardia [PJT]). The dysrhythmia results from rapid atrial or junctional depolarization that overrides the SA node. The impulse reenters the AV node with each revolution at the same time that it divides into a branch that is conducted to the ventricles (to produce the QRS complex). The cycle and the tachycardia continue until the reentry pathway is interrupted. PSVT is charac-

terized by repeated episodes (paroxysms) of atrial tachycardia, which often have a sudden onset (lasting minutes to hours) and an abrupt termination.

Etiology

In most cases, PSVT is a reentry tachycardia in which the electrical impulses are caught in a cycle that continuously circulates around the AV node. PSVT may occur at any age and is not commonly associated with underlying heart disease. It is rare in patients with myocardial infarction. Precipitating factors include stress, overexertion, tobacco use, and caffeine consumption. PSVT also is common in patients who have Wolff-Parkinson-White syndrome.

Rules for Interpretation (Lead II Monitoring)

QRS complex: Less than 0.12 second, provided no ventricular conduction disturbance is present.

P waves: The ectopic P waves differ from the normal sinus P waves. In lead II, the P waves may be normal and upright if the pacemaker site is near the SA node but inverted if they originate near the AV junction. The P waves frequently are buried in preceding T or U waves or QRS complexes and therefore cannot be identified.

Rate: 150 to 250 beats per minute.

Rhythm: Regular except at onset and termination.

PR interval: If P waves are discernible, the PR interval often is shortened but may be normal or, rarely, prolonged.

Clinical Significance

PSVT may occur in patients with healthy hearts and may be tolerated well for short periods. Frequently, the dysrhythmia is accompanied by palpitations, nervousness, and anxiety. Since a rapid ventricular rate may prevent the ventricles from filling com-

> **NOTE**
>
> The distinctions among VT, nonparoxysmal SVT, and PSVT may be difficult to make but are important. There are two critical points to remember: (1) If the patient displays serious signs and symptoms, particularly if the ventricular rate is greater than 150 beats per minute, prepare for immediate cardioversion; and (2) if the tachycardia complex appears wide, manage the rhythm as VT. These two clinical rules should help manage the most difficult tachydysrhythmias. Use of modified chest leads may help identify these rhythms.

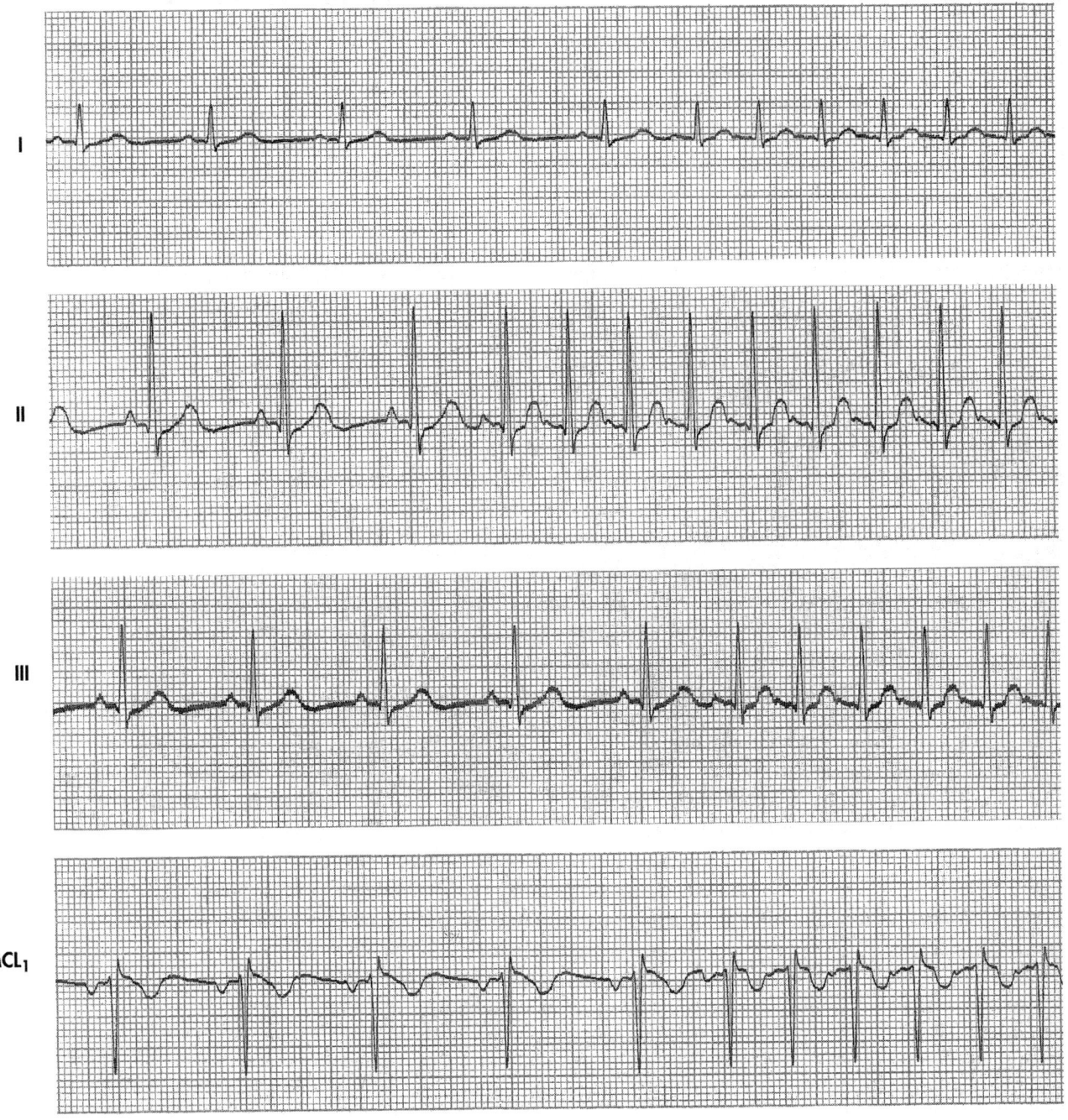

Fig. 28-47 PSVT.

pletely during diastole, PSVT can significantly compromise cardiac output in patients with underlying heart disease. Decreased perfusion may cause confusion, vertigo, lightheadedness, and syncope and may precipitate angina pectoris, hypotension, or congestive heart failure. In addition, PSVT increases the heart's oxygen requirement, which may increase myocardial ischemia and the frequency and severity of the patient's chest pain.

Management (Fig. 28-48)

Symptomatic PSVT should be managed promptly to reverse the consequences of the reduced cardiac output and increased workload on the heart. The

Narrow-QRS Tachycardia

Perform Primary ABCD Survey (Basic Life Support)
(Correct critical problems IMMEDIATELY as they are identified)
- Assess responsiveness, **A**irway, **B**reathing, **C**irculation, ensure availability of monitor/**D**efibrillator

Perform Secondary ABCD Survey (Advanced Life Support)
- Administer oxygen, establish IV access, attach cardiac monitor, administer fluids as needed (O_2, IV, monitor, fluids)
- Assess vital signs, attach pulse oximeter, and monitor blood pressure
- Obtain and review 12-lead ECG, portable chest x-ray
- Perform a focused history and physical exam

Is the patient stable or unstable?
Is the patient experiencing serious signs and symptoms due to the tachycardia?

Attempt to identify patient's cardiac rhythm using:
- 12-lead ECG, clinical information
- Vagal maneuvers
- Adenosine 6 mg rapid IV bolus over 1 to 3 sec. If needed, administer adenosine 12 mg rapid IV bolus over 1 to 3 sec after 1 to 2 minutes. May repeat 12 mg dose in 1 to 2 minutes if needed. Follow each dose immediately with 20-mL IV flush of NS. use of adenosine is relatively contraindicated in asthmatic patients. Decrease dose in patients on dipyridamole (Persantine) or carbamazepine (Tegretol); consider increasing dose in patients taking theophylline or caffeine-containing preparations.

IDENTIFY THE PATIENT'S CARDIAC RHYTHM

Junctional Tachycardia		Paroxysmal supraventricular tachycardia (PSVT) (includes AVNRT or AVRT)		Ectopic Atrial Tachycardia, Multifocal Atrial Tachycardia (MAT)	
STABLE PATIENT		STABLE PATIENT		STABLE PATIENT	
Normal Cardiac Function	**Impaired Cardiac Function**	**Normal Cardiac Function**	**Impaired Cardiac Function**	**Normal Cardiac Function**	**Impaired Cardiac Function**
Amiodarone (IIb) **OR** Beta-blocker (Indeterminate) **OR** Ca++ channel blocker (Indeterminate)	Amiodarone (IIb) Note: Impaired cardiac function = ejection fraction <40% or CHF	Priority order: Ca++ channel blocker (Class I) Beta-blocker (Class I) Digoxin (IIb) Sync cardioversion	Priority order: Sync cardioversion Digoxin (IIb) Amiodarone (IIb) Diltiazem (IIb)	Ca++ channel blocker (IIb) **OR** Beta-blocker (IIb) **OR** Amiodarone (IIb) **OR** Flecainide (IIb) **OR** Propafenone (IIb) **OR** Digoxin (Indeterminate) **Cardioversion ineffective**	Amiodarone (IIb) **OR** Diltiazem (IIb) **OR** Digoxin (Indeterminate) **Cardioversion ineffective**

UNSTABLE PATIENT

If hemodynamically unstable PSVT, perform synchronized cardioversion: 50 J, 100 J, 200 J, 300 J, 360 J (or equivalent biphasic energy.)

MEDICATION DOSING

Amiodarone[*,†,††] 150 mg IV over 10 minutes followed by an infusion of 1 mg/min for 6 hours and then a maintenance infusion of 0.5 mg/min. Repeat supplementary infusions of 150 mg as necessary for recurrent or resistant dysrhythmias. Maximum total daily dose 2 g.

Beta-blockers *Esmolol:* 0.5 mg/kg over 1 minute followed by a maintenance infusion at 50 mcg/kg/min for 4 minutes. If inadequate response, administer a second bolus of 0.5 mg/kg over 1 minute and increase maintenance infusion to 100 mcg/kg/min. The bolus dose (0.5 mg/kg) and titration of the maintenance infusion (addition of 50 mcg/kg/min) can be repeated every 4 minutes to a maximum infusion of 300 mcg/kg/min. *Metoprolol:* 5 mg slow IV push over 5 minutes x 3 as needed to a total dose of 15 mg over 15 minutes.

Calcium channel blockers[§] *Diltiazem* 0.25 mg/kg over 2 min (e.g., 15 to 20 mg). If ineffective, 0.35 mg/kg over 2 min (e.g., 20 to 25 mg) in 15 min. Maintenance infusion 5 to 15 mg/h, titrated to heart rate if chemical conversion successful. Calcium chloride (2 to 4 mg/kg) may be given slow IV push if borderline hypotension exists before diltiazem administration. *Verapamil:* 2.5 to 5.0 mg slow IV push over 2 min. May repeat with 5 to 10 mg in 15 to 30 min. Maximum dose 20 mg.

Digoxin Loading dose 10-to 15-mcg/kg lean body weight.

Flecainide, propafenone IV form not currently approved for use in the United States.

*Mehta AV et al: Ectopic automatic atrial tachycardia in children: clinical characteristics, management and follow-up, *J Am Coll Cardiol* 11:379, 1988.
†Holt P et al: Intravenous amiodarone in the acute termination of supraventricular arrhythmias, *Int J Cardiol*, 58:67, 1985.
††Kouvaras G et al: The effective treatment of multifocal atrial tachycardia with amiodarone, *Jpn Heart J* 30:301, 1989.
§Garratt C et al: Comparison of adenosine and verapamil for termination of paroxysmal junctional tachycardia, *Am J Cardiol* 64:1310, 1989.

Fig. 28-48 Narrow-QRS tachycardia (From Aehlert B: *ACLS quick review study guide*, ed 2, St Louis, 2002, Mosby.)

paramedic should attempt the following techniques to terminate PSVT.

Vagal maneuvers. Vagal maneuvers slow the heart and decrease the force of atrial contraction by stimulating postganglionic parasympathetic nerve fibers in the wall of the atria and specialized tissues of the SA and AV nodes via the vagus nerve. Vagal maneuvers may be used to terminate PSVT provided the patient is hemodynamically stable (conscious and normotensive without chest pain, congestive heart failure, or pulmonary edema).

Valsalva maneuver. Place the patient in a sitting or semisitting position with the head tilted down. In-

NOTE

Vagal maneuvers should be attempted only with authorization from medical direction. Continuous ECG monitoring and an IV line must be established before beginning these procedures. In addition, **atropine, lidocaine** (Xylocaine), and airway equipment should be readily available.

SEQUENCE OF CARE FOR NARROW-COMPLEX SUPRAVENTRICULAR TACHYCARDIAS

- Vagal maneuvers
- **Adenosine**
- Consider antidysrhythmics
  - Calcium Channel Blockers (Class I)
    - **Diltiazem** (Cardizem)
    - **Verapamil** (Isoptin)
  - Beta blockers (Class I)
    - Esmolol (Brevibloc)
    - **Metoprolol** (Lopressor)
  - **Digoxin** (Lanoxin) (Class II b)
  - **Amiodarone** (Cordarone) (Class II a)
  - **Procainamide** (Class II a)
  - **Flecainide** (Class II a)
  - Propafenone (Class II a)
  - Sotalol (Class II a)

struct the patient to take in a deep breath and to "bear down" as if to have a bowel movement. The forced expiration against a closed glottis stimulates the vagus nerve and may terminate the tachycardia. The procedure may be repeated if unsuccessful.

Ice-pack maneuver. Placing an ice pack on the patient's anterior neck may stimulate the vagus nerve because of the mammalian diving reflex (see Chapter 36). (In the pediatric patient, the application of this technique is performed with a washcloth soaked in ice water and placed across the patient's face, about to nostril level.)

NOTE

The ice-pack maneuver should not be attempted if ischemic heart disease is present or suspected. The procedure may be repeated (per medical direction) if unsuccessful.

Unilateral carotid sinus pressure. Carotid sinus pressure stimulates the carotid bodies located in the carotid arteries. This localized pressure is interpreted by the body as an increase in blood pressure. This activates the autonomic nervous system and stimulates the vagus nerve, and the heart rate slows in an attempt to lower blood pressure. The carotids should be auscultated for the presence of a bruit (described in Chapter 13) before applying carotid sinus pressure. Carotid sinus pressure should not be applied if bruits are present, if the patient is an older adult, or if there is known carotid artery disease or cerebral vascular disease. Possible complications from the procedure include cerebral emboli, stroke, syncope, sinus arrest, asystole, and increased degree of AV block.[1] The procedure for carotid sinus massage is as follows:

1. Position yourself behind the patient, who is lying supine with the neck extended and the head turned away from the side of the applied pressure.
2. Gently palpate each carotid artery to confirm the presence of equal pulses. If pulses are unequal,

---

CRITICAL POINTS TO REMEMBER

1. Administration of **verapamil** (Isoptin) to a patient with VT can be a lethal error.
2. Use the patient's signs and symptoms rather than ECG criteria to determine management modalities when distinguishing between PSVT with aberrant conduction and VT.
3. If the tachycardia complex is wide and difficult to distinguish, manage the rhythm like VT.

NOTE

If the complexes are wide and VT is suspected, consider **amiodarone** (Cordarone), **procainamide** (Pronestyl), or **lidocaine** (Xylocaine) (see Figs. 28-67 and 28-68).

---

or if one is absent, do not apply carotid sinus pressure.

3. Auscultate (while the patient holds his or her breath for 4 to 5 seconds) for the presence of bruits.
4. To apply carotid sinus pressure, place the index and middle fingers over the artery on the neck just below the angle of the jaw. Compress the artery firmly against the vertebral column while massaging the area. (Inform the patient that he or she may experience some pain or discomfort.) Maintain pressure no longer than 5 to 10 seconds. Discontinue the massage immediately if bradycardia or signs of heart block develop or if the tachycardia breaks. *Apply pressure to only one carotid sinus at a time.*
5. Observe the ECG monitor and run a strip during the procedure and obtain a tracing. Repeat the procedure in 2 to 3 minutes if it is ineffective.

? CRITICAL THINKING

What may happen if you perform carotid sinus massage on a patient with bruits or known carotid artery disease?

Pharmacological therapy. If vagal maneuvers fail or are contraindicated and the patient remains stable, administration of *adenosine* (Adenocard, the initial drug of choice), *verapamil* (Isoptin), *diltiazem* (Cardizem), or other antidysrhythmics may end PSVT.

The pharmacological regimen recommended by the American Heart Association for stable narrow-complex supraventricular tachycardias is struc-tured by rhythm diagnosis and then further directed by stability of the patient in terms of left ventricular function or **cardiac ejection fraction** (see Fig. 28-48). Without invasive hemodynamic monitoring, the paramedic can discern poor stroke volume or hemodynamic compromise by the presence of clinical signs and symptoms of congestive heart failure or poor perfusion. The patient's clinical condition, or hemodynamic status, directs treatment decisions.

Junctional tachycardia in adults is rare and is not paroxysmal in nature. Ectopic atrial tachycardia is also not paroxysmal and often will continue after pharmacological treatment to block conduction through the AV node. Unlike reentry dysrhythmias, ectopic atrial tachycardia, multifocal atrial tachycardia and sinus tachycardia are not responsive to electrical cardioversion.

For simplicity, in PSVT vagal maneuvers and *adenosine* should be used initially to terminate the tachydysrhythmia. With 'preserved ejection fraction', (a hemodynamically stable patient condition without evidence of congestive heart failure), the primary pharmacological treatment options include calcium channel blockers (Class I), beta blockers (Class I), *Amiodarone* (Class IIa), or digitalis (Class IIb).

Persistent or recurrent PSVT may be treated with antidysrhythmic agents such as **procainamide, amiodarone, flecainide, propafenone,** and **sotalol** (all are Class IIa). These agents will most probably be used after confirmed arrhythmia diagnosis and evaluation by a physician. As of yet, intravenous flecainide, propafenone and sotalol are not approved for use in the United States.

The consecutive use of calcium channel blockers, beta blockers, and primary antidysrhythmics is discouraged. The general rule is to use only one antidysrhythmic agent owing to their proarrhythmic and hypotensive actions when given serially. Furthermore, avoid negative inotropic drugs (*verapamil*, beta blockers, flecainide, *procainamide*, propafenone, flecainide, and sotalol) in hemodynamically unstable patients with impaired left ventricular function (poor ejection fraction).

Multiple pharmacological treatment modalities are available for narrow and wide complex tachycardias (ventricular rate >150). However, when serious signs and symptoms, evidence of clinical instability or poor perfusion accompany either form of tachycardia, synchronized electrical cardioversion is the treatment of choice. Cardioversion should commence with a synchronized shock of 50 joules. If this fails, the energy may be increased to 100, 200, 300 and finally 360 joules (see Fig. 28-70).

> **NOTE**
>
> Cardioversion encompasses vagal, pharmacological, and electrical therapy. The term, however, is ordinarily reserved to described electrical cardioversion.

Electrical therapy. If vagal maneuvers and pharmacological therapy fail to terminate PSVT or if the patient is or becomes hemodynamically unstable, synchronized cardioversion is indicated. Sedation should be considered before the cardioversion (if time permits).

> **? CRITICAL THINKING**
>
> *What properties of the drug midazolam (Versed) make it an ideal sedative before cardioversion?*

Atrial Flutter

Description

Atrial flutter (Fig. 28-49) is almost always a result of a rapid atrial reentry focus. Atrial flutter not slowed by preexisting AV block usually manifests a 2:1 AV conduction ratio (i.e., 50% of the atrial impulses are conducted through the ventricles) and may look like SVT. However, 3:1, 4:1, and greater conduction ratios are not uncommon, producing a discrepancy between atrial and ventricular rates. The conduction ratios may be constant or variable. Atrial flutter may be seen with atrial fibrillation ("atrial fib-flutter"). Rarely, particularly with accessory AV (bypass) tract, atrial flutter may conduct 1:1. This results in extremely rapid ventricular rates with rapid hemodynamic deterioration.

Etiology

Atrial flutter generally is seen in middle-aged and older patients with advanced cardiovascular disease. It also occasionally occurs in patients with healthy hearts. The dysrhythmia commonly is associated with:

- Cardiomyopathy
- Cardiac hypertrophy
- Digitalis toxicity (rare)
- Hypoxia
- Congestive heart failure
- Pericarditis
- Myocarditis

Rules for Interpretation (Lead II Monitoring)

QRS complex: Less than 0.12 second, unless ventricular conduction disturbance (aberrancy) is present.

P waves: Normal P waves are absent. The flutter waves (f waves) usually resemble a "sawtooth" or "picket fence" pattern. The flutter waves represent atrial depolarization in an abnormal direction that is followed by atrial repolarization.

> **NOTE**
>
> Flutter waves may be difficult to identify when there is a 2:1 ratio of atrial to ventricular complexes. The paramedic should suspect 2:1 flutter when the rhythm is regular and the ventricular rate is 150 beats per minute.

Rate: The atrial rate is 250 to 300 beats per minute; the ventricular rate is regular but often is less than the atrial rate.

Rhythm: The atrial rhythm is regular; the ventricular rate is usually regular but may be irregular if the AV conduction ratio varies.

PR interval: Usually is constant but may vary.

Clinical Significance

Provided there is a normal ventricular rate, atrial flutter usually is well tolerated by the patient. The signs and symptoms of decreased cardiac output from a rapid ventricular response are the same as those for atrial tachycardia. In addition, in some flutter rhythms (particularly a 2:1 atrial flutter), the atria do not regularly contract and empty before each ventricular contraction. The loss of the "atrial kick" results in incomplete filling of the ventricles and may further decrease cardiac output.

NOTE

The pulse rate of a patient with this dysrhythmia (and other tachydysrhythmias) might not reflect the electrical rate, because not all impulses are manifested as effective contractions with adequate output to create a palpable pulse.

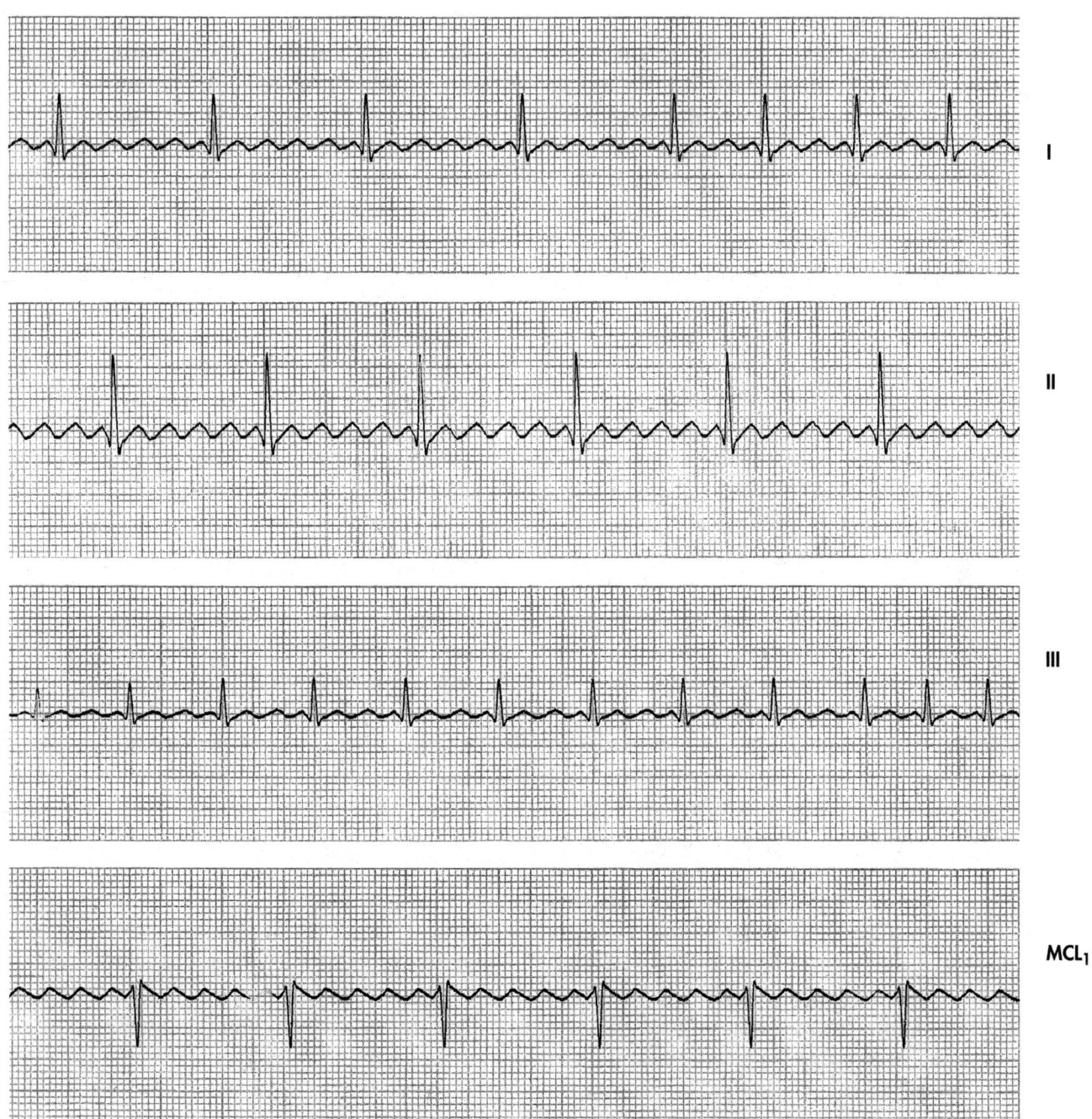

Fig. 28-49 Atrial flutter.

Atrial Fibrillation

Description

Atrial fibrillation (Fig. 28-50) results from multiple areas of reentry within the atria or from ectopic atrial pacemakers outside the SA node. (The activity of the SA node is completely suppressed by atrial fibrillation.) The electrical activity results in chaotic impulses too numerous for all to be conducted by the AV node through the ventricles. AV conduction is random, and ventricular response is irregular but usually rapid unless the patient is taking medication (e.g., *digoxin*) to slow the ventricular rate.

Etiology

Paroxysmal atrial fibrillation, which occurs in young adults after heavy alcohol ingestion (the "holiday heart" syndrome) or as a result of acute stress, is a self-limited phenomenon, usually resolv-

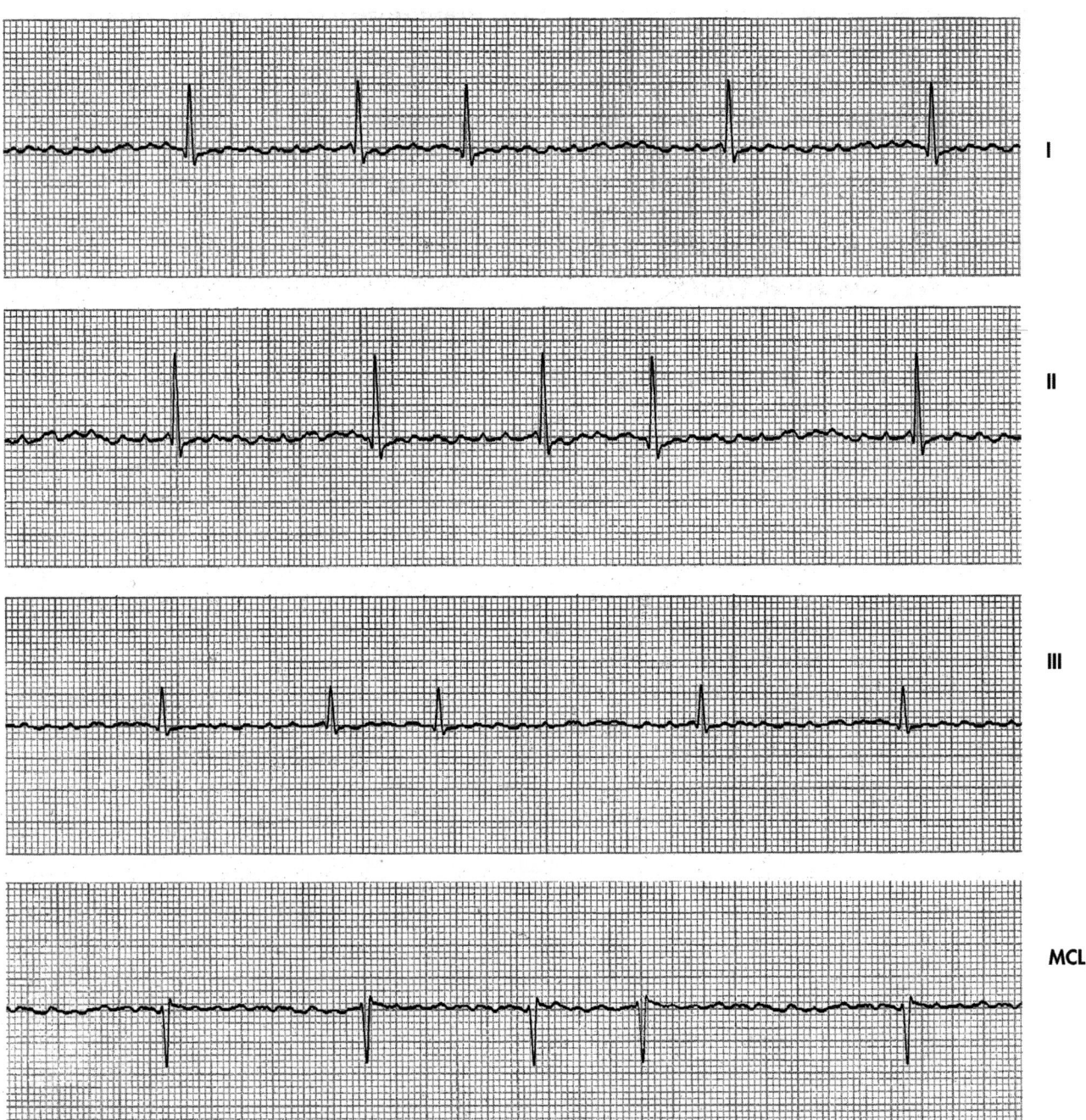

Fig. 28-50 Atrial fibrillation.

ing without management. Chronic atrial fibrillation may be intermittent and often is associated with rheumatic heart disease, congestive heart failure (atrial dilation), and atherosclerotic heart disease. Chronic atrial fibrillation usually requires digitalis (or calcium channel or beta blocker) therapy to slow the ventricular rate to 80 to 100 beats per minute. Less commonly, atrial fibrillation may occur in cardiomyopathy, acute myocarditis and pericarditis, and chest trauma. It rarely is caused by digitalis toxicity, but a very slow, regular ventricular response with atrial fibrillation should raise suspicion of digitalis toxicity.

Rules for Interpretation (Lead II Monitoring)

QRS complex: Less than 0.12 second, provided there is no ventricular conduction disturbance.

P waves: P waves and organized atrial contractions are absent. Fibrillation waves (f waves) may be "fine" (less than 1 mm) or "coarse" (greater than 1 mm). Fine f waves may be so small that they appear as a wavy or flat (isoelectric) line or absent. The f waves are irregularly shaped, rounded (or pointed), and dissimilar.

Rate: The atrial rate is 350 to 700 beats per minute (cannot be counted); the ventricular rate varies greatly, depending on conduction through the AV node (average 150 to 180 beats per minute, if uncontrolled).

Rhythm: Irregularly irregular.

PR interval: None.

> **NOTE**
>
> Irregularly irregular rhythms are most likely to be atrial fibrillation.

Clinical Significance

The "atrial kick" is lost in atrial fibrillation, which reduces cardiac output by as much as 15%. This, coupled with a rapid ventricular response, may cause cardiovascular decompensation (angina pectoris, myocardial infarction, congestive heart failure, or cardiogenic shock).

> **NOTE**
>
> Atrial fibrillation may be a stable rhythm that does not require management.

Management of Atrial Fibrillation/Atrial Flutter

The American Heart Association Tachycardia: Atrial Fibrillation and Atrial Flutter algorithm has three categories: atrial fibrillation or atrial flutter with normal heart function, impaired heart function, and WPW (Wolff Parkinson White syndrome described later in this chapter). Each condition is managed by controlling rate or converting rhythm (Fig. 28-51).

There is a risk of emboli formation when atrial fibrillation or atrial flutter has been present for more than 48 hours, increasing the risk of systemic embolization with conversion to sinus rhythm. The algorithm cautions against converting atrial fibrillation or atrial flutter without adequate anticoagulation. Electrical cardioversion and the use of antidysrhythmic agents that may convert the rhythm should be avioided unless the patient is unstable or hemodynamically compromised.[4]

Pharmacological rate control is the recommended initial treatment for stable, rapid atrial fibrillation or atrial flutter regardless of duration. Specific drug treatment is dependent on the patient's hemodynamically stability. Concurrent or serial administration of antidysrhythmic agents may have proarrhythmic potential. The paramedic should use only one pharmacological agent within the suggested spectrum of drugs.

In patients with a rapid atrial fibrillation or flutter and *preserved* left ventricular function, calcium channel blockers, beta blockers, and digitalis are recommended. Patients who are exhibiting signs of *impaired* heart function such as pulmonary congestion, diminished peripheral perfusion, or poor ejection fraction (<40%); digitalis, *diltiazem,* and *amiodarone* are recommended. Due to *amiodarone's* potential for rhythm conversion, it should be reserved for use within the first 48 hours of dysrhythmia onset when other medications for rate control have failed. Use of calcium channel blocking agents and beta blocking agents warrants caution in the presence of congestive heart failure due to their negative inotropic properties.

Patients with a known history of WPW experiencing rapid atrial fibrillation or atrial flutter for less than 48 hours may be treated with *amiodarone,* flecainide, *procainamide,* or propafenone. If the arrhythmia's duration is greater than 48 hours avoid nonemergent cardioversion unless anticoagulation precautions are taken. However, when serious signs or symptoms of hemodynamic or clinical instability related to the tachycardia occur (chest pain, shortness

Atrial Fibrillation/Atrial Flutter Algorithm

Perform Primary ABCD Survey (Basic Life Support)

(Correct critical problems IMMEDIATELY as they are identified)
- Assess responsiveness, **A**irway, **B**reathing, **C**irculation, ensure availability of monitor/**D**efibrillator

Perform Secondary ABCD Survey (Advanced Life Support)

- Administer oxygen, establish IV access, attach cardiac monitor, administer fluids as needed (O_2, IV, monitor, fluids)
- Assess vital signs, attach pulse oximeter, and monitor blood pressure
- Obtain and review 12-lead ECG, portable chest x-ray, perform a focused history and physical exam

Is the patient stable or unstable?
Is the patient experiencing serious signs and symptoms due to the tachycardia?
Is the patient's cardiac function normal or impaired?
Attempt to identify patient's cardiac rhythm using 12-lead ECG, clinical information.
Is Wolff-Parkinson-White syndrome (WPW) present? If yes, see WPW algorithm
Has atrial fibrillation/atrial flutter been present for more or less than 48 hours?

STABLE PATIENT			
Normal Cardiac Function		**Impaired Cardiac Function**	
Onset < 48 hours **Control Rate**	Onset > 48 hours **Control Rate**	Onset < 48 hours **Control Rate**	Onset > 48 hours **Control Rate**
Calcium channel blocker (Class I) **OR** Beta-blockers (Class I) **OR** Digoxin (IIb)	Calcium channel blocker (Class I) **OR** Beta-blocker (Class I) **OR** Digoxin (IIb)	Diltiazem (IIb) **OR** Amiodarone (IIb) **OR** Digoxin (IIb) Note: Impaired cardiac function = ejection fraction <40% or CHF	Diltiazem (IIb) **OR** Amiodarone (IIb) **OR** Digoxin (IIb)
Convert Rhythm	**Convert Rhythm**	**Convert Rhythm**	**Convert Rhythm**
Cardioversion **OR** Amiodarone (IIa) **OR** Procainamide (IIa) **OR** Ibutilide (IIa) **OR** Flecainide (IIa) **OR** Propafenone (IIa)	Delayed cardioversion **OR** Early cardioversion	Cardioversion **OR** amiodarone (IIb)	Delayed cardioversion **OR** Early cardioversion

Delayed cardioversion:

Anticoagulation therapy for 3 weeks before cardioversion, for at least 48 hours in conjunction with cardioversion, and for at least 4 weeks after successful cardioversion. Early cardioversion: IV heparin immediately, transesophageal echocardiography (TEE) to r/o atrial thrombus, cardioversion within 24 h, anticoagulation x 4 wks

Fig. 28-51 Atrial fibrillation/atrial flutter algorithm. (From Aehlert B: *ACLS quick review study guide,* ed 2, St Louis, 2002, Mosby.)

of breath, pulmonary congestion, decreased level of consciousness, hypotension), preparations should be made for immediate cardioversion. The initial attempt at cardioversion for atrial flutter should consist of a synchronized shock of 50 joules. If necessary, the energy may be increased to 100, 200, 300, and 360 joules. Since atrial fibrillation is a more difficult rhythm to convert and lower joule settings have been known to cause asystole, recommendations are to initially use a synchronized shock of 100 joules, followed by 200, 300, and 360 joules if necessary.[4]

? CRITICAL THINKING

What signs or symptoms would indicate hemodynamic instability in these patients?

Dysrhythmias Sustained or Originating in the AV Junction

When the SA node and the atria cannot generate the electrical impulses needed to begin depolarization because of factors such as hypoxia, ischemia, myo-

UNSTABLE PATIENT

If hemodynamically unstable, perform synchronized cardioversion: **Atrial fibrillation:** 100 J, 200 J, 300 J, 360 J, or equivalent biphasic energy. Atrial flutter: 50 J, 100 J, 200 J, 300 J, 360 J, or equivalent biphasic energy.

MEDICATION DOSING

Amiodarone*,† 150 mg IV bolus over 10 minutes followed by an infusion of 1 mg/min for 6 hours and then a maintenance infusion of 0.5 mg/min. Repeat supplementary infusions of 150 mg as necessary for recurrent or resistant dysrhythmias. Maximum total daily dose 2 g.

Beta-blockers *Esmolol:* 0.5 mg/kg over 1 minute followed by a maintenance infusion at 50 mcg/kg/min for 4 minutes. If inadequate response, administer a second bolus of 0.5 mg/kg over 1 minute and increase maintenance infusion to 100 mcg/kg/min. The bolus dose (0.5 mg/kg) and titration of the maintenance infusion (addition of 50 mcg/kg/min) can be repeated every 4 minutes to a maximum infusion of 300 mcg/kg/min. *Metoprolol:* 5 mg slow IV push over 5 minutes x 3 as needed to a total dose of 15 mg over 15 minutes. *Propranolol:* 0.1-mg/kg slow IV push divided in 3 equal doses at 2-3 minute intervals. Do not exceed 1 mg/min. Repeat after 2 minutes if necessary. *Atenolol:* 5 mg slow IV (over 5 min). Wait 10 min then give second dose of 5 mg slow IV (over 5 min).

Calcium channel blockers‡, § *Diltiazem* 0.25 mg/kg over 2 min (e.g., 15 to 20 mg). If ineffective, 0.35 mg/kg over 2 min (e.g., 20-25 mg) in 15 min. Maintenance infusion 5 to 15 mg/h, titrated to heart rate if chemical conversion successful. Calcium chloride (2 to 4 mg/kg) may be given slow IV push if borderline hypotension exists before diltiazem administration. *Verapamil*–2.5 to 5.0 mg slow IV push over 2 min. May repeat with 5 to 10 mg in 15 to 30 min. Maximum dose 20 mg.

Ibutilide Adults 60 kg: 1 mg (10-mL) over 10 min. May repeat x 1 in 10 min. Adults < 60 kg: 0.01 mg/kg IV over 10 min.

Procainamide‖ 100 mg over 5 minutes (20 mg/min). Maximum total dose 17 mg/kg. Maintenance infusion 1 to 4 mg/min.

Flecainide, propafenone IV form not currently approved for use in the United States

Sotaolol 1 to 1.5 mg/kg IV slowly at a rate of 10 mg/min

*Cotter G et al: Conversion of recent onset paroxysmal atrial fibrillation to normal sinus rhythm: the effect of no treatment and high-dose amiodarone: a randomized, placebo-controlled study [see comments], *Eur Heart J* 20:1833, 1999.
†Clemo HF et al: Intravenous amiodarone for acute heart rate control in the critically ill patient with atrial tachyarrhythmias, *Am J Cardiol* 81:594, 1998.
‡Ellenbogen KA et al: A placebo-controlled trial of continuous intravenous diltiazem infusion for 24-hour heart rate control during atrial fibrillation and atrial flutter: a multicenter study, *J Am Coll Cardiol* 18:891, 1991.
§Salerno DM et al: Efficacy and safety of intravenous diltiazem for treatment of atrial fibrillation and atrial flutter, *Am J Cardiol* 63:1046, 1989.
‖Chapman MJ et al: Management of atrial tachyarrhythmias in the critically ill: a comparison of intravenous procainamide and amiodarone, *Intensive Care Med* 19:48, 1993.

Fig. 28-51, cont'd Atrial fibrillation/atrial flutter algorithm.

cardial infarction, and drug toxicity, the AV node or the area surrounding the AV node may assume the role of the secondary pacemaker. Rhythms that start in the AV node or AV junctional area are considered junctional rhythms. A junctional rhythm usually is a benign dysrhythmia, but it must be assessed to determine the patient's tolerance of the rhythm disturbance. Dysrhythmias that originate in the AV junction include PJCs, junctional escape complexes or junctional escape rhythms, and accelerated junctional rhythm.

In junctional rhythms, electrical impulses travel in a normal pathway from the AV junction through the bundle of His and bundle branches to the Purkinje fibers, ending in the ventricular muscle. Because conduction through the ventricles proceeds normally, the QRS complex usually is within normal limits of 0.04 to 0.10 second. However, the impulse that depolarizes the atria travels in a backward or

retrograde motion. The retrograde depolarization of the atria results in one of the following three P-wave characteristics: (1) inverted P waves in lead II with a short PR interval, (2) absent P waves, or (3) retrograde P waves.

Premature Junctional Complex

Description

A premature junctional complex (PJC) (Fig. 28-52) results from a single electrical impulse originating in the AV junction, which occurs before the next expected sinus impulse.

Etiology

Isolated PJCs may occur in healthy individuals without apparent cause. However, they more commonly are a result of intrinsic cardiac disease or drug toxicity. The electrophysiological mechanism responsible

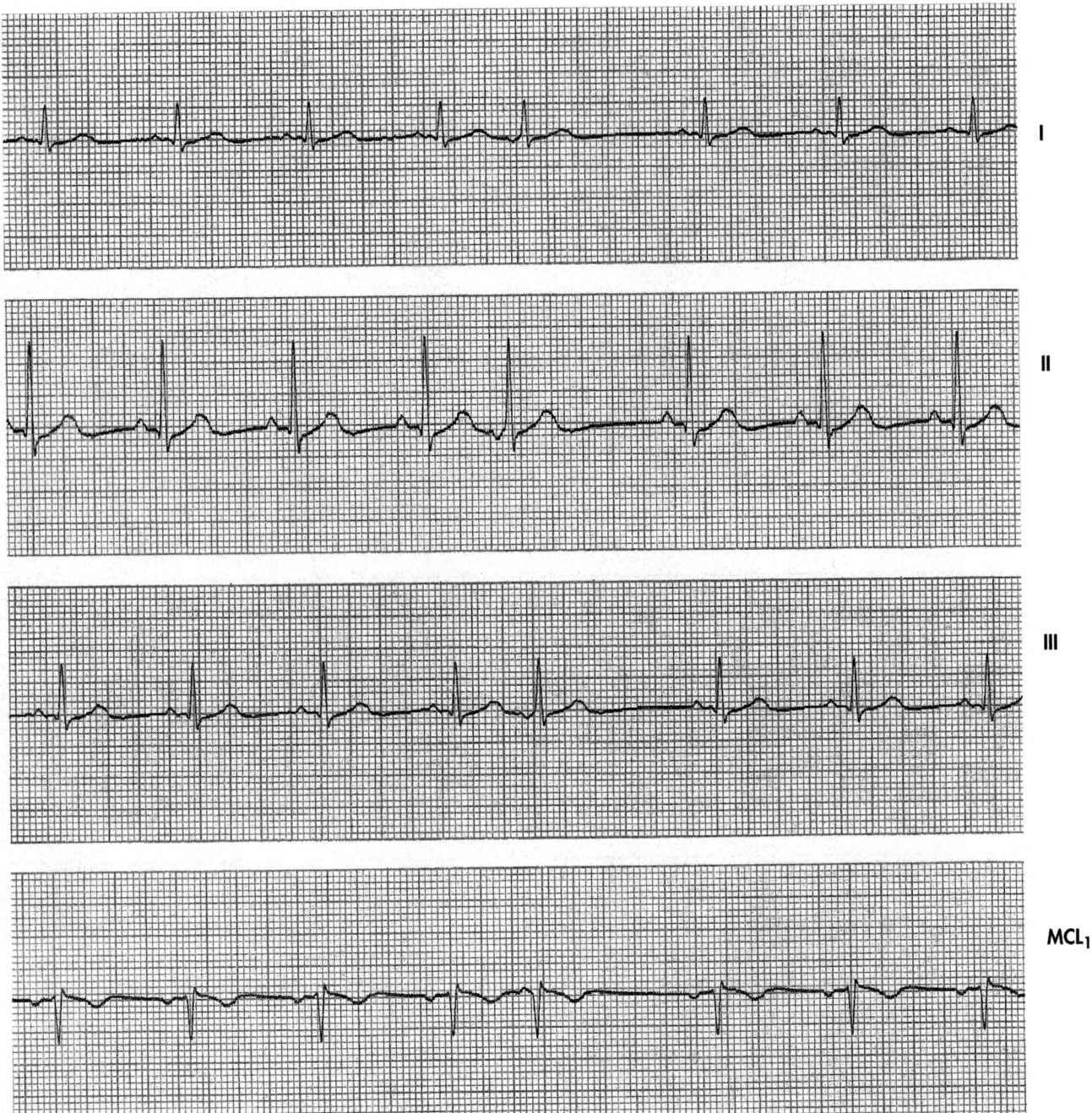

I

II

III

MCL₁

Fig. 28-52 PJCs.

for PJCs is thought to be enhanced automaticity or a reentry mechanism. PJCs have several causes:

- Digitalis toxicity
- Other cardiac medications (quinidine, *procainamide* [Pronestyl])
- Increased vagal tone on the SA node
- Sympathomimetic drugs (e.g., cocaine and methamphetamines)

- Hypoxia
- Congestive heart failure
- Damage to the AV junction

Rules for Interpretation (Lead II Monitoring)

QRS complex: Usually less than 0.12 second, provided there is no ventricular conduction disturbance.

P waves: May be associated with PJCs. P waves can occur before, during, or after the QRS complex or can be absent. If present, P waves are abnormal, differing in size, shape, and direction from normal P waves.

Rate: The heart rate is that of the underlying rhythm.

Rhythm: Usually regular, except when PJC(s) is present.

PR interval: Usually less than 0.12 second if the P wave precedes the QRS complex.

Clinical Significance

Isolated PJCs usually are not significant.

Management

No management is required.

Junctional Escape Complexes or Rhythms

Description

A junctional escape complex (isolated impulse) or rhythm (series of impulses) (Fig. 28-53) results when the rate of the primary pacemaker (usually the SA node) falls below that of the AV junctional area. The dysrhythmia also may occur when the electrical impulses from the SA node or atria fail to reach the AV junction because of SA or AV block. The escape complex or rhythm provided by the AV junction serves as a safety mechanism to prevent cardiac standstill. The AV junction is likely to assume pacemaker duties at its inherent firing rate of 40 to 60 beats per minute when an electrical impulse fails to be transmitted to the patient's AV junction within about 1.0 to 1.5 seconds.

Etiology

A junctional escape complex or a junctional escape rhythm is a normal response that may result from an increased vagal tone on the SA node, a pathological slowing of the SA discharge, or a complete AV block.

Rules for Interpretation (Lead II Monitoring)

QRS complex: Usually less than 0.12 second, provided no preexisting bundle branch block is present.

P waves: May be present (with or without relationship to QRS complex) or absent. If P waves are present, they may occur before, after, or during the QRS complex. Depending on the pacemaker site, P waves may differ from normal P waves in size, shape, and direction and may be upright or inverted.

Rate: Usually 40 to 60 beats per minute but may be less.

Rhythm: The ventricular rhythm usually is regular in junctional rhythm; may be irregular if an isolated junctional escape complex is present.

PR interval: If P waves precede the QRS complex, the PR interval commonly is shortened (less than 0.12 second) and constant.

Clinical Significance

Junctional bradycardias can cause decreased cardiac output. Therefore patients can exhibit signs and symptoms similar to those of other bradycardias (lightheadedness, hypotension, syncope). As a rule, patients tolerate junctional rhythms of 50 beats per minute or greater.

Management

Patients who are stable require no immediate intervention. If the patient is symptomatic or if ventricular irritability is present, pharmacological intervention (beginning with *atropine*) may be indicated. In severe cases and in patients unresponsive to *atropine*, external TCP may be necessary. If intrinsic disease is present in the SA node, the patient may ultimately require permanent pacemaker insertion (see Fig. 28-40).

Accelerated Junctional Rhythm

Description

Accelerated junctional rhythm (Fig. 28-54) results from increased automaticity of the AV junction, causing it to discharge faster than its intrinsic rate (40 to 60 beats per minute), overriding the primary (SA node) pacemaker. Technically, the rate of this dysrhythmia (usually 60 to 99 beats per minute) does not truly constitute a tachycardia, hence the term *accelerated junctional rhythm*. In this text, rapid junctional rhythms equal to or greater than 100 beats per minute (PJT or nonparoxysmal junctional tachycardia) and caused by a reentry mechanism are discussed with other SVTs.

Etiology

An accelerated junctional rhythm commonly is a result of digitalis toxicity. Other causes of this prob-

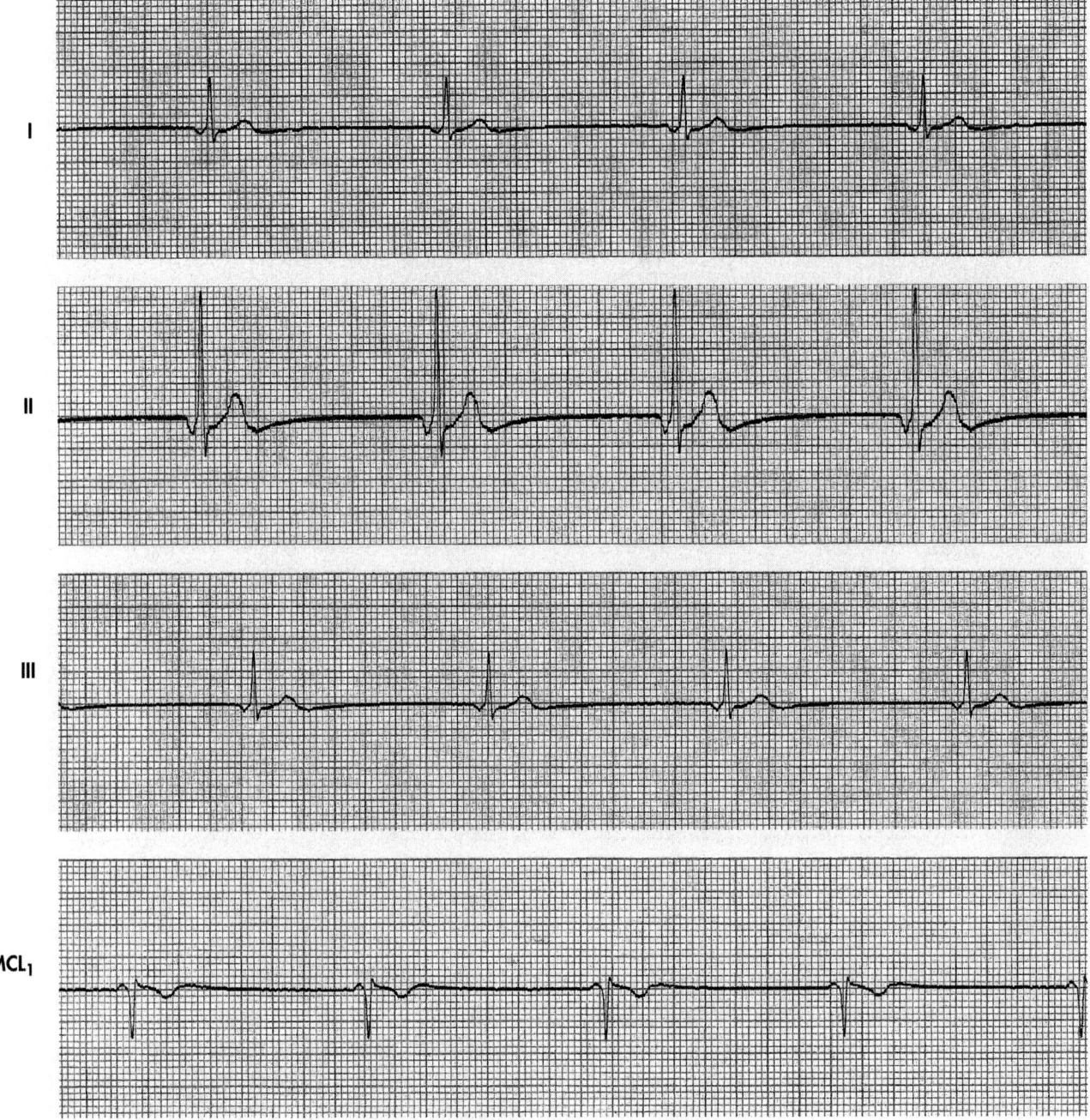

Fig. 28-53 Junctional escape complex or rhythm.

lem include excessive catecholamine administration, damage to the AV junction, inferior-wall myocardial infarction (described later in this chapter), and rheumatic fever.

Rules for Interpretation (Lead II Monitoring)

QRS complex: Usually is less than 0.12 second, provided there is no preexisting bundle branch block.

P waves: May be present (with or without relationship to the QRS complex), absent (retrograde AV block), or buried in the QRS complex. If present, P waves usually are inverted and appear before or after the QRS complex.

Rate: Usually 60 to 99 beats per minute.

Rhythm: Regular.

PR interval: If the P wave occurs before the QRS complex, the PR interval will be less than 0.12

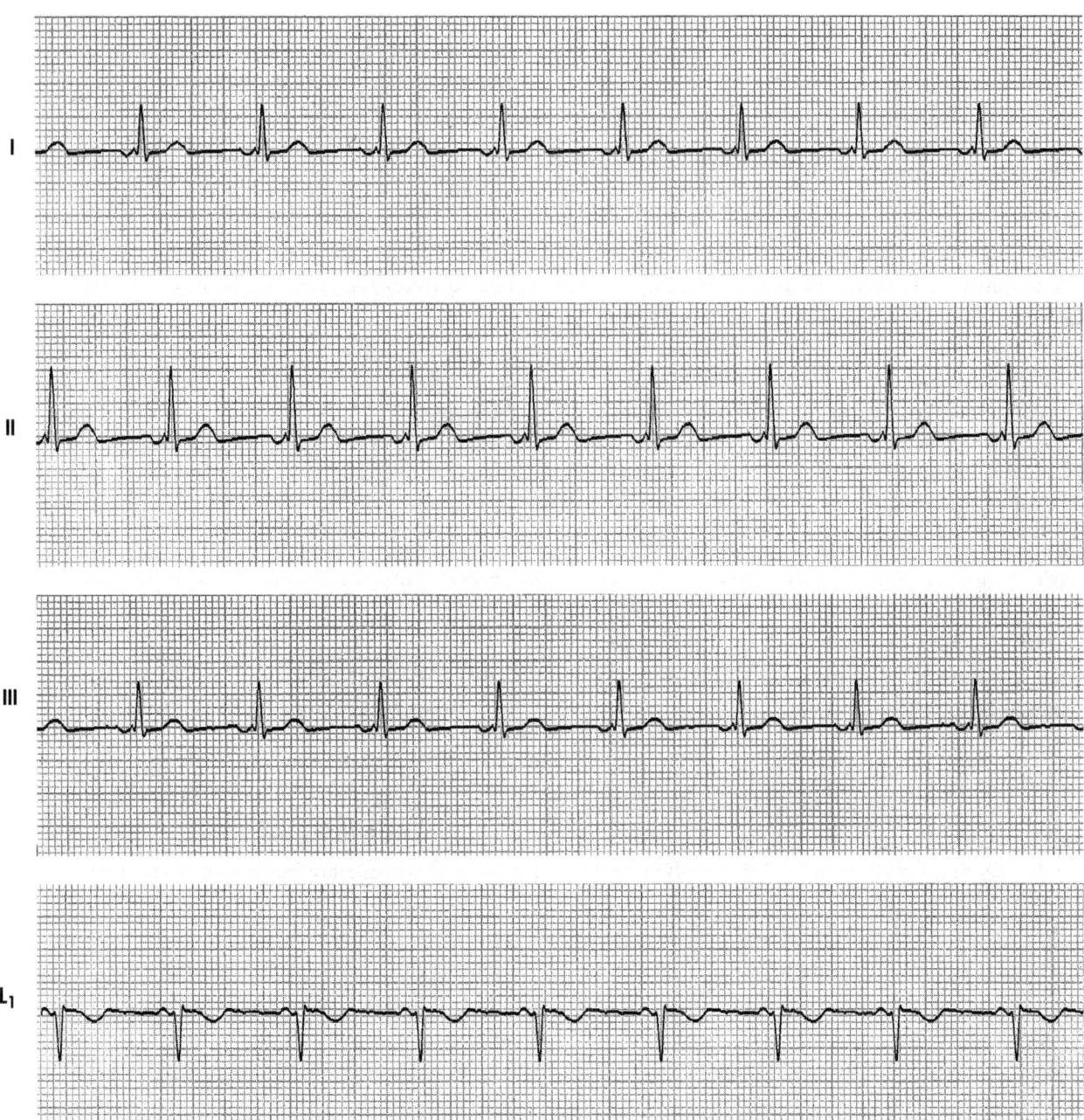

Fig. 28-54 Accelerated junctional rhythm.

second. If the P wave follows the QRS complex, it technically is an R-P interval and usually is less than 0.20 second.

Clinical Significance

Accelerated junctional rhythm usually is well tolerated by the patient. However, the presence of myocardial ischemia may predispose the patient to more serious dysrhythmias.

Management

Accelerated junctional rhythm generally requires no immediate intervention.

? CRITICAL THINKING

Do you need to start an IV line on these patients, since no drug therapy is indicated?

Dysrhythmias Originating in the Ventricles

Ventricular rhythms usually are considered to be life threatening. Ventricular rhythm disturbances generally result from failure of the atria, AV junction, or both, to initiate an electrical impulse, or they are secondary to enhanced automaticity or reentry phenomena in the ventricles. The latter group leads to PVC, VT, and even VF and often is associated with myocardial ischemia or infarction. The ventricle is the least efficient pacemaker of the heart, usually generating only 20 to 40 electrical impulses per minute. However, the ventricle can develop increased automaticity and may discharge at rates up to 99 impulses per minute (accelerated idioventricular rhythm) or even faster (VT). Dysrhythmias originating in the ventricles include ventricular escape complexes or rhythms, PVCs, VT, VF, asystole, and artificial pacemaker rhythm.

Because electrical impulses of ventricular origin start in the lower portion of the heart (the ventricular muscle, bundle branches, or Purkinje fibers), the electrical impulse must travel in a retrograde conduction pathway to depolarize the atria. It may travel in an antegrade direction to depolarize the ventricles, depending on the site of initiation of the impulse. Regardless of the direction of depolarization, the normal, rapid conducting pathways are bypassed, producing the following three ECG features:

1. QRS complexes are wide, bizarre in appearance, and 0.12 second or greater in duration.
2. P waves may be hidden in the QRS complex (since the atria are depolarized at about the same time as the ventricles) or superimposed on every second or third QRS complex when VT with **AV dissociation** (P waves that have no set relation to the QRS complexes) is present.
3. ST segments usually deviating from baseline and T waves are frequently slopped off in the opposite direction of the QRS complex.

Ventricular Escape Complexes or Rhythms

Description

A ventricular escape complex (isolated impulse) or rhythm (series of complexes), also known as *idioventricular rhythm* (Figs. 28-55 and 28-56), results

when impulses from higher pacemakers fail to fire or to reach the ventricles or when the rate of discharge of higher pacemakers falls to less than that of the ventricles. Like the junctional escape complex or rhythm, this dysrhythmia serves as a compensatory mechanism to prevent cardiac standstill.

Etiology

Ventricular escape rhythms occur when the rate of impulse formation of the dominant pacemaker (usually the SA node) and the escape pacemaker in the AV junction fails or falls below that of the escape pacemaker in the ventricles. This dysrhythmia frequently is seen as the first organized rhythm after defibrillation.

Rules for Interpretation (Lead II Monitoring)

QRS complex: Generally exceed 0.12 second and are bizarre in appearance. The shape of the QRS complex may vary in any given lead.

P waves: May be absent. If they are present and have no set relationship to the QRS complex, then a third-degree AV block should be suspected.

Rate: Usually 20 to 40 beats per minute; may be lower.

Rhythm: The ventricular rhythm usually is regular but may be irregular.

PR interval: If P waves are present, the PR interval is variable and irregular.

Clinical Significance

A ventricular escape rhythm generally is symptomatic. This dysrhythmia is manifested by hypotension, decreased cardiac output, and decreased perfusion of the brain and other vital organs, often resulting in syncope and shock. Patient assessment is essential because the escape rhythm may be perfusing or nonperfusing (PEA).

Management

If the rhythm is perfusing, management must be directed at increasing the heart rate by administering oxygen, TCP, and/or *dopamine.* Managing the escape rhythm with *lidocaine* (Xylocaine) would likely be lethal and is contraindicated. If the rhythm is nonperfusing, basic life support measures should be initiated and the treatment guidelines for PEA (pulseless electrical activity) should be followed (Fig. 28-57).

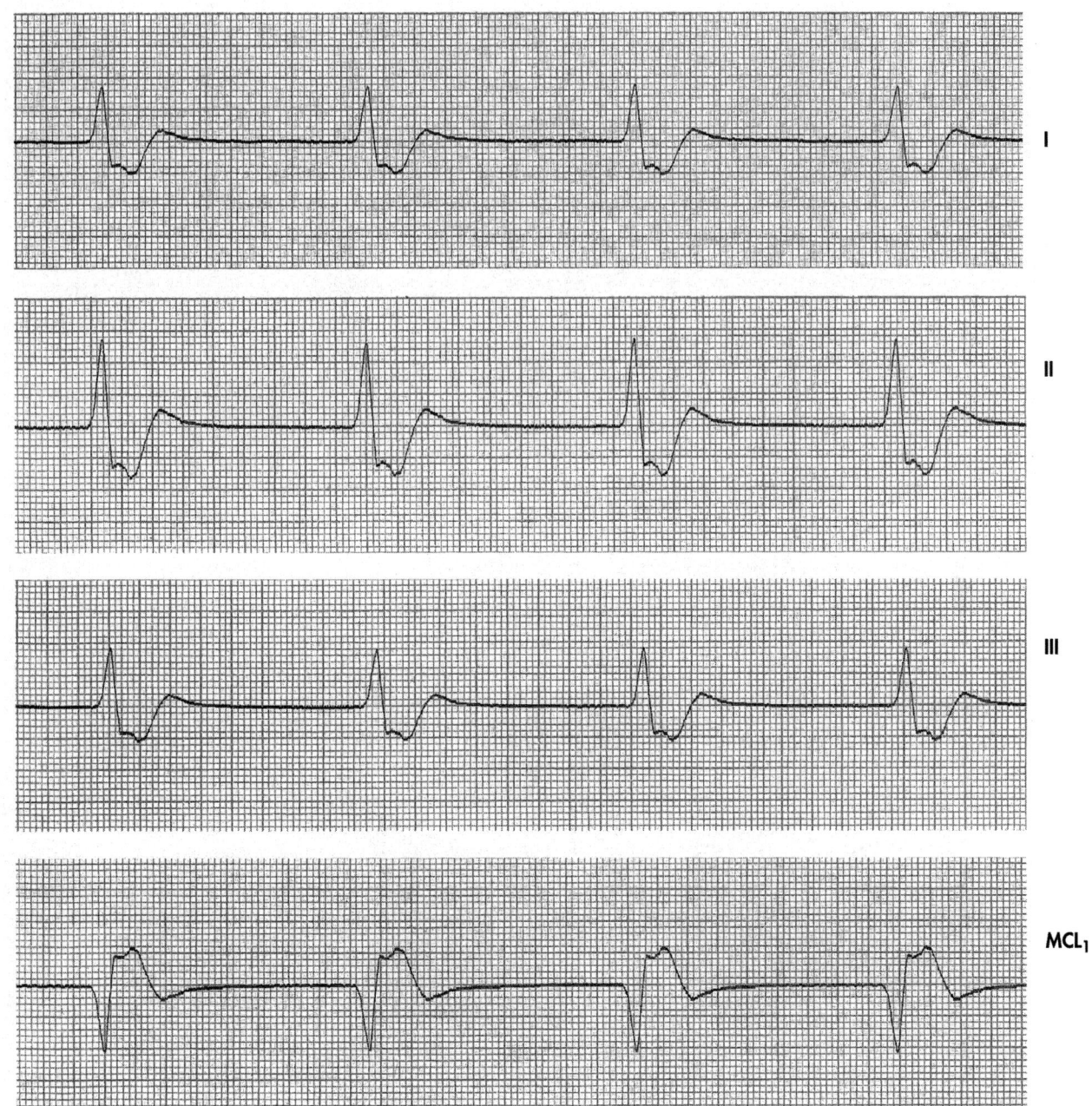

I

II

III

MCL₁

Fig. 28-55 Ventricular escape rhythm.

Premature Ventricular Complex

Description

A premature ventricular complex (PVC) (Fig. 28-58) is a single ectopic impulse arising from an irritable focus in either ventricle (bundle branches, Purkinje fibers, or ventricular muscle) that occurs earlier than the next expected sinus beat. It is a common dysrhythmia that can occur with any underlying cardiac rhythm and results from enhanced automaticity or a reentry mechanism.

When the ventricles initiate a PVC, the atria may or may not depolarize. If atrial depolarization does not occur, a P wave is not formed. If atrial depolarization does occur, the P wave often is hidden in the QRS complex because of the timing and large electrical force of ventricular depolarization compared

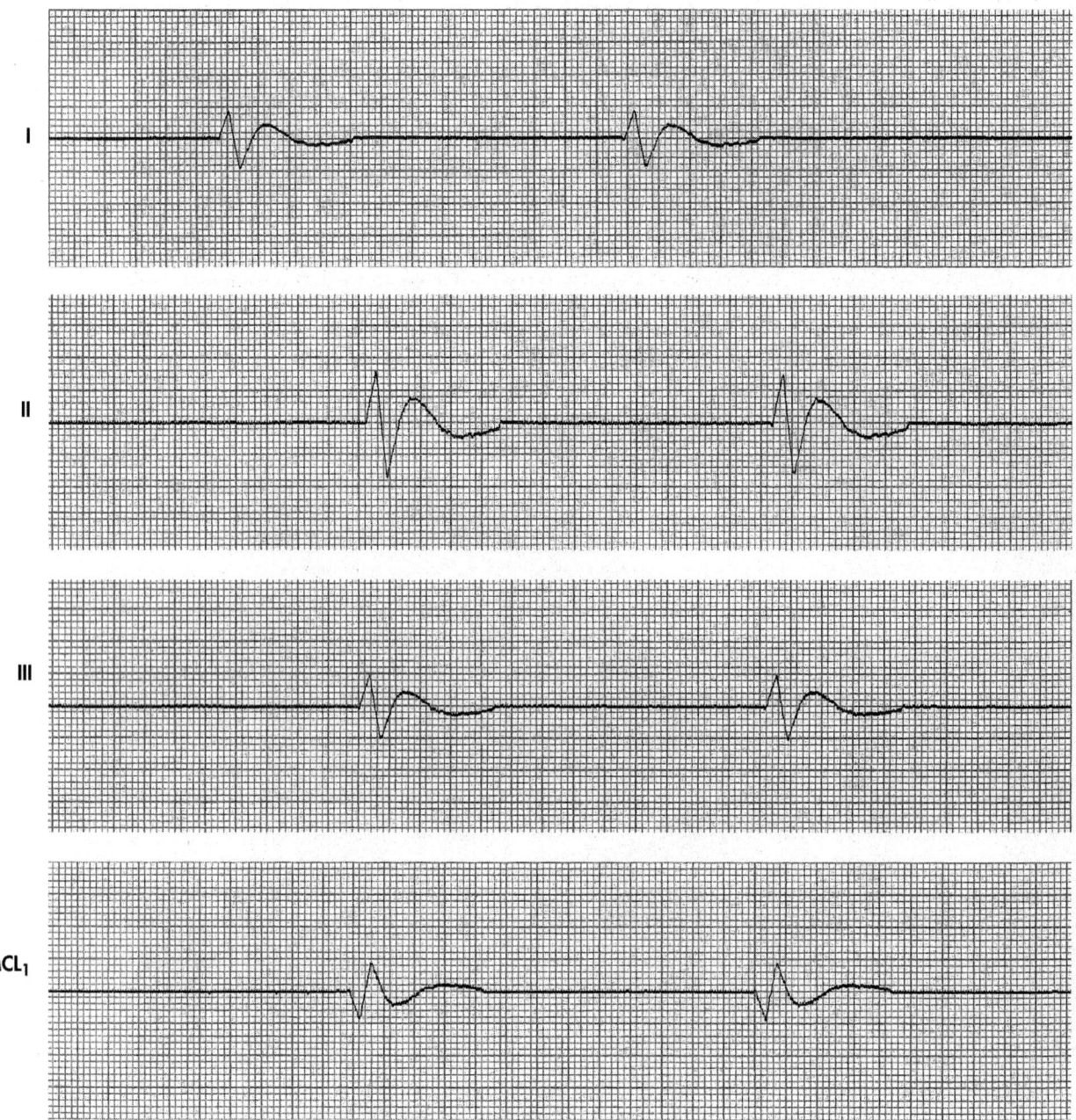

Fig. 28-56 "Dying heart" or agonal rhythm.

with atrial depolarization. The altered sequence of ventricular depolarization results in a wide, bizarre QRS complex that may be deflected in the opposite direction from the QRS complex in the underlying rhythm, or deflected in the same direction (depend-ing on the location of the focus and the lead selected). The T wave that immediately follows the PVC usually is deflected in the opposite direction from the QRS complex of the PVC because of the altered sequence of repolarization.

A PVC usually does not depolarize the SA node or interrupt its rhythm (i.e., the P wave of the underlying rhythm that follows the PVC occurs at its expected time but is obstructed by the PVC and finds the ventricles refractory). Therefore the ec-

? CRITICAL THINKING

Why is the QRS deflection opposite the underlying rhythm?

Pulseless Electrical Activity (PEA).

Basic Life Support

Perform Primary ABCD Survey
(Correct critical problems IMMEDIATELY as they are identified)
• Assess responsiveness
Call for help/call for defibrillator
Airway–open the airway
Breathing–deliver two slow breaths, administer oxygen as soon as it is available
Circulation–perform chest compressions
Ensure availability of monitor/**D**efibrillator–
On arrival of AED/monitor/defibrillator, perform
Secondary ABCD survey if rhythm is NOT pulseless VT/VF

Advanced Life Support

Possible causes of asystole:
PATCH-4-MD
Pulmonary embolism
Acidosis
Tension pneumothorax
Cardiac tamponade
Hypovolemia (most common cause)
Hypoxia
Heat/cold (hypo-/hyperthermia)
Hypo-/hyperkalemia (and other electrolytes)
Myocardial infarction
Drug overdose/accidents (cyclic antidepressants, calcium channel blockers, beta-blockers, digitalis)

Perform Secondary ABCD Survey
(ADVANCED) AIRWAY
Reassess effectiveness of initial airway maneuvers and interventions
Perform invasive airway management
BREATHING
Assess ventilation
Confirm ET tube placement (or other airway device) by at least two methods
Provide positive-pressure ventilation/Evaluate effectiveness of ventilations
Secure airway device in place with commercial tube holder (preferred) or tape
CIRCULATION
Establish IV access
Assess blood flow with Doppler
(If blood flow detected with Doppler, treat using hypotension/shock algorithm)
Administer appropriate medications
DIFFERENTIAL DIAGNOSIS
Search for and treat reversible causes (**PATCH-4-MD**)
(Fast narrow-QRS–consider hypovolemia, tamponade, pulmonary embolism, tension pneumothorax: Slow wide-QRS consider cyclic antidepressant overdose, calcium channel blocker, beta-blocker, or digitalis toxicity)

Epinephrine 1 mg (1:10,000 solution) IV every 3 to 5 minutes
(ET dose 2 to 2.5 mg diluted in 10-mL normal saline or distilled water)
• If the rate is slow, atropine 1 mg IV every 3 to 5 minutes to max 0.04 mg/kg (Class IIb)
  (ET dose 2 to 3 mg diluted in 10-mL normal saline or distilled water)

Consider sodium bicarbonate 1 mEq/kg:
• Known preexisting hyperkalemia (Class I)
• Cyclic antidepressant overdose (IIa)
• To alkalinize urine in aspirin or other drug overdoses (IIa)
• Patient that has been intubated + long arrest interval (IIb)
• On return of spontaneous circulation if long arrest interval (IIb)

Consider termination of efforts

Fig. 28-57 Pulseless electrical activity. (From Aehlert B: *ACLS quick review study guide*, ed 2, St Louis, 2002, Mosby.)

topic impulse usually is followed by a full compensatory pause. Compensatory pauses are confirmed by measuring the interval between the R wave before the PVC and the R wave after it. If the pause is compensatory, the distance is at least 2 times the R-R interval of the underlying rhythm. Occasionally, a PVC falls between two sinus beats without interrupting the rhythm (called an *interpolated PVC*) (Fig. 28-59).

PVCs may originate from a single ectopic pacemaker site (unifocal PVCs) or from multiple sites in the ventricles (multifocal PVCs) (Fig. 28-60). Unifocal PVCs that originate from a single site within the ventricles look alike. Multifocal PVCs that originate

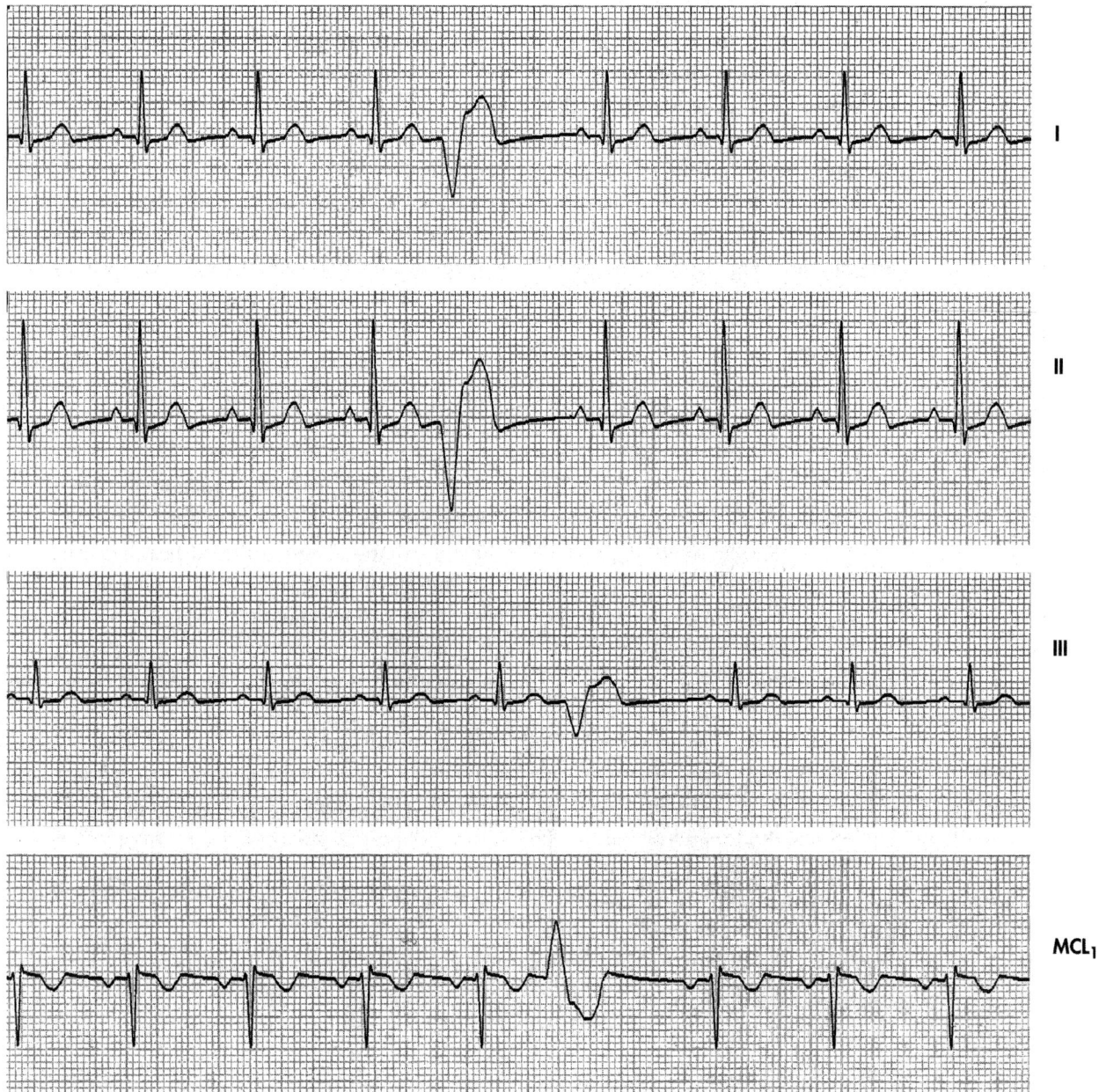

Fig. 28-58 PVCs.

from different ventricular sites have varying shapes and sizes.

Multifocal PVCs are considered more dangerous than unifocal PVCs, generally because they are a result of increased myocardial irritability. A PVC that occurs at about the same time as ventricular activation by the underlying rhythm can cause ventricular depolarization to occur simultaneously in two directions. This fusion beat results in a QRS complex that has the characteristics of the PVC and the QRS complex of the underlying rhythm (Fig. 28-61). The presence of a fusion beat helps confirm that the ectopic impulse is ventricular in origin rather than supraventricular with aberrant ventricular conduction.

> **NOTE**
>
> Usually, the fusion beat is recognized as having a similar (early) QRS pattern as the underlying rhythm, but the latter portion of the QRS becomes widened and bizarre as a result of the retrograde conduction.

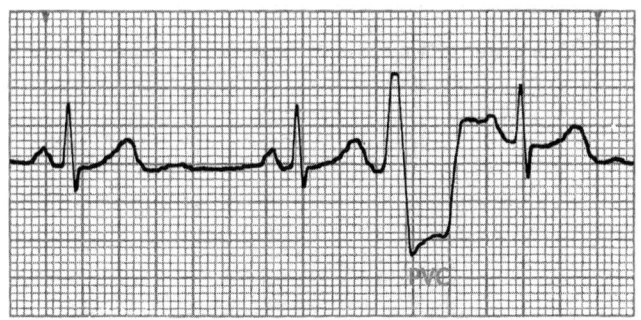

Fig. 28-59 Interpolated PVC. (From Huszar R: *Basic dysrhythmias*, ed 2, St Louis, 1994, Mosby.)

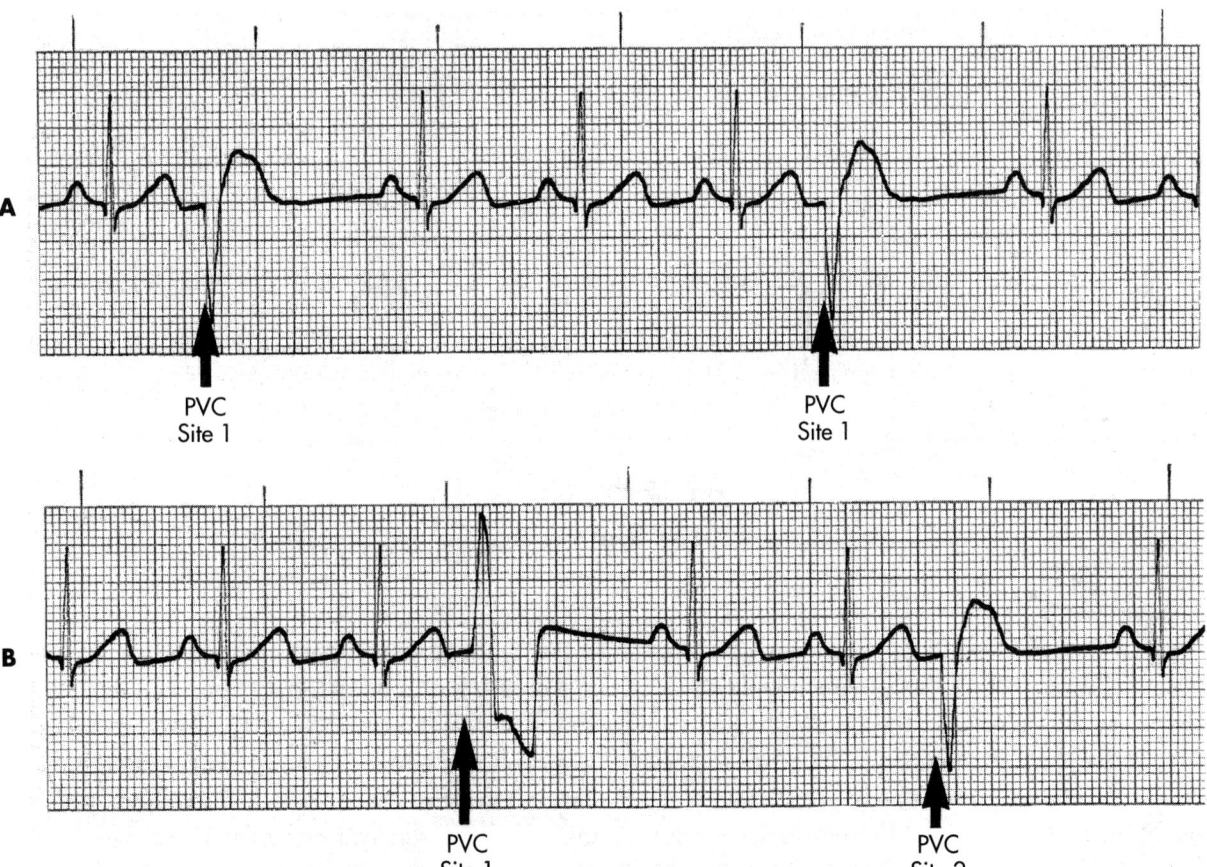

Fig. 28-60 A, Unifocal PVCs. **B,** Multifocal PVCs. (From Atwood S: *Introduction to basic cardiac dysrhythmias*, St Louis, 1990, Mosby.)

Frequently, PVCs occur in patterns of grouped beating: bigeminy occurs when every other complex is a PVC, trigeminy occurs when every third complex is a PVC, and quadrigeminy occurs when every fourth complex is a PVC (Fig. 28-62). Consecutive PVCs that are not separated by a complex of the underlying rhythm also can occur on the ECG: couplets, or salvos, are two PVCs in a row, and triplets are three PVCs in a row (a definition for VT). These terms also may be used to describe patterns of PACs and PJCs.

Like multifocal PVCs, frequently occurring PVCs usually indicate that the ventricles are highly irritable. These grouped beatings can trigger life-threatening repetitive discharge of the ventricles (VT and VF), particularly if they occur during the relative refractory phase of the cardiac cycle. This vulnerable period of ventricular repolarization is associated with the peak of the T wave. During this period, the heart muscle is at its greatest electrical nonuniformity.

During this period, some of the ventricular muscle fibers may be partially repolarized, others may

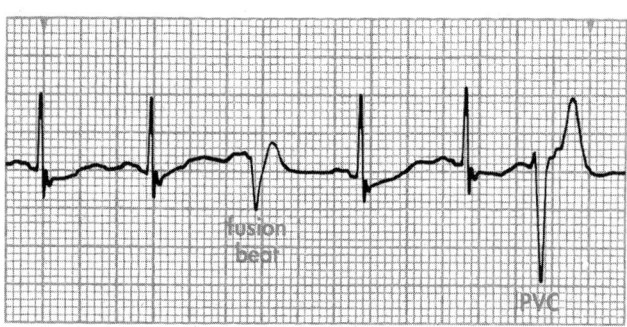

Fig. 28-61 Fusion beat with PVC. (From Huszar R: *Basic dysrhythmias*, ed 2, St Louis, 1994, Mosby.)

be completely repolarized, and still others may be completely refractory. Stimulation of the ventricles in the vulnerable period by an electrical impulse such as a PVC, cardiac pacemaker, or cardioversion may precipitate repetitive ventricular contractions, resulting in VT or VF. The occurrence of a ventricular depolarization during this vulnerable period of relative refractoriness is known as the **R-on-T phenomenon** (Fig. 28-63).

Etiology

PVCs do occur in healthy individuals without apparent cause and usually are of no significance. Pathological PVCs usually are a result of one or more of the following:

- Myocardial ischemia
- Hypoxia
- Acid-base and electrolyte imbalance
- Hypokalemia
- Congestive heart failure
- Increased catecholamine and sympathetic tone (as in emotional stress)
- Ingestion of stimulants (alcohol, caffeine, tobacco)
- Drug toxicity
- Sympathomimetic drugs (cocaine; stimulants such as phencyclidine, *epinephrine* [Adrenalin], *isoproterenol* [Isuprel])

Rules for Interpretation (Lead II Monitoring)

QRS complex: Equal to or greater than 0.12 second; frequently distorted and bizarre.

P waves: May be present or absent. If they are present, they usually are of the underlying rhythm and have no relationship to the PVC.

A

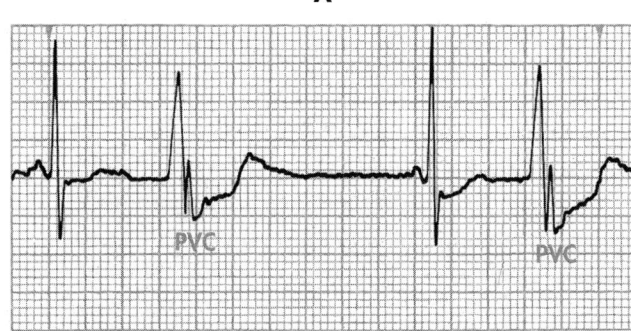

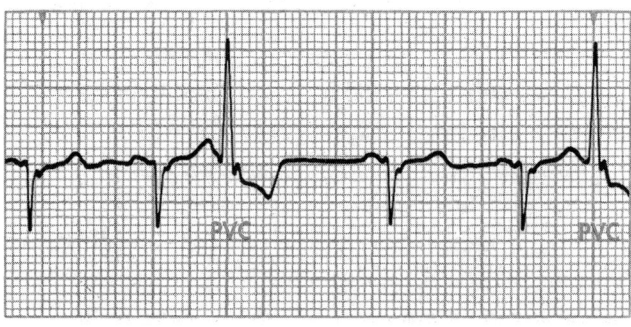

B

Fig. 28-62 A, Bigeminy (unifocal PVCs). **B,** Trigeminy (unifocal PVCs). (From Huszar R: *Basic dysrhythmias*, ed 2, St Louis, 1994, Mosby.)

Rate: Depends on the underlying rhythm and the number of PVCs.

Rhythm: PVCs interrupt the regularity of the underlying rhythm.

PR interval: None.

Clinical Significance

As previously stated, isolated PVCs that occur in patients without underlying cardiovascular disease usually are of no significance. These patients frequently experience the sensation of "skipped beats." PVCs that occur with myocardial ischemia may indicate the presence of enhanced automaticity, a reentry mechanism, or both, and may trigger lethal ventricular dysrhythmias. PVCs do not permit complete ventricular filling and may produce a diminished or nonpalpable pulse (nonperfusing PVC). If the PVCs are frequent enough and occur early enough in the cardiac cycle, cardiac output is compromised.

A number of warning signs of the potential development of serious ventricular dysrhythmias in patients with myocardial ischemia have been described. These include frequent PVCs, the presence of multifocal PVCs, early PVCs (R-on-T phenomenon), and patterns of grouped beating.

Management

PVCs that occur in asymptomatic patients without heart disease seldom require management. In patients with myocardial ischemia, frequent PVCs must be managed promptly with oxygen and antidysrhythmics (e.g., *lidocaine* [Xylocaine] and *procainamide* [Pronestyl]). The paramedic should follow local protocol or consult with medical direction.

> **? CRITICAL THINKING**
>
> *What signs and symptoms may the patient develop if a lidocaine drip is not regulated properly and infuses too rapidly?*

Ventricular Tachycardia

Description

Ventricular tachycardia (VT) (Fig. 28-64) is a dysrhythmia defined by three or more consecutive ventricular complexes occurring at a rate of more than 100 beats per minute, which overrides the primary pacemaker. The dysrhythmia generally starts suddenly, triggered by a PVC. During VT, the atria and ventricles are asynchronous. If the rhythm disturbance is sustained, the patient's condition may become unstable, possibly leading to unconsciousness and occasionally even to loss of a perfusing pulse. However, some patients in VT may be able to walk and talk. The misconception that VT cannot be associated with reasonable blood pressure may result in a patient being inappropriately managed. The electrophysiological mechanism responsible for VT is enhanced automaticity or reentry.

Etiology

Like PVCs, VT usually occurs in the presence of myocardial ischemia or significant cardiac disease. Other causes of VT include:

- Acid-base and electrolyte imbalance
- Hypokalemia
- Congestive heart failure
- Increased catecholamine and sympathetic tone (as in emotional stress)
- Ingestion of stimulants (alcohol, caffeine, tobacco)

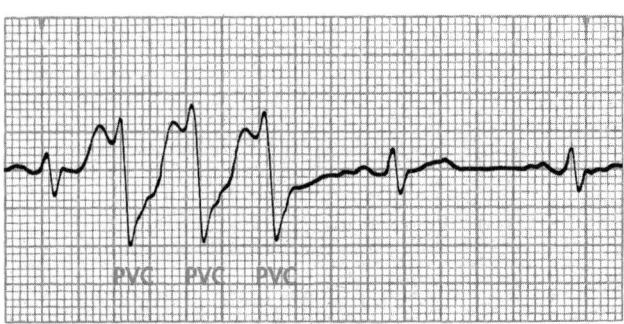

Fig. 28-63 R-on-T phenomenon (unifocal PVCs). (From Huszar R: *Basic dysrhythmias,* ed 2, St Louis, 1994, Mosby.)

- Drug toxicity (digitalis, tricyclic antidepressants)
- Sympathomimetic drugs (cocaine, methamphetamines)
- Prolonged QT interval (may be caused by drugs, metabolic problems, or be congenital)

> **NOTE**
>
> Patients who have had a previous myocardial infarction with subsequent tachycardias and who are now experiencing a wide-complex tachycardia very likely are in VT.

Rules for Interpretation (Lead II Monitoring)

QRS complex: Equal to or greater than 0.12 second and usually distorted and bizarre. The QRS complexes generally are identical, but if fusion beats are present, one or more QRS complexes may differ in size, shape, and direction.

P waves: May be absent. If present, P waves have no set relation to the QRS complex (AV dissociation).

> **NOTE**
>
> Torsades de pointes ("twisting around a point") is a form of VT characterized by QRS complexes that gradually change back and forth from one shape and direction to another over a series of beats (Fig. 28-65). Torsades de pointes usually is caused by one of a number of conditions that prolong the QT interval, including hypokalemia or hyperkalemia, hypomagnesemia, certain antidysrhythmic medications (quinidine or *procainamide* [Pronestyl]), and tricyclic antidepressant overdose.

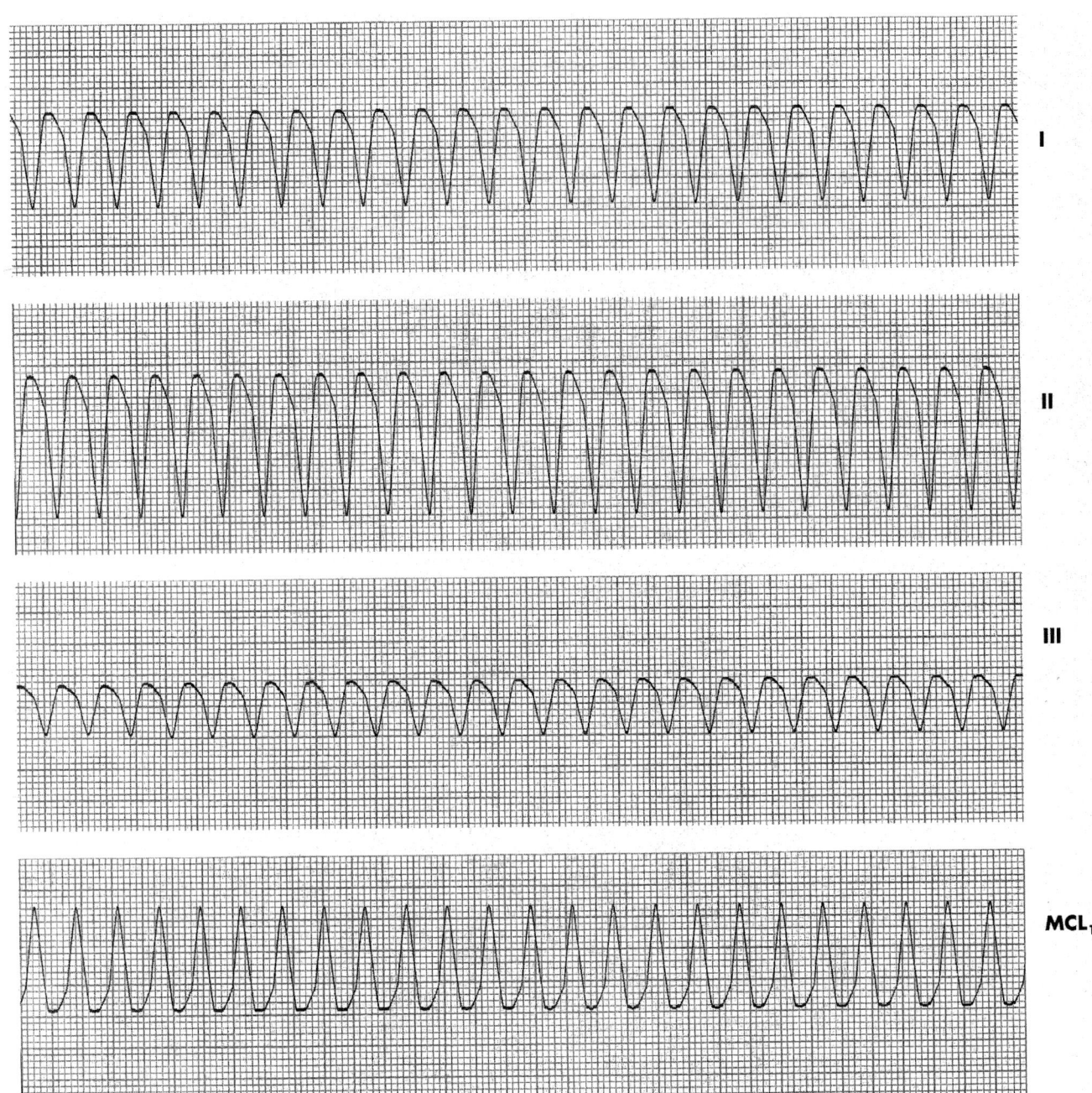

Fig. 28-64 Ventricular tachycardia.

P waves occur at a slower rate than the ventricular focus and are superimposed on the QRS complexes.

Rate: Usually between 100 and 250 beats per minute.

Rhythm: Usually regular but may be slightly irregular.

PR interval: If P waves are present, the PR interval varies widely.

NOTE

AV dissociation is diagnostic of VT.

NOTE

VT, unless drug induced, usually is very regular.

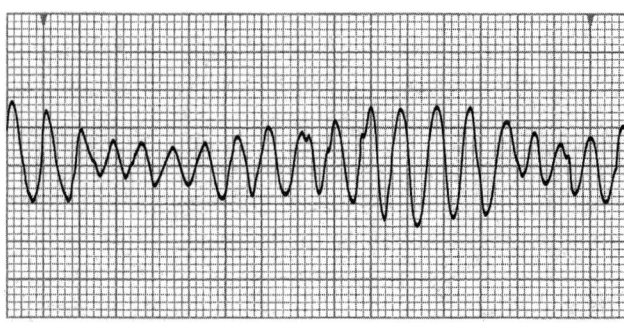

torsades de pointes

Fig. 28-65 Torsades de pointes.

SEQUENCE OF CARE FOR PERFUSING MONOMORPHIC VT

- Consider synchronized cardioversion
- Consider antidysrhythmics:
  - Normal Heart Function
    - ***Procainamide*** (Class II a)
    - Sotalol (Class II a)
    - ***Amiodarone*** (Class II b)
    - ***Lidocaine*** (Class Indeterminate)
  - Impaired Heart Function
    - ***Amiodarone***
    - ***Lidocaine***
    - Synchronized Cardioversion

> **NOTE**
>
> AV dissociation may precipitate cannon A waves (waves of pulse pressure that are visible in the jugular veins of a patient in VT). The cannon A waves result from the right atrium pumping against a closed tricuspid valve that in turn directs the waves of pressure into the jugular veins.

SEQUENCE OF CARE FOR PERFUSING POLYMORPHIC VT

- Consider synchronized cardioversion
- Treat ischemia and electrolyte imbalances
- Consider antidysrhythmics:
  - ***Amiodarone*** (Class II b)
  - ***Lidocaine*** (Class II b)
  - ***Procainamide*** (Class II b)
  - Sotalol (Class II b)
  - Beta Blockers (Class Indeterminate)
  - ***Phenytoin*** (Class Indeterminate)

If rhythm is suggestive of torsades de pointes:

- Discontinue any medications known to prolong the QT interval
- Correct electrolyte imbalances
- Consider antidysrhythmics:
  - ***Magnesium Sulfate*** (Class Indeterminate)
  - Overdrive pacing
    - Beta Blockers (as an adjunct to pacing)
  - ***Isoproterenol*** (temporary measure while overdrive pacing initiated)
  - ***Phenytoin*** (Class Indeterminate)
  - ***Lidocaine*** (Class Indeterminate)
- Severe hemodynamically unstable Polymorphic VT should be treated as pulseless VT using the VF/Pulseless VT algorithm

American Heart Association. Guidelines 2000 for Cardiopulmonary Resuscitation and Emergency Cardiovascular Care, International Consensus on Science. *Supplement to Circulation.* 2000;102(8): 115-116,159,163-165

Clinical Significance

VT usually indicates significant underlying cardiovascular disease. The rapid rate associated with VT and the concurrent loss of atrial kick result in compromised cardiac output and decreased coronary artery and cerebral perfusion. The severity of symptoms varies with the rate of the VT and the presence or absence of underlying myocardial dysfunction. VT may be perfusing or nonperfusing, and it may initiate or degenerate into VF.

Management

Treatment for patients with ventricular tachycardia is based on hemodynamic status and the presence or absence of torsades de pointes. Similar to supraventricular tachycardias, the paramedic is directed to obtain clinical history and identify a specific rhythm diagnosis (see Fig. 28-46). Management of wide-complex tachycardias of unknown type includes synchronized cardioversion, *amiodarone* or *procainamide* (Fig. 28-66). Confirmed ventricular tachycardia treatment guidelines are structured by monomorphic (having the same QRS morphology) or polymorphic (having varying QRS morphology) forms of ventricular tachycardia; furthermore, use of pharmacological agents is based on normal versus impaired cardiac function and short versus long QT intervals (Figs. 28-67 and 28-68). However, any

wide complex tachycardia that occurs with critical signs and symptoms of hemodynamic instability, such as chest pain, dyspnea, decreased level of consciousness, or hypotension, may require immediate synchronized cardioversion. Patients that present with a non-perfusing ventricular tachycardia rhythm should be managed as if it were ventricular fibrillation (Fig. 28-69).

Text continued on p. 838

Wide-Complex Tachycardia of Unknown Origin*

Perform Primary ABCD Survey (Basic Life Support)
(Correct critical problems IMMEDIATELY as they are identified)
• Assess responsiveness, **A**irway, **B**reathing, **C**irculation, ensure availability of monitor/**D**efibrillator

Perform Secondary ABCD Survey (Advanced Life Support)
• Administer oxygen, establish IV access, attach cardiac monitor
• Administer fluids as needed (O₂, IV, monitor, fluids)
• Assess vital signs, attach pulse oximeter, and monitor blood pressure
• Obtain and review 12-lead ECG, portable chest x-ray, perform a focused history and physical exam

Is the patient stable or unstable?
Is the patient experiencing serious signs and symptoms due to the tachycardia?

Use 12-lead ECG/clinical information to help clarify rhythm diagnosis

Rhythm confirmed as SVT Go to narrow-QRS tachycardia algorithm	Wide-Complex Tachycardia of Unknown Origin Stable Patient	Rhythm confirmed as VT Go to VT algorithm

	Normal Cardiac Function	**Impaired Cardiac Function**
	Sync cardioversion **OR** Procainamide (IIb) **OR** Amiodarone (IIb)	Sync cardioversion **OR** Amiodarone (IIb) Note: Impaired cardiac function = ejection fraction <40% or CHF

If medication therapy ineffective, perform synchronized cardioversion

UNSTABLE PATIENT

If hemodynamically unstable, sync 100 J, 200 J, 300 J, and 360 J or equivalent biphasic energy. If hypotensive (systolic BP < 90), unresponsive, or if severe pulmonary edema exists, defibrillate with same energy.

MEDICATION DOSING:

Amiodarone 150 mg IV bolus over 10 min. if chemical conversion successful, follow with IV infusion of 1 mg/min for 6 hours and then a maintenance infusion of 0.5 mg/min. Repeat supplementary infusions of 150 mg as necessary for recurrent or resistant dysrhythmias. Maximum total daily dose 2 g.

Procainamide† 100 mg over 5 min (20 mg/min). Maximum total dose 17 mg/kg. If chemical conversion successful, maintenance infusion 1 to 4 mg/min.

*The American Heart Association in Collaboration with the International Liaison Committee on Resuscitation (ILCOR). Part 7: Era of Reperfusion Section
†Ryan TJ et al: ACC/AHA guidelines for the management of patients with acute myocardial infarction: 1999 update: a report of the American College of Cardiology/American Heart Association Task Force on Practice Guidelines (Committee on Management of Acute Myocardial Infarction).

Fig. 28-66 Wide-complex tachycardia of unknown origin. (From Aehlert B: *ACLS quick review study guide*, ed 2, St Louis, 2002, Mosby.)

Monomorphic Ventricular Tachycardia[*,†]

Perform Primary ABCD Survey (Basic Life Support)

(Correct critical problems IMMEDIATELY as they are identified)
- Assess responsiveness, **A**irway, **B**reathing, **C**irculation, ensure availability of monitor/**D**efibrillator

Perform Secondary ABCD Survey (Advanced Life Support)

- Administer oxygen, establish IV access, attach cardiac monitor, administer fluids as needed (O_2, IV, monitor, fluids)
- Assess vital signs, attach pulse oximeter, and monitor blood pressure
- Obtain and review 12-lead ECG, portable chest x-ray, perform a focused history and physical exam

Is the patient stable or unstable?
Is the patient experiencing serious signs and symptoms due to the tachycardia?

Determine if the rhythm is monomorphic or polymorphic VT and determine patient's QT interval.

STABLE PATIENT	
Normal Cardiac Function	*Impaired Cardiac Function*

May proceed directly to synchronized cardioversion or use **one** of the following:

• Procainamide (IIa)	• Amiodarone (IIb)
• Sotalol (IIa)	• Lidocaine (Indeterminate)
• Amiodarone (IIb)	Note: Impaired cardiac function =
• Lidocaine (IIb)	ejection fraction <40% or CHF

If medication therapy ineffective, perform synchronized cardioversion

UNSTABLE VT WITH A PULSE

If hemodynamically unstable, sync 100 J, 200 J, 300 J, and 360 J (or equivalent biphasic energy)
If hypotensive (systolic BP < 90), unresponsive, or if severe pulmonary edema exists, defibrillate with same energy.

MEDICATION DOSING

Amiodarone[§‖¶] 150 mg IV bolus over 10 min. If chemical conversion successful, follow with IV infusion of 1 mg/min for 6 hours and then a maintenance infusion of 0.5 mg/min. Repeat supplementary infusions of 150 mg as necessary for recurrent or resistant dysrhythmias. Maximum total daily dose 2 g.

Lidocaine[#**‡‡§§] 1 to 1.5 mg/kg initial dose. Repeat dose is ½ the initial dose every 5 to 10 min. Maximum total dose 3 mg/kg. If chemical conversion successful, maintenance infusion 1 to 4 mg/min. If impaired cardiac function, dose = 0.5-0.75 mg/kg IV push. May repeat every 5 to 10 min. Maximum total dose 3 mg/kg. If chemical conversion successful, maintenance infusion 1 to 4 mg/min.

Procainamide[§§‖‖] 100 mg over 5 min (20 mg/min). Maximum total dose 17 mg/kg. If chemical conversion successful, maintenance infusion 1 to 4 mg/min.

Sotalol[¶¶] 1 to 1.5 mg/kg IV slowly at a rate of 10 mg/in

---

*Ryan TJ et al: ACC/AHA guidelines for the management of patients with acute myocardial infarction: 1999 update: a report of the American College of Cardiology/American Heart Association Task Force on Practice Guidelines (Committee on Management of Acute Myocardial Infarction).

†The American Heart Association in Collaboration with the International Liaison Committee on Resuscitation (ILCOR). Part 7: Era of Reperfusion Section 1: Acute Coronary Syndromes (Acute Myocardial Infarction): A Consensus on Science. *Circulation* 2000; 102 (suppl I):I-163.

††Maury P et al: Amiodarone therapy for sustained ventricular tachycardia after myocardial infarction: long-term follow-up, risk assessment and predictive value of programmed ventricular stimulation, *Int J Cardiol* 76(2-3):199, 2000.

§Leak D: Intravenous amiodarone in the treatment of refractory life-threatening cardiac arrhythmias in the critically ill patient, Am Heart J 111:456, 1986.

‖Remme WJ et al: Hemodynamic effects and tolerability of intravenous amiodarone in patients with impaired left ventricular function, *Am Heart J* 122:96, 1991.

¶Ryan TJ et al: ACC/AHA guidelines for the management of patients with acute myocardial infarction: 1999 update: a report of the American College of Cardiology/American Heart Association Task Force on Practice Guidelines (Committee on Management of Acute Myocardial Infarction).

#Nasir N Jr et al: Evaluation of intravenous lidocaine for the termination of sustained monomorphic ventricular tachycardia in patients with coronary artery disease with or without healed myocardial infarction, *Am J Cardiol* 74:1183, 1994.

**Gorgels AP et al: Comparison of procainamide and lidocaine in terminating sustained monomorphic ventricular tachycardia, *Am J Cardiol* 78:43, 1996.

‡‡Akhtar M et al: Wide QRS complex tachycardia: reappraisal of a common problem *Ann Intern Med* 109:905, 1988.

§§Pinter A, Dorian P: Intravenous antiarrhythmic agents, *Curr Opin Cardiol* 16(1):17, 2001.

‖‖Callans DJ, Marchlinski FE: Dissociation of termination and prevention of inducibility of sustained ventricular tachycardia with infusion of procainamide: evidence for distinct mechanisms, J Am Coll Cardiol 19:111, 1992.

¶¶Ho DS et al: Double-blind trial of lignocaine versus sotalol for acute termination of spontaneous sustained ventricular tachycardia [see comments], Lancet 344:18, 1994.

Fig. 28-67 Monomorphic ventricular tachycardia. (From Aehlert B: *ACLS quick review study guide,* ed 2, St Louis, 2002, Mosby.)

Polymorphic Ventricular Tachycardia[*, †]

Perform Primary ABCD Survey (Basic Life Support)

(Correct critical problems IMMEDIATELY as they are identified)

- Assess responsiveness, **A**irway, **B**reathing, **C**irculation, ensure availability of monitor/**D**efibrillator

Perform Secondary ABCD Survey (Advanced Life Support)

- Administer oxygen, establish IV access, attach cardiac monitor, administer fluids as needed (O$_2$, IV, monitor, fluids)
- Assess vital signs, attach pulse oximeter, and monitor blood pressure
- Obtain and review 12-lead ECG, portable chest x-ray, perform a focused history and physical exam

Is the patient stable or unstable?

Is the patient experiencing serious signs and symptoms due to the tachycardia?

Determine if the rhythm is monomorphic or polymorphic VT and determine patient's QT interval.

Polymorphic VT Normal QT interval		Polymorphic VT Prolonged QT interval (Suggests Torsades de Pointes)	
STABLE PATIENT		STABLE PATIENT	
Normal Cardiac Function	**Impaired Cardiac Function**	**Normal Cardiac Function**	**Impaired Cardiac Function**
Treat ischemia if present Correct electrolyte abnormalities	May proceed directly to electrical therapy or **use** one of the following: Amiodarone (IIb)	DC meds that prolong QT Correct electrolyte abnormalities	May proceed directly to electrical therapy or use the following: Amiodarone (IIb)
May proceed directly to electrical therapy or use **one** of the following: Amiodarone (IIb) Lidocaine (IIb) Procainamide (IIb) Sotalol (IIb) Beta-blockers (Indeterminate). (Indeterminate)	Lidocaine (indeterminate).	May proceed directly to electrical therapy or use **one** of the following: Magnesium (Indeterminate) Overdrive pacing with or without beta-blocker (Indeterminate) Phenytoin (Indeterminate) Lidocaine (Indeterminate)	Lidocaine (Indeterminate) Isoproterenol Note: Impaired cardiac function = ejection fraction <40% or CHF

If medication therapy ineffective, use electrical therapy.

Fig. 28-68 Polymorphic ventricular tachycardia. (From Aehlert B: *ACLS quick review study guide,* ed 2, St Louis, 2002, Mosby.)

UNSTABLE PATIENT

Sustained (>30 seconds or causing hemodynamic collapse) polymorphic VT should be treated with an unsynchronized shock using an initial energy of 200 J; if unsuccessful, a second shock of 200 to 300 J should be given, and, if necessary, a third shock of 360 J.*

MEDICATION DOSING

Amiodarone 150 mg IV bolus over 10 min. If chemical conversion successful, follow with IV infusion of 1 mg/min for 6 hours and then a maintenance infusion of 0.5 mg/min. Repeat supplementary infusions of 150 mg as necessary for recurrent or resistant dysrhythmias. Maximum total daily dose 2 g.

Beta-blockers *Esmolol:* 0.5 mg/kg over 1 minute followed by a maintenance infusion at 50 mcg/kg/min for 4 minutes. If inadequate response, administer a second bolus of 0.5 mg/kg over 1 minute and increase maintenance infusion to 100 mcg/kg/min. The bolus dose (0.5 mg/kg) and titration of the maintenance infusion (addition of 50 mcg/kg/min) can be repeated every 4 minutes to a maximum infusion of 300 mcg/kg/min. *Metoprolol:* 5 mg slow IV push over 5 minutes x 3 as needed to a total dose of 15 mg over 15 minutes. *Atenolol:* 5 mg slow IV (over 5 min). Wait 10 min then give second dose of 5 mg slow IV (over 5 min).

Isoproterenol Can be used as a temporizing measure until overdrive pacing can be instituted if no evidence of coronary artery disease, ischemic syndromes, or other contraindications. 2 to 10 mcg/min. Mix 1 mg in 500-mL NS or D5W.

Lidocaine 1 to 1.5 mg/kg initial dose. Repeat dose 1/2 the initial dose every 5 to 10 min. Maximum total dose 3 mg/kg. If chemical conversion successful, maintenance infusion 1 to 4 mg/min. If impaired cardiac function, dose = 0.5-0.75 mg/kg IV push. May repeat every 5 to 10 min. Maximum total dose 3 mg/kg. If chemical conversion successful, maintenance infusion 1 to 4 mg/min.

Magnesium‡ Loading dose of 1 to 2 g mixed in 50 to 100-mL over 5 to 60 min IV. If chemical conversion successful, follow with 0.5 to 1.0 g/h IV infusion.

Phenytoin 250 mg IV at a rate of 25-50 mg/min in NS using a central vein.

Procainamide 100 mg over 5 min (20 mg/min). Maximum total dose 17 mg/kg. If chemical conversion successful, maintenance infusion 1 to 4 mg/min.

Sotalol 1 to 1.5 mg/kg IV slowly at a rate of 10 mg/min

---

*Ryan TJ et al: ACC/AHA guidelines for the management of patients with acute myocardial infarction: 1999 update: a report of the American College of Cardiology/American Heart Association Task Force on Practice Guidelines (Committee on Management of Acute Myocardial Infarction).

†The American Heart Association in Collaboration with the International Liaison Committee on Resuscitation (ILCOR). Part 7: Era of Reperfusion Section 1: Acute Coronary Syndromes (Acute Myocardial Infarction): A Consensus on Science. *Circulation* 2000; 102 (suppl I):I-163.

‡Tzivoni D et al: Treatment of torsade de pointes with magnesium sulfate, *Circulation* 77:392, 1988.

Fig. 28-68, cont'd Polymorphic ventricular tachycardia.

Pulseless Ventricular Tachycardia (VT)/Ventricular Fibrillation (VF)

Basic Life Support   **Perform Primary ABCD Survey**

(Correct critical problems IMMEDIATELY as they are identified)
- Assess responsiveness
- Call for help/call for defibrillator

Airway–open the airway

Breathing–deliver two slow breaths, administer oxygen as soon as it is available

Circulation–perform chest compressions

Ensure availability of monitor/**D**efibrillator

On arrival of AED/monitor/defibrillator, evaluate caridac rhythm

If PEA or asystole, continue CPR and go to appropriate algorithm.

If pulseless VT/VF, shock up to three times (200 J, 200 to 300 J, 360 J, or equivalent biphasic energy).

Reevaluate cardiac rhythm

- If persistent or recurrent pulseless VT/VF, continue CPR and perform secondary ABCD survey

- If PEA or asystole, continue CPR and go to appropriate algorithm

- If return of spontaneous circulation (ROSC):
- Assess vital signs
- Maintain open airway
- Provide ventilation
- Administer medications for appropriate for rhythm, blood pressure, and heart rate

Advanced Life Support   **Perform Secondary ABCD Survey**

(ADVANCED) AIRWAY

Reassess effectiveness of initial airway maneuvers and interventions

Perform invasive airway management

Pattern becomes CPR-drug-shock or CPR-drug-shock-shock-shock

BREATHING

Assess ventilation

Confirm ET tube placement (or other airway device) by at least two methods

Provide positive-pressure ventilation / Evaluate effectiveness of ventilations

Secure airway device in place with commercial tube holder (preferred) or tape

CIRCULATION

Establish IV access and administer appropriate medications

DIFFERENTIAL DIAGNOSIS

Search for and treat reversible causes

Fig. 28-69 Pulseless ventricular tachycardia (VT)/ventricular fibrillation (VF). (From Aehlert B: *ACLS quick review study guide,* ed 2, St Louis, 2002, Mosby.)

Epinephrine (Class Indeterminate) 1 mg (1:10,000 solution) IV every 3 to 5 minutes
(ET dose 2-2.5 mg diluted in 10-mL normal saline or distilled water)
Vasopressin (Class IIb) 40 U IV bolus* (administered only once)
(If no response to vasopressin, may resume epinephrine after 10 to 20 min; epi dose 1 mg every 3 to 5 min)

Defibrillate with 360 J (or equivalent biphasic energy) within 30 to 60 seconds

Consider antiarrhythmics (avoid use of multiple antiarrhythmics because of potential proarrhythmic effects)

Amiodarone[†] (Class IIb) Initial bolus - 300 mg IV bolus diluted in 20 to 30-mL of NS or D5W. Consider repeat dose (150 mg IV bolus) in 3 to 5 minutes. If defibrillation successful, follow with 1 mg/min IV infusion for 6 hours (mix 900-mg in 500-mL NS), then decrease infusion rate to 0.5 mg/min IV infusion for 18 hours. Maximum daily dose 2 g IV/24 hours.

Lidocaine (Class Indeterminate) 1 to 1.5 mg/kg IV bolus, consider repeat dose (0.5 to 0.75 mg/kg) in 5 minutes; maximum IV bolus dose 3 mg/kg. (The 1.5 mg/kg dose is recommended in cardiac arrest). Endotracheal dose: 2 to 4 mg/kg. A single dose of 1.5 mg/kg is acceptable in cardiac arrest.

Magnesium (Class IIb if hypomagnesemia present) 1 to 2 g IV (2 to 4 mL of a 50% solution) diluted in 10-mL of D5W if Torsades de Pointes[†][§] or hypomagnesemia[||]

Procainamide[¶] (Class IIb for recurrent pulseless VT/VF; Class Indeterminate for persistent pulseless VT/VF) 20 mg/min; maximum total dose 17 mg/kg

Consider **sodium bicarbonate** 1 mEq/kg

---

*Chugh SS, Lurie KG, Lindner KH: Pressor with promise: using vasopressin in cardiopulmonary arrest, *Circulation* 96(7):2453, 1997.
[†]Kudenchuk PJ et al: Amiodarone for resuscitation after out-of-hospital cardiac arrest due to ventricular fibrillation, *N Engl J Med* 341:871, 1999.
[‡]Tzivoni D et al: Magnesium therapy for torsades de pointes, *Am J Cardiol* 53:528, 1984.
[§]Tzivoni D et al: Treatment of torsade de pointes with magnesium sulfate, *Circulation* 77:392, 1988.
[||]Cannon LA et al: Magnesium levels in cardiac arrest victims: relationship between magnesium levels and successful resuscitation, *Ann Emerg Med* 16:1195, 1987.
[¶]Stiell IG et al: Association of drug therapy with survival in cardiac arrest: limited role of advanced cardiac life support drugs, *Acad Emerg Med* 2:264, 1995.

Fig. 28-69, cont'd Pulseless ventricular tachycardia (VT)/ventricular fibrillation (VF).

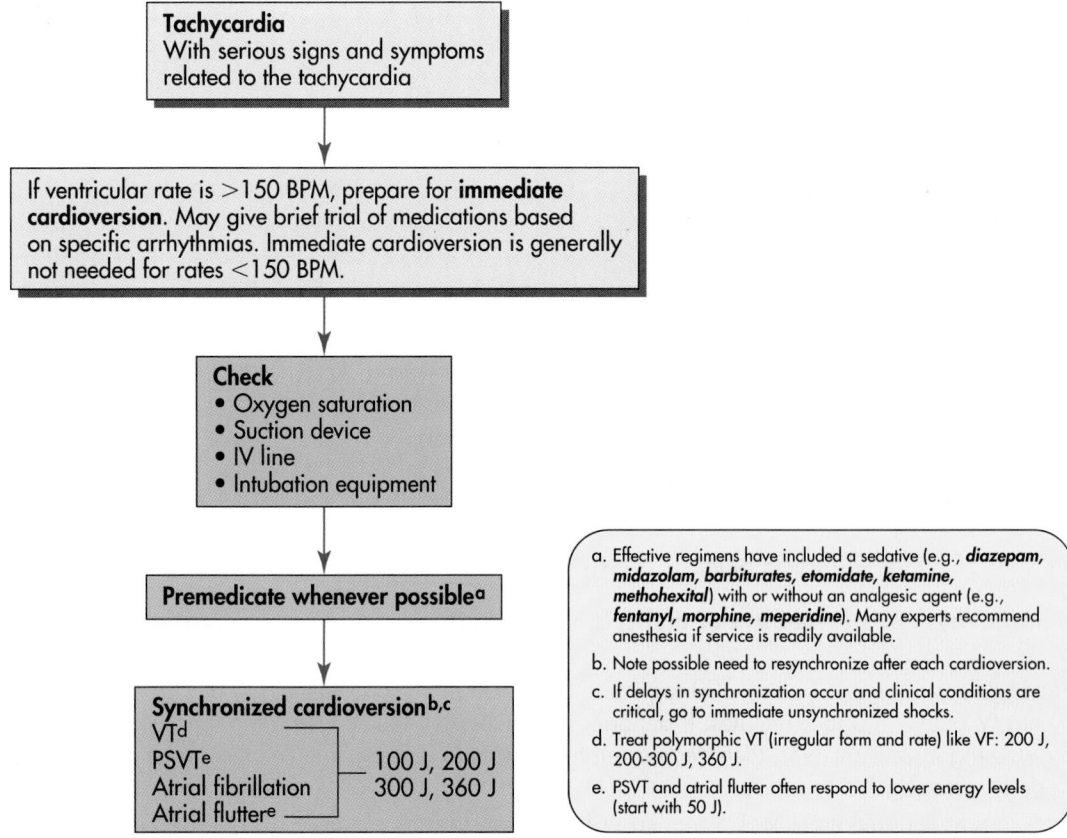

Fig. 28-70 Electrical cardioversion algorithm (with the patient not in cardiac arrest). (Reproduced with permission. CPR Issue of JAMA, Oct 28, 1992. Copyright © American Medical Association)

Synchronized cardioversion (Fig. 28-70) is an effective treatment for ventricular tachycardia; plus cardioversion is acceptable as the first treatment choice for all wide-complex tachycardias regardless of cardiac function. If synchronized cardioversion is not preferred as the first intervention, several pharmacological agents are available for chemical cardioversion.

Monomorphic ventricular tachycardia treatment guidelines are based on cardiac function (ejection fraction). Signs and symptoms of poor ejection fraction display as pulmonary congestion and decreased level of consciousness. Management of monomorphic ventricular tachycardia with preserved heart function is antidysrhythmic therapy with *procainamide,* sotalol, *amiodarone,* or *lidocaine.* Impaired heart function in the setting of monomorphic ventricular tachycardia requires administration of *amiodarone* or *lidocaine,* then if necessary, synchronized cardioversion.

Polymorphic ventricular tachycardia is usually hemodynamically unstable and is prone to degen-

erate into ventricular fibrillation quickly. With polymorphic VT it becomes a question of whether the patient is suffering from torsades de pointes, usually a product of a prolonged QT interval. If torsades de pointes is suspected, treatment needs to be expedient. The first directive is to discontinue any medications that may prolong the QT interval and correct any electrolyte imbalances present. Other interventions include intravenous *magnesium sulfate* and temporary overdrive pacing. *Isoproterenol* (Isuprel) may be administered as a temporary measure while pacing therapy is begun. Other medications include *phenytoin* and *lidocaine.*

Polymorphic ventricular tachycardia with a *prolonged* baseline QT interval, which is suggestive of torsades de pointes, is usually treated with intravenous magnesium and synchronized cardioversion beginning at 200 joules. Polymorphic ventricular tachycardia with a *normal* baseline QT interval can also be treated with synchronized cardioversion. In addition, pharmacological agents for treatment of polymorphic ventricular tachycardia (with a normal baseline QT interval) consist of *amiodarone, lidocaine, procainamide,* sotalol, beta-blockers, and *phenytoin.*

Antidysrhythmic agents may conversely be proarrhythmic. Sequential use of two or more antidysrhythmic drugs increases the incidence of bradycardias, hypotension, and torsades de pointes. It is strongly recommended to avoid using more than one antidysrhythmic agent in treating narrow or wide QRS complex tachydysrhythmias. In most circumstances, after an adequate dose of a single antidysrhythmic medication is unsuccessful in terminating the dysrhythmia, synchronized cardioversion is the next treatment intervention (see Fig. 28-70).

> **NOTE**
>
> - Torsades de pointes is a special form of VT that may not respond to the recommended antidysrhythmics **lidocaine** (Xylocaine) and **magnesium sulfate.** The first step is to stop medications known to prolong the QT interval, and correct any electrolyte or metabolic disorders. Overdrive pacing may be used in an attempt to control ventricular rate. **Isoproterenol** (Isuprel) sometimes is useful in abolishing torsades de pointes by decreasing repolarization rates and causing a sinus tachycardia overdrive. **Magnesium sulfate** also has been demonstrated to suppress runs of torsades de pointes. It therefore is important to search for an underlying cause of this rhythm and to institute corrective measures if possible.
> - Pulseless ventricular tachycardia is managed like ventricular fibrillation.

Monitored adult patients who become pulseless may be managed with a solitary precordial thump when a defibrillator is not readily available.[1] A precordial thump may terminate a dysrhythmia by causing ventricular depolarization and the resumption of an organized rhythm. To deliver a precordial thump, the arm and wrist should be parallel to the long axis of the sternum to avoid rib fractures and other injury. The thump is delivered to the midsternum with the heel of the fist from 10 to 12 inches above the patient's chest.

12-Lead Strategies for Wide-Complex Tachycardias

If an unstable patient's QRS complex is wide (greater than 0.12 seconds) and fast (greater than 150), immediate cardioversion may be indicated. If the patient is stable, however, the following steps in multi-lead assessments may help distinguish between VT and other wide-complex tachycardias[5]:

> **NOTE**
>
> These steps involve identifying the predominant direction of flow of impulses in the heart (axis), further described later in this chapter.

1. Assess leads I, II, III, MCL$_1$ (V$_1$), and MCL$_6$ (V$_6$). If the QRS complex is negative in leads I, II, and III and positive in MCL$_1$ (V$_1$), the rhythm indicates VT (Fig. 28-71). If these criteria are not met, proceed to step two.
2. Assess the QRS deflection in MCL$_1$ (V$_1$) and MCL$_6$ (V$_6$). Regardless of the QRS deflection in leads I, II, and III, positive QRS deflections with either a single peak, a taller left "rabbit ear," or an RS complex with a fat r wave or slurred s wave in MCL$_1$ (V$_1$) indicates VT. A negative QS complex, a negative rS complex, or any wide Q wave in MCL$_6$ (V$_6$) also indicates VT (Fig. 28-72).
3. A negative QRS complex in lead I; positive QRS complex in leads II and III and the QRS complex is negative in MCL$_1$ (V$_1$), the rhythm indicates VT (Fig. 28-73).
4. If all precordial leads (V leads) either are positive or negative (precordial concordance), the rhythm indicates VT (Fig. 28-74).
5. If the RS interval is greater than 0.10 second in any V lead (increased ventricular activation time), the rhythm indicates VT (Fig. 28-75).

> **NOTE**
>
> Non-VT precordial concordance may occur in patients who have Wolff-Parkinson-White syndrome and associated left bundle branch block.

? CRITICAL THINKING

Why is it important to distinguish between VT and wide-complex tachycardias in stable patients?

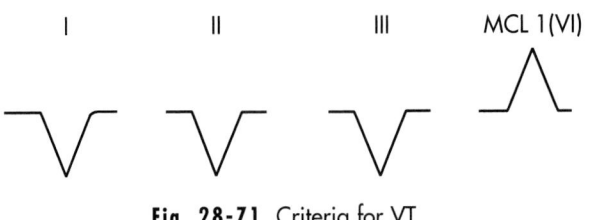

Fig. 28-71 Criteria for VT.

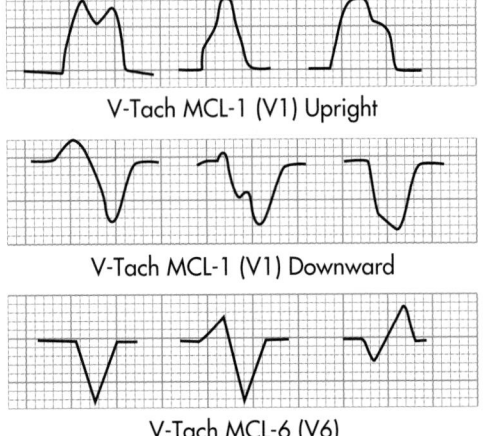

V-Tach MCL-1 (V1) Upright

V-Tach MCL-1 (V1) Downward

V-Tach MCL-6 (V6)

Fig. 28-72 Step 1: A QRS complex that is negative in leads I, II, III, and positive in MCL1 (V1) indicates VT. Step 2: Assess the QRS complex in MCL1 (V1) and MCL6 (V6). Step 3: Assess the QRS complex in leads I, II, III and MCL1 (V1). (From Multi-lead Medics, courtesy Bob Page, Springfield, Mo., 1997.)

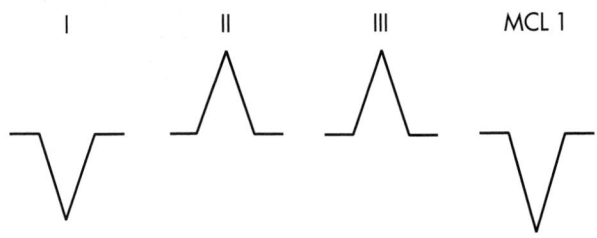

Fig. 28-73 Right axis deviation and a downward MCLI indicates VT.

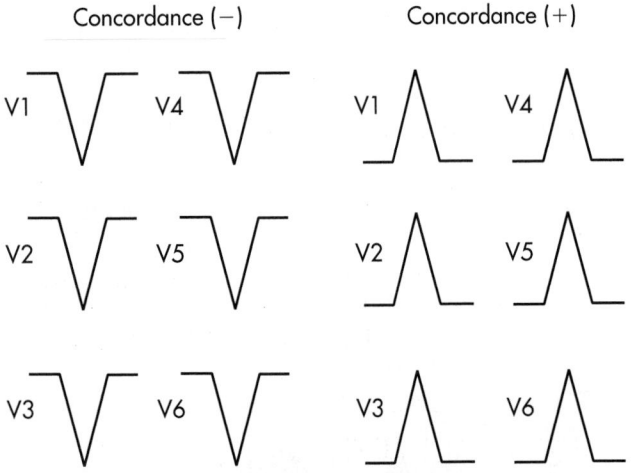

Concordance (−)   Concordance (+)

Fig. 28-74 VT-Concordance.

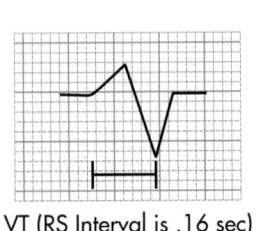

VT (RS Interval is .16 sec)

Fig. 28-75 RS interval. (From Multi-lead Medics, courtesy Bob Page, Springfield, Mo., 1997.)

? CRITICAL THINKING

How will you manage a patient with VT, chest pain, or difficulty breathing if you can't establish an IV?

Ventricular Fibrillation

Description

Ventricular fibrillation (VF) (Fig. 28-76) is a chaotic ventricular rhythm that results in quivering ventricular movements and pulselessness. The electrical impulses initiated by the multiple ectopic ventricular sites do not allow a sufficient mass of myocardium to fully depolarize and repolarize, so organized ventricular contraction does not occur. VF is the most common initial rhythm disturbance in sudden cardiac arrest. It results from multifocal reentry foci in the ventricles.

Etiology

VF most commonly is associated with significant cardiovascular system disease. The dysrhythmias also may be precipitated by PVCs, the R-on-T phenomenon (rarely), or a sustained VT. Other causes include the following:

- Myocardial ischemia
- AMI
- Third-degree AV block with a slow ventricular escape rhythm
- Cardiomyopathy
- Digitalis toxicity
- Hypoxia
- Acidosis
- Electrolyte imbalance (hypokalemia, hyperkalemia, submersion)
- Electrical injury
- Drug overdose or toxicity (cocaine, tricyclics)

Rules for Interpretation (All Leads)

QRS complex: Absent.

P waves: Absent.

Rate: No coordinated ventricular contractions are present. The unsynchronized ventricular impulses occur at rates from 300 to 500 beats per minute.

Rhythm: Irregularly irregular.

PR interval: Absent.

Because organized depolarizations of the atria and ventricles are absent, P waves, QRS complexes, ST segments, and T waves are absent. Ventricular fibrillatory waves (seen on the oscilloscope as bizarre, rounded or pointed, and markedly different in shape, varying at random from positive to negative) represent haphazard depolarization of small individual groups of muscle fibers. Fibrillatory waves less than 3 mm in amplitude are considered fine ventricular fibrillation, and those greater than 3 mm are considered coarse ventricular fibrillation (Fig. 28-77).

NOTE

Coarse VF usually indicates the recent onset of VF, which readily can be converted by prompt defibrillation. The presence of fine VF that approaches asystole often means that there has been a considerable delay since collapse, and successful defibrillation is more difficult.[2]

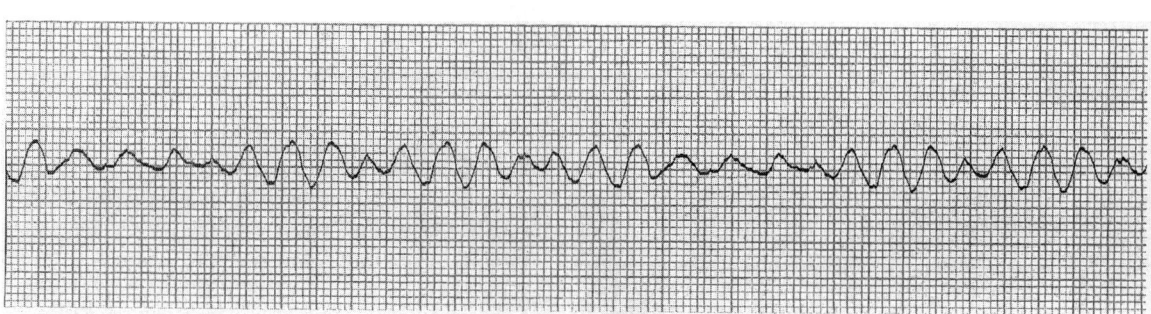

Fig. 28-76 Ventricular fibrillation.

The fibrillatory waves may be so fine that they appear isoelectric, resembling ventricular asystole.

Clinical Significance

VF causes all life-supporting physiological functions to cease because of lack of circulating blood flow. The dysrhythmia initially may result in lightheadedness, followed within seconds by loss of consciousness, apnea, and, if unmanaged, death.

Management (see Fig. 28-69)

For adult resuscitation, management of VF and pulseless VT is the most important sequence, since most adult cardiac arrests result from these two rhythm disturbances and the vast majority of successful resuscitations result from the appropriate management of these two dysrhythmias.[1] VF and nonperfusing VT are managed alike: basic life support (if a defibrillator is not immediately available), defibrillation, endotracheal intubation, and pharmacological therapy (*epinephrine* [Adrenalin], *lidocaine* [Xylocaine], and *bretylium* [Bretylol]), and in some cases *amiodarone* (Cordarone).

> **NOTE**
>
> If the monitor appears to show asystole, fine VF still may be the underlying rhythm. Asystole should be confirmed in two leads (90 degrees apart) to rule out fine VF so that the patient may be identified as "shockable."

> **SEQUENCE OF CARE FOR VF AND PULSELESS VT**
>
> Basic life support measures
> Defibrillation
> Endotracheal intubation/IV access
> **Epinephrine** (Adrenalin)
> **Vasopressin** (Pitressin)
> Antidysrhythmics
> **Amiodarone** (Cordarone)
> **Lidocaine** (Xylocaine)
> **Magnesium sulfate**
> **Procainamide** (Pronestyl)

Ventricular Asystole

Description

Ventricular asystole (cardiac standstill) (Fig. 28-78) refers to the absence of all ventricular activity.

Etiology

Ventricular asystole may be the primary event in cardiac arrest. It also may occur in complete heart block when there is no functional escape pacemaker. The dysrhythmia usually is associated with global myocardial ischemia or necrosis and often follows VT, VF, PEA, or an agonal escape rhythm in the dying heart. When faced with an isoelectric line on the monitor, the paramedic should confirm asystole as the rhythm by changing placement of the leads by 90 degrees or switching to a second lead on the monitor.

Rules for Interpretation (All Leads)

QRS complexes: Absent.
P waves: Absent or present.
Rate: Absent.
Rhythm: Absent.
PR Interval: Absent.

Clinical Significance

Ventricular asystole produces complete cessation of cardiac output. It is an ominous dysrhythmia, often representing a confirmation of death in which the prognosis for resuscitation is dismal.

Management (Fig. 28-79)

The management for ventricular asystole is basic life support, endotracheal intubation, and pharmacological therapy (*epinephrine* [Adrenalin], *atropine,* and possibly *sodium bicarbonate*). If fine VF is suspected, defibrillation is indicated. However, defibrillating asystole "just in case" is not recommended.[1] Cessation of resuscitation efforts in the prehospital setting after system-specific criteria and authorization from medical direction is indicated in this patient care situation.

> **NOTE**
>
> Potential causes of asystole that should be considered before cessation of resuscitative efforts include hypoxia, hyperkalemia, hypothermia, drug overdose, and acidosis.

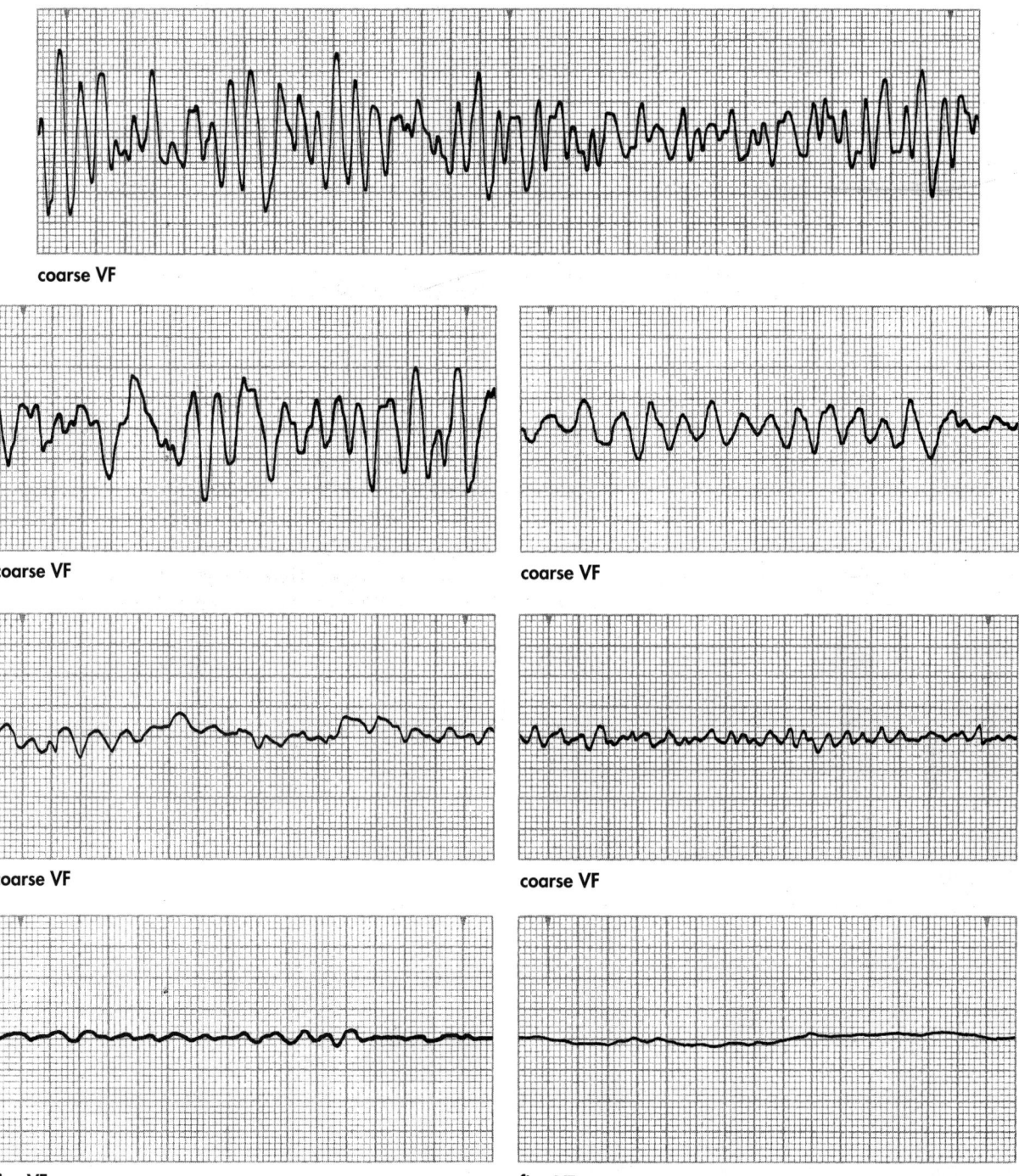

coarse VF

coarse VF

coarse VF

coarse VF

coarse VF

fine VF

fine VF

Fig. 28-77 Coarse and fine ventricular fibrillation. (From Huszar R: *Basic dysrhythmias,* ed 2, St Louis, 1994, Mosby.)

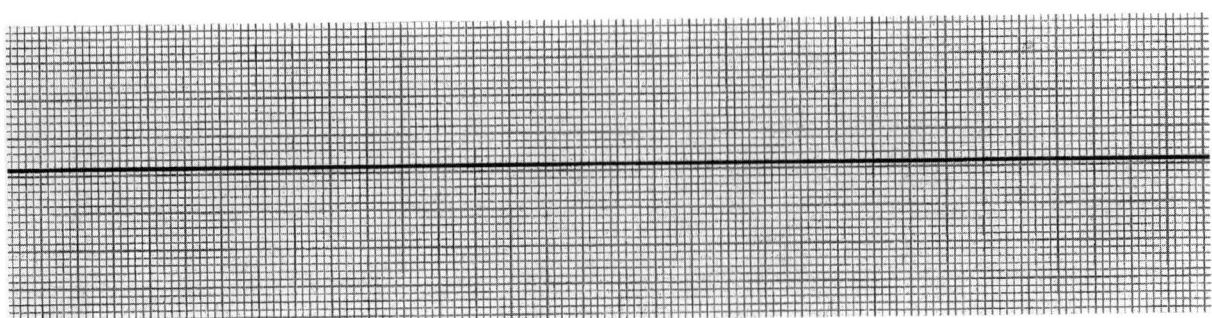

Fig. 28-78 Ventricular asystole.

SEQUENCE OF CARE FOR ASYSTOLE

Basic life support
Endotracheal intubation/IV access
TCP
Epinephrine (Adrenalin)
Atropine
Sodium bicarbonate (possibly)

? CRITICAL THINKING

What benefit is there to the community, and to the patient's family, when resuscitation is terminated in the field after following all appropriate guidelines?

Artificial Pacemaker Rhythms

Description

Artificial pacemakers generate a rhythm (Fig. 28-80) by regular electrical stimulation of the heart through an electrode implanted in the heart. The electrode is connected to a power source (a battery cell implanted subcutaneously, typically in the right or left pectoral region). The tip of the pacemaker wire commonly is positioned in the apex of the right ventricle (ventricular pacemaker), in the right atrium (atrial pacemaker), or in both locations (dual-chamber pacemaker). These devices are implanted most frequently in patients with complete heart block and in those who have episodes of severe symptomatic bradycardia.

Pacemakers that fire continuously at a preset rate without regard to the patient's own electrical activity are known as *fixed-rate* or *asynchronous pacemakers;* they rarely are used today. Pacemakers that fire only if the patient's own rate drops below the pacemaker's preset rate (acting as an escape rhythm) are known as *demand pacemakers.* Atrial and ventricular demand pacemakers "pace" the atria and/or ventricles when the intrinsic rate of the paced chamber drops dangerously low. *Atrial synchronous ventricular pacemakers* are synchronized with the patient's atrial rhythm. This type of pacemaker paces the ventricle at a preset time after the patient's intrinsic atrial depolarization. This pacemaker is useful in patients with normal sinus node activity but various degrees of AV block. *AV sequential pacemakers* pace the atria first and then the ventricles when spontaneous activity is absent or slowed in either or both. If intrinsic atrial activity is too slow, for example, then both chambers are paced sequentially to maintain the "atrial kick." If the atrial rate is adequate, the atrial pacer is suppressed. The ventricular pacemaker still fires if the ventricular rate is below a preset rate. This pacemaker is ideal for sick sinus syndrome and sinus arrest.

NOTE

Some implantable devices provide for pacemaker capability and defibrillation.

A class of newer pacemakers (rate-responsive pacemakers) can adjust their pacing rates to patient needs by sensing when cardiac output should be increased. Although there are several methods of

Asystole

Basic Life Support

Perform Primary ABCD Survey

(Correct critical problems IMMEDIATELY as they are identified)
- Assess responsiveness
- Call for help/call for defibrillator

Airway–open the airway
Breathing–deliver two slow breaths, administer oxygen as soon as it is available
Circulation–perform chest compressions
Ensure availability of monitor/**D**efibrillator–
On arrival of AED/monitor/defibrillator, perform secondary ABCD survey if rhythm is NOT pulseless VT/VF

Advanced Life Support

Possible causes of asystole:
PATCH-4-MD
Pulmonary embolism
Acidosis
Tension pneumothorax
Cardiac tamponade
Hypovolemia (most common cause)
Hypoxia
Heat/cold (hypo-/hyperthermia)
Hypo-/hyperkalemia (and other electrolytes)
Myocardial infarction
Drug overdose/accidents (cyclic antidepressants, calcium channel blockers, beta-blockers, digitalis)

Perform Secondary ABCD Survey

(ADVANCED) AIRWAY
Reassess effectiveness of initial airway maneuvers and interventions
Perform invasive airway management
BREATHING
Assess ventilation
Confirm ET tube placement (or other airway device) by at least two methods
Provide positive-pressure ventilation/Evaluate effectiveness of ventilations
Secure airway device in place with commercial tube holder (preferred) or tape
CIRCULATION
Confirm presence of asystole
(Check lead/cable connections, ensure power to monitor is on, correct lead is selected, gain turned up, confirm asystole in second lead)
Establish IV access and administer appropriate medications
DIFFERENTIAL DIAGNOSIS
Search for and treat reversible causes (**PATCH-4-MD**)

Consider immediate transcutaneous pacing
- **Epinephrine 1 mg (1:10,000 solution) IV every 3 to 5 minutes**
  (ET dose 2-2.5 mg diluted in 10-mL normal saline or distilled water)
- **Atropine*, † 1 mg IV every 3 to 5 minutes to maximum 0.04 mg/kg (Class IIb)**
  (ET dose 2 to 3 mg diluted in 10 -mL normal saline or distilled water)

Consider sodium bicarbonate 1 mEq/kg:
- Known preexisting hyperkalemia (Class I)
- Cyclic antidepressant overdose (IIa)
- To alkalinize urine in aspirin or other drug overdoses (IIa)
- Patient that has been intubated + long arrest interval (IIb)
- On return of spontaneous circulation if long arrest interval (IIb)

Consider termination of efforts
- Evaluate the quality of the resuscitation attempt
- Evaluate the resuscitation for atypical clinical features (e.g., hypothermia, reversible therapeutic or illicit drug use)
- Does support for cease-effort protocols exist?

*Brown DC, Lewis AJ, Criley JM: Asystole and its treatment: the possible role of the parasympathetic nervous system in cardiac arrest, JACEP 8:448, 1979.
†Coon GA, Clinton JE, Ruiz E: Use of atropine for brady-asytolic prehospital cardiac arrest, *Ann Emerg Med* 10:462, 1981.

Fig. 28-79 Asystole. (From Aehlert B: *ACLS quick review study guide,* ed 2, St Louis, 2002, Mosby.)

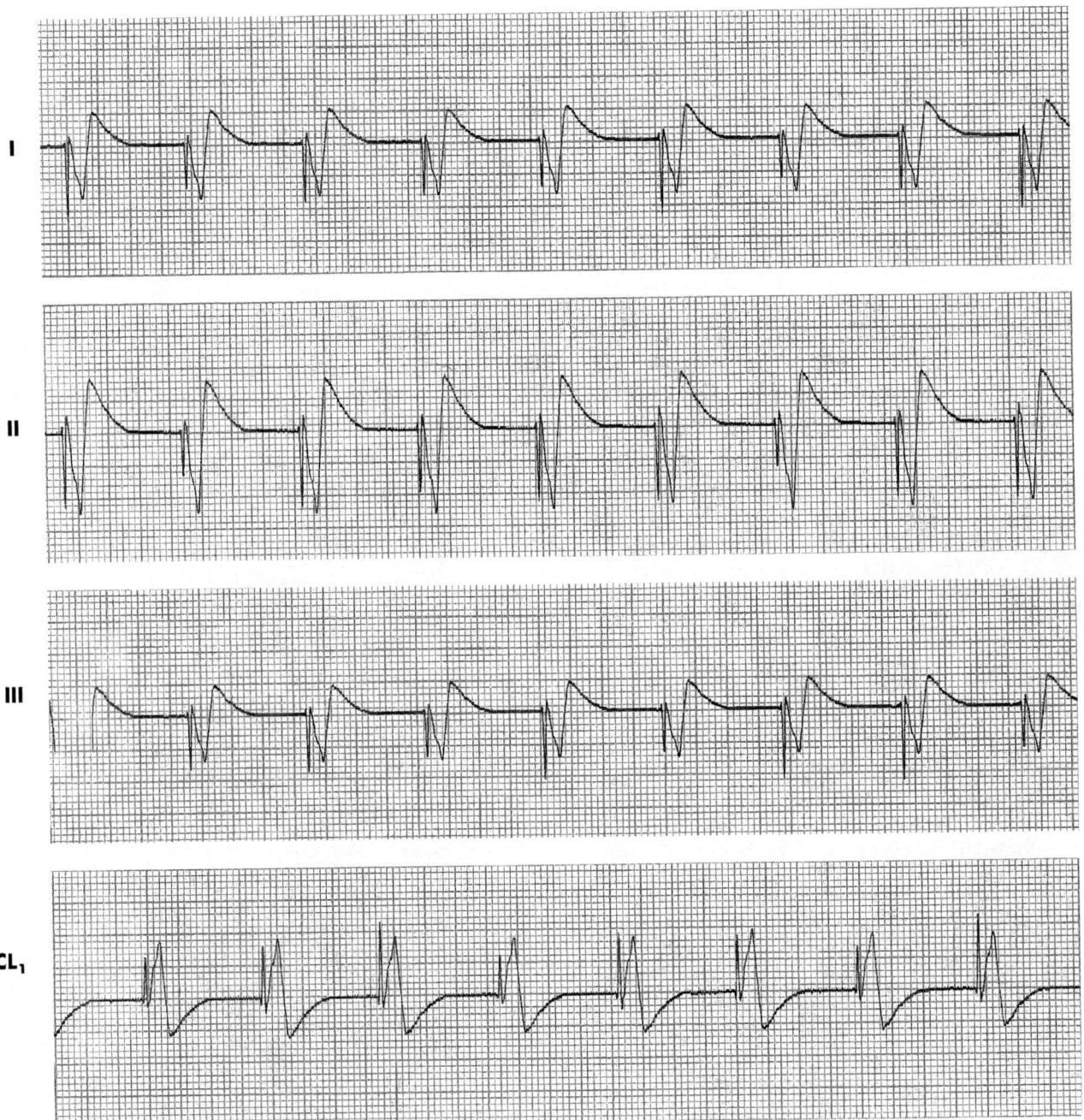

Fig. 28-80 Artificial pacemaker rhythms.

sensing metabolic activity, the most popular rate-responsive pacers detect patient movement to determine the optimum firing rate. These devices are popular because they can increase cardiac output and increase tolerance of physical activity. These pacemakers occasionally increase the patient's pacing rate inappropriately if they sense muscle movement that is not caused by increased patient activity.

Rules for Interpretation (Lead II Monitoring)

QRS complex: If pacemaker induced, QRS complexes are 0.12 second or greater. Their appearance usually is bizarre, resembling a PVC. The pacemaker is said to be "capturing" if each pacemaker spike elicits a QRS complex. If only the atria are being paced, the QRS complexes usually are normal, provided no bundle branch block is present. With demand pacemakers, some of the patient's own QRS complexes may be present. These normal QRS complexes occur without pacemaker spikes.

P waves: May be present or absent, normal or abnormal. The relationship of the P waves to the pacemaker (QRS) complex varies by type of artificial pacemaker. Pacemaker "spikes" precede QRS complexes induced by ventricular pacemakers, whereas dual-chambered pacemakers also produce an atrial spike followed by a P wave. The pacemaker spike is a narrow deflection on the oscilloscope and represents the electrical discharge of the pacemaker.

? CRITICAL THINKING

If the pacemaker fails, what rhythms might you see on the monitor?

NOTE

Pacemaker spikes indicate only that a pacemaker is discharging. They provide no information about ventricular contraction or perfusion.

Rate: Varies according to the preset rate of the pacemaker. Typically the rate is 60 to 80 beats per minute.

Rhythm: Regular if pacing is constant; irregular if pacing occurs only on demand.

PR interval: The presence and duration of PR intervals depend on the underlying rhythm and vary by the type of artificial pacemaker.

Clinical Significance

Pacemaker spikes indicate that the patient's heart rate is being regulated by an artificial pacemaker. Pacemaker spikes followed by QRS complexes indicate electrical capture. If spikes do not elicit a QRS complex, the pacemaker is not capturing the ventricle electrically, and there will be no ventricular contraction. A large percentage of pacemaker failures occur within the first month after implantation (see the box below).

FOUR POTENTIAL CAUSES OF PACEMAKER MALFUNCTION

1. Battery failure: Most implanted pacemakers today use a lithium-iodine cell power source that provides stable voltage output for about 80% to 90% of the life of the battery (5 to 10 years or more). Battery failure usually slows the pacemaker rate and decreases the spike amplitude. If the battery fails, the patient may have bradycardia or asystole.

2. Runaway pacemakers: Runaway pacemakers (pacemakers that develop very rapid discharge rates that may reach 300 beats per minute) occur rarely as the batteries decrease their voltage output. This type of failure seldom is seen in pacemakers used today because the newer power sources provide a gradual increase in rate as their batteries run low.

3. Failure of the sensing device in demand pacemakers: Demand pacemakers may fail to shut off when patients have an adequate rate of their own. When this occurs, there is competition between the natural and artificial pacemakers of the heart, and the pacemaker may discharge during the vulnerable period of the cardiac cycle, resulting in dysrhythmias.

4. Failure to capture: Failure of the pacemaker to capture may result from a variety of causes, including battery failure, loose or broken catheter electrode wires, inoperable electrodes, and a shift in the location of the catheter tip. In such cases, pacemaker spikes usually are present but are not followed by P waves or QRS complexes.

Management

Patients with artificial pacemakers require no special emergency care management. However, pacemaker failure is a true emergency that necessitates immediate recognition and rapid transport for definitive care (battery replacement or temporary pacemaker insertion). Therefore prolonged in-field stabilization of these patients is not recommended. The following five principles also are important in evaluating and managing patients with implanted pacemakers:

1. When examining an unconscious patient, be alert for battery packs implanted under the skin and for any medical alert information.
2. Manage all dysrhythmias per the appropriate algorithm.
3. Manage ventricular irritability with *lidocaine* (Xylocaine) without fear of suppressing ventricular response to a pacemaker rhythm.
4. Defibrillate the hearts of patients with artificial pacemakers in the usual manner, but do not discharge paddles directly over the implanted battery pack.
5. TCP, if indicated, may be used in the usual manner.

Besides pacemakers, implantable cardioverter-defibrillators (ICDs) also are becoming more common. The battery packs of these devices are located in the subcutaneous tissues of the abdominal wall. Emergency cardiac care may proceed in the usual manner. Although these devices present no danger to rescuers, gloves should be worn to help avoid unpleasant sensations when the device discharges. (ICDs will be further described later in this chapter.)

Dysrhythmias That are Disorders of Conduction

Partial delays or complete interruptions in cardiac electrical conduction are called *heart blocks.* Heart blocks can occur anywhere in the atria, between the SA node and the AV node, or in the ventricles between the AV node and the Purkinje fibers. These dysrhythmias of conduction may be caused by pathology in the conduction system or by a physiological block, as occurs in atrial fibrillation or atrial flutter. Causes of heart blocks include AV junctional ischemia, AV junctional necrosis, degenerative disease of the conduction system, electrolyte imbalances (e.g., hyperkalemia), and drug toxicity, especially with digitalis.

Classifications

Conduction blocks may be classified on the basis of several characteristics: site of block (e.g., left bundle branch block), degree of block (e.g., second-degree AV block), or category of AV conduction disturbances (e.g., type I). This text presents the dysrhythmias by degree and location. AV blocks are categorized by degree of block. It should be noted, however, that the term *degree* does not directly reflect gradients of clinical severity when applied to the classification of heart blocks. Any evaluation of heart block must consider the specific rates of the atria and ventricles, the patient's clinical presentation, and the findings of a complete history and physical examination before the clinical severity of AV conduction disturbances is determined. The dysrhythmias discussed in this section include first-degree AV block; second-degree AV block type I (or *Wenckebach*); second-degree AV block type II; third-degree AV block (complete heart block); and ventricular conduction disturbances, including bundle branch blocks and hemiblocks.

First-Degree AV Block

Description

First-degree AV block (Fig. 28-81) is not a true block but rather a delay in conduction, usually at the level of the AV node. First-degree AV block is not considered a rhythm in itself because it usually is superimposed on another rhythm. Therefore the underlying rhythm also must be identified (e.g., sinus bradycardia with first-degree AV block).

Etiology

First-degree AV block may occur for no apparent reason. The dysrhythmia sometimes is associated with myocardial ischemia, acute myocardial infarction, increased vagal (parasympathetic) tone, or digitalis toxicity.

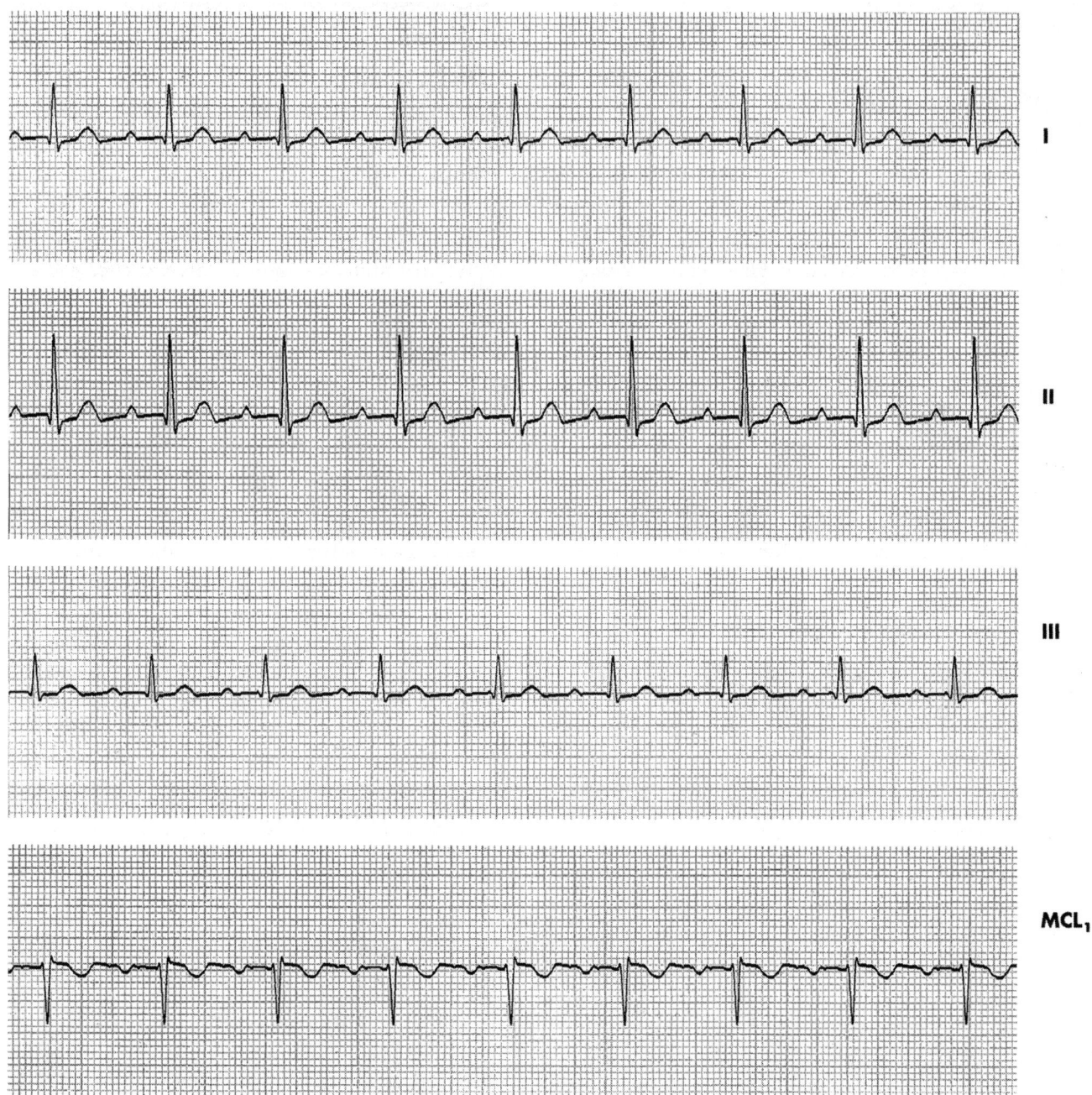

Fig. 28-81 First-degree AV block.

QRS complex: Typically normal (less than 0.12 second), with an AV conduction ratio of 1:1 (a QRS complex follows each P wave).

P waves: Present, identical waves that precede each QRS complex.

Rate: The rate is that of the underlying sinus or atrial rhythm.

Rhythm: The rhythm is that of the underlying rhythm.

PR interval: A prolonged (greater than 0.20 second), constant PR interval is the hallmark of first-degree AV block and often is the only alteration in the ECG.

Clinical Significance

As a general rule, first-degree AV block has little or no clinical significance because all of the impulses are conducted to the ventricles. Rarely, however, a newly developed first-degree AV block progresses to a more serious AV block.

Management

There is no definitive management.

Second-Degree AV Block Type I (or Wenckebach)
Description

Type I second-degree AV block (Fig. 28-82) is an intermittent block that usually occurs at the level of the AV node. The conduction delay progressively increases from beat to beat until conduction to the ventricle is blocked. This dysrhythmia produces a characteristic cyclical pattern in which the PR intervals get progressively longer until a P wave occurs that is not followed by a QRS complex. By the time the SA node fires again, AV conduction has had time to recover, and the sequence starts over.

Etiology

Type I second-degree AV block often occurs in acute myocardial infarction or acute myocarditis. Other causes include increased vagal tone, ischemia, drug toxicity (digitalis, *propranolol* [Inderal], *verapamil* [Isoptin]), head injury, and electrolyte imbalance.

Rules for Interpretation (Lead II Monitoring)

QRS complex: Usually less than 0.12 second. Commonly, the AV conduction ratio (P waves to QRS complexes) is 5:4, 4:3, 3:2, or 2:1; the pattern

may be constant or variable. A constant 2:1 block makes it difficult to distinguish between type I and type II blocks.

P waves: Are upright and uniform and precede the QRS complex when the QRS complex occurs.

Rate: The atrial rate is that of the underlying sinus or atrial rhythm. The ventricular rate may be normal or slow but always is slightly less than the atrial rate.

Rhythm: The atrial rhythm is regular; the ventricular rhythm is irregular (characteristic group beating).

PR interval: Progressively lengthens before the non-conducted P wave. The P-P interval is constant, but the R-R interval decreases until the dropped beat (producing grouping of QRS complexes).

> **NOTE**
>
> AV block, in which the PR interval before a dropped beat is prolonged and the PR interval after the dropped beat is shortened by comparison, is the most common form of second-degree block.

Clinical Significance

Type I second-degree AV block usually is a transient and reversible phenomenon but can progress to a more serious AV block. If dropped beats occur frequently, the patient may show signs and symptoms of decreased cardiac output.

Management

No management is required if the patient is asymptomatic. If the dropped beats compromise the heart rate and cardiac output, *atropine,* and/or TCP may be indicated (see Fig. 28-40).

Second-Degree AV Block Type II
Description

Type II second-degree AV block (Fig. 28-83) is an intermittent block that occasionally occurs when atrial impulses are not conducted to the ventricles. Unlike type I, this block is characterized by consecutive P waves being conducted with a constant PR interval before a dropped beat. This variation of AV block usually occurs in a regular sequence with the conduction ratios (P waves to QRS complexes), such as 2:1, 3:2, and 4:3 (Fig. 28-84). Type II second-degree AV block usually occurs below the bundle of His.

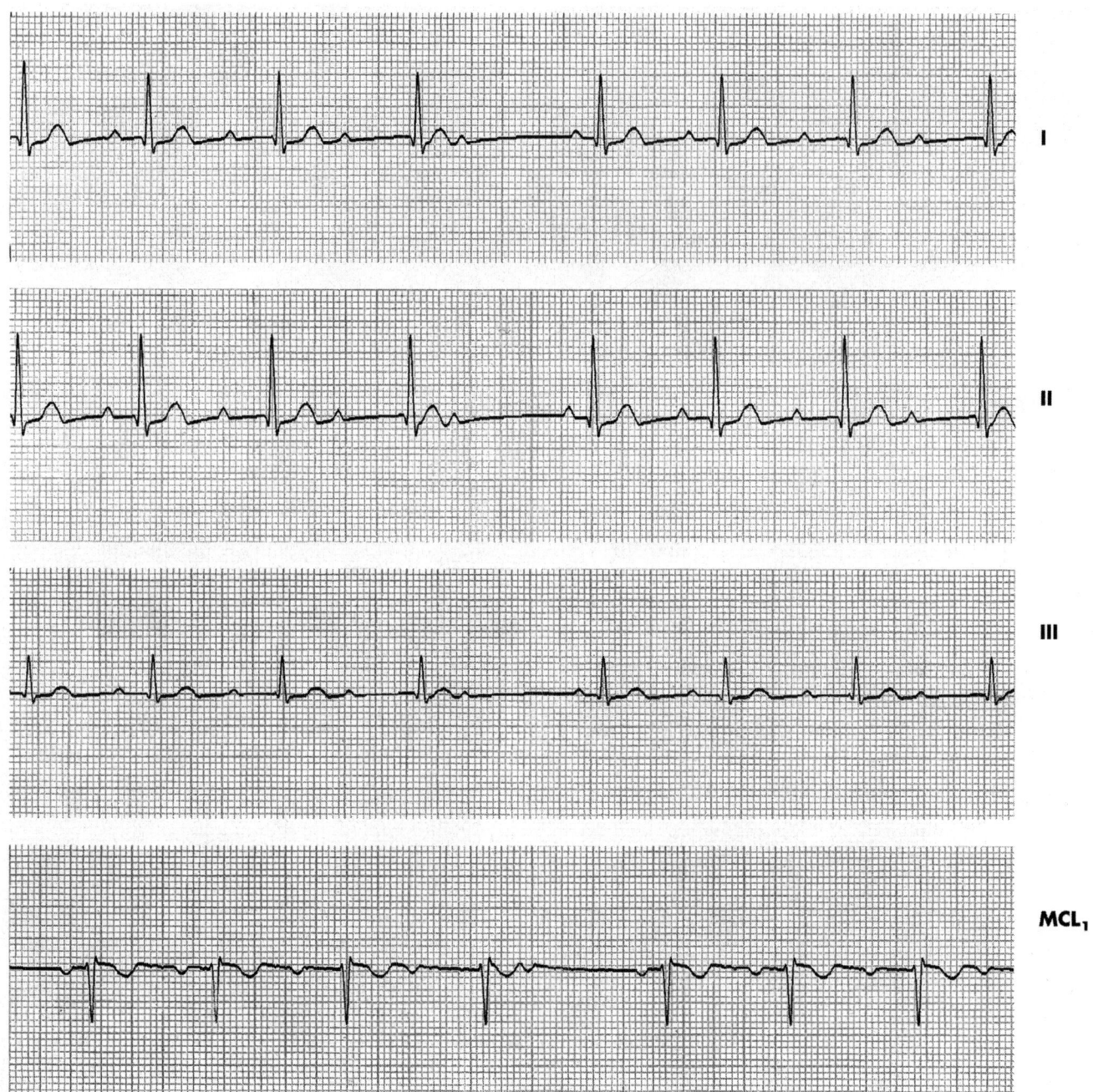

Fig. 28-82 Second-degree AV block, type I.

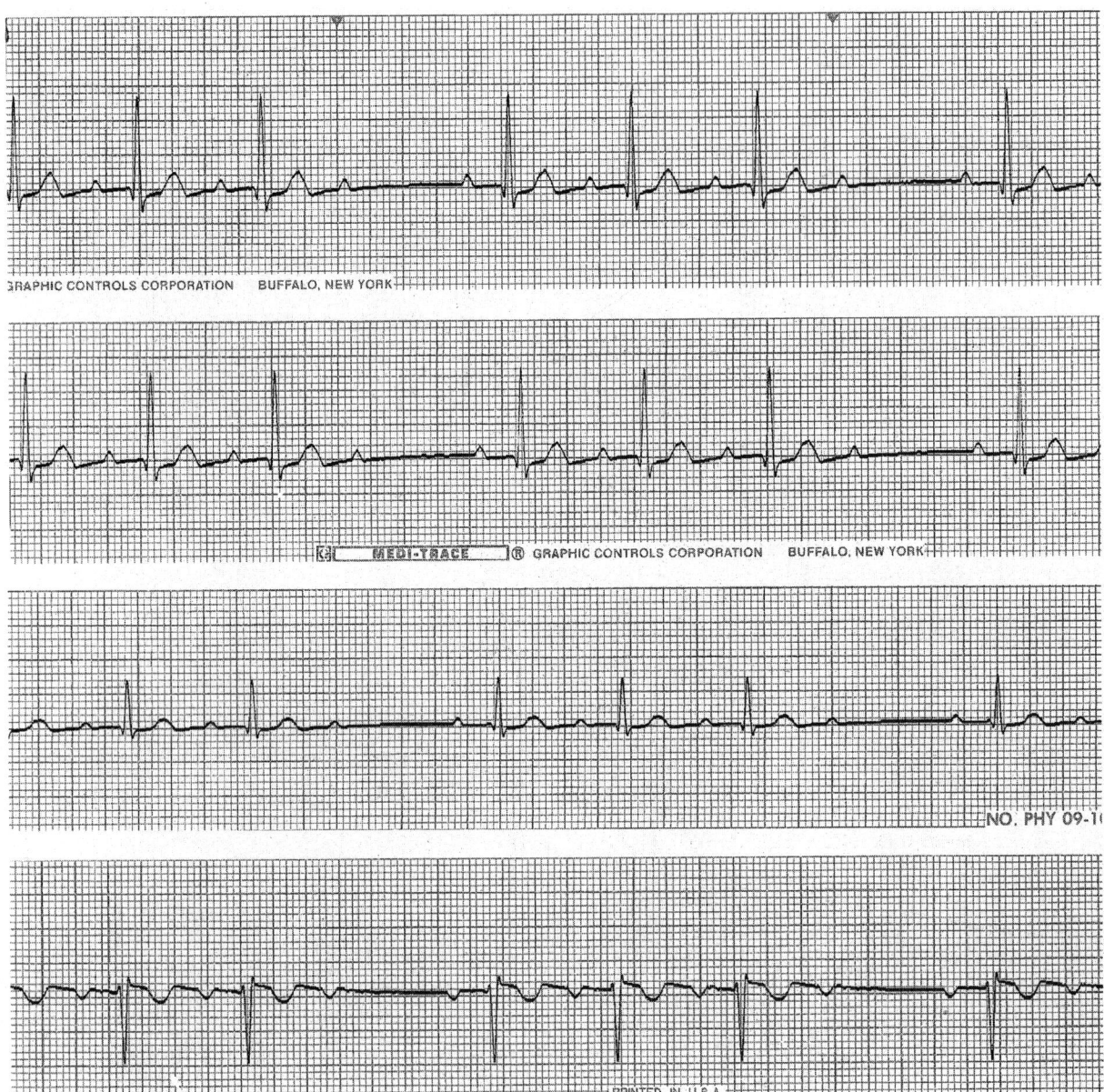

Fig. 28-83 Second-degree AV block, type II.

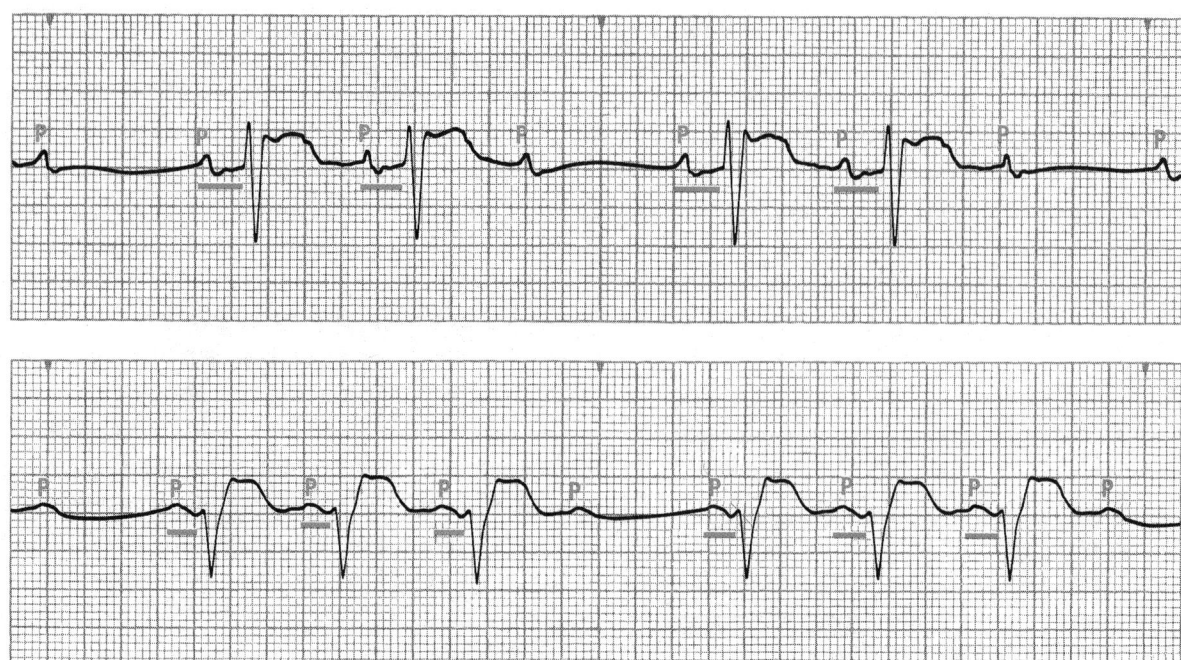

Fig. 28-84 A, 3:2 AV block. **B,** 4:3 AV block. (From Huszar R: *Basic dysrhythmias,* ed 2, St Louis, 1994, Mosby.)

When at least two consecutive impulses (atrial P waves) fail to be conducted to the ventricles, the AV block is referred to as a *high-grade AV block* (Fig. 28-85). Clinically, malignant high-grade AV blocks and those with a more favorable prognosis are distinguished by the underlying atrial and ventricular rates. A 2:1 block might be con-

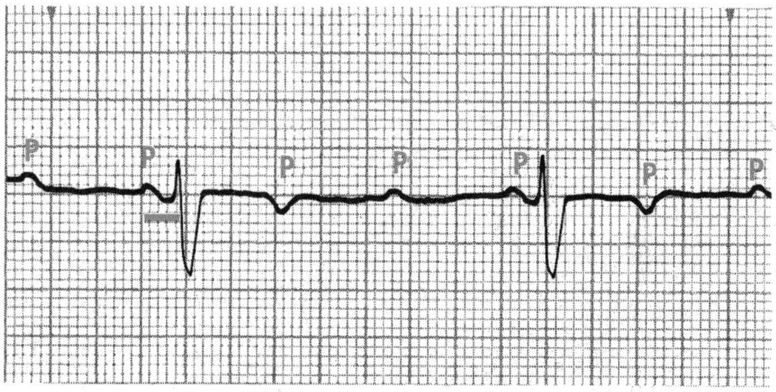

Fig. 28-85 3:1 high-grade AV block. (From Huszar R: *Basic dysrhythmias,* ed 2, St Louis, 1994, Mosby.)

sidered high grade (and certainly is clinically significant) when the patient's underlying atrial rate is 60 beats per minute, but it is of much less concern if the patient's atrial rate is 120 beats per minute.

Etiology

Type II second-degree AV block usually is associated with AMI and septal necrosis. Unlike type I second-degree AV block, type II normally does not result solely from increased parasympathetic tone or drug toxicity.

NOTE

A type II 2:1 AV block sometimes may be difficult to distinguish from a type I 2:1 AV block. When assessing a patient who has two atrial complexes for each QRS complex, the paramedic should evaluate the conducted cycle (the cycle with the P wave and the QRS complex together). If the conducted cycle has a prolonged PR interval (greater than 0.20 second), a narrow QRS complex (less than 0.12 second, indicating the absence of bundle branch block), and an adequate escape rate, the patient probably has a type I 2:1 AV block. If the conducted QRS complex has a normal PR interval, a wide QRS complex (greater than 0.12 second, which indicates the presence of a bundle branch block), and an adequate escape rate, a type II 2:1 AV block is most likely (Fig. 28-86).

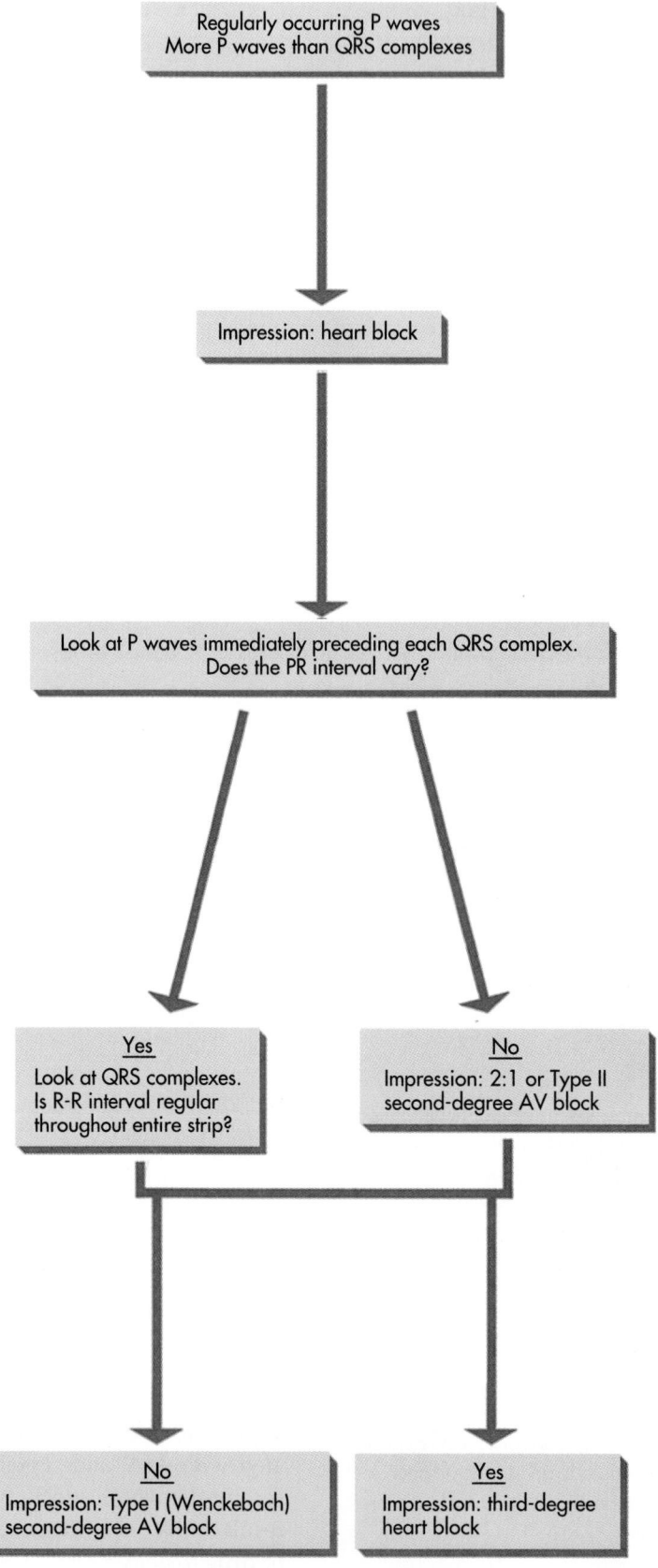

Fig. 28-86 Identifying heart blocks.

Rules for Interpretation (Lead II Monitoring)

QRS complex: May be abnormal (equal to or greater than 0.12 second) because of bundle branch block.

P waves: Are upright and uniform; some P waves will not be followed by QRS complexes.

Rate: The atrial rate is unaffected and is that of the underlying sinus, atrial, or junctional rhythm. The ventricular rate is less than that of the atrial rate and is often bradycardic.

Rhythm: Regular or irregular, depending on whether the conduction ratio is constant or variable.

PR interval: Usually is constant for conducted beats and may be greater than 0.20 second. (Refer to the preceding Note.)

Clinical Significance

Type II second-degree AV block is a serious dysrhythmia that is usually considered malignant in the emergency setting (unlike type I AV blocks, which usually are considered benign). Slow ventricular rates may result in signs and symptoms of hypoperfusion. This dysrhythmia may progress to a more severe heart block and even to ventricular asystole.

Management

Regardless of the patient's initial condition, pacemaker insertion is the definitive management. Prehospital care for symptomatic patients may consist of TCP and possibly the administration of *atropine* (see Fig. 28-40).

Third-Degree Heart Block

Description

Third-degree AV block (Fig. 28-87) results from complete electrical block at or below the AV node (infranodal). The dysrhythmia is said to be present

> **NOTE**
>
> ***Atropine*** should be used with caution in patients with complete heart block and wide-complex ventricular escape beats and also for patients with type II second-degree heart block.[1] (***Atropine*** may actually enhance the block or precipitate third-degree AV block.) Many of these patients cannot be effectively managed in the prehospital setting with only medication. Immediate transport to an emergency department is indicated.

when the opportunity for conduction between the atria and the ventricles is present but conduction does not occur. In this condition, the SA node serves as the pacemaker for the atria, and an ectopic focus serves as a pacemaker in the ventricles. The result is that P waves and QRS complexes occur rhythmically, but the rhythms are unrelated to each other (AV dissociation).

> **NOTE**
>
> The only electrical link between the atria and the ventricles is the AV node and bundle of His.

Etiology

Common causes of third-degree AV block include increased vagal tone (which may produce a transient AV dissociation), septal necrosis, acute myocarditis, digitalis, beta blocker or calcium channel blocker toxicity, and electrolyte imbalance. The dysrhythmia also may occur in older adults from chronic degenerative changes in the conduction system, such as those that occur with Lev's or Lenègre's disease.

Rules for Interpretation (Lead II Monitoring)

QRS complex: May be less than 0.12 second if the escape focus is below the AV node and above the bifurcation of the bundle branches or 0.12 second or greater if the escape focus is ventricular.

> **NOTE**
>
> When analyzing an ECG in which P waves and QRS complexes do not appear to be related to each other, the paramedic should look at the QRS-T–wave morphology. QRS-T–wave morphology that is altered by superimposed P waves suggests AV dissociation, and AV dissociation suggests third-degree AV block.

P waves: Are present but have no relationship to the QRS complexes. In cases of atrial flutter or fibrillation, complete heart block is manifested by a slow, regular ventricular response.

Rate: The atrial rate is that of the underlying sinus or atrial rhythm. The ventricular rate typically is 40 to 60 beats per minute if the escape focus is junctional and less than 40 beats per minute if the escape focus is in the ventricles.

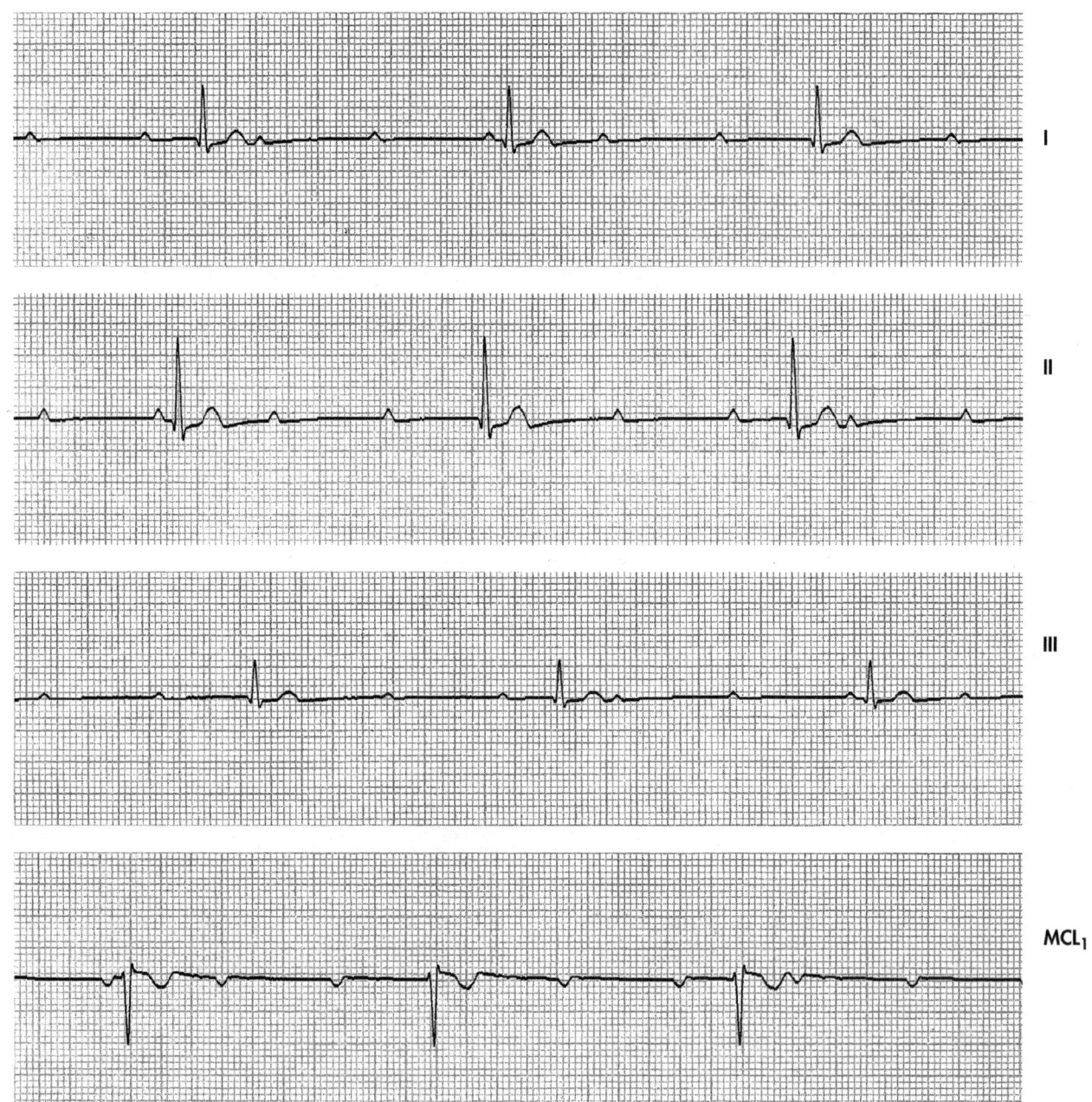

I

II

III

MCL₁

Fig. 28-87 Third-degree AV block.

A narrow QRS complex in third-degree block is less common than a wide QRS complex.

Rhythm: The atrial and ventricular rhythms usually are regular. The rhythms are independent of each other.
PR interval: There is no relation between atrial and ventricular activity (Fig. 28-88).

Clinical Significance

There may be signs and symptoms of severe bradycardia and decreased cardiac output because of the slow ventricular rate and asynchronous action of the atria and ventricles. Third-degree AV block associated with wide QRS complexes is an ominous sign. The dysrhythmia potentially is lethal, and patients with this rhythm often present as unstable.

NOTE

Complete AV block in the presence of atrial fibrillation often is caused by drug toxicity (usually digitalis). There is almost always some AV block with atrial fibrillation or flutter, but complete AV block is recognized by a slow, regular ventricular response (usually less than 60 beats per minute). The QRS complex may be normal if the escape focus is from above the bifurcation of the bundle branches.

Management

Pacemaker insertion is the definitive management for symptomatic third-degree AV block and for asymptomatic third-degree block with bundle branch block. Initial prehospital care includes TCP, *dopamine* (Intropin) to increase the ventricular rate if needed, *epinephrine* (Adrenalin), *isoproterenol* (Isuprel), and possibly *atropine* to stimulate AV conduction or to increase the rate of a junctional escape rhythm if sanctioned by medical direction.

? CRITICAL THINKING

What should you tell the patient before initiating TCP?

NOTE

TCP is a class I intervention for all symptomatic bradycardias and should be implemented as soon as possible if the bradycardia is severe and the patient's clinical condition is unstable (see Fig. 28-40).

NOTE

Atropine (a parasympatholytic) is unlikely to be effective in patients with complete heart block. Since the peripheral nervous system innervates the atria, and the focus controlling the heart in a third-degree block is most often in the ventricles, **atropine** will likely have no effect on the discharge rate of the ventricular focus.

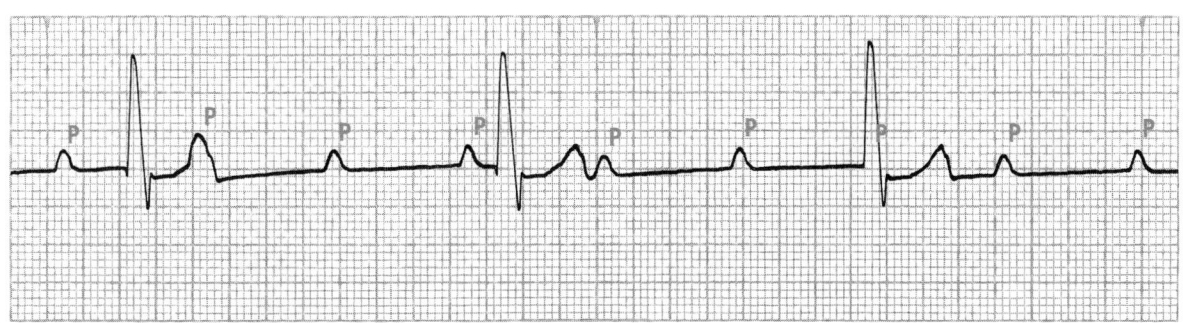

Fig. 28-88 Third-degree block demonstrating P waves superimposed on the QRS complex and T waves. (From Huszar R: *Basic dysrhythmias*, ed 2, St Louis, 1994, Mosby.)

Ventricular Conduction Disturbances

Ventricular conduction disturbances (bundle branch blocks and hemiblocks) are delays or interruptions in the transmission of electrical impulses that occur below the level of bifurcation of the bundle of His. Identifying these blocks can provide important information about a patient being at increased risk of developing severe bradycardia and third-degree heart block (especially when combined with other forms of AV block). Common causes of bundle branch block include:

- Ischemic heart disease
- Acute heart failure
- AMI
- Hyperkalemia
- Trauma
- Cardiomyopathy
- Aortic stenosis
- Infection (e.g., carditis)

Bundle Branch Anatomy

To review, the bundle of His begins at the AV node and divides to form the left and right bundle branches (Fig. 28-89). The right bundle branch continues toward the apex and spreads throughout the right ventricle. The left bundle branch subdivides into the anterior and posterior fascicles and spreads throughout the left ventricle. Conduction of electrical impulses through the Purkinje fibers stimulates the ventricles to contract.

With normal conduction, the first part of the ventricle to be stimulated is the left side of the septum. The electrical impulse then traverses the septum to stimulate the other side. Shortly thereafter, the left and right ventricles simultaneously are stimulated. Because the left ventricle is normally much larger and thicker than the right ventricle, its electrical activity predominates over that of the right ventricle.

Common ECG Findings

When an electrical impulse is blocked from passing through either the right or left bundle branch, one ventricle depolarizes and contracts before the other. Because ventricular activation no longer is simultaneous, the QRS complex widens (often with a slurred or notched appearance known as "rabbit ears"). The hallmark of bundle branch block is a QRS complex that is equal to or greater

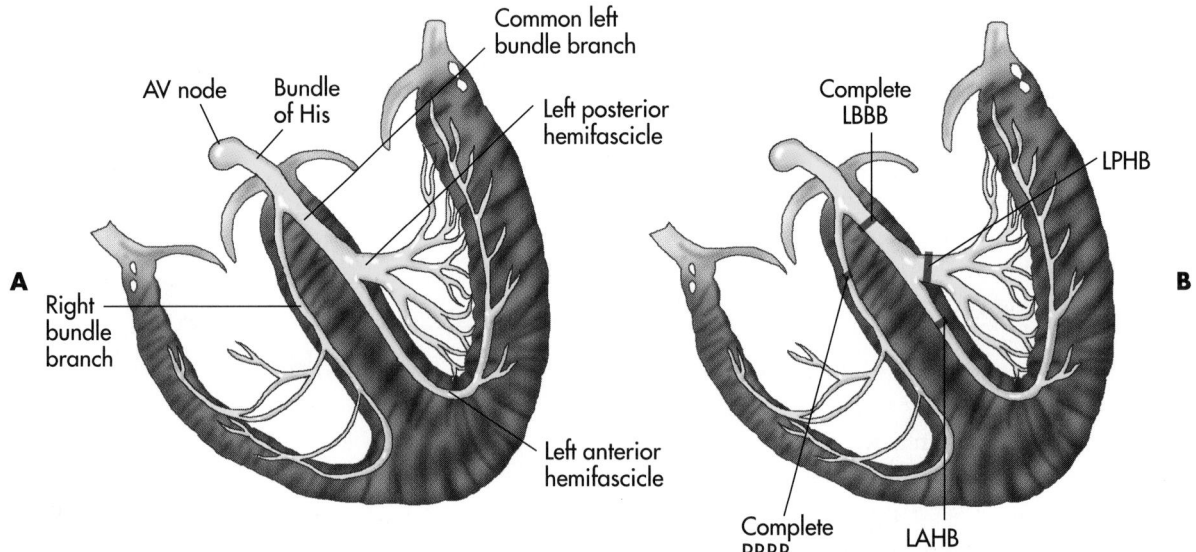

Fig. 28-89 A, Simplified illustration showing the major divisions of the ventricular conduction system. After passing through the AV node and the bundle of His, the electrical impulse is carried to the right and common left bundle branches. The latter structure divides into the left anterior and posterior hemifascicles. **B,** Possible sites of block and the conduction deficits that may be produced. (From Grauer K: *Practical guide to ECG interpretation,* St Louis, 1992, Mosby.)

Bundle branch block and hemiblock (fascicular block) are terms used to describe aberrant conduction in the ventricles where the focus originates from above the bundle branches. These patterns of aberrant conduction must be distinguished from beats of ventricular origin, which can have a similar QRS morphology.

than 0.12 second. The two criteria for bundle branch block recognition are:

- A QRS complex equal to or greater than 0.12 second
- QRS complexes produced by supraventricular activity

Ventricular conduction disturbances are best identified by monitoring leads MCL_1 and MCL_6 (or by monitoring V_1 and V_6 with a 12-lead machine). These leads permit the easiest differentiation of the right and left bundle branch blocks. For ECG evaluation, the paramedic should ensure that the electrodes are placed properly for leads I, II, and III. Lead MCL_1 looks at both right and left bundle branches and should be monitored during transport of these patients.[6]

NOTE

For the purpose of this discussion, the reader should assume that all MCL_1 descriptions can be applied to V_1 if using 12-lead monitoring.

Normal Conduction

In normal ventricular stimulation, the electrical impulse occurs first in the septum and then travels from the left endocardium through to the right endocardium of the septum (Fig. 28-90). This generates a small R wave in MCL_1. The remaining impulses primarily are conducted away from the MCL_1 electrode, yielding a negative deflection. Therefore during normal conduction, MCL_1 predominantly is negative and the QRS complex usually is 0.08 to 0.10 wide (the same as any other narrow QRS complex).

Right Bundle Branch Block

In right bundle branch block, the left bundle branch performs normally, thus activating the left

side of the heart before the right (Fig. 28-91). When the left ventricle is activated initially, the impulse travels away from the MCL_1 electrode, yielding a negative deflection (S wave). The electrical impulse then travels across the interventricular septum and activates the right ventricle. Since the impulse is coming back toward the MCL_1 electrode, a large positive deflection (R wave) occurs, resulting in the RSR' pattern seen in MCL_1 in patients with right bundle branch block. The QRS (or in this case, RSR) complex is at least 0.12 second.

NOTE

Whenever the two criteria for bundle branch block are met and MCL_1 displays an RSR' pattern, right bundle branch block should be suspected.

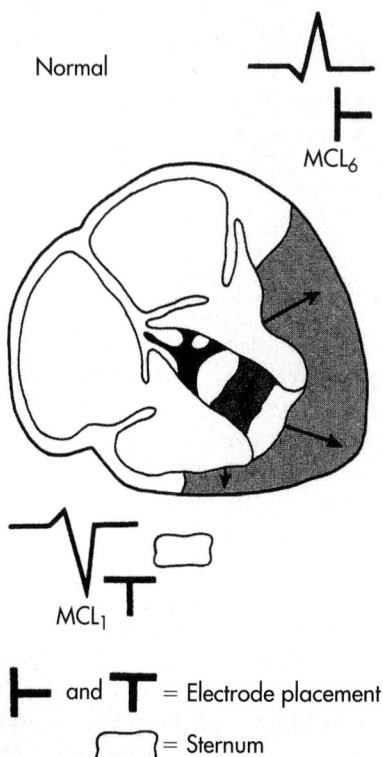

Fig. 28-90 Normal ventricular conduction. (From *JEMS*, pp 42-43, May 1990.)

RBBB

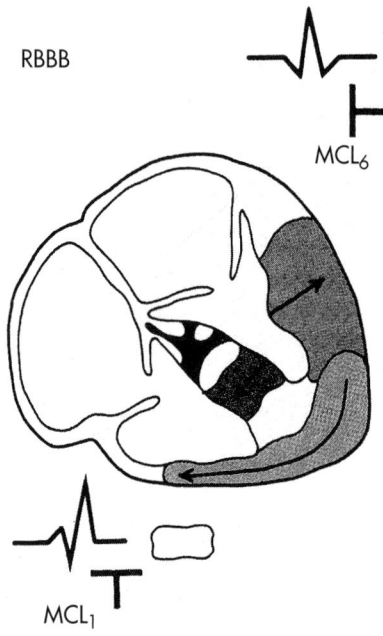

MCL₆

MCL₁

Fig. 28-91 Right bundle branch block. (From *JEMS,* pp 42-43, May 1990.)

LBBB

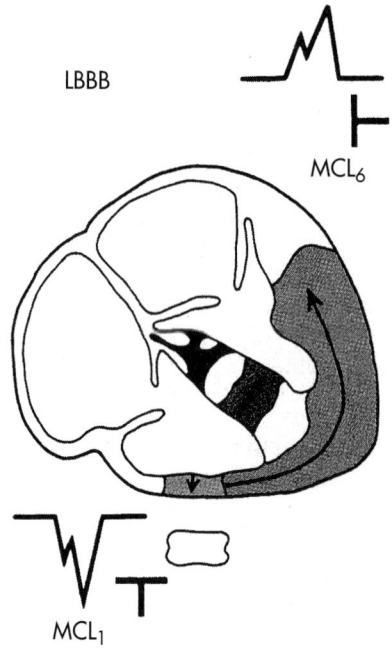

MCL₆

MCL₁

Fig. 28-92 Left bundle branch block. (From *JEMS,* pp 42-43, May 1990.)

BOX 28-3

DETERMINING RIGHT OR LEFT BUNDLE BRANCH BLOCK

When lead MCL_1 is monitored, the bundle branch block may be determined by the following procedure (see Fig. 28-93).
1. Find a QRS complex that is at least 0.12 second wide.
2. Draw a line backward from the J point (the point at which the QRS complex ends and the ST segment begins) into the QRS complex.
3. Fill in the triangle that is created by this line and the last portion of the QRS complex.
4. If the triangle points up it is a right bundle branch block.
5. If the triangle points down, it is a left bundle branch block.

Left Bundle Branch Block

In left bundle branch block, the fibers that usually fire the interventricular septum are blocked. This alters normal septal activation and sends it in the opposite direction (Fig. 28-92). This yields an initial Q wave in MCL_1 instead of the normal small R wave. The right ventricle is then activated, producing a

positive deflection R wave in MCL_1; this impulse travels across the interventricular septum to the left ventricle. Since the impulse is leading away from MCL_1, it shows a deep, wide S wave (QS pattern). As with right bundle branch block, the activation takes at least 0.12 second (Box 28-3).

NOTE

Whenever the two criteria for bundle branch block are met and a QS pattern is seen in MCL_1, a left bundle branch block should be suspected.

Anterior Hemiblock

Anterior hemiblocks (anterior hemifascicular blocks) occur more frequently than posterior hemiblocks (posterior hemifascicular blocks). The anterior fascicle of the left bundle branch is a longer and thinner structure, and its blood supply comes primarily from the left anterior descending (LAD) coronary artery. Anterior hemiblock is characterized by left axis deviation (described on p. 862) in a patient who has a supraventricular rhythm (Fig. 28-94). Other ECG findings associated with an anterior hemiblock

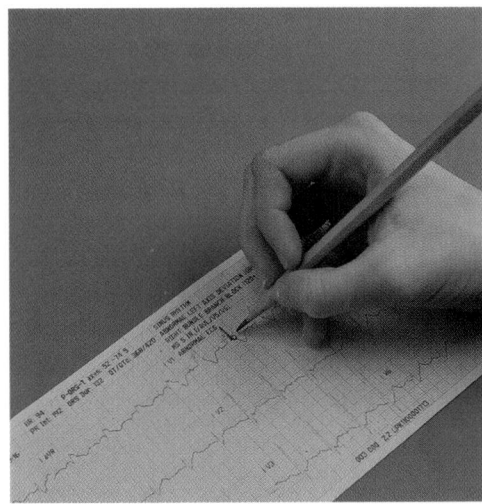

Fig. 28-93 To distinguish left from right bundle branch blocks, find the J point of the QRS complex, draw a line backward into the QRS complex, and fill in the triangle created by this line and the last portion of the QRS complex. The direction the triangle points distinguishes the two types of blocks.

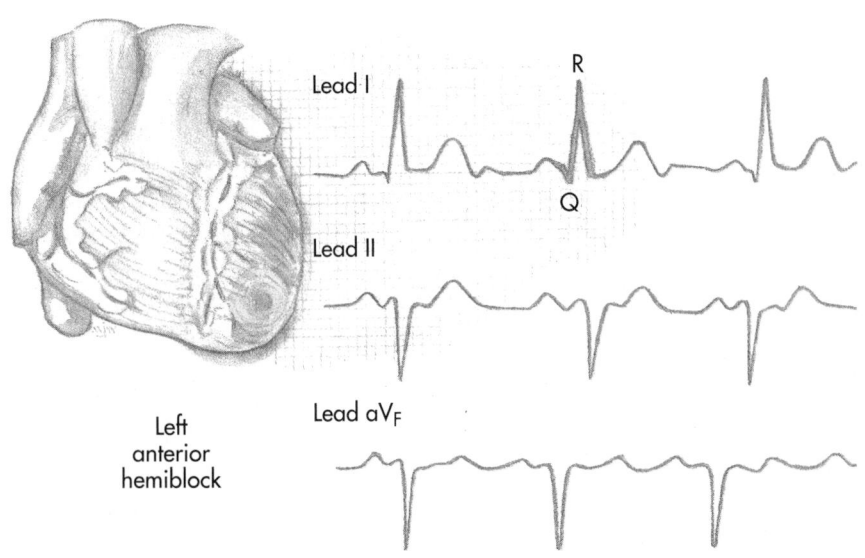

Lead I

Lead II

Left anterior hemiblock

Lead aV_F

Fig. 28-94 Anterior hemiblock.

include a normal QRS complex (less than 0.12 second) or a right bundle branch block, a small Q wave followed by a tall R wave in lead I, and a small R wave followed by a deep S wave in lead III. In a patient who has an anterior hemiblock with a right bundle branch block, impulses can only be conducted through the ventricles by way of the posterior fascicle of the left bundle branch. These patients are at high risk of developing complete heart block.

Posterior Hemiblock

The posterior fascicle of the left bundle branch does not become blocked as easily as the anterior fascicle and, consequently, posterior hemiblock occurs less frequently. Posterior hemiblock is identified by right axis deviation with a normal QRS complex or a right bundle branch block (Fig. 28-95). A definitive diagnosis for posterior hemiblock necessitates

? CRITICAL THINKING

What rhythms are produced by supraventricular activity?

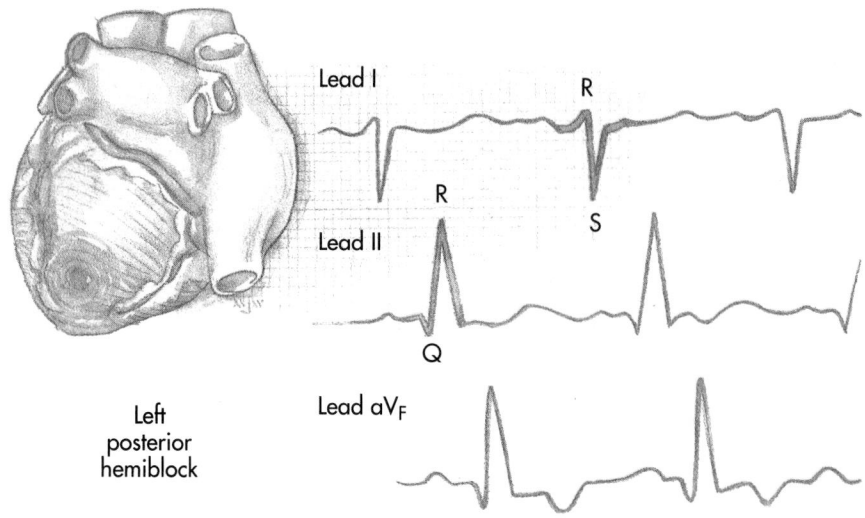

Fig. 28-95 Posterior hemiblock.

excluding right ventricular hypertrophy, which is difficult to do in the prehospital setting. For practical purposes, posterior hemiblock can be assumed in patients with right axis deviation and a QRS complex of normal width or with a right bundle branch block. (Other ECG findings that indicate the presence of a posterior hemiblock include a small R wave followed by a deep S wave in lead I and a small Q wave followed by a tall R wave in lead III.)

Bifascicular Block

Bifascicular block refers to the blockage of two out of three pathways for ventricular conduction. This condition occurs in the presence of right bundle branch block with anterior or posterior hemiblock and in left bundle branch block. Bifascicular block compromises myocardial contractility and cardiac output. Patients with this condition may develop complete heart block suddenly and without warning.

> **NOTE**
>
> As a rule, the more fascicles with impaired condition, the greater the chance a patient will develop complete AV block (especially in patients with AMI).

Multi-Lead Determination of the Axis and Hemiblocks

Identifying the axis (the direction of impulse flow in the heart that stimulates contraction) can be useful in determining the presence of hemiblocks (best evaluated by looking at the QRS complexes in leads I, II, and III). The axis is considered *normal* when the QRS deflection is positive (upright) in all bipolar leads; *physiological left* (which may be normal in some patients) when the QRS deflection is positive in leads I and II but negative (inverted) in lead III; *pathological left* when the QRS deflection is positive in lead I and negative in leads II and III (indicating an anterior hemiblock); *right axis* when the QRS deflection is negative in lead I, negative or positive in lead II, and positive in lead III (pathological in any adult and indicative of a posterior hemiblock); and *extreme right* ("no man's land") when the QRS deflection is negative in all three leads (indicating that the rhythm is ventricular in origin) (Table 28-2).

Management of Bundle Branch Blocks and Hemiblocks

There is no management per se for bundle branch blocks or hemiblocks except to say that if there are coexisting conditions (e.g., hypoxia, ischemia, electrolyte imbalance, drug toxicity) that may be causing a transient block in the ventricular conduction pathways, these conditions should be managed. Some emergency medications administered to cardiac patients (e.g., *procainamide* [Pronestyl], *digoxin* [Lanoxin], and *verapamil* [Isoptin] or *diltiazem* [Cardizem]) can impede electrical impulse conduction through the AV node. Thus to safely administer these medications, the paramedic must ensure that

TABLE 28-2   **IDENTIFYING AXIS BY QRS COMPLEX**

AXIS	QRS COMPLEX: LEAD I	LEAD II	LEAD III	INDICATIONS
Normal	Upright	Upright	Upright	May be normal
Physiological left	Upright	Upright	Inverted	May be normal
Pathological left	Upright	Inverted	Inverted	Anterior hemiblock
Right axis	Inverted	Inverted or upright	Upright	Posterior hemiblock
Extreme right	Inverted	Inverted	Inverted	Ventricular in origin

the patient is not at high risk of developing complete heart block. Those at such risk include:

- Any patient with type II AV block
- Any patient with evidence of disease in both bundle branches
- Any patient with two or more blocks of any kind (e.g., prolonged PR interval and anterior hemiblock, right bundle branch block and anterior hemiblock, type I AV block, and left bundle branch block)

Prehospital care for these patients should include management of any accompanying signs and symptoms, transport, constant ECG monitoring, and anticipation of the possible need for external pacing. Emergency pacing has been recommended for the following four indications[1]:

1. Hemodynamically compromising bradycardias
2. Bradycardias with malignant escape rhythms unresponsive to pharmacological therapy
3. Overdrive pacing of refractory supraventricular or ventricular tachycardia unresponsive to pharmacological therapy or cardioversion
4. Bradyasystolic cardiac arrest (in rare situations)

The AHA also recommends "pacing readiness" in the setting of AMI for patients with symptomatic sinus node dysfunction; type II second-degree block; third-degree heart block; or newly acquired left, right, or alternating bundle branch block or bifascicular block.[1]

Pulseless Electrical Activity

The term *pulseless electrical activity (PEA—also known as electromechanical dissociation [EMD])* (Fig. 28-96) is defined as the absence of a detectable pulse and the presence of some type of electrical activity other than VT or VF).[1] The prognosis for PEA invariably is poor unless an underlying cause can be identified and corrected. Therefore the highest priority of care is to maintain circulation for the patient with basic and advanced life support techniques while searching for a correctable etiology.

Correctable causes of PEA are cardiac tamponade, tension pneumothorax, hypoxemia, acidosis, hyperkalemia, hypothermia, and overdoses of, for example, tricyclic antidepressants, beta blockers, and digitalis. Other less correctable causes include massive myocardial damage from infarction, prolonged ischemia during resuscitation, profound hypovolemia, and massive pulmonary embolism. Patients in profound shock of any type (including anaphylactic, septic, neurogenic, and hypovolemic) may present with PEA. Tension pneumothorax should be managed with needle decompression; hypoxemia should be managed by improving oxygenation and ventilation. If acute hypovolemia is present (secondary to hemorrhage), fluid resuscitation with volume expanders should be initiated. Acidosis should be managed by ensuring adequate CPR and hyperventilation; if preexisting acidosis (e.g., diabetic ketoacidosis [DKA]) or hyperkalemia is suspected (e.g., a patient on home dialysis), the use of **sodium bicarbonate** may be indicated. **Calcium** is a specific therapy for hyperkalemia and calcium channel blocker toxicity, both of which can produce PEA. Besides calcium channel blockers, other drugs when taken in toxic amounts can produce wide-complex PEA. These overdoses can be managed with specific therapy, which may be effective in reestablishing a perfusing rhythm (see Fig. 28-58).

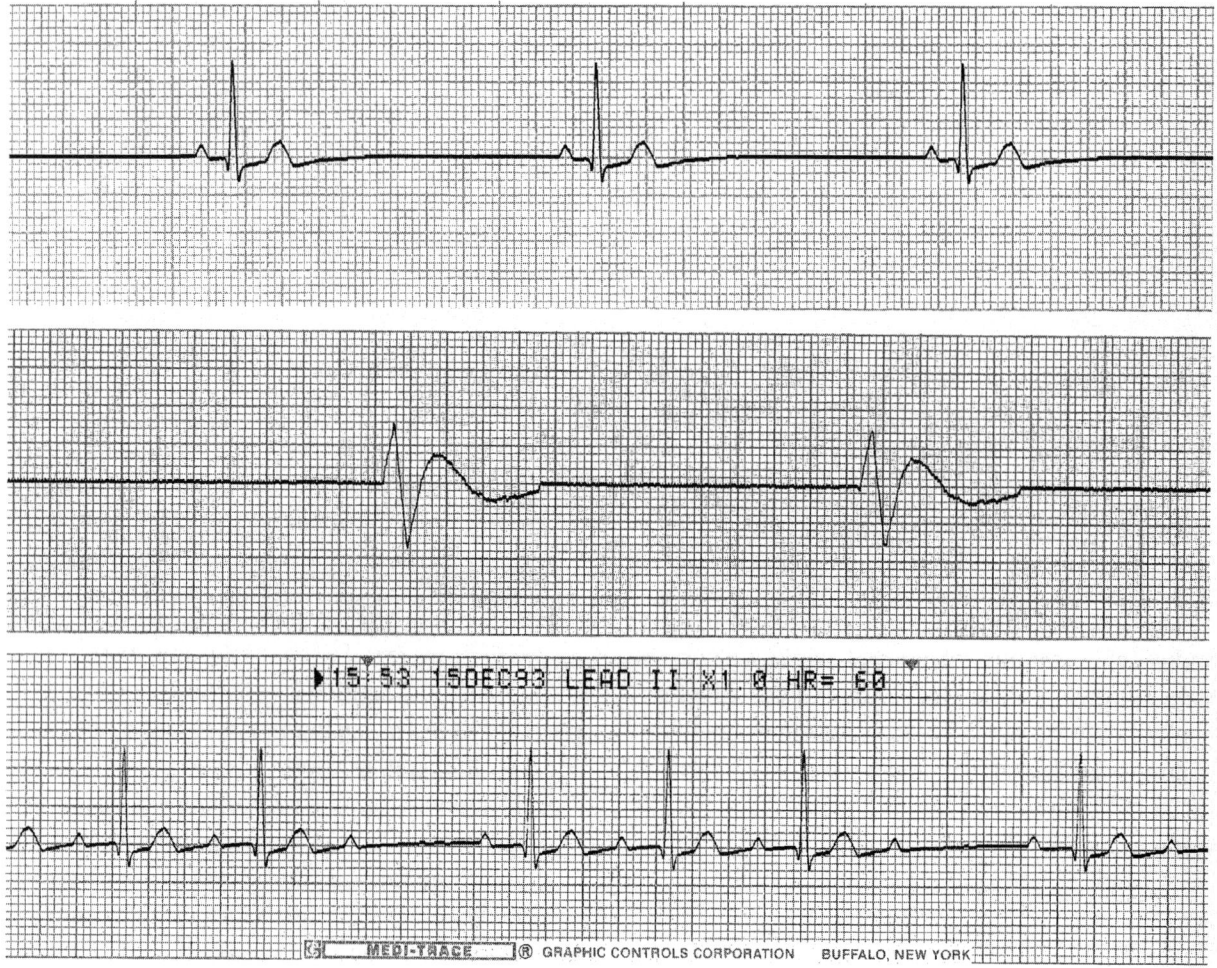

Fig. 28-96 Various PEA rhythms as seen in lead II.

What rhythms might you see on the monitor when a patient is in PEA?

What patient care measures should you take in this case?

Preexcitation Syndromes

Preexcitation syndrome (anomalous or accelerated AV conduction) is a clinical condition associated with an abnormal conduction pathway between the atria and ventricles that bypasses the AV node and/or bundle of His and allows the electrical impulses to initiate depolarization of the ventricles earlier than usual. This premature ventricular activation may occur through one of several accessory pathways. The most common preexcitation syndrome is Wolff-Parkinson-White (WPW) syndrome.

Wolff-Parkinson-White Syndrome
Description

In some hearts, an accessory muscle bundle (known as the **bundle of Kent** or the *Kent fibers*) connects the lateral wall of the atrium and the ventricle, bypassing the AV node. This anomaly is associated with early activation of the ventricle (WPW syndrome).[6] WPW syndrome is considered to be of minor clinical significance unless a tachycardia is present, in which case it can become life threatening.

	Normal conduction	WPW
A	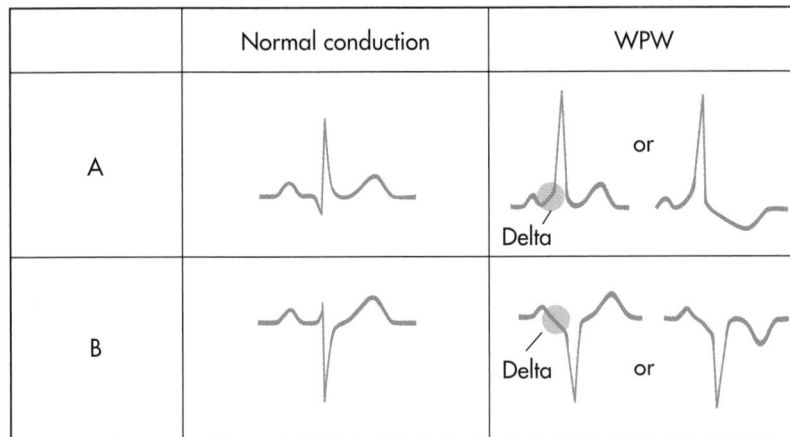	
B		

Fig. 28-97 Characteristic findings in WPW syndrome (short PR interval, QRS widening, and delta wave) compared with normal conduction. **A,** Usual appearance of WPW syndrome in leads where the QRS complex is predominantly upright. **B,** Appearance of WPW syndrome; the QRS complex is predominantly negative. (From Grauer K: *Practical guide to ECG interpretation,* St Louis, 1992, Mosby.)

Etiology

WPW syndrome may occur in young, healthy individuals (predominantly men) without apparent cause. The syndrome also may occur in multiple members of a family and may be present in successive generations.

Rules for Interpretation (Lead II Monitoring)

QRS complex: May be normal or wide (depending on whether conduction is retrograde or anterograde along the bundle of Kent). Conduction that occurs normally down the AV node and simultaneously in an anterograde fashion along the accessory pathway results in a meeting of the two waves or depolarization that forms a fusion (delta wave). A delta wave is evidenced by slurring or notching of the onset of the QRS complex and is a diagnostic finding in WPW syndrome. (Not all leads show the delta wave.)

> **NOTE**
>
> QRS widening may simulate right or left bundle branch block.

P waves: Normal.
Rate: Normal unless associated with rapid supraventricular tachycardia (SVT).
Rhythm: Regular.
PR interval: Usually less than 0.12 second, since the normal delay at the AV node does not occur.

The three characteristic ECG findings in WPW (Fig. 28-97) are a short PR interval, a delta wave, and QRS widening.

Clinical Significance

Patients with WPW syndrome are highly susceptible to bouts of PSVTs. This is because the accessory pathway provides a ready-made reentry circuit that allows continued transmission of the impulse from the atria to the ventricles. The majority of tachydysrhythmias seen in WPW syndrome occur with the wave of depolarization progressing from the AV node to the bundle of His to the accessory pathway, where it conducts in a retrograde direction to the atria. Therefore the majority of tachydysrhythmias seen in WPW syndrome are narrow complexes. Patients with WPW syndrome may have attacks of paroxysmal tachydysrhythmias for many years, but these attacks are not always benign. The AV node may be bypassed, and conduction rates can greatly exceed those in patients whose AV node is part of the reentry circuit. This leads to very rapid tachycardias, which can precipitate congestive heart failure and even death from VF.

Management (Fig. 28-98)

It is important to recognize WPW syndrome and differentiate it from VT and uncomplicated SVT. Many emergency drugs used to manage other reentry tachycardias are contraindicated in WPW syndrome because they can paradoxically facilitate conduction over the accessory pathway. Management must be based on the patient's clinical presentation. If the patient's heart rate is normal, no emergency care is required. If the patient presents with a symptomatic rapid tachycardia, emergency intervention is indicated to restore a normal

Wolff-Parkinson-White (WPW) Syndrome

Perform Primary ABCD Survey (Basic Life Support)

(Correct critical problems IMMEDIATELY as they are identified)

• Assess responsiveness, **A**irway, **B**reathing, **C**irculation, ensure availability of monitor/**D**efibrillator

Perform Secondary ABCD Survey (Advanced Life Support)

• Administer oxygen, establish IV access, attach cardiac monitor, administer fluids as needed (O₂, IV, monitor, fluids)
• Assess vital signs, attach pulse oximeter, and monitor blood pressure
• Obtain and review 12-lead ECG, portable chest x-ray, perform a focused history and physical exam

Is the patient stable or unstable?
Is the patient experiencing serious signs and symptoms due to the tachycardia?
Is the patient's cardiac function normal or impaired?

Attempt to identify patient's cardiac rhythm using 12-lead ECG, clinical information.

Is Wolff-Parkinson-White syndrome (WPW) present? (e.g., young patient, HR > 300, ECG: short PR interval, wide QRS, delta wave)
Has WPW been present for more or less than 48 hours?

NORMAL CARDIAC FUNCTION		IMPAIRED CARDIAC FUNCTION	
Onset < 48 hours	Onset > 48 hours	Onset < 48 hours	Onset > 48 hours
Control Rate	**Control Rate**	**Control Rate**	**Control Rate**
Cardioversion **OR** Amiodarone (IIb) **OR** Procainamide (IIb) **OR** Flecainide (IIb) **OR** Propafenone (IIb) **OR** Sotalol (IIb)	Use antiarrhythmics with extreme caution because of embolic risk	Cardioversion **OR** amiodarone (IIb) Note: Impaired cardiac function = ejection fraction <40% or CHF	Use antiarrhythmics with extreme caution because of embolic risk
Convert Rhythm	**Convert Rhythm**	**Convert Rhythm**	**Convert Rhythm**
Cardioversion **OR** Amiodarone (IIb) **OR** Procainamide (IIb) **OR** Flecainide (IIb) **OR** Propafenone (IIb) **OR** Sotalol (IIb)	Delayed cardioversion **OR** Early cardioversion	Cardioversion	Delayed cardioversion **OR** Early cardioversion

Delayed cardioversion:

Anticoagulation therapy for 3 weeks before cardioversion, for at least 48 hours in conjunction with cardioversion, and for at least 4 weeks after successful cardioversion. **Early cardioversion:** IV heparin immediately, transesophageal echocardiography (TEE) to r/o atrial thrombus, cardioversion within 24 h, anticoagulation x 4 wks

MEDICATION DOSING

Amiodarone* 150 mg IV bolus over 10 minutes followed by an infusion of 1 mg/min for 6 hours and then a maintenance infusion of 0.5 mg/min. Repeat supplementary infusions of 150 mg as necessary for recurrent or resistant dysrhythmias. Maximum total daily dose 2 g.

Procainamide 100 mg over 5 minutes (20 mg/min). Maximum total dose 17 mg/kg. Maintenance infusion 1–4 mg/min.

Flecainide, propafenone IV form not currently approved for use in the United States

Sotalol 1 to 1.5 mg/kg IV slowly at a rate of 10 mg/min

*Chapman MJ et al: Management of atrial tachyarrhythmias in the critically ill: a comparison of intravenous procainamide and amiodarone, *Intensive Care Med* 19:48, 1993.

Fig. 28-98 Wolff-Parkinson-White (WPW) syndrome algorithm. (From Aehlert B: *ACLS quick review study guide*, ed 2, St Louis, 2002, Mosby.)

rhythm by blocking conduction through the accessory pathways from the atria to the ventricles.

Prehospital care may include pharmacological therapy for specific dysrhythmias, vagal maneuvers for PSVT, *adenosine* (Adenocard), or cardioversion for severe clinical deterioration. *Verapamil* (Isoptin) is contraindicated in wide-QRS tachycardia because the drug may precipitate very rapid atrial-to-ventricular conduction down the accessory pathway (greater than 280 beats per minute) and may lead to VF and sudden death. Therefore in patients with wide-QRS tachycardia, the management of choice depends on the clinical impression and severity of symptoms. *Amiodarone* (Cordarone) or *Lidocaine* (Xylocaine) are the first drugs of choice for presumed VT, and *adenosine* (Adenocard) and *procainamide* (Pronestyl) are the initial choices for presumed SVT and SVT with aberrant conduction. Cardioversion should be performed without delay in patients with rapid ventricular rates (greater than 150 beats per minute) who are unstable.

SECTION SEVEN
SPECIFIC CARDIOVASCULAR DISEASES

Pathophysiology and Management of Cardiovascular Disease

Many true medical emergencies are cardiovascular in nature; they often result from atherosclerosis of the coronary arteries or peripheral arteries. The specific medical conditions in this section are:

- Atherosclerosis
- Angina pectoris
- Myocardial infarction
- Left ventricular failure and pulmonary edema
- Right ventricular failure
- Cardiogenic shock
- Cardiac tamponade
- Thoracic and abdominal aneurysm
- Acute arterial occlusion
- Noncritical peripheral vascular disorders
- Hypertension

Pathophysiology of Atherosclerosis

Atherosclerosis is a disease process characterized by progressive narrowing of the lumen of medium and large arteries (e.g., the aorta and its branches, cerebral arteries, coronary arteries). The process results in the development of thick, hard atherosclerotic plaque referred to as atheromas or *atheromatous lesions.* These lesions most commonly are found in areas of turbulent blood flow such as vessel bifurcations or in vessels with decreased lumen diameter.

Atherosclerosis is thought to be a result of the endothelial cell response to chronic mechanical or chemical injury. This response includes platelet adhesion and aggregation (secondary to the release of certain chemical mediators), and proliferation and migration of smooth muscle cells from the media (where they normally are found) into the intima, forming the atheroma. Over time, the atheromas become fibrotic and calcified, partially or totally obstructing the involved arteries. In most cases, some collateral circulation develops to compensate for the narrowed vessels.

Major Risk Factors

Atherosclerosis occurs to some extent in all middle-aged and older people and in some young people. The condition seems to have a heritable component and usually is seen at a younger age in men than in women. Associated risk factors include age, family history, and predisposing illness (e.g., diabetes). Risk factors that can be reduced or eliminated include cigarette smoking, obesity, hypertension, and hypercholesterolemia. Some research has shown that plaque formation is not only preventable but reversible.[1]

Effects

Atherosclerosis has two major effects on blood vessels: (1) the disease disrupts the intimal surface, causing a loss of vessel elasticity and an increase in thrombogenesis, and (2) the atheroma reduces the diameter of the vessel lumen and thus decreases the blood supply to tissues. Both effects result in an insufficient supply of nutrients to the tissue, particularly under conditions of increased demand.

The severity of this insufficiency is related to the extent of narrowing (stenosis) in the blocked arterial segment, the time interval during which the occlusion develops, and the patient's inherent ability to develop collateral circulation around the obstruction. For example, a patient who gradually develops an atherosclerotic occlusion in a distal artery of a lower extremity may compensate well for the vascular insufficiency through collateral circulation. The patient may experience only mild, intermittent pain during periods of exercise. In contrast, sudden-onset occlusion in a coronary artery (secondary to an acute thrombus) almost always results in ischemia, injury, and necrosis to the area of the myocardium supplied by the affected artery.

Angina Pectoris

Angina pectoris is a symptom of myocardial ischemia; the term literally means "choking pain in the chest." It is caused by an imbalance between myocardial oxygen supply and demand. The result is an accumulation of lactic acid and carbon dioxide in ischemic tissues of the myocardium. These metabolites irritate nerve endings that produce anginal pain. The most common cause of angina pectoris is atherosclerotic disease of the coronary arteries. A temporary occlusion caused by spasm of a coronary artery with or without atherosclerosis (Prinzmetal's angina) also can cause angina pectoris. Precipitating events for development of angina, particularly in patients with atherosclerosis, include emotional stress and any activity that increases myocardial oxygen demand. Myocardial ischemia may, in turn, predispose the patient to dysrhythmias.

> **NOTE**
>
> There are several noncardiac conditions that can mimic signs and symptoms of atherosclerotic disease and angina pectoris. These include cholecystitis, peptic ulcer disease, aneurysm, hiatal hernia, pulmonary embolism, pancreatitis, pleural irritation, and respiratory infection, among others (Box 28-4).

Angina pectoris generally is classified as *stable* or *unstable*. Stable angina usually is precipitated by physical exertion or emotional stress. The pain typically lasts 1 to 5 minutes but may last as long as 15 minutes and is relieved by rest, *nitroglycerin* (Nitrostat), or oxygen. Stable angina "attacks" usually are similar in nature and are always relieved by the same mode of therapy.

Unstable angina (preinfarction angina) denotes an anginal pattern that has changed in its ease of onset, frequency, intensity, duration, or quality. (This includes any "new onset" anginal chest pain.) It may occur during periods of light exercise or at rest. The pain usually lasts 10 minutes or more and is less promptly relieved with cessation of activity or *nitroglycerin* (Nitrostat) than the stable anginal pattern. Unstable angina mimics AMI, and the two are sometimes difficult to differentiate in the prehospital setting. Patients with unstable angina are at increased risk of AMI and sudden death.

> **NOTE**
>
> Many people do not describe anginal symptoms as pain, hence the question "Do you have chest pain?" may be answered in the negative.

The pain of angina usually is described by the patient as a pressure, squeezing, heaviness, or tightness in the chest. Although 30% of patients with angina feel pain only in the chest, others describe the pain as radiating to the shoulders, arms, neck, and jaw, and through to the back. Associated signs and symptoms include anxiety, shortness of breath, nausea or vomiting, and diaphoresis. The patient history often reveals previous attacks of angina. Many times, the patient will have taken *nitroglycerin* (Nitrostat) before EMS arrival. If so, the paramedic should determine the age of the *nitroglycerin* prescription (*nitroglycerin* is unstable and quickly loses its strength), the amount of *nitroglycerin* taken, and its effect. If the pain is not relieved by rest and medication, a myocardial infarction should be suspected.

Management

All patients with chest pain and signs and symptoms of myocardial ischemia should be managed as though an AMI were evolving. The goal of management is to increase the coronary blood supply, decrease the myocardial oxygen demand, or both. Management guidelines include the following:

1. Place the patient at rest physically and emotionally.
2. Administer oxygen.
3. Administer *aspirin* (per protocol).
4. Initiate IV therapy for any drugs that may be needed.

5. If pain is present on EMS arrival, use pharmacological therapy, which may include sublingual or topical *nitroglycerin* followed by *morphine*.
6. Monitor the ECG for dysrhythmias. Whenever possible (and if scene time is not excessively delayed), record and transmit a 3-lead and/or 12-lead ECG during pain. (The ECG may be normal during a pain-free period.) Also measure, record, and communicate any ST-segment changes.
7. Transport the patient for physician evaluation.

Myocardial Infarction

Acute myocardial infarction (AMI) occurs when there is a sudden and total occlusion or near-occlusion of blood flowing through an affected coronary artery to an area of heart muscle. This results in ischemia, injury, and necrosis to the area of the myocardium distal to the occlusion. AMI most often is associated with atherosclerotic heart disease (ASHD).

Precipitating Events

The process of myocardial infarction is dynamic and complex and generally begins with the formation of an atherosclerotic plaque involving the intimal layer of a coronary artery. The plaque disrupts the smooth arterial lining and results in an uneven surface, which creates turbulent blood flow. The plaque may rupture, exposing the injured tissue to circulating platelets, resulting in the formation of a thrombus that occludes the artery. As the thrombus enlarges, it further reduces blood flow in the coronary vessel.

Acute thrombotic occlusion generally is accepted as the precipitating event in the vast majority of myocardial infarctions. Other factors that may lead to AMI include coronary spasm, coronary embolism, severe hypoxia, hemorrhage into a diseased arterial wall, and reduced blood flow after any form of shock, all of which may result in an inadequate amount of blood reaching the myocardium.

Types and Locations of Infarcts

Infarction of the myocardium develops distal to the occluded artery. The size of the infarct is determined by the metabolic needs of the tissue supplied solely or predominantly by the occluded vessel, by the presence of collateral circulation, and by the duration of time until flow is reestablished. Therefore emergency care is directed at:

> ### BOX 28-4
>
> ### OTHER CONDITIONS THAT MAY MIMIC ANGINA PECTORIS
>
> Thoracic aortic dissection
> Pancreatitis
> Cholecystitis
> Hiatal hernia
> Esophageal disease
> Gastric reflux
> Pulmonary embolism
> Peptic ulcer disease
> Chest wall syndrome
> Costochrondritis
> Acromioclavicular disease
> Pleural irritation
> Respiratory infection
> Pneumothorax
> Dyspepsia
> Herpes zoster
> Chest wall tumors
> Chest wall trauma

- Increasing oxygen supply by administering supplemental oxygen
- Decreasing the metabolic needs and providing collateral circulation
- Reestablishing perfusion to the ischemic myocardium as quickly as possible after the onset of symptoms

The majority of AMIs involve the left ventricle or interventricular septum, which is supplied by either of the two major coronary arteries (although some patients sustain damage to the right ventricle). If the occlusion is in the left coronary artery, the result is an anterior, lateral, or septal wall infarction. Inferior wall infarction (of the inferior-posterior wall of the left ventricle) usually is a result of right coronary artery occlusion.

Infarction also can be classified into one of three ischemic syndromes based on the rupture of an unstable plaque in an epicardial artery: unstable angina, non–Q-wave myocardial infarction, and Q-wave myocardial infarction.[1] In unstable angina, the early thrombus has not completely obstructed coronary flow, causing an intermittent ischemic episode that may eventually result in complete occlusion and AMI. Non–Q-wave infarcts are evident

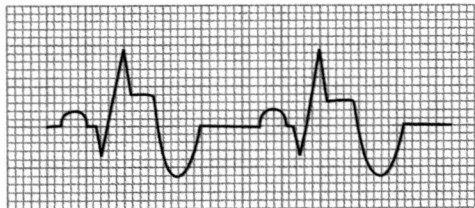

Fig. 28-99 Pathological Q waves.

only with ST-segment depression or T-wave abnormalities. Q-wave infarcts are diagnosed by the development of abnormal Q waves (Q waves greater than 5 mm in depth or greater than 0.04 second in duration) in two or more contiguous leads (Fig. 28-99).

> **NOTE**
>
> Unstable angina, non–Q-wave myocardial infarction, and Q-wave myocardial infarction represent a continuum of a similar disease process. All three of these acute coronary syndromes share common risk factors, and management overlaps considerably.

Death of Myocardium

When blood flow to the myocardium ceases, a cascade of events begins. Cells switch from aerobic to anaerobic metabolism, resulting in the release of lactic acid and increasing carbon dioxide tissue levels. This contributes to ischemic pain (angina). As cells lose their ability to maintain their electrochemical gradients, they begin to swell and depolarize. These initial changes are reversible, but within a few hours, if collateral flow and reperfusion are inadequate, much of the muscle distal to the occlusion dies. The area surrounding the necrotic tissue may survive because of collateral circulation, but it may become the origin of dysrhythmias (Fig. 28-100).

Scar tissue replaces the infarcted area in a process that takes about 8 weeks, starting with deposits of connective tissue on approximately the twelfth day. Although scar tissue is durable, it lacks elasticity, does not contract, and conducts the depolarization wave front poorly in the damaged area of the myocardium. The left ventricle, however, can lose as much as 25% of its muscle and still function as an effective pump. Areas with poor perfusion after a large myocardial infarction may not develop strong scar tissue, resulting in an aneurysmal area that can markedly diminish the effectiveness of ventricular

contractility and lead to the development of serious dysrhythmias.

The damaged myocardium is most vulnerable to rupture during the first 1 to 2 weeks after a myocardial infarction, since the scar tissue has not attained adequate tensile strength. For this reason, minimal activity and the prevention of hypertension and excitement usually are necessary during this period. Nonetheless, over the last several years, the length of hospitalization in patients with uncomplicated myocardial infarctions has progressively decreased. Today, most patients resume activity within 2 to 3 days and leave the hospital within 7 to 10 days. Many patients get a submaximal stress test before discharge to determine the patient's exercise tolerance level and whether there may be continued ischemia or a predisposition to dysrhythmias. The result of this test and clinical impression helps dictate what activities the patient may resume after discharge.

Deaths Secondary to Myocardial Infarction

Deaths secondary to myocardial infarction usually result from lethal dysrhythmias (VT, VF, and cardiac standstill), pump failure (cardiogenic shock and congestive heart failure), or myocardial tissue rupture (rupture of the ventricle, septum, or papillary muscle). Fatal dysrhythmias are the most common cause of death from myocardial infarction. Deaths that occur within the first 2 hours after the onset of illness or injury are sudden deaths. The majority of patients who suffer sudden death have no immediate premonitory symptoms.

> **NOTE**
>
> Sudden death is defined as a sudden dysrhythmic death that occurs within the first 2 hours of cardiac ischemic symptoms.[1] More than 50% of cardiac deaths occur with no evidence of infarction noted on postmortem examination when resuscitation attempts fail. Sudden death without infarction is a primary reason for the widespread availability of AEDs (in addition to the fact that the most common terminal dysrhythmia is VF).

Signs and Symptoms

Although some patients with AMI, particularly diabetic patients and those in the older age groups, have only symptoms of dyspnea, syncope, or confusion, substernal chest pain is present in 70% to 90%

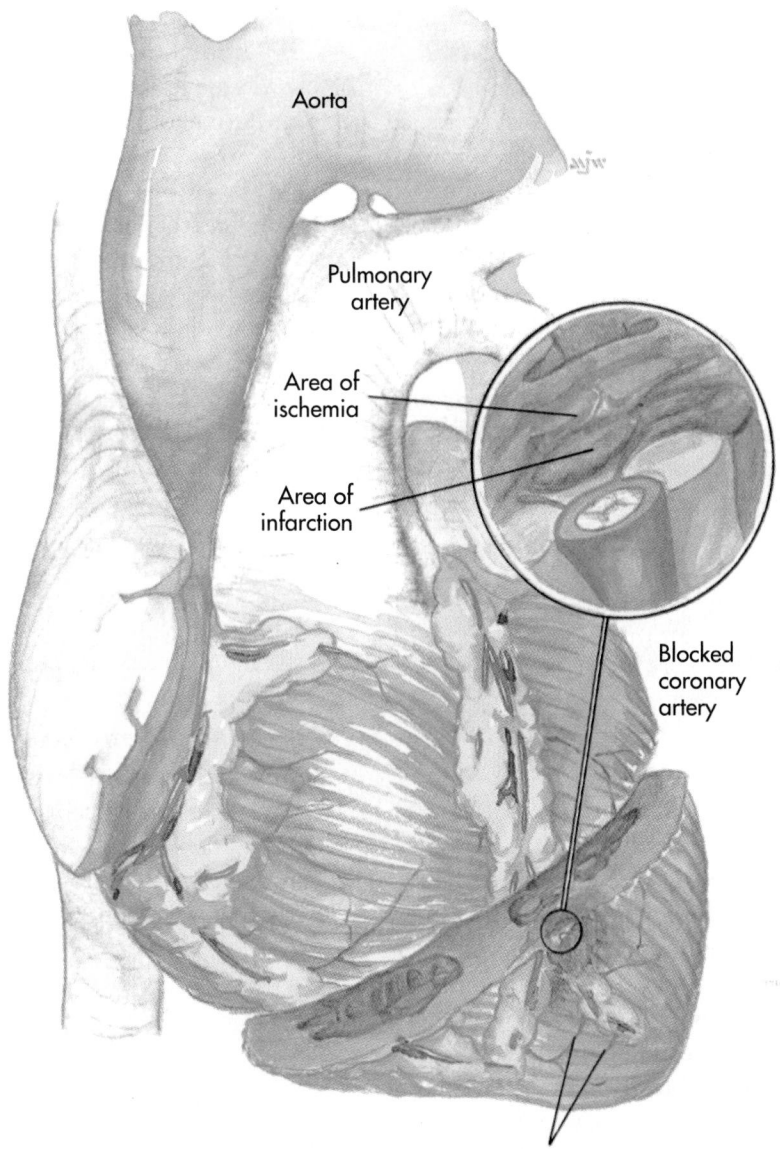

Aorta

Pulmonary artery

Area of ischemia

Area of infarction

Blocked coronary artery

Areas of collateral circulation

Fig. 28-100 Area of infarct.

of patients with AMI. The pain generally has the same characteristics and locations as anginal pain and may radiate to the arms, neck, jaw, or back. The following signs and symptoms may accompany the pain and occasionally are present even in the absence of pain ("silent myocardial infarction"):

- Dyspnea
- Anxiety
- Agitation
- Sense of impending doom
- Nausea and vomiting
- Diaphoresis
- Cyanosis
- Palpitations

The chest pain associated with AMI often is constant and is not altered or alleviated by *nitroglycerin* (Nitrostat) or other cardiac medications, rest, changes in body position, or breathing patterns. Unlike angina pectoris, which frequently occurs during periods of activity, the onset of pain in over half of all patients with AMI occurs during rest. Most patients have experienced warning anginal pains (preinfarction angina) hours or days before the attack. Many patients deny the possibility of an evolving myocardial infarction and attribute the chest pain or discomfort to unrelated causes such as fatigue or indigestion. This denial is a serious problem because it delays the request for EMS assistance during the most critical phase of the illness. According to the AHA, more than 50% of deaths from ischemic heart disease occur outside the hospital within the first 2 hours after the onset of pain.[1]

> **? CRITICAL THINKING**
>
> *How can the prehospital recognition of AMI affect the hospital care of the patient?*

> **? CRITICAL THINKING**
>
> *Why do you think patients deny that their signs and symptoms may be due to a heart attack?*

Vital signs vary, depending on the extent of damage to the heart muscle and conduction system, and the degree and type of autonomic nervous system response. (Inferior myocardial infarctions frequently present with a predominantly parasympathetic autonomic response, whereas anterior myocardial infarctions commonly present with a predominantly sympathetic autonomic response.) For example, the patient's blood pressure may be normal, elevated (sympathetic discharge), or low (parasympathetic discharge or pump failure); the pulse rate (which depends on the presence or absence of dysrhythmias) may be normal, tachycardic, bradycardic, regular, or irregular; and respirations may be normal or increased.

Common ECG Findings

When the heart muscle is damaged, the damaged area is unable to contract effectively and remains in a constant depolarized state. The flow of current between the pathologically depolarized and normally repolarized areas produces abnormal ST-segment elevation on the ECG tracing (Fig. 28-101). ST-segment elevation greater than 0.1 mV in at least two contiguous ECG leads indicates AMI. However, the initial ECG may not demonstrate ST-segment elevation in patients who are infarcting. Even if it is present, ST-segment elevation is a poor indicator of whether the infarction will be Q-wave or non–Q-wave infarction. ST-segment elevation also may be caused by conditions other than AMI, including the following:

- Left bundle branch block
- Some ventricular rhythms
- Left ventricular hypertrophy
- Pericarditis
- Ventricular aneurysm
- Early repolarization

> **NOTE**
>
> When ST-segment elevation is present in a patient suspected of having an AMI, the paramedic should notify the physician and transmit an ECG for evaluation (according to protocol).

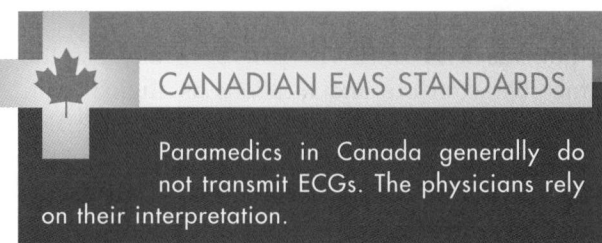

> **CANADIAN EMS STANDARDS**
>
> Paramedics in Canada generally do not transmit ECGs. The physicians rely on their interpretation.

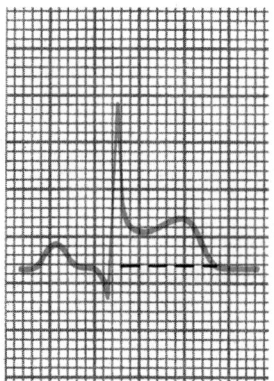

Fig. 28-101 ST-segment elevation likely to present with acute injury. (From Grauer K: *Practical guide to ECG interpretation*, St Louis, 1992, Mosby.)

Using a 12-Lead ECG to Assess Infarcts

Early recognition and management of AMI can sometimes salvage a damaged myocardium ("time is muscle"). Paramedics can play an important role in identifying these patients by using the five-step analysis for infarct recognition.[2]

Step 1: Identify rate and rhythm. Recognition and management of life-threatening rhythms takes precedence over 12-lead ECG monitoring for infarct location.

Step 2: Identify the area of infarct. ST-segment elevation is the most reliable marker during the first hours of infarction and may be recognized before serious tissue damage has occurred. If ST-segment elevation is present in a patient with chest pain, the paramedic should identify the degree of elevation and visualize cardiac anatomy to predict which coronary artery is occluded. A systematic approach for multi-lead assessment should be used. One method is to begin by monitoring the inferior leads (II, III, aV$_F$), followed by septal leads (V$_1$, V$_2$), anterior leads (V$_3$, V$_4$), and lateral leads (V$_5$, V$_6$, I, aV$_L$). The paramedic then evaluates each lead for ST-segment elevation (the most important sign of injury), deep symmetrically inverted T waves (a sign of ischemia), ST depression (a reciprocal change to ST elevation), and pathological Q waves (Table 28-3 and Fig. 28-102).

> **NOTE**
>
> The extent of the infarction sometimes can be gauged by the number of leads showing ST-segment elevation and the degree of ST-segment elevation. For example, large infarcts often will show an ST elevation of 7 mm or more in inferior leads and an ST elevation of 12 mm or more in anterior leads.

Step 3: Consider miscellaneous conditions. When evaluating the ECG, the paramedic must consider other conditions potentially responsible for ST-segment changes (as previously described). These "infarct impostors" also may be present in a patient who *is* experiencing AMI. With the exception of left bundle branch block (which makes the interpretation of myocardial infarction very difficult), left ventricular hypertrophy provides a less striking resemblance to infarction. Ventricular rhythms often produce both Q waves *and* ST-segment elevation and will not have reciprocal ST depression. ECG changes with pericarditis are very subtle, and early repolarization produces no clinical symptoms.

Step 4: Assess the patient's clinical presentation. An assessment of the patient's clinical condition is equally important as the ECG findings. Therefore

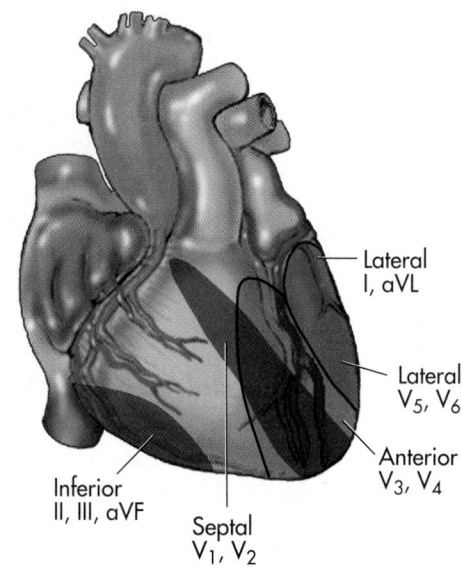

Fig. 28-102 Multilead assessment of the heart.

TABLE 28-3	ST-SEGMENT ELEVATION AND LOCATION OF INFARCT	
LEAD	**LOCATION OF INFARCT**	**CORONARY ARTERY INVOLVED**
II, III, aV$_F$	Inferior wall (most common)	Right
V$_1$, V$_2$	Septal wall	Left
V$_3$, V$_4$	Anterior wall (most lethal)	Left
I, aV$_L$, V$_5$, V$_6$	Lateral wall	Left
V$_4$, V$_5$, V$_6$	Right ventricle	Right

obtaining a thorough patient history and performing a physical examination should be incorporated into the ECG interpretation. Not all patients with AMI will present with classic signs and symptoms, so a high degree of suspicion should be maintained in the absence of pain (especially with diabetic patients, older adults, and postmenopausal women).

> **NOTE**
>
> A significant number of patients with AMI will have no early ECG changes. The clinical picture is therefore very important.

Step 5: Recognize the infarction and initiate care. When all indications point to AMI, the paramedic will need to take steps to speed the process of data collection, physician evaluation, and thrombolysis (when appropriate) to reduce the time from infarct to management.

> **NOTE**
>
> Suspicion of AMI that is based on clinical presentation and ECG findings must be confirmed by medical direction to determine the appropriateness of thrombolytic therapy.

Management of an Uncomplicated AMI (Fig. 28-103)

All patients with chest pain suggestive of angina are assumed to have an evolving myocardial infarction until proved otherwise. Any patient with chest pain should be transported to a medical facility for physician evaluation, regardless of the apparent severity on EMS arrival, the patient's age, or associated complaints. The primary goals of prehospital care are to relieve pain and apprehension, to prevent the development of serious dysrhythmias, and to limit the size of the infarct.

A thorough patient history should be obtained while conducting the physical examination and during initial patient care interventions. Because time is of the essence, the following components of patient care are a high priority:

1. Place the patient physically at rest or in a comfortable position to decrease anxiety and the heart rate, thereby decreasing oxygen demand.

2. Administer low-concentration oxygen (3 to 4 L per minute) via the nasal cannula. Patients with respiratory compromise need a higher oxygen concentration.

3. Initiate transport quickly (without audible or visual warning devices if the patient is stable).

4. Administer *aspirin* (according to protocol).

5. Consider the use of pulse oximetry.

6. Establish an IV line with normal saline or lactated Ringer's solution to keep the vein open.

7. Obtain baseline vital signs and repeat them frequently. Vital sign assessment should include auscultation of lungs for heart failure indicators (presence of crackles).

8. Attach ECG electrodes, document initial rhythm, and monitor for dysrhythmias.

9. Administer medications (by order of medical direction or according to protocol) for the relief of pain and the management of dysrhythmias:
   a. Medications that may be used for analgesia and to decrease preload and afterload include *nitroglycerin* and *morphine.*
   b. Medications that may be used to manage the various dysrhythmias include *lidocaine* (Xylocaine), *procainamide* (Pronestyl), *atropine, verapamil* (Isoptin), *adenosine* (Adenocard), *magnesium, propranolol* (Inderal), and *amiodarone* (Cordarone).

Fibrinolytic Therapy

Studies have shown that an acute intracoronary thrombus can be dissolved (thereby restoring blood flow to the ischemic area) with salvage of ischemic myocardium if a fibrinolytic agent is administered within 6 hours after the onset of symptoms.[1] Some EMS services are authorized by medical direction to administer these agents in the prehospital setting. However, the AHA recommends that prehospital systems focus on early diagnosis; field administration of fibrinolytics should occur in special circumstances when a physician is present or if transport time exceeds 90 minutes.[1]

Common thrombolytic agents include *streptokinase* (Streptase), *tissue plasminogen activator* (t-PA, alteplase), and *reteplase* (Retavase). All of these agents work through activation of the plasma protein plasminogen to dissolve the coronary thrombus. Plasminogen is converted to plasmin (the active form), which degrades fibrin, the basic component of a thrombus. *Aspirin* and *heparin* are part of the "fibrinolytic package."

A fibrinolytic agent can lyse beneficial and pathological thrombi, so the drug is administered selectively. Most EMS systems using fibrinolytic agents establish inclusion-exclusion criteria similar to the following[4]:

1. Patient inclusion criteria
   - Chest pain suggesting AMI for at least 20 minutes
   - Onset of symptoms less than 12 hours
   - Oriented and able to give informed consent
   - ST segment elevation $\geq$1 mm (0.1 mV) in 2 or more contiguous leads
   - Under 75 years of age
2. Patient exclusion criteria
   Absolute Contraindications
   - History of intracranial bleeding or stroke
   - Other stroke or CVA in less than 1 year

Initial Assessment and General Treatment of the Patient with an Acute Coronary Syndrome.

PREHOSPITAL	EMERGENCY DEPARTMENT

Initial Assessment (Goal: targeted clinical exam and 12-lead ECG within 10 minutes)

	RN triage for rapid care
• Obtain a brief, targeted history/physical exam (determine age, gender; S/S, pain presentation including location of pain, duration, quality, relation to effort, time of symptom onset; history CAD, CAD risk factors present?) History of Viagra use? Assess vital signs, determine oxygen saturation	• Targeted history - determine age, gender, S/S, pain presentation including location of pain, duration, quality, relation to effort, time of symptom onset; history CAD, CAD risk factors present? History of Viagra use? • Assess vital signs, determine oxygen saturation • Establish IV access, ECG monitoring • Obtain 12-lead ECG (present to physician for review)

If above consistent with possible or definite ACS:

	Physician evaluation

- Use checklist (yes-no); focus on eligibility for reperfusion therapy; evaluate contraindications to aspirin and heparin
- Establish IV access, ECG monitoring
- Administer aspirin 162 to 325 mg (chewed) if no reason for exclusion
- Obtain 12-lead ECG (machine interpretation or transmission of ECG to physician)
- Draw blood for initial serum cardiac marker levels (to lab on arrival in emergency department)

If above consistent with possible or definite ACS:
- Brief, targeted history/physical exam
- Evaluate eligibility for reperfusion therapy + contraindications to aspirin and heparin
- Administer aspirin 162 to 325 mg (chewed) if no reason for exclusion
- Administer nitroglycerin as indicated
- Evaluate 12-lead ECG—categorize patient into one of three groups: ST-elevation or new or presumably new LBBB; ST-depression/transient ST-segment/T wave changes; normal or nondiagnostic ECG
- Obtain serial ECGs in patients with history suggesting MI and nondiagnostic ECG
- Obtain baseline serum cardiac marker levels (CK-MB, Troponin T or I, myoglobin)
- Obtain lab specimens (CBC, lipid profile, electrolytes, coagulation studies)
- Obtain portable chest x-ray
- Evaluate results

Consider triage to facility capable of angiography and revascularization if any of the following are present:
- Signs of shock
- Pulmonary edema (rales > halfway up)
- Heart rate 100 beats/min and SBP 100 mm Hg

Routine Measures

- Oxygen 4 L/min by nasal cannula for first 2 to 3 hours (Class IIa)
- Oxygen 4 L/min by cannula, titrate if pulmonary congestion, SaO2 < 90% (Class I)
- Aspirin 162 to 325 mg–chewed (if hypersensitivity exists, ticlopidine); may administer via rectal suppository (325 mg) if nausea, vomiting, upper GI disorder present
- NTG SL or spray (ensure IV access, SBP > 90 mm Hg, HR > 50 beats/min, no RV infarction)
- Morphine 2 to 4 mg IV if pain not relieved with NTG; may repeat every 5 min (ensure SBP > 90 mm Hg)

Fig. 28-103 Acute myocardial infarction algorithm. (From Aehlert B: *ACLS quick review study guide*, ed 2, St Louis, 2002, Mosby.) *continued*

Management of ST-Segment Elevation MI.

ST-segment elevation 1 mm in two or more anatomically contiguous leads or new, or presumably new, LBBB
Confirm diagnosis by signs/symptoms, ECG, serum cardiac markers

All patients with ST-segment elevation MI should receive (if no contraindications):
- Antiplatelet therapy - aspirin 162–325 mg (chewed)
- Anti-ischemia therapy (beta-blockers, NTG IV if ongoing ischemia or uncorrected hypertension)
- Antithrombin therapy - heparin (if using fibrin-specific lytics)
- ACE inhibitors (after 6 hours or when stable)–especially with large or anterior MI, heart failure without hypotension (SBP > 100 mm Hg), previous MI

Symptom onset 12 hours?			Symptom onset > 12 hours?	
Patient Eligible for Reperfusion? Goals– • Fibrinolytics: Door-to-drug time < 30 min • Primary PCI: Door-to-dilation time 90 ± 30 min			Persistent Symptoms	Resolution of Symptoms
Yes		No	Consider reperfusion	Medical management
Signs of cardiogenic shock or contraindications in fibrinolytics?		Persistent or stuttering symptoms of EG changes?	Medical management	
Yes	No	Yes	No	
PCI Medical management	Can cath lab be mobilized within 60 min?	Cardiac cath, medical management	Medical management	
	Yes: PCI No: Fibrinolysis (alteplase, reteplase, streptokinase, anisteplase, or tenecteplase)			

Note: PCI = percutaneous coronary intervention (angioplasty ± stent).

Fig. 28-103, cont'd Acute myocardial infarction algorithm.

- Internal bleeding (menses excluded)
- Suspected aortic dissection

Relative Contraindications
- Pregnancy or postpartum state
- Uncontrolled hypertension
- Major surgery within 3 weeks
- Intracranial tumor
- Thoracic aortic aneurysm
- CPR in the nontrauma patient that has been in progress less than 10 minutes
- Trauma (within 2 to 4 weeks)
- Known bleeding disorder or current use of anticoagulants
- Terminal illness

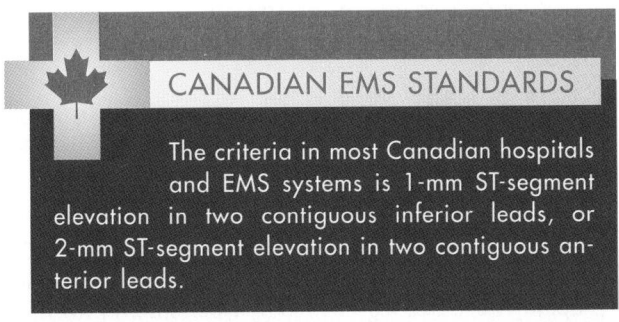

CANADIAN EMS STANDARDS

The criteria in most Canadian hospitals and EMS systems is 1-mm ST-segment elevation in two contiguous inferior leads, or 2-mm ST-segment elevation in two contiguous anterior leads.

Left Ventricular Failure and Pulmonary Edema

Left ventricular failure occurs when the left ventricle fails to function as an effective forward pump, caus-

Management of Unstable Angina/Non-ST-Segment Elevation MI

ECG changes in 2 or more anatomically contiguous leads:

ST-segment depression > 1 mm or T wave inversion > 1 mm or

Transient (<30 min) ST-segment/T wave changes > 1 mm with discomfort

Confirm diagnosis by signs/symptoms, ECG, serum cardiac markers

- Aspirin 162–325 mg (chewed) if not already administered (and no contraindications) (antiplatelet therapy)
- Heparin IV (antithrombin therapy)

If high-risk patient give:
- Aspirin + glycoprotein IIb/IIa inhibitors (i.e., Integrilin, Aggrastat, ReoPro) + IV heparin OR.
- Aspirin + glycoprotein IIb/IIa inhibitors + SC low molecular weight heparin

High-risk criteria
- Persistent ("stuttering") symptoms/recurrent ischemia; left ventricular (LV) dysfunction, CHF; widespread EG changes; prior MI, positive troponin or CK-MB

Anti-ischemic therapy
- Beta-blockers–if patient not previously on beta-blockers or inadequately treated on current dose of beta-blocker (if no contraindications)
- NTG sublingual tablet or spray, followed by IV NTG if symptoms persist despite sublingual NTG therapy and initiation of beta-blocker therapy (and SBP > 90 mm Hg)
- Morphine 2 to 4 mg IV (if discomfort is not relieved or symptoms recur despite antiischemic therapy)–may repeat every 5 min (ensure SBP > 90 mm Hg)

Assess clinical status–is patient clinically stable?

YES	NO
• Continue in-hospital observation • Consider stress testing	Cardiac cath • If anatomy suitable for revascularization–PCI, CABG • If anatomy unsuitable–medical management

Management of Patient with a Suspected Acute Coronary Syndrome and Nondiagnostic/Normal ECG.

Nondiagnostic or Normal ECG

Evaluate signs/symptoms, serial ECGs, serum cardiac markers

Aspirin + other therapy as appropriate

- Assess patient's clinical risk of death/nonfatal MI
- History and physical exam
- Obtain follow-up serum cardiac marker levels, serial ECG monitoring
- Continue evaluation and treatment in emergency department chest pain unit or monitored bed
- Consider radionuclide, echocardiography

Fig. 28-103, cont'd Acute myocardial infarction algorithm.

ing a back-pressure of blood into the pulmonary circulation. This condition may be caused by a variety of forms of heart disease, including ischemic, valvular, and hypertensive heart disease. If it remains unmanaged, significant left ventricular failure culminates in pulmonary edema.

In left ventricular failure, blood is delivered to the left ventricle but is not completely ejected from it. The increase in end-diastolic blood volume increases left ventricular end-diastolic pressure, which is transmitted to the left atrium and subsequently to the pulmonary veins and capillaries. As

BOX 28-5

SIGNS AND SYMPTOMS OF LEFT VENTRICULAR FAILURE

- Severe respiratory distress
  Orthopnea
  Spasmodic cough that may produce foamy, blood-tinged sputum
  History of paroxysmal nocturnal dyspnea (a sudden episode of dyspnea that occurs after lying down)
- Severe apprehension, agitation, confusion
- Cyanosis (if severe)
- Diaphoresis
- Adventitious lung sounds
  Bilateral crackles that do not clear with coughing (usually present at the base of the lungs and up to the level of the scapulae)
  Rhonchi (fluid in upper airways)
  Wheezes (reflex airway spasm, sometimes referred to as *cardiac asthma*)
- JVD (indicative of back-pressure through the right heart and into the venous system)
- Abnormal vital signs
  Blood pressure: possibly elevated
  Pulse rate: rapid to compensate for low stroke volume; possibly irregular if dysrhythmias are present
- Regular alterations of weak and strong beats without changes in the length of cycle (pulsus alternans)
  Respirations: rapid, labored
- Level of consciousness (Patient may be anxious, agitated, uncooperative, or obtunded because of poor cerebral perfusion or hypoxia.)
- Chest pain
  Presence or absence of pain
  Possible masking by respiratory distress

(particularly those with an abrupt onset) also should be suspected of having an AMI.

NOTE

Paroxysmal nocturnal dyspnea (PND) is an abnormal condition of the respiratory system, characterized by sudden attacks of shortness of breath, profuse sweating, tachycardia, and wheezing that awaken a person from sleep. It often is associated with left ventricular failure and pulmonary edema.

Left heart failure results in a reduction of stroke volume (SV), which initiates several compensatory mechanisms that restore cardiac output and organ perfusion (tachycardia, vasoconstriction, and activation of the renin-angiotensin-aldosterone system). These mechanisms often increase myocardial oxygen demand and thereby further decrease the functional capacity of the myocardium. Signs and symptoms of left heart failure and pulmonary edema are listed in Box 28-5.

Management (Fig. 28-104)
Pulmonary edema is an acute and critical emergency that may lead to death unless it is managed rapidly. Emergency management is directed at decreasing the venous return to the heart, improving myocardial contractility, decreasing myocardial oxygen demand, improving ventilation and oxygenation, and rapidly transporting the patient to a medical facility.

Emergency care entails patient positioning, oxygenation, ventilatory support as needed, and pharmacological therapy. As in any other true emergency, a complete but focused patient history and examination should be obtained while initiating management. Although no characteristic ECG changes are associated with pulmonary edema, an initial tracing should be obtained and the patient's rhythm continuously monitored for evidence of myocardial irritability and/or dysrhythmias.

The patient should be placed in a sitting position with the legs dependent. This increases lung volume and vital capacity, diminishes the work of respiration, and decreases venous return to the heart.

pulmonary capillary hydrostatic pressure increases, the plasma portion of blood is forced into the alveoli and mixes with air, resulting in the characteristic finding in pulmonary edema: foamy, blood-tinged sputum. If left unmanaged, the progressive fluid accumulation can cause death from hypoxia. Since myocardial infarction is a common cause of left ventricular failure, all patients with pulmonary edema

High-concentration oxygen should be administered with a well-fitted face mask, preferably a nonrebreather to optimize the fraction of inspired oxygen (FiO_2). Some patients may require (and will tolerate) positive-pressure assistance (including CPAP or BiPAP) to accelerate clearing of pulmonary edema and reduce the needed inspired oxygen concentration. If possible, a pulse oximeter should be used to ensure arterial oxygen saturation of at least 90%. If this cannot be achieved with 100% oxygen or if there are signs of cerebral hypoxia or progressive hypercapnia, endotracheal intubation and assisted ventilations may be indicated.

Pharmacological therapy. The following three medications may be used to decrease venous return, enhance contractile function of the myocardium, and reduce dyspnea:

1. *Nitroglycerin*
   a. Induction of peripheral vasodilation
   b. Possible reduction of preload and afterload, thereby reducing the myocardial workload and improving cardiac function
2. *Furosemide* (Lasix)
   a. Direct relaxant (dilating) effect on the venous system within 5 minutes

Management of Acute Pulmonary Edema.

Perform Primary ABCD Survey (Basic Life Support)
(Correct critical problems IMMEDIATELY as they are identified)
• Assess responsiveness, **A**irway, **B**reathing, **C**irculation, ensure availability of monitor/**D**efibrillator

Perform Secondary ABCD Survey (Advanced Life Support)
(Obtain arterial blood gas before oxygen administration if possible)
• Administer oxygen, establish IV access, attach cardiac monitor (O_2, IV, monitor)
• Assess vital signs, attach pulse oximeter, & monitor blood pressure
• Obtain & review 12-lead ECG, portable chest x-ray
• Perform a focused history and physical exam

If feasible and BP permits, place patient in sitting position with feet dependent
• Increases lung volume and vital capacity
• Decreases work of respiration
• Decreases venous return, decreases preload

If systolic BP > 100 mm Hg:
• Sublingual nitroglycerin–1 tablet or 2 sprays every 5 minutes (max 3 tablets) until IV nitroglycerin or nitroprusside can take effect
• Furosemide IV 0.5 to 1.0 mg/kg (typically 20 to 80 mg) can repeat in 30 minutes if symptoms persist and BP stable
• Consider morphine IV 2-4 mg

Consider additional preload/afterload reduction–nitroglycerin or nitroprusside IV, ACE inhibitors
• Nitroglycerin IV–start at 5 mcg/min and increase gradually until mean systolic pressure falls by 10% to 15%, avoid hypotension (SBP <90 mm hg)[11] **OR**
• Nitroprusside IV (If SBP > 100 mm Hg)–0.1 to 5 mcg/kg/min

Evaluate early for:
• Readily reversible cause and institute appropriate intervention (e.g., cardiac dysrhythmias, tamponade)
• Myocardial ischemia/infarction (Institute appropriate intervention–candidate for fibrinolytic therapy? PTCA?

If patient is refractory to above therapies, hypotensive, or in cardiogenic shock:
• Consider fluid or IV inotropic and/or vasopressor agents (e.g., dobutamine, dopamine, norepinephrine)
• Consider pulmonary and systemic arterial catheterization
• Obtain echocardiogram to assist in diagnosis, evaluation, and reparability of culprit lesion or condition
• Consider need for mechanical circulatory assistance (balloon pump)

Fig. 28-104 Acute pulmonary edema/hypotension/shock algorithm. (From Aehlert B: *ACLS quick review study guide,* ed 2, St Louis, 2002, Mosby.) continued

Management of Hypotension/Shock–Suspected Pump Problem.

Perform Primary ABCD Survey (Basic Life Support)

(Correct critical problems IMMEDIATELY as they are identified)
- Assess responsiveness, **A**irway, **B**reathing, **C**irculation, ensure availability of monitor/**D**efibrillator

Perform Secondary ABCD Survey (Advanced Life Support)

- Administer oxygen, establish IV access, attach cardiac monitor, administer fluids as needed (O_2, IV, monitor, fluids)
- Assess vital signs, attach pulse oximeter, and monitor blood pressure
- Obtain and review 12-lead ECG, portable chest x-ray,
- Perform a focused history and physical exam

Hypotension–suspected pump problem

If breath sounds are clear, consider fluid challenge of 250 to 500 -mL NS to ensure adequate ventricular filling pressure before vasopressor administration

Marked hypotension (systolic BP < 70 mm Hg)/cardiogenic shock

Pharmacologic management:[i]
- Norepinephrine infusion (0.5 to 30 mcg/min) until SBP 80 mm Hg
- Then attempt to change to dopamine 5 to 15 mcg/kg/min until SBP 90 mm Hg
- IV dobutamine (2 to 20 mcg/kg/min) can be given simultaneously in an attempt to reduce magnitude of dopamine infusion

Consider balloon pump or patient transfer to a cardiac interventional facility

Moderate hypotension (systolic BP 70 to 90 mm Hg)[ii]

- Dopamine 5 to 15 mcg/kg/min
- If BP remains low despite dopamine doses > 20 mcg/kg/min, may substitute norepinephrine in doses of 0.5 to 30 mcg/min
- Once SBP ≥ 90 with dopamine, add dobutamine 2 to 20 mcg/kg/min and attempt to taper off dopamine

Systolic BP 90 mm Hg[iii] [iv]

- Dobutamine 2 to 20 mcg/kg/min

Dosing:

Norepinephrine IV	0.5 to 30 mcg/min
Dopamine IV	5 to 15 mcg/kg/min
Dobutamine IV	2 to 20 mcg/kg/min

Fig. 28-104, cont'd Acute pulmonary edema/hypotension/shock algorithm.

  b. Diuretic effect that reduces intravascular volume

  c. May lead to electrolyte imbalance

3. *Morphine*

  a. Decrease of venous return by dilation of the capacitance vessels of the peripheral venous bed (reduces preload)

  b. Reduction of myocardial work

  c. Reduction of anxiety

? CRITICAL THINKING

What happens to the diffusion of oxygen and carbon dioxide in the lungs during this process?

NOTE

Care must be taken in patients with pulmonary edema and hypotension (blood pressure less than 100 mm Hg systolic), since any of these medications may lower blood pressure.

Right Ventricular Failure

Left ventricular failure produces elevated pressure in the pulmonary vascular system. This pressure causes resistance to pulmonary blood flow and an increase in the workload of the right side of the heart to overcome the resistance. Over time, the right ventricle is unable to keep up with the venous

Management of Hypotension/Shock–Suspected Volume Problem.

Perform Primary ABCD Survey (Basic Life Support)

(Correct critical problems IMMEDIATELY as they are identified)
- Assess responsiveness, **A**irway, **B**reathing, **C**irculation, ensure availability of monitor/**D**efibrillator

Perform Secondary ABCD Survey (Advanced Life Support)

- Administer oxygen, establish IV access, attach cardiac monitor, administer fluids as needed (O_2, IV, monitor, fluids)
- Assess vital signs, attach pulse oximeter, and monitor blood pressure
- Obtain and review 12-lead ECG, portable chest x-ray,
- Perform a focused history and physical exam

Hypotension–suspected volume (or vascular resistance) problem

Volume replacement

- Fluid challenge (250 to 500-mL IV boluses–reassess)
- Blood transfusion (if appropriate)
- If cause known, institute appropriate intervention (e.g., septic shock, anaphylaxis)
- Consider vasopressors, if indicated, to improve vascular tone if no response to fluid challenge(s)

Management of Hypotension/Shock–Suspected Rate Problem.

Perform Primary ABCD Survey (Basic Life Support)

(Correct critical problems IMMEDIATELY as they are identified)
- Assess responsiveness, **A**irway, **B**reathing, **C**irculation, ensure availability of monitor/**D**efibrillator

Perform Secondary ABCD Survey (Advanced Life Support)

- Administer oxygen, establish IV access, attach cardiac monitor, administer fluids as needed (O_2, IV, monitor, fluids)
- Assess vital signs, attach pulse oximeter, and monitor blood pressure
- Obtain and review 12-lead ECG, portable chest x-ray,
- Perform a focused history and physical exam

Hypotension - suspected rate problem

If rate too slow–bradycardia algorithm

If rate too fast–determine width of QRS, then use appropriate tachycardia algorithm

Fig. 28-104, cont'd Acute pulmonary edema/hypotension/shock algorithm.

return and begins to fail. As SV lessens, right atrial pressure rises and back-pressure is transmitted to the vena cava and the rest of the venous system. When the systemic venous pressure becomes too high, the plasma portion of the blood is forced out into the interstitial tissues of the body, resulting in edema, particularly in the dependent areas of the body (lower extremities and sacrum of patients who are bedridden). Signs and symptoms of right ventricular failure are listed in Box 28-6. When left and right ventricular failure occur together, signs and symptoms of each may be present.

Right ventricular failure occurs when the right ventricle fails as an effective forward pump, causing back-pressure of blood into the systemic venous circulation. Right-sided heart failure can result from several diseases, including chronic hypertension (in which left-sided heart failure usually precedes right-sided heart failure), chronic obstructive pulmonary disease (COPD), pulmonary embolism,

BOX 28-6

SIGNS AND SYMPTOMS OF RIGHT VENTRICULAR FAILURE

- Tachycardia
- Venous congestion
  Engorged liver, spleen, or both
  Venous distention: distention and pulsation of the neck veins
- Peripheral edema
  Lower extremities or entire body (anasarca)
  Sacral region in bedridden patients
  Pitting edema
- Fluid accumulation in serous cavities
  Abdominal cavity (ascites)
  Pericardium (pericardial effusion)

NOTE: Patients can often tolerate large quantities of effusion without compromise when the effusion develops over an extended period.

- History
  Often previous myocardial infarction in patients with chronic congestive failure
  Frequent medication history of digitalis and diuretics to control heart failure

NOTE

Hypotension secondary to right ventricular failure (often seen in right ventricular infarction) can mimic cardiogenic shock, except that fluid administration to help normalize left ventricular filling is crucial and resolves the hypotension, rather than worsening the heart failure associated with cardiogenic shock. Management may include 250-mL IV boluses of normal saline over 5 to 10 minutes to increase myocardial strength (Starling's law) and improve contractility. Close observation of the patient and vital signs is crucial.

valvular heart disease, and infarction of the right ventricle. Right ventricular failure most commonly results from left ventricular failure. Common signs and symptoms of acute right-sided heart failure include chest pain, hypotension, and distended neck veins.

Management

Right ventricular failure usually is not a medical emergency in itself unless it is associated with pulmonary edema or hypotension. The paramedic should be prepared to manage the patient for either complication. Patient management for right ventricular failure includes:

1. Placing the patient at rest in a sitting or semi-Fowler position (head elevated)
2. Administering high-concentration oxygen
3. Obtaining baseline vital signs and an ECG tracing
4. Initiating an IV line to keep the vein open or to manage hypotension
5. Monitoring the ECG
6. Managing symptoms of left ventricular failure, if present

Cardiogenic Shock

Cardiogenic shock is the most extreme form of pump failure. It occurs when left ventricular function is so compromised that the heart cannot meet the metabolic needs of the body. The result is a marked decrease in SV (resulting from ineffective myocardial contraction), cardiac output, and blood pressure, all of which result in an inadequate supply of blood to the body's organs. Cardiogenic shock occurs in 5% to 10% of patients with AMI.

By definition, cardiogenic shock is present when shock persists after correction of existing dysrhythmias, volume deficit, or decreased vascular tone. It usually is caused by extensive myocardial infarction, often involving more than 40% of the left ventricle, or by diffuse ischemia. Even with aggressive therapy, cardiogenic shock has a mortality rate of 70% or higher.[8]

In addition to the signs and symptoms of myocardial infarction, patients in cardiogenic shock show clinical evidence of hypoperfusion to vital organs and significant systemic hypotension similar to that found in other forms of shock (making it difficult to differentiate the exact etiology of shock). This evidence includes:

- Profound hypotension (systolic blood pressure usually less than 80 mm Hg)
- Pulmonary congestion (crackles)
- Hypoxemia
- Acidosis
- Altered level of consciousness
- Sinus tachycardia or other dysrhythmias
- Cool, clammy, cyanotic, or ashen skin
- Tachypnea

In early stages of cardiogenic shock, the patient's heart compensates by increasing the heart rate and, if possible, contractility and cardiac output. If the condition is inadequately managed, the heart progresses toward hypodynamic failure with depressed contractility, reduced SV, and subsequent hypoperfusion (see Chapter 19).

Management (See Fig. 28-104)

Patients in cardiogenic shock are severely ill and require rapid transport to a medical facility. (Prolonged in-field stabilization is not recommended.) Prehospital care should include airway management and ventilatory support with high-concentration oxygen, placement of the patient in a supine position (or semi-Fowler position, if the patient is dyspneic), insertion of an IV line with normal saline or lactated Ringer's solution to keep the vein open, ECG monitoring, correction of dysrhythmias, and frequent evaluation of vital signs (including auscultation of the lungs and observation for jugular venous distention). A patient in respiratory failure may require intubation and ventilatory support.

> **? CRITICAL THINKING**
>
> *How should you respond to unstable patients with signs and symptoms indicating cardiogenic shock when they ask you, "Am I going to die?"*

Pharmacological therapy may include inotropic agents such as *dopamine* (Intropin) or *dobutamine* (Dobutrex) to improve cardiac output. Use of vasodilators to increase forward flow by reducing afterload generally is reserved for in-hospital coronary care settings, where hemodynamics can be evaluated more accurately. If left-sided heart failure and pulmonary edema also are present, they should be managed concurrently.

> **? CRITICAL THINKING**
>
> *What dose of each of these drugs should be given for this condition?*

Cardiac Tamponade

Cardiac tamponade (described in Chapter 24) is defined as impaired diastolic filling of the heart caused by increased intrapericardial pressure and volume.[8] As the volume of pericardial fluid encroaches on the capacity of the atria and ventricles

to fill adequately, ventricular filling is mechanically limited and SV is decreased. The condition may have a gradual onset precipitated by neoplasm or infection, or it may be acute, resulting from trauma, including CPR. Cardiac tamponade also may occur secondary to renal disease or hypothyroidism. Signs and symptoms of cardiac tamponade include:

- Chest pain
- Tachycardia
- Ectopy
- Elevated venous pressure (an early sign) with associated jugular vein distention (JVD)
- Decreased systolic pressure (a late sign)
- Pulsus paradoxus
- Faint or muffled heart sounds
- ECG changes (usually inconclusive)
  Low-voltage QRS and T waves
  ST-segment elevation or nonspecific T-wave changes

> **? CRITICAL THINKING**
>
> *Why would large-volume fluid resuscitation not be indicated in this situation?*

> **NOTE**
>
> As described in Chapter 24, the most important reliable signs of cardiac tamponade are elevated venous pressure associated with hypotension and tachycardia (Beck's triad).

Management

After a thorough history to identify precipitating causes is obtained and a physical examination is performed, prehospital care is directed at ensuring an adequate airway and ventilatory support, and providing rapid transport for physician evaluation and possible pericardiocentesis. A fluid bolus may help support the circulatory system temporarily if the patient becomes hypotensive as a result of the intrapericardial pressure of the tamponade, but definitive

> **? CRITICAL THINKING**
>
> *Why is pericardiocentesis not routinely done in the prehospital setting?*

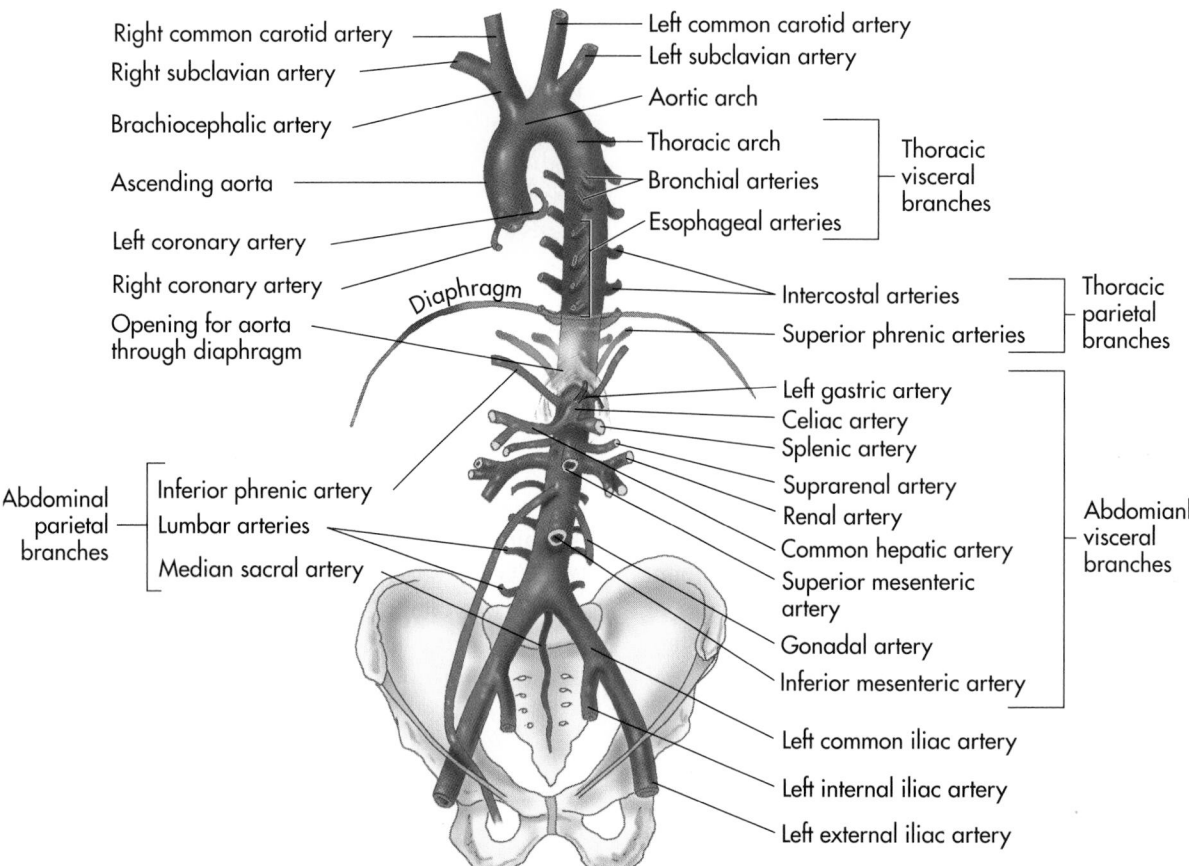

Fig. 28-105 Branches of the aorta: aortic arch, thoracic aorta, abdominal aorta, and their branches. (Illustrator David J. Mascaro and Associates.)

management requires drainage of the pericardial sac. Cardiac tamponade may result in death if the condition is not relieved.

Thoracic and Abdominal Aortic Aneurysms

Aneurysm is a nonspecific term meaning "dilation of a vessel." It may result from atherosclerotic disease (most common), infectious disease (primarily syphilis), traumatic injury, or certain genetic disorders (e.g., Marfan's syndrome). Fig. 28-105 illustrates the branches of the aorta. Abdominal aortic aneurysm and dissecting aneurysm of the aorta are presented here.

Most aneurysms develop at a weak point in the wall of an artery that results from degenerative changes in the medial layer. Weakening of the supportive elements of the vessel wall allows dilation, which causes turbulence and increasing lateral pressure. The aneurysm tends to enlarge over time

as the lateral pressure increases in the dilated segment. Eventually the aneurysm may rupture, producing life-threatening hemorrhage.

Abdominal Aortic Aneurysm

Abdominal aortic aneurysms affect about 2% of the population.[2] The most common site for an abdominal aortic aneurysm is below the renal arteries and above the bifurcation of the common iliac arteries. It is 10 times more common in men and is most prevalent between the ages of 60 and 70. An abdominal aneurysm usually is asymptomatic as long as it is stable. However, if the aneurysm begins to expand or leak, symptoms will indicate impending rupture (Box 28-7).

Rupture of an abdominal aortic aneurysm may begin with a small tear in the intima that allows blood to leak into the wall of the aorta. As the process continues with increasing pressure, the tear may extend through the outer layer of the vessel and cause bleeding into the retroperitoneal space. If bleeding is tamponaded by the retroperitoneal tissues, the patient may be normotensive on EMS arrival. If the rupture opens into the peritoneal cavity, however, massive fatal hemorrhage may follow. In either case, major blood loss results, and hypovolemic shock ensues.

NOTE

Fairly frequently a rupturing aneurysm will present with syncope followed by hypotension with bradycardia despite large-volume blood loss. The reason for bradycardia is that the aorta is wrapped with branches of the vagal nerve, which produces bradycardia (due to vagal effects) despite the hemorrhagic shock condition, which usually would produce hypotension and tachycardia.

Management. Patients with an expanding or a ruptured abdominal aneurysm usually appear acutely ill and require immediate operative repair of the vessel. A total of 20% of patients with an abdominal aortic aneurysm rupture their aneurysm before reaching the hospital, and 80% of these patients die.[10] Therefore early recognition and prompt transport are imperative to avert a fatal outcome.

In most cases, prehospital care should be limited to gentle handling, oxygen administration, cardiac monitoring (myocardial infarctions may be associated with advanced aneurysms), initiation of volume-expanding IV fluids while en route to the receiving hospital, and alerting the receiving facility to prepare for imminent surgery.

NOTE

Pulsatile masses (if present) are extremely fragile and in most cases membrane thin. The paramedic should avoid aggressive examination or deep palpation of the mass, which may cause rupture. Examination, if necessary, can be made by auscultation, which may reveal a sound similar to that of a systolic murmur or bruit.

The management of hypotension varies somewhat, depending on whether the aneurysm is leaking or ruptured. A patient with a suspected leaking aneurysm can be maintained with mildly hypotensive blood pressure to try to prevent frank rupture during transport. (The hypotension associated with small leaks is thought to be secondary to a compen-

---

BOX 28-7

SIGNS AND SYMPTOMS OF A LEAKING OR RUPTURED ABDOMINAL AORTIC ANEURYSM

- Unexplained hypotension (that results from either hemorrhage or a compensatory vasovagal response mechanism)
- Unexplained syncope (As the aneurysm ruptures, blood pressure drops transiently to zero, producing sudden cerebral hypoperfusion and syncope.)
- Sudden onset of abdominal or back pain (described as *tearing* or *ripping*) from the physical trauma itself or from inflammation
- Low back or flank pain (radiating to the thigh, groin, testicle, or perineum) that is unrelieved by rest or changes in position
- Signs of peritoneal irritation
- Urge to defecate (caused by retroperitoneal leakage of blood)
- Pulsatile, tender mass that may be palpated when greater than 5 cm and that is usually located above the umbilicus, left of the midline
- Distal pulses (femoral artery and below) that may be present or absent, depending on the patient's blood pressure, the occurrence of a dissection, and the degree of peripheral vascular disease
- Possible presentation as bleeding in the gastrointestinal tract if the aneurysm erodes into it

---

satory vasovagal mechanism.) In these patients, fluid resuscitation should be minimal and less aggressive than in patients who have a ruptured aneurysm.

If rupture has occurred, hypotension, tachycardia, and loss of the pulsating mass may suddenly develop, and the patient may become unresponsive. This often is followed by full cardiac and respiratory arrest. These patients require rapid and aggressive resuscitation (intubation, ventilation, fluid replacement, and rapid transport for surgical intervention).

Acute Dissecting Aortic Aneurysm

Acute dissection (separation of the arterial wall) is the most common aortic catastrophe, affecting 5 to 10 persons per million population each year (three times as many as ruptured abdominal aortic aneurysm).[7] Factors that can lead to the development of dissecting aneurysm are systemic hypertension,

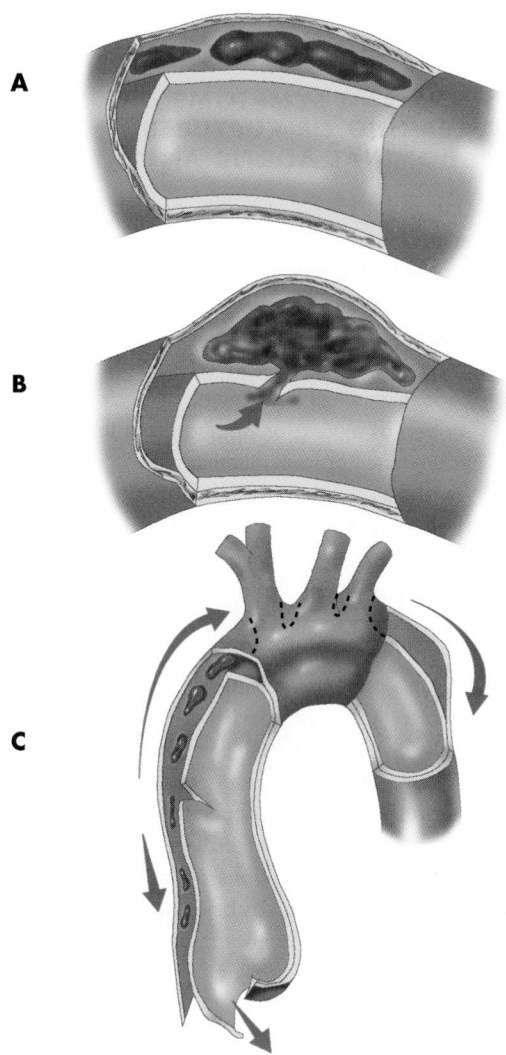

Fig. 28-106 Pathogenesis of dissecting aneurysms. **A**, Medial and intimal degeneration in anotic wall set stage. **B**, Hemodynamic forces acting on aortic wall produce intimal tear, directing bloodstream into diseased media. **C**, Resulting dissecting hematoma is propagated in both directions by pulse wave produced with each myocardial contraction.

atherosclerosis, congenital abnormalities, degenerative changes in the connective tissue of the aortic media (cystic medial necrosis), trauma, and pregnancy. The syndrome affects men twice as often as women and is more common in African-Americans.

A dissecting aneurysm of the aorta results from a small tear in the intimal layer of the vessel wall (Fig. 28-106). After the tear, the process of dissection begins. The tear in the inner wall allows blood to move between the inner and outer layers, creating a false passage between the layers of the vessel wall. Blood that enters the false passage results in the formation of a hematoma, which can subsequently rupture through the outer wall (adventitia) at any time, usually into the pericardial or pleural cavity.

Although any area of the aorta may be involved, in the majority of cases the site of a dissecting aneurysm is in the ascending aorta. Once begun, the aneurysm may extend distally or proximally to involve all of the thoracic and abdominal aorta and tributaries, the coronary arteries, the aortic valve, and the carotid and subclavian vessels. Any vessels (including the carotid and other aortic arch vessels) bypassed by the dissection have their blood flow compromised. As a result, aortic dissection may cause:

• Syncope
• Stroke
• Absent or reduced pulses
• Heart failure resulting from sudden aortic valve regurgitation
• Pericardial tamponade
• AMI

Signs and symptoms. The signs and symptoms of a dissecting aortic aneurysm depend on the site of the intimal tear (ascending or descending aorta) and the extent of dissection. More than 70% of patients with acute dissecting aneurysm of the aorta complain of severe pain in the back, epigastrium, abdomen, or extremities, which they often describe as the most intense pain they have ever experienced. The pain usually is sudden in onset and may be characterized by the patient as "ripping," "tearing," or "sharp and cutting, like a knife." It often originates in the back (between the scapulae) and possibly extends down into the legs. The patient with acute dissection may appear "shocky," with pallor, sweating, and peripheral cyanosis (from impaired perfusion), even when blood pressure is normal or elevated. If the patient is hypotensive, cardiac tamponade or aortic rupture should be suspected.

? CRITICAL THINKING

What other condition has signs and symptoms similar to abdominal aortic aneurysm?

NOTE

Blood pressure may differ significantly in the two arms if the dissection occludes the takeoff of either subclavian artery, leading to hypotension in the affected upper extremity.

Although it may be difficult to differentiate the pain of aortic dissection from that of myocardial infarction or pulmonary embolism in the prehospital setting, the following distinctive features may help:

1. Severity of pain is maximal from the onset (compared with crescendo pain characteristic of AMI).
2. Pain may migrate from the anterior portion of the chest or interscapular area downward as dissection progresses.
3. Significant differences in blood pressure occur between the left and right arm or between the arms and the legs.
4. Peripheral pulses are unequal.
5. Neurological deficits result from occlusion of a cerebral vessel.

Management. The goals of managing suspected aortic dissection in the prehospital setting are relief of pain and immediate transport to a medical facility. (Transport should not be delayed; analgesics should be administered en route to the hospital.) The EMS crew should be prepared to initiate intubation and to assist ventilation in case the patient begins to decompensate. Other prehospital care measures include:

- Gently handling the patient
- Decreasing anxiety
- Administering high-concentration oxygen
- Beginning a large-bore IV line of crystalloid solution (Fluids should be kept to a minimum unless severe hypotension is present.)
- Giving analgesia (e.g., *morphine, fentanyl* [Fentanyl]) per medical direction if the diagnosis is strongly suspected

Definitive in-hospital care generally includes reducing the myocardial contractile force to stop progressive dissection (with antihypertensives and beta blockers), monitoring of intraarterial pressure, and possibly surgical repair.

Acute Arterial Occlusion

Acute arterial occlusion is a sudden blockage of arterial flow, most commonly caused by trauma, embolus, or thrombosis. The severity of the ischemic episode depends on the site of occlusion and the quality of collateral circulation around the blockage. Vascular occlusion caused by thrombosis is a complication of atherosclerosis. Occlusions secondary to emboli may indicate an underlying disturbance in cardiac rhythm, particularly atrial fibrillation.

Arterial occlusion may follow blunt or penetrating trauma; it often is associated with long bone fractures. These injuries vary from intimal disruptions to complete transection. The occlusion usually is evident from decreased circulation distal to the injury.

An embolism occurs when a blood clot breaks away and enters the arterial system. It travels until it reaches a point of luminal narrowing, often a bifurcation of an artery. Since 90% of peripheral emboli originate in the heart, a history of cardiac disease (e.g., dysrhythmia, myocardial infarction, valvular heart disease) favors a diagnosis of embolic occlusion, particularly when the patient has an asymptomatic opposite extremity with normal pulses. The most common sites of embolic occlusion are the abdominal aorta, common femoral artery, popliteal artery, carotid artery, brachial artery, and mesenteric artery (Fig. 28-107).

Thrombosis usually results from atherosclerotic disease and occurs at a site of severe stenosis of a vessel. Unlike an embolus, thrombosis usually occurs gradually over a period of time. As the thrombosis propagates proximally, sources of collateral blood supply can become occluded, causing progressive ischemia. The location of the ischemic pain often is related to the site of occlusion:

- Terminal portion of the abdominal aorta: pain in both hips or lower limbs
- Iliac artery: pain in the buttocks or hip on the involved side
- Femoral artery: claudication (cramplike pain) in the calf of the involved leg
- Mesenteric artery: severe abdominal pain

If severe ischemia persists, muscle necrosis occurs. Thrombotic occlusion is seen most often in men, smokers, and those over 60 years of age. Common sites of atherosclerotic (thrombotic) occlusions are depicted in Fig. 28-108.

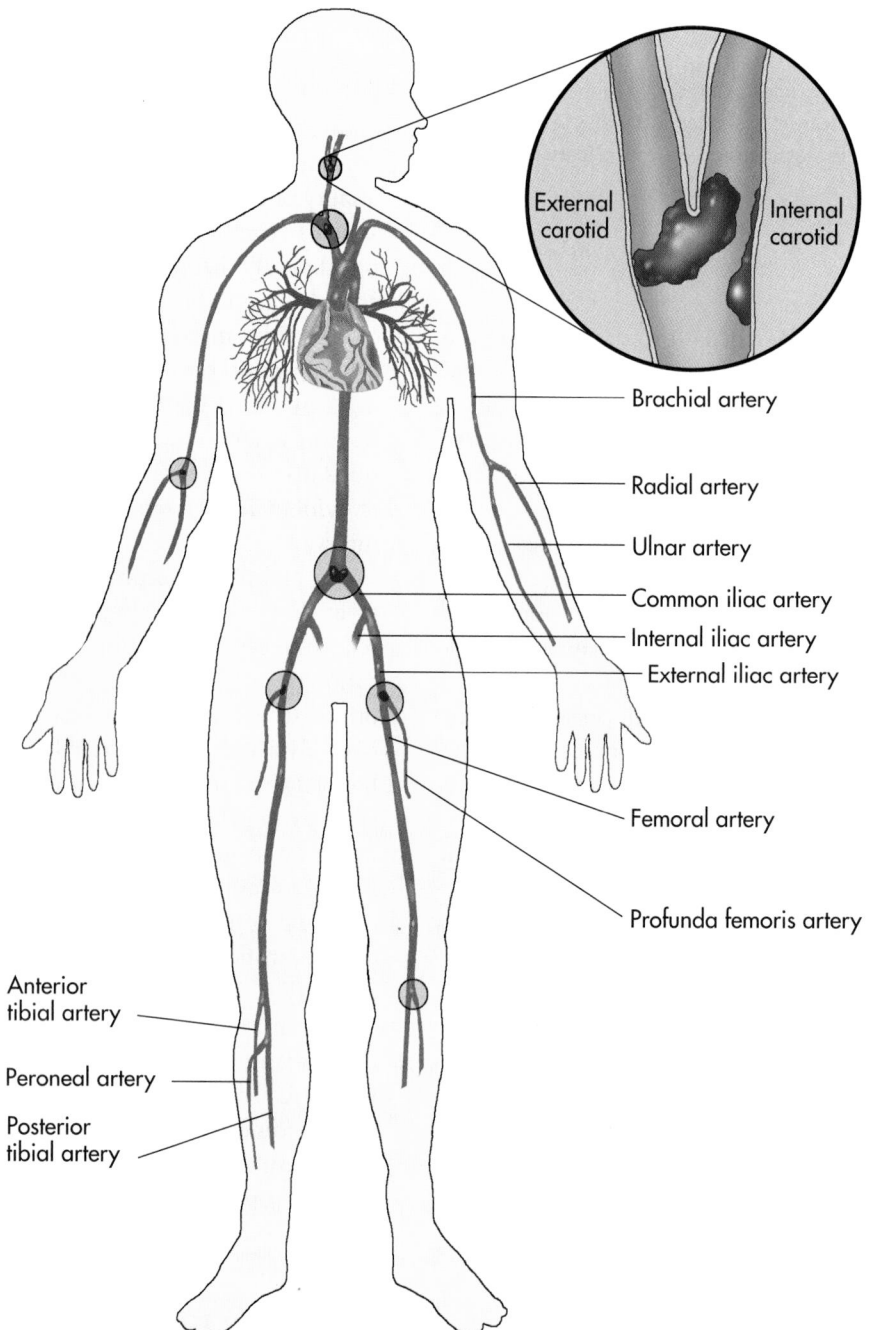

External
carotid

Internal
carotid

Brachial artery

Radial artery

Ulnar artery

Common iliac artery

Internal iliac artery

External iliac artery

Femoral artery

Profunda femoris artery

Anterior
tibial artery

Peroneal artery

Posterior
tibial artery

Fig. 28-107 Common sites of embolic arterial occlusion.

Signs and Symptoms

Regardless of the origin of the occlusion, the signs and symptoms of ischemia are the same. These include:

- Pain in the extremity that may be severe and sudden in onset or absent as a result of paresthesia
- Pallor (skin may also be mottled or cyanotic)

- Lowered skin temperature distal to the occlusion
- Changes in sensory and motor function
- Diminished or absent pulse distal to the injury
- Bruit over the affected vessel
- Slow capillary filling
- Sometimes shock (particularly in mesenteric occlusion)

NOTE

Some patients with vascular occlusion will have unequal blood pressure readings in the arms. Systolic readings in the arms that differ by 15 mm Hg or more suggest vascular disease. (A normal difference of 5 to 10 mm Hg exists between arms.)

Management

Acute arterial occlusion in an extremity is serious and painful and may be limb threatening if blood flow is not reestablished within 4 to 8 hours. The affected limb should be immobilized and protected, and the patient transported for physician evaluation. Patients with mesenteric occlusion should be managed for shock with oxygen and IV fluids. Analgesics also may be prescribed by medical direction to relieve pain. In-hospital, definitive care may include anticoagulant or thrombolytic therapy, transluminal arterial dilation using a balloon catheter, embolectomy, or vascular reconstruction.

Noncritical Peripheral Vascular Conditions

Noncritical peripheral vascular conditions include varicose veins, superficial thrombophlebitis (described in Chapter 7), and acute deep-vein thrombosis. Of these conditions, deep-vein thrombosis is the only one that can cause life-threatening pulmonary embolus. Predisposing factors to venous thrombosis include:

- History of trauma
- Sepsis
- Stasis or inactivity (e.g., bedridden patients, long air flights)
- Recent immobilization (e.g., leg fracture)
- Pregnancy
- Birth control pills
- Malignancy
- Coagulopathies
- Smoking
- Varicose veins (usually a benign condition)

? CRITICAL THINKING

Why does atrial fibrillation put the patient at increased risk for emboli?

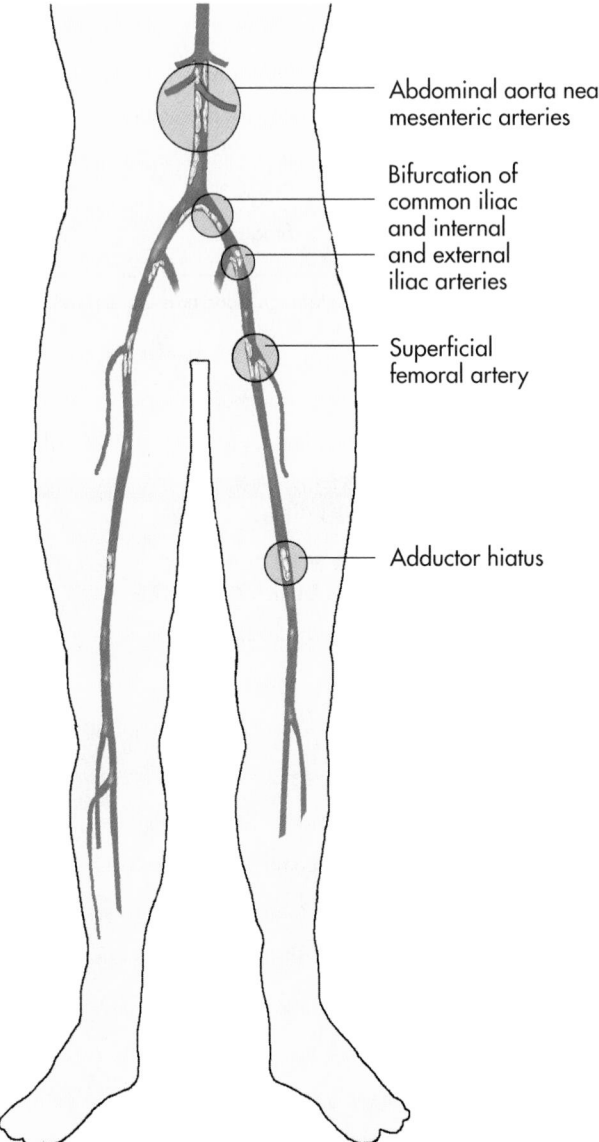

Fig. 28-108 Common sites of atherosclerotic occlusive disease.

Acute Deep-Vein Thrombosis

Occlusion of the deep veins is a serious, common problem. It may involve any portion of the deep venous system but is much more common in the lower extremities. Risk factors for deep-vein thrombosis include recent lower-extremity trauma, recent surgery, advanced age, recent myocardial infarction,

TABLE 28-4	CATEGORIES FOR BLOOD PRESSURE LEVELS IN ADULTS (AGE 18 YEARS AND OLDER)*		
		BLOOD PRESSURE LEVEL (MM HG)	
CATEGORY		**SYSTOLIC**	**DIASTOLIC**
Normal		<130	<85
High normal		130-139	85-89
High blood pressure			
Stage 1		140-159	90-99
Stage 2		160-179	100-109
Stage 3		≥180	≥110

*For those not taking medicine for high blood pressure and not having a short-term serious illness. These categories are from the National High Blood Pressure Education Program.

BOX 28-8

SIGNS AND SYMPTOMS OF HYPERTENSIVE EMERGENCIES

- Paroxysmal nocturnal dyspnea
- Shortness of breath
- Altered mental status
- Vertigo
- Headache
- Epistaxis
- Tinnitus
- Changes in visual acuity
- Nausea and vomiting
- Seizures
- ECG changes

NOTE

The presence of varicose veins usually is a benign condition caused by chronic increased venous pressure with a resultant dilation of superficial veins. The syndrome commonly is associated with veins of the lower extremities but also may occur in other parts of the body as hemorrhoids, esophageal varices, and varicocele (collections of varicose veins in the scrotum). With the exception of esophageal varices, which can lead to exsanguinating gastrointestinal hemorrhage, varicosities are a nuisance but rarely a serious problem.

---

inactivity, confinement to bed, congestive heart failure, cancer, previous thrombosis, oral contraceptive therapy, and obesity. Signs and symptoms of acute deep-vein thrombosis include:

- Pain
- Edema
- Warmth
- Erythema or bluish discoloration
- Tenderness

Management. Patients with acute deep-vein thrombosis require hospitalization. Prehospital care usually is limited to immobilization and elevation of the extremity and transport for physician evaluation. Deep-vein thrombosis in the calf of the leg usually is much less serious than deep-vein thrombosis of the thigh, which has a higher incidence of associated pulmonary embolus. Definitive care includes bed rest, administration of anticoagulants or occasionally thrombolytic agents, and, rarely, thrombectomy.

Hypertension

Hypertension is a common disorder, afflicting about 23% of the U.S. population, and is directly responsible for about 13,000 deaths per year.[11] Hypertension often is defined by a resting blood pressure consistently greater than 140/90 mm Hg.[12] There are several categories of hypertension based on the level of blood pressure, symptomatology, and urgency of need for intervention (Table 28-4 and Box 28-8). For the purpose of this textbook, two general categories are presented: chronic hypertension and hypertensive emergencies (including **hypertensive encephalopathy**).

> **NOTE**
>
> A common cause of hypertension is noncompliance with the medication regimen or other therapy.

Chronic Hypertension

Chronic hypertension has an adverse effect on the function of the heart and blood vessels, requiring the heart to perform more work than normal, leading to hypertrophy of the cardiac muscle and left ventricular failure. It increases the rate at which atherosclerosis develops, which in turn increases the probability of cardiovascular, cerebrovascular, and peripheral vascular disease and the risk of aneurysm formation. Conditions commonly associated with chronic, uncontrolled hypertension are cerebral hemorrhage and stroke, myocardial infarction, renal failure (secondary to vascular changes in the kidney), and development of thoracic and/or abdominal aortic aneurysm.

> **NOTE**
>
> Many persons with established hypertension have elevated peripheral resistance and elevated cardiac output (a function of Starling's law) that results from an increase in both the heart rate and SV.[7] The heart responds to the increased workload resulting from high peripheral resistance by becoming enlarged. Although the enlarged heart may be able to function effectively for many years, in time the heart will no longer be able to maintain adequate blood flow, and the patient will develop symptoms of pump failure.

Any hypertension-related problem, such as pulmonary edema, dissecting aortic aneurysm, toxemia of pregnancy, or stroke requires stabilization and prompt, appropriate management. The hypertension associated with these situations often is a result of a primary problem. Managing the primary problem (e.g., toxemia) often makes it easier to control the patient's blood pressure. However, the primary problem may not easily be correctable, and in situations such as dissecting aortic aneurysm, controlling the blood pressure is essential to managing the primary problem. A life-threatening problem that develops from unmanaged or partially managed hypertension may lead to a hypertensive emergency.

Hypertensive Emergencies

Hypertensive emergencies are conditions in which an increase in blood pressure leads to significant, irreversible end-organ damage within hours if not managed. The organs most likely to be at risk are the brain, heart, and kidneys. This now uncommon condition is experienced by 1% of all hypertensive patients whose illness is poorly controlled or unmanaged. As a rule, the diagnosis is based on altered end-organ function and the rate of the rise in blood pressure, not the level of blood pressure (although diastolic blood pressure usually is greater than 100 mm Hg). All hypertensive emergencies (except hypertension in ischemic stroke) require a 5% to 20% reduction in blood pressure within a few hours of discovery to avoid permanent organ damage.

> **NOTE**
>
> It is not uncommon for blood pressure readings to range from 220/120 mm Hg to 240/140 mm Hg in hypertensive emergencies.

Hypertensive emergencies include the following clinical conditions: (1) myocardial ischemia with hypertension, (2) aortic dissection with hypertension, (3) pulmonary edema with hypertension, (4) hypertensive intracranial hemorrhage, (5) toxemia, and (6) hypertensive encephalopathy. Although hypertension per se may not be the cause of the first five conditions, they all can be made worse by unremitting hypertension. The sixth condition, hypertensive encephalopathy, results solely from elevated blood pressure and, concurrently, raised intracranial pressure.

> **? CRITICAL THINKING**
>
> *What factors contribute to the failure of patients to take medicines prescribed for hypertension?*

Hypertensive encephalopathy. Unremitting hypertension produces hypertensive encephalopathy and cerebral hypoperfusion with loss of the integrity of the blood-brain barrier, which results in fluid exudation into the brain tissue. Hypertensive encephalopathy may progress over several hours from initial symptoms of severe headache, nausea, vomiting, aphasia, hemiparesis, and transient blindness to seizures, stupor, coma, and death. The condition is a true emergency that requires immediate transport to a medical facility for definitive care. The goal of therapy is controlled but rapid lowering of blood pressure to normalize cerebral blood flow. If blood pressure is lowered too fast, infarction of end organs (heart, kidney, brain) may occur. Prehospital management of these patients includes:

- Supportive care
- Calming the patient
- Oxygen therapy
- IV line to keep the vein open
- ECG monitoring
- Rapid transport

In most circumstances, pharmacological therapy for hypertensive emergencies is not instituted in the prehospital setting. However, in severe cases of hypertensive encephalopathy or if transport is delayed, medical direction may recommend administration of antihypertensives such as ***nitroglycerin*** or ***labetalol*** (Normodyne, an alpha and beta blocker) to induce arteriolar vasodilation.

> **? CRITICAL THINKING**
>
> *How will this fluid leak into the brain affect intracranial pressure and cerebral perfusion pressure?*

SECTION EIGHT
TECHNIQUES OF MANAGING CARDIAC EMERGENCIES

This section addresses various procedures, techniques, and equipment used in managing cardiac emergencies. These include basic life support, mechanical CPR devices, monitor-defibrillators (manual, fully automated, and semiautomated), defibrillation, automatic implantable cardioverter-defibrillators (ICDs), synchronized cardioversion, and transcutaneous cardiac pacing (TCP). This section also provides an overview of managing a cardiac arrest (the sudden cessation of cardiac output and effective circulation) as it applies to paramedics working within an advanced cardiac life support (ACLS) system. The reader is encouraged to review the dysrhythmias and pharmacological therapy presented previously in this text.

> **NOTE**
>
> Cardiac arrest most often is associated with cardiovascular disease and is precipitated by ventricular fibrillation or ventricular asystole. It also may result from noncardiac causes such as poisonings, drug overdose, toxic inhalation, trauma, and foreign body airway obstruction.

Basic Cardiac Life Support

Basic cardiac life support externally supports the circulation and respiration of a victim of cardiac arrest until ACLS is available. According to the AHA, "the highest hospital discharge rate—a measure of resuscitation success—is achieved in patients for whom CPR is initiated within 4 minutes of the time of the arrest and who, in addition, are provided with ACLS management within 8 minutes of their arrest. The victim whose heart and breathing have stopped for less than 4 minutes has an excellent chance for recovery if CPR is administered immediately. After 4 to 6 minutes without circulation, brain damage may occur; after 6 minutes . . . brain damage will almost always occur."[13]

> **NOTE**
>
> The passage of time drives all aspects of emergency cardiac care (ECC) and determines patient outcomes.

> **NOTE**
>
> CPR is intended to reverse acute disease such as electrocution, drowning, drug overdose, and sudden cardiac disease. It will not reverse end-stage chronic heart disease.

Physiology of Circulation via External Chest Compression

Two mechanisms are thought to be responsible for blood flow during CPR: (1) direct compression of the heart between the sternum and the spine, which increases pressure within the ventricles enough to provide blood flow to the lungs and body organs, and (2) increased intrathoracic pressure transmitted to all intrathoracic vascular structures, which produces an intrathoracic-to-extrathoracic pressure gradient that causes forward blood flow whereby the heart is merely a conduit. It is not known which mechanism contributes more to blood flow, and mechanisms not currently known also may be involved. Artificial circulation generates only about 20% to 30% of the normal output of the heart.[13]

Research has been conducted for many years on ways to improve CPR, including simultaneous chest compressions and ventilation, abdominal compression with synchronized ventilation, military antishock trousers–augmented CPR, interposed abdominal compression, continuous abdominal binding, and plunger mechanisms for chest compression that cause active compression and active expansion. However, no alternative method has been shown to unequivocally improve survival or circulation. The standards of CPR as recommended by the AHA and the American Red Cross (ARC) are presented in Table 28-5.

Mechanical CPR Devices

A number of mechanical devices provide external chest compression, and others provide chest compression with a system for synchronized ventilation in the patient with cardiac arrest (Fig. 28-109). These devices are designed to standardize CPR technique, eliminate rescuer fatigue, free other rescuers to participate in ACLS procedures, and ensure adequate compression during patient transport. In addition, these devices permit acceptable ECG recordings during compressions and defibrillation without interruption of CPR. The AHA recommends that use of mechanical CPR devices be limited to adult patients. The use of mechanical CPR devices requires special training and authorization from medical direction. EMS providers should follow the recommendations of the equipment manufacturers.

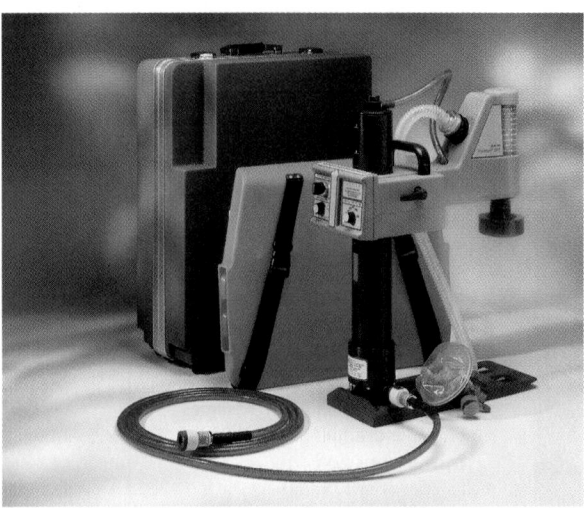

Fig. 28-109 Mechanical CPR device. (Courtesy Michigan Instruments, Grand Rapids, Michigan.)

Monitor-Defibrillators

Cardiac monitor-defibrillators are classified as manual or automated external defibrillators. The latter may be semiautomated or fully automated. The paramedic should be familiar with the monitor-defibrillators used in the local EMS system or community settings.

Manual Monitor-Defibrillators

Monitor-defibrillators are available from a number of equipment manufacturers and have a variety of designs and capabilities. All consist of:

- Paddle or patch electrodes (with "quick look" capability)
- Defibrillator controls
- Synchronizer switch
- Oscilloscope
- Patient cable and lead wires
- Controls for monitoring

In addition, some manual monitor-defibrillators contain special features such as data recorders, TCP capabilities, and 12-lead monitoring.

Automated External Defibrillators

Automated external defibrillators (AEDs) (Fig. 28-110) analyze multiple features of the surface ECG signal, including frequency, amplitude, and some

CPR/RESCUE BREATHING	SUMMARY OF ABCD MANEUVERS			
Establish unresponsiveness Activate EMS system or appropriate resuscitation team.	**MANEUVER**	**ADULT (8 YEARS OF AGE AND OLDER)**	**CHILD (1 TO 8 YEARS OF AGE)**	**INFANT (LESS THAN 1 YEAR OF AGE)**
A—Airway (head tilt–chin lift or jaw thrust).	Head tilt–chin lift (If trauma is present, use jaw thrust.)	Head tilt–chin lift (If trauma is present, use jaw thrust.)	Head tilt–chin lift (If trauma is present, use jaw thrust.)	Head tilt–chin lift (If trauma is present, use jaw thrust.)
B—Breathing (look, listen, and feel for no more than 10 seconds). • *If victim is breathing* or resumes effective breathing, place in the recovery position. • *If victim is not breathing*, give 2 slow breaths using pocket mask or bag-mask. Allow for exhalation between breaths.	Initial Subsequent Foreign-body airway obstruction	2 breaths at 2 sec/breath 10 to 12 breaths/min (approximate) Heimlich maneuver	2 breaths at 1 to 1½ sec/breath 20 breaths/min (approximate) Heimlich maneuver	2 breaths at 1 to 1½ sec/breath 20 breaths/min (approximate) Back blows and chest thrusts
C—Circulation (breathing, coughing, movement), *including pulse* for no more than 10 seconds. Carotid in child and adult; brachial or femoral in infant). • *If signs of circulation/pulse present but breathing is absent,* provide rescue breathing (1 breath every 4 to 5 seconds for adult, 1 breath every 3 seconds for infant or child). • *If signs of circulation/pulse absent,* begin chest compressions interposed with breaths. • *If signs of circulation/pulse present but <60 bpm in infant or child with poor perfusion,* begin chest compressions. **Continue basic life support** Integrate procedures appropriate for newborn resuscitation, pediatric advanced life support, or advanced cardiovascular life support at earliest opportunity	Pulse check* Compression landmarks Compression method Compression depth Compression rate Compression/ ventilation ratio	Carotid Lower half of sternum Heel of one hand, other hand on top 1½ to 2 inches Approximately 100/min 15:2 (Single rescuer or two rescuers. Pause for ventilation with unprotected airway.) 12-15 breaths/min (1 breath every 4-5 seconds) with asynchronous chest compressions with protected airway	Carotid Lower half of sternum Heel of one hand 1 to 1½ inches or approximately one third to one half the depth of chest Approximately 100/min 5:1 (Pause for ventilation until trachea is intubated.)	Brachial or femoral 1 finger's width below intermammary line 2 or 3 fingers or 2 thumb–encircled hands ½ to 1 inch or approximately one half the depth of chest At least 100/min (Newborn: 120/min) 5:1 (Pause for ventilation until trachea is intubated.) 3:1 for intubated newborn (2 rescuers)
D—Defibrillation Defibrillation using automated external defibrillators (AEDs) is now considered an integral part of adult basic life support by healthcare providers.	AED	Per local EMS protocol	Not yet recommended for use in infants and children	

From American Heart Association: *Guidelines 2000 for cardiopulmonary resuscitation and emergency cardiovascular care,* International Consensus on Science, Dallas, 2000, The Association.

*Note: Pulse check is performed by healthcare providers but is not expected of lay rescuers. Lay rescuers are taught to check for *signs of circulation* (eg, normal breathing, coughing, movement) in response to 2 rescue breaths given to the *unresponsive, nonbreathing victim.*

integration of frequency and amplitude (e.g., wave morphology). They are designed to be used by individuals with minimal training, increasing the range of personnel who can use a defibrillator in a cardiac arrest emergency.

> **NOTE**
>
> An increasing number of states have enacted legislation that permits community-based first-responder defibrillation programs using AEDs. These programs and others (e.g., AEDs located in airports and on public airlines) are supported by the AHA and other groups.

All AEDs are attached to the patient by two adhesive monitor-defibrillator pads (electrodes) and connecting cables. AEDs are available from a number of equipment manufacturers and have a variety of features and controls. Most units provide programmable modules, data recorders, and voice messages to the operator. All users should familiarize themselves with the AED device used in their system and follow the recommendations of the manufacturer and the guidelines provided by medical direction.

A fully automated defibrillator requires only that the operator attach the defibrillation pads and turn on the device. The rhythm is analyzed in the internal circuitry of the AED. If a shockable rhythm is detected, the AED charges capacitors and delivers a shock.

A semiautomated defibrillator requires the operator to press an "analyze" control to interpret the rhythm and a "shock" control to deliver the shock. The shock control is pressed only when the AED identifies a shockable rhythm and "advises" the operator to press the shock control.

? CRITICAL THINKING

What safety measure is still the responsibility of the AED operator?

AEDs have four safety features:

1. They can analyze multiple features of electrical activity.
2. They have built-in filters that check for QRS-like signals, radio transmission waves, 60-cycle interference, and loose or poor electrode contact.

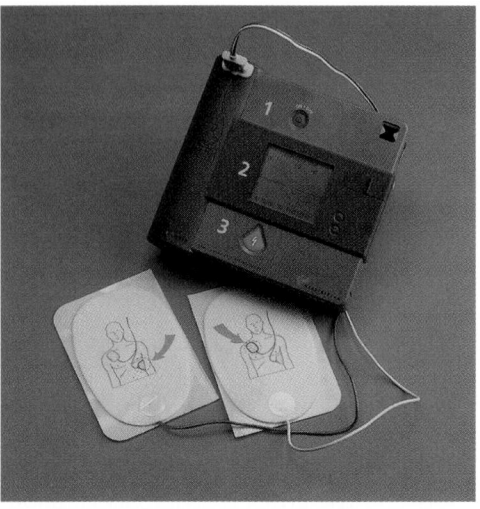

Fig. 28-110 R2 automated defibrillator. (Courtesy Darox Corporation, San Diego, Calif.)

3. Most are programmed to detect spontaneous patient movements, continued heartbeat and blood flow, and movement of the patient by others.
4. They make multiple evaluations of the rhythm before a shock advisory is made or a shock is delivered.

Biphasic Technology

Traditionally, defibrillation has been accomplished using monophasic waveforms where the current travels in only one direction—from positive pad to negative pad. These defibrillators require high energy to effectively defibrillate a patient and may deliver more energy than is necessary for some patients. These machines also require large batteries, energy storage capacitors, inductors, and large high-voltage mechanical devices.

Some of the newer AEDs (and most implantable defibrillators) use biphasic waveform technology that "predicts" a patient's energy requirements and chest wall impedance. The shock is then delivered by a current that travels in one direction, is stopped, and then reversed to travel in the opposite direction, allowing for effective defibrillation to occur with lower energy for most patients.[14] (Biphasic defibrillation of 115 and 130 joules appears to be as effective as 200 and 360 joules delivered with monophasic shocks.[15]) Since biphasic waveforms are more effective at lower energy than monophasic waveforms, AEDs (using smaller batteries) have become smaller, lighter, more durable, and less expensive to manufacture.

Defibrillation

Defibrillation is the delivery of electrical current through the chest wall for the purpose of terminating VF and pulseless VT. The shock depolarizes a large mass of myocardial cells at once. If about 75% of these cells are in the resting state (depolarized) after the shock is delivered, a normal pacemaker may resume discharging. Early defibrillation is supported by the following rationale[1]:

- The most frequent initial rhythm in sudden cardiac arrest is VF.
- The most effective management for VF is electrical defibrillation.
- The probability of successful defibrillation diminishes rapidly over time.
- VF tends to convert to asystole within a few minutes.

The modern defibrillator is designed to deliver an electrical shock via paddle, patches, or pads to the patient's chest. The defibrillator accepts the electrical charge from the battery source, stores it in the capacitor, and releases the current into the patient in a short, controlled burst (within 5 to 30 ms).

Paddle Electrodes

Paddle electrodes are designated by location of use as "apex" or "sternum" to allow the operator to view an approximation of lead II though the "quick look" function. (If the paddles are reversed in polarity or location, a negative QRS complex is noted.) With reference to defibrillation, however, the position of the paddles is unimportant.

The position of the paddles on the chest wall is extremely important during shock delivery (Fig. 28-111). The paddles should be placed so that the heart (primarily the ventricles) is in the path of the current and the distance between the electrodes and the heart is minimized. This helps ensure adequate

delivery of current through the heart. Bone is not a good conductor, and for that reason, the paddles should not be placed over the sternum. As recommended by the AHA, one paddle should be placed to the right of the upper sternum below the right clavicle, and the other to the left of the nipple in the midaxillary line.[1] (The anterior-posterior position also is acceptable.) Most manufacturers have both adult and pediatric paddles available. Adult paddles are usually 10 to 13 cm in diameter; pediatric paddles (used for children less than 1 year of age) are 4.5 cm in diameter.

The resistance to current that is offered by the chest wall is called *impedance*. The greater the resistance, the less current delivered. Dry, unprepared skin has high impedance. To reduce resistance, electrode gel, gel pads, or electrode paste should be placed between the paddles and the skin. The paddles should be held firmly in place with about 20 to 25 pounds of pressure. (Prepackaged self-adhesive monitor-defibrillator pads also may be used.) Whichever method is chosen to decrease impedance, care should be taken to prevent contact (bridging) between the two conductive areas on the chest wall. If contact between the two areas is made, superficial burns of the skin may result and the effective current may bypass the heart (arcing). Even when gels or pads and proper techniques are used, minor skin damage may occur.

Stored and Delivered Energy

Electrical energy is commonly measured in *joules* (watt seconds). One joule of electrical energy is the product of 1 volt (potential) multiplied by 1 ampere (current) multiplied by 1 second. Delivered energy is about 80% of stored energy because of losses within the circuitry of the defibrillator and resistance to the flow of current across the chest wall. As a rule, 80% of stored energy approximates the amount of joules delivered to the patient. The AHA currently recommends that initial defibrillation be attempted three times (200, 200 to 300, and 360 joules) and delivered in succession[1] (see the box on p. 898). The pediatric initial defibrillation generally is 2 joules/kg, followed by 4 joules/kg if needed.

Procedure

The following is the procedure for defibrillation as recommended by the AHA[1]:

1. Place the patient in a safe environment, away from pooled water or a metal surface under either the patient or the rescuer.
2. Apply appropriate conductive materials to hand-held electrodes or use monitor-defibrillator pads.
3. Turn on the defibrillator.
4. Select the energy level; 200 joules is recommended for the initial shock for VF.
5. Charge the capacitor.
6. Ensure proper placement of the electrodes on the chest: the apex—high right parasternal position is standard. If hand-held paddle electrodes are used, apply firm pressure on each. Do not lean on the paddles, because they may slip. Be sure that there is no smearing of coupling material between the paddles, or the current may preferentially follow this low-resistance pathway along the chest wall, "missing" the heart. Remove any transdermal medication patches.
7. Make sure that no personnel are directly or indirectly in contact with the patient. If ventilation via a bag-mask device or endotracheal tube is being performed, the rescuer should step back and momentarily release the bag. It is unnecessary to disconnect a bag from an endotracheal tube if the tube is well secured.
8. Deliver the electrical shock by depressing both discharge buttons simultaneously (or per manufacturer's instructions).

NOTE

The AHA recommends delivery of the first three shocks in succession without stopping to check a pulse if the monitor clearly demonstrates VF.

9. If defibrillation fails, continue with the management algorithm.

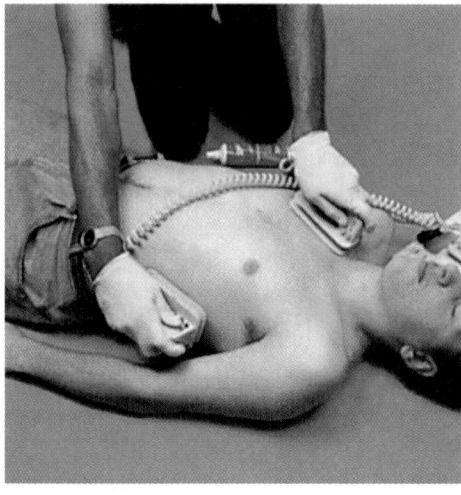

Fig. 28-111 Correct paddle placement for defibrillation.

Operator and Personnel Safety

The following 10 guidelines are designed to ensure safe defibrillator use[16]:

1. Make certain that all personnel are clear of the patient, bed, and defibrillator before making a defibrillation attempt.
2. Do not make contact with the patient except through the defibrillator paddle handles.
3. Do not use excessive gel or coupling material, which can become a contact between the patient's chest and the paddle handles. Do not discharge paddles over a pacemaker or ICD generator or *nitroglycerin* paste. Remove *nitroglycerin* patches before defibrillation.
4. To prevent gel from the patient's chest from being transferred to the paddle handles, do not have one person perform CPR and defibrillation alternately.
5. Apply gel or paste before turning on the defibrillator.
6. Do not "open air" discharge the defibrillator to get rid of an unwanted charge. Turn the defibrillator off to "dump" the charge.
7. Do not fire the defibrillator with the paddles placed together. This can cause pits on the paddles that can increase the risk of burns to the patient.
8. Treat equipment with respect. It is safe when used properly. Do not touch the metal electrodes or hold the paddles to your body when the defibrillator is on.

> ### CURRENT-BASED DEFIBRILLATION
>
> *Current-based defibrillation* (now under study) is an alternative to traditional defibrillation. With current-based defibrillation, the defibrillator operator selects electrical current (amps) versus energy (joules). This method avoids the problem of low-energy selection in the presence of high impedance (resulting in current flow that is too low and failure to defibrillate), or high-energy selection in the presence of low impedance (resulting in excessive current flow, myocardial damage, and failure to defibrillate). The optimal current for ventricular defibrillation appears to be 30 to 40 amps.[2]

9. Clean the paddles after use. Even dry gel presents a conductive pathway that could endanger the operator during a subsequent defibrillation attempt or equipment checkout procedure.
10. Routinely check the defibrillator (including batteries) to make sure the equipment is functioning properly. Follow the recommendations of the manufacturer.

Defibrillator Use in Special Environments

On occasion, a patient requires defibrillation in a special environment (e.g., in inclement weather). Although the guidelines in operator and personnel safety always apply, additional precautions are taken in special situations.

A patient can be defibrillated in wet conditions, such as near water, in rain, or in snowy weather. The patient's chest should be kept dry between the defibrillator electrode sites, and the operator's hands and the paddle handles should be kept as dry as possible. In a rainstorm, it would be safest to find shelter.

Depending on the defibrillator and its equipment specifications, the device may not be guaranteed to work properly in nonpressurized aircraft at certain altitudes or pressures. In addition, some electrical interference may occur between the radio equipment in the aircraft and the monitor-defibrillator or vice versa. This is affected by the distance and angle between the defibrillator and the radio equipment. Studies have demonstrated that defibrillation with current equipment would be expected to be safe in all types of rotary aircraft used for emergency medical transport.[17] Nonetheless, the medical crew should always inform the pilot(s) when electrical therapy is being used.

> **NOTE**
>
> When providing care in an aircraft, the paramedic should consult with the pilot(s) to make sure the flight instruments are well shielded from electromagnetic interference (EMI).

Implantable Cardioverter-Defibrillators

Implantable cardioverter-defibrillators (ICDs) commonly are implanted through a median sternotomy incision similar to that used for coronary artery bypass surgery, although left lateral thoracotomy, subcostal, and subxiphoid approaches also are used (Fig. 28-112). During implantation, the two defibrillation patches of the ICD are placed on the epicardium, usually opposite each ventricle to optimize the effectiveness of the device, which is tested intraoperatively. A pair of epicardial sensors also is attached to the left ventricle to monitor cardiac rhythm. The leads are connected to the biphasic defibrillator device, which is surgically placed in the left upper quadrant of the abdomen. (An outline of the generator usually can be felt or seen under the patient's skin.)

The ICD functions by monitoring the patient's cardiac rhythm, rate, and QRS morphology. When a monitored ventricular rate exceeds the preprogrammed rate, the ICD delivers a shock of about 6 to 30 joules through the patches to restore a normal sinus rhythm. The device requires 10 to 30 seconds to sense VT or VF and to charge the capacitor before delivering the shock. If defibrillation does not restore a normal sinus rhythm, the ICD will charge again and deliver up to four shocks. A complete sequence of five shocks, if required, may take up to 2 minutes. If the tachycardia or fibrillation persists after five shocks, no further shocks are delivered. Once a slower rhythm is restored (i.e., sinus or idioventricular) for at least 35 seconds, the device can deliver another series of up to five shocks if VT or VF recurs.

It is important to manage patients with ICDs as if they did not have a device. Standard ACLS proto-

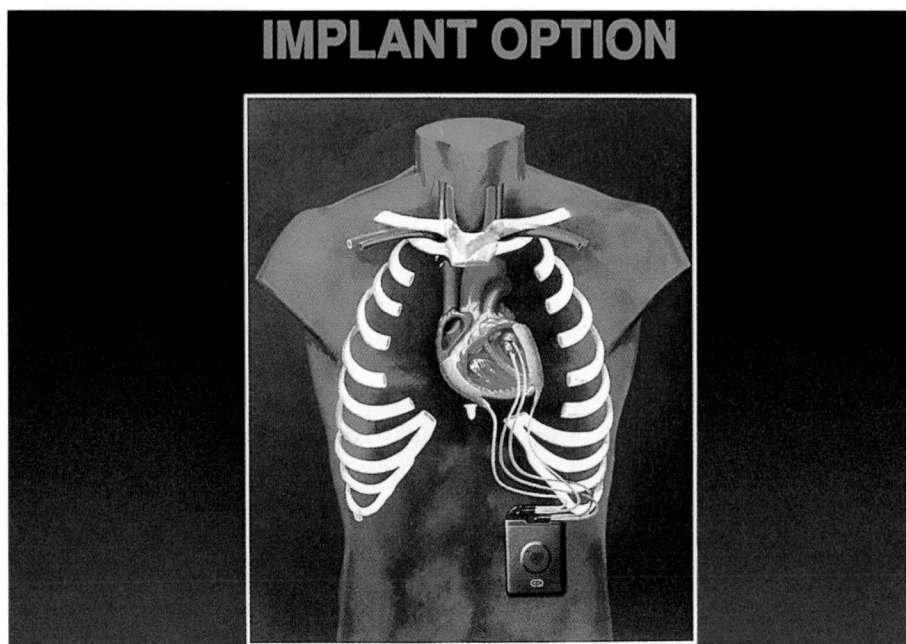

Fig. 28-112 Automatic ICD. (Courtesy Cardiac Pacemakers, Inc., St Paul, Minn.)

cols should be followed if the patient is in cardiac arrest or in any other way medically unstable. The AHA recommends the following four guidelines when caring for a patient with an ICD[1]:

1. If the ICD discharges while the rescuer is touching the victim, the rescuer may feel the shock, but it will not be dangerous. Personnel shocked by ICDs report sensations similar to contact with an electrical current.
2. ICDs are protected against damage from traditional transchest defibrillation shocks, but they require an ICD readiness check after external defibrillation occurs.
3. If VF or VT is present despite an ICD, an external shock should be given immediately because it is likely that the ICD failed to defibrillate the heart. After an initial series of shocks, the ICD will become operative again only if a period of nonfibrillatory rhythm occurs to reset the unit.
4. ICD units generally use patch electrodes that cover a portion of the epicardial surface, and these may reduce transcardiac current from transthoracic shocks. Thus, if transthoracic shocks of up to 360 joules fail to defibrillate a patient with an ICD, the chest electrode positions should be immediately changed (e.g., anterior-apex to anteroposterior) and the transthoracic shocks repeated. The different electrode posi-

tions could increase transthoracic current flow and facilitate defibrillation.

Since the ICD can be deactivated and activated with a magnet, patients with ICDs should be kept away from strong magnets to prevent accidental deactivation or reactivation of the device. The ability to use a magnet to deactivate and reactivate many of these devices can be useful when the unit is not functioning properly. However, use of a hand-held magnet to turn the unit off or back on should be considered only with the advice and under the direction of a physician.

? CRITICAL THINKING

What type of patients will have these devices?

Synchronized Cardioversion

Synchronized cardioversion (or countershock) is used to terminate dysrhythmias other than VF and pulseless VT. Unlike defibrillation (unsynchronized cardioversion), in which the current is delivered on the operator's command and with no regard as to where the shock occurs in the cycle of the underlying rhythm, synchronized cardioversion is designed

? CRITICAL THINKING

How can you minimize the discomfort and anxiety of a conscious patient whose device is repeatedly firing in response to the presence of a ventricular rhythm?

to deliver the shock about 10 ms after the peak of the R wave of the cardiac cycle (thus avoiding the "vulnerable" relative refractory period). Synchronization may reduce the energy required to end the dysrhythmia and decrease the potential for development of secondary complicating dysrhythmias.

Procedure

When the defibrillator is placed in the synchronized mode, the ECG displayed on the oscilloscope shows a "marker" denoting where in the cardiac cycle the energy will be discharged. This marker should appear on the R wave; if it does not, another lead should be selected. Adjustment of the ECG size may be needed if the marker does not appear. The procedure for synchronized cardioversion is as follows:

1. Turn on the defibrillator and select the synchronous mode.
2. Observe the oscilloscope to make certain that the R wave coincides with the marker.
3. Prepare the paddles or electrodes and place them on the patient's chest as previously described for defibrillation.
4. Set the energy level as prescribed by medical direction or protocol.
5. Call "clear" and visually ensure that the patient area is clear.
6. Depress the discharge buttons simultaneously and hold them in (or per manufacturer's instructions). The defibrillator will fire on the next identified R wave. After discharge, release the buttons.
7. If synchronization fails, follow the treatment algorithm. If a repeat attempt is required, it may be necessary to reselect the *synchronous mode* (depending on the defibrillator).

Transcutaneous Cardiac Pacing

Transcutaneous cardiac pacing (TCP) (also known as *external cardiac pacing*) is an effective emergency therapy for bradycardia, complete heart block, asystole, and suppression of some malignant ventricular tachydysrhythmias. These devices have been recognized by the AHA and are included in the management algorithms for bradycardia and asystole.

Artificial Pacemakers

Artificial pacemakers (Fig. 28-113) deliver repetitive electrical currents to the heart, substituting for a natural pacemaker that has become blocked or dysfunctional. The patient with severe sinus bradycardia, heart block, or idioventricular rhythm who is capable of generating a pulse with cardiac contractions may respond to an external pacing device and produce a perfusing pulse. Sinus bradycardia also may be paced but generally responds well to *atropine.* However, the majority of patients in cardiac arrest do not respond to pacing because the heart is metabolically compromised from inadequate perfusion and is therefore incapable of effective contractions.

The two modes of TCP are nondemand (asynchronous) pacing and demand pacing. Most devices provide both modes. An asynchronous pacemaker delivers timed electrical stimuli at a selected rate, regardless of the patient's intrinsic cardiac activity. These pacing devices are used less frequently than demand pacers because they have the potential to discharge during the vulnerable period of the cardiac cycle (producing the R-on-T phenomenon). The asynchronous mode generally is used only as a last resort and then usually in asystole. This mode also may be indicated when a significant artifact on the

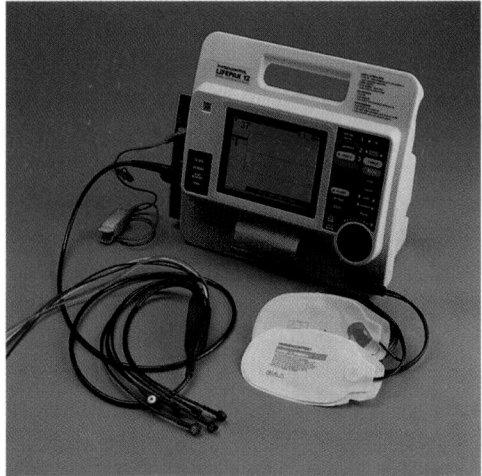

Fig. 28-113 Life Pack 12 3D Biphasic defibrillator/monitor. (Courtesy Medtronic Physio–Control.)

ECG signal interferes with the demand-mode sensing of intrinsic beats. Another use for asynchronous pacing is in overriding inherent prearrest tachydysrhythmias (e.g., torsades de pointes). However, this should be attempted only if other means of controlling the dysrhythmia have failed.

Demand pacing is designed to sense the patient's inherent QRS complex, delivering electrical stimuli only when needed. It is much safer to apply than the nondemand mode. When it senses an intrinsic beat, the pacemaker is inhibited. If no beats are sensed, the pacemaker delivers pacing stimuli at a selected rate. The device usually is set to discharge at a rate between 70 and 80 beats per minute. It is then increased in increments of 5 to 10 milliamps of electricity, and mechanical capture is achieved. Generally, the patient's clinical condition (blood pressure, level of consciousness, skin color, and temperature) improves at this point.

The paramedic should ensure that each pacemaker spike on the oscilloscope is followed by a QRS complex. If not, the current should gradually be increased until there is consistent capture. Unfortunately, motion artifact often makes ECG confirmation of electrical capture quite difficult. The only definitive method of monitoring mechanical capture by the pacing device is the presence of a pulse with each QRS complex. Therefore the patient requires constant monitoring of perfusion status.

> **NOTE**
>
> The patient's pulse rate and blood pressure should be assessed on the patient's right side to minimize interference from muscle artifact.

Procedure

1. Gather the required equipment.
2. Explain the procedure to the patient.
3. Connect the patient to a cardiac monitor and obtain a rhythm strip.
4. Obtain baseline vital signs.
5. Apply pacing electrodes (avoid large muscle masses) and attach the pacing cable and pacing device. (The electrodes should be placed in the anterior-posterior position, avoiding the diaphragm.)
6. Select the pacing mode.
7. Select the pacing rate (usually 80 beats per minute) and set the current (begin with 50 mil-

> **NOTE**
>
> As with synchronized cardioversion, selecting the "pacing mode" should result in the appearance of light markers on intrinsic beats. Paramedics should ensure that this occurs so that they know the demand mode is activated and functioning properly.

liamps, then increase until ventricular capture is obtained).
8. Activate the pacemaker, observing the patient and the ECG.
9. Obtain rhythm strips as appropriate.
10. Continue monitoring the patient and anticipate further therapy.

Indications and Contraindications

The primary indications for TCP in the prehospital setting are symptomatic bradycardia, heart block associated with reduced cardiac output that is unresponsive to *atropine,* pacemaker failure, and asystole. As previously stated, cardiac pacing seldom is effective in cardiac arrest. It also is ineffective in pulseless electrical activity (PEA) unless the underlying cause of PEA is corrected. Its use is contraindicated in patients with open wounds or burns to the chest and patients in a wet environment.

> **? CRITICAL THINKING**
>
> ***Why should patient movement be minimized during TCP?***

Electrode Placement

Proper electrode placement and polarity are important in providing effective external pacing (Fig. 28-114). The paramedic should apply the negative (anterior) electrode to the left of the sternum and centered as close as possible to the point of maximal cardiac impulse. The positive (posterior) electrode is placed directly behind the anterior electrode, to the left of the thoracic spinal column. In rare situations in which posterior placement cannot be used, the positive electrode can be placed in line with the patient's left nipple at the midaxillary line. (Anterior-anterior placement may produce pronounced pectoral muscle twitching.) The electrodes should be applied to clean, dry skin without localized trauma or infection.

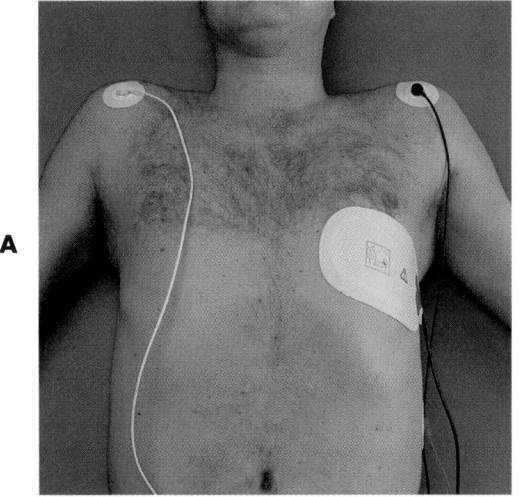

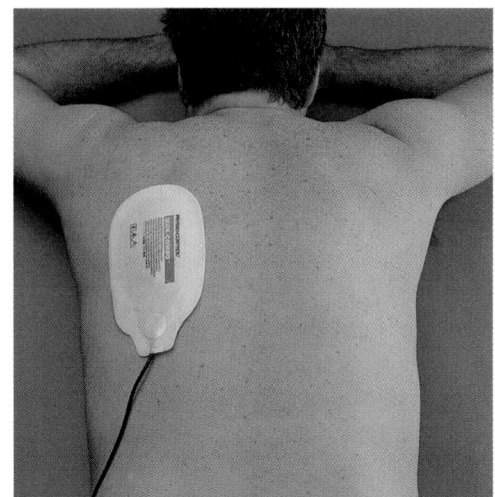

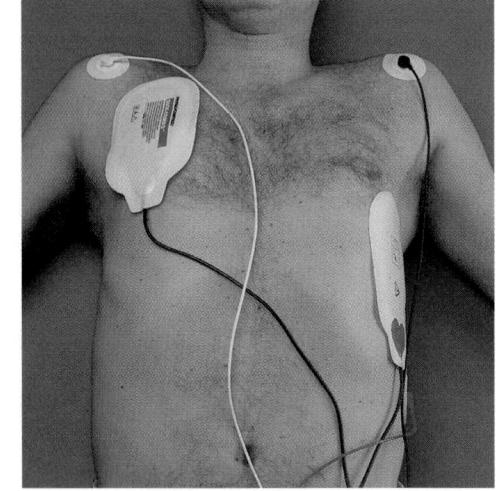

Fig. 28-114 Proper electrode attachment for external pacing. **A** and **B,** Preferred anterior-posterior placement. **C,** Alternative anterior-anterior placement.

The conscious patient probably will experience some pain and discomfort during TCP, which is directly correlated to the intensity of muscle contractions and the amount of applied current. Ideally, analgesia or sedation of the patient should be provided.

Cardiac Arrest and Sudden Death

It is becoming increasingly evident that patients who cannot be resuscitated in the prehospital setting rarely survive, even if they are resuscitated temporarily in the emergency department (Box 28-9). The patient's best chance for survival is to have rapid and appropriate interventions in the field. However, if various procedures needed for appropriate intervention (endotracheal intubation, IV access) cannot be successfully completed in a short period, main-

taining ventilation and compressions and rapidly transporting the patient to the nearest medical facility should be considered. Initial defibrillation should always be attempted as soon as possible, but prolonged field resuscitation in the face of procedural difficulties is almost always destined to fail.

There is much research underway in the area of emergency cardiac care. Some of this research deals with various drugs to improve cardiac and neu-

> **NOTE**
>
> As a rule, CPR should always be initiated in the presence of cardiac arrest unless there are obvious signs of death (e.g., rigor, fixed lividity, decapitation, open head injury with exposed cranial content) or legitimate prehospital advance directives.

rovascular resuscitation. Because of the fairly large number of patients who regain cardiac function but never regain consciousness, there is tremendous interest in how to improve cerebral perfusion after cardiac arrest and limit reperfusion injury. This research may lead to a variety of new drugs to be used by paramedics during resuscitation in future years.

Termination of Resuscitation

According to the AHA, health care professionals are expected to provide BLS and ACLS as part of their professional duty to respond, with the following exceptions[4]:

- When a person lies dead, with obvious clinical signs of irreversible death
- When attempts to perform CPR would place the rescuer at risk of physical injury
- When the patent or surrogate has indicated that resuscitation is not desired

It is further recommended that termination of resuscitative efforts in the prehospital setting follow system-specific criteria established by medical direction. This criteria should include consideration for advance directives and "no-CPR" orders (described in Chapter 4).

> **NOTE**
>
> If at any time paramedics are presented with an advance directive (e.g., a written directive, living will, durable power of attorney) that indicates a patient should not be resuscitated, they should follow established protocol or immediately consult with medical direction.

Criteria for Terminating Resuscitation

It may be appropriate to terminate resuscitation (in some circumstances) if asystole persists. The termination of resuscitative efforts should only occur after reviewing the quality of the resuscitation attempt and considering the presence of atypical clinical features. Questions about the resuscitation attempt to be considered include[4]:

- Has there been an adequate trial of BLS and ACLS?
- Has the patient's trachea been intubated?

> **BOX 28-9**
>
> ### RELATED TERMINOLOGY
>
> **Resuscitation:** To provide efforts to return spontaneous pulse and breathing to the patient in full cardiac arrest.
>
> **Survival:** Resuscitation of a patient who survives to hospital discharge.
>
> **Return of spontaneous circulation (ROSC):** Resuscitation of a patient to the point of having a pulse without CPR; may or may not have return of spontaneous respirations; the patient may or may not survive.

- Has effective ventilation been provided?
- If VF was present, was the patient defibrillated?
- Was IV access obtained?
- Were *epinephrine* (Adrenalin) and *atropine* administered?
- Have reversible causes been ruled out?
- Has the asystole been continuously documented for more than 5 to 10 minutes after all of the above have been accomplished?

Finally, the presence of atypical clinical features such as submersion or profound hypothermia, young age, toxins or electrolyte abnormalities, and drug overdose may be indicators that continued resuscitation is appropriate. Terminating resuscitation in the prehospital setting should be guided by medical direction.

Procedure for Termination of Resuscitation

The procedure for terminating resuscitation in the field will vary by protocol and must follow guidelines established by medical direction. When termination is considered to be appropriate, the paramedic should contact medical direction to convey the following information:

- Medical condition of the patient
- Known etiological factors
- Any therapy rendered
- Family's appraisal of the situation and any resistance or uncertainty

While gathering and presenting this information to medical direction, the paramedic should maintain continuous documentation of the event (including continuous ECG monitoring) to assist in the mandatory review of the call that commonly is performed for quality assurance in most EMS systems.

? CRITICAL THINKING

What resources can you contact to help the family after you have terminated resuscitation in the home?

Special Considerations

In addition to the needs of the patient, grief support for the family must be considered. Although this will vary by agency, often a paramedic (or other EMS personnel) will be assigned to stay with the family for a period of time, or a community agency referral will be arranged.

Law enforcement personnel may have additional duties at the scene as part of their professional responsibilities. These duties may include an on-scene determination that the patient be assigned to a medical examiner when the death or event is suspicious, or when a patient's private physician refuses or hesitates to sign the death certificate.

S U M M A R Y

- Persons at high risk for cardiovascular disease include those with diabetes, a family history of premature cardiovascular disease, and prior myocardial infarction. Prevention strategies include educational programs in community nutrition, cessation of smoking (smoking prevention for children), and screening for hypertension and high cholesterol.

- The left coronary artery carries approximately 85% of the blood supply to the myocardium, and the right coronary artery carries the remainder. The pumping action of the heart is a product of rhythmic, alternate contraction and relaxation of the atria and ventricles. The stoke volume is the amount of blood ejected from each ventricle with one contraction. Stroke volume depends on preload, afterload, and myocardial contractility. Cardiac output is the amount of blood pumped by each ventricle per minute.

- In addition to the body's intrinsic control in regulating the heart, extrinsic control by the parasympathetic and sympathetic nerves of the autonomic nervous system is a major factor influencing the heart rate, conductivity, and contractility. Sympathetic impulses cause the adrenal medulla to secrete epinephrine and norepinephrine into the blood.

- The major electrolytes that influence cardiac function are calcium, potassium, sodium, and magnesium. The electrical charge (potential difference) between the inside and outside of cells is expressed in millivolts. When the cell is in an unstimulated or "resting" state, the electrical charge difference is referred to as a resting membrane potential. The specialized sodium-potassium exchange pump actively pumps sodium ions out of the cell and potassium ions in. The cell membrane appears to have individual protein-lined channels that allow passage of a specific ion or group of ions.

- Nerve and muscle cells are capable of producing action potentials, a property known as *excitability.* An action potential at any point on the cell membrane stimulates an excitation process that is spread down the length of the cell and conducted across synapses from cell to cell.

- The fundamental contraction process for cardiac and skeletal muscle is believed to be activated by calcium ions, resulting in a binding between myosin and actin myofilaments.

- The conduction system of the heart is composed of two nodes (the sinoatrial [SA] node and the atrioventricular [AV] node) and a conducting bundle.

- Common chief complaints of the patient with cardiovascular disease include chest pain or discomfort, including shoulder, arm, neck, or jaw pain or discomfort; dyspnea; syncope; and abnormal heartbeat or palpitations. Patients suspected to have a cardiovascular disorder should be asked whether they take prescription medications, especially cardiac drugs; are being treated for any serious illness; have a history of myocardial infarction, angina, heart failure, hypertension, diabetes, or chronic lung disease; have any allergies; or have other risk factors for heart disease.

- After performing the initial assessment of the patient with cardiovascular disease, the paramedic should look for skin color, jugular venous distention, and the presence of edema or other signs of heart disease; listen for lung sounds, heart sounds, and carotid artery bruit; and feel for edema, pulses, skin temperature, and moisture.

- The electrocardiogram (ECG) is a diagnostic graphic representation of the heart's electrical activity generated by depolarization and repolarization of the atria and ventricles.

- Routine monitoring of cardiac rhythm in the prehospital setting is usually obtained in lead II or MCL_1 which are the best leads to monitor for dysrhythmias because of their ability to visualize P waves. A 12-lead ECG can be used to help identify changes relative to myocardial ischemia, injury, and infarction; distinguish ventricular tachycardia (VT) from supraventricular tachycardia (SVT); determine the electrical axis and the presence of fascicular blocks; and determine the presence of bundle branch blocks.

- The paper used to record ECGs is standardized to allow comparative analysis of an ECG wave.

- The normal ECG consists of a P wave, QRS complex, and T wave. The P wave is the first positive deflection on the ECG, representing atrial depolarization. The PR interval is the time it takes for an electrical impulse to be conducted through the atria and the AV node up to the instant of ventricular depolarization. The QRS complex represents ventricular depolarization. The ST segment represents the early part of repolarization of the right and left ventricles. The T wave represents repolarization of the ventricular myocardial cells and occurs during the last part of ventricular systole. The QT interval is the period from the beginning of ventricular depolarization (onset of the QRS complex) until the end of ventricular repolarization, or the end of the T wave.

- The steps in ECG analysis include analyzing the QRS complex, P waves, rate, rhythm, and PR interval.

- Dysrhythmias originating in the SA node include sinus bradycardia, sinus tachycardia, sinus dysrhythmia, and sinus arrest. Most sinus dysrhythmias result from increases or decreases in vagal tone.

- Dysrhythmias originating in the atria include wandering pacemaker, premature atrial complexes, paroxysmal supraventricular tachycardia, atrial flutter, and atrial fibrillation. Common causes of atrial dysrhythmias are ischemia, hypoxia, and atrial dilation caused by congestive heart failure or mitral valve abnormalities.

- When the SA node and the atria cannot generate the electrical impulses needed to begin depolarization because of factors such as hypoxia, ischemia, myocardial infarction, and drug toxicity, the AV node or the area surrounding the AV node may assume the role of the secondary pacemaker. Dysrhythmias originating in the AV junction include premature junctional complexes, junctional escape complexes or rhythms, and accelerated junctional rhythm.

- Ventricular dysrhythmias are usually considered to be life threatening. Ventricular rhythm disturbances generally result from failure of the atria, AV junction, or both, to initiate an electrical impulse, or they are secondary to enhanced automaticity or reentry phenomena in the ventricles. Dysrhythmias originating in the ventricles include ventricular escape complexes or rhythms, premature ventricular complexes, VT, ventricular fibrillation (VF), asystole, and, artificial pacemaker rhythm.

- Partial delays or complete interruptions in cardiac electrical conduction are called *heart blocks*. Causes of heart blocks include AV junctional ischemia, AV junctional necrosis, degenerative disease of the conduction system, and drug toxicity. Dysrhythmias that are disorders of conduction are first-degree AV block, type I second-degree AV block (Wenckebach), type II second-degree AV block, third-degree AV block, disturbances of ventricular conduction, pulseless electrical activity, and preexcitation (Wolff-Parkinson-White) syndrome.

- Atherosclerosis is a disease process characterized by progressive narrowing of the lumen of medium and large arteries. Atherosclerosis has two major effects on blood vessels: (1) the disease disrupts the intimal surface, causing a loss of vessel elasticity and an increase in thrombogenesis, and (2) the atheroma reduces the diameter of the vessel lumen and thus decreases the blood supply to tissues.

- Angina pectoris is a symptom of myocardial ischemia caused by an imbalance between myocardial oxygen supply and demand. Prehospital management includes placing the patient at rest, administering oxygen, initiating IV therapy, administering nitroglycerin and possibly morphine, monitoring the patient for dysrhythmias, and transporting the patient for physician evaluation.

- Acute myocardial infarction (AMI) occurs when there is a sudden cessation of blood flowing through an affected coronary artery to an area of heart muscle. This results in ischemia, injury, and necrosis to the area of myocardium supplied by the affected artery. Death secondary to myocardial infarction usually results from lethal dysrhythmias (VT, VF, and cardiac standstill), pump failure (cardiogenic shock and congestive heart failure), or myocardial tissue rupture (rupture of the ventricle, septum, or papillary muscle).

Although some patients with AMI, particularly those in the older age groups, have only symptoms of dyspnea, syncope, or confusion, substernal chest pain is usually present in patients with AMI (70% to 90% of patients). ST-segment elevation greater than 0.1 mV in at least two contiguous ECG leads indicates an AMI. However, some patients infarct without ST-segment elevation changes, and other conditions can produce ST-segment elevation. Prehospital management of the patient with a suspected myocardial infarction should include placing the patient at rest; administering oxygen at 3 to 4 L per minute via nasal cannula; frequently assessing vital signs and breath sounds; initiating an IV line with normal saline or lactated Ringer's solution to keep the vein open; monitoring for dysrhythmias; administering medications such as nitroglycerin, morphine, and aspirin; and screening for risk factors for thrombolytic therapy.

- Left ventricular failure occurs when the left ventricle fails to function as an effective forward pump, causing a back-pressure of blood into the pulmonary circulation, which may lead to pulmonary edema. Emergency management is directed at decreasing the venous return to the heart, improving myocardial contractility, decreasing myocardial oxygen demand, improving ventilation and oxygenation, and rapidly transporting the patient to a medical facility.

- Right ventricular failure occurs when the right ventricle fails as an effective forward pump, causing back-pressure of blood into the systemic venous circulation. Right ventricular failure is not usually a medical emergency in itself unless it is associated with pulmonary edema or hypotension.

- Cardiogenic shock is the most extreme form of pump failure. It is usually caused by extensive myocardial infarction and, even with aggressive therapy, has a mortality rate of 70% or higher. These patients require rapid transport to a medical facility.

- Cardiac tamponade is defined as impaired diastolic filling of the heart caused by increased intrapericardial pressure.

- Abdominal aortic aneurysms are usually asymptomatic, but signs and symptoms will signal impending or active rupture. If the vessel tears, bleeding may initially be tamponaded by the retroperitoneal tissues, and the patient may be normotensive on EMS arrival. If the rupture opens into the peritoneal cavity, however, massive fatal hemorrhage may follow.

- Acute dissection is the most common aortic catastrophe. Although any area of the aorta may be involved, in 60% to 70% of cases the site of a dissecting aneurysm is in the ascending aorta, just beyond the takeoff of the left subclavian artery. The signs and symptoms depend on the site of the intimal tear and the extent of dissection. The goals of managing suspected aortic dissection in the prehospital setting are relief of pain and immediate transport to a medical facility.

- Acute arterial occlusion is a sudden blockage of arterial flow, most commonly caused by trauma, an embolus, or thrombosis. The most common sites of embolic occlusion are the abdominal aorta, common femoral artery, popliteal artery, carotid artery, brachial artery, and mesenteric artery. The location of ischemic pain is related to the site of occlusion.

- Noncritical peripheral vascular conditions include varicose veins, superficial thrombophlebitis, and acute deep-vein thrombosis. Of these conditions, deep-vein thrombosis is the only one that can cause a life-threatening problem—pulmonary embolus.

- Hypertension is often defined by a resting blood pressure consistently greater than 140/90 mm Hg. Chronic hypertension has an adverse effect on the function of the heart and blood vessels, requiring the heart to perform more work than normal, leading to hypertrophy of the cardiac muscle and left ventricular failure. Conditions associated with chronic, uncontrolled hypertension are cerebral hemorrhage and stroke, myocardial infarction, and renal failure.

- Hypertensive emergencies are conditions in which a blood pressure increase leads to significant, irreversible end-organ damage within hours if not treated. The organs most likely to be at risk are the brain, heart, and kidneys. As a rule, the diagnosis is based on altered end-organ function and the rate of the rise in blood pressure, not the level of blood pressure.

- Basic cardiac life support externally supports the circulation and respiration of a victim of cardiac arrest until advanced cardiac life support is available. Two mechanisms are thought to be responsible for blood flow during CPR: (1) direct compression of the heart between the sternum and the spine, which increases pressure within the ventricles to provide blood flow to the lungs and body organs, and (2) increased intrathoracic pressure transmitted to all intrathoracic vascular structures, which produces an intrathoracic-to-extrathoracic pressure gradient that causes blood to flow out of the thorax. A number of mechanical devices provide external chest compression, and others provide chest compression with a system for synchronized ventilation in the cardiac arrest patient.

- Cardiac monitor-defibrillators are classified as manual or automated external defibrillators. Defibrillation is the delivery of electrical current through the chest wall for the purpose of terminating VF and certain other nonperfusing rhythms.

- Implantable cardioverter-defibrillators (ICDs) function by monitoring the patient's cardiac rhythm. When a monitored ventricular rate exceeds the preprogrammed rate, the ICD delivers a shock of approximately 6 to 30 joules through the patches to restore a normal sinus rhythm.

- Synchronized cardioversion is designed to deliver the shock approximately 10 ms after the peak of the R wave of the cardiac cycle (thus avoiding the relative refractory period). Synchronization may reduce the energy required to end the dysrhythmia and decrease the potential for development of secondary complicating dysrhythmias.

- Transcutaneous cardiac pacing is an effective emergency therapy for bradycardia, complete heart block, asystole, and suppression of some malignant ventricular dysrhythmias. Proper electrode placement and polarity are important in providing effective external pacing.

- It is becoming increasingly evident that patients who cannot be resuscitated in the prehospital setting rarely survive, even if they are resuscitated temporarily in the emergency department. Cessation of resuscitative efforts in the prehospital setting should follow system-specific criteria established by medical direction.

REFERENCES

1. American Heart Association: *Advanced cardiac life support,* Dallas, 1997, The Association.
2. Phalen T: *The 12-lead ECG in acute myocardial infarction,* St Louis, 1996, Mosby.
3. Marriott H, Conover M: *Advanced concepts in arrhythmias,* ed 2, St Louis, 1989, Mosby.
4. American Heart Association: *Guidelines 2000 for cardiopulmonary resuscitation and emergency cardiovascular care,* International Consensus on Science, Dallas, 2000, The Association.
5. Page B: *12-lead ECG interpretation workshop,* St Louis, 1998, Multi-lead Medics.
6. Taigman M, Cannon S: Reading bundle branch blocks, *JEMS* 15(5):41, 1990.
7. Little R, Little W: *Physiology of the heart,* ed 4, St Louis, 1989, Mosby.
8. Rosen P, Barkin R: *Emergency medicine: concepts and clinical practice,* ed 4, St Louis, 1998, Mosby.
9. US Department of Transportation, National Highway Traffic Safety Administration: *Paramedic national standard curriculum,* 1998, Washington, DC, The Department.
10. Grubbs T: The ultimate emergency: managing aortic aneurysms, *JEMS* 16(10):56, 1991.
11. National Center for Health Statistics: *Fastats: A to Z,* Atlanta, 1998, Centers for Disease Control and Prevention.
12. National Joint Committee on Hypertension: *The sixth report of the Joint National Committee on Prevention, Detection, Evaluation, and Treatment of High Blood Pressure,* Washington, DC, 1998, National Institutes of Health, National Heart Lung and Blood Institute.
13. American Heart Association: *Basic life support for healthcare providers,* Dallas, 1997, The Association.
14. *The forerunner biphasic waveform technical note,* Seattle, 1997, Heartstream.
15. Brady G et al: Multicenter comparison of trunicated biphasic shocks and standard damped sine wave monophasic shocks for transthoracic ventricular defibrillation, *PACE* 19:678, 1996.
16. Higgins S: *Defibrillation: what you should know,* Redmond, Tex, 1978, Physio-Control.
17. Dedrick D et al: Defibrillation safety in emergency helicopter transport, *Ann Emerg Med* 18(1):69, 1989.

29 *Neurology*

OBJECTIVES

Upon completion of this chapter, the paramedic student will be able to:

1. *Describe the anatomy and physiology of the nervous system.*
2. *Outline pathophysiological changes in the nervous system that may alter cerebral perfusion pressure.*
3. *Describe the assessment of a patient with a nervous system disorder.*
4. *Describe pathophysiology, signs and symptoms, and specific management techniques for each of the following neurological disorders: coma, stroke and intracranial hemorrhage, seizure disorders, headache, brain neoplasm and brain abscess, and degenerative neurological diseases.*

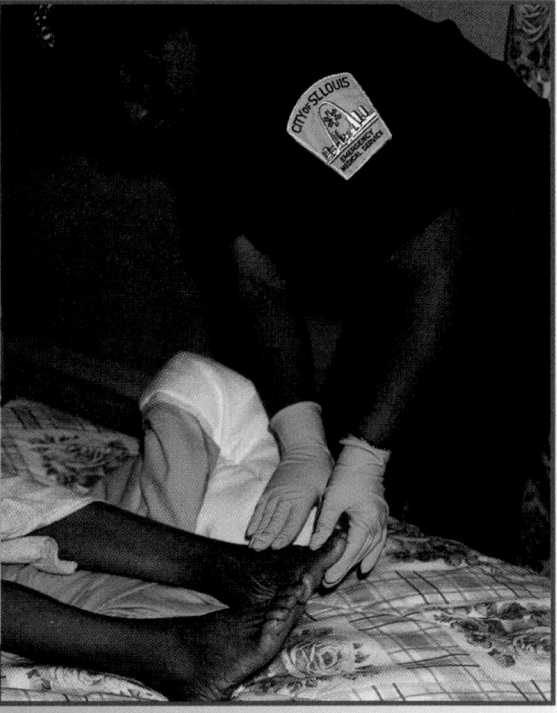

Acute disorders of the nervous system require rapid assessment and management. The paramedic's knowledge and skills, combined with appropriate and aggressive intervention, can help reduce mortality and morbidity and produce maximal potential for rehabilitation and recovery.

KEY TERMS

amyotrophic lateral sclerosis (ALS): One of a group of rare disorders in which the nerves that control muscular activity degenerate within the brain and spinal cord; also called *Lou Gehrig's disease.*

Bell's palsy: A condition in which there is paralysis of the facial muscles due to inflammation of the seventh cranial nerve; usually is one-sided and temporary and often develops suddenly.

central pain syndrome: Infection or disease of the trigeminal nerve (cranial nerve V).

cluster headache: A type of headache that occurs in bursts (clusters); also known as histamine headache.

dystonia: A condition characterized by local or diffuse alterations in muscle tone, resulting in painful muscle spasms, unusually fixed postures, and strange movement patterns.

epilepsy: A condition in which there is a tendency toward recurrent seizures (excluding those that arise from correctable or avoidable circumstances).

migraine: A severe, incapacitating headache that often is preceded by visual and/or GI disturbances.

multiple sclerosis (MS): A progressive disease of the central nervous system in which scattered patches of myelin in the brain and spinal cord are destroyed.

muscular dystrophy: An inherited muscle disorder of unknown cause in which there is a slow but progressive degeneration of muscle fibers.

myoclonus: A condition characterized by rapid and uncontrollable muscular contractions or spasms of muscles that occur at rest or during movement.

Parkinson's disease: A disease caused by degeneration or damage (of unknown origin) to nerve cells within the basal ganglia in the brain.

peripheral neuropathy: Diseases and disorders affecting the peripheral nervous system, including spinal nerve roots, cranial nerves, and peripheral nerves.

seizure: A temporary alteration in behavior or consciousness caused by abnormal electrical activity of one or more groups of neurons in the brain.

sinus headache: A headache characterized by pain in the forehead, nasal area, and eyes.

spina bifida: A congenital defect in which one part of one or more vertebrae fails to develop completely, leaving a portion of the spinal cord exposed.

status epilepticus: Continuous seizure activity lasting 30 minutes or longer or a recurrent seizure without an intervening period of consciousness.

tension headache: A headache caused by muscle contractions of the face, neck, and scalp.

Anatomy and Physiology of the Nervous System

As described in Chapter 6, the nervous system is divided into two parts: the central nervous system (CNS) and the peripheral nervous system (PNS). The human body's ability to maintain a state of homeostasis results primarily from the nervous system's regulatory and coordinating activities. To review, the CNS consists of the brain and spinal cord, both of which are encased in and protected by bone. A total of 43 pairs of nerves originate from the CNS to form the PNS: 12 pairs of cranial nerves originating from the brain and 31 pairs of spinal nerves originating from the spinal cord.

Cells of the Nervous System

The cells of the nervous system include neurons (the fundamental units of the nervous system) and connective tissue cells known as *neuroglia* (specialized cells that protect and hold functioning neurons together). Each neuron consists of three main parts: a neuron cell body, which contains a single, relatively large nucleus with a prominent nucleolus; one or more branching projections called dendrites; and a single, elongated projection known as an axon (Fig. 29-1). Dendrites transmit impulses to the neuron cell bodies, and axons transmit impulses away from the cell bodies. Axons are surrounded by supportive and protective sheaths formed by the cytoplasmic extensions of neuroglial cells in the CNS (unmyelinated axons) and by Schwann cells in the PNS (myelinated axons).

Bundles of parallel axons with their associated sheaths are white in color and are called *white matter.* The action potential, which is initiated in the neuron body, is propagated through the axons via conduction pathways or nerve tracts from one area of the CNS to another. In the PNS, bundles of axons and their sheaths are called *nerves.* Collections of nerve

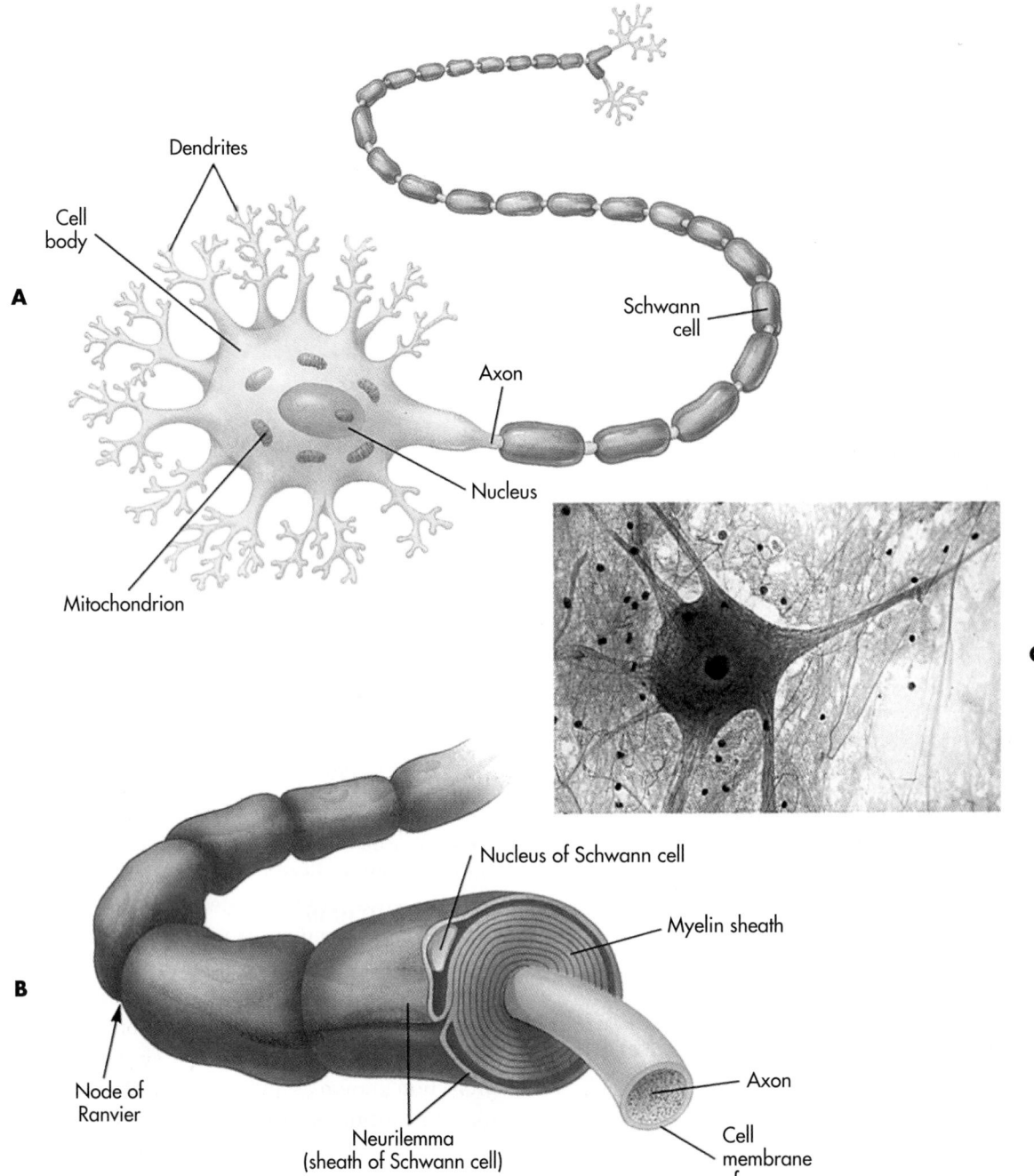

Fig. 29-1 Neuron. **A,** A typical neuron showing dendrites, a cell body, and an axon. **B,** Segment of a myelinated axon cut to show detail of the concentric layers of the Schwann cell filled with myelin. **C,** Photomicrograph of a neuron. (From Thibodeau GA: *Structure and function of the body,* ed 9, St Louis, 1992, Mosby.)

cells are more gray in color and are called *gray matter.* Gray matter is the site of integration within the nervous system. The outer surface of the cerebrum and the cerebellum consists of gray matter comprising the cerebral cortex and cerebellar cortex.

Types of Neurons

Based on the direction in which they transmit impulses, neurons are classified as *sensory neurons, motor neurons,* or *interneurons.* Sensory neurons transmit impulses to the spinal cord and brain from all parts of the body. Motor neurons transmit impulses in the opposite direction, away from the brain and spinal cord, and only to muscle and glandular epithelial tissue. Interneurons conduct impulses from sensory neurons to motor neurons. Sensory neurons also are called *afferent neurons,* motor neurons are called *efferent neurons,* and interneurons are called *central* or *connecting neurons.*

Impulse Transmission

The transmission of nerve impulses in the nervous system is similar to the conduction of electrical impulses through the heart. In its resting state, the neuron is positively charged on the outside and negatively charged on the inside. When stimulated by pressure, temperature, or chemical changes, the permeability of the neuron's membrane to sodium ions increases. As a result, positively charged sodium ions rush into the interior of the neuron. This inward movement begins a wave of depolarization that travels down the axon, resulting in the propagation of an action potential (Fig. 29-2).

? CRITICAL THINKING

Think of an example of a pressure, temperature, and chemical stimulus to a nerve.

In unmyelinated axons, action potentials are propagated along the entire axon membrane. Myelinated axons, however, have interruptions in the myelin sheaths known as *nodes of Ranvier.* These nodes allow nerve impulses to "jump" from one node to the next without propagation along the entire length of the cell (saltatory conduction). Therefore myelinated axons conduct action potentials more rapidly than unmyelinated axons.

Synapse

The membrane-to-membrane contact that separates the axon endings of one neuron (presynaptic neuron) from the dendrites of another neuron (postsynaptic neuron) is known as a *synapse.* The structures that compose a synapse are the presynaptic terminal, the synaptic cleft, and the plasma membrane of the postsynaptic neuron. Within each presynaptic

terminal are synaptic vesicles that contain neurotransmitter chemicals (Fig. 29-3).

Each action potential arriving at the presynaptic terminal initiates a series of specific events that results in the release of the neurotransmitter substance. The neurotransmitter chemical rapidly diffuses the short distance across the synaptic cleft and binds to specific receptor molecules on the postsynaptic membrane. After an impulse is generated and a conduction by postsynaptic neurons is initiated, neurotransmitter activity ends rapidly. Several substances have been identified as neurotransmitters, and others are suspected as neurotransmitters. Well-known neurotransmitters include acetylcholine, norepinephrine, epinephrine, and dopamine.

Reflexes

One type of route traveled by nerve impulses is known as a *reflex* or *reflex arc.* A reflex is the basic functional unit of the nervous system that is capable of receiving a stimulus and generating a response. Reflexes allow unidirectional conduction of impulses and have several basic components: a sensory receptor, a sensory neuron, interneurons, a motor neuron, and an effector organ. Individual reflexes vary in their complexity. Some function to remove the body from painful stimuli or prevent the body from suddenly falling or moving as a result of external forces. Others are responsible for maintaining a relatively constant blood pressure, body fluid pH, blood carbon dioxide level, and water intake. All reflexes are homeostatic; they function to maintain healthy survival.

Action potentials initiated in sensory receptors are propagated along sensory axons within the PNS to the CNS, where they synapse with interneurons. Interneurons synapse with motor neurons in the spinal cord, which send their axons out of the spinal cord and through the PNS to muscles or glands, causing the effector organ to respond. Fig. 29-4, which illustrates the neural pathway involved in the patellar reflex, shows the transmission of nerve impulses.

Blood Supply

The arterial blood supply to the brain comes from the vertebral arteries and the internal carotid arter-

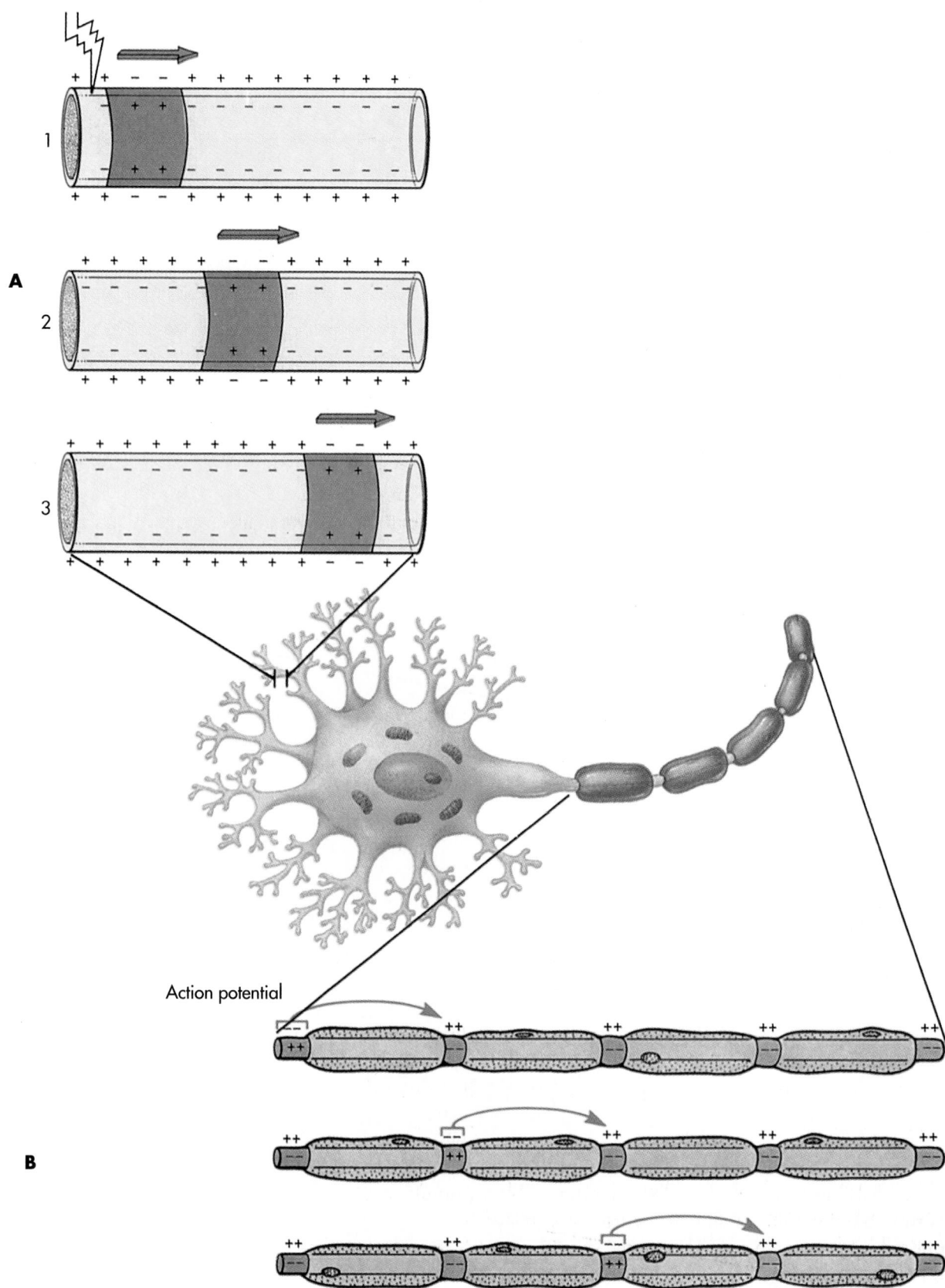

Fig. 29-2 Conduction of nerve impulses. **A,** In unmyelinated fiber, a nerve impulse (action potential) is a self-propagating wave of electrical disturbance. **B,** In myelinated fiber, the action potential "jumps" around the insulating myelin in a rapid type of conduction called saltatory conduction. (From Thibodeau GA: *Structure and function of the body,* ed 9, St Louis, 1992, Mosby.)

Action potential

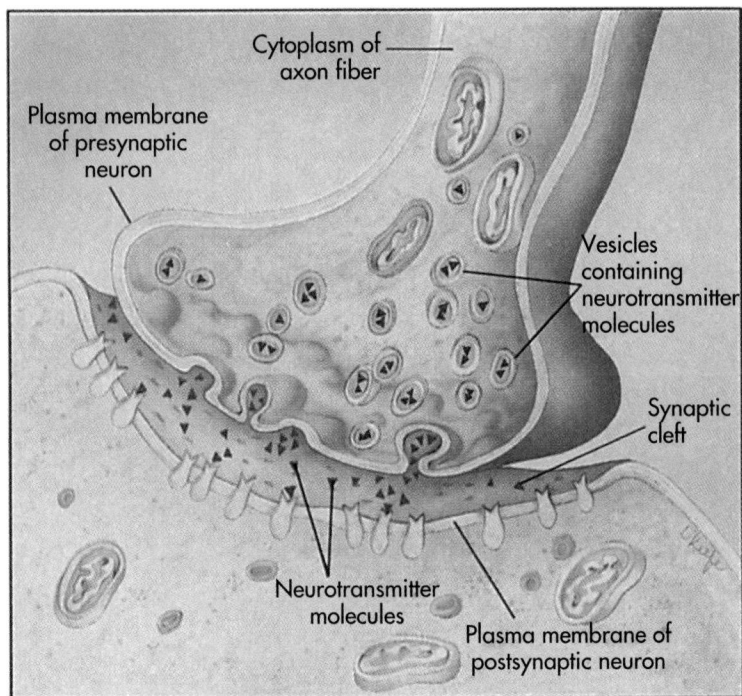

Fig. 29-3 Components of a synapse. Diagram shows axon terminal of a presynaptic neuron and a synaptic cleft. When an action potential arrives at the axon terminal of a presynaptic neuron, neurotransmitter molecules are released from vesicles in the axon terminal into the synaptic cleft. Combining neurotransmitter and receptor molecules in the plasma membrane of the postsynaptic neuron initiates impulse conduction in the postsynaptic neuron. (From Thibodeau GA: *Structure and function of the body,* ed 9, St Louis, 1992, Mosby.)

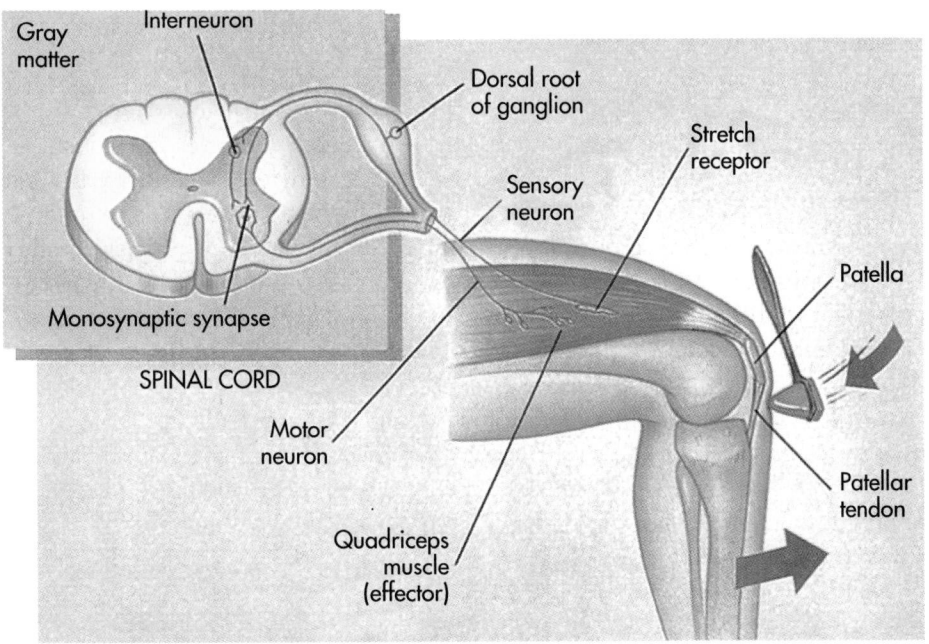

Fig. 29-4 The neural pathway involved in the patellar ("knee-jerk") reflex. (From Thibodeau GA: *Structure and function of the body,* ed 9, St Louis, 1992, Mosby.)

ies (Fig. 29-5). The right and left vertebral arteries (supplying the cerebellum) enter the cranial vault through the foramen magnum and unite to form the midline basilar artery. The basilar artery branches to supply the pons and cerebellum and bifurcates to form the posterior cerebral arteries, which supply the posterior portion of the cerebrum.

The internal carotid arteries enter the cranial vault through the carotid canals. These vessels give rise to the anterior cerebral arteries, which supply blood to the frontal lobes of the brain. They terminate by forming the middle cerebral arteries, which supply a large portion of the lateral cerebral cortex. A posterior communicating artery branches off each

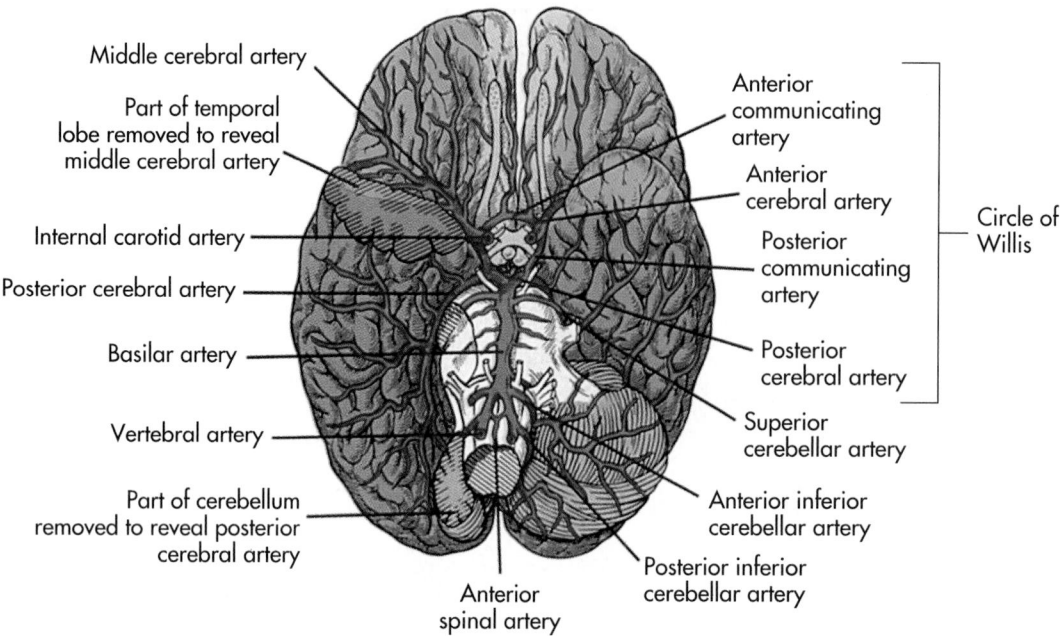

Fig. 29-5 Inferior view of the brain showing vertebral, basilar, and internal carotid arteries and their branches. (Sims/Illustrator: Karen Waldo.)

internal carotid artery and connects with the ipsilateral posterior cerebral artery. The two posterior cerebral arteries are connected at their common origin from the basilar artery. The anterior cerebral arteries are connected by an anterior communicating artery and thus complete a circle around the pituitary gland and the brain (circle of Willis). The circle of Willis provides an important safeguard to help ensure the supply of blood to all parts of the brain in the event of a blockage in the vertebral or internal carotid arteries.

The veins that drain blood from the head form the venous sinuses (spaces within the dura mater surrounding the brain) and eventually drain into the internal jugular veins (Fig. 29-6). These veins exit the cranial vault and receive several venous tributaries that drain the external head and face. The internal jugular veins join the subclavian veins on each side of the body.

Ventricles

Each cerebral hemisphere contains a large space filled with cerebrospinal fluid (CSF), known as a *lat-*

eral ventricle. The lateral ventricles are connected posteriorly, with the third ventricle located in the center of the diencephalon between the two halves of the thalamus. The two lateral ventricles communicate with the third ventricle through two interventricular foramina. The third ventricle communicates with the fourth ventricle (located in the superior region of the medulla) by way of a narrow canal known as the cerebral aqueduct. The fourth ventricle is continuous with the central canal of the spinal cord (Fig. 29-7).

> **? CRITICAL THINKING**
> *What happens if the flow in one of these canals becomes obstructed?*

Divisions of the Brain

As described in Chapter 6, the major divisions of the adult brain are the brain stem (medulla, pons,

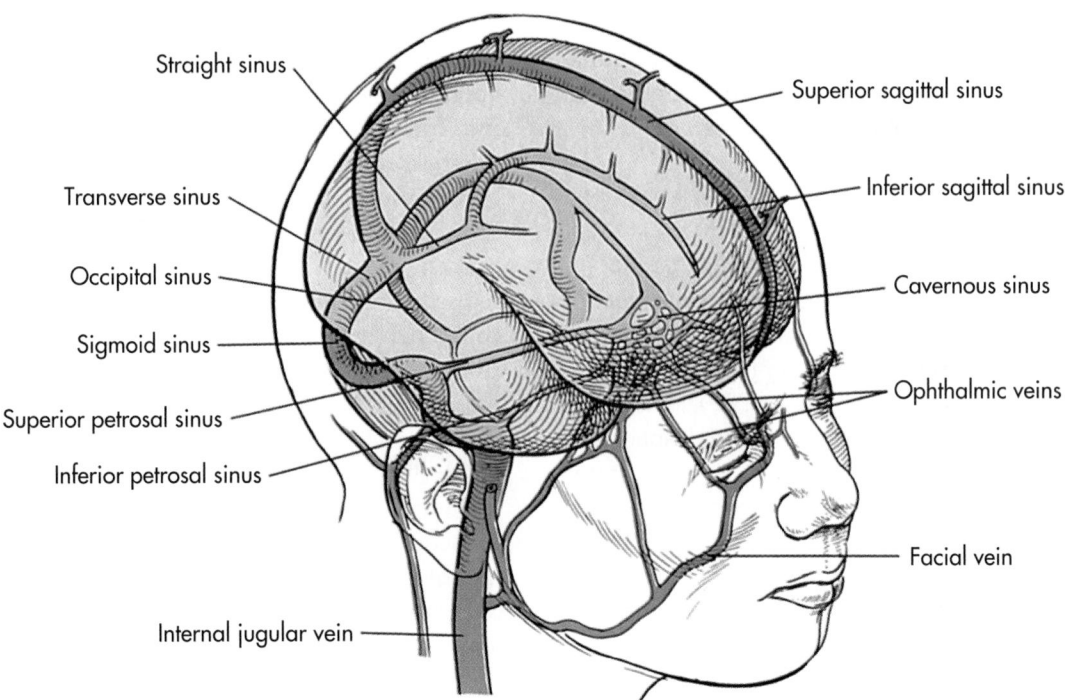

Fig. 29-6 Venous sinuses associated with the brain. (Sims/Illustrator: Karen Waldo.)

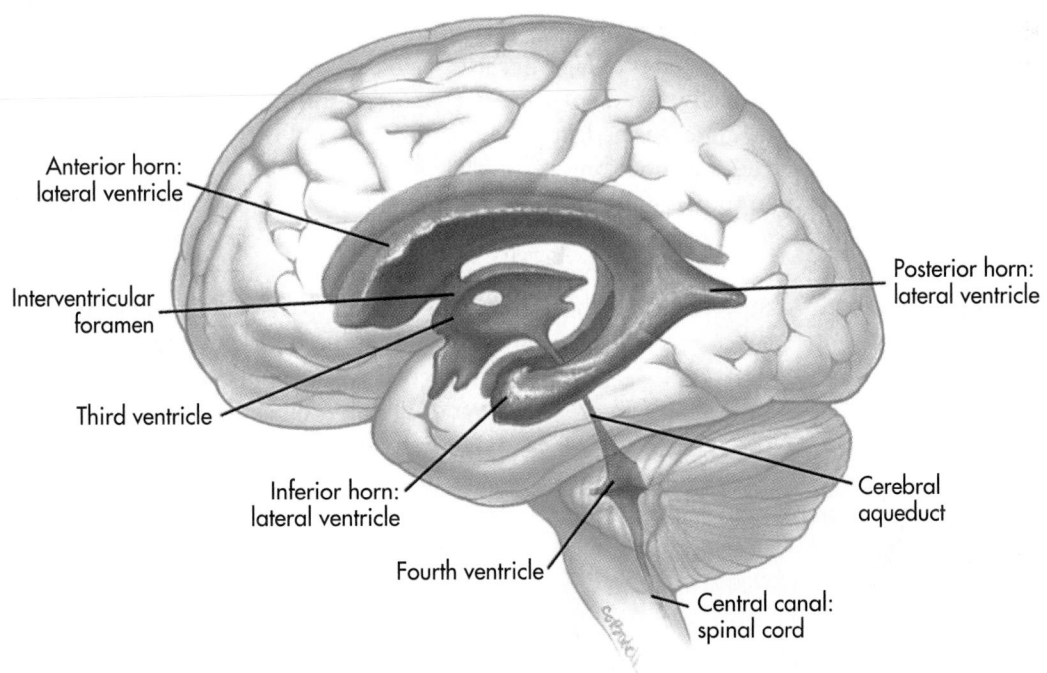

Fig. 29-7 Ventricles of the brain as seen from the left. (Sims/Illustrator: Scott Bodell.)

midbrain, and site of the reticular formation), cerebellum, diencephalon (hypothalamus and thalamus), and cerebrum. The reader should refer to that chapter for a review of these structures.

Neurological Pathophysiology

Some neurological emergencies are a consequence of structural changes or damage, circulatory changes, or alterations in intracranial pressure (ICP) that affect cerebral blood flow (CBF). The three structures that occupy the intracranial space are brain tissue, blood, and water. Brain tissue contains mostly water, both intracellular and extracellular. Blood is contained within the major arteries in the base of the brain; in arterial branches, arterioles, capillaries, venules, and veins within the substance of the brain; and in the cortical veins and dural sinuses. Water is located in the ventricles of the brain, in CSF, and in extracellular and intracellular fluid. Normally the volumes of brain tissue, blood, and water are such that the pressure inside the skull is maintained within a millimeter of mercury above atmospheric pressure.

Cerebral Perfusion Pressure

CBF depends on cerebral perfusion pressure (CPP), the pressure gradient across the brain. CBF remains constant when CPP is between 50 and 160 mm Hg. If CPP falls below 40 mm Hg, CBF declines and critically affects cerebral metabolism. As described in Chapter 22, CPP is estimated as mean arterial pressure (MAP) minus ICP. With mild to moderate elevation of ICP, MAP usually rises. The rise in MAP causes cerebral blood vessels to constrict and prevents the increase in blood volume and CBF that normally would occur.

> **? CRITICAL THINKING**
>
> *Relate the difficulty in cerebral blood flow with increased intracranial pressure to having someone pushing on a door from the outside as you are trying to open it from the inside. How much harder is it for you to open the door?*

Conversely, if MAP falls, the cerebral arteries dilate and increase CBF. Thus with an MAP between about 60 and 150 mm Hg, CBF may be maintained in a constant state. However, when ICP elevations are marked (greater than 22 mm Hg), perfusion of brain tissue often decreases despite a rise in systemic arterial pressure. Therefore if a mass or cerebral edema develops, there must be an immediate reduction in the volume of one or more of these components to prevent the ICP from rising and compressing brain tissue.

Assessment of the Nervous System

Although there are many similarities in the approaches to assessing traumatic and nontraumatic neurological deficits, the following discussion of patient assessment focuses on nontraumatic neurological emergencies. (Assessment of neurological trauma is addressed in Chapter 22.)

As with all patient encounters, care of a patient with a nontraumatic neurological emergency begins with the initial assessment. The paramedic should maintain a systematic approach in examining these patients to avoid overlooking signs and symptoms that may indicate the development of an urgent condition. Goals of emergency care are control of the airway, stabilization and support of the cardiovascular system, intervention to interrupt ongoing cerebral injury, and protection of the patient from further harm while at the scene and during transport to an appropriate medical facility.

Initial Assessment

The initial assessment should begin by determining the patient's level of consciousness and by ensuring an open and patent airway. If the patient is unconscious on EMS arrival and there is reason to suspect a cervical spine injury, the patient's airway should be opened with spinal precautions, and the cervical spine should be immobilized. The paramedic should remember that unconscious patients are unable to maintain their airways. Therefore airway adjuncts (including tracheal intubation with appropriate spinal precautions) may be indicated. The patient's airway also should be closely monitored for respiratory arrest, which may result from increased ICP, and for vomiting or aspiration of stomach contents. Suction should be readily available.

NOTE

The mantra of the cardiologist that "time is muscle" is echoed by many neurologists. Rapid stabilization of the patient and transport for definitive care may be the most prudent course of action in managing a patient with a neurological emergency.

Ventilatory support and supplemental oxygen administration should be provided for any patient experiencing a neurological emergency. Increased carbon dioxide pressure (PCO_2) or decreased oxygen pressure (PO_2) results in dilation of the blood vessels, presumably in response to greater cerebral metabolic needs. As PCO_2 is lowered, blood volume and flow to the brain are reduced. Therefore controlled hyperventilation may be indicated to maintain the patient's PCO_2 at about 30 mm Hg and PO_2 at greater than 80 mm Hg.

NOTE

The use of hyperventilation to reduce ICP is controversial. Medical direction may recommend hyperventilation only in a patient who shows ominous signs such as a fixed and dilated pupil or severe, abnormal posturing. The paramedic should follow protocols established by medical direction.

Physical Examination

The patient with neurological illness may be difficult to assess, particularly if the patient's mental function is impaired. Important elements of the physical examination that may provide clues to the nature of the neurological emergency include patient history and history of the event, vital signs, and respiratory patterns.

History. After any life-threatening problems have been identified and corrected, the paramedic should attempt to gather a thorough history of the event from the patient or from family members or bystanders. Six important elements of the patient history are:

1. The patient's chief complaint
2. Details of the presenting illness

3. Pertinent underlying medical problems
    a. Cardiac disease
    b. Lung disease
    c. Neurological disease (e.g., multiple sclerosis)
    d. Previous stroke
    e. Chronic seizures
    f. Diabetes
    g. Hypertension
4. Drug or alcohol use
5. Previous history of similar symptoms
6. Recent injury (particularly head trauma)

? CRITICAL THINKING

How could a history involving one of these problems cause an alteration in a patient's neurological status?

If loss of consciousness was involved, the paramedic should ascertain the events that preceded the unconscious state, such as patient position (sitting, standing, lying down), complaints of a headache, seizure activity, or a fall. When no history is available, the paramedic should assume that the onset of unconsciousness was acute and that an intracranial hemorrhage is likely. In addition, the paramedic should be alert to the presence of any environmental clues, such as evidence of current prescribed medications, medical alert identification, recreational drugs, or alcohol or drug paraphernalia.

Vital signs. Vital signs should be checked and recorded frequently because they often change rapidly in patients with a neurological emergency. The patient's ECG also should be monitored for dysrhythmias, which are common in these scenarios. In the early stages of increased ICP, there is an increase in systolic pressure, a widened pulse pressure, and a decrease in the pulse and respiratory rate (Cushing's triad). In the terminal stages, as ICP continues to rise and brain tissue is compressed, body temperature usually remains elevated, but the pulse rate generally decreases and the blood pressure falls, particularly after herniation occurs. Therefore hypotension is a late and ominous sign in patients with isolated neurological pathology.

Respiratory patterns. The respiratory pattern of a patient with a neurological emergency may be normal or abnormal. In the absence of respiratory arrest caused by CNS dysfunction of the lower respiratory centers in the medulla, abnormalities of respiratory rate and rhythm may give clues to the mechanisms responsible and the level of neurological dysfunction. Although apnea can occur with loss of consciousness even with relatively minor head trauma, acute respiratory arrest usually results from involvement of the medullary respiratory center (brain stem compression or infarct). Neural pathway involvement (anywhere from the cortex down to the medulla) is more often associated with disturbances of respiratory rhythm, not with respiratory arrest. Abnormal respiratory patterns (described in Chapter 11) include the following:

- Cheyne-Stokes respiration
- Central neurogenic hyperventilation
- Ataxic respiration
- Apneustic respiration
- Diaphragmatic breathing

? CRITICAL THINKING

Which respiratory control center is likely affected if the patient has ataxic or apneustic respirations?

Neurological Evaluation

Some neurological complications are obvious (such as paralysis), whereas others may be subtle (e.g., a decreasing sensorium). A sudden or rapidly worsening level of consciousness is the single most suggestive sign of a serious neurological condition.[1]

Use of the mnemonic device AVPU and the Glasgow Coma Scale (described in Chapter 22) are rapid, convenient ways to determine the patient's baseline neurological status and to allow comparisons during future management. Evaluation should be repeated and recorded frequently so that changes in the patient's mental state may be detected at the earliest possible time.

When evaluating a patient's neurological status, the paramedic should report and record patient information with descriptive terms specific to responses to certain stimuli (e.g., "the patient has no recall of the event"; "the patient moves on command"; "the patient does not open his or her eyes to painful stimuli"). Using clear descriptions of the pa-

tient's response permits others involved in the patient's care to follow the patient's progression.

Posturing, muscle tone, and paralysis. Significant neurological emergencies may be associated with abnormal or unusual posturing, paralysis of a limb or several limbs, or both. Generally, disturbances of posture result from flexor spasms, extensor spasms, or flaccidity. Abnormal flexor response of one or both arms with extension of the legs is called *decorticate rigidity.* This abnormal posturing is thought to result from structural impairment of certain cortical regions of the brain. Abnormal extensor response of the arms with extension of the legs is called *decerebrate rigidity.* Decerebrate rigidity has a worse prognosis than decorticate rigidity and is thought to result from impairment of certain subcortical regions of the brain. Flaccidity usually is caused by brain stem or cord dysfunction and carries a dismal prognosis.

Abnormal reflexes are not uncommon with decorticate or decerebrate rigidity. Associated with this may be a positive Babinski's sign (described in Chapter 23) and relaxation of sphincter tone with evacuation of the bowels and/or bladder.

Pupillary reflexes. Examination of the pupils is an important evaluation in the unconscious patient. Often, the diagnosis of drug intoxication can at least be suspected based on pupillary appearance and reaction (Fig. 29-8). If deviations from normal (in relative symmetry, size, and prompt reaction to light) are observed, it is important to note whether these deviations are unilateral or bilateral. If both pupils are dilated and do not react to light, the patient's brain stem has probably been affected, or the patient has suffered severe cerebral anoxia.

NOTE

The pupillary response must be taken into consideration with the patient's mental status. If the patient is awake, alert, and oriented and has unresponsive dilated pupils, this is most likely attributed to topical medications that have induced pupillary dilation.

Pupillary constriction is controlled by parasympathetic fibers that originate in the midbrain and accompany the oculomotor nerve (cranial nerve III). Pupillary dilation involves fibers that descend the

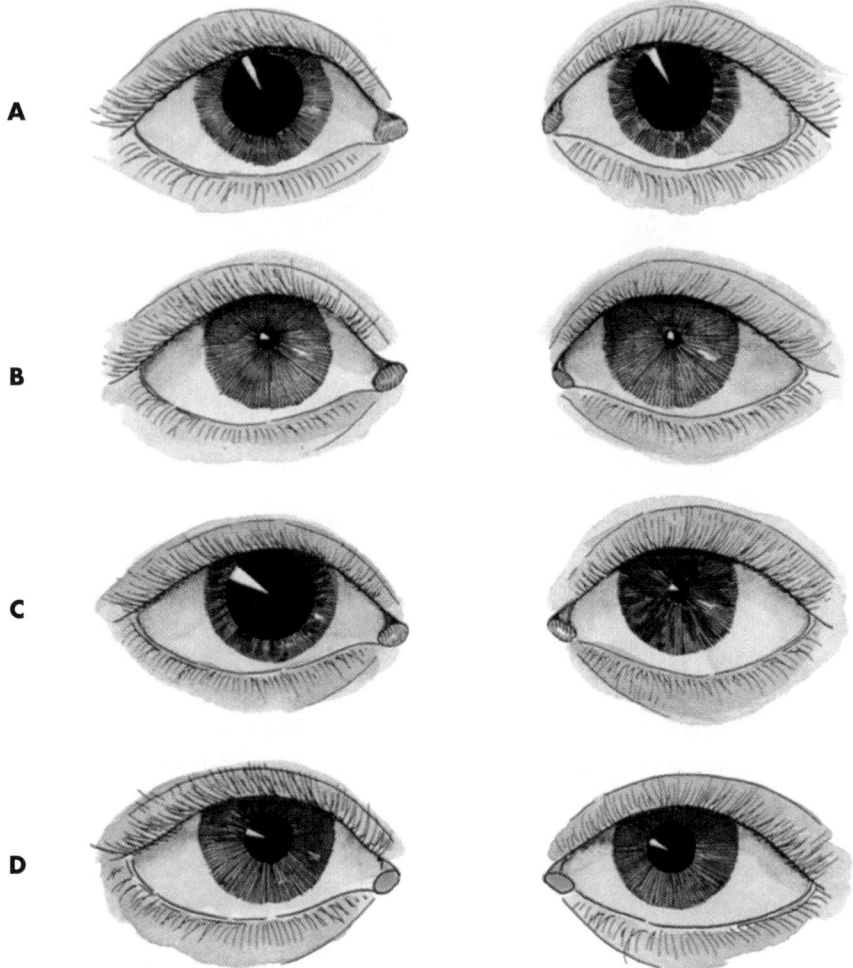

Fig. 29-8 Pupillary responses. **A,** Dilated. **B,** Pinpoint. **C,** Unequal. **D,** Normal. (From McSwain N: *The basic EMT: comprehensive prehospital patient care,* St Louis, 1996, Mosby.)

entire brain stem and ascend in the cervical sympathetic chains. Midbrain failure interrupts both pathways and generally results in fixed, midsize pupils. Third nerve compression interrupts parasympathetic tone and is manifested by a unilateral, fixed, dilated pupil. Any unconscious patient who suddenly develops a fixed, dilated pupil probably has suffered a significant brain event, which requires immediate transport to an appropriate medical facility.

Extraocular movements. Conscious patients should be able to move their eyes in full directional ranges. As described in Chapter 14, extraocular movements can be evaluated by requesting that the patient follow the finger movements of the paramedic: to the extreme left and then up and down and to the ex-

treme right and then up and down. Any deviations from normal should be recorded.

Deviation of both eyes to either side (conjugate gaze) at rest implies a structural lesion. The lesion may have an "irritative focus" in which the eyes look away from the lesion or a "destructive focus" in which the eyes look toward the lesion. Deviation of the eyes to opposite sides (dysconjugate gaze) at rest implies a structural brain stem dysfunction in the pathways that traverse the brain stem from the upper midbrain to at least the level of the lower pons (Fig. 29-9).

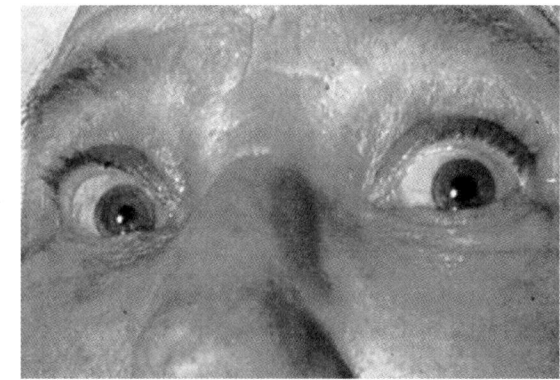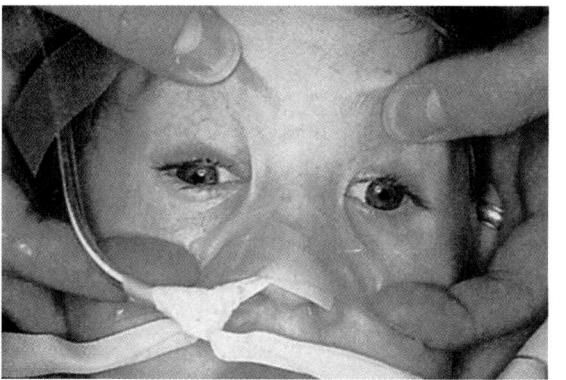

Fig. 29-9 A, Conjugate gaze. **B,** Dysconjugate gaze. (**A** from London: *A colour atlas of diagnosis after recent injury,* Ipswich, England, 1990, Wolfe Medical Publications, Ltd. **B** courtesy Gary Quick, M.D.)

Pathophysiology and Management of Specific CNS Disorders

There are numerous pathophysiologies associated with disorders of the nervous system. Specific abnormalities of the CNS discussed in this chapter include structural and metabolic coma, stroke and intracranial hemorrhage (including transient ischemic attack), seizure disorders, headaches, and brain neoplasm and brain abscess. Several degenerative neurological diseases also will be discussed in this section.

Coma

Coma is an abnormally deep state of unconsciousness from which the patient cannot be aroused by external stimuli. In general terms, only two mechanisms produce coma: (1) structural lesions (e.g., a tumor or abscess) that depress consciousness by destroying or encroaching on the ascending reticular activating system in the brain stem and (2) toxic metabolic states that involve the presence of circulating toxins or metabolites or the lack of metabolic substrate (e.g., oxygen or glucose). Either mechanism may cause diffuse depression of both cerebral hemispheres, with or without depression of the ascending reticular activating system. Within these two mechanisms there are six general causes of coma (Box 29-1). A mnemonic aid that may be useful in remembering the common causes of coma is AEIOU TIPS (Box 29-2).

Structural Versus Toxic-Metabolic Coma

Two major factors distinguish structural and toxic metabolic causes of coma. In patients with structural causes, there is a common association of focal (asymmetrical) neurological signs, whereas in patients with coma of toxic metabolic origin, the neurological findings are often symmetrical. In addition, coma of toxic metabolic origin often is slow in onset, whereas structural lesions occur acutely. Pupillary responses are perhaps the most important physical findings in helping to distinguish structural and toxic metabolic causes of coma. Preserved pupillary responses suggest that the origin of coma is toxic metabolic, whereas unresponsive or asymmetrical pupillary responses suggest a structural cause.

> **NOTE**
>
> Coma-like states can be mimicked by certain psychiatric conditions (e.g., "hysterical coma") in which the unconscious state has no organic origin. Patients who are experiencing a voluntary or involuntary psychogenic episode often vigorously blink and move the eyes and generally respond to noxious physical or verbal stimuli, whereas patients with organic sources of coma are unresponsive.

Unlike metabolic coma, structural coma follows a progressive pattern of deterioration caused by focal pressure or compression. The syndrome often is sudden in onset with an asymmetrical secondary examination (e.g., hemiparesis). As a rule, structural lesions affect the ascending reticular activating system by virtue of increased ICP and herniation and require rapid surgical correction. Distinguishing between toxic metabolic coma and structural coma can help prepare the paramedic to anticipate the course of the patient's condition.

BOX 29-1

SIX GENERAL CAUSES OF COMA

Structural Causes
- Intracranial bleeding
- Head trauma
- Brain tumor or other space-occupying lesions

Metabolic System
- Anoxia
- Hypoglycemia
- Diabetic ketoacidosis
- Thiamine deficiency
- Kidney and liver failure
- Postictal phase of seizure

Drugs
- Barbiturates
- Narcotics
- Hallucinogenics
- Depressants
- Alcohol

Cardiovascular System
- Hypertensive encephalopathy
- Shock
- Dysrhythmias
- Stroke

Respiratory System
- Chronic obstructive pulmonary disease
- Toxic inhalation (e.g., carbon monoxide poisoning)

Infection
- Meningitis
- Sepsis

BOX 29-2

AEIOU TIPS

A—Acidosis or alcohol
E—Epilepsy
I—Infection
O—Overdose
U—Uremia
T—Trauma
I—Insulin
P—Psychosis
S—Stroke

breaths per minute[1] with a target end-tidal CO_2 measurement of 25% to 28%. The trachea of the unconscious patient who has no gag reflex should be intubated. After the airway is secured, management of a patient in a coma of unknown origin includes the following:

1. Establish an IV line to keep the vein open or to manage hypotension (if present).
2. Monitor the patient's ECG.
3. Per protocol, draw a blood sample for laboratory analysis. If hypoglycemia is suspected, use a glucometer or other device to measure serum glucose levels (described in Chapter 30), and administer *dextrose 50%* if indicated (per protocol). If alcohol is suspected as the cause of coma, *thiamine* administration before glucose administration should be considered.

? CRITICAL THINKING

Why is thiamine indicated if you suspect an alcohol abuse problem?

NOTE

Thiamine is a B vitamin (B_1) usually found in adequate amounts in the normal diet. However, chronic alcoholism interferes with the intake, absorption, and utilization of thiamine and may result in the development of serious neurological disorders. The incidence of these alcohol-related neurological syndromes varies markedly in different regions of the United States. Therefore administration of *thiamine* may be a local consideration. The paramedic should follow established protocols and consult with medical direction.

Assessment and Management

Regardless of the cause of coma, prehospital care is directed at support of the patient's vital functions, prevention of further deterioration of the patient's condition, and administration of medications, IV fluids, or both, to manage potentially reversible causes of coma. As always, airway maintenance and ventilatory support with supplemental high-concentration oxygen are the first priorities in patient stabilization. Rapid transport for definitive care may be indicated.

If the patient's respirations are abnormally slow or shallow or if cerebral edema is suspected, the patient's lungs should be hyperventilated at 24 to 30

4. If there is no response to glucose administration, administer *naloxone* (Narcan) per protocol, (2 mg by slow IV infusion) to rule out or reverse narcotic depression.

> **NOTE**
>
> Patients who are physically dependent on narcotics may exhibit frank withdrawal symptoms. Therefore the paramedic should be prepared to restrain a patient who may become violent as the **naloxone** (Narcan) reverses narcotic effects. Repeated doses of **naloxone** (Narcan) may be necessary because the duration of some narcotics may be longer than that of **naloxone** (Narcan). Doses should be titrated to keep the patient awake, responsive, and free from respiratory depression.

5. If the patient remains in a comatose state, transport the patient in a lateral recumbent position (if not contraindicated) to facilitate drainage of secretions and to minimize the potential for aspiration of stomach contents. Closely monitor the patient's airway and have suction readily available. Protect the patient's eyes from corneal drying by gently closing them and covering the lids with moist gauze pads.

Stroke and Intracranial Hemorrhage

Stroke (also known as cerebovascular accident [CVA] or "brain attack") is a sudden interruption in blood flow to the brain that results in neurological deficit. Stroke is a serious disease that affects more than 500,000 Americans (and 50,000 Canadians) each year.[2] It is associated with a 30-day mortality of about 10% to 15%. It is the third leading cause of death in the United States and frequently leaves its survivors severely debilitated. According to the American Heart Association (AHA), patients who are more likely to suffer a stroke have prior risk factors that can be classified as modifiable and nonmodifiable:

Modifiable risk factors
- High blood pressure
- Cigarette smoking
- Transient ischemic attacks
- Heart disease
- Diabetes mellitus

- Hypercoagulopathy
- High red blood cell count and sickle cell anemia
- Carotid bruit

Nonmodifiable risk factors
- Age
- Gender (men are at greater risk than women)
- Race (African-Americans are at greater risk than Caucasians)
- Prior stroke
- Heredity

> **NOTE**
>
> The best way to prevent a stroke is to identify at-risk patients and to control as many risk factors as possible through modifying poor health habits and through drug therapy.

Pathophysiology

As previously described, blood reaches the brain through four major vessels: two carotid arteries (providing about 80% of CBF) and two vertebral arteries, which combine to form the single basilar artery (supplying the remaining 20% of CBF). These two systems are interconnected at various levels, the principal one being the circle of Willis. In addition, there are individual variations of extensive collateral blood flow supplied through facial anastomoses between scalp vessels and vessels of the dura and arachnoid. Beyond this, however, there is no collateral circulation in the depths of the brain. Therefore occlusion of any one of the more distal vessels may result in ischemia and infarction.

Normally, CBF is maintained through autoregulation of cerebral vessels that constrict or dilate to preserve perfusion pressure even with systemic hypotension. Cerebral perfusion also is regulated at the arteriolar level by the level of oxygen and glucose supplied (ischemia and acidosis are profound vasodilators). The sudden cessation of circulation to a portion of the brain that results from vessel occlusion or hemorrhage cannot be readily corrected by these autoregulatory mechanisms. The uncorrected ischemia that results within a short period of time leads to neuronal dysfunction and death. The onset and symptoms of the stroke depend on the area of the brain involved.

? CRITICAL THINKING

How much oxygen and glucose can the brain store for emergency situations?

Types of Stroke

Stroke is a general term that refers to the neurological manifestations of a critical decrease in blood flow to a portion of the brain, regardless of the cause. Strokes can be classified as ischemic strokes and hemorrhagic strokes. Determining the origin of a stroke often is difficult (and unnecessary) in the prehospital setting. However, understanding the various signs and symptoms of each type of stroke better prepares the paramedic to anticipate the course of patient care (Table 29-1). In addition, documenting a thorough history and physical examination helps others involved in the patient's care.

NOTE

Both forms of stroke can be life threatening. Ischemic stroke, however, rarely leads to death within the first hour. Hemorrhagic stroke can be rapidly fatal.[2]

Ischemic stroke. About 85% of strokes are ischemic and are caused by a cerebral thrombosis that occurs as a result of atherosclerotic plaques or extrinsic pressure from a mass within the brain itself. The onset of stroke from cerebral thrombosis usually is associated with a long history of vessel disease. Therefore the majority of these patients are older and have evidence of atherosclerotic disease in other areas of the body (angina pectoris, claudication, previous strokes). Signs and symptoms of thrombotic stroke usually are slower to develop than those of cerebral hemorrhage and include:

- Hemiparesis or hemiplegia on the side of the body opposite the lesion
- Numbness (decreased sensation) on the side of the body opposite the lesion
- Aphasia
- Confusion or coma
- Convulsions
- Incontinence
- Diplopia (double vision)
- Monocular blindness (painless visual loss in one eye)
- Numbness of the face
- Dysarthria (slurred speech)
- Headache
- Dizziness or vertigo
- Ataxia

Cerebral embolus. A stroke caused by an embolus results from an occlusion of any intracranial vessel by a fragment of a foreign substance arising outside of the CNS. Common sources of cerebral emboli include atherosclerotic plaques (originating from large vessels of the head, neck, or heart). Thrombi that develop on the valves or in the chambers of the heart are very common in patients with valvular heart disease and atrial fibrillation. Other, rare causes of cerebral emboli include air embolism after thoracic injury and fat embolism after long bone injury. Bacterial and fungal endocarditis also are capable of causing stroke from embolization. Women

TABLE 29-1	DIFFERENTIATING BETWEEN ISCHEMIC AND HEMORRHAGIC STROKES
ISCHEMIC STROKES	**HEMORRHAGIC STROKES**
Most common	Least common
Usually result from atherosclerosis or tumor within the brain	Usually result from cerebral aneurysms, AV malformations, hypertension
Develop slowly	Develop abruptly
Long history of vessel disease	Commonly occur during stress or exertion
May be associated with valvular heart disease and atrial fibrillation	May be associated with cocaine and other sympathomimetic amines
History of angina, previous strokes	May be asymptomatic before rupture

taking oral contraceptives and patients with sickle cell disease also are at increased risk of developing a stroke (both by thrombotic and perhaps embolic origin). Signs and symptoms of cerebral embolus are similar to those of thrombotic stroke, but usually they develop more quickly and often are associated with an identifiable cause (e.g., atrial fibrillation, valvular heart disease).

Hemorrhagic stroke. Cerebral hemorrhage accounts for 15% to 20% of all strokes. A hemorrhage may occur anywhere within the cranial vault, including the epidural, subdural, subarachnoid, intraparenchymal, and intraventricular spaces. The most common causes are cerebral aneurysms, arteriovenous (AV) malformations, and hypertension. Cerebral aneurysms and AV malformations are congenital anomalies that can be familial and often are asymptomatic until the time of rupture. Unlike thrombotic and embolic strokes, which have relatively high survival rates, cerebral hemorrhages are fatal in 50% to 80% of cases.[2]

Hemorrhagic strokes commonly occur during stress or exertion. Cocaine and other sympathomimetic amines also may contribute to intracranial hemorrhage by drug-induced rapid elevation of blood pressure. Presentation is abrupt and often begins with a headache (sometimes described as the worst headache of the patient's life) accompanied by nausea, vomiting, and progressive deterioration in mental status from alert to lethargic. Often, the patient loses consciousness or experiences a seizure at the time of the hemorrhage. As the hemorrhage expands and ICP increases, the patient becomes comatose, with increasing hypertension and bradycardia (Cushing's reflex).

? CRITICAL THINKING

Why do you think mortality is higher for hemorrhagic versus embolic stroke?

Transient Ischemic Attacks

Transient ischemic attacks (TIAs; often referred to as "little strokes") are episodes of focal cerebral dysfunction that last from minutes to several hours, from which the patient returns to normal within 24 hours without permanent neurological deficit. A TIA is thought to be the most important indication of impending stroke; about 5% of patients with a

TIA will develop a complete stroke within 1 month if untreated.[2]

NOTE

TIA is the most important forecaster of a brain infarction.

Signs and symptoms of a TIA are the same as those that characterize stroke and include weakness, paralysis, numbness of the face, and speech disturbances, all of which correspond to vascular occlusion of a specific cerebral artery. Most patients who experience a TIA are hospitalized for close observation, evaluation, and treatment of vascular disease (e.g., endarterectomy, anticoagulant therapy).

Role of EMS in Stroke Care

The role of EMS in stroke care is to rapidly identify a stroke event and to advise medical direction and quickly transport the patient to an appropriate facility where rapid hospital-based evaluation and treatment can take place. Key points in the management of stroke include the seven Ds: detection, dispatch, delivery, door, data, decision, and drug (see box on p. 927). (The first three Ds are the responsibility of the lay public and EMS providers.)

NOTE

About 85% of strokes occur at home. Public education programs focused on persons at risk for stroke, their friends, and family members, have been shown to reduce the time to arrival at the emergency department.[3] (See injury prevention strategies in Appendix C.)

Assessment

Initial examination of a patient who may have suffered a stroke (including TIA) follows the same sequence as for any other ill or injured patient in the emergency setting. Emergency care priorities are directed at maintaining a patent airway and providing adequate ventilatory support with supplemental high-concentration oxygen. If the patient is conscious and able to converse, a thorough history should be obtained. Important components of the patient history are:

- Previous neurological symptoms (TIAs)
- Previous neurological deficits

THE SEVEN Ds OF STROKE MANAGEMENT

Detection: Occurs when a patient, family member, or bystander recognizes the signs and symptoms of a stroke or TIA and activates the EMS system.

Dispatch: EMS dispatchers must prioritize the call for a suspected stroke patient and dispatch the appropriate EMS team with high transport priority.

Delivery: EMS providers must respond rapidly, confirm the signs and symptoms of stroke, and transport the patient *(delivery)* to an appropriate medical facility.

Door: An appropriate medical facility is a hospital that can provide fibrinolytic therapy within 1 hour after arrival at the ED *door.*

Data: Includes obtaining a computed tomography (CT) scan.

Decision: Made in identifying candidates eligible for fibrinolytic therapy.

Drug: Includes treating eligible patients with fibrinolytic therapy.

Note: The first three Ds are the responsibility of the lay public and EMS providers. The fourth D is the responsibility of EMS, and the last three Ds are performed in the hospital.

BOX 29-3

THE CINCINNATI PREHOSPITAL STROKE SCALE

Facial Droop (have patient show teeth or smile):
- Normal—both sides of face move equally well
- Abnormal—one side of face does not move as well as the other side

Arm Drift (patient closes eyes and holds both arms out):
- Normal—both arms move the same *or* both arms do not move at all (other findings, such as pronator grip, may be helpful)
- Abnormal—one arm does not move *or* one arm drifts down compared with the other

Speech (have the patient say "you can't teach an old dog new tricks"):
- Normal—patient uses correct words with no slurring
- Abnormal—patient slurs words, uses inappropriate words, *or* is unable to speak

---

- Initial symptoms and their progression
- Alterations in level of consciousness
- Precipitating factors
- Dizziness
- Palpitations
- Significant past medical history
  Hypertension
  Diabetes mellitus
  Cigarette smoking
  Oral contraceptive use
  Cardiac disease
  Sickle cell disease
  Previous stroke

Cincinnati Prehospital Stroke Scale. In addition to the abnormal neurological signs and symptoms previously described, other methods can be used to diagnose stroke. One such method is the *Prehospital Stroke Scale,*[4] developed in Cincinnati, that evaluates three major physical findings: facial droop, arm drift, and speech (Box 29-3). Using this scale can help the paramedic identify a stroke patient who requires rapid transport to a hospital, and enables prearrival notification of the receiving hospital.

Los Angeles Prehospital Stroke Screen. The Los Angeles Prehospital Stroke Screen (LAPSS) is another method that can be used to diagnose stroke. This screen requires the examiner to rule out other causes of altered level of consciousness (e.g., hypoglycemia, seizure), and then to identify asymmetry (right vs. left) in facial smile/grimace, grip, or arm strength (Table 29-2). Asymmetry in any category indicates a possible stroke. Like the Cincinnati Stroke Scale, the LAPSS can be performed quickly in the prehospital setting.

NOTE

Whenever possible, the paramedic should establish the time of onset of stroke signs and symptoms, which is important for potential therapy.

Management (Fig. 29-10)

Once the diagnosis of a stroke is suspected, *time in the field must be minimized* because there is limited time to initiate therapy. (Less than 3 hours from onset is required for use of fibrinolytics.[2]) Prehospital care is

TABLE 29-2	LOS ANGELES PREHOSPITAL STROKE SCREEN (LAPSS)

For evaluation of acute, noncomatose, nontraumatic neurological complaint: If items 1 through 6 are **ALL checked "yes"** (or "unknown"), notify the receiving hospital before arrival of the potential stroke patient. If any are checked "no," follow appropriate treatment protocol.

Interpretation: Ninety-three percent of patients with stroke will have positive findings (all items checked "yes" or "unknown") on the LAPSS (sensitivity = 93%), and 97% of those with positive findings will have a stroke (specificity = 97%). The patient may still be having a stroke if LAPSS criteria are not met.

CRITERIA	YES	UNKNOWN	NO
1. Age >45 years	[]	[]	[]
2. History of seizures or epilepsy **absent**	[]	[]	[]
3. Symptom duration <24 hours	[]	[]	[]
4. At baseline, patient is **not** wheelchair bound or bedridden	[]	[]	[]
5. Blood glucose between 60 and 400	[]	[]	[]
6. *Obvious asymmetry* (right vs left) in **any** of the following three categories **(must be unilateral)**	[]	[]	[]

	EQUAL	R WEAK	L WEAK
Facial smile/grimace	[]	[] Droop	[] Droop
Grip	[]	[] Weak grip	[] Weak grip
	[]	[] No grip	[] No grip
Arm strength	[]	[] Drifts down	[] Drifts down
	[]	[] Falls rapidly	[] Falls rapidly

directed at managing the patient's airway, breathing, and circulation, and monitoring vital signs.

> **NOTE**
>
> Aside from supporting vital functions, the most important element of prehospital care for a stroke victim is to identify the patient suffering from stroke and to rapidly transport the patient for definitive care.

? CRITICAL THINKING

> *How can you detect paralysis of the muscles of the throat, tongue, and mouth on your physical exam?*

Airway. Paralysis of the muscles of the throat, tongue, and mouth can lead to partial or complete airway obstruction (a major problem in acute stroke). Frequent suctioning of the oropharynx and nasopharynx is required to prevent aspiration of pooled saliva.

Breathing. Inadequate ventilation should be managed with supplemental oxygen (in hypoxic patients) and positive-pressure ventilation. Hypoxia and hypercarbia can occur from inadequate ventilation, contributing to cardiac and respiratory instability. Respiratory arrest from severe coma-producing brain injuries should be managed with intubation and assisted ventilations.

> **NOTE**
>
> Do not routinely administer supplemental oxygen to *nonhypoxic* (oxygen saturation >90%) stroke victims with minor or moderate strokes.[5]

Circulation. Cardiac arrest is uncommon but may follow respiratory arrest. Cardiac dysrhythmias are frequent; therefore the patient's ECG and blood pressure require constant monitoring. As described in Chapter 28, a difference in blood pressure readings in the upper extremities (of 10 mm Hg or more) may indicate aortic dissection and compromise of brain blood supply.

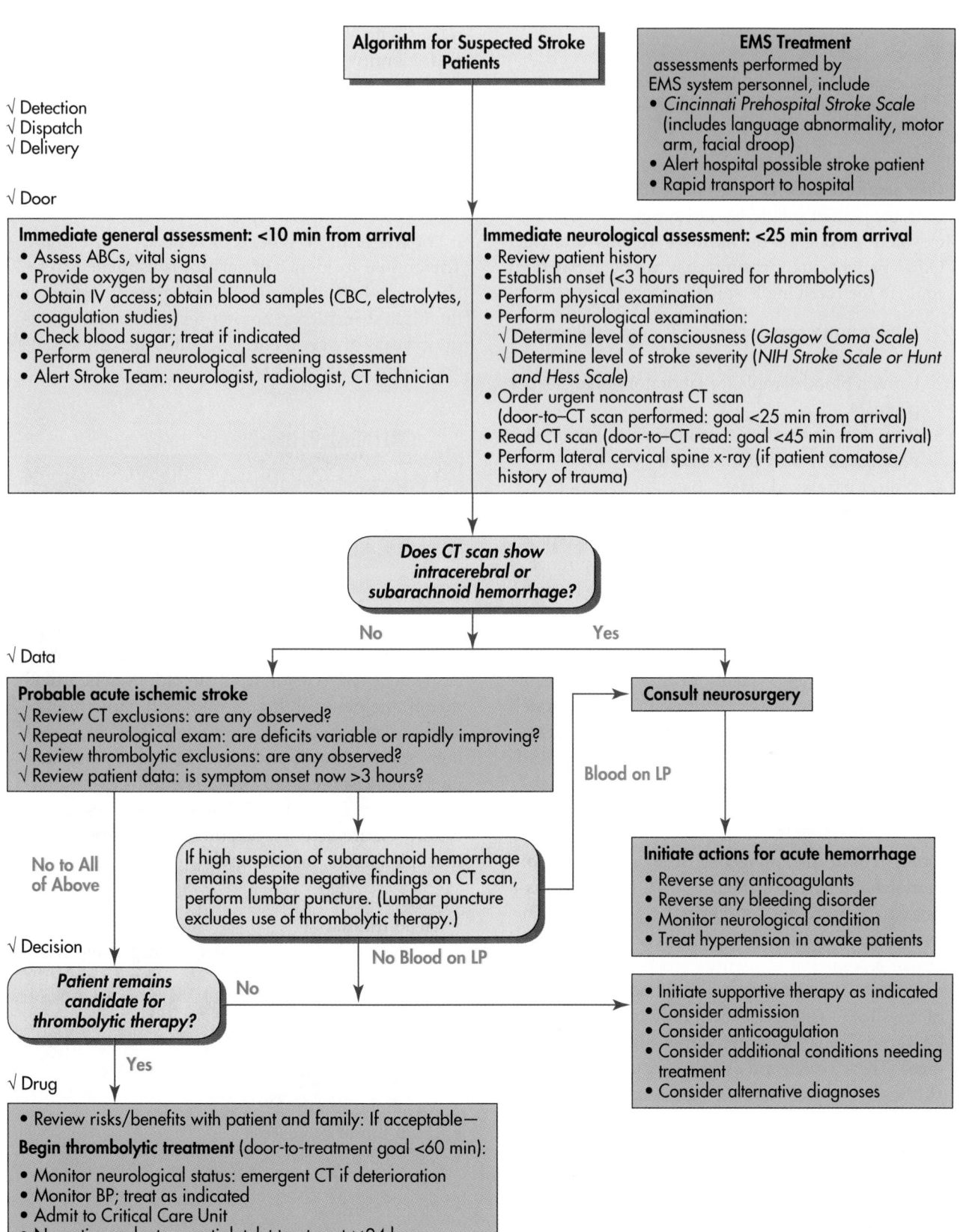

Fig. 29-10 Algorithm for suspected stroke patients. (From *CPR Issue of JAMA*, Oct. 28, 1992. Copyright © American Medical Association.)

NOTE

Management of hypertension in the prehospital setting is not recommended for suspected stroke patients.[2]

Other supportive measures. If the patient's condition permits, the patient should be kept supine with the head elevated 15 degrees to facilitate venous drainage. Other patient care measures that can be initiated en route to the receiving hospital are:

1. Initiate an IV line of lactated Ringer's solution or normal saline at 50 mL per hour.
2. Draw a blood sample for laboratory analysis per protocol.
3. Perform serum glucose analysis and administer ***dextrose 50%*** only if indicated.
4. Protect paralyzed extremities.
5. Maintain normal body temperature
6. Control any seizure activity with benzodiazepines.
7. Provide comforting measures and reassurance.
8. Provide gentle transport to the receiving hospital.

The paramedic should remember that stroke patients have experienced a catastrophic event that may seriously affect their quality of life. They often are frightened, embarrassed, confused, and frustrated with their inability to move or communicate. These patients have special physical and emotional needs and deserve a compassionate and caring approach.

In-Hospital Treatment

On arrival in the emergency department, the non-hemorrhagic stroke patient will be evaluated as a potential candidate for fibrinolytic therapy. This evaluation will include an emergency neurological stroke assessment to identify the patient's level of consciousness and the type, location, and severity of the stroke. This assessment is aided by use of the Glasgow Coma Scale and other standardized indices. These scales and other in-hospital diagnostic studies help measure neurological function that cor-

NOTE

Rapid neuroradiologic evaluation of the CT scan is imperative to ensure that the patient does not have an intracranial hemorrhage, which is a contraindication for fibrinolytic therapy.

relates with stroke severity and long-term outcome, and identify stroke patients who would benefit from fibrinolytic therapy.

Seizure Disorders

A **seizure** is a temporary alteration in behavior or consciousness caused by abnormal electrical activity of one or more groups of neurons in the brain. The annual incidence of seizure is estimated to be about one-half of 1% of the U.S. population, with the highest incidence among feverish children under 5 years of age. (Febrile seizures are further addressed in Chapter 42.)

? CRITICAL THINKING

What feelings may parents experience after witnessing their child having a febrile seizure? How should you respond to those feelings?

Although the underlying neuropathophysiology of seizures is not well understood, a seizure is generally believed to result from alterations in neuronal membrane permeability secondary to structural lesion or metabolic derangement. The increased membrane permeability to sodium and potassium ions enhances the ability of the neurons to depolarize and emit an electrical charge, sometimes resulting in seizure activity. Seizures may be caused by multiple factors, including:

- Stroke
- Head trauma
- Toxins, including alcohol or other drug withdrawal
- Hypoxia
- Hypoperfusion
- Hypoglycemia
- Infection
- Metabolic abnormalities
- Brain tumor or abscess
- Vascular disorders
- Eclampsia
- Drug overdose

In the prehospital setting, determining the origin of seizure activity is less important than managing the complications and recognizing whether the seizure is reversible with therapy (e.g., resulting from hypoglycemia). A tendency toward recurrent seizures (excluding those that arise from correctable or avoidable circumstances [e.g., alcohol withdrawal]) is called **epilepsy.**

Types of Seizures

All seizures are pathological. They may arise from almost any region of the brain and therefore have many clinical manifestations. The two most common seizure types are generalized and partial (focal).

Generalized seizures. As the name implies, generalized seizures do not have a definable origin (focus) in the brain, although focal seizures may progress to generalized seizures. This class includes petit mal (absence seizures) and grand mal (tonic-clonic) seizures. Petit mal seizures occur most often in children between the ages of 4 and 12. They are characterized by brief lapses of consciousness without loss of posture. Often there is no motor activity, although some children have eye blinking, lip smacking, or isolated clonic activity. These seizures usually last less than 15 seconds, during which time the patient is unaware of the surroundings, and are followed by the patient's immediate return to normal environmental contact. Most patients have remission by age 20 but may subsequently develop grand mal seizures.

? CRITICAL THINKING

> **What could cause death following a grand mal seizure?**

Grand mal seizures are common and are associated with significant morbidity and mortality. Grand mal seizures may be preceded by an aura (olfactory or auditory sensation), which often is recognized by the patient as a warning of the imminent convulsion. The seizure itself is characterized by a sudden loss of consciousness associated with loss of organized muscle tone and a tonic phase in which there is a sequence of extensor muscle tone activity (sometimes flexion) and apnea.

During the tonic phase of a grand mal seizure, tongue biting and bladder or bowel incontinence may occur. After the tonic phase, which lasts only seconds, the patient experiences a bilateral clonic phase (rigidity alternating with relaxation), which

usually lasts 1 to 3 minutes. During this phase of the seizure, there is a massive autonomic discharge that results in hyperventilation, salivation, and tachycardia. After the seizure, the patient usually experiences a period of drowsiness or unconsciousness resolving over minutes to hours. On regaining consciousness, the patient often is confused and fatigued and may demonstrate a transient neurological deficit. This phase of the seizure is known as the postictal phase. Grand mal seizures may be prolonged or recur before the patient regains consciousness. When this occurs, the patient is said to be in **status epilepticus** (see discussion on status epilepticus).

Partial seizures. In contrast to generalized seizures, in which a specific seizure focus is unknown, partial seizures arise from identifiable cortical lesions. Partial seizures may be classified as simple or complex. Simple partial seizures result mainly from seizure activity in the motor or sensory cortex. Simple motor seizures usually manifest as clonic activity limited to one specific body part (such as one hand, one arm or leg, or one side of the face). Simple sensory seizures result in symptoms such as tingling or numbness of a body part or abnormal visual, auditory, olfactory, or taste symptoms. Patients with partial seizures generally do not lose consciousness and maintain a relatively normal mental status. However, the seizure focus may subsequently spread and lead to a generalized tonic-clonic seizure. Partial seizure activity that spreads in an orderly fashion to surrounding areas is known as a *Jacksonian seizure.*

Complex partial seizures arise from focal seizures in the temporal lobe (psychomotor) and manifest primarily as changes in behavior. The classic complex partial seizure is preceded by an aura,

---

NOTE

A hysterical seizure can mimic a true seizure, but it stems from psychological causes. These seizures are not considered true seizures, because they have no organic origin and do not respond to normal management modalities. Hysterical seizures, or pseudoseizures, usually can be terminated by sharp commands or painful stimuli (e.g., a sternal rub). These maneuvers may help provide a differential aid in distinguishing between pathological and psychogenic seizure activity.

followed by abnormal repetitive motor behavior (automatisms), such as lip smacking, chewing, or swallowing, during which time the patient is amnestic. These seizures typically are brief (less than 1 minute), and the patient usually regains normal mental status quickly. Like simple partial seizures, complex partial seizures also may progress to a generalized tonic-clonic seizure.

Assessment

Prehospital assessment is determined by the patient's seizure status on EMS arrival. In most cases, the patient's seizure activity has ceased before the paramedic crew arrives. If possible, the assessment should include a thorough history and physical examination, including a neurological evaluation.

History. If the patient is postictal, information can be gathered from family members or bystanders who witnessed the event. Important components of the patient history include the following:

1. History of seizures
   a. Frequency
   b. Compliance in taking prescribed medications (e.g., *phenytoin* [Dilantin], phenobarbital [Luminal])
2. Description of seizure activity
   a. Duration of seizure
   b. Typical or atypical pattern of seizure for the patient
   c. Presence of aura
   d. Generalized or focal
   e. Incontinence
   f. Tongue biting
3. Recent or past history of head trauma
4. Recent history of fever, headache, nuchal rigidity (suggesting meningeal irritation)
5. Past significant medical history
   a. Diabetes
   b. Heart disease
   c. Stroke

Physical examination. In conducting the physical examination, maintaining a patent airway is always of primary importance. The paramedic also should be alert to signs of trauma (head and neck trauma, tongue injury, oral lacerations) that may have occurred before or during the seizure activity. In addition, the patient's gums should be inspected for gin-

gival hypertrophy (swelling of the gums), which is a sign of chronic *phenytoin* (Dilantin) therapy. Other components of the physical examination include:

- Level of sensorium, including presence or absence of amnesia
- Cranial nerve evaluation, particularly pupillary findings
- Motor and sensory evaluation, including coordination (Abnormalities may be caused by metabolic disturbances, meningitis, intracranial hemorrhage, and drug use.)
- An evaluation for hypotension and hypoxia
- Presence of urine or feces (suggesting bladder or bowel incontinence)
- Automatisms
- Cardiac dysrhythmias

> **? CRITICAL THINKING**
> *What are signs and symptoms of phenytoin toxicity?*

Syncope versus seizure. It may be difficult to determine whether the patient experienced a syncopal episode (described in Chapter 28) or a seizure, because the main differentiating characteristics are in the symptoms before and after the event. The factors listed in Table 29-3 may aid in the determination.

Management

The first step in managing a patient with seizure activity is to prevent the patient from sustaining physical injury. This is best accomplished by removing obstacles in the patient's immediate area or, if necessary, moving the patient to a safe environment such as a carpeted or soft, grassy area. *At no time should a patient with seizure activity be restrained, nor should objects be forced between the patient's teeth to maintain an airway.* Restraining activity may harm the patient or paramedic crew. Forcing objects into the oral cavity in an effort to secure an airway or prevent the patient from biting his or her tongue may evoke vomiting, aspiration, or spasm of the larynx.

Most patients with an isolated seizure can be appropriately managed in the postictal phase by being placed in a lateral recumbent position to allow drainage of oral secretions and to facilitate suction-

TABLE 29-3	DIFFERENTIATING CHARACTERISTICS OF SYNCOPE AND SEIZURE	
CHARACTERISTICS	**SYNCOPE**	**SEIZURE**
Position	The syncope usually starts in a standing position.	The seizure may start in any position.
Warning	There is usually a warning period of lightheadedness.	There is little or no warning.
Level of consciousness	The patient usually regains consciousness immediately on becoming supine; fatigue, confusion, and headache last less than 15 minutes.	The patient may remain unconscious for minutes to hours; fatigue, confusion, and headache last longer than 15 minutes.
Clonic-tonic activity	Clonic movements (if present) are of short duration.	Tonic-clonic movements occur during unconscious state.
ECG analysis	Bradycardia is caused by increased vagal tone associated with syncope.	Tachycardia is caused by muscular exertion associated with seizure activity.

ing (if needed). Supplemental oxygen should be administered via a nonrebreather mask, and the patient should be moved to a quiet environment (away from onlookers). Patients commonly are embarrassed or self-conscious after a seizure, particularly if incontinence has occurred. Therefore the paramedic should be sensitive to the physical and emotional needs of the patient.

Patients with a history of seizures who have experienced an atypical seizure or one that was complicated by an unusual event (e.g., trauma), and all others who have experienced a seizure for the first time should be transported to the emergency department for physician evaluation. Depending on the patient's status and seizure history, medical direction may recommend that an IV line be established if medication therapy becomes necessary. However, few patients who experience an isolated seizure require pharmacological agents in the prehospital setting.

Status epilepticus

Status epilepticus is continuous seizure activity lasting 30 minutes or longer or a recurrent seizure without an intervening period of consciousness. The condition is a true emergency; without immediate management, it can result in permanent neurological damage, respiratory failure, and death. Associated complications of status epilepticus include aspiration, brain damage, and fracture of long bones and the spine. The most common precipitating cause of this condition in adults is failure to take prescribed anticonvulsant medications.

Management. As in all patients with seizures, management priorities include managing the airway and providing ventilatory support, protecting the patient from injury, and, if indicated, transporting the patient to a medical facility for physician evaluation. In addition, management of a status seizure includes stopping the seizure activity with anticonvulsant medications (e.g., *diazepam* [Valium], *lorazepam* [Ativan], *phenytoin* [Dilantin]).

After the airway is secured with oral or nasal adjuncts (or intubation of the patient's trachea during the flaccid period between seizures), oxygen should be administered in high concentration and ventilation should be supported with a bag-valve device. An IV line should be established to keep the vein open, and secured well with tape and roller bandage. A sample of the patient's blood should be drawn for laboratory analysis (per protocol). With authorization from medical direction, administration of the following medications may be considered:

- ***Dextrose 50%*** by slow IV infusion (controversial unless hypoglycemia is suspected) to replace blood glucose lost during seizure activity or correct hypoglycemia that caused the seizure.

- Administration of *lorazepam* (Ativan) IV or *diazepam* (Valium) IV to stop the spread of the seizure focus; seizure activity may require *phenytoin* (Dilantin).

While administering anticonvulsants, the paramedic should closely monitor the patient's blood pressure and respiratory status and be prepared for aggressive airway control and ventilatory assistance. If the patient's blood pressure begins to fall or if the respiratory rate or effort decreases, drug therapy should cease and the paramedic should consult with medical direction.

Headache

Although headaches are painful and bothersome, most are minor health concerns and are easily managed with analgesics. Headaches are categorized according to their underlying cause as **tension headaches, migraines, cluster headaches,** and **sinus headaches.** Therapies that may be useful in managing these headaches include prescription and over-the-counter medications, herbal remedies, meditation, acupressure, aromatherapy, and others. Headache is an extremely common medical complaint; 40% of all Americans will have what they consider to be a serious headache at some time during their lives.[6]

> **NOTE**
>
> The pain associated with headaches arises from the meninges and from the scalp and its blood vessels and muscles.

Tension headaches are caused by muscle contractions of the face, neck, and scalp. They have a variety of causes, some of which include stress, persistent noise, eyestrain, and poor posture. The pain of tension headaches (usually described as dull, persistent, and nonthrobbing) may last for days or weeks and can cause variable degrees of discomfort. These headaches can be short-lived and infrequent, or chronic in nature. Most tension headaches can effectively be managed with analgesics such as *aspirin,* acetaminophen, or ibuprofen.

Migraines are severe, incapacitating headaches that often are preceded by visual and/or GI distur-

bances. These headaches usually begin with an intense, throbbing pain on one side of the head that may spread, and they often are accompanied by nausea and vomiting. The symptoms of migraines are associated with constriction and dilation of blood vessels that may be brought on by an imbalance of serotonin or hormone fluctuations. Migraines also can be triggered by excessive caffeine use, various foods, changes in altitude, and extremes of emotions. A wide range of medications are prescribed for migraines, including beta blockers, calcium channel blockers, antidepressants, and serotonin-inhibiting drugs.

> **NOTE**
>
> Many causes of headaches can be avoided. Examples include identifying triggers such as irregular meals, prolonged travel, noisy environments, and food additives in susceptible persons.

Cluster headaches are headaches that occur in bursts (clusters). They often begin several hours after a person falls asleep. The pain, which may be severe, usually is located in and around one eye and generally is accompanied by nasal congestion and tearing. The painful episode often lasts 30 minutes to 2 hours and then diminishes or disappears, recurring a day or so later. The headaches may occur every day for weeks or months before going into long periods of remission. Cluster headaches also are known as *histamine headaches*, since they are associated with the release of histamine from the body tissues and are marked by symptoms of dilated carotid arteries, fluid accumulation under the eyes, tearing or lacrimation, and rhinorrhea. Cluster headaches generally are managed with antihistamines, corticosteroids, and calcium channel blockers.

> **NOTE**
>
> Cluster headaches seem to be more common in heavy smokers than in nonsmokers. Alcohol consumption and certain foods also may be implicated. The vast majority of sufferers are men.

Sinus headaches are characterized by pain in the forehead, nasal area, and eyes. They often produce a feeling of pressure behind the face. Inflammation or infection of the membranes lining the sinus cavities or allergies usually are responsible for the discomfort. Sinus headaches are managed with medications that include analgesics, antihistamines, and antibiotics to manage infection.

Management

Headaches such as those described in the preceding paragraphs seldom require prehospital emergency care measures. A thorough history of the headache should be obtained, however, to help identify patients who may have a more serious cause of headaches (e.g., from aneurysm or stroke). Important assessment findings include:

- The patient's general health
- Previous medical conditions
- Medication use
- Previous experience with headaches
- Time of onset

After gathering a patient history and performing a neurological examination, prehospital care for patients with tension headaches, migraines, cluster headaches, and sinus headaches primarily is supportive. The paramedic should consult with medical direction to determine the appropriate disposition for the patient. Patient transport for physician evaluation may be indicated.

Brain Neoplasm and Brain Abscess

A brain tumor or, neoplasm, refers to a mass in the cranial cavity, which can be either malignant or benign. Brain tumors, which may have a heritable component, are associated with several risk factors that include exposure to radiation, tobacco use, dietary habits, some viruses, and use of some medications.[1] The effects of the tumor depend on the tumor's size, location, any evidence of hemorrhage or edema, and rate of growth. Brain tumors may cause local and generalized manifestations. Local effects are caused by the destructive action of the tumor on a particular site in the brain and by compression causing decreased CBF (Fig. 29-11). These effects are varied and may include[7]:

- Seizures
- Visual disturbances
- Unstable gait
- Cranial nerve dysfunction

Lesions inside the cranial vault produce pain by distending or stretching the arteries and other

> **NOTE**
>
> CNS tumors include both brain tumors and spinal cord tumors. The incidence of CNS tumors tends to increase up to age 70 and then decreases. These tumors represent the second most common group of tumors in children.[7]

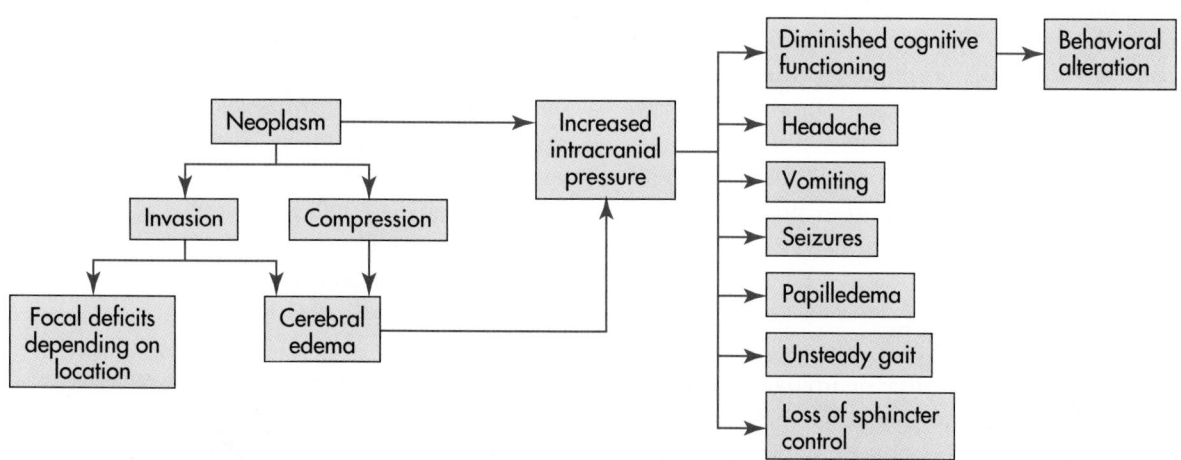

Fig. 29-11 Origin of clinical manifestations associated with an intracranial neoplasm. (From McCance KL, Huether SE: *Pathophysiology: the biologic basis for disease in adults and children,* ed 3, St Louis, 1998, Mosby.)

pain-sensitive structures of the head and neck. Headache may be present but often is a late finding in the absence of hemorrhage, which may cause a sudden onset of pain.[6] The principal treatment for a cerebral tumor is surgical or radiosurgical excision, or surgical decompression if total excision is not possible. Chemotherapy and radiation also may be used.

A brain abscess is an accumulation of purulent material (pus) surrounded by a capsule within the brain. It develops from a bacterial infection, often originating in the nasal cavity, middle ear, or mastoid cells. The condition also may follow surgery or penetrating cranial trauma, particularly when bone fragments are retained in cranial tissue. Clinical manifestations of a brain abscess are associated with intracranial infection (e.g., fever) and an expanding intracranial mass (e.g., nausea, vomiting, seizures, and alterations of mental status). Headache is the most frequent early symptom. Aspiration of the abscess or excision accompanied by antibiotic therapy generally is recommended to manage this disorder (controversial).

NOTE

The incidence of brain abscesses is about 1 per 100,000 hospital admissions. They are twice as common in men as in women. The median age for abscess formation is 30 to 40 years of age.[7]

Management

Prehospital care for a patient with a neoplasm or abscess in the brain may range from providing comfort and emotional support during patient transport to managing seizure activity and providing airway, ventilatory, and circulatory resuscitation. If the patient's condition permits, a focused history should be obtained and a neurological evaluation should be performed.

Degenerative Neurological Diseases

There are many degenerative neurological diseases, and the pathophysiology of many of these disorders is not fully understood. Some pathological processes may involve Schwann cells, the CSF, or axons of the CNS, and others may result from circulatory and immunological disorders and exposure to bacterial tox-

ins and chemicals. The specific neurological diseases discussed in this chapter include:

- Muscular dystrophy
- Multiple sclerosis
- Dystonia
- Parkinson's disease
- Central pain syndrome
- Bell's palsy
- Amyotrophic lateral sclerosis
- Peripheral neuropathy
- Myoclonus
- Spina bifida
- Polio

Muscular Dystrophy

Muscular dystrophy is an inherited muscle disorder of unknown cause in which there is a slow but progressive degeneration of muscle fibers. Different forms of the disease are classified by the age at which the symptoms appear, the rate at which the disease progresses, and the way in which it is inherited. Duchenne muscular dystrophy is the most common type, affecting about 1 or 2 in 10,000 male children. It is inherited through a recessive sex-linked gene, so that only males are affected and only females can pass on the disease.

Muscular dystrophy often is first diagnosed by the child's physician, who observes that the child is slow in learning to sit up and walk. The disease is confirmed through blood tests that reveal high levels of enzymes released from damaged muscle cells, through nerve conduction studies, and sometimes with muscle biopsy. Muscular dystrophy rarely is diagnosed before age 3. As the disease progresses, the child tends to walk with a waddle and has difficulty climbing stairs. Muscles (especially those in the calves) become bulky as wasted muscle is replaced by fat. By about age 12, affected children are no longer able to walk, and few will survive their teenage years. Death usually results from pulmonary infections and heart failure.

? CRITICAL THINKING

How can you determine a child's baseline level of functioning?

There is no effective treatment for muscular dystrophy. Parents or siblings of an affected child should receive genetic counseling. Some types of muscular dystrophy can be diagnosed before birth through blood analysis and amniocentesis.

Multiple Sclerosis

Multiple sclerosis (MS) is a progressive disease of the CNS in which scattered patches of myelin in the brain and spinal cord are destroyed. Although the cause of MS remains unknown, it is thought to be an autoimmune disease in which the body's defense system begins to treat the myelin in the CNS as foreign, gradually destroying it (demyelination), with subsequent scarring and nerve fiber damage.

MS is the most common acquired disease of the nervous system in young adults, affecting about 1 in every 1000 persons. The ratio of women to men sufferers is 3 to 2. The symptoms, which may be active briefly in early adult life and resume years later, vary according to the parts of the brain and spinal cord that are affected. Symptoms range from numbness and tingling to paralysis and incontinence and may last from several weeks to several months. Damage to the white matter in the brain may lead to fatigue, vertigo, clumsiness, unsteady gait, slurred speech, blurred or double vision, and facial numbness or pain. Some patients may have mild relapses and long symptom-free periods throughout life. Others may gradually become disabled from the first attack and are bedridden and incontinent in early middle life.

? CRITICAL THINKING

What is the patient who has been receiving long-term steroid therapy at risk for?

Diagnosis of the disease usually is by exclusion of all other possible conditions. Diagnostic tests that may be helpful in identifying MS include lumbar puncture, CT scanning, and MRI studies. Affected patients are managed with medications (e.g., corticosteroids, antidepressants, immunomodifers) to control symptoms of an acute episode and to prevent exacerbations, and with physical therapy to maintain mobility and independence. There is presently no cure for the disease.

Dystonia

Dystonia refers to local or diffuse alterations in muscle tone (usually abnormal muscle rigidity) that cause painful muscle spasms, unusually fixed postures, and strange movement patterns. Localized dystonia may result from torticollis (painful neck spasm) or scoliosis (abnormal curvature of the spine). More generalized dystonia results from various neurological disorders, including Parkinson's disease and stroke. It also may be a feature of schizophrenia or a side effect of some antipsychotic drugs. Following physician evaluation, dystonia sometimes is managed with medications such as benztropine (Cogentin) or *diphenhydramine* (Benadryl) to reverse the symptoms and to prevent recurrent symptoms.

Parkinson's Disease

Parkinson's disease is caused by degeneration or damage (of unknown origin) to nerve cells within the basal ganglia in the brain. The degeneration causes a lack of dopamine that prevents the basal ganglia from modifying nerve pathways that control muscle contraction. The result is muscles that are overly tense, causing tremor, joint rigidity, and slow movement. Parkinson's disease affects about 130 in 100,00 persons, with 50,000 new cases diagnosed in the United States each year.[1] Untreated, the disease progresses over 10 to 15 years to severe weakness and incapacity.

NOTE

Parkinson's disease is the leading cause of neurological disability in those over age 60. There are presently about 500,000 people in the United States with the disease.[1]

Parkinson's disease usually begins as a slight tremor in one hand, arm, or leg. In early stages, the tremor is worse while the limb is at rest. In later stages, the disease affects both sides of the body, causing stiffness, weakness, and trembling of the muscles. Other symptoms include an unusual walking pattern (shuffling) that may break into uncontrollable, tiny running steps; constant trembling of the hands, sometimes accompanied by shaking of the head; a permanent rigid stoop; and an unblinking, fixed facial expression. Late in the disease, intellect may be affected and speech becomes slow and hesitant. Depression is common.

Parkinson's disease initially is managed with counseling, exercise, and special aids in the home.

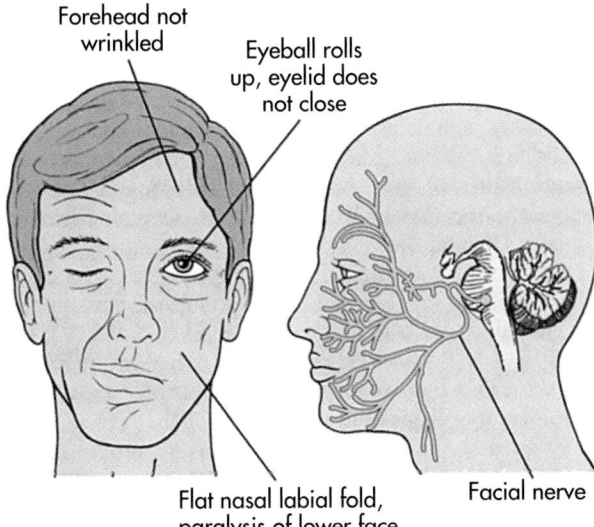

Forehead not wrinkled

Eyeball rolls up, eyelid does not close

Flat nasal labial fold, paralysis of lower face

Facial nerve

Fig. 29-12 Bell's palsy. (From Lewis S: *Medical-surgical nursing,* ed 4, St Louis, 1996, Mosby.)

As the disease progresses, management may include various combinations of drugs (e.g., levodopa [Dopar, L-Dopa], which is converted by the body into dopamine, and anticholinergic agents) to provide relief from specific symptoms. Other management modalities may include brain surgery to reduce tremor and rigidity, and transplantation of dopamine-secreting adrenal tissue (experimental).

Central Pain Syndrome

Central pain syndrome refers to infection or disease of the trigeminal nerve (cranial nerve V). A common form of the syndrome is *tic douloureux* (trigeminal neuralgia) in which patients complain of paroxysmal episodes of excruciating pain (often described as recurrent bursts of an electric shock) that affect the cheek, lips, gums, or chin on one side of the face. The episode usually is very brief, lasting only a few seconds to minutes, but may be so intense that the person is debilitated during the attack. The pain often causes wincing; hence the name tic douloureux (literally, "painful twitch"). Central pain syndrome is unusual in persons under age 50 but may be associated with MS in younger people. Attacks occur in bouts that may last weeks at a time.

The pain of trigeminal neuralgia usually begins from a "trigger point" on the face that can be brought

on by touching, washing, shaving, eating, drinking, or talking. Since the cause of the syndrome is uncertain, management is difficult. Management modalities include the use of drugs to inhibit nerve impulses (commonly carbamazepine [Epitol, Tegretol]) and sometimes surgery if the cause is a tumor or lesion.

Bell's Palsy

Bell's palsy (facial palsy) refers to paralysis of the facial muscles due to inflammation of the seventh cranial nerve (Fig. 29-12). It usually is one-sided and temporary and often develops suddenly. Bell's palsy is the most common cause of facial paralysis, affecting 1 in 60 to 70 persons in a lifetime.[1] The cause of inflammation is uncertain, but it has been associated with many past or present infectious processes that include Lyme disease, herpes viruses, mumps, and HIV infection.

> **? CRITICAL THINKING**
>
> *Should you diagnose and release a patient in the field who has Bell's palsy?*

Bell's palsy usually causes the eyelid and corner of the mouth to droop on one side of the face and sometimes is associated with numbness and pain. Depending on which branches of the nerve are affected, taste may be impaired or sounds may seem unusually loud. Management involves the use of corticosteroid drugs (controversial) to reduce inflammation of the nerve, along with analgesics. Recovery usually is complete within 2 weeks to 2 months. An important component of therapy is to protect the affected eye from corneal drying and injury that may result from paralysis of eyelid closure. This is best accomplished through the use of lubricating ointments and eye patches.

Amyotrophic Lateral Sclerosis

Amyotrophic lateral sclerosis (ALS), also called *Lou Gehrig's disease,* is one of a group of rare disorders (motor neuron disease) in which the nerves that control muscular activity degenerate within the brain and spinal cord. ALS usually affects people over age 50 and is more common in men than in women. One or two cases of ALS are diagnosed annually per 100,000 people in the United States.[7] About 10% of ALS cases are familial.

Motor neuron diseases may involve deterioration of both upper and lower neuron tracts. When only muscles of the tongue, jaw, face, and larynx are involved, the term *progressive bulbar palsy* is used. When only corticospinal processes are affected, the term *primary lateral sclerosis* is used. When only lower motor neurons are affected, the term *progressive spinal muscular atrophy* is used. *ALS* is used to describe neuron signs that predominate in the extremities and trunk.

Patients with ALS often first notice weakness in the hands and arms that is accompanied by involuntary quivering (fasciculations). The disease progresses to involve the muscles of all four extremities and those involved in respiration and swallowing. In the final stages of the disease, patients often are unable to speak, swallow, or move—even though awareness and intellect are maintained. Death usually follows in 2 to 4 years after diagnosis because of involvement of the respiratory muscles, aspiration pneumonia, and general inanition (starvation, failure to thrive). In some cases, life can be prolonged through the use of feeding tubes and ventilators. Care generally is aimed at providing emotional support and easing discomfort.

? CRITICAL THINKING

Why is there a tendency to treat these patients as though they have low intelligence?

Peripheral Neuropathy

As the name implies, **peripheral neuropathy** refers to diseases and disorders affecting the peripheral nervous system, including spinal nerve roots, cranial nerves, and peripheral nerves. Most neuropathies arise from damage or irritation either to the axons or to their myelin sheaths that slows or completely blocks the passage of electrical signals. The various types of peripheral neuropathy are classified according to the site and distribution of damage. For example, damage to sensory nerve fibers may cause numbness and tingling, sensations of cold, or pain that often starts at the hands and feet and spreads toward the central body. Damage

to motor nerve fibers may cause muscle weakness and muscle wasting. Damage that occurs to the nerves of the autonomic nervous system may result in blurred vision, impaired or absent sweating, fluctuations in blood pressure (and associated syncope), GI disorders, incontinence, and impotence.

Some peripheral neuropathies have no identifiable cause. Others may be related to specific causes that include:

- Diabetes
- Dietary deficiencies (especially of vitamin B)
- Alcoholism
- Uremia
- Leprosy
- Lead poisoning
- Drug intoxication
- Viral infection (e.g., Guillain-Barré syndrome)
- Rheumatoid arthritis
- Systemic lupus erythematosus
- Malignant tumors (e.g., lung cancer)
- Lymphomas
- Leukemias
- Inherited neuropathies (e.g., peronal muscular atrophy)

When possible, management is aimed at the underlying cause (e.g., blood glucose control in a diabetic patient, and correction of a nutritional deficiency). If management is successful and the cell bodies of the damaged nerves have not been destroyed, full recovery from the neuropathy is possible.

Myoclonus

Myoclonus refers to rapid and uncontrollable muscular contractions (jerking) or spasms of muscle(s) that occur at rest or during movement. The syndrome may be associated with disease of nerves and muscles or may be a symptom of a brain disorder (e.g., encephalitis) or seizure disorder. Myoclonus also may occur in healthy persons. An example is a limb jump that is sometimes experienced just before falling asleep.

Spina Bifida

Spina bifida is a congenital defect in which one part of one (or more) vertebra fails to develop completely, leaving a portion of the spinal cord exposed. The condition can occur anywhere on the spine but is most common in the lower back. Although the cause is unknown, spina bifida occurs in about 1 of every 1000 births.

Types of spina bifida. The severity of spina bifida depends on how much nerve tissue is exposed after neural tube closure. The four types of spina bifida are spina bifida occulta, meningocele, myelomeningocele, and encephalocele.

Spina bifida occulta is the most common and least serious form, with little external evidence of the defect. Meningocele is a type of spina bifida in which the nerve tissue of the spinal cord usually is intact and covered with a membranous sac of skin. Meningocele usually is without functional problems but requires surgical repair early in life. Myelomeningocele is the most severe form of spina bifida, often resulting in a child who is severely handicapped. With this type of spina bifida, there is a raw swelling over the spine and a malformed spinal cord that may or may not be contained in a membranous sac (Fig. 29-13). The legs of these children often are deformed, and there is partial or complete paralysis and loss of sensation in all areas below the level of the defect. Associated abnormalities of myelomeningocele include hydro-cephalus (excess CSF within the skull) with brain damage, cerebral palsy, epilepsy, and mental retardation. The fourth (and very rare) type of spina bifida is encephalocele in which the protrusion occurs through the skull. Severe brain damage is common with this condition.

Polio

Polio (poliomyelitis) is caused by poliovirus hominis. The virus attacks with variable severity ranging from unapparent infection, to a febrile illness without neurological sequela, to aseptic meningitis, and finally to paralytic disease (including respiratory paralysis) and possibly death. The incidence of polio has declined in the United States, Canada, and Europe since the development of the Salk and Sabin vaccines in the 1950s, but the disease may affect nonimmune adults and indigent (particularly immigrant) children. It remains a serious risk for anyone not vaccinated and traveling in southern Europe, Africa, or Asia.

?   CRITICAL THINKING

Ask your older friends or relatives about their memory of the polio epidemic. How did it affect their lives?

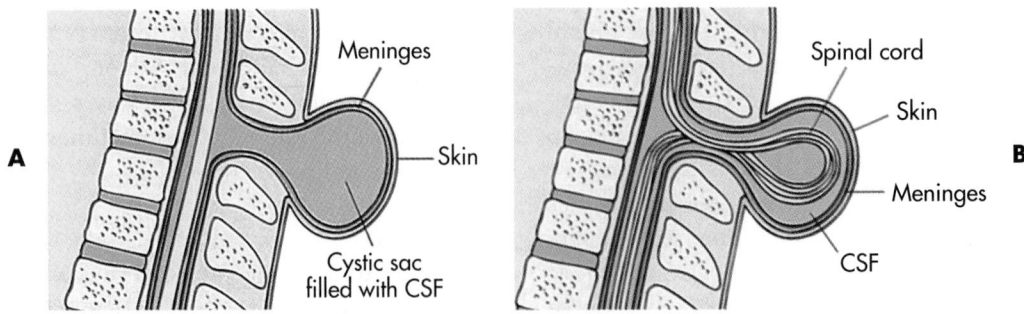

Fig. 29-13 A, Meningocele. **B,** Myelomeningocele. (From McCance KL, Huether SE: *Pathophysiology: the biologic basis for disease in adults and children,* ed 3, St Louis, 1998, Mosby.)

People infected with the poliovirus can pass large numbers of virus particles in their feces, where they may be spread directly or indirectly by fingers-to-food transmission to infect others, and by airborne transmission. Signs and symptoms of polio differ in the nonparalytic and paralytic forms. Although fever, headache, sore throat, and malaise are common to both forms, the paralytic form of polio also is associated with generalized pain, weakness, muscle spasms, and the paralysis of limbs and other muscles. If the infection spreads to the brain stem, the result may be difficulty or inability to swallow or breathe. Recovery from nonparalytic polio is complete. Of those who become paralyzed, more than half eventually make a full recovery. (Some patients may develop "postpolio deterioration" with new weakness and pain from recovered muscles.) The disease is confirmed though CSF analysis, throat culture, or sample of feces.

SUMMARY

- The human body's ability to maintain a state of homeostasis results primarily from the nervous system's regulatory and coordinating activities. The blood supply to the brain comes from the vertebral arteries and the internal carotid arteries.

- Some neurological emergencies are a consequence of structural changes or damage, circulatory changes, or alterations in intracranial pressure that affect cerebral blood flow.

- The initial survey should begin by determining the patient's level of consciousness and by ensuring an open and patent airway. Important elements of the physical examination that may provide clues to the nature of the neurological emergency include the patient history and history of the event, vital signs, and respiratory patterns.

- Coma is an abnormally deep state of unconsciousness from which the patient cannot be aroused by external stimuli. In general, two mechanisms produce coma: structural lesions or toxic metabolic states.

- Stroke is a sudden interruption in blood flow to the brain that results in a neurological deficit. Strokes can be classified as ischemic strokes and hemorrhagic strokes.

- A seizure is a temporary alteration in behavior or consciousness caused by abnormal electrical activity of one or more groups of neurons in the brain. In the prehospital setting, determining the origin of seizure activity is less important than managing the complications and recognizing whether the seizure is reversible with therapy.

- Four common types of headaches are tension headaches, migraines, cluster headaches, and sinus headaches.

- A brain tumor or neoplasm refers to a mass in the cranial cavity that can be either malignant or benign. Brain tumors, which may have a heritable component, are associated with several risk factors that include exposure to radiation, tobacco use, dietary habits, some viruses, and use of some medications.

- A brain abscess is an accumulation of purulent material (pus) surrounded by a capsule within the brain. It develops from a bacterial infection, often originating in the nasal cavity, middle ear, or mastoid cells.

- Muscular dystrophy is an inherited muscle disorder of unknown cause in which there is a slow but progressive degeneration of muscle fibers.

- Damage to the white matter of the brain in multiple sclerosis may lead to fatigue, vertigo, clumsiness, unsteady gait, slurred speech, blurred or double vision, and facial numbness or pain.

- Dystonia refers to local or diffuse alterations in muscle tone that cause painful muscle spasms, unusually fixed postures, and strange movement patterns.

- Parkinson's disease usually begins as a slight tremor in one hand, arm, or leg. In later stages, the disease affects both sides of the body, causing stiffness, weakness, and trembling of the muscles.

- Central pain syndrome refers to infection or disease of the trigeminal nerve.

- Bell's palsy refers to paralysis of the facial muscles due to inflammation of the seventh cranial nerve. It is usually one-sided and temporary and often develops suddenly.

- Amyotrophic lateral sclerosis, also called Lou Gehrig's disease, is one of a group of rare disorders in which the nerves that control muscular activity degenerate within the brain and spinal cord.

- Peripheral neuropathies usually arise from damage or irritation either to the axons or their myelin sheaths that slows or completely blocks the passage of electrical signals.

- Myoclonus refers to rapid and uncontrollable muscular contractions or spasms of muscles that occur at rest or during movement.

- Spina bifida is a congenital defect in which one part of one or more vertebrae fails to develop completely, leaving a portion of the spinal cord exposed.

- Polio is caused by a virus that attacks with variable severity ranging from unapparent infection, to a febrile illness without neurological sequela, to aseptic meningitis, and finally to paralytic disease and possibly death.

REFERENCES

1. US Department of Transportation, National Highway Traffic Safety Administration: *EMT-Paramedic national standard curriculum*, 1998, Washington, DC, The Department.
2. American Heart Association: *Advanced cardiac life support*, Dallas, 1997, The Association.
3. American Heart Association: Guidelines 2000 for cardiopulmonary resuscitation and emergency cardiovascular care, International Consensus on Science, *Circulation* 102 (8):204, 2000.
4. Kothari R et al: Early stroke recognition: developing an out-of-hospital stroke scale, *Acad Emerg Med* 4 (10):986, 1997.
5. American Heart Association: Guidelines 2000 for cardiopulmonary resuscitation and emergency cardiovascular care, International Consensus on Science, *Circulation* 102 (8):209, 2000.
6. Rosen P, Barkin R: *Emergency medicine: concepts and clinical practice*, ed 4, St Louis, 1998, Mosby.
7. McCance K, Huether S: *Pathophysiology: the biologic basis for disease in adults and children*, ed 2, St Louis, 1994, Mosby.

30 Endocrinology

OBJECTIVES

Upon completion of this chapter, the paramedic student will be able to:

1. *Describe how hormones secreted from endocrine glands function to assist the body to maintain homeostasis.*

2. *Describe the anatomy and physiology of the pancreas and how its hormones work to maintain normal glucose metabolism.*

3. *Discuss pathophysiology as a basis for key signs and symptoms, patient assessment, and patient management for diabetes and diabetic emergencies of hypoglycemia, diabetic ketoacidosis, and hyperosmolar hyperglycemic nonketotic coma.*

4. *Discuss pathophysiology as a basis for key signs and symptoms, patient assessment, and patient management for disorders of the thyroid gland.*

5. *Discuss pathophysiology as a basis for key signs and symptoms, patient assessment, and patient management of Cushing's syndrome and Addison's disease.*

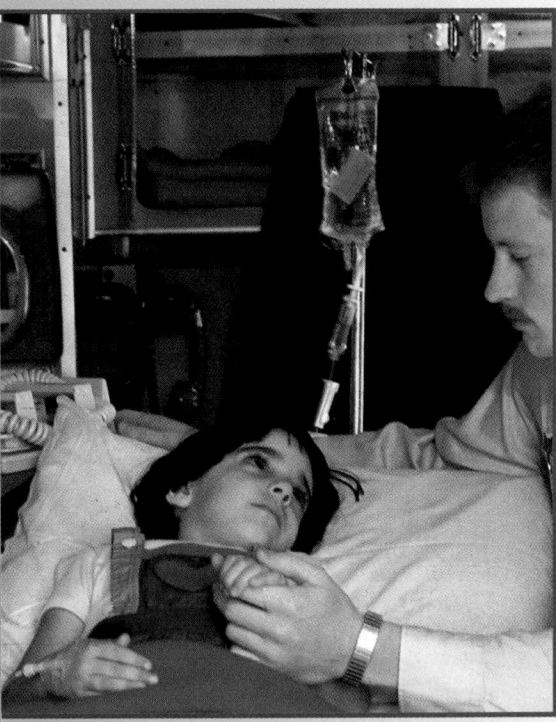

The endocrine system and the nervous system have evolved to allow the human body to regulate a multitude of functions and communicate among millions of cells. Paramedics will encounter patients with endocrine system disorders that range from a barely detectable variation from normal to life-threatening degrees of hypofunction or hyperfunction.

Addison's disease: A rare and potentially life-threatening disorder caused by a deficiency of the corticosteroid hormones normally produced by the adrenal cortex.

Cushing's syndrome: A condition caused by an abnormally high circulating level of corticosteroid hormones, produced naturally by the adrenal glands.

gluconeogenesis: The formation of glycogen from fatty acids and proteins rather than carbohydrates.

glycogenolysis: The breakdown of glycogen to glucose.

hyperosmolar hyperglycemic nonketotic (HHNK) coma: A diabetic coma in which the level of ketone bodies is normal; it is caused by hyperosmolarity of extracellular fluid and results in dehydration of intracellular fluid.

ketogenesis: The formation or production of ketone bodies.

myxedema: A condition that results from a deficiency in thyroid hormone.

thyrotoxicosis: A term that refers to any toxic condition that results from thyroid hyperfunction.

Anatomy and Physiology of the Endocrine System

As described in Chapter 6, the endocrine system is comprised of ductless glands and tissues that produce and secrete hormones. The major endocrine glands are the pituitary, thyroid, and parathyroid glands; the adrenal cortex and medulla; the pancreatic islets; and the ovaries and testes (Fig. 30-1). Other specialized groups of cells that secrete hormones are found in the kidneys and in the mucosa of the gastrointestinal (GI) tract.

Endocrine Gland Functions

Endocrine glands secrete their hormones directly into the bloodstream and exert a regulatory effect on various metabolic functions. Because the products of endocrine glands travel via the blood (or tissue fluids), they are able to exert their effects at widespread sites, often at some distance from their source of origin. The release of hormones occurs either in response to an alteration in the cellular environment or in the process of maintaining a regulated level of certain hormones or substances. This integrated chemical and coordination system enables reproduction, growth and development, and the regulation of energy. The specificity of this complex system is determined by the affinity of receptors on target organs and body tissues to a particular hormone.

? CRITICAL THINKING

How are hormones and their target organs like a lock and key?

Hormone Receptors

Most hormones can be categorized as proteins, polypeptides, derivatives of amino acids, or lipids. Each hormone may affect a specific organ or tissue or may have a general effect on the entire body. (Refer to Chapter 6 for a review of endocrine glands, hormones, and their functions.)

NOTE

Hormones also may be classified as steroid or nonsteroid. Steroid hormones are manufactured by endocrine cells from cholesterol and include cortisol, aldosterone, estrogen, progesterone, and testosterone. Nonsteroid hormones are synthesized primarily from amino acids and include insulin, parathyroid hormone, and others.

Hormones affect only cells with appropriate receptors and then act on these cells to initiate specific cell functions or activities. Hormone receptor sites may be on the cell membrane or in the interior of the cell. Cells with fewer receptor sites will bind with less hormone than cells with many receptor sites (Fig. 30-2). In addition, abnormalities in or the presence of specific hormone receptors can result in a pathological state as a result of complete rejection of that receptor's hormone by the target cells.

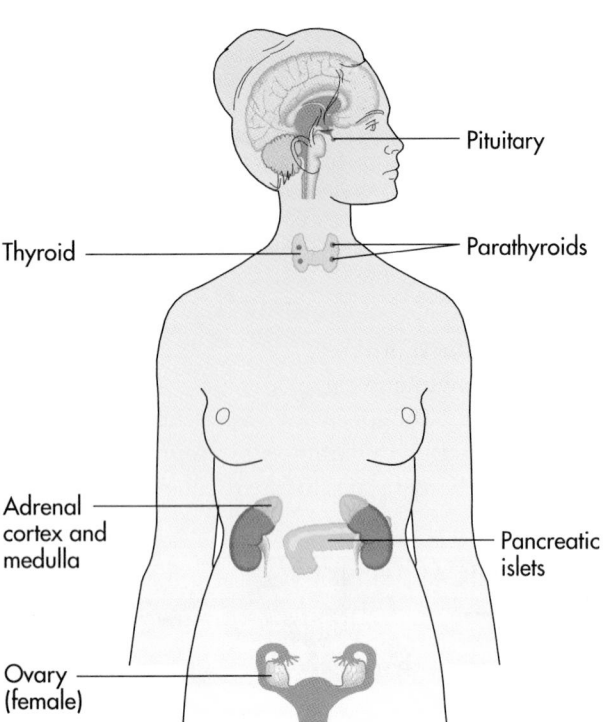

Fig. 30-1 Major endocrine glands.

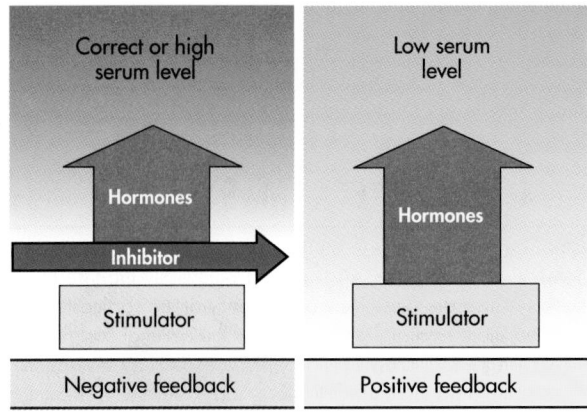

Fig. 30-3 Negative feedback.

Regulation of Hormone Secretion

All hormones operate within feedback systems (either positive or negative) to maintain an optimal internal environment. Negative feedback is the most common feedback mechanism and usually refers to an increase in the serum level of hormone or hormone-related substance that suppresses further hormone output. Conversely, hormone production is stimulated when the serum levels fall. Fig. 30-3 illustrates the negative feedback mechanism.

Specific Disorders of the Endocrine System

Disorders of the endocrine system arise from the effects of an imbalance in the production of one or more hormones or from the effects of an alteration in the body's ability to use the hormones produced. The clinical effects of endocrine gland function disturbances are determined by the degree of dysfunction and by the age and sex of the affected person. Specific disorders of the endocrine system presented in this chapter include the following:

- Diabetes mellitus
- Thyrotoxicosis
- Myxedema
- Cushing's syndrome
- Addison's disease

Diabetes Mellitus

Diabetes mellitus is a systemic disease of the endocrine system that usually results from pancreatic

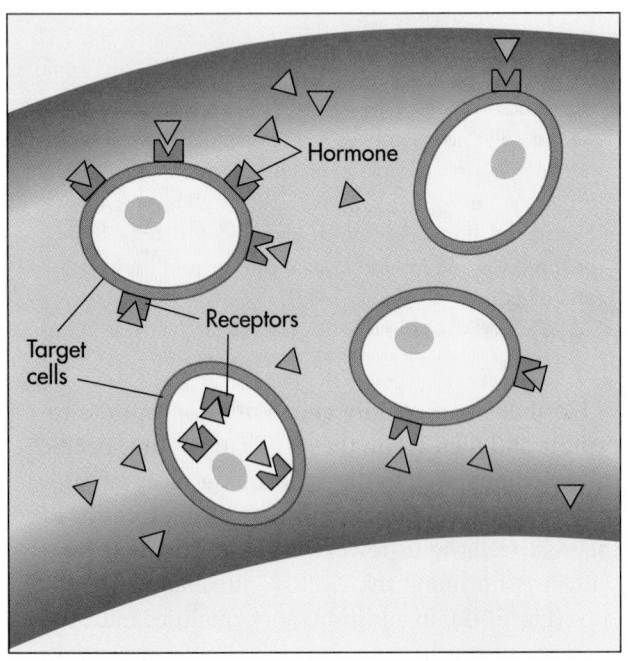

Fig. 30-2 The target cell concept. Cells with fewer receptor sites will bind with less hormone than cells with many receptor sites.

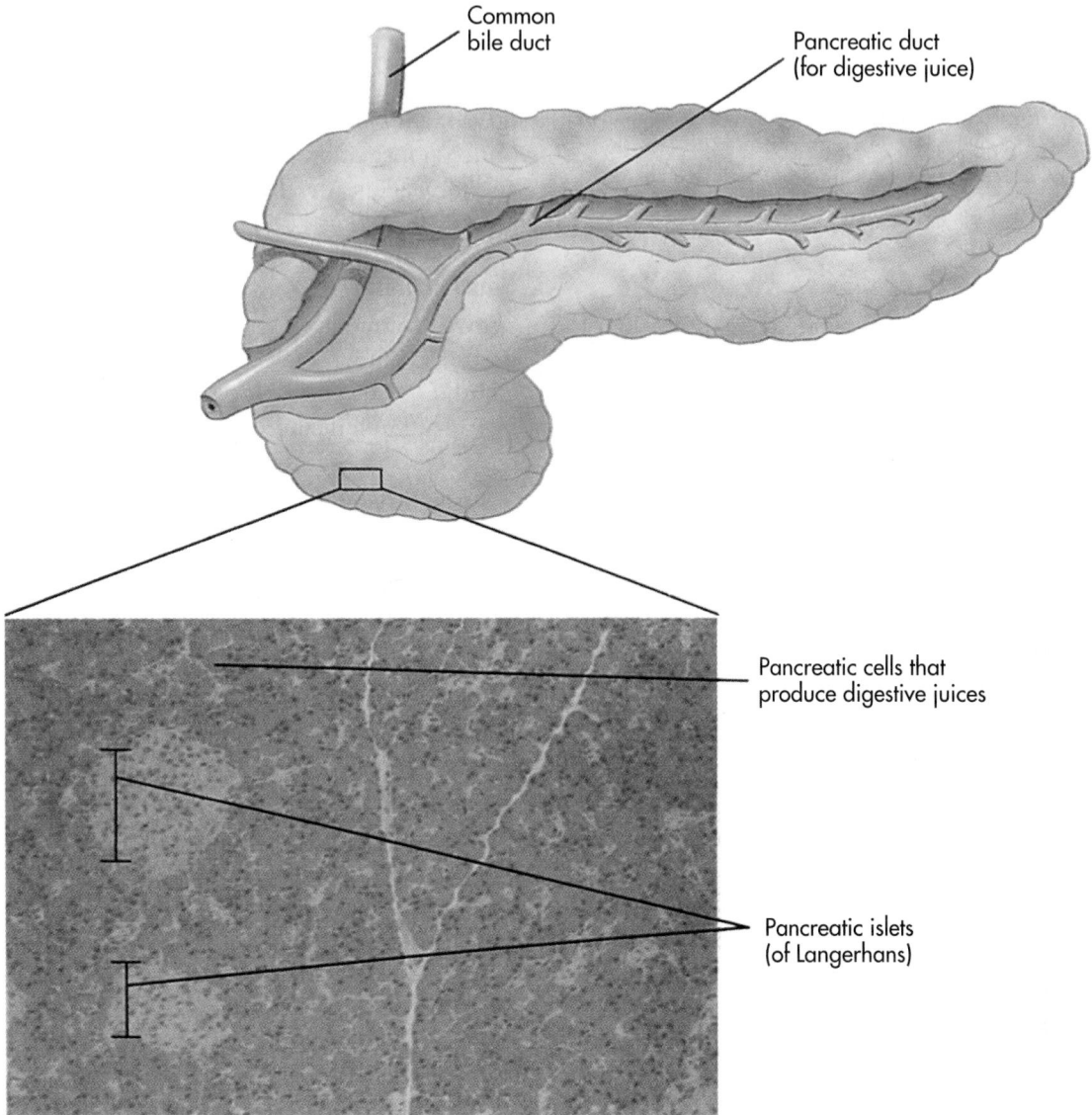

Fig. 30-4 Two pancreatic islets (of Langerhans) or hormone-producing areas are evident among the pancreatic cells that produce the pancreatic digestive juice. (From Thibodeau G: *Structure and function of the body,* ed 9, St Louis, 1992, Mosby.)

dysfunction. It is a complex disorder of fat, carbohydrate, and protein metabolism that affects more than 15.7 million Americans (both children and adults).[1] Diabetes mellitus is potentially lethal and can predispose the patient to several kinds of true medical emergencies.

Anatomy and Physiology of the Pancreas

The pancreas is important in the absorption and use of carbohydrates, fat, and protein; it is a principal regulator of blood glucose concentration. The pancreas is located retroperitoneally adjacent to the duodenum on the right and extending to the spleen on the left. The healthy pancreas has exocrine and endocrine functions. The exocrine portion consists of acini (glands that produce pancreatic juice) and a duct system that carries the pancreatic juice to the small intestine. The endocrine portion consists of pancreatic islets (islets of Langerhans) that produce hormones (Fig. 30-4).

Islets of Langerhans and Pancreatic Hormones

There are 500,000 to 1 million pancreatic islets dispersed among the ducts and the acini of the pancreas. Each islet is composed of beta cells that secrete insulin at a daily average of 0.6 units/kg of body weight, alpha cells that secrete glucagon, and other cells of questionable function, some of which are delta cells that secrete the hormone somatostatin, inhibiting the secretion of growth hormone. Nerves from both divisions of the autonomic nervous system innervate the pancreatic islets, and each islet is surrounded by a well-developed capillary network.

? CRITICAL THINKING

If part of the pancreas must be removed due to trauma, will the patient still be able to produce insulin and glucagon?

Insulin

Insulin is a small protein released by the beta cells when blood glucose levels rise. The primary functions of insulin are to increase glucose transport into cells, increase glucose metabolism by cells, increase liver glycogen levels, and decrease blood glucose concentration toward normal levels (Box 30-1). Many of the functions of insulin antagonize the effects of glucagon.

Glucagon

Glucagon is a protein released by the alpha cells when blood glucose levels fall. The two major effects of glucagon are to increase blood glucose levels by stimulating the liver to release glucose stores from glycogen and other glucose storage sites **(glycogenolysis)** and to stimulate **gluconeogenesis** (glucose formation) through the breakdown of fats and fatty acids, thereby maintaining a normal blood glucose level (Fig. 30-5).

Growth Hormone

Growth hormone (GH) is a polypeptide hormone produced and secreted by the anterior pituitary gland. GH secretion is triggered by many physiological stimuli, including exercise, stress, sleep, and hypoglycemia. GH acts as an insulin antagonist by decreasing insulin actions on cell membranes, reducing the capacity of muscles and adipose and liver cells to absorb glucose.

Regulation of Glucose Metabolism

Under normal conditions, the body maintains a range of serum glucose concentration that varies between 60 and 120 mg/dL. An understanding of food intake and digestion is required to understand glucose metabolism.

Dietary Intake

The three main organic components of food are carbohydrates, fats, and proteins. (Food also contains mineral and vitamins.) Carbohydrates, which are found in all sugary, starchy foods, are a ready source of near-instant energy and are the first food substances to enter the bloodstream after a meal is ingested. Carbohydrates yield the simple sugar glucose. If not "burned" for immediate energy, glucose is stored in the liver and muscles as glycogen for short-term energy needs or converted into fat by adipose tissue and stored for intermediate and long-term needs.

Process of Digestion

Before food compounds can be used by body cells, they must be digested and absorbed into the bloodstream. Digestion begins in the mouth and is accomplished by physical forces (chewing) and chemical (enzymatic) forces. This begins the process that reduces the food to soluble molecules and particles small enough to be absorbed. After food is swallowed, it enters the stomach, and various nutrients, including glucose, salts, water, and some other sub-

BOX 30-1

PRIMARY FUNCTIONS OF INSULIN

- To increase glucose transport into cells
- To increase glucose metabolism by cells
- To increase liver glycogen levels
- To decrease blood glucose concentration toward normal levels

stances (alcohol and certain other drugs) are absorbed into the circulatory system. The remaining material (chyme) is shunted from the stomach into the intestine for further digestion.

The duodenum signals the release of hormones that mobilize the pancreas to contribute its molecule-splitting enzymes and the gallbladder to release bile salts. These enzymes and salts neutralize acids and help emulsify fats. Carbohydrates are absorbed as simple sugars, fats as fatty acids and glycerol, and proteins as amino acids. These nutrients are then carried from the intestine to the liver by way of the portal vein. Water and remaining salts are absorbed from food residues reaching the colon. The liver synthesizes glycogen from the absorbed glucose, lipoproteins from the absorbed fatty acids, and many proteins required for health from absorbed amino acids.

Carbohydrate Metabolism

The secretion of insulin is contolled by chemical, neural, and hormonal means. An increased concentration of blood glucose, parasympathetic stimulation, and gastrointestinal hormones involved with

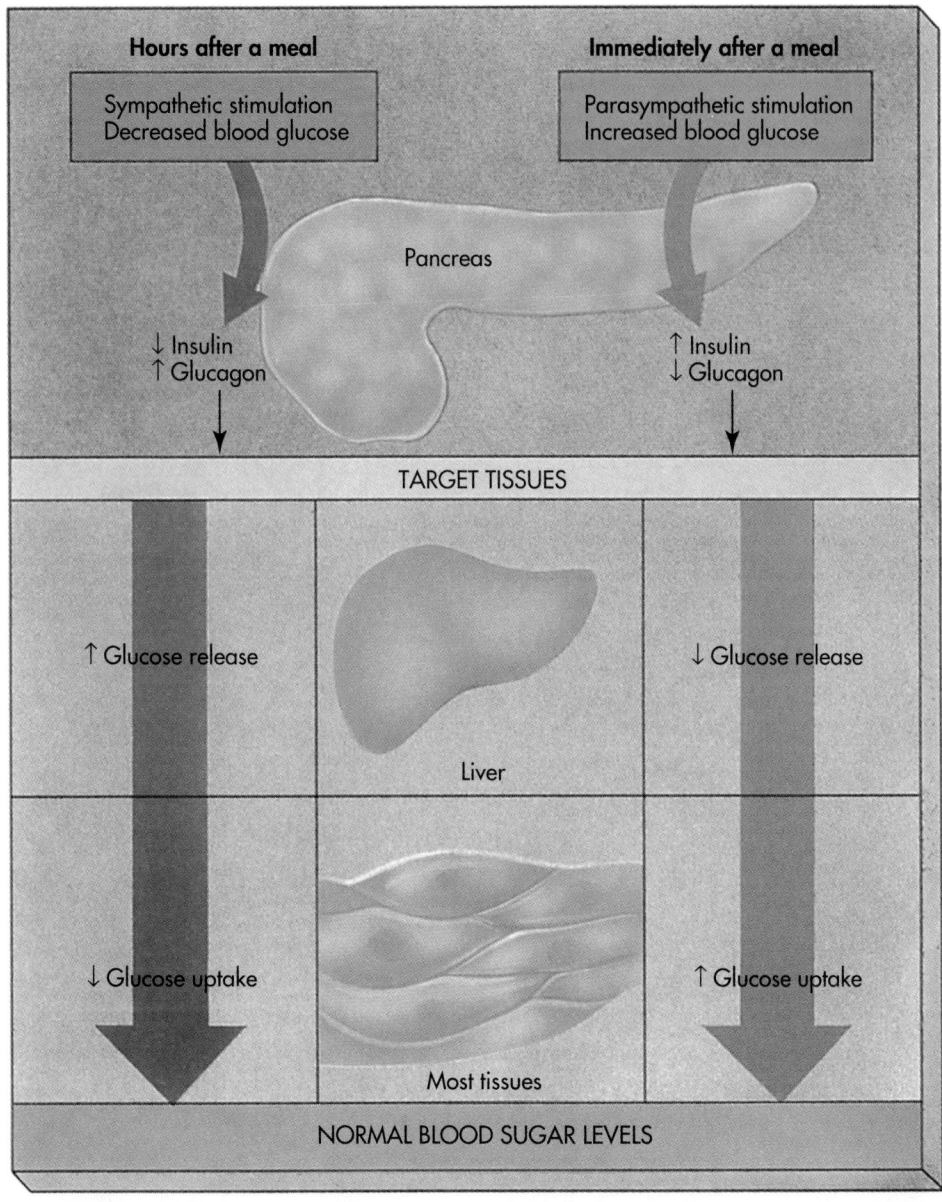

Fig. 30-5 Regulation of insulin and glucagon secretion. Sympathetic stimulation and decreasing concentrations of glucose increase the secretion of glucagon, which acts primarily on liver cells to increase the rate of glycogen breakdown and the secretion of glucose from the liver. The release of glucose from the liver helps maintain blood glucose levels. Increasing blood glucose levels has an inhibitory effect on glucagon secretion. Increasing concentrations of glucose and amino acids stimulate the beta cells of the islets to secrete insulin. In addition, parasympathetic stimulation causes insulin secretion. Insulin acts on most tissues to increase the uptake of glucose and amino acids. As the blood levels of glucose and amino acids decrease, the rate of insulin secretion also decreases. (From Seely R: *Anatomy and physiology,* ed 2, St Louis, 1992, Mosby.)

regulation of digestion cause beta cells of the pancreas to release insulin after dietary intake of carbohydrates. Insulin travels through the blood to target tissues, where it combines with specific chemical receptors on the surface of the cell membrane to permit glucose to enter the cell (Table 30-1). This allows the body cells to use glucose for energy, prevents the breakdown of alternative energy sources (proteins and fat cells), and promotes the uptake of glucose into the liver, where it is converted to glycogen for storage. This rapid uptake and storage of glucose normally prevents a large increase in blood glucose levels, even just after a normal meal.

? CRITICAL THINKING

Why do diabetics eat carbohydrates instead of protein or fat when they sense that their glucose level is too low?

When the blood glucose begins to fall, the liver releases glucose back into the circulating blood. Thus the liver removes glucose from the blood when it is in excess after dietary intake and returns it to the blood when it is needed between meals. Under normal circumstances, about 60% of the glucose in a meal is stored in the liver as glycogen and released later.

If the muscles are not exercised after a meal, much of the glucose transported into the muscle cells by insulin is stored as muscle glycogen. Muscle glycogen differs from liver glycogen in that it cannot be reconverted into glucose and released into the circulation. The stored glycogen must be used by the muscle for energy.

The brain is quite different from other body tissues with reference to glucose uptake. Insulin has little or no effect on the uptake or use of glucose by the brain; the cells of the brain do not have adequate storage capacities, and because the brain normally uses only glucose for energy, it cannot depend on stored supplies of glycogen. Therefore it is essential that serum glucose be maintained at a level that provides adequate energy to these tissues. When serum glucose falls too low, signs and symptoms of hypoglycemia can develop quickly. These include progressive irritability, altered mental states, fainting, convulsions, and even coma.

TABLE 30-1	EFFECTS OF INSULIN AND GLUCAGON ON TARGET TISSUES	
TARGET TISSUE	**RESPONSE TO INSULIN**	**RESPONSE TO GLUCAGON**
Skeletal muscle, cardiac muscle, cartilage, bone, fibroblasts, leukocytes, and mammary glands	Increased glucose uptake and glycogen synthesis; increased uptake of certain amino acids	Little effect
Liver	Increased glycogen synthesis; increased use of glucose for energy (glycolysis)	Causes rapid increase in the breakdown of glycogen to glucose (glycogenolysis) and release of glucose into the blood
		Increased formation of glucose (gluconeogenesis) from amino acids and, to some degree, from fats
		Increased metabolism of fatty acids, resulting in increased ketones in the blood
Adipose cells	Increased glucose uptake, glycogen synthesis, fat synthesis, and fatty acid uptake; increased glycolysis	High concentrations cause breakdown of fats (lipolysis); probably unimportant under most conditions
Nervous system	Little effect except to increase glucose uptake in the satiety center	No effect

From Seely R: *Anatomy and physiology,* ed 2, St Louis, 1992, Mosby.

Fat Metabolism

Because only a limited amount of glycogen can be stored in the liver and skeletal muscles, one third of any glucose passing through the liver is converted to fatty acids. Under the influence of insulin, fatty acids are converted to triglycerides (storable fats) and stored in adipose tissue. In the absence of insulin, the stored fat is broken down, and the plasma concentration of free fatty acids rapidly increases. Thus relative insulin deficiency can result in a high circulating concentration of triglycerides and cholesterol (in the form of lipoproteins) in the plasma and is thought to contribute to the development of atherosclerosis in patients with serious diabetes.

If needed (as in the absence of insulin), fatty acids in the liver can be metabolized and used for energy. A byproduct of the breakdown of fatty acids in the liver is acetate, which is converted to acetoacetic acid and beta-hydroxybutyric acid. These products are released into the circulating blood as ketone bodies (described in Chapter 7). These ketone bodies may cause acidosis and coma (diabetic ketoacidosis) in the diabetic patient.

Protein Metabolism

Insulin causes proteins, as well as carbohydrates and fats, to be stored. Amino acids (through the actions of GH and insulin) are actively transported into the various cells of the human body. Most amino acids are used as building blocks to form new proteins (protein synthesis), but some enter the metabolic cycle by being converted to glucose after their initial breakdown in the liver.

In the absence of insulin, protein storage stops, and protein breakdown (particularly in muscle) begins. This releases large quantities of amino acids into the circulation. The excess amino acids are used directly for energy or as substrates for gluconeogenesis. The degradation of the amino acids leads to increased urea excretion in the urine. This "protein wasting" has serious effects in diabetes mellitus because it leads to extreme weakness and dysfunction of many organs.

Glucagon and Its Functions

Glucagon has several functions opposite to those of insulin, the most important of which is to increase blood glucose concentration. The two major effects of glucagon on glucose metabolism are the breakdown of liver glycogen and increased gluconeogenesis.

As the serum glucose level returns to normal (several hours after dietary intake), insulin secretion is decreased with continued fasting, and the blood sugar level begins to drop. As a result, glucagon, cortisol, GH, and epinephrine (from sympathetic stimulation) are secreted, initiating the release of glucose from glycogen and other glucose-storage sites. Glycogen is converted back to glucose and released into the blood. Uptake of glucose by most tissues helps maintain blood glucose at levels necessary for normal function (Fig. 30-6).

In summary, the four mechanisms for achieving adequate blood glucose regulation are as follows:

1. The liver functions as a blood glucose-buffer system, removing glucose from the blood when it is in excess (and storing it as glycogen) and returning glucose to the blood when glucose concentration and insulin secretion decline.

? CRITICAL THINKING

What signs and symptoms will the patient have in response to the release of epinephrine when blood glucose falls?

2. Insulin and glucagon function as a feedback control system to maintain normal serum glucose concentrations. When serum glucose levels rise, insulin is secreted to lower them toward normal levels. Conversely, when serum glucose levels fall, glucagon is secreted to raise serum glucose toward normal levels.
3. Low serum glucose levels stimulate the sympathetic nervous system to secrete epinephrine. Epinephrine and, to a lesser degree, norepinephrine have a glucagon-like effect that promotes liver glycogenolysis.
4. GH and cortisol play a role in less immediate regulation of serum glucose levels. They are secreted in response to more prolonged hypoglycemic episodes (e.g., late overnight fast) and tend to increase the rate of glucose production (gluconeogenesis) and decrease the rate of glucose use.

Pathophysiology of Diabetes Mellitus

Diabetes mellitus is characterized by a deficiency of insulin or an inability of the body to respond to

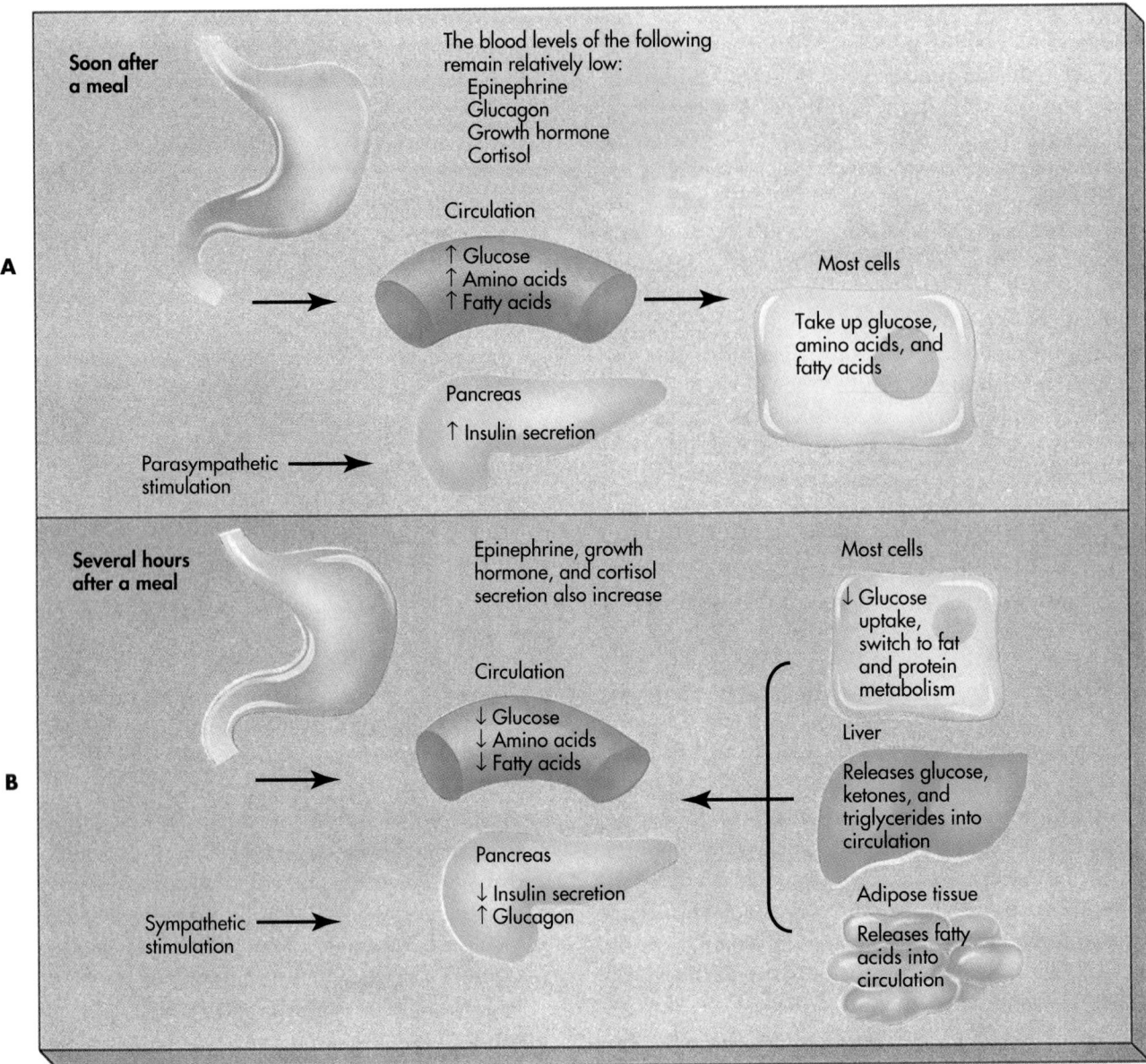

Fig. 30-6 **A**, Soon after a meal, glucose, amino acids, and fatty acids enter the bloodstream from the intestinal tract. Glucose and amino acids stimulate insulin secretion. Cells take up the glucose and amino acids and use them in their metabolism. **B**, Several hours after a meal, absorption from the intestinal tract decreases, the blood levels of glucose, amino acids, and fatty acids decrease. As a result, insulin secretion decreases, and glucagon, epinephrine, and GH secretion increases. Cell uptake of glucose decreases, and usage of fats and proteins increases. (From Seely R: *Anatomy and physiology*, ed 2, St Louis, 1992, Mosby.)

insulin. The disease often is associated with an increased intake of fluid (polydipsia), excretion of large quantities of urine-containing glucose (polyuria, glucosuria), and weight loss. Diabetes mellitus generally is classified as type 1 (insulin-dependent diabetes mellitus [IDDM]) or type 2 (noninsulin-dependent diabetes mellitus [NIDDM]).

NOTE

A new classification system endorsed by the American Diabetes Association and the World Health Organization identifies four types of diabetes: type 1, type 2, "other specific types," and gestational diabetes to address the continuum of hyperglycemia and insulin requirements.[2]

Type 1 Diabetes Mellitus

Type 1 diabetes is characterized by inadequate production of biologically effective insulin by the pancreas. This form of diabetes affects 1 in every 10 diabetics and may occur any time after birth, usually occurring in teenagers and young adults. Type 1 diabetes has a heritable component and appears to be an autoimmune phenomenon resulting from a genetic abnormality or susceptibility that causes the body to destroy its own insulin-producing cells. Type 1 diabetes requires lifelong treatment with *insulin* injections, exercise, and diet regulation. The symptoms of type 1 diabetes usually present suddenly and include polyuria; polydipsia; dizziness; blurred vision; and rapid, unexplained weight loss.

> **NOTE**
>
> Anyone with a parent or sibling who has type 1 diabetes has a 10% chance of developing the disease by age 50.[1]

Type 2 Diabetes Mellitus

Type 2 diabetes usually is characterized by a decreased production of insulin by the beta cells of the pancreas and diminished tissue sensitivity to insulin. The disease occurs most often in adults over 40 years of age and in those who are overweight. (Obesity predisposes a person to this form of diabetes because larger quantities of insulin are required for metabolic control in obese individuals than in those with normal weight.) Others at increased risk for this disease include Native Americans, Hispanics, and African-Americans.

> **? CRITICAL THINKING**
>
> *Would patients with type 1 or type 2 diabetes have an increased risk of complications related to this disease?*

> **NOTE**
>
> The American Diabetes Association estimates that 5.4 million people have diabetes and are unaware of it. Diabetes is the seventh leading cause of death in the United States.[1]

Most patients with type 2 diabetes require oral hypoglycemic medications, exercise, and dietary regulation to control their illness. A small number of patients require *insulin* injection. Warning signs (if present) are gradual and include all of those associated with type 1 diabetes. Fatigue; changes in appetite; and tingling, numbness, and pain in the extremities are also indicators.

Effects of Diabetes Mellitus

Most effects of diabetes mellitus can be attributed to one of the following three effects of decreased insulin levels:

1. Decreased use of glucose by the body cells, with a resultant increase in serum glucose
2. Markedly increased mobilization of fats from the fat storage areas, causing abnormal fat metabolism, which may result in the short term in ketoacidosis and in the long term in severe atherosclerosis
3. Depletion of protein in body tissues and muscle wasting

Loss of Glucose in the Urine

When the quantity of glucose entering the kidney tubules in the glomerular filtrate rises above the threshold for reabsorption of glucose by the tubules (typically 80 mg/dL), a significant portion of the glucose "spills" into the urine. The loss of glucose in the urine causes diuresis because the osmotic effect of glucose in the tubules prevents tubular reabsorption of fluid (osmotic diuresis). The effect is dehydration of the extracellular and intracellular spaces.

Acidosis in Diabetes

The shift from carbohydrate to fat metabolism results in the formation of ketone bodies (ketoacids). Ketone bodies are strong acids, and their continuous production leads to a metabolic acidosis, which is often at least partially compensated for by a respiratory alkalosis (manifested by Kussmaul's respirations). The body's mechanism for clearing the acid load by the kidneys is overwhelmed by the continuous production of ketone bodies, and profound acidosis eventually occurs. This acidosis, along with the usually severe dehydration secondary to the osmotic diuresis, can lead to death.

Treatment of this condition can be lifesaving. Diabetes mellitus is a systemic disease with many long-term complications, including the following:

*   Blindness
    5000 diabetics lose their sight each year
*   Kidney disease
    10% of all diabetics develop some form of kidney disease, including end-stage kidney failure, which requires dialysis or kidney transplant
*   Peripheral neuropathy that results in nerve damage to the hands and feet and increased incidence of foot infections
*   Autonomic neuropathy that causes damage to nerves controlling voluntary and involuntary functions and that may affect sexual function, bladder and bowel control, and blood pressure
*   Heart disease and stroke
    High blood glucose and blood fat contribute to atherosclerosis
    Diabetics are two to four times as likely to develop heart disease as nondiabetics and are two to six times as likely to have a stroke.
    Peripheral vascular disease (also secondary to atherosclerosis) resulting in the need for amputations

Management

The treatment of diabetes mellitus consists of drug therapy (*insulin* or oral hypoglycemic agents), diet regulation, and exercise. These therapies enable patients to control serum glucose levels and partially restore normal physiological metabolism.

> **NOTE**
>
> Pancreas transplants remain an experimental treatment for diabetes mellitus.

Insulin

Genetically engineered human *insulin* (Humulin) is available in rapid-, intermediate-, and long-acting preparations. (*Insulin* is administered by injection; it is a protein that would be digested if consumed orally.) An insulin-dependent diabetic usually self-administers one or two doses of one of the long-acting *insulin* preparations each day and additional quantities of a rapid-acting *insulin* (lasting only a few hours) for times when the serum glucose would be elevated (e.g., at meal times).

Another method for the patient to self-administer *insulin* is with an insulin-infusion pump. These devices administer a continuous dose of *insulin* and are adjusted so the level of blood glucose is constantly controlled. Regular glucose level monitoring by the patient is necessary to ensure adequate medication control. Medication balance is delicate. The same dosage of *insulin* that appears correct on one occasion may be too much or too little on another occasion, depending on various factors (e.g., exercise and infection).

> ✓ **TRICKS OF THE TRADE**
>
> Many diabetic patients (particularly older patients) "test their sugar" several times a day and consider themselves "experts" in managing their illness. Some are—and some aren't.

Oral Hypoglycemic Agents

Oral hypoglycemic agents stimulate the release of insulin from the pancreas. They are effective only in patients who have functioning beta cells (type 2 diabetes). Commonly prescribed oral hypoglycemic agents include chlorpropamide (Diabinese), tolazamide (Tolinase), tolbutamide (Orinase), acetohexamide (Dymelor), glipizide (Glucotrol), and glyburide (Micronase).

> **NOTE**
>
> New drugs have recently been developed and approved by the FDA to improve the metabolic defects found in type 2 diabetes. Pioglitazone (Actos) resensitizes patients' bodies to insulin. Glyburide and metformin HCl tablets (Glucovance) lower blood sugar by causing more of the body's own insulin to be released, by decreasing the production and absorption of blood sugar, and by helping the body use its own insulin more effectively. These newer drugs have important side effects and require careful patient monitoring (e.g., periodic tests for liver and kidney function).

Diabetic Emergencies

Three life-threatening conditions may result from diabetes mellitus: hypoglycemia (insulin shock), hyperglycemia (diabetic ketoacidosis [DKA]), and **hyperosmolar hyperglycemic nonketotic (HHNK) coma.**

Hypoglycemia

Hypoglycemia is a syndrome related to blood glucose levels below 80 mg/dL. Symptoms usually occur at levels less than 60 mg/dL or at slightly higher blood glucose levels if the fall has been rapid. The condition may occur in nondiabetic patients as well. It usually is a result of excessive response to glucose absorption, physical exertion, alcohol or drug effects, pregnancy and lactation, or decreased dietary intake. In diabetics, hypoglycemic reactions usually are caused by the following:

- Too much *insulin* (or oral hypoglycemic medication)
- Decreased dietary intake (a delayed or missed meal)
- Unusual or vigorous physical activity

TRICKS OF THE TRADE

If you are caring for an ill patient with diabetes who has been traveling in a car for some time (e.g., a person on vacation), suspect a diabetic reaction. These patients may not have considered the effects of prolonged physical inactivity as it relates to their disease and medication adjustments.

Less common causes and predisposing factors include the following:

- Chronic alcoholism (Alcohol depletes liver glycogen stores.)
- Adrenal gland dysfunction
- Liver disease (i.e., hepatic insufficiency or failure)
- Malnutrition
- Pancreatic tumor
- Cancer
- Hypothermia
- Sepsis
- Administration of beta blockers (e.g., *propranolol* [Inderal])
- Administration of salicylates in ill infants or children
- Intentional overdose with *insulin*, oral hypoglycemic agents, or salicylates

Signs and Symptoms

The signs and symptoms of hypoglycemia usually are rapid in onset (often within minutes) and related to a hyperadrenergic state that results from a compensatory increase in catecholamine secretion. In early stages, the patient may complain of extreme hunger and demonstrate one or more of the following signs and symptoms secondary to decreased glucose availability to the brain:

- Nervousness, trembling
- Irritability
- Psychotic (combative) behavior
- Weakness and incoordination
- Confusion
- Appearance of intoxication
- Weak, rapid pulse
- Cold, clammy skin
- Drowsiness
- Seizures
- Coma (in severe cases)

? CRITICAL THINKING

Why might this call be dispatched as a behavioral emergency?

NOTE

Hypoglycemia should be suspected in any diabetic patient with behavioral changes, confusion, abnormal neurological signs, or unconsciousness. This condition is a true emergency that requires immediate administration of glucose to prevent permanent brain damage or death.

Diabetic Ketoacidosis

DKA results from an absence of or resistance to insulin. The low insulin level prevents glucose from entering the cells and causes glucose to accumulate in the blood. As a result, the cells become starved for glucose and begin to use other sources of energy (principally fat). The metabolism of fat generates fatty acids and glycerol. The glycerol provides some energy to the cells, but the fatty acids are further metabolized to form ketoacids, resulting in acidosis.

Because any acidosis increases transport of potassium from the intracellular space into the intravascular space, the subsequent diuresis results in high potassium concentration in the urine and a total body potassium deficit (Box 30-2). In addition, the sodium concentration in the extracellular fluid usually decreases through osmotic dilution and is replaced by increased quantities of hydrogen ions, thus adding greatly to the acidosis. As blood sugar rises,

BOX 30-2

COMMON CAUSES OF DIABETIC KETOACIDOSIS

- Too-small *insulin* dose
- Failure to take *insulin*
- Infection
- Increased stress (trauma, surgery)
- Increased dietary intake
- Decreased metabolic rate
- Other less common predisposing factors, including significant emotional stress, alcohol consumption (often associated with hypoglycemia), and pregnancy

the patient undergoes massive osmotic diuresis, which combined with vomiting causes dehydration and shock. The associated electrolyte imbalances may cause cardiac dysrhythmias and altered neuromuscular activity, including seizures.

Signs and Symptoms

The signs and symptoms of DKA usually are related to diuresis and acidosis. They usually are slow in onset (over 12 to 48 hours) and include the following:

- Diuresis
  Warm, dry skin
  Dry mucous membranes
  Tachycardia, thready pulse
  Postural hypotension
  Weight loss
  Polyuria
  Polydipsia
- Acidosis
  Abdominal pain (usually generalized)
  Anorexia, nausea, vomiting
  Acetone breath odor (fruity odor)
  Kussmaul's respirations in an attempt to reduce carbon dioxide levels
  Decreased level of consciousness

? CRITICAL THINKING

How can you distinguish Kussmaul's respirations from hyperventilation?

NOTE

DKA patients seldom are deeply comatose. Patients who are unresponsive should be assessed for another cause, such as head injury, stroke, or drug overdose.

Hyperosmolar Hyperglycemic Nonketotic Coma

HHNK coma is a life-threatening emergency that frequently occurs in older patients with type 2 diabetes or in undiagnosed diabetics. The syndrome differs from DKA in that residual insulin may be adequate to prevent **ketogenesis** and ketoacidosis but not enough to permit glucose use by peripheral tissues or to decrease gluconeogenesis by the liver. The hyperglycemia produces CNS dysfunction, a hyperosmolar state followed by an osmotic diuresis, dehydration, and electrolyte losses. Therefore these patients typically have greater hyperglycemia because they are more dehydrated and less ketone formation because the presence of insulin in the liver directs free fatty acids into nonketogenic pathways, resulting in less acidemia than in patients with DKA (Fig. 30-7).

Precipitating factors and signs and symptoms of HHNK coma include the following:

- Precipitating factors
  Advanced age
  Preexisting cardiac or renal disease
  Inadequate insulin secretion or action (type 2 diabetes)
  Increased insulin requirements (stress, infection, trauma, burns, myocardial infarction)
  Medication use (thiazide and thiazide diuretics, glucocorticoids, *phenytoin* [Dilantin], sympathomimetics, *propranolol* [Inderal], immunosuppressives)
  Supplemental parenteral and enteral feedings
- Signs and symptoms
  Weakness
  Thirst
  Frequent urination
  Weight loss
  Extreme dehydration
  Flushed, dry skin
  Dry mucous membranes
  Decreased skin turgor
  Postural hypotension

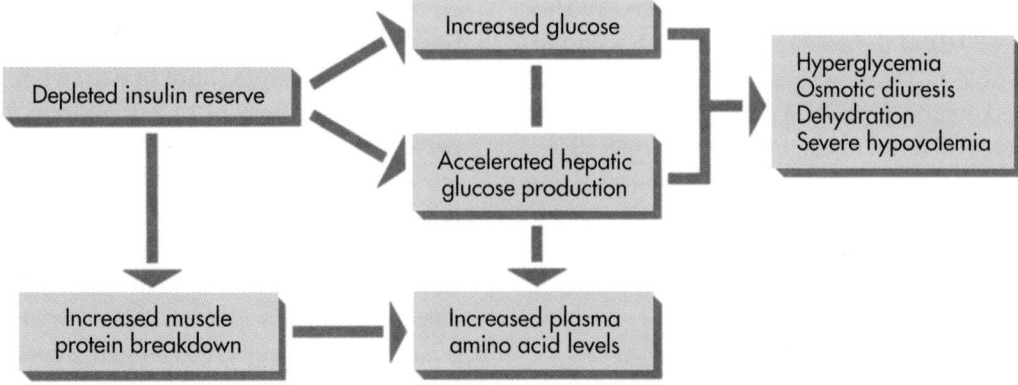

Fig. 30-7 Pathophysiology of HHNK coma.

Altered levels of consciousness
Tachycardia
Hypotension
Tachypnea

Assessment of the Diabetic Patient

A patient with a diabetic emergency may have a variety of signs and symptoms, many of which may mimic other more commonly encountered conditions. Therefore the paramedic must maintain a high degree of suspicion for diabetes-related illness.

In addition to the patient-assessment measures appropriate for any emergency patient encounter (initial assessment, physical examination, and treatment of life-threatening illness or injury), the paramedic should search for medical alert information, the presence of insulin syringes, and diabetic medications (*insulin* is often kept in a refrigerator). Important components of the patient history in assessing diabetic patients include onset of symptoms, food intake, *insulin* or oral hypoglycemic use, alcohol or other drug consumption, predisposing factors (exercise, infection, illness, stress), and any associated symptoms.

Management of the Conscious Diabetic Patient

If the diabetic patient is conscious and able to converse, the paramedic should obtain a pertinent history while assessing the patient's airway, breathing, and circulation. If appropriate, the patient should be given glucose.

Medical direction may recommend drawing a blood sample for laboratory analysis before administering glucose. Some EMS services use field glu-

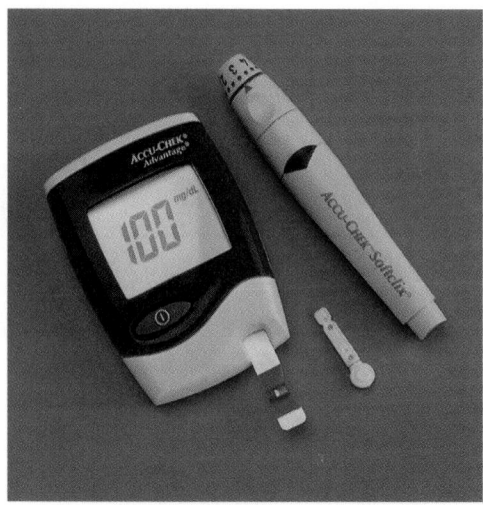

Fig. 30-8 Glucometer for measuring serum glucose levels.

cose testing with Dextrostix, Chemstrips, or a glucometer (Fig. 30-8). Any patient with a glucose reading of less than 80 mg/dL and signs and symptoms consistent with hypoglycemia should receive *dextrose.* Some patients who have experienced a diabetic reaction may be treated at the scene and released according to protocol. Others may need to be transported for physician evaluation. The paramedic should consult with medical direction or follow established protocol.

? CRITICAL THINKING

What steps should you take if the patient refuses transport (after treatment with dextrose), before leaving the scene?

Methods of glucose administration vary by protocol (Box 30-3). If the patient is alert with a gag reflex and able to swallow, sugar may be orally administered in the form of a candy bar, a glass of orange juice mixed with sugar, a nondiet soft drink, or by sublingual or buccal administration of a glucose gel preparation. An alternate method is to slowly administer **dextrose 50%** through a stable peripheral vein. (This dose may be repeated according to protocol.)

Management of the Unconscious Diabetic Patient

Prehospital management of any unconscious patient should be directed at airway management, high-concentration oxygen administration, and ventilatory and circulatory support. Depending on protocol, an IV line of a lactated Ringer's solution or a saline solution should be established to replenish fluids and electrolytes (the flow rate should be determined by the patient's blood pressure and heart rate). In addition, a blood sample should be drawn for laboratory analysis. If alcoholism or other drug abuse is suspected, medical direction may recommend the administration of **thiamine, naloxone** (Narcan), or both, before the administration of glucose.

If an IV line cannot be established, the administration of subcutaneous or intramuscular **glucagon** helps raise serum glucose levels by stimulating the breakdown of liver glycogen. However, **glucagon** is ineffective in chronic alcoholics and those with liver disease. Definitive treatment for patients with DKA or HHNK requires administration of **insulin,** fluid replacement, electrolyte monitoring, and in-hospital observation.

Differential Diagnosis

Differentiating the origin of a diabetic emergency sometimes is difficult in the prehospital setting. When the paramedic is not sure of the cause, all diabetic patients should receive glucose if indicated by testing. The findings in diabetic emergencies should assist in the differential diagnosis (Table 30-2).

✓ TRICKS OF THE TRADE

Always draw the blood sample *before* administering IV glucose.

NOTE

If the patient's age (over 50) and clinical history suggest a TIA or stroke, the administration of a concentrated glucose solution may exacerbate cerebral damage. (Consult with medical direction.) Otherwise, a patient in coma of unknown origin should receive dextrose (if indicated by testing), particularly if hypoglycemia cannot be ruled out.

BOX 30-3

CAUTIONS FOR ADMINISTERING INTRAVENOUS GLUCOSE

- **Dextrose 50%** should not be administered to infants or young children.
- The administration of **dextrose 50%** may precipitate neurological complications in alcoholics and other patients with thiamine deficiency. Therefore **thiamine** administration before or concurrent with the administration of **dextrose** should be considered in patients with suspected thiamine deficiency.

Thyrotoxicosis

Thyrotoxicosis is a term that refers to any toxic condition that results from thyroid hyperfunction. *Hyperthyroidism* and *thyrotoxicosis* are designations for common, milder forms of the disease. *Thyroid storm* is a heightened and life-threatening manifestation of thyroid hyperfunction and is a relatively rare

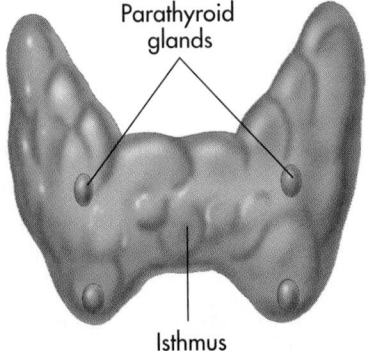

Fig. 30-9 Thyroid gland.

condition. The storm may occur spontaneously or may be precipitated by infection, stress, or a thyroidectomy. Most cases of thyroid storm are secondary to toxic diffuse goiter (Grave's disease).[3]

> **NOTE**
>
> Grave's disease is a type of excessive thyroid activity characterized by a generalized enlargement of the gland (goiter), leading to a swollen neck and often protruding eyes (exophthalmos). It most frequently occurs in young women and may result from an autoimmune process in which an antibody stimulates the thyroid cells.

Anatomy and Physiology of the Thyroid Gland

As described in Chapter 6, the thyroid gland is situated in the front of the neck, just below the larynx. It consists of two lobes, one on each side of the trachea, joined by a narrower portion of tissue called the *isthmus* (Fig. 30-9).

Thyroid tissue is composed of two types of secretory cells: follicular cells and parafollicular cells (or C cells). Follicular cells make up most of the gland. They are arranged in the form of hollow, spherical follicles and secrete the iodine-containing hormones thyroxine (T4) and triiodothyronine (T3). Parafollicular cells occur singly or in small groups in the spaces between the follicles and secrete the

TABLE 30-2　DIFFERENTIAL CONSIDERATIONS IN DIABETIC EMERGENCIES

FINDINGS	HYPOGLYCEMIA	HYPERGLYCEMIA	HHNK COMA
History			
Food intake	Insufficient	Excessive	Excessive
Insulin dosage	Excessive	Insufficient	Insufficient
Onset	Rapid	Gradual	Gradual
Infection	Uncommon	Common	Common
Gastrointestinal tract			
Thirst	Absent	Intense	Intense
Hunger	Intense	Absent	Intense
Vomiting	Uncommon	Common	Uncommon
Respiratory system			
Breathing	Normal or rapid	Deep or rapid	Shallow/rapid
Breath odor	Normal	Acetone smell	Normal
Cardiovascular system			
Blood pressure	Normal	Low	Low
Pulse	Normal, rapid, or full	Rapid or weak	Rapid or weak
Skin	Pale or moist	Warm or dry	Warm or dry
Nervous system			
Headache	Present	Absent	Absent
Consciousness	Irritability	Restless	Irritable
	Seizure or coma	Coma (rare)	Seizure or coma
Urine			
Sugar level	Absent	Present	Present
Acetone level	Usually absent	Usually present	Absent
Serum glucose levels	Less than 60 mg/dL	Greater than 300 mg/dL	More than 600 mg/dL
Treatment response	Immediate (after glucose) (NOTE: If the hypoglycemic episode is prolonged or severe, the response may be delayed and may require more than one dose.)	Gradual (within 6-12 hours after medication and fluid replacement)	Gradual (within 6-12 hours after medication and fluid replacement)

From Clark F et al: *Pharmacological basis of nursing*, ed 4, St Louis, 1993, Mosby.

hormone *calcitonin* that helps regulate the level of calcium in the body.

Thyroid hormones play an important role in controlling body metabolism and are essential in children for normal physical growth and mental development. The secretion of T3 and T4 is controlled by a feedback system involving the pituitary gland and hypothalamus. (The secretion of calcitonin is regulated directly by the level of calcium in the blood, independent of the pituitary gland or hypothalamus.)

Disorders of the Thyroid Gland

Disorders of the thyroid gland may be due to defects in the gland itself or may result from a disruption of the hypothalamic-pituitary hormonal control system (Box 30-4). The disease advances in a slow fashion (with nonspecific signs and symptoms over months to years), and may culminate in an acute episode. Nonspecific signs and symptoms of thyroid hyperfunction include fatigue, anxiety, palpitations, sweating, weight loss, diarrhea, and heat intolerance.

In acute episodes of thyroid storm, signs and symptoms are those related to adrenergic hyperactivity and may include the following:

- Severe tachycardia
- Heart failure
- Cardiac dysrhythmias
- Shock
- Hyperthermia
- Restlessness
- Agitation and paranoia
- Abdominal pain
- Delirium
- Coma

BOX 30-4

CAUSES OF THYROID GLAND DISORDERS

- Congenital defects
- Genetic disorders
- Infection (thyroiditis)
- Tumors (benign or malignant)
- Autoimmune disorders
- Hormonal disorders during puberty or pregnancy
- Nutritional disorders

? CRITICAL THINKING

What other medical emergencies could present with similar signs and symptoms?

NOTE

The paramedic should consider other causes of symptoms related to adrenergic hyperactivity—most notably the use of cocaine and amphetamines, hypoglycemia, and withdrawal from alcohol and other drugs.

Management

Mild hyperthyroidism requires no emergency therapy and is best managed with physician follow-up. By comparison, thyroid storm is a true emergency that requires immediate intervention. Emergency care efforts are directed at providing airway, ventilatory, and circulatory support and rapid transport to an appropriate medical facility. In-hospital care will focus on inhibiting hormone synthesis, blocking hormone release and the peripheral effects of thyroid hormone with antithyroid drugs, and providing general support of the patient's vital functions.

Myxedema

Myxedema is a condition that results from a deficiency in thyroid hormone. It may be associated with inflammation of the thyroid gland (e.g., Hashimoto's thyroiditis), atrophy of the thyroid gland, or it may be a consequence of treatment for hyperthyroidism. Myxedema causes the accumulation of mucinous material in the skin, resulting in thickening and coarsening of the skin and other body tissues (most notably the lips and nose of the face). The condition is most common in adults (especially women) over age 40.

Myxedema coma (a rare illness characterized by hypothermia, mental obtundation, and myxedema) is a medical emergency that may be precipitated by the following factors:

- Exposure to cold
- Infection (usually pulmonary)
- Congestive heart failure

- Trauma
- Drugs (sedatives, hypnotics, anesthetics)
- Stroke
- Internal hemorrhage
- Hypoxia
- Hypercapnia
- Hyponatremia
- Hypoglycemia

Management

Prehospital care is directed at managing life-threatening conditions (airway, ventilatory, and circulatory compromise) and providing rapid transport to an appropriate medical facility for physician evaluation. Once other causes of the coma are ruled out and the patient's vital functions are stabilized, treatment of myxedema involves the oral administration of thyroxine, which must be continued for life. Table 30-3 compares signs and symptoms resulting from thyroid gland disorders.

Cushing's Syndrome

Cushing's syndrome is caused by an abnormally high circulating level of corticosteroid hormones, produced naturally by the adrenal glands (Fig. 30-10). The condition may be produced directly by an adrenal gland tumor (causing excessive secretion of corticosteroids), by prolonged administration of corticosteroid drugs (used to treat conditions such as rheumatoid arthritis, inflammatory bowel disease, and asthma), or by enlargement of both adrenal glands due to a pituitary tumor. Cushing's syndrome is a rare condition and primarily affects women 30 to 50 years of age.

> **NOTE**
>
> The pituitary gland controls the activity of the adrenal gland by producing ACTH, which stimulates the cortex of the adrenal gland to grow.

People with Cushing's syndrome have a characteristic appearance (Fig. 30-11). The face appears round ("moon-faced") and red; the trunk tends to become obese from disturbances in fat metabolism; and the limbs become wasted from muscle atrophy. Acne develops and purple stretch marks may appear on the abdomen, thighs, and breasts. The skin often thins and bruises easily and weakened bones are at increased risk for fracture. Other features of the disease include the following:

- Increased body and facial hair
- Hump on the back of neck ("buffalo hump")
- Supraclavicular fat pads
- Weight gain
- Hypertension
- Psychiatric disturbances (depression, paranoia)
- Insomnia
- Diabetes mellitus

TABLE 30-3	**SIGNS AND SYMPTOMS OF THYROID DISORDERS**

HYPERTHYROIDISM	**HYPOTHYROIDISM**
Exophthalmos	Facial edema
Goiter	JVD (sometimes goiter)
Warm flushed skin	Cool skin
Fever	Exposure to cold
Agitation/psychosis	Coma
Hyperactivity	Weakness
Weight loss	Weight gain
Common Medications	
Iodine	Levothyroxine (Synthroid)
Methimazole (Tapazole)	Liothyronine (Cytomel)
Propylthiouracil (Propacil)	Liotrix (Euthroid)

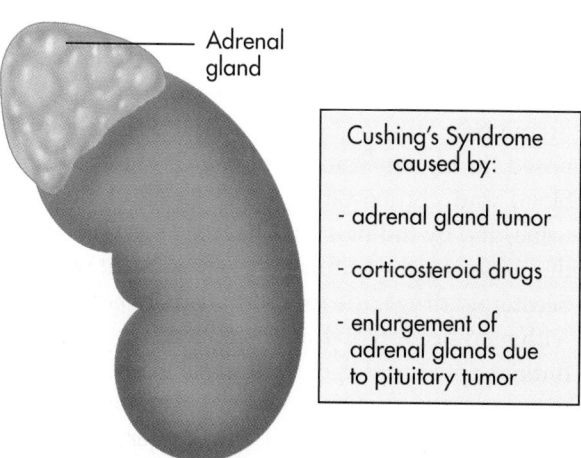

Fig. 30-10 Adrenal gland.

Adrenal gland

Cushing's Syndrome caused by:

- adrenal gland tumor
- corticosteroid drugs
- enlargement of adrenal glands due to pituitary tumor

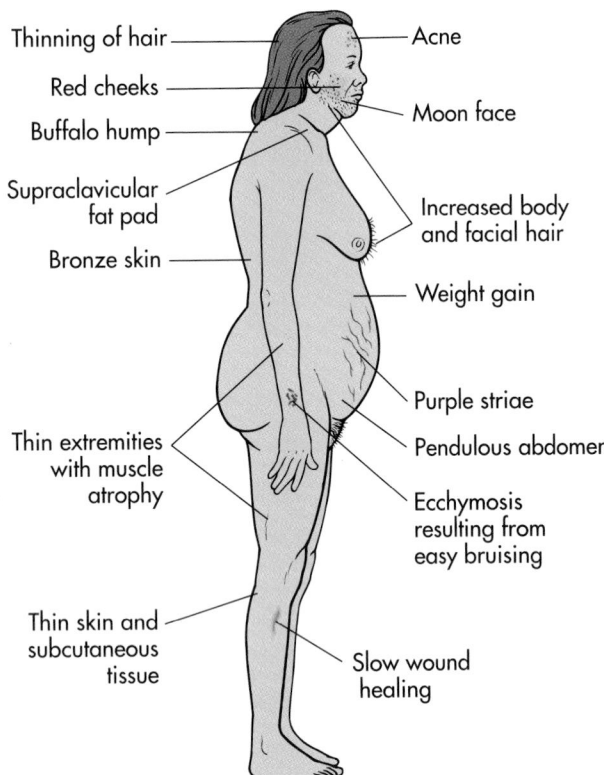

Thinning of hair

Red cheeks

Buffalo hump

Supraclavicular
fat pad

Bronze skin

Thin extremities
with muscle
atrophy

Thin skin and
subcutaneous
tissue

Acne

Moon face

Increased body
and facial hair

Weight gain

Purple striae

Pendulous abdomen

Ecchymosis
resulting from
easy bruising

Slow wound
healing

Fig. 30-11 Cushing's syndrome. (From Lewis SM, Collier IC, Heitkemper MM: *Medical-surgical nursing: assessment and management of clinical problems,* ed 4, St Louis, 1996, Mosby.)

? CRITICAL THINKING

How do you think patients who suffer from this disease feel about their body image?

Management

Prehospital care for patients with Cushing's syndrome primarily is supportive. The disease is diagnosed through measurement of ACTH levels in the blood and corticosteroid levels in the blood and urine, and by radiological imaging (e.g., CT scan). If the cause of the syndrome is overtreatment with corticosteroid drugs, the condition usually is reversible with modification of drug treatment. If the cause is a tumor or overgrowth of the adrenal gland, the gland may require surgical removal. If the tumor lies in the pituitary gland, it is treated with surgery or irradiation and medication. Successful treatment usually is

followed by regression of the clinical manifestation of the disease. Lifelong hormonal replacement therapy is required for these patients.

Addison's Disease

Addison's disease is a rare, potentially life-threatening disorder caused by a deficiency of the corticosteroid hormones *cortisol* and *aldosterone,* normally produced by the adrenal cortex. The condition can be caused by any disease process that destroys the adrenal cortices (e.g., adrenal hemorrhage or infarction, infections (TB, fungal, viral), and autoimmune diseases). However, the most common cause of Addison's disease is idiopathic atrophy of adrenal tissue whereby the production of corticosteroid hormones is inadequate to meet the metabolic requirements of the body. Signs and symptoms associated with this disease include the following:

- Progressive weakness
- Progressive weight loss
- Progressive anorexia
- Skin hyperpigmentation (caused by increased hormone production by the pituitary gland, which stimulates melanin)
- Hypotension
- Hyponatremia
- Hyperkalemia
- GI disturbances (nausea, vomiting, diarrhea)

Addison's disease generally has a slow onset and chronic course, with symptoms developing gradually over months to years. However, acute episodes (Addisonian crisis) may be precipitated by emotional and physiological stresses such as surgery, alcohol intoxication, hypothermia, myocardial infarction, severe illness, trauma, hypoglycemia, infection, and others. During these events, the adrenal glands cannot increase the production of the corticosteroid hormones to help the body cope with stress. As a result, blood glucose levels drop; the body loses the ability to regulate the content of sodium, potassium, and water in body fluids (causing dehydration and extreme muscle weakness); blood volume and blood pressure fall; and circulation may not be able to be maintained efficiently. In these situations, airway, ventilatory, and circulatory support will be required in the prehospital setting.

TABLE 30-4	SIGNS AND SYMPTOMS OF ADRENAL GLAND DISORDERS

CORTICOSTEROID EXCESS	ADRENAL INSUFFICIENCY
(Cushing's Syndrome)	(Addison's Disease)
Weight gain	Weight loss
Weakness	Weakness
Hump on back of neck	Hypotension
Slow healing	GI disorders
Increased body and facial hair	Skin hyperpigmentation

Common Medications

Aminoglutethimide (Cytadren)	Dexamethasone (Decadron)
Metyrapone (Metopirone)	Fludrocortisone (Florinef acetate)

Management

In-hospital care should be directed at maintaining the patient's vital functions and correcting the sodium deficiency and dehydration. After managing the life-threatening episode, the treatment of Addison's disease consists of administration of the deficient corticosteroids. The patient often is advised to increase the dosage of these drugs during times of emotional and physiological stress. Table 30-4 compares signs and symptoms resulting from disorders of the adrenal gland.

S U M M A R Y

- The endocrine system is comprised of ductless glands and tissues that produce and secrete hormones. Endocrine glands secrete their hormones directly into the bloodstream and exert a regulatory effect on various metabolic functions. All hormones operate within feedback systems (either positive or negative) to maintain an optimal internal environment.

- The pancreatic islets are composed of beta cells that secrete insulin, alpha cells that secrete glucagon, and other cells of questionable function. The primary functions of insulin are to increase glucose transport into cells, increase glucose metabolism by cells, increase liver glycogen levels, and decrease blood glucose concentration toward normal levels. The two major effects of glucagon are to increase blood glucose levels by stimulating the liver to release glucose stores from glycogen and other glucose storage sites (glycogenolysis) and to stimulate gluconeogenesis through the breakdown of fats and fatty acids, thereby maintaining a normal blood glucose level.

- Diabetes mellitus is characterized by a deficiency of insulin or an inability of the body to respond to insulin. Diabetes generally is classified as type 1 (insulin dependent) or type 2 (noninsulin dependent). Type 1 diabetes requires lifelong treatment with insulin injections, exercise, and diet regulation. Most patients with type 2 diabetes require oral hypoglycemic medications, exercise, and dietary regulation to control their illness.

- Hypoglycemia is a syndrome related to blood glucose levels below 80 mg/dL. The syndrome should be suspected in any diabetic patient with behavioral changes or unconsciousness. This condition is a true emergency that requires immediate administration of glucose to prevent permanent brain damage or death.

- Diabetic ketoacidosis results from an absence of or resistance to insulin. The signs and symptoms of DKA are related to diuresis and acidosis and usually are slow in onset.

- Hyperosmolar hyperglycemic nonketotic coma is a life-threatening emergency that frequently occurs in older patients with type 2 diabetes or in undiagnosed diabetics. The hyperglycemia produces a hyperosmolar state followed by an osmotic diuresis, dehydration, and electrolyte losses.

- Important components of the patient history in assessing diabetic patients include onset of symptoms, food intake, insulin or oral hypoglycemic use, alcohol or other drug consumption, predisposing factors, and any associated symptoms.

- Any patient with a glucose reading of less than 80 mg/dL and signs and symptoms consistent with hypoglycemia should receive dextrose.

- Thyrotoxicosis refers to any toxic condition that results from thyroid hyperfunction.

- Thyroid storm is a heightened and life-threatening manifestation of thyroid hyperfunction. Thyroid hormones play an important role in controlling body metabolism and are essential in children for normal physical growth and development.

- Myxedema is a condition that results from a deficiency in thyroid hormone. Myxedema coma is a rare illness characterized by hypothermia, mental obtundation, and myxedema and is a medical emergency.

- Cushing's syndrome is caused by an abnormally high circulating level of corticosteroid hormones, produced naturally by the adrenal glands.

- Addison's disease is a rare, potentially life-threatening disorder caused by a deficiency of the corticosteroid hormones cortisol and aldosterone, normally produced by the adrenal cortex.

REFERENCES

1. American Diabetes Association: *Diabetes facts and figures,* www.diabetes.org/ada/facts.asp.
2. American Diabetes Association: www.diabetes.org.
3. Rosen P, Barkin R: *Emergency medicine: concepts and clinical practice,* ed 4, St. Louis, 1998, Mosby.

31 *Allergies and Anaphylaxis*

OBJECTIVES

Upon completion of this chapter, the paramedic student will be able to:

1. *Describe the antigen-antibody response.*
2. *Differentiate between an allergic reaction and a normal immune response.*
3. *Describe signs and symptoms and management of local allergic reactions on the basis of an understanding of the pathophysiology associated with this condition.*
4. *Identify allergens associated with anaphylaxis.*
5. *Describe the pathophysiology, signs and symptoms, and management of anaphylaxis.*

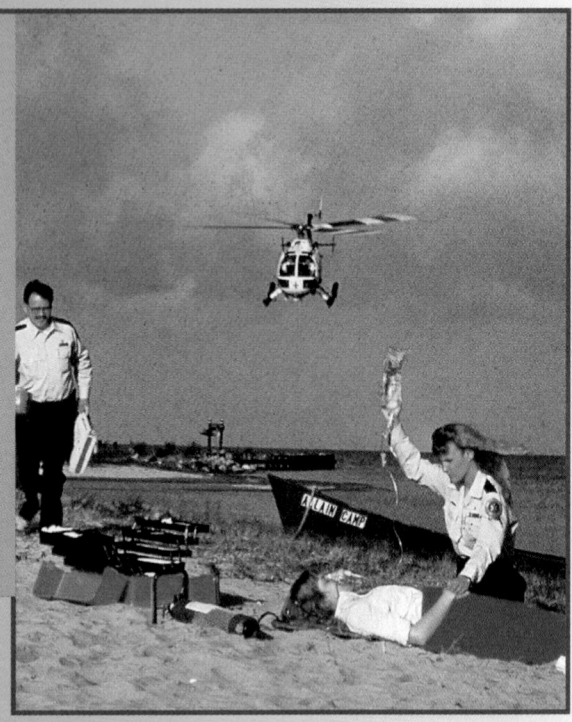

Anaphylaxis is an immediate, systemic, life-threatening allergic reaction associated with major changes in the cardiovascular, respiratory, and cutaneous systems. Prompt recognition and appropriate drug therapy in the prehospital phase are crucially important to patient survival.

- **eosinophil chemotactic factor of anaphylaxis:** A group of active substances, including histamine and leukotrienes, that are released during an anaphylactic reaction.
- **leukotrienes:** A class of biologically active compounds that occur naturally in leukocytes and that produce allergic and inflammatory reactions.
- **sensitization:** An acquired reaction in which specific antibodies develop in response to an antigen.
- **thromboxanes:** Antagonistic prostaglandin derivatives that are synthesized and released by degranulating platelets, causing vasoconstriction and promoting the degranulation of other platelets.

Antigen-Antibody Reaction

As described in Chapter 7, an antigen is a substance that induces the formation of antibodies. Antigens can enter the body by injection, ingestion, inhalation, or absorption. The antibodies bind to the antigen that produced them and facilitate antigen neutralization and removal from the body. This normal antigen-antibody reaction protects the body from disease by activating the immune response. The immune responses normally are protective; however, they can become oversensitive or be directed toward harmless antigens to which we often are exposed. When this occurs, the response is termed *allergic*. The antigen or substance causing the allergic response is called an *allergen*. Common allergens include drugs, insects, foods, animals, pollens and molds (see the box on p. 968).

> **NOTE**
>
> As described in Chapter 7, the healthy body responds to an antigen challenge through a collective defense system known as *immunity*. To review, immunity may be natural (present at birth), acquired (resulting from exposure to a specific antigenic agent or pathogen), or artificially induced through immunization.

Allergic Reaction

An allergic reaction is marked by an increased physiological response to an antigen after a previous exposure (sensitization) to the same antigen. The allergic reaction is initiated when a circulating antibody (IgG or IgM) combines with a specific foreign antigen, resulting in hypersensitivity reactions, or with antibodies bound to mast cells or basophils (IgE). As described in Chapters 7 and 8, hypersensitivity reactions are divided into four distinct types: *type I* (IgE-mediated allergic reactions), *type II* (tissue-specific reactions), *type III* (immune-complex-mediated reactions), and *type IV* (cell-mediated reactions). A type I or immediate hypersensitivity reaction is the most dramatic and may lead to life-threatening anaphylaxis. A sampling of agents that may cause hypersensitivity reactions (including anaphylaxis) can be found in Box 31-1. Patients who have known sensitivity to these or other agents should avoid exposure.

> **NOTE**
>
> *Anaphylactoid reactions* are allergic reactions that are not mediated by an antigen-antibody reaction. These reactions present exactly like anaphylaxis. The distinction is unimportant in relation to treatment of an acute attack.[1]

> **NOTE**
>
> Not all contact dermatitis associated with glove use indicates latex allergy. Other causes of contact dermatitis may result from frequent glove wearing and hand washing, and/or hypersensitivity to one or more chemicals used during the glove manufacturing process. (Allergy testing is necessary to confirm latex allergy.) If an allergy to latex is suspected, the paramedic should use latex-free gloves and obtain medical evaluation (according to protocol).

LATEX ALLERGIES

Today, there is significant concern about latex allergy, especially among health care workers. The first published account of contact urticaria related to glove use was published in 1979; however, latex allergy was relatively unknown until after the AIDS epidemic in the mid 1980s and the resulting tremendous increase in glove usage. The prevalence of **sensitization** to latex has been reported to range from 2.9% to 4.7% among health care workers, and from 7% to 10% among operating room staff. (In addition to latex gloves, health care workers and latex-sensitive patients can be exposed to latex on medical instruments, surgical equipment, and other appliances.) Those persons considered at high risk for latex allergy include the following:

- Individuals who have had significant and early exposure to latex (e.g., patients with spina bifida or genitourinary anomalies, and others who have had multiple surgeries and catheterizations)
- Persons with a genetic propensity to develop allergies
- Asthmatics
- Health care workers and law enforcement and fire service personnel who regularly use latex gloves
- Workers in some occupations (e.g., rubber manufacturing employees, hairdressers, food handlers, auto mechanics, tollbooth operators)

Symptoms of latex allergy can range from mild discomfort to life-threatening anaphylaxis. Most often, the first manifestation of a latex allergy is urticaria that typically is localized to the hands, but may be widespread. A type I latex allergy can manifest itself in symptoms that include rash, lacrimation, rhinitis, wheezing, bronchospasm, laryngeal edema, hypotension, dysrhythmia, and, very rarely, respiratory or cardiac arrest.

Many health care facilities, EMS agencies, and other public service agencies have addressed this issue by developing "latex safe" environments, and by using latex-free equipment for patients with latex allergy. For the health care provider, the need for education, early recognition, prevention strategies, and the implementation of safe and effective practice is essential. The National Institute for Occupational Safety and Health (NIOSH) and many professional organizations have recommended that health care workers wear low-protein, powder-free gloves when latex gloves are necessary, and synthetic gloves when the risk of exposure to bloodborne pathogens is low. Individuals not exposed to blood or body fluids (e.g., food handlers, maintenance workers) should avoid latex gloves altogether.

SOURCE: Korniewicz D: *Latex allergy: a current challenge,* Asepsis on the Web 20 (3), 1999, www.jnjmedical.com/asepsis/latex_allg.asp.

Localized Allergic Reaction

Localized allergic reactions (type IV) do not manifest multisystem involvement. In these situations, the sites of mast cell and basophil mediator release are limited. Common signs and symptoms of localized allergic reaction include the following:

- Conjunctivitis
- Rhinitis
- Angioedema
- Urticaria
- Contact dermatitis

Localized allergic reactions are best managed with drugs that compete at receptor sites with histamines to prevent their physiological actions. Common antihistamines include over-the-counter oral and nasal decongestants, and prescription and nonprescription *diphenhydramine* (Benadryl). Other medications that may be useful for some local reactions include steroids and topical creams.

> **NOTE**
>
> All patients should be questioned about latex allergy; persons with latex allergy should wear appropriate medical-alert identification. Sensitivity to latex should be documented on the patient care report, and this information should be conveyed to medical direction.

Anaphylaxis

The term *anaphylaxis* comes from Greek and means "against or opposite of protection." It is the most extreme form of an allergic reaction, accounting for 400 to 800 deaths per year.[2] Anaphylaxis has a mortality rate of 3%. Therefore rapid recognition and aggressive therapy are essential.

BOX 31-1

AGENTS THAT MAY CAUSE ALLERGIES AND ANAPHYLAXIS

Drugs and Biological Agents
Antibiotics
Local anesthetics
Cephalosporins
Chemotherapeutics
Aspirin
Nonsteroidal antiinflammatory agents
Opiates
Muscle relaxants
Anticancer agents
Vaccines
Insulin

Insect Bites and Stings
Wasps
Bees
Fire ants

Foods
Peanuts, soybeans
Cod, halibut, shellfish (e.g., shrimp)
Egg white
Strawberries
Food additives
Wheat and buckwheat
Sesame and sunflower seeds
Cottonseed
Milk
Mango

? CRITICAL THINKING

Based on the list of allergens in Box 31-1, what are some likely locations that you may be dispatched to, to care for a patient who is experiencing an anaphylactic reaction?

Causative Agents

Almost any substance can cause anaphylaxis. The antigenic agents most frequently associated with anaphylaxis are penicillin (by ingestion or injection), envenomation by stinging insects, and food (especially nuts and shellfish). Regardless of the offending antigen, the risk of anaphylaxis in sensitive individuals increases with the frequency of exposure and to a lesser extent the length of exposure or site of inoculation.

Pathophysiology

As described in Chapter 7, a person must first be exposed to a specific antigen to develop type I hypersensitivity. In the first exposure, the antigen enters the body by injection, ingestion, inhalation, or absorption and activates the immune system. In susceptible individuals, large amounts of IgE antibody are produced. IgE antibodies leave the lymphatic system and bind to the cell membranes of basophils circulating in the blood and to mast cells in tissues surrounding the blood vessels. They remain there and are inactive until the same antigen is introduced into the body a second time. With subsequent exposure to the specific antigen, the allergen crosslinks at least two of the cell-bound IgE molecules, resulting in degranulation (release of internal substances) of the mast cells and basophils and the onset of an anaphylactic reaction (Box 31-2).

NOTE

The manifestations of anaphylaxis are related to the release of chemical mediators from mast cells. The location and concentration of mast cells determine the organ(s) affected.

The degranulation of the target cell is associated with the release of pharmacologically active chemical mediators from inside the affected basophils and mast cells (described in Chapter 6). These chemicals include histamines, **leukotrienes**, **eosinophil chemotactic factor of anaphylaxis**, heparin, kinins, prostaglandins, and **thromboxanes**. All of these chemicals mediate or trigger an internal systemic response.

Histamines promote vascular permeability and cause dilation of capillaries and venules and contraction of nonvascular smooth muscle, especially in the gastrointestinal tract and bronchial tree. There is an associated increase in gastric, nasal, and lacrimal secretions, resulting in tearing and rhinorrhea. The increased capillary permeability allows plasma to leak into the interstitial space, decreasing the intravascular volume available for the heart to pump. The profound vasodilation that results further decreases cardiac preload, compromising stroke volume and cardiac output. These physiological effects lead to cutaneous flushing, urticaria, angioedema, and hypotension. The onset of action

of the histamines is very rapid, but their effects are short lived because they are quickly broken down by plasma enzymes. The pathophysiology of anaphylactic shock is illustrated in Fig. 31-1.

Leukotrienes are the most potent bronchoconstrictors, which cause wheezing. These chemical mediators also cause coronary vasoconstriction and increased vascular permeability. Leukotrienes were formerly known as *slow-reacting substances of anaphylaxis* because their effects were delayed relative to histamine. The duration of action of these chemicals, however, is much longer than that of histamines.

The process of anaphylaxis attracts eosinophils to the site of allergic inflammation by as yet unknown mechanisms. It is believed that eosinophils contain an enzyme that can deactivate leukotrienes. The remaining chemical mediators (heparin, neutrophil chemotactic factor, and kinins) exert varying effects that may include fever, chills, bronchospasm, and pulmonary vasoconstriction. These complex chemical processes can rapidly lead to upper airway obstruction and bronchospasm, dysrhythmias and cardiac ischemia, and circulatory collapse and shock.

Assessment Findings

An accurate history and physical assessment are necessary to differentiate severe allergic reactions from other medical conditions that may mimic anaphylaxis (Table 31-1). A flawed prehospital assess-

BOX 31-2

ANAPHYLAXIS

Three conditions must be met to sensitize an individual and generate an anaphylactic response:
1. An antigen-induced stimulation of the immune system with specific IgE antibody formation
2. A latent period after the initial antigenic exposure for sensitization of mast cells and basophils to occur
3. Subsequent reexposure to the same specific antigen

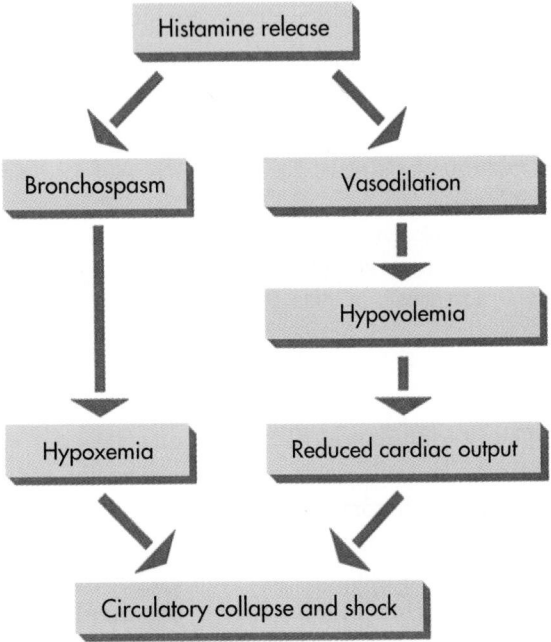

Fig. 31-1 Pathophysiology of anaphylactic shock.

TABLE 31-1	CONDITIONS THAT MAY MIMIC ANAPHYLAXIS	
SIGNS AND SYMPTOMS	**POSSIBLE CAUSES**	
Stridor	Upper airway obstruction Foreign body aspiration Epiglottitis, angioedema, ACE inhibitor use, some panic disorders	
Bronchospasm	Asthma, COPD, bronchitis	
Syncope	Vasovagal syncope Seizure Hypoglycemia Cardiac dysrhythmias	
Hypotension	Shock from any cause	
Urticaria	Infection, scombroid poisoning, angioedema	

ment in this group can have life-threatening consequences. Disease entities that may present similar signs and symptoms of anaphylaxis include:

- Severe asthma with respiratory failure
- Upper airway obstruction
- Toxic or septic shock
- Pulmonary edema (with or without myocardial infarction)
- Drug overdose
- Hypovolemic shock

Respiratory Effects

Initial signs of respiratory involvement associated with anaphylaxis may range from sneezing and coughing to complete airway obstruction (secondary to laryngeal and epiglottic edema) (Box 31-3). The patient may complain of throat tightness and dyspnea, and stridor or voice changes may be evident. Lower airway bronchospasm and associated hypersecretion of mucus caused by the actions of histamine, leukotriene, and prostaglandins may produce wheezing and significant respiratory distress. Symptoms can develop with startling rapidity.

TRICKS OF THE TRADE

A patient with an anaphylactic reaction is a scary situation for *you and the patient*. Keep your wits about you and monitor your patient closely.

Cardiovascular Effects

Cardiovascular manifestations of allergic reactions range from mild hypotension to vascular collapse and profound shock in anaphylaxis. Dysrhythmias are common and may be related to the severe hypoxia and intervascular hypovolemia inherent in this situation. The patient may complain of chest pain if myocardial ischemia is present.

? CRITICAL THINKING

Which of these effects has the potential to cause death first?

BOX 31-3

SIGNS AND SYMPTOMS OF ANAPHYLAXIS

Upper Airway
Hoarseness
Stridor
Laryngeal or epiglottic edema
Rhinorrhea

Lower Airway
Bronchospasm
Increased mucus production
Accessory muscle use
Wheezing
Decreased breath sounds

Cardiovascular System
Tachycardia
Hypotension
Dysrhythmias
Chest tightness

Gastrointestinal System
Nausea
Vomiting

Abdominal cramps
Diarrhea

Neurological System
Anxiety
Dizziness
Syncope
Weakness
Headache
Seizure
Coma

Cutaneous System
Angioedema
Urticaria
Pruritus
Erythema
Edema
Tearing of the eyes

Gastrointestinal Effects

Nausea, vomiting, diarrhea, and severe abdominal cramping may occur in a patient with an anaphylactic reaction. The increased gastrointestinal activity is related to smooth muscle contraction, increased mucus production, and outpouring of fluid from the gut wall into the intestinal lumen, initiated by the chemical mediators.

Nervous System Effects

Nervous system responses largely are caused by the impaired gas exchange and shock associated with anaphylaxis. Initially the patient may be agitated and speak of a sense of impending doom. As hypoxia and shock worsen, neurological function may deteriorate, resulting in confusion, weakness, headache, syncope, seizures, and coma.

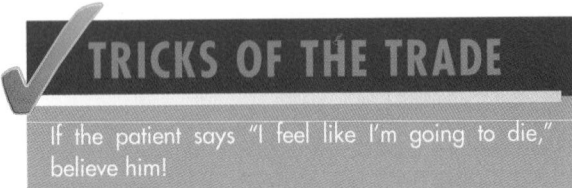

TRICKS OF THE TRADE

If the patient says "I feel like I'm going to die," believe him!

Cutaneous Effects

The physical findings on the skin are perhaps the most visible signs that distinguish anaphylaxis from other medical conditions. These signs are secondary to the vasodilation induced by histamine release from the mast cells. Initially the patient may complain of warmth and pruritus. Physical examination often reveals diffuse erythema and urticaria that result in well-circumscribed wheals of 1 to 6 cm, which may be more reddened or pallid than the surrounding skin and are often accompanied by

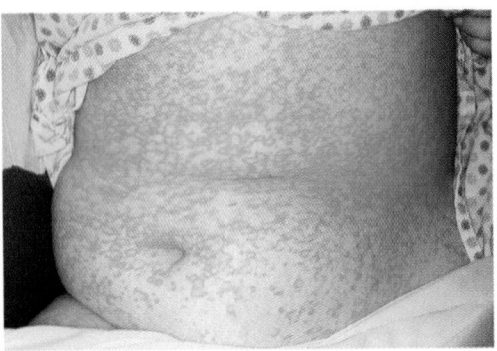

Fig. 31-2 Urticaria as a result of an allergic reaction. (Courtesy Gary Quick.)

severe itching (Fig. 31-2). Marked swelling of the face and tongue and angioedema also may be present, reflecting involvement of deeper capillaries of the skin and mucous membranes. As hypoxia and shock continue, cyanosis may be evident.

> **NOTE**
>
> Angioedema is a localized edematous reaction of the deep dermis or subcutaneous or submucosal tissues and appears in the form of giant wheals. Patients with angioedema are at high risk for rapid deterioration.

Initial Assessment

As in any critical emergency, initial patient care measures are directed at providing adequate airway, ventilatory, and circulatory support. Drug therapy often is the definitive treatment in anaphylaxis and therefore should be expedited.

? CRITICAL THINKING

How significant is stridor as a physical finding?

Airway assessment is critical because most deaths from anaphylaxis are directly related to upper airway obstruction. The conscious patient should be evaluated for voice changes, stridor, or a barking cough. Complaints of tightness in the neck and dyspnea should alert the paramedic of impending airway obstruction. The airway of an unconscious patient should be evaluated and secured. If airflow is impeded, endotracheal intubation should be performed. If there is severe laryngeal and epiglottic edema, surgical or needle cricothyrotomy (described in Chapter 11) may be indicated to provide airway access.

> **NOTE**
>
> Early, elective intubation is indicated for patients with hoarseness, lingual edema, and posterior or oropharyngeal swelling. If respiratory function deteriorates, medical direction may recommend tracheal intubation (with sedation) without paralytic agents.[3]

The patient should be closely monitored for signs of respiratory distress as indicated by pulse oximetry, skin color, accessory muscle use, wheezing, diminished breath sounds, and abnormal respiratory rates. Circulatory status also may deteriorate quickly. Therefore pulse quality, rate, and location should frequently be assessed.

History

A history may be difficult to obtain but can be critical to rule out other medical emergencies that may mimic anaphylaxis. The patient should be questioned regarding the chief complaint and the rapidity of onset of symptoms. Signs and symptoms of anaphylaxis usually appear within 1 to 30 minutes of introduction of the antigen. The onset of reaction can be delayed if the exposure is by the oral route.

Significant medical history to be elicited includes previous exposure and response to the suspected antigen. In addition, the method of introduction of the antigen should be ascertained, because injection frequently produces the most rapid and severe response. Other significant history includes chronic or concurrent illness and medication use. Preexisting cardiac disease or bronchial asthma should cause the paramedic to anticipate severe complications in these organ systems as a result of the allergic reaction. Use of certain drugs, such as beta-blocking agents, may diminish the patient's response to *epinephrine* (Adrenalin) and may necessitate administration of other medications. The paramedic should also determine whether the patient has been prescribed an emergency *epinephrine* (Adrenalin) drug kit (e.g., Epi Pen) and whether the medication was administered before the arrival of EMS personnel.

> **NOTE**
>
> Some patients with a history of allergic reaction may have taken an oral antihistamine (e.g., **diphenhydramine** [Benadryl]) or have used aerosolized **epinephrine** (e.g., Primatene Mist, Medinhaler Epi) before EMS arrival. The patient's use of these medications should be ascertained, if possible. Appropriate intervention, however, should not be delayed.

Physical Examination

Vital signs should be assessed frequently. In severe reactions, most patients initially are tachycardiac, tachypneic, and hypotensive if deterioration to cardiac arrest has not occurred. The patient's face and neck should be inspected for angioedema, hives, tear-

ing, and rhinorrhea. The presence of erythema or urticaria on other body regions should be noted. Along with vital signs, airway and lung sounds should frequently be assessed to evaluate the clinical progress of the patient and to monitor the effectiveness of interventions. Cardiac monitoring should be instituted as soon as possible to aid in patient evaluation.

Key Interventions to Prevent Arrest

Organ involvement in anaphylaxis varies and makes a standardized approach to patient management difficult. The following key interventions, however, are commonly used to manage anaphylaxis.[3]

1. Place the patient in position of comfort and elevate the legs until replacement fluids improve blood pressure.
2. Administer high-concentration oxygen.
3. Give *epinephrine* (Adrenalin) to all patients with clinical signs of shock, airway swelling, or difficulty breathing, using the following dose guidelines for adult patients:
   - IM dose: 0.3-0.5 mg (1:1000); may be repeated after 5 to 10 minutes if there is no clinical improvement.
   - SQ dose: Same as IM dose but absorption may be delayed with shock.
   - IV dose: 0.1 to 0.5 mg (1:10,000) over 5 minutes. IV *epinephrine* (Adrenalin) should be given only for profound, immediately life-threatening manifestations and when there are no delays in obtaining IV access. A continuous infusion at 1 to 4 mcg/min may avoid frequent repeat *epinephrine* injections.

> **NOTE**
>
> Complications of IV **epinephrine** are significant and include the development of uncontrolled systolic hypertension, vomiting, seizures, dysrhythmias, and myocardial ischemia. This route should be used only in patients with a critical life-threatening condition. It is performed with extreme caution in rare circumstances and only with authorization from medical direction.

4. Initiate IV therapy with normal saline solution if hypotension is present and does not respond

rapidly to *epinephrine* (Adrenalin). A rapid infusion of 1 to 2 L (up to 4 L) may be needed initially.

5. Transport the patient for physician evaluation. Most patients will be carefully observed in the hospital for up to 24 hours. Many do not respond promptly to therapy, and symptoms may recur in some patients.

? CRITICAL THINKING

How does epinephrine reverse the signs and symptoms of anaphylaxis?

Other Drug Therapy

Additional drug therapy may be helpful, but *epinephrine* (Adrenalin) is the only drug that can immediately reverse the life-threatening complications of anaphylaxis. Pharmacological agents that may be used with *epinephrine* (Adrenalin) include antihistamines to antagonize the effects of histamine, beta agonists to improve alveolar ventilation, corticosteroids to prevent a delayed reaction, *glucagon* (for patients unresponsive to *epinephrine*, especially those taking beta blockers) antidysrhythmics, and perhaps vasopressors to manage protracted hypotension (Box 31-4).

NOTE

Beta blockers may increase the incidence and severity of anaphylaxis and can produce a paradoxical response to *epinephrine*.[1] In these cases, *glucagon* may be effective.

Key Intervention During Arrest

Cardiac arrest from anaphylaxis may be associated with profound vasodilation, intravascular collapse, tissue hypoxia, and asystole. Special considerations for resuscitation of these patients are described below.[3]

Airway, Oxygenation, and Ventilation

Swelling of the airway can make bag-mask ventilation and endotracheal intubation difficult or ineffective in patients with anaphylaxis. In addition, the landmarks for needle cricothyrotomy may not be visible because of severe swelling in the soft tissues of the neck. Fiberoptic intubation or digital

BOX 31-4

ADDITIONAL DRUG THERAPY FOR ANAPHYLAXIS

Antihistamines
Diphenhydramine (Benadryl)
Hydroxyzine (Atarax, Vistaril)
Promethazine (Phenergan)
Cimetidine (Tagamet)
Ranitidine (Zantac)

Corticosteroids
Methylprednisolone (Solu-Medrol)
Hydrocortisone (Solu-Cortef)
Dexamethasone (Decadron)

Beta Agonists
Albuterol (Ventolin, Proventil)
Metaproterenol (Alupent)
Isoetharine (Bronkosol)

Antidysrhythmic
Amiodarone (Cordarone)
Lidocaine (Xylocaine) and others

Vasopressors
Dopamine (Intropin)
Norepinephrine (Levophed)

Glucagon

intubation are alternative methods to consider in these situations (see Chapter 11).

Support of Circulation

Circulatory support in cardiac arrest from anaphylaxis will require rapid and aggressive volume replacement (2 to 4 L) and the use of vasopressors to support blood pressure. *Epinephrine* (the drug of choice for treatment of both vasodilation and hypotension in cardiac arrest) also may need to be administered in high doses at 1 to 3 mg (3 minutes), 3 to 5 mg (3 minutes), and 4 to 10 mcg/min. In the presence of asystole or PEA (the most common arrest rhythms in anaphylaxis), the administration of *atropine* and TCP should be included in the algorithms (See Chapter 28). In addition, cardiac arrest from anaphylaxis may respond to prolonged periods of CPR, especially when the patient is young and has a healthy heart and cardiovascular system.

SUMMARY

- Antibodies bind to the antigen that produced them and facilitate antigen neutralization and removal from the body.

- Allergic reaction is an increased physiological response to an antigen after a previous exposure to the same antigen. Localized allergic reactions do not manifest multisystem involvement.

- Anaphylaxis is the most extreme form of allergic reaction. Rapid recognition and aggressive therapy are essential.

- Almost any substance can cause anaphylaxis. The risk of anaphylaxis increases with the frequency of exposure.

- Symptoms of anaphylaxis may include sneezing and coughing; airway obstruction; wheezing; hypotension or vascular collapse; chest pain; nausea, vomiting, or diarrhea; and weakness, headache, syncope, seizures, or coma.

 REFERENCE

1. American Heart Association: Guidelines 2000 for cardiopulmonary resuscitation and emergency cardiovascular care, International Consensus on Science, *Circulation* 102(8):241, 2000.

2. Rosen P, Barkin R: *Emergency medicine: concepts and clinical practice,* ed 4, St. Louis, 1998, Mosby.

3. American Heart Association: Guidelines 2000 for cardiopulmonary resuscitation and emergency cardiovascular care, International Consensus on Science, *Circulation* 102(8):243, 2000.

32 *Gastroenterology*

OBJECTIVES

Upon completion of this chapter, the paramedic student will be able to:

1. *Label a diagram of the abdominal organs.*
2. *Outline prehospital assessment of a patient who has abdominal pain.*
3. *Describe general prehospital management techniques for the patient with abdominal pain.*
4. *Describe signs and symptoms, complications, and prehospital management for the following gastrointestinal disorders: gastroenteritis, gastritis, colitis, diverticulosis, appendicitis, peptic ulcer disease, bowel obstruction, Crohn's disease, pancreatitis, esophagogastric varices, hemorrhoids, cholecystitis, and acute hepatitis.*

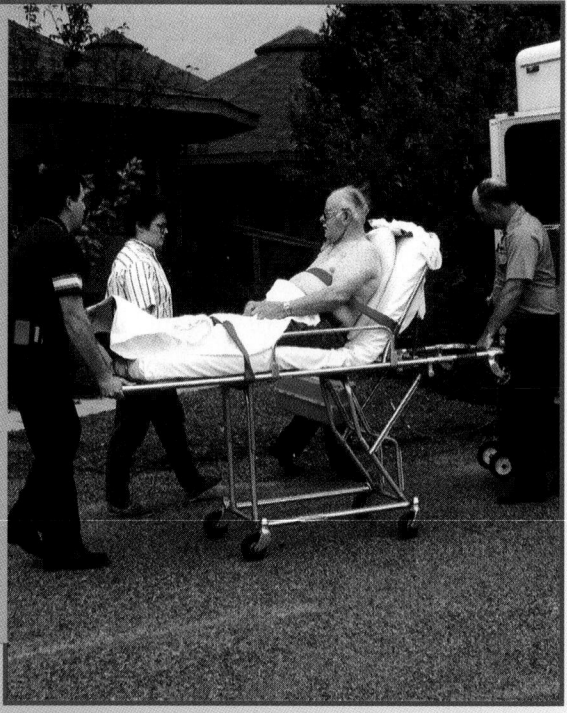

Acute abdominal pain is a common chief complaint in emergency care that may reflect serious illness. This chapter reviews gastrointestinal anatomy and disorders that produce gastrointestinal bleeding and/or abdominal pain. Appropriate evaluation and management in the prehospital phase of patient care may prevent the development of life-threatening complications.

KEY TERMS

appendicitis: An acute inflammation of the appendix.

bowel obstruction: An occlusion of the intestinal lumen that results in blockage of normal flow of intestinal contents.

cholecystitis: Inflammation of the gallbladder, most often associated with the presence of gallstones.

colitis: An inflammatory condition of the large intestine characterized by severe diarrhea and ulceration of the mucosa of the intestine.

Crohn's disease: A chronic, inflammatory bowel disease of unknown origin, usually affecting the ileum, the colon, or both structures.

diverticulitis: Inflammation of one or more diverticula.

diverticulosis: The presence of pouch-like herniations through the muscular layer of the colon.

esophagogastric varices: A complex of longitudinal, tortuous veins at the lower end of the esophagus that become large and swollen as a result of portal hypertension.

gastritis: Acute or chronic inflammation of the gastric mucosa that commonly results from hyperacidity, alcohol or drug ingestion, bile reflux, and *Helicobacter pylori* infection.

gastroenteritis: Inflammation of the stomach and intestines that accompanies numerous gastrointestinal disorders.

hemorrhoids: Swollen, distended veins (internal and/or external) in the rectoanal area.

hepatitis: An inflammatory condition of the liver associated with the sudden onset of malaise, weakness, anorexia, intermittent nausea and vomiting, and dull right-upper-quadrant pain, usually followed within 1 week by the onset of jaundice, dark urine, or both, characterized by jaundice.

pancreatitis: Inflammation of the pancreas, which causes severe epigastric pain.

peptic ulcer disease: Illness that results from a complex pathological interaction among the acidic gastric juice and proteolytic enzymes and the mucosal barrier.

referred pain: Visceral pain felt at a site distant from its origin.

somatic pain: Pain that arises from skeletal muscles, ligaments, vessels, or joints.

visceral pain: Deep pain that arises from smooth vasculature or organ systems.

NOTE

Acute abdominal pain accounts for about 5% of all visits to the emergency department each year. The most common diagnosis made in these patients is nonspecific abdominal pain or abdominal pain that has no clear origin.[1]

Gastrointestinal Anatomy

As described in Chapter 6, the gastrointestinal (GI) system provides the body with water, electrolytes, and other nutrients used by the cells. The major organs most commonly associated with the gastrointestinal system include the esophagus, stomach, small and large intestine, liver, gallbladder, and pancreas. To review GI anatomy, refer to Chapter 6 and Fig. 32-1.

NOTE

Genitourinary disorders also can produce abdominal pain and bleeding. These are described in Chapters 33 and 39.

Assessment of the Patient with Acute Abdominal Pain

After the initial survey to ensure adequacy of airway, breathing, and circulation, assessment of the patient with acute abdominal pain begins with a thorough history focused on the chief complaint. The paramedic should assess and document baseline vital signs and perform a systematic physical examination to help identify abdominal emergencies that may indicate the development of shock or the need for immediate transport for surgical intervention.

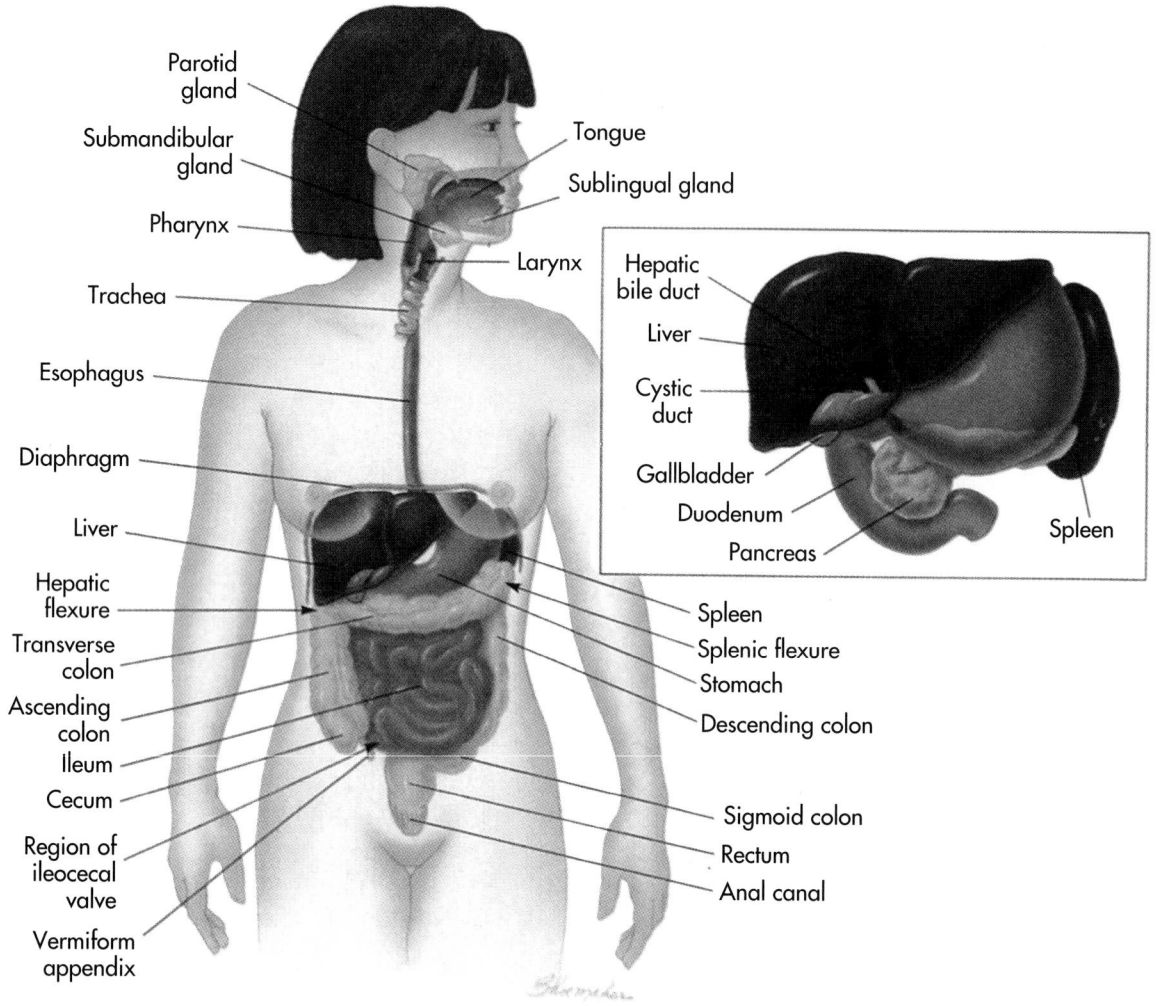

Fig. 32-1 Location of digestive organs. (From Thibodeau G: *Structure and function of the body,* ed. 9, St Louis, 1992, Mosby.)

History

When obtaining a history of abdominal pain, the paramedic should attempt to identify the location and type of pain and any associated signs and symptoms. Using the mnemonic OPQRST or a similar method can help in organizing this information. Sample questions that might be included in the OPQRST evaluation are listed below:

O (Onset): Was the onset of pain sudden? What were you doing when it started?

P (Provocative/ Palliative): What makes it better or worse?

Q (Quality): What does the pain feel like? Is it sharp, dull, burning, tearing?

R (Region): Where is the pain located? Does it radiate?

S (Severity): Is the pain mild, moderate, or severe? What is the degree of discomfort on a scale of 1 to 10?

T (Time): When did the pain begin? How long does it last?

Other important elements of a patient history include any recent illness and past significant medical history, such as hypertension, cardiac or respiratory disease that may manifest in abdominal pain, medication use, alcohol or other drug use, last bowel movement, and previous abdominal surgeries. Women of child-bearing age also should be ques-

---

BOX 32-1

LOCATION OF ABDOMINAL PAIN AND POSSIBLE ORIGINS

Right Upper Quadrant
Cholecystitis
Hepatitis
Pancreatitis
Perforated ulcer
Renal pain (right)

Left Upper Quadrant
Pancreatitis
Gastritis
Renal pain (left)

Right Lower Quadrant
Appendicitis
Abdominal aortic dissection or
  rupture
Ruptured ectopic pregnancy
Ovarian cyst (right)
Pelvic inflammatory disease
Urinary calculus
Hernia
Ovarian or testicular torsion

Left Lower Quadrant
Diverticulitis
Abdominal aortic dissection or rupture
Ruptured ectopic pregnancy
Ovarian cyst (left)
Pelvic inflammatory disease
Urinary calculus
Hernia
Ovarian or testicular torsion

Epigastric Pain
Gastritis
Esophagitis
Pancreatitis
Cholecystitis
Abdominal aortic aneurysm
Myocardial ischemia

Diffuse Pain
Intestinal obstruction
Perforation
Generalized peritonitis

---

tioned about menstrual activity (including regularity and last menstrual period), and the possibility of pregnancy.

NOTE

Do not permit a patient with abdominal pain to eat or drink before a physician's evaluation, because surgery may be indicated.

? CRITICAL THINKING

What factors can influence a patient's perception and description of pain?

Location and Type of Abdominal Pain

Recalling the anatomical location of gastrointestinal organs and structures provides a method for assessing a specific disorder. Location of abdominal pain and possible origins of illness are listed in Box 32-1. The types of abdominal pain that may result from

chronic or acute episodes may be classified as *visceral, somatic,* and *referred.*

NOTE

Persistent abdominal pain of any nature that lasts 6 hours or longer warrants patient transport for physician evaluation.

NOTE

Patients with abdominal pain seldom are given pain medication in the field. Analgesics can mask signs and symptoms that are critical for an accurate evaluation and determination of the cause of the patient's pain.

Visceral Pain

Visceral pain is caused by the stimulation of autonomic nerve fibers that surround a hollow viscus or by the distention or stretching of hollow viscus organs or ligaments. It usually is described by the patient as cramping or gas-type pain that varies in intensity, increasing to a high degree of severity and then subsiding. Visceral pain generally is diffuse and therefore difficult to localize. Often it is centered at the umbilicus or lower in the midline. Visceral pain frequently is associated with other symptoms of autonomic nerve involvement such as tachycardia, diaphoresis, nausea, or vomiting. Common causes of visceral abdominal pain include early appendicitis, pancreatitis, cholecystitis, and intestinal obstruction.

Somatic Pain

Somatic pain is produced by bacterial or chemical irritation of nerve fibers in the peritoneum (peritonitis). Unlike visceral pain, somatic pain usually is constant and localized to a specific area. The patient often describes it as sharp or stabbing. Patients with somatic abdominal pain generally are hesitant to move about and lie on their back or side with legs flexed to prevent additional pain from stimulation of the peritoneal area. These patients often exhibit involuntary guarding of the abdomen and rebound tenderness during the physical examination. Common causes of somatic pain are appendicitis and an inflamed or perforated viscus (ulcer, gallbladder, or small or large intestine).

Referred Pain

Referred pain is pain in a part of the body considerably removed from the tissues that cause the pain. This mechanism results from branches of visceral fibers that synapse in the spinal cord with the same second-order neurons that receive pain fibers from the skin. When these pain fibers are stimulated intensely, pain sensations spread, and the patient experiences the pain in areas distant from the original source.

✓ TRICKS OF THE TRADE

Pain in the shoulder associated with abdominal trauma or pain (Kehr's sign) may indicate peritoneal irritation, especially in a patient with an ectopic pregnancy or rupture of the appendix or other organ.

A knowledge of referred pain is important because many visceral ailments cause no other symp-

toms except referred pain. For example, cardiac pain may be referred to the neck and jaw, shoulders, pectoral muscles, and down the arms; biliary pain to the right subscapular area; renal colic to the genitalia and flank area; uterine and rectal pain to the low back; and a leaking aortic aneurysm to the lower back or buttocks. Surface areas of referred pain from visceral organs are illustrated in Fig. 32-2.

Signs and Symptoms

Although numerous signs and symptoms may be associated with acute abdominal pain, the following are the most common[2]:

1. Nausea, vomiting, anorexia
   Gastritis
   Appendicitis
   Pancreatitis
   Biliary tract disease
   High intestinal obstruction
2. Diarrhea
   Inflammatory process (gastroenteritis, ulcerative colitis)
3. Constipation
   Dehydration, obstruction, medication-induced decreased intestinal motility (codeine, *morphine*)
4. Change in stool color
   Biliary tract obstruction (clay-colored stools)
   Lower intestinal bleeding (black, tarry stools)
5. Chills and fever
   Bacterial infection
   Pyelonephritis
   Appendicitis
   Cholecystitis

Vital Signs

Vital sign assessment should be complete, including evaluation and documentation of the patient's blood pressure; pulse rate (including ECG assessment); respiratory rate; and skin color, moisture, temperature, and turgor. In addition, the presence or absence of orthostatic changes in the patient's pulse and blood pressure should be noted when possible. As described in Chapter 19, a rise from a recumbent position to a sitting or standing position associated with a fall in systolic pressure (after 1 minute) of 10 to 15 mm Hg and/or a concurrent rise in pulse rate (after 1 minute) of 10 to 15 beats per minute indicates a significant volume depletion

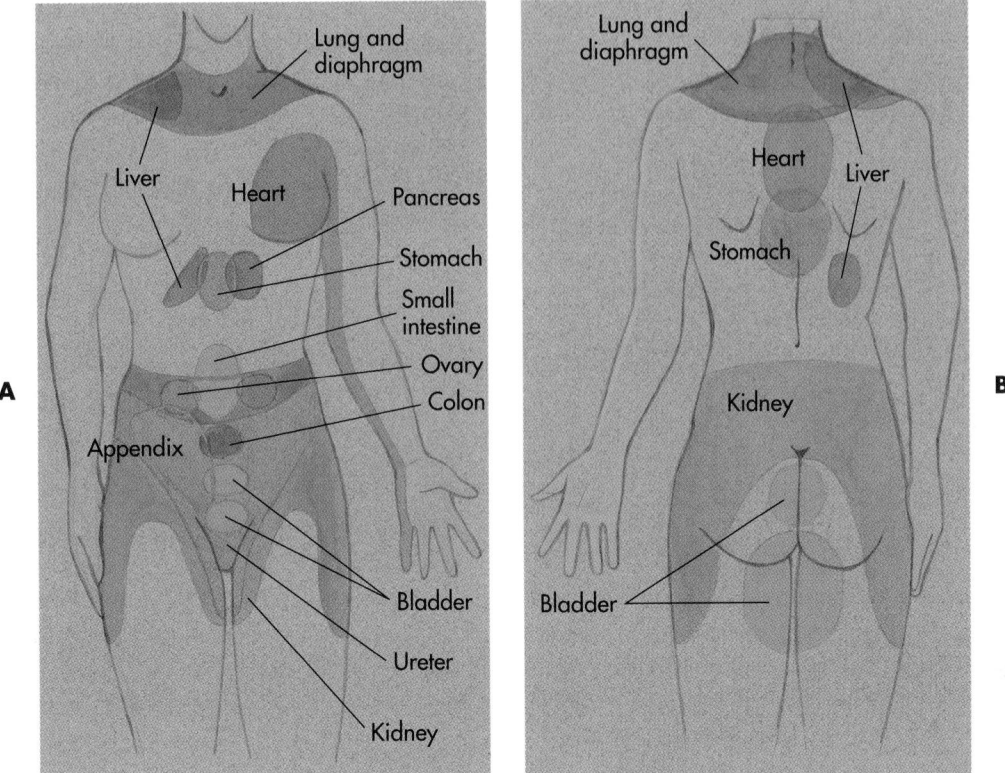

Fig. 32-2 Referred pain. **A,** Anterior view. **B,** Posterior view.

and a decrease in perfusion status. An assessment of blood pressure, pulses, and capillary refill in each extremity also should be performed as a consideration for aortic dissection (described in Chapter 28).

Physical Examination

The physical examination of a patient with acute abdominal pain includes the skills of inspection, auscultation, percussion, and palpation. If there is reason to suspect life-threatening illness that requires rapid stabilization and transportation of the patient, the examination should be completed en route to the receiving hospital. Physical examination of the patient's abdomen is described in Chapter 13, but the following discussion serves as a review. (Male and female physical examinations to evaluate genitourinary complaints are discussed in Chapter 33.)

Inspection

In the initial patient encounter, the paramedic should note the position in which the patient is lying. As previously stated, many patients with ab-dominal peritoneal irritation lie on their sides with their knees flexed and pulled in toward their chests. Other visual clues that may indicate abdominal pain are skin color, facial expressions such as grimacing, and the presence or absence of voluntary movement. The patient's clothing should be removed and the abdominal wall inspected for the presence of bruises, scars, ascites, abdominal distention, or abdominal masses.

Auscultation

Auscultation to confirm the presence or absence of bowel sounds usually is reserved for assessment in the emergency department. However, if auscultation is to be performed, it should be done for about 2 minutes in each quadrant before the examiner determines that bowel sounds are absent. (Auscultation should always precede palpation and percussion, which may alter the intensity of bowel sounds.) Bowel sounds that are increased in number, duration, or intensity indicate the possibility of gastroenteritis or intestinal obstruction. Bowel sounds that are markedly decreased in number and intensity (or their absence) may indicate peritonitis or ileus.

BOX 32-2

**EMERGENCY CARE FOR
ACUTE ABDOMINAL PAIN**

1. High-concentration oxygen administration
2. Adequate intravenous access with a crystalloid solution (Application of the pneumatic antishock garment for the treatment of shock with acute abdominal pain is controversial and should be authorized by medical direction.)
3. Electrocardiogram monitoring
4. Rapid and gentle transport to an appropriate medical facility

Palpation

The paramedic should begin palpation of the abdomen gently, avoiding the painful area until the remainder of the abdomen is examined. The paramedic should be alert to rigidity or spasm, tenderness or masses, and to the patient's facial expressions, which may provide clues about the severity of the pain. In addition, the paramedic should note whether the abdomen is soft or rigid.

Percussion

If time permits, a general assessment of tympany and dullness by percussion may be performed to detect the presence of fluid, air, or solid masses in the abdomen. A systematic approach should be used, moving either from side-to-side or in a clockwise direction, noting tenderness and abdominal skin temperature and color. To review, tympany is the major sound that should be noted during percussion because of the normal presence of air in the stomach and intestines. Dullness should be heard over organs and solid masses.

Management of the Patient with an Abdominal Emergency

Patients with acute abdominal pain or gastrointestinal bleeding cannot be definitively managed in the prehospital setting. The majority require extensive evaluation in the emergency department, including laboratory analysis, radiological imaging, fluid and medication therapy, and perhaps surgical intervention. The role of the paramedic (Box 32-2) is to support the patient's airway and ventilatory status; to perform and document an initial patient assessment, including a thorough history; to monitor vital signs and cardiac rhythm; to initiate IV therapy for fluid replacement or fluid resuscitation; and to rapidly transport the patient for physician evaluation.

Specific Abdominal Emergencies

Abdominal emergencies can result from inflammation, infection, and obstruction. Some disorders may be associated with upper GI bleeding (e.g., lesions, peptic ulceration, and esophagogastric varices), or lower GI bleeding (e.g., colonic lesions, diverticulosis, hemorrhoids). Others, such as pancreatitis and cholecystitis, more commonly are associated with acute abdominal pain in the absence of bleeding. The specific GI disorders discussed in this chapter are listed in Box 32-3.

Gastroenteritis

Gastroenteritis is inflammation of the stomach and intestines that accompanies numerous GI disorders. Symptoms include anorexia, nausea, vomiting, abdominal discomfort, and diarrhea. The condition may be caused by bacterial enterotoxins, bacterial or viral invasion, chemical toxins, and other conditions (e.g., lactose intolerance). Infectious forms of gastroenteritis often are transmitted through the fecal-oral route and by ingestion of infected food or nonpotable water. The condition is likely to affect travelers in endemic areas and populations in disaster areas where water supplies are contaminated. (Native populations in endemic areas generally are resistant.)

The onset of gastroenteritis may be slow, but more often is abrupt and violent, with rapid loss of fluids and electrolytes from persistent vomiting and diarrhea. Hypokalemia and hyponatremia, acidosis, or alkalosis may develop. Treatment primarily is supportive, employing IV fluid replacement, sedation, bed rest, and medications to control vomiting

? CRITICAL THINKING

What would be your primary concern for a patient with a history of severe gastroenteritis?

and diarrhea. Some forms of gastroenteritis can be treated with antibiotic therapy. EMS personnel who are working in disaster areas should observe the following guidelines[2]:

- Avoid patient contact if you are ill.
- Know the source of water supplies or drink hot beverages that have been brisk-boiled or disinfected.
- Avoid habits that facilitate fecal-oral/mucous membrane transmission.
- Observe body-substance isolation (BSI) precautions and effective hand washing procedures.

Gastritis

Gastritis is acute or chronic inflammation of the gastric mucosa; it commonly results from hyperacidity, alcohol or drug ingestion, bile reflux, and *Helicobacter pylori* infection. Signs and symptoms of gastritis include epigastric pain, nausea and vomiting (which may be severe), mucosal bleeding (erosive gastritis), and epigastric tenderness on palpation. The patient with gastritis may be hypovolemic as a result of prolonged bleeding with or without melena (abnormal maroon-colored or dark, tarry stools containing digested blood). The chronic use of alcohol, **aspirin** and other nonsteroidal or antiinflammatory medications, and *H. pylori* infection are the most common causes of gastrointestinal illness. Gastritis is treated with diet regulation, medications (e.g., antibiotics and antacids), and fluid replacement or fluid resuscitation if hypovolemia or dehydration occurs.

NOTE

Helicobacter pylori is a bacterium that resides in the human stomach between the epithelial cell surface and the overlying mucus. The bacterium is more prevalent in lower socioeconomic groups and may be spread in adults and children through the fecal-oral route. Its presence is believed to cause mucosal inflammation that disrupts the normal defense mechanisms of the stomach and leads to ulceration.

Colitis

Colitis is an inflammatory condition of the large intestine characterized by severe diarrhea and ulceration of the mucosa of the intestine (ulcerative colitis). Weight loss, significant pain, and grossly bloody

BOX 32-3

GASTROINTESTINAL DISORDERS

Gastroenteritis
Gastritis
Colitis
Diverticulosis
Appendicitis
Peptic ulcer disease
Bowel obstruction
Crohn's disease
Pancreatitis
Esophagogastric varices
Hemorrhoids
Cholecystitis
Acute hepatitis

stools are hallmarks of this condition. The disease affects all age groups, with the highest incidence in the third and fourth decades of life. A family history of the disease is present in 10% to 15% of cases. The cause of colitis is unknown; the condition usually is managed with steroids, electrolytes, antibiotics, and diet regulation.

NOTE

In patients with AIDS, the chronic diarrhea and diffuse colonic involvement of Kaposi's sarcoma (described in Chapter 37) may mimic chronic ulcerative colitis, as may otherwise undiagnosed manifestations of HIV infection itself. Surgical bowel resection sometimes is required in these patients.

Diverticulosis

A diverticulum is a sac or pouch that develops in the wall of the colon. It is a common development with advancing years and is associated with diets low in fiber. Diverticular outpouchings (a condition known as **diverticulosis**) tend to develop at the weakest point in the colon wall, where intraluminal vessels penetrate the circular muscular layer. Often there is a small artery or arteriole at the neck of the diverticulum from which subsequent bleeding may occur.

Serious complications of diverticular disease associated with perforation are massive, bright-red rectal bleeding, which can be brisk and commonly painless; peritonitis; and sepsis. Hemorrhage from a diverticulum is the most common cause of massive rectal bleeding in older patients. If the hemorrhage does not cease spontaneously, emergency surgery may be necessary.

Most patients with diverticula are completely asymptomatic. However, up to 30% of these patients experience **diverticulitis** when one or more diverticula become obstructed with fecal matter. Mild complications of diverticulitis include irregular bowel habits (alternating constipation and diarrhea), fever, and lower left quadrant pain. Recurrences of diverticulitis are common within the first 5 years after the onset of symptoms. Definitive care includes diet regulation, antibiotic therapy, and sometimes, surgical repair.

Appendicitis

Appendicitis is a common abdominal emergency that occurs when the opening between the lumen of the appendix and the cecum is obstructed by fecal material (fecalith) or as a result of inflammation from viral or bacterial infection. If the condition is allowed to persist, the inflamed organ eventually becomes gangrenous and ruptures within the peritoneal cavity, resulting in peritonitis (which may progress to shock), or evolution into a periappendiceal abscess.

The classic presentation of appendicitis is abdominal pain or cramping, nausea, vomiting, chills, low-grade fever, and anorexia. The pain initially is periumbilical and diffuse, later becoming intense and localized to the right lower quadrant just medial to the iliac crest (McBurney's point). If the appendix ruptures, the patient's pain diminishes before the development of peritoneal signs. The goal

? CRITICAL THINKING

What other illness presents similar signs or symptoms?

NOTE

Young children and older adults may have atypical illness caused by reduced inflammatory response associated with extremes of age; therefore appendicitis is more difficult to diagnose in these age groups.

of definitive care for appendicitis is surgical appendectomy before rupture.

Peptic Ulcer Disease

Peptic ulcer disease results from a complex pathological interaction among the acidic gastric juice and proteolytic enzymes and the mucosal barrier. The three most common causes of peptic ulcer disease are *H. pylori* infection, nonsteroidal inflammatory drug use, and increased circulatory gastrin from gastrin-secreting tumors (Zollinger-Eillison syndrome).[1] These factors are responsible for the formation of ulcers (an open wound or sore), usually in the stomach or duodenum. Ulcers cause disintegration and death of tissue as they erode the mucosal layers in the affected areas. If they are left untreated, massive hemorrhage or perforation may result.

The patient with a peptic ulcer usually is aware of the condition and often uses over-the-counter antacids. The ulcer pain often is described as a burning or gnawing discomfort in the epigastric region or left upper quadrant (in the case of gastric ulcer) that develops before meals (classically, early morning) or during stressful periods, when the production of gastric acids increases. The pain usually is sudden in onset and commonly is relieved by food intake, antacids, or vomiting. In addition to pain and vomiting of blood, the patient may experience melena as a result of hemorrhagic blood passing through the GI tract.

Prehospital care for patients with peptic ulcer disease includes obtaining a pertinent history, evaluating for hypotension, and providing circulatory support as needed. After physician evaluation, definitive care may involve antibiotics, antacids, H2-receptor antagonists or other medications, and occasionally, diet regulation (the benefit of which is controversial). Some patients with acute peptic ulcer disease require hospitalization for fluid or blood replacement, or for surgery if medications are not effective or blood loss is ongoing.

Bowel Obstruction

Bowel obstruction is an occlusion of the intestinal lumen that results in blockage of normal flow of intestinal contents. The condition may be caused by a number of factors, including adhesions, hernias, fecal impaction, polyps, and tumors. Obstructions can be closely mimicked by paralytic ileus (a decrease or absence of intestinal peristalsis), which may result from a number of localized or systemic conditions. Intestinal obstruction in the small bowel most often is caused by adhesions or hernia (see the box at the right). Large bowel obstructions commonly result from tumors or fecal impaction.

Signs and symptoms of intestinal obstruction include nausea and vomiting, abdominal pain, constipation, and abdominal distention. The speed of onset and degree of symptoms depend on the anatomical site of obstruction (small versus large bowel). The most significant danger of an obstructive condition is perforation with generalized peritonitis and sepsis.

The patient with bowel obstruction often presents with abdominal pain; dehydration may result from vomiting, decreased intestinal absorption, and fluid loss into the lumen and interstitium (bowel-wall edema). As the affected portion of the bowel distends, its blood supply is attenuated, and the segment becomes ischemic. The forces of distention and ischemia combine to produce perforation with secondary peritonitis. If the intestine becomes strangulated, blood or plasma also may be lost from the affected intestinal segment. Definitive care involves fluid replacement, antibiotics, placement of a nasogastric (NG) tube for decompression, and frequently surgery to correct the obstructing lesion. (NG tube insertion is described in the appendix to this chapter.)

? CRITICAL THINKING

Have you ever responded to a call for "constipation"? Did the paramedics consider this diagnosis a possibility? What was the attitude toward the patient?

Crohn's Disease

Crohn's disease is a chronic, inflammatory bowel disease thought to be of autoimmune etiology, usually affecting the ileum, the colon, or both structures. (The diseased segments associated with Crohn's disease may be separated by normal bowel segments or skip areas.) The formation of **fistulas** from the diseased bowel to the anus, vagina, skin surface, or other loops of bowel are common.

HERNIA

A hernia is the protrusion of a viscus from its normal position through a congenital or acquired opening, most commonly in the musculature of the groin or abdominal wall. Increases in intraabdominal pressure (e.g., those associated with straining, coughing, or lifting) can cause the peritoneum to push outward through such a defect. When this occurs, a sac is formed into which various organs within the peritoneal cavity may enter.

Most hernias are uncomplicated and can be manually reduced into the peritoneal cavity by a physician. If they cannot, however, the incarcerated contents of the peritoneal sac (usually a portion of bowel) can become strangulated. These patients frequently have acute abdominal pain and systemic signs such as fever and tachycardia. Incarcerated or strangulated hernias can lead to serious complications, including intestinal obstruction, perforation, and peritonitis. Definitive care for complicated hernias is in-hospital observation, IV rehydration, pain medication, and surgical repair.

Crohn's disease is characterized by frequent attacks of diarrhea, severe abdominal pain, nausea, fever, chills, weakness, anorexia, and weight loss. (Patients with Crohn's and similar diseases often suffer from depression because of the relentless and painful characteristics associated with these conditions.) The disease should be suspected in any patient with chronic inflammatory colitis and a history

NOTE

The incidence of Crohn's disease in the United States has been doubling every 10 years for the past three decades.[1]

NOTE

The term *irritable bowel syndrome* or spastic colon is used to describe abnormally increased motility of the small and large intestines. Unlike inflammatory bowel disease, the abdominal pain of irritable bowel syndrome generally is associated with emotional and physical stress and is relieved by bowel movement.

of anorectal problems such as fistulas or abscesses. These patients frequently are hospitalized. Once patients are stabilized, the condition may be managed with antibiotics, steroids, and antimotility agents to attempt to induce remission, and diet regulation.

Pancreatitis

Inflammation of the pancreas (**pancreatitis**) may cause severe epigastric pain. It frequently is associated with nausea, vomiting, and abdominal tenderness and distention. The abdominal pain often is described as severe, radiating from midumbilicus to the patient's back and shoulders. In severe cases, the patient has fever, tachycardia, and signs of generalized sepsis and shock. These patients often are hospitalized and treated with IV fluids, pain medication, and placement of a NG tube if there is vomiting.

Esophagogastric Varices

Esophagogastric varices are common with hepatic disease and often result from portal hypertension caused by cirrhosis of the liver. Obstruction to portal blood flow, produced by the fibrosis in the liver, increases portal pressure and dilates vessels that drain into the portal system. This subsequent dilation of thin-walled veins around the lower esophagus and upper end of the stomach produces esophagogastric varices. Varices are subject to rupture and result in life-threatening hemorrhage. Other causes of esophageal bleeding include esophagitis (associated with chronic use of alcohol and antiinflammatory nonsteroidal medications), malignancy, and episodes of prolonged, violent vomiting that produce a tear or laceration in the mucosa of the upper esophagus (Mallory-Weiss syndrome).

Clinically, a patient with esophageal bleeding has bright-red hematemesis, which may be severe. If bleeding is profuse, melena may be evident, and the patient may manifest the classic signs of shock. Variceal bleeding usually is massive and generally difficult to control. Therapeutic intervention includes ensuring a patent airway and fluid resuscitation. (The placement of a NG tube for gastric lavage is controversial.) Definitive care may include placement of a Sengstaken-Blakemore tube to tamponade bleeding vessels, surgical ligation of the bleeding varices, or transendoscopic injection of a sclerosing

agent into the bleeding vessels. The mortality rate for patients with variceal bleeding is about 25%.[1]

Hemorrhoids

Hemorrhoids are swollen, distended veins (internal and/or external) in the rectoanal area. They are present in 50% of all people by age 50, typically with blood streaking rather than life-threatening hemorrhage. Pain is infrequent unless thrombosis, ulceration, or infection is present. Slight bleeding is the most common symptom and usually occurs during or after defecation. Blood dripping into the toilet after defecation or blood-stained toilet tissue after wiping are common indications. Although blood loss usually is slight, recurrent episodes of bleeding may be significant enough to produce anemia. Definitive care includes conservative dietary management, stool softeners, tissue fixation techniques, and operative hemorrhoidectomy for severe cases.

> **NOTE**
>
> Anal fissure (a linear ulceration or laceration of the skin of the anus) or an abnormal opening of the cutaneous surface near the anus (anal fistula) also can produce bleeding and pain from the rectal region.

Cholecystitis

Cholecystitis is inflammation of the gallbladder, which most often is associated with the presence of gallstones (75% of which are cholesterol stones). The disease is very common in the United States and occurs more often in women 30 to 50 years of age than in men. On occasion, the gallstones totally obstruct the neck or cystic duct of the gallbladder. This is followed by a large increase in pressure within the organ. The increased pressure causes a sudden onset of pain (biliary colic), which radiates to the right upper quadrant or right scapula. Patients with gallbladder disease commonly have their pain episodes at night, and they generally are associated with recent ingestion of fried or fatty foods.

Other associated hallmarks of cholecystitis include previous episodes, a family history of gallbladder disease, low-grade fever, nausea, vomiting that may be bile stained and described as bitter (variable), and pain and tenderness on palpation in the right upper quadrant. Passage of stones into the common bile duct with subsequent obstruction may cause shaking chills, high fever, jaundice, and acute pancreatitis. Treatment may include hospitalization, IV fluid therapy, antibiotics, and placement of a NG tube. Definitive treatment is surgical removal of the gallbladder.

Acute Hepatitis

Hepatitis is inflammation of the liver. The condition is associated with the sudden onset of malaise, weakness, anorexia, intermittent nausea and vomiting, and dull right-upper-quadrant pain, usually followed within 1 week by the onset of jaundice, dark urine, or both. Although many viruses can infect the liver, the three classes of viruses that are of main concern as causes of acute infectious hepatitis are hepatitis A virus (HAV), hepatitis B virus (HBV), and hepatitis C virus (HCV), formerly known as *non-A/non-B hepatitis virus*. All types produce similar pathological alterations in the liver and stimulate an antibody response specific to the type of virus causing the disease (Box 32-4).

> **NOTE**
>
> Many hepatitis infections are subclinical and often present influenza-like symptoms.

The inflammation of hepatitis has many possible causes, including alcohol or other drug use, autoimmune disorders, and toxic bacterial, fungal, parasitic, and viral infections. Patients with hepatitis require medical evaluation to effectively manage the course of the disease. It is important for paramedics to receive appropriate immunizations and

---

BOX 32-4

RISK FACTORS FOR HEPATITIS

Hepatitis A
Health care practice without BSI precautions
Household or sexual contact with an infected person
Living in an area with HAV outbreak
Traveling to developing countries
Engaging in sex with infected partners and/or multiple partners
Drug use by injection

Hepatitis B
Health care practice without BSI precautions
Infant born to HBV infected mother
Engaging in sex with infected partners and/or multiple partners
Drug use by injection
Receiving hemodialysis

Hepatitis C
Health care practice without BSI precautions
Receiving blood transfusion before July 1992
Engaging in sex with infected partners and/or multiple partners
Drug use by injection
Receiving hemodialysis

---

to observe BSI procedures when caring for these patients. Hepatitis is discussed in depth in Chapter 37.

> **? CRITICAL THINKING**
>
> *Why do you think someone would refuse the opportunity to be vaccinated against this deadly disease?*

S U M M A R Y

- The major organs most commonly associated with the gastrointestinal system include the esophagus, stomach, small and large intestine, liver, gallbladder, and pancreas.

- After the initial survey, assessment of abdominal pain should begin with a thorough history. The physical examination may help to determine if the pain is visceral, somatic, or referred.

- Definitive treatment for abdominal pain will occur at the hospital. The paramedic should provide supportive treatment, manage life threats, and transport the patient to an appropriate facility.

- Gastroenteritis is inflammation of the stomach and intestines secondary to infectious agents, chemicals or other conditions.

- Gastritis is acute or chronic inflammation of the gastric mucosa that commonly results from hyperacidity, alcohol or other drug ingestion, bile reflux, and *Helicobacter pylori* infection.

- Colitis is an inflammatory condition of the large intestine characterized by severe diarrhea and ulceration of the mucosa of the intestine (ulcerative colitis).

- Diverticulosis may result in bright red rectal bleeding if perforation occurs.

- Diverticulitis results when a diverticulum becomes obstructed with fecal matter.

- Appendicitis occurs when the opening between the lumen of the appendix and cecum is obstructed by fecal material or by inflammation due to infection.

- Peptic ulcer disease occurs when open wounds or sores develop in the stomach or duodenum.

- Bowel obstruction is an occlusion of the intestinal lumen that results in blockage of the normal flow of intestinal contents.

- Crohn's disease is a chronic, inflammatory bowel disease of unknown origin.

- Inflammation of the pancreas (pancreatitis) causes severe abdominal pain.

- Esophagogastric varices result from obstruction of portal blood because of liver disease.

- Hemorrhoids are distended veins in the rectoanal area.

- Cholecystitis is inflammation of the gallbladder, most often associated with the presence of gallstones.

- Hepatitis is characterized by the sudden onset of malaise, weakness, anorexia, intermittent nausea and vomiting, and dull right-upper-quadrant pain, usually followed within 1 week by the onset of jaundice, dark urine, or both.

REFERENCES

1. Rosen P, Barkin R: *Emergency medicine: concepts and clinical practice*, ed. 4, St Louis, 1998, Mosby.
2. U.S. Department of Transportation National Highway Traffic Safety Administration: *EMT-Paramedic national standard curriculum*, Washington, DC, 1998, The Department.

Appendix

Nasogastric Tube Insertion

NG intubation may be indicated when the patient's stomach is severely distended or when evacuation of gastric contents by lavage is necessary. This procedure should be attempted only in conscious patients with an intact gag reflex or in unconscious patients whose airway is protected with an endotracheal tube.

Note: Passage of a NG tube is unpleasant under the most ideal of conditions and should be considered as a prehospital procedure only under unusual circumstances and under medical direction (Appendix Figs. 32-1 and 32-2).

Necessary Equipment

- Personal protective equipment (gloves, mask, face shield)
- Double-lumen Levin tube (large enough to evacuate desired material)
- Water-soluble lubricant
- Tape
- 50-mL irrigation syringe
- Cup of water or ice chips
- Emesis basin
- Intermittent suction equipment

Procedure

1. Explain the procedure to the patient.
2. Measure the length of tube to be inserted by placing the tip of the tube over the approximate area of the stomach and extending it to the patient's ear and from the ear to the tip of the nose. Note the marks on the tube used for measurement.
3. Lubricate the tip and the first 2 to 3 inches of the tube with a water-soluble lubricant.
4. Place the patient in a high Fowler's position and instruct the patient to lean forward and to flex his or her neck.
5. Instruct the patient to suck on ice chips or to take small sips of water (if not contraindicated) and to swallow on command during the procedure. This assists passage of the tube.
6. Insert the tube along the floor of an unobstructed nostril. If the patient has a deviated septum choose the nostril with the most open channel.
7. Gently and slowly advance the tube while having the patient continue to swallow until the tube is at the level previously noted by the marks. It is common for the patient to choke and cough during the procedure. If this occurs, hold the tube in place and allow the patient to rest. If choking and

coughing persist, remove the tube (it may have entered the trachea) and begin again.

8. After the tube has been fully inserted to its predetermined length, verify placement in the stomach by injecting 20 mL to 30 mL of air into the tube while auscultating the epigastric region for the sound of air movement. Leave the syringe attached to the tube until aspiration of stomach contents is initiated or intermittent suction is available.
9. Secure the tube with tape to the nose and forehead or cheek.
10. Lavage stomach contents by injecting 100-mL to 150-mL boluses of normal saline into the tube and allowing the return of gastric contents by aspiration or intermittent suction. Document the amount of fluid infused and returned by lavage.

Possible Complications

- Nasal hemorrhage
- Passage of the tube into the trachea
- Perforation of the esophagus
- Gastrointestinal bleeding
- Coiling of the tube in the posterior pharynx
- Obstruction of the passage resulting from septal deviation
- Passage of the tube intracranially (with cribriform plate fractures)

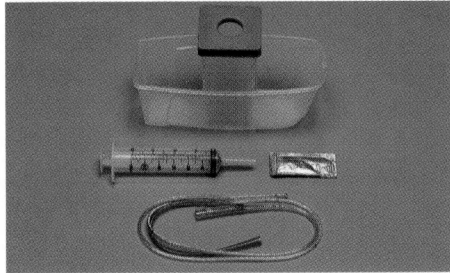

Appendix Fig. 32-1 Equipment for NG tube insertion.

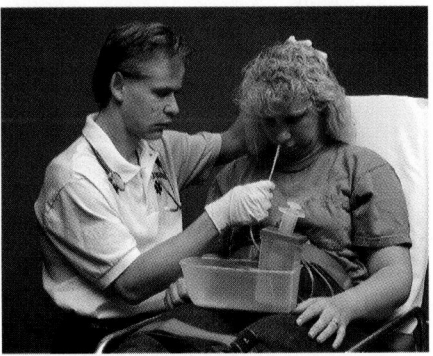

Appendix Fig. 32-2 NG tube insertion.

33 *Urology/Renal*

Upon completion of this chapter, the paramedic student will be able to:

1. *Label a diagram of the urinary system.*
2. *Describe pathophysiology, signs and symptoms, assessment, and prehospital management of the patient with urinary retention, urinary tract infection, pyelonephritis, urinary calculus, epididymitis, and testicular torsion.*
3. *Outline the physical examination for patients with genitourinary disorders.*
4. *Discuss general prehospital management for the patient with a genitourinary disorder.*
5. *Distinguish between acute and chronic renal failure.*
6. *Describe the signs and symptoms of renal failure.*
7. *Describe dialysis and emergent conditions associated with it, including prehospital management.*

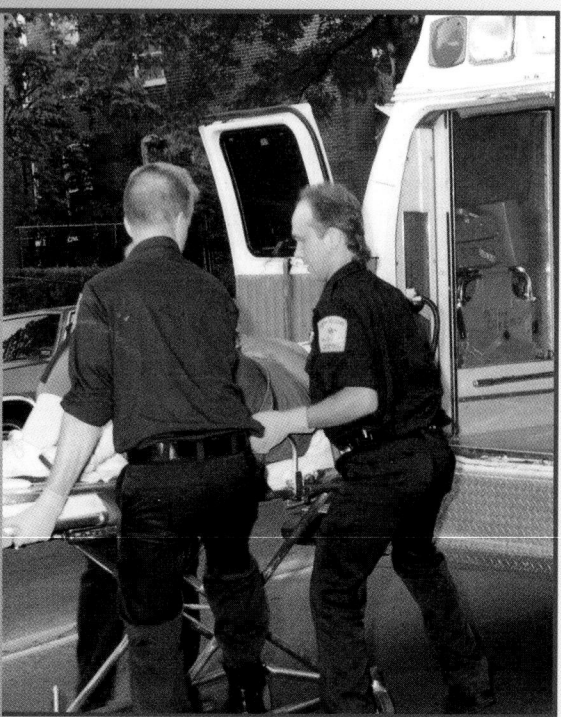

Like gastrointestinal disorders, many genitourinary disorders can produce acute abdominal pain and systemic illness. Management of patients with these disorders often begins in the prehospital setting, and successful outcomes often are determined in large part by the assessment skills of the paramedic.

KEY TERMS

acute renal failure: A clinical syndrome that results when there is a sudden and marked decrease in filtration through the glomeruli, leading to the accumulation of salt, water, and nitrogenous wastes within the body.

chronic renal failure: A progressive, irreversible systemic disease caused by kidney dysfunction that leads to abnormalities in blood counts and blood chemistry levels.

disequilibrium syndrome: A group of neurological findings that sometimes occur during or immediately after dialysis; thought to result from a disproportionate decrease in osmolality of the extracellular fluid compared to that of the intracellular compartment in the brain or cerebral spinal fluid.

epididymitis: An inflammation of the epididymis, a tubular section of the male reproductive system that carries sperm from the testicle to the seminal vesicles.

peritoneal dialysis: A dialysis procedure that uses the peritoneum as a diffusible membrane; performed to correct an imbalance of fluid or electrolytes in the blood or to remove toxins, drugs, or other wastes normally excreted by the kidney.

pyelonephritis: An inflammation of the kidney parenchyma associated with microbial infection.

uremia: The presence of excessive amounts of urea and other nitrogenous wastes produced in the blood.

urinary retention: The inability to urinate.

Anatomy and Physiology Review

As described in Chapter 6, the urinary system works with other body systems to maintain homeostasis by removing waste products from the blood and by helping to maintain a constant body fluid volume and composition. The urinary system comprises the kidneys, the ureters, the urinary bladder, and the urethra (Fig. 33-1). Genitourinary disorders that may cause acute pain include urinary retention,

> **NOTE**
>
> Like the pain associated with disorders of the abdomen, genitourinary disorders may produce visceral, somatic, and referred pain (see Chapter 32).

urinary tract infection (UTI), pyelonephritis, urinary calculus, epididymitis, and testicular torsion. (Other disorders specific to the female genitourinary system are addressed in Chapter 39.)

Urinary Retention

Urinary retention describes the inability to urinate. Possible causes include urethral stricture, an enlarged prostate (benign or malignant prostatic hypertrophy), central nervous system (CNS) dysfunction, foreign body obstruction, and use of certain drugs such as parasympatholytic or anticholinergic agents. Signs and symptoms include severe abdominal pain (except with CNS lesions) associated with

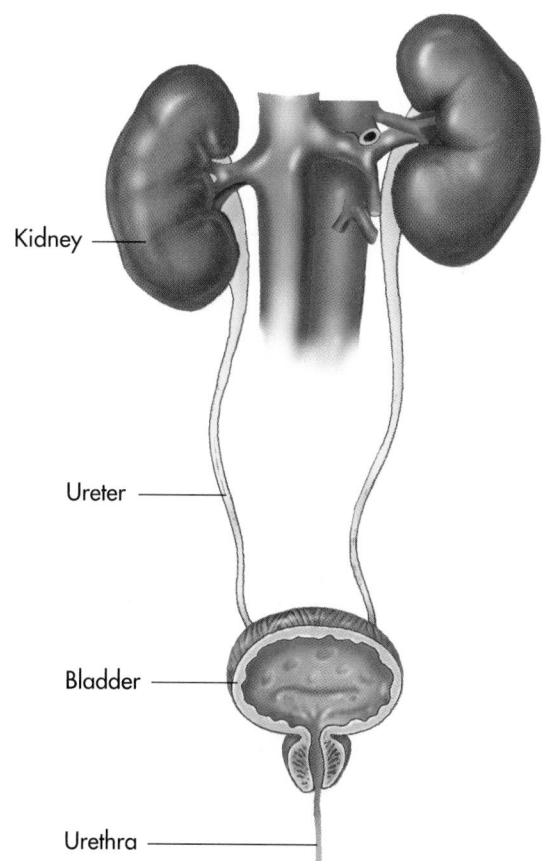

Kidney

Ureter

Bladder

Urethra

Fig. 33-1 Urinary system.

an urgent need to urinate and a distended bladder, which frequently is palpable. Patients with a progressive obstruction, such as prostatic hypertrophy, often have a history of urinary hesitancy, a poor urinary stream, a sense of incomplete emptying of the bladder, nocturia (excessive urination at night), and overflow incontinence (an overflow of urine from the bladder). In the emergency department, therapeutic intervention often requires passage of a urethral catheter to empty the bladder. Although urinary retention often is painful for the patient, prehospital care primarily is supportive. The cause of the retention should be sought, and if it is not easily correctable, the patient may require hospitalization.

? CRITICAL THINKING

Have you ever been in a situation when you needed to urinate very urgently but could not because of the circumstances? How did you feel?

Urinary Tract Infection

Urinary tract infections (UTIs) can involve the upper or lower urinary tract. Upper tract infections often are associated with pyelonephritis or intrarenal and perinephric abscesses. Infections of the lower urinary tract involve the bladder and urethra and are more common among women because the urethra is short and close to the vagina and rectum. The disease also occurs in men (as a result of urethritis, prostatitis, and cystitis) and children, although urethritis and prostatitis in young men most commonly result from a venereal disease rather than a true UTI.

NOTE

UTIs are secondary only to respiratory tract infections as a problem encountered by practicing physicians.[1]

Signs and symptoms of UTI include dysuria, urinary frequency, hematuria, and abdominal pain. Often the patient will reveal a history of UTI episodes. In addition, fever, chills, and malaise may be present. Diagnosis is confirmed in the hospital through urinalysis and microscopic examination for blood cells, sediment, and bacteria. UTIs generally are treated with antibiotic therapy.

Pyelonephritis

Pyelonephritis is inflammation of the kidney parenchyma (upper urinary tract). The disease is associated with microbial infection that reaches the kidneys from the hematogenous route or by ascending the ureters from the lower urinary tract. Pyelonephritis also is more common in women than men and in patients who have obstructive lesions along the genitourinary tract. Signs and symptoms include fever, chills, flank pain, nausea, and vomiting. Urinary frequency and dysuria often are absent in pyelonephritis. Therapeutic intervention consists primarily of antibiotics and fluid replacement and may include hospitalization. Pyelonephritis can progress to sepsis and result in renal failure.

? CRITICAL THINKING

How will you examine the patient for flank pain?

Urinary Calculus

Urinary calculi (kidney stones) are pathological concretions that originate in the renal pelvis. They result from supersaturation of the urine with insoluble salts (primarily calcium oxalate and uric acid) and most commonly occur in patients who are between the ages of 30 and 50. The disease is recurrent and is more common in men than women. Associated risk factors for this condition include dehydration, CNS disorders (absent sensory/motor impulses), drug use (anesthetics, opiates, psychotropic agents, some herbal medicines), and surgery (a postoperative complication).

NOTE

About 1% of the U.S. population will eventually form a urinary calculus.[2]

Signs and symptoms of urinary calculus vary according to location. Most stones obstruct the ureter at points of ureteral narrowing in their passage from kidneys to bladder, producing acute excruciating pain that originates in the flank area and radiates to the right or left lower abdominal quadrant, groin, and testes (in male patients). Renal or ureteral colic produces severe pain of a cyclical nature as the ureter attempts to use forceful contractions to push the stone into the bladder. This pain has often been described as having the same intensity as labor pain. The pain may be accompanied by restlessness, nausea and vomiting, urinary urgency or frequency, diaphoresis, low-grade fever, hematuria, dysuria, and increased blood pressure (secondary to pain). Definitive care includes analgesics (anesthetics, opiates, psychotropics), fluid replacement, antiemetics, and possible hospital admission. If the calculus does not pass spontaneously, surgical intervention may be required (see the box at the right).

? CRITICAL THINKING

Have you cared for or known someone who had a urinary calculus? How did that person describe the pain? What was the level of discomfort?

✓ TRICKS OF THE TRADE

Some persons who abuse narcotics will attempt to "fake" a kidney stone in order to obtain medication.

Epididymitis

Epididymitis is inflammation of the epididymis, a tubular section of the male reproductive system that carries sperm from the testicle to the seminal vesicles (see Chapter 6). Epididymitis commonly is caused by a bacterial infection associated with other structures of the genitourinary tract, and it tends to occur in sexually active young men. The most common type of epididymitis in young men results from venereal disease.[1]

Signs and symptoms of epididymitis include a gradual onset of unilateral scrotal pain that radiates to the spermatic cord. Sometimes tender swelling of the scrotum and testicle occurs, producing inflam-

✓ TRICKS OF THE TRADE

Patients with testicular pain often are embarrassed and will tell you it's "back pain."

► PREVENTION STRATEGIES FOR RECURRENT RENAL CALCULUS

The stone's composition will determine which prevention strategies are appropriate for a person with recurrent renal calculus. Patients may be advised to do the following:
- Increase water consumption
- Avoid foods containing calcium oxalate (e.g., chocolate, celery, grapes, strawberries, beans, asparagus)
- Take daily supplements of vitamin B_6 and magnesium (to reduce the formation of oxalates)
- Avoid foods that raise uric acid levels (e.g., anchovies, sardines)
- Reduce uric acid by eating a low-protein diet
- Limit salt intake to reduce the level of calcium oxalate in the urine

mation of one or both testes (orchitis). In addition, the patient may have a recent history of UTI, fever, and malaise. After physician evaluation, therapeutic intervention includes antibiotics, bed rest, analgesics, and elevation of the scrotum.

Testicular Torsion

Testicular torsion is a true urological emergency in which a testicle twists on its spermatic cord, disrupting its own blood supply. It may result from blunt trauma to the scrotal area, but it more commonly is spontaneous. The two peak periods in which torsion is likely to occur are the first year of life and at puberty, with a range in age from 5 months to 41 years, and an average of 16.2 years.[1]

Like epididymitis, testicular torsion results in a tender epididymis and painful swelling of the scrotal sac. Unlike epididymitis, however, the patient usually is afebrile. The pain is sudden in onset (often preceded by strenuous physical activity or an athletic event), severe (sometimes radiating to the ipsilateral left quadrant), unrelieved by rest or scrotal elevation, and often associated with nausea and vomiting. Testicular torsion must be diagnosed and treated within 6 hours to prevent loss of the testis from ischemic infarction.[1] Therapeutic intervention includes application of ice packs to the scrotum and manual manipulation by a physician to reduce the torsion. Because the patient must undergo surgical repair within 4 to 6 hours of onset of the torsion, rapid transport to the emergency department and efficient preoperative diagnosis are critical to a favorable outcome.

Physical Examination for Patients with Genitourinary Disorders

As described in Chapter 13, an assessment of the abdomen and genitalia of either sex can be awkward and uncomfortable for the patient and the paramedic. The patient's privacy should be protected with appropriate drapes. When possible, same-sex paramedics should perform these examinations, or a chaperon should be present. The examiner should proceed with a calm, caring, and competent attitude, and the patient and significant others should be kept informed of all actions. The examination is similar to that performed for abdominal pain (see Chapter 32) and should include the following:

- Initial assessment
- Focused history
    OPQRST
    Previous history of similar event
    Nausea or vomiting
    Change in bowel habits or stool (constipation, diarrhea)
    Change in urinary voiding pattern
    Weight loss
    Last oral intake
    Last bowel movement
- Physical examination
    Appearance
    Posture
    Level of consciousness
    Apparent state of health
    Skin color
    Vital signs
    Abdominal examination (inspection, auscultation, percussion, palpation)
    Genitalia examination (if indicated)

Management and Treatment Plan

The paramedic should manage patients with genitourinary disorders as any other patient with acute pain, including providing airway, ventilatory, and circulatory support; administering high-concentration oxygen (if indicated); ECG and vital sign monitoring; and rapid, gentle transportation for physician evaluation in the patient's position of comfort. The paramedic should not permit the patient to eat or drink, since surgery may be indicated. The administration of analgesics generally is avoided in these patients so that pain will not be masked before physician evaluation.

> **NOTE**
>
> All patients who have had persistent genitourinary pain or discomfort for more than 6 hours should be transported for physician evaluation.

Renal Failure

The kidneys play a major role in maintaining homeostasis by controlling extracellular fluid volume, maintaining proper electrolyte composition and blood pH, and eliminating waste products. If this organ system malfunctions, serious systemic consequences develop, including **uremia** with subsequent encephalopathy or pericarditis, hyperkalemia, acidosis, hypertension, and volume overload with subsequent congestive heart failure. Depending on the duration of renal failure and its potential for reversibility, the disease can be classified as *acute* or *chronic*.

> **? CRITICAL THINKING**
>
> *Think about why the patient would develop the complications just described.*

Acute Renal Failure

Acute renal failure is a clinical syndrome that results when there is a sudden and marked decrease in filtration through the glomeruli, leading to the accumulation of salt, water, and nitrogenous wastes (azotemia) within the body. Causes of acute renal failure are diverse and include trauma, shock, infection, urinary obstruction, and multisystem diseases. Acute renal failure can threaten the life of a patient, but if recognized early and treated appropriately, it may be readily reversible.

> **NOTE**
>
> Acute renal failure carries a 50% mortality rate.[3]

Acute renal failure may be classified as *prerenal, postrenal,* or *renal* in origin. Prerenal failure results from inadequate perfusion of the kidneys, which can be caused by hypovolemia, impaired cardiac output, or obstruction of renal arteries. Postrenal failure is caused by obstruction to urine flow from both kidneys. Postrenal failure may be caused by ureteral and urethral obstructions (bilateral calculi, prostatic enlargement, urethral strictures). Renal causes of acute renal failure include glomerular and other microvascular diseases, tubular diseases, and interstitial diseases that cause direct damage to the kidney parenchyma. Examples include hypertension, nephrotoxins, autoimmune diseases, and pyelonephritis.

Signs and Symptoms

The onset of acute renal failure can occur within hours. As normal kidney function rapidly deteriorates, urine output frequently decreases (oliguria) or stops completely (anuria). This results in generalized edema from water and salt retention, acidosis from failure of the kidneys to rid the body of normal acidic products, high concentrations of nonprotein nitrogens (especially urea) from failure of the body to excrete metabolic end products, and high concentrations of other products of renal excretion (such as uric acid and potassium). The resulting condition often is termed *uremia*.

If not recognized early and appropriately treated, renal dysfunction leads to the development of heart failure, volume overload, hyperkalemia, and metabolic acidosis. Definitive care is directed at restoring the normal homeostatic environment (usually by dialysis) and treating the underlying condition that has precipitated the renal failure.

Chronic Renal Failure

Chronic renal failure is a progressive, irreversible systemic disease that develops over months to years. It may be caused by congenital disorders or prolonged pyelonephritis, but in the industrialized world, it more commonly results from systemic diseases, such as diabetes and hypertension, and autoimmune disorders. This type of kidney dysfunction leads to progressive abnormality in blood counts and blood chemistry levels. In its final stages, chronic renal failure commonly requires treatment with dialysis (hemodialysis or **peritoneal dialysis**) or renal transplantation for continued patient survival. In addition to oliguria, the patient with chronic renal failure may exhibit the following six systemic manifestations:

1. Gastrointestinal manifestations
   a. Anorexia
   b. Nausea
   c. Vomiting
2. Cardiopulmonary manifestations
   a. Hypertension
   b. Pericarditis
   c. Pulmonary edema
   d. Peripheral, sacral, and periorbital edema
3. Nervous system manifestations
   a. Anxiety
   b. Delirium
   c. Progressive obtundation
   d. Hallucinations
   e. Muscle twitching
   f. Seizures
4. Metabolic or endocrine manifestations
   a. Glucose intolerance
   b. Electrolyte disturbances
   c. Anemia
5. Personality changes
   a. Fatigue
   b. Mental dullness
6. Signs of uremia
   a. Pasty, yellow skin discoloration and thin extremities from protein wasting
   b. Uremic frost caused by urea crystals that form on the skin (late finding)

Renal Dialysis

Dialysis is a technique used to normalize blood chemistry in patients with acute or chronic renal failure and to remove blood toxins in some patients who have taken a drug overdose. The two dialytic techniques are hemodialysis and peritoneal dialysis, which bring the patent's blood into contact with a semipermeable membrane across which water-soluble substances diffuse into a dialyzing fluid (dialysate). After an interval, equilibration of the patient's blood with the dialysate normalizes the electrolyte composition, and waste products are eliminated.

The amount of substance that transfers during dialysis depends on the difference in the concentrations of solutions on the two sides of the semipermeable membrane, the molecular size of the substance, and the length of time the blood and the dialysate remain in contact with the membrane. In patients with end-stage renal disease, hemodialysis usually is performed three times a week for 4 to 5 hours each time.

Hemodialysis

In hemodialysis, the patient's heparinized blood is pumped through a surgically constructed arteriovenous fistula, which is an internal anastomosis between an artery and a vein, or an arteriovenous graft, which is a synthetic material grafted to the patient's artery and vein (Fig. 33-2). These "internal shunts" usually are located in the inner aspect of the patient's forearm or much less commonly in the medial aspect of the lower extremity. Some patients may have an external dialysis catheter or a small, button-shaped device (Hemasite), usually located in the upper arm or proximal, anterior thigh. A Hemasite is similar to an AV graft but has an external rubber septum sutured to the skin through which a dialysis catheter is inserted for treatment (see Chapter 46).

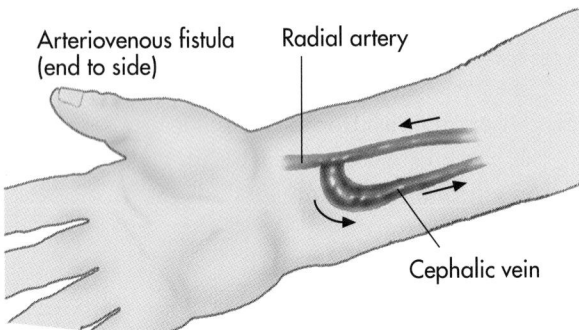

Arteriovenous fistula (end to side)   Radial artery

Cephalic vein

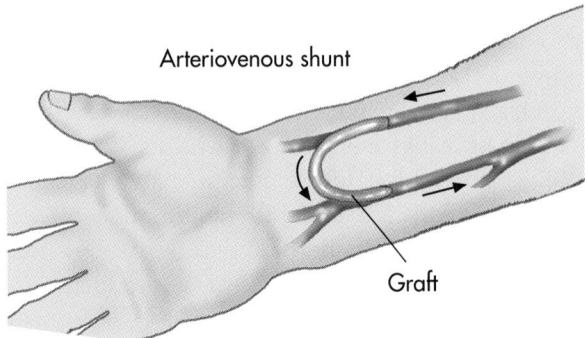

Arteriovenous shunt

Graft

Fig. 33-2 Arteriovenous shunts.

Peritoneal Dialysis

In peritoneal dialysis, the dialysis membrane is the patient's own peritoneum. The dialysate is infused into the peritoneal cavity by a temporary percutaneous or permanently implanted catheter. Fluid and solutes diffuse from the blood in the peritoneal capillaries into the dialysate. After 1 to 2 hours, when equilibration has occurred, the dialysate is drained and fresh fluid is infused. Peritoneal dialysis works considerably more slowly than hemodialysis, but over time, it is just as effective and does not require chronic blood access. A major complication of peritoneal dialysis is peritonitis, which usually results when the procedure is not performed with proper aseptic technique.

> **NOTE**
>
> Peritoneal dialysis may be carried out regularly in the home by the patient or family caregiver.

Dialysis Emergencies

Emergencies the paramedic may encounter when caring for a patient with acute or chronic renal failure may result from the disease process itself or from complications of dialytic therapy. For example, these patients may experience problems associated with vascular access, hemorrhage, hypotension, chest pain, severe hyperkalemia, **disequilibrium syndrome** (described hereafter), and the development of an air embolism. In addition, the paramedic should be aware of problems that may result from concurrent medical illness and its treatment. These include decreased ability to tolerate the stress of significant illness or trauma, inadvertent overadministration of IV fluid, and altered metabolism and unpredictable action of drugs.

> **? CRITICAL THINKING**
>
> *Which of these complications could cause an immediate life threat?*

Vascular Access Problems. Problems associated with vascular access are bleeding at the site of puncture for dialysis, thrombosis, and infection. Bleeding from the fistula or graft usually is minimal and generally can be controlled by direct pressure at the site. (However, excessive pressure can cause thrombosis in the graft or fistula.) A potential complication of an internal shunt is development of a pseudoaneurysm, which can rupture, causing a large hematoma and possible hypovolemia. If this occurs, direct pressure should be applied to the hematoma, and the patient should be assessed and treated for significant blood loss. This situation requires rapid transport for physician evaluation.

Fistulas and grafts that become occluded as a result of thrombus formation usually require surgical intervention or the administration of a thrombolytic agent to restore flow. Patients with a surgical anastomosis are instructed to periodically check for the presence of a bruit or "thrill" to verify unobstructed circulation. Attempts to clear the graft by irrigation or aspiration generally are not recommended. If thrombosis occurs while the patient is undergoing dialysis, the dialysis should be stopped and IV fluids initiated in an alternative site. Decreased blood flow is a common precipitating cause of thrombosis and is the main reason that blood pressure is not obtained in the arm with a vascular access.

Infection at the site of vascular access usually is the result of the puncture made during dialysis. Therefore meticulous sterile technique is mandatory when caring for these patients, and routine vascular access using the dialysis route should be discouraged. Vascular access infection should be considered when a dialysis patient has unexplained fever, malaise, or other signs of systemic infection.

> **NOTE**
>
> When obtaining vascular access for drawing blood or infusing IV fluids in a patient with a surgical anastomosis, the paramedic should choose an alternative site. In addition, blood pressure measurements and the use of tourniquets should be avoided in an extremity with an AV fistula or graft. Rarely, medical direction may recommend that the internal shunt be used to obtain vascular access. If so, the paramedic must be careful not to puncture the back wall of the vessel and to use careful aseptic technique throughout the procedure. IV infusions must be closely monitored to avoid a "runaway IV," and the IV catheter should be taped securely in place.

Hemorrhage. Patients receiving dialysis have an increased risk of hemorrhage because of their regular exposure to anticoagulants during hemodialysis and the decrease in their platelet function. Therefore a patient who experiences hemorrhage from trauma or a medical condition (e.g., gastrointestinal bleeding) should be closely monitored for signs of hypovolemia. Most patients on dialysis have a baseline anemia that lowers their reserves when they have acute hemorrhage. Any significant blood loss (whether external or internal) may manifest as dyspnea or angina. If hemorrhage from trauma occurs in an extremity with a fistula or graft, the paramedic should control the bleeding and immobilize the extremity, using special care to try to avoid obstructing circulation in the anastomosis.

Hypotension. Hypotension can occur with hemodialysis. This may result from the rapid reduction in intravascular volume, abrupt changes in electrolyte concentrations, or vascular instability that may occur during the procedure. In addition, the patient's compensatory mechanisms to cope with these physiological alterations may be impaired, resulting in an inability to maintain normal blood pressure. Patients with hypotension caused by dialysis must be cautiously managed with the administration of volume-expanding fluids. The paramedic should be careful not to produce a fluid overload, which may manifest as hypertension and the classic signs of congestive heart failure (Box 33-1). Most patients respond to a relatively small (200 to 300 mL) fluid challenge. If they do not, other potentially serious causes should be considered.

Chest Pain. The episodes of hypotension and mild hypoxemia that commonly occur during dialysis may

> **BOX 33-1**
>
> ### CLASSIC SIGNS OF CONGESTIVE HEART FAILURE
>
> Pulmonary edema
> Shortness of breath
> Crackles
> Engorged neck veins
> Liver congestion and engorgement
> Pitting edema

result in myocardial ischemia and chest pain. The patient also may complain of other symptoms associated with decreased oxygen delivery, such as headache and dizziness. Although these complaints may indicate an evolving myocardial infarction, they often are relieved with the administration of oxygen, fluid replacement, and antianginal medications. Regardless, all patients with chest pain should be treated as though a myocardial infarction has occurred.

Dysrhythmias resulting from myocardial ischemia also may be associated with dialysis. The most common ischemic rhythm disturbances are premature ventricular contractions (PVCs), which generally respond well to the administration of supplemental oxygen and *lidocaine* (Xylocaine). If dialysis is in progress, the procedure should be stopped, and the paramedic should consult with medical direction.

Severe Hyperkalemia. Severe hyperkalemia is a life-threatening emergency that can occur rapidly in patients with acute renal failure. The condition frequently results from poor dietary regulation and missed dialysis treatments. Patients with severe hyperkalemia may have weakness, although they frequently are relatively asymptomatic. Typical ECG changes initially demonstrate a tall or tented T wave. As the potassium levels rise, conduction slows, resulting in a prolonged PR interval, depressed ST segments, and sometimes the loss of P waves. This may be followed by a widened QRS complex and delayed conduction in the interventricular conducting system, producing patterns that resemble bundle branch blocks. Hyperkalemic disturbances may not become apparent until dangerous levels of potassium are present. Therefore any patient with renal failure who is in cardiac arrest should be suspected of having severe hyperkalemia. Based on patient history, medical direction may recommend separate infusions of *calcium* and *sodium bicarbonate* during resuscitation.

> **NOTE**
>
> Dialysis patients who have chronic renal failure tolerate increased potassium levels better than patients with normal kidney function.

Disequilibrium Syndrome. *Disequilibrium syndrome* refers to a group of neurological findings that sometimes occur during or immediately after dialysis. These symptoms are usually mild (e.g., headache, restlessness, nausea, fatigue), but they may be severe (including confusion, seizures, and coma). The syndrome is thought to result from a disproportionate decrease in osmolality of the extracellular fluid compared with that of the intracellular compartment in the brain or cerebrospinal fluid.[1] This results in an osmotic gradient between the blood and the brain, causing movement of water into the brain and subsequent cerebral edema and increased intracranial pressure. If seizures occur, *diazepam* (Valium) may be indicated.

Air Embolism. Negative pressure on the venous side of the dialysis tubing or a malfunction in the dialysis machine can allow an air embolism to enter the patient's bloodstream. If this occurs, the embolus may be carried to the right ventricle of the heart, blocking the passage of blood to the left myocardium. The patient may experience severe dyspnea, cyanosis, hypotension, and respiratory distress. A patient with an air embolus requires high-concentration oxygen administration and rapid transportation to a medical facility. In an effort to trap the embolism where it will be least likely to obstruct blood flow, the paramedic should position the patient on the left side and transport in the modified Trendelenburg position.

Management

To review, the prehospital management of patients with chronic or acute renal failure includes the following:

- Airway and ventilatory support with supplemental high-concentration oxygen administration
- Vascular access for fluid replacement, medication therapy (diuretics, antidysrhythmics, vasopressors), or fluid resuscitation if needed
- Meticulous aseptic technique if IV access is ordered by medical direction
- Electrocardiogram and other vital sign monitoring
- Rapid transport to an appropriate medical facility

S U M M A R Y

- The urinary system removes waste products from the blood and helps to maintain a constant body fluid volume and composition.

- Urinary retention is the inability to urinate.

- Urinary tract infections can involve the upper or lower urinary tract.

- Pyelonephritis is inflammation of the kidney parenchyma.

- Urinary calculi are pathological concretions that originate in the renal pelvis.

- Epididymitis is inflammation of the epididymis, a tubular section of the male reproductive system that carries sperm from the testicle to the seminal vesicles.

- Testicular torsion is a true emergency in which a testicle twists on its spermatic cord, disrupting its own blood supply.

- The physical examination for a urinary disorder is similar to that performed for abdominal pain. Patients with genitourinary pain should be managed as any other patient with acute pain.

- Renal failure may result in uremia, hyperkalemia, acidosis, hypertension, and volume overload with congestive heart failure. The classification of renal failure as acute or chronic depends on the duration and its potential for reversibility.

- Dialysis is a technique used to normalize blood chemistry in patients who have acute or chronic renal failure and to remove blood toxins. The two dialysis techniques are hemodialysis and peritoneal dialysis. Dialysis emergencies may include problems with vascular access, hemorrhage, hypotension, chest pain, severe hyperkalemia, disequilibrium syndrome, and air embolism.

REFERENCES

1. Rosen P, Barkin R: *Emergency medicine: concepts and clinical practice,* ed 4, St Louis, 1998, Mosby.
2. McCance K, Huether S: *Pathophysiology: the biologic basis for disease in adults and children,* ed 2, St Louis, 1994, Mosby.
3. US Department of Transportation National Highway Traffic Safety Administration: *EMT-Paramedic national standard curriculum,* Washington, DC, 1998, The Department.

34 Toxicology

OBJECTIVES

Upon completion of this chapter, the paramedic student will be able to:

1. Define poisoning.
2. Describe general principles for assessment and management of the patient who has ingested poison.
3. Describe the causative agents and pathophysiology of selected ingested poisons and management of patients who have taken them.
4. Describe how physical and chemical properties influence the effects of inhaled toxins.
5. Distinguish among the three categories of inhaled toxins: simple asphyxiants, chemical asphyxiants and systemic poisons, and irritants or corrosives.
6. Describe general principles of managing the patient who has inhaled poison.
7. Describe the signs, symptoms, and management of patients who have inhaled cyanide, ammonia, or hydrocarbon.
8. Describe the signs, symptoms, and management of patients injected with poison by insects, reptiles, and hazardous aquatic creatures.
9. Describe the signs, symptoms, and management of patients with organophosphate or carbamate poisoning.
10. Outline the general principles of managing patients with drug overdose.
11. Describe the effects, signs and symptoms, and specific management for selected drug overdose.
12. Describe the short- and long-term physiological effects of ethanol ingestion.
13. Describe signs, symptoms, and management of alcohol-related emergencies.
14. Identify general management principles for the most common toxic syndromes based on a knowledge of the characteristic physical findings associated with each syndrome.

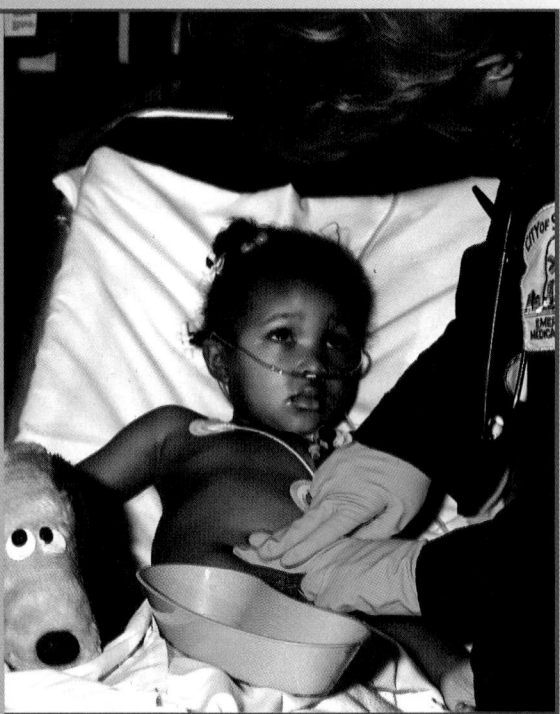

Our environment contains a large number of potentially harmful substances (natural and synthetic) that can be accidentally or deliberately introduced into the body. These include animal and plant toxins, industrial and household chemicals, therapeutic pharmaceuticals, and drugs of abuse. Early identification of these agents and prevention of systemic absorption are crucial to the successful management of patients with toxicological emergencies.

KEY TERMS

botulism: An often fatal form of food poisoning caused by the bacillus *Clostridium botulinum.*

delirium tremens: An acute and sometimes fatal psychotic reaction caused by cessation of excessive intake of alcohol over a long period of time; also known as DTs.

gastric lavage: Irrigation of the stomach with sterile water or normal saline.

Korsakoff's psychosis: A form of amnesia often seen in alcoholics, characterized by a loss of short-term memory and an inability to learn new skills.

Lyme disease: An acute, recurrent inflammatory infection transmitted by a tick.

nystagmus: Involuntary rhythmic movements of the eyes.

poison: Any substance that produces harmful physiological or psychological effects.

Rocky Mountain spotted fever: A serious tick-borne infectious disease, characterized by chills, fever, severe headache, mental confusion, and rash.

tick paralysis: A rare, progressive, reversible disorder caused by several species of ticks that release a neurotoxin that causes weakness, incoordination, and paralysis.

NOTE

Refer to the Injury Prevention section in Appendix C to review prevention strategies for toxic exposure.

? CRITICAL THINKING

How many substances that fit the definition of a poison are there in or around your home?

SECTION ONE
POISONINGS

Emergencies involving a **poison** (any substance that produces harmful physiological or psychological effects) are a significant cause of morbidity and mor-

tality in the United States. They are responsible for 10% of all emergency department visits, 9% of all ambulance patient transports, and 5% to 10% of all medical admissions to hospitals. According to the National Safety Council, poisoning by solids and liquids was the third leading cause of accidental death in the United States in 1996 and the second leading cause of accidental death for persons aged 20 to 54.[1]

Poison Control Centers

More than 70 poison control centers exist across the United States to help treat poisoning emergencies. Most are based in major medical centers or teaching hospitals, and each belongs to 1 of 41 regional poison control centers designated by the American Association of Poison Control Centers (AAPCC) (Box 34-1). Regional centers are staffed by medical professionals and offer 24-hour telephone access to population bases of at least 1 million. Each year, more than 2 million poisonings are reported to poison control centers throughout the United States. More than 90% of these poisonings happen in the home; 53% percent of poisoning victims are children younger than 6 years of age.[2] By helping people manage emergencies at home, these centers prevent about 50,000 hospitalizations and 400,000 visits to doctors' offices each year.[3]

By request, information and treatment advice is immediately provided by the poison control center through a comprehensive group of references on more than 350,000 toxic substances, including drugs (legal, illicit, foreign, and veterinary), chemicals, plants, animals, insects, fish, snakes, cosmetics, and hazardous materials. Each request for patient care information is followed up to determine effectiveness and confirm desired outcome. In addition, the centers are responsible for the following six elements of an organized poison system:

1. Treatment information and toxicological consultation with health care providers (e.g., hospitals,

BOX 34-1

CONTACTING A POISON CONTROL CENTER

Currently in the United States, poison control centers nationwide use more than 130 hotline numbers to answer calls for assistance. A new system (funded by a grant from the Centers for Disease Control and Prevention [CDC] is being developed so that calls made to one national toll-free number will be routed to the nearest local center. In Canada, the hotline numbers for poison control centers are:

Canadian Poison Control Centres

Alberta		*Ontario*	
Calgary	403-270-1414	Ottawa	613-737-1100
	800-332-1414		800-267-1373
		Toronto	416-813-5900
British Columbia			800-268-9017
Vancouver	604-682-5050		
	800-567-8911	*Prince Edward Island*	
		Halifax	800-565-8161
Manitoba		*Quebec*	
Winnipeg	204-787-2591	Sainte-Foy	418-656-8090
New Brunswick			800-463-5060
Moncton	506-857-5555		
Saint John	506-648-6222	*Saskatchewan*	
		Regina	306-766-4545
Newfoundland and Labrador			800-667-4545
St. John's	709-722-1110	Saskatoon	306-655-1010
			800-363-7474
Northwest Territories			
Yellowknife	403-920-4111	*Yukon*	
Calgary	403-270-1414	Whitehorse	403-667-8726
		Vancouver	604-682-5050
Nova Scotia			
Halifax	902-428-8161		

physicians, EMS agencies), and the public, using a toll-free number with linkage into various 911 systems
2. Professional education to train those involved in care of poisoned patients
3. Data collection on all poisonings in the region for epidemiological and evaluation purposes
4. Public education and prevention
5. Research
6. Regional EMS poison system development (e.g., patient classification criteria, triage and management protocols, and regional transfer agreements)

Use by EMS Agencies

Regional poison control centers are a ready source of information for any toxicological emergency. Depending on local communications protocol, poison control centers may be contacted directly by EMS providers (and other emergency personnel) through telephone, cellular phone, a dispatching center, or medical direction. The immediate determination of potential toxicity is based on the specific agent or agents; amount ingested; time of exposure; weight and medical condition of the patient; and any treatment rendered before EMS arrival. The poison center also can coordinate treatment protocol by notifying the receiving hospital while the patient is en route to the emergency department.

General Guidelines for Managing a Poisoned Patient

Poisons may enter the body through ingestion, inhalation, injection, and absorption. Three types of toxicological emergencies that may result in poisoning are listed in Box 34-2. Because most poisoned patients require only supportive therapy to recover (with few exceptions; e.g., the use of lifesaving antidotes), the poisoned patient often can be appropriately managed in the prehospital setting using the following guidelines:

1. Ensure adequate airway, ventilation, and circulation.
2. Obtain a thorough history and perform a focused physical examination.
3. Consider hypoglycemia in an unconscious or convulsing patient.
4. Administer *naloxone* (Narcan) or *nalmefene* (Revex) to a patient with respiratory depression.
5. If overdose is suspected, obtain an overdose history from the patient, family, or friends.
6. Consult with medical direction or a poison control center for specific management to prevent further absorption of the toxin (or antidote therapy).
7. Frequently reassess the patient; monitor vital signs and ECG.
8. Safely obtain any substance or substance container of a suspected poison and transport it with the patient.
9. Transport the patient for physician examination.

NOTE

When caring for a poisoned patient, personal safety is the top priority. A toxicological emergency response may involve hazardous materials or the possibility of patient behavior that is unpredictable or violent. If the scene is not safe, the paramedic crew should retreat to a safe staging area and wait until the scene has been secured by appropriate personnel.

Poisoning by Ingestion

About 80% of all accidental ingestion of poisons occurs in children 1 to 3 years of age. The most common poison exposures in this group result from household products such as petroleum-based agents, cleaning agents, and cosmetics; medications; toxic plants; and contaminated foods. Poisoning in adults, on the other hand, usually is intentional (although accidental poisoning from exposure to chemicals in the workplace also occurs). Deliberate poisonings often are an attempt at suicide or a result of recreational or experimental drug abuse. Intentional poisonings also may result from chemical warfare or acts of terrorism, or be a factor in assault and homicide.

BOX 34-2

TYPES OF TOXICOLOGICAL EMERGENCIES

Accidental Poisoning
Dosage errors
Idiosyncratic reactions
Childhood poisoning
Environmental exposure
Occupational exposure

Drug and Alcohol Abuse

Intentional Poisoning/Overdose
Chemical warfare
Assault/homicide
Suicide attempts

TRICKS OF THE TRADE

The poisoning/overdose patient may have a motive for the action, be it suicide, attention, or some other reason. These patients may intentionally mislead you about the amount or type of medication and the time it was ingested.

The toxic effects of ingested poisons may be immediate or delayed, depending on the substance ingested. For example, corrosive substances such as strong acids and alkalis may produce immediate tissue damage, as evidenced by burns to the lips, tongue, throat, and upper GI tract. Other substances, such as medications and toxic plants, usually require absorption and distribution through the bloodstream (and alterations by different organs) to produce toxic effects. Because only minimal absorption occurs in the stomach, poisons may take several hours to enter the bloodstream through the small intestine. Therefore early management of the ingested poisoning focuses on removing the toxin from the stomach or binding it to prevent absorption before the poison enters the intestines.

NOTE

Refer to Chapter 6 to review anatomy of the organs and structures that may affect toxic substances.

Assessment and Management

The primary goal of physical assessment of poisoned patients is to identify effects on the three vital organ systems most likely to produce immediate morbidity and mortality: the respiratory system, the cardiovascular system, and the central nervous system. A detailed history of the event and any past significant medical and/or psychiatric history also is important and may help direct patient management decisions in the field or in the emergency department.

Respiratory Complications

The first priority in managing a poisoned patient after ensuring scene safety is to secure a patent airway and provide adequate ventilatory support. This includes providing high-concentration oxygen and possibly aggressive airway management to protect against potential airway compromise or aspiration (see Chapter 11). Other respiratory complications that may be associated with poisoning include the early development of noncardiogenic pulmonary edema or the later development of adult respiratory distress syndrome (see Chapter 27). Bronchospasm may result from direct or indirect toxic effects.

Cardiovascular Complications

The most common cardiovascular complication of poisoning by ingestion is cardiac rhythm disturbances. Therefore the patient's circulatory status should be assessed and continually monitored by ECG and frequent blood pressure measurements. The presence of tachydysrhythmias or bradydysrhythmias may indicate serious metabolic disorders such as hypoxia and acidosis. Other cardiovascular complications include the development of hypotension (associated with decreased vascular tone) and, rarely, hypertension, which may lead to cerebral vascular hemorrhage. (Toxicology in emergency cardiac care is further addressed in the appendix at the end of this chapter.)

Neurological Complications

A baseline neurological examination should be performed and documented. Deviations from a normal sensorium may range from mild drowsiness and agitation to hallucinations, seizures, coma, and death. Neurological complications may result from the toxin itself, such as lead poisoning in children who have ingested paint chips, or be secondary to an underlying metabolic or perfusion disorder.

History

A thorough history of the exposure and any significant medical history should be obtained from the patient, family members, or bystanders. Although this information may be unreliable (as in cases involving pediatric patients, drug abuse, or suicide attempts), the following should be ascertained if possible:

- What was ingested? (Obtain the poison container and remaining contents unless doing so poses a threat to rescuer safety.)
- When was the substance ingested? (This may affect the decision to use *activated charcoal* or gastric lavage, to induce emesis, or to administer an antidote.)
- How much of the substance was ingested?
- Was an attempt made to induce vomiting?
- Has an antidote or *activated charcoal* been administered?
- Does the patient have a psychiatric history pertinent to suicide attempts or episodes of recent depression?

Gastrointestinal Decontamination

The goal of managing serious poisonings that occurred by ingestion is to prevent the toxic substance from reaching the small intestine, thereby limiting its absorption. This may be accomplished by gastrointestinal decontamination through the use of *activated charcoal*, and sometimes **gastric lavage** or *syrup of ipecac*. (Using *activated charcoal* alone for GI decontamination is considered equivalent or superior to other methods and has fewer complications.[4]) Before attempting gastrointestinal decontamination, the paramedic should consult with medical direction or a poison control center.

Activated Charcoal

Activated charcoal is an inert, nontoxic product of wood material that has been heated to extremely high temperature. The surface characteristics of *activated charcoal* enable it to *adsorb* (collect in a condensed form) molecules of many chemical toxins while in the intestinal tract, thereby inhibiting absorption of the poison by as much as 50% and preventing systemic toxicity.

Activated charcoal is considered a safe and effective treatment for most toxic ingestions (Box 34-3) and is administered in nearly all cases except when strong acid, strong alkali, or ethanol is the toxicant. Other agents not well adsorbed by *activated charcoal* include cyanide, ferrous sulfate, and methanol. If these substances have been ingested, *activated charcoal* should probably be withheld; consult with medical direction or a poison control center. It also may be withheld when specific oral antidotes (e.g., N-Acetylcysteine [Mucomyst] for acetaminophen overdose) are available and when the ingestion occurred 1 or more hours before presentation.

Activated charcoal comes mixed in an aqueous solution with or without a cathartic (an agent that causes bowel evacuation). A cathartic (most commonly sorbitol) decreases the transit time and expels the charcoal within a short period. Complications of *activated charcoal* therapy include poor patient acceptance and vomiting. EMS personnel should protect themselves, the patient, and the immediate area from the staining properties of *activated charcoal* and should use personal protective measures when administering this agent.

? CRITICAL THINKING

Why might a patient be reluctant to take activated charcoal?

Gastric Lavage

Gastric lavage is a method of gastrointestinal decontamination that has the advantage immediate recovery of a portion of gastric contents (if performed within 1 hour after ingestion). It also provides a method for the administration of *activated charcoal.*

NOTE

The first dose of *activated charcoal* sometimes is administered via lavage before actual lavage to allow immediate adsorption of toxins and before accidental passage of some stomach contents through the pylorus into the duodenum. In this case, the instilled charcoal may serve as a marker for lavage by continuing evacuation until charcoal clears (usually 2 to 3 L).

Gastric lavage generally is performed by using a large-bore orogastric tube (36 to 40 French in adults, 24 to 28 French in children) rather than a smaller nasogastric tube, which may be too narrow to empty

BOX 34-3

DOSAGE OF ACTIVATED CHARCOAL

1 to 2 g/kg body weight
   30 to 100 g in adults
   15 to 30 g in children
   Prepared in a slurry and administered orally or by gastric tube

the stomach if large particle or pill fragments are present. These large tubes should rarely be inserted nasally, because they may damage the mucosa or turbinates and result in epistaxis. The procedure for gastric lavage is as follows:

1. Place the conscious patient in a left lateral Trendelenburg's ("swimmer's") position to minimize the possibility of aspiration in case of emesis. Endotracheal intubation should precede gastric lavage in patients with a depressed level of consciousness or in those without an intact gag reflex.
2. Insert the tube through the mouth into the patient's esophagus and continue to advance the tube until it is placed in the stomach. If resistance to passage is noted, the procedure must cease.
3. Check tube placement before lavage by air insufflation into the stomach with a large syringe.
4. Aspirate gastric contents to confirm correct placement.
5. Infuse tap water or normal saline in amounts not to exceed 150 to 200 mL aliquots in adults or 50 to 100 mL aliquots in patients younger than 5 years of age.

NOTE

To prevent water absorption and resultant fluid-electrolyte derangements in pediatric patients, only normal saline should be infused.

6. Continue gastric lavage until the return fluid appears clear. The return fluid should be about the same amount as the fluid administered.

Gastric lavage is contraindicated in patients with unprotected airways and altered levels of consciousness and those who have ingested low-viscosity hydrocarbons or caustic agents. Gastric lavage can be performed in patients with depressed consciousness, but the airway should be protected with endotracheal intubation before the procedure. Potential complications include agitation of the patient (produced by the procedure), inadvertent tracheal intubation, esophageal perforation, aspiration pneumonitis, and as previously stated, fluid and electrolyte imbalances in pediatric patients.

> **NOTE**
>
> Gastric lavage is recommended only for patients who have ingested a potentially lethal amount of drug or toxin and who present within 1 hour after ingestion. In obtunded or comatose patients, rapid sequence intubation (RSI) should be performed before gastric lavage to prevent aspiration pneumonia.[4]

Syrup of Ipecac

Syrup of ipecac was once considered the treatment of choice in preventing absorption of poisons. However, studies have shown that ipecac-induced emesis reduces absorption by only about 30% and that its use may interfere with the efficacy of other methods of decontamination, such as *activated charcoal*. If *syrup of ipecac* is administered, it should be given within the first 20 minutes after ingestion of a poison and only in patients who are alert with a gag reflex (Box 34-4). Potential complications of ipecac-induced emesis include Mallory-Weiss tear of the esophagus, pneumomediastinum, fatal diaphragmatic or gastric rupture, and aspiration pneumonitis. Contraindications include the following:

- Altered level of consciousness
- Ingestion of caustic substances (the esophagus would be exposed to the agent twice)
- Loss of gag reflex
- Seizures
- Pregnancy
- Acute myocardial infarction
- Ingestion of:
  Acids
  Alkalis
  Ammonia
  Nontoxic agents
  Petroleum distillates (unless advised otherwise by medical direction or poison control)
  Rapidly acting CNS depressants (e.g., cyanide, tricyclic antidepressants)

Rapidly acting CNS irritants (e.g., strychnine)
Hydrocarbons (controversial)

Management of Specific Ingested Poisons

Specific ingested poisons discussed in this section include strong acids and alkalis, hydrocarbons, methanol, ethylene glycol, isopropanol, metals (iron, lead, and mercury), and poisons from food and plants. Because few effective antidotes can be used in poisoning situations, supportive and symptomatic management and prevention of absorption are the primary approaches in caring for the poisoned patient.

Strong Acids and Alkalis

Strong acids and alkalis (such as those found in toilet bowl cleaners, rust remover, ammonia, and most liquid drain cleaners [Box 34-5]) may cause burns to the mouth, pharynx, esophagus, and sometimes the upper respiratory and GI tracts. Perforation of the esophagus or stomach may result in vascular collapse, mediastinitis, or pneumoperitoneum. The frequency of caustic ingestions (most commonly lye) is highest in small children, accounting for 5000 to 8000 accidental exposures each year.[1]

Ingestions of caustic and corrosive substances generally produce immediate damage to the mucous membrane and the intestinal tract. Acids generally complete their damage within 1 to 2 minutes after exposure, whereas alkali, particularly solid alkali, may continue to cause liquefaction of tissue, and damage for minutes to hours. Therefore prehospital care usually is limited to airway and venti-

> **BOX 34-4**
>
> ### DOSAGE OF IPECAC
>
> **Patients 1 to 12 years**
> Contraindicated for patients less than 1 year old
> 15 mL of *ipecac* followed by two to three glasses of water
> May be repeated in 20 minutes if vomiting does not occur
>
> **Patients Over 12 years**
> 30 mL of *ipecac* followed by two to three glasses of water
> May be repeated in 20 minutes if vomiting does not occur

latory support, IV fluid replacement, and rapid transport to an appropriate medical facility.

In some situations, medical direction may recommend attempts to dilute the acid or alkali in a conscious patient with oral administration of milk or water (200 to 300 mL in the adult, 15 mL/kg maximum in a child). Efforts to neutralize the ingested agent with other fluids, such as fruit juice, lemon juice, or vinegar, are contraindicated because of the potential for intense exothermic reactions, which may produce severe thermal burns.

? CRITICAL THINKING

What is a risk of administering milk or water to a patient with this type of ingestion?

Hydrocarbons

Hydrocarbons are a group of saturated and unsaturated compounds derived primarily from crude oil, coal, or plant sources. Mixtures vary in their viscosity, surface tension, and volatility, which with other factors (such as the presence of other chemicals in the product, total amount, and route of exposure) determine the toxic effects of these agents.

Hydrocarbons are found in many household products (cleaning and polishing agents [mineral seal oil or signal oil], spot removers, paints, cosmetics, pesticides, hobby and craft materials) and in petroleum distillates (turpentine, kerosene, gasoline, lighter fluids, and pine-oil products). In addition, a large group of halogenated hydrocarbons (carbon tetrachloride, trichloromethane, trichloroethylene,

methyl chloride) and aromatic hydrocarbons (toluene, xylene, benzene) exist. Hydrocarbon poisonings are common, accounting for 7% of all ingestions in children under 5 years of age.[1] Most ingestions occur between May and September, when home use of petroleum products allows children the greatest amount of exposure.

The most important physical characteristic in the potential toxicity of ingested hydrocarbons is its viscosity: the lower the viscosity, the higher the risk of aspiration and associated complications. For example, an ingested hydrocarbon product with a low viscosity, such as gasoline or turpentine, rapidly disperses over the pharyngeal and glottic surfaces, the more volatile components becoming gases on contact with the warm mucous membranes. This exposure causes irritation, coughing, and possible aspiration, which may allow a toxic amount of hydrocarbons to enter the tracheobronchial tree. Chemical characteristics (aromatic, aliphatic, or halogenated) and the presence of toxic additives also are important in determining toxicity.

The clinical features of hydrocarbon ingestion vary widely, depending on the type of agent involved (Box 34-6). If the patient is asymptomatic on EMS arrival, the chances of serious complications usually are minimal. These patients generally are observed in the emergency department for several hours and often require no treatment. However, any patient suspected of hydrocarbon ingestion who coughs, chokes, cries, or has spontaneous emesis on swallowing should be assumed to have aspirated until proven otherwise. Hydrocarbon ingestion may involve the patient's respiratory, gastrointestinal, and neurological systems; clinical features may

---

BOX 34-5

COMMON ACID AND ALKALI SUBSTANCES

Acids
Hydrochloric acid
    Metal cleaners
    Swimming pool cleaners
    Toilet bowl cleaners
Sulfuric acid
    Battery acid
    Toilet bowl cleaners
Phenol
Acetic acid
Bleach disinfectants

Alkalis
Sodium or potassium hydroxide (lye)
    Washing powders
    Paint removers
Drainpipe and toilet bowl cleaners
Disk (button) batteries
Bleach
Ammonia
    Metal cleaners or polishes
    Hair dyes and tints
    Jewelry cleaners

BOX 34-6

CLINICAL FEATURES OF HYDROCARBON INGESTION

Immediate: Up to 6 Hours
Gastrointestinal system
Mucous membrane hyperemia
Irritation
Abdominal pain
Nausea and vomiting
Belching

Respiratory system
Cough and choking
Inspiratory stridor
Tachypnea
Cyanosis
Dyspnea

Neurological system
Lethargy
Coma
Seizures

Systemic factors
Fever
Malaise

Delayed: Days to Weeks
Gastrointestinal system
Diarrhea
Hepatic toxicity

Respiratory system
Bacterial pneumonia
Dyspnea
Sputum production
Atelectasis
Pulmonary edema

Systemic factors
Spontaneous hemorrhage
Hemolytic and aplastic anemias

---

be immediate or delayed in onset. Emergency care for symptomatic patients who have ingested hydrocarbon products includes the following:

1. Ensure a patent airway and provide adequate ventilatory and circulatory support as needed.
2. Identify the substance and contact medical direction or a poison control center.

3. Gastric decontamination generally is avoided in these patients to prevent potential aspiration pneumonitis. It is contraindicated with ingestion of mineral seal oil, signal oil, or polishing oils because of their low viscosity and the likelihood of aspiration. Medical direction may recommend gastric emptying of a petroleum product containing significant amounts (greater than 1 mL/kg) of camphor, benzene and its derivatives, organophosphates, halogenated hydrocarbons, and heavy metals such as arsenicals, lead, and mercury. In these situations, the chance of systemic toxicity is greater than the risk of aspiration. (The use of **activated charcoal** or diluents has not been shown to be effective in managing hydrocarbon ingestion.)
4. Initiate IV fluid therapy.
5. Monitor cardiac rhythm.
6. Transport for physician evaluation.

? CRITICAL THINKING

Will the potential lethal effects of this ingestion always be visible on the scene?

Methanol

Methanol (wood alcohol) is a common industrial solvent obtained from distillation of wood. It is a poisonous alcohol found in a variety of products, such as gas line antifreeze, windshield washer fluid, paints, paint removers, varnishes, canned fuels such as Sterno, and many shellacs. Methanol is a colorless liquid that has an odor distinct from that of ethanol, the form of alcohol designed for consumption. Poisonings may result from intentional or accidental ingestions, absorption through the skin, or inhalation. Examples include deliberate use of the agent by chronic alcoholics to maintain an inebriated state, accidental ingestion resulting from misuse or distribution of methanol for ethanol (as in contraband liquor), and accidental ingestions in children.

Methanol itself is no more toxic than ethanol, but its metabolites are extremely toxic. (Death has been reported after ingestion of 15 mL of a 40% solution.[4]) As the alcohol is absorbed, it rapidly is converted in the liver to formaldehyde and in minutes to formic acid. The accumulation of formic acid in the blood results in a group of symptoms relating to the central nervous system (depression), the gastrointestinal tract (pain, nausea, vomiting), the eyes (as little as 4 mL causing blindness), and the development of metabolic acidosis. The onset of symptoms after ingestion ranges from 40 minutes to 72 hours.

? CRITICAL THINKING

Do you think this could have been the origin of the expression "blind drunk"?

The symptoms of methanol poisoning correlate with the degree of acidosis and may include the following:

- CNS depression
  Lethargy
  Confusion
  Coma
  Seizures
- Gastrointestinal tract
  Nausea and vomiting
  Abdominal pain
- Visual complaints
  Photophobia
  Blurred or indistinct vision
  Pupils that are dilated and sluggish to react to light
  "Spots before the eyes"
  "Snow-filled vision"
  Blindness
- Metabolic acidosis
  Shortness of breath
  Tachypnea
  Shock
  Multisystem failure
  Death

Emergency care for methanol poisoning is as follows:

1. Supportive care: Secure a patent airway and provide adequate ventilatory and circulatory support as needed. Adequate ventilation is essential to ensure adequate oxygenation, help correct the profound metabolic acidosis, and maximize respiratory excretion. An IV line should be established, and the patient should be placed on a cardiac monitor to detect rhythm disturbances.
2. Gastrointestinal decontamination: If the patient is seen within 1 hour after ingestion, gastric lavage is indicated. The efficacy of **activated charcoal**

in adsorbing methanol is controversial. Consult with medical direction or a poison control center.
3. Correction of metabolic acidosis: Attempts to correct metabolic acidosis with **sodium bicarbonate** administration (1 mEq/kg) may be recommended by medical direction. Larger or repeated doses may be necessary. Although serum formic acid may be neutralized with bicarbonate administration, hemodialysis probably will be necessary to remove toxic levels of methanol and formate.
4. Prevention of the conversion of methanol to formic acid: The conversion of methanol to formic acid may be prevented by the administration of ethanol. (Ethanol has a nine-times-greater affinity for the enzyme that converts methanol to formic acid.) If the patient is conscious, give 30 to 60 mL of 80-proof ethanol by mouth or gastric lavage tube. Unconscious patients should have their airway protected with an endotracheal tube before gastric tube administration of ethanol.
5. Transport: Rapidly transport the patient to an appropriate medical facility for definitive treatment.

Ethylene Glycol

Ethylene glycol is a colorless, odorless, water-soluble liquid commonly used in windshield deicers, detergents, paints, radiator antifreeze, and coolants. Because of the brilliant coloring agents added to these preparations, their widespread availability, and the warm, sweet taste, accidental ingestion of ethylene glycol is common in young children. The agent also is commonly misused by alcoholics as a substitute for ethanol. As little as 60 mL has been reported lethal to an adult.[5]

Early signs and symptoms of CNS depression usually are caused by the ethanol-like effects of ethylene glycol. However, toxicity from ethylene glycol, as from methanol, is caused by the accumulation of intermediary metabolites, especially glycolic and oxalic acids after metabolism, which occurs primarily in the liver and kidneys. These metabolic intermediaries may affect the central nervous system and cardiopulmonary and renal systems and result in hypocalcemia (from the precipitation of oxalic acid as calcium oxalate). The signs and symptoms of ethylene glycol poisoning generally occur in three stages:

1. Stage One: Central nervous system effects occurring 1 to 12 hours after ingestion
   a. Slurred speech

b. Ataxia
c. Somnolence
d. Nausea and vomiting
e. Focal or generalized convulsions
f. Hallucinations
g. Stupor
h. Coma

? CRITICAL THINKING

What could the effects in stage one of ethylene glycol poisoning be mistaken for?

2. Stage Two: Cardiopulmonary system effects occurring 12 to 36 hours after ingestion
   a. Rapidly progressive tachypnea
   b. Cyanosis
   c. Pulmonary edema
   d. Cardiac failure
3. Stage Three: Renal system effects occurring 24 to 72 hours after ingestion
   a. Flank pain
   b. Cluster of urological symptoms (oliguria, crystalluria, proteinuria, anuria, hematuria, uremia)

Emergency care for ethylene glycol poisoning is similar to that used in managing methanol poisoning and includes the following:

1. Ensure a patent airway and provide adequate ventilatory and circulatory support as needed. Monitor the patient for dysrhythmias.
2. Use gastric lavage if the patient is seen within 1 hour after ingestion. Administer **activated charcoal,** which has been shown to decrease gastrointestinal absorption of ethylene glycol by 50%.
3. Initiate IV fluid therapy with a volume-expanding fluid to maintain adequate urine output.
4. Administer IV **sodium bicarbonate** (per protocol) to correct acidosis.
5. Administer 80-proof ethanol (30 to 60 mL) by mouth or gastric tube to block the conversion of ethylene glycol into toxic metabolites. Unmetabolized ethylene glycol is excreted by the lungs and kidneys.
6. Rapidly transport the patient for definitive treatment, which may include hemodialysis and continued ethanol administration.

In addition, the paramedic should anticipate orders from medical direction or a poison control center for the following medications:

- **Thiamine** to degrade glycolic acid to nontoxic metabolites
- **Calcium gluconate** or **calcium chloride** to manage hypocalcemia
- **Diazepam** (Valium) to control seizure activity

Isopropanol

Isopropanol (isopropyl alcohol) is a volatile, flammable, colorless liquid with a characteristic odor and bittersweet taste. Rubbing alcohol is the most common household source of this agent. It also is used in disinfectants, degreasers, cosmetics, industrial solvents, and cleaning agents. Common routes of toxic exposure to isopropanol include intentional ingestion as a substitute for ethanol, accidental ingestion, and inhalation of high concentrations of local vapor, as from alcohol sponging of febrile children (a harmful and inappropriate procedure). Isopropanol is more toxic than ethanol but less toxic than methanol or ethylene glycol. A potentially lethal dose in adults is 150 to 240 mL.[5] In children, any amount of ingestion should be considered potentially toxic.

After ingestion, the majority of isopropanol (80%) is metabolized to acetone. The rest is excreted unchanged by the kidneys. The acetone is excreted by the kidneys and to a lesser extent by the lungs. Isopropanol poisoning affects several body systems, including the central nervous, gastrointestinal, and renal systems. Signs and symptoms frequently occur within 30 minutes after ingestion and include central nervous system and respiratory depression (isopropanol is two to three times more potent a CNS depressant than ethanol), abdominal pain, gastritis, hematemesis, and hypovolemia. Although isopropanol poisoning causes acetonemia and ketonuria, there usually is no associated metabolic acidosis unless the patient manifests hypotension.

Emergency care for isopropanol poisoning primarily is supportive and includes airway and ventilatory support to ensure adequate respiratory elimination of acetone, gastric lavage (isopropanol also is secreted by the salivary glands and stomach), fluid resuscitation as needed, and rapid transport to an appropriate medical facility, where dialysis may be necessary. Administration of ethanol has not proven to inhibit the toxic metabolite to the same degree as in methanol or ethylene glycol poisoning.

Metals

Infants and children are high-risk groups for accidental iron, lead, and mercury poisoning due to their immature immune systems or increased absorption as a function of age.

Iron poisoning. About 10% of the ingested iron (mainly ferrous sulfate) is absorbed each day from the small intestine. After absorption, the iron is converted, stored in iron storage protein, and transported to the liver, spleen, and bone marrow for incorporation into hemoglobin. When ingested iron exceeds the body's ability to store it, the free iron circulates in the blood and is deposited into other tissues.

> **NOTE**
>
> Most iron poisonings result from the ingestion of pediatric multivitamins by children under 6 years of age.[2]

Accidental or intentional ingestion of iron may have lethal complications. Ingested iron is corrosive to gastrointestinal tract mucosa and may produce GI hemorrhage, bloody vomitus, painless bloody diarrhea, and dark stools. In severe cases (ingestion of more than 20 mg/kg), iron toxicity can produce cardiovascular collapse and death 12 to 48 hours after ingestion.

Prehospital care includes supportive measures and rapid transport for physician evaluation and possible gastrointestinal decontamination to prevent further absorption. The administration of *activated charcoal* generally is not recommended, because it adsorbs iron poorly. Most patients with iron poisoning survive the episode, and the long-term prognosis is favorable.

Lead poisoning. Metallic lead has been used by humans for more than 5000 years but was not widely recognized as a potential health hazard until 1978 when it was banned from household paints in the United States (Box 34-7). Children are the most common victims of lead poisoning; an estimated 889,000 children in the United States have levels of lead in their bloodstream of 10 mg/dL or greater.[6] Most pediatric poisonings results from ingestion of lead-based paint chips and contaminated house dust. Lead toxicity in adults most commonly results from exposure by inhalation. If not detected early, children with high levels of lead in their bodies can suffer from damage to the brain and nervous system, behavioral and learning problems, hyperactivity, slowed growth, hearing problems, and headaches. Adults can suffer from a number of problems including the following:

- Difficulties during pregnancy
- Reproductive problems
- Hypertension
- GI disorders
- Nerve disorders
- Memory and concentration problems
- Muscle and joint pain

> **NOTE**
>
> Even children who appear healthy can have dangerous levels of lead in their bodies.

BOX 34-7

PLACES WHERE LEAD CAN BE FOUND

Homes in the city, country, or suburbs

Apartments, single-family homes, and both private and public housing painted before 1978

Soil around a home (soil contaminated from exterior paint, or other sources such as past use of leaded gasoline in cars)

Painted windows and window sills

Doors and door frames

Stairs, railings, and banisters

Porches and fences

Paint surfaces that have been scraped, dry-sanded, or heated (lead dust)

Old painted toys and furniture

The air after vacuuming or sweeping contaminated surfaces

Food and liquid stored in lead crystal or lead-glazed pottery or porcelain

Lead smelters or other industries

Hobbies that use lead (e.g., making pottery or stained glass)

Folk remedies ("greta" or "azarcon" used to treat an upset stomach)

Most lead poisoning is slow in onset (from chronic ingestion or inhalation), eventually resulting in toxicity. The metal is excreted by the body very slowly and tends to accumulate in body tissues (primarily bone). Lead causes the most significant pathophysiology in the hematopoietic, neurological, and renal systems; however, it also affects the reproductive, GI, skeletal, hepatic, and cardiovascular systems. Signs and symptoms of chronic exposure generally are nonspecific and may include malaise, mental disturbances, incoordination, abdominal pain, diarrhea, and vomiting. If the intoxication is acute, anemia, weakness or paralysis of the limbs, seizures, and death may result. (If symptoms progress to include seizure and coma, the risk of death is high. Patients who survive are likely to sustain brain damage.) Prehospital care is focused on recognizing the potential for lead poisoning and transporting the patient for physician evaluation.

Lead poisoning is diagnosed from the patient's condition and history, from blood tests to measure lead levels, from x-rays of the bones and abdomen that may reveal lead deposits, and with urine tests to measure the level of lead breakdown products. Following GI decontamination, whole bowel irrigation may be indicated after an acute lead ingestion when evidence exists of lead in the stomach or small bowel. Many adults and children who have high lead levels from chronic exposure require in-hospital and outpatient chelation therapy to detoxify the lead and help the body excrete the metal at a faster rate. All patients must be discharged to a lead-free environment.

> ### ? CRITICAL THINKING
>
> *Aside from emergency management of lead poisoning, what other role can paramedics play in the management of this problem?*

Mercury poisoning. Mercury is the only metallic element that is liquid at room temperature. It is used in thermometers, sphygmomanometers, and dental amalgam (dental fillings). Various compounds of mercury also are used in some paints, pesticides, cosmetics, drugs, and in certain industrial processes. All forms of mercury (except dental amalgam) are poisonous. Some, however, are absorbed into the body more readily than others and therefore are more dangerous.

Liquid mercury is highly volatile and mercury vapor readily is absorbed into the body via the lungs. Inhalation of mercury vapor (the most common route of poisoning) may cause shortness of breath and lung damage. Mercury also may be absorbed through the skin (causing severe inflammation) or intestines after ingestion, resulting in nausea, vomiting, diarrhea, and abdominal pain. After mercury enters the body, it passes into the bloodstream and later accumulates in various organs (principally the brain and kidneys), causing a wide range of symptoms that may include the following:

- Malaise
- Incoordination
- Excitability
- Tremors
- Numbness in the limbs
- Vision impairment
- Nausea and emesis (symptoms of renal failure)
- Mental status changes

Prehospital care primarily is supportive. Following physician evaluation, patients are managed with GI decontamination (if the ingestion was recent) and chelating agents. In severe cases, hemodialysis may be indicated.

Food Poisoning

Food poisoning is a term used for any illness of sudden onset (usually associated with stomach pain, vomiting, and diarrhea) suspected of being caused by food eaten within the previous 48 hours. Food poisoning can be classified as *infectious*, resulting from bacteria or virus, or *noninfectious*, resulting from toxins or pollutants. Some foods also can cause poisoning of either type (e.g., shellfish such as mussels, clams, and oysters, which may be contaminated by viruses or bacteria or by toxins or chemical pollutants in water).

Infectious (bacterial) types. One of the common types of bacteria responsible for food poisoning is salmonella, an organism found in many animals (especially poultry) as well as humans. Salmonella bacteria also may be transferred to food from the excrement of infected animals or humans and by food handling by an infected person. Other bacteria (e.g., strains of staphylococcal bacteria) cause formation of toxins, which may be difficult to destroy even with thorough cooking. Other bacteria that commonly cause diarrhea are certain strains of *Escherichia coli* (traveler's diarrhea) and *Campylobacter* and *Shigella* organisms.

Botulism is a rare but life-threatening form of food poisoning that may result from eating improperly canned or preserved food contaminated with the bacterium *Clostridium botulinum*. This is found in soil and untreated water in most parts of the world and is harmlessly present in the intestinal tracts of many animals, including fish. Its spore-forming properties resist boiling, salting, smoking, and some forms of pickling, allowing the bacterium to thrive in improperly preserved or canned foods.

Although botulism is rare, the disease is more common in the United States than elsewhere in the world because of the popularity of preserving food in the home. Botulism is associated with severe CNS symptoms that appear in a characteristic head-to-toe progression: headache, blurred or double vision, dysphagia, respiratory paralysis, and quadriplegia. Death from respiratory failure occurs in about 70% of untreated cases. *Pseudomembranous colitis* (associated with long-term administration of certain antibiotics) is another life-threatening form of diarrhea, often caused by *Clostridium difficile*.

Infectious (viral) types. The viruses that most commonly cause food poisoning are Norwalk virus, a common contaminant of shellfish, and rotavirus. These agents may be responsible for illness when raw or partly cooked foodstuffs have been in contact with water contaminated by human excrement.

Noninfectious types. Noninfectious types of food poisoning may result from consuming mushrooms and toadstools or from eating fresh foods and vegetables accidentally contaminated with large amounts of insecticide. Chemical food poisoning also may result from eating food stored in a contaminated container (e.g., a container previously used to store poison) and from improperly preparing and cooking various exotic foods. Drugs or medications also can cause diarrhea. Quinidine, certain antacids, some antibiotics, and stool softeners or laxatives may cause diarrhea.

Management guidelines. The onset of signs and symptoms from food poisoning varies by cause and by how heavily the food was contaminated. As a rule, symptoms usually develop within 30 minutes in the

case of chemical poisoning, in 1 to 12 hours in the case of bacterial toxins, and in 12 to 48 hours with viral and bacterial infections. General principles of management for patients with suspected food poisoning include the following:

- Use precautions to avoid contamination of self (gloves, gown if appropriate) and equipment.
- Ensure adequate airway, ventilatory, and circulatory support.
- Gather a complete history, including time and onset of symptoms, recent travel, the relation of symptoms to ingestion of a particular food, and effects on others who ate the same food. In addition, information on the consistency, frequency, and odor of stool (including the presence of mucus or blood) should be obtained, and fever should be noted. Any patient history also should include significant past medical history, allergies, and use of medications.
- Initiate IV therapy with a crystalloid solution to manage dehydration and electrolyte disturbances resulting from vomiting and diarrhea.
- Transport the patient for physician evaluation.

Plant Poisoning

Toxic plant ingestion is a frequently reported category of poisonings, second only to ingestion of cleaning substances.[1] The majority of these exposures occur in children under 6 years of age.

> **? CRITICAL THINKING**
>
> *What features of a plant would make it attractive for children to eat?*

Signs and symptoms. The toxic manifestations of major poisonous plant ingestions are predictable and are categorized by the chemical and physical properties of the plant. Most human physiological responses tend to be consistent with the type of major toxic chemical component in the plant, although some disparities exist. For example, anticholinergic crisis may result from ingestion of certain alkaloid components (jimsonweed and lantana), manifesting in tachycardia, dilated pupils, hot dry skin, decreased bowel sounds, altered vision, and abnormal mental status; cholinergic symptoms may result from ingestion of certain mushroom species, which usually is manifested by bradycardia, miosis, salivation, hyperactive bowel sounds, and diarrhea; and nicotinic alkaloids (poison hemlock and delphinium) may initially act as stimulants but generally are soon followed by depression and weakness. Most signs and symptoms appear within several hours after ingestion, but some symptoms may be delayed 1 to 3 days. Box 34-8 lists common poisonous plants. Paramedics should be familiar with common poisonous plant life in their response area.

Management. Several hundred species of green plants and more than 100 varieties of mushrooms in the United States contain toxic compounds. Many similar species of plants and mushrooms have widely varying potencies and combinations of toxins, and such factors as the age of the plant and soil conditions may influence the severity of toxic symptoms. Management guidelines should therefore be customized to the patient's symptoms rather than to a particular type of ingestion. Although it is important to identify the plant if possible, the inability to do so should not delay management. As always, the paramedic should consult with medical direction or a poison control center regarding appropriate emergency care procedures. Principles in the management of toxic plant ingestion generally include the following:

1. Ensure adequate airway, ventilatory, and circulatory support.
2. In patients with a depressed gag reflex, unresponsiveness, or seizures, secure the airway with an endotracheal tube, and then use orogastric decontamination. Medical direction or a poison control center may recommend administration of **activated charcoal** in place of gastric emptying or after it.
3. Initiate IV fluid therapy with a volume-expanding solution.
4. Monitor the patient's vital signs and cardiac rhythm.
5. Obtain a sample of the suspected plant or mushroom (if possible).
6. Transport the patient for physician evaluation. Most patients are hospitalized for observation and treatment as indicated for the toxin involved. Dialysis has not been shown to be effective in removing most plant toxins.

BOX 34-8

COMMON POISONOUS PLANTS, TREES, AND SHRUBS

House Plants
Dieffenbachia
Hyacinth
Narcissus
Mistletoe
Oleander
Poinsettia

Flower-Garden Plants
Daffodil
Foxglove
Iris
Larkspur
Lily of the valley

Ornamental Plants
Azaleas
Daphne
Jessamine
Rhododendron
Wisteria

Other Plants
Buttercups
Jack-in-the-pulpit
Mayapple
Nightshade
Water and poison hemlock

Trees and Shrubs
Elderberry
Oaks
Wild and cultivated cherries

Poisoning by Inhalation

Accidental or intentional inhalation of poisons can lead to a life-threatening emergency. The type and location of injury caused by toxic inhalation depend on the specific actions and behaviors of the chemical involved.[7]

✓ **TRICKS OF THE TRADE**

Respiratory difficulty may not appear for several hours after exposure to toxic fumes and/or smoke. Use all of your persuasive skills to encourage the patient to be examined at the hospital, even if the patient feels fine.

Physical Properties

The concentration of a chemical in the air and the duration of exposure help determine the severity of inhalation injury. At low concentrations and with brief exposure, the chemical may be removed from the air before reaching the tracheobronchial tree, whereas large concentrations or prolonged exposure are more likely to cause contact with the lungs and damage to lung tissue. As a rule, increasing the concentration of the chemical or the duration of exposure increases the dose received.

Solubility also influences inhalation injury. For example, soluble chemicals such as chlorine and anhydrous ammonia can be converted to hydrochloric acid and ammonium hydroxide, respectively, when they contact moisture in the respiratory tract mucus, producing injury in the nasopharynx and conducting airways. In contrast, insoluble chemicals such as phosgene and nitrogen dioxide may have little impact on the upper airways but can produce severe damage to the alveoli and respiratory bronchioles.

Chemicals may be inhaled as gases and vapors, mists, fumes, or particles. Gases and vapors mix with air and distribute themselves freely throughout the lung and its airways. Mists are liquid droplets dispersed in air. Their toxic effects depend on droplet size (the larger the size, the greater the exposure). Fumes contain fine particles of dust dispersed in air. Large particles are likely to be trapped in the nasopharynx and conducting airways, whereas small particles (1 to 5 microns) are more likely to penetrate the lower airways.

Chemical Properties

The ability of a chemical to interact with other chemicals and body tissue is called its *reactivity*. As a rule, highly reactive chemicals cause more severe and rapid injury than less-reactive chemicals. Four potential properties of chemicals that determine reactivity are the following:

1. Chemical pH: The likelihood for severe injury from alkaloid or acid exposure increases as the pH approaches its extremes: a pH of less than 2 for acidic substances and greater than 11.5 for alkaline substances.
2. Direct-acting potential of chemicals: Direct-acting chemicals are capable of producing injury without first being transformed or changed. An example is hydrofluoric acid, which causes severe corrosive burns on contact with mucous membranes of the upper airways.
3. Indirect-acting potential of chemicals: Indirect-acting chemicals must be transformed before they can produce injury. An example is phosgene, a gas that may cause acidic burns of the alveolar membranes after conversion to hydrogen chloride (a process that may take up to several hours).
4. Allergic potential of chemicals: Some reactive chemicals bind with proteins to form structures that stimulate allergic reactions. For example, formaldehyde can cause severe asthmatic and anaphylactic reactions after even a small exposure. In general, the allergic potential of a chemical is related to its reactivity.

> **? CRITICAL THINKING**
>
> *Do you think that situations involving toxic gas inhalation are likely to involve single patients or multiple patients? Why?*

Classifications

Toxic gases can be classified in three categories: simple asphyxiants, chemical asphyxiants, and irritants/corrosives. Simple asphyxiants (methane, propane, and inert gases) cause toxicity by displacing or lowering ambient oxygen concentration. Chemical asphyxiants (carbon monoxide and cyanide) possess intrinsic systemic toxicity manifested after absorption into the circulation. Irritants/corrosives (chlorine and ammonia) cause cellular destruction and inflammation as they come into contact with moisture. Table 34-1 provides an overview of toxic gases and their clinical manifestations.

General Management

The general principles of managing patients who have inhaled poisons are the same as for any other hazardous materials incident (see Chapter 51). These include the following:

1. Scene safety
2. Personal protective measures (protective clothing and appropriate respiratory protective apparatus)
3. Rapid removal of the patient from the poison environment
4. Surface decontamination

CLASS OF TOXIN	TOXIN	SOURCE	CLINICAL FEATURES	MANAGEMENT
Simple asphyxiants	Propane Methane Carbon dioxide Inert gases (nitrogen, argon)	Cooking gas Cooking gas All fires Industry (especially welding)	Displacement of normal air and lower fractional inspired oxygen concentration, symptoms of hypoxemia without airway irritation	Remove patient from source; give oxygen.
Chemical asphyxiants	Carbon monoxide	Fires	Formation of carboxyhemoglobin; inhibition of oxygen transport (Headache is earliest symptom.)	Give 100% oxygen.
	Hydrocyanic acid	Industry, burning plastics, furniture, fabrics	Highly toxic cellular asphyxiant	Use cyanide antidote.
	Hydrogen sulfide	Liquid manure pits, decaying organic materials	Highly toxic cellular asphyxiant similar to cyanide; sudden collapse; ability to smell characteristic odor of rotten eggs; rapid fatigue	Use sodium nitrite for cyanide (makes sulmethemoglobin). *Do not use thiosulfate.*
Irritants High solubility in water	Chlorine gas Hydrochloric acid	Industry, swimming pool chemicals, bleach mixed with acid at home	Early onset of lacrimation, sore throat, stridor, tracheobronchitis; with heavy exposure, pulmonary edema in 2 to 6 hours	Use humidified oxygen, bronchodilators, and airway management.
	Ammonia	Industry, burning fabrics		
Low solubility in water	Nitrogen dioxide	Burning cellulose, fabrics Grain silos (acrid red gas)	Sweet "electric" smell; delayed onset (12-24 hours) of tracheobronchitis, pneumonitis, and pulmonary edema; late chronic bronchitis	Give oxygen: observe for 24 to 48 hours; give ateroids (controversial).
	Ozone	Inert gas arc welding, industry		
	Phosgone	Burning of chlorinated organic material		
Allergenic	Toluene dilsocyanate	Manufacture of polyurethanes	Reactive bronchoconstriction; possible long-term effects (chronic obstructive pulmonary disease) in susceptible persons	Use bronchodilators.
Metal fumes	Zinc Copper Tin Teflon	Welding (especially galvanized metal welding)	"Metal fumes fever"; chills, fever, myalgias, headache, nonproductive cough, leukocytosis 4 to 8 hours after exposure	Self-limited (12-24 hours)
	Arsine	Burning arsenic-containing ores, electronics industry	Highly toxic effect; hemolysis, pulmonary edema, renal failure; chronic arsenic toxicity	Exchange transfusion; use dimercaprol (BAL) for chronic arsenic toxicity only.
	Mercury Lead	Industry, welding	See specific metals	

From Ho MT: *Current emergency diagnosis and treatment,* ed 3, Norwalk, Conn, 1990, Appleton and Lange.

5. Adequate airway, ventilatory, and circulatory support
6. Initial assessment and physical examination
7. Irrigation of the eyes (as needed)
8. IV line with a saline solution
9. Regular monitoring of vital signs and cardiac rhythm by ECG
10. Rapid transport to an appropriate medical facility

Management of Specific Inhaled Poisons

The specific inhaled poisons discussed in this section include cyanide, ammonia, and hydrocarbons. Carbon monoxide poisoning is described in Chapter 21.

Cyanide

Cyanide refers to any of a number of highly toxic substances that contain the cyanogen chemical group. Because of its toxicity, cyanide has few applications. The agent sometimes is used in industry in electroplating, ore extraction, and fumigation of buildings and as a fertilizer. It has been used in gas chambers as a means of execution. Cyanide is one of the products of combustion from burning nylon and polyurethane and is therefore a potential hazard in fire environments.

Cyanide poisoning may result from the inhalation of cyanide gas; ingestion of cyanide salts, nitriles, or cyanogenic glycosides (e.g., amygdalin, a substance found in the seeds of cherries, apples, pears, and apricots, and the principal constituent of laetrile); or the infusion of nitroprusside (Nitropress). Cyanide also can be absorbed across the skin. Regardless of the route of entry, cyanide is a rapidly acting poison that combines and reacts with ferric ions (Fe^3) of the respiratory enzyme cytochrome oxidase to inhibit cellular oxygenation. The cytotoxic hypoxia produces a rapid progression of symptoms from dyspnea to paralysis, unconsciousness, and death (Box 34-9). Large doses usually are fatal within minutes from respiratory arrest.

NOTE

Cyanide poisoning may produce a characteristic odor of bitter almonds on the patient's breath or body.

? CRITICAL THINKING

What type of protective equipment will you need to care for a patient with cyanide poisoning?

After ensuring personal safety, emergency care for a patient with cyanide poisoning begins with securing a patent airway and providing adequate ventilatory support with high-concentration oxygen. Oxygen competitively displaces cyanide from cytochrome oxidase and enhances the efficacy of drug administration. After these measures, the principal treatment of cyanide poisoning is to convert (oxidize) ferrous ions in hemoglobin (Fe^2) to ferric ions (Fe^3), forming methemoglobin, hemoglobin with ferrous ion in the oxidized (Fe^3) state. Cyanide, which has a greater affinity for iron in the ferric state, is released from the cytochrome oxidase and combines with methemoglobin, thus allowing cytochrome oxidase to resume its function in normal cellular respiration. Cyanide antidotes, such as those found in the Pasadena cyanide antidote kit (formerly the *Lily Cyanide Poison Kit*), are thought to be effective because they induce methemoglobin (Box 34-10).

Methemoglobin cannot transport oxygen and must therefore be reconverted to hemoglobin by sodium thiosulfate. This is accomplished in a three-step process, which includes administration of (1) *amyl nitrite* by inhalation (converting about 5% of hemoglobin to methemoglobin); (2) sodium nitrite (300 mg IV), which results in methemoglobinemia approaching 25% to 30%; and (3) sodium thiosulfate (12.5 mg IV).

BOX 34-9

EARLY AND ADVANCED SIGNS AND SYMPTOMS OF CYANIDE POISONING

Early Effects
Agitation
Anxiety
Confusion
Dyspnea
Hypertension with reflex bradycardia

Advanced Effects
Hypotension
Acidosis
Seizures
Pulmonary edema
Dysrhythmias
Intractable hypotension
Lactic acidosis
Coma

BOX 34-10

CYANIDE ANTIDOTE KIT

Two *Amyl Nitrite* Inhalants in Gauze
Administer by inhalation 15 of every 30 seconds

3% Sodium Nitrite (Stop *Amyl Nitrite*)
Adults: 10-mL slow intravenous administration over
   2 to 4 minutes
Children 0.2 mL/kg (up to 10 mL) slow intravenous
   administration over 5 minutes
**NOTE: If hypotension develops, stop nitrite, treat
for shock, and consider administration of *dopamine*
(per medical direction).**

25% Sodium Thiosulfate
Adults: 50-mL intravenous bolus
Children: 5 mL sodium thiosulfate per 1 mL sodium
   nitrite given

Prehospital care for patients with cyanide poisoning is as follows:

1. Don personal protective equipment as needed to prevent rescuer contamination.
2. Remove the patient from the cyanide source. Rapid decontamination and removal of any contaminated clothing is essential.
3. Ensure a patent airway and provide adequate ventilatory support.
4. Administer high-concentration oxygen.
5. If using the Pasadena cyanide antidote kit, consult with medical direction or a poison control center and follow the instructions provided by the manufacturer.
6. If an antidote kit is not available, a pearl of *amyl nitrite* should be crushed and held under the patient's nose for 15 of every 30 seconds, followed by continuation of supplemental oxygen. If the patient's respirations are being assisted, place

NOTE

Hypotension should be anticipated as a consequence of antidote therapy. The patient should remain supine if possible, and the blood pressure must be closely monitored. If hypotension develops, medical direction may recommend administration of vasopressors.

the crushed pearl under the intake valve of a bag-valve device.
7. Initiate IV fluid therapy with a volume-expanding solution.
8. Monitor cardiac rhythm by ECG.
9. Rapidly transport the patient for physician evaluation.

Ammonia Inhalation

Ammonia is a toxic irritant that causes local pulmonary complications after inhalation. Exposure to ammonia vapors results in inflammation, irritation, and in severe cases, erosion of the mucosal tissue of all respiratory structures as the ammonia vapor combines with water, producing a highly caustic alkaline compound. Patients usually develop coughing, choking, congestion, burning and tightness in the chest, and a feeling of suffocation. These respiratory symptoms often are accompanied by burning of the eyes and lacrimation. In severe cases, bronchospasm and pulmonary edema may ensue. In addition to the general management principles, emergency care may include positive-pressure ventilation and the administration of diuretics and bronchodilators.

Hydrocarbon Inhalation

The hydrocarbons that pose the greatest risk for injury have a low viscosity, a high volatility, and a high surface tension or adhesion of molecules along a surface. These characteristics combine to allow hydrocarbons to enter the pulmonary tree, causing aspiration pneumonitis and the potential for systemic effects such as CNS depression and liver, kidney, or bone marrow toxicity.

Most hydrocarbon inhalations result from "recreational use" of halogenated hydrocarbons such as carbon tetrachloride and methylene chloride or aromatic hydrocarbons such as benzene and toluene. These agents may produce a state of inebriation or euphoria through "sniffing" or "huffing" (placing the solvent on a rag and inhaling the vapors through a plastic bag). The onset of these effects usually is rapid (occurring within seconds) and may be followed by CNS depression, respiratory failure, or cardiac dysrhythmias. Other signs and symptoms of hydrocarbon inhalation include the following:

- Burning sensation on swallowing
- Nausea and vomiting

- Abdominal cramps
- Weakness
- Anesthesia
- Hallucinations
- Changes in color perception
- Blindness
- Seizures
- Coma

Emergency care for hydrocarbon inhalation generally is supportive and includes airway, ventilatory, and circulatory support; IV fluid therapy; vital sign and ECG monitoring; and transport for physician evaluation.

Poisoning by Injection

Human poisonings from injection may result from drug abuse or therapeutic misadventure (described later in this chapter) and from arthropod bites and stings, reptile bites, and hazardous aquatic life. In contrast to most chemical compounds previously described, injected poisons are mixtures of many different substances, which may produce several different toxic reactions in humans. The paramedic must therefore be prepared to manage reactions in many organ systems simultaneously.

Arthropod Bites and Stings

Approximately 900,000 species of arthropods exist throughout the world. Some arthropods bite, some sting, and a few bite and sting. Arthropod venoms are complex and diverse in their chemistry and pharmacology and may produce major toxic reactions such as anaphylaxis and upper airway obstruction in sensitized individuals. The various reactions to venoms are classified as local, toxic, systemic, and delayed (Box 34-11).[8]

Hymenoptera

Hymenoptera venom is used for defense and subjugation of prey. Medically important venoms are mixtures of protein or polypeptide toxins, enzymes, and other compounds such as histamines, serotonin, acetylcholine, and dopamine. Hymenoptera stings most commonly are inflicted on the head and neck followed by the foot, leg, hand, and arm. The mouth, pharynx, and esophagus may be stung when bees or yellow jackets in soft drink or beer containers are accidentally ingested.

A single wasp, bee, or ant sting in an unsensitized individual usually causes instant pain followed by a wheal-and-flare reaction with variable edema. Large local reactions can spread more than 15 cm beyond the sting site and persist for more than 24 hours. Anaphylaxis is the most serious complication of hymenoptera stings. An estimated 0.4% of the U.S. population has some degree of chemical allergy to insect venoms; 40 to 100 deaths caused by anaphylaxis from hymenoptera stings are reported annually.[5] Individuals with a history of allergic reactions to stings often wear medical alert identification and carry an emergency kit containing a preloaded syringe of *epinephrine* (Epi-Pen).

The ant species of greatest concern in the United States is the imported fire ant, whose venom is primarily an alkaloid. The fire ant is the only hymenopteran species whose venom results in necrotic activity, and sterile pustules at the sting site are not uncommon. Stings or bites from fire ants may produce systemic reactions and are managed like other hymenoptera stings. Secondary infection may occur (requiring antibiotic therapy), and extensive scarring may require skin grafts (very rare).

Management. Prehospital care for mild hymenoptera stings should include close observation for signs or symptoms of an allergic reaction. If an extremity is involved, immobilization and elevation can help limit the reaction's duration. If physician evaluation is warranted, as evidenced by signs of anaphylaxis or vigorous reaction, an antihistamine may be prescribed.

Honey bees (and other hymenoptera) frequently leave their stingers in the wound. If a stinger is present, it should be scraped or brushed off. Stingers should not be removed with forceps, because squeezing the attached venom sac may worsen the injury. Severe allergic reactions should be managed as described in Chapter 31. Hypovolemia (if present) should be treated in the conventional manner with a volume-expanding crystalloid infusion.

Arachnida

Eleven types of Arachnida exist; however, this discussion is limited to spiders, scorpions, and ticks.

BOX 34-11

TYPES OF REACTIONS TO VENOMS

Local Reaction
- Marked and prolonged edema at the sting site
- Possible involvement of one or more neighboring joints
- Possible occurrence in the mouth or throat, producing airway obstruction
- Severe local reactions that may increase the likelihood of future systemic reactions (controversial)
- Symptoms that usually subside within 24 hours

Toxic Reaction*
- Gastrointestinal disturbances:
  Vomiting
  Diarrhea
  Lightheadedness
- Other symptoms:
  Syncope (common finding)
  Headache
  Fever
  Involuntary muscle spasms
  Edema without urticaria
  Convulsions (rare)
- Symptoms that usually subside within 48 hours

Systemic (Anaphylactic) Reaction†
- Reactions that can progress to death within minutes

- Immediate symptoms:
  Itching eyes or generalized itching
  Facial flushing
  Generalized urticaria
- Subsequent symptoms:
  Respiratory failure, cardiovascular collapse, or both
  Hypotension
  Chest or throat constriction or both
  Wheezing
  Dyspnea
  Cyanosis
  Nausea and vomiting
  Chills and fever
  Laryngeal stridor
  Shock
  Loss of consciousness
  Loss of bowel or bladder control
  Bloody and frothy sputum production

Delayed Reaction‡
- Serum sickness symptoms:
  Fever
  Malaise
  Headache
  Urticaria
  Polyarthritis

*Should be considered with a history of 10 or more stings.
†May occur in response to single or multiple stings.
‡Usually occurs 10 to 14 days after a sting.

Spider bites. About 20,000 species of spiders are found in the United States, and all, with the exception of two small groups (Uloboriade and Liphistiidae), have venom glands. The two major types of reactions that occur from spider venom are neurotoxic reactions resulting from the black widow bite and local tissue necrosis from the bites of most other spiders.

Black widow spider. The black widow is the most notorious spider in North America. Although a number of variations exist in the species, the typical mature female (who often devours her mate, thus the name *black widow*) is shiny and black with a red hourglass marking on the undersurface of the abdomen (Fig. 34-1). The size of the female varies with age but rarely exceeds 2.5 cm overall. (The male is about half the size of the female, brown, and non-

venomous to humans.) The spider generally is found in undisturbed areas (under stones, logs, and clumps of vegetation) and rarely inhabits occupied dwellings. Most black widow bites occur in rural and suburban areas of southern and western states between April and October.

The bite of a black widow usually occurs when the spider has been disturbed. It generally is described by patients as a slight pinprick that is initially painless. As a rule, the only physical findings are two small fang marks about 1 mm apart surrounded by a small papule. Multiple bites usually rule out any type of spider envenomation, because spiders rarely bite more than once. Within 1 hour of envenomation, the neurotoxin produces characteristic muscle spasms and cramps, which may result in abdominal rigidity (in the absence of palpable tenderness) and intense pain.

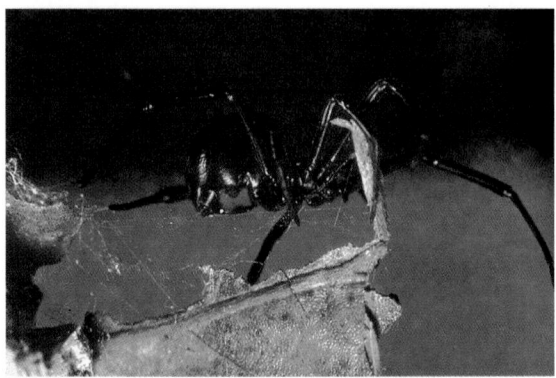

Fig. 34-1 Black widow spider. (Courtesy Saint Louis Zoo, St Louis, Mo.)

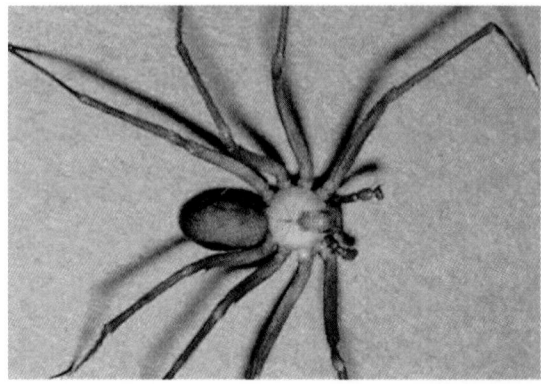

Fig. 34-2 Brown recluse spider. (From Auerbach PS: *Management of wilderness and environmental emergencies*, ed 2, St Louis, 1989, Mosby.)

Abdominal rigidity in the absence of palpable tenderness is an important finding that helps distinguish envenomation from an acute abdominal condition. Associated symptoms include paresthesia (frequently described as a burning sensation in the soles of the feet or entire body); pain in the muscles of the shoulders, back, and chest; headache; dizziness; nausea and vomiting; edema of the eyelids; and increased perspiration and salivation. Emergency care for a patient with a black widow bite primarily is supportive and includes the following:

1. Ensure adequate airway, ventilatory, and circulatory support.
2. Clean the affected area with saline, cover with a sterile dressing, and intermittently apply ice. Obstruction tourniquets or suction devices are not helpful in delaying absorption. A commercially prepared antivenin is available but should be administered only in the emergency department and only after appropriate sensitivity testing.
3. Moderate-to-severe symptoms require aggressive management. Per medical direction, muscle spasm, severe headache, vomiting, and paresthesia may be managed with 5 mg of *diazepam* (Valium) and pain medication (e.g., *morphine*). Severe hypertension may be managed with antihypertensive agents.
4. Transport the patient for physician evaluation. Most patients recover completely within 36 to 72 hours. Those at greatest risk for morbidity are the very young, older adults, and those with underlying hypertension or other medical problems.

Brown recluse spider. The brown recluse spider (also known as the fiddle-back spider) is most prevalent in the Mississippi-Ohio-Missouri river basin and the southwestern United States. The species prefers hot, dry, and abandoned environments, such as vacant buildings; it frequently is found in clothing closets. The spider is fawn to dark brown in color and is between and 1 and 2 cm long (Fig. 34-2). Identifying characteristics of the brown recluse are six white eyes arranged in a semicircle on the head (versus the usual eight eyes of most other spiders) and the presence of a dark, violin-shaped marking on the top of the cephalothorax (the combined head and thorax). The brown recluse is considered shy and generally does not attack unless threatened. Like black widows, these spiders are most active from April to October.

The venom of the brown recluse manifests in a broad spectrum of reactions. Initially the bite causes little pain and often is overlooked by the victim. Some 1 to 2 hours later, localized pain and erythema develop (Fig. 34-3). This transient irritation often is followed within 1 to 2 days by a blister or vesicle. The lesion may be surrounded by an ischemic ring that is further outlined by an irregular erythematous halo, producing the classical "bull's-eye" appearance. Over the next 24 to 72 hours, the area often becomes larger, and necrosis may occur, the center of the lesion yielding a purple or black eschar. The eschar eventually sloughs within 2 to 5 weeks, leaving an ulcer of variable size and depth. The tissue defect may extend to include underlying muscle and typically is slow to heal (often visible for months to years after the bite). Occasionally, ex-

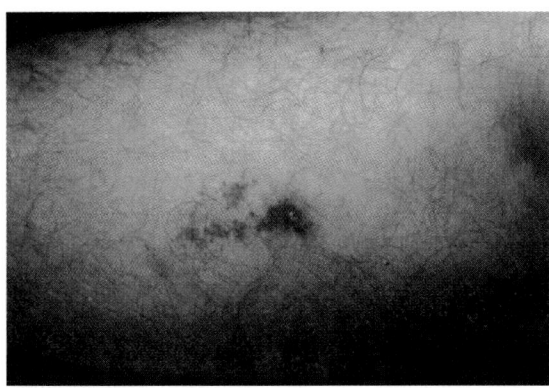

Fig. 34-3 Brown recluse spider bite at approximately 6 hours, with central hemorrhagic vesicle and gravitational pattern spread of venom. (From Auerbach PS: *Management of wilderness and environmental emergencies*, ed 2, St Louis, 1989, Mosby.)

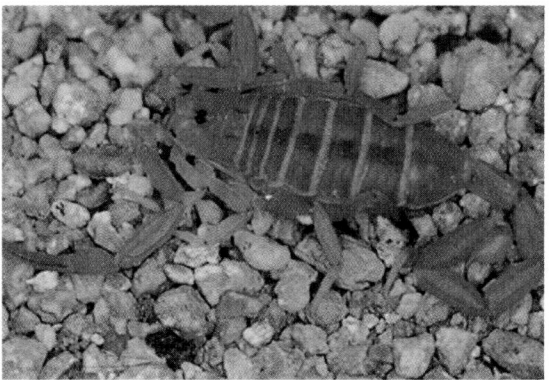

Fig. 34-4 The sculptured scorpion commonly found in the deserts of Arizona, New Mexico, and California. (From Auerbach PS: *Management of wilderness and environmental emergencies*, ed 2, St Louis, 1989, Mosby.)

cision and skin grafting are necessary. Systemic involvement may occur with signs and symptoms that include fever, chills, malaise, nausea and vomiting, generalized rash, and the development of hemolytic anemia, hemoglobinuria, and hypotension. Death occasionally occurs, usually from disturbance of the coagulation system or hepatic injury.

Emergency care for patients with a brown recluse bite generally is supportive. Cold compresses and sterile dressings should be applied to the lesion, and the patient should be transported for physician evaluation. As a rule, pharmacological therapy is not indicated in the prehospital setting. In-hospital therapy may include ice, antibiotics, and consideration of dapsone, a leukocyte inhibitor (controversial). Although an antivenin has been used in research, it is not widely clinically available. Most patients do well with outpatient management.

> **? CRITICAL THINKING**
>
> **For which type of spider bite is a patient most likely to call an ambulance? Why?**

Scorpion stings. More than 650 species of scorpions exist, but only a few produce human envenomation. In North America, the sculptured or bark scorpion, found in the southwestern United States and Mexico, is the only species that is dangerous to humans. The scorpion is nocturnal and favors wooded areas along the edges of desert washes, where generally it clings upside down in its hideouts. It may

be found under the bark of the eucalyptus and cottonwood trees. Occasionally the scorpion invades homes, especially adobe houses. The sculptured scorpion is small (2 to 7.5 cm) and yellow to brown in color, and some have tail stripes (Fig. 34-4). The species is most active from April to August, hibernating during the winter.

The scorpion's venom is delivered by a stinger on the telson and is used for both defense and food acquisition. The venom is a mixture of proteins with complex effects on cellular sodium channels. It acts at the presynaptic terminal of the neuromuscular junction, releasing acetylcholine, which results in depolarization of the junction. The venom also stimulates sympathetic nerves and directly stimulates the CNS, causing hyperactivity. This particular scorpion venom does not contain enzymes that cause tissue destruction, so local inflammation is not a feature. If swelling, ecchymosis, or erythema is present, the scorpion was not of the neurotoxic type. Signs and symptoms of sculptured scorpion envenomation are listed in Box 34-12.

Despite the potential for life-threatening systemic effects, the vast majority of scorpion envenomations, especially in adults, produce symptoms that reach maximum severity within 5 hours. As a rule, mild analgesics, cool compresses, and in-hospital observation are all that are required for these patients. The use of antivenin for scorpion bites is reserved for severe cases. Prehospital care is supportive, airway control being the highest priority. The patient should be transported for physician evaluation.

Tick bites. Although tick bites seldom require emergency care, ticks are capable of causing human disease by transmitting microorganisms or by secreting toxins or venoms. In North America, hard ticks are the most familiar type, although soft ticks also are common to western states. Hard ticks have a leathery exterior that makes them resistant to environmental stresses. They are relatively free of natural enemies. They can regenerate lost parts and have been known to survive without feeding for more than 4 years.[8] Local reactions to tick bites vary from the formation of a small pruritic nodule to development of extensive areas of ulceration that may be accompanied by fever, chills, and malaise unrelated to infection. Some of the more important diseases for which ticks are vectors include **Rocky Mountain spotted fever** (RMSF), **Lyme disease**, and **tick paralysis**.

Rocky Mountain spotted fever. RMSF is an infectious disease transmitted from rabbits and other small mammals to humans by the bites of the wood tick and dog tick. The disease occurs more commonly on the Atlantic seaboard, and accounts for more than 40 deaths in the United States each year. Signs and symptoms usually develop within 5 to 7 days of the tick bite and include headache, high fever, and loss of appetite. Usually within 2 to 3 days after the onset of symptoms, small pink spots appear on the wrists and ankles. Eventually the rash spreads over the entire body, and the spots darken and enlarge and become petechial. In mild cases, recovery occurs within 20 days. The mortality rate, if untreated, is between 8% and 25%.

Lyme disease. Lyme disease is the most commonly reported tick-borne disease in the United States. The disease is caused by a spirochete transmitted by the bite of an Ixodes tick known to infect deer and dogs. The course of the disease follows several stages. Initially a red dot appears at the site of the tick bite. This gradually expands into a reddened annular rash, often with central clearing. During this stage, fever, lethargy, muscle pain, and general malaise may develop. This stage may be followed by a second stage about 4 to 6 weeks later, manifested by cardiac abnormalities (including various AV blocks) and neurological effects (including cranial nerve palsies). About 10% of infected patients go on to the second stage. Still later, a third stage

---

BOX 34-12

SIGNS AND SYMPTOMS OF SCORPION ENVENOMATION

Hyperesthesia at the site of bite
Pain, tingling and a burning sensation radiating along the nerves at the location of the bite
SLUDGE: salivation, lacrimation, urination, defecation, gastrointestinal distress, and emesis
Initial bradycardia followed by tachycardia
Cardiac dysrhythmias
Muscle twitching
Convulsions
Roving eye movements (cranial nerve dysfunction)
Temporary blindness

---

may develop, with arthritis as the primary symptom. Unless the disease is diagnosed and treated, symptoms may continue for several years, gradually declining in severity.

Tick paralysis. Tick paralysis results from a prolonged bite by a female wood tick. The disease occurs sporadically during the spring and summer months and is caused by a neurotoxin secreted from the tick's salivary glands during a blood meal. Tick paralysis develops in humans within 6 days after the tick attaches to the host. Initially the patient presents with restlessness and complaints of paresthesia in the hands and feet. Over the next 24 to 48 hours, an ascending, symmetrical flaccid paralysis may develop with loss of deep tendon reflexes. In severe cases, death may result from respiratory paralysis. Removal of the tick usually results in rapid improvement and complete resolution within several days. If undiagnosed, the disease may be fatal, particularly in young and older patients.

? CRITICAL THINKING

How can you distinguish tick paralysis from other conditions that cause progressive paralysis?

Management. The principal treatment of tick bites is proper removal of the tick. The tick should be grasped as close to the skin surface as possible with forceps, tweezers, or protected fingers and pulled out with steady pressure. Care should be taken not to crush or squeeze the body of the tick, which can transmit disease from infective tick fluid. Other methods of tick removal, such as applying fingernail polish, isopropanol, or a hot match head, should be avoided. These traditional methods are ineffective and may induce the tick to salivate or regurgitate into the wound. After removal, the bite should be disinfected with soap and water and covered with a sterile dressing.

Reptile Bites

The AAPCC National Data Collection System listed a total 5715 bites from poisonous and nonpoisonous snakes in 1997.[2] Of these exposures, 1579 were known to be poisonous, and 1638 were bites from unidentified snakes. According to these records, two deaths were reported, reflecting the high morbidity and low mortality rates associated with snake venom poisoning. Of the 115 species of snakes in the United States, only 19 are venomous. The two main families of venomous snakes indigenous to the United States are pit vipers and coral snakes.

Pit Vipers

The pit viper family that inhabits the United States consists of rattlesnakes (15 species), the cottonmouth (water) moccasin, the copperhead, the pigmy rattlesnake, and the massasauga rattlesnake. The vast majority of snakebites in the United States are caused by the rattlesnake family (Fig. 34-5).

The general term *pit viper* is derived from a depression or pit in the maxillary bone of these snakes, which is believed to be a heat-sensing organ that detects warm-blooded prey or enemies. The pit

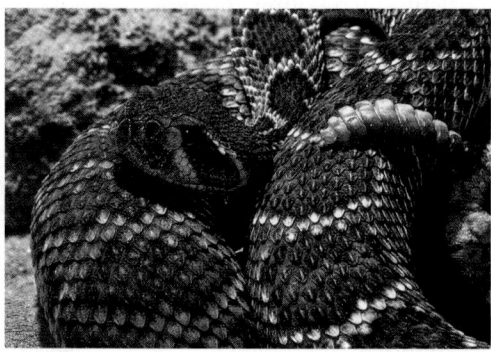

Fig. 34-5 Pit viper. (Courtesy Saint Louis Zoo, St Louis, Mo.)

guides the direction of the strike and possibly determines the amount of venom released, based on the size and heat emission of the prey. Other identifying characteristics of the pit viper are vertical elliptical pupils and a triangular head that is distinct from the rest of the body. The rattlesnake is further characterized by "rattles" (interlocking horny segments formed on the tail) that sometimes vibrate in direct relation to environmental temperatures.

The venom apparatus of pit vipers consists of a gland and a duct connected to one or more elongated hollow fangs on each side of the head. The venom is composed of a variety of proteins designed to immobilize, kill, and digest prey. Depending on the species and the amount of venom injected, these proteins may be capable of producing various toxic effects on blood and other tissues, including hemolysis, intravascular coagulation, convulsions, and acute renal failure (Box 34-13). Bleeding secondary to coagulation defects and massive swelling can lead to hypovolemic shock. On any given strike, the snake may release a quantity of venom varying from little or none to almost the entire content of the glands. (A total of 20% of bites do not result in envenomation.[8])

BOX 34-13

SIGNS AND SYMPTOMS OF PIT VIPER ENVENOMATION

Mild Envenomation
Presence of one or more fang marks
Local swelling and pain
Lack of systemic symptoms

Moderate Envenomation
Presence of one or more fang marks
Pain and edema beyond the site
Systemic signs and symptoms
    Weakness
    Diaphoresis
    Nausea and vomiting
    Paresthesias

Severe Envenomation
Presence of one or more fang marks
Massive edema
Subcutaneous ecchymosis
Severe systemic symptoms
Shock

Coral Snakes

Two members of the coral snake family are found in the United States: the Arizona coral snake and the Eastern coral snake. In contrast to the pit viper, the coral snake has round pupils and small, fixed fangs located near the anterior end of the maxilla. Most coral snakes have a three-color pattern with red, black, and yellow or white bands that completely encircle the body, along with a black snout (Fig. 34-6). Many nonpoisonous snakes in the United States mimic the appearance of the coral snake. The coral snake is identified by the sequence of colors: red bands bordered by yellow indicate a venomous species. Thus "red on yellow, kill a fellow; red on black, venom lack."

Most coral snakes are shy and docile and seldom bite unless threatened. The snake's small mouth and fangs make it difficult to bite anything larger than a finger, toe, or fold of skin. The coral snake tends to hang on and chew rather than to strike and release like the pit viper. The venom of the coral snake primarily is neurotoxic and has a blocking action on acetylcholine receptor sites. The bite generally produces little or no pain and no necrosis or edema. Early signs and symptoms of a coral snake bite are slurred speech, dilated pupils, and dysphagia (usually delayed several hours after the bite). If untreated, the venom produces flaccid paralysis and death (within 8 to 24 hours) by respiratory failure, secondary to nervous system dysfunction.

Management of Snake Envenomation

Venom, like any drug or toxin, has absorption, distribution, and elimination phases. Tissue damage increases as venom spreads into the lymphatics and blood. Therefore emergency care is directed at retarding the systemic spread of the venom. Prehospital management of snake bites includes the following:

1. Stay clear of the snake's striking range (about the length of the snake), and move the patient to a safe area. If the snake has been destroyed before EMS arrival, it should be transported in a closed container to the emergency department with the patient. No attempt should be made by EMS personnel to capture or destroy the snake; doing so may result in a second envenomation. It is not absolutely necessary to identify the snake to manage the patient appropriately.

2. Provide adequate airway, ventilatory, and circulatory support to the patient as needed. Continually monitor vital signs and the ECG and establish an IV line in an unaffected extremity with a volume-expanding fluid.

3. When practical, immobilize the bitten extremity in a neutral position. Immobilization by splinting may delay systemic absorption and diminish local tissue necrosis. Every effort should be made to keep the patient at rest.

4. Prepare the patient for immediate transport to an appropriate medical facility.

5. Additional measures in the management of snake envenomation, such as incision and suction or use of a lymphatic-venous constriction band or pressure device, are controversial and potentially harmful. The paramedic should consult with medical direction and follow local protocol. Application of ice or chemical cold packs should be avoided because their use may further damage tissue. In severe cases, in-hospital administration of antivenin to neutralize the venom may be required after appropriate sensitivity testing.

? CRITICAL THINKING

What strategies can you use to calm the emotional state of a patient who has sustained a snake bite?

Hazardous Aquatic Life

The marine animals most likely to be involved in human poisonings in U.S. coastal waters are the coelenterates, echinoderms, and stingrays. The

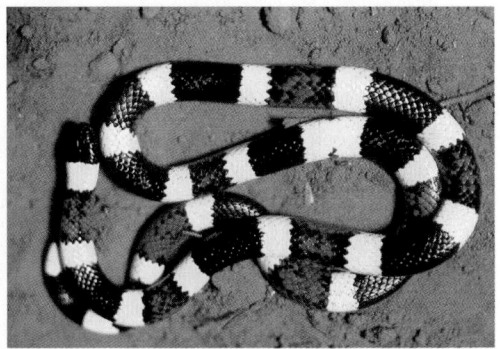

Fig. 34-6 Coral snake. (Courtesy Saint Louis Zoo, St Louis, Mo.)

specialized venom apparatuses of these animals are used for defense and for capturing prey. In addition to venom produced by the animal, aquatic life may contain other poisonous substances as a result of toxic ingestions. Exposures to hazardous aquatic life result from recreational, industrial, scientific, and military oceanic activities.

Coelenterates

Coelenterates are a group of more than 9000 species that may be encountered in the ocean (Fig. 34-7). Those that carry venomous stinging cells (nematocysts) are known as *cnidaria*. The nematocyst is venom filled and contains a long, coiled, hollow, threadlike tube that serves as a tiny hypodermic needle. Many types of nematocysts exist; an individual coelenterate may have more than one type. The severity of envenomation is related to the toxicity of the venom (which may contain various fractions), the number of nematocysts discharged, and the physical condition of the victim.

Jellyfish, of which the Portuguese man-of-war is the largest, occur throughout the Atlantic and Pacific oceans, usually near the coastline. Their nematocyst-bearing tentacles may be up to 100 feet long, and a single envenomation may involve several hundred thousand nematocysts. A swimmer who comes into contact with the tentacles of the jellyfish may suffer sufficient envenomation to produce systemic signs and symptoms. Nematocysts frequently remain embedded in the tissues of the victim. Detached tentacle fragments can retain their potency for months.

Sea anemones are colorful bottom dwellers (sometimes found in tidal pools) that have a flower-like appearance. They possess slender projections used to sting and paralyze passing fish. Their modifications of nematocysts are capable of producing mild-to-moderate pain in humans.

Fire corals are not true (stony) corals but rather ocean-bottom dwellers that are widely distributed in tropical waters. They often are mistaken for seaweed because they frequently are found attached to rocks, shells, and corals. These stinging corals may grow to 2 m in height and have a razor-sharp exoskeleton with thousands of protruding nematocyst-bearing tentacles.

Management. Coelenterate envenomation ranges in severity from irritant dermatitis to excruciating pain, respiratory depression, and life-threatening cardiovascular collapse. Envenomation most often is mild, characterized by stinging, paresthesias, pruritus, and reddish-brown linear wheals or "tentacle prints." If a potent venom or a large body surface area is involved, systemic symptoms may include nausea, vomiting, abdominal pain, headache, bronchospasm, pulmonary edema, hypotension, and respiratory arrest. Emergency care is directed at

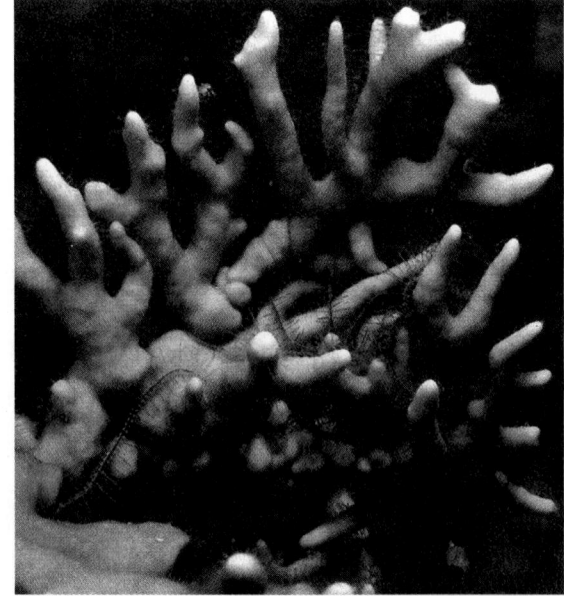 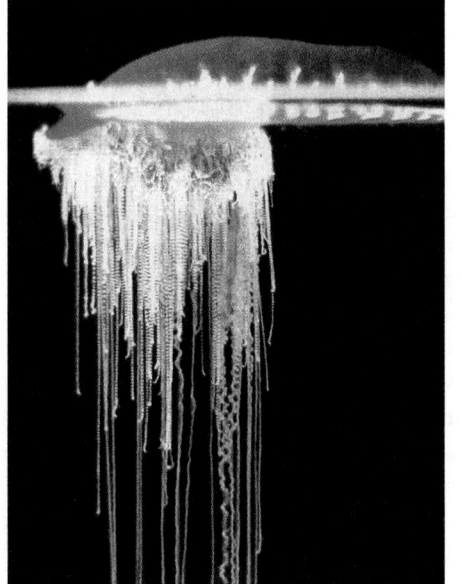

A   B

Fig. 34-7 Colenterates. **A,** Fire coral. **B,** Man-of-war. (From Auerbach PS: *A medical guide to hazardous marine life,* ed 2, St Louis, 1991, Mosby.)

stabilizing the patient and counteracting the effects of the venom.

1. Stabilize the patient.
   a. Provide adequate airway, ventilatory, and circulatory support as needed.
   b. Continually monitor the patient's vital signs and ECG. Be prepared to provide aggressive airway management if systemic reactions develop.
2. Counteract effects of the venom.
   a. Remove visible tentacle fragments with forceps. Avoid self-contamination.
   b. Immediately rinse the patient's wound with seawater. (Wet sand or fresh water usually causes the nematocysts to discharge their venom and therefore is contraindicated.)
   c. Apply copious amounts of isopropanol and then a baking soda slurry to inactivate the nematocysts. (Isopropanol "fixes" nematocytes from firing. Baking soda helps remove them.)
   d. Apply a lather of shaving cream and gently shave the affected area to remove invisible nematocysts.
   e. Rinse again until pain is largely alleviated. If necessary, consult medical direction regarding administration of analgesics.
   f. Transport the patient for physician evaluation.

Echinoderms

Echinoderms include the sea urchins, starfish, and sea cucumbers (Fig. 34-8). Sea urchins have a globular, dome-shaped body and are found on rocky bottoms or burrowed in sand or crevices. These animals have tiny spines, some of which are venomous. Between the spines of some sea urchins are small pincer-like organs that also are thought to discharge a poisonous substance. The spines are extremely dangerous to handle and may break off easily in the flesh, lodging deeply and making removal very difficult.

Some starfish are covered with thorny spines of calcium carbonate crystals that secrete toxins. As the spine enters the skin, it carries venom into the wound with immediate pain, copious bleeding, and mild edema. Multiple puncture wounds may result in acute systemic reactions.

Sea cucumbers are sausage-shaped animals found in shallow and deep water. They produce a liquid toxin in a tentacle-shaped organ that can be projected and extended anally. Generally the substance is secreted into the surrounding ocean, producing only a minor dermatitis or conjunctivitis in swimmers and divers.

Management. Emergency management for echinoderm envenomation usually involves caring for puncture wounds caused by spines and inactivating the venom. Embedded spines should be removed with forceps. Protective gloves should be worn, and the paramedic should be careful to avoid self-contamination. Larger spines may require surgical removal by a physician.

Echinoderm toxins may cause immediate intense pain, swelling, redness, aching in the affected extremity, and nausea. Delayed toxic effects may include respiratory distress, paresthesia of the lips and face, and in severe cases, respiratory paralysis and complete atonia. The paramedic must therefore be prepared to deal with a variety of physical reactions.

Most marine venoms lose their toxicity when exposed to changes in temperature or humidity. The recommended management for stable patients is to immerse the affected area (usually the foot or hand) in extremely warm water before and during transport. The water should be as hot as can be tolerated without scalding (no warmer than 45° C, 113° F). As a safety precaution, it generally is recommended that both hands or feet not be immersed simultaneously to protect against thermal injury that may go unnoticed by the patient because of numbness or pain in the affected part.

Stingrays

Stingrays are responsible for about 1800 injuries each year in the United States. These marine animals vary in size from 2 inches to 14 feet and often are found half-buried in mud or sand in shallow water (Fig. 34-9). The venom organ of stingrays consists of two to four venomous stings on the dorsum of a whiplike tail. Envenomation generally occurs from stepping on the sand-buried ray, which causes the tail to thrust up and forward, driving the sting into the victim's leg or foot. The sting (which is

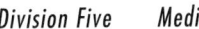

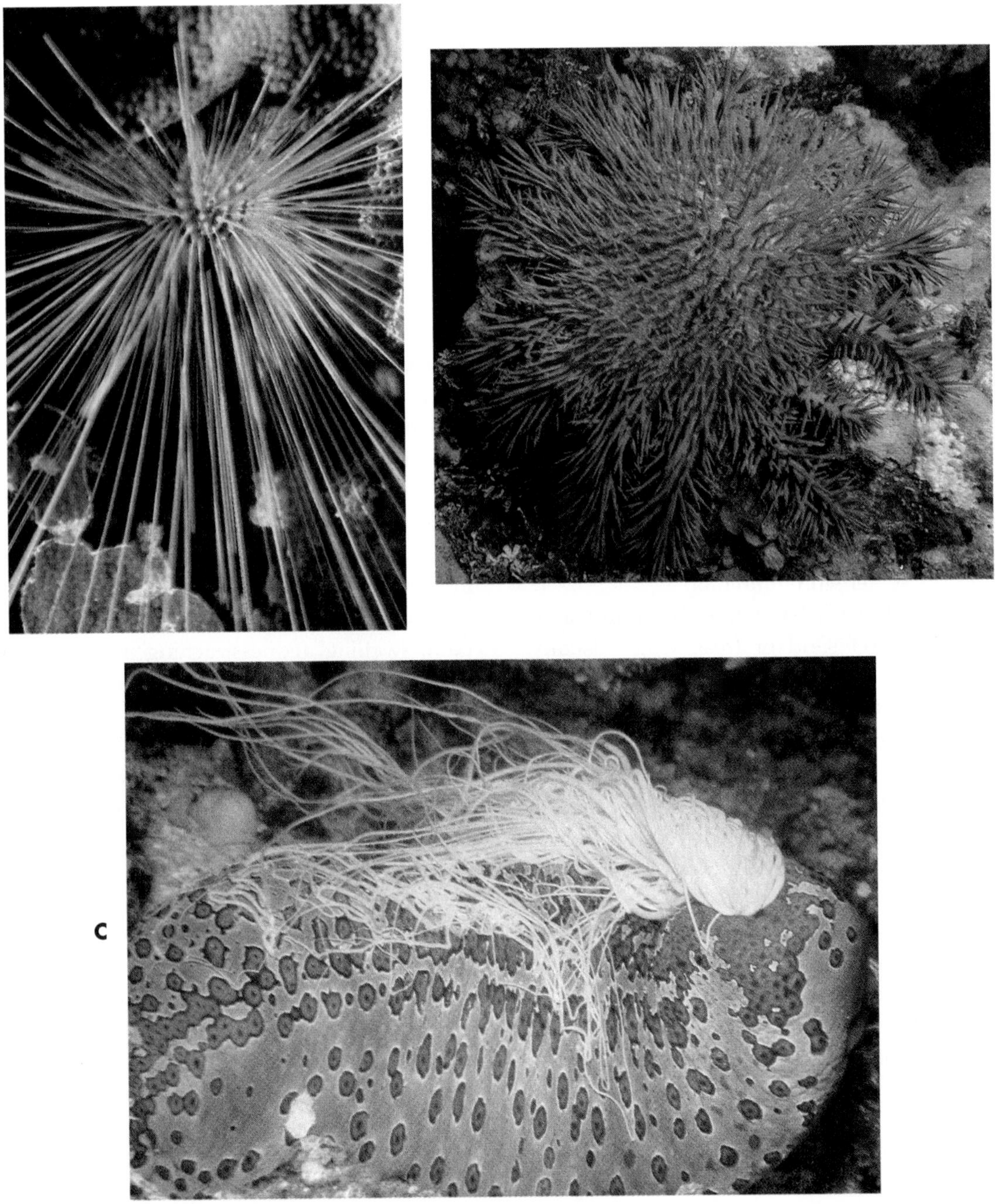

Fig. 34-8 Echinoderms. **A,** Black sea urchin. **B,** Crown-of-thorns starfish. **C,** Sea cucumber with extended tentacles. (From Auerbach PS: *A medical guide to hazardous marine life,* ed 2, St Louis, 1991, Mosby.)

purely defensive) produces a large, severe laceration that may be more than 15 to 20 cm long. In addition to injecting venom into the wound, the entire spine tip of the venom apparatus sometimes is broken and embedded in the tissue.

Stingray venom has local and systemic complications. Locally, it produces a traumatic injury that causes immediate, intense pain; edema; variable bleeding; and necrosis. Systemic manifestations include weakness, nausea, vomiting, diarrhea, vertigo, seizures, cardiac conduction abnormalities, paralysis, hypotension, and death.

Management. Prehospital care is directed to life support, alleviation of pain, inactivation of venom, and prevention of infection.

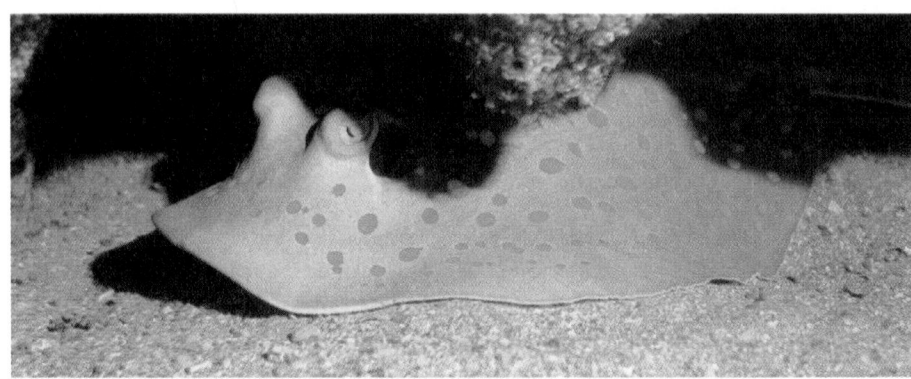

Fig. 34-9 Stingray. (From Auerbach PS: *A medical guide to hazardous marine life*, ed 2, St Louis, 1991, Mosby.)

1. Ensure adequate airway, ventilatory, and circulatory support. Continually monitor the patient's vital signs and ECG.
2. Copiously irrigate the wound with normal saline or fresh water. If the venom apparatus is visible, it should be removed. Avoid self-contamination.
3. Immerse the affected part in very warm water as previously described. Immersion should continue until pain subsides or until the patient reaches the emergency department.
4. Medical direction may recommend administration of analgesics.
5. Transport the patient for physician evaluation.

Poisoning by Absorption

Although many poisons may be absorbed through the skin, more than 75,000 cases of pesticide poisoning are reported to the American Association of Poison Control Centers (AAPCC) each year.[2] A large number of these poisonings results from exposure to organophosphates and carbamates that are available for commercial and public use in the form of pet, home, and commercial insecticides. Because of the widespread availability of such products, paramedics must be aware of the nature of these chemicals, necessary precautions for personal safety, and the immediate management that may be required before symptoms or signs of illness occur.

Organophosphates and carbamates are among the most toxic chemicals currently used in pesticides and are well absorbed by ingestion, inhalation, and dermal routes. Both classes of compounds have similar pharmacological actions, inhibiting the effects of acetylcholinesterase. This enzyme degrades acetylcholine at nerve terminals; however, organophosphates have a stronger bond to this enzyme than carbamates. Carbamate poisoning is easier to manage effectively than organophosphate intoxication. Acetylcholine is a cholinergic neurotransmitter for preganglionic autonomic fibers, postganglionic parasympathetic fibers, somatic nerves to skeletal muscle, and many synapses in the central nervous system. When acetylcholinesterase is inhibited, acetylcholine accumulates at the synapses, and a cholinergic "overdrive" occurs with resulting signs and symptoms characteristic of organophosphate and carbamate poisoning.

Signs and Symptoms

Early signs and symptoms of organophosphate or carbamate poisoning may be nonspecific, including headache, dizziness, weakness, and nausea. However, as overstimulation and subsequent disruption of transmission in the central and peripheral nervous systems occur, signs and symptoms begin to manifest in a spectrum of physiological and metabolic derangements (Box 34-14). The rapidity and sequence in which these signs and symptoms develop depend on the particular compound and the amount and route of exposure. The onset of symptoms is probably quickest after inhalation and slowest (possibly delayed for several hours) after a

---

NOTE

Organophosphates were used in the development of military nerve agents (such as sarin and soman) during World War II and were considered a potential threat to troops who served in the Gulf War. Military personnel in the Gulf War were prophylactically treated with pyridostigmine (an acetylcholinesterase inhibitor) to counteract the effects of these poisonous agents.

BOX 34-14

SIGNS AND SYMPTOMS OF ORGANOPHOSPHATE OR CARBAMATE POISONING

Cardiovascular System
Bradycardia
Variable blood pressure (usually hypotensive)

Respiratory System
Rhinorrhea
Bronchoconstriction
Wheezing
Dyspnea

Gastrointestinal System
Cramps
Emesis
Defecation
Increased bowel sounds

Vision
Miosis
Rapidly changing pupil size

Lacrimation
Blurred vision

Central Nervous System
Anxiety
Dizziness
Coma
Convulsions
Respiratory depression

Musculoskeletal System
Fasciculations
Flaccid paralysis

Skin
Diaphoresis

Other
Salivation
Urination

primary skin exposure. A helpful mnemonic to recognize the signs of poisoning is *SLUDGE* (salivation, lacrimation, urination, defecation, gastrointestinal cramping, and emesis).

? CRITICAL THINKING

If a person did not suspect poisoning, what condition may they think they are suffering from with this clinical presentation?

NOTE

Rapidly changing pupils with miosis are very common with vapor exposure of organophosphates, and muscle fasciculations can rapidly follow. Focal muscle fasciculation can be associated with liquid contact and local skin absorption at the site.

Management

Emergency care begins with scene safety, personal protection, and decontamination procedures (see Chapter 51). After these measures, patient care can be initiated. The general principles of management for poisoning by absorption include respiratory support, drug administration, and ECG monitoring. Although organophosphates and carbamates produce similar physiological effects, carbamates have a shorter duration of action and therefore a more rapid decrement of effect.

Respiratory Support

Respiratory tract symptoms usually are first to appear after exposure to organophosphates or carbamates, and respiratory paralysis may occur suddenly without clear warning signs. The need for aggressive airway management and ventilatory support should therefore be anticipated throughout the patient care encounter. Copious bronchial secretions may require suctioning, and bronchoconstriction may necessitate positive-pressure ventilation and positive end-expiratory pressure.

Drug Administration

Drug therapy in organophosphate or carbamate poisoning is directed at blocking the effects of acetylcholine, separating cholinesterase from the chemical compound, and suppressing seizure activity (if present). The drugs currently used as antidotes include *atropine*, *pralidoxime chloride* (2-PAM Chloride), and *diazepam* (Valium).

Atropine reverses the muscarinic effects (bradycardia, bronchoconstriction, respiratory secretions, and miosis) of moderate-to-severe organophosphate or carbamate poisoning. The drug competitively antagonizes the actions of acetylcholine, resulting in a decrease in the hyperactivity of smooth muscles and glands. The initial dose is 2 to 5 mg IV push every 5 to 15 minutes is required to dry the patient's secretions and to decrease pulmonary resistance to ventilation. The pediatric dose is 0.05 mg/kg, repeated every 15 minutes as necessary. (Medical direction may recommend that *atropine* be administered intramuscularly during the decontamination process before establishing an IV line.) Because potentially hypoxic patients may require administration of large doses of *atropine*, ECG monitoring for signs of dysrhythmias (other than tachycardia) and provision of supplemental oxygen must be undertaken to minimize the risk of ventricular fibrillation. *Atropine* is the drug of choice for carbamate poisonings.

Pralidoxime (2-Pam Chloride) is the treatment of choice for organophosphate poisoning after administration of *atropine*, and should be used for nearly all patients with clinically significant exposures, particularly those with muscular fasciculations and weakness. *Pralidoxime* (2-Pam Chloride) is one of a few drugs that correct a biochemical lesion. *Pralidoxime* (2-Pam Chloride) has the primary effect of reversing the phosphorylation-acetyl-cholinesterase bond, thus freeing and reactivating acetylcholinesterase. The initial adult dose of *pralidoxime* (2-PAM Chloride) is 600 mg IM or 1 to 2 g IV over 15 to 30 minutes. The pediatric dose is 20 to 50 mg/kg IV over 15 to 30 minutes. Subsequent doses may be repeated within 1 to 2 hours.

Diazepam (Valium) may be indicated if seizures are present. If the need for *diazepam* (Valium) arises before decontamination is complete, the drug should be administered IM in 2-mg increments as necessary to control seizure activity. (IV therapy should not be initiated in a patient in a contaminated area.) The paramedic should be alert to the possibility of respiratory and CNS depression.

? CRITICAL THINKING

If you give diazepam for seizures in this situation, will that eliminate the need for atropine?

ECG Monitoring

ECG monitoring may reveal a variety of abnormalities, including idioventricular rhythms, multifocal PVCs, VT, torsades de pointes, VF, complete heart block, and asystole (see the appendix at the end of this chapter). These dysrhythmias usually occur in two phases, beginning with a transient episode of intense sympathetic tone that results in sinus tachycardia and followed by a period of extreme parasympathetic tone that may manifest as sinus bradycardia, AV block, and ST-segment and T-wave abnormalities. Significant ventricular bradydysrhythmias that do not respond to conventional therapy may need to be managed with overdrive pacing (see Chapter 28).

SECTION TWO
DRUG ABUSE

The term *drug abuse* refers to the use of prescription drugs for nonprescribed purposes or the use of drugs that have no prescribed medical use (Box 34-15). Emergencies resulting from drug abuse include adverse effects caused by the drug or impurities or

BOX 34-15

DRUG ABUSE TERMINOLOGY

Drug abuse: Self-medication or self-administration of a drug in chronically excessive amounts, resulting in psychological and/or physical dependence, functional impairment, and deviation from approved social norms

Drug dependence: Condition marked by an overwhelming desire to continue taking a drug for its desired effect, usually an altered mental activity, attitude, or outlook

Psychological dependence: Emotional reliance on a drug (Manifestations range from a mild desire for a drug to craving and drug-seeking behavior to repeated compulsive use of a drug for its subjectively satisfying or pleasurable effects.)

Physical dependence: An adaptive physiological state occurring after prolonged use of many drugs (discontinuation causes withdrawal syndromes that are relieved by readministering the same drug or a pharmacologically related drug).

Tolerance: A tendency to increase drug dosage to experience the same effect formerly produced by a smaller dose

Withdrawal syndrome: A predictable set of signs and symptoms that occurs after a decrease in the amount of the usual dose of a drug or its sudden cessation

ILLICIT DRUG USE IN THE UNITED STATES

A survey conducted by Health and Human Services' Substance Abuse and Mental Health Services Administration (SAMSHA) in 1998 revealed the following statistics:

- An estimated 13.6 million Americans currently use illicit drugs.
- An estimated 1.8 million Americans are frequent cocaine users.
- An estimated 2.3 million Americans regularly use marijuana.
- An estimated 730,000 Americans used cocaine for the first time in 1997.
- An estimated 81,000 Americans used heroin for the first time in 1997.
- An estimated 1.1 million Americans began using hallucinogens in 1997.
- An estimated 4.3 million women of childbearing age are illicit drug users; more than 1.6 million have children living with them, including 390,000 with at least one child under 2 years of age.

From HHS News: *Summary findings from the 1998 national household survey on drug abuse,* US Department of Health and Human Services, 1999, http://www.samhsa.gov

? CRITICAL THINKING

Why might a patient (or their friends) delay calling for help in a situation involving drug overdose?

Toxic Effects of Drugs

EMS personnel frequently encounter people suffering from the toxic effects of drugs as the result of an overdose, a potential suicide, polydrug administration, or an accident (accidental ingestion, miscalculation, changes in drug strength). The drugs discussed in this chapter are listed in Box 34-16.

✓ TRICKS OF THE TRADE

Acute dystonic reactions are caused by reactions to psychotropic medications. Because the face is distorted and speech may be affected, Bell's palsy may come to mind. Always ask the patient about *any* medication that may have been taken.

contaminants mixed with the drug, life-threatening infections from intravenous or intradermal injection of drugs with unsterile equipment, accidents during intoxication, and drug dependence or withdrawal syndrome resulting from the habit-forming potential of many drugs (see Chapter 8).

No single cause or set of conditions clearly leads to drug abuse. It is widespread and common among all socioeconomic, cultural, and ethnic groups. Drug abuse is a major medical, social, and interpersonal problem that affects individuals from all backgrounds and of all ages (see the box in the right column). Because of the widespread use and misuse of drugs, the paramedic should maintain a high degree of suspicion and consider the possibility for a drug-related problem in any patient who has seizures, behavioral changes, stupor, or coma. In addition, consideration of the visibility, accessibility, and careful handling of all medications carried on an EMS vehicle should be a part of any EMS policy and procedure.

TRICKS OF THE TRADE

About 98% of clandestine drug labs manufacture methamphetamine. If you come upon a suspected drug lab, retreat from the scene and request backup with a hazardous materials team and/or bomb squad.

NOTE

Common drugs of abuse (along with their names and uses) vary widely in different geographical areas and frequently change over time. Table 34-2 is a partial list of common drugs of abuse, their street names, and miscellaneous terminology relating to drug use.

General Management Principles

The general principles for managing drug abuse and the overdose that may result are listed below:

1. Ensure scene safety and be prepared for unpredictable patient behavior. (Consider the need for law enforcement assistance.)
2. Ensure adequate airway, ventilatory, and circulatory support as needed.
3. Obtain a history of the event (including the self-administration of other drugs that may have been taken by another route) and any significant past medical or psychiatric history.
4. Identify the substance and consult with medical direction or a poison control center.
5. Perform a thorough focused physical examination. Continually monitor the patient's vital functions and ECG.
6. Initiate IV therapy. Draw a blood sample for laboratory analysis and administer appropriate pharmacological antidotes such as *naloxone* (Narcan) if an opiate overdose is suspected. Personal protective measures should be given special attention because many of these patients are at high risk of harboring infectious disease.
7. Prevent further absorption of an orally administered drug by the administration of *activated charcoal* (per protocol).
8. Rapidly transport the patient for physician evaluation.

BOX 34-16

COMMON AGENTS INVOLVED IN POISONING

Opioids
Sedatives-hypnotics
Stimulants
Phencyclidine (PCP)
Hallucinogens
Tricyclic antidepressants (TCAs)
Lithium
Cardiac medications
MAO inhibitors
Nonprescription pain medicines
Salicylates
Acetaminophen
Drugs abused for sexual purposes/sexual gratification
Metals (iron, lead, and mercury)

NOTE

When examining any patient suspected of abusing drugs, the paramedic should always look for "track marks" (in the antecubital space, under the tongue, on top of the feet). The possibility of "body packing" (concealing packets of drugs in body cavities of the stomach, rectum, and vagina) or "body stuffing" (swallowing drugs to avoid arrest) also should be considered when a person who abuses drugs appears ill for no apparent reason.

? CRITICAL THINKING

For what illnesses is the patient who uses IV narcotics at risk?

Opioid Overdose

Heroin accounts for about 90% of the opioid abuse in the United States. Pure heroin is a bitter-tasting white powder that is usually adulterated or "cut" for street distribution with various agents such as lactose, sucrose, baking soda, powdered milk, starch, magnesium silicate (talc), procaine, quinine, and recently with scopolamine. A typical "bag" is the single-dose unit of heroin and may weigh 100 mg, which on average is only 20% to 30% pure. Other opioid drugs include *morphine*, hydromorphone, methadone,

TABLE 34-2 COMMONLY ABUSED DRUGS—STREET NAMES FOR DRUGS OF ABUSE

SUBSTANCE	EXAMPLES OF PROPRIETARY OR STREET NAMES	MEDICAL USES	ROUTE OF ADMINISTRATION	DEA SCHEDULE*	PERIOD OF DETECTION
Stimulants					
Amphetamine	Biphetamine, Dexedrine; black beauties, crosses, hearts	Attention deficit hyperactivity disorder (ADHD), obesity, narcolepsy	Injected, oral, smoked, sniffed	II	1-2 days
Cocaine	Coke, crack, flake, rocks, snow	Local anesthetic, vasoconstrictor	Injected, smoked, sniffed	II	1-4 days
Methamphetamine	Desoxyn; crank, crystal, glass, ice, speed	ADHD, obesity, narcolepsy	Injected, oral, smoked, sniffed	II	1-2 days
Methylphenidate	Ritalin	ADHD, narcolepsy	Injected, oral	II	1-2 days
Nicotine	Habitrol patch, Nicorette gum, Nicotrol spray, Prostep patch; cigars, cigarettes, smokeless tobacco, snuff, spit tobacco	Treatment for nicotine dependence	Smoked, sniffed, oral, transdermal	Not scheduled	1-2 days
Hallucinogens and Other Compounds					
LSD	Acid, microdot	None	Oral	I	8 hours
Mescaline	Buttons, cactus, mesc, peyote	None	Oral	I	2-3 days
Phencyclidine and Analogs	PCP; angel dust, boat, hog, love boat	Anesthetic (veterinary)	Injected, oral, smoked	I, II	2-8 days
Psilocybin	Magic mushroom, purple passion, shrooms	None	Oral	I	8 hours
Amphetamine variants	DOB, DOM, MDA, MDMA; adam, ecstasy, STP, XTC	None	Oral	I	1-2 days
Marijuana	Blunt, grass, herb, pot, reefer, sinsemilla, smoke, weed	None	Oral, smoked	I	1 day-5 weeks
Hashish	Hash	None	Oral, smoked	I	1 day-5 weeks
Tetrahydrocannabinol	Marinol, THC	Antiemetic	Oral, smoked	I, II	1 day-5 weeks
Anabolic steroids	Testosterone (T/E ratio), stanazolol, nandrolene	Hormone replacement therapy	Oral, injected	III	Oral: up to 3 weeks (for testosterone and others); injected: up to 3 months (Nandrolene up to 9 months)
Opioids and Morphine Derivatives					
Codeine	Tylenol w/codeine, Robitussin A-C, Empirin w/codeine, Fiorinal w/codeine	Analgesic, antitussive	Injected, oral	II, III, IV	1-2 days
Heroin	Diacetylmorphine; horse, smack	None	Injected, smoked, sniffed	I	1-2 days
Methadone	Amidone, Dolophine, Methadose	Analgesic, treatment for opiate dependence	Injected, oral	II	1 day-1 week
Morphine	Roxanol, Duramorph	Analgesic	Injected, oral, smoked	II, III	1-2 days
Opium	Laudanum, Paregoric; Dover's powder	Analgesic, antidiarrheal	Oral, smoked	II, III, V	1-2 days
Depressants					
Alcohol	Beer, wine, liquor	Antidote for methanol poisoning	Oral	Not scheduled	6-10 hours
Barbiturates	Amytal, Nembutal, Seconal, Phenobarbital; Barbs	Anesthetic, anticonvulsant, hypnotic, sedative	Injected, oral	II, III, IV	2-10 days
Benzodiazepines	Activan, Halcion, Librium, Rohypnol, Valium; roofies, tranks, Xanax	Antianxiety, anticonvulsant, hypnotic, sedative	Injected, oral	IV	1-6 weeks
Methaqualone	Quaalude; ludes	None	Oral	I	2 weeks

*Drug Enforcement Administration (DEA) Schedule I and II drugs have a high potential for abuse. They require greater storage security and have a quota on manufacture among other restrictions. Schedule I drugs are available for research only and have no approved medical use. Schedule II drugs are available only through prescription, cannot have refills and require a form for ordering. Schedule III and IV drugs are available with prescription, may have five refills in 6 months, and may be ordered orally. Most Schedule V drugs are available over the counter.

Information about NIDA send e-mail to *Information@lists.nida.nih.gov*. This page last updated Wednesday, September 29, 1999.

http://www.nih.gov/ For additional information about NIDA send e-mail to *Information@lists.nida.nih.gov.* This page last updated Wednesday, September 29, 1999.

meperidine (Demerol), codeine, oxycodone, propoxyphene, and "designer opiates" that have been chemically modified such as alpha methyl fentanyl ("China white").

Depending on the preparation, these drugs may be taken orally, injected intradermally ("skin popping") or intravenously ("mainlining"), taken intranasally ("snorted"), or smoked. All opioids are CNS depressants and can cause life-threatening respiratory depression. In severe intoxication, hypotension, profound shock, and pulmonary edema may be present. Signs and symptoms of narcotic/opiate overdose include the following:

- Euphoria
- Arousable somnolence ("nodding")
- Nausea
- Pinpoint pupils (except with *meperidine* [Demerol], hypoxia, or in combination with other types of drugs)
- Coma
- Seizures

Antidote Therapy

As described in Chapter 8, *naloxone* (Narcan) is a pure opioid antagonist effective for virtually all opioid and opioid-like substances. The drug reverses the triad of symptoms of opioid overdose (respiratory depression, coma, and miosis) and should be considered for administration when opioid intoxication is suspected or when a coma of unknown origin is present. The EMS crew should be prepared to restrain the patient, whose behavior may be unpredictable when the effects of the drug are reversed and the patient experiences withdrawal symptoms. Medical direction may recommend that the *naloxone* (Narcan) administration be titrated to keep the patient responsive and free from respiratory depression but somewhat docile during transport.

> **NOTE**
>
> Two other pure opioid antagonists are available: Naltrexone (Trexan) is an oral medication used in long-term programs for opioid addiction. **Nalmefene** (Revex) appears to be as effective as *naloxone* (Narcan) in acute opioid intoxications and has a longer duration of action (4 to 8 hours) than *naloxone* (Narcan).

Some opiates (e.g., heroin), have a longer duration than *naloxone* (Narcan). Therefore the patient must be closely monitored during antidote therapy, and repeated doses of *naloxone* (Narcan) may be necessary. In communities where abuse of naloxone-resistant opiates or where China white use is prevalent, larger initial doses of *naloxone* (Narcan) may be needed.[4]

> **NOTE**
>
> The desired end points of opiate reversal are adequate airway reflexes and ventilations—not complete arousal.[4]

Naloxone (Narcan) can precipitate a withdrawal syndrome in opioid-dependent patients. This is seldom life threatening and usually can be managed by symptomatic and supportive care. Signs and symptoms of opioid withdrawal are listed in Box 34-17.

Sedative-Hypnotic Overdose

Sedative-hypnotic agents include benzodiazepines and barbiturates. These drugs usually are taken orally but may be diluted and injected intravenously. Use with alcohol markedly increases their effects. Sedative-hypnotic drugs commonly are known as *downers*.

Benzodiazepines are among the best-known and most widely prescribed drugs used to control symptoms of anxiety, stress, and insomnia. In addition, these drugs sometimes are used to manage alcohol withdrawal and control seizure disorders. Benzodiazepines promote sleep and relieve anxiety by depressing brain function; they frequently are abused for their sedative effects. Individually, these

> **BOX 34-17**
>
> ### SIGNS AND SYMPTOMS OF OPIOID WITHDRAWAL
>
> Gooseflesh
> Tachycardia
> Diaphoresis
> Irritability
> Insomnia
> Abdominal cramps
> Tremors
> Nausea and vomiting
> Anorexia
> Cold sweats or chills
> Fever
> Diarrhea
> General malaise

drugs are relatively nontoxic, but they may accentuate the effects of other sedative-hypnotic agents. Common benzodiazepines are *diazepam* (Valium) and chlordiazepoxide (Librium).

Barbiturates are general CNS depressants that inhibit impulse conduction in the ascending reticular activating system. These drugs once were widely used to treat anxiety and insomnia. Their addictive properties and potential for abuse have led to their replacement by benzodiazepines and other nonbarbiturate drugs. Barbiturates that commonly are abused include phenobarbital (Luminal), amobarbital (Amytal), and secobarbital (Secogen).

Signs and symptoms of sedative-hypnotic overdose chiefly are related to the central nervous and cardiovascular systems. Adverse effects include excessive drowsiness, staggering gait, and in some cases, paradoxical excitability. In cases of severe toxicity, the patient may become comatose, with respiratory depression, hypotension, and shock. Pupils may be constricted but often become fixed and di-

lated even in the absence of significant brain damage. Airway control and ventilatory management are the essential points in managing significant sedative-hypnotic overdose. *Flumazenil* (Romazicon), a benzodiazepine antagonist, can be used to reverse the effects of benzodiazepines. The drug, however, can produce seizure activity and is not routinely recommended.[4]

Stimulant Overdose

Commonly abused stimulant drugs are those of the sympathomimetic family (e.g., Benzedrine, Dexedrine, cocaine, methamphetamine) (see the box below).

Sympathomimetic drugs frequently are used to produce general mood elevation, improve task performance, suppress appetite, and prevent sleepiness. Structurally, the amphetamines are similar to the endogenous catecholamines (epinephrine and norepinephrine) but differ in their more pronounced effects on the central nervous system. Adverse effects include tachycardia, increased blood pressure, tachypnea, agitation, dilated pupils, tremors, and disorganized behavior. In severe intoxication, the patient may exhibit psychosis and paranoia and experience hallucinations. Sudden withdrawal or cessation of amphetamine use may result in a "crash"

NOTE

Flumazenil (Romazicon) is contraindicated in patients who are prone to seizures and in those with tricyclic antidepressant overdose.

METHAMPHETAMINE

Methamphetamine is a synthetically manufactured CNS stimulant. Although it is legally manufactured for medicinal purposes (methedrine and desoxyn), its illicit production as a street drug in the United States is on the rise. Common names for methamphetamine include *meth, speed, crank, crystal, water,* or *ice.*

Illegal methamphetamine can be inexpensively produced in clandestine "meth labs" with common chemical methods (hydriodic acid, phenyl-2-propane, sodium ammonia, thiony-chloride). The drug can then be smoked, injected, snorted, or taken orally. Once methamphetamine enters the body, it can produce skeletal muscle tremors, sleeplessness, and euphoria that can last up to 10 days. During these drug-induced sleepless "binges," users may become hostile and paranoid followed by a "crash" (an emotionally depressed state) that can last for several days.

In addition to ensuring personal safety when dealing with these patients, the paramedic crew should be

keenly aware of potential hazards associated with clandestine labs. These hazards include the production of highly explosive toxic gases (e.g., phosphine) that can be readily absorbed through the skin in quantities that can be fatal; an oxygen-depleted environment; the use of toxic solvents that can lead to lab explosions; and exposure to other dangerous chemicals. Any time a meth lab is suspected, the EMS crew should withdraw and patients and bystanders should be evacuated. Law enforcement and specialized hazardous materials personnel should be summoned to the scene. Drug-making paraphernalia that should alert the paramedic to the presence of a meth lab include the following:*

- Amber stains on walls, furniture, and counters
- Equipment that has a red or amber color
- Two large, round-bottom flasks (with stoppers) connected by a hose
- Pyrex-type meatloaf container
- Various measuring and funnel devices
- A heat source

*From Goss J: Meth labs, *JEMS* 23:1, 1998.

stage in which the patient becomes depressed, suicidal, incoherent, or near coma. As a rule, these agents are taken orally, but they also may be smoked or injected for a rapid onset of action. Amphetamines commonly are known as *speed* or *uppers*.

Cocaine

Cocaine is one of the most popular illegal drugs in the United States. Cocaine is a fine, white crystalline powder. Like heroin, street forms of cocaine usually are adulterated and vary in purity from 25% to 90%; doses vary from near 0 to 200 mg. This form of cocaine generally is taken intranasally by snorting a "line" containing 10 to 35 mg of the drug (depending on purity). After absorption through the mucous membranes, the effects of the drug begin within minutes. Peak effects occur 15 to 60 minutes after use, with a half-life of 1 to 2½ hours. Cocaine also is used parenterally by the subcutaneous, intramuscular, and IV routes; the IV route provides immediate absorption and intense stimulation (peak occurs within 5 minutes with a half-life of about 50 minutes).

> **NOTE**
>
> *Speed-balling* refers to an injection of a cocaine-heroin combination.

Freebase or "crack" cocaine is a more potent formulation of the drug that is prepared by mixing powdered street cocaine with an alkaline solution and then adding a solvent such as ether. The combination separates into two layers, the top layer containing the dissolved cocaine. Evaporation of the solvent results in pure cocaine crystals, which are smoked and absorbed via the pulmonary route. Cocaine in this form is called *rock* or *crack* because of the popping sound produced when the crystals are heated. Freebase cocaine generally is combined with marijuana or tobacco and smoked in a pipe or a cigarette. The reactions are similar to those experienced in IV use, with equal intensity and effects.

Cocaine is a major CNS stimulant that causes profound sympathetic discharge. The increased levels of circulating catecholamines result in excitement, euphoria, talkativeness, and agitation. The effects of the drug can precipitate significant cardiovascular and neurological complications such as cardiac dysrhythmias, myocardial infarction, seizures, intracranial hemorrhage, hyperthermia, and psychiatric disturbances. Cocaine overdose can

occur with any form of the drug and any route of administration. The adult fatal dose is thought to be about 1200 mg (1.2 g), but fatalities from cocaine-induced cardiac dysrhythmias have been reported with single doses of as little as 25 to 30 mg.[5]

Prehospital management of the cocaine-intoxicated patient may be complex; the toxicity may range from minor symptoms to life-threatening overdose. Emergency care may require a full spectrum of basic and advanced life-support measures, including aggressive airway management, ventilatory and circulatory support, pharmacological therapy (benzodiazepines are the mainstay of treatment initially in cocaine toxicity), and rapid transport to an appropriate medical facility (see the appendix at the end of this chapter).

Phencyclidine (PCP) Overdose

PCP is a dissociative analgesic (originally used as a veterinary tranquilizer) with sympathomimetic and CNS stimulant and depressant properties. It is a potent psychoactive drug illegally sold in liquid, tablet, or powder form to be taken orally, intranasally, IV/IM, or with other drugs to be smoked (a "Sherman"). Most tablets contain about 5 mg of PCP. As a rule, PCP in its powder form is relatively pure (50% to 100% PCP). Chronic use can result in permanent memory impairment and loss of higher brain functions. The pharmacological effects are dose related and can be divided into low-dose and high-dose toxicity.

> **NOTE**
>
> Ketamine is a derivative of PCP and has identical actions. It is now as popular as PCP.

Low-Dose Toxicity

In low doses (less than 10 mg), PCP intoxication produces an unpredictable state that can resemble drunkenness; the user may have a sense of euphoria or confusion, disorientation, agitation, or sudden rage. An intoxicated patient often has a blank stare and a stumbling gait and is in a dissociative state. The patient's pupils generally are reactive; the patient may experience flushing, diaphoresis, facial grimacing, hypersalivation, and vomiting. **Nystagmus** with a burst-like quality is characteristic of low-dose PCP use. In this range of toxicity, death usually is related to behavioral disturbances resulting from spatial disorientation, drug-induced immobility, and insensitivity to pain. This insensitivity to pain leads to Herculean acts of strength, because the normal muscle activity limitation resulting from pain is inhibited.

> **? CRITICAL THINKING**
>
> *What characteristics of this type of intoxication make the patient high risk for injury?*

Low-dose toxicity is best managed by keeping sensory stimulation to a minimum (verbal and physical stimuli exacerbate the clinical symptoms). Violent and combative patients require protection from self-injury while safeguards are provided for the emergency crew and bystanders. Vital signs and level of consciousness should be closely monitored, and the patient should be observed for increasing motor activity and muscle rigidity, which may precede seizures.

High-Dose Toxicity

Patients with high-dose PCP intoxication (more than 10 mg) may be in a coma, which may last from hours to several days, and thus often are unresponsive to painful stimuli. Respiratory depression, hypertension, and tachycardia also may be present, depending on the dosage. In severe cases, a hypertensive crisis causing cardiac failure, hypertensive encephalopathy, seizures, and intracerebral hemorrhage may result. Prehospital care is directed at managing life-threatening complications such as respiratory and cardiac arrest and status epilepticus and rapidly transporting the patient for physician evaluation.

Phencyclidine Psychosis

PCP psychosis is a true psychiatric emergency that may mimic schizophrenia. The psychosis usually is of acute onset and may not become apparent until several days after ingestion. It can occur after a single low-dose exposure to PCP and may last from several days to weeks. The clinical syndromes range from a catatonic and unresponsive state to bizarre and violent behavior. The patient frequently appears agitated and suspicious and often experiences auditory hallucinations and paranoia. Appropriate management usually requires involuntary hospitalization, control of violent behavior, and administration of antipsychotic agents. When dealing with these patients in the prehospital setting, personal safety is of paramount importance; law enforcement should be summoned for assistance.

Hallucinogen Overdose

Hallucinogens are substances that cause perceptual distortions. The most common hallucinogen in use today is lysergic acid diethylamide (LSD). Other hallucinogens include mescaline, found in the buttons of peyote cactus, which can be used legally in some religious settings; psilocybin mushrooms, found in the United States and Mexico; marijuana, the active agent of the plant *Cannabis sativa;* morning glory plant; nutmeg; mace; and some amphetamines, such as MDMA ("Ecstasy") and MDEA ("Eve").

Depending on the agent, the effects of hallucinogens may range from minor visual to more serious complications (associated with LSD use) such as respiratory and central nervous system depression (rare). Prehospital management usually is limited to supportive care, minimal sensory stimulation, calming measures, and transportation to a medical facility. After arrival at the emergency department, these patients generally are observed in a quiet environment.

Tricyclic Antidepressant Overdose

Tricyclic antidepressants (TCAs) commonly are prescribed in the management of depression and certain pain syndromes. These drugs work by blocking the uptake of norepinephrine and serotonin into the presynaptic neurons and by altering the sensitivity of brain tissue to the actions of these chemicals. Serious TCA toxicity results from sodium-channel blockade in the myocardium. Other toxicities include potassium efflux blockade and blockade of blood vessels, anticholinergic effects, and seizures. Commonly prescribed antidepressant drugs include the TCAs amitriptyline (Amitril), imipramine (Apo-Imipramine), and nortriptyline (Aventyl). The newer *selective serotonin reuptake inhibitors* (SSRIs) such as fluoxetine (Prozac), sertraline (Zoloft), and paroxetine (Paxil) are chemically unrelated to TCAs and are considered extremely safe and effective when compared with TCAs.

Early symptoms of TCA overdose are dry mouth, blurred vision, confusion, inability to concentrate, and occasionally visual hallucinations. More severe symptoms include delirium, depressed respirations, hypertension, hypotension, hyperthermia, hypothermia, seizures, and coma (Box 34-18). Cardiac effects may range from tachycardia to bradycardia and various dysrhythmias secondary to atrioventricular block. A prolonged QRS complex, a Glasgow coma scale less than 8, or both, are characteristic findings that should alert the paramedic to a major toxicity with potentially serious complications. Sudden death from cardiac arrest may occur several days after an overdose.

Little effective prehospital management exists for major toxicity of a TCA overdose. Basic supportive care and rapid transport should be instituted. A total of 25% of patients who ultimately die as a result of the overdose are alert and awake, and 75% have normal sinus rhythm when EMS personnel arrive.[2] Tachycardia, especially with a wide QRS complex greater than 100 ms, is an early sign of toxicity. *Sodium bicarbonate*, 1 to 2 mEq/kg given IV per medical direction, may begin to reverse cardiac toxicity. Any patient with a history of TCA ingestion should receive airway, ventilatory, and circulatory support; IV access; ECG monitoring; and rapid transport for physician evaluation. More definitive treatment for specific problems (e.g., seizures, ventricular dysrhythmias) is complex, using a combination of alkalinization and anticonvulsants when appropriate. Rapid transport to the emergency department is the most prudent course of action.

? CRITICAL THINKING

How can you ensure rapid transport of these patients?

Lithium

Lithium is a mood-stabilizing drug that sometimes is prescribed for the management of bipolar disorders (see Chapter 38). Because the drug has a very low toxic-to-therapeutic dose ratio, lithium overdose is common.

> **NOTE**
> Patients who are prescribed lithium have frequent blood tests to monitor the level of lithium in the body.

Lithium helps to prevent "mood swings" by interfering with hormonal responses to cyclic adenosine monophosphate and by augmenting the reuptake of norepinephrine (producing an antiadrenergic effect). As a result of these actions, lithium has multiple ef-

> **BOX 34-18**
>
> ### FIVE SIGNS OF MAJOR TCA TOXICITY
>
> Coma
> Cardiac dysrhythmias
> GI disturbances
> Respiratory depression
> Hypotension or hypertension

fects on the body that include muscle tremor, thirst, nausea, increased urination, abdominal cramping, and diarrhea. With toxic ingestion, signs and symptoms may include the following:

- Muscle weakness
- Slurred speech
- Severe trembling
- Blurred vision
- Confusion
- Seizure
- Apnea
- Coma

Prehospital care for patients with suspected lithium overdose should focus on airway management, ventilatory and circulatory support, and the control of seizure activity (if present). (*Activated charcoal* does not effectively bind lithium.) In-hospital care may include restoring intravascular volume, maintaining urine output, correcting hyponatremia, and sometimes dialysis.

Cardiac Medications

Cardiac drugs are a common cause of poisoning fatalities in children and adults. The drugs responsible for the majority of these fatalities are *digoxin* (Lanoxin), beta blockers, and calcium channel blockers (Box 34-19; also see the appendix at the end of this chapter).

> **NOTE**
> As in all other cases of poisoning, patients with toxic ingestion of cardiac drugs require high-concentration oxygen administration, IV access, and careful monitoring of vital signs and ECG.

Digoxin (Lanoxin) exerts direct and indirect effects on SA and AV nodal fibers. At toxic levels, the

BOX 34-19

TOXIC EFFECTS OF COMMON CARDIAC DRUGS

Digoxin
Bigeminal and multifocal PVCs
First- and second-degree AV block
Sinus bradycardia
Atrial fibrillation
Atrial tachycardia
VT/VF

Beta Blockers
Bradycardia
Hypotension
Unconsciousness
Respiratory arrest
Seizure
VT/VF (rare)

Calcium Channel Blockers
Hypotension
Sinus bradycardia
Sinus arrest
AV dissociation
Asystole
Respiratory depression
Pulmonary edema
ARDS
Confusion
Slurred speech
Coma
Lactic acidosis
Mild hyperglycemia/hyperkalemia

drug can halt impulses in the SA node, depress conduction through the AV node, and increase sensitivity of the SA and AV nodes to catecholamines.[5] *Digoxin* (Lanoxin) also affects the Purkinje fibers by decreasing the resting potential and action potential duration and by enhancing automaticity, which can lead to an increase in PVC formation. Unlike most cardiovascular drugs, *digoxin* (Lanoxin) can produce most any dysrhythmia or conduction block. In addition to dysrhythmias, common signs and symptoms of *digoxin* (Lanoxin) toxicity include nausea, anorexia, fatigue, visual disturbances, and a variety of disorders of the GI, ophthalmological, and neurological systems. Oral overdoses generally are managed with *activated charcoal* and drugs to manage life-threatening dysrhythmias. Severe

overdoses are managed with IV *digoxin-specific FAB* (Digibind), a binding compound that decreases the morbidity and mortality associated with *digitalis* (Lanoxin) overdose.

? CRITICAL THINKING

Why is it possible that this type of overdose would not be detected immediately?

Beta blockers are rapidly absorbed after ingestion. Toxicity impairs SA and AV node function, leading to bradycardias and AV blocks. The associated depression in ventricular conduction and sodium channel blockade makes these patients susceptible to wide QRS complexes and, occasionally, ventricular dysrhythmias (rarely VT or VF). Other signs and symptoms include CNS and respiratory depression, hypotension, and seizures. Emergency care for patients with beta blocker overdose includes *activated charcoal*, and drugs to manage hypotension and dysrhythmias. In-hospital care may include infusions of *glucagon* and various catecholamines, and possible hemodialysis (depending on the particular agent involved).

Toxic ingestion of calcium channel blockers can lead to myocardial depression and peripheral vasodilation with negative inotropic, chronotropic, dromotropic, and vasotropic effects. Hypotension and bradycardia are early manifestations of toxicity. Overdose may result in serious dysrhythmias that include AV block of all degrees, sinus arrest, AV dissociation, junctional rhythm, and asystole. (Calcium channel blockers have little effect on ventricular conduction; ventricular dysrhythmias are uncommon.) Other signs and symptoms of calcium channel toxicity include nausea and vomiting, hypotension, and CNS and respiratory depression. In addition to airway, ventilatory, and circulatory support, emergency care may include the use of antidysrhythmics, vasopressors, and *activated charcoal*.

MAO Inhibitors

As described in Chapter 8, MAO inhibitors block the breakdown of monoamines (norepinephrine, dopamine, serotonin). These CNS transmitters are widely distributed throughout the body, with the highest concentration in the brain, liver, and kidneys. MAO inhibitors are prescribed as antidepressants, antineoplastics, antibiotics, and antihypertensives. Some MAO inhibitors (e.g., the antidepressants phenelzine and tranylcypromine) have active metabolites. Signs of MAO inhibitor toxicity usually are delayed (6 to 24 hours after ingestion), and the duration of effects may last for several days (Box 34-20). These effects include CNS depression and various neuromuscular and cardiovascular system manifestations.

Prehospital care is primarily supportive and includes airway, ventilatory, and circulatory support; cardiac medications as needed; and rapid transport for physician evaluation. *Activated charcoal* is recommended for all patients if awake.

Nonsteroidal Antiinflammatory Drugs

Nonsteroidal antiinflammatory drugs (NSAIDs) are a group of agents that have an analgesic and antipyretic action and also reduce inflammation of joints and soft tissues, such as muscles and ligaments. They work by blocking the production of prostaglandins, chemicals that cause inflammation and trigger transmission of pain signals to the brain. NSAIDs are widely used to relieve symptoms caused by types of arthritis (rheumatoid arthritis, osteoarthritis, gout) and in the treatment of back pain, menstrual pain, headaches, minor postoperative pain, and soft tissue injuries. Common NSAIDs include difunisal (Dolobid), fenoprofen (Nalfon), ibuprofen (Advil, Motrin), and naproxen (Aleve).

> **NOTE**
>
> Ibuprofen and naproxen are available in over-the-counter forms and are promoted as safer and more effective alternatives to salicylates and acetaminophen in the management of fever and mild to moderate pain.

Ibuprofen Overdose

Ibuprofen (Advil, Motrin) is the most commonly ingested NSAID in overdose. The effects usually are reversible and seldom life threatening (although significant toxicity may result in coma, seizure, hypotension, and acute renal failure). Common symptoms of chronic and acute ingestion (more than 300 mg/kg) include mild GI and CNS disturbances that usually resolve within 24 hours after ingestion. Other less common effects include mild metabolic acidosis, muscle fasciculations, chills, hyperventila-

> **BOX 34-20**
>
> ### EFFECTS OF MAO INHIBITOR TOXICITY
>
> CNS depression
> Neuromuscular system manifestations
>   Agitation
>   Rigidity
>   Hyperflexia
>   Nystagmus
>   Hallucinations
>   Seizure
> Cardiovascular system manifestations
>   Sinus tachycardia
>   Hypotension with vascular collapse
>   Hypertension
>   Bradysystolic rhythms

tion, hypotension, and asymptomatic bradycardia. Emergency care for patients who have ingested toxic amounts of ibuprofen consists of gastric decontamination with *activated charcoal*, and careful monitoring for secondary complications, such as hypotension and dysrhythmias.

Salicylate Overdose

Salicylates are widely available in prescription and over-the-counter products such as acetylsalicylic acid (*aspirin*), many cold preparations, and oil of wintergreen (methyl salicylate) and in combination with some analgesics such as propoxyphene and oxycodone. Table 34-3 contains general guidelines for salicylate toxicity.

> **NOTE**
>
> At one time, ingestion of colorful and tasty children's *aspirin* was the most common cause of pediatric poisoning. In response to this problem, the number of tablets now is limited to 36 per container. Because of the association of *aspirin* with Reye's syndrome, *aspirin* is not recommended for children younger than 16 years of age who have viral symptoms.

The mechanism of toxicity with salicylate poisoning is complex and includes direct CNS stimulation, interference with cellular glucose uptake, and inhibition of Krebs cycle enzymes that affect energy

TABLE 34-3	TOXICITY GUIDELINES TO SALICYLATE	
TOXICITY	**AMOUNT INGESTED**	
Mild	Less than 150 mg/kg	
Moderate to severe	150 to 300 mg/kg	
Severe	Greater than 300 mg/kg	
Fatal	Greater than 500 mg/kg	

From Clark J: *Pharmacological basis of nursing*, ed 4, St Louis, 1993, Mosby.

production and amino acid metabolism. The volume of distribution is dose dependent and usually small; with toxic ingestion, however, redistribution of the drug into the CNS occurs and prolongs elimination of the drug from the body. Complications that may result from chronic or acute ingestion of salicylates include CNS stimulation, gastrointestinal irritation, glucose metabolism, fluid and electrolyte imbalance, neurological symptoms, and coagulation defects.

Central Nervous System Stimulation

Salicylates initially produce direct stimulation of the respiratory center in the CNS, causing an increased rate and depth of respiration. This early respiratory alkalosis is followed by a compensatory elimination of bicarbonate ions by the kidneys and a subsequent compensatory metabolic acidosis. After this period, intermediate acids accumulate and are involved in energy metabolism, leading to profound metabolic acidosis. Confusion, lethargy, convulsions, respiratory arrest, coma, and brain death all can occur in severe salicylate poisoning.

? CRITICAL THINKING

Would you predict a tachypnea or bradypnea in these patients? Why?

Gastrointestinal Irritation

Salicylates have irritant effects on the gastric mucosa, which can lead to nausea, vomiting, and hematemesis. They also can cause pylorospasm delaying gastric emptying.

Glucose Metabolism

Interference with cellular glucose uptake causes accumulation of serum glucose. Eventually, cellular

glucose is depleted, and the patient can demonstrate tissue effects of hypoglycemia (particularly in CNS tissue). Patients who die from salicylate poisoning frequently demonstrate primary central nervous system tissue toxicity and severe cerebral edema.

Fluid and Electrolyte Imbalance

Total body fluids are adversely affected by hypermetabolism. Fluid and electrolyte losses occur via gastrointestinal fluids, emesis, and renal clearance. Acid-base disturbances may result in hypokalemia and hyperchloremia. Cardiac dysrhythmias, including PVCs, VT, and VF are possible.

Neurological Symptoms

Mild neurological effects such as tinnitus (a symptom of salicylism on the cranial nerve VIII) and lethargy are common. Severe intoxication may result in hallucination, seizure, and coma.

Coagulation Effects

Salicylates alter normal platelet function and often lead to coagulation disorders when taken in toxic amounts. Therefore these patients are at increased risk of significant bleeding. Patients who take anticoagulants are at even greater risk for hemorrhage after salicylate ingestion.

In addition to general supportive measures, prehospital care for salicylate poisoning may include administration of *activated charcoal* for intestinal decontamination and IV glucose to manage hypoglycemia. Salicylates are weak acids excreted by the kidney. Therefore medical direction may recommend the administration of *sodium bicarbonate* to produce an alkaline urine. Definitive care includes in-hospital intensive care observation, continued support of vital functions, and perhaps hemodialysis.

✓ TRICKS OF THE TRADE

Always be alert when the patient has taken an acetaminophen overdose. Many times these suicide attempts are cries for help with the patient believing that something over-the-counter couldn't possibly kill them. Deaths from acetaminophen overdose are hideous and violent.

Acetaminophen Overdose

Acetaminophen is a commonly prescribed analgesic and antipyretic agent available in many prescription and nonprescription preparations (e.g., Tylenol, Panadol). Its widespread availability accounts for its high incidence in accidental and intentional poisoning. Acetaminophen overdose can cause life-threatening hepatic toxicity from formation of a hepatotoxic intermediate metabolite if not managed within 16 to 24 hours of ingestion. As few as 30 standard-size (325 mg) acetaminophen tablets are toxic in an average adult. Acetaminophen also is present in many drug combinations including Darvocet-N, Excedrin, and Sinutab.

> **NOTE**
>
> Acetaminophen is 1 of 10 most commonly used drugs for intentional self-poisoning and is associated with significant morbidity and mortality.[5]

The toxic effects of acute acetaminophen ingestion (doses of 140 mg/kg or greater) can be classified in four stages (Box 34-21). The course of toxicity begins with mild symptoms that may be overlooked or masked by more dramatic effects of other agents followed by transient clinical improvement and finally peak liver abnormalities. (If acetaminophen was the sole ingestant and a dangerously high dose was ingested, the first two stages may be asymptomatic.) If antidote management is started within 8 hours of ingestion, complete recovery should occur.

> **? CRITICAL THINKING**
>
> *Do you think most nonmedical personnel realize that acetaminophen overdose can be lethal?*

Emergency care includes respiratory, cardiac, and hemodynamic support in critically ill patients. If ingestion is recent (within 1 hour) and the patient is alert, medical direction may recommend the administration of *activated charcoal*. Definitive care for patients with progressive acetaminophen toxicity is in-hospital administration of the antidote, N-acetylcysteine (Mucomyst).

> **BOX 34-21**
>
> ### STAGES OF ACETAMINOPHEN POISONING
>
> **Stage I: Gastrointestinal Irritability (0 to 24 hours)**
> Anorexia
> Nausea
> Vomiting
> General malaise
> Pallor
> Diaphoresis
>
> **Stage II: Abnormal Laboratory Findings (24 to 48 hours)**
> Resolution of stage 1 symptoms
> Possible abdominal pain and tenderness in the right abdominal quadrant
>
> **Stage III: Hepatic Damage (72 to 96 hours)**
> Hepatotoxicity with significant increase in hepatic enzymes
> Vomiting
> Lethargy
> Jaundice
> Hypoglycemia
> Dysrhythmias
>
> **Stage IV: Recovery (4 to 14 days) or Progressive Hepatic Failure**
> Resolution of hepatic dysfunction
> Lack of permanent effects in patients who recover
> NOTE: The percentage of patients who recover in stage IV depends on the amount of acetaminophen ingested and whether effective therapy (*activated charcoal*, acetylcysteine [Mucomyst], or both) was given. Patients with serum levels in the hepatotoxic range have mortality rates up to 25% if untreated.

Drugs Abused for Sexual Purposes/Sexual Gratification

Drugs that are abused for sexual purposes or for sexual gratification commonly are classified by users as "uppers," "downers," and those that have more than one primary effect ("all-arounders"). A sampling of these drugs is listed in Box 34-22. As previously described, uppers are CNS stimulants and downers are CNS depressants. The third category encompasses drugs such as anesthetics and mood-altering agents. They generally are taken

BOX 34-22

UPPERS, DOWNERS, AND ALL-AROUNDERS

Uppers
Ecstasy
Speed/meth/crystal
Coke/crack
Anabolic steroids

Downers
Alcohol
Heroin
Benzodiazepines (diazepam/temazepam/rohypnol)
Gamma hydroxybutyrate (GHB)

All-Arounders
Ketamine
Cannabis/skunk
Poppers (alkyl nitrates)
LSD

---

alone or in combination to produce one or more of the following effects:

- A sense of euphoria
- Excitation ("rush")
- Relaxation ("blissed out")
- A loss of inhibition

Each of these drugs has different chemical structures, mechanisms of action, and side effects. Therefore the problems associated with their use can vary greatly. Signs and symptoms of abuse can range from mild nausea and vomiting to life-threatening respiratory depression, hypotension, methemoglobinemia, coma, and death. Emergency care for these patients primarily is supportive and includes airway, ventilatory, and circulatory support, and rapid transport for physician evaluation. As with all other cases of patients who use mood-altering agents, personal safety is of primary importance.

SECTION THREE
ALCOHOLISM

Alcohol and related illness continue to be a major problem in the United States. In 1998, 113 million

Americans (52% of the population) age 12 years and older reported current use of alcohol; 33 million (29.2% of the population) admitted to binge drinking; and 12 million (10.6% of the population) reported drinking five or more drinks per occasion on 5 or more days per month.[9] In addition, alcohol is a key factor in 40% of vehicle fatalities, 68% of manslaughters, 62% of assaults, 54% of murder attempts, and 48% of robberies. The economic cost of alcohol and other drug-related crime is $61.8 billion annually.[1]

? CRITICAL THINKING

How many calls have you been on that involved patients intoxicated with alcohol? What kinds of calls were they?

Alcohol Dependence

Alcohol dependence is a disorder characterized by chronic, excessive consumption of alcohol that results in injury to health or in inadequate social function and the development of withdrawal symptoms when the patient stops drinking suddenly. There are an estimated 5 million alcohol-dependent persons in the United States (1 in 50) and another 7 million have difficulty controlling their consumption of the drug. Alcohol dependence should be considered a chronic, progressive, potentially fatal disease characterized by remissions, relapses, and cures.

No single cause of alcohol dependence exists; however, it is believed that three causative factors interact in development of the illness: personality, environment (widespread social acceptance and availability of alcohol), and the addictive nature of the drug. In some cases, genetic and hormonal factors also may play a role in causing dependence. However, it generally is believed that any person, regardless of environment, genetic background, or personality traits, can become chemically dependent on alcohol when the drug is consumed for long periods.

The development of alcohol dependence can be divided into four main stages, which merge imperceptibly. The time frame of these stages may range from 5 to 25 years, but the average is about 10 years. In the first stage, tolerance of the drug develops in the heavy social drinker, allowing the individual to consume larger quantities of alcohol before experiencing its ill effects. On entering the second stage, the drinker experiences memory lapses relating to events occurring during the drinking episodes. The third stage is characterized by loss or lack of control over alcohol; the drinker can no longer be certain of discontinuing alcohol consumption at will. The final stage begins with prolonged binges of intoxication with associated mental and physical complications. Some drinkers halt their consumption temporarily or permanently during one of the first three stages.

Ethanol

The active ingredient in all alcoholic beverages is ethanol, a colorless, flammable liquid produced from the fermentation of carbohydrates by yeast. All alcoholic drinks are rated based on their ethanol percentage. The alcohol content of beer and wine is measured as a percentage by weight or volume. United States beers contain 2.3% to 5.1% alcohol by volume. Wines vary in content up to 14% to 16%. Distilled liquors are subjected to a rating process called *proof* (see the box in the right column).

Metabolism

A total of 80% to 90% of ingested alcohol is absorbed within 30 minutes (20% in the stomach, the remainder in the small intestine). Once absorbed, the drug is rapidly distributed throughout the vascular space and reaches virtually every organ system. About 3% to 5% of alcohol is excreted unchanged via the lungs and kidneys; the rest is metabolized in the liver to carbon dioxide and water. The actual rate at which alcohol is metabolized depends on individual variation (e.g., physical and mental state, body weight, size) and whether the drinker is alcohol dependent. Alcohol generally is metabolized at a constant rate of about 20 mg/dL per hour (in nonalcoholics), regardless of its concentration. The rate of metabolism may be increased in alcoholics.

Blood Alcohol Content

The alcohol content of blood is measured in terms of weight (milligrams) of alcohol per given volume of blood (deciliter). The time it takes for the alcohol concentration to peak in the blood depends on a number of factors, including the rate at which the

"PROOF"

Proof was initially based on a test in which gunpowder moistened with a distilled product was ignited. Ignition was "proof" that the alcohol content of the product was at least 50%. Although the ignition test has been replaced with modern techniques to determine alcohol percentage, the term has been retained. A product containing 50% alcohol is considered 100 proof.

alcohol is consumed, the amount of food present in the stomach before drinking, and physical characteristics of the drinker. Although blood alcohol content is widely used to evaluate the CNS status of an intoxicated person, individual variation is considerable in blood alcohol content and degree of intoxication. In many states the legal limit of intoxication is 100 mg/dL (equivalent to 0.10%).

NOTE

Some states have legislation that permits paramedics to assist in conducting breathalyzer or blood tests to detect alcohol or drug intoxication. EMS personnel should be well versed in the laws of their state before assisting with these tests and should carefully follow established protocols.

? CRITICAL THINKING

Can you use an alcohol prep to prepare the site before drawing a blood alcohol specimen? Why?

Medical Consequences of Chronic Alcohol Ingestion

Because alcohol affects nearly every organ system, people who consume large quantities of alcohol are susceptible to numerous physical and mental disorders. Through a variety of direct and indirect mechanisms, alcohol causes multiple systemic effects, including neurological disorders, nutritional deficiencies, fluid and electrolyte imbalances, gastrointestinal disorders, cardiac and skeletal muscle myopathy, and immune suppression. In addition, alcohol may affect a patient's ability to tolerate traumatic injury.

Neurological Disorders

Alcohol is a potent CNS depressant. When consumed in moderate amounts, the drug reduces anxiety and tension and provides most drinkers with a feeling of relaxation and confidence. The clinical manifestations of alcohol are dose dependent and progress predictably as the level of consumption increases and blood alcohol content rises (Table 34-4). Initial feelings of well-being give way to impaired judgment and discrimination, prolonged reflexes, and incoordination and drowsiness, which may ultimately progress to stupor and coma. The long-term neurological effects of chronic alcohol abuse are similar to those of the aging process and include short-term memory deficit, problems with coordination, and difficulty with concentration and abstraction.

Nutritional Deficiencies

Alcohol can temporarily satisfy the body's caloric requirements and also decreases a drinker's appetite through an irritant effect on the stomach. Although it provides satiation, alcohol does not have essential vitamins, proteins, or fats. Therefore alcohol-dependent persons have a potential for decreased dietary intake and malabsorption, leading to multiple vitamin and

TABLE 34-4		ALCOHOL INTAKE AND ITS BEHAVIORAL EFFECTS	
ALCOHOL CONTENT (OZ)	**BEVERAGE INTAKE IN 1 HR***	**BLOOD ALCOHOL LEVEL (MG/DL) IN A 150-LB MAN**	**BEHAVIORAL EFFECTS**
$\frac{1}{2}$	1 oz 100-proof spirits 1 glass wine 1 can beer	0.025	No noticeable effect
1	2 oz 100-proof spirits 2 glasses wine 2 cans beer	0.050	Lower alertness, impaired judgment, good feeling, and less inhibition
2	4 oz 100-proof spirits 4 glasses wine 4 cans beer	0.100	Slow reaction time, impaired motor function, and less cautious; should not drive; may activate vomiting reflex
3	6 oz 100-proof spirits 6 glasses wine 6 cans beer	0.150	Large increase in reaction times
4	8 oz 100-proof spirits 8 glasses wine 8 cans beer	0.200	Marked depression of sensory and motor abilities
5	10 oz 100-proof spirits 10 glasses wine 10 cans beer	0.250	Severe depression of sensory and motor abilities
6	12 oz 100-proof spirits 12 glasses wine 12 cans beer	0.300	Stuporous and unconscious of surroundings
7	14 oz 100-proof spirits 14 glasses wine 14 cans beer	0.350	Unconscious
8	16 oz 100-proof spirits 16 glasses wine 16 cans beer	0.400	Lethal dose in 50% of the population
12	24 oz 100-proof spirits 24 glasses wine 24 cans beer	0.600	Lethal dose in 95% of the population

*Because only $\frac{1}{4}$ to $\frac{1}{3}$ oz of alcohol is metabolized each hour, alcohol rapidly accumulates.

mineral deficiencies. Clinical manifestations associated with these deficiencies include the following:

- Altered immunity
- Anorexia
- Cardiac dysrhythmias
- Coma
- Irritability and disorientation
- Muscle cramps
- Paresthesias
- Poor wound healing
- Seizures
- Tremor and ataxia

Wernicke-Korsakoff Syndrome

Alcohol-dependent persons are at particular risk of developing Wernicke-Korsakoff syndrome, a disease that results from chronic thiamine (vitamin B_1) deficiency combined with an inability to utilize thiamine from a heritable disorder or from a reduction in intestinal absorption and metabolism of thiamine by alcohol. Wernicke-Korsakoff syndrome affects the brain and nervous system by disrupting central and peripheral nerve function. The disease may consist of two stages: Wernicke's encephalopathy and **Korsakoff's psychosis**, or a combination of the two.

Wernicke's encephalopathy usually develops suddenly with the clinical manifestations of ataxia, ocular changes (nystagmus), disturbances of speech and gait, signs of neuropathy (paresthesias, impaired reflexes), stupor, or coma (rare). Because the body uses thiamine stores to metabolize sugar, the syndrome may be precipitated in the malnourished patient by the IV administration of glucose or glucose-containing fluids. Wernicke's encephalopathy also is the cause of coma in 1% of all alcoholics. Therefore medical direction may recommend the IV administration of *thiamine* before IV administration of glucose in patients with altered mental status or coma of unknown origin.

> **? CRITICAL THINKING**
>
> *Why do you think recognizing this syndrome is delayed in alcoholic patients?*

After administration of *thiamine*, patients with Wernicke's encephalopathy usually become more alert and attentive, but gait and mental difficulties often persist for days or months; fewer than half of the affected patients recover completely. Many chronic alcoholic patients also display signs of Korsakoff's psychosis, a mental disorder often found with Wernicke's encephalopathy. These signs include apathy, poor retentive memory, retrograde amnesia, confabulation (invention of stories to make up for gaps in memory), and dementia. Korsakoff's psychosis usually is considered irreversible, leaving the patient permanently handicapped by memory loss and in need of continual supervision.

Fluid and Electrolyte Imbalances

Urinary output increases (over and above that expected from the amount of fluid ingested) after alcohol consumption. This diuresis results from an inhibition of antidiuretic hormone secretion, which can lead to dehydration as well as electrolyte imbalances.

Gastrointestinal Disorders

The effects of alcohol on the GI system can produce several types of alcohol-related illnesses and diseases. The alcohol-related GI disorders most likely to initiate an EMS response include gastrointestinal hemorrhage, cirrhosis, and acute or chronic pancreatitis.

Gastrointestinal Hemorrhage

Four primary causes of gastrointestinal hemorrhage in patients who drink alcohol are gastritis, ulcer formation, esophageal tear (Mallory-Weiss syndrome), and variceal hemorrhage. Gastritis results from the toxic effects of ethanol on the gastric mucosa, which leads to diffuse or localized areas of erosion. In the chronic form of gastritis, blood may continually ooze from the mucosal lining, and ulcers may develop.

Esophageal tears of the gastroesophageal junction, stomach, or esophagus usually follow severe or protracted vomiting or retching. The injury results when gastric contents are forced against an unrelaxed gastroesophageal junction, which produces a sudden increase in pressure and a mucosal tear with subsequent bleeding. The bleeding can be exacerbated by clotting abnormalities, which are common in patients with alcoholic liver disease.

Varices are a result of portal hypertension caused by cirrhosis. Any of these thin-walled, blood-engorged veins are subject to rupture and hemorrhage, although the most common site is the varices of the esophagus. Bleeding esophagastric varices remain one of the most difficult conditions to manage. Severe hematemesis requires aggressive supportive care through large-bore IV lines and fluid resuscitation.

Cirrhosis

Cirrhosis of the liver is caused by chronic damage to liver cells that results in inflammation and eventually necrosis. In this disease process, bands of fibrosis (scar tissue) develop and break up the normal structure of the liver. The distortion and fibrosis of the liver lead to portal hypertension, with the resultant complications of ascites, splenomegaly, and bleeding esophageal and gastric varices. In addition, cirrhosis may lead to hepatic encephalopathy caused by the accumulation of toxic metabolic waste products, which normally would be detoxified by a healthy liver. It is estimated that 1 in 70 Americans dies as a direct result of chronic liver disease and cirrhosis, accounting for 30,000 deaths each year.

Acute or Chronic Pancreatitis

Alcohol is the most common cause of acute and chronic pancreatitis. Although the exact mechanism by which alcohol produces pancreatic inflammation is not clear, it may be caused at least in part by activation of pancreatic proenzymes, obstruction of pancreatic ducts, and stimulation of enzymatic secretion. A direct toxic effect may result, as has been demonstrated for the liver. Chronic pancreatitis usually produces the same symptoms as the acute form (described in Chapter 32). The pain, however, may last from several hours to several days, and the attacks become more frequent as the condition progresses. Other effects of chronic pancreatitis include malabsorption (a result of a deficiency of pancreatic enzymes), electrolyte imbalances such as hypocalcemia, and diabetes mellitus (caused by insufficient insulin production). Complications of pancreatitis are hemorrhagic pancreatitis, sepsis, and pancreatic abscess and are associated with high mortality.

Cardiac and Skeletal Muscle Myopathy

Cardiac and skeletal muscle myopathy is thought to result from a direct toxic effect of alcohol or its metabolites. The pathological changes associated with these alcoholic muscle syndromes include in-

tracellular edema, formation of lipid droplets, excessive cellular glycogen, and deranged sarcoplasmic reticula and mitochondria. In heart muscle, these changes result in a decreased force of contraction (negative inotropic effect), dysrhythmias, and a tendency to develop congestive heart failure. In skeletal muscle, the major symptoms are weakness and muscle wasting.

Immune Suppression

Long-term alcohol abuse renders the immune system less effective by suppressing bone marrow production of white blood cells; red blood cells and platelet production also are often decreased. Alcohol has direct, specific effects on lung tissue, which impair macrophage mobilization and mucociliary function. As a result, the body's ability to fight pulmonary infection is altered, making the alcoholic more susceptible to viral and bacterial pneumonia, which may occur secondary to aspiration during alcoholic stupor or for other reasons. Although the exact mechanism is unknown, the incidence of cancer is increased in alcoholic patients, which may also be related to immune suppression.

> **? CRITICAL THINKING**
>
> *For what other pulmonary disease is the immune-suppressed alcoholic patient at risk?*

Trauma

Alcohol suppresses clotting factors produced in the liver. This blood-clotting deficiency makes alcoholics susceptible to bruising and internal hemorrhage and adds to the frequency of subdural bleeding, even after relatively minor head trauma.

Alcohol Emergencies

In addition to the clinical conditions previously described, several other conditions caused by consumption or abstinence from alcohol may require emergency care. These include acute alcohol intoxication, alcohol withdrawal syndromes, and disulfiram-ethanol reaction. Alcohol-induced ketoacidosis and hypoglycemia are discussed in Chapter 30.

Acute Alcohol Intoxication

The ingestion of alcohol may cause acute poisoning if consumed in sufficiently large amounts over a relatively short period. The clinical features are similar to those induced by sedative-hypnotic agents and can be correlated to a degree with blood alcohol content. At toxic levels, hypoventilation (including respiratory arrest), hypotension, and hypothermia may develop. The patient who has signs and symptoms of acute alcohol intoxication should be carefully considered for occult trauma and coexisting medical conditions such as hypoglycemia, cardiac myopathy and dysrhythmias, GI bleeding, polydrug abuse, and ethylene glycol or methanol ingestion. Because of the patient's susceptibility to injury and potential for numerous secondary disease processes, the paramedic should never assume that an intoxicated patient is merely inebriated.

Management

A patient who is mildly intoxicated should be transported for physician evaluation. In most cases, management requires patient observation in the emergency department only until he or she is sober. The patient's vital signs and level of consciousness should be carefully monitored en route. A thorough physical examination is warranted to rule out illness or injury masked by alcohol ingestion.

Management of the acutely intoxicated patient is directed at protecting the patient from further injury and maintaining vital functions. If the patient is conscious and agitated, it may be necessary to use restraints to protect the patient and various health care providers from bodily harm. If physical restraint becomes necessary, police should be summoned. After scene safety has been established, initial assessment and resuscitation should include the following:

1. Rapidly evaluate airway patency with spinal precautions and ventilatory and hemodynamic status while obtaining a patient history. The patient's account of the history of the event may be unreliable as a result of alcohol ingestion.
2. Initiate IV therapy. Draw blood samples for laboratory analysis. Per protocol, administer *thiamine*, *dextrose 50%* (if hypoglycemia is likely or confirmed), and *naloxone* (Narcan), if opiate overdose is suspected.
3. Continually monitor the patient's airway and provide adequate ventilatory and circulatory support as needed. Be prepared to provide suction and aggressive airway management.
4. Monitor ECG for dysrhythmias.
5. Rapidly transport the patient for physician evaluation.

Alcohol Withdrawal Syndromes

A period of relative or absolute abstinence from alcohol may cause withdrawal in an alcoholic. The severity of these syndromes depends on the magnitude of blood alcohol content (serum ethanol level), the length of time the level was maintained, the abruptness of cessation, the tissue tolerance to alcohol, and the general physical and psychological condition of the patient. Although the pathophysiological mechanism of alcohol withdrawal remains largely undefined, it is thought to result from central nervous system hyperexcitability (as the CNS depressant is removed) and from biochemical changes such as respiratory alkalosis and hypomagnesemia. Alcohol withdrawal syndromes can be divided into four general categories: minor reactions, hallucinations, alcohol withdrawal seizures, and **delirium tremens**.

Minor Reactions

Minor reactions begin about 6 to 8 hours after cessation or reduction of alcohol intake. These symptoms peak within 24 to 36 hours and may persist for 10 to 14 days. When alcohol withdrawal is confined to minor reactions, the prognosis for full recovery is excellent with appropriate management. Minor reactions include the following:

- Sudden and unexpected startle
- Flushed face and diaphoresis
- Anorexia
- Nausea and vomiting
- Insomnia
- General muscle weakness
- Slight disorientation
- Generalized tremor (worsened by agitation)
- Mild tachycardia, hypertension, and hyperreflexia

? CRITICAL THINKING

What kinds of feelings do you think the patient and the patient's family may be having during withdrawal reactions?

Hallucinations

Hallucinations usually occur 24 to 36 hours after cessation of alcohol. Disorders of perception are common and may vary from auditory and visual illusions to frank hallucinations, which can produce agitation, fear, and panic. During this period, the patient may show signs of suicidal and homicidal tendencies, and minor reactions may be more pronounced. The prognosis for hallucinations is the same as for minor reactions with appropriate management.

Alcohol Withdrawal Seizures

Alcohol withdrawal seizures (or "rum fits") usually occur 7 to 48 hours after ethanol cessation. These seizures may occur singly or in groups of two to six. They most often are grand mal of short duration; status seizures are rare. Alcohol withdrawal seizures are associated with varying degrees of tremor, anorexia, hallucinations, and autonomic hyperactivity. This category of withdrawal may be self-limiting or may progress to delirium tremens with or without a lucid interval.

Because of the drug tolerance level of the alcoholic patient, seizure activity may require IV administration of large doses of *diazepam* (Valium), 5 mg every 5 minutes up to 30 mg or more. *Diazepam* (Valium) may synergistically interact with any ethanol still in the patient's system, so vital signs, respirations, and mental status should be closely monitored.

Delirium Tremens

Delirium tremens (DTs) is the most dramatic and serious form of alcohol withdrawal. It affects about 5% of all alcoholics hospitalized for withdrawal. It usually occurs 72 to 96 hours after cessation of alcohol but may be delayed up to 14 days. The syndrome is characterized by psychomotor, speech, and autonomic hyperactivity; profound confusion; disorientation; delusion; vivid hallucinations; tremor; agitation; and insomnia. A single episode may last 1 to 3 days and, with multiple recurrences, may last up to 1 month.

Autonomic hyperactivity is the most distinguishing feature of DTs. It is characterized by tachycardia, fever, hypertension, dilated pupils, and profuse diaphoresis. In severe cases, cardiovascular collapse may be present. DTs is a true medical emergency with a mortality rate as high as 15%. Associated al-cohol-related illnesses such as pneumonia, pancreatitis, and hepatitis are frequent contributing causes of death.

Management

Prehospital care for patients experiencing alcohol withdrawal syndromes primarily is supportive. After scene safety is ensured, the patient's airway, ventilatory, and circulatory status should be carefully monitored. IV therapy should be initiated with a saline solution for rehydration. Pharmacological therapy may be indicated for an altered level of consciousness, dysrhythmias, or seizure activity. In addition, these patients need calm reassurance and frequent reorientation. All patients with signs and symptoms of alcohol withdrawal syndrome require physician evaluation.

Disulfiram-Ethanol Reaction

Disulfiram (tetraethylthiuram disulfide or Antabuse) is a medication prescribed to some alcoholic patients to help them abstain. The drug works by inhibiting ethanol metabolism and by allowing the accumulation of the metabolite acetaldehyde. Acetaldehyde produces ill effects on the gastrointestinal, cardiovascular, and autonomic nervous systems and is the metabolic product thought to be responsible for the common "hangover." Patients who take disulfiram and then ingest ethanol experience an unpleasant and potentially life-threatening physiological response. A disulfiram-like reaction also can occur in patients taking metronidazole (Flagyl) for *Trichomonas* and other types of infection.

The disulfiram-ethanol reaction begins 15 to 30 minutes after ingestion of two to five alcoholic drinks and continues for 1 to 2 hours. The reaction causes the patient to experience vertigo, headache, vomiting, flushing (which may give the skin a "lobster-red" appearance), dyspnea, diaphoresis, abdominal pain, and sometimes chest pain. More serious reactions include hypotension, shock, and dysrhythmias. Sudden death, myocardial and cerebral infarction, and cerebral hemorrhage also have been reported after as little as one drink of ethanol in patients taking disulfiram.

Management

Prehospital care for a disulfiram-ethanol reaction involves airway, ventilatory, and circulatory support;

the administration of IV fluids to manage hypotension; pharmacological therapy as needed to manage dysrhythmias; and rapid transport for physician evaluation. Most episodes are self-limiting. Supportive care and in-hospital observation are usually all that are required.

MANAGING TOXIC SYNDROMES

General Management Principles for Toxic Syndromes

As stated earlier in this chapter, most poisoned patients (regardless of the toxic agent) require only supportive therapy to recover (Box 34-23). Grouping toxicologically similar agents and physical findings into toxic syndromes, however, can give the paramedic important clues to narrow a differential diagnosis and to more easily remember assessment and management strategies (Table 34-5). The five toxic syndromes presented in this chapter are the following[2,11]:

1. Cholinergic
2. Anticholinergic
3. Hallucinogen
4. Opiate
5. Sympathomimetic

NOTE

Toxic syndrome classification does not consider how or why the toxin was introduced into the body. The paramedic should therefore consider route of entry in addition to specific treatments.

Cholinergics

Exposure to cholinergics is uncommon. However, it is important to recognize so that lifesaving management can be initiated. Causative agents include pesticides (organophosphates, carbamates) and nerve agents (e.g., sarin, Soman). Assessment findings include headache, dizziness, weakness, bradycardia, nausea, and a "wet" presentation manifested by profound salivation, lacrimation, urination, defecation, GI upset, and emesis (SLUDGE). In severe cases, coma and convulsions may be present. In addition to airway, ventilatory, and circulatory support and decontamination, drug therapy may include *atropine*, *pralidoxime* (2-PAM Chloride), *diazepam* (Valium), and *activated charcoal*.

Anticholinergics

Exposure to anticholinergics is fairly common because so many medications and plants have anticholinergic properties. Signs and symptoms include tachycardia, dry flushed skin, dilated pupils, and facial flushing. This "dry" patient presentation usually is managed with airway, ventilatory, and circulatory support, and rarely the administration of physostigmine (Antilirium) in the absence of TCA overdose.

Hallucinogens

Common hallucinogens include LSD, PCP, peyote, mushrooms, and mescaline. Depending on the

BOX 34-23

GENERAL MANAGEMENT GUIDELINES FOR THE POISONED PATIENT

1. Ensure scene and personal safety.
2. Provide adequate airway, ventilation, and circulation.
3. Obtain a thorough history and perform a focused physical examination.
4. Consider hypoglycemia in an unconscious or convulsing patient.
5. Administer **naloxone** (Narcan) or **nalmefene** (Revex) to a patient with respiratory depression and suspected opioid ingestion.
6. If overdose is suspected, obtain an overdose history from the patient, family, or friends.
7. Consult with medical direction or a poison control center for specific treatment to prevent further absorption of the toxin (or antidote therapy).
8. Frequently monitor vital signs and ECG.
9. Safely obtain any substance or substance container of a suspected poison and transport it with the patient.
10. Transport the patient for physician evaluation.

TABLE 34-5 TOXICOLOGICAL SYNDROMES

COMMON SIGNS	CAUSATIVE AGENTS	SPECIFIC TREATMENT
Cholinergic ("Wet" Patient Presentation)		
Confusion, CNS depression, weakness, SLUDGE (salivation, lacrimation, urination, defecation, GI upset, emesis), bradycardia, wheezing, bronchoconstriction, miosis, coma, convulsion, diaphoresis, seizures	Organophosphate and carbamate insecticides, nerve agents, some mushrooms	*Atropine, pralidoxine* (2-PAM Chloride), *diazepam* (Valium), *activated charcoal*
Anticholinergic ("Dry" Patient Presentation)		
Delirium, tachycardia, dry, flushed skin, dilated pupils, seizures, and dysrhythmias (in severe cases)	Antihistamines, antiparkinson medications, atropine, antipsychotic agents, antidepressants, skeletal muscle relaxants, many plants (e.g., jimson weed and *Amanita muscaria*)	*Diazepam* (Valium), *activated charcoal,* rarely physostigmine (Antilirium)
Hallucinogen		
Visual illusions, delusions, bizarre behavior, flashbacks, respiratory and CNS depression	LSD, PCP, mescaline, some mushrooms, marijuana, jimsonweed, nutmeg, mace, some amphetamines	Minimal sensory stimulation and calming measures, *diazepam* (Valium) if necessary
Opioids		
Euphoria, hypotension, respiratory depression/arrest, nausea, pinpoint pupils, seizures, coma	Heroin, *morphine,* codeine, *meperidine* (Demerol), propoxyphene, fentanyl	*Naloxone* (Narcan), *nalmefene* (Revex)
Sympathomimetic		
Delusions, paranoia, tachycardia or bradycardia, hypertension, diaphoresis; seizures, hypotension, and dysrhythmias in severe cases	Cocaine, amphetamine, methamphetamine, over-the-counter decongestants	Minimal sensory stimulation and calming measures, *diazepam* (Valium) if necessary

agent and dose, signs and symptoms may include CNS stimulation and/or depression, behavioral disturbances, delusions, hypertension, chest pain, tachycardia, seizures, and respiratory and cardiac arrest. Prehospital care for these patients is focused on ensuring personal safety, and providing airway, ventilatory, and circulatory support.

Opiates

The opiate syndrome carries a hallmark triad of depressed level of consciousness, respiratory depression, and pinpoint pupils. Common causative agents include heroin, *morphine*, codeine, *meperidine* (Demerol), propoxyphene, and fentanyl. Drugs in this class frequently are mixed with alcohol or other drugs (e.g., bendoziapines), leading to increased respiratory depression, hypotension, and bradycardia. Other signs and symptoms may include euphoria, nausea, pinpoint pupils, and seizures. In addition to ensuring airway, ventilatory, and circulatory support, drug therapy may include the administration of *naloxone* (Narcan) or another opiate-specific antidote agent.

Sympathomimetic

The sympathomimetic syndrome usually results from acute overdose of amphetamines or cocaine. Signs and symptoms include elevated blood pressure, tachycardia, dilated pupils, and altered mental status (including paranoid delusions). In severe cases, cardiovascular collapse can occur. Management consists of ensuring personal safety and providing airway, ventilatory, and circulatory support.

? CRITICAL THINKING

Why is it important to be able to identify these toxic syndromes?

S U M M A R Y

- A poison is any substance that produces harmful physiological or psychological effects.

- The toxic effects of ingested poisons may be immediate or delayed, depending on the substance ingested. The primary goal of physical assessment of poisoned patients is to identify effects on the three vital organ systems most likely to produce immediate morbidity and mortality: the respiratory system, the cardiovascular system, and the central nervous system. The goal of managing serious poisonings by ingestion is to prevent the toxic substance from reaching the small intestine, thereby limiting its absorption.

- Strong acids and alkalis may cause burns to the mouth, pharynx, esophagus, and sometimes the upper respiratory and GI tracts. Prehospital care is usually limited to airway and ventilatory support, IV fluid replacement, and rapid transport to the appropriate medical facility.

- The most important physical characteristic in the potential toxicity of ingested hydrocarbons is its viscosity: the lower the viscosity, the higher the risk of aspiration and associated complications. Hydrocarbon ingestion may involve the patient's respiratory, gastrointestinal, and neurological systems; clinical features may be immediate or delayed in onset.

- Methanol is a poisonous alcohol found in a variety of products. Methanol itself is no more toxic than ethanol, but its metabolites (formaldehyde and formic acid) are extremely toxic. Ingestion can affect the central nervous system, the gastrointestinal tract, and the eyes, and cause development of metabolic acidosis.

- Ethylene glycol toxicity is caused by the accumulation of intermediary metabolites, especially glycolic and oxalic acids after metabolism, which occurs primarily in the liver and kidneys. This may affect the central nervous system and cardiopulmonary and renal systems and result in hypocalcemia.

- The majority of isopropanol (isopropyl alcohol) is metabolized to acetone after ingestion. Isopropanol poisoning affects several body systems, including the central nervous, gastrointestinal, and renal systems.

- Infants and children are high-risk groups for accidental iron, lead, and mercury poisoning because of their immature immune systems or increased absorption as a function of age. Ingested iron is corrosive to gastrointestinal tract mucosa and may produce lethal GI hemorrhage, bloody vomitus, painless bloody diarrhea, and dark stools.

- Food poisoning is a term used for any illness of sudden onset (usually associated with stomach pain, vomiting, and diarrhea) suspected of begin caused by food eaten within the previous 48 hours. Food poisoning can be classified as infectious, resulting from a bacterium or virus, or noninfectious, resulting from toxins and pollutants.

- The toxic manifestations of major poisonous plant ingestions are predictable and are categorized by the chemical and physical properties of the plant. Most responses are consistent with the type of major toxic chemical component in the plant.

- The concentration of a chemical in the air and the duration of exposure help determine the severity of inhalation injury. Solubility also influences inhalation injury. Highly reactive chemicals cause more severe and rapid injury than less-reactive chemicals. Properties that determine chemical reactivity are chemical pH; direct-acting potential of chemicals; indirect-acting potential of chemicals; and allergic potential of chemicals.

- Cyanide refers to any of a number of highly toxic substances that contain the cyanogen chemical group. Regardless of the route of entry, cyanide is a rapidly acting poison that combines and reacts with ferric ions of the respiratory enzyme cytochrome oxidase to inhibit cellular oxygenation. This produces a rapid progression from dyspnea to paralysis, unconsciousness, and death.

- Ammonia is a toxic irritant that causes local pulmonary complications after inhalation. In severe cases, bronchospasm and pulmonary edema may ensue.

- Hydrocarbon inhalation may cause aspiration pneumonitis and the potential for systemic effects such as CNS depression and liver, kidney, or bone marrow toxicity.

- Simple asphyxiants cause toxicity by lowering ambient oxygen concentration. Chemical asphyxiants possess intrinsic systemic toxicity manifested after absorption into the circulation. Irritants or corrosives cause cellular destruction and inflammation as they come into contact with moisture.

- The general principles of managing inhaled poisons are the same as for any other hazardous materials incident.

- *Hymenoptera* and *Arachnida* cause the highest incidence of need for emergency care. Arthropod venoms are complex and diverse in their chemistry and pharmacology and may produce major toxic reactions such as anaphylaxis and upper airway obstruction in sensitized individuals.

- The two main families of venomous snakes indigenous to the United States are pit vipers and coral snakes. Pit viper venom can produce various toxic effects on blood and other tissues, including hemolysis, intravascular coagulation, convulsions, and acute renal failure. The venom of the coral snake is primarily neurotoxic. Signs and symptoms range from slurred speech, dilated pupils, and dysphagia to flaccid paralysis and death.

- The marine animals most likely to be involved in human poisonings in U.S. coastal waters are coelenterates, echinoderms, and stingrays. Coelenterate envenomation ranges in severity from irritant dermatitis to excruciating pain, respiratory depression, and life-threatening cardiovascular collapse. Echinoderm toxins may cause immediate intense pain, swelling, redness, aching in the affected extremity, and nausea. Delayed effects may include respiratory distress, paresthesia of the lips and face, and in severe cases, respiratory paralysis and complete atonia. Locally stingray venom produces a painful traumatic injury that may cause bleeding and necrosis. Systemic manifestations range from weakness and nausea to seizures, paralysis, hypotension, and death.

- Organophosphates and carbamates inhibit the effects of acetylcholinesterase. A mnemonic aid that may help recognize this type of poisoning is *SLUDGE* (salivation, lacrimation, urination, defecation, gastrointestinal upset, and emesis). The most specific findings, however, are miosis, rapidly changing pupils, and muscle fasciculation.

- General principles for managing drug abuse and overdose include scene safety; ensuring adequate airway, breathing, and circulation; history; substance identification; focused physical exam; initiation of an IV; administration of an antidote if needed; prevention of further absorption; and rapid transport.

- Narcotics are CNS depressants and can cause life-threatening respiratory depression. In severe intoxication, hypotension, profound shock, and pulmonary edema may be present. Naloxone is a pure narcotic antagonist effect for virtually all narcotic and narcotic-like substances.

- Sedative-hypnotic agents include benzodiazepines and barbiturates. Signs and symptoms of sedative-hypnotic overdose are chiefly related to the central nervous and cardiovascular symptoms. Flumazenil (Romazicon), a benzodiazepine antagonist, is useful in reversing the effects of these agents.

- Commonly used stimulant drugs are those of the amphetamine family. Adverse effects include tachycardia, increased blood pressure, tachypnea, agitation, dilated pupils, tremors, and disorganized behavior. With sudden withdrawal, the patient becomes depressed, suicidal, incoherent, or near coma.

- Phencyclidine (PCP) is a dissociative analgesic with sympathomimetic and CNS stimulant and depressant effects. In low doses, PCP intoxication produces an unpredictable state that can resemble drunkenness (and rage). High-dose intoxication may cause coma, which may last from several hours to several days. Respiratory depression, hypertension, and tachycardia may be present. PCP psychosis is a psychiatric emergency that may mimic schizophrenia.

- Hallucinogens are substances that cause perceptual distortions. Depending on the agent, overdose may range from visual hallucinations and anticholinergic syndromes, to more serious complications, including psychosis, flashbacks, and respiratory and CNS depression.

- Tricyclic antidepressant toxicity is thought to result from central and peripheral, atropine-like anticholinergic effects and direct depressant effects on myocardial function. A prolonged QRS complex, a GCS less than 8, or both, should alert the paramedic to a major TCA toxicity.

- Lithium is a mood-stabilizing drug. Toxic ingestion can include CNS effects that can range from blurred vision and confusion to seizure and coma.

- Cardiac drugs are a common cause of poisoning fatalities in children and adults. The drugs responsible for the majority of these fatalities are digitalis, beta blockers, and calcium channel blockers.

- MAO inhibitors block or diminish the activity of the monoamines (norepinephrine, dopamine, serotonin). Toxic effects include CNS depression and various neuromuscular and cardiovascular system manifestations.

- Nonsteroidal antiinflammatory drugs (NSAIDs) work by blocking the production of prostaglandins. The effects of overdose of ibuprofen are usually reversible, are seldom life-threatening, and include mild GI and CNS effects. Salicylate poisoning may cause CNS stimulation, GI irritation, glucose metabolism, fluid and electrolyte imbalance, and coagulation defects.

- Acetaminophen overdose may cause life-threatening hepatotoxicity from formation of a hepatotoxic intermediate metabolite if not managed within 16 to 24 hours of ingestion.

- Drugs that are abused for sexual purposes or for sexual gratification are commonly classified by users as "uppers," "downers," and those that have more than one primary effect ("all-arounders"). Problems associated with their use vary widely.

- Alcohol dependence is a disorder characterized by chronic, excessive consumption of alcohol that results in injury to health or in inadequate social function and the development of withdrawal symptoms when the patient stops drinking suddenly. Alcohol causes multiple systemic effects, including neurological disorders, nutritional deficiencies, fluid and electrolyte imbalances, gastrointestinal disorders, cardiac and skeletal muscle myopathy, and immune suppression. Several conditions caused by consumption or abstinence from alcohol that may require emergency care are acute alcohol intoxication, alcohol withdrawal syndromes, and disulfiram-ethanol reaction.

• The most common toxic syndromes are cholinergic, anticholinergic, hallucinogen, opiate, and sympathomimetic. Using these classifications allows the paramedic to group toxicologically similar agents and to more easily remember assessment and management strategies.

REFERENCES

1. National Safety Council: *Injury facts*, Chicago, 1999, The Council.
2. Litovitz TL et al: 1996 annual report of the American Association of Poison Control Centers Toxic Exposure Surveillance System, *Am J Emerg Med* 15:447, 1997.
3. Miller TR, Lestina DC: Costs of poisoning in the United States and savings from poison control centers: a benefit-cost analysis, *Ann Emerg Med* 29:239, 1997.
4. American Heart Association: Guidelines 2000 for cardiopulmonary resuscitation and emergency cardiovascular care, International Consensus on Science, *Circulation* 102(8): 223, 2000.
5. Rosen P, Barkin R: *Emergency medicine: concepts and clinical practice*, ed 4, St Louis, 1998, Mosby.
6. American Academy of Pediatrics: *Handbook of pediatric environmental health: reducing risk at home, school, and play!* Washington, DC, 1999, The Academy.
7. Borak J et al: *Hazardous materials exposure*, Englewood Cliffs, NJ, 1991, Brady.
8. Auerbach PS, editor: *Wilderness medicine*, ed 3, St Louis, 1995, Mosby.
9. U.S. Department of Health and Human Services: 1998 annual national drug survey results, SAMHSA Press Office, http://wasigate.hhs.gov/cgi-bin.
10. National Clearinghouse for Alcohol and Drug Information: Violence and crime and alcohol and other drugs, http://www.health.org/makelink/ml-violc.htm.
11. U.S. Department of Transportation National Highway Traffic Safety Administration: *EMT-Paramedic national standard curriculum*, Washington, DC, 1998, The Department.

Appendix

Toxicology in Emergency Cardiac Care

Guidelines have been developed by the American Heart Association (AHA) to provide guidance in the management of severe poisonings when standard emergency cardiac care guidelines may not be optimum or appropriate.[4] The following summarizes the AHA guidelines. The paramedic should follow established protocol and should provide care to these patients with the advice of medical direction or a poison control center (Appendix Tables 1 and 2).

Drug-Induced Hemodynamically Significant Bradycardia (HSB)

- *Atropine* is seldom helpful, but it is not harmful.
- *Atropine* (starting dose of 2 to 4 mg for adults) is lifesaving in organophosphate or carbamate poisoning.
- *Isoproterenol* (Isuprel) may induce or aggravate hypotension and ventricular dysrhythmias and should not be given unless there is a massive beta-blocker poisoning (in which cases high doses of *isoproterenol* [Isuprel] may be effective).
- Electrical cardiac pacing is often effective in cases of mild-to-moderate drug-induced HSB.
- HSB that is resistant to atropine and pacing should be managed with vasopressors with greater beta-agonist activity

Drug-Induced Hemodynamically Significant Tachycardia (HST)

- HST may induce myocardial ischemia, myocardial infarction, or ventricular dysrhythmias and may lead to high-output heart failure and shock.
- Avoid routine therapy with *adenosine* (Adenocard) and synchronized cardioversion (tachycardia is likely to recur or to be refractory).
- *Diltiazem* (Cardizem) and *verapamil* (Isoptin) are relatively contraindicated in patients with borderline hypotension as they may cause more severe shock.
- Drug therapy is preferred when rate control is necessary.
- *Diazepam* (Valium) or *lorazepam* (Ativan) in doses that do not produce a decreased level of consciousness or respiratory depression are generally safe and effective in patients with HST.

- Cautious use of nonselective beta blockers (e.g., *propranolol* [Inderal]) may be effective when HST is due to sympathomimetic poisoning.

Drug-Induced Hypertensive Emergencies

- These emergencies are often short-lived and do not require aggressive therapy (important because hypertension may occur in later cases of severe stimulant poisoning).
- Benzodiazepines are first-line therapy; short-acting agents (e.g., nitroprusside [Nitropres]) are second-line therapy; carefully titrated doses of *labetalol* (Normodyne) are third-line therapy (effective with sympathomimetic poisoning).
- *Propranolol* (Inderal) may block B_2 receptors (leaving a-adrenergic stimulation unopposed and worsening hypertension) and is contraindicated.

Drug-Induced Acute Coronary Syndromes

- Treatment is similar to drug-induced hypertensive emergencies.
- Benzodiazepines and *nitroglycerin* are first-line agents; phentolamine (Regitine) is a second-line agent; *propranolol* (Inderal) is contraindicated.
- Fibrinolytics are contraindicated with uncontrolled, severe drug-induced hypertension.

Drug-Induced VT and VF

- Drug-induced VT may be difficult to distinguish from drug-induced impaired conduction (wide complex).
- Drug-induced VT is likely and should be cardioverted when a sudden conversion to wider-complex rhythm occurs with hypotension.
- Antidysrhythmics are indicated in hemodynamically stable drug-induced VT.
- *Procainamide* (Pronestyl) is contraindicated in TCA poisoning and in poisonings with drugs that have similar antidysrhythmic properties.
- *Lidocaine* (Xylocaine) is safe and effective in cases of cocaine poisoning and is the drug of choice in monomorphic VT or VF.
- *Magnesium* may be effective in some cases of drug-induced VT but may also aggravate drug-induced hypotension.
- Correctable factors (hypoxemia, hypokalemia, hypomagnesemia) should be considered in the presence of torsades de pointes; the rhythm may respond to electrical and pharmacological

| TABLE 1 | SYMPATHOMIMETIC AND CARDIOTOXIC DRUGS |

DRUG CLASS	CARDIOVASCULAR SIGNS OF TOXICITY*	THERAPY TO CONSIDER
Stimulants, Sympathomimetic		
Amphetamines	Tachycardia	α-Blockers
Methamphetamine	Supraventricular and ventricular arrhythmias	Benzodiazepines
Cocaine	Impaired conduction	Lidocaine
Phencyclidine (PCP)	Hypertensive emergencies	Sodium bicarbonate
	Acute coronary syndromes	
	Shock, cardiac arrest	
Calcium Channel Blockers		
Verapamil	Bradycardia	Mixed α-/β-agonists
Nifedipine	Impaired conduction	Pacemakers
Diltiazem	Shock	Calcium infusions
	Cardiac arrest	Insulin euglycemia
β-Adrenergic Receptor Antagonists		
Propanolol	Bradycardia	Pacemakers
Atenolol	Impaired conduction	Mixed α-/β-agonists
	Shock	Glucagon, insulin
	Cardiac arrest	Insulin euglycemia
Tricyclic Antidepressants		
Amitriptyline	Tachycardia	Sodium bicarbonate
Desipramine	Bradycardia	Mixed α-/β-agonists or α-agonists
Nortriptyline	Ventricular arrhythmia	Lidocaine
	Impaired conduction	Procainamide is contraindicated
	Shock, cardiac arrest	
Cardiac Glycosides		
Digoxin	Bradycardia	Digoxin-specific Fab fragments
Digitoxin	Supraventricular and ventricular arrhythmias	(Digibind)
Foxglove	Impaired conduction	Magnesium
Oleander	Shock, cardiac arrest	Pacemakers
Anticholinergics		
Diphenhydramine	Tachycardia	Physostigmine
Doxylamine	Supraventricular and ventricular arrhythmias	
	Impaired conduction	
	Shock	
	Cardiac arrest	
Cholinergics		
Carbamates	Bradycardia	Atropine
Nerve agents	Ventricular arrhythmias	Decontamination
Organophosphates	Impaired conduction, shock	Pralidoxime
	Pulmonary edema, bronchospasm	Obidoxime
	Cardiac arrest	
Opiates		
Heroin	Hypoventilation (slow, shallow respirations)	Naloxone
Fentanyl	Bradycardia, hypotension	Nalmefene
Methadone		
Isoniazid		
	Lactic acidosis with or without seizures	Pyridoxine (vitamin B_6)
	Tachycardia or bradycardia	
	Shock, cardiac arrest	
Sodium Channel Blockers		
Type 1_A antiarrhythmics,	Impaired conduction	Sodium bicarbonates
propranolol, verapamil,	Bradycardia	Pacemakers
TCAs	Ventricular arrhythmias	α-/β-Agonists, high dose
	Seizures	if necessary
	Shock, cardiac arrest	Hypertonic saline

*Unless stated otherwise, assume that all altered vital signs (bradycardia, tachycardia, tachypnea) are "hemodynamically significant."

TABLE 2	DRUG-INDUCED CARDIOVASCULAR EMERGENCIES AND ALTERED VITAL SIGNS	

| | THERAPY | |
DRUG-INDUCED EMERGENCY	INDICATED	CONTRAINDICATED
Bradycardia*	Pacemaker (TC, IV) Mixed α-/β-agonists For OD of calcium channel blocker: calcium For OD of β-blocker: glucagon or β-agonist	Isoproterenol if hypotensive Prophylactic TV pacing
Tachycardia	Benzodiazepines Selective β_1-blockers Mixed α-/β-blockers	Cardioversion Adenosine, verapamil, diltiazem For OD of TCA: physostigmine
Impaired conduction, ventricular arrhythmias	Sodium bicarbonate Lidocaine	For OD of TCA: type 1_A antiarrhthmics (procainamide)
Hypertensive emergency	Benzodiazepines Mixed α-/β-blockers Nitroprusside	Nonselective β-blockers (propranolol)
Acute coronary syndrome	Benzodiazepines Nitroglycerin α-Blocker	Nonselective β-blockers (propranolol)
Shock	Mixed α-/β-agonists (high dose if necessary) For OD of calcium channel blocker: calcium, insulin† For OD of β-blocker; glucagon, insulin† If refractory to *maximal* medical therapy: circulatory assist devices	Isoproterenol
Acute cholinergic syndrome	Atropine Pralidoxime/obidoxime	Succinylcholine
Acute anticholinergic syndrome	Physostigmine	Antipsychotics or other anticholinergics
Opiate poisoning	Naloxone Nalmefene	

TC, Transcutaneous; *IV*, intravenous; *TV*, transvenous; and *OD*, overdose.
*Unless stated otherwise, assume all altered vital signs (bradycardia, tachycardia, tachypnea) are "hemodynamically significant."
†Administer to achieve euglycemia.

therapy: *magnesium, lidocaine* (Xylocaine); electrical or pharmacological overdrive pacing; and perhaps potassium supplementation.

Drug-Induced Impaired Conduction

- Prolonged ventricular conduction predisposes the heart to monomorphic VT.
- Hypertonic saline and systemic alkalinization can reverse adverse electrophysiological effects, preventing or terminating VT secondary to poisoning from sodium channel blocking agents (hypertonic *sodium bicarbonate* is particularly valuable).
- Respiratory alkalosis can be a temporary measure until the appropriate degree of metabolic alkalosis can be achieved with *sodium bicarbonate* (repeat boluses of 1 to 2 mEq/kg for a goal arterial pH of 7.50 to 7.55).

Drug-Induced Shock

- Drug-induced shock usually results when the drug induces decreases in intravascular volume, falls in systemic vascular resistance (SVR), diminished myocardial contractility, or a combination of these factors.
- For drug-induced hypovolemic shock, give fluid challenge to correct hypovolemia and optimize preload; if ineffective give *dopamine* (Intropin); then high-dose vasopressors (with central hemodynamic monitoring) if needed.
- For drug-induced distributive shock, potent vasoconstrictors (e.g., *norepinephrine* [Levophed] may be needed; *dobutamine* (Dobutrex) and *isoproterenol* (Isuprel) decrease SVR and are contraindicated; high-dose vasopressors should be given until shock is adequately treated or adverse effects (e.g., ventricular dysrhythmias) develop.
- For drug-induced cardiogenic shock, inotropic agents (e.g., *calcium, amrinone* [Inocor], *glucagon, insulin, isoproterenol* [Isuprel], and *dobutamine* [Dobutrex]) are often required (sometimes in combination); concomitant use of a vasopressor may be needed.

Drug-Induced Cardiac Arrest

- Electrical cardioversion or defibrillation is appropriate for pulseless drug-induced VT/VF.
- The cost-benefit ratio of *epinephrine* (Adrenalin) in sympathomimetic poisoning with refractory VF is unknown; if used, increase the interval between standard-amount doses (avoid high-dose *epinephrine* [Adrenalin]); *propranolol* (Inderal) is contraindicated in sympathomimetic poisoning.
- Resuscitation is usually terminated after 20 to 30 minutes of ACLS unless there are signs that the CNS is viable; prolonged resuscitation and CPR (sometimes up to 3 to 5 hours) have been associated with good recovery and may be warranted in some poisoned patients.
- When resuscitation is unsuccessful, organ donation may still be an option.

35 *Hematology*

OBJECTIVES

Upon completion of this chapter, the paramedic student will be able to:

1. *Describe the physiology of blood and its components.*
2. *Discuss pathophysiology and signs and symptoms of specific hematological disorders.*
3. *Outline general assessment and management of patients with hematological disorders.*

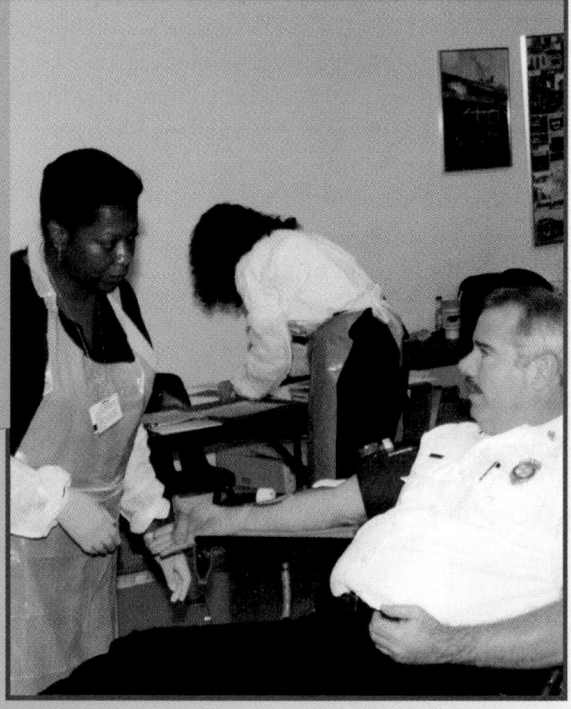

The blood and blood-forming organs comprise the hematological system. Dysfunction in the system can profoundly affect other body systems, resulting in a variety of clinical manifestations that characterize hematological disorders. Although prehospital care for most patients with hematological disorders is primarily supportive, the paramedic's knowledge of these diseases enhances assessment skills and provides an understanding of treatment strategies required for these patients.

Blood and Blood Components

As described in Chapter 6, blood is composed of cells and formed elements surrounded by plasma. About 95% of the volume of formed elements consists of red blood cells (RBCs; erythrocytes). The remaining 5% consists of white blood cells (WBCs; leukocytes) and cell fragments (platelets) (Fig. 35-1 and Table 35-1). The continuous movement of blood keeps the formed elements dispersed throughout the plasma, where they are available to carry out their chief functions[1]: (1) delivery of substances needed for cellular metabolism in the tissues, (2) defense against invading microorganisms and injury, and (3) acid-base balance.

All types of blood cells are formed within the red bone marrow, which is present in all tissues at birth. In the adult, the red bone marrow primarily is found in membranous bone such as the vertebrae, pelvis, sternum, and ribs. Yellow marrow produces some white cells but is composed mainly of connective tissue and fat. Other blood-forming organs include the following:

- Lymph nodes, which produce lymphocytes and antibodies

- The spleen, which stores large quantities of blood and produces lymphocytes, plasma cells, and antibodies
- The liver, a blood-forming organ only during intrauterine life, which plays an important role in the coagulation process

Plasma

Plasma, the clear portion of blood, is about 92% water. It contains three important proteins: albumin, globulins, and fibrinogen. Albumin, the most plentiful protein, is similar to egg white and gives blood its gummy texture. These large proteins keep the water concentration of blood low so that water diffuses readily from tissues into the blood. The globulins (alpha, beta, and gamma) transport other proteins and provide immunity to disease. Fibrinogen is responsible for blood clotting. Plasma proteins perform various functions that include maintaining blood pH (acting as either an acid or a base); transporting fat-soluble vitamins, hormones, and carbohydrates; and allowing the body to digest them temporarily for food. Plasma also contains salts, metals, and inorganic compounds.

Red Blood Cells

RBCs are the most abundant cells in the body and primarily are responsible for tissue oxygenation. They appear as small rounded disks with nearly hollowed-out centers (Fig. 35-2) and are comprised of mainly water and the red protein hemoglobin. RBC production continues throughout life to replace blood cells that grow old and die, are killed by disease, or are lost through bleeding. After RBC production occurs in the bone marrow, the new cell divides until there are 16 RBCs. The cells produce hemoglobin protein until the concentration of the protein becomes 95% of the dry weight of the cell, at which time the cell expels its nucleus, giving the cell its characteristic "pinched" look. The new shape of the RBC increases the cell's surface area and thus its

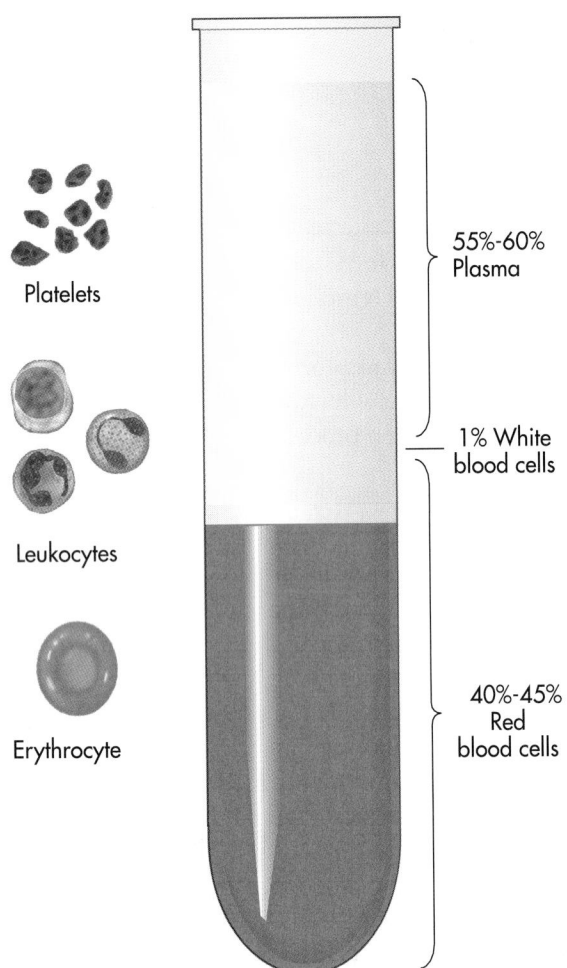

Platelets

Leukocytes

Erythrocyte

55%-60% Plasma

1% White blood cells

40%-45% Red blood cells

Fig. 35-1 Blood will settle into three distinct, proportional layers when treated with salt. The transparent yellow layer at the top is plasma, the liquid portion of blood through which solid elements travel. White blood cells (WBCs) settle in the narrow white band in the center, and red blood cells (RBCs), which give blood its crimson color, fall to the bottom of the flask. RBCs outnumber WBCs 600 to 1.

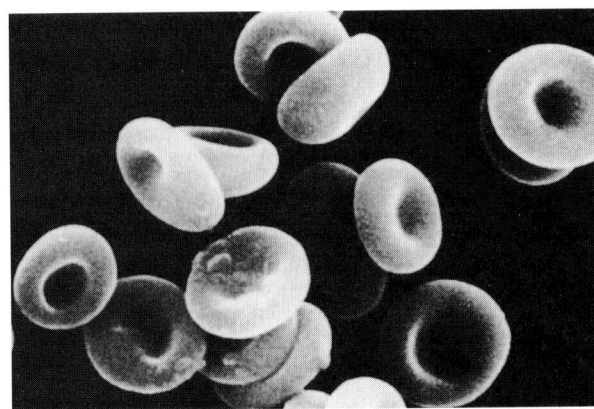

Fig. 35-2 Mature erythrocytes. (Courtesy Dennis Kunkel, PhD, MicroVision, Kailua, Hawaii.)

BOX 35-1

LABORATORY TESTS

- *Hematocrit* (Hct) is the fraction of the total volume of blood that consists of red blood cells (RBCs), normally about 45%. For example, a value of 46% implies that there are 46 mL of RBCs in 100 mL of blood. The normal hematocrit for males is 40% to 54%, and in females a normal hematocrit is 38% to 47%.
- *Hemoglobin* (Hgb) is reported in grams per 100 mL of blood. The normal hemoglobin for males is 13.5 to 18 g/100 mL, and in women a normal hemoglobin is 12 to 16 g/100 mL.
- *Reticulocyte count* provides information about the rate of RBC production. A reticulocyte count of less than 0.5% of the RBC count usually indicates a slowdown in the process of RBC formation. A reticulocyte count greater than 1.5% usually indicates an acceleration of RBC formation.

---

oxygen-carrying potential. RBCs have a life span of about 120 days. As the cells age, their internal chemical machinery weakens; they lose elasticity; and they become trapped in small blood vessels in the bone marrow, liver, and spleen. They are then destroyed by specialized WBCs (macrophages).

NOTE

Most components of destroyed hemoglobin molecules are used again. However, some are broken down to the waste product bilirubin.

Each RBC contains about 270 million hemoglobin molecules, and each hemoglobin molecule carries 4 oxygen molecules. The normal amount of hemoglobin in blood is about 15 g/100 mL and normally is a little higher in males than in females. The number of RBCs is about 4.2 to 6.2 million cells/mm^3 (Box 35-1).

White Blood Cells

As described in Chapter 7, WBCs arise from the bone marrow and are released into the bloodstream. WBCs destroy foreign substances (e.g., bacteria and

TABLE 35-1		CELLULAR COMPONENTS OF THE BLOOD		
CELL	**STRUCTURAL CHARACTERISTICS**	**NORMAL AMOUNTS OF CIRCULATING BLOOD**	**FUNCTION**	**LIFESPAN**
Erythrocyte (red blood cell)	Nonnucleated cytoplasmic disk containing hemoglobin	4.2-6.2 million/mm^3	Gas transport to and from tissue cells and lungs	80-120 days
Leukocyte (white blood cell)	Nucleated cell	5000-10,000/mm^3	Bodily defense mechanisms	See below
Lymphocyte	Mononuclear immunocyte	25% to 33% of leukocyte count (leukocyte differential)	Humoral and cell-mediated immunity	Days or years depending on type
Monocyte and macrophage	Large mononuclear phagocyte	3% to 7% of leukocyte differential	Phagocytosis; mononuclear phagocyte system	Months or years
Eosinophil	Segmented polymorphonuclear granulocyte	1% to 4% of leukocyte differential	Phagocytosis, antibody-mediated defense against parasites, allergic reactions, associated with Hodgkin disease, recovery phase of infection	Unknown
Neutrophil	Segmented polymorphonuclear granulocyte	57% to 67% of leukocyte differential	Phagocytosis, particularly during early phase of inflammation	4 days
Basophil	Segmented polymorphonuclear granulocyte	0% to 0.75% of leukocyte differential	Unknown, but associated with allergic reactions and mechanical irritation	Unknown
Platelet	Irregularly shaped cytoplasmic fragment (not a cell)	140,000 to 340,000/mm^3	Hemostasis after vascular injury; normal coagulation and clot formation/retraction	8-11 days

From McCance KL, Huether SE: *Pathophysiology: the biologic basis for disease in adults and children,* ed 3, St Louis, 1998, Mosby.

viruses) and clear the bloodstream of debris. Leukocyte production increases in response to infection, causing an elevated WBC count in the blood.

NOTE

Chapters 7, 31, and 37 provide a discussion of blood groups, the inflammatory process, and the immune response.

The bone marrow and lymph glands continually produce and maintain a reserve of WBCs. However, there are not many WBCs in the healthy bloodstream. The normal WBC count is about 5000 to 10,000 cells/mm^3. Monocytes make up about 5% of the total WBC count and increase with chronic infections. Lymphocytes account for about 27.5%, neutrophils about 65%, and eosinophils and basophils together about 2.5% of the total WBC count. A rise in the number of WBCs aids in the diagnosis

CLOTTING MEASUREMENTS

Clotting time is normally about 7 to 10 minutes. The patient bleeds if the clotting time is prolonged, and the patient develops intravascular clots if the clotting time is less than normal. Prothrombin (PT) time measures the integrity of the intrinsic clotting cascade. Partial thromboplastin (PTT) time measures the integrity of the extrinsic clotting cascade, which is affected by warfarin (Coumadin). A newer test, the *International Normalized Ratio (INR)*, is routinely used to assess clotting efficiency of patients taking warfarin.

of some diseases because WBCs are somewhat specific for various illnesses.

? CRITICAL THINKING

What body functions are impaired if the WBC number or function is diminished?

NOTE

The differential count identifies the different types of leukocytes (WBCs) present in blood. RBC and platelet morphology also are evaluated in this way.

Platelets

Platelets (thrombocytes) are small, sticky cells that play an important role in blood clotting. When a blood vessel is cut, platelets travel to the site and swell into odd, irregular shapes and adhere to the damaged vessel wall. Platelets "plug" the leak and allow other cells to stick to them and to form a clot. However, if the damage to the vessel is too great, the platelets will chemically signal the complex clotting process, the clotting cascade (described in Chapter 20). Platelets repair millions of ruptured capillaries on a daily basis, often making the rest of the clotting cascade unnecessary (Box 35-2).

Specific Hematological Disorders

Hematological disorders presented in this chapter are anemia, leukemia, lymphomas, polycythemia,

disseminated intravascular coagulopathy (DIC), hemophilia, sickle cell disease, and multiple myeloma.

Anemia

Anemia is a condition in which the concentration of hemoglobin or erythrocytes in the blood is below normal. Precipitating causes of anemia include chronic or acute blood loss, decreased production of erythrocytes, and increased destruction of erythrocytes.[2] Two common forms of anemia are iron-deficiency anemia and hemolytic anemia.

NOTE

Anemia is not a disease, but rather a symptom of an underlying disease process. Some forms of anemia are self-limiting but must be confirmed by laboratory diagnosis.

Iron-Deficiency Anemia

Iron is the critical part of a hemoglobin molecule's ability to bind oxygen (Fig. 35-3). The lack of iron in iron-deficiency anemia prevents the bone marrow from making sufficient hemoglobin for the RBCs. The RBCs produced are small and pale-centered and have a reduced oxygen-carrying capacity. The most common cause of iron-deficiency anemia in adults is blood loss from menstrual bleeding or intestinal bleeding.[3] A diet low in iron usually is the cause of iron-deficiency anemia in children.

? CRITICAL THINKING

Can you predict the signs and symptoms of anemia?

NOTE

Vitamin deficiencies also can produce anemia. Lack of folic acid (one of the B vitamins) is the most common form of vitamin-deficiency anemia.

Hemolytic Anemia

Premature destruction of RBCs in the blood (hemolysis) causes hemolytic anemia. It can result from an inherited disorder inside the RBC or from a disorder outside the cell and usually is acquired later in life.

Inherited disorders. Hemolysis can occur as a result of abnormal rigidity of the cell membrane. This rigidity causes the cell to become trapped at an early stage of its life span in the smaller blood vessels (usually of the spleen) where it is destroyed by macrophages. This type of anemia can occur from a genetic defect in the hemoglobin within the cell (e.g., sickle cell anemia and thalassemia) or from a defect in one of the cell's enzymes that help protect the cell from chemical damage during infectious illness. A deficiency of one of the enzymes, glucose-6-phosphate dehydrogenase, is common in African-Americans.

Acquired disorders. Acquired hemolytic anemia results from one of three conditions:

1. Disorders in which normal RBCs are disrupted as a result of mechanical forces (e.g., abnormal blood vessel linings or blood clots)
2. Autoimmune disorders, which can destroy RBCs with antibodies that are produced by the immune system (e.g., an incompatible blood transfusion)
3. Conditions that can cause hemolytic anemia when RBCs are destroyed by microorganisms in the blood (e.g., malaria).

Signs and Symptoms of Anemia

All forms of anemia share signs and symptoms, including fatigue and headaches, sometimes a sore mouth or tongue, brittle nails, and in severe cases, breathlessness and chest pain (Table 35-2). Other patient complaints are related to an abnormal decrease in the number of WBCs (leukopenia) or a reduction in platelets (thrombocytopenia) and may include the following:

- Fatigue
- Lethargy
- Fever
- Cutaneous bleeding
- Bleeding from mucous membranes

Diagnosis and Treatment

The patient's signs and symptoms, the patient's history, and examination of the patient's blood through blood tests and bone marrow biopsy indicate a diagnosis of most forms of anemia. For example, iron-deficiency anemia usually reveals RBCs that are smaller than normal, and hemolytic anemia shows RBCs that are immature and abnormally shaped. Treatment should be indicated to correct, modify, or

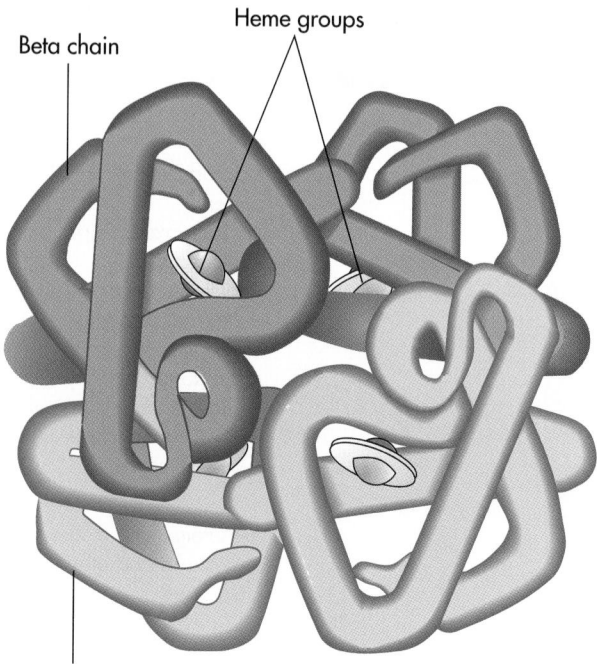

Fig. 35-3 The four-chained hemoglobin molecule is made from more than 10,000 atoms. Yet, when fully laden, the molecule will carry only 4 pairs of oxygen atoms. Hemoglobin is built around 4 atoms of iron that act like oxygen magnets. Each RBC holds 300 million of these vital protein molecules.

diminish the mechanism or process that is leading to defective RBC production or reduced RBC survival.

> **NOTE**
>
> A bone marrow biopsy specimen taken from the sternum or pelvis provides information about the various components of blood and the presence of cells foreign to the marrow. Bone marrow biopsy is useful in diagnosing many hematological disorders such as anemia, leukemia, and certain infections. A bone marrow transplantation sometimes is used in the treatment of these and other diseases.

Leukemia

Leukemia refers to any of several types of cancer in which there usually is a disorganized proliferation of WBCs in the bone marrow. The proliferation of leukemic cells crowds and impairs the normal production of RBCs, WBCs, and platelets. Leukemia is more common in males than in females, and it is more common in Caucasians than in African-Americans. About 30,000 cases are diagnosed in the United States each year.[4]

TABLE 35-2	CAUSES, SIGNS AND SYMPTOMS, AND TREATMENT FOR SPECIFIC FORMS OF ANEMIA		
FORM OF ANEMIA	**CAUSES**	**SIGNS AND SYMPTOMS**	**TREATMENT**
Iron-deficiency anemia	• Insufficient intake of iron • GI disorders (e.g., ulcer disease) • External and/or internal bleeding • Prolonged aspirin or NSAID therapy • Gastrectomy (surgical removal of part or all of the stomach)	• Those related to the underlying cause (e.g., bleeding) • Those common to all forms of anemia	• Correction of the underlying cause • Supplemental iron tablets or injections
Hemolytic anemia	• Genetic RBC disorder • Autoimmune disorders • Malaria and other infections	• Jaundice • Those common to all forms of anemia	• Splenectomy • Immunosuppressant drugs • Avoidance of drugs or foods that precipitate hemolysis • Antimalarial drugs • Blood transfusions

GI, Gastrointestinal; *NSAID,* nonsteroidal antiinflammatory drug; *RBC,* red blood cell.

The exact cause of leukemia is not known; however, genetics may play a role. Abnormal chromosomes associated with congenital disorders (for example, Down's syndrome) and HIV-type viruses are associated with a rare form of this disease. Other factors that may play a role in the development of leukemia include exposure to radiation, viral infections, immune defects, and various chemicals in home and work environments.[2]

Classifications

Leukemia is classified as *acute* or *chronic*. Cancer cells in acute leukemia begin proliferating at an early stage of their development (arrested as immature cells). Chronic leukemia implies an abnormal proliferation of more mature but not fully differentiated cells. Leukemias are further classified according to the type of WBC involved. Two common forms of leukemia are acute lymphoblastic leukemia, which affects mostly children (sometimes called *childhood leukemia*), and *acute myeloblastic leukemia,* which affects mostly middle-age adults. Acute myeloblastic leukemia is one of the most intractable blood cancers. In both types, abnormal WBCs are produced in such large amounts that they eventually accumulate in the body's vital organs (liver, spleen, lymph, and brain), impeding their function and leading to death.

NOTE

Chronic forms of leukemia can develop slowly, often over many years. Cases frequently are discovered "by chance" during routine blood analysis.

Signs and Symptoms

The proliferation of leukemic cells or the resulting inadequate production of other normal blood cells makes the patient highly susceptible to serious infections, anemia, and bleeding episodes. Signs and symptoms of leukemia include the following:

• Fatigue
• Bone pain
• Elevated body temperature and diaphoresis
• Heat intolerance
• Abdominal fullness
• Bleeding
• Frequent bruising
• Headache

- Weight loss
- Night sweats
- Enlargement of lymph nodes
- Enlargement of the liver, spleen, and testes

? CRITICAL THINKING

If a child presents with a lot of unusual bruises, what would you suspect if a diagnosis of leukemia is not known?

Diagnosis and Treatment

The diagnosis of leukemia is confirmed by bone marrow biopsy. The severity of the disease is assessed by the degree of liver and spleen enlargement, anemia, and lack of platelets in the blood. Treatment for acute leukemia can include the transfusion of blood and platelets, antibiotic therapy to manage anemia and infection, and the use of anticancer drugs and sometimes radiation to destroy the leukemic cells. In some cases the leukemia is treated with bone marrow transplantation. Clients with chronic leukemia can be effectively managed with medication, and many require no treatment in its early stages.

Lymphomas

Lymphoma is a general term applied to any neoplastic disorder of the lymphoid tissue. Hodgkin's disease is one type; all others, despite their diversity, are called *non-Hodgkin's lymphomas*. All lymphomas are malignant.

Hodgkin's Disease

Hodgkin's disease is characterized by painless, progressive enlargement of lymphoid tissue found mainly in the lymph nodes and spleen. Left unchecked, these cancer cells multiply and eventually displace healthy lymphocytes, suppressing the immune system. Signs and symptoms include swollen lymph nodes in the neck, armpits, or groin; fatigue; chills; and night sweats. Some patients also experience severe itching, persistent cough, weight loss, shortness of breath, and chest discomfort.

Hodgkin's disease is a relatively rare cancer of unknown etiology that may have a heritable component. It is more common in males than in females, with a peak incidence in people in their twenties

BONE MARROW TRANSPLANTATION FOR LYMPHOMA

In bone marrow transplantation for lymphoma, a small amount of the patient's bone marrow is removed, chemically treated to kill the cancer cells, and placed in cold storage. After the patient's radiation treatment and sometimes chemotherapy, the stored cancer-free bone marrow is returned to the patient by intravenous infusion to allow immature blood cells in the replacement bone marrow to multiply and "regrow" healthy bone marrow. During this "regrowth period," the patient's immune system is severely suppressed, making the possibility of infection a serious health threat.

and in people between 55 and 70 years of age.[1] The disease is confirmed by the identification of Reed-Sternberg cells in lymph nodes or organs affected by the cancer. Treatment depends on the level of lymph node and organ system involvement (the *stage* of the disease) and can consist of radiation and chemotherapy with anticancer drugs. Hodgkin's disease is one of the most curable cancers.

Non-Hodgkin's Lymphomas

Non-Hodgkin's lymphomas vary in their malignancy according to the nature and activity of the abnormal cells. At least 10 types of non-Hodgkin's lymphoma have been identified, and each is ranked as low, intermediate, or high grade based on how aggressively the disease behaves. Low-grade diseases usually progress slowly and tend not to spread beyond the lymphatic system. High-grade diseases can spread to distant organs within a few months. Signs and symptoms include painless swelling of one or more groups of lymph nodes, enlargement of the liver and spleen, fever, and in rare cases, abdominal pain and gastrointestinal bleeding.

The cause of these cancers is largely unknown. One form, Burkitt's lymphoma, is strongly associated with infection by Epstein-Barr virus, commonly found in Africa. Other types have been linked to infection by HIV-type viruses and other conditions that affect the immune system (e.g., organ transplantation, radiation and chemotherapy, lupus, and rheumatoid arthritis). Treatment consists of radiation therapy, anticancer drugs, and sometimes bone marrow transplantation (see the box above).

BOX 35-3

HEREDITARY CHARACTERISTICS OF HEMOPHILIA

Chromosomes from the mother link with an equal number from the father, and each pair determines the type of information that genes carry. Females have two X chromosomes, and males have an X and a Y chromosome. The mother passes on the X chromosome to her child, and the father passes on either an X or a Y. Two X chromosomes produce a female child, an X and a Y produce a male child.

Hemophilia stems from an abnormal gene on the X chromosome. A female with an abnormal X chromosome usually is spared the disease because, although she received one abnormal X chromosome from one parent, the normal X chromosome passed on from her other parent counteracted the abnormal gene. However, she is a "carrier" of the disease and can pass it on to her children. A woman can have hemophilia only if her mother is a carrier and her father has hemophilia, which is rare. Affected males do not pass the defective gene to sons, but they pass it on to all of their daughters. A male, however, receives only one X chromosome. If his mother is a carrier, the male child will have a 50% chance of having hemophilia.

Polycythemia

Polycythemia is an increase in the total RBC mass of the blood. The condition may be a natural response to hypoxia (secondary polycythemia), or it may occur for unknown reasons (primary polycythemia).

NOTE

Polycythemia also can result from dehydration (apparent polycythemia), in which the RBC production does not exceed the upper limits of normal.

Secondary Polycythemia

Secondary polycythemia can be naturally present in people who live in or visit areas of high altitude because of reduced air pressure and low oxygen. When oxygen supply to the blood is reduced, the kidneys produce the hormone *erythropoietin*, which stimulates RBC production in the bone marrow to

compensate for the reduced oxygen supply. The result is an increase in the oxygen-carrying efficiency of the blood. The RBC numbers return to normal when the person returns to sea level.

NOTE

Secondary polycythemia also can be present in heavy smokers and can be caused by chronic bronchitis and conditions that increase erythropoietin production (e.g., liver cancer and some kidney disorders).

Primary Polycythemia

Primary polycythemia, also known as *polycythemia vera*, is a rare disorder of the bone marrow in which the increased production of RBCs causes the blood to thicken. This condition primarily develops in people over 50 years of age[2] and can lead to several physiological problems that include the following:

- Headache
- Dizziness
- Blurred vision
- Generalized itching
- Red hands and feet; red-purple complexion
- Hypertension
- Splenomegaly

Other complications that are associated with primary polycythemia include platelet disorders, which cause bleeding or clot formation; stroke; and the development of other bone marrow diseases (e.g., leukemias). Treatment consists of phlebotomy (the slow removal of blood through a vein) and anticancer drug therapy to control the overproduction of RBCs in the marrow.

Disseminated Intravascular Coagulopathy

Disseminated intravascular coagulopathy (DIC) (described in Chapter 19) is a complication of severe injury, trauma, or disease. DIC is a relatively common abnormal clotting disorder, most often seen in the critical care setting. It disrupts the balance among procoagulants, inhibitors, thrombus formation, and lysis. Signs and symptoms of DIC include dyspnea, bleeding, and those associated with hypotension and hypoperfusion.

DIC occurs in two phases.[2] The first phase is characterized by free thrombin in the blood, fibrin deposits, and aggregation of platelets. The second phase is characterized by hemorrhage caused by depletion of clotting factors. The clinical consequences of these processes predispose the patient to multiple-system organ failure from bleeding and coagulation disorders caused by the following:

- Loss of platelets and clotting factors
- Fibrinolysis
- Fibrin degradation interference
- Small vessel obstruction, tissue ischemia, RBC injury, and anemia from fibrin deposits

Management

Once DIC is confirmed though laboratory tests, treatment is aimed at reversing the underlying illness or injury that triggered the event. In an effort to control the depletion of clotting factors, initial care includes the replacement of platelets, coagulation factors, and blood while attempts are made to manage the primary process.

Hemophilia

Hemophilia, meaning "love of blood," is a group of inherited bleeding disorders (Box 35-3). Hemophilia A is due to a deficiency in factor VIII, which is essential to the process of blood clotting (Table 35-3). Another less common form of hemophilia, caused by a deficiency of factor IX, is known as *hemophilia B*, or Christmas disease (named for a man first diagnosed with the disease in 1952). All types of hemophilia present with similar problems, but the specific factor involved determines the severity of bleeding.

Bleeding from hemophilia can occur spontaneously, after even minor injury, or during some medical procedures (e.g., tooth extraction). Hemorrhage can occur anywhere in the body, but bleeding into joints, deep muscles, the urinary tract, and intracranial sites is the most common. Head trauma is potentially life threatening. Central nervous system (CNS) bleeding is the major cause of death for hemophilia patients in all age groups.[4]

Hemophilia is controlled by infusions of concentrates of factor VIII that can be self-administered by the patient. However, serious or unusual bleeding episodes often require hospitalization. Clients with hemophilia are cautioned to avoid activities (e.g., contact sports) that expose them to increased risk of injury. Most patients with hemophilia are knowledgeable about their disease and seek emergency

TABLE 35-3	CLOTTING FACTORS AND SYNONYMS
FACTOR	**SYNONYMS**
I	Fibrinogen
II	Prothrombin
III	Thromboplastin
IV	Calcium
V	Proaccelerin
VI	None in use
VII	Serum prothrombin conversion accelerator (SPCA)
VIII	Antihemophilic globulin (AHG) Antihemophilic factor (AHF)
IX	Plasma thromboplastin component (PTC) Christmas factor
X	Stuart factor
XI	Plasma thromboplastin antecedent (PTA)
XII	Hageman factor
XIII	Fibrin-stabilizing factor

care only when complicated problems and trauma-related difficulties arise.

? CRITICAL THINKING

What should you do if you are caring for a patient with hemophilia who has fallen 15 feet from a ladder and refuses care and transportation?

NOTE

Factor VIII is made from large pools of donor blood. During the first few years of the acquired immunodeficiency syndrome (AIDS) epidemic, many people with hemophilia and their sexual partners became infected with human immunodeficiency virus (HIV) through factor VIII infusions. Even with careful screening protocols for blood, infusions still carry a very small risk of transmitting hepatitis B virus (HBV), hepatitis C virus (HCV), and HIV to factor VIII recipients. Another factor VIII product, recombinant factor VIII (Recombinate), is produced by inserting cloned factor VIII into animal tissues. Recombinate is not made from human plasma, is the purest form of factor VIII, does not transmit viral contamination, and is as effective as plasma-derived factor VIII.[5]

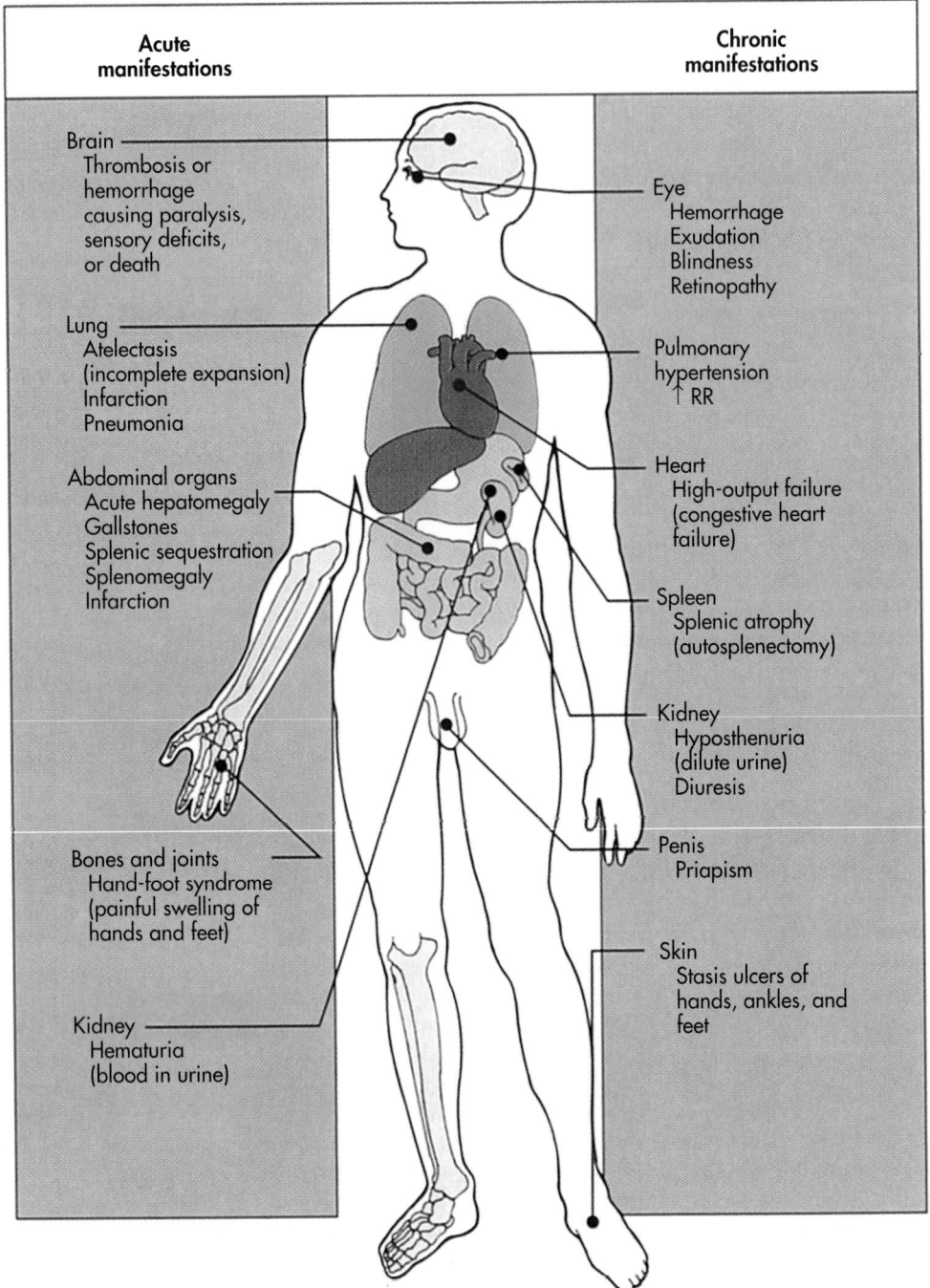

Acute manifestations

Brain
 Thrombosis or
 hemorrhage
 causing paralysis,
 sensory deficits,
 or death

Lung
 Atelectasis
 (incomplete expansion)
 Infarction
 Pneumonia

Abdominal organs
 Acute hepatomegaly
 Gallstones
 Splenic sequestration
 Splenomegaly
 Infarction

Bones and joints
 Hand-foot syndrome
 (painful swelling of
 hands and feet)

Kidney
 Hematuria
 (blood in urine)

Chronic manifestations

Eye
 Hemorrhage
 Exudation
 Blindness
 Retinopathy

Pulmonary
hypertension
 ↑ RR

Heart
 High-output failure
 (congestive heart
 failure)

Spleen
 Splenic atrophy
 (autosplenectomy)

Kidney
 Hyposthenuria
 (dilute urine)
 Diuresis

Penis
 Priapism

Skin
 Stasis ulcers of
 hands, ankles, and
 feet

Fig. 35-4 Clinical manifestations of sickle cell disease. (From McCance KL, Huether SE: *Pathophysiology: the biologic basis for disease in adults and children,* ed 3, St Louis, 1998, Mosby.)

Sickle Cell Disease

Sickle cell disease (also known as *sickle cell anemia*) is a debilitating and unpredictable recessive genetic illness that affects persons of African descent (and less commonly, persons of Mediterranean origins). It is estimated that 1 in 12 African-Americans suffer from sickle cell disease. Approximately 1 in 12 African-Americans has *sickle cell trait.*[6] (See the box at the bottom of p. 1073.) Signs and symptoms of sickle cell disease include: (see Fig. 35-4)

- Jaundice
- Stroke

- Delayed growth, development, and sexual maturation in children
- Priapism in adolescent and adult males
- Splenomegaly

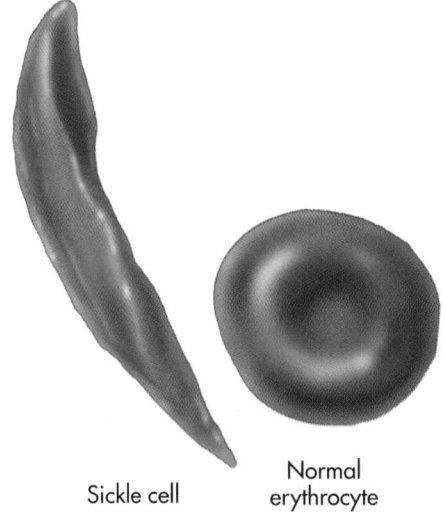

Sickle cell   Normal erythrocyte

Fig. 35-5 Sickle cell versus normal erythrocyte.

> **NOTE**
>
> More than 70,000 Americans of different ethnic origins have sickle cell disease.[6]

Pathophysiology

Sickle cell anemia produces an abnormal type of hemoglobin, called *hemoglobin S*, that has an inferior oxygen-carrying capacity. When hemoglobin S is exposed to low oxygen states, it crystallizes, distorting the RBCs into a sickle shape (Fig. 35-5). The sickle-shaped cells are fragile and easily destroyed. They also are unable to pass easily through tiny blood vessels and block flow to various organs and tissues, causing a vasoocclusive sickle cell crisis that can be life threatening. As fewer RBCs pass through congested vessels, tissues and joints become starved for oxygen and other nutrients, causing excruciating pain. Other signs and symptoms of sickle cell anemia are listed in Box 35-4.

> **NOTE**
>
> Three less common types of sickle cell crisis are aplastic, hemolytic, and splenic sequestration. In aplastic crisis the bone marrow temporarily stops producing RBCs. In hemolytic crisis the RBCs break down too rapidly to be replaced adequately. Splenic sequestration usually is a childhood difficulty that occurs when blood becomes trapped in the spleen, causing the organ to enlarge and possibly leading to death.

> **? CRITICAL THINKING**
>
> *How do you think a client with such chronic pain must feel at the beginning of a sickle cell crisis?*

CHARACTERISTICS OF SICKLE CELL TRAIT

A person must inherit two sickle cell genes—one from each parent—to develop sickle cell disease. When only one gene is present, the condition is known as a *sickle cell trait*. Persons with sickle cell trait generally do not experience symptoms except occasionally under low-oxygen conditions (e.g., scuba diving or traveling at high altitudes). However, these persons can pass the gene, and possibly the disease, on to their children. If both parents have sickle cell trait, there is a 25% chance that the child will develop the disease, a 50% chance the child will have sickle cell trait, and a 25% chance that the child will have neither.

BOX 35-4

SIGNS AND SYMPTOMS OF SICKLE CELL DISEASE

Increased weakness
Aching
Chest pain with shortness of breath
Sudden, severe abdominal pain
Bony deformities
Icteric (jaundice) sclera
Fever
Arthralgia (joint pain)

BOX 35-5

PATIENT COMPLAINTS ASSOCIATED WITH MULTIPLE MYELOMA

Weakness
Skeletal pain
Hemorrhage
Hematuria
Lethargy
Weight loss
Frequent fractures

Sickle cell crisis can occur in any part of the body and can vary in intensity from one person to the next and from one crisis to the next. Over time the crises can destroy the spleen, kidneys, gallbladder, and other organs. Sickle cell crisis may occur for no apparent reason or be triggered by conditions such as the following:

• Dehydration
• Infection
• Stress
• Trauma
• Exposure to extremes in temperature
• Lack of oxygen
• Strenuous physical activity

NOTE

Genetic counseling should be considered for carriers of the disease who plan to become parents. Many states require sickle cell screening of newborns.

Management

Currently no cure exists for sickle cell disease. Because of the eventual damage that occurs to the spleen, patients with sickle cell disease are at increased risk for septicemia if infected by certain types of bacteria. Children with the disease should be current with all immunizations. When in crisis, these patients require prompt treatment with oxygen, intravenous (IV) therapy to manage dehydration, antibiotics to manage infection, and analgesics to manage pain. In severe cases, a blood transfusion may be indicated to effect a temporary replacement of hemoglobin S.

NOTE

Blood transfusions can be recommended during pregnancy to reduce the risk of a crisis, which can be fatal to both the mother and fetus, and before surgery since anesthesia can be hazardous to those with the disease.

Multiple Myeloma

Multiple myeloma is a malignant neoplasm of the bone marrow. The tumor, composed of plasma cells, destroys bone tissue (especially in flat bones), causing pain, fractures, hypercalcemia, and skeletal deformities. In myeloma the neoplastic cells produce large amounts of protein (M-protein) that affect the viscosity of the blood. Masses of coagulated protein can accumulate within the tissues and impair function. Some patients with this disease die of kidney failure from the accumulation of proteins that infiltrate the kidneys and block the renal tubules.

? CRITICAL THINKING

Which are the flat bones?

NOTE

In many ways, multiple myeloma resembles leukemia, but the plasma cell proliferation generally is confined to the bone marrow.

Other disorders associated with multiple myeloma include proteinuria, anemia, weight loss, pulmonary complications secondary to rib fracture, and recurrent infections from suppression of the immune system (from unknown factors secreted from the malignant plasma cells) (Box 35-5). Multiple myeloma occurs rarely before 40 years of age and then occurs increasingly with age. It is more common in males than in females and may have a heritable component.[1] Multiple myeloma is diagnosed though x-ray examination, blood studies, and tumor biopsy. Treatment consists of chemotherapy with anticancer drugs, radiation, plasma exchange, and bone marrow transplantation.

General Assessment and Management of Patients with Hematological Disorders

As previously stated, most patients with hematological disorders are knowledgeable about their disease. Often they summon emergency medical services (EMS) to help manage a "change" in their condition or to arrange for transportation to an emergency department for physician evaluation. Situations that initiate a call for emergency care vary by patient and disease.

> ✓ **TRICKS OF THE TRADE**
>
> Many patients with hematological disorders are "experts" about their disease. Listen to them, and respect their level of knowledge.

Common chief complaints can be classified by body system and include the following:

- Central nervous system
  Altered level of consciousness
  Increased weakness
- Integumentary system
  Prolonged bleeding
  Bruising
  Itching
  Pallor
  Jaundice
- Visual disturbances
- Epistaxis
- Gastrointestinal system
  Bleeding or infected gums
  Ulceration

  Melena
  Liver disease
  Pain
- Musculoskeletal system
  Bone or joint pain
  Fracture
- Cardiorespiratory system
  Dyspnea
  Chest pain
  Hemoptysis
  Tachycardia
- Genitourinary system
  Hematuria
  Amenorrhagia (absence of menstruation)
  Infections

Emergency Care

In many cases emergency care is primarily supportive. As with any other patient care encounter, the paramedic should ensure adequate airway, ventilatory, and circulatory support. Vital signs and a detailed physical examination help determine the appropriateness of emergency transportation. Calming measures and emotional support for both the patient and family are particularly important because some of these patients will be gravely ill. Other prehospital care measures include IV fluid replacement, the use of antidysrhythmics, and the administration of analgesics for pain management.

> ✓ **TRICKS OF THE TRADE**
>
> Patients with hematological disorders often have complicated medical histories. Whenever possible, you should transport them to their primary hospital where they usually receive their medical care.

SUMMARY

- Blood is composed of cells and formed elements surrounded by plasma. About 95% of the volume of formed elements consists of red blood cells (RBCs; erythrocytes). The remaining 5% consists of white blood cells (WBCs; leukocytes) and cell fragments (platelets).

- Anemia is a condition in which the concentration of hemoglobin or erythrocytes in the blood is below normal. Two common forms of anemia are iron-deficiency anemia and hemolytic anemia. All forms of anemia share signs and symptoms, including fatigue and headaches, sometimes a sore mouth or tongue, brittle nails, and in severe cases, breathlessness and chest pain. Diagnosis is made by history and from blood tests and bone marrow biopsy.

- *Leukemia* refers to any of several types of cancer in which there usually is a disorganized proliferation of WBCs in the bone marrow. The proliferation of leukemic cells crowds and impairs the normal production of RBCs, WBCs, and platelets. Leukemia is classified as acute or chronic. The proliferation of leukemic cells makes the patient highly susceptible to serious infections, anemia, and bleeding episodes. The diagnosis is confirmed by bone marrow biopsy.

- *Lymphoma* refers to a group of diseases that range from slowly growing chronic disorders to rapidly evolving acute conditions. Hodgkin's disease is one type; all others are called *non-Hodgkin's lymphomas.*

- Polycythemia is characterized by an unusually large number of RBCs in the blood as a result of their increased production by the bone marrow. Polycythemia may be a natural response to hypoxia (secondary polycythemia), or it may occur for unknown reasons (primary polycythemia).

- Disseminated intravascular coagulopathy (DIC) is a complication of severe injury, trauma, or disease. It disrupts the balance among procoagulants, thrombin formation, inhibitors, and lysis. Signs and symptoms of DIC include dyspnea, bleeding, and those associated with hypotension and hypoperfusion. Treatment is aimed at reversing the underlying illness or injury that triggered the event.

- Hemophilia A is caused by a deficiency of a blood protein called *factor VIII,* and hemophilia B is caused by a deficiency of factor IX. Bleeding from hemophilia can occur spontaneously, after even minor injury, or during some medical procedures.

- Sickle cell disease is a debilitating and unpredictable recessive genetic illness that affects persons of African descent and, less commonly, persons of Mediterranean origin. Sickle cell anemia produces an abnormal type of hemoglobin, called *hemoglobin S*, that has an inferior oxygen-carrying capacity. Complications of sickle cell disease include episodes of severe pain, fatigue, pallor, jaundice, stroke, delayed growth, hematuria, priapism, and splenomegaly.

- Multiple myeloma is a malignant neoplasm of the bone marrow. The tumor destroys bone tissue (especially flat bones), causing pain, fractures, hypercalcemia, and skeletal deformities.

- In many cases of hematological disorders, prehospital treatment is supportive and includes ensuring adequate airway, ventilatory, and circulatory support.

REFERENCES

1. McCance KL, Huether SE: *Pathophysiology: the biologic basis for disease in adults and children,* ed 3, St Louis, 1998, Mosby.
2. US Department of Transportation, National Highway Traffic Safety Administration: *EMT-Paramedic national standard curriculum,* Washington, DC, 1998, The Department.
3. Rosen P, Barkin R: *Emergency medicine: concepts and clinical practice,* ed 4, St Louis, 1998, Mosby.
4. *The medical advisor,* Alexandria, VA, 1996, Time-Life Books.
5. Hemophilia Health Services: *About hemophilia,* 1999. Available at www.hemophiliahealth.com/Hemophilia/hemophilia.html.
6. American Institute for Preventive Medicine: *Sickle cell anemia,* 1995. Available at www.healthy.net/hwlibrary-books/healthyself/sicklecell.htm.

36 *Environmental Conditions*

OBJECTIVES

Upon completion of this chapter, the paramedic student will be able to:

1. **Describe the physiology of thermoregulation.**

2. **Discuss the risk factors, pathophysiology, assessment findings, and management of specific hyperthermic conditions.**

3. **Discuss the risk factors, pathophysiology, assessment findings, and management of specific hypothermic conditions and frostbite.**

4. **Discuss the risk factors, pathophysiology, assessment findings, and management of submersion and drowning.**

5. **Identify mechanical effects on the body based on a knowledge of basic properties of gases.**

6. **Discuss the risk factors, pathophysiology, assessment findings, and management of diving emergencies and high-altitude illness.**

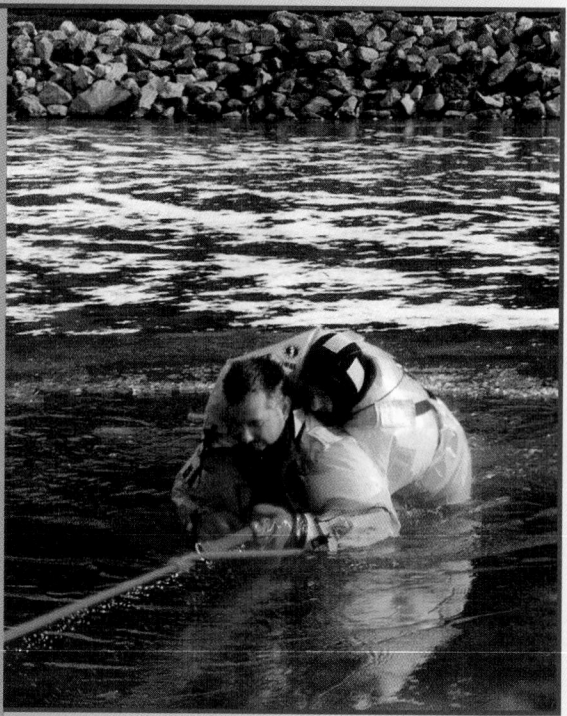

Many medical emergencies can result from physical exposure to environmental elements. The paramedic must be prepared to recognize and manage these conditions by understanding their causative factors and distinctive underlying pathophysiology.

KEY TERMS

acute mountain sickness: A common high-altitude illness that results from rapid ascent of an unacclimatized person to high altitudes.

core body temperature: The temperature of deep structures of the body as compared with temperatures of peripheral tissues.

decompression sickness: A multisystem disorder that results when nitrogen in compressed air converts back from solution to gas, forming bubbles in the tissues and blood.

drowning: A mortal event in which a submersion victim is pronounced dead at the scene of the attempted resuscitation, or within 24 hours after arrival in the emergency department (ED) or hospital.

frostbite: A localized injury that results from environmentally induced freezing of body tissues.

heat cramps: Brief, intermittent, and often severe muscular cramps that frequently occur in muscles fatigued by heavy work or exercise.

heat exhaustion: A form of heat illness characterized by minor aberrations in mental status, dizziness, nausea, headache, and mild to moderate core body temperature elevation.

heat stroke: A syndrome that occurs when the thermoregulatory mechanisms normally in place to meet the demands of heat stress break down entirely, resulting in body temperature elevated to extreme levels and producing multisystem tissue damage and physiological collapse.

high-altitude pulmonary edema: A high-altitude illness thought to be caused at least in part by increased pulmonary artery pressure that develops in response to hypoxia.

high-altitude cerebral edema: The most severe form of acute high-altitude illness, characterized by a progression of global cerebral signs in the presence of acute mountain sickness.

nitrogen narcosis: An illness associated with scuba diving in which nitrogen becomes dissolved in solution as a result of greater-than-normal atmospheric pressure; also known as rapture of the deep.

submersion: An incident in which a person experiences some swimming-related distress that is sufficient to require support in the prehospital setting and transportation to a medical facility for further observation and treatment.

thermogenesis: Production of heat, especially by the cells of the body.

thermolysis: Dissipation of heat by radiation, evaporation, conduction, or convection.

Thermoregulation

A thermoregulatory center in the posterior hypothalamus regulates body temperature. This center receives input from central thermoreceptors in or near the anterior hypothalamus and from peripheral thermoreceptors located in the skin and some mucous membranes. Peripheral thermoreceptors are nerve endings usually categorized as cold receptors, which are stimulated by a lower skin-surface temperature, and warm receptors, which are stimulated by higher temperatures. There are up to 10 times as many cold receptors as warm ones in many parts of the skin. Information from these receptors is transmitted via afferent nerves and ascending pathways to the posterior hypothalamus, which responds with appropriate efferent output to decrease heat loss and increase heat production (cold-receptor stimulation) or increase heat loss and decrease heat production (warm-receptor stimulation).

> **? CRITICAL THINKING**
>
> *Why do you think the body has so many more cold receptors than heat receptors?*

Central thermoreceptors are temperature-sensitive neurons that react directly to alterations in the temperature of blood. These neurons innervate skeletal muscle through descending pathways and somatic motor nerves. They affect vasomotor tone, sweating, and metabolic rate through sympathetic nerve output to skin arterioles, sweat glands, and the adrenal medulla.

As discussed in Chapter 13, the thermoregulatory center has an inherent set point, which maintains a relatively constant **core body temperature** (CBT) of 98.6° F (37° C). To maintain an optimum environment for normal cell metabolism (homeostasis), it is necessary to keep the CBT fairly constant, notwithstanding the external and internal conditions that tend to raise or lower it. The body temperature can be increased or decreased in two ways: through regulation of heat production (**thermogenesis**) and regulation of heat loss (**thermolysis**).

Regulating Heat Production

The body can generate heat in response to cold through mechanical, chemical, metabolic, and endocrine activities. Several physiological and biochemical factors, such as the individual's age, general health, and nutritional status, affect the direction and magnitude of these compensatory responses.

Heat production is controlled chemically by cellular metabolism (oxidation of energy sources). Every tissue contributes to this type of heat production, but in humans, skeletal muscles produce the largest amount of heat, particularly when shivering occurs. Along with shivering, which is often associated with chattering of teeth, the body undergoes vasoconstriction to conserve as much heat as possible. Shivering is the body's best defense against cold and can increase heat production by as much as 400%.

Endocrine glands also regulate heat production through the release of hormones from the thyroid gland and adrenal medulla. Sympathetic discharge of epinephrine and norepinephrine and the activity of sympathetic nerves that lead to adipose tissue increase the basal metabolic rate and thereby augment heat production.

Regulating Heat Loss

Heat is lost from the body to the external environment through the skin, lungs, and excretions. The skin is the most important of these in regulating heat loss. Radiation, conduction, convection, and evaporation are the major sources of heat loss.

The surface of the human body constantly emits heat in the form of infrared rays. The temperature of the radiating surface determines the rate of emissions. Thus if the surface of the body is warmer than the average of the various surfaces in the environment, net heat is lost because the rate depends di-

> ? CRITICAL THINKING
>
> **What fuels does the body need for heat production to increase by shivering?**

TABLE 36-1   **COOLING POWER OF WIND ON EXPOSED FLESH EXPRESSED AS AN EQUIVALENT TEMPERATURE (UNDER CALM CONDITIONS)**

ESTIMATED WIND SPEED (IN MPH)	ACTUAL THERMOMETER READING (°F)											
	50	40	30	20	10	0	−10	−20	−30	−40	−50	−60
	EQUIVALENT CHILL TEMPERATURE (°F)											
Calm	50	40	30	20	10	0	−10	−20	−30	−40	−50	−60
5	48	37	27	16	6	−5	−15	−26	−36	−47	−57	−68
10	40	28	16	4	−9	−24	−33	−46	−58	−70	−83	−95
15	36	22	9	−5	−18	−32	−45	−58	−72	−85	−99	−112
20	32	18	4	−10	−25	−39	−53	−67	−82	−96	−110	−124
25	30	16	0	−15	−29	−44	−59	−74	−88	−104	−118	−133
30	28	13	−2	−18	−33	−48	−63	−79	−94	−109	−125	−140
35	27	11	−4	−21	−35	−51	−62	−82	−98	−113	−129	−145
40	26	10	−6	−21	−37	−53	−69	−85	−100	−116	−132	−148

(Wind speeds greater than 40 mph have little additional effect.)	Little danger. In <5 hr with dry skin. Maximum danger is false sense of security.	Increasing danger. Danger from freezing of exposed flesh within 1 minute	Great danger. Flesh may freeze within 30 seconds.
	Trenchfoot and immersion foot can occur at any point on this chart.		

Measure local temperature and wind speed if possible. If not, *estimate*. Enter table at closest 5° F interval along the top and with appropriate wind speed along left side. Intersection gives approximate equivalent chill temperature (i.e., the temperature that would cause the same rate of cooling under calm conditions). Note that regardless of cooling rate, you do not cool below the actual air temperature unless wet.
From Sheehy S: *Emergency nursing*, ed 3, St Louis, 1992, Mosby.

rectly on the temperature difference between the environment and the body (thermal gradient).

Conduction is the exchange of heat that occurs simply by the transfer of thermal energy. Heat moves down a concentration gradient from higher to lower temperature. Therefore the body surface loses or gains heat by direct contact with cooler or warmer surfaces, including air. If ambient air temperature is lower than skin temperature, body heat is lost to the surrounding air by conduction.

Convection is the process whereby air or water next to the body is heated, moves away, and is replaced by cool air or water, which repeats the same pattern. Convection can be greatly facilitated by external forces such as wind or fans and aids conductive heat exchange by continuously maintaining a supply of cool air. Factors that contribute to the cooling effects of convection are the velocity of air currents and the temperature of the air. The windchill chart calculates the cooling effects of the ambient temperature based on thermometer readings and wind speed (Table 36-1).

> **? CRITICAL THINKING**
>
> *How does wearing the fully encapsulated hazardous materials suit affect your body's ability to regulate temperature?*

Evaporation of any fluid absorbs heat from surrounding objects and air. Ambient temperature and relative humidity greatly affect evaporative heat loss from moisture on the skin or lining membranes of the respiratory tract. The relative humidity is the ratio of the actual amount of moisture in the air to the greatest amount that the air can hold at a specified temperature. The relative humidity is 100% when, at a given temperature, the air is fully saturated with moisture. Diaphoresis can markedly increase evaporative heat loss provided that the relative humidity is low enough that the sweat can evaporate. At humidity levels above 75%, evaporation decreases, and at levels approaching 90%, evaporation essentially ceases.

Maintenance of Thermoregulation

The balance between heat loss and heat production is constantly changing because of changes in metabolic rate or changes in the external environment.

The extent to which the hypothalamus initiates and integrates physiological activity to maintain body temperature is not fully understood. However, several hyperthermic and hypothermic compensatory responses are the basis for maintaining thermoregulation (Box 36-1).

External Environmental Factors

External environmental factors that can contribute to a medical emergency and affect rescue and transportation considerations include the climate, season, weather, atmospheric pressure, and terrain. When the potential for an environmental emergency exists, the paramedic must consider the following:

- Localized prevailing weather norms and any deviations
- Characteristics of seasonal variation to climate
- Weather extremes (wind, rain, snow, humidity)
- Barometric pressure (e.g., at altitude or under water)
- Terrain that can complicate injury or rescue

The patient's general health also is a factor related to environmental stressors and can exacerbate

> **BOX 36-1**
>
> **HYPERTHERMIC AND HYPOTHERMIC COMPENSATION**
>
> **Hyperthermic Compensation**
> *Increased heat loss*
> Vasodilation of skin vessels
> Sweating
>
> *Decreased heat production*
> Decreased muscle tone and voluntary activity
> Decreased hormone secretion
> Decreased appetite
>
> **Hypothermic Compensation**
> *Decreased heat loss*
> Peripheral vasoconstriction
> Reduction of surface area by body position (or clothing)
> Piloerection (not effective in humans)
>
> *Increased heat production*
> Shivering
> Increased voluntary activity
> Increased hormone secretion
> Increased appetite

other medical or traumatic conditions. Examples include the patient's age, predisposing medical conditions, use of prescription and over-the-counter medications, use of alcohol or recreational drugs, and previous rate of exertion.

Hyperthermia

Heat illness results from one of two basic causes:

1. The normal thermoregulatory mechanisms are overwhelmed by environmental conditions such as heat stress or, more commonly, by excessive exercise in moderate to extreme environmental conditions.
2. Failure of the thermoregulatory mechanisms, as in older adults or ill or debilitated patients.

Either cause can result in heat illness such as heat cramps, heat exhaustion, and heat stroke.

Heat Cramps

Heat cramps are brief, intermittent, and often severe muscular cramps that occur in muscles fatigued by heavy work or exercise. They are caused primarily by a rapid change in extracellular fluid osmolarity resulting from sodium and water loss.

Persons who suffer from heat cramps sweat profusely and drink water without adequate salt. During environmental heat stress, 1 to 3 L of water per hour can be lost through sweating. Each liter contains between 30 and 50 mEq of sodium chloride. The water and sodium deficiency combine to cause muscle cramping, which normally occurs in the most heavily exercised muscles, including the calves and arms (although any muscle can be involved). These patients usually are alert with hot sweaty skin, tachycardia, and normotension, but they have a normal CBT. Heat cramps are easily

managed by removal of the patient from the hot environment and replacement of sodium and water. In more serious cases, medical direction may recommend intravenous (IV) infusion of a balanced sodium chloride solution.

Heat Exhaustion

Heat exhaustion is a more severe form of heat illness characterized by minor aberrations in mental status (e.g., irritability and poor judgment), dizziness, nausea, headache, and mild to moderate CBT elevation (less than 103° F [39° C]). In severe cases, orthostatic dizziness (which occurs when rising from a lying position to a sitting or standing position) resulting from significant intravascular volume loss and syncope may occur.

Like heat cramps, heat exhaustion more commonly is associated with hot ambient temperature and results in profuse sweating. With water and salt deficiency, electrolyte imbalance and vasomotor regulatory disturbances contribute to inadequate peripheral and cerebral perfusion, the signs of which are characteristic of this illness. Rapid recovery generally follows removal from the hot environment and fluid administration. Patients with significant fluid abnormalities or orthostatic hypotension may require IV administration of a balanced sodium chloride solution. Heat exhaustion can progress to heat stroke if left untreated.

Heat Stroke

Heat stroke occurs when the thermoregulatory mechanisms normally in place to meet the demands of heat stress break down entirely. This failure results in body temperature elevated to 105.8° F (41° C) or higher, producing multisystem tissue damage and physiological collapse. Heat stroke is a true medical emergency. The syndrome is classified

---

NOTE

Oral salt additives (e.g., salt tablets) can cause gastrointestinal irritation, ulceration, and vomiting, which exacerbates electrolyte imbalance. The paramedic should generally avoid the use of oral salt additives in managing heat-related illness and should follow local protocol regarding oral rehydration with a salt-containing fluid-replacement beverage (e.g., Gatorade and PowerAde).

NOTE

Increased body temperature caused by failure of the thermoregulatory mechanisms should not be confused with fever associated with an inflammatory response. In fever the effect on the hypothalamus is caused by endogenous pyrogens that are released by phagocytic leukocytes. Antipyretic drugs can reverse these effects, returning the set point of the hypothalamus to normal.

into two types: classic heat stroke and exertional heat stroke.

Classic heat stroke occurs during periods of sustained high ambient temperatures and humidity. The illness commonly affects the young, older adults, and those who live in poorly ventilated homes without air conditioning. Examples include young children left in an enclosed automobile on a hot afternoon and older persons confined to a hot room during a heat wave. Classic heat stroke victims also frequently suffer from chronic diseases such as diabetes, heart disease, alcoholism, or psychiatric disorders, which predispose them to the syndrome. Many patients with classic heat stroke take prescribed medications such as diuretics, antihypertensives, psychotropics (antipsychotics, antihistamines, phenothiazines), and anticholinergics, which further impair their ability to tolerate heat stress. In these patients the illness develops from poor dissipation of environmental heat.

> **NOTE**
>
> The autoimmune neuropathy associated with diabetes can interfere with vasodilation, perspiration, and thermoregulatory input. Some cardiac medications (e.g., diuretics and beta blockers) can predispose a patient to dehydration, interfere with vasodilation, and reduce the capacity to increase heart rate in response to a volume loss.

In contrast to patients with classic heat stroke, patients with exertional heat stroke are usually young and healthy. Commonly afflicted groups include athletes and military recruits who exercise in hot and humid conditions. In these situations, heat accumulates more rapidly in the body than it can be dissipated into the environment. Preventive measures to reduce the risk for exertional heat illness for all age groups include the following:

- Avoiding or limiting exercise in hot environments
- Maintaining adequate fluid intake
- Acclimatization that results in more perspiration with lower salt concentration, thereby increasing fluid volume in the body

Clinical Manifestations

As previously described, the hypothalamic temperature regulatory centers receive their information largely from the temperature of circulating blood in the deep and superficial veins and from peripheral thermoreceptors in the skin. In response to hypothalamic stimulation, the respiratory rate quickens to increase heat loss through exhaled air, cardiac output increases to provide additional blood flow through skin and muscle to enhance heat radiation, and sweat gland activity increases to enhance evaporative heat loss. These compensatory mechanisms require a normally functioning central nervous system (CNS) to integrate thermal inputs and initiate appropriate thermoregulatory responses and an intact cardiovascular system to transport excess heat from the core to the periphery. Dysfunction in either or both of these systems leads to a rapidly increasing CBT.

CNS manifestations. The CNS manifestations of heat stroke vary. Some patients may be in frank coma, whereas others may exhibit confusion and irrational behavior before collapse. Convulsions are common and can occur early or late in the course of the illness. Since the brain stores little energy, it depends on a constant supply of oxygen and glucose. Decreased cerebral perfusion pressure results in cerebral ischemia and acidosis, and increased temperatures markedly increase the metabolic demands of the brain. The extent of cerebral damage depends on the severity and duration of the hyperthermic episode.

> **? CRITICAL THINKING**
>
> *What other conditions can present with these types of mental status changes?*

> **NOTE**
>
> Fever from illness (e.g., infection) and increased CBT from heat stroke can have similar presentations, including neurological symptoms. The paramedic should obtain a thorough history (if available) to differentiate between the two syndromes. If unsure of the etiology, the paramedic should manage the patient for heat stroke.

Cardiovascular manifestations. A rise in skin temperature reduces the thermal gradient between the core and the skin and evokes an increase in skin blood flow (peripheral vasodilation) that results in cutaneous flushing. About 25% of exertional heat stroke cases have persistent sweating that results from increased catecholamine release, although in the classic form of heat stroke sweating usually is absent because of dehydration, drug use that impairs sweating, direct thermal injury to sweat glands, or sweat gland fatigue. Therefore the presence of sweating does not preclude the diagnosis, and cessation of sweating is not the cause of heat stroke.

Peripheral vasodilation results in decreased vascular resistance and shunting as the illness progresses. High-output cardiac failure is common, manifested by extreme tachycardia and hypotension. Cardiac output can initially be four to five times that of normal, although as temperatures continue to rise, myocardial contractility begins to decrease and patients can demonstrate an elevated central venous pressure. In any age group, the presence of hypotension and decreased cardiac output indicates a poor prognosis.

Other systemic manifestations. Other systemic manifestations associated with heat stroke include pulmonary edema (plus concomitant systemic acidosis, tachypnea, hypoxemia, and hypercapnia), myocardial dysfunction, gastrointestinal bleeding, aberrations in renal function (secondary to hypovolemia and hypoperfusion), hepatic injury, clotting disorders, and electrolyte abnormalities.

Management

Heat stroke almost invariably culminates in death if untreated. The factors most important to a successful outcome are initiation of basic life support (BLS) and advanced life support (ALS) measures, rapid recognition of the heat illness, and rapid cooling of the patient. After ensuring adequate airway, ventilatory, and circulatory support, the paramedic should manage the patient with heat stroke as follows:

1. Move the patient to a cool environment and remove all clothing. If available, use hyperthermic thermometers (e.g., rectal probes) to monitor CBT. Take and record the temperature at least every 5 minutes during the cooling process to ensure adequate rates of cooling and to avoid rebound hypothermia. Rebound hypothermia can best be avoided by stopping the cooling measures when the patient's CBT reaches about 102° F (39° C).

2. Begin cooling by fanning the patient while keeping the skin wet. The paramedic should continue lowering the body temperature by this method en route to the receiving hospital. If transportation is to be delayed, complete immersion or spraying of tepid water (60° F [16° C]) over the body surface is recommended. The paramedic should avoid ice-water submersion or cold-water cooling because these methods can precipitate shivering, frank shaking, peripheral vasoconstriction, and convulsions that will act to increase CBT as the body temperature is being lowered.

3. If hypovolemia is present, give the patient an initial fluid challenge of 500 mL over 15 minutes. In most patients the blood pressure rises to a normal range during the cooling process as large volumes of blood in the cutaneous vessels shift back to the central circulation (rapid cooling improves cardiac output directly). Be extremely cautious with fluid replacement, and closely monitor the patient for signs of fluid overload. Vigorous fluid administration can precipitate pulmonary edema, especially in older adults.

4. Administer pharmacological agents as prescribed by medical direction. Depending on the patient's status and response to cooling methods, these drugs may include ***diazepam*** (Valium) for sedation and seizure control, ***mannitol*** (Osmitrol)

TABLE 36-2	PROGRESSION OF CLINICAL SIGNS AND SYMPTOMS OF HYPOTHERMIA		
	CORE TEMPERATURE		
CLASS	**°C**	**°F**	**SIGNS AND SYMPTOMS**
Mild	36°	96.8°	Increased metabolic rate, maximum shivering, thermogenesis
	34°	93.2°	Impaired judgment, slurred speech
Moderate	30°	86.0°	Respiratory depression, myocardial irritability, bradycardia, atrial fibrillation, Osborn waves
Severe	<30°	<86.0°	Basal metabolic rate that is 50% of normal, loss of deep tendon reflexes, fixed and dilated pupils, spontaneous ventricular fibrillation

to promote renal blood flow and diuresis, and glucose to manage hypoglycemia.

Hypothermia

Hypothermia (CBT less than 95° F [35° C]) can result from a decrease in heat production, an increase in heat loss, or a combination of the two factors. Although hypothermia can result from metabolic, neurological, traumatic, toxic, and infectious causes, it most commonly is seen in cold climates and during periods of exposure to extreme environmental conditions. Failure to recognize and properly manage hypothermia can increase the rate of morbidity and mortality.

Pathophysiology

Cold exposure produces a cascade of physiological events to conserve core heat. Initially there is immediate vasoconstriction in the peripheral vessels and a simultaneous increase in sympathetic nervous discharge, catecholamine release, and basal metabolism. In addition, the blood pressure and the heart and respiratory rates increase dramatically. As cold exposure continues, preshivering muscle tone increases, and the body generates heat in the form of shivering. Shivering continues until the CBT reaches about 86° F (30° C), glucose or glycogen is depleted, or insulin is no longer available for glucose transfer. When shivering stops, cooling is rapid and there is a general decline in all physiological responses.

With continued cooling, respirations decline slowly, pulse rate and blood pressure decrease, and there are significant decreases in blood pH and commonly electrolyte imbalances. Hypovolemia can develop from a shift of fluid out of the vascular space, with increased loss of fluid through urination (cold diuresis). After early tachycardia, progressive bradycardia develops that often is refractory to *atropine.* Significant electrocardiograph (ECG) changes occur, including prolonged PR, QRS, and QT intervals; obscure or absent P waves; and ST-segment and T-wave abnormalities. In addition, the J point (Osborn wave) may be present at the junction of the QRS complex and ST segment (see Chapter 28). These events generally are followed by cardiac and respiratory arrest as the CBT approaches 68° F (20° C).

The progression of clinical signs and symptoms of hypothermia is divided into three classes based on CBT[1]: mild, moderate, and severe (Box 36-2). Characteristics of the three classes of hypothermia are listed in Table 36-2.

Those at increased risk for developing accidental hypothermia are outdoor enthusiasts (e.g., campers, hikers, hunters, and fishermen), older adults, the very young, and individuals with concurrent medical or psychiatric illness. Thermoregulatory mechanisms also can be impaired by brain damage resulting from trauma, hemorrhage, hypoxia, and CNS depression from drug overdose or intoxicants. Drugs known to impair thermoregulation include alcohol, antidepressants, antipyretics, phenothiazines, sedatives, and various pain medicines (including *aspirin,* acetaminophen, and nonsteroidal antiinflammatory drugs [NSAIDs]). Acid-base imbalances such as those that occur during ketoacidosis also can affect thermostability by decreasing heat production or increasing heat loss.

> **? CRITICAL THINKING**
>
> *What group of people is especially vulnerable to hypothermia as a result of their environmental, medical, and social situation?*

Management

The first step in managing accidental hypothermia is to maintain a high degree of suspicion for its presence. When the exposure is obvious (e.g., a victim involved in an avalanche or cold water immersion), diagnosis is simple. However, in some situations, signs and symptoms may be subtle (e.g., hunger, nausea, chills, and dizziness). When hypothermia is suspected, the paramedic's immediate action is to

---

BOX 36-2

CLASSIFICATIONS OF HYPOTHERMIA

Mild: CBT between 93.2° and 96.8° F (34° and 36° C)

Moderate: CBT between 86° and 93° F (30° and 34° C)

Severe: CBT below 86° F (30° C)

CBT, Core body temperature.

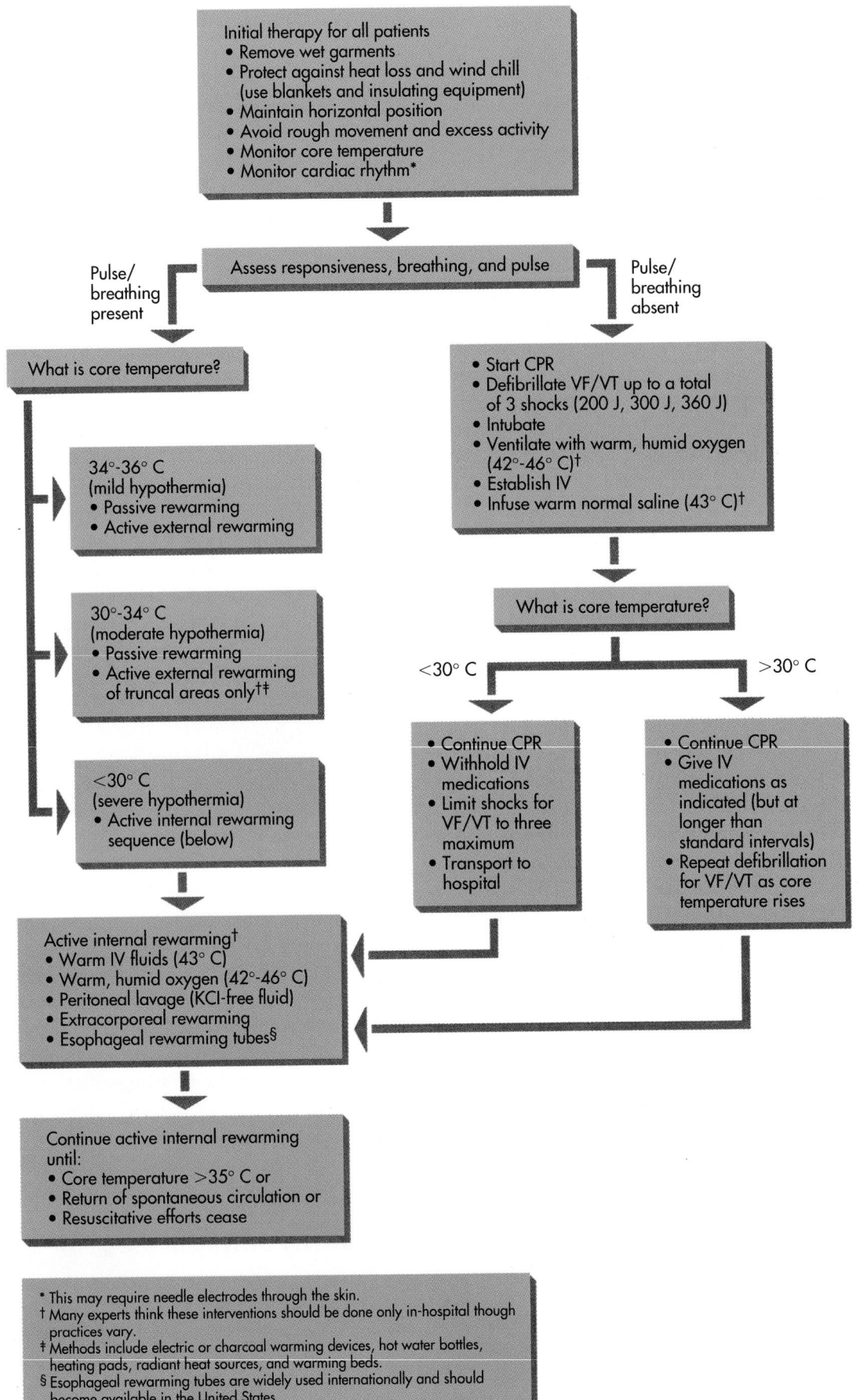

Fig. 36-1 Algorithm for the treatment of hypothermia. (Reproduced with permission, CPR Issue of *JAMA*, Oct 28, 1992;268:2199-2275. Copyright © American Medical Association.)

extricate and evacuate the patient to a site of warm shelter; expose the patient and remove cold, wet clothing; prevent a further drop in the victim's CBT; survey for traumatic injuries; cover the patient with warm blankets and increase the temperature in the ambulance; and rapidly transport the patient for definitive care. Fig. 36-1 presents a treatment algorithm for hypothermia.

> **NOTE**
>
> There often is no reliable correlation between clinical signs and symptoms and specific CBT.[2]

Mild to Moderate Hypothermia

In mild to moderate cases of hypothermia, removal of the victim from the cold environment and passive rewarming may be all that is necessary to manage the cold exposure. The paramedic can accomplish this by removing wet clothing (wet clothes allow five times as much heat loss as dry clothes) and wrapping the victim in a dry blanket to prevent further chilling and help retain endogenously produced heat. If the victim is conscious, warm drinks and sugar sources can support a gradual rise in CBT and help correct any dehydration present. The paramedic should not give the patient alcoholic beverages, which produce peripheral vasodilation and increase heat loss from the skin, and caffeine-containing beverages, which cause vasoconstriction and diuresis. These patients may be lethargic and somewhat dulled mentally but generally are oriented with no marked mental derangements.

External application of hot packs (covered with towels to avoid burns) to the neck, armpits, and groin is considered a safe and effective way to rewarm these patients. IV fluid therapy may be warranted to correct a drop in blood pressure caused by heat-stimulated peripheral vasodilation. If possible, the paramedic should administer heated, humidified oxygen. Patients with mild to moderate hypothermia generally improve rapidly with proper treatment. However, close monitoring and transportation for physician evaluation are indicated.

Moderate to Severe Hypothermia

At CBTs below 90° F (32° C), mental derangements are invariably present and include disorientation, confusion, and lethargy proceeding to stupor and coma. Patients with moderate to severe hypother-

mia usually have lost their ability to shiver, and their uncoordinated physical activity renders them unable to perform meaningful tasks.

Management of patients with moderate to severe hypothermia begins with ensuring adequate airway, ventilatory, and circulatory support and maintaining body temperature. The paramedic should not permit these patients to move about independently or physically exert themselves. Even minor physical activity can bring about dysrhythmias, including ventricular fibrillation. The paramedic should manage moderate hypothermia with external heat application (e.g., heat packs, heat guns, and heat lights); heated, humidified oxygen administration; IV fluid therapy (warmed, if possible); and rapid and gentle transportation for definitive care. Careful monitoring of the patient's mental status, ECG, and vital functions is imperative. If low-reading thermometers (e.g., tympanic membrane sensors, rectal probes) are available, the paramedic should use them to measure the patient's CBT at 5-minute intervals.

If the patient's CBT is below 82.4° F (28° C), he or she usually is unconscious. The paramedic should gently move the patient to a warm environment if vital signs are present. The paramedic should institute passive external rewarming and administer heated, humidified oxygen during transportation to a medical facility. The paramedic should begin airway management with basic manual procedures (head-tilt, chin-lift) and slow ventilatory assistance. The use of oral or nasal adjuncts, including intubation, can induce ventricular dysrhythmias, and therefore, if required, the most experienced paramedic should perform these gently. Overzealous ventilatory assistance can induce hypocapnia and resultant ventricular irritability.[1] However, when indicated the paramedic should not withhold these procedures. Medical direction may recommend the administration of *thiamine*, *dextrose 50%*, *naloxone* (Narcan), and an initial fluid challenge of 250 to 500 mL of D_5W or normal saline. The paramedic should avoid use of lactated Ringer's solution because the cold liver may not be able to metabolize the lactate.

> **NOTE**
>
> The paramedic should move patients with severe hypothermia in the horizontal position to avoid aggravating hypotension through orthostatic mechanisms.[1]

Severely hypothermic patients have no vital signs, including respiratory effort, pulse, and blood pressure. Depending on core temperature, cyanosis, fixed and dilated pupils, and stiff and rigid muscles (simulating rigor mortis) may be present. Prolonged resuscitation can be beneficial in severely hypothermic patients, and cardiopulmonary resuscitation (CPR) is indicated even if signs of death are present. Hypothermic patients cannot be presumed dead until a CBT of 94° to 95° F (34° to 35° C) has been achieved and resuscitation efforts are still unsuccessful. The paramedic should confirm a nonperfusing rhythm (VF, pulseless VT, or asystole) by ECG monitor for a minimum of 30 to 45 seconds, and he or she should institute CPR only if there are absolutely no vital signs.

> **NOTE**
>
> ET intubation is required if the hypothermic victim is unconscious or if ventilation is inadequate. The intubation will serve two purposes: (1) it will enable provision of effective ventilation with warm, humidified oxygen; and (2) it will isolate the airway to reduce the likelihood of aspiration.[4]

> **NOTE**
>
> Resuscitation in the prehospital setting may be withheld if the victim has obvious lethal injuries or if the body is frozen so completely that chest compression is impossible and the nose and mouth are blocked with ice.[3]

If the patient in cardiac arrest fails to respond to three defibrillation attempts, the paramedic should administer subsequent defibrillations or additional cardiac life support medications at extended intervals or avoid them until the patient has been rewarmed in the emergency department. These patients need to be rapidly transported to a facility that can institute internal core rewarming techniques. In patients with vital signs, the rewarming technique of choice is to place the patient on cardiopulmonary bypass (active core rewarming) to sustain perfusion and to rewarm the patient concurrently. In-hospital peritoneal and pleural lavage and esophageal rewarming techniques also have been used to successfully manage patients with profound hypothermia and cardiac arrest.

> **NOTE**
>
> The administration of medications including **epinephrine** (Adrenalin), **lidocaine** (Xylocaine), and **procainamide** (Pronestyl) can accumulate to toxic levels in the peripheral circulation if they are administered repeatedly in the severely hypothermic patient. For these reasons IV drugs often are withheld when the CBT is less than <30° C. If CBT is >30° C, IV drugs may be given, but with increased intervals between doses.[4] IV drug therapy in these patients should be guided by medical direction.

Most authorities agree that active rewarming methods other than the administration of heated, humidified oxygen are inappropriate field care for severe hypothermia.[1] Rewarming methods such as hot water immersion can cause hypotension from peripheral vasodilation (rewarming shock) and a sudden return of cold, acidotic blood and waste products to the body's core (afterdrop phenomenon). Therefore the paramedic generally should avoid active field rewarming techniques unless patient transportation is to be delayed.

Frostbite

Frostbite is a localized injury that results from environmentally induced freezing of body tissues. It frequently occurs in the lower extremities (particularly the toes and feet) and less commonly in the upper extremities (particularly the fingers and hands). Frostbite also occurs in the ears, nose, and other body areas that are unprotected from environmental extremes.

Pathophysiology

Frostbite occurs as ice crystals form in tissue, producing macrovascular and microvascular abnormalities and direct cellular injury. The freezing depth depends on the intensity and duration of cold exposure. Severe freezing can also occur in tissue exposed to volatile hydrocarbons at low temperatures.

Under most conditions of frostbite, ice crystals form in the extracellular tissue. This draws water out of the cells into the extravascular spaces, allowing the electrolyte concentration within the cell to reach toxic levels. These crystals can also expand

and cause direct mechanical destruction of tissue. This phenomenon leads to damage of blood vessels (particularly the endothelial cells), partial shrinkage and collapse of the cell membrane, loss of vascular integrity, local edema, and disruption of nutritive blood flow. Ischemia often produces the most damaging effects of frostbite.

When frozen tissue thaws, capillary patency is initially restored, but blood flow declines within minutes after thawing through vasoconstriction of arterioles and venules and the release of emboli that course through microvessels. Ultimately there is progressive tissue loss from thrombosis and hypoxia. This vascular injury damages the endothelium and results in deterioration of the microvasculature and dermal necrosis. Thawing and refreezing is more dangerous to tissue than allowing the frostbitten part to remain frozen until it can be warmed with minimal risk of refreezing. In addition to extreme temperature, wind, and humidity, predisposing factors to frostbite include the following:

- Lack of protective clothing
- Poor nutrition
- Preexisting injury or medical or psychiatric illness
- Fatigue
- Decrease in local tissue perfusion
- Tobacco use
- Atherosclerosis
- Tight, constrictive clothing
- Increase in vasodilation
- Alcohol consumption
- Medications
- History of previous cold injury

Classifications and Symptoms

There are numerous classifications for cold injury. A common classification separates cold injury into two categories: superficial frostbite (also known as frostnip) and deep frostbite. In superficial frostbite there is at least some minimal tissue loss, whereas in deep frostbite there is significant tissue loss even with appropriate therapy. Superficial frostbite usually involves the dermis and shallow subcutaneous layers, whereas deep frostbite is associated with subdermal layers and deep tissues.

The initial evaluation of severity is difficult because the injury does not always reflect underlying vascular changes. Regardless of the depth of injury, the area may appear to be frozen; palpation may distinguish between superficial and deep injury. In superficial injury the underlying tissue springs back on compression, whereas in deep injury the underlying tissue is hard and not compressible.

> **NOTE**
>
> Frozen tissue should not be massaged in an attempt to improve circulation.

Superficial Frostbite

In most patients with superficial frostbite, the initial symptoms are coldness and numbness in the affected area, followed by extreme pain (tingling and throbbing) during rewarming. After rewarming, edema usually appears within 3 hours, followed by the formation of vesicles within 3 to 24 hours (Fig. 36-2). These blisters begin to resolve within 1 week, after which the skin blackens into a hard eschar. Eventually the blackened tissue peels away (demarcation), revealing shiny, red skin beneath. This tissue is sensitive to heat and cold and, for unknown reasons, remains unusually susceptible to repeated frostbite injury.

> **NOTE**
>
> Trenchfoot (immersion foot) is similar to frostbite but occurs at temperatures above freezing. The signs and symptoms of this condition are similar to frostbite and include pain and the formation of blisters upon rewarming. The paramedic should cover the affected area with sterile dressings and keep it dry and warm.

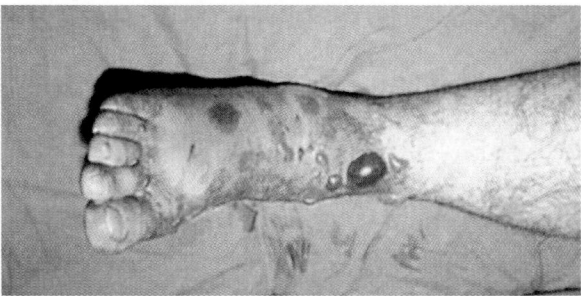

Fig. 36-2 Edema and blister formation 24 hours after frostbite injury in an area covered by a tightly fitted boot. (From Auerbach PS: *Management of wilderness and environmental emergencies*, ed 2, St Louis, 1989, Mosby.)

Deep Frostbite

In deep frostbite the disrupted nutritional capillary flow is never restored to the patient's damaged tissue. The affected area remains cold, mottled, and blue or gray after rewarming. During the first 9 to 15 days, severely frostbitten skin forms a black, hard eschar. In contrast to superficial frostbite, edema is slow to develop. Deep blisters with purple blood-containing fluid may appear within 1 to 3 weeks. Within 22 to 45 days, definite lines of demarcation between the eschar and viable tissue develop. Eventually, nonviable skin and deep structures mummify and slough (Fig. 36-3).

Management

Prehospital care for frostbite is limited to supporting the patient's vital functions, elevation and protection of the affected extremity, pain management, and rapid transportation to a medical facility. Vigorous rubbing is ineffective and potentially harmful, and partial, slow rewarming with blankets or other warm objects is injurious. If frostbite involves the client's lower extremities, the paramedic should not permit the patient to walk. During transportation, the paramedic should remove all restrictive and wet clothing from the patient and replace it with warm, dry clothing and blankets to guard against hypothermia. The paramedic should prohibit the patient from consuming alcohol and smoking tobacco. Rapid rewarming of the frozen part by immersion in hot water (104° F [40° C] maximum) is the most effective therapeutic measure for preserving viable tissue. The paramedic should not attempt this method of rewarming in the prehospital setting because of the risk of refreezing.

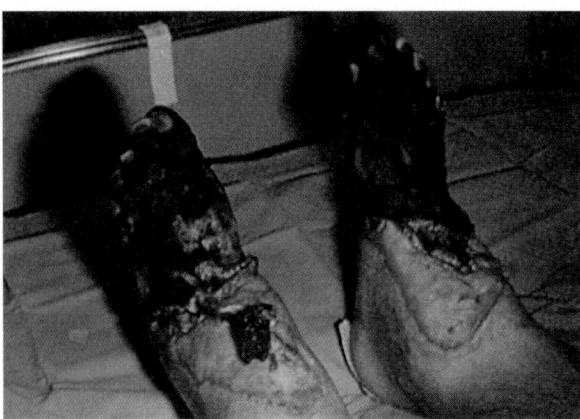

Fig. 36-3 Gangrenous necrosis 6 weeks after a frostbite injury. (From Auerbach PS: *Management of wilderness and environmental emergencies*, ed 2, St Louis, 1989, Mosby.)

Submersion

Drowning was the fourth leading cause of accidental death in the United States in 1996, accounting for more than 2500 deaths. In addition, there are about 80,000 submersion incidents reported each year. Of these, 85% of victims are male, and two thirds of the victims are nonswimmers.[6]

Classifications

There are numerous classifications of submersion incidents. This text defines **submersion** as an incident in which a person experiences some swimming-related distress that is sufficient to require support in the prehospital setting and transportation to a medical facility for further observation and treatment. **Drowning** is defined as a "mortal" event in which a submersion victim is pronounced dead at the scene of the attempted resuscitation, or within 24 hours after arrival in the emergency department (ED) or hospital. If death occurs after 24 hours, it is considered a *drowning-related death*.[5] Victims of submersion incidents usually fall into one of two categories:

1. Conscious patients, such as nonswimmers, exhausted swimmers, river canoeists who become trapped by roots or strong currents, persons who have fallen overboard or off a dock, and motor vehicle crash victims trapped in submerged vehicles
2. Unconscious patients, such as those who have suffered a stroke or cardiac arrest while swimming and those who have fallen into water and succumbed to hypothermia

Pathophysiology

Drowning begins with intentional or accidental submersion. After submersion, the victim realizes that a drowning may ensue (e.g., a nonswimmer who panics or a swimmer who tires). The sequence of events that leads to drowning begins with the conscious victim taking in several deep breaths in an attempt to store oxygen before breath-holding (Fig. 36-4). The victim holds the breath until reflex inspiratory efforts override the breath-holding effort. As water is aspirated, laryngospasm occurs. Laryngospasm and aspiration produce severe hypoxia. The resultant profound hypoxemia and acidosis lead to cardiac dysrhythmias and CNS anoxia. In 15% of drownings, the laryngospasm is severe enough that very little fluid is aspirated ("dry drowning"); in the remaining 85% of drownings, fluid enters the lungs ("wet drowning"). The physiological events that follow are partially determined by the type and amount of water aspirated. Regardless of the type of water aspirated, the pathophysiology of drowning is characterized by hypoxia, hypercapnia, and acidosis, which result in cardiac arrest.

> **NOTE**
>
> The duration of hypoxia is the critical factor in determining the victim's outcome.[5]

> **? CRITICAL THINKING**
>
> **Do other swimmers or onlookers often "hear" a person who is drowning?**

Drowning can occur in almost any type of water. Victims of submersion aspirate salt water or fresh water, tap water, or contaminated water (such as water containing sewage, chemicals, algae, bacteria, or sand). Although there are theoretical differences between the effects of different submersion fluids, they are not clinically significant and should not be considered in the initial management of submersion incidents. The single most important factor is the duration of submersion and the duration and severity of hypoxia.[5]

Pulmonary Pathophysiology Secondary to Near Drowning

Respiratory failure and ischemic neurological injury from hypoxia and acidosis are the life-threatening complications of submersion. Hypoxia can result from the following factors:

- Fluid in the alveoli and interstitial spaces
- Loss of surfactant
- Contaminant particles in the alveoli and tracheobronchial tree
- Damage to the alveolar-capillary membrane and vascular endothelium

Poor perfusion and hypoxemia lead to metabolic acidosis in most patients. In those who survive the incident, acute respiratory failure (including adult respiratory distress syndrome [ARDS]) may follow, with a reduction in compliance and an increase in ventilation-perfusion mismatching and intrapulmonary shunting. The onset of symptoms can be delayed for as long as 24 hours after the submersion.

In addition to having pulmonary effects, submersion can affect other body systems. For example, cardiovascular derangements can occur secondary to hypoxia and acidosis, resulting in dysrhythmias and decreased cardiac output. CNS dysfunction and neuronal damage commonly are caused by cerebral edema and anoxia. The paramedic also must be suspicious of concurrent spinal injury in submersion victims. Renal dysfunction is unusual but can progress to acute renal failure as a result of hypoxic injury or hemoglobinuria, leading to acute tubular necrosis.

Factors that Affect Clinical Outcome

The following four factors can affect clinical outcome after a submersion incident:

1. *Temperature of the water*: Submersion in cold water can have beneficial and deleterious effects on survival. The rapid development of hypothermia can

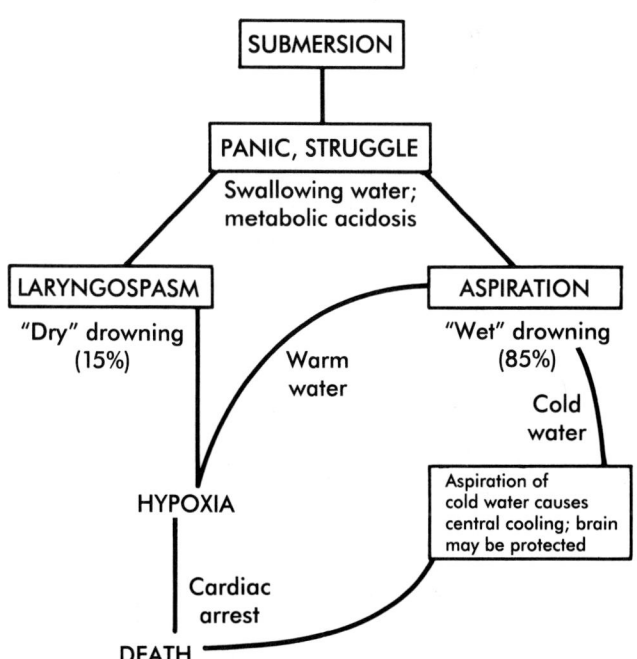

Fig. 36-4 Progression of the drowning incident. (From Auerbach PS: *Management of wilderness and environmental emergencies,* ed 2, St Louis, 1989, Mosby.)

serve a protective function, particularly regarding brain viability in patients with prolonged submersion. The survival of a child submerged for 66 minutes in a creek with a water temperature of 37° F (5° C) is the longest documented submersion with good neurological outcome.[7] The exact mechanism of this phenomenon is not understood; in the past it was attributed to a "mammalian diving reflex" found in seals and lower mammals. Hypothermia, which may be organ protective, also contributes to neurological recovery after prolonged submersion, probably by decreasing the metabolic needs of the brain. The relative contributions of these two mechanisms are not clear. The adverse effects of cold-water submersion include severe ventricular dysrhythmias.

> **NOTE**
>
> Hypothermia also may develop as a secondary complication of the submersion and subsequent heat loss through evaporation during attempted resuscitation. In these circumstances, the hypothermia is not protective.

2. *Duration of submersion*: The longer the duration of submersion, the less likely the patient is to survive. When rescue operations have been in progress for more than 30 minutes, victims retrieved from warm water in summer months or in warm southern waters usually are considered nonviable. Because cold-water submersion for up to 60 minutes has been associated with neurological recovery, most patients rescued from cold-water drowning should receive resuscitative life-support measures. Resuscitation is indicated unless there is physical evidence of death (e.g., putrefaction, dependent lividity, and rigor mortis).[1]

> **NOTE**
>
> Submersion victims who have spontaneous circulation and breathing when they reach the hospital usually recover with good outcomes.[5]

3. *Cleanliness of the water*. Contaminants in water have an irritant effect on the pulmonary system, leading to bronchospasm and an increased tendency toward poor gas exchange. They also can cause a secondary pulmonary infection with delayed severe respiratory compromise.

4. *Age of the victim*. The younger the patient or victim, the better the chance for survival.

Management

Safety at the scene and of the EMS crew are of paramount importance at the site of a submersion incident, and only personnel trained in water rescue should attempt emergency intervention (see Chapter 50). Depending on the type and duration of submersion, patients may vary from an asymptomatic presentation to cardiac arrest. After gaining access to the victim, the paramedic should take spinal precautions while the victim is still in the water (see Chapter 23) and initiate rescue breathing (if needed) as soon as possible. The use of subdiaphragmatic thrusts to remove water from the airways is controversial and generally is not recommended unless foreign body airway obstruction is suspected.[1] (Chest thrusts can be used as an alternative to the Heimlich maneuver.)

After extrication from the water, the paramedic should evaluate the patient to ensure an adequate airway and provide ventilatory and circulatory support as needed. Other forms of initial patient care management include high-concentration oxygen administration, ECG monitoring, and establishment of an IV line. The paramedic should manage patients who are in cardiac arrest with standard BLS and ALS protocols and rapid transportation to the receiving hospital.

Victims of submersion incidents often are at risk from immersion hypothermia; heat loss in water can be up to 32 times greater than in air. Hypothermia can make resuscitation more difficult and requires special consideration with reference to gentle handling, use of pharmacological agents, and defibrillation. As with all other hypothermic patients, the paramedic should remove wet clothing and dry and wrap the patient in blankets to maintain body heat. The paramedic should consider external warming and the administration of heated, humidified oxygen at the scene and during transportation. The paramedic should manage all patients with suspected hypothermia as described previously and outlined in Fig. 36-1.

Asymptomatic patients also require transportation for physician evaluation. The paramedic should supply these patients with oxygen and carefully monitor them to guard against aspiration pneumonia and undetected hypoxia that can result from the submersion incident. Oxygen is the most important treatment required by submersion victims.

Diving Emergencies

There are more than 4 million recreational scuba divers in the United States, and over 400,000 new sport divers are certified each year.[8] The medical emergencies unique to pressure-related diving include those caused by the mechanical effects of pressure (barotrauma), air embolism, and breathing compressed air (**decompression sickness** and **nitrogen narcosis**).

> **NOTE**
>
> *Scuba* (self-contained underwater breathing apparatus) is equipment worn by divers for breathing underwater. Scuba gear typically consists of one or two compressed air tanks strapped to the back of the diver and connected by a hose to a mouthpiece.

Mechanical Effects of Pressure

When a scuba diver submerges under water, the ambient pressure to which the diver is exposed increases because of the weight of the water. Water is much denser than air, so pressure changes are greater under water, even at reasonably shallow depths. Since body tissues are composed mostly of water, which is not compressible, they are not directly affected by pressure changes. However, gases are compressible, and gas-filled organs of the body are directly affected by pressure changes.

> **NOTE**
>
> Every 33 feet of water adds 1 atmosphere (14 pounds per square inch). Therefore at the depth of 33 feet, there is a pressure of 2 atmospheres—1 from the air and 1 from the 33 feet of water.

Basic Properties of Gases

The laws pertaining to the basic properties of gas responsible for all pressure-related diving emer-

gencies and some high-altitude illnesses are Boyle's law, Dalton's law, and Henry's law. The following properties of gas help the paramedic understand these laws: increased pressure dissolves gases into blood; oxygen metabolizes and nitrogen dissolves.

> **NOTE**
>
> The fact that gas expands with an increase in altitude applies to increases in altitude that occur during air transportation. For example, the patient can experience expansion of gas in the respiratory system, gastrointestinal system, or sinuses. Medical equipment (e.g., endotracheal [ET] tube cuffs and the pneumatic antishock garment [PASG]) also can be affected by an increased volume of air.

Boyle's law states that, at a constant temperature, the volume of gas is inversely related to its pressure. This is expressed by $PV = K$, where P is pressure, V is volume, and K is a constant. Thus when the pressure is doubled, the volume of gas is halved, and vice versa. This principle is the basic mechanism for all types of barotrauma: gas volume expands as pressure decreases.

Dalton's law states that the pressure exerted by each gas in a mixture of gases is the same as it would exert if it alone occupied the same volume. Alternatively, the total pressure of a mixture of gases equals the sum of the partial pressures of the component gases. This law is expressed by the equation $Pt = P_{O_2} + P_{N_2} + Px$ where Pt is the total pressure, P_{O_2} is the partial pressure of oxygen, P_{N_2} is the partial pressure of nitrogen, and Px is the partial pressure of the remaining gases in the mixture. The principles of this law explain problems caused by breathing compressed air: gas expansion causes the partial pressure of oxygen to drop as gas molecules move farther apart, decreasing available oxygen.

Henry's law states that, at a constant temperature, the solubility of a gas in a liquid solution is proportionate to the partial pressure of the gas. The law is expressed by the equation $\%X = Px/Pt \times 100$, where $\%X$ is the amount of gas dissolved in a liquid, Px is the partial pressure of gas x, and Pt is the total atmospheric pressure. This law explains why more nitrogen, which makes up almost 80% of air, dissolves in the diver's body as ambient pressure increases with descent. This dissolved nitrogen is then released from tissues on ascent as pressure decreases.

Barotrauma

Barotrauma is tissue damage that results from compression or expansion of gas spaces when the gas pressure in the body or its compartments differs from ambient pressure. The type of barotrauma depends on whether the diver is in descent or ascent. Barotrauma is the most common affliction of scuba divers.

Barotrauma of Descent

Barotrauma of descent (also known as *squeeze*) results from the compression of gas in enclosed spaces as the ambient pressure increases with descent under water. Air trapped in noncollapsible chambers is compressed, leading to a vacuum-type effect that results in severe, sharp pain caused by the distortion; vascular engorgement; edema; and hemorrhage of the exposed tissue (Box 36-3). As a rule, squeeze usually results from a blocked eustachian tube or from failure of the diver to clear (open) the eustachian tube with exhalation during descent. The ears and paranasal sinuses are most likely to be affected. Squeeze occurs in the ears, sinuses, lungs and airways, gastrointestinal tract, thorax, teeth (pulp decay, recent extraction sockets or fillings), or added air spaces (face mask or diving suit).

Management of barotrauma of descent begins with the diver performing a gradual ascent to shallower depths. Prehospital care largely is supportive. After physician evaluation, definitive care may include bed rest with the head elevated, avoidance of strain and strenuous activity, use of decongestants and possibly antihistamines and antibiotics, and perhaps surgical repair.

? CRITICAL THINKING

What preexisting illness can make a diver more susceptible to squeeze?

Barotrauma of Ascent

Barotrauma of ascent occurs through the reverse process of descent ("reverse squeeze"). Assuming that the air-filled cavities of the body have equalized pressure during the diver's descent, the volume of air trapped in this pressurized space expands as ambient pressure decreases with ascent (Boyle's law). If air is not allowed to escape because of obstruction (e.g., breath-holding, bronchospasm, or mucus plug), the expanding gases distend the tissues surrounding them. The most common cause of this type of barotrauma is breath-holding during ascent because of running out of air at depth or of panic.

NOTE

The compressed gas at 33 feet (2 atmospheres) doubles in volume when the diver moves to the surface (1 atmosphere) because the pressure is half of 33 feet. The last 6 feet of ascent have the greatest potential for volume expansion and is considered the most dangerous depth.

Although problems from reverse squeeze are rare, pulmonary overpressurization syndrome (POPS) resulting from expansion of trapped air in the lungs occurs. POPS can lead to alveolar rupture and extravasation of air into extraalveolar locations (see Box 36-3). The clinical syndromes associated with barotrauma of ascent include pneumomediastinum, subcutaneous emphysema, pneumopericardium, pneumothorax, pneumoperitoneum, and systemic arterial air embolism. Except for tension pneumothorax (a rare complication that may require needle or tube decompression) and air embolism that may require hyperbaric recompression therapy, POPS usually requires only oxygen administration, observation, and transportation for physician evaluation.

Air Embolism

Air embolism is the most serious complication of pulmonary barotrauma and is a major cause of death and disability among sport divers. Divers risk this injury when they ascend too rapidly or when they hold their breath during ascent.

Air embolism results as the expanding air disrupts tissues and air is forced into the circulatory system. The air bubbles pass through the left side of the heart and become lodged in small arterioles, occluding distal circulation. The syndrome usually presents as the diver surfaces and exhales, releasing the high intrapulmonic pressure that resulted from lung overexpansion. With the decrease in intrathoracic pressure, bubbles advance into the left side of

NOTE

The most common presentation of air embolism is similar to that of stroke and includes vertigo, confusion, loss of consciousness, visual disturbances, and focal neurological deficits.

the heart and enter the systemic arterial supply, resulting in a dramatic presentation, with clinical manifestations that depend on the site of systemic arterial occlusion (see Box 36-3).

The paramedic should suspect air embolism when a diver suddenly loses consciousness immediately after surfacing. The paramedic should institute BLS and ALS measures and rapidly transport the patient for recompression treatment. If endotracheal intubation is necessary, the paramedic should fill the balloon with normal saline, not air, to avoid inadvertent extubation during recompression. In addition, the paramedic should thoroughly evaluate the patient for signs of POPS, such as a pneumothorax.

The paramedic should transport the patient with a suspected air embolism in a left lateral recumbent position with a 15-degree elevation of the thorax if not contraindicated by injury. Some medical direction agencies recommend that the paramedic transport the patient in a supine position to avoid aggravating cerebral edema that may develop. (The paramedic should always follow local protocol.) If air trans-portation is to be used, the paramedic should transport the diver by aircraft pressurized to sea level or by rotary wing aircraft that fly at low altitude so that existing intraarterial air bubbles do not expand further. The flight altitude must be as low as possible (ideally never over 1000 feet above sea level) if internal cabin pressure cannot be maintained at sea level.

Recompression

Management of the patient with an air embolism consists of rapidly increasing ambient pressure (recompression) in a hyperbaric chamber. Hyperbaric chambers allow for the administration of oxygen at a greater-than-normal atmospheric pressure. The technique is used to overcome the natural limit of oxygen solubility in blood, thereby reducing

? CRITICAL THINKING

Where is the nearest hyperbaric chamber in your area?

BOX 36-3

SIGNS AND SYMPTOMS OF DIVING-RELATED CONDITIONS

Squeeze
Pain
Sensation of fullness
Headache
Disorientation
Vertigo
Nausea
Bleeding from the nose or ears

POPS
Gradually increasing chest pain
Hoarseness
Neck fullness
Dyspnea
Dysphagia
Subcutaneous emphysema

Air Embolism
Focal paralysis or sensory changes (strokelike symptoms)
Aphasia
Confusion
Blindness or other visual disturbances
Convulsions
Loss of consciousness

Dizziness
Vertigo
Abdominal pain
Cardiac arrest

Decompression Sickness
Shortness of breath
Itch
Rash
Joint pain
Crepitus
Fatigue
Vertigo
Paresthesias
Paralysis
Seizures
Unconsciousness

Nitrogen Narcosis
Impaired judgment
Sensation of alcohol intoxication
Slowed motor response
Loss of proprioception
Euphoria

intravascular bubble volume and restoring tissue perfusion. Slow decompression is calculated to avoid the re-formation of bubbles. The paramedic should be familiar with the location of the nearest hyperbaric treatment facility and follow protocol established by medical direction.

Decompression Sickness

Decompression sickness is also known as the *bends, dysbarism, caisson disease,* and *diver's paralysis.* It is a multisystem disorder that results when nitrogen in compressed air (dissolved into tissues and blood from the increase in its partial pressure at depth) converts back from solution to gas, forming bubbles in the tissues and blood. The syndrome occurs when the ambient pressure decreases (Henry's law) and results from an ascent that is too rapid, in which equilibrium between the dissolved nitrogen in tissue and blood and the partial pressure of nitrogen in the inspired gas cannot be established.

The most significant mechanical effect of bubbles is vascular occlusion that impairs arterial venous flow. Since the bubbles can form in any tissue, lymphedema (the accumulation of lymph in soft tissues), cellular distention, and cellular rupture also can occur (see Box 36-3). The net effect of all these processes is poor tissue perfusion and ischemia. The joints and the spinal cord are the anatomic areas most often affected.

The paramedic should suspect decompression sickness in any patient who has symptoms within 12 to 36 hours after a scuba dive that cannot adequately be explained by other conditions. An example is a patient with unexplained joint pain who had been diving within the previous 24 hours. Prehospital care includes support of vital functions, high-concentration oxygen administration, fluid resuscitation, and rapid transportation for recompression. The paramedic should use the patient transporta-

tion and air evacuation guidelines described for air embolism when caring for these patients.

Nitrogen Narcosis

Nitrogen narcosis ("rapture of the deep") is a condition in which nitrogen becomes dissolved in solution as a result of a greater-than-normal partial pressure of nitrogen. Dissolved nitrogen crosses the blood-brain barrier and produces neurodepressant effects similar to those of alcohol. This can significantly impair the diver's discrimination, leading to potentially lethal errors in judgment (see Box 36-3). Symptoms of nitrogen narcosis usually become evident at depths between 75 and 100 feet. At depths over 300 feet with standard air (oxygen-nitrogen mixture), unconsciousness ensues. Nitrogen narcosis affects all divers but is better tolerated by experienced divers. Helium-oxygen mixtures are used to improve the nitrogen complication for deep dives.

The narcotic effects of nitrogen are reversed with ascent. The syndrome is a common precipitating factor in diving incidents and may be responsible for memory loss. Prehospital care primarily is supportive. The paramedic should assess the patient for injuries that may have occurred during the diving episode and transport the patient for physician evaluation.

High-Altitude Illness

High-altitude illness principally occurs at altitudes of 8000 feet or more above sea level[2] and is attributed directly to exposure to reduced atmospheric pressure (described previously), resulting in hypobaric hypoxia. Activities associated with these syndromes include mountain climbing, aircraft or glider flight, and use of hot-air balloons and low-pressure or vacuum chambers.

The high-altitude syndromes discussed in this chapter are **acute mountain sickness** (AMS), **high-altitude pulmonary edema** (HAPE), and **high-altitude cerebral edema** (HACE). Emergency care for all forms of high-altitude illness includes airway, ventilatory, and circulatory support and descent to a lower altitude. In addition, a physician should evaluate all patients with high-altitude illness. Strategies for preventing high-altitude illness include the following:

- Gradual ascent (days)
- Limited exertion

NOTE

Exposure to high altitude can exacerbate chronic medical conditions, even without induced altitude sickness. Examples include angina pectoris, congestive heart failure (CHF), chronic obstructive pulmonary disease (COPD), and hypertension. These medical conditions occur as a result of low partial pressure of oxygen; therefore less oxygen is inhaled with each normal respiratory volume.

HYPERBARIC OXYGEN THERAPY

Manipulating the surrounding air pressure for medicinal purposes is a practice that dates back to the seventeenth century when "fevers and inflammations" were treated in crude chambers that were pressurized using hand bellows. Today, hyperbaric oxygen therapy (HBOT) is carried out in single-person (monoplace) chambers or in larger multiplace chambers that can accommodate several patients together with attending hyperbaric health care workers. HBOT has proven to be effective in the treatment of a wide variety of medical disorders that include air embolism and decompression sickness; carbon monoxide poisoning and smoke inhalation; carbon monoxide poisoning complicated by cyanide poisoning; clostridial myonecrosis (gas gangrene); crush injury, compartment syndrome, and other acute traumatic ischemias; intracranial abscesses; thermal burns; and enhancement of healing in selected problem wounds.

- Decreased sleeping at altitude
- High carbohydrate diet
- Medications (all are controversial)
- Acetazolamide (to speed acclimatization and decrease incidence of AMS)
- Nifedipine (Procardia; used solely by those with a history of HAPE to prevent recurrence upon ascent)
- Steroids

Acute Mountain Sickness

AMS is a common high-altitude illness that results from rapid ascent of an unacclimatized person to high altitudes. The illness in susceptible individuals usually develops within 4 to 6 hours of reaching high altitude, attains maximal severity within 24 to 48 hours, and abates on the third or fourth day after exposure with gradual acclimatization (Box 36-4).

Physical findings are variable and include tachycardia, bradycardia, postural hypotension, and ataxia (an impaired ability to coordinate movement). Ataxia is the most useful sign for recognizing the progression of the illness. As AMS becomes severe, the victim may experience alterations in consciousness, disorientation, and impaired judgment. Coma may ensue within 24 hours after onset of ataxia. Emergency care includes oxygen administration and descent to as low an altitude as necessary to achieve relief. Definitive treatment after physician evaluation may involve the use of diuretics to treat fluid retention associated with AMS, steroids to reduce associated cerebral edema, and hyperbaric therapy.

High-Altitude Pulmonary Edema

HAPE is caused at least in part by increased pulmonary artery pressure that develops in response to hypoxia. The increased pressure results in the release of leukotrienes, which increase pulmonary arteriolar permeability, and in leakage of fluid into extravascular locations. Initial symptoms of HAPE usually begin 24 to 72 hours after exposure to high altitudes and often are preceded by strenuous exercise (see Box 36-4).

Physical findings in patients include hyperpnea, crackles, rhonchi, tachycardia, and cyanosis. Emergency care includes oxygen administration to increase arterial oxygenation and reduce pulmonary artery pressure and descent to lower altitude. After

SIGNS AND SYMPTOMS OF HIGH-ALTITUDE ILLNESS

AMS

Headache (most common symptom) attributed to subacute cerebral edema or to spasm or dilation of cerebral blood vessels secondary to hypocapnia or hypoxia

Malaise

Anorexia

Vomiting

Dizziness

Irritability

Impaired memory

Dyspnea on exertion

HAPE

Shortness of breath

Dyspnea

Cough (with or without frothy sputum)

Generalized weakness

Lethargy

Disorientation

HACE

Headache

Ataxia

Altered consciousness

Confusion

Hallucinations

Drowsiness

Stupor

Coma

NOTE

Portable hyperbaric chambers (e.g., the Gamow Bag and Gamow Tent) are commercially available to reverse the effects of high-altitude pulmonary and cerebral edema and are used by some EMS systems located in high-risk areas.

physician evaluation, the patient may be hospitalized for observation.

High-Altitude Cerebral Edema

HACE is the most severe form of acute high-altitude illness. It is characterized by a progression of global cerebral signs in the presence of AMS that probably are related to increased intracranial pressure from cerebral edema and swelling. Therefore the distinctions between AMS and HACE are inherently blurred. The progression from mild AMS to unconsciousness associated with HACE can be as fast as 12 hours but usually requires 1 to 3 days of exposure to high altitudes (see Box 36-4).

Management of HACE must be prompt because the syndrome rapidly progresses to stupor, coma, and death without treatment. Like other forms of high-altitude illness, emergency care is focused on airway, ventilatory, and circulatory support and descent to a lower altitude.

SUMMARY

- Body temperature is regulated by a thermoregulatory center in the posterior hypothalamus. The body temperature can be increased or decreased in two ways: through regulation of heat production (thermogenesis) and regulation of heat loss (thermolysis).

- Heat illness results from one of two basic causes: (1) the normal thermoregulatory mechanisms are overwhelmed by environmental conditions such as heat stress or, more commonly, by excessive exercise in moderate to extreme environmental conditions; and (2) failure of the thermoregulatory mechanism, as in older adults or ill or debilitated patients. Heat cramps are brief, intermittent, and often severe muscular cramps that occur in muscles fatigued by heavy work or exercise. Heat exhaustion is characterized by minor aberrations in mental status, dizziness, nausea, headache, and mild to moderate core body temperature (CBT) elevation (less than 103° F [39° C]). Heat stroke occurs when the thermoregulatory mechanisms break down entirely. This failure results in body temperature elevated to 105.8° F (41° C) or higher, producing multisystem tissue damage and physiological collapse.

- Hypothermia (CBT less than 95° F [35° C]) can result from a decrease in heat production, an increase in heat loss, or a combination of the two factors. The progression of clinical signs and symptoms of hypothermia is divided into three classes based on CBT: mild (CBT between 93.2° and 96.8° F [34° and 36° C]), moderate (CBT between 86° and 93° F [30° and 34° C]), and severe (CBT below 86° F [30° C]). Severely hypothermic patients have no vital signs, including respiratory effort, pulse, and blood pressure.

- Frostbite is a localized injury that results from environmentally induced freezing of body tissues, which leads to damage of blood vessels. Ischemia often produces the most damaging effects of frostbite. In deep frostbite this can include mummification and sloughing of nonviable skin and deep structures.

- Drowning is a mortal event in which a submersion victim is pronounced dead at the scene of the attempted resuscitation, or within 24 hours after arrival in the emergency department (ED) or hospital. Near drowning is submersion with at least temporary survival. Regardless of the type of water aspirated, the pathophysiology of drowning is characterized by hypoxia, hypercapnia, and acidosis, which result in cardiac arrest.

- The laws pertaining to the basic properties of gas responsible for all pressure-related diving emergencies are Boyle's law, Dalton's law, and Henry's law. Increased pressure dissolves gases into blood; oxygen metabolizes and nitrogen dissolves.

- Barotrauma is tissue damage that results from compression or expansion of gas spaces when the gas pressure in the body differs from ambient pressure. The type of barotrauma depends on whether the diver is in descent or ascent. Air embolism is the most serious complication of pulmonary barotrauma and is a major cause of death and disability among sport divers.

- High-altitude illness is attributed directly to exposure to reduced atmospheric pressure resulting in hypobaric hypoxia. Forms of high-altitude illness include acute mountain sickness, high-altitude pulmonary edema, and high-altitude cerebral edema.

■ REFERENCES

1. American Heart Association: *Advanced cardiac life support*, Dallas, 1997, The Association.
2. U.S. Department of Transportation, National Highway Traffic Safety Administration: *EMT-Paramedic national standard curriculum*, Washington, DC, 1998, The Department.
3. American Heart Association: Guidelines 2000 for cardiopulmonary resuscitation and emergency cardiovascular care, International Consensus on Science, *Circulation* 102(8):232, 2000.
4. American Heart Association: Guidelines 2000 for cardiopulmonary resuscitation and emergency cardiovascular care, International Consensus on Science, *Circulation* 102(8):231, 2000.
5. American Heart Association: Guidelines 2000 for cardiopulmonary resuscitation and emergency cardiovascular care, International Consensus on Science, *Circulation* 102(8):233, 2000
6. National Safety Council: *Injury facts*, Itasca, Ill, 1999, The Council.
7. Callaham M: *Current practice of emergency medicine*, ed 2, Philadelphia, 1991, BC Decker.
8. Auerbach PS: *Wilderness medicine*, ed 3, St Louis, 1995, Mosby.

37 Infectious and Communicable Diseases

OBJECTIVES

Upon completion of this chapter, the paramedic student will be able to:

1. Identify general public health principles relative to infectious diseases.

2. Describe the chain of elements necessary for an infectious disease to occur.

3. Explain how internal and external barriers affect susceptibility to infection.

4. Distinguish among the four stages of infectious disease: the latent period, the incubation period, the communicability period, and the disease period.

5. Describe the mode of transmission, pathophysiology, prehospital considerations, and personal protective measures to be taken for HIV, hepatitis, tuberculosis, meningococcal meningitis, and pneumonia.

6. Describe the mode of transmission, pathophysiology, signs and symptoms, and prehospital considerations for patients who have rabies or tetanus.

7. List the signs, symptoms, and potential secondary complications of selected childhood viral diseases.

8. List the signs, symptoms, and potential secondary complications of influenza and mononucleosis.

9. Describe the mode of transmission, pathophysiology, prehospital considerations, and personal protective measures for sexually transmitted diseases.

10. Identify signs and symptoms and prehospital considerations related to lice and scabies.

11. Outline the reporting process for exposure to infectious or communicable diseases.

12. Discuss the paramedic's role in preventing disease transmission.

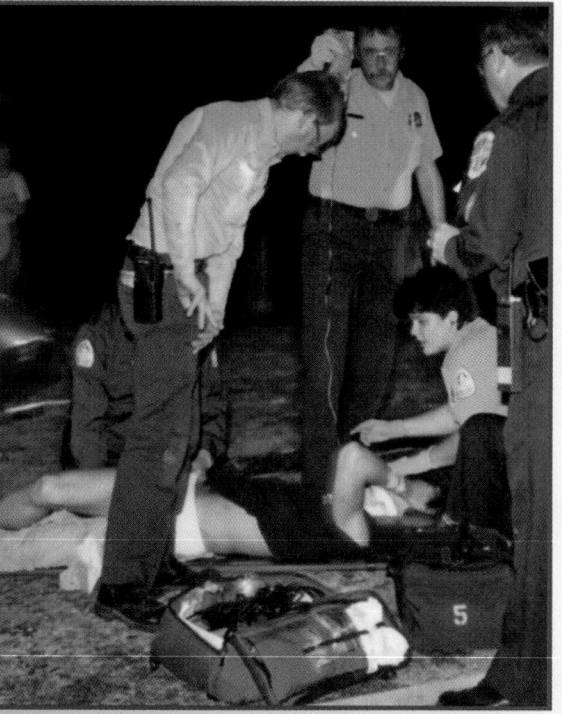

Emergencies involving infectious and communicable diseases are common in the prehospital setting and can pose a significant health risk to EMS providers. This chapter addresses the responsibilities of the paramedic and EMS agencies to ensure personal protection, the pathophysiology of infectious and communicable disease, and special aspects of providing care.

KEY TERMS

communicability period: A stage of infection that begins when the latent period ends and continues as long as the agent is present and can spread to other hosts.

disease period: A stage of infection that follows the incubation period; the duration of which varies with the disease.

incubation period: A stage of infection during which an organism reproduces and which begins with invasion of an agent and ends when the disease process begins.

latent period: A stage of infection that begins with the pathogenic invasion of the body and ends when the agent can be shed or communicated.

> **NOTE**
>
> An *infectious disease* refers to any illness that is caused by a specific microorganism. *Communicable disease* is an infectious disease that can be transmitted from one person to another.

Public Health Principles Relative to Infectious Diseases

Infectious (communicable) diseases affect entire populations of humans. Therefore the paramedic must consider the demographic characteristics of the population (e.g., location, age, socioeconomic considerations) and the relationships between populations when considering the dynamics of infectious diseases (see the box on p. 1102). In addition, populations display varying susceptibilities to infection, and conversely, varying degrees of susceptibility. Factors that affect the life cycle of an infectious agent include the following:

- Demographics of the host
- Population and their ability to move internationally
- Age distributions
- Socioeconomic considerations
- Population settling and migration dictated by religion

- Genetic factors
- Efficacy of therapeutic interventions once infection has been established

> **NOTE**
>
> A disease cluster is a discrete population that is infected in a defined span of time in defined geographical areas. Although it is usually regional, a disease cluster may lead to an international infection.

When dealing with infectious disease, paramedics should consider the needs of the patient, and the potential consequences of the disease on public health and on their person-to-person contacts with family members and friends. When a disease "outbreak" occurs, local, state, private, and federal health agencies and organizations become involved in prevention and management (Box 37-1).

> **? CRITICAL THINKING**
>
> *Have you had an "outbreak" of a communicable disease in your region? How was it controlled?*

Agency Responsibility Relative to Infectious Agent Exposure

National concerns regarding communicable disease and infection control have resulted in public law, guidelines, standards, and recommendations to protect health care providers and emergency responders from infectious diseases. The components of a health care agency Exposure Control Plan include[1]:

- Health maintenance and surveillance
- Appointing a Designated Officer (DO) to serve as a liaison between the agency and community health agencies involved in monitoring and responding to communicable diseases

THE EMERGENCE OF AIDS–AN OUTBREAK OF DISEASE

The presence of HIV is suggested to have been identified as early as 1959 in Zaire. The virus, however, did not become epidemic until 20 to 30 years later. The outbreak may have resulted from the migration of poor and young sexually active individuals from rural areas to urban centers in developing countries, with subsequent return migration and, internationally, because of civil wars, tourism, business travel, and drug trade.

AIDS was first identified in the United States in 1981 when young, previously healthy homosexual men in New York and California were found to have an unusual clustering of rare diseases (most notably Kaposi's sarcoma, *Pneumocystis carinii* pneumonia, and unexplained persistent lymphadenopathy). (Retrospective sera examination for antibodies to HIV sug-

gests that the virus entered the U.S. population in the late 1970s.) Between June 1981 and December 1998, more than 688,000 cases of AIDS had been reported to the CDC.* It is estimated that between 650,000 and 900,000 people are living with HIV in the United States. Based on estimates from the United Nations AIDS program (UN-AIDS), approximately 47 million people worldwide have been infected with HIV since the start of the global epidemic. Through December 1998, an estimated 14 million children and adults died from the disease, and more than 33 million people are living with HIV infection or AIDS. UNAIDS also estimates 5.8 million new HIV infections occurred in 1998, representing almost 16,000 new cases per day. Worldwide, an estimated 2.5 million adults and children died of HIV/AIDS in 1998.

*Source: *HIV/AIDS Surveillance Report, UNAIDS AIDS Epidemic Update: December 1998.* Centers for Disease Control and Prevention, Atlanta, http://www.cdc.gov/hiv/pubs

• Identification of job classifications, and in some cases, specific tasks where possibility exists for exposure to bloodborne pathogens
• A schedule detailing when and how the provisions of bloodborne pathogen standards will be implemented
• Personal protective equipment (PPE)
• Body substance isolation (BSI)
• Procedures for evaluating exposure and postexposure counseling (e.g., the Ryan White Act)
• Interfacing with and notifying local health authorities and state and federal agencies
• Personal, building, vehicular, equipment disinfection and storage
• Education of employees regarding disinfection agents
• After-action analysis of agency response
• Correct disposal of needles and sharps in appropriate containers
• Correct handling of body fluid-tinged linens and supplies used in patient care
• Identification of agency and/or contracted personnel for counseling, authorization of acute medical care, and documentation

Guidelines, Recommendations, Standards, and Laws

To protect against infection, OSHA requires that PPE be available to all employees considered at high risk

for exposure to infectious diseases and that all employees be offered preexposure prophylaxis to hepatitis by inoculation with hepatitis vaccines.[2] The Centers for Disease Control and Prevention (CDC) and National Fire Protection Association (NFPA) have established similar guidelines, recommendations, and standards regarding the protection of health care workers and emergency providers from bloodborne pathogens, including regular testing for tuberculosis and vaccination for measles in nonimmune individuals (Box 37-2).

The *Ryan White Comprehensive AIDS Resources Emergency Act of 1990* (PL 101-381) requires that emergency responders be notified if they have been exposed to infectious diseases. It also requires that employers name a DO to coordinate communications between the hospital and emergency response organization in case of an exposure. Notification must occur no later than 48 hours after determining the presence of the disease (Box 37-3).

? CRITICAL THINKING

What rights do you think paramedics had to get infectious disease information before the Ryan White law?

AGENCIES AND ORGANIZATIONS INVOLVED IN DISEASE OUTBREAKS

Private sector

  Regional and national health care providers

  Laboratories (hospital and private)

  Local and national health maintenance organizations

  Infection control/disease specialist

  Influences protocols and guidelines for dealing with disease surveillance/response to outbreaks

Local (municipal/city/county public health agencies)

  First line of defense in disease surveillance

  First line of defense in disease outbreaks

State health agencies

  Regulate and enforce federal guidelines

  Required by statute or law to meet or exceed federal guidelines and recommendations

Federal and national organizations

  U.S. Congress plays a role in national health policy through public laws and drafting of the federal budget

  U.S. Department of Labor (OSHA rules and guidelines)

  U.S. Department of Health and Human Services (CDC, NIOSH guidelines)

  U.S. Department of Defense and Federal Emergency Management Agency (FEMA guidelines)

  National Fire Protection Association (NFPA standards), U.S. Fire Protection Administration (USFPA) and International Association of Firefighters (IAFF)

RECOMMENDED IMMUNIZATIONS FOR EMS PROVIDERS

HBV vaccination (OSHA requirement)

Diphtheria

Measles

Mumps

Rubella

Tetanus

Polio

Testing for TB is required at time of initial employment, and then annually thereafter.

REPORTING REQUIREMENTS

The CDC has classified infectious disease into two types: airborne and bloodborne. The primary airborne disease is listed as infectious tuberculosis. The primary bloodborne pathogen diseases are HBV, HCV, and HIV. The CDC also lists less common infectious diseases, which include diphtheria, hemorrhagic fevers, meningococcal disease, plague, and rabies.

At present, no requirement exists for medical facilities to test patients for any infectious disease. If paramedics suspect a possible exposure has occurred, they may submit a written notification to the DO who must in turn submit a written request to the medical facility who treated the patient. The act requires that the medical facility attempt to identify the patient in question and review the results of diagnostic tests performed and any signs and symptoms the patient may have had that are compatible with the CDC list of infectious diseases. After determining that a paramedic may have been exposed (or was not exposed) to an infectious disease, the medical facility must notify the DO within 48 hours after receiving the request.

Personal Responsibilities Relative to Infectious Agent Exposure

The paramedic should be familiar with laws, regulations, and national standards that address issues of infectious disease and should take personal protective measures against being exposed to these pathogens. Table 37-1 and the box on p. 1105 provides an overview of CDC guidelines designed to help prevent the transmission of infectious disease to public safety and emergency response workers. Paramedics should follow local protocol regarding similar or additional precautions concerning personal protection and should be aware of their individual responsibilities, including[1]:

- A proactive attitude relative to infection control

- Maintenance of personal hygiene and prevention of offensive body odors (esthetics of patient care)
- Attention to wounds and maintenance of integument (external barrier to infection)
- Effective hand washing after every patient contact using warm water and antiseptic cleanser or waterless antiseptic cleanser when portable water is unavailable
- Washing or disposal of work garments before entering the home

TABLE 37-1	PERSONAL EQUIPMENT FOR PROTECTION AGAINST TRANSMISSION OF HIV AND HEPATITIS B VIRUS			
ACTIVITY	**DISPOSABLE GLOVES**	**GOWN**	**MASK**	**PROTECTIVE EYEWEAR**
Bleeding control (spurting blood)	Yes	Yes	Yes	Yes
Bleeding control (minimal blood)	Yes	No	No	No
Emergency childbirth	Yes	Yes	Yes*	Yes*
Intravenous therapy	Yes	No	No	No
Endotracheal intubation	Yes	No	Yes*	Yes*
Oral or nasal suctioning	Yes	No	No	No
Administration of an injection	No	No	No	No

*If splashing is likely.
Adapted from Centers for Disease Control, *Examples of recommended personal protective equipment for worker protection against HIV and HBV transmission in prehospital setting,* February 1989.

BOX 37-4

CDC/FDA CLARIFICATIONS FOR USE OF UNIVERSAL PRECAUTIONS

Body fluids to which universal precautions apply
Blood and other body fluids containing visible blood
Semen and vaginal secretions
Human tissue
Human fluids (cerebrospinal fluid, synovial fluid, pleural fluid, peritoneal fluid, pericardial fluid, amniotic fluid)

Body fluids to which universal precautions do not apply (in the absence of blood)
Feces
Nasal secretions
Sputum
Sweat
Tears
Urine
Vomitus

Precautions for other body fluids in special settings
Human breast milk in mothers infected with HBV (e.g., milk banking procedures)
Saliva in some persons infected HBV or HIV (e.g., human bites [remote], dental procedures)

Source: Perspectives in disease prevention and health promotion update: universal precautions for prevention of transmission of human immunodeficiency virus, hepatitis B virus, and other bloodborne pathogens in health-care settings, *MMWR* 37(24):377-388, June 24, 1988.

- Handling uniforms in accordance with their agency's definition of PPE
- Proper handling and laundering of work clothes soiled with body fluids, with consideration for bathing and showering after work shift and before returning home
- Preparing food and eating in appropriate areas
- Maintenance of general physiological and psychological health to prevent distress, which can immunocompromise a healthy individual
- Proper disposal of needles and sharps into appropriate containers
- Proper disposal of body fluid-tinged linens and supplies
- An awareness and avoidance of tendencies to wipe face and/or rub eyes, nose, and mouth with gloved hands
- Knowledge of general classifications of exposure to determine the extent of the infection-control measures applied to the health care worker

Body Substance Isolation

In 1987, the CDC published the *Recommendations for Prevention of HIV Transmission Guidelines in Health-Care Settings,* which recommended that body fluid precautions (Universal [Standard] Precautions recommended by the CDC in 1983) be extended and consistently used for all patients regardless of their bloodborne infection status.[3] Since then, the FDA and CDC have worked together to identify further those body fluids to which universal precautions apply (Box 37-4).

The Universal/Standard Precautions (mainly applicable to clinical and research facilities) for EMS personnel are superceded by BSI guidelines (an

GUIDELINES FOR PREVENTION OF TRANSMISSION OF HIV AND HEPATITIS B VIRUS TO HEALTH CARE AND PUBLIC SAFETY WORKERS

The general principles presented here have been developed from existing principles of occupational safety and health in conjunction with data from studies of health care workers in hospital settings. The basic premise is that workers must be protected from exposure to blood and other potentially infectious body fluids in the course of their work activities. There is a paucity of data concerning the risks these worker groups face, however, which complicates development of control principles. Thus the guidelines presented here are based on principles of prudent public health practice.

Fire and emergency medical services personnel are engaged in delivery of medical care in the prehospital setting. The following guidelines are intended to assist these personnel in making decisions concerning use of personal protective equipment and resuscitation equipment, as well as for documentation, disinfection, and disposal procedures.

Personal Protective Equipment

Appropriate personal protective equipment should be made available routinely by the employer to reduce the risk of exposure. For many situations, the chance that the rescuer will be exposed to blood and other body fluids to which universal precautions apply can be determined in advance. Therefore if the chance of being exposed is high (for example, cardiopulmonary resuscitation, intravenous line insertion, trauma, and childbirth), the worker should put on protective attire before beginning patient care. (This list is not intended to be all-inclusive.)

1. Gloves: Disposable gloves should be a standard component of emergency response equipment and should be donned by all personnel before initiating any emergency patient care tasks involving exposure to blood or other body fluids to which universal precautions apply. Extra pairs should always be available. Considerations in the choice of disposable gloves should include dexterity, durability, fit, and the task being performed. Thus there is no single type or thickness of glove appropriate for protection in all situations. For situations in which large amounts of blood are likely to be encountered, it is important that gloves fit tightly at the wrist to prevent blood contamination of hands around the cuff. For multiple trauma victims, gloves should be changed between patient contacts, if the emergency situation allows.

Greater personal protective equipment measures are indicated for situations in which broken glass and sharp edges are likely to be encountered, such as extricating a person from an automobile wreck. Structural firefighting gloves that meet the federal OSHA requirements for firefighter gloves (as contained in 29 Code of Federal Register [CFR] 1910.156 or National Fire Protection Association Standard 1973, *Gloves for Structural Fire Fighters*) should be worn in any situation in which sharp or rough surfaces are likely to be encountered.

While wearing gloves, avoid handling personal items, such as combs and pens, that could become soiled or contaminated. Gloves that have become contaminated with blood or other body fluids to which universal precautions apply should be removed as soon as possible, taking care to avoid skin contact with the exterior surface. Contaminated gloves should be placed and transported in bags that prevent leakage and should be disposed of or, in the case of reusable gloves, cleaned and disinfected properly.

2. Mask, eyewear, and gowns: Mask, eyewear, and gowns should be present on all emergency vehicles that respond or potentially respond to medical emergencies or victim rescues. These protective barriers should be used in accordance with the level of exposure encountered. Minor lacerations or small amounts of blood do not merit the same extent of barrier use as required for exsanguinating victims or massive arterial bleeding. Management of the patient who is not bleeding and who has no body fluids present should not routinely require use of barrier precautions. Masks and eyewear (for example, safety glasses) should be worn together, or a face shield should be used by all personnel before any situation in which splashes of blood or other body fluids to which universal precautions apply are likely to occur. Gowns or aprons should be worn to protect clothing from splashes with blood. If large splashes or quantities of blood are present or anticipated, impervious gowns or aprons should be worn. An extra change of work clothing should be available at all times.

3. Resuscitation equipment: No transmission of hepatitis B virus or HIV infection during mouth-to-mouth resuscitation has been documented. However, because of the risk of salivary transmission of other infectious diseases (for example, herpes simplex, *Neisseria meningitidis*) and theoretical risk of HIV and hepatitis B virus transmission during artificial ventilation of trauma victims, disposable airway equipment or resuscitation bags should be used. Disposable resuscitation equipment and devices should be used once and disposed of or, if reusable, thoroughly cleaned and disinfected after each use according to the manufacturer's recommendations.

Mechanical respiratory assist devices (for example, bag-valve masks, oxygen demand-valve resuscitators) should be available on all emergency vehicles and to all emergency response personnel who respond or potentially respond to medical emergencies or victim rescues.

Pocket mouth-to-mask resuscitation masks designed to isolate emergency response personnel (that is, double-lumen systems) from contact with victims' blood and blood-contaminated saliva, respiratory secretions, and vomitus should be provided to all personnel who provide or potentially provide emergency treatment.

From U.S. Department of Health and Human Services, Centers for Disease Control, National Institute of Occupational Safety and Health: *Guidelines for prevention of transmission of human immunodeficiency virus and hepatitis B virus to health-care and public-safety workers,* Washington, DC, 1989, DHHS, CDC, NIOSH.

enhanced version of Universal/Standard Precautions). BSI is based on the premise that *all* exposures to body fluids, under any circumstances, are potentially infectious.[1]

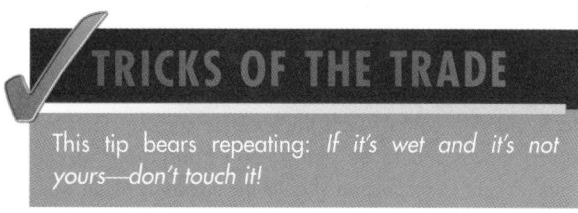

TRICKS OF THE TRADE

This tip bears repeating: *If it's wet and it's not yours—don't touch it!*

Pathophysiology of Infectious Disease

Infectious (communicable) disease is the fifth most common cause of death in the United States.[4] The development and/or manifestations of clinical disease are dependent on several factors, including virulence (degree of pathogenicity), number of infectious agents (dose), resistance (immune status) of the host, and the correct mode of entry. These factors all rely on an intact "chain of elements" to produce an infectious disease (Fig. 37-1). These elements include[5]:

- The pathogenic agent
- A reservoir
- A portal of exit from the reservoir
- An environment conducive to transmission of the pathogenic agent
- A portal of entry into the new host
- Susceptibility of the new host to the infectious disease

NOTE

Even in the presence of all necessary elements, exposure does not mean that a person will become infected.

Pathogenic Agent

As described in Chapter 7, pathogens are organisms that can create pathological processes in the human host. They are classified according to morphology, chemical composition, growth requirements, and viability. Pathogens rely on a host to supply their nutritional requirements.

NOTE

Some viruses such as HIV and HBV can survive for several hours outside of hosts. This is why blood products can be infectious.

Some pathogens (such as certain bacteria) are metabolically equipped so that they can survive outside a host, whereas others (such as certain viruses) can only survive in the human cell (Box 37-5). Most bacteria are susceptible to certain drugs (antibiotics), which kill them or inhibit their growth. Viruses, however, are more difficult to treat because they reside in cells for most of their life cycle and become intricately enmeshed in the host cell's deoxyribonucleic acid (DNA). The factors that affect a pathogen's ability to create pathological processes include the following:

- Ability to invade and reproduce within a host and the mode in which it does so

Fig. 37-1 Chain of transmission for infection. The chain must be intact for an infection to be transmitted to another host. Transmission can be controlled by breaking any link in the chain.

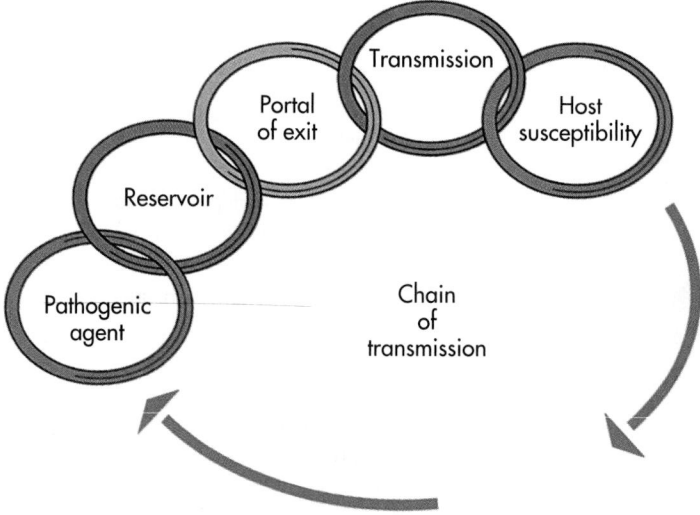

- Speed of reproduction, ability to produce a toxin, and the extent of tissue damage that it causes
- Potency
- Ability to induce or evade an immune response in the host

Reservoir

Pathogens may live and reproduce in a human or other animal host, an arthropod, a plant, soil, water, food, or some other organic substance, or a combination of these reservoirs. When infected, the human host may exhibit signs of clinical illness or may be an asymptomatic carrier (i.e., transmitting the pathogen to others). The life cycle of the infectious agent depends on the demographics of the host, genetic factors, and the efficacy of therapeutic interventions once infection has been established.

Portal of Exit

The method by which a pathogenic agent leaves one host to invade another involves a "portal of exit." The portal of exit from the human host depends on the agent. The portal may be single or multiple, involving the genitourinary (GU) tract, intestinal tract, oral cavity, respiratory tract, an open lesion, or any wound through which blood escapes. The time during which an actively infectious pathogen escapes to produce disease in another organism coincides with the period of communicability (described later in this chapter), which varies with each disease.

Transmission

The portal of exit and the portal of entry determine the mode of transmission, which may be direct or indirect. Direct transmission results from physical contact between the source and the victim. Examples of direct transmission include oral transmission and transmission by airborne mucus droplets, fecal contamination, and sexual contact.

In indirect transmission, the organism survives on animate or inanimate objects for a period without a human host. Diseases can be transmitted indirectly by air, food, water, soil, or biological matter.

Portal of Entry

Portal of entry refers to the method used by the pathogenic agent to enter a new host. The portal of

? CRITICAL THINKING

Think of a precaution or intervention that could break each of the links in this chain of disease transmission.

entry may be by ingestion, inhalation, percutaneous injection, crossing of a mucous membrane, or crossing of the placenta. The duration of exposure to the pathogen and the number of organisms required to initiate the infectious process vary with the disease

---

BOX 37-5

REVIEW OF INFECTIOUS AGENTS AND THEIR PROPERTIES

Bacteria

Prokaryotic (nuclear material is not contained within a distinctive envelope)

Self-reproducing without host cell

Signs and symptoms depend on the cells and tissues affected

Produce toxins (are often more lethal than the bacterium itself)

Endotoxins (chemicals, usually proteins) are integral parts of a bacteria's outer membrane and steadily shed from living bacteria

Exotoxins (proteins released by bacteria that can cause disease symptoms by acting as neurotoxins or enterotoxins)

Lysis of bacteria may release endotoxins

Can cause localized or systemic infection

Viruses

Living organisms without a nucleus

Must invade host cells to reproduce

Many cannot survive outside a host cell

May contain other microorganisms

Fungi

Eukaryotic (nuclear material is contained within a distinct envelope)

Has protective capsules that surround the cell wall to protect the fungi from phagocytes

Protozoa

Single-celled microorganisms

More complex than bacteria

Helminths (worms, including tapeworms, roundworms)

Pathogenic parasites

Not necessarily microorganisms

BOX 37-6

FACTORS THAT INFLUENCE HOST SUSCEPTIBILITY

Human characteristics
    Age
    Gender
    Ethnic group
    Heredity
General health status
    Nutrition
    Hormonal balance
    Presence of concurrent disease
    History of previous disease
Immune status
    Prior exposure to disease (conferring resistance)
    Effective immunization against disease (conferring host immunity)
Geographical and environmental conditions
Cultural behaviors
    Eating habits
    Personal hygiene
    Sexual behaviors

and host susceptibility. Exposure to an infectious agent does not always produce infection.

Host Susceptibility

Host susceptibility is influenced by a person's immune response (described in Chapters 7 and 31) and by several other factors—some of which are listed in Box 37-6.

Physiology of the Human Response to Infection

Although the human body is constantly exposed to pathogens capable of producing illness, most people do not succumb to infectious disease. This protection is provided by external and internal barriers that act as lines of defense against infection.

External Barriers

The first line of defense against infection is the surface of the body, which is exposed to the environment. These surfaces, inhabited by an indigenous flora (agents that could produce disease if allowed access to the interior of the body), include the skin

and the mucous membranes of the digestive, respiratory, and GU tract. These surfaces form a continuous closed barrier between the internal organs and the environment (Fig. 37-2).

Flora

Nearly the whole body surface is inhabited by normal microbial flora, which enhance the effectiveness of the surface barrier by interfering with the establishment of pathogenic agents in several ways. Indigenous flora compete with pathogens for space and nutrients. They maintain a pH optimal for their own growth, which can be incompatible with that needed for many pathogenic agents to survive. Some flora also secrete germicidal substances and are thought to stimulate the immune system.

Although resident (normal) flora play an important role in defense, some indigenous flora can be pathogenic under certain conditions. For example, flora can be responsible for infection when the skin or mucous membranes are interrupted or when flora are displaced from their natural habitat to another area of the body (a common cause of urinary tract infection after catheterization of the bladder).

Skin

Intact skin defends against infection by preventing penetration and by maintaining an acidic pH level that inhibits growth of pathogenic bacteria. In addition, microbes are sloughed from the skin's surface with dead skin cells, and oil and sweat wash microorganisms from the skin's pores.

GI System

The resident bacterial flora in the GI system provide competition between colonies of microorganisms for nutrients and space and help prevent proliferation of pathogenic organisms. In addition, stomach acid may destroy some microorganisms or deactivate their toxic products. The digestive system also eliminates pathogens through feces.

Upper Respiratory Tract

The sticky membranes of the upper airway protect against pathogens by trapping large particles, which may then be swallowed or expelled by coughing or sneezing. Coarse nasal hairs and cilia also trap and filter foreign substances in inspired air and thereby prevent the pathogens from reaching the lower respiratory tract. In addition, the lymph tissues of the tonsils and adenoids permit a rapid local immuno-

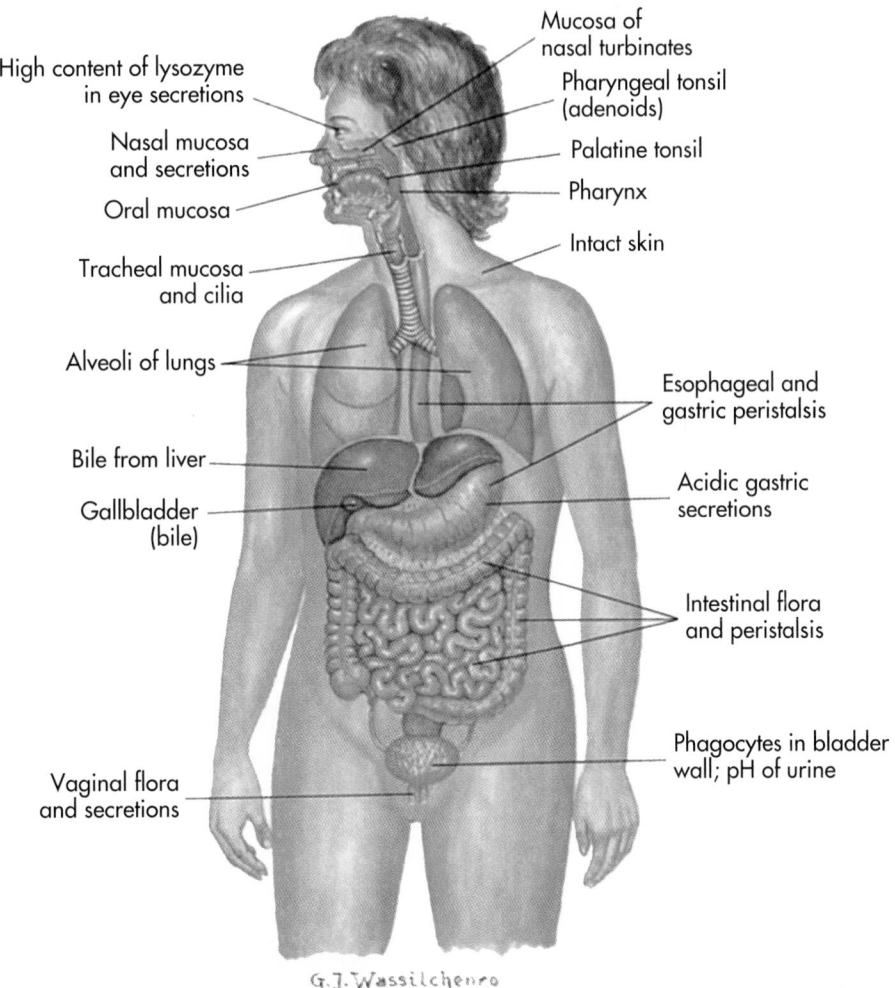

Fig. 37-2 First line of defense: external barriers. (From Grimes D: *Infectious diseases,* St Louis, 1991, Mosby.)

logical response to pathogenic organisms that may enter the respiratory tract.

Genitourinary Tract

The natural process of urination and the bacteriostatic properties of urine help prevent the establishment of microorganisms in the GU tract. Antibacterial substances in prostatic fluid and the presence of vaginal flora also help prevent infection in the GU system.

Internal Barriers

Internal barriers protect against pathogenic agents when the external lines of defense are breached. Internal barriers include the inflammatory response and the immune response, which share many of the same processes and cellular components.

Inflammatory Response

Inflammation (described in Chapter 7) is a local reaction to cellular injury: a response that may be initiated by microbial infection. When invasion occurs, this line of defense is activated to prevent further invasion of the pathogen by isolating, destroying, or neutralizing the microorganism as illustrated in Fig. 37-3.

Although the inflammatory response generally is protective and beneficial, it may initiate destruction of the body's own tissue if the response is sustained or directed against the host's own antigens. To review, the inflammatory response may be divided into three separate stages: cellular response to injury, vascular response to injury, and phagocytosis.

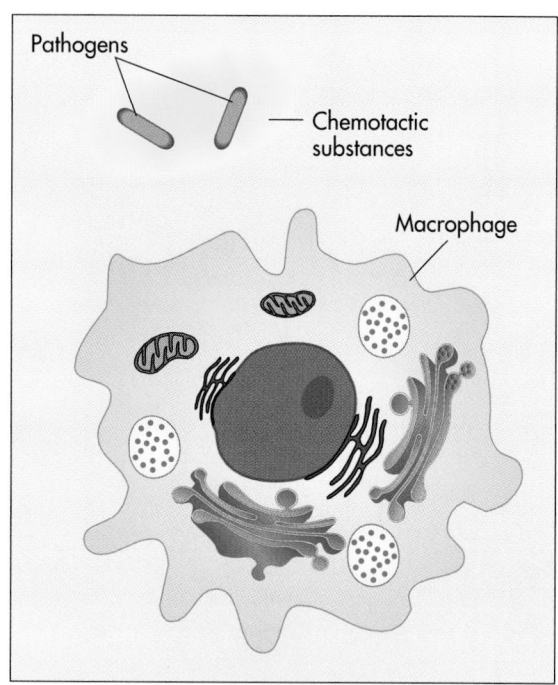

1. Injured area produces chemotactic exudate that attracts macrophages in area.

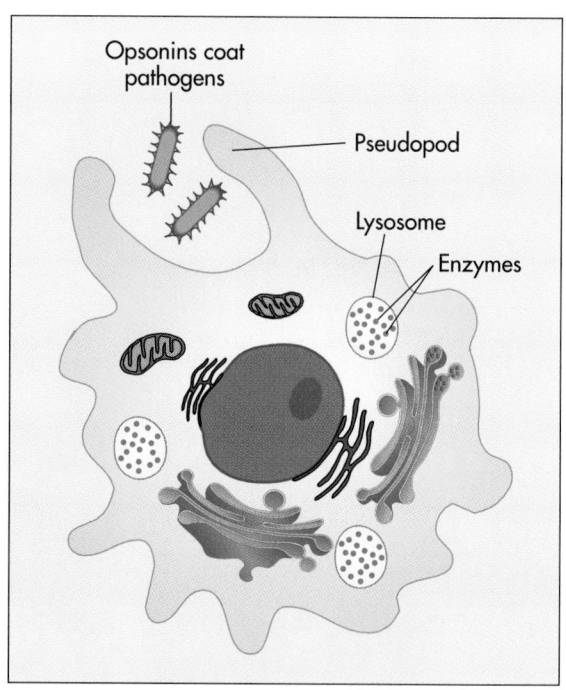

2. Opsonins facilitate phagocytosis.

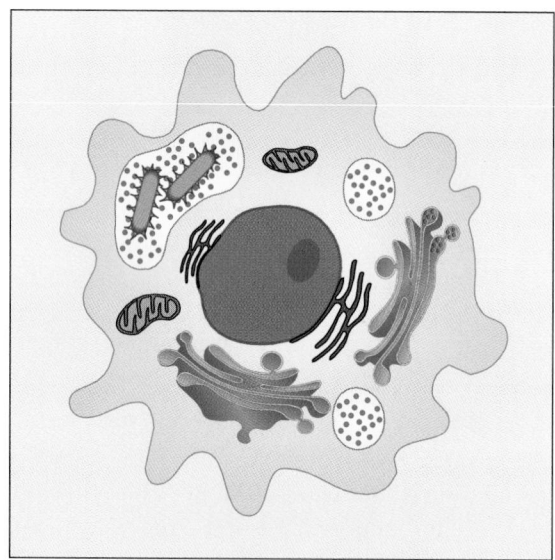

3. The engulfed pathogen becomes digested by enzymes in the lysosomes.

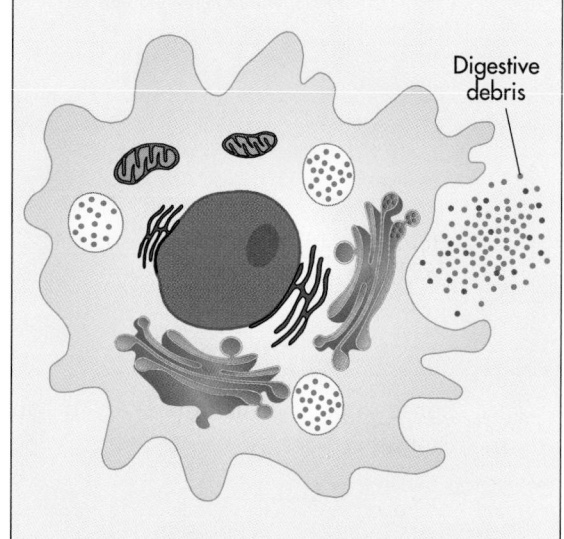

4. The macrophage expels debris after digestion is complete, including prostaglandins, interferon, and complement components. These elements continue the immune response.

Fig. 37-3 Second line of defense: inflammatory response. (From Grimes D: *Infectious diseases,* St Louis, 1991, Mosby.)

Cellular Response to Injury

As described in Chapter 7, there are various types of cellular response to injury, and the precise biological processes responsible for cellular injury are complex. When cells that are the target of specific inflammatory mediators (e.g., leukotrienes, histamine) are injured, the cell's aerobic respiration and oxidative phosphorylation may lead to decreasing energy reserves. When the energy sources are depleted, an accumulation of sodium ions causes the cell to swell, which along with increasing acidosis, further impairs enzyme function and leads to deterioration of the cell membranes.

Eventually, the membranes of the cellular organelles begin to leak, contributing to cellular destruction, autolysis, and stimulation of the inflammatory response in surrounding tissues.

Vascular Response to Injury

Localized hyperemia develops after cellular injury. The associated increase in filtration pressure and capillary permeability produces edema. Leukocytes collect along the vascular endothelium where they release chemotactic factors that eventually migrate to the injured tissue.

Phagocytosis

Through phagocytosis, leukocytes engulf, digest, and destroy the invading pathogens, and circulating macrophages clear the area of dead cells and other debris. The ingestion of bacteria and dead cell fragments (internal phagocytosis) stimulates the release of chemicals that induce lysis of the leukocytes.

Immune Response

The first two lines of defense against infection use identical nonspecific mechanism to respond to pathogens, but the immune response is specific to individual pathogens. The immune system has four unique characteristics:

1. It possesses "self-nonself" recognition and therefore normally responds only to foreign antigens.
2. It produces antibodies, which are antigen specific and can produce new antibodies in response to new antigens.
3. Some of the antibody-producing lymphocytes become "memory cells" that allow a more rapid response to subsequent invasions by the same antigen.
4. It is self-regulated to activate only when there is an invading pathogen. This ability to activate or deactivate the immune response prevents the destruction of healthy tissues. When this regulatory function goes awry, autoimmune disease (e.g., rheumatoid arthritis, active glomerulonephritis, and systemic lupus erythematous) can occur. The immune system may require extrinsic regu-

? CRITICAL THINKING

Why would a person's internal defenses be weakened after splenectomy for trauma?

BOX 37-7

TYPE OF T CELLS

Sensitized T cells develop into distinct subsets, each with a specific set of functions that coordinate the activity of other components of the immune system:

Killer T cells (like B cells) are sensitized and stimulated to multiply by the presence of antigens present on abnormal body cells. Unlike B cells, killer T cells do not produce antibodies.

Helper T cells "turn on" the activities of killer (cytotoxic) cells and control other aspects of the immune response.

Suppressor T cells "turn off" the action of the helper and killer T cells, preventing them from causing harmful immune reactions.

Inflammatory T cells stimulate allergic reactions, anaphylaxis, and autoimmune reactions.

lation using certain medications in patients with transplanted organs or with severe autoimmune diseases.

The immunological response to an invading pathogen depends partly on the size and antigenic properties of the pathogen. Often, peripheral phagocytic cells encounter a pathogen first, but circulating B and T cells (described in Chapter 6) also play a reconnaissance role (Box 37-7). Complex interactions occur among neutrophils, macrophages, and B and T cells. These cellular components assist each other in processing antigen so that it is recognizable and effective in neutralizing the invading organism.

The B cell's role is to produce antibody (humoral immunity), which coats the pathogen and facilitates phagocytosis. Antibody can also fix complement—a protein cascade that often results in the death of the organism and in the production of chemotactic factors. The T cell not only processes antigen for the B cell, but also has a subpopulation of "killer cells,"

NOTE

Humoral- and cell-mediated immunity are time-consuming responses. Both require previous exposure to mobilize specialized white cells, which eventually differentiate between antibodies and coordinate an attack on the foreign material. By comparison, the complement system recognizes and kills invaders on first sight. It does not take time to mobilize specialized responses.

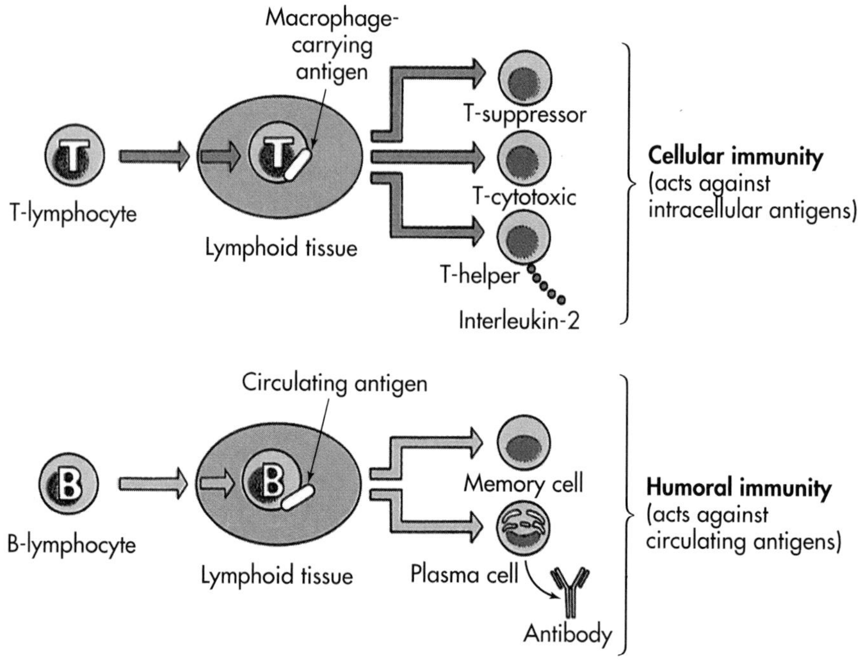

Fig. 37-4 Cellular and humoral immunity. Cellular immunity results from activation of T cells by contact with intracellular organisms. Activated T cells differentiate and proliferate. Humoral (antibody-mediated) immunity results from activating B cells. (From Grimes D: *Infectious diseases*, St Louis, 1991, Mosby.)

which are a major component of cell-mediated immunity (Fig. 37-4).

The Reticuloendothelial System

The reticuloendothelial system (RES), described in Chapter 7, works in conjunction with the lymphatic system to dispose of debris that results from the immune system attack on invading organisms. The RES is composed of immune cells in the spleen, lymph nodes, liver, bone marrow, lungs, and intestines. These structures store mature B and T cells until the immune system is activated.

Stages of Infectious Disease

The progression from exposure to an infectious agent to the onset of clinical disease follows specific stages. The duration of each stage and the potential outcomes vary, depending on the infectious agent and individual host factors. These stages include the **latent period,** the **incubation period,** the **communicability period,** and the **disease period** (Table 37-2).

> **NOTE**
>
> The risk of infection may be theoretical where the possibility of transmission is acknowledged to have a potential to occur, or measurable (known or deduced from reported data).

The latent period begins with pathogenic invasion of the body and ends when the agent can be "shed" or communicated. During the latent period, the infectious agent cannot be transmitted to another host or cause clinically significant symptoms.

> **NOTE**
>
> The window phase is the period after infection in which antigen is present, but there is no detectable antibody.

The incubation period (during which the organism reproduces) begins with invasion of the agent and ends when the disease process begins. This time interval occurs between exposure to an infectious agent and the first appearance of symptoms.

The communicability period begins when the latent period ends and continues as long as the agent is present and can spread to other hosts. (Clinically significant symptoms from the infection may manifest during this period.) This stage is variable and often is the major determining factor in ease of transmission. The communicable period and the method of transmission can be altered in some diseases (e.g., tuberculosis, syphilis, gonorrhea), depending on the stage of the disease and the primary site of infection.

The disease period follows the incubation period and is of variable disease-specific duration. This

TABLE 37-2	STAGES OF INFECTIOUS DISEASE	
STAGE OF DISEASE	**BEGINS**	**ENDS**
Latent period	With invasion	When the agent can be shed
Incubation period	With invasion	When the disease process begins
Communicability period	When the latent period ends	Continues as long as the agent is present and can spread to others
Disease period	Follows incubation period	Of variable duration

stage may be subclinical or produce overt symptoms, which can arise directly from the invading organism or from the host's physiological responses. During the disease period, the pathological process may resolve completely or the organism may become incorporated and quiescent inside certain cells. The infection is then considered to be in a latent stage. Several viruses (e.g., HIV and hepatitis) can lead to latent infection.

? CRITICAL THINKING

Which of these stages can overlap? What problems can the overlap(s) pose?

NOTE

Resolution of symptoms does not mean that the infectious agent is destroyed.

HIV

HIV is present in blood and serum-derived body fluids (semen, vaginal or cervical secretions) of individuals infected with the virus. The disease is directly transmitted person to person through anal or vaginal intercourse, across the placenta, or by contact with infected blood or body fluids on mucous membranes or open wounds. It can also be indirectly transmitted by transfusion with contaminated blood or blood products, transplanted tissues and organs, and use of contaminated needles or syringes. Occurrence is highest in persons with the following risk factors:

- High-risk sexual behavior
- Intravenous drug abuse
- Transfusion recipient between 1978 and 1985

- Hemophilia or other coagulation disorders requiring blood products
- Infant born from HIV-positive mother

Other factors that may affect susceptibility to HIV include coexisting sexually transmitted diseases (especially with ulceration) and penile foreskin. Race and gender do not appear to be risk factors.[1]

Pathophysiology

HIV results from one of two retroviruses: a group of viruses that convert genetic ribonucleic acid (RNA) to DNA after entering the host cell (referred to as *HIV-1* and *HIV-2*). Once the retrovirus is inside the cell, the cell's genetic material is altered into a hybrid composition of part virus and part cell. The virus essentially commandeers the cell's machinery to make more viral particles. When sufficient quantities of the virus are produced, the host cell ruptures, destroying the cell and releasing the virus into the blood to seek new target cells. The cell receptor sought by HIV is called *CD4+ T cell* (a type of lymphocyte used to determine how active the disease is [very low counts suggest severe disease]). It is found on the surface of T-4 cells (T helper cells, T-4 cells), certain nerve cells, and monocytes and macrophages, which probably carry the virus to other parts of the body. Even though the body develops antigen-specific antibodies to HIV, they do not protect against HIV. Secondary complications generally are caused by opportunistic infections, which develop as the immune system deteriorates. These infections include the following:

- Pulmonary tuberculosis
- Recurrent pneumonia
- *Pneumocystis carinii* pneumonia
- Kaposi's sarcoma
- Wasting syndrome
- HIV dementia

- Sensory neuropathy
- Toxoplasmosis of the CNS

> **NOTE**
>
> Although both HIV types 1 and 2 (HIV-1 and HIV-2) are serologically and geographically distinct, they do share similar epidemiological characteristics. HIV-1 is much more pathogenic than HIV-2, and most cases worldwide and in the United States are caused by HIV-1. HIV-2 seems to be more restricted to West Africa.[1] Some screening blood tests only test for HIV-1.

Classification and Categories

The average time from HIV transmission to serious complications in the absence of treatment is about 10 years, although there is considerable variation (Table 37-3).

The CDC has devised a classification system for HIV (revised in 1993), which uses three categories of CD4+ T cell counts[6]: category 1—more than or equal to 500 cells per mL; category 2—200 to 499 per microliter (μL); and category 3—less than 200 per μL. (As the number of CD4+ T cells decreases, the risk and severity of opportunistic illness increase.) After viral transmission, the progression of HIV in adolescents and adults can be divided into three clinical categories: A, B, and C.

Category A

- Acute retroviral infection: This syndrome generally occurs 2 to 4 weeks after exposure. Clinical features include an infectious mononucleosis-like illness with fever, adenopathy, and sore throat.

The febrile illness is self-limited, usually lasting 1 to 2 weeks. During this stage, a transient decrease is observed in CD4+ T cell counts.
- Seroconversion: The serological response with antigen-specific antibodies to HIV generally occurs between 6 and 12 weeks after transmission. During this stage, CD4+ T cell counts will return to normal levels.

> **? CRITICAL THINKING**
>
> *What will likely happen if a blood test for HIV antibodies is drawn at the third week after exposure?*

- Asymptomatic infection: The person with HIV may have persistent generalized lymphadenopathy (enlarged lymph nodes involving two noncontiguous sites other than inguinal nodes) and a gradual decline in the CD4+ T cell count.

Category B

- Early symptomatic HIV: The usual CD4+ T cell count in this group is 100 to 300 per μL. At this stage, common complications include localized Candida infections (thrush, *Candida esophagitis*, *Candida vaginitis*), oral lesions, shingles, pelvic inflammatory disease, peripheral neuropathy, and constitutional symptoms such as fever or diarrhea lasting more than 1 month.

Category C

- Late symptomatic HIV: This stage represents all AIDS-defining diagnoses found primarily with CD4+ T cell counts of 0 to 200 per μL, including

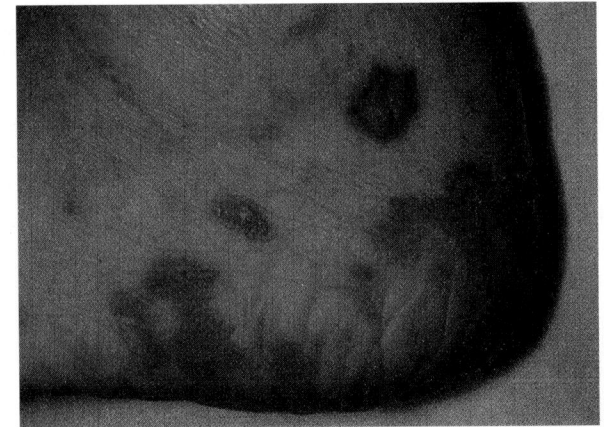
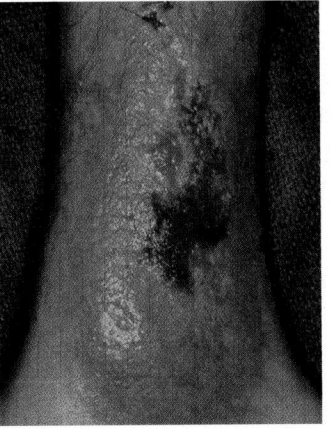

Fig. 37-5 A, Kaposi's sarcoma of the heel and lateral foot. **B,** Kaposi's sarcoma of the distal leg and ankle. (Courtesy The Centers for Disease Control, 1990. In Grimes D: *Infectious diseases*, St Louis, 1991, Mosby.)

TABLE 37-3	INCUBATION AND COMMUNICABILITY PERIODS

INCUBATION PERIOD	COMMUNICABILITY PERIOD
Childhood Diseases	
Chickenpox 2 to 3 weeks (average 13 to 17 days)	Occurs 1 to 2 days before the onset of rash and until lesions have crusted over and not more than 6 days after the appearance of vesicles
Mumps 2 to 3 weeks (average 18 days)	Occurs 6 days before parotid symptoms to 9 days after; disease is most communicable 48 hours after parotid swelling.
Pertussis 7 to 14 days, commonly 7 to 10 days	Occurs 7 days after exposure to 3 weeks after onset; highly communicable in early stage before cough; not communicable after 3 weeks, even though cough may be present
Rubella 14 to 23 days (average 16 to 18 days)	Occurs from 1 week before and 4 days after appearance of rash; infants with congenital rubella syndrome may shed virus for months after birth.
Rubeola Commonly 10 days, 8 to 13 days until fever, 14 days until rash	Occurs a few days before the fever to 5 to 7 days after the appearance of the rash
Hantavirus 3 days to 6 weeks	No known transmission from human to human
Hepatitis Virus	
HAV 15 to 50 days (28 to 30 days average)	Usually occurs in the latter half of the incubation period and continues for several days after the onset of jaundice
HBV 45 to 180 days (60 to 90 days average)	Occurs during incubation period and throughout clinical course (Carrier state may persist for years.)
HCV 2 weeks to 6 months (average 6 to 9 weeks)	Occurs 1 or more weeks before symptom onset and indefinitely during chronic and carrier states
HIV Variable (6 to 12 weeks from exposure to seropositivity, up to 20 years for symptomatic immune suppression and to diagnosis of AIDS)	Is lifelong from presence of HIV in serum until death; the degree of communicability may vary during the course of the HIV
Influenza 24 to 72 hours	Occurs three days from onset of symptoms; infection produces immunity to specific strain of virus, but duration of immunity varies
Meningitis 2 to 10 days	Is variable; lasts as long as infectious agents remain in the nasal and oral secretions; microorganisms disappear from the upper respiratory tract within 24 hours of antibiotic therapy.

Continued

TABLE 37-3	INCUBATION AND COMMUNICABILITY PERIODS—*cont'd*
INCUBATION PERIOD	**COMMUNICABILITY PERIOD**
Mononucleosis 4 to 6 weeks	Prolonged; pharyngeal excretion may persist for years; 15% to 20% of adults are carriers
Pneumonia 1 to 3 days	Occurs until organisms are not present in respiratory discharges; 24 to 48 hours after antibiotic treatment
Rabies Usually 2 to 16 weeks	Human-to-human transmission by bite or scratch or aerosol has not been documented; theoretical transmission from contact with secretions of infected person
Sexually transmitted diseases *Chlamydia* 5 to 10 days	Is unknown
Gonorrhea 2 to 7 days	Occurs for months if disease is untreated
Herpesvirus HSV-1: 2 to 12 days	Occurs when lesions are present; virus is found in saliva as long as 7 weeks after recovery of lesions; transient shedding of virus is common
HSV-2: 2 to 12 days (average 6 days)	Occurs in 7 to 12 days with lesion; transient shedding of virus in the absence of lesions probably occurs
Syphilis 10 days to 10 weeks (average 3 weeks)	Is variable; occurs during primary and secondary stages and in mucocutaneous recurrences (2 to 4 years if untreated)
Tetanus 3 to 21 days, commonly 10 days	Not directly transmitted; recovery from tetanus does not confer permanent immunity
Tuberculosis 4 to 12 weeks after exposure or any time the disease is in a latent stage	Occurs as long as bacilli are in the sputum, sometimes intermittently for years

severe opportunistic infections; bacterial pneumonia (e.g., *Pneumocystis carinii* pneumonia); pulmonary tuberculosis; debilitating diarrhea; tumors in any body system, including Kaposi's sarcoma (Fig. 37-5); HIV-associated dementia; and neurological manifestations.

• Advanced HIV: This stage applies to individuals with CD4+ T cell counts of 0 to 50 per μL. These patients have a limited life expectancy, and most of these patients die from AIDS-related complications.

Personal Protection

Strict compliance with universal precautions is the only prophylactic measure health care workers can

take to protect themselves against HIV. However, the chance of EMS personnel acquiring this disease by exposure to infected blood appears to be low (0.2% to 0.44%).[1] Hepatitis B virus (HBV) poses a much greater occupational hazard.[7] Health care worker risks increase when:

1. The exposure involves a large quantity of blood as when a device is visibly contaminated with

NOTE

Health care workers suffer between 600,000 and 1 million injuries from conventional needles and sharps each year.[8]

blood; when care of the patient involves placing a needle in a vein or artery; and in deep injuries. Needle size, type (hollow bore vs. suture), and depth of penetration influences volume transferred to the skin.

2. The exposure involves a source patient with a terminal illness, possibly reflecting a higher dose of HIV in the late course of AIDS.

> **NOTE**
>
> The risk of exposure needs to be understood in terms of how the exposure occurred and what factors were involved. Although the potential may appear high, the probability may actually be quite low.

✓ TRICKS OF THE TRADE

Here's a reason to remember how important effective hand washing is: Any soap will kill HIV.

? CRITICAL THINKING

Why would testing within 2 to 3 weeks of exposure be needed?

Postexposure Prophylaxis

If a known or possible exposure occurs, the paramedic should immediately notify the DO (per protocol), so that elective postexposure prophylaxis (PEP) can begin. Information regarding primary HIV indicates that systemic infection does not occur immediately, leaving a brief "window of opportunity" during which postexposure antiretroviral intervention may modify viral replication.[9] Several antiretroviral agents from at least three classes of drugs are available for treating HIV. Examples include the nucleoside analogue reverse transcriptase inhibitors (NRTIs), nonnucleoside reverse transcriptase inhibitors (NNRTIs), and protease inhibitors (PIs). Among these drugs, ZDV (an NRTI) is the only agent shown to prevent HIV transmission in humans.[9] Following PEP, testing for HIV is again performed 2 to 3 weeks after the exposure, and again at 6 weeks, 3 months, 6 months, and 1 year.

> **NOTE**
>
> An important goal of PEP is to encourage and facilitate compliance with a 4-week PEP regimen. All antiretroviral drugs have been associated with side effects (primarily gastrointestinal). In addition, some of these drugs (especially PIs) have potentially serious drug interactions when used with certain other drugs. Paramedics should receive postexposure counseling regarding evaluation and treatment protocols.

> **NOTE**
>
> Paramedics should follow local protocol regarding reporting and notification of significant exposures to any infectious disease.

Psychological Reactions to HIV

HIV is almost invariably a progressive disease with morbid late consequences. Throughout the course of the infection, HIV-infected persons are likely to feel and express anger regarding many aspects of their illness, including pain, dying prematurely and without dignity, and the social rejection and prejudice that they may experience. Patient care should include helping these patients feel that they can obtain acceptance and compassion from health care workers.

> **NOTE**
>
> When caring for patients with HIV, isolation is unnecessary, ineffective, and unjustified.

Although no immunization exists for HIV, new treatments are evolving rapidly. Despite current limitations, progression of the illness can be delayed with drug therapy and other strategies, permitting access to new therapeutic options.

Hepatitis

As described in Chapter 32, hepatitis is a viral disease that produces pathological alterations in the liver. The three main classes of hepatitis viruses are hepatitis A (viral hepatitis), HBV (serum hepatitis), and hepatitis C (non-A/non-B hepatitis) (Table 37-4).

> **NOTE**
>
> Hepatitis non-ABC is a fourth class of hepatitis caused by infection from the hepatitis D virus and the newer hepatitis viruses (E and G). The routes of transmission for these viruses are similar to those for HBV and often are mistaken for HBV.

Hepatitis A Virus

Hepatitis A (HAV) is the most common type of viral hepatitis in the United States. The disease is acquired by ingesting HAV-contaminated food or drink or by the fecal–oral route. The virus localizes in the liver, reproduces, enters the bile, and is carried to the intestinal tract, where it is shed in the feces. (Fecal shedding usually occurs before the onset of clinical symptoms.) Antibodies (anti-HAV) develop during acute disease and later during convalescence. Once infected, the person is immune to HAV for life. Hepatitis A is the only hepatitis virus that does not lead to chronic liver disease or a chronic carrier state. Many HAV infections are subclinical and often present with influenza-like symptoms. About 1 in 100 patients with HAV suffer from a fulminant infection that may require a liver transplant.[10]

Immune globulin (IG) can provide a temporary immunity to the virus for 2 to 3 months if given before exposure to HAV or within 2 weeks after contact. Hepatitis A vaccines approved for persons 2 years of age and older are recommended for the following groups:

- Persons who have close physical contact with people who live in areas with poor sanitary conditions or who are traveling or working in developing countries
- Men who have sex with other men
- Users of illicit drugs
- Children in populations that have repeated epidemics of hepatitis A (Alaska Natives, Native Americans, Pacific Islanders, and certain closed religious communities)
- Persons who have chronic liver disease or clotting factors disorders

> **NOTE**
>
> Safety of the vaccine has not been determined during pregnancy.

Hepatitis B Virus

Infectious HBV particles are found in blood and in secretions containing serum (e.g., oozing, cutaneous lesions), or in secretions derived from serum (e.g., saliva, semen, vaginal secretions). Like other viral types of hepatitis, HBV affects the liver and causes the signs and symptoms previously described. The virus may produce chronic infection that can lead to cirrhosis and other complications. Although HBV usually lasts less than 6 months, the carrier state may persist for years.

The effects of HBV vary from low-grade fever and malaise (influenza-like illness) with complete resolution of symptoms to extensive liver necrosis that may lead to death. Other complications associated with HBV include coagulation defects, impaired protein production, impaired bilirubin elimination, pancreatitis, and hepatic cancer. Exposure generally occurs in one of five ways:

1. Direct percutaneous inoculation of infectious serum or plasma by needle or transfusion of infected blood or blood products
2. Indirect percutaneous introduction of infective serum or plasma (e.g., skin cuts or abrasions, tattoo/body piercing)
3. Absorption of infective serum or plasma through mucosal surfaces (such as those of the eyes or mouth), transplacentally, or through contamination from the mother's infective blood at birth

> **NOTE**
>
> Hepatitis B virus is stable on environmental surfaces and can remain infective in visible blood for more than 7 days.[1]

> **? CRITICAL THINKING**
>
> *Why is this information significant to paramedics?*

TABLE 37-4	THE ABC OF HEPATITIS				
	HEPATITIS A (HAV)	**HEPATITIS B (HBV)**	**HEPATITIS C (HCV)**	**HEPATITIS D (HDV)**	**HEPATITIS E (HEV)**
What is it?	HAV is a virus that causes inflammation of the liver. It does not lead to chronic disease.	HBV is a virus that causes inflammation of the liver. It can cause liver cell damage, leading to cirrhosis and cancer.	HCV is a virus that causes inflammation of the liver. It can cause liver cell damage, leading to cirrhosis and cancer.	HDV is a virus that causes inflammation of the liver. It only infects those persons with HBV.	HEV is a virus that causes inflammation of the liver. It is rare in the United States. There is no chronic state.
Incubation Period	2 to 7 weeks Average 4 weeks	6 to 23 weeks. Average 17 weeks.	2 to 25 weeks. Average 7 to 9 weeks.	2 to 8 weeks.	2 to 9 weeks. Average 40 days.
How is it Spread?	Transmitted by fecal/oral route, through close person-to-person contact or ingestion of contaminated food and water	Contact with infected blood, seminal fluid, vaginal secretions, contaminated needles, including tattoo and body-piercing tools. Infected mother to newborn. Human bite. Sexual contact.	Contact with infected blood, contaminated IV needles, razors, and tattoo or body-piercing tools. Infected mother to newborn. NOT easily spread through sex.	Contact with infected blood, contaminated needles. Sexual contact with HDV infected person.	Transmitted through fecal/oral route. Outbreaks associated with contaminated water supply in other countries.
Symptoms	May have none. Others may have light stools, dark urine, fatigue, fever, nausea, vomiting, abdominal pain, and jaundice.	May have none. Some persons have mild flulike symptoms, dark urine, light stools, jaundice, fatigue, and fever.	Same as HBV	Same as HBV	Same as HBV
Treatment of Chronic Disease	Not applicable	Interferon and Lamivudine with varying success.	Interferon and combination therapies with varying success.	Interferon with varying success.	Not applicable.
Vaccine	Two doses of vaccine to anyone over 2 yrs of age or older	Three doses may be given to persons of any age.	None	HBV vaccine prevents HDV infection.	None
Who is at Risk?	Household or sexual contact with an infected person or living in an area with HAV outbreak. Travelers to developing countries, persons engaging in anal/oral sex, and injection drug users.	Infants born to infected mother, having sex with an infected person or multiple partners, injection drug users, emergency responders, health care workers, persons engaging in anal/oral sex, and hemodialysis patients.	Blood transfusion recipients before 1992, health care workers, injection drug users, hemodialysis patients, infants born to infected mother, multiple sex partners.	Injection drug users, persons engaging in anal/oral sex and those having sex with an HDV infected person.	Travelers to developing countries, especially pregnant women.
Prevention	Immune globulin within 2 wks of exposure. Vaccination. Washing hands with soap and water after going to the toilet. Use household bleach (10 parts water to 1 part bleach) to clean surfaces contaminated with feces, such as changing tables. Safe sex.	Immune globulin within 2 wks of exposure. Vaccination provides protection for 18 years. Clean up infected blood with household bleach and wear protective gloves. Do not share razors, toothbrushes, or needles. Safe sex.	Clean up spilled blood with household bleach. Wear gloves when touching blood. Do not share razors, toothbrushes, or needles with anyone. Safe sex.	Hepatitis B vaccine to prevent HBV infection. Safe sex.	Avoid drinking or using potentially contaminated water.

From Hepatitis Foundation International On-Line, http://hepfi.org

4. Absorption of infective secretions (such as saliva or semen) through mucosal surfaces, as might occur during vaginal, anal, or oral sexual contact (but never fecal transmission)

5. Transfer of infective serum or plasma via inanimate environmental surfaces

Preexposure Prophylaxis

Following regulatory and legislative efforts and OSHA's *Bloodborne Pathogen Standard*, cases of HBV in health care workers have dropped from 17,000 annually to about 400 annually.[11] (The exposure risk for health care providers to HBV-positive patients is estimated to be between 2% and 40%.) Even with this decline, HBV is a serious concern to all health care workers.

NOTE

The CDC recommends and OSHA requires that HBV vaccines be offered to all health care workers. The vaccine sometimes is given to newborns, and several states now require immunization of middle school-age children.

Blood is the most important potential source of HBV in the workplace. The risk of infection is directly proportional to the probability that the blood contains HBV, the immunity status of the recipient, and the efficacy of transmission. Hepatitis B virus vaccinations are available that provide protection

---

ANTIVIRAL THERAPY WITH INTERFERONS

Interferons are proteins produced naturally by body cells in response to viral infection and other stimuli. Interferon alpha (Intron A and others) is effective in controlling the spread of common colds caused by rhinoviruses and may be effective in treating chronic HBV, HCV, and HIV.

Interferons work by attaching to the membranes of host cells and stimulating them against viral attack. If a virus invades a cell primed by interferon, enzymes are produced that impair viral copying, nullifying the virus. Interferons also increase the activity of natural killer cells to stop or shorten the effects of the virus. Side effects of interferon include fever, malaise, headache, fatigue, hair loss, and bone marrow suppression.

---

for 18 years in those who respond to the inoculation.[10] The HBV vaccination schedule generally requires three intramuscular (deltoid) doses over 6 months. For optimal protection against HBV, the vaccination series should be completed before an exposure occurs. Vaccinations currently available include Recombivax HB and Engerix-B.

Postexposure Prophylaxis

Postexposure prophylaxis may be indicated if a nonvaccinated person or an individual who has not completed the vaccination schedule is exposed to HBV. Before treatment, a blood test is performed to determine immunity to HBV. Seronegative candidates generally receive the HBV vaccine and hepatitis B immune globulin, an antibody used in postexposure patients to provide passive immunity to HBV.

Hepatitis C Virus

Hepatitis C virus (HCV) is a bloodborne virus that causes a disease similar to HBV. The virus was associated with receipt of contaminated blood during transfusion before 1992 (accounting for more than 90% of posttransfusion hepatitis in the United States). At present, approximately 4 million Americans are believed to be infected with the virus. Hepatitis C virus is the most frequent infection resulting from needlestick and sharps injury.[12] Of health care workers who become infected, 85% become chronic carriers. About one half to two thirds of those infected with HCV develop chronic hepatitis; one in five suffer severe liver disease such as cirrhosis and liver cancer. There is no available HCV vaccine.

Although transmission of HCV occurs in the same manner as other forms of hepatitis, it is not easily spread through sexual contact. When they occur, signs and symptoms of the disease are similar to those of other types of hepatitis. Most persons infected with HCV are asymptomatic.

Signs and Symptoms

Infection with any of the causative viruses may be symptomless or may cause a typical hepatitis with an abrupt onset of flulike illness followed by jaundice, dark urine, or both. A patient is most infectious during the first week of symptoms (see Table 37-3). Within 2 to 3 months after infection, the patient generally will develop nonspecific symptoms such as anorexia, nausea and vomiting, fever, joint pain, and generalized rashes. (Approximately 1% of patients hospitalized with HBV develop full-blown liver crisis and die.)

Patient Management and Protective Measures

Patient management for out-of-hospital care primarily is supportive for maintenance of circulatory status and prevention of shock (see the box on p. 1120). All health care workers involved in the patient's care must observe personal protective measures, including effective hand washing and proper care in the use of diagnostic and therapeutic equipment (e.g., high-level disinfection of laryngoscope blades and the appropriate disposal of sharps).

Tuberculosis

Eight million new tuberculosis (TB) cases occur each year worldwide, and 3 million people die of the disease.[13] Although reports of TB in the United States declined continually after the turn of the century, in 1985 this trend reversed. The reversal is attributed to the epidemic of HIV and to the following factors:

- Immigration of persons from areas with a high prevalence of TB
- Transmission of TB in high-risk environments, such as correctional facilities, homeless shelters, hospitals, and nursing homes
- Deterioration of the TB public health care infrastructure

> **NOTE**
>
> The rate of TB for patients with HIV is 40 times the rate for people who are not infected with HIV.[14]

> **?**   **CRITICAL THINKING**
>
> *Why is TB more prevalent in this patient group?*

Pathophysiology

As described in Chapter 27, TB is a chronic pulmonary disease acquired by inhalation of a dried-droplet nucleus containing tubercle bacilli (*Myco-*

bacterium tuberculosis, M. bovis, or a variety of atypical mycobacteria). The infection is transmitted primarily from infected persons coughing or sneezing the bacteria into the air or from contact with sputum that contains virulent TB bacilli. (Persons who share the same airspace with persons infected with infectious TB are at greatest risk for infection.) Although less common, transmission may occur by ingestion or invasion of the skin or mucous membranes.

> **NOTE**
>
> Reservoirs for TB include some primates, cattle, badgers, and swine.

The pathology of TB is related to the production of inflammatory lesions throughout the body and to the ability of the TB bacillus to break through the body's natural defenses, leading to the formation of caseating granulomas (necrotic inflammatory cells) and TB cavities, which may cause chronic and debilitating lung disease. Susceptibility to mycobacterial infection generally is highest in children younger than 3 years of age; in adults older than 65; and in chronically ill, malnourished, and immunosuppressed or immunocompromised individuals. The infection may remain dormant for an indefinite time (often not causing disease) or may lead to active disease that is contagious.

Tuberculosis is characterized by stages of early infection (frequently asymptomatic), latency, and a potential for recurrent postprimary disease (see Table 37-3). Signs and symptoms of TB include cough, fever, night sweats, weight loss, fatigue, and hemoptysis. Organ systems and associated complications include:

- Cardiovascular
  Pericardial effusions
  Lymphadenopathy (cervical lymph nodes are usually involved)
- Skeletal
  Intervertebral disk deterioration
  Chronic arthritis of one joint
- Central nervous system (CNS)
  Subacute meningitis
  Brain granulomas
- Systemic miliary TB (extensive dissemination by the bloodstream of tubercle bacilli)

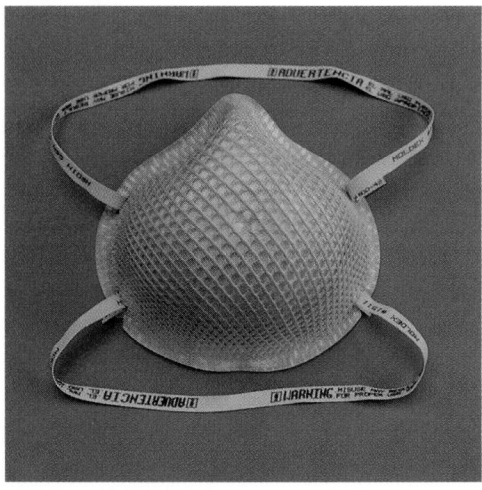

Fig. 37-6 HEPA respirator.

NOTE

In the United States, an estimated 10 to 15 million persons are infected with *Mycobacterium tuberculosis.* Without intervention, approximately 10% of these people will develop TB disease at some point in their lives.[13] Paramedics should maintain a high degree of suspicion for TB in persons with undiagnosed pulmonary disease, especially in patients who are HIV seropositive.

TB Testing

Although the signs and symptoms of initial infection may be minimal, early infection can be detected using the Mantoux tuberculin skin test (purified protein derivative [PPD]). A positive reaction to the PPD test indicates past infection and the presence of antibodies. Patients who test positive generally will receive a chest x-ray and an acid-fast bacilli (AFB) sputum culture before treatment. Counseling and HIV-antibody testing should be offered to all TB-infected persons, because medical management may be altered in the presence of HIV. By law, tuberculosis reporting is required in every state.

NOTE

A negative TB skin test does not absolutely rule out TB infection, especially in persons with TB-like symptoms, HIV, or AIDS. In these cases, a repeat skin test may be warranted 10 weeks postexposure.

NOTE

Because identification and early treatment of TB are important, all health care workers should receive a routine evaluation consisting of PPD, and in some cases, chest x-ray and AFB.[1] A negative immune response does not preclude reinfection with subsequent exposure.

Patient Care and Protective Measures

Prehospital care for patients with infectious TB primarily is supportive. As with any other infectious disease, universal precautions (including respiratory barriers for patient and paramedic) should be taken during the patient-care encounter. Paramedics should be aware of those populations with a significant prevalence of active TB in their jurisdictions (as reported by local public health authorities) and use National Institute of Occupational Safety and Health (NIOSH)-approved particulate filter respirators (Fig. 37-6 and the box on p. 1123, left column). After each call, disinfection should be practiced at all levels. Other methods for preventing exposure to droplet nuclei during patient transport include enhancing ventilation by opening windows on both sides of the ambulance and operating the vehicle's air-conditioning system on a nonrecirculating cycle.[15] A mask should be placed on the patient during transport to minimize exposure risk to the paramedic.

NOTE

A surgical mask is insufficient for preventing tuberculosis bacteria from escaping or from being inhaled.

Treatment

Tuberculosis usually is curable if effective treatment is instituted without delay. Because of the increase in multidrug-resistant TB (see the box on p. 1123, right column), most persons with TB are started on a lengthy four-drug regimen of isoniazid (INH), rifampin (RIF), pyrazinamide (PZA), and ethambutol (EMB) or streptomycin (SM) until the drug susceptibility results are known. (Patients given preventative therapy should be monitored for drug side effects, especially for signs and symptoms of hepatitis.) Positive-to-negative sputum conversion and results of culture are usually available 3 to 8 weeks after beginning therapy.

TB-PROTECTIVE RESPIRATORS

OSHA (in conjunction with CDC guidelines) currently requires the use of respirators and is enforcing their use while developing specific standards for preventing TB exposure to health care workers. The required NIOSH-certified respirator must have a disposable (or replaceable), high-efficiency particulate air (HEPA) filter capable of trapping airborne particles. Whenever respirators (including disposables) are required, a complete respiratory protection program must be implemented in accordance with 29 CFR 1910.134. Elements of the required respiratory protection program include:

1. Permissible practices for respirator use
2. Respirator program administration
3. Respiratory selection
4. Inspection of respirators
5. Cleaning and maintenance of respirators
6. Storage of respirators
7. Training in respiratory protection
8. Fit testing of respirators (ensuring accurate sizing)
9. Respirator program evaluation
10. Medical surveillance of respirator users

Source: *NIOSH guide to the selection and use of particulate respirators certified under 42 CFR 84*, DHHS (NIOSH) Publication No. 96-101, 1996.

NOTE

Patients with TB may be noncompliant with medication therapy and may remain infected or develop resistant strains of the disease.

Prophylactic INH

Prophylactic INH is recommended for persons less than 35 years of age who are PPD skin-test positive and have not previously been treated. Isoniazid is not routinely recommended for persons younger than 35 years old because of its hepatic complications, unless one or more of the following is present[1]:

- Recent infection as evidenced by PPD skin test conversion
- Close or household contact with a known case of infectious TB
- Abnormal chest x-ray

MULTIDRUG-RESISTANT TUBERCULOSIS

During the resurgence of TB in the United States, outbreaks of multidrug-resistant TB (MDR-TB) occurred in hospitals and prisons, resulting in high death rates and transmission to health care workers.

Multidrug-resistant TB is resistant to conventional drugs (isoniazid and rifampin) and is an extremely serious aspect of TB because there is limited preventive therapy. Persons at high risk for MDR-TB include:

- Those recently exposed to MDR-TB (especially if they are immunocompromised)
- Tuberculosis patients who fail to take medications as prescribed
- Tuberculosis patients who were prescribed an ineffective treatment regimen
- Patients previously treated for TB

A major cause of treatment failure and drug-resistant TB is nonadherence to treatment. This threatens the health of TB patients and poses a serious public health risk, leading to prolonged infectiousness and the spread of TB within the community.

- Prolonged therapy with immunosuppressant drugs
- HIV or other immunosuppressive disease

Patients receiving INH should avoid alcohol to decrease the likelihood of chemical- or drug-induced hepatitis. (Patients receiving INH should also avoid pregnancy.) Side effects of INH include paresthesias, seizures (toxic reaction), orthostatic hypotension, nausea and vomiting, hepatitis, and hypersensitivity to the drug.

Meningococcal Meningitis

Meningococcal meningitis (also known as *spinal meningitis*) refers to inflammation of the membranes that surround the spinal cord and brain. It can be caused by a variety of different bacteria, viruses, and other microorganisms (see Table 37-3). A major cause of bacterial meningitis is *Neisseria meningitidis*, which like *M. tuberculosis*, is spread by airborne pathogens. The usual mode of transmission is prolonged, direct contact with upper respiratory secretions (discharge from the nose and throat) from an infected person or carrier. Once inhaled, the bacteria invade the respiratory passages and travel by way of blood to the brain and spinal cord. As the infecting agent spreads to additional organs, it causes toxic manifestations in the involved organ system.

> **NOTE**
>
> An estimated 2% to 10% of the population may carry meningococci at any one time.[1] The pathogen generally is prevented from invading the meninges and gaining access to the cerebrospinal fluid by the throat's epithelial lining. Although the conversion from carrier to clinical disease is rare in developed countries, outbreaks of disease in the United States have increased since the 1990s partly because of increased rates of disease in persons who may have a common organizational affiliation or who live in the same community.[16]

Other Infectious Agents Known to Cause Meningitis

Other common pathogens that cause meningitis include *Streptococcus pneumoniae* and *Haemophilus influenza*e type b (Hib), and some viruses. *Streptococcus pneumoniae* is the second most common cause of bacterial meningitis in adults, the most common cause of pneumonia in adults, and the most common cause of otitis media (middle ear infection) in children. This bacteria is spread by droplets, prolonged personal contact, or contact with linen soiled with respiratory discharges. (Episodic contact rarely results in infection.)

H. influenza has the same mode of transmission as *N. meningitidis*. Before the introduction of vaccines for children in 1981, *H. influenza* was the leading cause of bacterial meningitis in children aged 6 months to 3 years. (This bacteria is also responsible for conditions such as pediatric epiglottitis, septic arthritis, and generalized sepsis.) Although this type of meningitis can be treated effectively with antibiotics, 50% of all infected children with bacterial meningitis specific to *H. influenza* will have long-term neurologic sequelae.

> **NOTE**
>
> Fortunately, none of the bacteria that cause meningitis are as contagious as the common cold or flu. In addition, they are not spread by casual contact or by simply breathing the air where a person with meningitis has been.[16]

Viral meningitis (aseptic meningitis) is a syndrome generally associated with an existing systemic viral disease (e.g., enterovirus, HSV, mumps, and, less commonly, influenza). Toxic and meningeal symptoms are similar to those of bacterial meningitis (described below), but usually are less severe. In most cases, viral meningitis is self-limited with complete recovery. The patient may experience muscle weakness and malaise during prolonged convalescence. Viral meningitis is not considered to be communicable.

Signs and Symptoms

Signs and symptoms of meningitis depend on the age and general health of the patient. In infants, for example, signs of meningeal irritation may be absent or include only irritability, poor feeding or vomiting, a high-pitched cry, and fullness of the fontanelle. (Maternal antibodies generally protect neonates to 6 months of age.) In older infants and children, signs of meningitis may include the presence of malaise, low-grade fever, projectile vomiting, petechial rash, headache, and stiff neck from meningeal irritation (nuchal rigidity) (Box 37-8). If there is extensive meningeal involvement in a toxic or debilitated patient, the illness may be accompanied by acute adrenal insufficiency, convulsions, coma, and disseminated intravascular coagulation (Waterhouse-Friderichsen syndrome), associated with hemorrhage into the adrenal glands causing adrenal insufficiency; death can ensue in 6 to 8 hours. Other conditions and long-term complications associated with severe cases of meningitis include blindness and deafness (from cranial nerve damage), arthritis, myocarditis, and pericarditis. Death can follow overwhelming infection.

> **? CRITICAL THINKING**
>
> *What does a petechial rash look like?*

> **NOTE**
>
> The risk of bacterial meningitis is most significant in neonates and children between 6 months and 2 years of age. However, infection should be suspected in any patient with fever, headache, stiff neck, altered mental status, or underlying health problems (e.g., recent neurosurgery, trauma, or immunocompromise).

Immunization and Control Measures

Vaccines are available for Hib, some strains of *N. meningitidis,* and many types of *S. pneumoniae.* The vaccines against Hib are very safe and highly effective. By 6 months of age, infants should have received at least 3 doses of an Hib vaccine; a fourth dose ("booster") is recommended between 12 and 18 months of age. Vaccine against some strains of *N. meningitidis* is not routinely used in the United States and is not effective in children under 18 months of age.[16] However, the vaccine is sometimes used to control outbreaks of some types of meningococcal meningitis. Vaccines to prevent meningitis caused by *S. pneumoniae* also can prevent other forms of infection due to the bacterium. Although this vaccine is ineffective for children under 2 years of age, it is recommended for all persons over age 65 (and younger persons with certain chronic medical problems).

> **NOTE**
>
> Vaccines against meningitis have been instrumental in preventing outbreaks of the disease among military recruits in the United States, which before 1971, was a common occurrence.[1]

Patient Management and Protective Measures

Patient management is focused on ensuring adequate airway, ventilatory, and circulatory support. The paramedic should use protective measures when caring for patients who have signs and symptoms suggestive of meningitis. Universal and BSI precautions (with surgical masks applied to the patient) are indicated during care and transport. Post-EMS exposure activities should be addressed as part of an agency Exposure Control Plan.

Early diagnosis and treatment of bacterial meningitis is very important. The diagnosis usually is confirmed by identifying the type of bacteria responsible from a sample of spinal fluid obtained through a spinal tap (lumbar puncture). The disease

> **NOTE**
>
> Meningitis should always be considered a true medical emergency. A primary goal of emergency treatment is to administer an appropriate antibiotic agent 30 to 60 minutes after arriving at the emergency department.

> **BOX 37-8**
>
> ### DIAGNOSTIC SIGNS OF MENINGITIS IN OLDER CHILDREN
>
> *Brudzinski's sign:* An involuntary flexion of the arm, hip, and knee when the neck is passively flexed.
>
> *Kernig's sign:* Loss of the ability of a seated or supine patient to completely extend the leg when the thigh is flexed on the abdomen. The patient, however, usually can extend the leg completely when the thigh is not flexed on the abdomen.

is then treated using several antibiotics. Prophylactic drug treatments are available for individuals who may have intimate contact with the patient (e.g., family members).

Pneumonia

As described in Chapter 27, pneumonia is an acute inflammatory process of the respiratory bronchioles and alveoli. Routes of transmission include droplet spread and direct and indirect contact with respiratory secretions (see Table 37-3). Etiologic agents responsible for this disease may be bacterial (*S. pneumoniae, M. pneumoniae, Staphylococcus. aureus, H. influenzae, Klebsiella pneumoniae, Moraxella catarrhalis, Legionella*), viral, or fungal. These organisms may affect several body systems, including the respiratory system (pneumonia); the CNS (meningitis); and the ears, nose, and throat (otitis, pharyngitis media). The signs and symptoms of pneumonia include the following:

- Sudden onset of chills, high-grade fever, chest pain with respirations, dyspnea
- Tachypnea and chest retractions (an ominous sign in children)
- Congestion from the development of purulent alveolar exudates in one or more lobes
- A productive cough with yellow-green phlegm

Susceptibility and Resistance

Susceptibility to pneumonia is increased by processes such as smoking, pulmonary edema, influenza, exposure to inhaled toxins, chronic lung disease, and aspiration from any form (postalcohol ingestion, near-drowning, regurgitation caused by gastric distention from gag-valve mask ventilation). Extremes of age also appear to increase susceptibility to the disease (e.g., elderly persons, infants with low birth weight and/or malnourishment). Other high-risk groups for pneumonia include persons with the following:

- Sickle cell disease
- Cardiovascular disease
- Asplenia (congenital absence or surgical removal of a spleen)
- Diabetes
- Chronic renal failure (or other kidney disease)
- HIV
- Organ transplantation
- Multiple myeloma, lymphoma, Hodgkin's disease

Patient Management and Protective Measures

Prehospital care for patients with pneumonia includes providing airway support, oxygen, ventilatory assistance (as needed), IV fluids, cardiac monitoring, and transport for physician evaluation. Bacterial pneumonia is usually managed using analgesics, decongestants, expectorants, and antibiotic therapy. Patient isolation generally is not warranted except in clinical facilities where a patient with a resistant strain of pneumonia may be in contact with other patients who have increased susceptibility to infection.

> **? CRITICAL THINKING**
> *Which locations in your area are at high risk for influenza outbreaks?*

Measures for protecting health care workers include BSI precautions and effective hand washing. Although immunizations exist for some causes of pneumonia, they generally are not recommended for persons who come in contact with patients who have the disease.

Tetanus

Tetanus is a serious, sometimes fatal, disease of the CNS caused by infection of a wound with spores of *Clostridium tetani*. Although tetanus spores live mainly in soil and manure, they are also found in the human intestine. If the spores enter tissue (e.g., via a puncture wound or burn), they multiply and produce a toxin that acts on the nerves controlling muscular activity. (Dead or necrotic tissue is a favorable environment for *C. tetani*.) Approximately 500,000 cases of tetanus occur worldwide each year, with a mortality rate of 45%—often from wounds that appear too trivial for medical evaluation. Only about 100 cases of tetanus are reported annually in the United States (they occur most often in patients 50 years of age or older). The relatively low number of tetanus cases in the United States is a result of immunizing the general population with tetanus vaccines.[17]

Signs and Symptoms

The most common symptom of tetanus is trismus (stiffness of the jaw); it is also known as "lockjaw," because of the accompanying difficulty in opening the mouth. Other symptoms include:

- Muscular tetany (muscle spasms and twitching)
- Painful muscular contractions in the neck, moving to the trunk
- Abdominal rigidity (often the first sign in pediatric patients)
- Painful spasms (contortions) of the face (*risus sardonicus*), producing a grotesque smile
- Respiratory failure

Patient Management and Protective Measures

Prehospital care goals are to support vital functions, which may include aggressive airway management (intubation and surgical or needle cricothyrotomy). Muscle spasms should be treated with *diazepam* (Valium), benzodiazepines, or paralytic agents (as per medical direction). Drugs that may also be indicated to manage a patient with tetanus include IV

> **NOTE**
>
> Patients who have experienced a recent wound should be counseled regarding postinjury tetanus prophylaxis and effective wound care. All patients should be questioned regarding their tetanus immunization status. (Boosters should be given every 10 years—5 years for a "dirty" wound.) A subsequent recovery from infection does not confer immunity.

fluids, *magnesium sulfate*, narcotics, and antidysrhythmics. After physician evaluation and stabilization, care for patients with tetanus will include administration of antitoxin (tetanus immunoglobulin [TIG]) to provide postexposure passive immunity, treatment to eliminate the toxin, active immunization with tetanus toxoid, and wound care. Most patients recover completely after receiving prompt treatment.

Immunization

Immunization against tetanus generally is begun during childhood using DPT vaccination—a combined immunization against diphtheria (laryngitis, pharyngitis with discharge), pertussis (whooping cough), and tetanus. The initial immunization is followed by a booster before entry into elementary school and thereafter every 10 years.

Rabies

Rabies (also known as *hydrophobia*) is an acute viral infection of the CNS. Although the disease primarily affects animals, it can be transmitted from an infected animal to a human through virus-laden saliva (e.g., via a bite or scratch). (Transmission from person to person is theoretical but has never been documented.[1]) In the United States, wildlife rabies is common in skunks, raccoons, bats, foxes, dogs, wolves, jackals, mongooses, and coyotes. Hawaii is the only rabie-free state in the United States.

Humans are highly susceptible to the rabies virus after being exposed to saliva from a bite or scratch of an infected animal. Several factors govern the severity of infection, including:

- Severity of the wound
- Richness of nerve supply close to the wound
- Distance from the wound to the CNS
- Amount and strain of the virus
- Degree of protective clothing

Signs and Symptoms

The incubation period between bite and appearance of symptoms varies from 9 days to 7 years[1] (see Table 37-3). Initial symptoms include low-grade fever, headache, loss of appetite, hyperactivity, disorientation, and in some cases, seizures. Often, the patient will have intense thirst, but attempts to drink will induce violent and painful spasms in the throat (thus the name *hydrophobia*). Eye and facial muscles may become paralyzed as the disease progresses. Without medical intervention, the disease lasts 2 to 6 days, often resulting in death secondary to respiratory failure.

Patient Management and Protective Measures

After evaluation by a physician, signs and symptoms of the disease are treated with respiratory and cardiovascular support (as needed), and the administration of sedatives and analgesics. Thorough debridement of the wound without sutures (if possible) is

> **NOTE**
>
> Airborne spread of rabies virus has been documented in bat caves (rare). Transmission from vampire bats who bite domestic animals is common in Latin America.

> **NOTE**
>
> Healthy, wild animals (e.g., skunks) are seldom seen by casual observance. A high degree of suspicion for rabies is indicated for all animals found outside of their natural habitat.

> **NOTE**
>
> If given within 2 days of the bite, immunizations will almost always prevent rabies.

indicated to permit free bleeding and drainage. Passive immunization may be given with human rabies immune globulin, and a rabies vaccine (Human Diploid Rabies Vaccine, Rabies Vaccine) is given by a course of injections lasting several weeks. (Injections are no longer administered in the stomach.) Tetanus prophylaxis and antibiotics may be indicated for the bite wound.

Most cases of rabies in humans are the result of dog bites from a rabid dog. The possibility of rabies, however, must be considered with *all* mammal bites. Scene safety and use of BSI precautions during wound management are paramount. Contact law enforcement personnel and animal-control authorities to assist in scene control. Immunizations should be given for contact with open wounds or for exposure of mucous membranes to saliva. Immunizations also should be given to persons with high probability of contact with animal reservoirs (e.g., animal care workers, animal shelter personnel, and outdoor workers). If an animal is suspected of being rabid, it should be killed by proper authorities, and its brain should be examined for the presence of rabies inclusion bodies. In the absence of these inclusion bodies, the patient's rabies treatment will be stopped.

Hantavirus

Hantavirus was previously known to be associated with hemorrhagic fever with renal syndrome that occurs in Asia. Hantaviruses also are associated with a syndrome of severe respiratory distress and shock occurring in persons in several areas of the United States.[17] The virus is carried by rodents and is transmitted via inhalation of aerosols of material contaminated with rodent urine and feces (see Table 37-3). Many forms of this disease occur in specific geographical areas.

> **NOTE**
>
> In 1994, a previously unknown hantavirus, thought to be transmitted from the deer mouse, was identified in the southwestern United States. It caused a pulmonary syndrome associated with tachycardia, hemoconcentration, and leukocytosis, and had a mortality rate that exceeded 50%.

Hantavirus can cause significant disease in humans. Patients are typically healthy adults who experience an onset of fever and malaise, followed several days later by respiratory distress. (The severity of the illness is determined by the strain of the virus.) Other signs and symptoms may include fever, chills, headache, and GI upset, and capillary hemorrhage. With severe infection, oliguria, kidney failure, and hypotension ensue. Death typically occurs from depressed cardiac output and eventual cardiovascular collapse. Treatment primarily is supportive and should be guided by medical direction. Body substance or BSI isolation precautions are indicated because of the infectious nature of these viruses.

Viral Diseases of Childhood

The childhood infectious diseases presented in this chapter include rubella (German measles), rubeola (red measles or hard measles), mumps (parotitis), chickenpox (varicella), and pertussis (whooping cough). These infectious diseases are preventable with immunization for chickenpox and with the triple immunization measles, mumps, and rubella (MMR) vaccine. The incidence of these childhood infectious diseases has decreased secondary to widespread immunization of children. Immunization provides long-lasting immunity and is known to be 98% to 99% effective.

> **NOTE**
>
> All health care workers should use personal protective measures when caring for children with viral infections. Protective immunization, effective hand washing, BSI (including the use of surgical masks for both the paramedic and the patient), and being cautious about handling linens, supplies, and equipment that may be contaminated are important in preventing the spread of these diseases.

Rubella

Rubella is a mild, febrile, and highly communicable viral disease (caused by the *Rubella virus*), characterized by a diffuse punctate macular rash (Fig. 37-7). The disease usually is transmitted by direct contact with nasopharyngeal secretions or droplet spray from an infected person. It also may be transmitted transplacentally (producing active infection in the fetus) and by contact with articles contaminated with blood, urine, or feces. After inoculation, the virus invades the lymph system. From there, it enters the blood and produces an immune response, and the subsequent rash spreads from forehead to face to torso to extremities (lasting 3 days). Maximal communicability appears to be the first few days before and 5 to 7 days after the onset of rash. Although complications from the disease are rare, young females sometimes develop a self-limiting arthritis (see Table 37-3).

NOTE

A rash that lasts more than 3 days indicates the presence of rubeola.

NOTE

Immunization is not recommended for pregnant women because of the theoretical risk of the vaccine causing developmental defects.

? CRITICAL THINKING

Is there any way for a paramedic to avoid rubella other than immunization?

Congenital rubella syndrome (CRS) affects approximately 90% of infants born to women who were infected with rubella during the first trimester of pregnancy.[1] The disease is associated with multiple congenital anomalies, mental retardation, deafness, and an increased risk of death from congenital heart disease and sepsis during the first 6 months of life. The CDC recommends that all health care providers receive immunization if they are not immune from previous rubella infection to reduce the risk of exposure to themselves and those they treat.

NOTE

Infants with CRS shed large quantities of virus in their secretions.

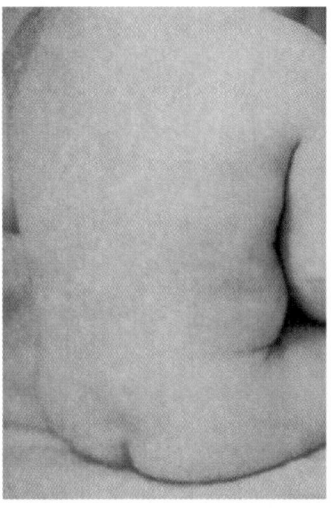

Fig. 37-7 Acquired rubella (German measles) in an 11-month-old infant. (Courtesy The Centers for Disease Control, 1990. In Grimes D: *Infectious diseases,* St Louis, 1991, Mosby.)

As a precaution, pregnant EMS providers should not be exposed to patients with rubella.

Rubeola

Rubeola (caused by the measles virus) is an acute, highly communicable viral disease characterized by fever, conjunctivitis, cough, bronchitis, and a blotchy red rash (Fig. 37-8). The virus is found in the blood, urine, and pharyngeal secretions. The disease usually is transmitted directly or indirectly through contact with infected respiratory secretions. After exposure, the virus invades the respiratory epithelium and spreads via the lymph system. Rubeola may predispose to secondary bacterial complications such as otitis media, pneumonia, and myocarditis. The most serious life-threatening complication is subacute sclerosing panencephalitis (a slowly progressing neurological disease marked by deterioration of mental capacity and muscle coordination).

Early (prodromal) symptoms that mark the onset of disease include high fever, nasal discharge, conjunctivitis, photophobia, and cough (see Table 37-3). A day or two before the rash, patients with rubeola usually have white spots on the internal cheek (Koplik's spots). The dermal rash begins a few days after respiratory tract involvement and is red, maculopapular, and spreads from the forehead to the face, neck, torso, and eventually to feet by

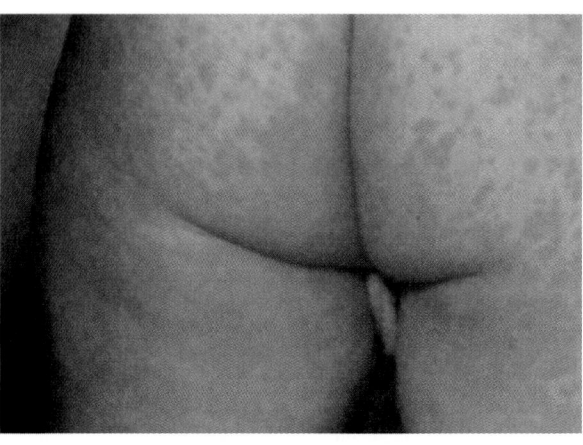

Fig. 37-8 Rubeola (measles) rash on the third day. (Courtesy The Centers for Disease Control, 1990. In Grimes D: *Infectious diseases,* St Louis, 1991, Mosby.)

the third day. (The onset of rash coincides with the production of serum antibodies.) Uncomplicated cases of rubeola usually last 6 days. Immunity acquired after illness is lifelong.

Mumps

Mumps (caused by the mumps virus) is an acute, communicable systemic viral disease characterized by localized unilateral or bilateral edema of one or more of the salivary glands (usually the parotid), with occasional involvement of other glands (Fig. 37-9). The virus is transmitted via direct contact with the saliva droplets of an infected person (see Table 37-3).

The virus invades and multiplies in the parotid gland or epithelium of the upper respiratory passages. From there, it enters the blood and localizes in glandular or nervous tissue. The parotid, testes, and pancreas are the most frequently involved glands. When mumps occurs after the onset of puberty, it may cause a painful inflammation of the testicle (orchitis) and testicular atrophy; however, sterility is rare. The intensity of symptoms in mumps is variable; 30% of infections are asymptomatic. Immunity after clinical and subclinical disease is lifelong. Placental transfer of antibodies sometimes occurs.

? CRITICAL THINKING

Why are selected cases of these diseases still seen despite community immunization?

Chickenpox

Chickenpox (caused by the varicella-zoster virus) is a common childhood disease. The illness is caused by a member of the herpesvirus family and is transmitted by direct and indirect contact with droplets (mainly airborne) from respiratory passages of an infected person. (Exposure to linen tainted with vesicle or mucous membrane discharges of infected persons has been implicated.[1])

Chickenpox is highly communicable (see Table 37-3) and is characterized by a sudden onset of low-grade fever, mild malaise, and a skin eruption that is maculopapular for a few hours and vesicular for 3 to 4 days, leaving a granular scab (Fig. 37-10). Initially, the skin lesions appear on the trunk and usually progress to the extremities. The crops of skin eruptions (each associated with itching) generally are more abundant on covered areas of the body; the scalp, conjunctivae, and upper respiratory tract may also be affected. The appearance of crops of vesicles (fresh vesicles appearing while other lesions are scabbed) differentiates chickenpox from smallpox, which has vesicles of the same age. Treatment is symptomatic, and the disease is self-limited. Complications may include secondary bacterial infections, aseptic meningitis, mononucleosis, and Reye syndrome.

NOTE

Children with chickenpox should be isolated from schools, medical offices, emergency departments, and public places until all lesions are crusted and dry.

After recovery, the virus is thought to remain in the body in an asymptomatic latent stage (possibly localized in the dorsal root ganglia). The virus may reactivate during periods of stress or immunosuppression, producing an illness known as shingles. The vesicles associated with shingles are restricted to the skin area supplied by the sensory nerves of a single group or associated groups of dorsal root ganglia. Unlike chickenpox, shingles is not transmitted through respiratory droplets, but it can cause chickenpox in susceptible individuals who are in contact with open (not yet scabbed) skin lesions.

Antiviral drugs may shorten the duration of symptoms and pain in older patients. EMS workers who have not had chickenpox should consider receiving the chickenpox vaccine. Data indicate that

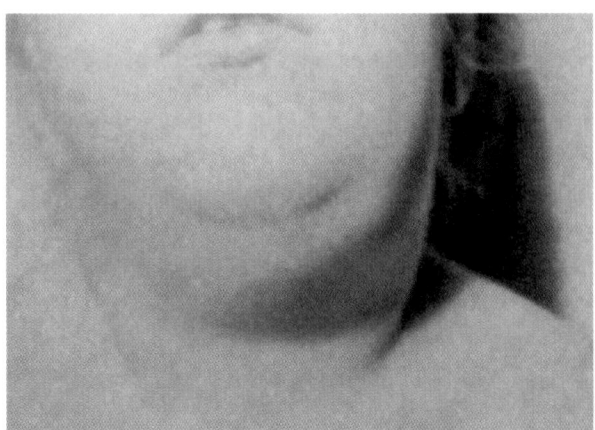

Fig. 37-9 Submaxillary mumps in an infant. (Courtesy The Centers for Disease Control, 1990. In Grimes D: *Infectious diseases*, St Louis, 1991, Mosby.)

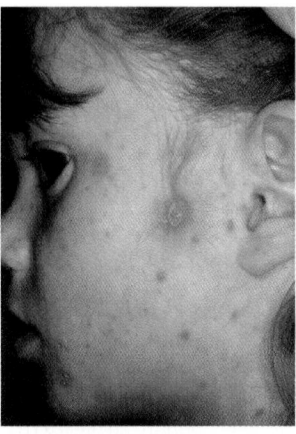

Fig. 37-10 Chickenpox skin lesions. (Courtesy Gary Quick, M.D.)

adult antibody production occurs in 82% of patients after one dose and in 92% of patients after two doses. (Vaccine should not be given to persons receiving high doses of systemic steroids in the previous month.) Approximately 5% of patients who receive the vaccine develop rash, and some develop frank chickenpox, which is very debilitating in adults. Varicella zoster immune globulin (VZIG) is recommended for pregnant women with significant exposure to chickenpox (without history of previous exposure) to protect the fetus.

Pertussis

Pertussis (caused by *Bordetella pertussis*) is an infectious disease that mainly affects infants and young children (see Table 37-3). It is spread by direct contact by discharges from mucous membranes contained in airborne droplets. The disease causes inflammation of the entire respiratory tract and an insidious onset of cough that becomes paroxysmal in 1 to 2 weeks and lasts for 1 to 2 months. The coughing episodes are violent (sometimes without an intervening inhalation), causing the high-pitched inspiratory "whoop," and end with expulsion of clear mucus and vomiting. (The whoop often is not present in children younger than 6

> **NOTE**
>
> Pertussis vaccine usually is given in combination with diphtheria and tetanus (DPT) vaccines to children at 2, 4, and 6 months of age; a booster dose is given at age 5.

months of age.) Before the introduction of a vaccine against pertussis in the 1950s, the disease killed more children in the United States than all other infectious diseases combined.[18]

The communicability for pertussis is thought to be greatest before the onset of paroxysmal coughing (thus the need for BSI and surgical mask protection for paramedic and patient). Although erythromycin is known to decrease the communicability period, it can only reduce symptoms if given during the incubation period (before the onset of paroxysmal cough). Infection with pertussis generally confers immunity; however, subsequent attacks after immunization in older children and adults indicate that immunity may wane over time.

Other Viral Diseases

Other viral diseases easily transmitted during the course of patient care include influenza, mononucleosis, and herpes simplex type 1 (described later in this chapter). Like all other contacts with patients who may have infectious disease, BSI precautions are indicated during patient-care encounters.

Influenza

As described in Chapter 27, influenza is a respiratory infection spread by influenza viruses A, B, and C (see Table 37-3). The disease is popularly known as "the flu" and is spread by virus-infected droplets that are coughed or sneezed into the air. Influenza

INFLUENZA VIRUS A, B, AND C

Persons infected with certain strains or influenza type A or B acquire immunity to that strain. The A- and B-type viruses, however, occasionally alter to produce new strains, leading to a new infection. Although type-B virus is relatively stable, it occasionally alters to overcome resistance and may lead to small outbreaks of infection. Type A-virus is highly unstable and has caused worldwide flu epidemics. These variants are named for geographical site and year of isolation (e.g., the Spanish flu in 1918, Asian flu in 1957, and the Hong Kong flu in 1968) and the culture number (e.g., A/Japan/305/57). Type C-virus stimulates antibodies that provide immunity for life.

zanamivir (Relenza) may be given to hospitalized patients to protect against influenza A. Despite advances in prevention and treatment, approximately 20,000 people die each year in the United States from influenza and its complications.[19]

NOTE

Health care workers should be immunized in the fall of each year with the current influenza vaccine.

? CRITICAL THINKING

Will you get the influenza vaccine? What influenced your decision?

usually occurs in small outbreaks, or every few years in epidemics. Resistance is normally conferred after recovery, but only to the specific strain or variant (Box 37-9).

Signs and symptoms typically include chills, fever, headache, muscular aches, loss of appetite, and fatigue. These symptoms are followed by upper respiratory infection and cough (which often is severe and protracted) lasting for 2 to 7 days. Patient management primarily is supportive, and mild cases of the virus generally are not treated. Severe cases (particularly in the elderly and those with lung or heart disease) may result in secondary bacterial infection (e.g., *S. pneumonia*) and can be fatal.

NOTE

Other viral respiratory diseases that can lead to bacterial complications include acute afebrile viral respiratory disease (excluding influenza) and acute febrile respiratory disease. Both diseases may cause illnesses in the upper and lower respiratory tract, including pharyngitis, laryngitis, croup, bronchitis, and bronchiolitis.

Antiinfluenza vaccines (containing killed strains of type A and B virus currently in circulation) may help prevent infection. Immunity, however, is short-lived, and the vaccine must be repeated each year just before the start of "flu season" (November to March in the United States). Amantadine (Symmetrel, Symadine), rimantadine (Flumadine), or

Mononucleosis

Mononucleosis (often referred to as "mono") is caused either by Epstein-Barr virus (EBV) or by cytomegalovirus (CMV)—both members of the herpesvirus family (see Table 37-3). Mononucleosis is spread from person to person via the oropharyngeal route and saliva (thus the name *kissing disease*). (Although blood transfusions also can be a mode of transmission, resultant clinical disease is rare.) Most people with a healthy immune system are able to fend off the infection, even after significant exposure. Transmission from care providers to young children is common.[1]

NOTE

Approximately 90% of people over age 35 have antibodies to the CMV or EBV virus in their blood, probably as a result of mild, childhood infection (often passed off as a common cold or the flu). Previous infection by EBV generally confers a high degree of resistance to future exposures.

Signs and symptoms appear gradually and are characterized by fever (which may last for weeks), sore throat, oropharyngeal discharges, lymphadenopathy (especially posterior cervical), and splenomegaly with abdominal tenderness. Approximately 10% of people will also develop a generalized rash or darkened areas in the mouth, which resemble bruises. Although recovery usually occurs in a few weeks, some people take months to regain their former level of energy. The patient may remain a carrier for several months after symptoms disappear. Immunization for mononucleosis is not available.

Sexually Transmitted Diseases

Sexually transmitted diseases (STDs) are a group of disease syndromes that can be transmitted sexually, regardless of whether the disease has genital pathological manifestations. More than 20 etiological agents have been identified as belonging to this group of diseases (including HBV and HIV). Other common STDs include syphilis, gonorrhea, chlamydia, and herpesvirus infections.

Several pathogenic agents are responsible for the host of STDs, including bacteria, viruses, protozoa, fungi, and ectoparasites. These pathogens can produce multiple disease syndromes, and patients with STD syndromes frequently have multiple STDs. These infections usually result in a short-lived cellular immune response and a longer-lasting humoral antibody response—neither of which protects against future exposures.

Syphilis

Syphilis is a systemic disease characterized by a primary lesion, a secondary eruption involving skin and mucous membranes, long latency periods, and late seriously disabling lesions of the skin, bone, viscera, CNS, and cardiovascular system. The disease is caused by penetration of *Treponema pallidum* into intact mucous membranes or abraded skin. Common modes of transmission include direct contact with exudate from lesions on skin and mucous membranes, blood transfusions/needle sticks (rare), and congenital transmission. After penetration, the organisms travel (within hours) to lymph nodes, where they are disseminated throughout the body. After the initial infection, syphilis follows well-defined stages of disease (see Table 37-3). Syphilis is treatable with antibiotic therapy. No immunization is available.

NOTE

Estimates are that 30% of exposures result in infection.

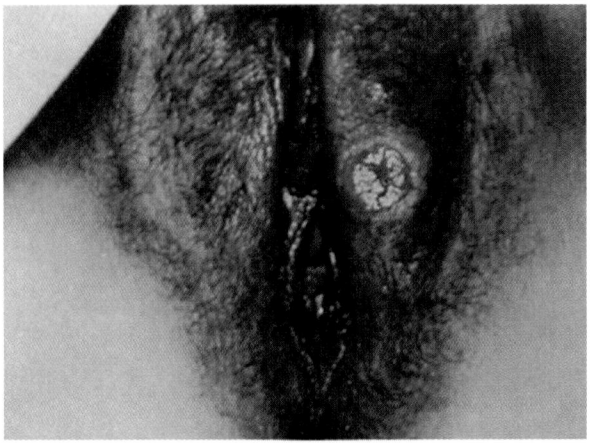

Fig. 37-11 Primary syphilis chancre on the labia.

Primary Stage

Within 10 to 90 days after exposure, a primary lesion or chancre develops at the site of initial invasion (Fig. 37-11). The surface of the chancre is usually crusted or ulcerated and varies in size from 1 to 2 cm in diameter. The lesion usually is single and painless, and it generally heals spontaneously within 1 to 5 weeks. Syphilis is highly communicable during this stage.

Secondary Stage

The secondary stage begins about 2 to 10 weeks after the appearance of the primary lesion and lasts for 2 to 6 weeks. This stage is heralded by systemic symptoms, including headache, malaise, anorexia, fever, sore throat, lymphadenopathy, and bald spots in the area of infection. In addition, the patient may develop a rash, which usually is bilaterally symmetrical and frequently involves the palms and soles. Painless, wartlike regions (*condyloma latum*), which are extremely infectious, may also be found in moist, warm sites (e.g., the inguinal area). The CNS, eyes, bones, joints, or kidneys may be affected during this stage.

? CRITICAL THINKING

Why do you think a patient at this stage of syphilis calls EMS?

Latency

A latency period (ranging from 1 to 40 years or more) follows the secondary stage in untreated persons. During latency, recurrent episodes of secondary-stage symptoms (in about 25% of cases) with subclinical infection may occur. Approximately 33% of these patients will progress to tertiary syphilis; the remainder will remain asymptomatic. Tertiary syphilis is infectious involvement of the skin, CNS, and cardiovascular systems and may include the following manifestations:

- Skin
  Granulomatous lesions (gummas) on skin (painless) and bone (painful)
- CNS
  Paresis
  Tabes dorsalis (spinal column degeneration characterized by wide gait and ataxia: "syphilitic shuffle")
  Loss of reflexes, pain, and temperature sensation
  Meningitis
  Psychosis
- Cardiovascular
  Cerebrovascular occlusion
  Dissecting aneurysm of ascending aorta
  Myocardial insufficiency; aortic necrosis (which can lead to aortic rupture and death)

Gonorrhea

Gonorrhea is caused by the sexually transmitted bacterium *Neisseria gonorrhoeae*, which is communicated by a purulent exudate from mucous membranes of an infected person. Other modes of transmission include maternal infection during pregnancy and transmission of the pathogen during birth. The disease occurs in men and women but differs in course, severity, and ease of recognition. Although gonorrhea often is treatable with antibiotics, some strains brought into the United States from other countries have resisted conventional antibiotic therapy. Immunization is not available.

> **NOTE**
>
> Antibodies develop after exposure, but only to the specific strain of gonorrhea that caused the infection. Subsequent reinfection by other strains can therefore occur.

Affected areas of the male anatomy are the urethra, Littre's gland, Cowper's gland, prostate gland, seminal vesicles, and epididymis. A sudden onset of dysuria, urgency, and frequency is seen several days after exposure (see Table 37-3). The associated urethral discharge rapidly becomes purulent and profuse. Direct spread of the infection may result in prostatitis, epididymitis, and seminal vesiculitis. Primary gonorrheal infections may also affect the pharynx, conjunctivae, and anus.

Affected areas of the female anatomy are the Bartholin glands, Skene glands, urethra, cervix, and fallopian tubes. More than 50% of infected women remain asymptomatic; others have a mucopurulent discharge that varies from scant to profuse. Contiguous spread of the disease may lead to endometritis, salpingitis, and parametritis (pelvic inflammatory disease) and the formation of tuboovarian abscesses. Complete or partial occlusion of the fallopian tubes may result in sterility and increased risk for ectopic pregnancy.

Between 1% and 3% of gonococcal infections become disseminated in the blood. This extension of the disease may produce septicemia, arthritis, endocarditis, meningitis, and skin lesions. In the bacteremic stage, the patient may complain of fever, chills, and malaise. Erythematous lesions are common, especially on the extremities, and may occur in clusters or singly.

Chlamydia

Chlamydia trachomatis is a major cause of sexually transmitted nonspecific urethritis (NSU) or nongonococcal genital infection. The disease is the most common sexually transmitted disease in the United State (an estimated 25% of men are carriers) and is the world's leading cause of preventable blindness.[1] Signs and symptoms are similar to gonorrhea, making differentiation difficult. No immunization is available.

In men, NSU may cause a penile discharge and complications such as swelling of the testes, which, if untreated, may lead to infertility. In women, NSU usually is symptomless but may cause a vaginal discharge or pain with urination, salpingitis, and cervicitis. Transmission occurs secondary to direct contact with exudates—either sexually or during birth (see Table 37-3). Chlamydial infections are treated with antibiotics.

Herpesvirus Infections

The herpes simplex virus (HSV) is one of four herpesviruses. The others include CMV, which is associated with mononucleosis, hepatitis, and severe systemic disease in the immunosuppressed host; EBV, which causes mononucleosis; and varicella-zoster virus, which causes chickenpox and shingles. This section of the text addresses only the HSVs associated with STDs.

Herpes Simplex Virus

The two antigenically distinct herpes simplex viral agents responsible for STDs are herpes simplex virus type 1 (HSV-1) and herpes simplex virus type 2 (HSV-2). Both pathogens may lead to herpes infection, and both can produce infection anywhere in the body. As a rule, HSV-1 most often is associated with herpes above the waist, whereas HSV-2 generally is associated with genital herpes. However, either type can cause disease in the genital area. Immunization is not available for either virus.

Herpes simplex virus is common in the United States, producing 300,000 to 500,000 new infections each year. (It is estimated that 70% to 90% of adults have antibodies against HSV-1.) The mode of transmission for HSV is strictly by skin-to-skin contact with an infected area of the body. The virus enters through a break in the skin or through mucous membranes. Sexual contact is not required for transmission. For example, touching the herpes virus may result in finger infection (herpetic whitlow), and many young children who experience oral herpes (HSV-1) probably contract the virus from a casual kiss from a parent or relative. The virus also may be spread to other external body sites by autoinoculation (e.g., lip to finger to genitalia). Initial HSV-1 transmission usually occurs by 4 years of age and is manifested by gingivostomatitis ("cold sores" or "fever blisters"). Initial HSV-2 transmission generally occurs during sexual activity and is manifested by painful vesicular lesions of the cervix, vulva, penis, rectum, anus, and mouth (depending on sexual practices).

? CRITICAL THINKING

Why do you think the incidence of herpetic whitlow in health care workers has declined over the last 10 years?

Once it is present in tissue, HSV produces an acute infection with self-limited tissue destruction. This "primary infection" produces a vesicular le-sion (blister) that heals spontaneously from the periphery without residual scarring. The virus, however, remains viable in the body despite circulating antibodies (see Table 37-3).

After the primary infection, the HSV enters the CNS (nearest the site of initial infection) and travels along sensory nerve pathways to a sensory nerve ganglion, where it remains in a latent stage until reactivated. When triggered by another infectious disease, menstruation, emotional stress, trauma, or immunosuppression, the virus reaches the epidermis by way of peripheral nerves and reproduces a recurrent infectious disease state that usually lasts from 4 to 10 days. The lesions generally appear in the area of initial inoculation. The number of lesions a person might experience during any given episode varies considerably.

Herpes simplex virus can remain dormant indefinitely. It is unknown why many infected people never exhibit the disease, whereas others experience a lifetime of periodic outbreaks. Antiviral agents such as acyclovir (Zovirax) may shorten the disease episode and may be useful as prophylactic agents in instances of frequent recurrence.

Lice and Scabies

Lice and scabies are potential health hazards for all health care providers. Both are medically important as potential vectors of communicable skin disease and systemic illness, as well as dermatitis and discomfort. (Other vector-borne illnesses [e.g., Lyme disease] are described in Chapter 34.)

Lice

Lice are small, wingless insects that are ectoparasites of birds and mammals. Most are host specific. Two of the species are human parasites: *Phthirus pubis*, the pubic or crab louse, and *Pediculus humanus*, which comes in two varieties—*P. h. capitis* (the head louse) and *P. h. corporis* (the body louse, which was involved in outbreaks of epidemic typhus and trench fever in WWI) (Fig. 37-12). There is a three-stage life cycle for lice: the eggs hatch in 7 to 10 days; the nymph stage lasts 7 to 13 days; and the egg-to-egg cycle lasts about 3 weeks.

Lice subsist on blood from the host and have mouths modified for piercing and sucking. During biting and feeding, secretions from the louse cause

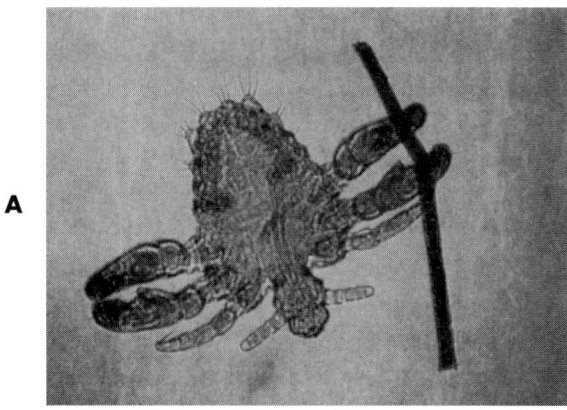
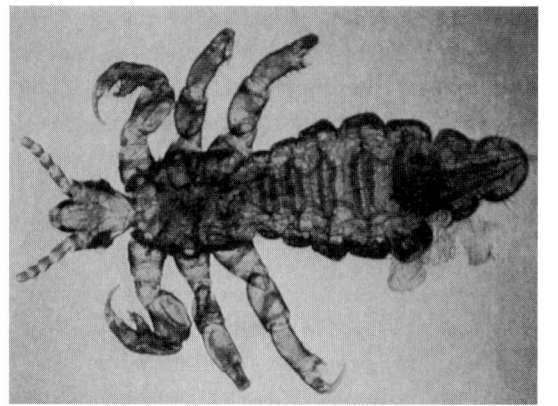

Fig. 37-12 A, The pubic or crab louse. **B,** Male of the human head louse.

a small, red macule and pruritus. Long infestation periods may bring a decrease in pruritus and often impart a thick, dry, scaly appearance to the skin. In severe cases, oozing and crusting may be present. If sensitization to lice saliva and feces occurs, inflammation may develop. Secondary infection may result from scratching of lesions. Lice spread through close personal contact and sharing of clothing and bedding may produce outbreaks (e.g., at school, daycare facilities, and within families).

Pubic lice have a distinctive appearance, suggestive of a miniature crab. Grayish-blue spots may be observed on the abdomen and thighs of infested patients. The eggs (nits or ova) often are evident on the shaft of pubic hairs and sometimes in eyelashes, eyebrows, and axillary hairs. Pubic lice usually are acquired during sexual activity or from unchanged bedding where egg-infested pubic hairs have been shed. Although primary bite lesions seldom are evident, the patient normally complains of intense pruritus and pubic scratching.

Head lice have an elongated body with a head that is slightly narrower than the thorax. Each louse has three pairs of legs, which possess delicate hooks at the distal extremities. The white ova of head lice (usually one nit to a shaft) are easily mistaken for dandruff, but the nits cannot be brushed out. These parasites most frequently affect children.

Body lice are slightly larger than head lice and concentrate around the waist, shoulders, axillae, and neck. Body lice and their nits usually are found in seams and on fibers of clothing. The lesions from their bites begin as small, noninflammatory red spots, which quickly become papular wheals that resemble linear scratch marks (parallel scratch

marks on the shoulders are a common finding). Head lice and body lice interbreed.

The treatment for all types of lice is designed to eradicate the parasites and nits and to prevent reinfestation. Patients usually are advised to wash thoroughly all clothing, bedding, and personal articles in hot water and to wash the infected body area with gamma benzene hexachloride shampoo (Kwell), crotamiton (Eurax), Rid, or Nix. (Overtreatment should be avoided to prevent toxicity.)

Scabies

The human scabies mite (*Sarcoptes scabiei var. hominis*) is a parasite that completes its entire life cycle in and on the epidermis of its host. Although scabies infestation resembles that of lice, scabies bites generally are concentrated around the hands and feet, especially between the webs of the fingers and toes. Other common infestation areas include the face and scalp of children, the nipples in females, and the penis in males. The scabies mite usually is passed by intimate contact or from infested bedding, furniture, and clothing. The mite can burrow into the skin in 2.5 minutes.[1]

Scabies infestation often is manifested by severe nocturnal pruritus, although it takes 4 to 6 weeks for sensitization to develop and itching to begin. The adult female mite is responsible for symptoms. After impregnation, she burrows into the epidermis to lay her eggs and remains in the burrow for a life span of about 1 month. Although vesicles and papules form at the surface, they often are disguised by the results of scratching. In severe cases (e.g., Norwegian scabies), oozing, crusting, and secondary infection may result. Susceptibility is general, but people with a previous exposure usually develop fewer mites on successive exposures and experience symptoms earlier (in 1 to 4 days).

Treatment is similar to that prescribed for lice infestation. Symptoms may persist for more than 1 month until the mite and mite products are shed with the epidermis. (Mites are communicable until all mites and eggs are destroyed.) Because reinfestation is common, the patient should be reexamined if the itching has not abated after several weeks. Antibiotic therapy may be needed to treat secondary bacterial infection. Immunization is not available (Box 37-10).

Reporting an Exposure to an Infectious/Communicable Disease

As previously discussed, all suspected exposures to an infectious or communicable disease must be reported to the DO (Box 37-11). Reporting a possible exposure is important for the following reasons[1]:

1. It permits immediate medical follow up, permitting identification of infection and immediate intervention.

2. It enables the DO to evaluate the circumstances surrounding the incident and to implement engineering or procedural changes to avoid future exposures.
3. It facilitates follow-up testing of the source individual if permission for testing can be obtained.

NOTE

Under provisions of the Ryan White Act, an exposed employee has the right to request the infection status of the source patient from the patient's health care provider, but neither the agency nor the employee can force testing of the source individual. As part of an effective exposure control plan, employees must know what to do if an exposure incident occurs.

✓ TRICKS OF THE TRADE

If you think you may have been exposed to a communicable disease, report it! It's your responsibility—it's *your* health!

? CRITICAL THINKING

How do you think you would feel, if after being stuck by a contaminated needle, a patient refused HIV testing?

NOTE

Reporting also ensures that if the health care worker converts to a positive communicable disease status, it can be appropriately documented that the injury occurred from a work-related exposure.

Whom To Report To

The Ryan White Act stipulates that an employer will designate a person or officer within the organization to whom exposed employees will report. That officer will then initiate those elements of the exposure control plan to comply with standards and guidelines relative to the exposure and follow any local reporting requirements.

Medical Evaluation and Follow-Up

By law, employers must provide free medical evaluation and treatment to exposed employees to include the following:

- Counseling regarding the risks, signs and symptoms, probability of developing clinical disease, and how to prevent future spread of the potential infection
- Appropriate treatment in line with current U.S. Public Health Service recommendations
- A discussion of medications offered and their side effects and contraindications
- Evaluation of any reported illness to determine whether the symptoms are related to HIV or hepatitis

Steps Involved

Blood tests of exposed employees are always contingent on employee agreement. Employees have the option to provide blood samples but can refuse permission for HIV testing at the time the sample is drawn. The employer must maintain the blood samples for 90 days in case employees change their mind regarding testing if HIV- or hepatitis-like symptoms develop.

As an agent of the employer, a health care provider (1) must provide counseling to the employee based on test results, (2) must provide informed consent regarding prophylaxis to therapeutic regimens, and (3) must implement those regimens after receiving approval from the employee. Vaccines also should be made available to all employees who are occupationally exposed to blood and other potentially infectious materials.

Written Report and Confidentiality

The health care provider will provide a written report to the DO of the employer, which identifies whether a vaccination was offered to the exposed employee and whether the employee received it. The written report also must note that the employee was informed of the results of the evaluation and told of any medical conditions resulting from the occupational exposure that may require further evaluation or treatment. A copy of this report must be provided to the employee and to the DO for the agency's files.

All other elements of the employee's medical record are confidential and cannot be supplied to the employer. The employee must give written consent for anyone to view the records. The records must be maintained for the duration of employment, plus 30 years, to comply with OSHA standards regarding access to employee exposure and medical records.

The Paramedic's Role in Preventing Disease Transmission

Because paramedics deal with infectious disease emergencies, they must be vigilant regarding consequences to themselves and to their patients and coworkers. Part of this professional responsibility in preventing the spread of disease is knowing when *not* to go to work. A health care worker should not go to work if the following conditions are present:

- Fever
- Diarrhea
- Draining wound or any type of wet lesions
- Jaundice
- Mononucleosis
- Treatment with a medication and/or shampoo for lice or scabies
- Strep throat (unless antibiotics have been taken for longer than 24 hours)
- Cold (unless the paramedic wears a surgical mask)

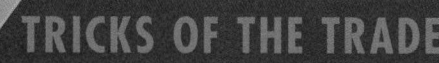

✔ TRICKS OF THE TRADE

You aren't doing yourself, your co-workers, or your patients any favors if you go to work when you are sick.

? CRITICAL THINKING

Have you come to school or work with any of these conditions?

The health care worker also should ensure that personal immunization status is current for MMR, hepatitis, DPT, polio, chickenpox, and influenza.

Other Considerations in Disease Prevention

When providing emergency care duties, the paramedic should always approach the scene with caution and be aware that an uncontrolled scene increases the likelihood for transmission of body fluids. Body substance or BSI isolation guidelines should be observed at all times and include wearing gloves, protective eyewear, face shield, and gown (if splash or spray is possible) and wearing an appropriate particulate mask when airborne disease is suspected. As mentioned previously, BSI is based on the premise that all body fluids, in any situation, may be infectious.

As a rule, if a patient has a cough, headache, general weakness, recent weight loss, nuchal rigidity, or high fever, the paramedic should immediately suspect an infectious process. Regardless of the patient's infectious status, however, the paramedic should do the following:

- Provide the same level of care to all patients.
- Disinfect equipment and the patient compartment with appropriate disinfectant solution.
- Practice effective hand washing procedures.
- Report any infectious exposure to the agency's DO.

? CRITICAL THINKING

Imagine that you are on a call and get a small splash of blood in your eyes. What do you think would prevent you from reporting it immediately so that your postexposure care could begin?

S U M M A R Y

- National concerns regarding communicable disease and infection control have resulted in public law, standards, guidelines, and recommendations to protect health care providers and emergency responders against infectious diseases. The paramedic must be familiar with these guidelines and must take personal protective measures against exposure to these pathogens.

- The chain of elements needed to transmit an infectious disease includes the pathogenic agent, a reservoir, a portal of exit from the reservoir, an environment conducive to transmission of the pathogenic agent, a portal of entry into the new host, and susceptibility of the new host to the infectious disease.

- The human body is protected from acquiring infectious disease by external and internal barriers, which serve as lines of defense against infection. External barriers include the skin, GI system, upper respiratory tract, and genitourinary tract. Internal barriers include the inflammatory response and the immune response.

- Progression of infectious disease from exposure to an infectious agent to the onset of clinical symptoms follows four stages: the latent period, the incubation period, the communicability period, and the disease period.

- Human immunodeficiency virus is directly transmitted person to person through anal or vaginal intercourse, across the placenta, by contact with infected blood or body fluids on mucous membranes or open wounds, through blood transfusion, tissue transplant, or use of contaminated needles or syringes. The virus affects the CD4$^+$ T cells. Secondary complications are usually related to opportunistic infections that arise as the immune system deteriorates. The disease progression can be categorized into category A (acute retroviral infection, seroconversion, and asymptomatic infection); category B (early symptomatic HIV); and category C (late symptomatic HIV and advanced HIV). Paramedics should observe strict compliance with universal precautions for protection against HIV. Patient care should include helping these patients feel that they can obtain acceptance and compassion from health care workers.

- Hepatitis is a viral disease that produces pathologic changes in the liver. The three main classes of hepatitis virus are hepatitis A, hepatitis B, and hepatitis C.

- Tuberculosis is a chronic pulmonary disease acquired by inhaling dried-droplet nucleus containing a tubercle bacilli. The infection is transmitted primarily by infected persons coughing or sneezing the bacteria into the air or from contact with sputum that contains virulent TB bacilli. The infection is characterized by stages of early infection (frequently asymptomatic), latency, and a potential for recurrent postprimary disease.

- Meningococcal meningitis refers to inflammation of the membranes that surround the spinal cord and brain. It can be caused by bacteria, viruses, and other microorganisms.

- Pneumonia is an acute inflammatory process of the respiratory bronchioles and alveoli. Agents responsible for this disease may be bacterial, viral, or fungal.

- Tetanus is a serious, sometimes fatal, disease of the CNS caused by infection of a wound with spores of the bacterium *Clostridium tetani*. The most common symptom is trismus, which makes it difficult to open the mouth.

- Rabies is an acute viral infection of the CNS. Humans are highly susceptible to the rabies virus after being exposed to saliva from a bite or scratch of an infected animal.

- Hantaviruses are carried by rodents and transmitted via inhalation of aerosols of material contaminated with rodent urine and feces. Many forms of this disease occur in specific geographical areas.

- Rubella is a mild, febrile, and highly communicable viral disease characterized by a diffuse punctate macular rash. The CDC recommends that all health care providers receive immunization if they are not immune from previous rubella infection.

- Rubeola (caused by the measles virus) is an acute, highly communicable viral disease characterized by fever, conjunctivitis, cough, bronchitis, and a blotchy red rash.

- Mumps is an acute, communicable systemic viral disease characterized by localized unilateral or bilateral edema of one or more of the salivary glands, with occasional involvement of other glands.

- Chickenpox is highly communicable and is characterized by a sudden onset of low-grade fever, mild malaise, and a maculopapular skin eruption for a few hours and vesicular for 3 to 4 days, leaving a granular scab. The virus may reactivate during periods of stress or immunosuppression, producing an illness known as *shingles*.

- Pertussis is an infectious disease that leads to inflammation of the entire respiratory tract and causes an insidious cough that becomes paroxysmal in 1 to 2 weeks and lasts for 1 to 2 months.

- Influenza is primarily a respiratory infection spread by influenza viruses A, B, and C.

- Mononucleosis is caused either by the Epstein-Barr virus or cytomegalovirus—both members of the herpesvirus family.

- Syphilis is a systemic disease characterized by a primary lesion; a secondary eruption involving skin and mucous membranes; long latency periods; and eventual seriously disabling lesions of the skin, bone, viscera, CNS, and cardiovascular system.

- Gonorrhea is caused by the sexually transmitted bacterium *Neisseria gonorrhoeae*. Although gonorrhea is treatable with antibiotics, some strains brought into the United States from other countries have resisted conventional antibiotic therapy.

- Chlamydia is a major cause of sexually transmitted nonspecific urethritis or genital infection. Signs and symptoms are similar to gonorrhea.

- Herpes simplex virus is transmitted by skin-to-skin contact with an infected area of the body. The primary infection produces a vesicular lesion (blister) that heals spontaneously. After the primary infection, the virus travels to a sensory nerve ganglion where it remains in a latent stage until reactivated.

- Lice are small, wingless insects that are ectoparasites of birds and mammals. During biting and feeding, secretions from the louse cause a small, red macule and pruritus.

- The human scabies mite is a parasite that completes its life cycle in and on the epidermis of its host. Scabies bites are usually concentrated around the hands and feet, especially between the webs of the fingers and toes.

- Reporting a possible communicable disease exposure permits immediate medical follow-up, enables the DO to evaluate the circumstances of the exposure to assess the need for procedural changes or engineering controls to prevent further occurrences, and facilitates source patient evaluation and testing if appropriate.

- Part of the paramedic's professional responsibility related to infectious disease transmission is to know when not to go to work. Paramedics also have an obligation to use appropriate BSI at all times.

■ REFERENCES

1. *EMT-Paramedic national standard curriculum,* U.S. Department of Transportation National Highway Traffic Safety Administration, Washington, DC, 1998, The Department.
2. *Final rule on protecting health care workers from occupational exposure to bloodborne pathogens* (29 CFR 1910.1030), March 1993.
3. CDC: Perspectives in disease prevention and health promotion update: universal precautions for prevention of transmission of immunodeficiency virus, hepatitis B virus, and other bloodborne pathogens in health care settings, *MMWR* 37(24):377, 1988.
4. McCance K, Huether S: *Pathophysiology: the biologic basis for disease in adults and children,* ed 2, St Louis, 1994, Mosby.
5. Grimes D: *Infectious diseases,* St Louis, 1991, Mosby.
6. *1993 revised classification system for HIV infection and expanded surveillance case definition for AIDS among adolescents and adults,* National Center for Infectious Diseases of HIV/AIDS, http://aepo-xdv-www.epo.cdc.gov.
7. Recommendations for preventing transmission of human immunodeficiency virus and hepatitis B virus to patients during exposure-prone invasive procedures, *MMWR,* 40 (RR08):1-9, July 12, 1991.
8. Evaluation of safety devices for preventing percutaneous injuries among healthcare workers during phlebotomy procedures, *MMWR* 46:21, 1997.
9. Public health service guidelines of the management of health-care worker exposures to HIV and recommendations for postexposure prophylaxis, *MMWR,* 47:1, 1998.
10. Hepatitis International On-Line, Cedar Grove, NJ, 1999, http://hepfi.org.

11. Mahoney F et al: Progress toward elimination of hepatitis B virus transmission among health care workers in the United States, *Arch Intern Med* 157:2601, 1997.

12. Recommendations for prevention and control of hepatitis C virus (HCV) infection and HCV-related chronic disease, *MMWR* 47:1, 1998.

13. *TB facts for health care workers: tuberculosis–yes it's still a problem,* Centers for Disease Control and Prevention, Atlanta, 1999.

14. TB (Tuberculosis), *New Mexico AIDS InfoNet Fact Sheet* (No. 515), New Mexico AIDS Education and Training Center, National Library of Medicine and New Mexico Department of Health, October 10, 1998.

15. Personal respiratory protection against tuberculosis, *TB 2000,* Francis J. Curry National Tuberculosis Center, San Francisco, 1997.

16. Control and prevention of meningococcal disease and control and prevention of serogroup C meningococcal disease: evaluation and management of suspected outbreaks: recommendations of the advisory committee on immunization practices (ACIP), *MMWR,* 46(RR-5):13, February 14, 1997.

17. Rosen P, Barkin R: *Emergency medicine: concepts and clinical practice,* ed 4, St Louis, 1998, Mosby.

18. *Home medical encyclopedia,* American Medical Association, New York, 1989, Rand House.

19. *The medical advisor,* 1996, Alexandria, VA, 1996, Time-Life Books.

38 *Behavioral and Psychiatric Disorders*

OBJECTIVES

Upon completion of this chapter, the paramedic student will be able to:

1. **Define what constitutes a behavioral emergency.**

2. **Identify potential causes for behavioral and psychiatric illness.**

3. **List three critical principles that should be considered in the prehospital care of a patient with a behavioral emergency.**

4. **Outline key elements of the prehospital patient examination during a behavioral emergency.**

5. **Describe effective techniques for interviewing a patient during a behavioral emergency.**

6. **Distinguish between key symptoms and management techniques for selected behavioral/psychiatric disorders.**

7. **Identify factors that must be considered when assessing suicide risk.**

8. **Formulate appropriate interview questions to determine suicidal intent.**

9. **Explain prehospital management techniques for the patient who has attempted suicide.**

10. **Describe assessment of the potentially violent patient.**

11. **Outline measures that may be used in an attempt to safely diffuse a potentially violent patient situation.**

12. **List situations when patient restraint can be used.**

13. **Discuss key principles in patient restraint.**

14. **Describe safety measures to be taken when patient violence is anticipated.**

15. **Explain variations in approach to behavioral emergencies in children.**

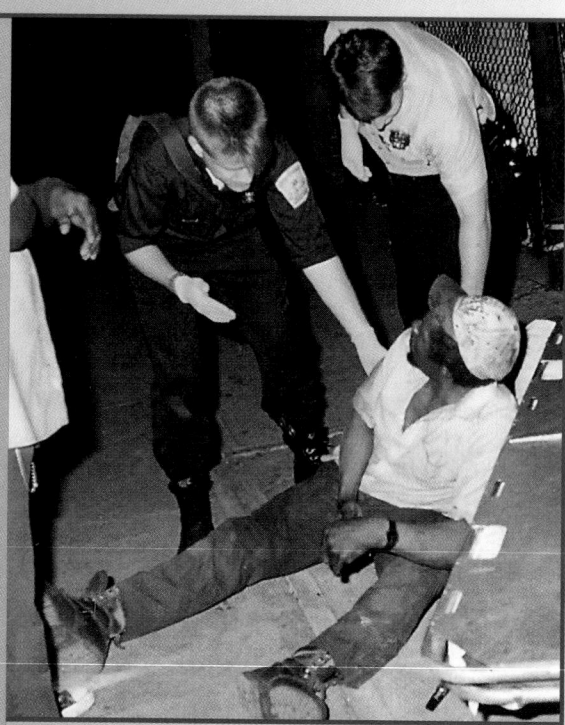

Behavioral and psychiatric emergencies require a different approach than medical or trauma-related calls. There are no scientific tools to assess the situation and no firm protocols to ensure a positive outcome. Fortunately, most behavioral emergencies require only excellent communication skills and supportive measures to prevent the escalation of a crisis. The paramedic's primary role often is to provide understanding, compassion, and direction for people with temporary turmoil. Emergency Medical Services (EMS) personnel must be oriented to helping and protecting these patients until they are able to gain self-control or other therapeutic skills can be applied.

KEY TERMS

NOTE

Mental illness accounts for 4 of the 10 leading causes of disability in established market economies worldwide. The cost of mental illness in the United States (including days lost from work) exceeds 148 billion dollars each year.[1]

Understanding Behavioral Emergencies

Although there is no clear agreement or ideal model for "normal" behavior, it generally is considered to be adaptive behavior that is accepted by society (which can vary by culture and ethnic group). The concept of abnormal (maladaptive) behavior also is defined by society when behavior:

- Deviates from society's norms and expectations
- Interferes with well being and ability to function
- Is harmful to the individual or group

? CRITICAL THINKING

Can you think of a time in your life when either you, a family member, or close friend had a behavior that fit this definition? How did it make you feel?

A **behavioral emergency** can be defined as a change in mood or behavior that cannot be tolerated by the involved person or others and requires imme-

diate attention (Box 38-1). Behavioral emergencies may range from disordered and disturbed patients who are dangerous to themselves and others to less intense situations in which a patient has a transient inability to cope with stress or anxiety. Most behavioral emergencies result from biological/organic, psychosocial, or sociocultural causes. (Common misconceptions about mental illness are listed in Box 38-2.)

NOTE

It has been estimated that as much as 20% of the U.S. population has some form of mental health problems and that one person out of every seven will require treatment at some point in their life for an emotional disturbance. Mental health problems incapacitate more people in the United States than all other health problems combined.[2]

BOX 38-1

TERMS AND DEFINITIONS

Affect: An outward manifestation of a person's feelings or emotions.

Anger: A feeling of displeasure resulting from injury, mistreatment, or opposition.

Anxiety: A state or feeling of apprehension, uneasiness, agitation, uncertainty, and fear resulting from the anticipation of some threat or danger.

Confusion: A state of disorder or failure to distinguish between things.

Depression: A mood disturbance characterized by feelings of sadness, despair, and discouragement.

Fear: A feeling of anxiety and agitation caused by the presence or nearness of danger or pain.

Mental status: The degree of competence shown by a person in intellectual, emotional, psychological, and personality function.

Open-ended questions: Questions that encourage a person to answer in detail.

Posture: The position or carriage of the body.

BOX 38-2

COMMON MISCONCEPTIONS ABOUT MENTAL ILLNESS

- Abnormal behavior is always bizarre.
- All patients with mental illness are unstable and dangerous.
- Mental disorders are incurable.
- Having a mental disorder is cause for embarrassment and shame.

Biological/Organic Causes

Physical or biochemical disturbances (which may have a heritable component) can result in significant changes in behavior. Examples of organic causes of behavioral emergencies have been discussed throughout this text and include substance abuse, trauma, illness (e.g., diabetes, electrolyte imbalance), infections, tumors, and dementia. It is important to consider the possibility of organic causes in all behavioral emergencies (Box 38-3).

Psychosocial Causes

Psychosocial mental illness may have many causes; it may be the result of childhood trauma, parental deprivation, or a dysfunctional family structure. Most conditions are characterized by **neurosis** (a restricted ability to achieve optimal functioning in social life) or **psychosis** (maladaptive behavior that involves major distortions of reality). The behavioral changes associated with these illnesses manifest in a wide range of psychological and physiological responses; these include:

- Depression
- Withdrawal
- Catatonic state
- Violence or homicidal acts
- Suicidal acts
- Paranoid reactions
- Phobias
- Disorientation or disorganization

Sociocultural Causes

Most people maintain a delicate balance among emotions, thoughts, and actions. When this equilib-rium shifts rapidly, a person may experience emotional turmoil that results in crisis. Changes in behavior caused by interpersonal or situational stress frequently are linked to a specific incident or series of incidents. Examples include environmental violence (e.g., war, riots, rape, assault), death of a loved one, and economic and employment problems.

Assessment and Management of Behavioral Emergencies

The first step in assessing a behavioral emergency is to evaluate the scene for possible danger. Most EMS services operate under protocol that includes law enforcement response for any behavioral emergency. If a dangerous situation is suspected, the EMS crew should not approach the patient until police are present and the potential for danger is controlled. Four general principles when dealing with behavioral emergencies are:

1. Ensure scene safety.
2. Contain the crisis.
3. Render appropriate emergency medical care.
4. Transport the patient to an appropriate health care facility.

Assessment

Patient assessment should begin with gathering the information necessary for immediate management of life-threatening conditions. On arrival, the scene should be surveyed for patient care information such as evidence of violence, substance abuse, or a suicide attempt. Other information can be volunteered by the patient, obtained from the patient interview, or provided by family, bystanders, and first-responders. The paramedic should limit the number of people around the patient (or isolate the patient if necessary) and must stay alert to signs of possible danger (e.g., patient rage, hostility). During the patient assessment, an attempt should be made to gather the following data (see Chapter 14):

- Patient's mental state (alertness, orientation, and ability to communicate)
- Patient's name and age
- Significant past medical history
- Medications that have been taken

BOX 38-3

COMMON MEDICAL CONDITIONS PRESENTING AS BEHAVIORAL DISORDERS

Metabolic Disorders
Glucose, sodium, calcium, or magnesium imbalance
Acid-base imbalance
Acute hypoxia
Renal failure
Hepatic failure

Endocrine Disorders
Thyroid disease
Parathyroid disease
Adrenal hormone imbalance

Infectious Diseases
Encephalitis
Meningitis
Brain abscess
Severe systemic infection

Trauma
Concussion
Intracranial hematoma (especially subdural hematoma)

Cardiovascular Disorders
Cardiac dysrhythmia
Hypotension

Transient ischemic attack
Cerebrovascular accident (or stroke)
Hypertensive encephalopathy

Neoplastic Diseases
Central nervous system tumors or metastases

Degenerative Diseases
Dementia of the Alzheimer's type
Other dementias

Drug Abuse
Alcohol
Barbiturates
Sedative-hypnotics
Amphetamines and other stimulants
Hallucinogens

Drug Reactions
Beta-adrenergic blockers
Antihypertensives
Cardiac drugs
Bronchodilators
Beta-adrenergic agonists
Anticonvulsants

- Past psychiatric problems
- Precipitating situation or problem

NOTE

It sometimes is necessary to have relatives, bystanders, and others removed from the patient assessment area in order to provide uninterrupted patient care. Law enforcement personnel should be summoned if needed.

Interview Techniques

After any life-threatening illness or injury has been managed, alert and communicative patients should be interviewed. The paramedic should not ask for more information than is necessary, but a limited and supportive interview strengthens the paramedic's rapport with the patient and can help establish and maintain a relationship during the patient encounter (see box on p. 1148). Effec-

tive interviewing techniques include active listening, being supportive and empathetic, limiting

? CRITICAL THINKING

Think about interviewing techniques that you've seen EMS crews use when caring for patients with behavioral emergencies. Were they effective? Could they have improved their patient care by using any of these techniques?

NOTE

Asking patients to rate their mood on a scale of 1 to 10 is often helpful. This provides a baseline measurement of how patients perceive their level of anxiety. If a patient takes medications for behavior modification or psychiatric disease, the paramedic should ascertain whether the medications have been taken as prescribed.

TEN USEFUL INTERVIEWING SKILLS FOR BEHAVIORAL EMERGENCIES

1. Listen to the patient in a caring concerned, and receptive manner. Be aware of nonverbal communications such as eye contact, facial expression, and posture, which can reassure the patient that you are responding with empathy.

2. Elicit feelings as well as facts to help develop a more accurate impression of the patient. If the patient is anxious, encourage him or her to share information relevant to that feeling.

3. Respond to the patient's feelings by acknowledging and labeling them (e.g., "You seem angry"). This may help validate and legitimize the patient's intense and sometimes overwhelming feelings.

4. Correct cognitive misconceptions or distortions. If a distorted sense of reality is producing fear or anxiety, offer a simple and correct explanation.

5. Provide information on the nature of the intervention or the care the patient can expect after arrival at the hospital.

6. Offer honest and realistic reassurance and support. Providing this support helps calm the patient and establishes rapport.

7. Ask effective questions. When seeking immediate information, ask closed-ended questions such as "Are you thinking of hurting yourself?" and "What medicines did you take?" More open-ended questions are appropriate after identifying problems that require immediate attention; such questions permit the individual to develop answers that usually help the paramedic completely understand the problem.

8. Avoid questions that may lead the person to say things he or she did not intend.

9. Structure the interview to develop a pattern rather than permitting a natural flow of information. Chronologically reported histories or sequences of events usually permit more complete understanding of the patient's problem (particularly causal relationships) and help the patient to organize thoughts. Keep the patient's responses focused by comments such as "What happened next?" and "Was that before or after what you were just telling me about?"

10. Conclude the interview. After obtaining relevant information, encourage the patient to describe other important events or feelings.

From Bassuk E et al: *Behavioral emergencies: a field guide for EMTs and paramedics,* Boston, 1983, Little, Brown.

---

interruptions, and respecting a patient's personal space by limiting physical touch. Important assessment findings during the interview include the following:

- Physical/somatic complaints
- Intellectual functioning (orientation, memory, concentration, judgment)
- Thought content (disordered thoughts, delusions, hallucinations, unusual worries/fears)
- Language (speech pattern and content)
- Mood (anxiety, depression, elation, agitation, alertness, distractibility)
- Appearance (personal hygiene, dress)
- Psychomotor activity

Difficult Patient Interviews

Some patients with behavioral or psychiatric disorders are difficult to interview. For example, a patient may refuse to talk to the paramedic (especially if the family requested EMS assistance without the patient's consent), may be extremely talkative with disorganized speech, or may be confrontational. If a patient refuses to be interviewed, the paramedic should speak to the patient in a quiet voice, avoid questions that may be interpreted by the patient as an "interrogation," and allow extra time for the patient to respond. Patients who are too talkative will need to be focused on the interview (e.g., by calling out their names, raising your hand to get their attention). A patient who is confrontational may require additional manpower at the scene to ensure scene safety; the patient may sometimes require restraint (described later in this chapter).

Other Patient Care Measures

After the initial assessment and history taking, the remainder of the examination is determined by the patient's overall condition and the nature of the psychiatric problem. The benefits of a thorough physical examination must be weighed against the risks involved in an encounter that the patient may construe as a physical violation. If there is reason to suspect an organic cause and the patient demonstrates no apprehension or disapproval, the examination should be performed. Otherwise, prehospital management may be limited to maintaining an effective rapport with the patient during transfer to the hospital.

Elements of the physical examination that may be associated with a behavioral emergency include abnormal pupillary size and reactivity (indicating toxic ingestion or an intracranial process), a breath odor of alcohol, needle tracks on the extremities, and unilateral weakness or loss of sensation.

Specific Behavioral/ Psychiatric Disorders

More than 250 psychiatric conditions have been identified by mental health workers. Common classifications of psychiatric illness discussed in this chapter include the following:

- Cognitive disorders
- Schizophrenia and other psychotic disorders
- Anxiety disorders
- Substance-related disorders
- Somatoform disorders
- Factitious disorders
- Dissociative disorders
- Eating disorders
- Impulse control disorders
- Personality disorders

Prehospital care for most behavioral emergencies primarily is supportive and includes protecting the patient and others from harm (including possible use of restraints), assessing and managing coexisting emergency medical problems, and transporting the patient for physician evaluation.

Cognitive Disorders

Cognitive disorders may have an organic etiology (e.g., a disease process) or may be a result of physical or chemical injury (e.g., trauma, drug abuse). All cognitive disorders result in a disturbance of cognitive functioning, which may manifest as delirium or dementia (see Chapter 43).

Delirium

Delirium is an abrupt disorientation of time and place, usually with delusions and hallucinations. The symptoms vary according to personality, environment, and the severity of illness. Common signs and symptoms of delirium include inattention, memory impairment, disorientation, clouding of consciousness, and vivid visual hallucinations. Treatment of delirium is aimed at correcting the underlying physical disorder to reduce anxiety. Sedatives may be required to manage the patient. The exact occurrence rate of delirium is unknown because it often is overlooked. However, some groups are more susceptible to delirium than others. These groups include the following:

- Older adults
- Children
- Burn patients
- Patients who have had major heart surgery
- Patients with previous brain damage (e.g., stroke)
- AIDS patients

Dementia

Dementia is a clinical state characterized by loss of function in multiple cognitive domains.

It is a slow, progressive loss of awareness for time and place, usually with an inability to learn new things or remember recent events. Although about 75 different types of dementia have been identified (Box 38-4), the majority of cases result from cerebrovascular disease (including stroke) and Alzheimer's disease (an irreversible, gradual loss of brain cells and shrinkage of brain tissue). Dementia is a major health problem in the United States because of long lifespans, affecting some 10% of those over age 65 and 20% of those over age 75. The personal habits of patients with dementia often deteriorate, speech may become incoherent, and many of these patients may revert to a "second childhood"

NOTE

Delirium and dementia may be difficult to tell apart, because both may cause disorientation and impaired memory, thinking, and judgment. Dementia usually occurs in people without diminished alertness. Dementia appears gradually and gets worse over time. Sleeping and waking problems occur less frequently in people with dementia than with delirium. People with dementia may have difficulty with short- and long-term memory, impaired judgment, and abstract thinking. Sometimes delirium may occur at the same time as dementia, especially in older adults or people with chronic illnesses.

BOX 38-4

A SAMPLING OF DISORDERS THAT CAUSE DEMENTIA

Degenerative Diseases
Huntington's disease
Parkinson's disease (not in all cases)
Cerebellar degenerations
Amyotrophic lateral sclerosis (not in all cases)
Rare genetic and metabolic diseases

Vascular Dementia
Multi-infarct dementia
Micro-infarct dementia
Large infarct dementia
Cerebral embolic disease

Anoxic Dementia
Cardiac arrest
Cardiac failure (severe)
Carbon monoxide poisoning

Traumatic Dementia
Dementia pugilistica (Boxer's dementia)
Head injury (open or closed)

Infectious Dementia
AIDS dementia
Opportunistic infection

Post-encephalitic dementia
Herpes dementia
Fungal meningitis or encephalitis
Bacterial meningitis or encephalitis
Parasitic encephalitis
Brain abscess
Neurosyphilis (general paresia)

Space-Occupying Lesions
Chronic or acute subdural hematoma
Primary brain tumor
Metastatic tumor

Autoimmune Disorders
Disseminated lupus erythematosus
Vasculitis

Toxic Dementia
Alcohol dementia
Metallic dementia (e.g., from lead, mercury, arsenic)
Organic poisons (e.g., solvents, some insecticides)

From FYI: *Disorders causing dementia*, Alzheimer's Association, Northern Virginia Chapter, www.alz-nova.org/fyi.htm.

and require total care for their feeding, toilet, and physical activities. Treatment of certain illnesses may be effective in arresting the mental decline associated with this disease.

Schizophrenia

Schizophrenia is a group of disorders characterized by recurrent episodes of psychotic behavior, which may include abnormalities of thought process, thought content (delusions), perception (auditory hallucinations are particularly common), and judgment. A family history of schizophrenia often exists, and the disorder usually becomes apparent during adolescence or early adulthood (Box 38-5).[1]

Many schizophrenic patients function quite well with medication therapy; others function poorly between frank psychotic episodes (which are often due to medication noncompliance). Most require lifelong management with antipsychotic drugs and agents that block the action of the brain chemical

dopamine. Compliance with drug therapy usually is effective in suppressing obvious symptoms of the disease but may result in side effects, especially dyskinesia (abnormal muscular movements) and tremor. The management of paranoid reactions associated with schizophrenia should include[2]:

1. Clearly identifying yourself as a paramedic and expressing the intent to provide help.
2. Exhibiting an attitude that is friendly yet somewhat distant and neutral. Kindness and warmth may be interpreted by a patient as an attempt to gain the patient's confidence for ulterior motives.
3. Never responding to a patient's anger.
4. Not speaking with family members or bystanders in hushed or secretive tones.
5. Using tact and firmness in persuading a patient to be transported to the hospital.
6. Remembering that paranoid reactions can lead to violent behavior. Precautions regarding personal safety must be a priority.

FACTS ABOUT SCHIZOPHRENIA

- More than 2 million adult Americans are affected by schizophrenia.
- In men, schizophrenia usually appears in the late teens or early twenties.
- In women, schizophrenia usually appears in the twenties to early thirties.
- Schizophrenia affects men and women with equal frequency.
- Most people with schizophrenia suffer chronically throughout their lives.
- One of every ten people with schizophrenia eventually commits suicide.
- Schizophrenia costs the nation more than $32 billion annually.

? CRITICAL THINKING

Besides auditory hallucinations, think of other sensory hallucinations that may be possible in these patients.

Anxiety Disorders

A certain amount of anxiety is useful and necessary in adapting constructively to stress (see Chapter 2). However, a patient who suffers from an anxiety disorder displays a persistent, fearful feeling that cannot be consciously related to reality (Box 38-6).[1] This type of illness may be disabling as the patient withdraws from daily activities in a usually unsuccessful attempt to avoid the episodes of intense activity. Severe anxiety disorders may manifest in a panic disorder ("panic attack") with the following signs and symptoms (Box 38-7)[1]:

- Hyperventilation
- Feeling of breathlessness or smothering
- Blurred vision
- Perioral and hand and foot paresthesias
- Fear of losing control
- Fear of dying
- Somatic complaints
- Chest discomfort
- Palpitations or tachycardia
- Dyspnea
- Choking

FACTS ABOUT ANXIETY DISORDERS

- More than 16 million adults ages 18 to 54 in the United States suffer from anxiety disorders.
- Anxiety disorders frequently are complicated by depression, eating disorders, or substance abuse.
- Anxiety disorders cost the nation more than 46 billion dollars annually.

FACTS ABOUT PANIC DISORDERS

- Panic disorders affect about 2.4 million people in the United States each year.
- Panic disorders typically strike in young adulthood; about half of those affected develop the condition before age 24.
- Women are twice as likely as men to develop a panic disorder.
- People with panic disorder also may suffer from depression and substance abuse. About 30% of people with panic disorder abuse alcohol; 17% abuse other drugs (e.g., cocaine, marijuana).
- About one third of people with panic disorder develop agoraphobia.

- Faintness
- Syncope
- Vertigo
- Trembling and sweating
- Urinary frequency and diarrhea

Patient management primarily is supportive. The paramedic should assure these patients that although they may feel like they are dying, they are not, and that effective treatment is available. Panic attacks may mimic a number of medical emergencies, including myocardial infarction. Therefore any patient who exhibits the signs and symptoms previously described should be thoroughly assessed at the scene and transported for physician evaluation (sedation may be required). Patients with anxiety disorders should not be left alone.

Phobia

A **phobia** is a type of anxiety disorder and describes a patient who has transferred anxiety onto a situation or object in the form of an irrational, intense fear (e.g., fear of heights, closed spaces, water, other people). As the object or situation comes closer to the person, the anxiety increases. If the crisis is allowed to continue, the patient's anxiety may escalate into a panic attack. These patients generally recognize that their fear is unreasonable, but they cannot prevent the phobia. In some cases, the phobia did not initiate the EMS response but becomes a secondary complication in emergency care. An example is a submerged motor vehicle crash in which a patient who is phobic of water is trapped in the automobile.

> **? CRITICAL THINKING**
>
> *Do you know someone with an intense fear of a situation or object? How do they behave when subjected to the object of their phobia?*

When caring for these patients, the paramedic should be careful to explain each step involved in an emergency or rescue procedure. A careful rehearsal with the patient, explaining exactly what and how care will be accomplished, is important. In addition, the EMS crew should show patience and understanding of the phobia and assure the patient

---

BOX 38-8

FACTS ABOUT POSTTRAUMATIC SYNDROME

- About 5.2 million people in the United States have posttraumatic syndrome during the course of a given year.
- Posttraumatic syndrome can develop at any age, including childhood.
- Posttraumatic syndrome is more common in women than men.
- About 30% of men and women who spent time in war zones experience this disorder.
- Posttraumatic syndrome frequently occurs after violent personal assaults, such as rape, mugging, or domestic violence; terrorism; natural or human-caused disasters; and accidents.
- Depression, alcohol or other substance abuse, or another anxiety disorder often accompanies posttraumatic syndrome.

---

that no forceful steps will be taken to place the patient in an unwilling position.

Posttraumatic Syndrome

Posttraumatic syndrome (posttraumatic stress disorder) is an anxiety reaction to severe psychosocial events (Box 38-8).[1] These events often are life threatening (e.g., events associated with military service, rape) and associated with repetitive, intrusive memories. Manifestations of this illness may include depression, sleep disturbances, nightmares, and survivor guilt. The syndrome frequently is complicated by substance abuse.

> **NOTE**
>
> EMS personnel and other emergency responders may be subject to posttraumatic syndrome as a result of their work. Examples include responding to major incidents with large numbers of injured persons, the death of a co-worker, a sudden infant death syndrome (SIDS) death, and the stress associated with responding to emergency calls (see Chapter 2).

Mood Disorders

The term *mood disorder* is used to describe the illnesses of depression and bipolar disorder. Both of these conditions are associated with an increased risk for suicide.

Depression

Depression is an impairment of normal functioning. It is one of the most prevalent major psychiatric conditions, affecting 10% to 15% of the general population (Box 38-9).[1,2] Depression is characterized as episodic (usually lasting longer than 1 month) with periods of remission and is known to have a gradual or rapid onset and, occasionally, a clustering of episodes. The depressed patient may show feelings of hopelessness, extreme isolation, tenseness, and irritability. In severe cases, the depression may be followed by anhedonia (an inability to feel pleasure or happiness from experiences that ordinarily are pleasurable), insomnia or hypersomnia, weight loss (from decreased appetite) or gain, decreased libido, and deep feelings of worthlessness and guilt.

Depression is associated with an increased risk for suicide (described later in this chapter). Care for these patients is directed at quietly talking to the patient about things that appear to be of interest and attempting to gain responsiveness. Depression may be treated with antidepressant drug therapy (described in Chapter 8), counseling, psychotherapy, and, in a small number of cases, electroconvulsive therapy (ECT).

Bipolar Disorder

Bipolar disorder is a biphasic emotional disorder in which depressive and manic episodes alternate with one another (Fig. 38-1). Mania is characterized by excessive elation, talkativeness, flight of ideas, motor activity, irritability, accelerated speech, and, frequently, delusions that center around personal grandeur. Bipolar disorders sometimes begin gradually, but they may occur abruptly and be precipitated by a single event. The manic phase can be very brief or last weeks to months. Compared with depression, mania is rare. The most frequent age for initial episodes is between 20 and 35 years, with initial attacks of depression occurring about 10 years later (Box 38-10).[1]

? CRITICAL THINKING

Do you think patients would be at higher risk for suicide during the depressive or manic phase of their illness? Why?

BOX 38-9

FACTS ABOUT DEPRESSION

- More than 19 million adult Americans suffer from a major depressive illness each year. Many will be unnecessarily incapacitated for weeks or months because their illness is untreated.
- Twice as many women (12%) as men (7%) are affected by depressive illness each year.
- Depression is a frequent and serious complication of heart attack, stroke, diabetes, and cancer.
- Depression increases the risk of heart attack.
- Depression costs the nation more than 30 billion dollars per year in direct and indirect costs.
- Major depression is the leading cause of disability worldwide.

Prehospital care should consist of calm, firm emotional support and transport for physician evaluation. If this is the patient's first manic episode, the paramedic should consider the possibility of drug abuse. It generally is recommended to keep sensory stimulation to a minimum. If the patient's condition permits, EMS transport should proceed without audible or visual warning devices.

Suicide and Suicide Threats

A threat of suicide is an indication that a patient has a serious crisis that requires immediate intervention. In many cases, suicide attempts are a cry for help or a form of direct or indirect communication (statements such as "I don't want to live" or "I am angry with you") (see the box on p. 1155). Other suicide attempts are an effort by the patient to manipulate relationships so that he or she is surrounded by individuals ready and willing to provide advice and support. In assessing the risk of suicide, the paramedic should consider these seven facts:

1. Suicide is the third leading cause of death in people 15 to 25 years of age and the fourth leading cause of death in people between the ages of 25 and 45.
2. The highest suicide rates in the United States are found in white men over age 85.
3. Women *attempt* suicide more often than men.
4. Men *commit* suicide more often than women.
5. Men use more violent means (guns, knives) than women (pills, razor blades).
6. About 60% of people who successfully commit suicide have a history of a previous attempt.
7. The more specific and detailed the suicide plan, the greater the suicide potential.

BOX 38-10

FACTS ABOUT BIPOLAR DISORDER

- More than 23 million Americans ages 18 and over (about 1% of the U.S. population) suffer from bipolar disorder.
- As many as 20% of people with bipolar disorder die by suicide.
- Men and women are equally likely to develop bipolar disorder.

The balance of emotions

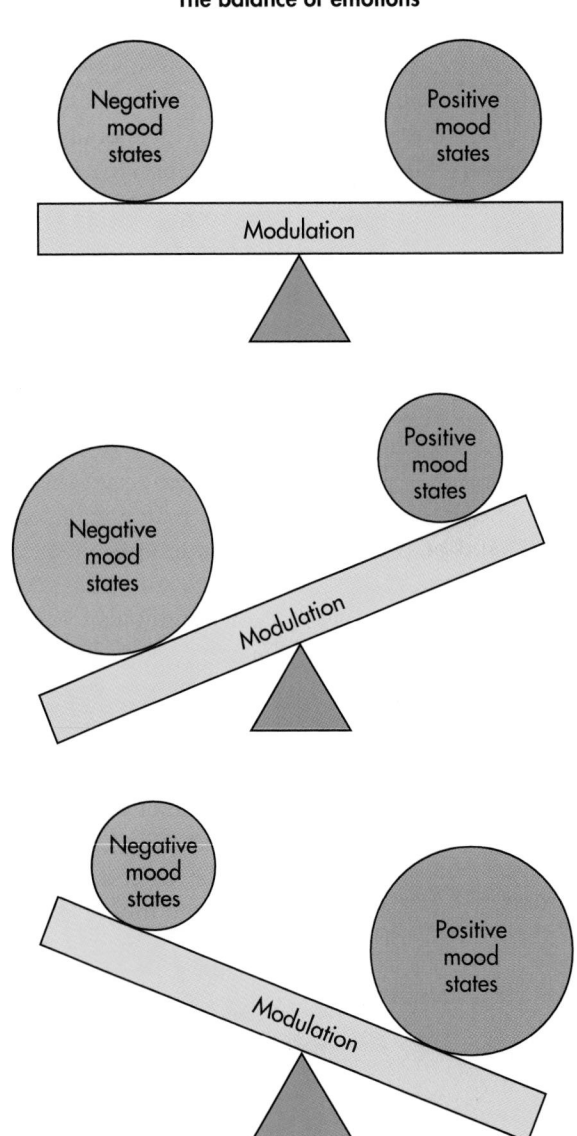

Fig. 38-1 Bipolar disorder.

Other factors associated with suicide threats include recent death of a loved one or loss of a significant relationship, financial setback or job loss, chronic or debilitating illness, social isolation, alcohol or other drug abuse, depression, and schizophrenia. If a suicide attempt is suspected, the paramedic should discuss these intentions with the patient. Questions such as "Do you have thoughts about killing yourself or others?" or "Have you ever tried to kill yourself?" are appropriate; many depressed patients are willing to discuss their suicidal (or homicidal) thoughts.

? CRITICAL THINKING

How would you feel about asking a patient, "Have you ever thought about killing yourself?"

NOTE

During the patient interview, the paramedic should try to ascertain if the patient has a plan (how and when the suicide will be done), if the plan is intended to be successful, and if the patient has the available means or method to follow through with the plan.

MYTHOLOGY OF SUICIDE

MYTH: People who talk about killing themselves rarely commit suicide.

FACT: Most people who commit suicide have given some clue or warning of their intent; therefore suicidal threats and attempts should always be treated seriously.

MYTH: The tendency toward suicide is inherited and passed from generation to generation.

FACT: Although suicide does tend to "run in families," it appears that it is not transmitted genetically.

MYTH: All suicidal people are deeply depressed.

FACT: Although depression is often associated with suicidal feelings, not all people who kill themselves are obviously depressed. In fact, some suicidal people appear to be happier than they have been in quite a while because they have decided to "resolve" all of their problems at the same time.

MYTH: There is a very low correlation between alcoholism and suicide.

FACT: Alcoholism and suicide often go hand in hand. Alcoholics are prone to suicide, and even people who do not normally drink often ingest alcohol shortly before killing themselves.

MYTH: Suicidal people are mentally ill.

FACT: Although many suicidal people are depressed and distraught, most of them would not be diagnosed as mentally ill.

MYTH: If someone attempts suicide, he or she will always entertain thoughts of suicide.

FACT: Most people who are suicidal are that way for only a brief period in their lives. If the attempter receives the proper assistance and support, he or she will probably never be suicidal again. Only about 10% of attempters later complete the act.

MYTH: If you ask the person about his or her suicidal intentions, you will encourage the person to kill himself or herself.

FACT: Actually, the opposite is true. Asking someone directly about suicidal intent often lowers the anxiety level and acts as a deterrent to suicidal emotions.

MYTH: Suicide is more common among the lower classes.

FACT: Suicide crosses all socioeconomic groups, and no one class is more susceptible to it than another.

MYTH: Suicidal people rarely seek medical attention.

FACT: Research has consistently shown that about 75% of suicidal people visit a physician within 3 months before they kill themselves.

MYTH: Suicide is basically a problem limited to young people.

FACT: The suicide rate rises with age and reaches a peak among older white men.

MYTH: Professional people do not kill themselves.

FACT: Physicians, lawyers, dentists, and pharmacists may have high suicide rates.

MYTH: When a person's depression lifts, there is no longer any danger of suicide.

FACT: The greatest danger of suicide exists during the first 3 months after a person recovers from a deep depression.

MYTH: Suicide is a spontaneous activity that occurs without warning.

FACT: Most people plan their self-destruction and then present clues indicating that they have become suicidal.

MYTH: Because it includes the Christmas season, December has a high suicide rate.

FACT: There is not a rash of suicides at Christmas, and December has the lowest rate of any month.

The Mythology of Suicide, Denver, 1987, Suicide Prevention Allied Regional Effort (SPARE).

When responding to a suicide attempt, the paramedic should request police protection before approaching the scene. After scene safety is ensured and access to the patient is gained, the scene should be evaluated for the presence of dangerous objects (see Chapter 52).

The first priority in patient management is medical care. Unconscious patients should be managed with airway, ventilatory, and circulatory support

NOTE

Armed patients must be considered homicidal as well as suicidal.

and rapid transport. If the patient is conscious, developing rapport within a relatively short period is essential. The paramedic should conduct a brief interview to assess the situation and determine the need and direction for further action. The following six steps are helpful in reducing the potential for suicide:

1. Provide support and honest assurance about the patient's well being.
2. Provide for physical safety as well as emotional security. Establish protective limits and measures to prevent injury to the patient or others. This conveys to patients that the paramedic will help them control their behavior until they can gain self-control.
3. Listen to the person, even if the speech seems bizarre, inappropriate, or unrealistic. Do not feel that every statement must be answered or that advice or opinions must be given. During the interview, acknowledge the patient's feelings and do not argue with the patient's wish to die. Explain alternatives to suicide that the patient may not have considered.
4. Determine the patient's support system or significant others when possible. Others may be better able to communicate with and calm the patient.
5. Encourage and reassure the patient throughout the crisis.
6. Transport the patient to an appropriate facility for emergency intervention.

Substance-Related Disorders

Substance-related disorders were described previously (see Chapter 34). Psychiatric illness and behavioral problems associated with these disorders often are a result of drug dependence, drug abuse, and intoxication from use/misuse of the following:

- Narcotics and opiates
- Sedative-hypnotics
- Stimulants (e.g., cocaine)
- Phencyclidine (PCP)
- Hallucinogens
- Tricyclic antidepressants
- Drugs abused for sexual purposes/sexual gratification
- Alcohol

Somatoform Disorders

Somatoform disorders are a group of conditions in which there are physical symptoms for which no physical cause can be found and there is definite or strong evidence that the underlying cause is psychological. Two of the most common disorders in this group are somatization disorder and conversion disorder. Both are associated with anxiety, depression, and threats of suicide. Treatment for both disorders often requires psychotherapy to address the emotional conflicts that manifest in these illnesses.

Somatization Disorder

Somatization disorder is a condition in which an individual has complaints (lasting several years) of various physical problems for which no physical cause can be found (Box 38-11).[3] The condition is more common in women than men, and it sometimes results in unnecessary surgery and other treatments. Symptoms most commonly complained of include:

- Neurological
  Double vision
  Seizure
  Weakness
- Gynecological
  Painful menstruation

BOX 38-11

FACTS ABOUT SOMATIZATION DISORDERS

- The lifetime prevalence rate for somatization disorder is 0.2% to 2% of the U.S. population.
- Somatization disorders are rare in men.
- Somatization disorders tend to run in families, occurring in 10% to 20% of the primary female relatives of somatization disorder patients.
- Most somatization disorders begin in adolescence or early adulthood and are chronic in nature.
- Symptoms sometimes increase and decrease in severity over time, but usually there are few symptom-free episodes.
- Anxiety and depression often accompany the disorder.
- Suicide threats are common in these patients, but suicide is rarely completed.

Painful intercourse
• Gastrointestinal
  Abdominal pain
  Nausea

Conversion Disorder

Conversion disorder is a mental illness in which painful emotions are repressed and unconsciously converted into physical symptoms (Box 38-12).[4] There may be a loss of sensory, motor, or special senses. For example, the person suddenly cannot speak, hear, see, or feel, or an arm or leg is paralyzed. In many cases, the areas of the body affected do not correspond to the actual arrangement of neural pathways. The symptoms also may come and go or appear at different times and in different areas of the body.

Management

The paramedic should manage symptoms of somatoform disorders as if they are real, because it may be difficult to differentiate them from an organic ailment. The paramedic should recognize that these patients are not "faking"; they believe their illness or loss of function to be factual. These patients require physician evaluation.

Factitious Disorders

Factitious disorders are a group of disorders in which symptoms mimic a true illness but actually have been invented and are under the control of the patient for the purpose of receiving attention. The most common disorder in this group is Munchausen's syndrome, in which the patient makes habitual pleas for treatment and hospitalization for a symptomatic but imaginary, acute illness (Box 38-13). The symptoms (which often are dramatic but plausible) usually resolve with treatment, after which the person seeks further treatment for another imaginary disease. Once the factitious disorder is diagnosed, treatment is aimed at protecting these people from unnecessary surgeries and treatments.

> **NOTE**
>
> Munchausen's syndrome by proxy is a psychological disorder in which persons injure or induce illness in others (usually children) in order to gain sympathy.

Dissociative Disorders

Dissociative disorders are a group of psychological illnesses in which a particular mental function is separated (dissociated) from the mind as a whole (Box 38-14). The illness usually is associated with emotional conflicts that are so repressed that a split in the personality occurs, resulting in an altered state of consciousness or a confusion in identity. The condition also may be caused by an inability to cope with severe stress or conflict, where dissociation occurs suddenly after a catastrophic event (e.g., the traumatic death of a child or spouse). People with dissociative disorders often are unable to remember their names or personal histories, but they can still speak, read, and learn new material. Treatment may include antianxiety medications, hypnosis, and psychotherapy.

BOX 38-12

FACTS ABOUT CONVERSION DISORDER

• True conversion disorder is rare in the United States.
• The disorder is seen more commonly in lower socioeconomic groups and may be more common in military personnel exposed to combat situations.
• Conversion disorder may present at any age but is rare before age 10 or after age 35.
• In pediatric patients, the incidence of conversion is increased after physical or sexual abuse. The incidence also increases in those children whose parents are seriously ill or have chronic pain.
• About 64% of adult patients with conversion disorder have evidence of organic brain disorder.

BOX 38-13

A SAMPLING OF FACTITIOUS DISORDERS

• Bereavement
• Cushing's syndrome
• Dental problems
• HIV infection
• Hypoglycemia
• Munchausen's syndrome
• Stroke

BOX 38-14

A SAMPLING OF DISSOCIATIVE DISORDERS

Dissociative amnesia: A disorder characterized by a blocking out of critical personal information, usually of a traumatic or stressful nature. Dissociative amnesia, unlike other types of amnesia, does not result from other medical trauma.

Dissociative fugue: A rare disorder in which an individual suddenly and unexpectedly takes physical leave of the surroundings.

Dissociative identity disorder: A disorder that has been called *multiple personality disorder*.

Depersonalization disorder: A condition marked by a feeling of detachment or distance from one's own experience, body, or self.

BOX 38-15

FACTS ABOUT EATING DISORDERS

- More than 5 million Americans suffer from eating disorders.
- Anorexia, bulimia, and binge-eating disorders are diseases that affect the mind and body simultaneously.
- Three percent of adolescent and adult women and one percent of men have an eating disorder.
- A young woman with anorexia is 12 times more likely to die than another woman her age without anorexia.
- Fifteen percent of young women have substantially disordered eating attitudes and behaviors.

Eating Disorders

The two most common eating disorders considered to be forms of psychiatric illness are anorexia nervosa and bulimia nervosa (Box 38-15).[5] Both of these eating disorders can result in starvation and death. They are best managed with supervision and regulation of eating habits, psychotherapy, and, sometimes, antidepressants. Most patients require hospitalization.

Anorexia Nervosa

Anorexia nervosa is an eating disorder characterized by intense fear of being obese, severe weight loss, malnutrition, and, eventually, amenorrhea. A patient feels intensely hungry, even though hunger pains are denied. Signs and symptoms include weight loss, obsession with exercise, fatigue, binge eating, induced vomiting and use of laxatives to promote weight loss. The condition primarily is seen in adolescents (predominantly girls) and usually is associated with emotional stress or conflict. It frequently is difficult to identify an exact underlying cause of this disease.

Bulimia Nervosa

Bulimia nervosa (sometimes considered a variant of anorexia) is an insatiable craving for food, often resulting in episodes of binge eating followed by purging (through self-induced vomiting or use of laxatives), depression, and self-deprivation. Like anorexia, bulimia is most common in adolescent girls and young women. Anorexic and bulimic patients often are highly distressed about their com-

pulsive behavior and, as a result, may become depressed and suicidal.

> **NOTE**
>
> Anorexia and bulimia can lead to serious dehydration, starvation, and electrolyte imbalances, which may cause critical illness or death.

Impulse Control Disorders

Impulse control disorders are a group of psychiatric conditions characterized by the inability to resist an impulse or a temptation to perform some act that is unlawful, socially unacceptable, or self-harmful. Examples of this disorder include pathological gambling, kleptomania (an impulse to steal), and pyromania (an impulse to set fires). These disorders often are difficult to treat; incarceration is not unusual.

Obsessive-Compulsive Disorder

Obsessive-compulsive disorder (OCD) is a psychiatric disorder in which people feel stress or anxiety about thoughts or rituals over which they have little control (Box 38-16).[1] The disorder can take many forms, which include excessive hand washing or showering and thoughts or mental images of an up-

> **NOTE**
>
> Clinical depression, panic attacks, or both are common in individuals with an OCD.

BOX 38-16

FACTS ABOUT OBSESSIVE-COMPULSIVE DISORDER

- About 3.3 million American adults have OCD in a given year.
- OCD affects men and women with equal frequency.
- The nation's social and economic loss due to OCD totals more than 8 billion dollars each year.

setting nature (e.g., of violence, vulgarities, harm to self or others). Obsessions also may involve special numbers, colors, single words or phrases, and sometimes melodies.

Although most adults realize in part that these obsessions and compulsions are senseless, they have great difficulty stopping them. (Children with OCD may not realize their behavior is unusual.) OCD affects men and women equally, can start at any age, and may have a heritable component. Persons with OCD often cleverly hide their condition from family, friends, and co-workers. Medications (e.g., antidepressants) and behavior therapy give many patients significant relief from OCD.

Personality Disorders

Personality disorders are a large group of conditions characterized by a general failure to learn from experience or adapt appropriately to changes, resulting in personal distress and impairment of social functioning. These disorders (which may have an environmental or heritable component) often produce behavior that is especially obvious during times of stress. The symptoms generally are first recognized in adolescence and continue through life. (Depression and anxiety are common in adolescents.) The maladaptive behavior patterns associated with these conditions impair a person's ability to function in society, severely limiting adapting potential. Examples of personality disorders include eccentric behavior, paranoia, narcissism (intense self-love), and obsessive-compulsive behavior. Treatment involves behavior modification techniques, counseling, and individual psychotherapy.

Special Behavioral Problems

In addition to assessing a suicidal patient, other special problems include assessing potentially violent patients and behavioral problems in children.

Assessing the Potentially Violent Patient

Only a small proportion of persons with mental health problems are potentially violent. Nonetheless, assessment and management of the potentially violent patient should be part of an EMS protocol. The following four factors may help determine the potential for a violent episode[6]:

1. Past history (Has the patient exhibited hostile, aggressive, or violent behavior?)
2. Posture (Is the patient sitting or standing? Does the patient appear to be tense or rigid?)
3. Vocal activity (Loud, obscene, and erratic speech indicates emotional distress.)
4. Physical activity (Is the patient pacing or agitated or displaying protection of physical boundaries?)

If any of these signs of potentially violent behavior are present, the paramedic should attempt to reduce the effect of the stress but avoid confrontation and prepare a way to cope with the crisis that reduces the potential for a life-threatening incident or psychologically damaging consequences.

> **NOTE**
>
> If a paramedic anticipates violence that threatens personal safety or the safety of the crew, the paramedic should retreat from the scene and wait for law enforcement personnel to make the scene safe.

Controlling Violent Situations

Severely disturbed patients who pose a threat to themselves or others may need to be restrained, transported, and hospitalized against their will. Each state has a statute covering the criteria for involuntary commitment, and the paramedic should be familiar with all applicable laws. The premise on which most state laws are based suggests that one person may restrain another to protect life or prevent injury.

When a psychiatric patient refuses care in the prehospital setting, EMS personnel should consult with medical direction. The decision to restrain, treat, or release the patient is a medical direction decision. If violent behavior must be contained, "reasonable force" to restrain the patient should be used as humanely as possible. In most cases, the restraint duty (if necessary) should be given to law enforcement personnel. As in all other aspects of health care, details of the incident should be carefully recorded for future reference. When dealing with a patient who may require restraint, the paramedic should do the following:

1. Ensure a safe environment.
2. Gather a pertinent medical and psychiatric history.
3. Attempt to gain the patient's cooperation.
4. Be confident but not confrontational.

? CRITICAL THINKING

Have you ever seen an EMS or law enforcement person lose control of their own behavior when dealing with a violent patient? How did it affect the patient's physical or psychological state?

Restraint Guidelines

- If the patient is homicidal, do not attempt restraint without law enforcement assistance. If the patient is armed, move everyone out of range, retreat from the scene, and wait for law enforcement personnel.
- Remember that the patient may not be responsible for his or her actions.
- Plan the restraining action to include a backup plan in case the initial action fails.
- Be sure that adequate help is available. Make certain that a minimum of four capable individuals are available to help restrain an adult patient.
- Remember that the potential for personal injury and legal liability is always present.

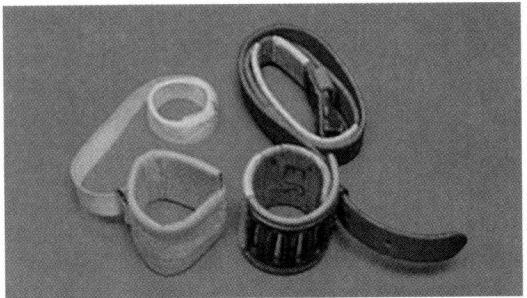

Fig. 38-2 Restraint devices.

NOTE

The dignity of the patient should be respected as much as possible during the restraint.

Restraint Methods

A number of restraint methods can be used to manage a violent patient. The techniques used to contain violent behavior should begin with a gentle, nonthreatening, low-profile approach and progress to more direct intervention as needed. The options of physical restraint should always be explained to the patient before applying force. If the patient is still unwilling to cooperate, he or she should be advised that restraint is necessary to protect against injury and ensure the safety of others.

Before approaching a violent patient, the paramedic should be aware of the patient's surroundings. Seemingly harmless items, including ashtrays, lighted cigarettes, hot coffee, letter openers, soda bottles, cans, and furniture, should be noted. The paramedic should make no attempt to enter the patient's physical space (usually considered to be one arm's length) until the other members involved in the restraint action are ready to proceed.

The paramedic should consider the patient's muscle groups and potential range of motion before initiating restraint procedures. The paramedic should plan to position the patient in a way that limits the effectiveness of strength and range of motion. Each member of the restraint team should be assigned a specific body part or responsibility before actual restraint activity.

The paramedic must be familiar with the restraint devices available and should be able to improvise if the need arises. The preferred method is to use commercially manufactured wrist/waist/ankle padded leather or Velcro straps, or full jacket restraints (Fig. 38-2). Effective restraints also may be improvised using common materials such as:

- Small towels that can be wrapped around the patient's wrists and ankles and secured with tape to the stretcher
- Cravats
- Webbed straps ordinarily used to secure patients to spine boards
- Roller bandage
- Blanket roll

Regardless of the types of restraint used, they should be strong enough to produce the desired effect without compromising circulatory or respiratory status.

Sequence of Restraint Actions

Trained personnel can use many restraint techniques. The following sequence is an example of a restraint action that may be used to contain violent behavior:

1. The paramedic offers the patient one final opportunity to cooperate.
2. If there is no response, a minimum of two rescuers move swiftly toward the patient and position themselves close to and slightly behind the patient. Each rescuer should then position an inside leg in front of the patient's leg to force the patient to the ground if needed (Fig. 38-3). Swift movement by two or more rescuers minimizes the patient's ability to focus on restraint actions and decreases the accuracy of kicks or blows. During the restraint procedure, the patient should be continually reassured by a rescuer not involved in the physical maneuver.
3. If the patient calms and agrees to be transported without restraints, the paramedic positions the patient lateral or supine on a stretcher (if not contraindicated by mechanism of injury or medical condition) and secures the patient with straps to limit range of motion (Fig. 38-4). If the patient be-

comes dangerous en route to the hospital, restraints should be used.
4. Once applied, restraints should not be removed until the patient is delivered to the emergency department or there are adequate resources to control the situation. Restrained limbs should be checked periodically for adequacy of circulation and the presence of any soft tissue injury. If a change in the restraints is required, adequate assistance must be available and only one limb should be repositioned at a time.

> **NOTE**
>
> The patient's respiratory and circulatory status should frequently be assessed (and documented) to ensure the restraint action has not compromised vital functions.

Restraint procedures should be thoroughly documented on the patient care report. Attempts at negotiations and the sequence of patient behavior that led to the need for restraint should be clearly described. Documentation also should verify that circulatory evaluation and continued monitoring of the patient were performed after restraint. Again, physical restraint is recommended only when all verbal and nonverbal techniques have been exhausted and only when an individual presents a danger to self or others.

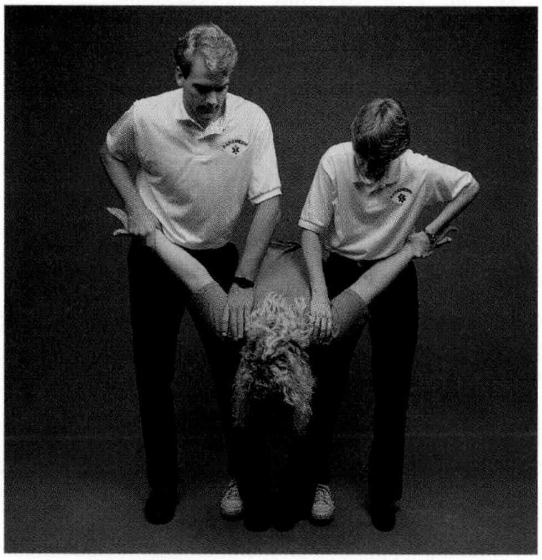

Fig. 38-3 Control position. Rescuers face the same direction. Inside legs are placed in front of the patient. Rescuers' outside hands hold patient's wrists. Rescuers' inside hands form a C on the patient's shoulders.

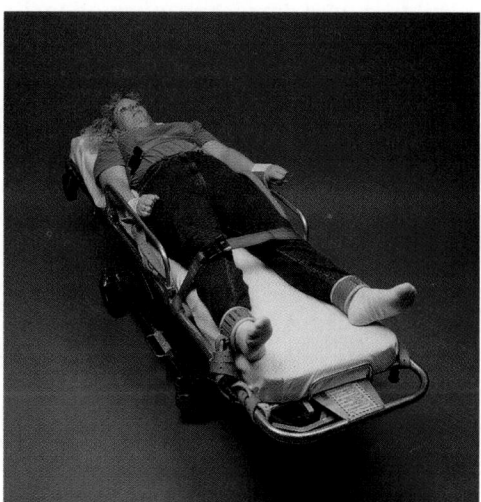

Fig. 38-4 Patient restrained in supine position.

Personal Safety

Although personal safety should be considered in any emergency response, behavioral emergencies are more likely to require that the paramedic protect himself or herself and the crew from hostile injury. The following methods to avoid personal injury should be considered:

- When possible, remain at a safe distance from the patient.
- Do not allow the patient to block the exit.
- Keep large furniture between you and the patient. Do not allow a single paramedic to remain alone with the patient.
- Avoid threatening statements.
- Use folded blankets or cushions to absorb the impact of thrown objects.

Various training programs have been developed to provide safety and security to the rescuer and the violent patient. Nonviolent personal protection maneuvers should be learned and practiced under the supervision of someone trained in these procedures.

? CRITICAL THINKING

Do you use the same safety guidelines when responding to a behavioral emergency that involves a child or adolescent that you would use with an adult?

Behavioral Problems in Children

Young children who are victims of emotional crisis need to be managed with techniques that differ from those used to care for older children and adults. The following suggestions may be helpful when dealing with some children:

1. Gain the child's trust and try to convince the child that you are a friend who can help.
2. Make it clear that you are strong enough to be in control but will not hurt the child.
3. Keep the interview questions brief; the child's attention span may be extremely short.
4. Never lie; be honest.
5. Use all available resources to communicate (e.g., drawing pictures, telling stories).
6. Involve parents or caregivers in the interview or examination (if appropriate).
7. Take any threat of violence seriously.

CHEMICAL RESTRAINT

Chemical restraint refers to the use of drugs to control behavior. Pharmacological treatment will vary, but it is generally intended to provide sedation. Two groups of drugs that are effective for chemical restraint include benzodiazepines and antipsychotics. (See Chapter 8 and the Emergency Drug Index.)

Benzodiazepines are drugs that bind to specific receptors in the cerebral cortex and limbic system (a major integrating system that governs emotional behavior). These drugs are popular because of their very high therapeutic index. They have four main actions: anxiety-reducing, sedative-hypnotic, muscle relaxing, and anticonvulsant. Benzodiazepines that are commonly used for chemical restraint include *diazepam* (Valium), *midazolam* (Versed), and *lorazepam* (Ativan).

Antipsychotics are a group of drugs that block dopamine receptors in specific areas of the central nervous system. The primary use of these drugs is to treat schizophrenia and other conditions that exhibit disturbed behavior (e.g., Tourette's syndrome and senile dementia associated with Alzheimer's disease). Two well known antipsychotics that can be used for chemical restraint are *droperidol* (Inapsine) and *haloperidol* (Haldol). The short-term use of antipsychotics rarely produces extrapyramidal reactions (e.g., pseudoparkinsonism, akathisia, and dystonias). If these reactions occur, however, the administration of *diphenhydramine* (Benadryl) can reverse these side effects.

Benzodiazepines and antipsychotics can be very effective in controlling hostile or combative patients. Like all other restraint methods, the paramedic should consult with medical direction, follow established protocol, and carefully document the event.

If the child's behavior or physical condition makes restraint necessary, the paramedic should use only reasonable force (with sufficient help) to ensure the patient's safety and the safety of the EMS crew. If calming measures fail to work, wrapping the child in a full body blanket secured to the stretcher with straps often is sufficient during transport for physician evaluation. As with any method of restraint, the paramedic should monitor and ensure that the child's airway and circulation are not compromised. Documentation should be thorough and complete.

S U M M A R Y

- A behavioral emergency is a change in mood or behavior that cannot be tolerated by the involved person or others and requires immediate attention.

- Physical or biochemical disturbances can result in significant changes in behavior. Psychosocial mental illness is often the result of childhood trauma, parental deprivation, or a dysfunctional family structure.

- Changes in behavior caused by interpersonal or situational stress are frequently linked to specific incidents, such as environmental violence, death of a loved one, economic or employment problems, or prejudice and discrimination.

- When dealing with behavioral emergencies, the paramedic should contain the crisis, render appropriate emergency care, and transport the patient to an appropriate health care facility.

- During the patient assessment, an attempt should be made to determine the patient's mental state, name and age, significant past medical history, medications (and compliance with medications), and past psychiatric problems, as well as the precipitating situation or problem.

- Effective interviewing techniques include active listening, being supportive and empathetic, limiting interruptions, and respecting the patient's personal space.

- All cognitive disorders result in a disturbance of cognitive functioning that may manifest as delirium or dementia.

- Schizophrenia is characterized by recurrent episodes of psychotic behavior that may include abnormalities of thought process, thought content, perception, and judgment.

- Anxiety disorders may cause a panic attack. Anxiety disorders include phobias, obsessive-compulsive disorders, and posttraumatic syndrome.

- Depression is an impairment of normal functioning in which an individual may demonstrate feelings of hopelessness, loss of appetite, decreased libido, and feelings of worthlessness and guilt.

- Bipolar disorder is a manic-depressive illness in which depressive and manic episodes alternate with one another.

- Somatoform disorders are conditions in which there are physical symptoms for which no physical cause can be found and the cause is thought to be psychological. These include somatization disorder and conversion disorder.

- Factitious disorders are disorders in which symptoms mimic a true illness but have been invented and are under the control of the patient.

- Dissociative disorders are a group of psychological illnesses in which a particular mental function is separated from the mind as a whole.

- The most common eating disorders considered to be forms of psychiatric illness are anorexia nervosa and bulimia nervosa.

- Impulse control disorders are characterized by the inability to resist an impulse or temptation to do some act that is unlawful, socially unacceptable, or self-harmful.

- Personality disorders are a group of conditions characterized by a general failure to learn from experience or adapt appropriately to changes, resulting in personal distress and impairment of social functioning.

- A threat of suicide is an indication that a patient has a serious crisis that requires immediate intervention.

- Questions that determine the patient's ideation, plan, intent, and means to commit suicide should be asked.

- After ensuring scene safety, the first priority in patient management after a suicide attempt is medical care. If the patient is conscious, developing rapport as soon as possible is essential.

- Assessment of a potentially violent patient should include past history of violence, posture, vocal activity, and physical activity.

- When attempting to diffuse a situation involving a potentially violent patient, the paramedic should ensure a safe environment, gather the patient's history, try to gain the patient's cooperation, avoid threats, and explain the paramedic's role in providing care.

- Severely disturbed patients who pose a threat to themselves or others may need to be restrained.

- Reasonable force to restrain a patient should be used as humanely as possible. An adequate number of personnel is needed to ensure patient and rescuer safety during restraint. The potential for personal injury and legal liability is always present.

- Personal safety measures while responding to a behavioral emergency should include not allowing the patient to block the exit, keeping large furniture between you and the patient, working as a team, avoiding threatening statements, and using soft objects to absorb the impact of thrown objects.

- When caring for children with behavioral emergencies, the paramedic should attempt to gain their trust, tell them they won't be hurt, keep questions brief, be honest, involve parents (if appropriate), and take threats of violence seriously.

REFERENCES

1. National Institute of Mental Health: *The numbers count: mental illness in America*, NIH Publication No. NIH 99-4584, Bethesda, Md, National Institute of Mental Health.
2. U.S. Department of Transportation National Highway Traffic Safety Administration: *EMT-Paramedic national standard curriculum*, Washington, DC, 1998, The Department.
3. *Conversion and somatization disorders*, Vanderbilt Medical Center, www.mc.vanderbilt.edu.
4. Dufel S: *Conversion disorder*, e-medicine.com, www.emedicine.com/emerg/topic112.htm.
5. *Facts about eating disorders*, Harvard Eating Disorders Center, www.hedc.org/info.html.
6. Judd R, Peszke M: Psychological and behavioral emergencies, *Top Emerg Med* 4(4):7, 1983.

39 Gynecology

OBJECTIVES

Upon completion of this chapter, the paramedic student will be able to:

1. *Describe the physiological processes of menstruation and ovulation.*

2. *Describe the pathophysiology of the following nontraumatic causes of abdominal pain in females: pelvic inflammatory disease, ruptured ovarian cyst, cystitis, dysmenorrhea, mittelschmerz, endometriosis, ectopic pregnancy, vaginal bleeding.*

3. *Describe the pathophysiology of traumatic causes of abdominal pain in females, including vaginal bleeding and sexual assault.*

4. *Outline the prehospital assessment and management of the female with abdominal pain.*

5. *Outline specific assessment and management for the patient who has been sexually assaulted.*

6. *Describe specific prehospital measures to preserve evidence in sexual assault cases.*

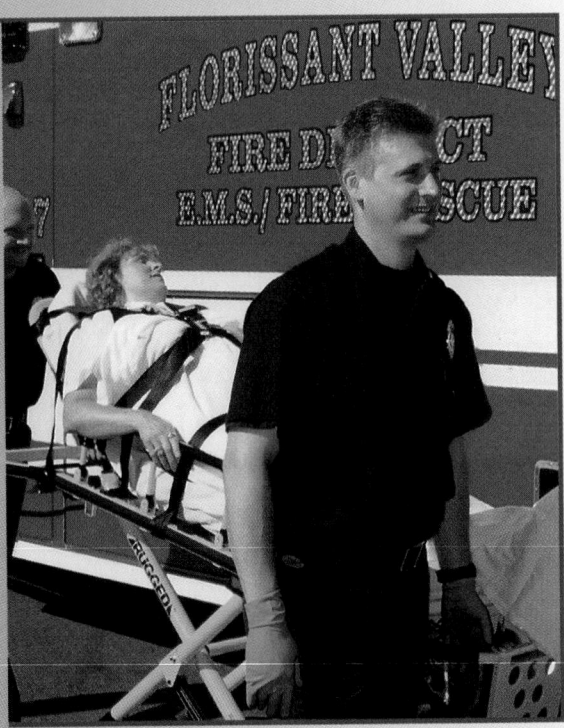

A number of disorders can occur in the female reproductive system, some of which lead to gynecological emergencies. This chapter explains the etiology and emergency care measures for common problems associated with the female reproductive system.

Organs of the Female Reproductive System

The female reproductive organs were illustrated and described in Chapter 6. They include the ovaries, fallopian tubes, uterus, vagina, external genital organs, and mammary glands. (Fig. 39-1 serves as a review of these structures.)

Menstruation and Ovulation

Menstruation

Menstruation is the normal, periodic discharge of blood, mucus, and cellular debris from the uterine mucosa. The normal menstrual cycle lasts approximately 28 days and occurs at more or less regular intervals from puberty to **menopause** (except during pregnancy and lactation). The average menstrual flow of 25 to 60 milliliters (mL) usually lasts 4 to 6 days and is fairly constant from cycle to cycle. The onset of menses (**menarche**) generally begins between ages 12 and 13 and ends permanently (menopause) at an average age of 47 years, with wide variation. Depending on the individual, normal menopause may occur from ages 35 to 60.

Follicle and Oocyte Development

By the fourth prenatal month, the ovaries contain about 5 million cells from which oocytes (immature ova) develop. At birth, there are about 2 million primary oocytes, which decline in number to 300,000 to 400,000 at puberty. Of these primary oocytes,

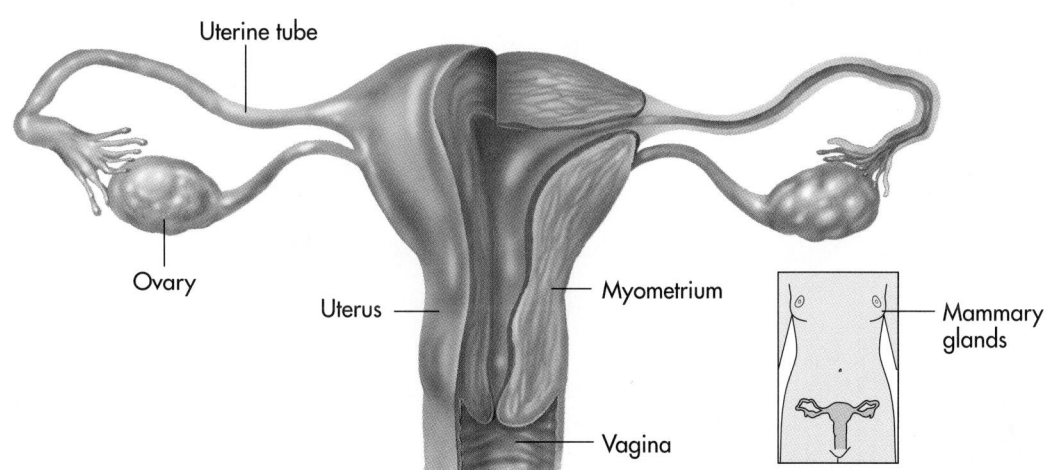

Fig. 39-1 Female organs.

only about 400 are eventually released from the ovary. Oocytes are surrounded by a layer of cells (granulosa cells), and the entire structure is known as a primary follicle (Fig. 39-2).

The menstrual cycle is associated with hormonal changes that stimulate some of the primary follicles to continue development and become secondary follicles. A secondary follicle continues to enlarge, forming a lump on the surface of the ovary. The fully mature follicle is known as the vesicular, or graafian, follicle.

Ovulation

Cellular secretions of the graafian follicle cause it to swell more rapidly than can be accommodated by follicular growth. The follicle expands and ruptures, forcing a small amount of blood and follicular fluid out of the vesicle. Shortly after this initial burst of fluid, an oocyte escapes from the follicle. The release of this secondary oocyte is termed **ovulation.**

After ovulation, the follicle is transformed into a yellow glandular structure called the corpus luteum, whose cells secrete large amounts of proges-

terone and some estrogen. If pregnancy occurs, the fertilized oocyte (zygote) begins releasing a hormonelike substance (chorionic gonadotropin) that keeps the corpus luteum from degenerating. As a result, blood levels of estrogen and progesterone do not decrease, and the menstrual period does not occur. In the absence of pregnancy, the corpus luteum degenerates, and the secondary oocyte passes out of the system with the menstrual flow.

Hormonal Control of Ovulation and Menses

Hormones released from the hypothalamus and anterior pituitary control ovulation and menses. Follicle-stimulating hormone (FSH) stimulates development of the follicle, including the cells that produce estrogen. Before ovulation, these cells release estrogen and cause a surge in the pituitary production of luteinizing hormone (LH), initiating the ovarian cycle (and leading to ovulation), which in turn regulates the uterine cycle (Fig. 39-3). Under the influence of the ovarian hormones, the lining of the uterus (**endometrium**) goes through two phases of development: the proliferative and secretory phases.

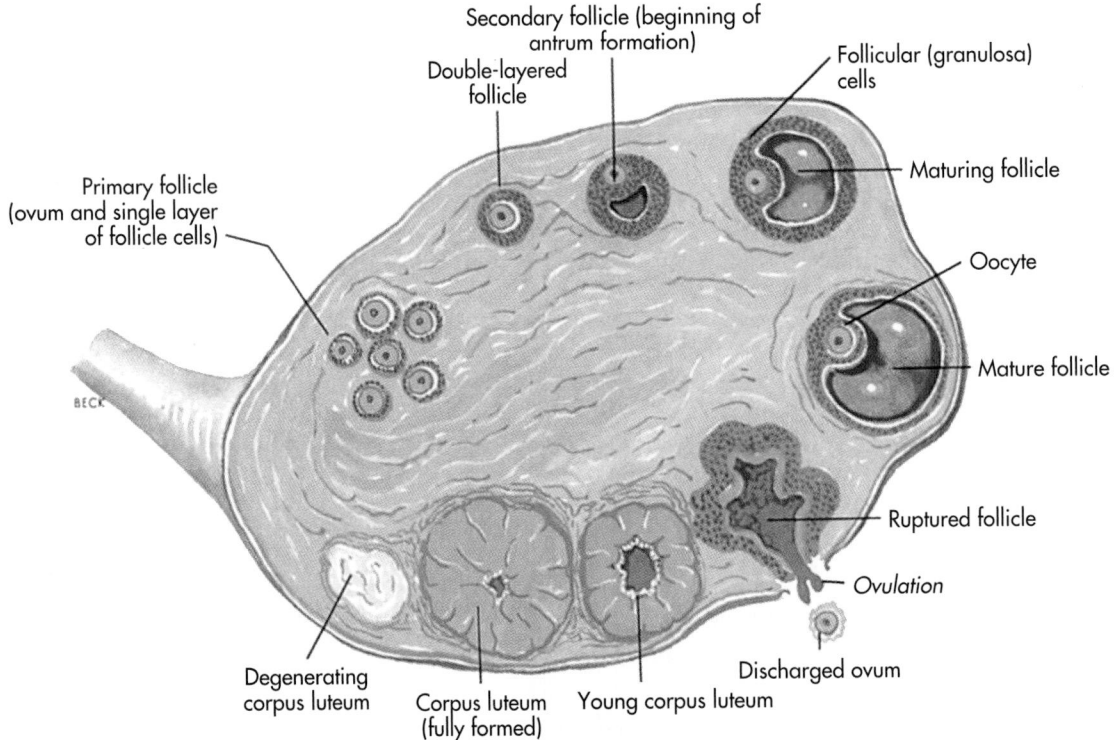

Secondary follicle (beginning of antrum formation)
Double-layered follicle
Follicular (granulosa) cells
Maturing follicle
Primary follicle (ovum and single layer of follicle cells)
Oocyte
Mature follicle
Ruptured follicle
Ovulation
Discharged ovum
Degenerating corpus luteum
Corpus luteum (fully formed)
Young corpus luteum

Fig. 39-2 Diagram of ovary and oogenesis. Cross-section of mammalian ovary shows successive stages of ovarian (graafian) follicle and ovum development. Begin with the first stage (primary follicle) and follow around clockwise to the final stage (degenerating corpus luteum). (From Thibodeau G: *Structure and function of the body,* ed 11, St Louis, 2000, Mosby.)

? CRITICAL THINKING

What could happen to the menstrual cycle if the hormonal balance was off?

The proliferative phase is initiated and maintained by increasing amounts of estrogen produced by the maturing follicle. Estrogen stimulates the endometrium to grow and increase in thickness, preparing the uterus for implantation of a fertilized ovum. The secretory phase begins after ovulation and is under the combined influence of estrogen and progesterone. During this phase, tortuous secretory glands and spiral vessels develop to prepare the endometrium for implantation of the fertilized ovum. Within 7 days after ovulation (about day 21 of the menstrual cycle), the endometrium is ready to receive the developing embryo if fertilization has occurred.

In the absence of fertilization, the ovum can survive only 6 to 24 hours, after which the hormone levels drop and the endometrium is shed as menstrual flow. This process normally occurs on day 28 of the menstrual cycle (about 14 days after ovulation). The

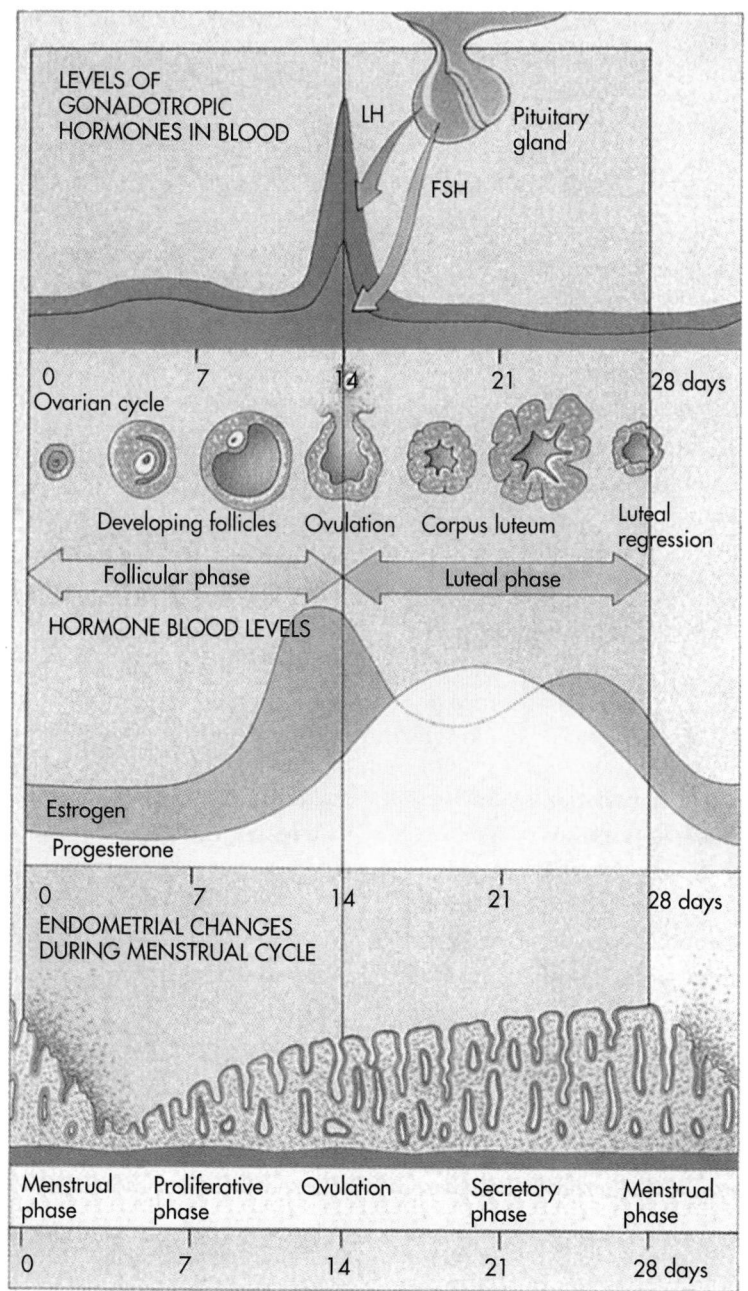

Fig. 39-3 Human menstrual cycle. The interrelationship of pituitary, ovarian, and uterine functions throughout the usual 28-day cycle. A sharp increase in LH levels causes ovulation, whereas menstruation (sloughing of the endometrial lining) is initiated by lower levels of progesterone. (From Thibodeau G: *Structure and function of the body*, ed 11, St Louis, 2000, Mosby.)

oocyte is capable of being fertilized for up to 24 hours after ovulation (see Chapter 40).

Specific Gynecological Emergencies

Gynecological emergencies are classified into 3 groups: nontraumatic, traumatic, and sexual assault (Box 39-1).

Nontraumatic Emergencies

In addition to GI causes of abdominal pain (described in Chapter 32), acute or chronic infection involving a patient's uterus, ovaries, fallopian tubes,

---

BOX 39-1

CLASSIFICATION OF GYNECOLOGICAL EMERGENCIES

Nontraumatic Abdominal Emergencies
Pelvic inflammatory disease
Ruptured ovarian cyst
Cystitis
Mittelschmerz
Endometritis
Endometriosis
Ectopic pregnancy
Vaginal bleeding

Traumatic Abdominal Emergencies
Vaginal bleeding

Sexual Assault

---

and adjacent structures may be a source of severe abdominal pain. The scope of abdominal pain associated with the female reproductive system may range from benign episodes of difficult menstruation to a potentially life-threatening hemorrhage from a ruptured ovarian cyst or ectopic pregnancy.

Pelvic Inflammatory Disease

Pelvic inflammatory disease (PID) affects about 1 million women annually and is responsible for more than 250,000 hospitalizations each year.[1] The disease results from infection of the cervix, uterus, fallopian tubes, and ovaries and their supporting structures (Fig. 39-4). It usually is caused by sexually transmitted bacteria, most commonly *Neisseria gonorrhoeae* and *Chlamydia trachomatis* (chlamydia). Staphylococci, streptococci, and other pathogens also may cause infection, but these organisms usually are transmitted by doctor's instruments during medical procedures.

Ascending infection from the vaginal area may infect the cervix (cervicitis) initially, followed by infection of the uterus proper (endometritis) and fallopian tubes (salpingitis), and finally the associated contiguous supporting structures around the uterus and fallopian tubes (parametritis). The infection is polymicrobial in etiology, producing diffuse lower abdominal pain associated with low-grade fever (variable), vaginal discharge, and dyspareunia (pain with sexual intercourse). The inflammation frequently follows the onset of menstrual bleeding by 7 to 10 days, when reproductive organs are especially vulnerable to bacterial infection from the presence of relatively avascular endometrial tissue that sloughs during menstruation.

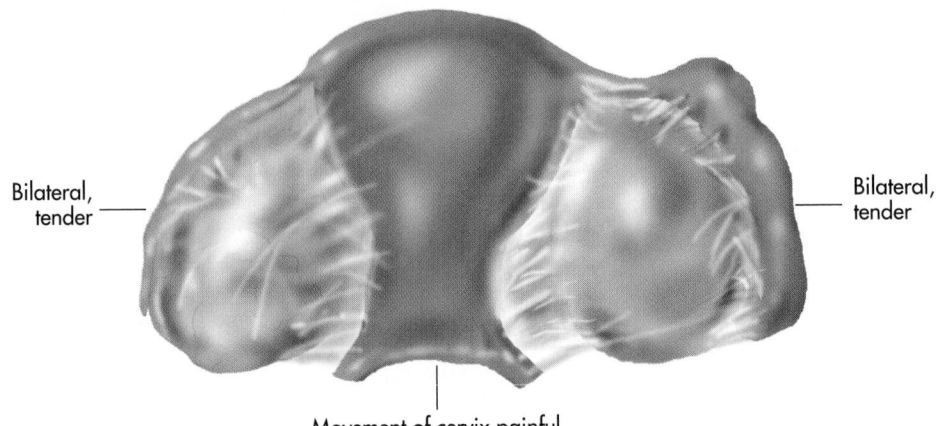

Bilateral, tender

Bilateral, tender

Movement of cervix painful

Fig. 39-4 Pelvic inflammatory disease.

PID often is accompanied by pain on ambulation, with the patient bent forward; taking short, slow steps; and often guarding the abdomen (the "PID shuffle"). Consequences include secondary infertility, ectopic pregnancies, and tuboovarian abscesses. In severe cases, reproductive organs may require surgical removal. Definitive treatment usually consists of antibiotic therapy to eradicate the infection and preserve fallopian tube structure and function.

Ruptured Ovarian Cyst

A ruptured ovarian cyst is a gynecological emergency that can result in significant internal hemorrhage. An ovarian cyst is a thin-walled, fluid-filled sac located on the surface of the ovary (Fig. 39-5). The abdominal pain caused by an ovarian cyst may result from rapid expansion, torsion that produces ischemia, or acute rupture. The type of cyst most prone to rupture is known as the *corpus luteum cyst*, which forms as a result of hemorrhage in a mature corpus luteum. Since the corpus luteum develops after ovulation (day 14 of the 28-day cycle), most ruptures occur about 1 week before menstrual bleeding is to begin. However, some patients with a ruptured ovarian cyst have vaginal bleeding or report a late or missed period at the time of rupture.

> **? CRITICAL THINKING**
>
> *How will you assess for the possibility of bleeding in a patient who you suspect has a ruptured ovarian cyst?*

A ruptured ovarian cyst can result in localized, unilateral lower abdominal pain or generalized signs of peritonitis if massive hemorrhage has occurred. The onset of pain frequently is associated with minimal abdominal trauma, sexual intercourse, or exercise.

Cystitis

Cystitis is inflammation of the inner lining of the bladder, usually caused by a bacterial infection. Although both sexes can develop infection, cystitis in women is more common because the urethra is shorter, making it easier for infectious agents from the vagina or rectum to pass from the mucous membrane around the urethral opening into the bladder. The main symptom of cystitis is a frequent urge to pass urine, with only a small amount of urine passed each time. Other signs and symptoms may include painful (burning) urination, fever, chills, and lower abdominal pain. The urine may occasionally be foul smelling or contain blood. Prompt treatment of cystitis with antibiotics usually settles the infection within 24 hours.

> **NOTE**
>
> Cystitis also can occur from structural abnormality of the ureters (common in children), compression of the urethra (e.g., an enlarged prostate gland in men), or indwelling urinary catheters.

Dysmenorrhea and Mittelschmerz

Many women experience dysmenorrhea during menstruation. Dysmenorrhea is characterized by painful menses but also may be associated with headache, faintness, dizziness, nausea, diarrhea, backache, and leg pain. In severe cases, chills, headache, diarrhea, nausea, vomiting, and syncope can occur. Occurrence is more common in unmarried women and women who have not borne children. The lower abdominal

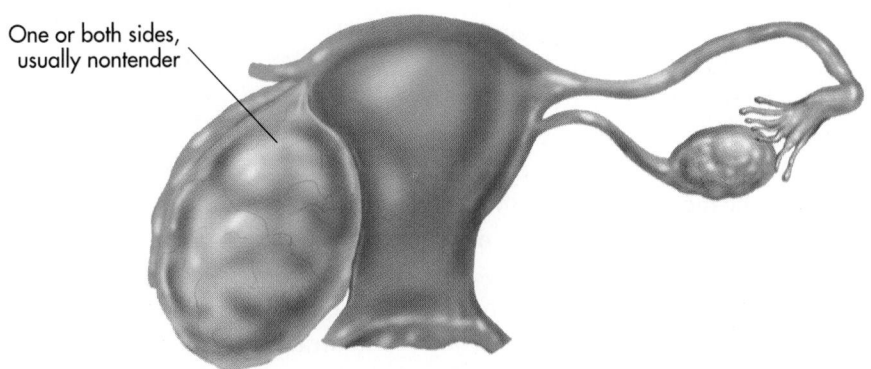

One or both sides, usually nontender

Fig. 39-5 Ovarian cyst.

pains associated with dysmenorrhea are thought to be related to muscular contraction of the myometrium (the muscular layer of the uterus), mediated by local prostaglandins. Other factors associated with dysmenorrhea include infection, inflammation, and the presence of an intrauterine contraceptive device (IUCD).

Mittelschmerz (German for "middle pain") is another cause of pain, possibly from the rupture of the graafian follicle and bleeding from the ovary during the menstrual cycle. Mittelschmerz is characterized by right or left lower quadrant abdominal pain that occurs in the normal midcycle of a menstrual period (after ovulation). Duration is about 24 to 36 hours. The hormones produced by the ovary also may produce slight endometrial bleeding and low-grade fever. Dysmenorrhea and mittelschmerz are not life-threatening conditions, but physician evaluation is required to rule out more serious causes of menstrual pain and differentiate the pain from that of appendicitis.

Endometritis

Endometritis (inflammation of the uterine lining) usually is a result of infection; it occurs most often after childbirth or abortion and is caused by retained placental tissue. (The condition also is a feature of PID and other sexually transmitted infections.) Endometritis may affect the uterus and fallopian tubes, and if untreated, result in sterility, sepsis, and death. Signs and symptoms of endometritis include fever, purulent vaginal discharge, and lower abdominal pain. Treatment includes removal of any foreign tissue and antibiotic therapy.

Endometriosis

Endometriosis is an abnormal gynecological condition characterized by ectopic growth and functioning of endometrial tissue. The disease is thought to result from fragments of endometrium being regurgitated backward (during menstruation) through the fallopian tubes into the peritoneal cavity, where they attach and grow as small cystic structures. The endometrial tissue of endometriosis functions cyclically and undergoes periodic menstrual breakdown that results in bleeding within cysts, stretching of the cyst wall, and pain.

Endometriosis is more common in women who defer pregnancy. The average age of women found to have endometriosis is 37 years. Characteristic

? CRITICAL THINKING

Why do you think these patients tend to be infertile?

symptoms of endometriosis are pain (particularly dysmenorrhea), painful defecation, and suprapubic soreness. Other common symptoms include premenstrual vaginal staining of blood, and infertility. After physician evaluation, treatment may consist of medication with analgesics or hormones and sometimes surgery.

Ectopic Pregnancy

An ectopic pregnancy is one that develops outside of the uterus (most commonly in the fallopian tube, but sometimes in the ovary or [rarely] the abdominal cavity or cervix). Most ectopic pregnancies are discovered in the first 2 months, often before the woman realizes she is pregnant. Signs and symptoms include severe abdominal pain and vaginal "spotting." If rupture occurs, internal hemorrhage, sepsis, and shock may develop. Once confirmed, the ectopic pregnancy is treated with surgery to remove the developing fetus, placenta, and any damaged tissue at the site of the pregnancy. Ectopic pregnancy is common (occurring in 19.7 out of every 1000 pregnancies[1]) and should be considered in any female of reproductive age with abdominal pain. (Ectopic pregnancy is further described in Chapter 40.)

NOTE

Torsion of an ovary around its vascular pedicle (ovarian torsion) may produce severe sudden pain (usually right sided) or a dull ache with sharp exacerbations. This condition may be associated with nausea, vomiting, and low-grade fever, and it often presents similarly to ectopic pregnancy, urinary tract infection, or appendicitis. Ovarian torsion is a surgical emergency that can lead to infection and necrosis of the ovary, resulting in peritonitis and shock.

Vaginal Bleeding

Vaginal bleeding refers to the loss of blood from the uterus, cervix, or vagina. The most common source of nontraumatic vaginal bleeding is menstruation (which rarely results in a request for emergency care). Possible causes of serious nonmenstrual bleeding include:

- Spontaneous abortion
- Disorders of the placenta
- Hormonal imbalances (especially menopause)
- Lesions
- PID
- Onset of labor

The paramedic should never assume that vaginal hemorrhage is due to *normal* menstruation. Some causes of vaginal bleeding may be life threatening and lead to hypovolemic shock and death. (The vaginal passage of clots usually indicates bleeding at a rate greater than menstrual flow.)

Traumatic Emergencies

Traumatic abdominal pain in a female patient usually is associated with vaginal bleeding or sexual assault.

Vaginal Bleeding

Traumatic causes of vaginal bleeding are described in Chapter 25 and include straddle injuries, blows to the perineum, and blunt forces to the lower abdomen. Other causes include foreign bodies inserted into the vagina, injury during intercourse, abortion attempts, and soft tissue injuries resulting from sexual assault. Complications of vaginal bleeding that results from trauma may cause organ rupture of any or all of the pelvic organs and can lead to life-threatening hypovolemia and shock. Treatment is consistent with severe internal injuries and often requires surgical repair.

Assessment and Management

Precise diagnosis of lower abdominal pain in females is difficult because many gynecological conditions produce common clinical characteristics. For example, ruptured ectopic pregnancy, ruptured ovarian cyst, and PID can have identical presentations (Table 39-1). The goal of prehospital care is to quickly identify conditions that require aggressive therapy and rapid transport for surgical intervention. Prehospital care includes obtaining a history of the present illness (including a thorough gynecological history); providing airway, ventilatory, and circulatory support as needed; and transporting the patient for physician evaluation.

History of Present Illness and Obstetric History

A history of the present illness should be obtained to better understand the patient's chief complaint (see Chapter 12). Important associated symptoms include the presence of fever, diaphoresis, syncope, diarrhea, constipation, and abdominal cramping. In addition to gathering information appropriate for all patients, the interview should be expanded to

TABLE 39-1	CHARACTERISTICS OF ABDOMINAL PAIN IN GYNECOLOGICAL EMERGENCIES				
ONSET	**LOCATION**	**QUALITY**	**RADIATION**	**VAGINAL DISCHARGE**	**MENSTRUAL HISTORY**
Ruptured Ectopic Pregnancy					
Rapid (can become generalized)	Unilateral (can generalize)	Cramplike, then steady	Shoulder (may indicate intra-peritoneal bleeding)	Vaginal bleeding (75% of cases)	Amenorrhea, 6 weeks or more since last period
Ruptured Ovarian Cyst					
Sudden	Unilateral (can generalize)	Steady	Shoulder (may indicate intra-peritoneal bleeding)	Possible vaginal bleeding	Usually 1 week before period
PID					
Gradual (can become generalized)	Diffuse, bilateral	Steady ache	Right upper quadrant	Water, foul-smelling discharge	Usually within 1 week after period

include a thorough obstetric history. The obstetric history includes 10 components[2]: (See Chapter 40.)

1. Pregnancy
   a. Total number of pregnancies (gravida)
   b. Number of pregnancies carried to term (para)
2. Previous cesarean deliveries
3. Last menstrual period
   a. Date
   b. Duration
   c. Normalcy
   d. Bleeding between periods
   e. Regularity
4. Possibility of pregnancy
   a. Missed or late period
   b. Breast tenderness
   c. Urinary frequency
   d. Morning sickness (nausea and/or vomiting)
   e. Unprotected sexual activity
5. History of previous gynecological problems
   a. Infections
   b. Bleeding
   c. Dyspareunia
   d. Miscarriage
   e. Abortion
   f. Ectopic pregnancy
6. Present blood loss
   a. Color
   b. Amount (number of pads soaked per hour)
   c. Duration
7. Vaginal discharge
   a. Color
   b. Amount
   c. Odor
8. Use and type of contraceptive
   a. Birth control pills
   b. Intrauterine device (IUD)
   c. Spermicides
   d. Condoms
   e. Withdrawal or rhythm method
   f. Tubal ligation
   g. Contraceptive systems (e.g., Norplant, Depo-Provera)
9. History of trauma to the reproductive system
10. Degree of emotional distress

Physical Examination

A physical examination should be conducted with a comforting and professional attitude. The paramedic should attempt to protect the patient's modesty, maintain privacy, and be considerate of reasons for patient discomfort. When evaluating the potential for serious blood loss, the paramedic should assess the patient's skin and mucous membranes for color, cyanosis, or pallor. Vital sign assessment should include orthostatic measurements. If indicated, the vaginal area should be inspected for bleeding or discharge, noting the color, amount, and presence of clots and/or tissue. The abdomen should be auscultated (if time permits) and palpated to assess for masses, areas of tenderness, guarding, distention, and rebound tenderness.

Patient Management

Patient management includes support of the patient's vital functions and administration of high-concentration oxygen during transport. IV access usually is not necessary unless the patient is demonstrating signs of impending shock or has excessive vaginal bleeding. Many patients prefer to be transported in a left-lateral recumbent, knee-chest position, or in a hips-raised, knees-bent position for comfort.

NOTE

Vaginal bleeding should be controlled with application of sanitary pads or trauma dressings. The vagina should never be packed with dressings or tampons. The number of soaked pads should be counted and documented on the patient care report.

During transport, the patient should be monitored for the onset of serious bleeding. If this occurs or the patient's condition begins to deteriorate, one or two large-bore intravenous (IV) lines should be established with normal saline or lactated Ringer's solution. At this point, electrocardiograph (ECG) and pulse oximetry monitoring are indicated. Drug therapy (e.g., analgesics) may mask important symptoms and generally should not be administered prior to physician evaluation.

Sexual Assault

Sexual assault is a crime of violence with serious physical and psychological implications. Anyone of either gender at any age can be sexually assaulted (see Chapter 44). However, women and girls are most often the victims. It is estimated that one in three women will be raped during their lifetimes and that only 16% of these crimes will be reported.[3] Often, the paramedic is first to encounter these patients. Tact, kindness, and sensitivity during the patient care episode are essential.

> **? CRITICAL THINKING**
>
> *How do you feel about rape, and how would you manage a patient who has been raped?*

A victim of sexual assault should be initially cared for like any other injured patient. After the management of life-threatening injury, however, the paramedic's approach to the patient should be somewhat modified with reference to history taking and the physical examination. Before gathering a history or performing a physical examination, the patient should be moved to a private area. If possible, the patient should be given the opportunity to be interviewed and examined by a paramedic of the same sex.

History Taking

As a rule, victims of sexual assault should not be questioned in detail about the incident in the prehospital setting. The history should be limited to the elements necessary to provide emergency medical care. For example, questions regarding penetration or inquiries about the patient's sexual history or practices are irrelevant to prehospital care and only add to the patient's emotional stress. The patient should be allowed to speak openly if he or she wishes, and all information should be recorded ac-curately and thoroughly. Common reactions to sexual assault may range from anxiety to withdrawal and silence. Denial, anger, and fear also are normal behavior patterns.

Assessment

The purpose of the physical examination is to identify any physical trauma, outside of the pelvic area, for which the patient needs immediate attention. It is not uncommon to find facial fractures, human bites of the hands and breasts, long bone fractures, broken ribs, or trauma to the abdomen. The paramedic should examine the genitalia only if severe injury is present or suspected. When possible, all procedures should be explained to the patient before the examination takes place. All observations of the physical examination should be documented, including the patient's emotional state, condition of the patient's clothing, obvious injuries, and any patient care rendered. The paramedic should maintain a nonjudgmental and professional attitude during the patient care encounter. Personal feelings and prejudices about the victim or the assault should not affect the delivery of patient care.

Management

After managing life-threatening injury, emotional support is the most important patient care procedure that can be offered to a victim of sexual assault. The paramedic should provide a safe environment for the patient and respond appropriately to the victim's physical and emotional needs. Paramedics also should be aware of the need to preserve evidence from the crime scene (further described in Chapter 52). Special considerations include the following:

- Handle clothing as little as possible.
- Do not clean wounds unless absolutely necessary.
- Do not allow the patient to drink or brush teeth.
- Do not use plastic bags for bloodstained articles.
- Bag each clothing item separately.
- Ask the victim not to change clothes or bathe.
- Disturb the crime scene as little as possible.

SUMMARY

- Menstruation is the normal, periodic discharge of blood, mucus, and cellular debris from the uterine mucosa. The release of a secondary oocyte from the ovary is termed *ovulation*.

- Pelvic inflammatory disease (PID) results from infection of the cervix, uterus, fallopian tubes, and ovaries and their supporting structures.

- Ruptured ovarian cyst occurs when a thin-walled, fluid-filled sac located on the ovary ruptures. This can cause significant internal hemorrhage.

- Cystitis is inflammation of the inner lining of the bladder, usually caused by a bacterial infection.

- Dysmenorrhea is characterized by painful menses and may be associated with headache, faintness, dizziness, nausea, diarrhea, backache, and leg pain.

- Mittelschmerz causes abdominal pain, possibly from rupture of the graafian follicle and bleeding from the ovary during the menstrual cycle.

- Endometritis is inflammation of the uterine lining. Endometriosis is characterized by ectopic growth and functioning of endometrial tissue.

- An ectopic pregnancy is one that develops outside the uterus.

- Vaginal bleeding is the loss of blood from the uterus, cervix, or vagina.

- Traumatic causes of vaginal bleeding include straddle injuries, blows to the perineum, blunt forces to the lower abdomen, foreign bodies in the vagina, injury during intercourse, abortion attempts, and soft tissue injuries from sexual assault.

- The goal of prehospital care of lower abdominal pain in the female is to obtain a history (including a gynecological history); provide airway, ventilatory, and circulatory support as needed; and provide transport for physician evaluation.

- Sexual assault is a crime of violence with serious physical and psychological implications.

- Paramedics should be aware of the need to preserve evidence from a sexual assault crime scene.

REFERENCES

1. Rosen P, Barkin R: *Emergency medicine: concepts and clinical practice*, ed 4, St Louis, 1998, Mosby.
2. U.S. Department of Transportation National Highway Safety Administration: *EMT—Paramedic national standard curriculum*, Washington, DC, 1998, The Department.
3. *Rape and sexual assault fact sheet*, DC Rape Crisis Center, www.dcrcc.org/facts.html.

40 Obstetrics

OBJECTIVES

Upon completion of this chapter, the paramedic student will be able to:

1. Describe the organization and function of the specialized structures of pregnancy.
2. Outline fetal development from ovulation through adaptations at birth.
3. Explain normal maternal physiological changes that occur during pregnancy and how they influence prehospital patient care and transportation.
4. Describe appropriate information to be elicited during the obstetrical patient's history.
5. Describe specific techniques for assessment of the pregnant patient.
6. Describe general prehospital care of the pregnant patient.
7. Discuss the implications of prehospital care after trauma to the fetus and mother.
8. Describe the assessment and management of patients with preeclampsia and eclampsia.
9. Explain the pathophysiology, signs and symptoms, and management of the processes that cause vaginal bleeding in pregnancy.
10. Outline the physiological changes that occur during the stages of labor.
11. Describe the role of the paramedic during normal labor and delivery.
12. Compute an Apgar score.
13. Describe assessment and management of postpartum hemorrhage.
14. Discuss the identification, implications, and prehospital management of complicated deliveries.

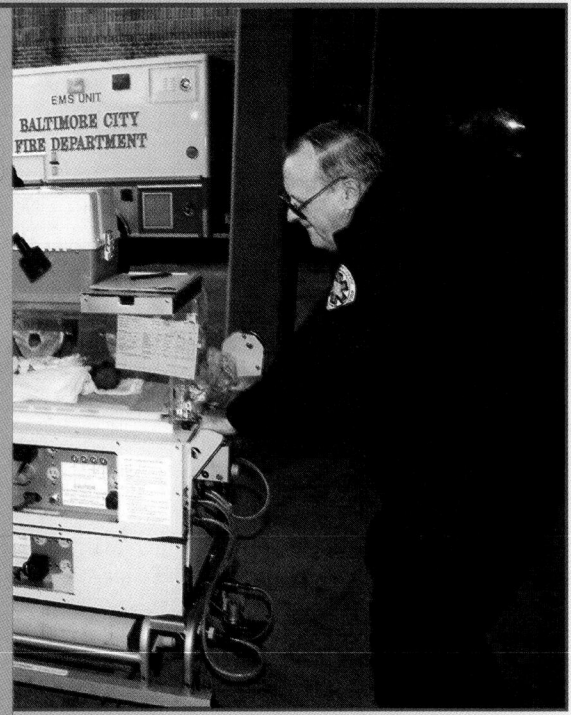

Childbirth is common in the prehospital setting. Most often, EMS personnel only assist in this natural process and provide appropriate care for the mother and newborn. However, obstetrical emergencies can develop suddenly and become life threatening. The paramedic must be prepared to recognize and manage these events and sometimes assist in abnormal deliveries. This chapter presents the etiology and treatment of obstetrical emergencies and the normal and abnormal events associated with childbirth.

KEY TERMS

Apgar score: The evaluation of a newborn's physical condition, usually performed at 1 minute and 5 minutes after birth, including heart rate, respiratory effort, muscle tone, reflex irritability, and color.

crowning: The phase at the end of labor in which the fetal head is seen at the opening of the vagina.

gestation: The period from fertilization of the ovum until birth.

gravida: The number of all current and past pregnancies.

para: The number of past pregnancies that have remained viable to delivery.

placenta: A highly vascular fetal-maternal organ through which the fetus absorbs oxygen, nutrients, and other substances and excretes carbon dioxide and other wastes.

Normal Events of Pregnancy

As described in Chapter 39, fertilization occurs in the fallopian tube when the head of a sperm penetrates a mature ovum. After penetration the nuclei of the sperm and ovum fuse, and the newly fertilized ovum becomes a zygote. The zygote undergoes repeated cell divisions as it passes down the fallopian tube. After a few days of rapid cell division, a ball of cells called a *morula* is formed, it develops into a blastocyst, and it becomes implanted in the uterus (Fig. 40-1). Implantation begins within 7 days after fertilization and is completed when the trophoblast cells make contact with the maternal circulation (about day 12).

Specialized Structures of Pregnancy

Specialized structures of pregnancy include the placenta, the umbilical cord, and the amniotic sac and its fluid. These structures transport metabolic fuel and raw materials for the developing embryo and are part of fetal circulation.

Placenta

The trophoblast cells continue to develop and form the placenta for about 14 days after ovulation. The **placenta** is a disklike organ composed of interlocking fetal and maternal tissues. It is the organ of exchange between the mother and fetus and is responsible for the following five functions:

1. *Transfer of gases.* The diffusion of oxygen and carbon dioxide through the placental membrane is similar to the diffusion that occurs through the pulmonary membranes. Dissolved oxygen in maternal blood passes through the placenta into fetal blood as a result of the pressure gradient between the blood of the mother and fetus. Conversely, as fetal carbon dioxide pressure (Pco_2) accumulates, a low pressure gradient of carbon dioxide develops across the placental membrane and carbon dioxide diffuses from fetal blood to maternal blood.

> **? CRITICAL THINKING**
>
> **What happens to diffusion of gases if the mother becomes hypoxic?**

2. *Transport of nutrients.* Other metabolic substrates that the fetus needs diffuse into fetal blood in the same manner as oxygen. For example, glucose levels in fetal blood are about 20% to 30% lower than those in maternal blood, which results in a rapid diffusion of glucose to the fetus. Diffusion also transports other substrates, such as fatty acids, potassium, sodium, and chloride. The placenta also actively absorbs some nutrients from maternal blood.

3. *Excretion of wastes.* Waste products such as urea, uric acid, and creatinine diffuse from fetal blood into maternal blood, where they are excreted with the waste products of the mother. Wastes transfer from fetal circulation to maternal circulation in the same manner as carbon dioxide does.

Uterine (Fallopian) tube

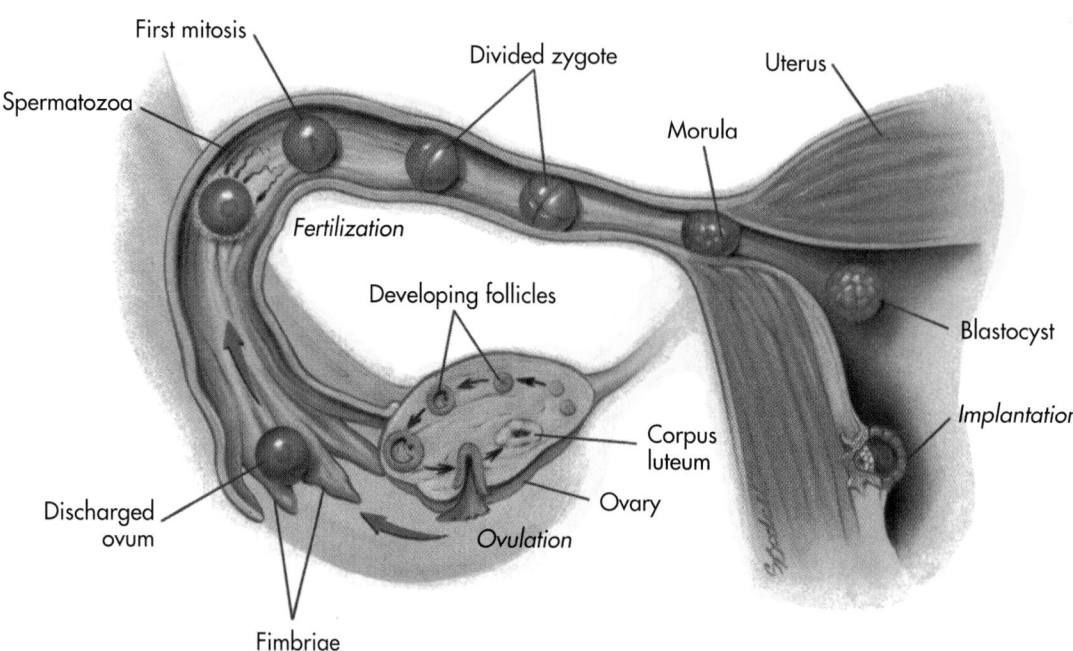

Fig. 40-1 Fertilization and implantation. At ovulation the ovary releases an ovum, which begins its journey through the uterine tube. While in the tube, sperm fertilizes the ovum to form the single-celled zygote. After a few days of rapid cell division, a ball of cells called a *morula* forms. After the morula develops into a hollow ball (blastocyte), implantation occurs. (From Thibodeau G: *Structure and function of the body*, ed 9, St Louis, 1992, Mosby.)

4. *Hormone production.* The placenta becomes a temporary endocrine gland, secreting sufficient quantities of estrogen and progesterone so that by the third month of fetal development the corpus luteum on the ovary no longer is necessary to sustain the pregnancy. Estrogen, progesterone, and other hormones maintain the uterine lining, prevent the occurrence of menses, and stimulate changes in the pregnant woman's breasts, vagina, cervix, and pelvis that prepare her body for delivery and lactation.

5. *Formation of a barrier.* The placenta provides a barrier against some harmful substances and chemicals in the mother's circulation. The placental barrier is incomplete and only partially selective and therefore does not totally protect the fetus. Among the medications that easily transport across the placenta are steroids, narcotics, anesthetics, and some antibiotics.

Umbilical Cord

Blood flows from the fetus to the placenta through two umbilical arteries carrying deoxygenated blood, and oxygenated blood returns to the fetus through the umbilical vein (Fig. 40-2). The blood remains in a closed system independent of and separated from the maternal circulation. Other structures unique to fetal circulation are the ductus venosus, the foramen ovale, and the ductus arteriosus. The ductus venosus is a continuation of the umbilical cord that serves as a shunt to allow most blood returning from the placenta to bypass the immature liver of the embryo and empty directly into the inferior vena cava. The foramen ovale and the ductus arteriosus allow blood to bypass the nonfunctional lungs, which remain collapsed until birth.

The foramen ovale shunts blood from the right atrium directly into the left atrium, and the ductus arteriosus connects the aorta and the pulmonary

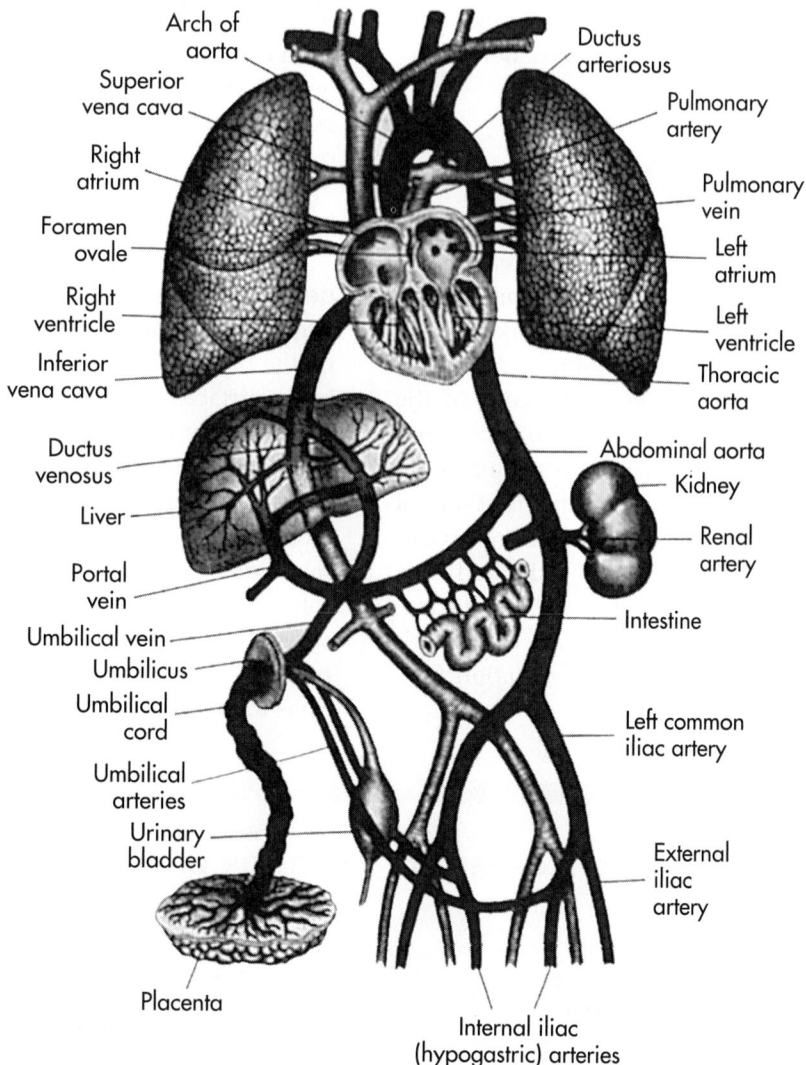

Fig. 40-2 Fetal circulation. (From McCance KL, Huether SE: *Pathophysiology: the biologic basis for disease in adults and children,* ed 3, St Louis, 1998, Mosby.)

artery. Thus the well-oxygenated blood from the placenta enters the left side of the heart rather than the right side, and the left ventricle pumps the oxygenated blood mainly into vessels of the head and forelimbs. The blood entering the right atrium from the superior vena cava progresses downward through the tricuspid valve into the right ventricle. Most of this blood is deoxygenated blood from the head region of the fetus and is pumped by the right ventricle into the pulmonary artery. The deoxygenated blood passes from the pulmonary artery, through the ductus arteriosus, into the descending aorta, through the two umbil-ical arteries, and into the placenta for oxygena-tion. At birth the various arteriovenous shunts close in most infants.

Amniotic Sac and Amniotic Fluid

The amniotic sac is a fluid-filled cavity that com-pletely surrounds and protects the embryo. Amniotic fluid originates from several fetal sources, including fetal urine and secretions from the respiratory tract, skin, and amniotic membranes. The fluid accumu-lates rapidly and amounts to about 175 to 225 mL by the fifteenth week of pregnancy and about 1 L at birth. The rupture of the amniotic membranes produces the watery discharge at the time of delivery.

Fetal Growth and Development

The developing ovum is called an *embryo* during the first 8 weeks of pregnancy, and thereafter until birth it is called a *fetus*. The period during which intrauterine fetal development takes place, known as **gestation,** usually averages 40 weeks from the time of fertilization to delivery of the newborn. The progress of gestation usually consists of 90-day periods, or trimesters. Since conception occurs about 14 days after the first day of the last menstrual period, the obstetrician can calculate fetal development and the estimated date of confinement (EDC), or delivery date, with reasonable reliability. Rapid fetal growth and development characterize the period of gestation (Fig. 40-3 and Box 40-1).

Adjustments of the Infant to Extrauterine Life

Birth results in the infant's loss of the placental connection with the mother and therefore loss of metabolic support. The infant's immediate need to obtain oxygen and excrete carbon dioxide are especially important. This requires circulatory adjustments that permit adequate blood flow through the lungs.

After a normal delivery by a mother who is not depressed with anesthetics, a newborn ordinarily begins to breathe spontaneously when the chest exits the birth canal or with minimal stimulation. At birth, surface tension of the viscid fluid that fills the alveoli holds the walls of the alveoli together. The newborn needs to create more than 25 mm Hg of negative pressure to oppose the effects of this surface tension, allowing the alveoli to open for the first time. The initial inspirations of the newborn can create as much as 50 mm Hg of negative pressure in the intrapleural space. These powerful first breaths open the alveoli and allow further respirations to occur with much less effort.

BOX 40-1

EMBRYO AND FETAL DEVELOPMENT IN UTERO FOR EACH LUNAR MONTH (28 DAYS)

First Lunar Month
- Foundations form for the nervous system, genitourinary system, skin, bones, and lungs.
- Buds of arms and legs begin to form.
- Rudiments of eyes, ears, and nose appear.

Second Lunar Month
- The head is disproportionately large because of brain development.
- Gender differentiation begins.
- The centers of bones begin to ossify.

Third Lunar Month
- Fingers and toes are distinct.
- The placenta is complete.
- Fetal circulation is complete.

Fourth Lunar Month
- Gender is differentiated.
- Rudimentary kidneys secrete urine.
- Heartbeat is present.
- Nasal septum and palate close.

Fifth Lunar Month
- Fetal movements are felt by the mother.
- Heart sounds are perceptible with a fetoscope.

Sixth Lunar Month
- The skin appears wrinkled.
- Eyebrows and fingernails develop.

Seventh Lunar Month
- The skin is red.
- The pupillary membrane disappears from the eyes.
- If born, the infant cries and breathes but frequently dies.

Eighth Lunar Month
- The fetus is viable if born.
- The eyelids open.
- Fingerprints are set.
- Vigorous fetal movement occurs.

Ninth Lunar Month
- The face and body have a loose, wrinkled appearance because of subcutaneous fat deposits.
- Amniotic fluid decreases somewhat.

Tenth Lunar Month
- Skin is smooth.
- Eyes are uniformly slate colored.
- The bones of the skull are ossified and nearly together at sutures.

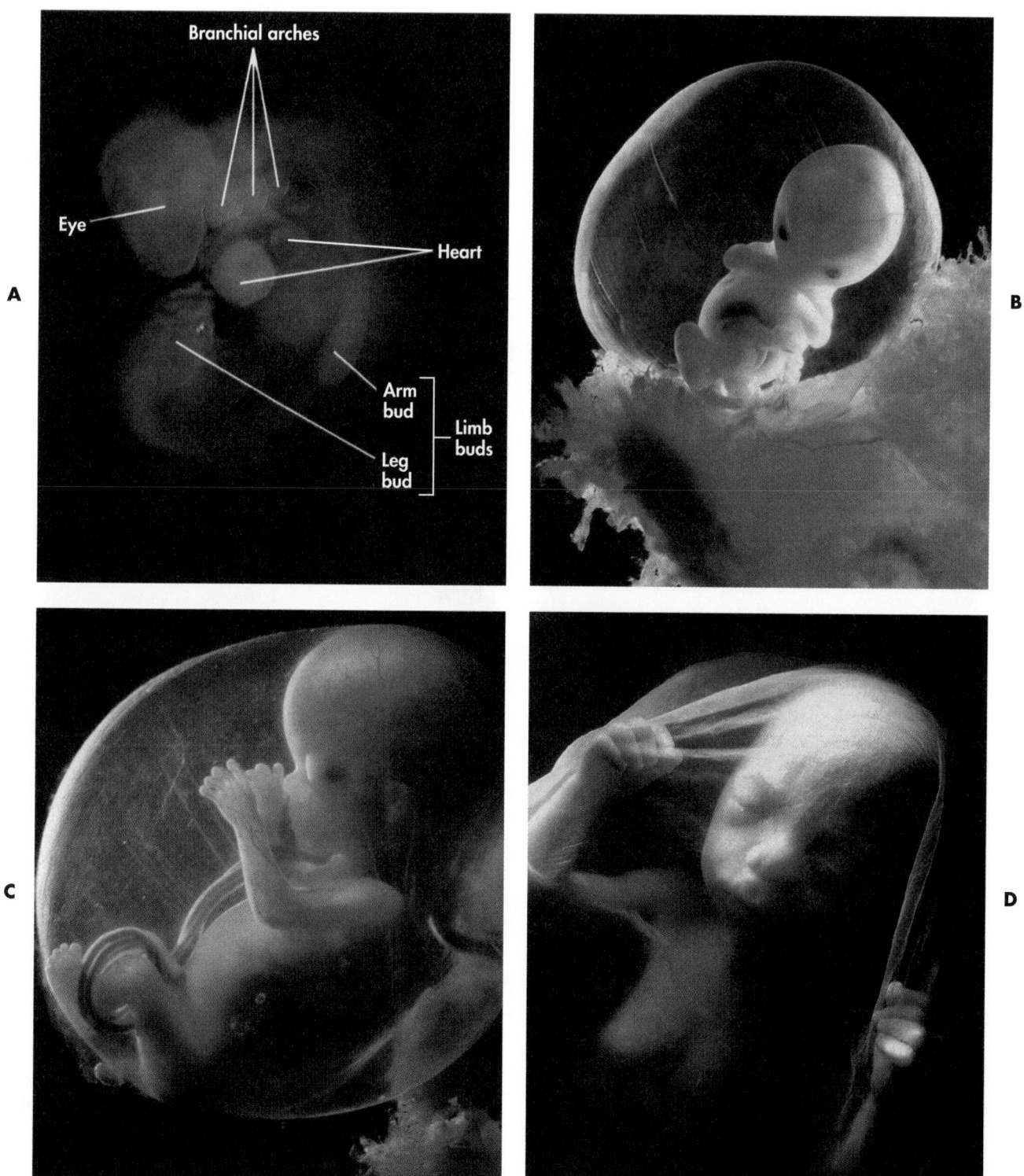

Fig. 40-3 Human embryos and fetuses. **A,** At 35 days. **B,** At 49 days. **C,** At the end of the first trimester. **D,** At 4 months. (From Thibodeau G: *Structure and function of the body,* ed 9, St Louis, 1992, Mosby.)

The ductus venosus, ductus arteriosus, and foramen ovale bypass the immature liver and nonfunctional lungs of the developing fetus. When blood flow through the placenta ceases at birth, there is a resultant increase in systemic vascular resistance and in aortic, left ventricular, and left atrial pressures. In addition, pulmonary vascular resistance decreases greatly because of expansion of the lungs, which reduces the pulmonary arterial, right ventricular, and right atrial pressures. As a result of these changes in pressure gradients, the arteriovenous shunts close normally within a few hours after birth and eventually occlude as a result of growth of fibrous tissue, a change that certain chemical mediators trigger.

? CRITICAL THINKING

Do fetal heart tones sound normal if you auscultate them immediately after birth?

Obstetrical Terminology

Pregnant patients are described by their gravid and parous states. The term **gravida** refers to the number of all of the woman's current and past pregnancies; **para** refers only to the number of the woman's past pregnancies that have remained viable to delivery. For example, a woman who is pregnant for the first time is gravida 1, para 0 (Box 40-2).

Patient Assessment

The paramedic must be familiar with the normal physiological changes that occur in the pregnant woman to adequately assess a pregnant patient.

Maternal Changes During Pregnancy

In addition to cessation of menstruation and the obvious enlargement of the uterus, the pregnant woman undergoes many other physiological changes. These changes affect the genital tract, breasts, gastrointestinal (GI) system, cardiovascular system, respiratory system, and metabolism.

Genital Tract

Uterus

- Uterine size increases from 70 g (nongravid) to 1000 g by term.
- The uterus triples in size and weight by the second month of pregnancy.
- The uterus occupies the entire pelvic cavity and may be palpated suprapubically by the third month of pregnancy.
- The uterus becomes an abdominal organ and the top of the uterus (fundus) reaches the level of the umbilicus by the fourth month of pregnancy.
- The uterine fundus recedes a little when the fetus descends into the pelvis in the last trimester.

Cervix

Increased uterine blood and lymphatic flow cause pelvic congestion and edema. This results in softening and bluish discoloration of the cervix (Chadwick's sign).

Vagina

- The vagina develops a characteristic violet color from increased vascularity.
- The vaginal walls prepare for labor, and the vaginal mucosa increases in thickness.
- Vaginal secretions increase, and the pH decreases to about 3.5 because of increased production of lactic acid from glycogen in the vaginal epithelium. Acidic pH helps keep the vaginal area relatively free of pathogens.

Bladder

Frequency of urination occurs from pressure of the expanding uterus on the bladder. Frequency disappears when the uterus rises out of the pelvis and returns when the fetal head engages in the pelvis near term.

Breasts

- The breasts become tender in the early weeks of pregnancy.
- The breasts increase in size as a result of hypertrophy of the mammary alveoli by the second month of pregnancy.
- The nipples become larger, more deeply pigmented, and more erectile early in pregnancy.
- As breast glands proliferate, they begin to secrete a clear fluid by the tenth week of pregnancy.

Gastrointestinal System

- Morning sickness and nausea may occur at any time, usually beginning by the sixth and abating by the fourteenth week of pregnancy. The cause of morning sickness is related to the high serum levels of chorionic gonadotropin in early pregnancy.
- The enlarging uterus displaces the patient's stomach and intestines upward and laterally. This displacement may cause indigestion and can increase the risk for aspiration in unconscious patients.

? CRITICAL THINKING

What are problems associated with these GI changes for the unconscious pregnant woman who has sustained trauma?

- The liver is displaced backward, upward, and to the right.
- The tone and motility of the GI tract decrease, leading to prolonged gastric emptying and relaxation of the pyloric sphincter. Heartburn and constipation are common.

Cardiovascular System

Heart

- Elevation of the diaphragm displaces the heart to the left and upward. Flat or negative T waves may be present in lead III on the electrocardiogram (ECG).
- Cardiac output increases by 30% by the thirty-fourth week of pregnancy.
- The pulse rate may increase 15 to 20 beats/min above baseline late in the third trimester (variable).
- Pulmonic systolic and apical systolic murmurs are common because lowered blood viscosity and increased flow lead to turbulence in the great vessels.

Circulation

- Total blood volume increases by 30%, and plasma volume increases by 50%.
- Blood pressure decreases 10 to 15 mm Hg during the second trimester because of the reduction in peripheral resistance but gradually increases to prepregnancy levels toward term.
- The enlarged uterus interferes with venous return from the legs.

BOX 40-2

OBSTETRICAL TERMINOLOGY

Antepartum: the maternal period before delivery

Grand multipara: a woman who has had seven deliveries or more

Multigravida: a woman who has had two or more pregnancies

Multipara: a woman who has had two or more deliveries

Nullipara: a woman who has never delivered

Perinatal: occurring at or near the time of birth

Postpartum: the maternal period after delivery

Prenatal: existing or occurring before birth

Primigravida: a woman who is pregnant for the first time

Primipara: a woman who has given birth only once

Term: a pregnancy that has reached 40 weeks' gestation

- Hemorrhoids, slight edema of the ankles, and varicose veins may be present.
- The supine position may cause the uterus to compress the inferior vena cava, producing decreased cardiac filling and decreased cardiac output (supine hypotension syndrome). The patient may become faint and hypotensive while lying on her back after the first or second trimester.

Hematology

- Increased plasma volume results in a decrease in hemoglobin and hematocrit concentrations.
- The leukocyte count increases.
- Fibrinogen levels increase by 50% because of the influence of estrogen and progesterone.

Respiratory System

- Tidal volume and minute ventilation increase by 30% to 40% in late pregnancy.
- Functional residual capacity decreases by about 25%.
- The respiratory rate may be normal or may increase because of elevation of the diaphragm by the uterus.

- P_{CO₂} normally decreases because of the increased respiratory rate (30 torr vs. 40 torr, which provides a gradient for fetal carbon dioxide). This may cause dizziness and a sensation of shortness of breath.

Metabolism

- The mother experiences a normal weight gain of 9.1 kg (20 lb).
- Increased water retention produces increased intracapillary hydrostatic pressure, which favors filtration from the vascular bed and resultant edema.
- The metabolic rate and caloric demand (especially for protein) increase.
- Glucose escapes into urine as a result of increased glomerular filtration.
- Maternal gestational diabetes mellitus (GDM) may result from an impaired ability to metabolize carbohydrates, which usually is caused by a deficiency of insulin. Generally GDM disappears after delivery, but in some cases it returns years later.
- Fetal demands for calcium and iron may deplete maternal stores if the patient does not supplement them through diet.

History

When obtaining a history from an obstetrical patient, the paramedic should first gather information on the chief complaint, which may not be related to the pregnancy. Paramedics should solicit information regarding the onset of signs and symptoms in confidence, and they should provide privacy for the physical examination. After ruling out life-threatening illness or injury, the paramedic should interview the patient to obtain relevant data, including the following eight points:

1. Obstetrical history
   a. Length of gestation
   b. Parity and gravidity
   c. Previous cesarean delivery
   d. Maternal lifestyle (alcohol or other drug use, smoking history)
   e. Infectious disease status
   f. History of previous gynecological or obstetrical complications (e.g., eclampsia, GDM, premature labor, or ectopic pregnancy)
2. Presence of pain
   a. Onset (gradual or sudden)
   b. Character
   c. Duration and evolution over time
   d. Location and radiation
3. Presence, quantity, and character of vaginal bleeding
4. Presence of abnormal vaginal discharge
5. Presence of "show" (expulsion of the mucous plug in early labor) or rupture of membranes
6. Current general health and prenatal care (none, physician, nurse, midwife)

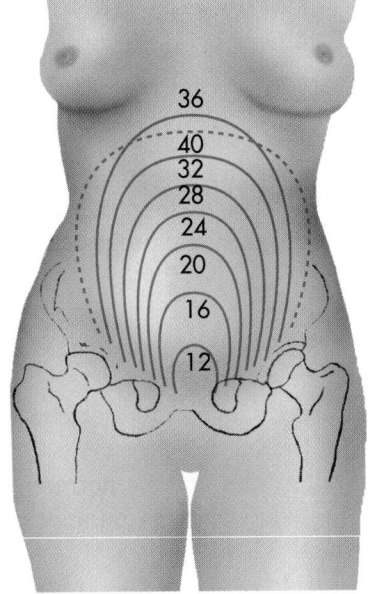

Fig. 40-4 Changes in fundal height during pregnancy. *Weeks 10 to 12:* The uterus is within the pelvis, and fetal heartbeat can be detected with a Doppler probe. *Week 12:* The uterus is palpable just above the symphysis pubis. *Week 16:* The uterus is palpable just between the symphysis pubis and umbilicus. *Week 20:* The uterine fundus is at the lower border of the umbilicus. A fetal heartbeat can be auscultated with a fetoscope. *Weeks 24 to 26:* The uterus becomes ovoid in shape, and the fetus is palpable. *Week 28:* The uterus is approximately halfway between the umbilicus and xiphoid process, and the fetus is easily palpable. *Week 32:* The uterus fundus is just below the xiphoid. *Week 40:* Fundal height drops as the fetus begins to engage in the pelvis. (From Seidel HM et al: *Mosby's guide to physical examination,* ed 2, St Louis, 1991, Mosby.)

7. Allergies and medications taken (especially the use of narcotics in the last 4 hours)
8. Maternal urge to bear down or sensation of imminent bowel movement, indicating imminent delivery

Physical Examination

The patient's chief complaint determines the extent of the physical examination. The prehospital objective in examining an obstetrical patient is to rapidly identify acute surgical or life-threatening conditions or imminent delivery and take appropriate management steps.

The patient's general appearance and skin color should be evaluated. If she is markedly pale, hemorrhage should be suspected. Sunken cheeks, cracked lips, or hollow eyes with a history of vomiting indicate dehydration. Vital signs should be frequently monitored throughout the patient encounter. Orthostatic vital signs may indicate the early presence of significant bleeding or fluid loss. The paramedic should recall that normal physiological changes in the pregnant patient can produce variations in vital signs, such as mild tachycardia, a slight fall in systolic and diastolic blood pressures, and an increase in respiratory rate.

The patient's abdomen should be examined for previous scars and gross deformities, such as those caused by a hernia or marked abdominal distention. Gentle palpation may reveal the presence of masses, enlarged organs, intestinal distention, or a distended bladder, but in late pregnancy, it may be difficult to recognize these abnormalities. During the physical examination, it may be possible to discern peritoneal irritation, which is diagnosed by the presence of tenderness, guarding, or rebound tenderness. If the patient is obviously pregnant, the paramedic may need to evaluate uterine size and monitor the fetus.

Evaluation of Uterine Size

The uterine contour usually is irregular between 8 and 10 weeks' gestation. Therefore early uterine enlargement may not be symmetrical, and the uterus may be deviated to one side. The uterus is above the symphysis pubis at 12 to 16 weeks' gestation, at the level of the umbilicus at 24 weeks, and near the xiphoid process at term. Fig. 40-4 shows changes in fundal height at the various weeks of gestation.

Fetal Monitoring

Fetal heart sounds can be auscultated between 16 and 40 weeks' gestation by use of a stethoscope, fetoscope, or Doppler probe (Fig. 40-5). The benefits of fetal monitoring include ascertaining the presence or absence of fetal circulation and providing baseline measurements for use in evaluating fetal or maternal distress. Fetal heart rate and maternal vital signs should be monitored every 5 to 10 minutes.

When auscultating the fetal heart rate, the high-intensity diaphragm of the stethoscope (the bell of the fetoscope or the microphone of the Doppler probe) should be positioned firmly on the mother's abdominal wall. The diaphragm is then moved in a circular pattern about 6 to 8 inches in diameter around the woman's umbilicus until fetal heart tones can be heard (Fig. 40-6). Once the paramedic locates the tones, the fetal heart rate is measured in beats per minute.

The normal fetal heart rate is 120 to 160 beats/min. A persistent fetal heart rate above 160 (fetal tachycardia) or below 120 beats/min (fetal bradycardia) is an early sign of fetal distress and fetal or maternal hypoxia. Intermittent, short-term acceleration or deceleration of the fetal heart rate usually is normal and can occur at any time. Short-term periodic changes in fetal heart rate are common during fetal sleep, fetal movement, and contractions associated with labor and delivery.

General Management of the Obstetrical Patient

If birth is not imminent, prehospital care for the healthy patient should be limited to basic treatment modalities (airway, ventilatory, and circulatory support) and transportation for physician evaluation. In the absence of distress or injury, the patient should be transported in a comfortable position (usually left lateral recumbent). The paramedic may need to monitor ECG, administer high-concentration oxygen, and monitor the fetus based on patient assessment and vital sign determinations. Medical direction may recommend intravenous (IV) access in some patients. Medications usually are inappropriate because

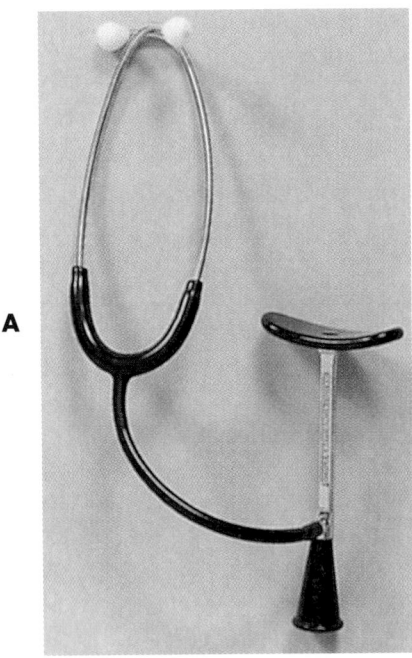

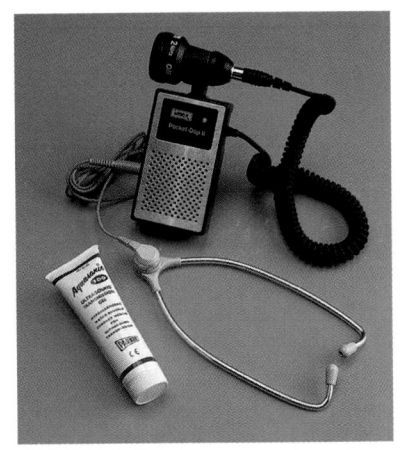

Fig. 40-5 A, Fetoscope. **B,** Doppler probe. (From Seidel HM et al: *Mosby's guide to physical examination,* ed 2, St Louis, 1991, Mosby.)

they may mask symptoms of a deteriorating condition.

Complications of Pregnancy

Complications associated with pregnancy can result from trauma, medical conditions or prior disease processes that the pregnancy can aggravate or mask, the pregnancy itself (vaginal or intraperitoneal hemorrhage), spontaneous abortion, or problems associated with labor and delivery. Often the patient with gynecological or obstetrical complaints is embarrassed, apprehensive, and if pregnant, concerned about the unborn child. Tact, understanding, and a caring, supportive attitude from the paramedic are important when managing these patients.

Trauma During Pregnancy

Poor fetal outcome is related to increasing severity of maternal injury. When the mother sustains life-threatening injuries, 40.6% of fetuses die compared with only 1.6% in nonlife-threatening cases.[1] Anatomical and physiological changes associated with pregnancy can alter the patient's response to

injury, requiring modified assessment, treatment, and transportation strategies.

> **NOTE**
>
> Mortality related to the pregnancy itself is rare, occurring in an estimated 1 of every 30,000 deliveries.[2]

Maternal Injury

The causes of maternal injury in decreasing order of frequency are vehicular crashes, falls, and penetrating objects. These injuries can result in trauma to the gravid uterus and to the maternal bladder, liver, and spleen. In addition, an injury that results in a pelvic fracture can produce massive hemorrhage and damage to the fetal skull. As described in Chapter 18, the severity of any injury depends on many factors and may involve multiple organ systems.

During pregnancy, the fetus is well protected within the uterus; amniotic fluid surrounds the fetus and serves as an excellent shock absorber. Because of this protection, the fetus rarely experiences physical trauma except as a result of direct penetrating wounds or extensive blunt trauma to the maternal abdomen. The greatest risk of fetal death is from fetal distress and intrauterine demise caused

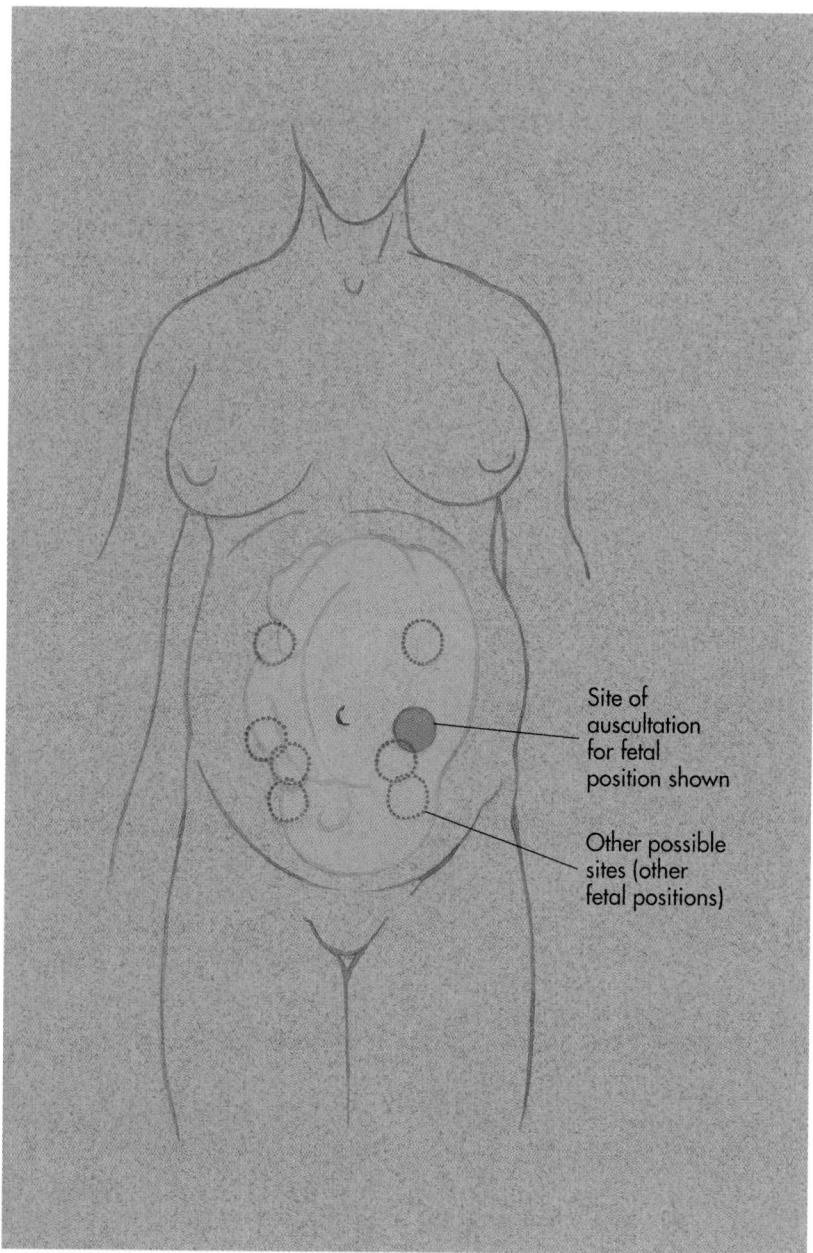

Site of auscultation for fetal position shown

Other possible sites (other fetal positions)

Fig. 40-6 Sites for auscultation of fetal heart tones.

by trauma to the mother or her death. Therefore when dealing with a pregnant trauma patient, the paramedic should promptly assess and intervene on behalf of the mother. Severe abdominal injury can result in premature separation of the placenta, premature labor or abortion, rupture of the uterus, and fetal death. Causes of fetal death from maternal trauma include death of the mother, separation of the placenta, maternal shock, uterine rupture, and fetal head injury.

Assessment and Management

Priorities in assessing and managing a pregnant trauma patient are the same as for a nongravid patient: adequate airway, ventilatory, and circulatory support with spinal precautions; hemorrhage control; and rapid assessment, stabilization, and rapid transportation to a medical facility. Resuscitating the mother is the key to survival of both mother and fetus. Therefore during the initial stages of assessment and management, the paramedic should focus on the mother's status. Regardless of the severity of injury, all pregnant trauma patients should be transported for physician evaluation.

The physical examination should be thorough. The paramedic must detect, identify, and manage injuries that contribute to hypovolemia or hypoxia. With the normal increase in maternal blood volume, the mother can tolerate more blood loss before demonstrating signs and symptoms of hypoperfusion. A 30% to 35% reduction in blood volume can produce minimal changes in blood pressure but reduce uterine blood flow by 10% to 20%.[1] Thus the mother may achieve homeostasis at the expense of the fetus, and the true magnitude of blood loss may be difficult to discern. Fetal monitoring is the best available indicator of fetal well-being after trauma. However, patient transport should never be delayed to assess fetal heart rate.

Accelerations of fetal heart rate above baseline are associated with fetal movement and contractions but also may be an early sign of fetal distress. Decreased fetal movement and increased fetal heart rate can indicate maternal shock.

Decelerations of fetal heart rate below the baseline are associated with a decrease in cardiac output and the presence of hypoxia. A hypoxic fetus in metabolic acidosis cannot accelerate his or her heart rate and thus becomes bradycardic (a heart rate of less than 120 beats/min). Sustained fetal bradycardia (lasting 10 minutes or more) may be a response to increased parasympathetic tone, which the fetus can only tolerate for a short time before becoming acidotic. Fetal bradycardia usually is a late occurrence from maternal hypoxia and decreased maternal circulating volume.

? CRITICAL THINKING

How do you think the traumatized pregnant patient feels emotionally?

Special Management Considerations

Special considerations in managing the pregnant trauma patient include oxygenation, volume replacement, and hemorrhage control. Labor also is a complication of trauma in pregnancy, so the EMS crew should be prepared to manage imminent delivery or spontaneous abortion.

Cardiac arrest can occur in pregnant women from a number of causes (Box 40-3). However, many cardiovascular problems associated with pregnancy are related to anatomy interacting with gravity that decreases the return of venous blood.[2] Key prehospital interventions to prevent cardiac arrest in a distressed or compromised pregnant patient include placing the patient in the left lateral position or *manually* and *gently* displacing the uterus to the left, administering 100% oxygen, and giving a fluid bolus.

NOTE

The key to resuscitation of the child is resuscitation of the mother. The mother cannot be resuscitated until blood flow to her right ventricle is restored.

If cardiac arrest occurs, the paramedic should institute cardiopulmonary resuscitation with a few modifications[2]:

- Relieve aortocaval compression by manually displacing the gravid uterus or by using wedge-shaped cushions, pillows, or overturned chairs to displace the uterus (Fig. 40-7).
- Generally perform chest compressions higher on the sternum (that ensures a palpable pulse wave) to adjust for the shifting of the pelvic and abdominal contents toward the head.
- Address the need for left-lateral tilt of the torso to prevent compression or blockage of the vena cava. This can be accomplished with wedge-shaped pillows that support the tilted torso during chest com-

BOX 40-3

CAUSES OF CARDIAC ARREST ASSOCIATED WITH PREGNANCY

Events that occur at the time of delivery
Amniotic fluid embolism
Eclampsia
Drug toxicity (e.g., due to magnesium sulfate or epidural anesthetic)

Events that occur from complex physiological changes associated with pregnancy
Congestive cardiomyopathy
Aortic dissection
Pulmonary embolism
Hemorrhage from a pregnancy-related pathological condition

pression, or by using the angled backs of several chairs and the angled thighs of several rescuers.

An aggressive resuscitation effort is justified in patients near term to allow for emergency cesarean delivery at the emergency department. Fetal survival is good if the interval between maternal death and delivery is less than 5 minutes and poor if longer than 20 to 25 minutes. Advance notice to the receiving emergency department of impending emergency cesarean delivery is paramount.

Oxygenation

- Adequate airway maintenance and oxygenation are essential to prevention of fetal hypoxemia.
- Oxygen requirements are 10% to 20% greater than in the nongravid patient. Fetal hypoxia may occur with even small changes in maternal oxygenation. The paramedic should administer high-concentration oxygen.
- If available, the paramedic should use pulse oximetry to monitor oxygen saturation.

Volume replacement

- Signs and symptoms of hypovolemia may not be present until a blood loss is large.
- Blood is preferentially shunted from the uterus to preserve maternal blood pressure.
- Bleeding also may occur inside the uterus. The pregnant uterus can sequester up to 2000 mL of blood after separation of the placenta with little or no evidence of vaginal bleeding.[1]
- The paramedic initiates crystalloid fluid replacement, even in normotensive patients.
- Application of pneumatic antishock garment (PASG) is controversial. If the PASG is to be applied, only the leg compartments should be inflated because use of the abdominal compartment may increase blood loss from disrupted vasculature of the pelvis. The paramedic may rarely inflate the abdominal compartment when maternal and fetal death are imminent (by order of medical direction).
- Vasopressors generally are not recommended because they decrease uterine blood flow and fetal oxygen delivery.

Hemorrhage control

- External hemorrhage should be controlled as in a nonpregnant patient.

- Vaginal bleeding may indicate placental separation or uterine rupture.
- Avoid a vaginal examination. It may increase bleeding and precipitate delivery, especially if unsuspected placenta previa is present.
- Document the amount and color of vaginal bleeding.
- Collect and transport any expelled tissue with the patient to the medical facility.

Transportation Strategies

Pregnant patients after 3 to 4 months' gestation should not be transported in a supine position because of the potential for supine hypotension. In the absence of suspected spinal injury, transport the patient in a left lateral recumbent position. If spinal injury is suspected, prepare the patient for transportation in the following manner:

1. Fully immobilize the patient on a long spine board.
2. After immobilization, carefully tilt the board on its left side by log-rolling the secured patient 10 to 15 degrees.
3. Place a blanket, pillow, or towel under the right side of the board to move the uterus to the left side.

? CRITICAL THINKING

Are facilities in your community equipped to manage high-risk deliveries?

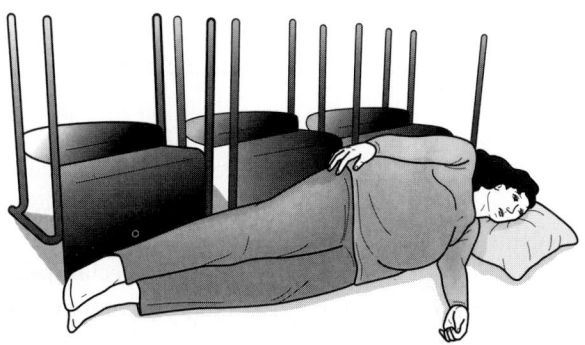

Fig. 40-7 Using chairs and patient positioning to displace the uterus.

Medical Conditions and Disease Processes

Pregnancy can mask or aggravate some medical conditions and disease processes, including acute appendicitis, acute cholecystitis, hypertension, diabetes, infection, neuromuscular disorders, and cardiovascular disease. Two hypertensive disorders, preeclampsia and eclampsia (toxemia of pregnancy), are specific to pregnancy. Hypertensive disorders occur in about 5% of pregnancies in the United States and increases the risk to both the mother and the fetus.[1]

Preeclampsia and Eclampsia

Preeclampsia is a disease of unknown origin that primarily affects previously healthy, normotensive primigravidae. The disease occurs after 20 weeks' gestation, often near term. The pathophysiology of preeclampsia, which does not reverse until after delivery, is characterized by vasospasm, endothelial cell injury, increased capillary permeability, and activation of the clotting cascade. The signs and symptoms of preeclampsia result from hypoperfusion to the tissue or organs involved (Box 40-4). Eclampsia is characterized by the same signs and symptoms with the addition of seizures or coma.

The criteria for diagnosis of preeclampsia are based on the presence of the "classic triad," which includes hypertension (blood pressure greater than 140/90 mm Hg, an acute rise of 20 mm Hg in systolic pressure, or a rise of 10 mm Hg in diastolic pressure over prepregnancy levels), proteinuria, and excessive weight gain with edema.[3] Besides nulliparity, factors predisposing to preeclampsia include advanced maternal age, chronic hypertension, chronic renal disease, vascular diseases such as diabetes and systemic lupus, and multiple gestation. Preeclampsia is a clinical diagnosis that can be confirmed by postpartum renal biopsy. When preeclampsia is suspected, most patients are hospitalized or confined to bed rest at home until delivery.

Management. Not all hypertensive patients have preeclampsia, and not all preeclamptic patients have hypertension. Because of the potentially devastating course of the illness, the paramedic should always suspect preeclampsia or eclampsia when hypertension is present in late pregnancy. If preeclampsia or eclampsia is suspected, prehospital care is directed at preventing or controlling seizures and treating hypertension.

Seizure activity in eclampsia is similar to generalized grand mal seizures of other etiologies and is characterized by tonic-clonic activity (described in Chapter 29). The seizure often begins around the mouth in the form of facial twitching. Eclampsia may be associated with apnea during the seizure. Labor can begin spontaneously and progress rapidly. The regimen for managing severe preeclampsia is as follows:

1. Place the patient in a left lateral recumbent position to maintain or improve uteroplacental blood flow and to minimize risk of insult to the fetus.

BOX 40-4

SIGNS AND SYMPTOMS OF PREECLAMPSIA

Cerebrum
Headache
Hyperreflexia
Dizziness
Confusion
Seizures
Coma

Retina
Blurred vision
Diplopia

Gastrointestinal System
Nausea
Vomiting
Right upper quadrant or epigastric pain and tenderness

Renal System
Proteinuria
Azotemia
Oliguria
Anuria
Hematuria
Hemoglobinuria

Vasculature or Endothelium
Hypertension
Edema
Activation of the clotting cascade

Placenta
Abruptio placentae
Fetal distress

2. Handle the patient gently and minimize sensory stimulation (e.g., darken the ambulance) to avoid precipitating seizures.
3. Administer high-concentration oxygen and assist respirations as needed.
4. Initiate IV therapy per protocol.
5. Anticipate seizures at any moment, and be prepared to provide airway, ventilatory, and circulatory support.
6. Be prepared to administer the following medications per medical direction and local protocol:
   a. *Magnesium sulfate* 10%. The antidote *(calcium gluconate)* should be close at hand to treat respiratory depression.
   b. *Diazepam* (Valium)
      (1) *Diazepam* may precipitate a fall in blood pressure.
      (2) *Diazepam* may jeopardize fetal circulation.
      (3) Closely monitor vital signs.
7. Gently transport the patient to an appropriate medical facility.

Vaginal Bleeding

Vaginal bleeding during pregnancy can result from abortion (miscarriage), ectopic pregnancy, abruptio placentae, placenta previa, uterine rupture, or postpartum hemorrhage. Patients with vaginal bleeding develop varying degrees of blood loss, and some require aggressive resuscitation.

> **? CRITICAL THINKING**
>
> **As the mother loses blood from vaginal hemorrhage, what effect does that have on the fetus?**

Abortion. Abortion is the termination of pregnancy from any cause before 20 weeks' gestation (after which it is known as a *preterm birth*). Abortion is the most frequent cause of vaginal bleeding in pregnant women and occurs in about 1 in 10 pregnancies. Box 40-5 lists common classifications of abortion.

> **NOTE**
>
> A criminal abortion is an intentional ending of any pregnancy under any condition not allowed by law.

Most abortions occur in the first trimester, usually before the tenth week. The patient often is anxious and apprehensive and complains of vaginal bleeding, which may be slight or profuse. In addition, the patient may have suprapubic pain referred to the lower back and described as "cramp-like" and similar to the pain of labor or menstruation. When obtaining a history, the paramedic should ascertain the time of onset of pain and bleeding, amount of blood loss (a soaked sanitary pad suggests 20 to 30 mL of blood loss), and whether the patient passed any tissue with the blood. If the patient passed tissue during bleeding episodes, it should be collected and transported with the patient for analysis.

Management. The assessment of all first-trimester emergencies should include close observation for signs of significant blood loss and hypovolemia. Vital signs (including orthostatic vital signs) should be measured frequently during transportation. Depending on the patient's hemodynamic status, IV fluid therapy may be indicated. All patients with suspected abortion should receive oxygen, emotional support, and transportation for physician evaluation.

> **BOX 40-5**
>
> **CLASSIFICATIONS OF ABORTION**
>
> **Complete abortion:** an abortion in which the patient has passed all of the products of conception.
>
> **Incomplete abortion:** an abortion in which the patient has passed some but not all of the products of conception.
>
> **Induced abortion:** an abortion in which the pregnancy is intentionally terminated.
>
> **Missed abortion:** the retention of the fetus in utero for 4 or more weeks after fetal death.
>
> **Spontaneous abortion:** an abortion that usually occurs before the twelfth week of gestation (the lay term is *miscarriage*). (Predisposing factors include acute or chronic illness in the mother, abnormalities in the fetus, and abnormal attachment of the placenta. Often the cause is unknown.)
>
> **Therapeutic abortion:** a pregnancy legally terminated for reasons of maternal well-being.
>
> **Threatened abortion:** an abortion in which a patient has some uterine bleeding with an intrauterine pregnancy in which the internal cervical os is closed. A threatened abortion may stabilize and end in normal delivery or progress to an incomplete or complete abortion.

Ectopic pregnancy. An ectopic pregnancy occurs when a fertilized ovum implants anywhere other than the endometrium of the uterine cavity. Ectopic gestation occurs in 1 of every 200 pregnancies; it is the leading cause of first-trimester death and accounts for more than 11% of all maternal deaths in the United States.[1] Death from ectopic pregnancy usually results from hemorrhage.

Although ectopic pregnancy has numerous causes, most involve factors that delay or prevent passage of the fertilized ovum to its normal site of implantation. Predisposing factors include pelvic inflammatory disease (PID), adhesions from previous surgery, tubal ligation, previous ectopic pregnancy, and possibly the presence of intrauterine contraceptive devices (IUCDs). Thus it is important to obtain a thorough gynecological history. Although the time from fertilization varies, most ruptures occur by 2 to 12 weeks' gestation.

The signs and symptoms of ectopic pregnancy often are difficult to distinguish from those of a ruptured ovarian cyst, PID, appendicitis, or abortion (thus the name the *great imitator*). The classic triad of symptoms includes abdominal pain, vaginal bleeding, and amenorrhea; however, vaginal bleeding may be absent, spotty, or minimal, and amenorrhea may be replaced by oligomenorrhea (scanty flow). The variable presentation of ectopic pregnancy is one reason for its high-risk profile. Other symptoms of ectopic pregnancy include signs of early pregnancy, referred pain to the shoulder, nausea, vomiting, syncope, and the classic signs of shock.

Management. A ruptured ectopic pregnancy is a true emergency that requires initial resuscitation measures and rapid transportation for surgical intervention. The patient may deteriorate rapidly and become hemodynamically unstable. If the paramedic suspects an ectopic pregnancy, he or she should manage the patient like any victim of hemorrhagic shock—with airway, ventilatory, and circulatory support and aggressive IV fluid resuscitation.

Third-trimester bleeding. Third-trimester bleeding occurs in 3% of all pregnancies and is never normal. The majority of bleeding episodes are a result of abruptio placentae, placenta previa, or uterine rupture. Table 40-1 differentiates among abruptio placentae, placenta previa, and uterine rupture.

Abruptio placentae. Abruptio placentae is partial or complete detachment of a normally implanted placenta at more than 20 weeks' gestation. It occurs in up to 2% of all pregnancies and is severe enough to result in fetal death in 1 in 400 cases of abruption.[1] Predisposing factors to abruptio placentae include maternal hypertension, preeclampsia, multiparity, trauma, and previous abruption.

TABLE 40-1	DIFFERENTIATION OF ABRUPTIO PLACENTAE, PLACENTIA PREVIA, AND UTERINE RUPTURE			
HISTORY	**BLEEDING**	**ABNORMAL PAIN**	**ABDOMINAL EXAMINATION**
Abruptio Placentae Association with toxemia of pregnancy and hypertension of any cause	Single attack of scant, dark vaginal bleeding (often concealed) that continues until delivery	Present	Localized uterine tenderness Labor Absent fetal heart tones (often)
Placenta Previa Lack of association with toxemia of pregnancy	Repeated "warning" hemorrhages over days to weeks	Usually absent	Lack of uterine tenderness (usually) Labor (rare) Fetal heart tones (usually)
Uterine Rupture Previous cesarean section	Possible bleeding	Usually present and associated with sudden onset of nausea and vomiting	Diffuse abdominal tenderness Sudden cessation of labor Possible fetal heart tones

? CRITICAL THINKING

Why is abruptio placentae associated with such a high fetal death rate?

The common presentation of abruptio placentae is sudden third-trimester vaginal bleeding and pain. The vaginal bleeding may be minimal and often is out of proportion to the degree of shock because much of the hemorrhage may be concealed. The more extensive the abruption, the greater the uterine irritability, resulting in a tender abdomen and rigid uterus. Contractions may be present. In severe abruptio placentae, fetal heart sounds are absent because fetal death is likely.

Placenta previa. Placenta previa is placental implantation in the lower uterine segment encroaching on or covering the cervical os. It occurs in about 1 in 300 deliveries, and the incidence is higher in preterm births. The condition is characterized by painless, bright red bleeding without uterine contraction. The bleeding may occur in repetitive episodes and be slight to moderate, becoming more profuse if active labor ensues. Fetal heart rate often is diminished because of placental insufficiency and hypoxia.

Placenta previa is associated with increasing maternal age, multiparity, previous cesarean section, and previous placenta previa episodes. Recent sexual intercourse can precipitate bleeding.

Uterine rupture. Uterine rupture is a spontaneous or traumatic rupture of the uterine wall that may result from re-opening of a previous uterine scar (e.g., a previous cesarean section), a prolonged or obstructed labor, or direct trauma. It occurs in about 1 in 1400 deliveries and has a 5% to 15% maternal mortality rate and a 50% fetal mortality rate.[1]

Uterine rupture is characterized by sudden abdominal pain described as steady and "tearing," active labor, early signs of shock (complaints of weakness, dizziness, anxiety), and vaginal bleeding, which may not be visible. On examination, the abdomen usually is rigid with diffuse pain, and fetal parts may easily be palpated through the abdominal wall.

Management of third-trimester bleeding. Prehospital management of a patient with third-trimester bleeding is aimed at preventing shock. The paramedic should not attempt to examine the patient vaginally; doing so may increase hemorrhage and pre-cipitate labor. Emergency care measures should include the following:

1. Provide adequate airway, ventilatory, and circulatory support as needed (with spinal precautions if indicated).
2. Place patient in left lateral recumbent position.
3. Begin transportation immediately.
4. Initiate IV therapy with volume-expanding fluid.
5. Apply a fresh perineal pad and note the time of application to assess bleeding during transportation.
6. Check fundal height and document it for baseline measurement.
7. Closely monitor the patient's vital signs en route to the medical facility.

Labor and Delivery

Parturition is the process by which the infant is born. Near the end of pregnancy the uterus becomes progressively more irritable and exhibits occasional contractions, which become stronger and more frequent until parturition begins. During and as a result of these contractions, the cervix begins to dilate. As uterine contractions increase, complete cervical dilation occurs to about 10 cm; the amniotic sac ruptures; and the fetus, and shortly thereafter the placenta, are expelled from the uterus through the vaginal canal (Fig. 40-8).

Stages of labor. Labor follows several distinct stages. The lengths of these stages vary, depending on whether the mother is nullipara or multipara (Box 40-6). Therefore the paramedic should use the stages

---

BOX 40-6

STAGES OF LABOR

Stage I (Dilation Stage)
- Onset of regular contractions to complete cervical dilation
- Average time: 12.5 hours in primipara, 7 hours in multipara

Stage II (Expulsion Stage)
- Full dilation of cervix to delivery of the newborn
- Average time: 80 minutes in primipara, 30 minutes in multipara

Stage III (Placental Stage)
- Immediately after delivery of the infant until expulsion of the placenta
- Average time: 5 to 20 minutes

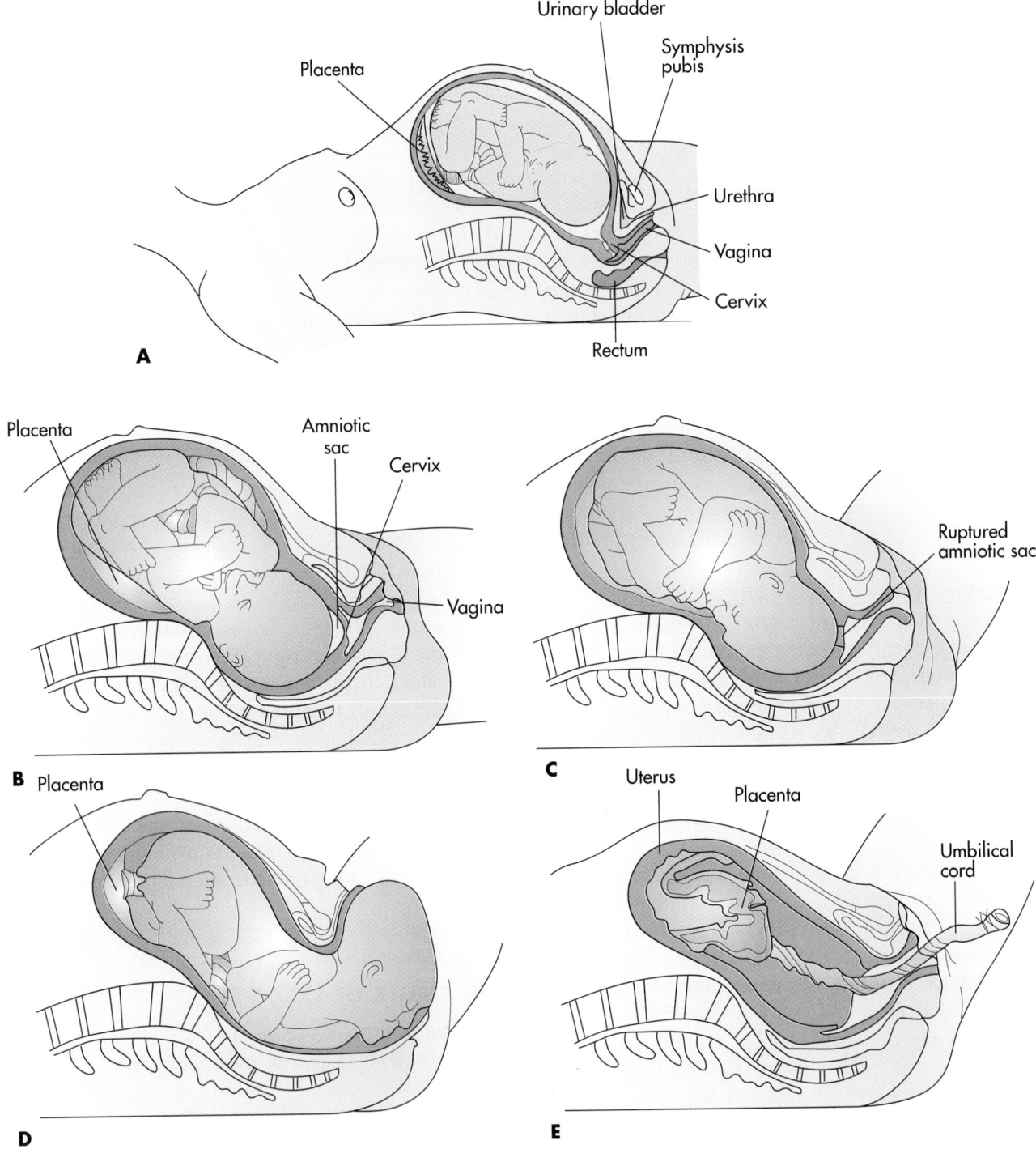

Fig. 40-8 Parturition. **A,** The relation of the fetus to the mother. **B,** The fetus moves into the birth canal. **C,** Dilation of the cervix is complete. **D,** The fetus is expelled from the uterus. **E,** The placenta is expelled.

of labor only as a guideline in estimating labor progression in the average pregnancy. About 2 to 3 weeks before the onset of active labor, while the cervix undergoes the process of softening, effacement (thinning), and dilation, the uterus begins to become a contractile organ. Braxton-Hicks contractions, which before 30 weeks' gestation were uncoordinated and of low intensity, begin to steadily increase in intensity and duration. The patient may not notice the contractions or may perceive them as

NOTE

There is a great deal of individual variation in the perception and tolerance of uterine contractions. Some mothers experience relatively painless contractions even with the onset of labor, whereas others are uncomfortable from the earlier and less intense Braxton-Hicks contractions. In the former group, delivery may be more imminent than anticipated; members of the latter group may develop "false labor" several days to weeks before term.

a slight uterine hardening. The contractions eventually strengthen and increase in frequency and duration, heralding the onset of clinical labor.

Labor begins with a prodromal stage that marks the infant's descent into the birth canal. The fetal descent is characterized by a relief of pressure in the upper abdomen and a simultaneous increase in pressure in the pelvis. During this stage a mucous plug (sometimes mixed with blood, thus the name *bloody show*) is expelled from the dilating cervix and discharged from the vagina. The mother may not notice the prodromal stage.

The first stage of labor begins with the onset of regular contractions and ends with complete dilation of the cervix. The uterine contractions generally occur at 5- to 15-minute intervals and are characterized by cramplike abdominal pains that radiate to the small of the back. As the uterus contracts, the cervix becomes soft and thinned (effaced), and the less muscular segment of the uterus is pulled upward over the presenting part. The first stage usually lasts 8 to 12 hours in the nullipara mother and about 6 to 8 hours in the multipara mother. In most pregnancies the amniotic sac ruptures (rupture of membranes) toward the end of the first stage of labor.

? CRITICAL THINKING

What comfort measures can you use during transportation for the patient who is in the first stage of labor?

The second stage of labor is measured from full dilation of the cervix to delivery of the infant. During the second stage the fetal head enters the birth canal, and the mother's pain and contractions become more intense and frequent (usually 2 to 3 minutes apart). Often the mother becomes diaphoretic and tachycardiac during this stage. She experiences an urge to bear down with each contraction and may express the need to have a bowel movement (a normal sensation caused by pressure of the fetal head against the mother's rectum). The presenting part of the fetus (usually the head) emerges from the vaginal opening. This process, known as **crowning,** indicates that delivery is imminent. The second stage of labor usually lasts 1 to 2 hours in the nullipara mother and 30 minutes or less in the multipara mother.

The third stage of labor begins with delivery of the infant and ends when the placenta is expelled and the uterus has contracted. The length of this stage varies from 5 to 60 minutes, regardless of parity.

Signs and symptoms of imminent delivery. The following signs and symptoms indicate that delivery is imminent and that the paramedic should prepare for childbirth at the scene.

- Regular contractions last 45 to 60 seconds at 1- to 2-minute intervals. Intervals are measured from the beginning of one contraction to the beginning of the next. If contractions are more than 5 minutes apart, there generally is time to transport the mother to a receiving hospital.
- The mother has an urge to bear down or has a sensation of a bowel movement.
- There is a large amount of bloody show.
- Crowning occurs.
- The mother believes that delivery is imminent.

If any of these signs and symptoms are present, the EMS crew should prepare for delivery. With the exception of cord presentation (described later in this chapter), the paramedic should not attempt to delay delivery. If complications are anticipated, or an abnormal delivery occurs, medical direction may recommend expedited transportation of the patient to a medical facility.

Preparation for delivery. When preparing for delivery in the prehospital setting, the paramedic should attempt to provide an area of privacy. The mother should be positioned on a bed, stretcher, or table that has a surface long enough to project beyond the mother's vagina. The delivery area should be as clean as possible and covered with absorbent material to guard against staining and contamination by blood and fecal material.

The mother should be placed on her back with her knees flexed and widely separated (or in another position preferred by the mother) and the vaginal area draped appropriately. If delivery occurs in an automobile, the mother should be instructed to lie on her back across the seat with one leg flexed on the seat and the other leg resting on the floorboard. A pillow or blanket, if available, should be placed beneath the mother's buttocks to facilitate delivery of the infant's head. The paramedic should evaluate the mother's vital signs for baseline measurements and monitor fetal heart rate for signs of fetal distress. Per protocol and medical direction, the paramedic should consider maternal oxygen administration and IV access for volume expansion or postdelivery administration of *oxytocin* (Pitocin) if needed.

The mother should be coached to bear down and push during contractions and to rest between contractions to conserve strength. If the mother finds it difficult to refrain from pushing, she should be encouraged to breathe deeply or "pant" through her mouth between contractions to prevent glottic closure. Deep breathing and panting help decrease the force of bearing down and promote rest.

Delivery equipment. Prehospital delivery equipment ("OB kit") generally includes the following components (Fig. 40-9):

- Surgical scissors
- Cord clamps or umbilical tape
- Towels
- Surgical masks
- 4 × 4 gauze sponges
- Sanitary napkins

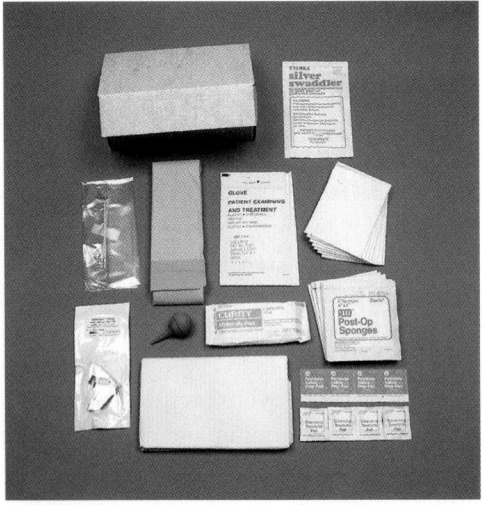

Fig. 40-9 Prehospital delivery equipment.

- Bulb syringe and DeLee suction kit
- Baby blanket and baby stocking cap
- Plastic bag for placental transportation
- Neonatal resuscitation equipment
- IV fluid supplies

Personal protective measures and sterile technique should be used before handling this equipment.

Assistance with delivery. In most cases the paramedic only assists in the natural events of childbirth. The primary responsibilities of the EMS crew are to prevent an uncontrolled delivery and protect the infant from cold and stress after the birth. The following are steps to be taken in assisting the mother with a normal delivery (Fig. 40-10):

1. Don sterile gloves and other personal protective equipment.
2. When crowning occurs, apply gentle palm pressure to the infant's head to prevent an explosive delivery and tearing of the perineum. If membranes are still intact, tear the sac with finger pressure to allow escape of amniotic fluid.
3. After delivery of the head, examine the infant's neck for a looped umbilical cord. If the cord is looped around the neck, gently slip it over the infant's head.
4. Suction the infant's mouth and nose with a bulb syringe to clear the airway. Perform suction after the head appears but before the next contraction, which delivers the shoulders and chest. The birth canal prevents chest expansion and minimizes the risk of aspiration if suction is performed well before the first breath, which usually occurs on delivery of the chest and shoulders.
5. Support the infant's head as it rotates for shoulder presentation. Most infants present face down, after which the infant rotates to the left so that the shoulders present in an anterior-posterior position.
6. With gentle pressure, guide the infant's head downward to deliver the anterior shoulder and then upward to release the posterior shoulder. The remainder of the infant is delivered quickly by smooth uterine contraction.
7. Be careful to grasp and support the infant as he or she emerges. Use care because the infant

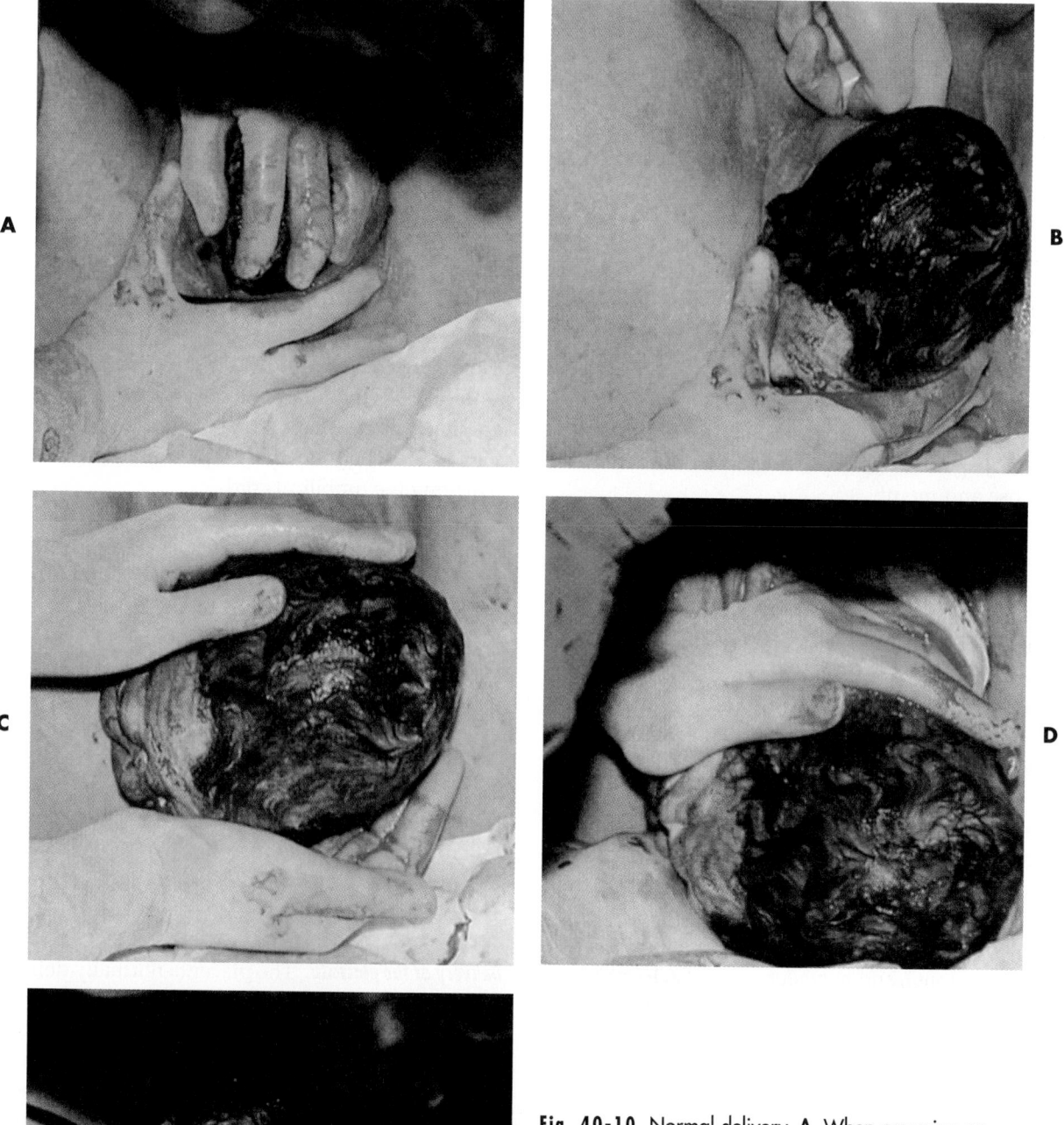

Fig. 40-10 Normal delivery. **A,** When crowning occurs, apply gentle palm pressure to the infant's head. **B,** Examine the neck for the presence of a looped umbilical cord. **C,** Support the infant's head as it rotates for shoulder presentation. **D,** Guide the infant's head downward to deliver the anterior shoulder. **E,** Guide the infant's head upward to release the posterior shoulder. (From Al-Azzawi F: *Color atlas of childbirth and obstetric techniques,* London, 1990, Wolfe.)

is very slippery. Hold the infant firmly with his or her head dependent to facilitate drainage of secretions. Maintain the infant's position at or slightly above the level of the mother's vagina to prevent overtransfusion or undertransfusion of blood from the umbilical cord.

? CRITICAL THINKING

How do you think you will feel after delivering a healthy infant?

8. Clear the infant's airway of any secretions with sterile gauze, and repeat suction of the infant's nose and mouth.
9. Dry the infant with sterile towels, and cover the infant (especially the head) to reduce heat loss.
10. Record the infant's gender and time of birth.

Evaluation of the infant. After delivery the newborn should be dried and covered to prevent heat loss, positioned on the side or with padding under the back, the airway cleared, and tactile stimulation should be provided to initiate respirations. Suction should be continued as necessary. If there is no need for resuscitation, the paramedic should assign an **Apgar score** at 1 minute and 5 minutes (Table 40-2) to evaluate in the infant. Criteria for computing the Apgar score include *appearance* (color), *pulse* (heart rate), *grimace* (reflex irritability to stimulation), *activity* (muscle tone), and *respiratory effort*. Each criterion is rated on a basis of 0 to 2, and the numbers are added for a total Apgar score.

NOTE

The paramedic should never delay or interrupt resuscitation efforts to assign an Apgar score.

An Apgar score of 10 indicates that the infant is in the best possible condition, 7 to 9 indicates that the infant is slightly depressed (near normal), 4 to 6 indicates that the infant is moderately depressed, and 0 to 3 indicates that the infant is severely depressed. Most newborns have an Apgar score of 8 to 10 at 1 minute after birth. Newborns with an Apgar score of less than 6 generally require resuscitation; however, *the Apgar score should not be used to determine the need for resuscitation.*[4] (Neonatal resuscitation is presented in Chapter 41.)

Cutting of the umbilical cord. After the paramedic delivers and evaluates the infant, he or she should clamp (or tie with umbilical tape) and cut the umbilical cord (Fig. 40-11). The following steps should be taken in managing the umbilical cord:

1. Clamp the cord about 4 to 6 inches away from the infant in two places. Do not strip or milk the cord; doing so may lead to red blood cell destruction, polycythemia, and hyperbilirubinemia.
2. Cut between the two clamps with sterile scissors or a scalpel.
3. Examine the cut ends of the cord to ensure that there is no bleeding. If the cut end attached to the infant is bleeding, clamp the cord proximal to the previous clamp and reassess for bleeding. Do not remove the first clamp.
4. Handle the cord carefully at all times because it can tear easily.

Delivery of the placenta. The placenta normally delivers within 20 minutes of the infant. Therefore there is no need to delay transportation for placental delivery. Sometimes referred to as the fourth stage of labor, placental delivery is characterized by episodes of contractions, a palpable rise of the uterus within the abdomen, lengthening of the umbilical cord protruding from the vagina, and a sudden gush of vaginal blood.

TABLE 40-2	THE APGAR SCORING SYSTEM		
SIGN	**0**	**1**	**2**
Appearance (skin color)	Blue, pale	Body pink, blue extremities	Completely pink
Pulse rate (heart rate)	Absent	<100/minute	>100/minute
Grimace (irritability)	No response	Grimace	Cough, sneeze, cry
Activity (muscle tone)	Limp	Some flexion	Active motion
Respirations (respiratory effort)	Absent	Slow, irregular	Good, crying

As the placenta delivers, the mother should be advised to bear down with contractions. The paramedic should hold the placenta with both hands and gently twist it as it delivers to facilitate complete separation from the uterine wall. (Never pull on the umbilical cord to assist with placental delivery.) When the placenta is expelled, it should be placed in a plastic bag or other container and transported with the mother and infant to the receiving hospital, where it will be examined for abnormality and completeness. Pieces of placenta retained in the uterus can cause persistent hemorrhage and infection.

After placental delivery, the perineum should be evaluated for tears. If tears are present, they should be managed by applying sanitary napkins to the area and maintaining direct pressure. The paramedic should monitor the mother closely during transportation for signs of hemorrhage or shock. Fundal massage should be initiated to promote uterine contraction. In addition, medical direction may prescribe the administration of *oxytocin* (Pitocin) to manage postpartum hemorrhage.

Postpartum hemorrhage. Postpartum hemorrhage is characterized by more than 500 mL of blood loss after delivery of the newborn. It frequently occurs within the first few hours after delivery but can be delayed up to 24 hours. Postpartum hemorrhage occurs in about 5% of all deliveries and often results from ineffective or incomplete contraction of the interlacing uterine muscle fibers. Other causes of postpartum hemorrhage include retained pieces of placenta or membranes in the uterus and vaginal or cervical tears incurred during delivery (rare). Risk factors associated with postpartum hemorrhage include uterine atony (lack of tone) from prolonged or tumultuous labor, grand multiparity, twin pregnancy, placenta previa, and a full bladder.

Management. Postpartum hemorrhage can occur in the prehospital setting after a field delivery, home delivery, or delivery at an independent birthing center. Assessment and management are similar to those previously described for third-trimester bleeding. In addition, the following six measures should be taken to encourage uterine contraction:

1. *Control external hemorrhage.* Manage external bleeding from perineal tears with firm pressure.

2. *Massage the uterus.* Palpate the uterus for firmness or loss of tone. If the uterus does not feel firm, apply fundal pressure by supporting the lower uterine segment with the edge of one hand just above the symphysis and massaging the fundus with the other hand. Continue massaging until the uterus feels firm. Reevaluate the patient every 10 minutes; note the location of the fundus in relation to the level of the umbilicus, the degree of firmness, and vaginal flow.

3. *Encourage the infant to breast feed.* If the mother and infant are stable, place the newborn to her breast and encourage the infant to breast-feed. Stimulation of the breasts may promote uterine contraction.

4. *Administer oxytocin* (Pitocin). Per medical direction and after ensuring that a second fetus is not present in the uterus, add 10 units of *oxytocin* (Pitocin) to 1000 mL lactated Ringer's solution and infuse at 20 to 30 drops/min via microdrip tubing (titrated to the severity of hemorrhage and uterine response or as ordered by medical direction). Continue with fluid resuscitation as indicated by the patient's hemodynamic status.

5. Do not attempt a vaginal examination or vaginal packing to control hemorrhage.

6. Rapidly transport the patient for physician evaluation.

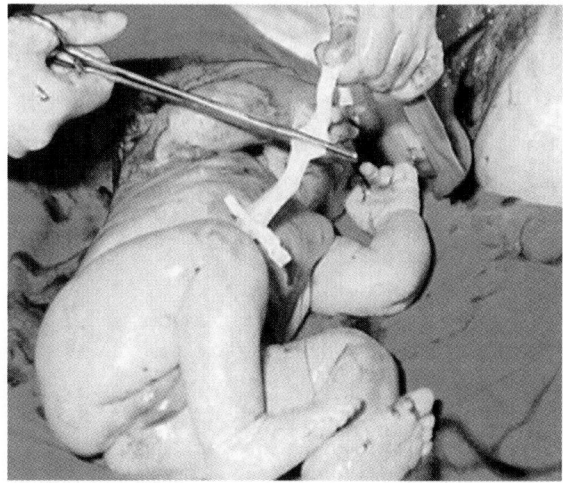

Fig. 40-11 After delivery and evaluation of the infant, the paramedic clamps and cuts the cord. (From Al-Azzawi F: *Color atlas of childbirth and obstetric techniques,* London, 1990, Wolfe.)

Delivery Complications

As stated previously, most women have routine pregnancies. Prehospital deliveries seldom present any significant problems for the mother, newborn, or emergency crew. The delivery complications discussed in this chapter include cephalopelvic disproportion, abnormal presentation, premature birth, multiple gestation, precipitous delivery, uterine inversion, pulmonary embolus, and fetal membrane disorders. Box 40-7 lists factors that should alert the paramedic to anticipate an abnormal delivery.

Cephalopelvic Disproportion

Cephalopelvic disproportion is a condition in which the newborn's head is too large or the mother's birth canal is too small to permit normal labor or birth. The mother often is primigravida and experiencing strong, frequent contractions for a prolonged period. Definitive care is cesarean delivery because uterine rupture and fetal demise are possible. Prehospital care is limited to maternal oxygen administration, IV access for fluid resuscitation if needed, and rapid transportation to the receiving hospital.

Abnormal Presentation

Most infants are born head first (cephalic or vertex presentation). However, sometimes a presentation is abnormal, as in a breech presentation, shoulder dystocia, shoulder presentation, and a cord presentation (prolapsed umbilical cord).

Breech Presentation

In breech presentations, the largest part of the fetus (the head) is delivered last. Breech presentation occurs in 3% to 4% of deliveries at term and is more frequent with multiple births and when labor occurs before 32 weeks' gestation. Fig. 40-12 illustrates three types of breech presentation (Box 40-8).

BOX 40-7

FACTORS ASSOCIATED WITH HIGH RISK OF ABNORMAL DELIVERY

Maternal Factors
• Maternal age: very young or very old
• Absence of prenatal care
• Maternal lifestyle: alcohol, tobacco, or drug usage
• Preexisting maternal illness, including diabetes, chronic hypertension, or Rh sensitization
• Previous obstetric history
  Premature delivery or miscarriage
  Perinatal loss
  Previous malformed neonate
  Previous multiple births
  Previous cesarean delivery
• Intrapartum disorders
  Preeclampsia
  Prolonged rupture of membranes
  Prolonged labor
  Abnormal presentation
  Abruptio placentae
  Placenta previa

Fetal Factors
• Lack of fetal well-being
  History of decreased fetal movement
  History of heart rate abnormalities
  Evidence of fetal distress
• Fetal immaturity: prematurity as established by dates, ultrasound, uterine size, amniocentesis
• Fetal growth: history of poor intrauterine growth or postdate delivery
• Specific fetal malformation detected by ultrasound: diaphragmatic hernia or omphalocele

---

?   CRITICAL THINKING

What resources can you use to assist in an abnormal presentation delivery?

BOX 40-8

CATEGORIES OF BREECH PRESENTATION

• Front or frank breech: The fetal hips are flexed and the legs extend in front of the fetus. The buttocks are the presenting part. Frank breech accounts for approximately 60% of breech presentations.
• Complete breech: The fetus has both knees and hips flexed. The buttocks are the presenting part. Complete breech accounts for approximately 5% of breech presentations.
• Incomplete breech: The fetus has one or both hips incompletely flexed, resulting in presentation of one or both lower extremities (often a foot). Incomplete breech accounts for approximately 30% of breech presentations.

Management. An infant in a breech presentation is best delivered in a hospital where emergency cesarean section is a possible alternative to vaginal delivery. However, sometimes the paramedic must assist in a breech delivery in the prehospital setting. If delivery is imminent, the EMS crew should proceed as follows:

1. Prepare the mother for delivery as described previously.
2. Provide supplemental oxygen and IV access, and continuously monitor the fetal heart rate.
3. Allow the fetus to deliver spontaneously up to the level of the umbilicus. If the fetus is in a front presentation, gently extract the legs downward after the buttocks are delivered.
4. After the infant's legs are clear, support his or her body with the palm of the hand and volar surface of the arm.
5. After the umbilicus is visualized, gently extract a 4- to 6-inch loop of umbilical cord to allow delivery without excessive traction on the cord. Gently rotate the fetus to align the shoulders in an anterior-posterior position. Continue with gentle traction until the axilla is visible.
6. Gently guide the infant upward to allow delivery of the posterior shoulder.
7. Gently guide the infant downward to deliver the anterior shoulder.
8. Ensure that the fetal face or abdomen is turned away from the maternal symphysis.
9. Be aware that the head often is delivered without difficulty after shoulder delivery. Be careful to avoid excessive head and spine manipulation or traction.

If the head does not deliver immediately, action must be taken to prevent suffocation of the infant. The paramedic should place a gloved hand in the vagina with the palm toward the infant's face, forming a V with the index and middle fingers on either side of the infant's nose. The vaginal wall should be gently pushed away from the infant's face until the head is delivered. If the head does not deliver within 3 minutes, the paramedic should maintain the infant's airway with the V formation and rapidly transport the mother to the receiving hospital.

Shoulder Dystocia

Shoulder dystocia occurs when the fetal shoulders impact against the maternal symphysis pubis, block-ing shoulder delivery. In this presentation, the head delivers normally but then pulls back tightly against the maternal perineum. The incidence of shoulder dystocia is small but increases significantly with increasing birth weight (up to 10% incidence with birth weights of 10 or more pounds). Complications include brachial plexus damage, fractured clavicle, and fetal anoxia from cord compression.

Management. Shoulder dystocia delivery entails dislodging one shoulder and rotating the fetal shoulder girdle into the wider oblique pelvic diameter. Because of the potential for cord compression, the paramedic should deliver the anterior shoulder immediately after the head (before suctioning of the nares and mouth). Several maneuvers can help the paramedic successfully deliver an infant when shoulder dystocia arises. The following steps constitute a reasonable field approach to shoulder dystocia:

1. Position the mother on her left side in a dorsal-knee-chest position to increase the diameter of the pelvis.
2. Attempt to guide the infant's head downward to allow the anterior shoulder to slip under the symphysis pubis. Avoid excessive force or manipulation.
3. Gently rotate the fetal shoulder girdle into the wider oblique pelvic diameter. The posterior shoulder usually delivers without resistance. Medical direction may recommend that the paramedic attempt delivery of the posterior shoulder first. The paramedic can accomplish this by rotating the posterior shoulder downward and into the left posterior quadrant. The anterior shoulder usually follows.

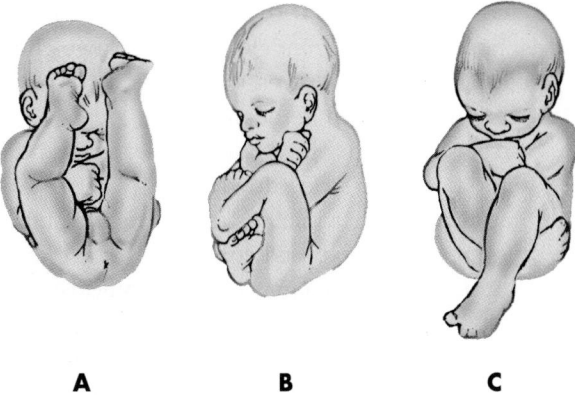

A   **B**   **C**

Fig. 40-12 Types of breech presentation. **A,** Front or back. **B,** Complete. **C,** Incomplete.

4. After delivery, continue with resuscitative measures as needed.

Shoulder Presentation

Shoulder presentation (transverse presentation) results when the long axis of the fetus lies perpendicular to that of the mother. This position usually results in the fetal shoulder lying over the pelvic inlet. The fetal arm or hand may be the presenting part. This abnormal delivery occurs in only 0.3% of deliveries but occurs in 10% of second twins.

Management. Spontaneous delivery of a shoulder presentation is not possible. The paramedic should provide the mother with adequate oxygen, ventilatory and circulatory support, and rapid transportation to the receiving hospital. Cesarean section is required whether the fetus is viable or nonviable.

Cord Presentation

Cord presentation occurs when the cord slips down into the vagina or presents externally after the amniotic membranes have ruptured. The umbilical cord is compressed against the presenting part, diminishing fetal oxygenation from the placenta. A prolapsed cord occurs in about 1 in every 200 pregnancies and should be suspected when fetal distress is present. Predisposing factors include breech presentation, premature rupture of membranes, a large fetus, multiple gestation, a long cord, and preterm labor.

Management. Fetal asphyxia can rapidly ensue if circulation through the cord is not reestablished and maintained until delivery. If the paramedic can see or feel the umbilical cord in the vagina, the following steps should be taken:

1. Position the mother with hips elevated as much as possible. The Trendelenburg or knee-chest position may relieve pressure on the cord.
2. Administer oxygen to the mother.
3. Instruct the mother to "pant" with each contraction to prevent bearing down.
4. If assistance is available, apply moist sterile dressings to the exposed cord to minimize temperature changes that may cause umbilical artery spasm.
5. With a gloved hand, gently push the infant back into the vagina and elevate the presenting part to relieve pressure on the cord. The cord may spontaneously retract, but the paramedic should not attempt to reposition the cord.
6. Maintain this hand position during rapid transportation to the receiving hospital. The definitive treatment is cesarean section.

Other Abnormal Presentations

Other abnormal presentations include face or brow presentation and occiput posterior presentation, in which the infant's head is delivered face up instead of face down. Nonvertex presentations result in increased perinatal morbidity and mortality as a result of difficult labor and delivery and associated abnormalities. These presentations may require cesarean section. Therefore early recognition of potential complications, maternal support and reassurance, and rapid transportation for definitive care are the goals of prehospital management.

Premature Birth

A premature infant is born before 37 weeks' gestation. Low birth weight (less than 2.5 kg [5.5 pounds]) also determines prematurity, although the conditions are not synonymous. Premature deliveries occur in 6% to 9% of all pregnancies. After a preterm labor, the newborn is at increased risk for hypothermia because of a large surface-mass ratio and for cardiorespiratory distress because the cardiovascular system is premature. Therefore these infants require special care and observation. After delivery, prehospital management for a premature infant includes the following:

- Keep the infant warm. Dry the infant, wrap the infant in a warm blanket, place the infant on the mother's abdomen, and cover the mother and infant.
- Frequently suction the infant's mouth and nares.
- Carefully monitor the cut end of the umbilical cord for oozing. If bleeding is present, manage as described previously.
- Administer humidified free-flow oxygen through a makeshift oxygen tent. Aim oxygen flow toward the top of the tent; do not allow it to flow directly into the infant's face.

- Protect the infant from contamination. Don a mask and gown and minimize family member and bystander contact with the infant.
- Gently transport the mother and infant to the receiving hospital.

> **? CRITICAL THINKING**
>
> *Do you have enough supplies on your ambulance to manage more than one delivery?*

Multiple Gestation

A multiple gestation is a pregnancy with more than one fetus. Twins occur in 1 in 80 to 90 (Box 40-9) births, and triplets occur in 1 in 8000 births.[1] Multiple gestation places additional stress on the maternal system and is accompanied by an increased complication rate. Associated complications include premature labor and delivery (30% to 50% of twin deliveries are premature), premature rupture of membranes, abruptio placentae, postpartum hemorrhage, and abnormal presentation. A mother who has not had prenatal care is often unaware of her multiple pregnancy.

Delivery Procedure

First-twin delivery is identical to single delivery with the same presentation. However, up to 50% of second-twin deliveries are in nonvertex presentation. Because fetuses are smaller in multiple births, the breech presentation of the second twin usually does not pose significant delivery problems.

After delivery of the first twin, the paramedic should cut and clamp (or tie) the umbilical cord in the usual fashion, as described previously. Within 5 to 10 minutes after delivery of the first twin, uterine contractions begin again. Delivery of the second twin usually occurs within 30 to 45 minutes. Medical direction may recommend transportation before delivery of the second twin. Usually both twins are born before placental delivery.

Infants in multiple births often are smaller than infants in single term births. The paramedic should give special attention to keeping these infants warm, well oxygenated, and free from unnecessary contamination as described for premature infants. Postpartum hemorrhage may be more severe after multiple births, requiring fluid resuscitation, uterine massage, and *oxytocin* (Pitocin) infusion.

Precipitous Delivery

A precipitous delivery is a rapid spontaneous delivery with less than 3 hours from onset of labor to birth. It results from overactive uterine contractions and little maternal soft tissue or bony resistance. A precipitous delivery most frequently occurs in a mother who is grand multipara. It can be associated with soft tissue injury and uterine rupture (rare) and has an increased perinatal mortality rate secondary to trauma and hypoxia. The primary danger to the fetus during a precipitous delivery is from cerebral trauma or tearing of the umbilical cord.

If the paramedic anticipates a precipitous delivery, he or she should attempt to prevent an explosive delivery by providing gentle counterpressure to the infant's head; however, no attempt should be made to detain fetal head descent. After the delivery, the infant should be kept dry and warm to prevent heat loss; the mother should be examined for perineal tears that often accompany a rapid birth.

Uterine Inversion

Uterine inversion is an infrequent but serious complication of childbirth, occurring in about 1 in 2100 deliveries, in which the uterus turns "inside out."

> **BOX 40-9**
>
> **TWIN TERMINOLOGY**
>
> **Fraternal twins** result from the fertilization of two ova by two spermatozoa. Each fraternal twin has a separate placenta and is separated by individual amniotic membranes. Fraternal twins are not identical in appearance and are often of different gender.
>
> **Identical twins** result from the fertilization of a single ovum; they may share a common placenta and amniotic sac or have separate placental structures. Identical twins are less common than fraternal twins (occurring in one out of three twin conceptions). Unlike fraternal twins, identical twins look alike, are of the same gender, and are genetically identical.

It may occur spontaneously after a contraction or with increased abdominal pressure caused by coughing or sneezing. However, uterine inversion is more often iatrogenic (caused by medical personnel or a medical procedure) secondary to excessive cord traction and fundal pressure, particularly when fundal implantation of the placenta has occurred. Uterine inversion is incomplete if the uterine fundus does not extend beyond the cervix and complete if the entire uterus protrudes through the cervical ring. Signs and symptoms of uterine inversion include postpartum hemorrhage, which may be profuse, and sudden and severe lower abdominal pain. Hypovolemic shock may develop quickly.

Management

Prehospital care for a patient with uterine inversion includes airway, ventilatory, and circulatory support and rapid transportation for physician evaluation. Medical direction may recommend that the paramedic attempt manual replacement of the uterus only if the cervix has not yet constricted. The technique for manual replacement is as follows:

1. Place the patient in a supine position.
2. Do not attempt to remove the placenta, which will increase hemorrhage.
3. Apply pressure with the fingertips and palm of a gloved hand and push the fundus upward and through the cervical canal. If this is ineffective, cover all protruding tissues with moist sterile dressings and rapidly transport the patient.

NOTE

Manual replacement of the uterus may be very painful to the patient. Medical direction may indicate the use of analgesics, and the paramedic should explain the need for the procedure to the patient.

Pulmonary Embolism

The development of pulmonary embolism during pregnancy, labor, or the postpartum period is one of the most common causes of maternal death. The embolus frequently is the result of a blood clot in the pelvic circulation (venous thromboembolism) and is more commonly associated with cesarean section than vaginal delivery. The patient often has classic signs and symptoms, including sudden dyspnea; sharp, focal chest pains; tachycardia; tachypnea; and occasionally hypotension. If the embolism occurs in the prehospital setting, emergency care should be focused on airway, ventilatory, and circulatory support; ECG monitoring; and rapid transportation for physician evaluation (see Chapter 27).

Fetal Membrane Disorders

The fetal membrane disorders discussed in this chapter include premature rupture of membranes and amniotic fluid embolism. Another fetal membrane disorder, meconium staining, is described in Chapter 41.

Premature Rupture of Membranes

Premature rupture of the membranes is a rupture of the amniotic sac before the onset of labor, regardless of gestational age. Premature rupture occurs in about 1 in 10 pregnancies. At term, 70% of patients are in labor within 12 hours of premature rupture of the membranes and 85% are in labor within 24 hours.[1] Signs and symptoms include a history of a "trickle" or sudden gush of fluid from the vagina. The paramedic should transport patients for physician evaluation. The medical facility will make delivery preparations if the patient enters the advanced stages of labor or if an infection of fetal membranes (chorioamnionitis) is diagnosed.

Chorioamnionitis is associated with premature rupture of membranes of greater than 24 hours' duration or with prolonged labor. The infection generally is accompanied by maternal fever, chills, and uterine pain and is treated with antibiotic therapy. The definitive treatment for chorioamnionitis is delivery of the fetus.

Amniotic Fluid Embolism

An amniotic fluid embolism may occur when amniotic fluid gains access to maternal circulation during labor or delivery or immediately after delivery. Probable routes of entry include lacerations of the endocervical veins during cervical dilation, the lower uterine segment or placental site, and uterine veins at sites of uterine trauma. Particulate matter in the amniotic fluid (e.g., meconium, lanugo hairs, and fetal squamous cells) forms an embolus and obstructs the pulmonary vasculature. Amniotic fluid embolism is rare, occurring in 1 in 20,000 to 30,000 deliveries.[1] The condition most commonly is seen in multiparous women late in the first stage of labor. Other conditions that can increase the incidence of this severe complication are placenta previa, abruptio placentae, and intrauterine fetal death. The maternal mortality rate is near 90%.

Signs and symptoms of amniotic fluid embolism are the same as those described for pulmonary embolism and may include cardiopulmonary arrest. These patients are managed with airway, ventilatory, and circulatory support; fluid resuscitation; and rapid transportation.

S U M M A R Y

- The placenta is a disklike organ composed of interlocking fetal and maternal tissues. It is the organ of exchange between the mother and fetus. Blood flows from the fetus to the placenta through two umbilical arteries carrying deoxygenated blood, and oxygenated blood returns to the fetus through the umbilical vein. The amniotic sac is a fluid-filled cavity that completely surrounds and protects the embryo.

- The developing ovum is known as an *embryo* during the first 8 weeks of pregnancy, and thereafter until birth it is called a *fetus*. Gestation (fetal development) usually averages 40 weeks from the time of fertilization to delivery of the newborn.

- The pregnant woman undergoes many physiological changes that affect the genital tract, breasts, gastrointestinal system, cardiovascular system, respiratory system, and metabolism.

- The patient history should include obstetrical history; presence of pain; presence, quantity, and character of vaginal bleeding; presence of abnormal vaginal discharge; presence of "bloody show"; current general health and prenatal care; allergies and medicines taken; and maternal urge to bear down.

- The prehospital objective in examining an obstetrical patient is to rapidly identify acute surgical or life-threatening conditions or imminent delivery and take appropriate management steps. In addition to the routine physical examination, the paramedic should assess the abdomen, uterine size, and fetal heart sounds.

- If birth is not imminent, the paramedic should limit prehospital care for the healthy patient to basic treatment modalities and transportation for physician evaluation.

- Causes of fetal death from maternal trauma include death of the mother, separation of the placenta, maternal shock, uterine rupture, and fetal head injury.

- Preeclampsia occurs after 20 weeks' gestation, and criteria for diagnosis include hypertension, proteinuria, and excessive weight gain with edema. Eclampsia is characterized by the same signs and symptoms with the addition of seizures or coma.

- Vaginal bleeding during pregnancy can result from abortion (miscarriage), ectopic pregnancy, abruptio placentae, placenta previa, uterine rupture, or postpartum hemorrhage. Abortion is the termination of pregnancy from any cause before 20 weeks' gestation. Ectopic pregnancy occurs when a fertilized ovum implants anywhere other than the endometrium of the uterine cavity. Abruptio placentae is partial or complete detachment of a normally implanted placenta at more than 20 weeks' gestation. Placenta previa is placental implantation in the lower uterine segment encroaching on or covering the cervical os. Uterine rupture is a spontaneous or traumatic rupture of the uterine wall.

- The first stage of labor begins with the onset of regular contractions and ends with complete dilation of the cervix. The second stage of labor is measured from full dilation of the cervix to delivery of the infant. The third stage of labor begins with delivery of the infant and ends when the placenta is expelled and the uterus has contracted.

- The primary responsibilities of the EMS crew are to prevent an uncontrolled delivery and protect the infant from cold and stress after birth.

- Criteria for computing the Apgar score include appearance (color), pulse (heart rate), grimace (reflex irritability), activity (muscle tone), and respiratory effort.

- Postpartum hemorrhage is characterized by more than 500 mL of blood loss after delivery of the newborn. It often results from ineffective or incomplete contraction of the interlacing uterine muscle fibers.

- Paramedics should be alert to factors that indicate a possible abnormal delivery.

- Cephalopelvic disproportion produces a difficult labor because of the presence of a small pelvis, an oversized uterus, or fetal abnormalities. Most infants are born head first (cephalic or vertex presentation). However, sometimes a presentation is abnormal. In breech presentation, the largest part of the fetus (the head) is delivered last. Shoulder dystocia occurs when the fetal shoulders impact against the maternal symphysis pubis, blocking shoulder delivery. Shoulder presentation (transverse presentation) results when the long axis of the fetus lies perpendicular to that of the mother. The fetal arm or hand may be the presenting part. Cord presentation occurs when the cord slips down into the vagina or presents externally.

- A premature infant is born before 37 weeks' gestation.

- A multiple gestation is a pregnancy with more than one fetus and is accompanied by an increased complication rate.

- A precipitous delivery is a rapid spontaneous delivery with less than 3 hours from onset of labor to birth. The primary danger to the fetus is from cerebral trauma or tearing of the umbilical cord.

- Uterine inversion is an infrequent but serious complication of childbirth in which the uterus turns "inside out."

- The development of pulmonary embolism during pregnancy, labor, or the postpartum period is one of the most common causes of maternal death.

- Premature rupture of the membranes is a rupture of the amniotic sac before the onset of labor, regardless of gestational age.

- An amniotic fluid embolism may occur when amniotic fluid gains access to maternal circulation during labor or delivery or immediately after delivery.

■ REFERENCES

1. Rosen P, Barkin R: *Emergency medicine: concepts and clinical practice,* ed 4, St Louis, 1998, Mosby.
2. American Heart Association: Guidelines 2000 for cardiopulmonary resuscitation and emergency cardiovascular care, International Consensus on Science, *Circulation* 102(8):247, 2000.
3. U.S. Department of Transportation, National Highway Traffic Safety Administration: *EMT-Paramedic national standard curriculum,* Washington, DC, 1998, The Department.
4. American Heart Association: *Pediatric advanced life support,* Dallas, 1997, The Association.

Division Six ——————→

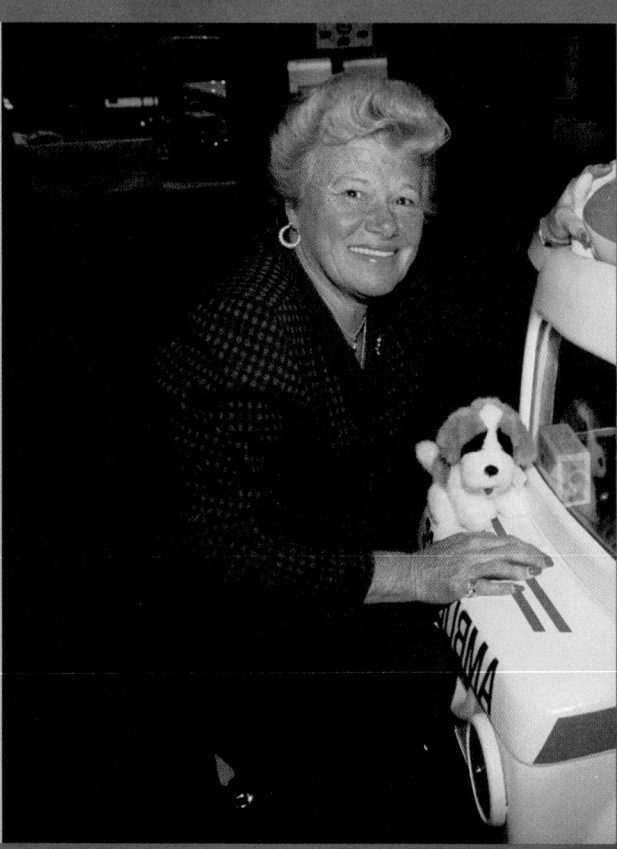

**Bobbie Dilworth,
EMT-P, AHA-IT
Owner, MEDIC
(Medical Education
Dedicated to Industry
and Community)
Fiesta, Texas**

*"A special challenge for me is when
we get a call for a child who isn't
accompanied by parents or family.
You have to really work with the child,
calm him down, and get him to trust
you so you can help him."*

Special Considerations

IN THIS DIVISION

41 Neonatology

OBJECTIVES

Upon completion of this chapter, the paramedic student will be able to:

1. Identify risk factors associated with the need for neonatal resuscitation.
2. Describe physiological adaptations at birth.
3. Outline the prehospital assessment and management of the neonate.
4. Describe resuscitation of the distressed neonate.
5. Discuss postresuscitative management and transport.
6. Describe signs and symptoms and pre-hospital management of specific neonatal resuscitation situations.
7. Identify injuries associated with birth.
8. Describe appropriate interventions to manage the emotional needs of the neonate's family.

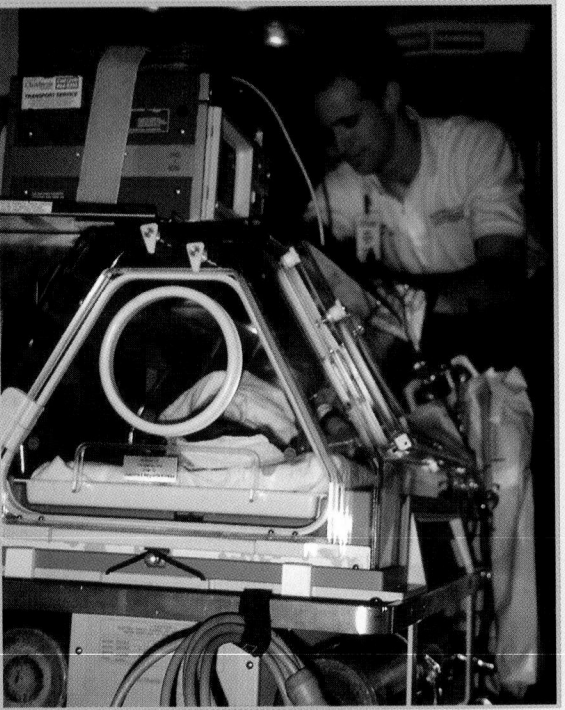

About 6% of infants born in U.S. hospitals require resuscitation immediately after birth, and this figure is thought to be much higher in the prehospital setting.[1] This chapter addresses risk factors associated with the need for resuscitation and the initial care and postresuscitation that may be required for the newborn and neonate.

antepartum: The period before labor and delivery.
intrapartum: The period during labor and delivery.
meconium staining: The inhalation of meconium by the fetus or newborn; this can block air passages and result in failure of the lungs to expand or cause other pulmonary dysfunction.
neonate: An infant in the first 28 days of life.
newborn: An infant in the first few hours of life.

> **NOTE**
>
> **Newborn** is used to describe a recently born infant in the first few hours of life. **Neonate** refers to infants in the first 28 days of life.

Risk Factors Associated with the Need for Resuscitation

The vast majority of term newborns require no resuscitation beyond maintenance of temperature, suctioning of the airway, and mild stimulation.[2] The incidence of complications, however, increases as birth weight decreases. In fact, resuscitation is required for about 80% of the 30,000 babies who weigh less than 1500 grams (3.12 pounds) at birth.[3] Causes of low birth weight include premature birth, undernourishment in the uterus, and maternal fac-

> **NOTE**
>
> *Premature infant* refers to a baby born before 37 weeks of gestation. (The weight of these newborns often is between 0.6 to 2.2 kilograms [kg] [1.5 to 5 pounds].) Premature infants have an increased risk for respiratory depression, hypothermia, and head and brain injury. Most will have a large trunk, short extremities, and skin that appears translucent. *Resuscitation should be attempted if the infant has any signs of life.* Transportation to a facility with special services for low-birth-weight newborns may be indicated.

tors such as preeclampsia and cigarette smoking during pregnancy.

> **NOTE**
>
> The average term newborn weighs about 3600 g (7.5 pounds). The baby's birth weight depends on a number of factors, including the size and racial origin of the parents. For example, small parents tend to have small babies, and Asian babies tend to be smaller than Caucasian babies. Newborn boys usually weigh about 8 ounces more than baby girls.

In addition to low birth weight, various **antepartum** (before labor and delivery) and **intrapartum** (during labor and delivery) risk factors may affect the need for resuscitation; these include the following[1]: (The obstetric history is presented in Chapter 40.)

- Antepartum
  Multiple gestation
  Inadequate prenatal care
  Mother's age (less than age 16 or older than age 35)
  History of perinatal morbidity or mortality
  Postterm gestation
  Drugs/medications
  Toxemia, hypertension, diabetes
- Intrapartum
  Premature labor
  Meconium-stained amniotic fluid
  Rupture of membranes greater than 24 hours before delivery
  Use of narcotics within 4 hours of delivery
  Abnormal presentation
  Prolonged labor or precipitous delivery
  Prolapsed cord
  Bleeding

When any of the above risk factors are present during delivery or imminent delivery, the paramedic should prepare equipment and drugs that may be required for neonatal resuscitation (Box 41-1). Medical

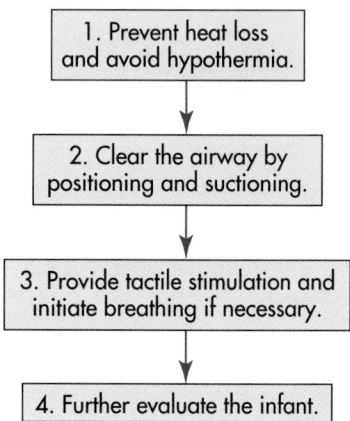

1. Prevent heat loss and avoid hypothermia.

↓

2. Clear the airway by positioning and suctioning.

↓

3. Provide tactile stimulation and initiate breathing if necessary.

↓

4. Further evaluate the infant.

Fig. 41-1 Steps in neonatal resuscitation.

? CRITICAL THINKING

Does your ambulance have equipment appropriately sized for neonatal resuscitation?

direction also should be advised of the situation so the appropriate destination hospital can be determined.

Congenital Anomalies

The presence of some congenital anomalies also may be a factor in the need for neonatal resuscitation. Some of the more common congenital anomalies include choanal atresia, cleft lip, cleft palate, diaphragmatic hernia, and Pierre Robin syndrome. (A brief description of each of these congenital anomalies can be found in Box 41-2.)

Physiological Adaptations at Birth

At birth, newborns make three major physiological adaptations necessary for survival: (1) emptying fluids from their lungs and beginning ventilation, (2) changing their circulatory pattern, and (3) maintaining body temperature.[4]

During vaginal delivery, the newborn's chest is usually compressed, which forces fluid from the lungs into the mouth and nose. As the chest wall recoils, air is drawn into the lungs and the newborn takes the first breath in response to chemical changes and changes in temperature.

When the cord is cut and placental circulation shuts down, the circulatory system must become an

BOX 41-1

NEONATAL RESUSCITATION EQUIPMENT AND DRUGS

In addition to a standard obstetrics kit, neonatal resuscitation equipment should include the following:
- Endotracheal tube stylets
- Endotracheal tubes (2.5, 3.0, 3.5, 4.0)
- Meconium aspirator attachment
- Laryngoscope blades (straight, 0, and 1)
- Laryngoscope handles
- Face masks (premature, newborn, and infant sizes)
- Orogastric/nasogastric tubes
- Multiple blankets
- Medications and fluids
  Dextrose 10%
  Epinephrine (Adrenalin) 1:10,000
  Naloxone (Narcan)
  Sodium bicarbonate (0.5 mEq/mL; 4.2% solution)
  Volume expanders (normal saline, lactated Ringer's solution)
- Self-inflating bag (450 mL to 750 mL)
- Umbilical vessel catheterization equipment
- Suction catheters (5F, 8F, 10F)
- Syringes (1, 3, 10, and 20 mL)
- Three-way stopcocks

independently functioning unit. This involves the immediate and permanent closure of the pathways that allowed the fetus to receive oxygen without the use of lungs (described in Chapter 40). As the lungs expand with initial breaths, the resistance to blood flow in the lungs decreases, and the newborn's blood begins to be oxygenated. Newborns are very sensitive to hypoxia, and permanent brain damage will occur from prolonged hypoxemia. Causes of hypoxia include compression of the cord, difficult labor and delivery, maternal hemorrhage, airway obstruction, hypothermia, newborn blood loss, and immature lungs in the premature newborn.

Newborns are at great risk for rapidly developing hypothermia and should be delivered in a warm, draft-free area. This is due to their larger body surface area (BSA), decreased tissue insulation, and immature temperature regulatory mechanisms. The cool, wet environment of birth also increases heat loss for the newborn. Newborns attempt to conserve body heat through vasoconstriction and increasing their metabolism, placing them at risk for hypoxemia, acidosis, bradycardia, and hypoglycemia.

BOX 41-2

CONGENITAL ANOMALIES

Choanal atresia: A bony or membranous occlusion that blocks the passageway between the nose and pharynx; can result in serious ventilation problems in the neonate.

Cleft lip: One or more fissures that originate in the embryo; a vertical, usually off-center split in the upper lip that may extend to the nose.

Cleft palate: A fissure in the roof of the mouth that runs along its midline; may extend through both the hard and soft palates into the nasal cavities.

Diaphragmatic hernia: The protrusion of a part of the stomach through an opening in the diaphragm; in some cases the intestines may herniate into the chest, displacing the heart and resulting in severe respiratory distress; occurs in 1 in 2200 live births, most commonly on the left side of the body.

Pierre Robin syndrome: A complex of anomalies including a small mandible, cleft lip, cleft palate, other craniofacial abnormalities, and defects of the eyes and ears.

Assessment and Management of the Neonate

The initial steps of neonatal resuscitation (with the exception of infants born through meconium, described later in this chapter) are listed below.[3] Following these steps enables the paramedic to immediately recognize an infant in need of resuscitation and leads to efficient and effective emergency care delivery (Fig. 41-1):

1. Prevent heat loss and avoid hypothermia.
2. Clear the airway by positioning and suctioning.
3. Provide tactile stimulation and initiate breathing if necessary.
4. Further evaluate the infant.

NOTE

Body substance isolation (BSI) precautions are recommended during delivery of a newborn. Gloves and other appropriate protective barriers (including gowns and goggles) should be worn when handling the newborn or contaminated equipment.

Prevention of Heat Loss and Hypothermia

Even healthy term newborns are limited in their ability to conserve heat when exposed to a cold environment and are subject to developing hypothermia. Therefore, immediately after delivery, the infant's body and head should be dried to prevent evaporative heat loss and metabolic problems that may be brought on by cold stress (cold stress can increase oxygen consumption and impede effective resuscitation). Care also should be taken to remove any wet coverings from the infant and cover the infant with dry wrappings. The majority of heat loss can be prevented by covering the newborn's head (which accounts for 20% of the newborn's BSA).

? CRITICAL THINKING

What other measures can you take to warm the infant?

NOTE

Hypothermia can be associated with perinatal respiratory depression.

NOTE

The act of drying also provides gentle stimulation, which may initiate or help maintain respirations.

Opening the Airway

After the newborn has been dried and covered, the next step is to establish an open airway by correctly positioning the infant and suctioning the mouth and nose. The neonate should be placed on the back or side with the head in a neutral (or slightly extended) position. Care should be taken to prevent hyperextension or underextension, which may compromise the airway (as described in Chapter 11). Placing a blanket or towel under the infant's shoulders (thereby elevating the torso ¾ to 1 inch) can help maintain the correct position.

? CRITICAL THINKING

Do infants breathe through their noses or mouths?

Once the infant has been properly positioned, the mouth and nose should be suctioned with a bulb syringe or mechanical suction. It is preferable to suction the mouth first to prevent aspiration in case the infant gasps when the nose is cleared of secretions. Each application of suction should last no more than 5 seconds to prevent hypoxia.

The paramedic should be careful to avoid deep or vigorous suctioning because stimulation of the posterior pharynx can produce a vagal response with resulting bradycardia, apnea, or both. The newborn's heart rate should be monitored during suctioning, and time should be provided during suction attempts for spontaneous ventilation or assisted ventilation with 100% oxygen. Like drying, suctioning provides a degree of tactile stimulation that may initiate respirations.

? CRITICAL THINKING

> *Why would you want to intubate and suction meconium before the infant's first breath?*

Meconium Staining

Meconium staining is the presence of fetal stool in the amniotic fluid (occurring either in utero or intrapartum). The condition occurs in about 12% of all deliveries, becoming more common in postterm and small-for-gestational-age newborns. Meconium staining is associated with increased perinatal mortality, hypoxemia, aspiration pneumonia, pneumothorax, and pulmonary hypertension. Depending on the amount of meconium particles and amniotic fluid, the staining may range from a slight yellow or light green to a thick "pea-soup" appearance (Fig. 41-2). When thick meconium is present in amniotic fluid, there is a chance the particles will be aspirated into

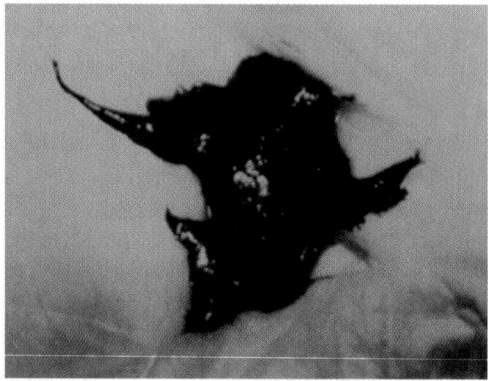

Fig. 41-2 Meconium-stained birth. (Courtesy Nellcor Puritan Bennett, Minneapolis, Minnesota.)

the infant's mouth and potentially into the trachea and lungs (this is known as *meconium aspiration syndrome*), which leads to atelectasis and the development of pneumothorax. Death may result from hypoxia, hypercapnia, and acidosis.

> **NOTE**
>
> When amniotic fluid is meconium-stained, the mouth, pharynx, and nose should be suctioned as soon as the head is delivered, regardless of whether the meconium is thin or thick.[5]

> ✓ **TRICKS OF THE TRADE**
>
> Meconium can be used to test for maternal drug use. It has a greater sensitivity than urine and positive findings that persist longer. If time permits, a specimen should be collected and delivered to the emergency department.

After meconium is observed in the amniotic fluid, intervention is aimed at preventing or minimizing the risk of aspiration by the newborn. Because the presence of meconium can only be determined after the membranes have ruptured, it is important that the proper equipment be readily available and the Emergency Medical Services (EMS) crew be organized to act instantly. Emergency care includes the following steps:

1. Prepare the necessary equipment (e.g., intubation equipment, bulb syringe and DeLee suction, 12-French or larger suction catheter, portable suction and irrigation solution, gauze pads, infant bag-valve device).

> **NOTE**
>
> Intubation equipment should include padding for patient positioning, stethoscope, number 0 and number 1 laryngoscope blades, endotracheal (ET) tubes (2.5, 3.0, 3.5, 4.0), stylet, meconium aspirator, and oxygen tubing. (The procedure for intubation is described in Chapter 11.)

2. As the baby's head is delivered (and before shoulder delivery), clear the infant's airway and thoroughly suction the nose, mouth, and pharynx.

3. After delivery of the infant, remove residual meconium in the hypopharynx by suction under direct visualization.

4. If the neonate is depressed (absent or depressed respirations, decreased muscle tone, heart rate <100 bpm) perform direct ET suctioning using the ET tube as a suction catheter. Quickly intubate the trachea (preferably before the baby has taken its first breath). Apply suction to the proximal end of the ET tube while withdrawing the tube. During intubation and suction, aim 100% oxygen toward the infant's face and monitor the fetal heart rate for bradycardia. If bradycardia develops, ventilate the infant's lungs using a bag-valve device after suctioning to prevent persistent bradycardia and hypoxia.

5. Repeat the intubation-suction-extubation cycle until no further meconium is obtained. Do not ventilate between intubations.

6. After tracheal suction is complete, continue resuscitative measures as needed. If respirations are adequate, manage the infant's airway in the normal fashion. Medical direction may recommend that an 8F orogastric tube that is aspirated with a syringe and left open to air be placed to prevent aspiration of gastric contents after resuscitation is complete.

Provision of Tactile Stimulation

If drying and suctioning do not induce respirations in the infant, additional tactile stimulation should be provided. The two safe and appropriate methods of tactile stimulation are slapping or flicking the soles of the infant's feet and rubbing the infant's back. If the infant remains apneic after a brief period (5 to 10 seconds) of stimulation, positive-pressure ventilation should be initiated immediately with a pediatric bag-valve device and supplemental oxygen (at 40 to 60 ventilations/minute).

Evaluation of the Infant

Drying, positioning, suctioning, and stimulating are necessary in every infant at birth and are used to clear the airway and initiate respirations. The next step in the resuscitation process depends on evaluation of the infant's respiratory effort, heart rate, and color. The following steps are suggested for monitoring and evaluating the newborn (Fig. 41-3):

1. Observe and evaluate the infant's respirations. If they are normal (e.g., crying), continue the evaluation. If respirations are inadequate or gasping is present, positive-pressure ventilation should be initiated immediately. If the respiratory response is slow or shallow, a brief period of stimulation may be attempted while 100% oxygen is administered. If no response is noted after 5 to 10 seconds of stimulation and oxygen administration, positive-pressure ventilation should begin.

2. Evaluate the infant's heart rate by stethoscope or palpation of the pulse in the base of the umbilical cord. If it is above 100 beats/minute, continue the evaluation. If it is less than 100 beats/minute, initiate positive-pressure ventilation. If the heart rate is less than 60 beats/minute and does not increase despite 30 seconds of positive-pressure ventilation, coordinate chest compressions with ventilations at a ratio of 3:1 at a rate of 120 events/minute to achieve approximately 90 compressions and 30 breaths/minute. Administer *epinephrine* (adrenalin) if the heart rate remains <60 bpm despite 30 seconds of assisted ventilations and chest compressions.[6]

> **NOTE**
>
> As described in Chapter 28, the two thumb-encircling hands chest compression is the preferred technique for chest compressions for newly born infants and older infants when size permits. Compressions should be performed on the lower third of the sternum. Depth of compression should be about one-third of the anterior-posterior diameter of the chest and should be sufficiently deep to generate a palpable pulse.[6]

> **? CRITICAL THINKING**
>
> *Why would compressions be initiated when the infant still has a pulse?*

3. Evaluate the infant's color. If central cyanosis, bradycardia, or other signs of distress are present in a newborn infant with spontaneous respirations and an adequate heart rate, administer 100% oxygen while determining the need for additional intervention. Free-flow oxygen can be given through a face mask and flow-inflating bag, an oxygen mask, or a hand cupped around oxygen tubing (held ½ inch from the infant's nose)

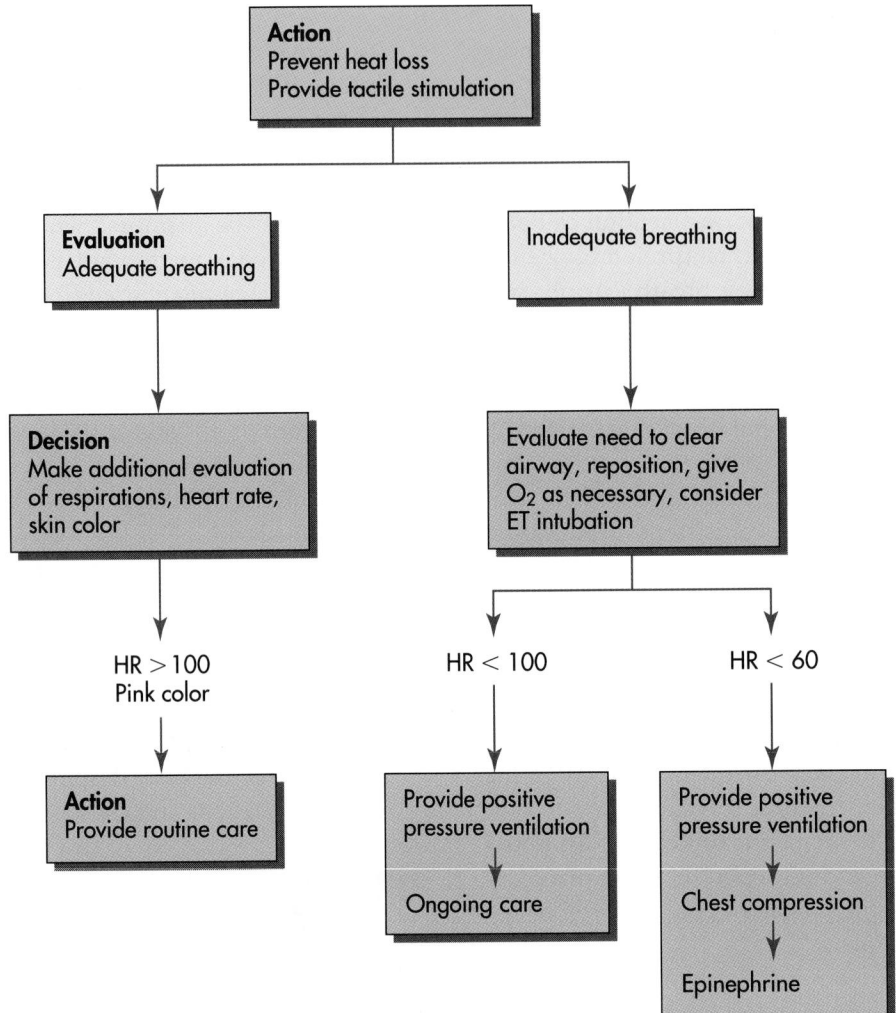

Fig. 41-3 Action-evaluation-decision cycle.

using an oxygen flow rate of at least 5 L/minute.[7] Sufficient oxygen should be administered to achieve pink color in the mucous membranes.

> **NOTE**
>
> Hypoxia is nearly always present in a newly born infant who requires resuscitation.[7]

> **NOTE**
>
> Oxygen administration is not indicated for newborns with peripheral cyanosis (acrocyanosis). This condition is common in the first few minutes of life and not indicative of hypoxemia.

> **NOTE**
>
> If oxygen is needed during resuscitation of the newborn, 100% oxygen should be used without concern for its potential long-term hazards (e.g., retinopathy).

Apgar Score

The Apgar score (described in Chapter 40) enables rapid evaluation of a newborn's condition at specific intervals after birth. It routinely is assessed at 1 and 5 minutes of age. Although the Apgar score is a useful tool to evaluate the newborn, it should not be used alone in determining the need for resuscitation.

Resuscitation of the Distressed Newborn

As previously described, risk factors associated with the need for resuscitation include premature delivery, maternal health problems, complicated pregnancies, and delivery complications. If with continued assisted ventilations the infant's condition continues to deteriorate or fails to improve, the infant may require ET intubation and the administration of drugs (Fig. 41-4). Before the paramedic considers intubation or pharmacological therapy, two components of the resuscitation process should be reevaluated:

1. Is chest movement adequate? Check for the adequacy of chest expansion and auscultate for bilateral breath sounds.
   a. Is the bag valve face mask seal tight? A relatively large mask should be turned upside down for a better fit.
   b. Is the airway blocked from improper head position or secretions in the nose, mouth, or pharynx? Reassess head position and reexamine the airway for the presence of secretions.
   c. Is adequate ventilatory pressure being used? A bag-valve mask pop-off valve may need to be disabled to allow for higher inspiratory pressures, especially for premature or meconium-aspiration delivery.[2]
   d. Is air in the stomach interfering with chest expansion? Consider nasogastric or orogastric decompression per protocol.
2. Is 100% oxygen being administered?
   a. Is the oxygen tubing attached to the bag and flowmeter?
   b. If using a self-inflating bag, is the oxygen reservoir attached?

NOTE

ET intubation may be indicated at several points during neonatal resuscitation.[8] These include:

- When tracheal suctioning for meconium is required
- If bag-mask ventilation is ineffective or prolonged
- When chest compressions are performed
- When tracheal administration of medications is desired
- Special resuscitation circumstances (e.g., congenital diaphragmatic hernia, extremely low birth rate)
- Tube placement should be verified with primary and secondary confirmation methods (see Chapter 11)

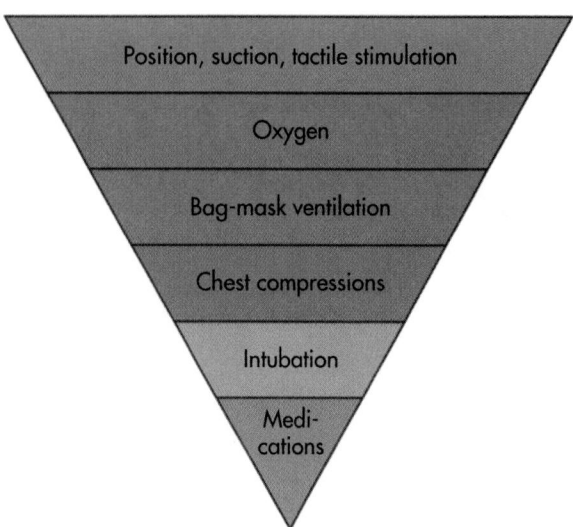

Fig. 41-4 Inverted pyramid reflecting the approximate relative frequency of neonatal resuscitative efforts. Note that a majority of infants respond to simple measures. (Reproduced with permission. CPR Issue of JAMA, Oct 28, 1992. Copyright © American Medical Association)

NOTE

The laryngeal mask airway (LMA) may be used to establish an airway in a newborn if bag-mask ventilation is ineffective or tracheal intubation has failed (Chapter 11).[6]

Routes of Drug Administration

Drugs are rarely indicated in the resuscitation of the newly born infant. As a rule, drugs should be administered only if the heart rate remains <60 bpm, despite adequate ventilation with 100% oxygen and chest compressions.[8] The tracheal route (described in Chapter 9) is generally the most rapidly accessible route for drug administration during resuscitation; the umbilical vein is the most rapidly accessible venous route. Peripheral sites (scalp or peripheral vein) may be adequate but are usually more difficult to cannulate. The intraosseous (IO) route is not commonly used in newborns because the umbilical vein is more accessible, the small bones are fragile, and the IO space is small in a premature infant.

Accessing the Umbilical Vein

As described in Chapter 40, the umbilical cord contains three vessels: two arteries and one vein. The vein in the umbilical cord has a thin wall and is larger than the arteries, which are thick walled and usually paired. To gain access to the umbilical vein, the paramedic should take the following steps (Fig. 41-5):

1. Set up intravenous (IV) fluid (per protocol) and tubing with a three-way stopcock.

2. Select a 3.5-French or 5-French umbilical catheter.

3. Connect the catheter to the stopcock and purge the air from the catheter.

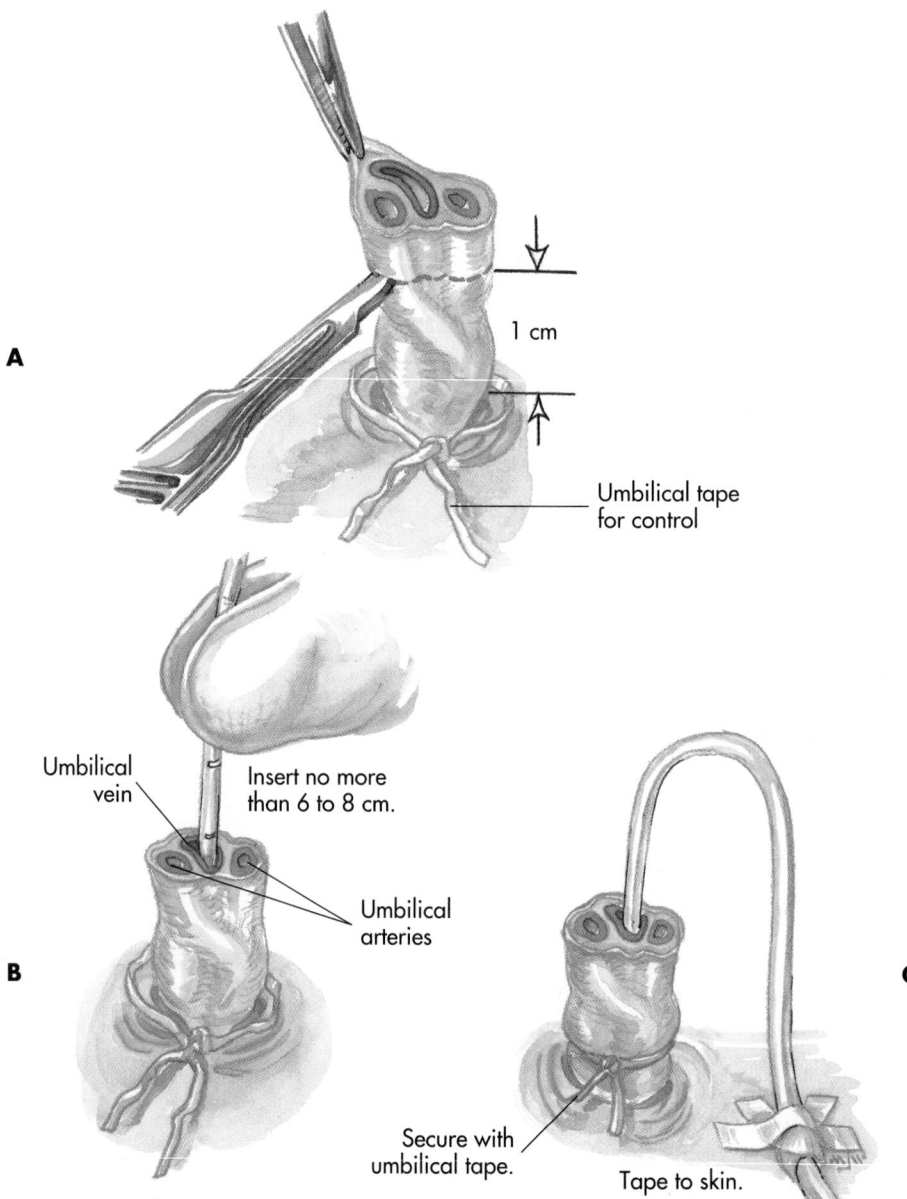

Fig. 41-5 Umbilical vein cannulation procedure. **A,** Identify the umbilical vein after trimming the cord. **B,** Insert the umbilical catheter or angiocatheter into the vein. **C,** Secure the base of the cord to hold the catheter in place and stabilize the catheter with tape.

A

1 cm

Umbilical tape for control

Umbilical vein

Insert no more than 6 to 8 cm.

Umbilical arteries

B

Secure with umbilical tape.

Tape to skin.

C

4. Cleanse the umbilical stump and surrounding skin with antibacterial solution.

5. Loosely tie umbilical tape around the cord near the body so that pressure can be applied to control bleeding.

6. Hold the umbilical stump firmly and trim (with a scalpel) the cord several centimeters (cm) above the abdomen.

7. Locate the umbilical vein and insert the catheter until blood is freely obtained. Do not insert the catheter more than 6 to 8 cm. If the catheter is inserted farther, there is a risk of infusing solutions directly into the liver rather than the systemic circulation. Take care to avoid introduction of air emboli into the umbilical vein.

8. Draw blood for a sample, if needed.

9. Start the infusion and regulate the fluid flow per medical direction.

10. Secure the catheter in place with tape and cover with a sterile dressing.

11. Document the procedure.

The umbilical cord also may be cannulated by using a typical IV catheter. Insert the catheter-over-needle through the side of the proximal end of the cord into the vein and advance it upward through the translucent wall. Start the infusion, adjust the fluid flow per medical direction, and secure the catheter in place with tape.

Medications Used in Neonatal Resuscitation

Medications most frequently used during neonatal resuscitation are *epinephrine* (Adrenalin), volume expanders, and *naloxone* (Narcan). (Table 41-1 lists the medications recommended by the American Heart Association and the American Academy of Pediatrics.) The box in the left column reviews important points in neonatal resuscitation.

Postresuscitation Care

The three most common complications of the postresuscitation period are ET tube migration (including dislodgement), tube occlusion by mucus or meconium, and pneumothorax.[2] These complications should be suspected in the presence of:

- Decreased chest wall movement
- Diminished breath sounds
- Return of bradycardia
- Unilateral decrease in chest expansion
- Altered intensity to pitch of breath sounds
- Increased resistance to hand ventilation

> **NOTE**
>
> Exhaled CO_2 devices are useful for monitoring tracheal tube placement.

Corrective management in the field for these postresuscitative complications may include adjustment of the ET tube, reintubation, and suction. Needle decompression to manage a suspected pneumothorax must be carefully guided by medical direction.

> **? CRITICAL THINKING**
>
> *How much movement would it take to dislodge an ET tube from a neonate?*

Neonatal Transport

During transport of the neonate, it is important to maintain body temperature and prevent hypother-

---

IMPORTANT POINTS TO REMEMBER IN NEONATAL RESUSCITATION

- Prevent heat loss and avoid hypothermia.
- In the newly born infant with a heart rate <100 bpm and unresponsive to stimulation, the primary concern is to establish adequate ventilation.
- When meconium is observed in the amniotic fluid, deliver the head and suction the meconium from the hypopharynx on delivery of the head. If the neonate is distressed, perform direct tracheal suctioning to remove meconium from the airway.
- Provide chest compressions if the heart rate is absent or remains <60 bpm despite adequate assisted ventilation with 100% oxygen for 30 seconds.
- Coordinate chest compressions with ventilations at a ratio of 3:1 and at a rate of 120 events per minute to achieve approximately 90 compressions and 30 breaths per minute.
- Administer *epinephrine* (Adrenalin) when the heart remains <60 bpm despite 30 seconds of effective assisted ventilation and chest compressions.

TABLE 41-1	MEDICATIONS FOR NEONATAL RESUSCITATION				
MEDICATIONS	**DOSE/ROUTE**	**CONCENTRATION**	**WT (kg)**	**TOTAL (mL)**	**PRECAUTIONS**
Epinephrine	0.01–0.03 mg/kg IV, or ET*	1:10,000	1 2 3 4	0.1–0.3 0.2–0.6 0.3–0.9 0.4–1.2	Give rapidly Repeat every 3-5 min
Volume expanders — Normal saline — Lactated Ringer's	10 mL/kg IV over 5 to 10 minutes		1 2 3 4	10 20 30 40	Reassess after each bolus
Naloxone	0.1 mg/kg IV, ET, or IM/SQ if perfusion is adequate	0.4 mg/mL	1 2 3 4	0.25 0.50 0.75 1.0	Repeat doses may be needed to prevent apnea
		1.0 mg/mL	1 2 3 4	0.1 0.2 0.3 0.4	Do not give to if mother is suspected of abusing narcotics

IM, Intramuscular; *ET,* endotracheal tube; *IV,* intravenous; *SQ,* subcutaneous.
*Note: ET dose may not result in effective plasma concentration of drug, so vascular access should be established as soon as possible.
*ET drugs should be diluted to volume of 3 to 5 mL before instillation.

mia, oxygen administration, and ventilatory support. In the initial prehospital phase of care, transport strategies usually are limited to providing a warm ambulance, free-flow oxygen administration, and warm blankets. Specialized transport equipment such as isolettes and radiant heating units often are used for interhospital transfers and require special training. Highly trained neonatal transport teams consisting of paramedics, nurses, respiratory therapists, and physicians are part of several well-organized regional referral systems throughout the United States (Fig. 41-6).

Specific Situations

Specific situations that may require advanced life support for the neonate include respiratory disorders (e.g., apnea, respiratory distress, cyanosis), cardiovascular disorders (e.g., bradycardia, cardiac arrest), hypovolemia, gastrointestinal disorders (e.g., vomiting, diarrhea), seizures, fever, hypothermia, and hypoglycemia.

Respiratory Disorders

As previously described, respiratory insufficiency in the neonate generally is managed with stimulation and positioning of the airway, prevention of heat loss and hypothermia, oxygenation and ventilation, suction, and intubation with ventilatory support (if needed). Pharmacological therapy that may be appropriate in managing some infants with respiratory disorders (per medical direction) includes the administration of *sodium bicarbonate* for prolonged resuscitation (unresponsive to other therapy), *dextrose* if hypoglycemia is suspected or confirmed, and *naloxone* (Narcan) for reversal of respiratory depression in a newborn whose mother received narcotics within 4 hours of delivery.[8]

Apnea

Apnea (respiratory pauses that exceed 20 seconds) is a common finding in preterm infants and, if

> **NOTE**
>
> Primary apnea is a self-limited condition (controlled by PCO_2 levels) that is common immediately after birth. Secondary apnea describes respirations that are absent and do not begin again spontaneously.

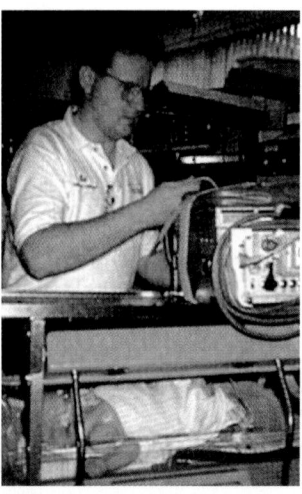

Fig. 41-6 Neonatal transport.

prolonged, can lead to hypoxemia and bradycardia. The condition usually is a result of hypoxia or hypothermia, but it also may be due to causes that include:

- Narcotics or CNS depressants
- Airway and respiratory muscle weakness
- Oxyhemoglobin dissociation curve shift
- Septicemia
- Metabolic disorders
- Central nervous system (CNS) disorders

Respiratory Distress and Cyanosis

Prematurity is the single most common factor influencing respiratory distress and cyanosis in the neonate. The condition occurs most frequently in infants less than 1200 g (2.5 pounds) and 30 weeks of gestation, and it may be related to the infant's immature central respiratory control center, which is easily affected by environmental or metabolic changes. Other risk factors for respiratory distress and cyanosis include:

- Lung or heart disease
- Primary pulmonary hypertension
- CNS disorders
- Mucous obstruction of nasal passages
- Spontaneous pneumothorax
- Choanal atresia
- Meconium aspiration
- Amniotic fluid aspiration
- Lung immaturity
- Pneumonia
- Shock and sepsis

- Metabolic acidosis
- Diaphragmatic hernia

The pathophysiology of respiratory distress and cyanosis can lead to cardiac arrest and requires immediate intervention to support respirations. Assessment findings may include tachypnea, paradoxical breathing, intercostal retractions, nasal flaring, expiratory grunting, and central cyanosis.

? CRITICAL THINKING

Should you be concerned if a baby's hands and feet are blue, but the baby is centrally pink?

Cardiovascular Disorders

A neonate's heart generally is healthy and strong; however, disorders in the heart's conduction system can and do occur, most commonly as a result of hypoxemia and respiratory arrest. All neonates with cardiovascular disorders should therefore be assessed for treatable causes of hypoventilation.

Bradycardia

Bradycardia (a heart rate less than 100 beats/minute) most commonly is caused by hypoxia, but it also may be the result of increased intracranial pressure (ICP), hypothyroidism, and acidosis. Bradycardia is considered a minimal risk to life in neonates if it is corrected quickly (see Table 41-1). (Guidelines for managing bradycardia are presented in Chapter 42.)

Cardiac Arrest

Asystole and pulseless arrest are uncommon in children and, like bradycardia, usually are the result of hypoxia. Other risk factors associated with cardiac arrest in the newborn include:

- Intrauterine asphyxia
- Drugs administered to or taken by the mother
- Congenital neuromuscular disease
- Congenital malformations
- Intrapartum hypoxemia

Emergency care for neonates with asystole or pulseless arrest includes airway, ventilatory, and circulatory support; pharmacological therapy; and rapid transport to an appropriate facility (see Table 41-1). (Guidelines for managing cardiac arrest are presented in Chapter 42.)

Hypovolemia

Hypovolemia in infants may result from dehydration, hemorrhage, trauma, or sepsis, and it may be associated with myocardial dysfunction (see Chapter 7). Signs and symptoms of hypovolemia include mottled or pale color, cool skin, tachycardia, diminished peripheral pulses, and delayed capillary refill despite normal ambient temperature. Shock may be present despite a "normal" blood pressure. Prompt and effective treatment of early signs of compensated shock may prevent the development of hypotension (decompensated shock) and associated high morbidity and mortality.[2] Prehospital care is always directed at ensuring adequate airway, ventilatory, and circulatory support (including control of external hemorrhage) and providing rapid transport to an appropriate medical facility.

When signs of hypovolemia are present, a fluid bolus (10 milliliters [mL]/kg over 5 to 10 minutes of isotonic crystalloid immediately after IV access is obtained) should be administered, and the infant should be reassessed. If signs of shock persist, a second 10-mL/kg bolus should be given, and additional boluses should be infused as indicated by repeated reassessments of the patient under the guidance of medical direction.

Gastrointestinal Disorders

Occasional vomiting or diarrhea is not unusual in the neonate. For example, vomiting mucus (that may occasionally be streaked with blood) is common in the first few hours of life, and five to six stools per day is considered normal, especially if the infant is breast feeding. Persistent vomiting and/or diarrhea, however, should be considered warning signs of serious illness.

Vomiting

Persistent vomiting in the first 24 hours of life suggests obstruction in the upper digestive tract or perhaps increased ICP. Vomit that contains non–bile-stained fluid is a sign of anatomical or functional obstruction at or above the first portion of the duodenum, or it may be indicative of gastroesophageal reflux. Bile-stained vomit may result from obstruction below the opening of the bile duct. Assessment findings may include a distended stomach and signs of infection, dehydration, and increased ICP. The paramedic also should consider the possibility of vomiting as a result of drug withdrawal (from the mother's drug use).

> **NOTE**
>
> Vomit that contains dark blood usually is a sign of life-threatening illness.

Prehospital care usually is limited to maintaining a patent airway that is clear of vomit and ensuring adequate oxygenation. In severe cases, medical direction may recommend that IV fluid therapy be initiated prior to transport to treat dehydration and any bradycardia that may develop from vagal stimulation. If possible, infants should be transported on their sides to help prevent aspiration.

Diarrhea

Persistent diarrhea can lead to serious dehydration and electrolyte imbalances in the neonate. The diarrhea often is associated with a bacterial or viral infection. Other possible causes include:

- Gastroenteritis
- Rotavirus
- Lactose intolerance
- Phototherapy (a treatment for hyperbilirubinemia and jaundice in the newborn)
- Neonatal abstinence syndrome (drug withdrawal)
- Thyrotoxicosis
- Cystic fibrosis

Assessment findings often include the presence of loose stools, decreased urinary output, and signs of dehydration. Treatment consists of supporting the infant's vital functions, IV fluid therapy (per medical direction), and rapid transport to the receiving hospital.

Seizures

Seizures occur in a very small percentage of newborns and, when present, usually are a sign of an underlying abnormality (Box 41-3). Prolonged seizure activity or frequent seizures may result in metabolic changes and cardiopulmonary difficulties.

Types of Seizures

Seizures in neonates generally are fragmented and not well sustained. They have been classified as *subtle seizures, tonic seizures, multifocal seizures, focal clonic seizures,* and *myoclonic seizures.*[1]

Subtle seizures involve eye deviation, blinking, sucking, swimming movements of the arms, and peddling movements of the legs. Apnea may be present during subtle seizures. Tonic seizures usually involve extension of the limbs and, less commonly, flexion of upper extremities and extension of lower extremities. This type of seizure is more common in premature infants, especially those with intraventricular hemorrhage. Multifocal seizures usually involve clonic activity in one extremity that may randomly migrate to another area of the body. This type of seizure primarily occurs in full-term infants. Focal clonic seizures involve clonic, localized jerking and have been known to occur in both full-term and premature newborns. Myoclonic seizures involve flexion and jerking of the upper or lower extremities. These seizures may occur singly or in a series of repetitive jerking cycles.

Emergency care for managing neonatal seizures includes providing airway, ventilatory, and circulatory support and maintaining the infant's body temperature. Pharmacological therapy that may be prescribed by medical direction includes *dextrose* to treat hypoglycemia, anticonvulsant agents, and perhaps benzodiazepines (for status epilepticus). Seizure activity is always considered pathological; rapid transport for physician evaluation is indicated.

> **BOX 41-3**
>
> ### CAUSES OF NEONATAL SEIZURES
>
> - Hypoglycemia
> - Hypoxic-ischemic encephalopathy
> - Intracranial hemorrhage
> - Metabolic disturbances
> - Meningitis or encephalopathy
> - Developmental abnormalities
> - Drug withdrawal

Fever

Fever in neonates (a rectal temperature greater than 100.4° Farenheit [F] [38.0° Celsius (C)]) generally is a cause for concern and often is a response to an acute viral or bacterial infection. It also may result from an alteration in the infant's limited ability to control body temperature or be an effect of dehydration. The rise in core temperature is associated with increased oxygen demand and an increase in glucose metabolism, which may lead to metabolic acidosis. Assessment findings may include mental status changes (e.g., irritability, somnolence), a history of decreased intake, and warm or hot skin.

> **NOTE**
>
> Term newborns will produce beads of sweat on their brow but not over the rest of their bodies. Premature infants generally will have no visible sweat.

Prehospital care for febrile infants primarily is supportive. As a rule, cooling procedures and the use of antipyretics will be delayed until the child has arrived in the emergency department. Febrile seizures usually affect children between 6 months and 5 years of age and generally are not a concern in caring for this age group (see Chapter 42).

> **NOTE**
>
> All febrile neonates require immediate transport for physician evaluation. These patients should be presumed to have systemic sepsis until it is proven otherwise.

Hypothermia

Hypothermia (as described in Chapter 36) is a core body temperature below 95° F (35° C) that may result from a decrease in heat production, an increase in heat loss (through evaporation, conduction, convection, or radiation), or a combination of both. Neonates are particularly sensitive to the effects of hypothermia because of their increased surface-to-volume ratio, especially when they are wet (e.g., after delivery). The associated increase in metabolic demand to maintain body temperature can cause metabolic acidosis, pulmonary hypertension, and hypoxemia. Hypothermia also may be an indicator of sepsis in the neonate. Assessment findings may include:

- Pale color
- Cool skin (especially in the extremities)
- Respiratory distress
- Apnea
- Bradycardia
- Central cyanosis
- Irritability (initially)
- Lethargy (in the late stage)
- Absence of shivering (variable)

> **NOTE**
>
> Infants may die of cold exposure at temperatures that adults find comfortable.

Prehospital care for these patients may include provision of both basic and advanced cardiac life support (depending on the severity of hypothermia) and rapid transport to an appropriate facility. Other therapeutic measures include ensuring the child is dry and warm and perhaps the administration of *dextrose* to treat hypoglycemia and IV therapy with warm fluids. The patient should be transported in a heated ambulance (76° F to 80° F [24° C to 26.5° C]).

> ✓ **TRICKS OF THE TRADE**
>
> It is not known whether newborns shiver. They generate heat mainly by nonshivering thermogenesis.

Hypoglycemia

A blood glucose measurement less than 40 mg/dL in the infant indicates hypoglycemia (described in Chapter 31).[6] The condition (which should be determined by blood glucose screening on all sick infants) may be due to inadequate glucose intake or increased utilization of glucose. Risk factors associated with hypoglycemia include asphyxia, toxemia, being the smaller twin, CNS hemorrhage, and sepsis. Assessment findings may include:

- Twitching or seizure
- Limpness
- Lethargy
- Eye rolling

- High-pitched crying
- Apnea
- Irregular respirations
- Cyanosis (possibly)

> **NOTE**
>
> Small infants and chronically ill children have limited glycogen stores that may rapidly be depleted during stress events. If allowed to persist, hypoglycemia can depress myocardial function and may have catastrophic effects on the brain.

Prehospital care is directed at ensuring adequate airway, ventilatory, and circulatory support; maintaining body temperature; providing rapid transport; and perhaps IV administration of *dextrose 10%* (per medical direction) (Box 41-4). The glucose level determination should be repeated if the infant fails to respond to initial resuscitative measures. All infants with an altered level of consciousness and those who are hypoglycemic and fail to respond to the administration of *dextrose* should be immediately transported to an appropriate medical facility.

> **NOTE**
>
> *Dextrose* that is administered to infants is *always* of a lower concentration (e.g., 5%, 10%) than standard dextrose.

Common Birth Injuries

About 2% to 7% of every 1000 live births result in avoidable and unavoidable mechanical and anoxic trauma during labor and delivery.[1] An uncontrolled, explosive delivery is the greatest risk factor for birth injuries. Injuries that sometimes occur to the infant during childbirth include:

- Cranial injuries
  Molding of the head and overriding of the parietal bones
  Soft-tissue injuries from forceps delivery
  Subconjunctival and retinal hemorrhage
  Subperiosteal hemorrhage
  Skull fracture
- Intracranial hemorrhage (from trauma or asphyxia)

> **BOX 41-4**
>
> ### GLUCOSE ADMINISTRATION
>
> Dose: 0.5 to 1.0 g/kg IV over 20 minutes
> Preparation: Dilute dextrose 50% (D50) 1:1 with sterile water, resulting in D25W; administer 2 to 4 mL/kg
>
> *or*
>
> Dilute dextrose 50% (D50) 1:4 with sterile water, resulting in D10W; administer 5 to 10 mL/kg
> Precautions: Hypertonic glucose is very hyperosmolar and may sclerose peripheral veins.

NOTE: Some sterile water has preservatives containing alcohol. This solution should not be used as it can cause profound hypoglycemia and death when administered to infants.

- Spine and spinal cord injury (from strong traction or lateral pull)
- Peripheral nerve injury
- Liver or spleen injury
- Adrenal hemorrhage
- Clavicle or extremity fracture
- Hypoxia-ischemia

> **NOTE**
>
> Of every 100,000 infants, 5 to 8 die of birth trauma; 25 out of every 100,000 die of anoxic injuries. Together these account for 2% to 3% of infant deaths.[1]

Assessment findings vary by the nature of the injury and may range from minor soft tissue trauma to paralysis to life-threatening cardiorespiratory compromise and shock. The goal of prehospital care is to support the newborn's vital functions and rapidly transport the infant to an appropriate medical facility for definitive care.

> **? CRITICAL THINKING**
>
> *How will you feel if you deliver a critically ill or dead infant?*

Psychological and Emotional Support

It is important for the paramedic to be aware of the normal feelings and reactions of parents, siblings, other family members, and caregivers while providing emergency care to an ill or injured child. (These events also are often highly charged and emotional for the emergency crew.) Those at the scene should be kept abreast of all procedures being performed and informed of the necessity of the procedures.

> **NOTE**
>
> After delivery, the mother continues to be a patient herself, with physical and emotional needs.

As a rule, emergency responders should never discuss the infant's chances of survival with a parent or family member, nor give "false hopes" about the infant's condition. The paramedic should assure the family that everything that can be done for the child is being done, and that their baby will receive the best possible care during transport and while at the emergency department. The receiving hospital will have appropriate support personnel available to assist family members and loved ones.

SUMMARY

- Premature infants have an increased risk of respiratory suppression, hypothermia, and head and brain injury. In addition to low birth weight, various antepartum and intrapartum risk factors may affect the need for resuscitation.

- Some of the more common congenital anomalies include choanal atresia, cleft lip, diaphragmatic hernia, and Pierre Robin syndrome.

- At birth, newborns make three major physiological adaptations necessary for survival: (1) emptying fluids from their lungs and beginning ventilation, (2) changing their circulatory pattern, and (3) maintaining body temperature.

- The initial steps of neonatal resuscitation (except for those born through meconium) are to prevent heat loss, clear the airway by positioning and suctioning, provide tactile stimulation and initiate breathing if necessary, and further evaluate the infant.

- If with oxygenation and continued ventilations the infant's condition deteriorates or fails to improve, the infant may require ET intubation and administration of drugs. Medications most frequently used during neonatal resuscitation are epinephrine, volume expanders, and naloxone.

- The three most common complications during the postresuscitation period are endotracheal position change (including dislodgement), tube occlusion by mucus or meconium, and pneumothorax. During transport of the neonate, it is important to maintain body temperature, oxygen administration, and ventilatory support.

- Specific situations that may require advanced life support for the neonate include respiratory disorders (e.g., apnea, respiratory distress, cyanosis), cardiovascular disorders (e.g., bradycardia, cardiac arrest), gastrointestinal disorders (e.g., vomiting, diarrhea), seizures, fever, hypothermia, and hypoglycemia.

- About 2% to 7% of every 1000 live births result in avoidable and unavoidable mechanical and anoxic trauma during labor and delivery.

- The paramedic should be aware of the normal feelings and reactions of parents, siblings, other family members, and caregivers while providing emergency care to an ill or injured child.

■ REFERENCES

1. U.S. Department of Transportation National Highway Traffic Safety Administration: *EMT—Paramedic national standard curriculum*, Washington, DC, 1998, The Department.
2. American Heart Association: *Pediatric advanced life support*, Dallas, 1997, The Association.
3. American Heart Association: *Textbook of neonatal resuscitation*, Dallas, 1995, American Academy of Pediatrics.
4. Eichelberger M et al: *Pediatric emergencies*, Englewood Cliffs, NJ, 1992, Prentice-Hall.
5. Hoekelman R et al: *Primary pediatric care*, ed 3, St Louis, 1997, Mosby.
6. American Heart Association: Guidelines 2000 for cardiopulmonary resuscitation and emergency cardiovascular care, International Consensus on Science, *Circulation* 102 (8):343, 2000.
7. American Heart Association: Guidelines 2000 for cardiopulmonary resuscitation and emergency cardiovascular care, International Consensus on Science, *Circulation* 102 (8):349, 2000.
8. American Heart Association: Guidelines 2000 for cardiopulmonary resuscitation and emergency cardiovascular care, International Consensus on Science, *Circulation* 102 (8):352, 2000.

42 Pediatrics

OBJECTIVES

Upon completion of this chapter, the paramedic student will be able to:

1. *Identify the role of the Emergency Medical Services for Children program.*

2. *Identify modifications in patient assessment techniques that assist in the examination of patients at different developmental levels.*

3. *Identify common age-related illnesses and injuries in pediatric patients.*

4. *Outline the general principles of assessment and management of the pediatric patient.*

5. *Describe the pathophysiology, signs and symptoms, and management of selected pediatric respiratory emergencies.*

6. *Describe the pathophysiology, signs and symptoms, and management of shock in the pediatric patient.*

7. *Describe the pathophysiology, signs and symptoms, and management of selected pediatric dysrhythmias.*

8. *Describe the pathophysiology, signs and symptoms, and management of pediatric seizures.*

9. *Describe the pathophysiology, signs and symptoms, and management of hypoglycemia and hyperglycemia in the pediatric patient.*

10. *Describe the pathophysiology, signs and symptoms, and management of infectious pediatric emergencies.*

11. *Identify common causes of poisoning and toxic exposure in the pediatric patient.*

12. *Describe special considerations for assessment and management of specific injuries in children.*

13. *Outline the pathophysiology and management of sudden infant death syndrome.*

14. *Describe the risk factors, key signs and symptoms, and management of injuries or illness resulting from child abuse and neglect.*

15. *Identify prehospital considerations for the care of infants and children with special needs.*

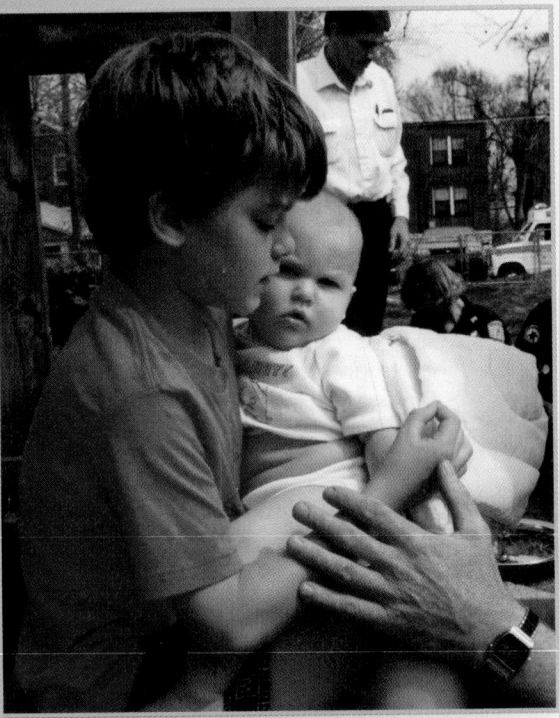

Emergencies involving pediatric patients account for a about 10% or fewer of emergency medical service (EMS) responses.[1] However, caring for these patients presents unique challenges related to size, physical and intellectual maturation, and diseases specific to neonates, infants, and children. This chapter addresses the anatomical and physiological mechanisms of growth and development, medical emergencies common to children, and initial assessment and management strategies that often are critical in the patient's survival.

KEY TERMS

bacterial tracheitis: A bacterial infection of the upper airway and subglottic trachea that may arise after a viral illness.

child abuse: The physical, sexual, or emotional maltreatment of a child.

shunt: A surgical procedure performed to relieve abnormal fluid pressures from excess cerebrospinal fluid (CSF) around the brain in children with hydrocephalus or in the portal veins in patients with portal hypertension.

sudden infant death syndrome (SIDS): The unexpected and sudden death of an apparently normal and healthy infant that occurs during sleep.

NOTE

Paramedics play an important role in the care of infants and children through both prehospital care (primary transport) and interfacility transfer (secondary transport). It is important to improve one's knowledge and clinical skills through continuing education programs and clinical application specific to this age group (Box 42-1).

Emergency Medical Services for Children

In 1985 the Emergency Medical Services for Children (EMSC) Demonstration Program was established through grants provided by the Maternal and Child Health Bureau of the U.S. Department of Health and Human Services and by the National Highway Traffic Safety Administration, a division of the U.S. Department of Transportation. This program, which was designed to enhance and expand emergency medical services for acutely ill and injured children, defined 12 basic components of an effective EMSC system[2]:

1. System approach
2. Education
3. Data collection
4. Quality improvement
5. Injury prevention
6. Access
7. Prehospital care
8. Emergency care
9. Definitive care
10. Rehabilitation
11. Finance
12. Continual health care from birth to young adulthood

? CRITICAL THINKING

Are you familiar with any EMSC injury prevention programs in your area?

Through the funding of EMSC grants and the efforts of organizations dedicated to improving emergency care for children, specific programs targeted to prehospital care providers have been developed.

BOX 42-1

SOURCES OF CONTINUING EDUCATION AND CLINICAL APPLICATION

Continuing Education
Advanced Pediatric Life Support (APLS)
Neonatal Resuscitation Program (NRP)
Pediatric Advanced Life Support (PALS)
Pediatric Basic Trauma Life Support (PBTLS)
Pediatric Emergencies for Paramedics (PEP)
Regional conferences and seminars
Teaching Resources for Instructors of Prehospital Pediatrics (TRIPP)
Textbooks and journals

Clinical Application
Pediatric emergency department
Pediatric hospital
Pediatric department of a community hospital
Pediatrician's office
Prevention programs

These include continuing education programs, educational resources for instructors, equipment guidelines, protocols for prehospital management, quality improvement procedures for evaluating prehospital care for children, and designation of facilities with special capabilities for pediatric care. As stated in *Emergency Medical Service for Children: A Report to the Nation*, published in 1991 by the National Center for Education in Maternal and Child Health, "The lives of many infants, children, and young adults . . . can be saved through implementation of emergency medical services for children (EMSC). Outcomes for critically ill and injured children can be influenced by the provision of timely care by health care professionals who are well trained and equipped for pediatric emergency and critical care."[3]

NOTE

Paramedics can play a significant role in the reduction of mortality and morbidity for children through becoming active participants in school, community, and parent education programs and injury prevention programs and by providing thorough documentation appropriate for prehospital trauma registries, epidemiological research, and surveillance. (See the section on Injury Prevention in Appendix C.)

? CRITICAL THINKING

How comfortable are you with the "normal" well child?

BOX 42-2

PEDIATRIC AGE CLASSIFICATIONS

Newborn: First few hours of life
Neonate: First 28 days of life
Infant: Up to 1 year of age
Toddler: 1 to 3 years of age
Preschooler: 3 to 5 years of age
School age: 6 to 12 years of age
Adolescence: The period between the end of childhood (beginning of puberty) and the start of adulthood (18 years of age). Adolescence is highly child specific; in boys the average age of onset is 13 years; in girls, it is 11 years. Adolescence may be further subdivided as *early* (puberty), *middle* (middle school/high school), and *late* (high school/college age).

Growth and Development Review

Children have unique anatomical, physiological, and psychological characteristics, which change during their development (see Appendix A). Box 42-2 lists the various age classifications for children; the box on p. 1233 presents the developmental stages of children and the special considerations that must be taken into account when caring for a pediatric patient. Appendix 42-1 provides a review of pediatric anatomy and physiology and associated implications in caring for children. The reader should refer to these areas for a review.

? CRITICAL THINKING

Why is it important to know what injuries and illnesses are commonly encountered in specific age groups?

Illness and Injury by Age Group

Some childhood diseases and disabilities are predictable by age group. Illnesses and injuries in the following seven age groups frequently are encountered by prehospital providers:

1. Neonate (first 28 days of life)
   Respiratory distress
   Jaundice
   Vomiting
   Fever
   Sepsis
   Meningitis
   Physical and sexual abuse
2. Infant (1 to 5 months old)
   Respiratory distress
   Fever
   Sudden infant death syndrome (SIDS)
   Vomiting and diarrhea with dehydration
   Sepsis
   Meningitis
   Physical and sexual abuse
3. Infant (6 to 12 months old)
   Fever, febrile seizures
   Vomiting and diarrhea with dehydration
   Bronchiolitis
   Croup
   Sepsis
   Meningitis

DEVELOPMENTAL STAGES AND APPROACH STRATEGIES FOR PEDIATRIC PATIENTS

Infants

Major fears
Separation and strangers

Approach strategies
Provide consistent caretakers.
Reduce parents' anxiety, because it is transmitted to the infant.
Minimize separation from parents.

Toddlers

Major fears
Separation and loss of control

Characteristics of thinking
Primitive
Unable to recognize views of others
Little concept of body integrity

Approach strategies
Keep explanations simple.
Choose words carefully.
Let toddler play with equipment (stethoscope).
Minimize separation from parents.

Preschoolers

Major fears
Bodily injury and mutilation
Loss of control
The unknown and the dark
Being left alone

Characteristics of thinking
Highly literal interpretation of words
Unable to abstract
Primitive ideas about the body (e.g., fear that all blood will "leak out" if a bandage is removed")

Approach strategies
Keep explanations simple and concise.
Choose words carefully.
Emphasize that a procedure will help the child be healthier.
Be honest.

School-Age Children

Major fears
Loss of control
Bodily injury and mutilation
Failure to live up to expectations of others
Death

Characteristics of thinking
Vague or false ideas about physical illness and body structure and function
Able to listen attentively without always comprehending
Reluctant to ask questions about something they think they are expected to know
Increased awareness of significant illness, possible hazards of treatments, lifelong consequences of injury, and the meaning of death

Approach strategies
Ask children to explain what they understand.
Provide as many choices as possible to increase the child's sense of control.
Reassure the child that he or she has done nothing wrong and that necessary procedures are not punishment.
Anticipate and answer questions about long-term consequences (e.g., what the scar will look like, how long activities may be curtailed).

Adolescents

Major fears
Loss of control
Altered body image
Separation from peer group

Characteristics of thinking
Able to think abstractly
Tendency toward hyperresponsiveness to pain (reactions not always in proportion to event)
Little understanding of the structure and workings of the body

Approach strategies
When appropriate, allow adolescents to be a part of decision making about their care.
Give information sensitively.
Express how important their compliance and cooperation are to their treatment.
Be honest about consequences.
Use or teach coping mechanisms such as relaxation, deep breathing, and self-comforting talk.

Respiratory distress (bronchiolitis, foreign body
  aspiration, croup)
Physical and sexual abuse
Foreign body airway obstruction
Falls
Injuries from motor vehicle crashes

It is estimated that 40,000 to 50,000 children are injured permanently each year and that at least 1 million seek medical care because of unintentional
injuries.[4]

4. Child (1 to 3 years old)
   Fever, febrile seizure
   Vomiting and diarrhea with dehydration
   Respiratory distress (asthma, bronchiolitis, foreign
     body aspiration, croup)
   Sepsis
   Meningitis
   Ingestions
   Foreign body airway obstruction
   Falls
   Injuries from motor vehicle crashes
   Physical and sexual abuse
5. Child (3 to 5 years old)
   Croup
   Asthma
   Febrile seizures
   Sepsis
   Meningitis
   Burns
   Drowning, near-drowning
   Injuries from motor vehicle crashes
   Physical and sexual abuse
6. Child (6 to 12 years old)
   Drowning, near-drowning
   Injuries from motor vehicle crashes
   Injuries from bicycle accidents
   Fractures
   Falls
   Sports injuries
   Burns
   Physical and sexual abuse
7. Adolescent (12 to 15 years old)
   Asthma
   Injuries from motor vehicle crashes

Sports injuries
Alcohol or other drug use
Suicide gestures
Physical and sexual abuse
Pregnancy
Physical and sexual abuse

General Principles of Pediatric Assessment

Many components of the initial patient evaluation
for children can be taken care of by observing the
patient and by involving the child's parent or
guardian in the initial assessment (see Chapter 14).
The parent or guardian often can help make the
child more comfortable during the assessment and
usually can provide valuable information about the
child's medical history and whether certain aspects
of the child's behavior or response to the illness or
injury is normal or abnormal.

TRICKS OF THE TRADE

Some paramedics feel uncomfortable when caring
for pediatric patients. Learning a little "pediatric pop
culture" helps establish a rapport; examples include
Barney, Teletubbies, and other popular TV characters
and children's toys.

Scene Assessment

As with all other patient care encounters, the
paramedic should begin the physical examination
with a quick scene survey, noting any hazards or
potential hazards and any visible mechanism of
injury or illness. For example, the presence of
pills, medicine bottles, or household chemicals
may indicate the possibility of toxic ingestion; injury and a history that does not coincide with the
mechanism of injury may indicate **child abuse.** In
addition, the paramedic should observe the relationship between the parent, guardian, or caregiver and the child and determine the appropriateness of their interaction. For example, does the
interaction demonstrate concern or is it angry or
indifferent? Other important assessments that can

be made during the scene survey include the orderliness, cleanliness, and safety of the home and the general appearance of other children in the family.

> ? CRITICAL THINKING
>
> **Would you want to make a comment to the parents about an unsafe situation on the scene before transport? Why or why not?**

Initial Assessment

The initial assessment begins with the paramedic formulating a general impression of the patient. The initial assessment should focus on the information most valuable for ascertaining if life-threatening conditions exist. The *Pediatric Assessment Triangle* (Fig. 42-1) is a paradigm that can be used for assessing a child. Following are the three components of the Pediatric Assessment Triangle:

- Appearance
  Mental status
  Muscle tone
- Work of breathing
  Respiratory rate
  Respiratory effort
- Circulation
  Skin signs
  Skin color

> ? CRITICAL THINKING
>
> **Think about one abnormal finding in each area of the assessment triangle. Would that single finding influence your triage decision?**

Using the pediatric assessment triangle or a similar method allows the paramedic to make initial triage decisions: If the child's condition is urgent, care should proceed with rapid assessment of airway, breathing, and circulation; management; and rapid transport. If the child's condition is not urgent, care can proceed with a focused history and detailed physical examination.

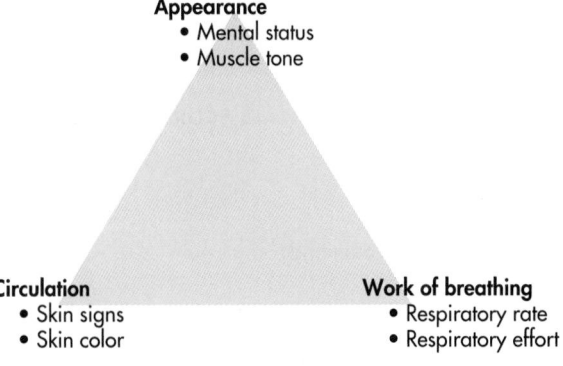

Fig. 42-1 Pediatric assessment triangle.

Vital Functions

The AVPU scale or the *Modified Glasgow Coma Scale* (Table 42-1) can be used to determine the child's level of consciousness and to assess for signs of inadequate oxygenation.

Airway and breathing. The child's airway should be patent, and breathing should proceed with adequate chest rise and fall. Signs of respiratory distress include the following:

- Tachypnea
- Use of accessory muscles
- Nasal flaring
- Grunting
- Bradypnea
- Irregular breathing pattern
- Head bobbing
- Absent breath sounds
- Abnormal breath sounds

Circulation. Circulation is assessed by comparing the strength and quality of central and peripheral pulses, measuring blood pressure (in children over 3 years of age), evaluating skin color, temperature, moisture, and turgor and capillary refill, and looking for visible hemorrhage. A review of normal vital signs for each age group is provided in Table 42-2.

Transition Phase

The transition phase is integrated throughout assessment and is used to allow the child to become more familiar with the paramedic crew and medical

TABLE 42-1	PEDIATRIC MODIFICATION OF GLASGOW COMA SCALE (GCS) BY AGE OF PATIENT*

GLASGOW COMA SCALE SCORE		**PEDIATRIC MODIFICATION**	
Eye Opening			
≥1 year		*birth-1 year*	
4 Spontaneously		4 Spontaneously	
3 To verbal command		3 To shout	
2 To pain		2 To pain	
1 No response		1 No response	
Best Motor Response			
≥1 year		*0-1 year*	
6 Obeys		5 Localizes pain	
5 Localizes pain		4 Flexion withdrawal	
4 Flexion withdrawal		3 Flexion abnormal (decorticate)	
3 Flexion abnormal (decorticate)		2 Extension (decerebrate)	
2 Extension (decerebrate)		1 No response	
1 No response			
Best Verbal Response			
>5 years	*birth-2 years*		*2-5 years*
5 Oriented and converses	5 Cries appropriately, smiles, coos		5 Appropriate words and phrases
4 Disoriented and converses	4 Cries		4 Inappropriate words
3 Inappropriate words	3 Inappropriate crying/screaming		3 Cries/screams
2 Incomprehensible sounds	2 Grunts		2 Grunts
1 No response	1 No response		1 No response

*The GCS score is the sum of the individual scores from eye opening, best verbal response, and best motor response, using age-specific criteria. A GCS score of 13 to 15 indicates mild head injury, a score of 9 to 12 indicates moderate head injury, and a score of 8 or lower indicates severe head injury.

equipment (e.g., "get to know you" conversations, playing with stethoscope) (see Chapter 13). Use of the transition phase depends on the seriousness of the patient's condition and is appropriate only for a conscious child who is not acutely ill. If the patient is unconscious or acutely ill, management should proceed directly to emergency care and transport.

TRICKS OF THE TRADE

If your service handles a lot of pediatric patients, consider investing in an inexpensive watch with Tweety Bird, Elmo, or a Pokémon character on the watch face. This can be a great icebreaker!

Focused History

When obtaining the focused history for an infant, a toddler, or a preschooler, the paramedic often must elicit information from the parent, guardian, or caregiver. School-age and adolescent patients can provide most information and should be questioned in private (away from parents or family members) about sexual activity, pregnancy, alcohol or other drug use, or suspicion of child abuse. The focused history (described in Chapter 12) should include the following:

1. Chief complaint
   Nature of illness or injury
   The length (duration) of illness or injury
   Last meal
   Presence of fever
   Effects on behavior
   Vomiting or diarrhea
   Frequency of urination
2. Medications and allergies
3. Past medical history
   Physician care
   Chronic illnesses

TABLE 42-2   VITAL SIGNS BY AGE GROUP

GROUP	AGE	RESPIRATORY RATE		PULSE RATE		BLOOD PRESSURE	
		BREATHS/MIN	SUSPECT POSSIBLE ↓ IN MINUTE VOLUME AND NEED FOR VENTILATORY ASSIST WITH BVM	BEATS/MIN	ASSUME A SERIOUS PROBLEM EXISTS (BRADYCARDIA OR TACHYCARDIA)	EXPECTED MEAN FOR BLOOD PRESSURE (SYSTOLIC/DIASTOLIC)	LOWER LIMIT OF SYSTOLIC BLOOD PRESSURE
Newborn	Birth-6 weeks	30-50	↓ 30 or ↑ 50	120-160	↓ 100 or ↑ 150	74-100 mm Hg/50-68 mm Hg	↓ 70 mm Hg
Infant	7 weeks-1 year	20-30	↓ 20 or ↑ 30	80-140	↓ 80 or ↑ 120	84-106 mm Hg/56-70 mm Hg	↓ 70 mm Hg
Toddler	1-2 years	20-30	↓ 20 or ↑ 30	80-130	↓ 60 or ↑ 110	98-106 mm Hg/50-70 mm Hg	↓ 70 mm Hg
Preschool	2-6 years	20-30	↓ 20 or ↑ 30	80-120	↓ 60 or ↑ 110	98-112 mm Hg/64-70 mm Hg	↓ 70 mm Hg
School age	6-13 years	(12-20)-30	↓ 20 or ↑ 30	(60-80)-100	↓ 60 or ↑ 110	104-124 mm Hg/64-80 mm Hg	↓ 80-90 mm Hg
Adolescent	13-16 years	12-20	↓ 12 or ↑ 20	60-100	↓ 60 or ↑ 100	118-132 mm Hg/70-82 mm Hg	↓ 80-90 mm Hg

BVM, Bag-valve-mask device.
Modified from the National Association of Emergency Medical Technicians: *Basic and advanced prehospital trauma life support,* 1998, The Association.

Detailed Physical Examination

The detailed physical examination should be performed as described in Chapter 14. It should proceed from head to toe in older children and from toe to head in younger children (under 2 years of age). Depending on the patient's condition, some or all of the following assessments may be appropriate:

- Pupils
- Capillary refill (most accurate in patients under 6 years of age)
- Hydration (skin turgor, sunken or flat fontanelles in infants, presence of tears and saliva)
- Pulse oximetry
- Electrocardiographic (ECG) monitoring

Continuous Assessment

Continuous assessment is appropriate for all patients and should be performed throughout the patient care encounter. The purpose of continuous assessment is to monitor the patient for changes in respiratory effort, skin color and temperature, mental status, and vital signs (including pulse oximetry measurements). Measurement tools (e.g., blood pressure cuffs, electrodes) should be appropriate for the size of the child.

? CRITICAL THINKING

Why is continuous examination especially important in the young child?

General Principles of Patient Management

The principles of patient management depend on the patient's condition and may include the following:

1. Basic airway management
   Manual positioning
   Removal of foreign body airway obstruction with basic clearing methods
   Suction
   Oxygenation
   Airway adjuncts (nasal and oral)
   Ventilation with bag-valve device

2. Advanced airway management
   Removal of foreign body airway obstruction with advanced clearing methods
   Endotracheal (ET) intubation
   Needle cricothyroidotomy (per medical direction)

NOTE

Basic and advanced airway procedures and the use of airway adjuncts are described in Chapter 11.

3. Circulation
   Vascular access (intravenous [IV] and intraosseous [IO])
   Fluid resuscitation
4. Pharmacological
   Pain management
   Rapid sequence intubation (per medical direction)
   Respiratory, cardiac, endocrinological, and neurological medications
5. Nonpharmacological
   Spine immobilization for trauma patients
   Hemorrhage control
   Bandaging and splinting
   Fever control

✓ TRICKS OF THE TRADE

If a young child with an extremity injury has a special toy, such as Big Bird or Cookie Monster, do to the toy what you need to do to the child. Splinting Big Bird's leg or arm first often improves the child's cooperation.

6. Transport considerations
   Appropriate mode (rapid transport versus on-scene care)
   Appropriate facility (e.g., pediatric trauma facility)
7. Psychological support and communication strategies
   Approach strategies

NOTE

Approach strategies specific for pediatric patients and their caregivers are described in Chapter 10. The reader should refer to that chapter for review.

Specific Pathophysiology, Assessment, and Management

The conditions discussed in this section are respiratory compromise, shock, dysrhythmias, seizure, hypoglycemia and hyperglycemia, infection, poisoning and toxic exposure, trauma, sudden infant death syndrome (SIDS), and child abuse and neglect.

Respiratory Compromise

Several conditions manifest chiefly as respiratory distress in children. These include upper and lower foreign body airway obstruction, upper airway disease (croup, bacterial tracheitis, and epiglottitis), and lower airway disease (asthma, bronchiolitis, and pneumonia). Most cases of cardiac arrest in children occur secondary to respiratory insufficiency.[5] For this reason, respiratory emergencies require rapid prehospital assessment and management.

> **NOTE**
>
> The paramedic should attempt to calm and reassure a child with respiratory compromise. It is important not to agitate the conscious patient or lay the child down (supine) because doing so may aggravate the airway condition and lead to life-threatening airway obstruction. When possible, allow the parent or other caregiver to remain with the child. The receiving hospital should be advised of the patient's status as soon as possible so that arrangements can be made for appropriate medical personnel.

Upper and Lower Foreign Body Airway Obstruction

Obstruction of the upper or lower airway by a foreign body may cause a partial or complete airway obstruction. These events usually occur in toddlers and preschoolers (1 to 4 years of age), and commonly are caused by food (hard candy, nuts, seeds, hot dogs) or small objects (e.g., coins, balloons). Complete airway obstruction requires immediate intervention to relieve the obstruction. Basic and advanced methods of clearing the airway are presented in Chapter 11.

Signs and symptoms of airway obstruction include anxiety, inspiratory stridor, muffled or hoarse voice, drooling, pain in the throat, decreased breath sounds, rales, rhonchi, and wheezing. There may be a history of choking (observed by an adult). The paramedic should suspect foreign body aspiration in an otherwise healthy child with sudden onset of respiratory compromise. If a complete airway obstruction cannot be relieved with basic and advanced methods of clearing, tracheal intubation may be indicated.

> **NOTE**
>
> If a child with a partial airway obstruction is conscious and has adequate movement of air, the paramedic should not agitate the child but rather provide continuous respiratory monitoring and immediate transportation to the receiving hospital. Agitation or attempts to relieve a partial airway obstruction may cause movement of a foreign body and lead to complete obstruction.

Croup

Croup (laryngotracheobronchitis) is a common inflammatory respiratory illness in children. It is a viral infection of the upper airway that usually occurs in children between the ages of 6 months and 4 years, often during the late fall and early winter months. The responsible organism usually is the parainfluenza virus, although respiratory syncytial virus (RSV), rubeola, and adenovirus have been implicated. Croup may involve the entire respiratory tract, but the symptoms are caused by inflammation in the subglottic region (at the level of the larynx extending to the cricoid cartilage).

A child with croup usually has a history of recent upper respiratory tract infection and a low-grade fever. The patient may have hoarseness, inspiratory stridor (from subglottic edema), and a "barking" cough. Wheezing may be present if the lower airways are involved. Commonly, the emergency episode occurs at night after the child has gone to bed. On arrival of paramedics, a patient with severe croup may exhibit all the classic signs of respiratory distress. The child may be sitting upright and leaning forward to facilitate breathing (variable), and nasal flaring, intercostal retraction, and cyanosis (a late sign of respiratory insufficiency) may be present.

Children with severe croup are at risk of serious airway obstruction from the narrowed diameter of the trachea. Differentiating croup from epiglottitis in the prehospital setting may be difficult. Table 42-3 lists the different characteristics of croup and epiglottitis.

Prehospital management of croup includes airway maintenance, administration of cool mist or humidified or nebulized oxygen, and transportation in a position of comfort. Symptoms may improve dramatically in patients with croup after the child is exposed to cool, humidified air (e.g., after moving the patient from the residence to the emergency vehicle). The paramedic should make all efforts to keep the child comfortable and at ease.

Bacterial Tracheitis

Bacterial tracheitis is an infection of the upper airway and subglottic trachea that may occur after a viral illness. It generally occurs in infants and toddlers (1 to 5 years of age) but can also occur in older children. The signs and symptoms of bacterial tracheitis are those of respiratory distress or failure (depending on the severity) and may include the following:

- Agitation
- High-grade fever
- Inspiratory and expiratory stridor
- Cough that produces pus or mucus
- Hoarseness
- Throat pain

Emergency care is directed at providing airway, ventilatory, and circulatory support and rapid transport for evaluation by a physician. If airway obstruction or respiratory failure (inability of the cardiopulmonary system to maintain the adequate exchange of oxygen and carbon dioxide) or respiratory arrest develops, tracheal intubation is required with tracheal suction to remove mucus or pus. (Bag-valve-mask [BVM] ventilation may require high pressures.) In-hospital care includes administration of intravenous antibiotics specific for the causative organism after the child's airway has been stabilized.

Epiglottitis

Epiglottitis is a rapidly progressive, life-threatening bacterial infection. It most often affects children between 3 and 7 years of age but can occur at any age. The disease usually is associated with *Haemophilus influenzae* type B, but *Streptococcus, Pneumococcus,* and *Staphylococcus* organisms also have been implicated. The bacterial infection causes edema and swelling of the epiglottis and supraglottic structures (pharynx, aryepiglottic folds, and arytenoid cartilage). Epiglottitis is a true emergency that requires prompt, expert airway management.

> **NOTE**
>
> The *H. influenzae* type B (Hib) vaccine has dramatically reduced the number of cases of epiglottitis in children.[4]

Epiglottitis usually begins suddenly (within 6 to 8 hours). Commonly, the child goes to bed asymptomatic and wakes up complaining of a sore throat and pain on swallowing. The child may have fever, a muffled voice (from edema of the mucosal covering of the vocal cords), and drooling from the pooled saliva that occurs secondary to dysphagia (an ominous sign of impending airway obstruction).

On arrival of the paramedics, a child with epiglottitis typically is found sitting upright and leaning forward with the head hyperextended to facilitate breathing (tripod position). The tongue may be protruding, or the child may have inspiratory stridor. These children usually do not cry or strug-

TABLE 42-3	COMPARISON OF THE SYMPTOMS OF CROUP AND EPIGLOTTITIS
CHARACTERISTICS	**CROUP**	**EPIGLOTTITIS**
Occurrence	6 months–4 years	3-7 years
Onset	Slow	Rapid
Comfortable position	Patient may lie down or sit upright	Patient prefers to sit upright
Cough	Barking cough	No barking cough; may have inspiratory stridor
Drooling	No drooling	Drooling, pain on swallowing
Temperature	Under 104° F	Over 104° F

gle because all available attention and energy is being expended to maximize air exchange. Inspiratory stridor with a characteristic "rattle" often is present, and the child may be gasping or gulping for air. Classic signs of respiratory distress usually are present. Definitive care for epiglottitis is in-hospital intubation and parenteral antibiotic therapy.

? CRITICAL THINKING

What other childhood respiratory problems (traumatic and nontraumatic) can manifest with stridor?

Children with acute epiglottitis are in danger of progressing to complete airway obstruction and respiratory arrest (absence of breathing). Occlusion can occur suddenly and may be precipitated by minor irritation of the throat, aggravation, and anxiety. For these reasons, it is very important that a child suspected of having epiglottitis be handled gently. The following guidelines in prehospital management should be observed:

- Make no attempt to lay the child down or to change the position of comfort.
- Make no attempt to visualize the airway if the child is still ventilating adequately.
- Advise medical direction of the suspicion of epiglottitis so that appropriate personnel and resources can be made available.
- Administer 100% humidified oxygen by mask unless it provokes agitation.
- Do not attempt vascular access.
- Have appropriate-sized emergency airway equipment selected and immediately available.
- Transport the child to the receiving hospital in the position of comfort.

If the patient progresses to respiratory arrest before arrival at the emergency department, field intubation must be attempted. The child's lungs should be hyperventilated and preoxygenated with a bag-valve device before intubation. After the airway has been established, IV access should be obtained if time permits.

The paramedic should be prepared for a difficult intubation because the vocal cords are likely to be obscured by the swollen supraglottic tissues. An uncuffed ET tube one to two sizes smaller than normal should be used. The paramedic should locate the laryngeal inlet by looking for mucus bubbles in the cleft between the edematous aryepiglottic folds and the swollen epiglottis. (Chest compressions during glottic visualization may produce a bubble at the tracheal opening.) In the rare instance that intubation cannot be achieved and the child cannot be adequately ventilated by a bag-valve device, medical direction may recommend needle cricothyroidotomy.

NOTE

Very often a child can be ventilated through the occlusive crisis of epiglottitis by BVM ventilation using a tight facial seal. This may require two people—one to maintain the seal and the other to ventilate.

Asthma

Asthma, which is obstruction of the lower airways, is characterized by inflammation and bronchoconstriction that results from autonomic dysfunction or sensitizing agents (see Chapter 27). The hallmarks of an acute exacerbation are anxiety, dyspnea, tachypnea, and audible expiratory wheezes with a prolonged expiratory phase. (A silent chest indicates impending respiratory failure.) Asthma is common among children over 2 years of age and affects 5% to 10% of those under 10 years of age. An acute exacerbation may be triggered by infection, changes in temperature, physical exercise, and emotional response.

? CRITICAL THINKING

What other signs or symptoms would lead you to believe that a child with asthma is decompensating?

NOTE

Bronchiolitis and asthma are different illnesses, but both are characterized by wheezing.

The goals of prehospital management include ventilatory assistance, administration of humidified

PHARMACOLOGICAL TREATMENT OF ASTHMA

Oxygen (Preferably Humidified)

- Simple face mask (6 L/min)
- Nonrebreather mask (15 L/min)

Aerosolized Beta₂-Adrenergic Agonists

- Albuterol
  Metered dose inhaler (MDI): 1 to 2 inhalations (90-180 μg) every 4 to 6 hours (with 5 minutes between inhalations)
  Solution: 0.01-0.03 mL (0.05-0.15 mg)/kg/dose to maximum of 0.5 mL/dose diluted in 2 mL of 0.9% NS; may be repeated every 20 minutes three times
- Metaproterenol (for children over 12 years of age)
  MDI: 2 to 3 inhalations every 3 to 4 hours (with 2 minutes between inhalations)
  Solution: 5 to15 inhalations of 5% solution

Subcutaneous Beta₂-Adrenergic agonists

- Epinephrine
  0.01 mL/kg (1:1000), maximum 0.3 mL

Corticosteroids

- Methylprednisolone
  1-2 mg/kg IV bolus
- Hydrocortisone
  4-6 mg/kg IV bolus

oxygen, reversal of the bronchospasm, and rapid transport for evaluation and treatment. Severe asthma exacerbations may be life threatening and can rapidly progress to respiratory failure. The paramedic should be prepared to initiate aggressive airway management along with ventilatory and circulatory support. Depending on local protocol, prior medication use, and the recommendations of medical direction, pharmacological therapy may include administration of aerosolized bronchodilators (*albuterol* [Proventil], *metaproterenol* [Alupent]), subcutaneous *epinephrine* (Adrenalin) with severe respiratory distress or failure, and occasionally corticosteroids during prolonged transports (Box 42-3).

Bronchiolitis

Bronchiolitis is a viral disease frequently caused by RSV infection of the lower airway that usually affects children under 2 years of age. It commonly occurs in the winter months and generally is associated with an upper respiratory infection. Bronchiolitis manifests with tachypnea and wheezing. The illness is caused by infection and the inflammation of the distal airway and is sometimes unresponsive to therapy aimed at relieving bronchospasm. Important features that may aid in differential diagnosis are listed in Table 42-4.

Bronchiolitis generally is benign and self-limiting, but it may be life threatening. Infants are at greater risk of developing respiratory failure because of the relatively small diameter of the bronchioles. Prehospital care for a patient with bronchiolitis is aimed at providing ventilatory support with humidified oxygen and rapid transport for evaluation by a physician. A therapeutic trial of *albuterol* (Proventil) via nebulizer may greatly reduce respiratory distress.

Pneumonia

Pneumonia (described in Chapter 27) is an acute infection of the lower airway and lungs that involves either the alveolar walls or the alveoli. It is commonly caused by a bacterial or viral infection. Children with pneumonia may have a history of recent airway infection. They also may have respiratory distress or failure (depending on the severity) and any of the following:

- Anxiety
- Decreased breath sounds
- Rales
- Rhonchi (localized or diffuse)
- Pain in the chest
- Fever

Most children with pneumonia have only mild disease and require no immediate stabilization or airway support. In cases of respiratory distress, stabilization of the airway is the highest priority. In severe cases, pharmacological therapy with bronchodilators may be indicated, and assisted ventilations via bag-valve device or intubation of the trachea may be necessary.

Shock

Shock (described in Chapter 7) is an abnormal condition characterized by inadequate delivery of oxygen and metabolic substrates to meet the metabolic demands of tissues. It may occur with increased, normal, or decreased blood pressure. The condition is further categorized as *compensated* (shock without hypotension) or *decompensated* (shock with

TABLE 42-4	DIFFERENTIATION OF BRONCHIOLITIS AND ASTHMA		
CLINICAL FEATURES	**BRONCHIOLITIS**		**ASTHMA**
Occurrence	Usually <18 months		Any age
Season	Winter, spring		Any time
Family history of asthma	Usually absent		Usually present
Etiology	Virus		Allergy, infection, exercise
Response to drugs	Some reversal of bronchospasm with beta agonists		Reversal of bronchospasm

TABLE 42-5	SYSTOLIC BLOOD PRESSURE CHARACTERIZING HYPOTENSION IN THE PEDIATRIC PATIENT	
AGE		**SYSTOLIC BLOOD PRESSURE**
Term neonates (0 to 28 days of age)		<60 mm Hg
Infants (1 month to 12 months)		<70 mm Hg
Children (1 year to 10 years)		<70 mm Hg + (2 × age in years)
Beyond 10 years		<90 mm Hg

hypotension). Compensated shock is detected by evaluation of heart rate, the presence and strength of peripheral pulses, and adequacy of end organ perfusion (assessed in the prehospital setting by mental status, capillary refill, and skin temperature).[5]

NOTE

In some children with shock, the pulses may be readily palpable and the skin may feel warm.

Shock may be classified as noncardiogenic (resulting from hypovolemia or distributive causes) and cardiogenic (resulting from cardiomyopathy or dysrhythmias).

Special Considerations for Pediatric Patients in Shock

Several special considerations must be taken into account when caring for a child in shock. These include circulating blood volume, body surface area and hypothermia, cardiac reserve, respiratory fatigue, vital signs, and assessment.

Circulating blood volume. In adults, blood volume accounts for 5% to 6% of total body weight, or 70 mL/kg of body weight; in children, blood volume accounts for 7% to 8% of total body weight, or 88 mL/kg of body weight. Although the percentage of circulating blood volume in a child is greater than that in an adult, a child's absolute blood volume is considerably lower than an adult's. Therefore a relatively small loss of blood may be devastating. For example, a blood loss of 100 mL in an adult is a 2% loss; a 100 mL loss in an infant is a 15% to 20% loss, resulting in shock.

A child with a volume deficit will maintain stable hemodynamics until all compensatory mechanisms fail (i.e., the blood pressure may be normal or only slightly decreased) (Table 42-5). At that point, shock progresses rapidly, with catastrophic deterioration. Because these efficient compensatory mechanisms can mask a potentially life-threatening condition, the paramedic must maintain a high degree of suspicion. Early recognition, stabilization (airway control, fluid replacement), and rapid transport to an appropriate medical facility are especially important when caring for children in shock.

? CRITICAL THINKING

How comfortable are you with starting an IV on an infant or young child?

Body surface area and hypothermia. Children have a relatively large body surface area in proportion to body weight, and their compensatory mechanisms (e.g., shivering) are not well developed. Children in shock quickly can develop hypothermia from exposure and concurrent metabolic acidosis, increased vascular resistance, respiratory depression, and myocardial dysfunction. Because hypothermic states can make resuscitation and medication therapy less effective, the paramedic should maintain the patient's body temperature by using blankets, covering the child's head with towels, and using warming devices for IV fluids.

Cardiac reserve. Because of their already high metabolic needs, infants and children have less cardiac reserve than adults for stressful situations such as shock. It is important to reduce the energy and oxygen requirements of a child in shock as much as possible. This can be accomplished by providing ventilatory support, reducing anxiety, and maintaining moderate ambient temperatures.

Respiratory fatigue. Respiratory muscle fatigue may lead to hypoventilation, hypoxemia, and respiratory failure or arrest. Like other compensatory mechanisms of the child, respiratory compensation in shock syndrome generally is at a maximum until it is depleted, at which time deterioration can be sudden. For this reason, airway control and supplemental oxygen are essential in all children who are seriously ill or injured.

Vital signs and assessment. Many variables must be considered when evaluating a child's vital signs. For example, blood pressure and pulse rate vary greatly with age, body temperature, and degree of agitation. Therefore these parameters should be measured as baseline assessments; they may be of limited value in assessing the circulation of a child in shock. The most

effective assessment is constant monitoring of the child's mental and physical status and the response to therapy. The following nine evaluation components should be noted when assessing a child in shock.

1. Level of consciousness
   Anxiety
   Agitation
   Ability to make eye contact
   Ability to recognize family members
2. Skin
   Temperature
   Moisture
   Color
   Turgor
   Capillary refill (in children under 6 years of age)
3. Mucous membranes
   Color
   Moisture
4. Nail beds
   Capillary refill (in children younger than 6 years of age)
   Color
5. Peripheral circulation
   Collapse
   Distention
6. Cardiac
   ECG findings
   Rate
   Rhythm
   Quality of pulses
   Location of pulses
7. Respiration
   Rate
   Depth
8. Blood pressure (in children over 3 years of age)
9. Body temperature

> **NOTE**
>
> Sustained tachycardia in the absence of known causes such as fever or pain may be an early sign of cardiovascular compromise. Bradycardia, on the other hand, may be a preterminal cardiac rhythm indicating advanced shock and is often associated with hypotension.[5]

Hypovolemia

Hypovolemia results from intravascular volume depletion (vomiting, diarrhea, burns) and blood loss (trauma, internal bleeding).

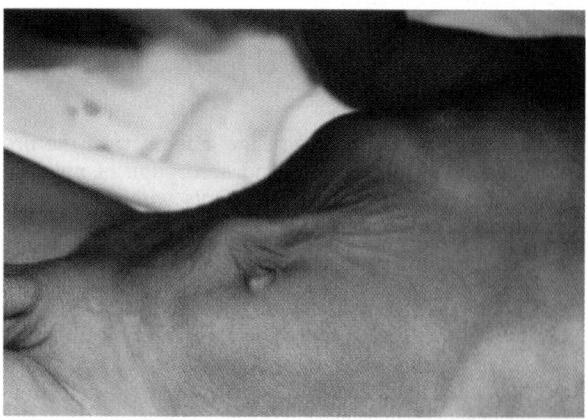

Fig. 42-2 Severe dehydration. (From Zitelli BJ, Davis HW: *Atlas of pediatric physical diagnosis*, ed 3, St Louis, 1997, Mosby-Wolfe.)

Dehydration. Profound fluid and electrolyte imbalances can occur in children as a consequence of diarrhea, vomiting, poor fluid intake, fever, or burns. Dehydration compromises cardiac output and systemic perfusion if the child loses the fluid equivalent of 5% or more total body weight or if the adolescent loses 5% to 7% of total body weight (Fig. 42-2). If allowed to progress, dehydration can result in renal failure, shock, and death. The severity of the dehydration and fluid volume deficit can be estimated from a history of the child's weight loss and the physical examination. Physical findings depend on the type of dehydration (isotonic, hypotonic, hypertonic). Table 42-6 provides signs and symptoms related to degrees of dehydration.

After provision of airway and ventilatory support, the initial management of dehydration in the child is directed at restoring and maintaining intravascular volume and systemic perfusion. IV therapy should be initiated (per medical direction) with isotonic crystalloids such as lactated Ringer's solution or normal saline. A fluid bolus of 20 mL/kg (administered in less than 20 minutes)[6] should be administered and may be repeated until the patient's systemic perfusion improves and an appropriate blood pressure has been obtained. After physician evaluation and initial shock resuscitation, the fluid administration rate and type of fluid

replacement are determined by the volume and type of fluid deficit and the patient's response to therapy.

Hemorrhage. As previously stated, even a relatively small amount of blood loss can be quite serious for the pediatric patient (Table 42-7). After controlling external hemorrhage (if present), securing the patient's airway, and providing high-concentration oxygen, the child's circulatory status may require support with IV therapy (per medical direction).

Like with other causes of hypovolemia, volume replacement to manage blood loss should be initiated using isotonic crystalloid solutions such as normal saline or lactated Ringer's solution. The first bolus should be 20 mL/kg. If the volume loss is in the 20% range, physiological measurements should improve after this infusion. If physiological parameters improve, IV therapy should be continued at maintenance rate during patient transport. If there is little response to the first bolus (slight improvement in color and capillary refill and decreased heart rate) or if the patient does not respond to the

?	CRITICAL THINKING

What are some ways to determine the child's weight for fluid and drug dosing?

> **NOTE**
>
> Establishing an IV line in children through a peripheral vein (described in Chapter 9) can be difficult even in the most controlled settings. Accordingly, medical direction may recommend that the child in shock have an IO line established, or be stabilized without establishing venous access and rapidly transported to an appropriate medical facility.

TABLE 42-6	ASSESSMENT OF DEGREE OF DEHYDRATION IN ISOTONIC FLUID LOSS

CLINICAL PARAMETERS	MILD	MODERATE	SEVERE
Body weight loss			
Infant	5% (50 mL/kg)	10% (100 mL/kg)	15% (150 mL/kg)
Adult	3% (30 mL/kg)	6% (60 mL/kg)	9% (90 mL/kg)
Skin turgor	Slightly ↓	↓↓	↓↓↓
Fontanelle	Possibly flat or depressed	Depressed	Significantly depressed
Mucous membranes	Dry	Very dry	Parched
Skin perfusion	Warm with normal color	Cool (extremities)	Cold (extremities)
		Pale	Mottled or gray
Heart rate	Mildly tachycardic	Moderately tachycardic	Extremely tachycardic
Peripheral pulses	Normal	Diminished	Absent
Blood pressure	Normal	Normal	Reduced
Sensorium	Normal or irritable	Irritable or lethargic	Unresponsive

TABLE 42-7	CLASSIFICATION OF HEMORRHAGIC SHOCK IN PEDIATRIC TRAUMA PATIENTS BASED ON SYSTEMIC SIGNS			
SYSTEM	VERY MILD HEMORRHAGE*	MILD HEMORRHAGE†	MODERATE HEMORRHAGE‡	SEVERE HEMORRHAGE§
Cardiovascular	Normal or mildly increased heart rate	Tachycardia	Significant tachycardia	Severe tachycardia
	Normal pulse rate	Peripheral pulses may be diminished	Thready peripheral pulses	Thready central pulses
	Normal blood pressure	Normal blood pressure	Hypotension	Significant hypotension
	Normal pH	Normal pH	Metabolic acidosis	Significant acidosis
Respiratory	Normal rate	Tachypnea	Moderate tachypnea	Severe tachypnea
Central nervous system	Slight anxiousness	Irritability, confusion	Irritability or lethargy	Lethargy
		Combative affect	Diminished pain response	Coma
Skin	Warm, pink color	Cool extremities, mottling	Cool extremities, mottling or pallor	Cold extremities, pallor or cyanosis
	Brisk capillary refill	Delayed capillary refill	Prolonged capillary refill	Prolonged capillary refill
Kidneys	Normal urine output	Oliguria, increased specific gravity	Oliguria, increased blood urea nitrogen level	Anuria

*<15% blood volume loss.
†15% to 25% blood volume loss.
‡25% blood volume loss.
§40% blood volume loss.

initial infusion, a second bolus of 20 mL/kg should follow immediately (Fig. 42-3).

Distributive Shock

Distributive (vasogenic) shock is used to refer to septic shock, neurogenic shock, and anaphylactic shock. It is relatively uncommon in children, resulting in peripheral pooling due to loss of vasomotor tone. Signs and symptoms are those of compensated or decompensated shock (hypotension), depending on severity. In addition, each type of shock has characteristic findings described in Box 42-4.

Emergency care is directed at ensuring the patient's vital functions though airway, ventilatory, and circulatory support, and rapid transport to an appropriate medical facility. Medical direction may recommend IV fluid therapy and pharmacological agents to manage specific forms of distributive shock (e.g., *dopamine* [Intropin] for neurogenic shock; *epinephrine* [Adrenalin] for anaphylaxis).

> **NOTE**
>
> Aids that commonly are used to calculate drug and fluid doses for pediatric patients were described in Chapter 9 and include the Pedi-Wheel (see Fig. 9-5) and the Broselow tape (Fig. 42-4).

Cardiomyopathy. *Cardiomyopathy* refers to any disease of the heart muscle that causes a reduction in the force of heart contractions and a resultant decrease in the efficiency of circulation of blood throughout the lungs and to the rest of the body. In children, the condition usually is the result of viral infection or congenital abnormalities that affect both ventricles of the heart. Symptoms include fatigue, chest pain, dysrhythmias and, in severe cases, signs of heart failure and cardiogenic shock, such as the following:

- Tachycardia
- Tachypnea

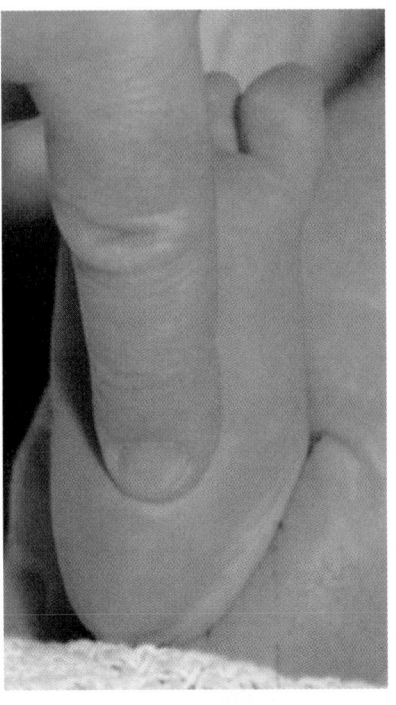 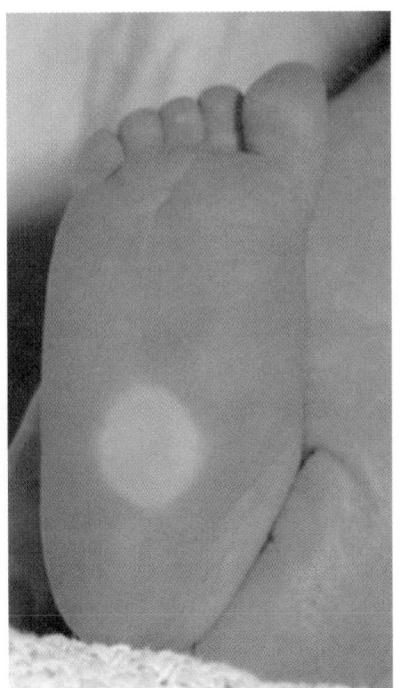 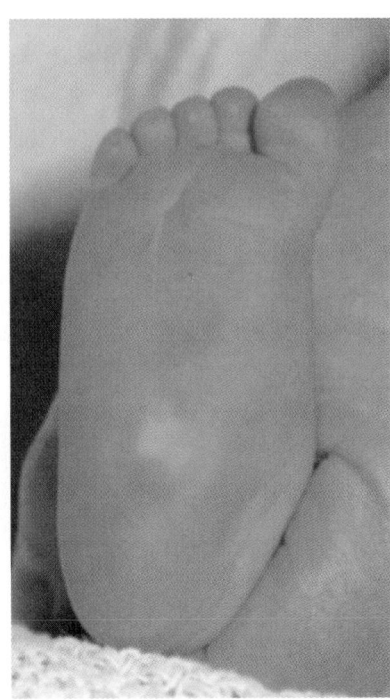

Fig. 42-3 Capillary refill in a child in shock. (From Beattie T: *Pediatric emergencies*, London, 1997, Mosby-Wolfe.)

BOX 42-4

CHARACTERISTIC FINDINGS IN DISTRIBUTIVE SHOCK

Septic Shock
Early stages (skin is warm)
Late stages (skin is cool)

Neurogenic Shock
Warm skin
Bradycardia
Impaired neurological function

Anaphylactic Shock
Allergic rash, erythema
Airway swelling, wheezing
Angioedema
Gastrointestinal upset

- Crackles
- Hypotension
- Jugular vein distention (difficult to determine in young children)
- Peripheral edema

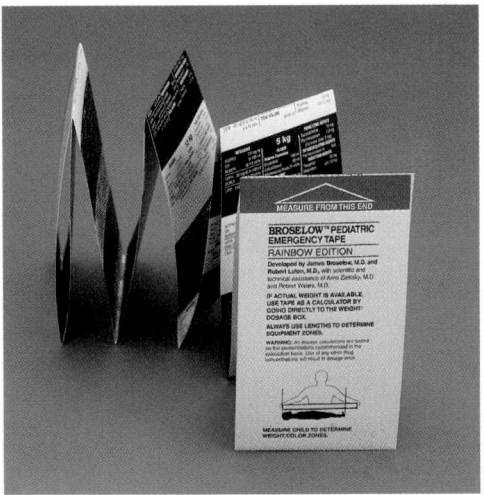

Fig. 42-4 Pediatric Broselow tape.

Patients in stable condition are managed with supportive care, administration of oxygen, and transport for evaluation by a physician. Children who are hypotensive and show other signs and symptoms of decompensation may require vascular access for administration of drugs (e.g., antidysrhythmics, diuretics, vasopressors). Intravenous fluid therapy should be restricted in these patients to avoid volume overload.

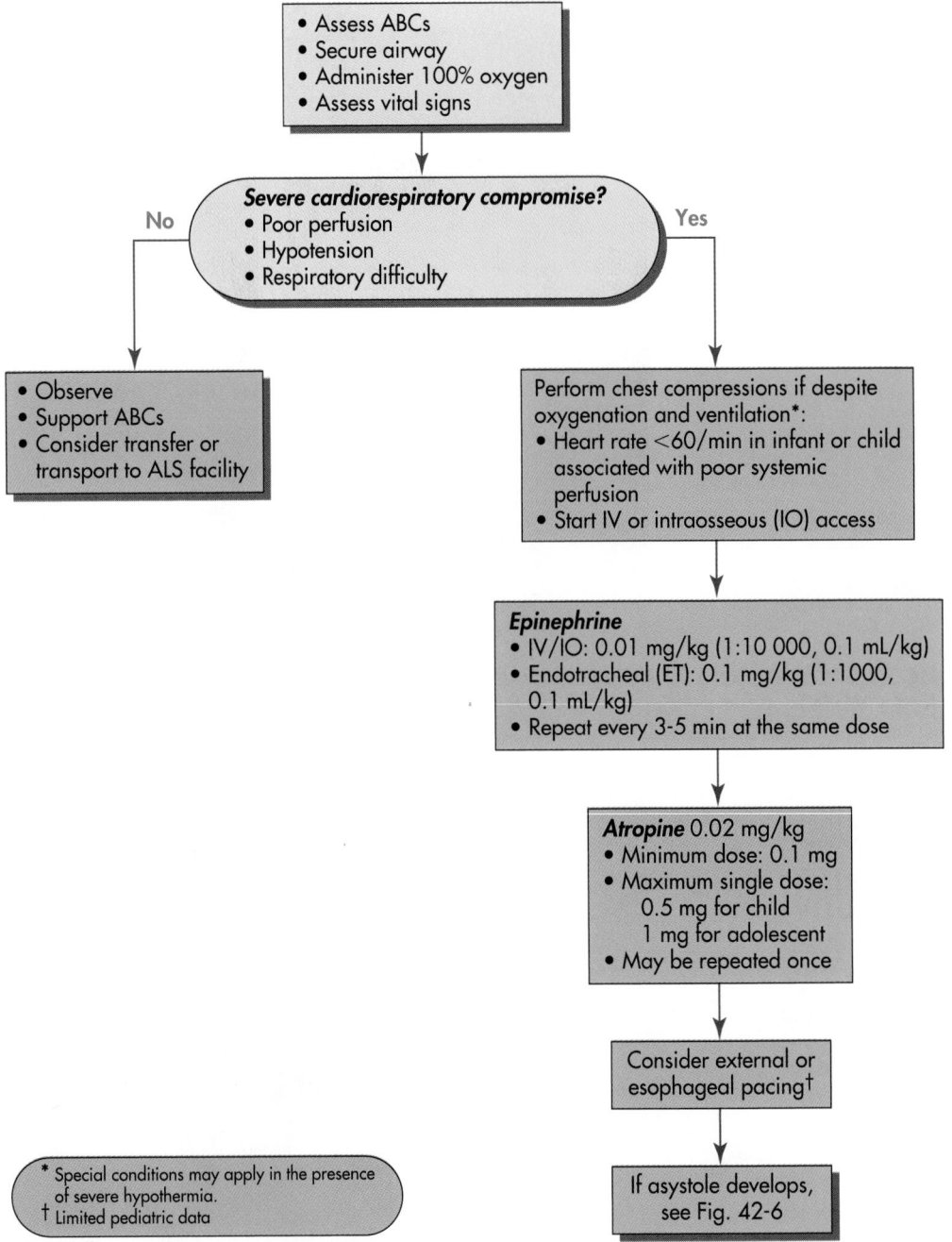

Fig. 42-5 Algorithm for bradycardia in a pediatric patient. (Reproduced with permission. CPR Issue of JAMA, Oct 28, 1992. Copyright © American Medical Association)

Rhythm Disturbances

As discussed in Chapter 41, most children have healthy hearts. When rhythm disturbances occur, they usually are the result of hypoxia, acidosis, hypotension, or structural heart disease.[5] The most common dysrhythmias in pediatric patients are sinus tachycardia, SVT, bradycardia, and asystole. Ventricular tachycardia and ventricular fibrillation are not common but do occur.[2] The recommended management for these dysrhythmias is outlined in Figures 42-5 to 42-8. The various drugs and preparations that may be administered and specific guidelines for use of airway equipment during pediatric life support are listed in Tables 42-8 and 42-9.

Dysrhythmias and basic and advanced life support procedures (including CPR) are addressed in

Text continued on p. 1253

Pulseless Arrest Algorithm

Basic Life Support   **Perform Primary ABCD Survey**

(Correct critical problems IMMEDIATELY as they are identified)
- Assess responsiveness
- Call for help/call for defibrillator

Airway—open the airway

Breathing—deliver two slow breaths, administer oxygen as soon as it is available

Circulation—perform chest compressions

Ensure availability of monitor/**D**efibrillator—

On arrival of AED/monitor/defibrillator, evaluate cardiac rhythm

If PEA or asystole, continue CPR and administer epinephrine.

If pulseless VT/VF, shock up to three times (2J/kg, 2 to 4 J/kg, 4J/kg, or equivalent biphasic energy).

Reevaluate cardiac rhythm

• If persistent or recurrent pulseless VT/VF, continue CPR and perform secondary ABCD survey	• If PEA or asystole, continue CPR and administer epinephrine	• If return of spontaneous circulation (ROSC): • Assess vital signs • Maintain open airway • Provide ventilation • Administer medications for appropriate for rhythm, blood pressure, and heart rate

Advanced Life Support   **Perform Secondary ABCD Survey**

(ADVANCED) AIRWAY

Reassess effectiveness of initial airway maneuvers and interventions

Perform invasive airway management

BREATHING

Pattern becomes CPR-drug-shock or CPR-drug-shock-shock-shock

Assess ventilation

Confirm ET tube placement (or other airway device) by at least two methods

Provide positive-pressure ventilation / Evaluate effectiveness of ventilations

Secure airway device in place with commercial tube holder (preferred) or tape

CIRCULATION

Establish IV access and administer appropriate medications

DIFFERENTIAL DIAGNOSIS

Search for and treat reversible causes

Epinephrine (Class Indeterminate) 0.01 mg/kg (1:10,000; 0.1 mL/kg) IV/IO every 3 to 5 minutes

ET dose 0-0.1 mg/kg (1:1000; 0.1 mL/kg); higher doses may be required for second and subsequent doses

Defibrillate with 4 J/kg (or equivalent biphasic energy) within 30 to 60 seconds after each medication dose

Consider antiarrhythmics (avoid use of multiple antiarrhythmics because of potential proarrhythmic effects)

Amiodarone (Class IIb) 5 mg/kg bolus IV/IO

Lidocaine (Class Indeterminate) 1 mg/kg bolus IV/IO

Magnesium (Class IIb if hypomagnesemia is present) 25 to 50 mg/kg IV/IO (max 2 g) for torsades de pointes or hypomagnesemia

Fig. 42-6 PALS pulseless arrest algorithm.

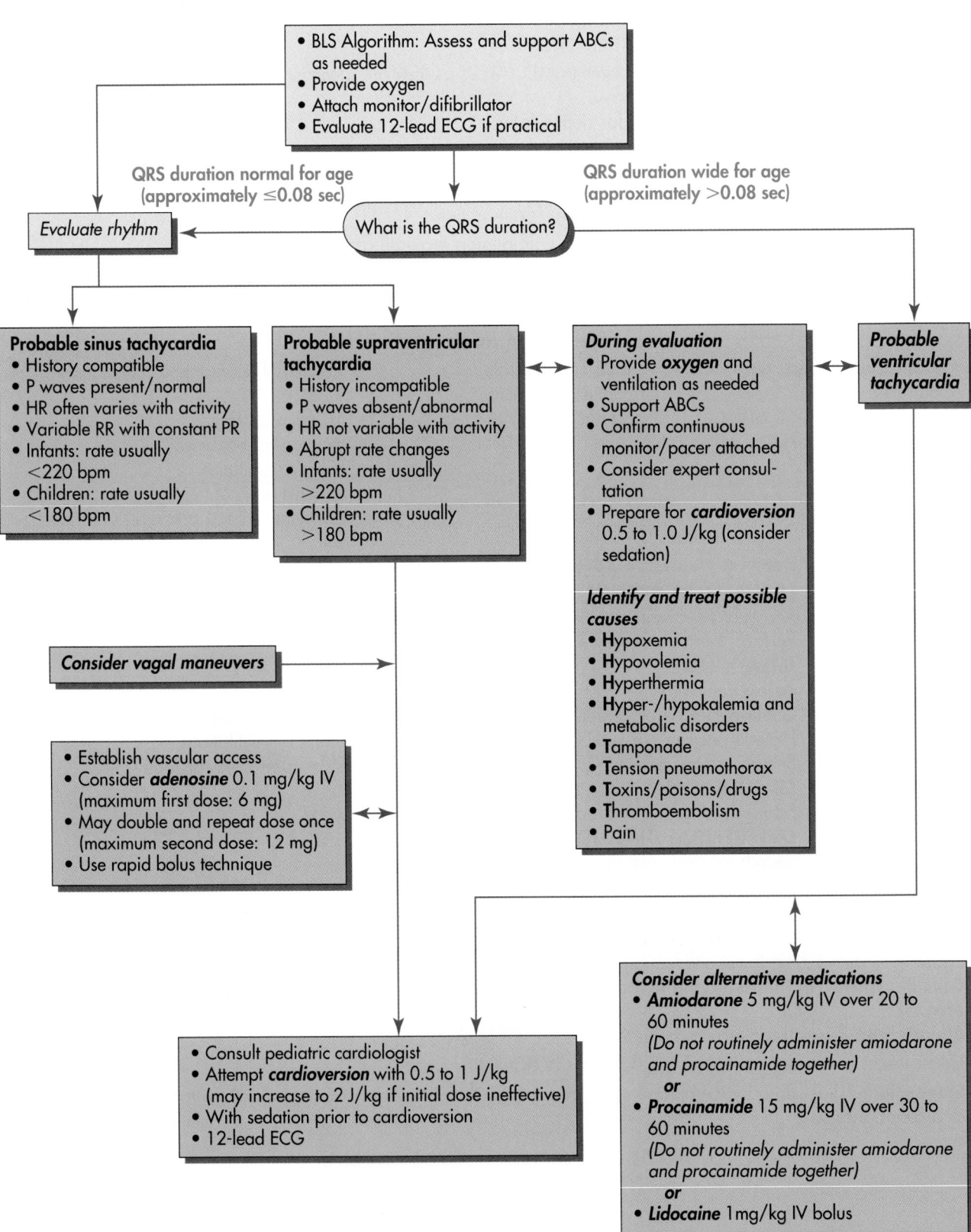

Fig. 42-7 PALS tachycardia algorithm for infants and children with rapid rhythm and adequate perfusion.

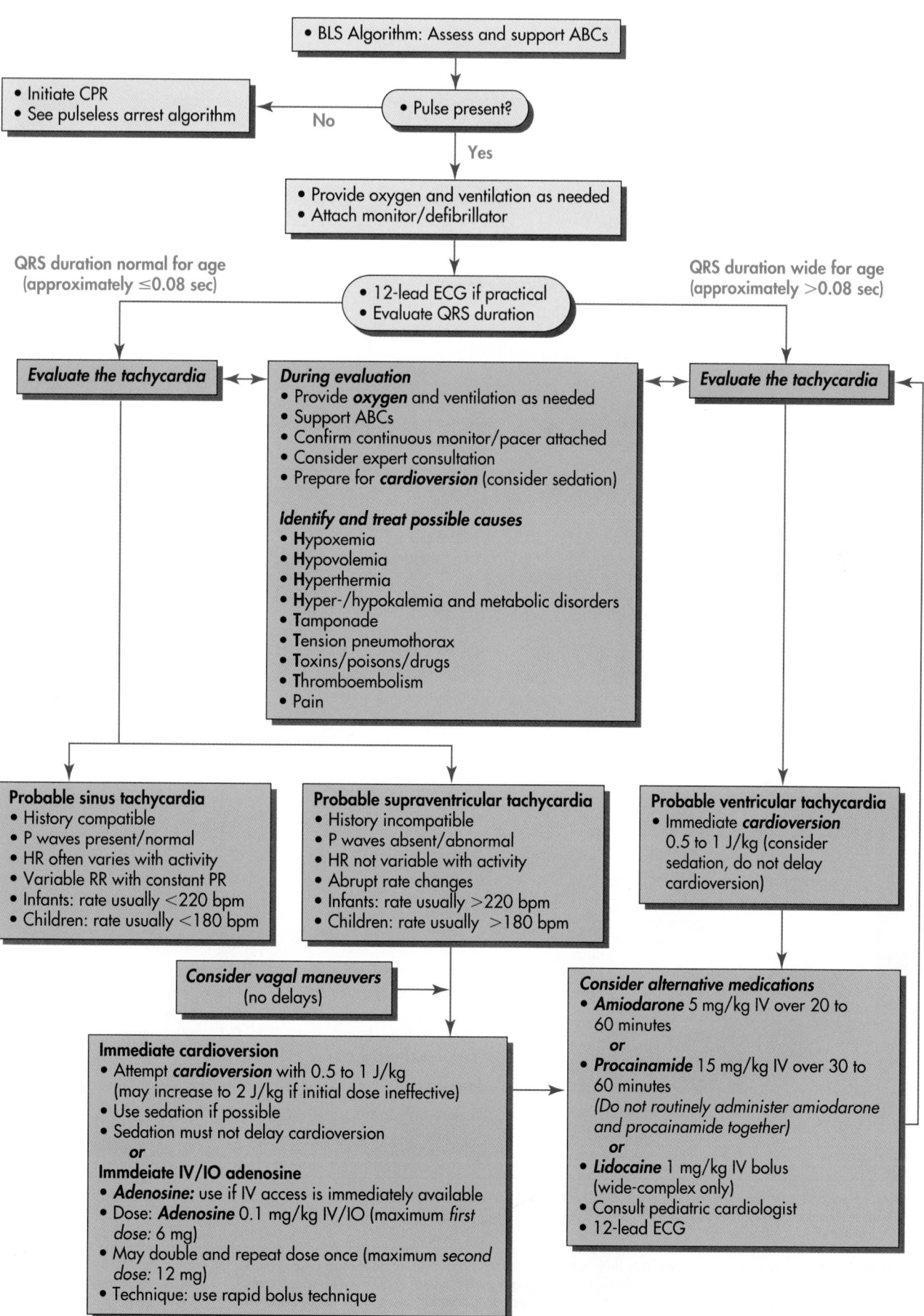

Fig. 42-8 PALS tachycardia algorithm for infants and children with rapid rhythm and evidence of poor perfusion.

TABLE 42-8	PALS MEDICATIONS TO MAINTAIN CARDIAC OUTPUT AND FOR POSTRESUSCITATION STABILIZATION		
MEDICATION	**DOSE RANGE**	**COMMENT**	**PREPARATION***
Amrinone	IV/IO loading dose: 0.75–1 mg/kg IV over 5 minutes; may repeat 2 times IV/IO infusion: 5–10 μg/kg per minute	Inodilator	6 × body weight (in kg) = No. of mg diluted to total 100 mL; then 1 mL/h delivers 1 μg/kg per minute
Dobutamine	IV/IO infusion: 2–20 μg/kg per minute	Inotrope; vasodilator	6 × body weight (in kg) = No. of mg diluted to total 100 mL; then 1 mL/h delivers 1 μg/kg per minute
Dopamine	IV/IO infusion: 2–20 μg/kg per minute	Inotrope; chronotrope; renal and splanchnic vasodilator in lower doses; pressor in higher doses	6 × body weight (in kg) = No. of mg diluted to total 100 mL; then 1 mL/h delivers 1 μg/kg per minute
Epinephrine	IV/IO infusion: 0.1–1 μg/kg per minute	Inotrope; chronotrope; vasodilator in lower doses and pressor in higher doses	0.6 × body weight (in kg) = No. of mg diluted to total 100 mL; then 1 mL/h delivers 0.1 μg/kg per minute
Lidocaine	IV/IO loading dose: 1 mg/kg IV/IO infusion: 20–50 μg/kg per minute	Antidysrhythmic, mild negative inotrope. Use lower infusion rate if poor cardiac output or poor hepatic function.	60 × body weight (in kg) = No. of mg diluted to total 100 mL; then 1 mL/h delivers 10 μg/kg per minute *or* **alternative premix** 120 mg/100 mL at 1 to 2.5 mL/kg per hour
Milrinone	IV/IO loading dose: 50–75 μg/kg IV/IO infusion: 0.5–0.75 μg/kg per minute	Inodilator	0.6 × body weight (in kg) = No. of mg diluted to total 100 mL; then 1 mL/h delivers 0.1 μg/kg per minute
Norepinephrine	IV/IO infusion: 0.1–2 μg/kg per minute	Vasopressor	0.6 × body weight (in kg) = No. of mg diluted to total 100 mL; then 1 mL/h delivers 0.1 μg/kg per minute
Prostaglandin E_1	IV/IO infusion: 0.05–0.1 μg/kg per minute	Maintains patency of ductus arteriosus in cyanotic congenital heart disease. Monitor for apnea, hypotension, and hypoglycemia.	0.3 × body weight (in kg) = No. of mg diluted to total 50 mL; then 1 mL/h delivers 0.1 μg/kg per minute
Sodium nitroprusside	IV/IO infusion: 1–8 μg/kg per minute	Vasodilator Prepare only in dextrose in water	6 × body weight (in kg) = No. of mg diluted to total 100 mL; then 1 mL/h delivers 1 μg/kg per minute

From American Heart Association: Guidelines 2000 for cardiopulmonary rersuscitation and emergency cardiovascular care, International Consensus on Science, *Circulation* 102(8):328, 2000.
IV, Intravenous; *IO,* intraosseous.
*Most infusions may be calculated on the basis of the "Rule of 6" as illustrated in the table. Alternatively, a standard concentration may be used to provide more dilute or more concentrated drug solution, but then an individual dose must be calculated for each patient and each infusion rate as follows: Infusion rate (mL/h) = (weight [kg] × dose [μg/kg per minute] × 60 min/h)/concentration (μg/mL). Diluent may be 5% dextrose in water, 5% dextrose in half-normal saline, normal saline, or lactate Ringer's unless noted otherwise.

TABLE 42-9	PEDIATRIC TRACHEAL TUBE AND SUCTION CATHETER SIZES*	
APPROXIMATE AGE/SIZE (WEIGHT)	**INTERNAL DIAMETER OF TRACHEAL TUBE, mm**	**SUCTION CATHETER SIZE, F**
Premature infant (<1 kg)	2.5	5
Premature infant (1–2 kg)	3.0	5 or 6
Premature infant (2–3 kg)	3.0 to 3.5	6 or 8
0 month to 1 year/infant (3–10 kg)	3.5 to 4.0	8
1 year/small child (10–13 kg)	4.0	8
3 years/child (14–16 kg)	4.5	8 or 10
5 years/child (16–20 kg)	5.0	10
6 years/child (18–25 kg)	5.5	10
8 years/child to small adult (24–32 kg)	6.0 cuffed	10 or 12
12 years/adolescent (32–54 kg)	6.5 cuffed	12
16 years/adult (50+ kg)	7.0 cuffed	12
Adult female	7.0 cuffed	12 or 14
Adult male	7.0–8.0 cuffed	14

From American Heart Association: Guidelines 2000 for cardiopulmonary rersuscitation and emergency cardiovascular care, International Consensus on Science, *Circulation* 102(8):328, 2000.
*These are approximations and should be adjusted on the basis of clinical experience. Tracheal tube selection for a child should be based on the child's size or age. One size larger and one size smaller should be allowed for individual variation. Color-coding based on length or size of the child may facilitate approximation of correct tracheal tube size.

Chapter 28; the reader should refer to that chapter for review. The following discussions outline the unique aspects of abnormal rhythms in children.[5]

Bradydysrhythmias

Bradydysrhythmias may be caused by hypoxemia, acidosis, hypotension, hypoglycemia, CNS injury, or excessive vagal stimulation (e.g., from ET intubation). In infants and children, sinus bradycardia, sinus node arrest with slow junctional or idioventricular rhythm, and AV block are the most common preterminal rhythms. The paramedic should consider drug-induced causes (e.g., digitalis toxicity) and myocarditis with bradycardia due to heart block. Infants and children with a history of heart surgery may have injury at the AV node or conduction system, producing sick sinus syndrome or heart block. All hemodynamically significant bradycardias require treatment. Important ECG findings include:

- Heart rate that is less than 60 bpm
- P waves may or may not be visible
- QRS duration may be normal or prolonged
- The P wave and QRS complex often are unrelated

NOTE

Clinically significant bradycardia is defined as a heart rate less than 60 bpm (or a rapidly dropping heart rate) despite adequate oxygenation and ventilation associated with poor systemic perfusion.

Treatment (see Fig. 42-5)

The initial management of bradycardia is aimed at ensuring adequate breathing with supplemental oxygen. If drug therapy is required, *epinephrine* (Adrenalin) is the drug of choice for hemodynamically significant bradycardia. Bradycardia caused by heart block or increased vagal tone should be managed with *atropine.* In cases where bradycardia is caused by dysfunction in the sinus node, external cardiac pacing may be lifesaving.

NOTE

External cardiac pacing is very uncomfortable. Its use in children is reserved for profound symptomatic bradycardia refractory to ALS and BLS.

Pulseless Electrical Activity (PEA)

PEA often represents a preterminal condition that immediately precedes asystole and usually is caused from prolonged periods of hypoxia, ischemia, or hypercarbia. Reversible causes of PEA include the *4 Hs* (hypovolemia, hypoxemia, hypothermia, and hyperkalemia) and the *4 Ts* (tension pneumothorax, pericardial tamponade, toxins, and thromboembolus), described in Chapter 28. Important ECG findings include:

- A slow, wide-complex rhythm
- The presence of some electrical activity (other than VT/VF) and the absence of a detectable pulse

Treatment (see Fig. 42-6)

PEA is managed in the same manner as asystole with drug therapy (*epinephrine* [Adrenalin]) and CPR. Reversible causes of the condition (the *4 Hs* and *4 Ts*) should be considered and corrected if possible. Early recognition and treatment of PEA that results in a return of spontaneous circulation before arrival in the emergency department is associated with improved survival.

> **NOTE**
>
> Defibrillation is not effective in the treatment of asystolic arrest.[5]

Supraventricular Tachycardia (SVT)

SVT is the most common nonarrest dysrhythmia during childhood and is the most common dysrhythmia that produces cardiovascular instability during infancy.[5] Factors that can help distinguish SVT from sinus tachycardia due to shock include patient history (e.g., dehydration or hemorrhage associated with shock) and heart rate. (Sinus tachycardia is usually <220 bpm in infants and <180 bpm in children, and greater than those rates with SVT.) Important ECG findings in SVT include:

- Heart rate is >220 bpm infants and >180 bpm in children
- The rhythm usually is regular because associated atrioventricular (AV) block is rare
- P waves may not be identifiable, especially when the ventricular rate is high. If present, P waves usually are negative in leads II, III, and aVF.

- QRS duration is normal in most children. SVT with aberrant conduction (wide-complex SVT) may be difficult to distinguish from VT (but this form of VT is rare in infants and children).

Treatment (see Figs. 42-7 and 42-8)

Signs and symptoms during SVT are affected by the child's age, duration of SVT, prior ventricular function, and ventricular rate. If the child is hemodynamically stable and cooperative, vagal maneuvers such as ice water being applied to the child's face, blowing through a straw, and carotid sinus massage may be successful in terminating the rhythm. Unstable SVT is best managed with synchronized cardioversion or drug therapy (*adenosine* [Adenocard] is the drug of choice).

Wide-complex tachycardias associated with hemodynamic instability (evidenced by signs of compromised tissue perfusion and impaired level of consciousness) require immediate care and should be treated as if they are VT. Urgent treatment includes synchronized cardioversion if pulses are present, and defibrillation if pulses are absent.

Ventricular Tachycardia (VT) and Ventricular Fibrillation (VF)

As previously stated, VT and VF are uncommon in children. If present, the paramedic should consider causes of these dysrhythmias that include congenital heart disease, cardiomyopathies, myocarditis, reversible causes (e.g., drug toxicity), metabolic causes (e.g., hypoglycemia), or hypothermia. Important ECG findings include:

<u>VT</u>

- Ventricular rate at least 120 bpm and regular
- Wide QRS complex
- P waves that often are not identifiable

<u>VF</u>

- No identifiable P, QRS, or T wave
- VF waves may be coarse or fine

> **NOTE**
>
> Data suggest that AEDs can accurately detect VF in children of all ages but may not correctly identify tachycardic rhythms in infants. Therefore, AEDs should be considered for rhythm identification purposes only in children 8 years or older, but they are not recommended for younger children or infants.[5]

Treatment (see Figs. 42-6 through 42-8)

Hemodynamically stable VT should be managed cautiously and under the advice of medical direction. Initial efforts are directed at determining the origin of the tachycardia and obtaining a thorough history. Drug therapy generally is delayed in the stable patient until arrival in the emergency department where *amiodarone* (Cordarone), *procainamide* (Pronestyl) or *lidocaine* (Xylocaine) may be considered. VT that is associated with a palpable pulse and signs of shock (low cardiac output, poor perfusion) require immediate synchronized cardioversion. Pulseless VT and VF are managed with immediate defibrillation, CPR, intubation with ventilatory support, and drug therapy (e.g., *epinephrine* [Adrenalin] and *vasopressin* [Pitressin], *amiodarone* [Cordarone], *lidocaine*, [Xylocaine], and *procainamide* [Pronestyl]). See the box in the right column.

? CRITICAL THINKING

Are you comfortable using the pediatric paddles on the defibrillators you will be using in clinicals and on the ambulance?

NOTE

Infant paddles (4.5 cm) generally should be used during defibrillation for infants up to about 1 year of age or 10 kg. Adult paddles (8 to 13 cm) generally should be used for patients older than 1 year of age or more than 10 kg.[6]

Postresuscitation Stabilization

The postresuscitation phase begins after initial stabilization of the patient with shock or respiratory failure or after return of spontaneous circulation in a patient who was in cardiac arrest. The goals of postresuscitation stabilization are to[5]:

- Preserve brain function
- Avoid secondary organ injury
- Seek and correct causes of illness
- Enable the patient to arrive at an appropriate care facility in the best possible physiological state

Postresuscitation stabilization continues assessment and support of the ABCs and focuses on preservation of neurological function and the avoidance of multisystem organ failure (Table 42-10). It requires knowledge and experience in the evaluation of all organ systems and includes stabilizing the

---

TERMINATING RESUSCITATIVE EFFORTS

Most children who experience a cardiac arrest will not survive—even with a transient return of spontaneous circulation. In the absence of recurring or refractory VF or VT, history of toxic drug exposure, or a primary hypothermic insult, medical direction may advise that resuscitative efforts be discontinued if there is no return of spontaneous circulation despite 30 minutes of ALS interventions.[5] When family members are present during resuscitation, one person should be assigned to the family to answer questions and provide comfort measures.

---

airway and supporting oxygenation, ventilation, and perfusion; performing a thorough secondary assessment; and obtaining a medical history.

Seizure

A seizure (described in Chapters 29 and Chapter 41) is an episode of sudden abnormal electrical activity in the brain that results in abnormalities in motor, sensory, or autonomic function usually associated with abnormal behavior, alterations in level of consciousness, or both. Common causes of seizure in adults and children include noncompliance with a drug regimen for the treatment of epilepsy, head trauma, intracranial infection, metabolic disturbance, or poisoning. The most common cause of new onset of seizure in children is fever.

Febrile Seizures

A febrile seizure is a seizure associated with fever but without evidence of intracranial infection or other definable cause; such seizures usually occur between the ages of 6 months and 5 years. About 2% to 5% of children under 7 years of age experience a febrile seizure, and about 30% of those who have one experience a recurrence. More than half of febrile seizures occur in children age 9 to 20 months. In 60% of cases, a family history of febrile seizures is a factor.[4]

Febrile seizures usually are associated with an underlying viral infection (most often of the upper respiratory tract), gastroenteritis, roseola, otitis media, or another febrile illness. The seizures generally occur in vulnerable patients during a rapid rise in body temperature, but the intensity of the seizure is not related to the severity of the fever.

TABLE 42-10	SUMMARY OF POSTRESUSCITATION CARE
	INTERVENTION
Airway	Tracheal intubation with confirmation of tube position and repeat confirmation on movement/transport Secure tube before transport Gastric decompression
Breathing	100% inspired oxygen Provide mechanical ventilation targeting normal ventilation goals (PCO_2 35 to 40 mm Hg) Monitor continuous pulse oximetry and exhaled CO_2 (or capnography) if available
Circulation	Ensure adequate intravascular volume (volume titration) Optimize myocardial function and systemic perfusion (inotropes, vasopressors, vasodilators) Monitor capillary refill, blood pressure, continuous ECG, urine output; measure arterial blood gas and lactate to assess degree of acidosis, if available Ideally maintain two routes of functional vascular access
Disability	Perform rapid secondary survey including brief neurological assessment Avoid hyperglycemia, treat hypoglycemia (monitor glucose) If seizures are observed, medicate with anticonvulsant agents Obtain laboratory studies (if available): arterial blood gases, glucose, electrolytes, hematocrit, chest radiograph
Exposure	Avoid and correct hyperthermia (monitor temperature) Avoid profound hypothermia <33°C

From American Heart Association: Guidelines 2000 for cardiopulmonary rersuscitation and emergency cardiovascular care, International Consensus on Science, *Circulation* 102(8):328, 2000.
Be sure to communicate interventions and status of the patient to family and to transport and receiving providers.

Febrile seizures may manifest with generalized tonic-clonic activity, or they may have a more subtle presentation. As a rule, classic febrile seizures are of short duration (usually lasting less than 5 minutes) and have an uncomplicated and short postictal period. Seizures that last longer than 20 minutes require extensive investigation and should never be considered benign. Regardless of the suspected etiology, all children who have suffered a seizure should be transported for evaluation by a physician per protocol.

Assessment and management. In most cases the seizure has stopped before EMS arrival, and in many instances the child is in a postictal state. As in any emergency, the first priorities are airway management and ventilatory and circulatory support. This includes airway positioning, suctioning of the airway, and administration of oxygen. Repeated assessment of the adequacy of ventilation is necessary, with special emphasis on respiratory rate and depth. If the airway cannot be maintained with manual maneuvers, airway adjuncts should be used.

After initial stabilization of the patient's condition, vital signs should be assessed and a history should be obtained. Important elements of the history include the following:

- Previous seizures
- Number of seizures in this episode
- Description of seizure activity
- Presence of vomiting during the seizure (aspiration risk)
- Condition of the child when first found
- Recent illness
- Potential for toxic ingestion
- Potential head injury (as primary etiology or secondary complication)
- Significant medical problems
- Recent headache or stiff neck (which may suggest meningitis)
- Medication use and compliance with anticonvulsant medication

During transport to the emergency department, the child should be continuously monitored and the paramedic should be alert for recurrent seizures. Medical direction may recommend that a febrile patient be given an antipyretic if alert to reduce the fever en route to the receiving hospital.

Status Epilepticus

Status epilepticus (continuous seizure activity lasting 30 minutes or longer or a recurrent seizure without an intervening period of consciousness) is a true emergency that can lead to hypotension and cardiovascular, respiratory, and renal failure, in addition to permanent brain damage. Children in status epilepticus should be managed with the following initial interventions:

1. Provide adequate airway, ventilatory, and circulatory support. Intubation for airway protection or mechanical ventilation seldom is necessary and should be withheld unless the child fails to respond to initial management.
2. Per protocol, obtain vascular access through an IV or IO route and measure the blood glucose level to screen for hypoglycemia. If the value is below 60 mg/dL (40 mg/dL in an infant[4]), administer *dextrose* 10%, 25%, or 50% (per medical direction). If seizures do not stop, consult medical direction regarding IV, IO, or rectal administration of the anticonvulsants *diazepam* (Valium) or *lorazepam* (Ativan).
3. Attach a cardiac monitor and observe for rhythm or conduction abnormalities that may suggest hypoxia.

> **NOTE**
>
> Hypoglycemia also can be treated with an intramuscular (IM) injection of **glucagon** if IV or IO access cannot be established.

Diazepam. *Diazepam* (Valium) breaks active seizures in 75% to 90% of cases.[7] The drug has a short duration of action (15 minutes) and may require repeat administration to a maximum of three doses. In addition, the paramedic should be prepared for unpredictable sudden respiratory depression or hypotension associated with use of this drug. If IV or IO access cannot be obtained, *diazepam* (Valium) may be administered rectally (Box 42-5).

BOX 42-5

PROCEDURE FOR ADMINISTRATION OF RECTAL DIAZEPAM

1. Carefully restrain the child. If possible, place the child in a knee-chest or decubitus position with the legs flexed at the hip and knee.
2. Draw the calculated diazepam dose into a syringe. A higher dose of 0.5 mg/kg is required because absorption is incomplete.
3. Introduce a lubricated 1-mL syringe just beyond the external sphincter (aimed just above the junction of the skin and mucous membranes and directed toward the rectal wall).
4. Inject the solution into the rectum and clear the syringe with 1 mL of normal saline.
5. Facilitate drug retention by squeezing the buttocks together with manual pressure.
6. Transport the patient for evaluation by a physician. Remove excessive clothing and cool the patient with tepid water if the child is febrile. En route, continually monitor the patient for recurrent seizures and the need for airway, ventilatory, and circulatory support.

Lorazepam. An alternative to IV or IO administration of *diazepam* (Valium) is *lorazepam* (Ativan), which some physicians prefer over *diazepam* (Valium). *Lorazepam* (Ativan) may be injected intramuscularly or given intravenously, intraosseously, or rectally. Side effects resemble those of *diazepam* (Valium) in terms of cardiorespiratory and central nervous system (CNS) depression. The paramedic should be alert for these complications.

Hypoglycemia and Hyperglycemia

Hypoglycemia and hyperglycemia (discussed in Chapter 30) should be suspected whenever a child shows an altered level of consciousness that has no explainable cause. Signs and symptoms of hypoglycemia can be classified as *mild, moderate,* and

> **NOTE**
>
> Severe hypoglycemia is a medical emergency that requires prompt treatment with **dextrose** to prevent brain damage.

BOX 42-6

SIGNS AND SYMPTOMS OF HYPOGLYCEMIA AND HYPERGLYCEMIA

Hypoglycemia

Mild

Hunger, weakness, tachypnea, tachycardia

Moderate

Sweating, tremors, irritability, vomiting, mood swings, blurred vision, stomachache, headache, dizziness

Severe

Decreased level of consciousness, seizure

Hyperglycemia

Early

Increased thirst, increased hunger, increased urination, weight loss

Late (dehydration/early ketoacidosis)

Weakness, abdominal pain, generalized aches, loss of appetite, nausea, vomiting, signs of dehydration (except urinary output), fruity breath odor, tachypnea, hyperventilation, tachycardia; Kussmaul respirations and coma (if untreated)

BOX 42-7

SIGNS AND SYMPTOMS OF INFECTION IN PEDIATRIC PATIENTS

Fever
Hypothermia (neonates)
Chills
Tachycardia
Cough
Sore throat
Nasal congestion
Malaise
Tachypnea
Cool or clammy skin
Respiratory distress
Poor feeding
Vomiting or diarrhea (or both)
Dehydration
Hypoperfusion
Seizure
Severe headache
Irritability
Lethargy
Stiff neck
Bulging fontanelle (infants)

---

severe; they are designated as *early* and *late* for hyperglycemia (Box 42-6).

Prehospital care is directed first at ensuring adequate airway, ventilatory, and circulatory support. In any child with an altered level of consciousness that has no explainable cause, a blood glucose measurement should be obtained. Conscious children who are mildly hypoglycemic should receive an oral glucose solution or paste; unconscious children or those with moderate or severe hypoglycemia require IV/IO dextrose or IM *glucagon,* followed by a repeat blood glucose measurement in 10 to 15 minutes. Children who are hyperglycemic may require IV fluid therapy if signs of dehydration are present, in addition to in-hospital administration of *insulin.* Any child with hypoglycemia or hyperglycemia should be transported for evaluation by a physician.

NOTE

About 10 in 100,000 children develop type I diabetes; 1 in 200 children die at onset of the disease.[8]

? CRITICAL THINKING

Why do you think type I diabetes may go undetected until a child is seriously ill?

Infection

Children with infection may have a variety of signs and symptoms, depending on the source and extent of infection and the length of time since the patient was exposed (Box 42-7). Often the parent or caregiver provides a history of recent illness (e.g., fever, upper respiratory tract infection, otitis media) (Fig. 42-9).

NOTE

When caring for any patient who may have an infectious disease, BSI must be strictly adhered to because of the unknown etiology of the infection.

Most children with infection need only supportive care while being transported for evaluation by a physician. In severe cases the patient may require airway, ventilatory, and circulatory support. If signs of decompensated shock are present, IV therapy may be warranted (per medical direction). Active seizure activity may require the administration of anticonvulsant agents. When possible, children in stable condition should be transported in their position of comfort in the company of the parent or caregiver.

Poisoning and Toxic Exposure

As discussed in Chapter 34, most poisoning events in the United States involve children. Common sources of poisoning (accidental and intentional) include the following[2]:

- Alcohol
- Barbiturates
- Sedatives
- Anticholinergics
- Acetaminophen
- *Aspirin*
- Corrosives
- Digitalis, beta blocker agents
- Hydrocarbons
- Narcotics
- Organic solvents (inhaled)
- Organophosphates

> **NOTE**
> Poisoning is the major cause of preventable death in children under 5 years of age.[9]

Signs and symptoms of an accidental poisoning vary, depending on the toxic substance and the length of time since the child was exposed. These signs and symptoms may include cardiac and respiratory depression, CNS stimulation or depression, GI irritation, and behavioral changes. Emergency care should first be directed at ensuring adequate airway, ventilatory, and circulatory support (see the box on p. 1260). Medical direction and the poison control center should be contacted to obtain directions for specific treatments. All pills, substances, and contain-

> **? CRITICAL THINKING**
> *For what critical signs or symptoms of poisoning should you be alert?*

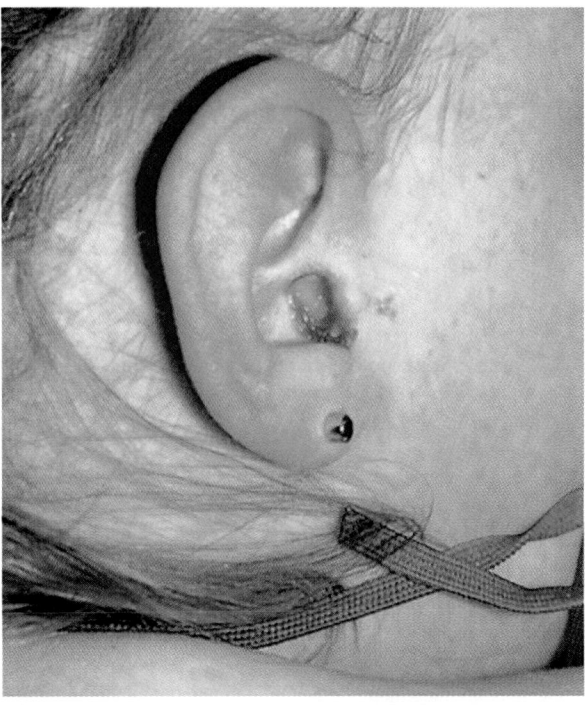

Fig. 42-9 Otitis media. (From Beattie T: *Pediatric emergencies,* London, 1997, Mosby-Wolfe.)

ers associated with the poisoning event should be transported with the child to the receiving hospital.

Pediatric Trauma

Blunt and penetrating trauma is a predominant cause of injury and death in children.[9] The following facts and figures about common trauma events emphasize the importance of injury prevention programs[2]:

1. Falls
   - Single most common cause of injury in children
   - Serious injury or death resulting from truly accidental falls is relatively uncommon unless from a significant height

> **? CRITICAL THINKING**
> *Why are children at risk for injuries related to falls?*

2. Motor vehicle crashes
   - Leading cause of permanent brain injury
   - Leading cause of death and serious injury in children

The most important agents associated with cardiac arrest or requiring advanced life support in children are cocaine, narcotics, TCAs, calcium-channel blockers, beta-adrenergic blockers, and opioids.[5] Regardless of the drug, the initial approach in toxicological emergencies is to ensure adequate oxygenation, ventilation, and circulation. Subsequent priorities include reversing the adverse effects of the toxin (if possible), and preventing further absorption of the agent (see Chapter 34). This is an overview of these drugs, their effects, and specific treatment that may be required in the prehospital setting. (NOTE: All drug therapy referenced in this box is based on patient presentation and should be guided by medical direction.)

Cocaine
Effects are complex and are related to route of administration and form of cocaine used

Signs and Symptoms
May include tachycardia, tremor, diaphoresis, mydriasis, mood elevation, movement disorders, hypertension, and acute coronary syndrome (chest pain and dysrhythmias)

Specific Treatment
Oxygen administration and ventilatory support
Continuous ECG monitoring
Benzodiazepines (**diazepam** [Valium] or **lorazepam** [Ativan]) for anticonvulsant and CNS depressant effect
Aspirin and **heparin** to reverse platelet activating effects of cocaine
Nitroglycerin to reduce coronary vasoconstriction
Sodium bicarbonate and **lidocaine** (Xylocaine) for ventricular dysrhythmias and cocaine-induced myocardial infarction
Epinephrine (Adrenalin) to increase coronary perfusion pressure during CPR

TCAs (and other sodium-channel blocking agents)
Effects result from inhibition of fast sodium channels in the brain and myocardium

Signs and Symptoms
May include cardiac rhythm disturbances, including preterminal sinus bradycardia and heart block with junctional or ventricular wide-complex escape beats

Specific Treatment
Oxygen administration and ventilatory support
Continuous ECG monitoring
Sodium bicarbonate and **lidocaine** (Xylocaine) to increase myocardial contractility and to manage ventricular dysrhythmias
Normal saline boluses (10 mL/kg) to manage hypotension
Vasopressors (**norepinephrine** [Levophed] or **dopamine** [Intropin]) to maintain vascular tone and blood pressure

Calcium-Channel Blockers
Effects result from inhibiting the influx of calcium into cells leading to bradydysrhythmias and hypotension

Signs and Symptoms
May include bradycardia, hypotension, and altered mental status (including syncope, seizure, coma) from cerebral hypoperfusion

Specific Treatment
Oxygen administration and ventilatory support
Continuous ECG monitoring
Normal saline boluses (5 to 10 mL/kg) to manage hypotension (avoid pulmonary edema)
Calcium chloride 10% (controversial) to overcome channel blockade
High-dose vasopressor therapy with **norepinehrine** (Levophed) or **epinephrine** (Adrenalin) to treat bradycardia and hypotension
Insulin-glucose therapy to maintain serum glucose concentration (avoid hypoglycemia)

Beta-Adrenergic Blockers
Effects result from competition at B-adrenergic receptors resulting in bradycardia and decreased cardiac contractility

Signs and Symptoms
May include hypotension with bradycardia, varying degrees of heart block, and altered mental status (including seizures and coma)

Specific Treatment
Oxygen administration and ventilatory support
Continuous ECG monitoring
Treat for shock
Epinephrine (Adrenalin) infusions and **glucagon** may be effective in managing B-adrenergic blockade and overdose
Insulin-glucose therapy to maintain serum glucose concentration (avoid hypoglycemia)
Sodium bicarbonate to manage intraventricular conduction delay
Calcium chloride to improve heart rate if **glucagon** and catecholamine are not effective (controversial)

Opioids
Effects produce CNS depression

Signs and Symptoms
May include altered level of consciousness, hypoventilation, apnea, and respiratory failure

Specific Treatment
Oxygen administration and ventilatory support
Continuous ECG monitoring
Naloxone (Narcan) to reverse narcotic toxicity (normalize partial pressure of P_{CO_2} with ventilations before administration)

3. Pedestrian-vehicle collisions
   - Particularly lethal form of trauma in children
   - Initial injury caused by impact with vehicle (extremity or trunk)
   - Child is thrown from force of impact, causing additional injury (head, spine) upon impact with other objects (e.g., ground, another vehicle, light standard)
4. Drowning/submersion
   - Third leading cause of injury or death in children between birth and 4 years of age
   - Causes about 2000 deaths annually
   - Severe, permanent brain damage occurs in 5% to 20% of hospitalized children for submersion
5. Penetrating injuries
   - A significant problem in adolescence
   - Higher incidence in inner city (mostly intentional), but significant incidence in other areas (mostly unintentional)
   - Risk of death from firearm injuries increases with age
   - Stab wounds and firearm injuries account for about 10% to 15% of all pediatric trauma admissions
   - Visual inspection of external injuries cannot determine the extent of internal involvement
6. Burns
   - Leading cause of accidental death in the home for children under 14 years of age
   - Burn survival is a function of burn size, inhalation injury, and concomitant injuries
   - Modified "rule of nines" is used to determine percentage of surface area involved

? CRITICAL THINKING

What types of situations cause burn injuries to children in the home?

7. Physical abuse
   - Includes physical abuse, sexual abuse, emotional abuse, and child neglect
   - Social phenomena such as increased poverty, domestic disturbances, younger-aged parents, substance abuse, and community violence have been attributed to increase of abuse; however, abuse occurs in all social strata
   - Document all pertinent findings, treatments, and interventions (for legal purposes)

NOTE

The reader should refer to Appendix C for injury prevention strategies.

Special Considerations for Specific Injuries

Special considerations for managing pediatric injury were addressed in the chapters of Division Four. The specific injuries reviewed here include traumatic brain injury, head and neck injury, chest injury, abdominal injury, extremity injury, and burns.

? CRITICAL THINKING

What are some early signs of increasing intracranial pressure (ICP) in a child?

NOTE

Drugs that may be used to manage some forms of pain and to alter the emotional response in pediatric patients include **meperidine** (Demerol), **morphine**, and **ketorolac** ([Toradol] in the absence of hemorrhage).[4] Pain medicine can mask signs and symptoms of illness or injury and should be administered only under medical direction.

Head and Neck Injury

1. Larger relative mass of the head and lack of neck muscle strength provide increased momentum in acceleration-deceleration injuries.
2. Fulcrum of cervical mobility in the younger child is at the C2 to C3 level (60% to 70% of fractures in children occur in C1 or C2).
3. Head injury is the most common cause of death in pediatric trauma victims.
4. Diffuse head injuries are common in children; focal injuries are rare.
5. Soft tissues, skull, and brain are more compliant in children than in adults.
6. Because of open fontanelles and sutures, infants up to 12 months of age may be more tolerant to increased ICP and can have delayed signs.
7. Subdural bleeding in an infant can produce hypotension (extremely rare).
8. Significant blood loss can occur through scalp lacerations, and such bleeding should be controlled immediately.

9. The modified Glasgow Coma Scale (GCS) should be used for assessing infants and young children.

Traumatic Brain Injury

1. Early recognition and aggressive management can reduce mortality and morbidity.
2. May be classified as *mild* (GCS score of 13 to 15), *moderate* (GCS of 9 to 12), or *severe* (GCS of 8 or lower).
3. Signs of increased ICP include elevated blood pressure, bradycardia, irregular respirations progressing to Cheyne-Stokes respirations, and bulging fontanelle in infants.
4. Signs of herniation include asymmetrical pupils and abnormal posturing.
5. Management
   a. Administer high-concentration oxygen for mild to moderate head injury (GCS score of 9 to 15).
   b. Intubate and ventilate at normal breathing rate with 100% oxygen for severe head injury (GCS score of 3 to 8).
   c. Administer *lidocaine* (Xylocaine) per medical direction to blunt rise in ICP (controversial) before intubation.
   d. Hyperventilate only with signs of increased ICP.

Chest Injury

1. Chest injuries in children under 14 years of age usually are the result of blunt trauma.
2. Because of the thoracic compliance of the chest wall, severe intrathoracic injury can be present without signs of external injury.
3. Tension pneumothorax is poorly tolerated and is an immediate threat to life.
4. Flail segment is an uncommon injury in children; when noted without a significant mechanism of injury, child abuse should be suspected.
5. Many children with cardiac tamponade have no physical signs of tamponade other than hypotension.

Abdominal Injury

1. Musculature is minimal and poorly protects the viscera.
2. Organs most commonly injured are the liver, kidneys, and spleen.
3. Onset of symptoms may be rapid or gradual.
4. Because of the small size of the abdomen, palpation should be performed in one quadrant at a time.

5. Any child who is hemodynamically unstable without an obvious source of blood loss should be considered to have an abdominal injury until it is proven otherwise.

Extremity Injury

1. Relatively more common in children than adults.
2. Growth plate injuries are common.
3. Compartment syndrome is an emergency in children.
4. Any sites of active bleeding must be controlled.
5. Splinting should be performed to prevent further injury and blood loss.
6. Pneumatic antishock garment (PASG) may be useful for an unstable pelvic fracture with hypotension (per protocol).

Burns

1. Burns may be thermal, chemical, or electrical.
2. Management priorities
   a. Prompt management of the airway is required because swelling can develop rapidly.
   b. If intubation is indicated, an ET tube one half size smaller than expected may be required.
   c. Suspect musculoskeletal injuries in electrical burn patients and perform spine immobilization.

Trauma Management Considerations for Pediatric Patients

In addition to the general patient care guidelines appropriate for all injured people, injured children require special consideration for airway control, immobilization techniques, and fluid management. The following discussion reviews the highlights of management guidelines presented in the chapters of Division Four.

Airway Control

The airway of an injured child should be maintained in an in-line or neutral position (rather than the sniffing position, which is appropriate for older children and adults). (Padding may need to be placed under the shoulders in some children to maintain a neutral airway position.) High-concentration oxygen should be provided to all patients while the airway is kept patent through jaw-thrust positioning and suction (if needed). Endotracheal intubation (followed by insertion of a gastric tube) should be performed when airway and ventilation remain inadequate. Needle cricothyroidotomy rarely is indicated for traumatic upper airway obstruction.

> **NOTE**
>
> Even though ET intubation is recommended under specific conditions, all paramedics who provide care for infants and children must be able to provide effective oxygenation and ventilation using the bag-mask technique.

> **NOTE**
>
> Tracheal tube placement should be confirmed by monitoring exhaled CO_2, especially in children with a perfusing rhythm.

Immobilization

Spinal immobilization devices must be appropriately sized for infants and children. Equipment that may be used includes the following:

- Rigid cervical collar
- Towel/blanket roll
- Child safety seat
- Pediatric immobilization device
- Vest-type/short spine board
- Long spine board
- Straps, cravats
- Tape
- Padding

The patient should be placed supine and immobilized in a neutral in-line position. This is most effectively achieved by using a backboard with a recess for the head or by using a roll under the back from the shoulders to the buttocks.[5]

Fluid Management

Management of the child's airway and breathing takes priority over management of circulation because circulatory compromise is less common in children than adults. When vascular access is indicated, the paramedic should consider the following:

- Large-bore IV catheters should be inserted into large peripheral veins.
- Transport should not be delayed to obtain vascular access.
- IO access in children can be used if IV access fails.
- An initial fluid bolus of 20 mL/kg of lactated Ringer's solution or normal saline should be given to manage volume depletion.

- Vital signs should be reassessed and the bolus repeated if needed; vital signs that do not improve after a second bolus indicate the need for rapid surgical intervention.

Sudden Infant Death Syndrome

Sudden infant death syndrome (SIDS) is the leading cause of death in American infants under 1 year of age.[7] The syndrome is defined as the sudden death of an apparently healthy infant that remains unexplained by history and a thorough autopsy. SIDS occurs an average of 1.1 times for every 1000 live births and is responsible for more than 7000 deaths in the United States each year.[4] The syndrome cannot be predicted or prevented, although positioning during sleep may be a factor (see the box on the next page).

SIDS occurs during periods of sleep, usually between midnight and 6 AM. The typical age for SIDS is the first year of life, but most SIDS deaths (85%) occur within the first 6 months.[4] The seasonal distribution for SIDS is October through March (during cool weather worldwide). The infant often has a history of minor illness, such as a cold, within 2 weeks before death. Classic signs that usually are present include lividity; frothy, blood-tinged drainage from the nose and mouth; and rigor mortis. With most SIDS cases no external signs of injury are found. Often evidence indicates that the baby was active just before the death (e.g., rumpled bed clothes, unusual position or location in the bed).

Pathophysiology

The cause of SIDS is unknown. Studies have failed to confirm a number of physiological, environmental, genetic, and social factors as causes. The studies have confirmed, however, that SIDS is not caused by external suffocation, regurgitation or aspiration of vomitus, hereditary factors, or allergies. (A small percentage of SIDS deaths are thought to be abuse related.[2]) Various physiological aspects that have been suggested to explain SIDS include immaturity of the central nervous system secondary to a prenatal event, idiopathic apnea, brain stem abnormalities, upper airway obstruction, hyperactive upper airway reflexes, cardiac conduction disorders, abnormal responses to hypoxia and hypercarbia, abnormal responses to hyperthermia, and alterations in fat metabolism. Although no specific cause has

SLEEP POSITIONS AND OTHER FACTORS THAT MAY REDUCE THE RISK OF SUDDEN INFANT DEATH SYNDROME (SIDS)

In 1994 the Association of SIDS and Infant Mortality Programs (ASIP) joined with the U.S. Public Health Service, the American Academy of Pediatrics, the SIDS Alliance, and others to launch a national public health campaign titled *Back to Sleep* to reduce the risk of sudden infant death syndrome. This initiative was based on research reports from Australia, New Zealand, England, Norway, and the United States. The data indicated that placing healthy newborns to sleep on the back or side was a means of reducing the risk of SIDS. In 1996 this recommendation was revised to endorse "back sleeping" as the best position for infants. Since the inception of this campaign, the SIDS rate has declined 30% to 40% in the United States, the greatest decline in the SIDS rate since statistics began to be compiled. Although such a dramatic decline suggests that a change in the sleeping position to back sleeping may reduce the risk of SIDS, it also has demonstrated that sleeping position, in and of itself, is not a cause of SIDS. Other recommendations for reducing the risk include the following:

- Starting medically recommended prenatal care early
- Avoiding drugs, alcohol, and smoking during pregnancy
- Forbidding smoking around the infant
- Breast-feeding when possible
- Avoiding overdressing or overheating the baby
- Maintaining regular well-baby health visits
- Obtaining immunizations on schedule
- Maintaining immunizations
- Placing the baby to sleep on a firm mattress and avoiding the use of beanbag cushions, waterbeds, soft, fluffy blankets, comforters, sheepskins, pillows, stuffed toys, or other soft materials

NOTE: Paramedics can play an important role in prevention by conveying this information to parents, other caregivers, and family members.
From Infant Sleep Positioning and SIDS: Counseling Implications, Association of SIDS and Infant Mortality Programs, www.asip1.org/isp.html.

been identified, several risk factors have been associated with the syndrome, including the following:

- Maternal smoking
- Young maternal age (under age 20)
- Infants of mothers who received poor or no prenatal care
- Social deprivation
- Premature births and low-birth-weight infants
- Infants of mothers who used cocaine, methadone, or heroin during pregnancy

SIDS is confirmed by excluding other causes of death. Autopsy findings that occur in most SIDS deaths include smooth muscle thickening in small pulmonary arteries and right ventricular hypertrophy, both thought to occur secondary to hypoxia and constriction of the pulmonary vasculature. Other findings include brain stem tumors, which may be associated with respiratory center dysfunction, and neuroepithelial bodies in the tracheobronchial tree, along with distal atelectasis. About 80% of SIDS victims also have intrathoracic petechiae, especially on the thymus, pleura, and pericardium.[4]

Management

EMS providers can do little to help the SIDS infant. The primary role of the paramedic is to provide emotional support for parents or other caregivers and loved ones. If the infant is potentially or questionably viable, resuscitation should proceed as for any other infant in cardiac arrest. Even though resuscitation probably will be unsuccessful, it is important for the parents or other caregivers to see that everything possible is being done for their child. The paramedic should follow pediatric resuscitation protocols and obtain medical direction about decisions to initiate or continue resuscitation efforts.

The paramedic should expect a variety of grief reactions from those who witness the event (parents, family members, neighbors, babysitters). These reactions may vary from shock and disbelief to anger, rage, and self-blame. Arrangements should be made for a relative or neighbor to stay with the family or accompany them to the hospital so that they are not left alone. Many areas have SIDS resource services that provide immediate counseling and support for the family of a SIDS infant.

Because of the mysterious nature of SIDS deaths and classic signs such as postmortem lividity and frothy fluid in the infant's nose and mouth, SIDS victims may appear to have been abused or neglected. Regardless of the circumstances, the paramedic should avoid comments or questions that may imply a suspicion of inappropriate child care. Determining the cause of death is not the responsibility of the EMS crew (although careful scene observation is crucial). The paramedic should document all findings objectively, accurately, and completely. Medical direction and other authorities (per protocol) should be advised if inappropriate child care is suspected.

NOTE

The death of an infant has a powerful effect on all involved, and it is common for rescuers to experience a range of emotional reactions after a SIDS death. Some emergency medical services, in conjunction with medical direction and SIDS resource agencies, provide counseling and formal debriefing programs by trained professionals. If these services are not available, the EMS crew should discuss the event openly with others involved in the response (e.g., co-workers, law enforcement officers) to help relieve normal feelings of anxiety and stress.

Child Abuse and Neglect

More than 2.4 million cases of suspected child abuse and neglect are reported each year in the United States,[7] resulting in about 4000 deaths. Paramedics should follow local protocol in reporting suspected abuse and discuss any suspicions of child abuse or neglect with medical direction. Agencies that may be involved in cases of child abuse or neglect include state, regional, and local child protection services and hospital social service departments.

NOTE

Child abuse and neglect is a crime that is reportable under law in all 50 states and the Canadian provinces. In some states there is a legal duty to report child abuse or neglect (mandate reporter). Failure to report these cases may result in criminal prosecution and may be punishable by fine or imprisonment, or both. As a rule, reporting in good faith provides immunity from legal liability as a consequence of reporting, which may be raised as a defense if one is sued for negligent reporting.

Elements of Child Abuse

Child abuse and neglect is the maltreatment of children by their parents, guardians, or other caregivers. Forms of maltreatment include infliction of physical injury ("battered child syndrome," "shaken baby syndrome"), sexual exploitation, and infliction of emotional pain and neglect (medical neglect, safety neglect, and nutritional deprivation). A number of factors are implicated in the potential for child abuse. These include a caregiver with the potential to abuse, a child with particular characteristics that place him or her at risk for abuse, and an element of crisis.

Characteristics of Abusers

Child abuse usually reflects a pattern of maladjusted behavior rather than an isolated act of violence. In many cases the abuser is the child's parent, although other caregivers (e.g., family members, a boyfriend of the child's mother, an unrelated babysitter, a sibling of the abused child) may be responsible. In the case of physical abuse, most abusers tend to be unhappy, angry adults under tremendous stress. They usually are isolated and incapable of using support agencies or an extended family in times of crisis. Often the abusers experienced physical or emotional abuse themselves as children. Abusers come from all ethnic, geographical, religious, educational, occupational, and socioeconomic groups. Other factors characteristic of abusers include impoverishment (low socioeconomic conditions) and alcohol or other drug dependence.

Characteristics of an Abused Child

Abused children often have certain characteristics that increase their risk for abuse. Common traits include demanding and difficult behavior, decreased level of functioning (e.g., a handicapped child or preterm infant requiring extra parenting), hyperactivity, and precociousness with intellectual ability equal to or superior to the parent. Often the parent sees the abused child as "special" or "different" from other siblings. Other factors that tend to increase the potential for child abuse are age (the child is usually under 5 years old), gender (boys are involved more often than girls), and illegitimacy.

Crises That May Precipitate Abuse

Physical abuse or neglect can occur constantly during a child's life. More often, however, it is intermittent and unpredictable. The abuse frequently is precipitated by stressors in the adult caregiver's life, particularly when the caregiver expects the child to fill emotional needs created by the stress. Failure of the child to respond in an ideal way to the caregiver's needs may lead to an abusive episode. Common crises associated with an episode of child abuse include the following:

- Financial stress
- Loss of employment
- Eviction from housing
- Marital or relationship stress
- Physical illness in a child that leads to intractable crying
- Death of a family member
- Diagnosis of an unwanted pregnancy
- Birth of a sibling

History of Injuries Suspicious for Abuse

Physical abuse or neglect often is difficult to determine. The ultimate diagnosis usually begins with suspicions based on unexplained injuries, discrepant history, delays in seeking medical care, and repeated episodes of suspicious injuries. If at any time an injured child indicates that a particular adult caused him or her physical harm, the paramedic should take this report seriously, advise medical direction, and contact the appropriate authorities. In many cases these accusations are true. The following are 15 indicators of possible abuse[10]:

1. Any obvious or suspected fractures in a child under 2 years of age
2. Injuries in various stages of healing, especially burns and bruises
3. More injuries than are usually seen in other children of the same age
4. Injuries scattered on many areas of the body
5. Bruises or burns in patterns that suggest intentional infliction
6. Suspected increased intracranial pressure in an infant
7. Suspected intraabdominal trauma in a young child
8. Any injury that does not fit the description of the cause

9. An accusation that the child injured himself or herself intentionally
10. Long-standing skin infections
11. Extreme malnutrition
12. Extreme lack of cleanliness
13. Inappropriate clothing for the situation
14. Child who withdraws from parent
15. Child who responds inappropriately to the situation (e.g., quiet, distant, withdrawn)

Physical Findings Suggestive of Abuse

Some physical findings, such as multiple, widely dispersed bruises; welts; and burns are suggestive of nonaccidental trauma. Such physical findings, in conjunction with a vague history or delays in seeking medical care for the child, should alert the paramedic to the possibility of abuse or neglect (Fig. 42-10).

Bruises (Table 42-11)

- Bruises that predominate on the buttocks or lower back are almost always related to punishment.
- Genital area or inner thigh bruises usually are inflicted for toileting mishaps.
- Facial bruises or numerous petechiae on the ear lobe usually are caused by slapping.
- Bruises of the upper lip and labial frenulum usually are caused by forced feedings or from

? CRITICAL THINKING

Where would you expect to see "normal" bruises on an infant under 3 months of age based on the physical capabilities of this age group?

TABLE 42-11	DATING OF BRUISES BY COLOR
COLOR OF BRUISE	**AGE OF BRUISE**
Reddish blue or purple	Less than 24 hours
Dark blue to purple	1 to 5 days
Green	5 to 7 days
Yellow	7 to 10 days
Brown	10 to 14 days or longer
Resolution	2 to 4 weeks

jamming a pacifier into the mouth of a screaming infant.
- Human hand marks resulting from squeezing are pressure bruises in shapes resembling fingertips, fingers, or the entire hand of the abuser.
- Human bite marks result in paired, crescent-shaped bruises that often contain individual teeth marks. The size of the arc distinguishes adult bites from child bites.

Welts

- Strap marks 1 to 2 inches wide are almost always caused by a belt.
- Bizarre-shaped welts or bruises usually are inflicted by a blunt object that resembles its shape (e.g., a toy or shoe).
- Choke marks may be seen on the neck.

- Circumferential bruising or abrasions on the ankles or wrists may be caused by rope, cord, or a dog leash.

Burns

- Cigarette burns often are found on the palms, soles, or abdomen.
- A lighted cigarette, a hot match, or burning incense sometimes is applied to the hand to stop the child from sucking the thumb or to the genital area to discourage masturbation.
- Burns may be inflicted with lighters or other sources of open flame (e.g., a gas stove) to teach a child not to play with fire.
- Dry contact burns may result from forcibly holding a child against a heating device (e.g., a radiator, hot iron, or electric hot plate).

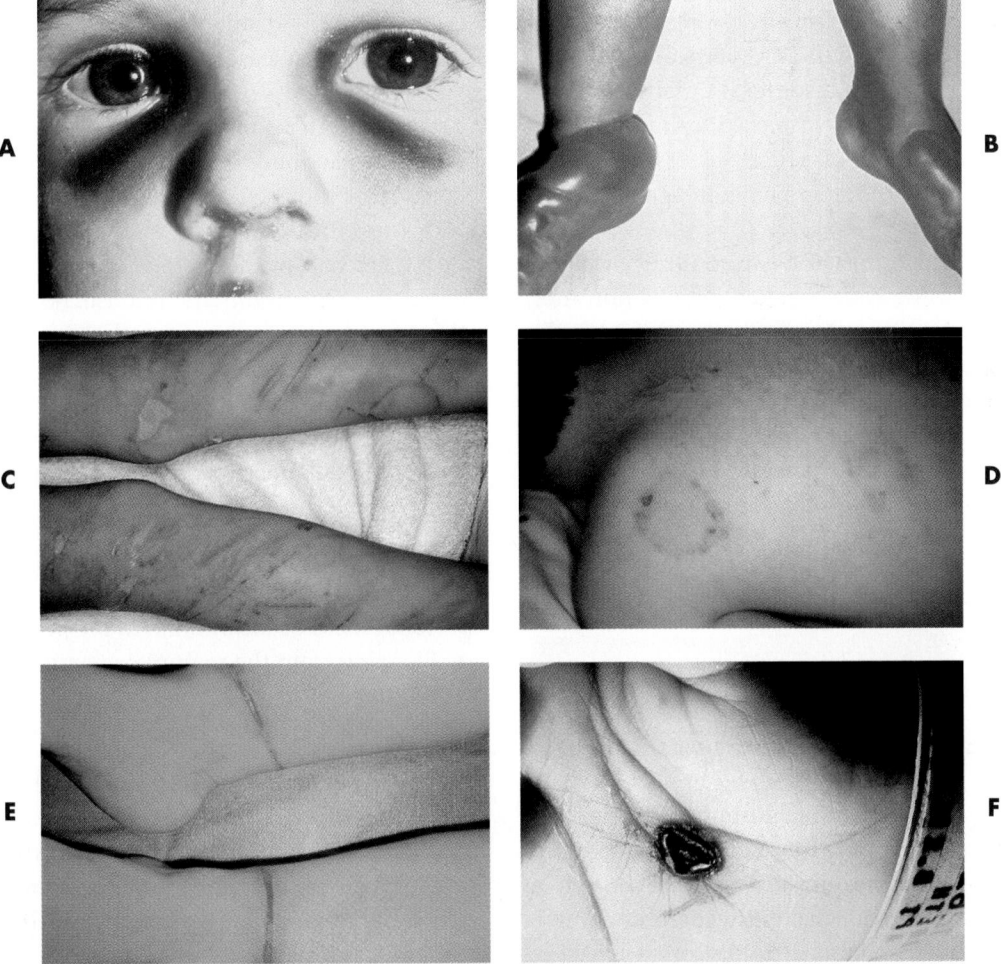

Fig. 42-10 Cutaneous manifestations of child abuse. **A,** "Raccoon eyes," or periorbital bruising, possible indication of anterior fossa skull fracture. **B,** "Dunking" burns of the feet. **C,** Welts and abrasions to legs as a result of an electrical cord. **D,** Human bites. **E,** Fresh abrasions of restraint injury. **F,** Fresh cigarette burn to palm. (Courtesy Gary Quick, MD.)

- The most common hot-water burns or scalds occur from forcible immersion of the hands, feet, or buttocks in scalding water. These injuries often involve both arms or both legs, or they may be circular burns restricted to the buttocks; such burns are incompatible with falling or stepping into a tub of hot water.

Other less visible injuries that may indicate child abuse include brain injury, abdominal visceral injury, and bone fractures.

Subdural hematoma. Brain injury is the leading cause of death in battered children. The various pathological lesions include cerebral contusions, intraparenchymal hemorrhage, and subdural or even epidural hematomas. Subdural hematomas are among the most common pathological abnormalities associated with intentionally inflicted head injury in children. They should be suspected in any young child who is in a coma or having convulsions, particularly if there is no history of seizure disorder. In many cases intracranial bleeding is associated with skull fractures or scalp bruises caused by a direct blow from a caregiver's hand or by the child being hit against a wall or door.

Subdural hematomas also can result from vigorous shaking of the child (shaken baby syndrome). The acceleration and deceleration forces on the brain associated with shaking cause tearing of the bridging cerebral veins, with bleeding into the subdural space. Signs and symptoms of the shaken baby syndrome include retinal hemorrhages, irritability, altered level of consciousness, vomiting, and a full fontanelle.

> **? CRITICAL THINKING**
>
> *Why is it particularly important that your documentation be clear, objective, and complete in cases of suspected abuse?*

Abdominal visceral injury. Intraabdominal injuries are the second most common cause of death in battered children. These injuries usually are produced by a blunt force such as a punch or blow to the abdomen. Children with an abdominal injury often have recurrent vomiting, abdominal distention, absent bowel sounds, and localized tenderness with or without abdominal bruising. Caregivers routinely deny a history of trauma to the child's abdomen in these cases.

Bone injury. More than 20% of physically abused children have a positive result on radiological bone survey from previous abusive episodes.[7] Injuries that may be obvious only through radiography include fractures of the ribs, lateral portion of the clavicle, scapula, sternum, and extremities. Multiple fractures in various stages of healing are highly suspicious for physical abuse.

Injuries from Sexual Abuse

Sexual abuse of a child is a symptom of a seriously disturbed family relationship usually associated with physical or emotional neglect or abuse. Often the sexually abusive adult experienced similar abuse as a child and justifies this maladaptive behavior subconsciously. Family relationships are complex, and silent complicity by at least one parent often is involved.

Injuries from sexual abuse may be physical and psychological. Sexual abuse may include vaginal intercourse, sodomy (anal intercourse), oral-genital contact, or molestation (fondling, masturbation, or exposure). In many cases the victimized child is a girl. Over half of the victims are under 12 years of age at the time of the first offense. Because many of these incidents are chronic and occur without force, an EMS response seldom is initiated. If, however, a physical injury results from the abuse, emergency care may be summoned. Physical findings suggestive of sexual abuse include the following:

- Pregnancy or venereal disease in a child 12 years of age or younger
- Painful urination or defecation
- Tenderness or lacerations to the perineal area
- Bleeding from the rectum or vagina
- Presence of dried blood, semen, or pubic hair in the genital area of a child

Emergency care for child victims of sexual abuse should be limited to managing life-threatening injury and providing emotional support during transport to the receiving hospital. These children undergo extensive interviews and examination by the emergency department physician and others. The paramedic should carefully document any statements made by the patient, family member, or caregiver, and any findings should be reported to medical direction. These children require compassionate support. A sexually abused child should never receive the impression that she or he is responsible for any of the abuse or that discussion of the event is inappropriate. If possible, the child should be interviewed and cared for by a paramedic of the same sex.

Infants and Children with Special Needs

Some infants and children are born with or develop conditions that pose special needs and require special medical equipment to sustain life. Examples of these conditions include infants born prematurely, those who have altered functions from birth, and those who have chronic or acute disease of the lung, heart, or central nervous system. Often these children are cared for at home by family and home health services; many are technologically dependent on special medical equipment such as tracheostomy tubes, home artificial ventilators, central venous lines, gastrostomy tubes, and shunts (see Chapter 46).

> **? CRITICAL THINKING**
>
> *How can an EMS agency prepare crews to care for these special needs children before a call is even received?*

> **NOTE**
>
> The parents and other family members of a child with special medical needs often are "experts" in caring for the child and maintaining the required medical equipment. Their knowledge, skills, and experience are valuable and should be used when managing these emergencies.

Tracheostomy Tubes

A patient with a complete tracheostomy has had the airway surgically interrupted so that the larynx is no longer connected to the trachea. Modern tracheostomy tubes are flexible and relatively comfortable for the patient and have few associated risks (Fig. 42-11). Complications that can occur with the tracheostomy tube include obstruction, air leak, bleeding, dislodgment, and infection, all of which may lead to inadequate ventilation. Aseptic technique and respiratory support are always high priorities in caring for these patients.

> **NOTE**
>
> Bleeding around a tracheostomy usually occurs within 24 hours of the surgical procedure and is not commonly seen in the prehospital setting.

Management

Should the tracheostomy tube fail to provide a patent airway because of obstruction or dislodgment, it must be cleaned with sterile water or saline or removed and reinserted as described in Chapter 11. (Medical direction may recommend that a tracheostomy tube be replaced with an ET tube as a temporary measure.) Tracheal suctioning (using sterile technique) may be necessary to remove secretions and mucus. If tracheal intubation becomes necessary in these patients, it must be performed via the stoma.

> **NOTE**
>
> Tracheal suctioning is a difficult procedure and a traumatic experience for the patient. It can easily lead to hypoxia. Tracheal suctioning should be performed only when absolutely necessary and only for a period of 10 to 15 seconds after which high-concentration supplemental oxygen should be administered by mask to stoma or via a bag-valve mask.

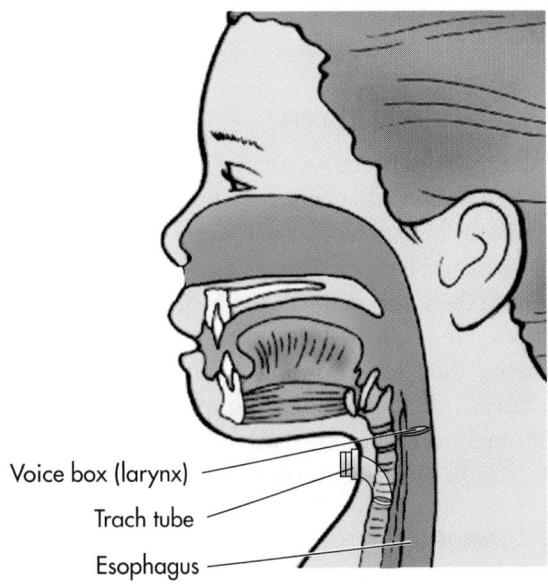

Voice box (larynx)

Trach tube

Esophagus

Fig. 42-11 Pediatric tracheostomy tube.

TABLE 42-12	COMPLICATIONS SEEN WITH HOME ARTIFICIAL VENTILATORS
COMPLICATION	**POSSIBLE CAUSE**
Airway obstruction	Bronchospasm, mucus or secretions, tracheostomy or endotracheal (ET) tube malfunction, patient cough, fear, anxiety
Barotrauma	
Pneumothorax	High-pressure volumes
Atelectasis	Improper deep breathing, pneumothorax
Cardiovascular impairment	Reduction in venous return to the heart caused by positive intrathoracic pressure, which compresses pulmonary circulation
Gastrointestinal (GI) complications	Swallowing air, GI bleeding, gastric distention
Tracheal trauma	Cuff pressure on trachea
Respiratory infection	Bypass of upper airway's natural defenses, poor aseptic technique
Oxygen toxicity	High concentration of oxygen over prolonged periods

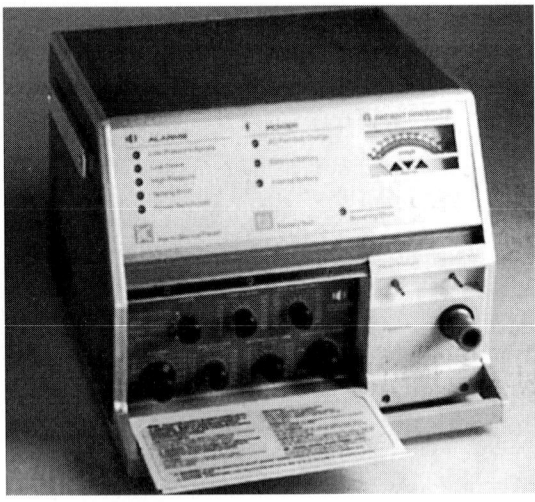

Fig. 42-12 Home ventilator. (Courtesy Puritan-Bennett LP6 from Mallinckrodt, St Louis, Mo.)

Home Artificial Ventilators

When a patient needs help breathing, the child may be put on a mechanical ventilator, which can simulate the normal bellows action usually provided by the diaphragm and thoracic cage. The type of home ventilator used depends on the patient's specific needs. Ventilators are classified by function based on the variables they deliver during certain phases of the respiratory cycle (Fig. 42-12). Complications can occur from malfunction of the machine and alarms, airway obstruction, and respiratory distress (Table 42-12).

Management

Because the numerous types of artificial ventilators operate differently, the paramedic should never try to "troubleshoot" a ventilator problem or adjust the machine's settings. Rather, the EMS crew should always treat the patient and not try to correct the machine's malfunction. Steps in managing a patient with a home artificial ventilator problem are presented in Chapter 46.

Central Venous Lines

Some patients with chronic illnesses require prolonged and frequent access to venous circulation for drug or fluid therapy. This is made possible through vascular access devices (VADs) that may frequently be encountered in the prehospital setting in both child and adult patients who are cared for in the home (Fig. 42-13). These devices include surgically implanted medication delivery devices (e.g., Mediports), peripheral vascular access devices (e.g., peripherally inserted central catheters [PICCs], Intracath), and central venous access devices (e.g., Hickman, Groshong) (see Chapters 9 and 46). Complications that may occur with VADs include a cracked line, air embolism, bleeding, obstruction, and local infection.

> **NOTE**
>
> Patients with VADs often have a serious illness such as cancer or acquired immunodeficiency syndrome (AIDS). The effects of these illnesses may complicate the assessment and management of emergencies associated with central venous lines.

Management

A torn or leaking catheter (cracked line) may allow fluids or medications to infiltrate into the surround-

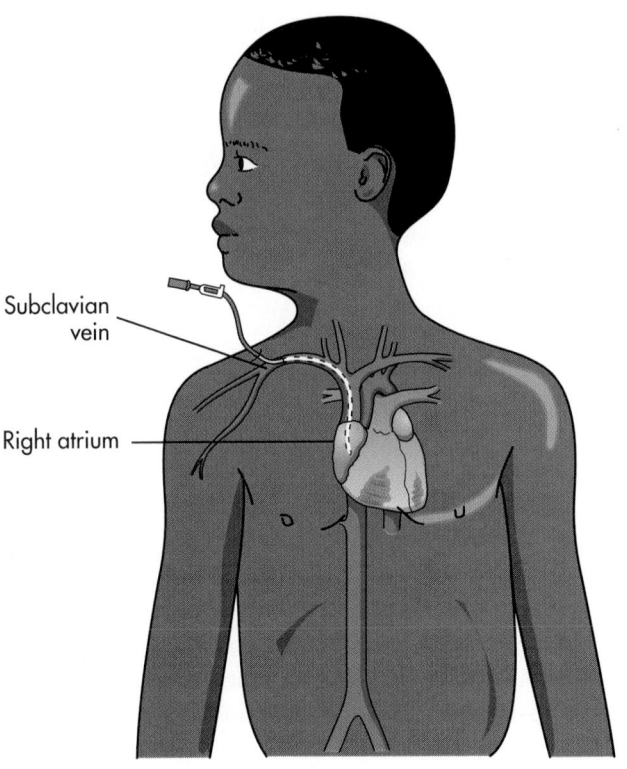

Subclavian
vein

Right atrium

Fig. 42-13 Central venous line.

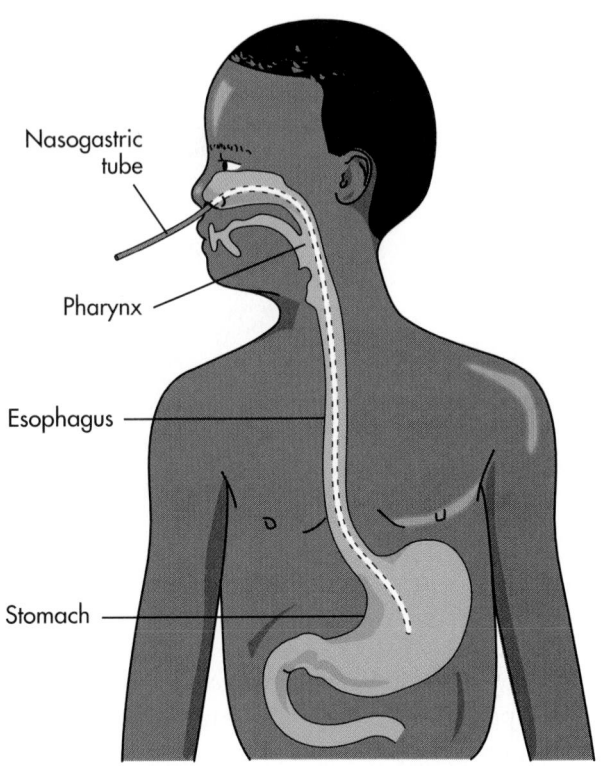

Nasogastric
tube

Pharynx

Esophagus

Stomach

Fig. 42-14 Nasogastric tube.

ing tissues and can lead to an air embolism. If a torn catheter is suspected (evidenced by leaking fluid, a complaint of a burning sensation, or swollen and tender skin near the insertion site), the infusion should be stopped immediately and the catheter clamped between the tear and the patient. The patient who develops an altered level of consciousness (indicating a possible air embolism) should be positioned on the left side with the head slightly lowered to help prevent the embolism from traveling to the brain. High-concentration oxygen, IV access, and rapid transport for evaluation by a physician are indicated. Any bleeding at the site should be controlled with direct pressure.

Occasionally, the lumen port will become obstructed by a blood clot that disrupts the flow of fluids or medications. (Signs and symptoms of obstruction include a sluggish flow and swelling and tenderness at the site.) When this occurs, the patient should be transported to the hospital so that the catheter can be cleared with thrombolytics or replaced. Attempts to clear a VAD require special training and authorization from medical direction. The technique is described in Chapter 46.

Gastric Tubes and Gastrostomy Tubes

A gastric tube (Fig. 42-14) is used as a temporary measure to provide liquid feeding to a patient who cannot swallow or absorb nutrients (often used for feeding premature infants). They are inserted through the nose or mouth into the stomach and can cause irritation to the nasal and mucous membranes. They are designed for short-term use.

A gastrostomy tube (Fig. 42-15) provides a permanent route for gastric feeding in patients who usually cannot be fed by mouth (e.g., a patient with facial burns or paralysis). The tube is surgically placed into the stomach and can be visualized in the upper left quadrant of the abdomen. The opening (stoma) has a flexible, silicone "button" (covered with a protective cap) that allows for regular feedings.

Management

Serious complications with gastric or gastrostomy tubes are rare and seldom require emergency care. Potential complications include obstruction, pulmonary aspiration, GI disturbances (vomiting and diarrhea), irritation to the mucous membrane, and electrolyte imbalances. All can result in inadequate

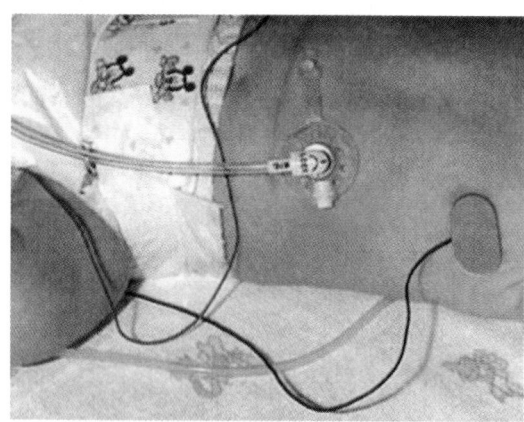

Fig. 42-15 Gastrostomy tube.

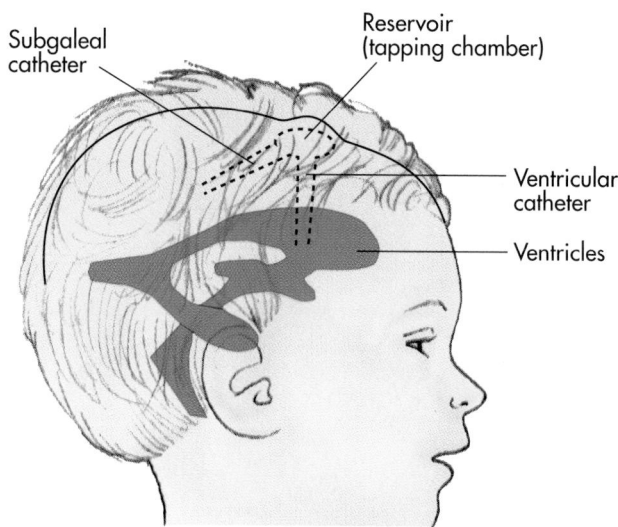

Fig. 42-16 Shunt.

nutrition and fluid needs. Emergency care primarily is supportive and may include transportation for evaluation by a physician. If not contraindicated, the patient will be most comfortable lying on the right side with the head elevated.

Shunts

A **shunt** is a surgical procedure performed to relieve abnormal fluid pressures from excess cerebrospinal fluid (CSF) around the brain in children with hydrocephalus (ventricular shunt) or in the portal veins in patients with portal hypertension. The shunt for hydrocephalus consists of two catheters, a reservoir, and a valve to prevent backflow (Fig. 42-16). The first catheter is inserted through the skull to drain fluid from the ventricles of the brain. The second catheter is passed into another body cavity (usually the abdomen or right atrium of the heart through the jugular vein), where the excess fluid is absorbed. The reservoir usually can be palpated over the mastoid area, just behind the ear.

Management

Complications from this procedure include the need for catheter replacement as the child grows

(requiring several surgeries in the first 10 years of life), obstruction from clotted blood or fluid, and catheter displacement. Infection is a complication that occurs within several weeks of surgical placement. Signs and symptoms of obstruction or displacement are those of increased ICP and include the following:

- Headache
- Nausea and vomiting
- Visual disturbances
- Cushing's triad (elevated systolic pressure, irregular respirations, bradycardia)

Children who have a complication from a ventricular shunt are surgical emergencies and require immediate care to prevent brain stem herniation. The paramedic should first ensure adequate airway, ventilatory, and circulatory support for these patients. Medical direction may recommend additional therapies that include endotracheal intubation and hyperventilation to lower ICP, along with IV access. These patients are prone to respiratory arrest and require immediate transportation to an appropriate facility for evaluation by a physician. If possible, the patient's head should be elevated during transport.

SUMMARY

- The Emergency Medical Services for Children (EMSC) program was designed to enhance and expand emergency medical services for acutely ill and injured children. It has defined 12 basic components of an effective EMSC system.

- Children have unique anatomical, physiological, and psychological characteristics, which change during their development.

- Some childhood diseases and disabilities are predictable by age group.

- Many components of the initial patient evaluation for children can be done by observing the patient and by involving the child's parent or guardian in the initial assessment. The three components of the Pediatric Assessment Triangle are appearance, work of breathing, and circulation.

- Obstruction of the upper or lower airway by a foreign body usually occurs in toddlers or preschoolers and may cause a partial or complete obstruction.

- Croup is a common inflammatory respiratory illness usually seen in children between the ages of 6 months and 4 years. Symptoms are caused by inflammation in the subglottic region.

- Bacterial tracheitis is an infection of the upper airway and subglottic trachea often seen in infants and toddlers; it often occurs with or after croup.

- Epiglottitis is a rapidly progressive, life-threatening bacterial infection that causes edema and swelling of the epiglottis and supraglottic structures. It often affects children between 3 and 7 years of age.

- Asthma, common in children over 2 years of age, is characterized by bronchoconstriction that results from autonomic dysfunction or sensitizing agents.

- Bronchiolitis is a viral disease frequently caused by RSV infection of the lower airway; it usually affects children age 6 to 18 months of age.

- Pneumonia is an acute infection of the lower airway and lung that involves either the alveolar walls or the alveoli.

- Several special considerations must be taken into account when caring for a child in shock. These include circulating blood volume, body surface area and hypothermia, cardiac reserve, and vital signs and assessment. A child with a volume deficit maintains stable hemodynamics until all compensatory mechanisms fail. At that point, pediatric shock progresses rapidly, with catastrophic deterioration.

- When dysrhythmias occur in children, they usually are the result of hypoxia or structural heart disease.

- The most common causes of seizure in adult and pediatric patients is noncompliance with a drug regimen for the treatment of epilepsy, in addition to head trauma, intracranial infection, metabolic disturbance, or poisoning. The most common cause of new onset of seizure in children is fever.

- Hypoglycemia and hyperglycemia should be suspected whenever a child has an altered level of consciousness with no explainable cause.

- Children with infection may have a variety of signs and symptoms, depending on the source and extent of infection and the length of time since the patient was exposed.

- Most poisoning events in the United States involve children. Signs and symptoms of accidental poisoning vary, depending on the toxic substance and the length of time since the child was exposed.

- Blunt and penetrating trauma is a predominant cause of injury and death in children. Head injury is the most common cause of death in pediatric trauma patients. Early recognition and aggressive management can reduce morbidity and mortality secondary to traumatic brain injury in children.

- Because of the thoracic compliance of the chest wall, severe intrathoracic injury can be present without signs of external injury. The liver, kidneys, and spleen are the most frequently injured abdominal organs. Extremity injuries are more common in children than adults.

- Sudden infant death syndrome (SIDS) is the leading cause of death in American infants under 1 year of age. The syndrome is defined as the sudden death of an apparently healthy infant that remains unexplained by history and a thorough autopsy.

- Child abuse and neglect is the maltreatment of children by their parents, guardians, or other caregivers. Forms of maltreatment include infliction of physical injury, sexual exploitation, and infliction of emotional pain and neglect.

- Some infants and children are born with or develop conditions that pose special needs and require special medical equipment to sustain life. Often these children are cared for at home; many are technologically dependent on specialized medical equipment such as tracheostomy tubes, home artificial ventilators, central venous lines, gastrostomy tubes, and shunts.

■ REFERENCES

1. Tsai A, Kallsen G: Epidemiology of pediatric prehospital care, *Ann Emerg Med* 16:284, 1987.
2. U.S. Department of Transportation, National Highway Traffic Safety Administration: *EMT-Paramedic national standard curriculum*, Washington, DC, 1998, The Department.
3. National Center for Education in Maternal and Child Health: *Emergency medical services for children: a report to the nation*, Washington, DC, 1991, The Center.
4. Hoekelman R et al: *Primary pediatric care*, ed 3, St Louis, 1997, Mosby.
5. American Heart Association: *Guidelines 2000 for cardiopulmonary resuscitation and emergency cardiovascular care*, International Consensus on Science, Dallas 2000, The Association.
6. American Heart Association: *Pediatric advanced life support*, Dallas, Texas, 1997, The Association.
7. Rosen P, Barkin R: *Emergency medicine: concepts and clinical practice*, ed 4, St Louis, 1998, Mosby.
8. Volugaropoulos C: *Type 1 diabetes in childhood: before and after diagnosis*, Pediatric Endocrinology and Diabetes Care, St Louis, 1998, Unity Health Systems.
9. National Safety Council: *Injury facts*, Itasca, Ill, 1999, The Council.
10. Touloukian R: *Pediatric trauma*, ed 2, St Louis, 1990, Mosby.

ANATOMY AND PHYSIOLOGY REVIEW FOR PEDIATRIC PATIENTS

A. Head
1. Proportionally larger size
2. Larger occipital region
3. Fontanelles open in infancy
4. Face smaller compared with size of head
5. Paramedic implications
   a. Higher proportion of blunt trauma involves the head.
   b. Different airway positioning techniques
      (1) Place thin layer of padding under back of seriously injured child to obtain neutral position.
   c. Condition of fontanelle in infants
      (1) Bulging fontanelle suggests increased intracranial pressure (ICP).
      (2) Sunken fontanelle suggests dehydration.

B. Airway
1. Airway is narrower at all levels.
2. Infants are obligate nasal breathers.
3. Jaw is posteriorly smaller in young children.
4. Larynx is higher (C3-C4) and more anterior.
5. Cricoid ring is the narrowest part of the airway in young children.
6. Tracheal cartilage is softer.
7. Trachea is smaller in both length and diameter.
8. Epiglottis
   a. Omega shaped in infants
   b. Extends at a 45-degree angle into airway
   c. Epiglottic folds have softer cartilage and are more floppy, especially in children
9. Paramedic implications
   a. Keep nares clear in infants under 6 months of age.
   b. Narrower upper airways are more easily obstructed from the following:
      (1) Flexion or hyperextension
      (2) Particulate matter
      (3) Soft tissue swelling (injury, inflammation)
   c. Intubation techniques and modifications
      (1) Use gentler touch.
      (2) Use straight blade.
      (3) Lift epiglottis.
      (4) Use uncuffed tube up to age 8.
      (5) Ensure precise placement.

C. Chest and lungs
1. Ribs are positioned horizontally.
2. Ribs are more pliable and offer less protection to organs.
3. Chest muscles are immature and fatigue easily.
4. Lung tissue is more fragile.
5. Mediastinum is more mobile.
6. Thin chest wall allows for easily transmitted breath sounds.
7. Paramedic implications
   a. Infants and children are diaphragmatic breathers.
   b. Infants and children are prone to gastric distention.
   c. Rib fractures are less common but not uncommon in child abuse and trauma.
   d. Greater energy is transmitted to underlying organs with trauma (significant internal injury can be present without external signs).
   e. Pulmonary contusions are more common in major trauma.
   f. Lungs are prone to pneumothorax with barotrauma.
   g. Mediastinum has greater shift with tension pneumothorax.
   h. Transmitted breath sounds make it easy to miss a pneumothorax or misplaced intubation.

D. Abdomen
1. Immature abdominal muscles offer less protection.
2. Abdominal organs are closer together.
3. Liver and spleen are proportionally larger and more vascular.
4. Paramedic implications
   a. Liver and spleen are more frequently injured.
   b. Multiple organ injuries are common.

E. Extremities
1. Bones are softer and more porous until adolescence.
2. Injuries to growth plate may disrupt bone growth.
3. Extremities are a site for intraosseous (IO) access.
4. Paramedic implications
   a. Any sprain or strain must be immobilized because it is likely a fracture.
   b. The growth plate should not be pierced during IO needle insertion.

F. Skin and body surface area
1. Skin is thinner and more elastic.
2. Thermal exposure results in a deeper burn.
3. Less subcutaneous fat is present.
4. The surface area to body mass ratio is larger.
5. Paramedic implications
   a. Children are more easily and deeply burned.
   b. Children experience greater losses of fluid and heat.

APPENDIX 42-1

ANATOMY AND PHYSIOLOGY REVIEW FOR PEDIATRIC PATIENTS—*cont'd*

G. Respiratory system
 1. Tidal volume is proportionally smaller than that of adolescents and adults.
 2. Metabolic oxygen requirements of infants and children are about double those of adolescents and adults.
 3. Children have proportionally smaller functional residual capacity and therefore proportionally smaller oxygen reserves.
 4. Paramedic implications
   a. Hypoxia develops rapidly because of increased oxygen requirements and decreased oxygen reserves.
H. Cardiovascular system
 1. Cardiac output is rate dependent in infants and small children.
 2. The cardiovascular reserve is vigorous but limited.
 3. Bradycardia is a response to hypoxia.
 4. Children can maintain blood pressure longer than adults.
 5. Circulating blood volume is proportionally larger than in adults.
 6. Absolute blood volume is smaller than in adults.
 7. Paramedic implications
   a. Smaller volumes of fluid and blood loss can cause shock.
   b. Hypotension is a late sign of shock.
   c. A child may be in shock despite having normal blood pressure.
   d. Shock assessment is based on clinical signs of tissue perfusion.
   e. Careful assessment for shock is necessary if tachycardia is present.
   f. Careful monitoring is necessary for development of hypotension.
   g. Early intervention is necessary to prevent decompensation.
I. Nervous system
 1. Develops throughout childhood.
 2. Developing neural tissue is more fragile.
 3. Brain and spinal cord are less well protected by skull and spinal column.
 4. Fontanelles are open in early months.
 5. Paramedic implications
   a. Brain injuries are more devastating in young children.
   b. Greater force is transmitted to the underlying brain of young children.
   c. Spinal cord injury can occur without spinal column injury.
J. Metabolic differences
 1. Infants and children have limited glycogen and glucose stores.
 2. Blood glucose can drop low in response to stressors.
 3. Significant volume loss can result from vomiting and diarrhea.
 4. Children are prone to hypothermia because of their increased body surface area.
 5. Newborns and neonates are unable to shiver to maintain body temperature.
 6. Paramedic implications
   a. Children should be kept warm during treatment and transport.
   b. The head should be covered to minimize heat loss.
   c. If prolonged stress state exists, the child should be assessed for hypoglycemia.

APPENDIX 42-2

Recommended Childhood Immunization Schedule
United States, January-December 2001

Vaccines[1] are listed under routinely recommended ages. Bars indicate range of recommended ages for immunization. Any dose not given at the recommended age should be given as a "catch-up" immunization at any subsequent visit when indicated and feasible. Ovals indicate vaccines to be given if previously recommended doses were missed or given earlier than the recommended minimum age.

Age ▶ Vaccines ▼	Birth	1 mo	2 mos	4 mos	6 mos	12 mos	15 mos	18 mos	24 mos	4-6 yrs	11-12 yrs	14-16 yrs
Hepatitis B[2]		Hep B #1	Hep B #2			Hep B #3					Hep B[2]	
Diphtheria, Tetanus, Pertussis[3]			DTaP	DTaP	DTaP		DTaP[3]			DTaP	Td	
H. influenzae type b[4]			Hib	Hib	Hib	Hib						
Inactivated Polio[5]			IPV	IPV		IPV[5]				IPV[5]		
Pneumococcal Conjugate[6]			PCV	PCV	PCV	PCV						
Measles, Mumps, Rubella[7]						MMR				MMR[7]	MMR[7]	
Varicella[8]						Var					Var[8]	
Hepatitis A[9]									Hep A—in selected areas[9]			

Approved by the Advisory Committee on Immunization Practices (ACIP), the American Academy of Pediatrics (AAP), and the American Academy of Family Physicians (AAFP).

1. This schedule indicates the recommended ages for routine administration of currently licensed childhood vaccines, as of 11/1/00, for children through 18 years of age. Additional vaccines may be licensed and recommended during the year. Licensed combination vaccines may be used whenever any components of the combination are indicated and its other components are not contraindicated. Providers should consult the manufacturers' package inserts for detailed recommendations.

2. **Infants born to HBsAg-negative mothers** should receive the 1st dose of hepatitis B (Hep B) vaccine by age 2 months. The 2nd dose should be at least one month after the 1st dose. The 3rd dose should be administered at least 4 months after the 1st dose and at least 2 months after the 2nd dose, but not before 6 months of age for infants.

Infants born to HBsAg-positive mothers should receive hepatitis B vaccine and 0.5mL hepatitis B immune globulin (HBIG) within 12 hours of birth at separate sites. The 2nd dose is recommended at 1-2 months of age and the 3rd dose at 6 months of age.

Infants born to mothers whose HBsAg status is unknown should receive hepatitis B vaccine within 12 hours of birth. Maternal blood should be drawn at the time of delivery to determine the mother's HBsAg status; if the HBsAg test is positive, the infant should receive HBIG as soon as possible (no later than 1 week of age).

All children and adolescents who have not been immunized against hepatitis B should begin the series during any visit. Special efforts should be made to immunize children who were born in or whose parents were born in areas of the world with moderate or high endemicity of hepatitis B virus infection.

3. The 4th dose of DTaP (diphtheria and tetanus toxoids and acellular pertussis vaccine) may be administered as early as 12 months of age, provided 6 months have elapsed since the 3rd dose and the child is unlikely to return at age 15-18 months. Td (tetanus and diphtheriatoxoids) is recommended at 11-12 years of age if at least 5 years have elapsed since the last dose of DTP, DTaP or DT. Subsequent routine Td boosters are recommended every 10 years.

4. Three *Haemophilus influenzae* type b (Hib) conjugate vaccines are licensed for infant use. If PRP-OMP (PedvaxHIB® or ComVax®[Merck]) is administered at 2 and 4 months of age, a dose at 6 months is not required. Because clinical studies in infants have demonstrated that using some combination products may induce a lower immune response to the Hib vaccine component, DTaP/Hib combination products should not be used for primary immunization in infants at 2, 4 or 6 months of age, unless FDA-approved for these ages.

5. An all-IPV schedule is recommended for routine childhood polio vaccination in the United States. All children should receive four doses of IPV at 2 months, 4 months, 6-18 months, and 4-6 years of age. Oral polio vaccine (OPV) should be used only in selected circumstances. (See MMWR *Morb Mortal Wkly Rep* May 19, 2000/49(RR-5);1-22).

6. The heptavalent conjugate pneumococcal vaccine (PCV) is recommended for all children 2-23 months of age. It also is recommended for certain children 24-59 months of age. (See MMWR *Morb Mortal Wkly Rep* Oct. 6, 2000/49(RR-9);1-35).

7. The 2nd dose of measles, mumps, and rubella (MMR) vaccine is recommended routinely at 4-6 years of age but may be administered during any visit, provided at least 4 weeks have elapsed since receipt of the 1st dose and that both doses are administered beginning at or after 12 months of age. Those who have not previously received the second dose should complete the schedule by the 11-12 year old visit.

8. Varicella (Var) vaccine is recommended at any visit on or after the first birthday for susceptible children, i.e. those who lack a reliable history of chickenpox (as judged by a health care provider) and who have not been immunized. Susceptible persons 13 years of age or older should receive 2 doses, given at least 4 weeks apart.

9. Hepatitis A (Hep A) is shaded to indicate its recommended use inselected states and/or regions, and for certain high risk groups; consult your local public health authority. (See MMWR *Morb Mortal Wkly Rep* Oct. 1, 1999/48(RR-12); 1-37).

For additional information about the vaccines listed above, please visit the National Immunization Program Home Page at www.cdc.gov/nip or call the National immunization Hotline at 800-232-2522 (English) or 800-232-0233 (Spanish)

43 *Geriatrics*

OBJECTIVES

Upon completion of this chapter, the paramedic student will be able to:

1. **Explain the physiology of the aging process as it relates to major body systems and homeostasis.**

2. **Describe general principles of assessment specific to older adults.**

3. **Describe the pathophysiology, assessment, and management of specific illnesses that affect selected body systems in the geriatric patient.**

4. **Identify specific problems with sensations experienced by some geriatric patients.**

5. **Discuss effects of drug toxicity and alcoholism in the older adult.**

6. **Identify factors that contribute to environmental emergencies in the geriatric patient.**

7. **Discuss prehospital assessment and management of depression and suicide in the older adult.**

8. **Describe epidemiology, assessment, and management of trauma in the geriatric patient.**

9. **Identify characteristics of elder abuse.**

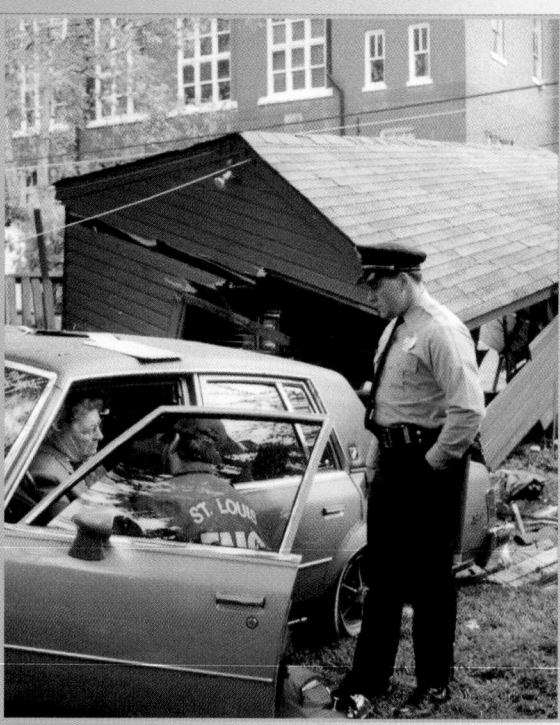

The progressive "graying" of American society includes the prospect that the health care needs of older adults will continue to increase in all areas, including prehospital care. Approximately 25% of Americans will be 65 years of age or older by the year 2030 and will represent 70% of all ambulance transports[1] (see the box on p. 1280). This chapter addresses anatomical and physiological changes that accompany the aging process, special considerations in assessing and managing geriatric patients, and common emergencies that may result from normal aging and chronic illness.

KEY TERMS

elder abuse: The infliction of physical pain, injury, debilitating mental anguish, unreasonable confinement, or willful deprivation by a caregiver of services necessary to maintain the mental and physical health of a geriatric patient.

gerontology: The study of the problems of all aspects of aging.

NOTE

The Injury Prevention section in Appendix C provides strategies that can help prevent medical illness and traumatic injury in the elderly population and other age groups.

NOTE

Many older Americans enjoy independent living with the help of spousal or family support and home health care programs. Others live dependently in nursing care facilities, assisted living environments, and nursing homes. The elderly often receive assistance in independent and dependent living environments through local, state, and national programs and other resource agencies (Box 43-1). The paramedic should be familiar with various programs in his or her community that provide assistance to the elderly.

Physiological Changes of Aging

Gerontology is the study of the problems of all aspects of aging. The aging process proceeds at different rates in different people, and organ systems age at differing rates within the individual. However, in certain areas predictable functional declines occur in all people with increasing age. As a rough guideline, these changes begin to occur at a rate of 5% to 10% for each decade of life after 30 years of age. Although all body systems are affected by the aging process, the effects on specific organ systems particularly relevant to the older adult occur in the respiratory, cardiovascular, renal, nervous, and musculoskeletal systems (Table 43-1).

? CRITICAL THINKING

What age-related changes have you noticed in family members and friends who are in their forties, sixties, or eighties?

Respiratory System Changes

Respiratory function in the older adult generally is compromised as a result of changes in pulmonary physiology that accompany the aging process. Reduced pulmonary capacity is related to alterations in lung and chest wall compliance. With aging, the chest wall becomes increasingly stiff as the bony thorax becomes more rigid, and lung elastic recoil decreases. Despite the loss of elasticity, which would tend to increase total lung capacity, total lung capacity remains unchanged because of the opposing loss of chest wall compliance and weakened respiratory muscles. Variable increases in alveolar diameter and the tendency for distal airways to collapse on expiration lead to an increase in residual

BOX 43-1

SAMPLING OF SUPPORT AND ASSISTANCE PROGRAMS FOR THE GERIATRIC PATIENT

State and national aging organizations
State advisory councils
Community-based services
In-home services
Institutional services
Home health care services
Hospice programs
Religious and pastoral services
Nutrition services
Multipurpose senior centers
Volunteer organizations

THE CHALLENGE: THE AGING OF THE U.S. POPULATION

More than 34 million Americans (12% of the U.S. population) are 65 years of age or older, and the size of this group has soared during the last 100 years. At the same time, fertility rates in the United States have dropped, meaning that there will be fewer people under 65 years of age to support the costs of health care and living expenses of those over 65 years of age. By the year 2050, nearly 25% of Americans will be eligible for Medicare, and the population over 85 years of age will grow from 4 million to 19 million in 2050. This creates challenges as society attempts to provide quality, cost-effective health care and support the increasing health and living expenses for the elderly. To properly meet the needs of this aging population, society must accomplish the following:

• The public must become better educated about the needs of the elderly population because caregiving responsibilities often fall to families and friends.

• Current and new health care professionals must be educated regarding the special needs of the aging

population. Older adults have unique characteristics that differentiate them from younger populations, such as a higher level of adverse drug reactions and urinary incontinence. Thus health care professionals need special training to treat the aging population.

• The aging of the U.S. population demands continued and expanded research efforts into chronic diseases that affect the aging and their families.

• Health care professionals need to reform heath care financing, delivery, and administrative structures to accommodate the predominance of chronic illness among the aging population.

• Health care professionals must develop solutions for the long-term care needs of the growing aging population that addresses the emotional and financial needs of older adults and their families and the financial influence of long-term care in the United States.

Modified from American Geriatrics Society Foundation for Health in Aging: *2000-2010 decade of health in aging: the challenge: the aging of the U.S. population,* accessed April 10, 2000. Available at www.healthinaging.org/the challenge.html.

volume and a decrease in vital capacity. Consequently, by 75 years of age, vital capacity may decrease by as much as 50%, maximum breathing capacity by as much as 60%, and maximum work rate and maximum oxygen uptake by as much as 70%.[2]

Arterial oxygen pressure (PaO_2) also slowly decreases with age, but arterial carbon dioxide pressure ($PaCO_2$) remains unchanged (probably related to the much greater reserve in carbon dioxide elimination than in oxygen absorption). At 30 years of age the PaO_2 of a healthy person breathing ambient air at sea level is about 90 torr, whereas at 70 years of age the expected PaO_2 is 70 torr. These findings, combined with the normal decline in central and peripheral chemoreceptor function, produce a diminished ventilatory response to hypoxic and hypercapnic challenge.

Other factors affecting the respiratory system are the loss of cilia in the airways and a diminished cough reflex and impaired gag reflex, which can impair the body's defense against inhaled bacteria and particulate matter. The decline in pulmonary defense mechanisms makes infectious pulmonary diseases of the older adult more common and more difficult to eradicate.

Cardiovascular System Changes

Cardiac function declines with age as a result of nonischemic physiological changes and the high incidence of atherosclerotic coronary artery disease.[3] It is difficult to sort out changes that are solely due to aging from those associated with ischemia because coronary artery disease is so prevalent in the older adult. However, even with aging alone, structural and physiological changes that limit cardiac function occur in the cardiovascular system. These changes include a diminished ability to raise the heart rate even in response to exercise or stress, a decrease in compliance of the ventricle, a prolonged duration of contraction, and a decreased responsiveness to catecholamine stimulation. Between 30 and 80 years of age, resting cardiac output decreases about 30%. Combined with the progressive increase in peripheral vascular resistance that occurs after 40 years of age, this decrease in cardiac output yields a significant drop in organ perfusion.[2] Myocardial hypertrophy, coronary artery disease, and hemodynamic changes predispose the geriatric patient to dysrhythmias, heart failure, and sudden cardiac arrest when the cardiovascular system is placed under unexpected stress.

TABLE 43-1	PHYSIOLOGICAL CHANGES OF AGING

CHANGE	RESULT
Overall Appearance	
Skin	
Loss of elasticity	Wrinkling
Loss of collagen	Wrinkling, thinning of skin
	Increased susceptibility to injury
Shrinking of sweat glands	Dryness
Pigment deposition	Age spots
Sun damage	Senile keratosis
Eyes	
Clouding of lens	Cataracts (decreased visual acuity)
	Poor peripheral vision
Pigment deposition	Arcus senilis (bluish circle that forms around the outer edge of the iris of the eye)
Cardiovascular	
Increased internal thickening of arteries	Hypertension
	Increased risk of stroke or heart attack
	Varicosities and clots
	Dysrhythmias
Increased cholesterol deposits (atherosclerotic heart disease)	Coronary artery disease and peripheral vascular disease
Decreased rate of cardiac hypertrophy	Decreased cardiac output
Decreased cardiac output	Loss of exercise tolerance
	Diminished activity
	Increased work to heart
	Increased risk of myocardial infarction
Pulmonary	
Decreased elasticity	Diminished breathing capacity
Decreased compliance and surface area	Decreased maximal oxygen uptake
Decreased ciliary activity	Increased risk of infection/toxicity
GI Tract	
Decreased hydrochloric acid production	Difficulty with digestion
Delay in intestinal motility	Food absorption problems and constipation
	Feeling full early, causing weight loss
Decreased saliva flow	Dry mouth, difficulty chewing
Fewer taste buds	Loss of food enjoyment, decreased appetite
Gum atrophy (shrinkage)	Tooth loss
Decreased liver function	Risk of toxicity from drugs
	Alcohol damage
	Loss of blood clotting
CNS	
Decreased cortical cell count	Memory impairment (dementia)
Increased synapse time (ST)	Decreased complex learning
Decreased nerve conduction velocity	Slower psychomotor skills
	Increased reflex time leading to risk of falling
Brain atrophy (shrinkage)	Prone to subdural hematomas
Vision	
Growth of lens	Decreased focusing ability
Cataract deposition	Hyperopia (farsightedness)
	Opacification of vision
Decreased pupil size	Decreased acuity and color perception
Loss of accommodation (focusing ability)	Decreased depth perception
	All cause increased risks of accidents and falls

From MedicAlert: *Geriatric emergencies: an EMT teaching manual,* Turlock, Calif, 1994, MedicAlert Foundation.

TABLE 43-1 ▷ PHYSIOLOGICAL CHANGES OF AGING—*cont'd*

CHANGE	RESULT
Hearing	
Ossicle degeneration	Loss of high frequency range of hearing
Atrophy (shrinkage) of auditory meatus	Loss of high frequency range of hearing
Atrophy (shrinkage) of cochlear hair cells and auditory neurons	Decreased acuity and pitch discrimination
	Decreased sense of balance
	All cause increased risks of accidents and falls
Renal Function	
Decreased glomerular function	Decreased renal clearance
Decreased renal blood flow	Increased risk of toxicity from all drugs and toxins processed in the kidneys
Genitourinary	
Loss of bladder control	Urinary infections
Prostate enlargement	Tumors and urinary retention
Endocrine Function	
Decrease in thyroid, ovarian, and testicular function	Decreased energy, decreased metabolic rate
	Decreased heat/cold tolerance
	Decreased reproductive function
Increased insulin	Predisposition for hypoglycemia
Musculoskeletal	
Decreased muscle mass	Loss of strength
Increased joint/tendon breakdown	Arthritis, stiffness, loss of flexibility
	Increased risk of falls
Bone demineralization	Loss of bone strength and size
	Increased risk of fracture
Psychological/Social	
Loss of physical function	Decreased activity
Loss of friends/family	Depression
Loss of social support	Increased isolation and anxiety
	Increased risk of suicide attempts
Immune System	
Loss of T-cell function	Increased infection

Changes also occur in the heart's electrical conduction pathways as functional cells are lost in the sinoatrial (SA) and atrioventricular (AV) nodes and the rest of the conduction system. These physiological changes often lead to dysrhythmias, including chronic atrial fibrillation, sick-sinus syndrome, and various types of bradycardias and heart blocks, all of which can contribute to the decline in cardiac output.

? CRITICAL THINKING

What life-style choices can retard these physiological changes of aging?

Renal System Changes

Structural and functional changes in the kidneys occur during the aging process. For example, renal blood flow falls an average of 50% between 30 and 80 years of age.[2] This reduction in renal blood flow is associated with a proportional decrease in the glomerular filtration rate of about 8 mL/min/decade. Renal mass decreases by about 20% between 40 and 80 years of age. The steady decline in kidney function places the geriatric patient at greater risk for renal failure from trauma, obstruction, infection, and vascular occlusion.

As the patient ages, significant impairment develops in renal concentrating ability, sodium conservation, free water clearance (diuresis), glomerular filtration, and renal plasma flow. Hepatic blood flow also decreases, limiting the effectiveness of liver metabolism. These decreases in renal and hepatic function, combined with changes in lean body mass and body water, make the geriatric patient more susceptible than young adults to electrolyte abnormalities or toxic manifestations in response to medications or drugs.

Nervous System Changes

Although it was long thought that mental dysfunction in the geriatric patient was caused solely by senility, it is now well known that intellectual functioning deteriorates selectively and may result from many organic causes.[4] For example, beginning at about 30 years of age, the total number of neurons in certain cortical areas decreases gradually, so by 70 years of age, a 10% reduction in brain weight has occurred.[2] These factors, decreased cerebral blood flow, and alterations in the location and amounts of specific neurotransmitters probably contribute to alterations in the central nervous system (CNS). The velocity of nerve conduction in the peripheral nervous system also decreases with aging. This may lead to changes in motor or position sense and delays in reaction time and motor responses. Other gradual alterations in the patient's nervous system can result in decreased visual and auditory acuity and changes in sleep patterns.

Toxic or metabolic factors that can affect mental functioning include the use of medications (e.g., anticholinergics, antihypertensives, antidysrhythmics, and analgesics); electrolyte imbalances; hypoglycemia; acidosis; alkalosis; hypoxia; liver, kidney, and lung failure; pneumonia; congestive heart failure (CHF); cardiac dysrhythmias; infection; and neoplastic syndromes.

Musculoskeletal System Changes

As the body ages, muscles shrink, muscles and ligaments calcify, and intervertebral disks become thin. Osteoporosis is common in geriatric patients (especially women), and an estimated 68% of geriatric patients show some degree of kyphosis ("humpback posture"). These musculoskeletal changes result in a decrease in total muscle mass, a decrease in height of 2 to 3 inches, widening and weakening of certain bones, and a posture that impairs mobility and alters the body's balance. As a result, falls are common and often are associated with significant morbidity and mortality.

> **? CRITICAL THINKING**
>
> *What aspects of care may you have to alter to immobilize the spine of a patient who has significant kyphosis?*

Other Physiological Changes

Other physiological changes that occur with aging include alterations in body mass and total body water, a decreased ability to maintain internal homeostasis, a decrease in the function of immunological mechanisms, nutritional disorders, and decreases in hearing and visual acuity.

As an individual approaches 65 years of age, lean body mass may decrease as much as 25% and fat tissue may increase as much as 35%.[2] These changes in body composition can influence the dosage and frequency of administration of fat-soluble drugs because there is more drug per weight of metabolically active tissue and a larger reservoir for accumulation of the drug. Similarly, the decrease in total body water is likely to increase the concentration of water-soluble drugs.

The body's ability to maintain internal homeostasis through normal thermoregulatory mechanisms declines over time in a linear fashion beginning at about 30 years of age. This and other factors predispose the geriatric patient to cold- and heat-related conditions such as hypothermia, heat exhaustion, and hyperthermia. Several factors contribute to the increased risk of thermoregulatory disorders, including impaired sympathetic nervous system function causing decreased capacity for peripheral vasoconstriction, lowered metabolic rate, poor peripheral circulation, and chronic illness. Because of the progressive decline in homeostatic control, including blood pressure, cardiac output, and temperature regulation, specific illness or injury often puts the geriatric patient "over the edge," presenting as a generalized deterioration in the patient's condition.

Aging causes a decrease in primary antibody response and cellular immunity and elevations in the amount of abnormal immunoglobulins and immune complexes.[2] These physiological changes increase the risk of infection, autoimmune disorders, and perhaps cancer. In addition, infections may not manifest in a classical manner.

Many geriatric patients consume less than the minimum daily requirement of most vitamins,[5] which may be a result of loneliness and depression, decreased sensitivity to taste, decreased appetite, financial difficulties, physical infirmity, decreased vision, or a combination of these elements, all of which may act to reduce the motivation to shop for and prepare fresh food. Other factors associated with poor nutrition are poor dentition and reduced mastication, decreased esophageal motility, frequent hypochlorhydria, and decreased intestinal secretions that reduce absorption. Geriatric patients easily can become victims of malnutrition, causing dehydration and hypoglycemia.

? CRITICAL THINKING

What effects can poor nutrition have on body function?

NOTE

About one in eight deaths in geriatric patients results from cancer.[6] Unlike younger patients, in whom cancer often is the main or only disease, geriatric patients frequently have concurrent disease processes and disabilities. Therefore signs and symptoms such as a change in bowel habits, rectal bleeding, malaise, fatigue, weight loss, and anorexia may result from other maladies. Treatment with chemotherapy frequently results in immunosuppression, which increases the risk of infection and often masks the typical signs and symptoms associated with infection.

General Principles in Assessment of the Geriatric Patient

Normal physiological changes and underlying acute or chronic illness may make evaluation of an ill or injured geriatric patient a challenge. In addition to the components of a normal physical assessment (described in Chapter 14), the paramedic

should consider special characteristics of geriatric patients that can complicate the clinical evaluation[7]:

- Geriatric patients are likely to suffer from concurrent illness.
  - Chronic problems can make assessment for acute problems difficult.
  - Signs or symptoms of chronic illness can be confused with signs or symptoms of an acute problem.
- Aging can affect an individual's response to illness or injury.
  - Pain may be diminished or absent.
  - The patient or paramedic can underestimate the severity of a condition.
- Social and emotional factors may have a greater influence on health in geriatric patients than in any other age group.
  - The patient fears losing autonomy.
  - The patient fears the hospital environment.
  - The patient has financial concerns about health care.

Patient History

Gathering a history from a geriatric patient usually requires more time than with younger patients (see Chapter 12). In addition to a longer medical history because of the patient's advanced age, chronic illness, and medication use, the geriatric patient may have physical impediments such as hearing loss and visual impairment. Questioning a patient who is fatigued or easily distracted also may lengthen the interview process. The paramedic should use the following techniques when communicating with geriatric patients:

- Always identify yourself.
- Speak at eye level to ensure that the patient can see you as you communicate.
- Locate a hearing aid, eyeglasses, and dentures (if needed).
- Turn on lights.
- Speak slowly, distinctly, and respectfully.
- Use the patient's surname, unless he or she requests otherwise.
- Listen closely.
- Be patient.
- Preserve dignity.
- Use gentleness.

Physical Examination

When conducting the physical examination of a geriatric patient, the paramedic should consider the following six points:

1. The patient may fatigue easily.
2. Geriatric patients commonly wear many layers of clothing for warmth, which may hamper the examination.
3. Respect the patient's modesty and need for privacy unless it interferes with care procedures.
4. Explain actions clearly before examining all geriatric patients, especially those with diminished sight.
5. Be aware that the patient may minimize or deny symptoms through fear of being bedridden or institutionalized or losing self-sufficiency.
6. Try to distinguish symptoms of chronic disease from acute immediate problems.

If time permits, the paramedic should evaluate the geriatric patient's immediate surroundings for evidence of alcohol or medication use (e.g., insulin syringes, "vial of life," or medic-alert information), presence of food items, general condition of housing, and signs of adequate personal hygiene. These and other observations help provide information to the physician regarding the patient's general health and ability for self-care after release from the hospital. If friends or family members are available, the paramedic should ask them about the patient's appearance and responsiveness *now* versus his or her normal appearance, responsiveness, and other char-

acteristics. The paramedic should ensure gentle handling and adequate padding for patient comfort if ambulance transportation is necessary.

System Pathophysiology, Assessment, and Management

The pathophysiology, assessment, and management of specific illnesses described in this section include those of the pulmonary system (see Chapter 27), cardiovascular system (see Chapter 28), CNS (see Chapter 29), endocrine system (see Chapter 30), gastrointestinal (GI) system (see Chapter 32), integumentary system (see Chapter 6), musculoskeletal system (see Chapter 26), and problems associated with special senses. Toxicology (see Chapter 34), environmental considerations (see Chapter 36), behavioral and psychiatric disorders (see Chapter 38), trauma (see Division Four), and elder abuse (see Chapter 44) are also discussed in this section.

Pulmonary System

Bacterial Pneumonia

Pneumonia is a leading cause of death in the geriatric age group and often is fatal in frail adults.[7] In addition, geriatric patients are more likely to develop bacteremia and are more susceptible to several respiratory pathogens (e.g., gram-negative bacilli). This susceptibility, associated with the presence of chronic disease, impairs respiratory tract clearance and allows pharyngeal colonization by pathogens that may be aspirated into the lungs. Because of the decreased pulmonary reserve in geriatric patients, pneumonia may commonly be associated with respiratory failure. Risk factors for bacterial pneumonia include institutionalized environments, chronic diseases, and immune compromise.

Unlike in younger patients with bacterial pneumonia, the usual clinical picture of pyrexia, productive cough, pleurisy, and signs of pulmonary consolidation often is absent in the geriatric patient. This atypical presentation is responsible for the common delay in diagnosis. The following are possible signs and symptoms:

- Fever (variable)
- Cough
- Shortness of breath
- Alterations in mental status
- Tachycardia
- Tachypnea

NOTE

Geriatric patients with pneumonia may be too weak to effectively cough or produce sputum and may not be able to breathe deeply. Therefore breath sounds may be misleading because of preexisting emphysema or chronic CHF. Tachycardia and tachypnea often are the most reliable indicators of bacterial pneumonia in the prehospital setting.

The paramedic focuses emergency care for geriatric patients with bacterial pneumonia on managing life threats, maintaining oxygenation, and providing transportation for physician evaluation. Bacterial pneumonia is associated with a high rate of hospital admission and generally is managed with specific antibiotic agents.

? CRITICAL THINKING

Why is influenza season associated with an increase in the incidence of pneumonia in geriatric patients?

Chronic Obstructive Pulmonary Disease

Chronic obstructive pulmonary disease (COPD) in the geriatric patient is a major health problem in the United States. COPD is a common finding in the geriatric patient with a history of cigarette smoking and usually is associated with various disease processes (e.g., asthma, emphysema, and chronic bronchitis) that result in reduced expiratory air flow. An exacerbation of COPD often follows an acute respiratory infection that causes airway edema, bronchial smooth muscle irritability, and increased

mucus secretion. These airway abnormalities may lead to factors associated with acute decompensation, including the following:

- Limited air flow
- Increased work of breathing
- Dyspnea
- Ventilation-perfusion mismatching
- Hypoxemia
- Respiratory acidosis
- Hemodynamic compromise

Signs and symptoms of COPD in the geriatric patient include cyanosis, wheezing, and abnormal or diminished breath sounds associated with marked dyspnea and the use of accessory muscles. Other signs and symptoms include dysrhythmias, paradoxical breathing, jugular vein distention, decreased oxygen saturation levels (per pulse oximetry), and extreme anxiety. The paramedic should obtain a thorough history of the event (including a history of intubation or steroid therapy) and be prepared for aggressive airway management. The paramedic focuses emergency management of COPD on correcting life-threatening hypoxemia and improving air flow. The paramedic accomplishes these approaches in the prehospital setting through the use of airway and ventilatory support with supplemental oxygenation and administration of bronchodilators by inhalation or injection (per medical direction).

NOTE

Failure to initiate aggressive management to correct the acidosis and hypoxia from COPD can lead to progressive deterioration.

Pulmonary Embolism

Pulmonary embolism is a life-threatening cause of dyspnea that is associated with venous stasis, heart failure, COPD, malignancy, and immobilization, all of which are common in older adults. Most pulmonary emboli in geriatric patients arise indirectly from the leg veins with propagation to the iliofemoral veins. The clinical presentation of pulmonary embolism often is misleading in geriatric patients and frequently is misdiagnosed.[2]

Signs and symptoms of pulmonary embolism may range from a presentation of left ventricular failure with sudden tachypnea, unexplained tachycardia (a hallmark sign), and atrial fibrillation to signs and symptoms solely of the underlying venous thrombosis (calf discomfort without tenderness, mild calf or ankle edema, increased warmth, and dilation of superficial veins in one foot or leg). Pulmonary embolism can precipitate CHF and also may masquerade as bacterial pneumonia in geriatric patients.

? CRITICAL THINKING

What other conditions present with similar cardiovascular signs and symptoms?

The paramedic focuses emergency care on ensuring adequate airway, ventilatory, and circulatory support; immobilizing and elevating an affected extremity; and rapidly transporting the patient for physician evaluation. In-hospital care may include analgesics, bed rest, hemodynamic stabilization with intravenous (IV) fluids and vasopressors to support blood pressure, and efforts to prevent further embolization. The physician may give some patients thrombolytics to lyse the thrombus and place them on a regimen of anticoagulant therapy.

Cardiovascular System

Myocardial Infarction

Chest pain as a symptom of myocardial infarction (MI) becomes less frequent by 70 years of age, and only 45% of patients over 85 years of age with MI have this complaint. Lack of typical chest pain can cause MI to go unrecognized in the geriatric patient.[3] The following are six major risk factors that the paramedic should evaluate when assessing a patient for MI:

1. Previous MI
2. Angina
3. Diabetes
4. Hypertension
5. High cholesterol level
6. Smoking

NOTE

The mortality rate associated with acute MI doubles after 70 years of age.[7]

Although some geriatric patients have chest pain or discomfort, many complain only of vague symptoms such as dyspnea (the most common sign in patients over 85 years of age), abdominal or epigastric distress, and fatigue. For many geriatric patients the event is completely "silent," which may be a result of decreased visceral sensory function or a higher incidence of mental deterioration in this age group. Silent MIs are almost always marked by an atypical complaint, such as fatigue, breathlessness, nausea, or abdominal pain.

? CRITICAL THINKING

What hormonal change in older women increases their risk for heart disease?

NOTE

The paramedic must maintain a high index of suspicion for MI in patients with unusual or absent warning signs or symptoms.

Emergency care includes airway, ventilatory, and circulatory support; oxygen administration and pain management therapy; management of serious dysrhythmias according to advanced life support (ALS) protocol; and rapid and gentle transportation for physician evaluation.

Heart Failure

Heart failure is more frequent in geriatric patients and has a larger incidence of noncardiac causes. It occurs when the ventricular output is insufficient to meet the metabolic demands of the body. Heart failure often is caused by ischemic heart disease, valvular heart disease, cardiomyopathy, dysrhythmias, hyperthyroidism, and anemia. The following are common signs and symptoms of heart failure:

- Dyspnea
- Fatigue (often the first symptom of left-sided heart failure)
- Orthopnea
- Dry, hacking cough progressing to productive cough with frothy sputum
- Dependent edema due to right-sided heart failure

- Nocturia
- Anorexia, hepatomegaly, ascites

> **NOTE**
>
> Differentiating among the causes of dyspnea is difficult (but important) in the prehospital setting. If the patient has had acute episodes of heart failure in the past, the current emergency event also is likely to be heart failure.[8] A thorough patient history is important.

The paramedic must reverse the conditions associated with heart failure as soon as possible to prevent cardiac damage. In addition to oxygen administration and electrocardiograph (ECG) monitoring, management may include intubation, IV therapy, and drug therapy (*furosemide* [Lasix], *nitroglycerin, morphine*).

> **? CRITICAL THINKING**
>
> *How do furosemide, nitroglycerin, and morphine work to relieve the signs and symptoms of heart failure?*

> **BOX 43-2**
>
> ### SIGNS AND SYMPTOMS OF ABDOMINAL AND THORACIC ANEURYSM
>
> Unexplained hypotension
> Sudden onset of abdominal or back pain
> Syncope
> Low back pain or flank pain
> Pulsatile, tender mass
> Diminished distal pulses
> Chest pain
> Syncope
> Stroke
> Hypotension
> Absent or reduced pulses
> Heart failure
> Pericardial tamponade
> Acute myocardial infarction

Dysrhythmias

The most common cause of dysrhythmias in the geriatric patient is hypertensive heart disease,[7] although any condition that decreases myocardial blood flow also can produce cardiac rhythm disturbances. When assessing dysrhythmias in the geriatric patient, the paramedic should consider the following:

- Premature ventricular contractions (PVCs) frequently are present in most adults over 80 years of age.
- Atrial fibrillation is the most common dysrhythmia.
- Dysrhythmias may result from electrolyte imbalances.

In addition to the serious implications of some dysrhythmias, associated complications may include traumatic injury from falls that result from cerebral hypoperfusion, transient ischemic attacks (TIAs), and heart failure. The paramedic should focus emergency care on ensuring adequate airway, ventilatory, and circulatory support; administering oxygen; and transporting the patient for physician evaluation. The paramedic should manage serious dysrhythmias as described in Chapter 28.

Abdominal and Thoracic Aneurysm

Atherosclerotic disease is a common cause of abdominal and thoracic aneurysm. Abdominal aortic aneurysm affects about 2% to 4% of the U.S. population over 50 years of age.[4] Acute dissecting aortic aneurysm is more common than abdominal aneurysm and is associated with a high mortality rate. Signs and symptoms vary according to the site of rupture or extent of dissection (Box 43-2).

The goals of prehospital care are relief of pain and immediate transportation to a medical facility. Airway, ventilatory, and circulatory support may be required if the patient decompensates. Other prehospital care measures include the following:

- Gentle handling of the patient
- Decreasing anxiety
- High-concentration oxygen administration
- Large-bore IV access to restrict fluids unless severe hypotension is present
- Pain medication per medical direction

Hypertension

The incidence of hypertension in the geriatric patient increases when atherosclerosis is present. Associated risk factors include advanced age, diabetes, and obesity. Hypertension often is defined by a resting blood pressure consistently greater than 140/90 mm Hg.[9] (Blood pressure greater than 160/95 mm Hg doubles the mortality rate in men.[7]) Chronic hypertension is associated with many medical conditions, including the following:

- Myocardial ischemia and infarction
- Cardiac hypertrophy and left ventricular failure
- Kidney failure
- Blindness
- Stroke
- Peripheral vascular disease
- Aneurysm formation

Hypertension in the geriatric patient often presents as memory loss.[7] Other signs and symptoms that may indicate chronic hypertension include epistaxis, tremors, and nausea and vomiting. Prehospital care primarily is supportive. In severe cases, medical direction may recommend the administration of antihypertensives (e.g., *labetalol* [Normodyne]). The physician evaluates the patient with chronic hypertension and often manages him or her with oral medications, dietary sodium reduction, weight loss, and exercise.

Neurology

Cerebral Vascular Disease

Stroke is the third leading cause of death in most countries and the leading cause of brain injury in adults.[3] The neurological impairment is caused by either an ischemic or hemorrhagic interruption in the blood supply to the brain. Associated risk factors for cerebral vascular disease in the older adult include smoking, hypertension, diabetes, atherosclerosis, hyperlipidemia, polycythemia, and heart disease. Box 43-3 provides a review of the signs and symptoms of stroke and TIA (see Chapter 28).

Once the paramedic suspects stroke, he or she must *minimize time in the field* because there is limited time to initiate therapy (less than 3 hours from onset is recommended for fibrinolytic therapy). The paramedic should focus prehospital care on managing the patient's airway, breathing, and circulation, and monitoring vital signs. Aside from supporting vital functions, the most important element of prehospital care for a stroke victim is identification of the patient with stroke and rapid transportation of the patient to a stroke center that can provide treatment within 1 hour after arrival at the emergency department door.[10]

? CRITICAL THINKING

What factors can cause a delay between the onset of signs and symptoms of stroke in the geriatric patient and when an emergency telephone call is made?

Delirium

Delirium is an abrupt disorientation to time and place, usually with illusions and hallucinations. The patient's mind may "wander," speech may be incoherent, and the patient may be in a state of mental confusion or excitement. Delirium commonly is a result of physical illness. Signs and symptoms vary according to personality, environment, and severity of illness. Causes of delirium are associated with organic brain dysfunction and include the following:

- Tumor
- Metabolic disorders
- Fever
- Drug reactions
- Alcohol intoxication or withdrawal

Delirium is potentially life threatening and requires emergency care. The condition may be reversible if diagnosed early but can progress to chronic mental dysfunction. Prehospital care includes the following measures[8]:

BOX 43-3

SIGNS AND SYMPTOMS OF STROKE AND TRANSIENT ISCHEMIC ATTACK

Unilateral paralysis
Numbness
Language disturbance
Visual disturbance
Monocular blindness
Vertigo
Diplopia
Ataxia

1. Ensure adequate airway, breathing, and circulatory support.
   a. Manage hypoxia with oxygen.
   b. Manage hypotension with IV fluids if appropriate.
2. Reduce agitation and anxiety.
3. Avoid patient injury, and ensure personal safety.
   a. Restrain if necessary per protocol.
   b. Sedate as a last resort.
4. Consider hypoglycemia or a narcotic state.
   a. Measure blood glucose level.
   b. Administer *dextrose 50%* or *naloxone* (Narcan) per protocol.
5. Assess for CNS injury (e.g., trauma or stroke), and perform a careful neurological examination.
6. Look for signs of CNS infection (e.g., encephalitis).
7. Transport the patient for physician evaluation.

Dementia

Dementia is a slow, progressive loss of awareness of time and place, usually with an inability to learn new things or remember recent events. This condition often is a result of brain disease caused by strokes, genetic or viral factors, and Alzheimer's disease. Dementia generally is considered irreversible and eventually results in total dependence on others as a result of the progressive loss of cognitive functioning. During the course of the disease, patients often attempt to "cover up" their memory loss by *confabulation* (making up stories to fill gaps in memory). Sudden outbursts or embarrassing behavior may be the first obvious signs of dementia. Some patients eventually regress to a "second childhood" and require total care for feedings, toileting, and physical activity.

> **NOTE**
>
> Dementia is present in about 50% of nursing home residents and affects, to some degree, about 20% of those over 80 years of age.[4]

Dementia can be difficult to differentiate from delirium in the prehospital setting. The key difference between the two conditions is that delirium is "new" with rapid onset and dementia is progressive (Table 43-2). Therefore a history of the event from a reliable witness (e.g., friend or family member) is the best source of information because a history provided by the patient is unreliable. If a reliable witness is not available, the paramedic should manage the patient for delirium that may be a life-threatening emergency.

Alzheimer's Disease

Alzheimer's disease is a condition in which nerve cells in the cerebral cortex die and the brain substance shrinks. It is the single most common cause of dementia and is responsible for the majority of cases in persons over 75 years of age.[2] Alzheimer's disease does not directly cause death; patients ultimately stop eating and become malnourished and immobilized so that they are prone to intercurrent infections. The cause of Alzheimer's disease is not known. The following are possible causes:

- Abnormalities in glutamate metabolism
- Chronic infection
- Toxic poisoning by metals
- Reduction in brain chemicals (e.g., acetylcholine)
- Genetics

> **NOTE**
>
> Atherosclerosis is *not* a cause of Alzheimer's disease. The primary disorder is in the nerve cells, not the blood vessels.

Early symptoms of Alzheimer's disease primarily are related to memory loss, especially the ability to make and recall new memories. As the disease progresses, agitation, violence, and impairment of

TABLE 43-2	DIFFERENTIAL DIAGNOSIS FOR DELIRIUM AND DEMENTIA	
DELIRIUM		**DEMENTIA**
Abrupt		Gradual
Reduced attention span		Impaired recent memory
Disorganized thinking		Regression
Hallucinations		Poor judgment

abstract thinking commence. Judgment and cognitive abilities begin to interfere with work and social interactions. In advanced stages of Alzheimer's disease, patients often become bedridden and totally unaware of their surroundings. Once the patient is bedridden, bedsores, feeding problems, and pneumonia shorten life expectancy.

No specific treatment exists for Alzheimer's disease apart from the provision of nursing and social care for the patient and relatives. In the prehospital setting, the paramedic manages patients with Alzheimer's disease as previously described for dementia.

Parkinsons's Disease

As described in Chapter 29, Parkinson's disease is a brain disorder (caused by degeneration of or damage to nerve cells in the basal ganglia) that causes muscle tremor, stiffness, and weakness. Characteristic signs of Parkinson's disease are trembling (usually beginning in one hand, arm, or leg), a rigid posture, slow movements, and a shuffling, unbalanced walk. If left untreated, the disease progresses over 10 to 15 years to severe weakness and incapacity. Parkinson's disease affects about 1 person in 200 (mostly older adults), with 50,000 new cases diagnosed in the United States each year.[7]

Emergency care for these patients primarily is supportive and includes airway, ventilatory, and circulatory support and transportation for physician evaluation. Although there is no cure for Parkinson's disease, counseling, exercise, special aids in the home, and drug therapy can improve the patient's morale, mobility, and quality of life.

Endocrinology

Diabetes

About 20% of older adults have diabetes, and almost 40% have some impaired glucose tolerance.[7] Type II (non–insulin-dependent) diabetes is most common in geriatric patients, especially when the person is overweight. The following are associated risk factors for complications related to diabetes:

- Decreased ability to care for self
- Living alone
- Intercurrent illness
- Decline in renal function
- Polydrug use

NOTE

Hyperglycemic hyperosmolar nonketotic coma (HHNK) is a serious complication of elderly type II diabetics with a mortality rate of 20% to 50%.[2] The paramedic often finds the type II diabetic patient comatose or complaining of profound polydipsia and polyuria from the osmotic diuresis, leading to dehydration and electrolyte loss. Predisposing factors that make the geriatric patients susceptible to HHNK include infection, noncompliance with medications, polydrug use, pancreatitis, stroke, hypothermia, heat stroke, and MI. If the paramedic suspects HHNK, he or she should vigorously search for an underlying cause; ensure adequate airway, ventilatory, and circulatory support; initiate IV therapy; and rapidly transport the patient for physician evaluation.

? CRITICAL THINKING

What prehospital assessment finding that is present in the patient with diabetic ketoacidosis is absent in the patient with HHNK?

A combination of dietary measures, weight reduction, and oral hypoglycemic agents can usually keep type II diabetes under control. In most cases, insulin injections are not required for type II diabetes. However, if uncontrolled, diabetes can lead to complications that include retinopathy, peripheral neuropathy (ulcers on the feet are common), and kidney damage. Diabetics also have a higher-than-average risk of atherosclerosis, hypertension and other cardiovascular disorders, and cataracts. Emergency care for diabetic patients is outlined in Chapter 30 and includes airway, ventilatory, and circulatory support; blood glucose screening; IV *dextrose* (if indicated and in the absence of cerebral damage); and transportation for physician evaluation.

Thyroid Disease

Thyroid disease is more common in geriatric patients and may be related to the aging process. The classic signs and symptoms of thyroid disorders (described in Chapter 30) often are not present in the geriatric patient. Therefore the paramedic should suspect thyroid dysfunction in any geriatric patient who is ill. The following are thyroid diseases and their signs and symptoms common to the geriatric patient:

1. Hyperthyroidism
   a. Weight loss
   b. Mental status changes
   c. CHF
   d. Tachydysrhythmias
   e. Lethargy
   f. Constipation
2. Hypothyroidism
   a. Weight loss
   b. Nonspecific musculoskeletal complaints
   c. CHF
   d. Anemia
   e. Altered mental status (e.g., dementia, depression, coma, or seizures)
   f. Hyponatremia

Emergency care primarily is supportive to ensure vital functions. The physician evaluates the patient with thyroid disease and treats him or her with various thyroid drugs, radioactive iodine treatments, and sometimes surgery. Severe complications from thyroid disease include thyroid storm and myxedema coma (described in Chapter 30), which may be complicated by coexisting coronary artery disease.

Gastroenterology

Gastrointestinal Hemorrhage

GI bleeding most commonly affects patients between 60 and 90 years of age and has a mortality rate of about 10%. The older the patient, the higher the risk of death. This higher risk is because of the following characteristics of geriatric patients[8]:

- Less able to compensate for acute blood loss
- Less likely to feel symptoms and therefore seek treatment at later stages of disease
- More likely to be taking *aspirin* or nonsteroidal antiinflammatory drugs (NSAIDs), which places them at higher risk for ulcer disease and bleeding

> **NOTE**
>
> The paramedic should always consider abdominal pain a serious complaint in a geriatric patient. Life-threatening causes of abdominal pain in this age group include abdominal aortic aneurysm, GI hemorrhage, ruptured viscus, dead or ischemic bowel, and acute bowel obstruction.

- At higher risk for colon cancer, intestinal vascular abnormalities, and diverticulitis
- More likely to be on blood-thinning medications

Signs and symptoms of GI bleeding include vomiting of blood or coffee-ground emesis; blood-tinged stools or black, tarry stools; and weakness, syncope, or pain. If the paramedic suspects or confirms bleeding in a patient with signs and symptoms of shock, he or she should initiate measures to ensure adequate airway, ventilatory, and circulatory support and rapidly transport the patient for definitive care.

Bowel Obstruction

Bowel obstruction generally occurs in patients with prior abdominal surgeries or hernias and in those with colonic cancer. Most complain of constipation, abdominal cramping, and an inability to pass gas. Other signs and symptoms include protracted vomiting of foodstuffs or bile and vomiting of fecal material. The patient's heart rate and blood pressure often are in normal ranges, and the abdomen may be mildly distended and tender in all four quadrants (abdominal pain is variable).

Prehospital care primarily is supportive to ensure vital functions. The physician evaluates the patient and treats him or her conservatively with bowel rest, nasogastric suction, and hydration. The patient sometimes needs surgery to lyse the offending adhesions, which may result in a cycle of new scarring and obstruction, or for hernia repair (most commonly in men).

Problems with Continence

Continence is the ability to control bladder or bowel function. It requires anatomically correct GI and genitourinary (GU) tracts, competent sphincter mechanisms, cognitive and physical function, and motivation. Some factors associated with continence are affected by age and include a decrease in bladder capacity, involuntary bladder contractions, decreased ability to postpone voiding, and medications that can affect bladder and bowel control. *Incontinence* of urine or bowel is abnormal at any age. The following are causes of incontinence:

1. Bladder incontinence
   a. Injury or disease of the urinary tract
   b. Prolapse of the uterus

c. Decline in sphincter muscle control surrounding the urethra (common in geriatric patients)

d. Damage to the brain or spinal cord with seizures

e. Pelvis fracture

f. Prostate cancer

g. Dementia

2. Bowel incontinence

a. Fecal impaction

b. Severe diarrhea

c. Injury to anal muscles (e.g., from childbirth or surgery)

d. Damage to the brain or spinal cord with seizures

e. Dementia

Urinary incontinence can vary in severity from mild incontinence (the escape of small amounts of urine) to total incontinence (the complete loss of bladder control). Bowel incontinence in the geriatric patient usually is the result of fecal impaction. Feces that are lodged in the rectum irritate and inflame the lining and may allow fecal fluid and small feces to pass involuntarily. All forms of incontinence usually are embarrassing for the patient and, if chronic, can lead to skin irritation, tissue breakdown, and urinary tract infection. Some cases of incontinence are managed surgically to restore sphincter function. Patients with mild cases often wear absorptive undergarments to relieve discomfort and embarrassment.

? CRITICAL THINKING

How can you minimize the incontinent patient's embarrassment and discomfort?

Problems with Elimination

Causes of difficulty in urination usually result from enlargement of the prostate (in men), urinary tract infection, urethral strictures, and acute or chronic renal failure. Difficulty in bowel elimination often is associated with diverticular disease, constipation, and colorectal cancer. Problems with elimination can cause extreme pain and anxiety for geriatric patients, and the paramedic should take their complaints seriously. These conditions require physician evaluation to identify the cause and to select an appropriate therapy.

✓ TRICKS OF THE TRADE

Difficulties in "moving the bowels" or "passing water" often are serious concerns for the geriatric patient. The paramedic should not make light of these complaints.

Integumentary Changes

As people age, the skin gradually becomes dry, transparent, and wrinkled. These integumentary changes are associated with a loss of elasticity, uneven pigmentation, and various benign and malignant lesions. In addition, aging results in a gradual decrease in epidermal cellular turnover and a reduced rate of nail and hair growth. The associated loss of deep, dermal vessels and capillary circulation leads to common complaints such as dry, itchy skin; alterations in thermal regulation; and skin-related complications, including the following:

• Slow healing
• Increased risk of secondary infection
• Increased risk of fungal or viral infections
• Increased susceptibility to abrasions and tears

The paramedic should always be gentle with the skin of a geriatric patient when performing medical procedures. Examples include use of aseptic technique during wound management, gentle placement and removal of ECG electrodes, and employment of careful taping procedures when securing IV catheters or tubing.

? CRITICAL THINKING

How do these changes influence the recovery of a geriatric patient who has a burn injury?

Pressure Ulcers

Pressure ulcers are common in geriatric patients (Fig. 43-1). They often develop on the skin of patients who are bedridden or immobile (e.g., *decubitus ulcers*). Most pressure ulcers occur in the lower legs, back, and buttocks, and over bony areas such as the greater trochanter or the sacrum. They commonly affect victims of stroke or other illnesses that result in a loss or alteration in the sensation of pain.

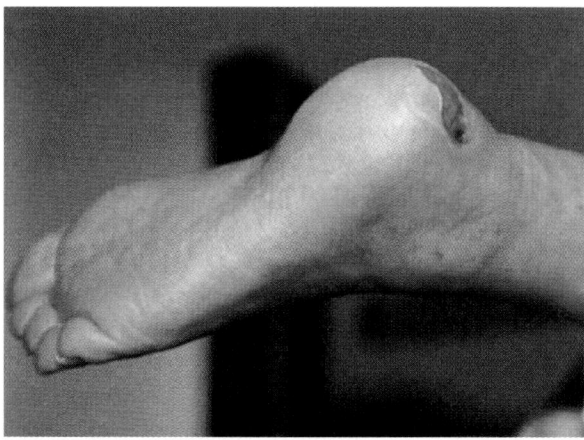

Fig. 43-1 Pressure ulcer. (From Potter PA, Perry AG: *Fundamentals of nursing,* ed 4, St Louis, 1997, Mosby.)

Skin exposure to moisture (e.g., from incontinence), poor nutrition, and friction or shear also may be factors for developing pressure ulcers. Other causes of pressure ulcers in geriatric patients include vascular and metabolic disorders (e.g., venous stasis and diabetes), trauma, and cancer.

Pressure ulcers result from tissue hypoxia. They generally start as red, painful areas that become purple before the skin breaks down, developing into open sores. Once integrity of the skin has been breached, the sores often become infected, after which they are slow to heal. The paramedic should cover pressure ulcers with sterile dressing using aseptic technique. The paramedic should then transport the patient for physician evaluation and wound care to facilitate healing.

Musculoskeletal Changes
Osteoarthritis

Osteoarthritis (degenerative arthritis) is a common form of arthritis in geriatric patients that results from cartilage loss and wear and tear on the joints. The condition leads to pain, stiffness, and occasionally loss of function of the affected joint. Often the affected joint becomes large and distorted from outgrowths of new bone (*osteophytes*) that tend to develop at the margins of the joint surface. Osteoarthritis evolves in middle years and occurs to some extent in almost all people over 60 years of age, although some have no symptoms. After physician evaluation, treatment may include medications (analgesics, NSAIDs, corticosteroids), physical therapy, and sometimes joint-replacement surgery.

> **NOTE**
>
> Newer drugs *(COX-2 inhibitors)* relieve the inflammation and pain associated with arthritis with less risk of causing stomach irritation than traditional medications such as **aspirin,** NSAIDs, and ibuprofen. Examples of these newer drugs include celecoxib (Celebrex) and rofecoxib (Vioxx).

Osteoporosis

Osteoporosis is a natural part of aging. It especially is common in older women after menopause because of a decrease in the estrogen hormone that helps maintain bone mass. Osteoporosis is present in most people by 70 years of age, by which time the density of the skeleton has diminished by one third. Most people with osteoporosis have some degree of kyphosis.

The loss of bone density causes bones to become brittle and easily fractured, which often is the first sign of osteoporosis. Typical sites for fractures are just above the wrist, at the head of the femur, and at one of several vertebrae (often a spontaneous fracture). Osteoporosis is treated with preventive measures, such as a diet high in calcium, calcium supplements, exercise, and hormone replacement therapy after menopause.

Special Problems with Sensations

As people age, they may experience problems with vision, hearing, and speech.

Problems with Vision

Vision changes begin to occur at around 40 years of age and gradually increase over time. Vision impairments can severely limit daily activities and lead to a loss of independence in geriatric patients. The following are some effects of aging on vision:

- Reading difficulties
- Poor depth perception
- Poor adjustment of the eyes to variations in distance
- Altered color perception
- Sensitivity to light
- Decreased visual acuity

Two common eye conditions that develop with age are cataracts and glaucoma. A cataract is a loss of transparency of the lens of the eye that results from changes in the delicate protein fibers within the lens. A cataract never completely causes blindness, but clarity and detail of an image progressively are lost. Cataracts usually occur in both eyes, but in most cases one eye is affected more severely than the other. Almost everyone over 65 years of age has some degree of cataract, and most persons over 75 years of age have minor visual deterioration from the disorder. Surgery to remove the cataract is a common procedure in the United States.

Glaucoma is a condition in which intraocular pressure increases and causes damage to the optic nerve. The result is nerve fiber destruction and partial or complete loss of peripheral and central vision. Glaucoma may result from aging (rarely seen before 40 years of age), a congenital abnormality, or trauma to the eye. It is the most common major eye disorder in persons over 60 years of age and is the leading cause of preventable blindness in the United States.[11] Symptoms of acute glaucoma include dull, severe, aching pain in and above the eye; fogginess of vision; and the perception of "rainbow rings" (halos) around lights at night. Testing for glaucoma is part of most eye examinations in adults. If detected early, the condition can be treated with oral medications and eye drops to relieve intraocular pressure.

? CRITICAL THINKING

What prehospital cardiac medication should not be given to the patient who has glaucoma?

Problems with Hearing

Although not all geriatric patients have hearing loss, overall hearing tends to decrease with age from degeneration of the hearing mechanism (*sensorineural* deafness). *Meniere's disease* (increased fluid pressure in the labyrinth), certain drugs, tumors, and some viral infections also can cause hearing problems. Hearing loss can interfere with the ability to perceive speech and thereby limit the ability to communicate. Hearing aid devices and surgical implants can sometimes restore or improve hearing.

Tinnitus can occur as a symptom of many ear disorders. The noise in the ear (e.g., ringing, buzzing, or whistling) sometimes may change in nature and intensity. However, in most cases it is present at all times with intermittent awareness by the person. Tinnitus is almost always associated with hearing loss, especially hearing loss that develops from aging.

? CRITICAL THINKING

What common analgesic, when taken excessively, can cause tinnitus?

Problems with Speech

Speech is the most frequently used method of human communication. Common problems with speech in geriatric patients often are associated with difficulty in word retrieval, decreased fluency of speech, slowed rate of speech, and changes in voice quality. These disorders may occur from damage to the language centers of the brain (usually as a result of stroke, head injury, or brain tumor), degenerative changes in the nervous system, hearing loss, disorders of the larynx, and poor-fitting dentures.

Toxicology

As described in Chapter 8 and Chapter 34, geriatric patients are at increased risk for adverse drug reactions because of age-related alterations in body composition and drug distribution, because of metabolism and excretion, and because they are often prescribed multiple drugs. The following are drugs that commonly cause toxicity in the geriatric patient:

- *Lidocaine* (Xylocaine)
- Beta blockers
- Antihypertensives
- Diuretics
- Digitalis
- Psychotropics
- Antidepressants

The adverse reactions associated with these and other drugs often result from "accidents" or "mishaps" in the prescribed drug regimen. Box 43-4 provides common reasons for drug-induced illness in the geriatric patient. Box 43-5 provides drugs that elicit symptoms related to drug toxicity and adverse drug reactions in the geriatric patients.[8] Emergency care for geriatric patients with adverse drug reactions may vary from "transport only" to full advanced cardiac life support measures.

BOX 43-4

COMMON CAUSES OF DRUG-INDUCED ILLNESS IN THE GERIATRIC PATIENT

Noncompliance
Confusion
Vision impairment
Self-selection of drugs
Forgetfulness
Multiple prescriptions from more than one physician
Improper resumption of old medications in addition to newly prescribed ones
Excessive dosing of over-the-counter drugs with synergistic or cumulative effects
Changes in habits regarding alcohol, diet, and exercise that may affect drug metabolism
Dispensing error

BOX 43-5

SYMPTOMS OF DRUG TOXICITY AND ADVERSE DRUG REACTIONS IN THE GERIATRIC PATIENT

Acute delirium
Akathisia
Altered vision
Bradycardia
Cardiac dysrhythmias
Chorea
Confusion
Constipation
Coma
Fatigue
Glaucoma
Hypokalemia
Orthostatic hypotension
Paresthesias
Psychological disturbances
Pulmonary edema
Severe bleeding
Tardive dyskinesia
Urinary hesitancy

Alcohol Abuse

Alcohol abuse is a common problem in the geriatric patient and often is attributed to severe stress as the primary risk factor.[7] Signs and symptoms of alcohol abuse may be very subtle, including the following:

- Mood swings
- Denial
- Hostility
- Confusion
- Frequent falling
- Anorexia
- Insomnia

NOTE

Ingestion of even small amounts of alcohol by the geriatric patient can cause intoxication.

If the paramedic suspects alcohol abuse, he or she should discretely interview friends and family members about the patient's alcohol or other drug use. Identification of these patients and appropriate referral by a physician for treatment are the cornerstones of therapy. Treatment of the acutely intoxicated patient is described in Chapter 34 and may include resuscitative measures to manage the patient's airway, ventilation, and circulation. In addition, the paramedic should carefully assess the geriatric patient who has signs and symptoms of acute alcohol intoxication for occult trauma and coexisting medical conditions such as hypoglycemia, cardiomyopathy and dysrhythmias, GI bleeding, polydrug abuse (especially barbiturates and tranquilizers), and ethylene glycol or methanol ingestion.

Environmental Considerations

Hypothermia

Unlike younger patients who experience hypothermia often from environmental extremes, the geriatric patient may develop hypothermia while indoors as a result of cold surroundings and/or accompanying illness that alter heat production or conservation. This is due in part to the following characteristics of older adults:

- They are less able to compensate for environmental heat loss.
- They have a decreased ability to sense changes in ambient temperature.
- They have less total body water to store heat.
- They are less likely to develop tachycardia to increase cardiac output in response to cold stress.
- They have a decreased ability to shiver to increase body heat.

In addition to physiological factors, geriatric patients are more prone to develop hypothermia as a result of socioeconomical factors such as fixed incomes to pay for the cost of heat in the home. This often results in lower ambient temperatures in the home, inefficient insulation (cool and drafty homes), and poorly functioning furnaces. Malnutrition and an associated decrease in fat stores also may be factors in hypothermia in geriatric patients who live alone. The following are other medical causes of hypothermia in geriatric patients:

- Arthritis
- Drug overdose
- Hepatic failure
- Hypoglycemia
- Infection
- Parkinson's disease
- Stroke
- Thyroid disease
- Uremia

The signs and symptoms of hypothermia may be subtle and include an altered mental state, slurred speech, ataxia, and dysrhythmias. In severe cases, coma without signs of life may be present. Hypothermia in the geriatric patient carries a high mortality rate. The paramedic should manage these patients as described in Chapter 36. Rapid and gentle transportation for in-hospital rewarming and life-support measures is crucial for the patient's survival.

Hyperthermia

Hyperthermia in the geriatric patient is less common than hypothermia but carries a significant mortality rate. The condition most likely results from exposure to high environmental temperatures that continue for several days (e.g., during a heat wave). As in hypothermia, the thermoregulatory mechanisms of geriatric patients render them unable to control body temperature even in moderate environmental heat. Hyperthermia also may result from medical conditions such as hypothalamic dys-

BOX 43-6

COMMON CAUSES OF DEPRESSION IN THE GERIATRIC PATIENT

Physiological
Dehydration
Electrolyte imbalance
Fever
Hyponatremia
Hypoxia
Metabolic disturbances
Medications
Organic brain disease
Reduced cardiac output
Thyroid disease

Psychological
Fear of dying
Financial insecurity
Loss of a spouse
Loss of independence
Significant illness

function and spinal cord injury. Certain medications (e.g., antidysrhythmics, beta blockers, and cyclic antidepressants) can lead to hyperthermia by inhibiting heat dissipation, increasing motor activity, and impairing cardiovascular function.

As described in Chapter 36, hyperthermic illness may present as heat cramps, heat exhaustion, or heat stroke. The paramedic focuses emergency care on removing the patient from the warm environment, cooling the patient, and ensuring the patient's vital functions through airway, ventilatory, and circulatory support. Rapid transportation for physician evaluation is indicated to manage the systemic manifestations that may result from serious heat-related illness.

Behavioral and Psychiatric Disorders

Depression

Depression is common in geriatric patients and can result from physiological and psychological causes. Examples include cognitive disorders with organic etiology (e.g., dementia) and various mood disorders such as bipolar disease (described in Chapter 38). Box 43-6 provides common causes of depression in geriatric patients.

Signs and symptoms of depression vary by individual and may include the following:

- Feelings of hopelessness
- Extreme isolation
- Loss of energy (fatigue)
- Irritability
- Sleeplessness
- Loss of appetite
- Significant weight loss
- Decreased libido
- Deep feelings of worthlessness and guilt
- Recurrent thoughts of death
- Suicide attempts

? CRITICAL THINKING

What endocrine disorder can produce signs or symptoms similar to those of depression?

A major goal of prehospital care is to identify the patient who may be depressed so that the paramedic can provide appropriate resources (e.g., physician evaluation and counseling). After determining that there are no physical threats to life, the paramedic should try to establish a rapport with these patients so that he or she can evaluate their mood. If possible the paramedic should interview family members to gather information about the patient's mental state and any history of depression.

NOTE

Depression is a serious illness that requires physician evaluation.

Suicide

The rate of completed suicides for geriatric patients is higher than that of the general population, and most of these people visited their primary care physician in the month before the suicide.[12] Most were suffering from their first episode of major depression, which was only moderately severe, yet the depressive symptoms went unrecognized and untreated. The paramedic should therefore be aware of the increased risk for suicide when evaluating geriatric patients who are depressed.

NOTE

The highest rate of completed suicide occurs in white men over 65 years of age. White men 85 years of age and older have a suicide rate that is six times the overall national rate.[12]

As described in Chapter 38, there is no evidence that questions about suicidal thoughts and feelings increase the risk of suicide. Many depressed people are willing to discuss their suicidal thoughts; therefore the paramedic should question the patient about suicidal thoughts if he or she suspects that the patient is at high risk. The following questions are appropriate for the paramedic to ask the patient:

1. Do you have thoughts about killing yourself?
2. Have you ever tried to kill yourself?
3. Have you thought about how you might kill yourself?

NOTE

Safety of the scene and EMS crew is a priority when caring for a patient with suicidal tendencies. When indicated, law enforcement personnel should be available at the scene.

After assessing the risk for suicidal tendencies, the paramedic should transport the patient for physician evaluation. While en route to the hospital, the paramedic should encourage the patient to discuss his or her feelings and reassure the patient that he or she can be helped through the crisis.

Trauma

Trauma is the fifth leading cause of death for persons over 65 years of age. One third of traumatic deaths in people 65 to 74 years of age are secondary

✔ TRICKS OF THE TRADE

Do not be surprised if a geriatric patient suffers an injury while jogging or playing tennis. Not all older adults limit their physical activity to watching television, knitting, and baby-sitting their grandchildren.

to vehicular trauma, and 25% result from falls. In those older than 80 years of age, falls account for 50% of injury-related deaths.[13] Burns also are a major cause of disability and death in geriatric patients.

Vehicular Trauma

More than 15 million licensed drivers are over 65 years of age. In 1996, more than 3000 deaths in this age group were attributed to motor vehicle crashes.[13] Most of these vehicle collisions are not related to high speed or alcohol but rather to errors in perception or judgment or to delayed reaction time. In addition, although a large number of older adults are injured as drivers or passengers in moving vehicles, more than 2000 pedestrian fatalities among older adults occur each year in the United States, accounting for 20% of all pedestrian deaths from trauma.

The risk of fatality from multiple trauma is estimated to be three times greater at 70 years of age than at 20 years of age. This is primarily because the geriatric patient is more susceptible to serious injury from equivalent degrees of trauma and less capable of an appropriate, protective physiological response. Prompt identification of injuries and sources of hemorrhage is critical in any trauma patient, especially the geriatric patient, who has much less cardiac reserve and who will succumb more quickly to shock.

Head Trauma

Head injury with loss of consciousness in geriatric patients often is associated with poor outcome. Among other physiological changes, the aging process may be associated with cerebral atrophy that produces a notable distance between the surface of the brain and the inner tables of the skull. As bridging veins stretch across this subdural space, they more easily are torn, resulting in subdural hematomas. The extra space within the cranial vault often allows a geriatric patient to sustain a significant amount of internal hemorrhage before the volume-pressure relationship of the cranium is exceeded and symptoms are manifested.

> **? CRITICAL THINKING**
>
> *What home medications can also lead to an increased risk of intracerebral bleeding in geriatric patients with head trauma?*

Geriatric patients also are particularly susceptible to injuries of the cervical spine because of progressive arthritic and degenerative changes associated with aging. These structural alterations lead to increased stiffening and decreased flexibility of the spine with narrowing of the spinal canal, which renders the spinal cord much more susceptible to damage from relatively minor trauma.

Chest Injuries

The paramedic must consider a mechanism of injury that suggests thoracic trauma in a geriatric patient potentially lethal. The aged thorax is less elastic and more susceptible to injury, and the pulmonary system has marginal reserve because of a reduced alveolar surface area, decreased patency of small airways, and diminished chemoreceptor response.

Injuries to the heart, aorta, and major vessels are a greater risk to geriatric patients than younger adults, again because of decreased functional reserve and anatomical alterations that make injury in these areas more likely of greater significance. Myocardial contusion may be a complication of blunt injury to the chest and, if severe, may result in pump failure or life-threatening dysrhythmias. Rarely, cardiac tamponade occurs after blunt thoracic trauma. Cardiac rupture, valvular injury (e.g., flail valves), and aortic dissection also may occur with significant blunt chest injury. The first two entities are rare but rapidly fatal. The paramedic should always consider dissecting aortic aneurysm when the mechanism of injury produces rapid deceleration. Aortic dissections often are not immediately fatal, and proper evaluation and treatment can be lifesaving (see Chapter 28).

> **? CRITICAL THINKING**
>
> *What specific physical findings may the paramedic detect in the patient who has a dissecting aortic aneurysm?*

Because of impaired coronary response to increased oxygen demands and commonly occurring underlying conduction disturbance, geriatric patients may develop ischemia and dysrhythmias from significant trauma, even if the heart has not been directly affected. These patients need meticulous attention to their oxygenation and circulatory status.

Abdominal Injuries

Abdominal injuries in geriatric patients have more serious sequelae than those in any other anatomical site. Abdominal injuries often are less apparent, requiring a high degree of suspicion. The geriatric patient also is less likely to tolerate surgery and is more susceptible to postoperative pulmonary and septic complications.

Musculoskeletal Injuries

The osteoporotic bones of geriatric patients are vulnerable to fracture with even mild trauma. Pelvic fractures are highly lethal in this age group, causing severe hemorrhage and associated soft tissue injury. When evaluating for skeletal trauma, the paramedic should remember that the geriatric patient may have decreased pain perception and often surprisingly little tenderness with major fractures. Even with appropriate care, the mortality rate for geriatric patients with musculoskeletal injury is increased by delayed complications such as adult respiratory distress syndrome (ARDS), sepsis, renal failure, and pulmonary embolism.

Falls

Falls are a major cause of morbidity and mortality in older adults, accounting for about 10,000 deaths each year.[13] Approximately one third of older adults living at home fall each year, and 1 in 40 of these persons is hospitalized. A major cause of falls in older adults results from the use of prescribed sedative-hypnotics that affect balance and postural control, such as alprazolam (Xanax), *diazepam* (Valium), chlordiazepoxide (Librium), and flurazepam (Dalmane).

? CRITICAL THINKING

What complications may contribute to an increased mortality rate in geriatric patients who have fallen?

Fractures are the most common fall-related injuries, the hip being the fracture that most often results in hospitalization. In those who survive hip fracture, most will have significant mobility problems and may become more functionally dependent. Falls that do not result in physical injury may lead to self-imposed immobility resulting from the fear of falling again. When immobility is strict and prolonged, joint contractures, pressure sores, urinary tract infection, muscle atrophy, depression, and functional dependency may result.

Assessment. The paramedic should assume that any fall indicates an underlying problem until proved otherwise. The paramedic should attempt to uncover the medical, psychological, and environmental factors that may have been responsible for the fall. For the paramedic to obtain as much information as possible about the falling episode, the patient history should include a comprehensive review of all medical problems and medications and a precise recounting of the fall (history of falling, time of fall, location, symptoms experienced, activity in which the victim was engaged, use of devices, and presence of witnesses). The paramedic should also evaluate the patient's cardiovascular, neurological, and musculoskeletal systems.

Burns

More than 1000 older adults die from fires and burns in the United States each year.[13] The increased risk of morbidity and mortality from burn trauma in older adults is due to preexisting disease, skin changes that result in increased burn depth, altered nutrition, and decreased ability to fight infection. After initial care and resuscitation (described in Chapter 21), geriatric patients with thermal injury require special considerations in fluid therapy to prevent renal tubular damage. The paramedic assesses hydration in the initial hours after burn injury by monitoring pulse and blood pressure and striving to maintain a urine output of at least 50 to 60 mL per hour.

Trauma Management Considerations

Priorities of trauma care for geriatric patients are similar to those for all trauma patients described in Division Four. However, the paramedic should give special consideration to transportation strategies and the geriatric patient's cardiovascular, respiratory, and renal systems.

Cardiovascular system

- Recent or past MI contributes to the risk of dysrhythmias and congestive heart failure.
- Adjustment of heart rate and stroke volume may be decreased in response to hypovolemia.
- Geriatric patients may require higher arterial pressures than younger patients for perfusion of vital organs because of atherosclerotic peripheral vascular disease.

- Rapid IV fluid administration to geriatric patients may precipitate volume overload. The paramedic must take care not to overhydrate these patients because older adults as a group are more susceptible to congestive heart failure; however, hypovolemia and hypotension are also poorly tolerated. The paramedic should consider hypovolemia in any geriatric patient whose systolic blood pressure is less than 120 mm Hg. Tachycardia may not occur if the patient takes beta blockers. The paramedic should monitor lung sounds and vital signs carefully and frequently during fluid administration.

Respiratory system

- Physical changes decrease chest wall compliance and movement and thus diminish vital capacity.
- PaO_2 decreases with age.
- Lower PO_2 at the same fractional inspired oxygen concentration occurs with each passing decade.
- All organ systems have less tolerance to hypoxia.
- COPD (common in geriatric patients) requires that the paramedic carefully adjust airway management and ventilation support for appropriate oxygenation and carbon dioxide removal. High-concentration oxygen may suppress hypoxic drive in some patients, but the paramedic should never withhold this therapy from a patient with clinical signs of cyanosis. (The paramedic may need to remove dentures for adequate airway and ventilation management.)

Renal system

- The kidneys have decreased ability to maintain normal acid-base balance and to compensate for fluid changes.
- Preexisting renal disease may further decrease renal ability to compensate.
- Decreased renal function (along with decreased cardiac reserve) places the injured geriatric patient at risk for fluid overload and pulmonary edema secondary to IV fluid therapy.

Transportation strategies

- Positioning, immobilization, and transportation of a geriatric trauma patient may require modifications to accommodate physical deformities (e.g., arthritis or spinal abnormalities).
- Packaging should include bulk and extra padding to support and provide comfort for the patient.
- The paramedic can prevent hypothermia by keeping the patient warm.

Elder Abuse

Elder abuse refers to the infliction of physical pain, injury, debilitating mental anguish, unreasonable confinement, or willful deprivation by a caregiver of services that are necessary to maintain mental and physical health of a geriatric patient. Elder abuse has become increasingly recognized as a growing problem in the United States, affecting more than 1 million older adults in 1996[14] (see Chapter 44).

Elder abuse is classified as physical abuse, psychological abuse, financial or material abuse, and neglect. All 50 states have elder abuse statutes, and reporting of suspected elder abuse is mandatory under law in most states. If the paramedic suspects abuse or neglect of an older adult, he or she should advise medical direction and follow the procedures established by local protocol. In addition to suspicious physical injuries, some warning signs that a geriatric patient may be the victim of abuse or neglect include the following:

- An upset or agitated state
- Dehydration, malnutrition, or poor personal hygiene
- Hazardous or unsafe living conditions
- Unsanitary and unclean living conditions

SUMMARY

- The aging process proceeds at different rates in different people. Respiratory function in the older adult generally is compromised as a result of changes in pulmonary physiology that accompany the aging process. Cardiac function declines with age as a result of nonischemic physiological changes and the high incidence of atherosclerotic coronary artery disease. Renal blood flow falls an average of 50% between 30 and 80 years of age. A gradual decrease in neurons, decreased cerebral blood flow, and alterations in the location and amounts of specific neurotransmitters probably contribute to alterations in the central nervous system (CNS). As the body ages, muscles shrink, muscles and ligaments calcify, and the intervertebral disks become thin. Other physiological changes that occur with aging include alterations in body mass and total body water, a decreased ability to maintain internal homeostasis, a decrease in the function of immunological mechanisms, nutritional disorders, and decreases in hearing and visual acuity.

- Normal physiological changes and underlying acute or chronic illness may make evaluation of an ill or injured geriatric patient a challenge.

- Pneumonia is a leading cause of death in the geriatric age group and often is fatal in frail adults. Chronic obstructive pulmonary disease (COPD) is a common finding in the geriatric patient who has a history of cigarette smoking and usually is associated with various disease processes that result in reduced expiratory airflow. Pulmonary embolism is a life-threatening cause of dyspnea that is associated with venous stasis, heart failure, COPD, malignancy, and immobilization, all of which are common in older adults.

- Lack of typical chest pain can cause myocardial infarction (MI) to go unrecognized in the geriatric patient. Heart failure is more frequent in geriatric patients and has a larger of noncardiac causes. The most common cause of dysrhythmias in the geriatric patient is hypertensive heart disease. Abdominal aortic aneurysm affects 2% to 4% of the U.S. population over 50 years of age and is most prevalent between 60 and 70 years of age. The incidence of hypertension in the geriatric patient increases when atherosclerosis is present.

- Risk factors for cerebral vascular disease in the older adult include smoking, hypertension, diabetes, atherosclerosis, hyperlipidemia, polycythemia, and heart disease.

- Delirium is an abrupt disorientation of time and place, commonly a result of physical illness.

- Dementia is a slow, progressive loss of awareness of time and place, usually with an inability to learn new things or remember recent events. This condition often is a result of brain disease. Alzheimer's disease, the most common cause of dementia, is a condition in which nerve cells in the cerebral cortex die and the brain substance shrinks.

- Parkinson's disease is a brain disorder that causes muscle tremor, stiffness, and weakness.

- About 20% of older adults have diabetes, and almost 40% have some impaired glucose tolerance. Hyperglycemic hyperosmolar nonketotic coma (HHNK) is a serious complication of elderly type II diabetics with a mortality rate of 20% to 50%. Thyroid disease is more common in geriatric patients and may not present in the classic manner.

- Gastrointestinal (GI) bleeding most commonly affects patients between 60 and 90 years of age and has a mortality rate of about 10%. Bowel obstruction generally occurs in patients with prior abdominal surgeries or hernias and in those with colonic cancer. Some geriatric patients also may experience difficulties with continence or problems with elimination.

- Aging results in a gradual decrease in epidermal cellular turnover and loss of deep, dermal vessels, and capillary circulation leads to alterations in thermal regulation and skin-related complications.

- Osteoarthritis is a common form of arthritis in geriatric patients that results from cartilage loss and wear and tear on the joints. The loss in bone density due to osteoporosis causes bones to become brittle and easily fractured.

- As people age, they may experience problems with vision, hearing, and speech.

- Geriatric patients are at increased risk for adverse drug reactions because of age-related alterations in body composition and drug distribution, because of metabolism and excretion, and because they are often prescribed multiple drugs. Alcohol abuse is a common problem in geriatric patients.

- The geriatric patient may develop hypothermia while indoors as a result of cold surroundings and/or accompanying illness that alter heat production or conservation. Hyperthermia most likely results from exposure to high environmental temperatures that continue for several days.

- Depression is common in geriatric patients and can result from both physiological and psychological causes. The rate of completed suicides for geriatric patients is higher than that of the general population.

- One third of traumatic deaths in people 65 to 74 years of age are secondary to vehicular trauma, and 25% result from falls. In those older than 80 years of age, falls account for 50% of injury-related deaths. The risk of fatality from multiple trauma is estimated to be three times greater at 70 years of age than at 20 years of age.

- Elder abuse is classified as physical abuse, psychological abuse, financial or material abuse, and neglect.

◼ REFERENCES

1. U.S. Senate Special Committee on Aging: *Aging America: trends and projections*, Washington, DC, 1988, U.S. Department of Health and Human Services.
2. Bosker G et al: *Geriatric emergency medicine*, St Louis, 1990, Mosby.
3. American Heart Association: *Advanced cardiac life support*, Dallas, 1997, The Association.
4. Rosen P, Barkin R: *Emergency medicine: concepts and clinical practice*, ed 4, St Louis, 1998, Mosby.
5. Family health almanac: fitness, food, and medicine, *US News and World Report*, 1998.
6. National Centers for Health Statistics, Centers for Disease Control and Prevention: *Health, United States, 1999 with health and aging chartbook*, accessed April 10, 2000. Available at www.cdc.gov/nchs/data/hus99.pdf.
7. U.S. Department of Transportation, National Highway Traffic Safety Administration: *EMT-Paramedic national standard curriculum*, Washington, DC, 1998, The Department.
8. Hogan T: *Geriatric emergencies*, Turlock, Calif, 1994, Medic Alert Foundation.
9. Joint National Committee on Hypertension: *The sixth report of the Joint National Committee on prevention, detection, evaluation, and treatment of high blood pressure*, Washington, DC, 1998, National Institutes of Health, National Heart Lung and Blood Institute.
10. American Heart Association: Guidelines 2000 for cardiopulmonary resuscitation and emergency cardiovascular care, International Consensus on Science, *Circulation* 102(8):204, 2000
11. The Glaucoma Foundation: *About glaucoma*, accessed April 10, 2000. Available at www.glaucoma-foundation. org/about.htm.
12. National Institute of Mental Health: *Frequently asked questions about suicide*, December, 1999. Available at www.nimh.nih.gov/research/suicidefaq.cfm.
13. National Safety Council: *Injury facts*, Chicago, 1999, The Council.
14. Tatara T et al: *Domestic elder abuse information series*, Washington, DC, 1997, National Center on Elder Abuse.

44 Abuse and Neglect

OBJECTIVES

Upon completion of this chapter, the paramedic student will be able to:

1. Define battering.
2. Describe the characteristics of abusive relationships.
3. Outline findings that indicate a battered patient.
4. Describe prehospital considerations when responding to and caring for battered patients.
5. Identify types of elder abuse.
6. Discuss legal considerations related to elder abuse.
7. Describe characteristics of abused children and their abusers.
8. Outline the physical examination of the abused child.
9. Describe the characteristics of sexual assault.
10. Outline prehospital patient care considerations for the patient who has been sexually assaulted.

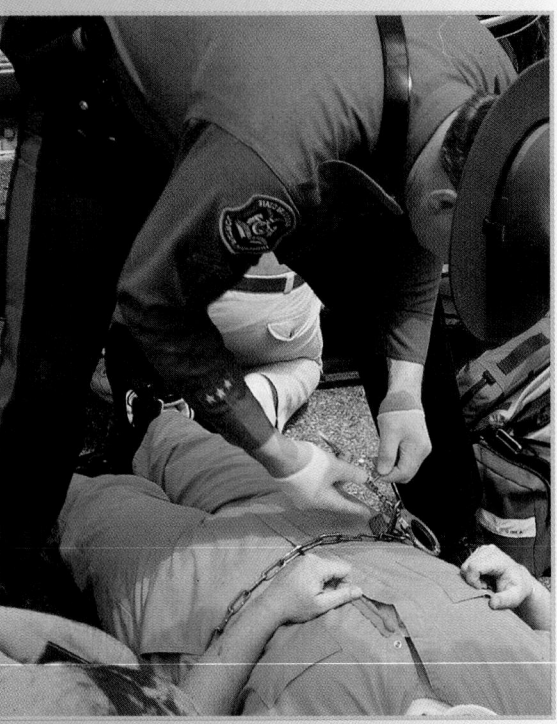

Spouse, elder, and child abuse are growing problems in the United States. Abuse and neglect can result in mental and physical illness or injury and even death. This chapter addresses the types of abuse and neglect, the personality traits of those who abuse, and legal considerations in providing emergency care.

battering: A form of domestic violence that describes the establishment of control and fear in a relationship through violence and other forms of abuse.

patterned injuries: Injuries that result from an identifiable object.

self-neglect: A type of elder abuse; behaviors of an older adult that intentionally threaten personal health or safety (e.g., poor nutrition or noncompliance with medication regimens).

> **NOTE**
>
> Paramedics encounter victims of domestic violence and other forms of abuse in the course of their careers. Education programs for emergency medical services (EMS) personnel must incorporate information about these violent crimes, including identification of victims, special aspects of care, scene safety, and documentation requirements.

Battering

Battering, a form of domestic violence, is the establishment of control and fear in a relationship through violence and other forms of abuse.[1] The batterer uses acts of violence and a series of behaviors, including intimidation, threats, psychological abuse, and isolation, to coerce and control the other person (Box 44-1). The violence may not happen often, but it is a hidden and constant terrorizing factor in some relationships. Over time the beatings

> **NOTE**
>
> Medical expenses from domestic violence total at least $3 to $5 billion in the United States each year. Businesses forfeit another $100 million in lost wages, sick leave, absenteeism, and nonproductivity.

generally become more severe and more frequent and often occur without provocation. If children are present in a marriage or relationship, often the violence eventually turns toward them.[2]

Domestic violence follows a cycle of three phases[3] (Fig. 44-1). Phase one involves arguing and verbal abuse; phase two progresses to physical and sexual abuse; and phase three consists of denial and apologies (the "honeymoon phase"). The paramedic best accomplishes intervention in phase two or three. The cycle repeats itself without intervention, usually increasing in frequency and severity. Understanding this cycle of violence will help the paramedic assess the situation and care for the victim.

> **NOTE**
>
> Persons involved in abusive relationships often fail to see alternatives and feel powerless to change.

Battered Women

A woman is battered by her husband, boyfriend, or live-in partner approximately every 15 seconds in

> **BOX 44-1**
>
> ### TYPES OF ABUSE AND NEGLECT
>
> *Physical abuse.* Use of physical force that may result in bodily injury, physical pain, or impairment
>
> *Sexual abuse.* Nonconsensual sexual contact of any kind
>
> *Emotional abuse.* Infliction of anguish, pain, or distress through verbal or nonverbal acts
>
> *Financial/material exploitation.* Illegal or improper use of funds, property, or assets
>
> *Neglect.* Refusal or failure of the caregiver to fulfill obligations or duties to a person

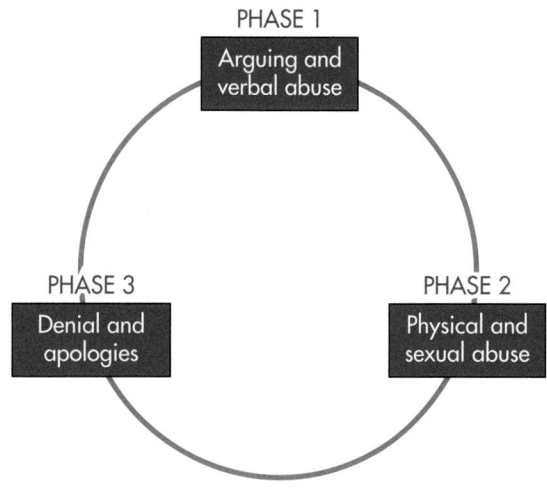

Fig. 44-1 Cycle of violence.

the United States[4] (see the box on p. 1307). Less than 10% of women report battering incidents for reasons that include the following[2]:

1. Personal fear or fear for her children
2. Belief that the offender's behavior will change (abusers often appear charming and loving after the battering incident)
3. Lack of financial and/or emotional support
4. Belief that she is the cause of the violent behavior
5. Belief that battering is "part of the marriage" and must be endured to keep the family together

> **NOTE**
>
> Women who leave their batterers are at a 75% greater risk of being killed by the batterer than those who stay in the abusive relationship.[5]

Women of all cultures, races, occupations, income levels, and ages are battered by their husbands, boyfriends, and lovers (opposite- and same-sex partners). Domestic violence is the leading cause of injury to women between 15 and 44 years of age in the United States.

Battered Men

In about 95% of domestic assaults the batterer is a man.[3] However, women are not the only battering victims. More than 150,000 men in the United States each year are victims of physical violence by a spouse or partner (from both opposite- and same-sex relationships).[6] Men report physical violence by a spouse or partner less frequently than women, probably as a result of humiliation, guilt, fear to admit loss of control, or societal issues.

> **NOTE**
>
> Society seems to be less empathetic toward battered men than battered women and has allocated fewer resources for support.

Characteristics of Persons in Abusive Relationships

Certain personality traits may predispose people to abusive relationships. The following are characteristics of one or both persons in an abusive relationship[2]:

1. Intense need for love and affection
2. Low self-esteem
3. Alcohol or other drug dependence
4. Difficulty in finances, job security, and possible legal issues
5. Background of physical, emotional, or sexual abuse
6. Belief that abuse is demonstrating discipline
7. Fear of being "out of control"
8. Uncontrolled temper, extreme jealousy, and insecurity
9. Inability to set and enforce personal boundaries
10. Unrealistic expectations of a relationship
11. Difficulty in expressing anger
12. Loyalty to the abuser that takes precedence over emotional or physical safety
13. Repeated attempts to leave the relationship
14. Clinical depression
15. Suicidal ideation or attempts

DOMESTIC VIOLENCE: FACTS AND STATS

- Battered women often are severely injured. At least one third of all emergency department visits by women are caused by battering.
- Every year an estimated 4 to 6 million women are beaten by a spouse or partner, which is more than are hurt in auto crashes, rapes, and muggings combined.
- One half of all homeless women and children are homeless as a result of domestic violence.
- About 15% to 25% of pregnant women are battered.
- Battered women are more likely to suffer miscarriages and give birth to infants with low birth weights.
- Living in suburban and rural areas does not decrease a woman's risk of experiencing an act of violence by a spouse or partner.
- Up to 75% of domestic assaults reported to law enforcement agencies were inflicted after separation of the couples.
- Between 50% and 70% of the men who batter their spouse or partner also abuse their children.

- About 63% of young men between 11 and 20 years of age who are serving time for homicide have killed their mother's abuser.
- Domestic violence is the sixth most dangerous call for law enforcement officers killed in the line of duty.
- There are nearly three times as many animal shelters in the United States as there are shelters for battered women and their children.
- Compared with males, females experience over 10 times as many incidents of violence by a spouse or partner annually.
- Children are present in 40% to 55% of homes when police intervene in domestic violence calls.
- In 85% to 90% of domestic homicides, the police had been called to the home at least once during the 2 years before the incident. In more than half of these cases the police had been called five times or more.
- Almost six times as many women victimized by spouses or partners as those victimized by strangers did not report their violent victimization to police because they feared reprisal from the offender.

From Federal Bureau of Investigation; National Coalition Against Domestic Violence; National Woman Abuse Prevention Project; United States Senate; Committee on the Judiciary; U.S. Department of Justice; Bureau of Justice Statistics, May 1999.

NOTE

Abusers often are survivors of abuse.

Identification of the Battered Patient

The paramedic may have difficulty identifying the battered patient. Often the description of the injuries may be incorrect, inaccurate, and protective of the attacker. Accidental injuries often involve the extremities and periphery of the body, whereas injuries from domestic violence often involve contusions and lacerations of the face, head, neck, breast, and abdomen. Bruises and lacerations may appear to be "old" since many victims of abuse do not seek medical attention for their injuries. Box 44-2 provides other clues of domestic violence.

Scene Safety

The paramedic must ensure scene and personal safety in domestic violence disputes. If dispatch information reveals that the scene involves domestic violence, the paramedic should summon law en-

forcement personnel and the EMS crew should not enter the scene until it has been secured. If the paramedic does not suspect domestic violence until after he or she arrives at the scene, he or she should remove the victim from the scene as soon as possible. Violence is commonly directed toward EMS personnel, particularly if the abuser feels that the paramedic is directing too much empathy toward the victim. Therefore the paramedic should not question the victim regarding possible violence and should make no display of sympathy until the victim is in the ambulance or has been separated from the suspected perpetrator.

Care of the Victim

The paramedic should manage physical injuries according to standard practice protocols, directing

? CRITICAL THINKING

If you suspect abuse, what can you say to invite the victim to talk about it?

special attention toward the emotional needs of the victim. The abuser often is unwilling to allow the victim to give a history or allow the victim to be alone with EMS personnel. Therefore the paramedic should question the patient privately about the incident when possible.

The paramedic should attempt to gather information about events that led to physical injury by using direct questions. Often the patient will avoid eye contact and be hesitant or evasive about details of an injury. Some may offer clues by saying "Things haven't been going well lately," or "There have been problems at home." The paramedic should convey to the patient his or her awareness that the injuries may have resulted from battering. The patient may be relieved to know that someone else is aware of the abuse. The paramedic should remember the following key points during the patient interview:

1. Maintain a nonjudgmental attitude (avoid comments such as "How awful," or "Why don't you leave?").
2. Maintain a supportive attitude.
   a. Listen attentively.
   b. Provide emotional support and encouragement.

TRICKS OF THE TRADE

What the patient says to you may be admissible in a court of law. Document carefully!

---

3. Return control to the patient when possible.
   a. Encourage the patient to gain control of his or her life.
   b. Encourage the patient to identify what he or she wants and the needs of the children.
4. Provide access to community resources, such as battered spouse programs and victim-witness assistance programs.

? CRITICAL THINKING

How would you feel if you respond to a call in which a woman has been injured by a batterer but chooses not to leave?

---

5. Discuss safety precautions.
   a. Help the patient identify a quick way out (e.g., where to go and whom to call).
   b. Provide an approved, written list (or small card that the victim can easily hide from the abuser) of community resources, including shelters and hotline numbers, to patients who elect not to be transported for physician evaluation.

NOTE

Community resources vary widely. The paramedic should be knowledgeable of available resources and support agencies. Many communities have state funded and federally funded programs for abused victims and their families (see the box at the left).

Some patients who have suffered abuse eventually leave the abusive relationship. This often is made possible by health care providers and support agency personnel who do the following:

- Treat the victim in a sensitive and sympathetic manner.
- Confirm that the victim is not at fault and does not deserve to be abused.

NATIONAL DOMESTIC VIOLENCE HOTLINE

In 1996 the U.S. government established a nationwide, 24-hour, toll-free domestic violence hotline through the Violence Against Women Act (VAWA) of 1994. The voice number for the hotline is 1-800-799-SAFE, and the TDD number for the hearing impaired is 1-800-787-3224. The hotline is available 365 days a year and operates throughout the United States, Puerto Rico, and the Virgin Islands. It is staffed by trained advocates who offer crisis intervention, support, and referrals to local services in the caller's community.

Other components of VAWA include the allocation of funds for training prosecutors and police, maintaining shelters, and providing educational programs in schools and communities. These programs work with the hotline to treat domestic violence as a serious crime and help prevent domestic violence before it starts.

- Ensure the victim's safety.
- Become "agents of change" in helping provide the support needed for the victim to leave the abusive environment.

Legal Considerations

Physical assault is a crime that may be a misdemeanor or a felony, depending on state law, the amount of injury inflicted, and devices that the attacker uses during the assault. Often the attacker is arrested but is released from custody within hours on his or her own recognizance. If early release from custody is likely, the patient must be made aware of this and encouraged to take personal safety precautions.

Most states do not have mandatory reporting requirements for acts of domestic violence. Paramedics should be aware of reporting requirements in their state. EMS personnel are professionally responsible to advise medical direction of their suspicions and observations about acts of violence (see the box below).

TRICKS OF THE TRADE

In all cases of suspected abuse, be careful about what you say and what you put in writing. Objectively document your findings, but make no accusations.

PRESERVING THE SCENE

Any act of physical abuse against a spouse, partner, elder, or child is a crime. Therefore the paramedic must treat the scene as a crime scene. Paramedics should be careful not to disturb the scene or destroy possible evidence. Documentation is important and should include a precise recording of injuries, reported mechanisms of injuries, and a description of the behavior of the victim and alleged abuser. Using body diagrams in the patient care report may be helpful, and the paramedic should record the victim's own words in the narrative when possible. The paramedic should also record the names of police officers and witnesses at the scene. This information is important in cases of litigation.

Elder Abuse

As described in Chapter 43, elder abuse is a prevalent medical and social problem in the United States. There are between 820,000 and 1,860,000 abused elders in the United States, yet the true national prevalence of incidence of elder abuse is not known today.[7] Factors that contribute to elder abuse include the following:

- Increased life expectancy
- Physical and mental impairment
- Decreased productivity
- Increased dependence
- Limited resources for care of the elderly
- Economic factors
- Stress of the middle-age caregiver responsible for two generations

? CRITICAL THINKING

Do you think that the problem of elder abuse will increase or decrease during your career in EMS? Why?

Types of Elder Abuse

Elder abuse is classified into four categories: physical abuse, psychological abuse, financial or material abuse, and neglect (passive and active) (Box 44-3). Elder abuse also is classified by where it occurs—domestic settings and institutions.

NOTE

Self-neglect also is a type of elder abuse. This type of neglect describes behaviors of an older adult that intentionally threaten personal health or safety (e.g., poor nutrition and noncompliance with medication regimens).

Domestic Settings

The average victim of elder abuse in domestic settings is about 78 years of age with multiple, chronic health conditions that make him or her dependent on others for care. Widows over 75 years of age carry the greatest risk of elder abuse. Unexplained trauma is the most common finding. Evidence suggests that elder abuse is associated more with the personality

BOX 44-3

TYPES OF ELDER ABUSE

Physical Abuse
Hitting
Biting
Sexually molesting
Physically restraining

Psychological Abuse
Threatening verbally
Causing fear
Isolating
Name calling
Humiliating
Intimidating
Insulting

Financial or Material Abuse
Stealing or misusing money
Stealing or misusing property
Forcing relocation from one dwelling to another

Neglect (active and passive)
Withholding medication, food, exercise, companionship, or bathroom assistance
Ignoring the person

BOX 44-4

PERCENTAGE OF THOSE WHO ABUSE ELDERS

Adult children: 32.5%
Grandchildren: 4.2%
Spouse: 14.4%
Sibling: 2.5%
Other relative: 12.5%
Friend or neighbor: 7.5%
All others: 18.2%
Unknown: 2.0%

From *EMT-Paramedic national standard curriculum,* U.S. Department of Transportation National Highway Traffic Safety Administration, Washington, D.C., 1997, The Department.

3. A "cycle of violence" commonly occurs in elder abuse. The cycle begins with on-going tension that escalates in a crisis in which abuse occurs. The abuse generally is followed by a period of calm, reconciliation, and denial, after which the cycle repeats.
4. Abusers of older adults often have more personal problems (e.g., job insecurity and financial difficulties) than nonabusers.

NOTE

Older adults often are repeatedly abused by family members, and the abusers most often are the children of the abused. Because of this familial relationship, many older adults do not report the abuse or seek medical care for their injuries.

of the abuser or the caregiver than with the burden of caring for a sick, dependent person. The National Aging Resource Center on Elder Abuse provides percentages of who the perpetrators are most likely to be in domestic settings[2] (Box 44-4).

NOTE

Neglect is the most common form of elder abuse in domestic settings.

Major theories of causes of domestic elder abuse. Four major theories of causes of domestic elder abuse are as follows[2]:

1. Elder abuse occurs in settings where the caregiver is under a great amount of stress as a result of personal problems and/or a lack of knowledge about how to provide care to an older adult.
2. Mental and/or physical impairments common in many older adults make them more likely to be abused than older adults who are in good health.

Institutional Abuse

More than 1.5 million people are currently residents in nursing homes and other heath care facilities. These individuals are at risk for intentional harm, physical violence, verbal aggression, or neglect from other residents and paid caregivers, staff, and professionals. Clues that may indicate institutional abuse include the following:

- Physical abuse
  - Open wounds, cuts, bruises, welts, or discoloration
  - Caregiver who cannot adequately explain the victim's condition
  - Victim's sudden change in behavior
  - Loss of weight
  - Burns caused by cigarettes, caustics, or acids

- Emotional abuse
  - Victim who is emotionally upset or agitated
  - Victim who is extremely withdrawn and non-communicative
  - Unusual behavior by the victim (sucking, biting, or rocking)
- Neglect
  - Dehydration, malnutrition, or pressure sores
  - Victim with poor personal hygiene
  - Victim who is begging for food
  - Unsanitary and unclean conditions (dirt, soiled bed, or fecal or urine odor)

Legal Considerations

All 50 states have elder abuse statutes, and reporting of suspected elder abuse is mandatory under law in most states. If the paramedic suspects abuse or neglect, he or she should carefully document all findings; advise medical direction; and follow procedures established by local protocol.

Child Abuse

In 1996, child protective service agencies investigated more than 2 million reports alleging maltreatment of more than 3 million children, and these agencies determined that almost 1 million children were victims of substantiated or indicated abuse or neglect.[8] As described in Chapter 42, various forms of child abuse, including physical injury, sexual exploitation, infliction of emotional pain, and neglect, can result in physical or emotional impairment.

✓ TRICKS OF THE TRADE

Caring for a child who has been abused is a "tough call" for the EMS crew. Openly discuss your feelings with co-workers after the call, and do not hesitate to seek professional guidance.

Neglect is the most common form of child abuse, although many children suffer more than one type of maltreatment. Neglect is the failure to provide physical care (e.g., medical care, nutrition, shelter, and clothing) or the failure to provide emotional care (i.e., indifference and disregard).

BOX 44-5

CHARACTERISTICS OF CHILD ABUSERS

- Demonstrate immature behavior
- Show personal preoccupation (self-centeredness)
- Have little perception of how a child feels (physically or emotionally)
- Are critical of the child
- Seldom touch or look at the child
- Are unconcerned about the child's injury, treatment, or prognosis
- Show no feeling of guilt or remorse
- Blame the child for the injury or illness

NOTE

Most substantiated reports of child abuse or neglect come from professional sources (educators, social services, law enforcement, and medical personnel). Persons in the family of the victim report only 18% of child abuse cases.

Characteristics of Abusers

The characteristics of abusers are not related to social class, income, or level of education. Most child abusers are the child's parents (77%), and 11% are other relatives of the victim. Most perpetrators are under 40 years of age, and two thirds are female (usually the child's mother). People who are in other caregiving relationships to the victim (e.g., child care providers, foster parents, and facility staff) account for only 2% of perpetrators. About 10% of all abusers are noncaregivers or unknown. Neglect often is attributed to female perpetrators, whereas sexual abuse most often is attributed to males.[8] Box 44-5 provides other characteristics of child abusers.

NOTE

Children in alcohol-abusing families are 4 times more likely to be maltreated, 5 times more likely to be physically abused, and 10 times more likely to be emotionally neglected than children in non–alcohol-abusing families. About 50% to 80% of all child abuse cases involve some degree of substance abuse by the child's parents.[9]

? CRITICAL THINKING

How does it make you feel when you hear a story about child abuse on the news? Think about how you will manage those feelings when you are at a scene with such a child.

A family history of rigorous discipline accounts for the cyclical nature of child abuse.[2] Since many abusers were severely punished and beaten as children by their parents, they often prefer to use other forms of discipline for their children. However, the stresses associated with child rearing eventually culminate in some parents regressing to the earliest patterns of discipline that they experienced as a child. The abusive adult sometimes is aware of this cyclical nature and tries to seek help to prevent abusive behavior toward their children. This is known as the "pre-abuse state," during which the following pattern often occurs[2]:

1. The adult makes several calls for help within a 24-hour period to 911 or support agencies.
2. The adult frequently calls EMS for inconsequential symptoms.
3. The adult begins to demonstrate behavior of being unable to handle an impending crisis.

NOTE

The pre-abuse state is important in identifying the potential for abuse. The pattern is often repetitive and results in frequent EMS calls to the patient's home. The paramedic should remember that this behavior indicates the adult's awareness that child abuse is likely to occur and that he or she is actively seeking help to prevent the abuse.

Characteristics of the Abused Child

Abused children often exhibit behavior that provides important clues about abuse and neglect (see the box on p. 1313). Although this behavior may be age-related, the paramedic should carefully observe the child under 6 years of age who is excessively passive, the child over 6 years of age who is excessively aggressive, and the child with the following characteristics:

- Does not mind (at any age) if his or her parents leave the room

- Cries hopelessly during treatment or cries very little
- Does not look at parents for reassurance
- Is wary of physical contact
- Is extremely apprehensive
- Appears constantly on the alert for danger
- Constantly seeks favors, food, or comfort items (e.g., blankets, toys)

Physical Examination

Injuries during childhood are common, and most are unintentional and not the result of abuse. Distinguishing between an intentional and unintentional injury can be challenging for the paramedic. The paramedic obtains the most important clues by observing the child and his or her relationship with the parent or caregiver and by matching the history of the event to the injury. If the child volunteers the history of the event without hesitation and matches the history that the parent provides (and the history is suitable for the injury), child abuse is unlikely.[2]

Legal Considerations

When possible, the paramedic should perform the physical examination of a child who is a suspected victim of abuse with another colleague. This will help verify that the recording of information is objective and that assumptions and personal perceptions do not taint findings in the examination. The report must be succinct and legible, and the paramedic should document all pertinent findings and observations.

NOTE

Child abuse is a crime that is reportable under law in all 50 states. Paramedics should follow local protocol in reporting suspected child abuse and discuss any suspicions of child abuse or neglect with medical direction.

Common Types of Injuries

See Chapter 42 for a detailed discussion of the types of injuries suffered as a result of child abuse. This section provides an outline of these types of injuries.

Soft tissue injuries
- Most common injuries
- Found most frequently in early abuse and may present in various forms

- Multiple bruises and ecchymosis, especially if bruises are extensive and/or a mixture of "old" and "new" bruises
- Defense wounds, injuries on multiple body planes, patterned injuries, and scalds (common form of abuse in the young and old)

> **NOTE**
>
> **Patterned injuries** result from an identifiable object. Examples include bites, loop marks from a cord or belt, distinct cigarette burns, and bristle marks from a hairbrush.

Fractures
- Second most common injury
- Possibly caused by abusive force (twisting and jerking)
- Rib fractures and multiple fractures
- Fractures of different ages (fresh and healed), indicating repeated injury

Head injuries
- Most common cause of death
- Greater amount of permanent disability
- Progression of injuries often beginning at trunk and extremities and moving toward the head
- Possible scalp wounds, skull fractures, subdural or subgaleal hematomas, repeated concussions

Abdominal injuries
- Not as common but very serious
- Possible rupture of liver and injuries to intestines and mesentery

Children Who Die from Abuse and Neglect

About 4000 children die from child abuse and neglect in the United States each year.[10] Fatal injuries from maltreatment result from many different acts, including the following:

- Severe head trauma
- Shaken baby syndrome
- Trauma to the abdomen and/or thorax
- Scalding
- Drowning
- Suffocation
- Poisoning

> **WHO ARE THE CHILD VICTIMS OF ABUSE?**
>
> - More than 50% are 7 years of age or younger.
> - 25% are younger than 4 years of age.
> - 25% are 8 to 12 years of age.
> - 21% are 13 to 18 years of age.
> - 52% are female.
> - 23% of sexual abuse victims are boys.
> - Children younger than 4 years of age account for 76% of fatalities from abuse.

From National Clearinghouse on Child Abuse and Neglect Information, Washington, DC, 1998.

> **NOTE**
>
> Shaken baby syndrome (SBS) is a serious form of child abuse that describes injuries to infants that occur after being violently shaken. These rapid shakes can cause cerebral hemorrhage, brain damage, blindness, paralysis, and death. SBS most often occurs before 1 year of age and less often between 1 and 2 years of age. The shaking episode usually results from inconsolable crying.

> **? CRITICAL THINKING**
>
> *How can you calm yourself after caring for a child killed by abuse so that you will be able to write a patient care report that will likely be called to court?*

Types of neglect that can result in death include the following:

1. *Supervision neglect* includes death that involves a critical moment in which the parent or caregiver is absent and the child is killed by a suddenly arising danger (e.g., leaving a child unattended in a bathtub).
2. *Chronic neglect* includes death caused by slowly building problems (e.g., malnutrition).
3. Deaths that result from *child physical abuse* involve fatal parental assaults on infants and children that are "triggered" by events such as inconsolable crying, feeding difficulties, failed toilet training, and the parent's exaggerated perceptions of acts of "disobedience." Parents may have unrealistic expectations for the child's behavior for his or her developmental level.

Another factor that increases a child's risk of being killed is living in a home where spouse or partner abuse occurs. Acts of domestic violence often are transferred to children living in the household. Studies have shown that frequently the following characteristics identify an abusive parent who kills a child[11]:

- Is a young male in his mid-twenties
- Lives near or below poverty level
- Has not finished high school
- Is depressed and unable to cope with stress
- Has experienced violence first hand

Sexual Assault

Sexual assault is one of the fastest growing and most serious crimes in the United States. More than 500,000 women and about 49,000 men report sexual assault each year.[12] About 1 in 5 women is sexually assaulted by 21 years of age. Sexual assault is more frequently committed than other forms of abuse and can result in mental or physical injury and death.

> **NOTE**
>
> Most states use the gender-neutral term *sexual assault* instead of the traditional term *rape*.

Legal Aspects of Sexual Assault

Each state has different interpretations of sexual assault. The term generally refers to any genital, anal, oral, or manual penetration of the victim's body by way of force and without the victim's consent.

> **NOTE**
>
> Lack of consent includes the inability to give consent as a result of impaired mental function caused by alcohol and/or other drugs, sleep, or unconsciousness.

In many cases, sexual assault is a felony crime that must be proved by evidence. Legal considera-tions for providing care to a patient who has been sexually assaulted include the following:

1. Take steps to preserve evidence.
2. Discourage the patient from urinating or defecating, douching, or bathing.
3. Do not remove evidence from any part of the body that was subjected to sexual contact unless necessary to provide urgent medical care.
4. Notify law enforcement personnel as soon as possible.
5. Be aware that there will be a "chain of evidence" with specific requirements of proof.
6. Follow local and state requirements in reporting these cases. Consult with medical direction and follow established protocols.

Characteristics of Sexual Assault

Anyone can be a victim of sexual assault at any age. The highest incidence of sexual assault occurs in women who live alone in isolated areas. The victim frequently knows the assailant and sometimes feels shame and personal responsibility for the attack. The methods that the assailant uses to gain control over both male and female victims include entrapment, intimidation, and physical force. The assailant commonly uses threats of physical harm and exhibition of a weapon to gain submission. Male victims are more likely to suffer significant physical trauma from sexual assault by other men than are female victims (see the box on p. 1315). The following are common injuries that result from sexual assault:

- Abrasions and bruises on the upper limb, head, and neck
- Forcible signs of restraint (e.g., rope burns and mouth injuries)
- Petechiae of the face and conjunctiva secondary to choking
- Broken teeth, swollen jaw or cheekbone, and eye injuries from being punched or slapped in the face

> **? CRITICAL THINKING**
>
> *How do you feel when you hear people say, "That rape victim brought it on herself?"*

- Muscle soreness or stiffness in the shoulder, neck, knee, hip, or back from restraint in postures that allow sexual penetration

Psychosocial Aspects of Care

The trauma of sexual assault creates physical and psychological disorganization. Victims may behave in various ways. Some may be surprisingly calm and seem in control of their emotions, whereas others may be agitated, apprehensive, distraught, or tearful. After managing all threats to life, the paramedic should proceed with care by providing emotional support to the victim. As described in Chapter 39, the paramedic should not question victims of sexual assault in detail about the incident in the prehospital setting. The paramedic should limit the patient history to elements that are necessary to provide emergency medical care. The initial contact with the victim should include the following:

- Nonjudgmental and supportive attitude
- Empathetic and sensitive comments
- Quiet speech
- Slow movements
- Considerate gestures (ensure privacy and respect modesty)

TRICKS OF THE TRADE

Only ask questions that are relevant to provide emergency care. The patient will be questioned many times about the "specifics" of the incident at the hospital.

The paramedic should move the patient to a safe and quiet environment to avoid further exposure and embarrassment. When possible, a paramedic of the same sex should provide any required medical care. If this is not possible, a chaperone should be present. The paramedic should not leave the patient alone and should ask for permission to call a friend, family member, or sexual assault crisis advocate. The paramedic should relay concerns of the victim about pregnancy and contracting human immunodeficiency virus (HIV) and other sexually transmitted diseases to medical direction. After the patient recovers from physical injury, the goal of treatment is for the patient

FIVE MYTHS AND MISCONCEPTIONS ABOUT SEXUAL ASSAULT

Myth. All victims of sexual assault are women, and all perpetrators are men.

Fact. Most sexual assaults are perpetrated by men. However, men can be assaulted by other men, and women sometimes perpetrate sexual assaults against men and other women.

Myth. Rape is an impulsive act.

Fact. 58% to 71% of rapes are clearly planned.

Myth. Rape is motivated by sexual desire.

Fact. Rape is a crime of violence, motivated by anger and the desire for power and control.

Myth. Most women are raped by strangers.

Fact. Most women are victims of "acquaintance rape" by a known trusted assailant.

Myth. According to the law, a husband cannot be charged with rape against his wife.

Fact. The law stipulates circumstances in which the husband can be charged with rape against his wife.

to regain control of his or her life. Often this requires long-term counseling and support.

Child Victims

Children are particularly vulnerable to sexual assault and usually have frequent contact with the assailant. Often the assault occurs in a trusted person's home. Most involve a male assailant and female victim.[2] About 30% of acquaintance sexual assaults occur when the victim is between 11 and 17 years of age. Many young victims do not think of their experience as a sexual assault since they often are fondled or physically explored without intercourse. Consequently, they rarely report the attack and often assume that they are to blame. Victims involved in a same-sex assault also are unlikely to report the incident because of confusion or embarrassment. For these reasons, most victimized children do not receive appropriate medical treatment, including prophylaxis and counseling.

NOTE

Children often conceal sexual assault out of fear of punishment.

Assessment and Patient Care Considerations

Assessment for children of sexual assault should proceed as previously described for other victims and include age-related considerations appropriate for all children. The paramedic should be aware of the following symptoms that may indicate behavior or physical manifestations as a result of sexual assault:

- Abrupt behavior changes
- Sleep difficulties, sleep disorders, and nightmares
- Withdrawal from and avoidance of friends and family
- Low self-esteem or desire to be invisible
- Phobias related to the offender
- Hostility
- Self-destructive behaviors
- Mood swings, depression, and anxiety
- Regression (e.g., bed wetting)
- Truancy
- Eating disorders
- Alcohol or other drug use

Emotional influence. The attitude and behavior of adults, including health care providers, greatly influences a child's impression of the assault. The paramedic should attempt to lessen the emotional influence of the assault by reassuring the child that he or she is not responsible for the attack and that he or she did nothing wrong. The paramedic should encourage the child to talk openly about the assault and any sexual concerns that he or she may have.

Legal Considerations

If the paramedic suspects or confirms sexual assault, he or she must follow laws that apply to the crime. Local and state laws affect the confidentiality of children, and paramedics should be aware of regulations in their community and consult with medical direction.

SUMMARY

- Battering is the establishment of control and fear in a relationship through violence and other forms of abuse.

- Domestic violence follows a cycle of three phases. Phase one involves arguing and verbal abuse, phase two progresses to physical and sexual abuse, and phase three consists of denial and apologies. Certain personality traits may predispose people to abusive relationships.

- The paramedic may have difficulty identifying the battered patient. Injuries from domestic violence often involve contusions and lacerations of the face, neck, head, breast, and abdomen.

- The paramedic must ensure scene and personal safety in domestic violence disputes. The paramedic should manage physical injuries according to standard practice protocols, directing special attention toward the emotional needs of the victim.

- Elder abuse is classified into four categories: physical abuse, psychological abuse, financial or material abuse, and neglect.

- All 50 states have elder abuse statutes, and reporting of suspected elder abuse is mandatory under law in most states.

- Most child abusers are the child's parents (77%), and 11% are other relatives of the victim. Abused children often exhibit behavior that provides important clues about abuse and neglect. The paramedic should carefully observe the child under 6 years of age who is excessively passive or the child over 6 years of age who is excessively aggressive.

- If the child volunteers the history of the event without hesitation and matches the history that the parent provides (and the history is suitable for the injury), child abuse is unlikely.

- Injuries may include soft tissue injuries, fractures, head injuries, and abdominal injuries.

- *Sexual assault* generally refers to any genital, anal, oral, or manual penetration of the victim's body by way of force and without the victim's consent. The highest incidence of sexual assault occurs in women who live alone in isolated areas.

- After managing all threats to life, the paramedic should proceed with care by providing emotional support to the victim. The paramedic should deliver care in a manner that considers preservation of evidence.

REFERENCES

1. Federal Bureau of Investigation: *Uniform crime reports,* Washington, DC, 1990, The Bureau.
2. U.S. Department of Transportation, National Highway Traffic Safety Administration: *EMT-Paramedic national standard curriculum,* Washington, DC, 1998, The Department.
3. American College of Emergency Physicians: *Guidelines for the role of EMS personnel in domestic violence,* Policy resource and education paper, May, 1999. Available at www.acep.org/POLICY/PR400168.HTM.
4. U.S. Department of Justice, Bureau of Justice Statistics: *Violence against women: a national crime victimization report,* Washington, DC, 1994, The Department.
5. Hart B: *Myths and facts,* National Coalition Against Domestic Violence, 1988.
6. Department of Justice, Centers for Disease Control and Prevention: *Third annual report on the national violence against women survey,* Washington, DC, 1998, The Department.
7. Tatara T et al: *The basics: domestic elder abuse information series,* Washington, DC, 1997, National Center on Elder Abuse.
8. U.S. Department of Health and Human Services: *Child maltreatment 1996: reports from the states to the national child abuse and neglect data system,* Washington, DC, 1998, U.S. Government Printing Office.
9. U.S. Department of Health and Human Services, National Center on Child Abuse and Neglect: *A report on child maltreatment in alcohol-abusing families,* Washington, DC, 1993, U.S. Government Printing Office.
10. Rosen P, Barkin R: *Emergency medicine: concepts and clinical practice,* ed 4, St Louis, 1998, Mosby.
11. National Clearinghouse on Child Abuse and Neglect Information: *Child fatalities fact sheet,* accessed 4/19/00. Available at www.calib.com/nccanch/pubs/factsheets/fatality.htm.
12. American Academy of Pediatrics, Committee on Adolescence: Sexual assault and the adolescent, *Pediatrics* 94:761, 1994.

45 *Patients with Special Challenges*

OBJECTIVES

Upon completion of this chapter, the paramedic student will be able to:

1. *Identify considerations in prehospital management related to physical challenges such as hearing, visual, and speech impairments; obesity; and patients with paraplegia or quadriplegia.*

2. *Identify considerations in prehospital management of patients who have mental illness; are developmentally disabled; or are emotionally or mentally impaired.*

3. *Describe special considerations for prehospital management of patients with selected pathological challenges.*

4. *Outline considerations in management of culturally diverse patients.*

5. *Describe special considerations in the prehospital management of terminally ill patients.*

6. *Identify special considerations in management of patients with communicable diseases.*

7. *Describe special considerations in the prehospital management of patients with financial challenges.*

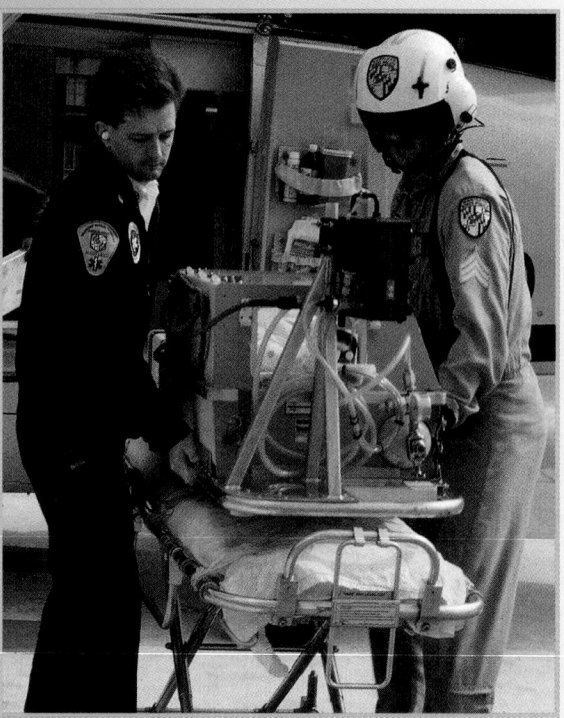

Paramedics frequently provide care to patients with special challenges. The patient groups to be discussed in this chapter include those who have physical, emotional, or pathological challenges; patients who are culturally diverse, have terminal illness, and communicable diseases; and those with financial challenges that may hinder access to health care.

KEY TERMS

cerebral palsy: A general term for nonprogressive disorders of movement and posture.

deafness: A complete or partial inability to hear.

diversity: Differences of any kind: race, class, religion, gender, sexual preference, personal habitat, and physical ability.

emotional/mental impairment: Impaired intellectual functioning that results in an inability to cope with normal responsibilities of life.

mental illness: Any form of psychiatric disorder.

myasthenia gravis: An autoimmune disorder in which muscles become weak and tire easily.

paraplegia: A weakness or paralysis of both legs and sometimes, part of the trunk.

quadriplegia: A weakness or paralysis of all four extremities and the trunk.

terminally ill patients: Patients with advanced stage of disease with an unfavorable prognosis and no known cure.

Physical Challenges

Patients who are physically challenged may require special considerations in patient assessment and management. The physical challenges presented in this chapter include hearing, visual, and speech impairments; obesity; and patients with paraplegia or quadriplegia.

Hearing Impairments

Deafness is a complete or partial inability to hear. Total deafness is rare and usually congenital. Partial deafness may range from mild to severe and most commonly is the result of an ear disease, injury, or degeneration of the hearing mechanism that occurs with age. All deafness is either conductive or sensorineural.

Conductive deafness refers to the faulty transportation of sound from the outer to the inner ear. This type of deafness often is curable. In adults, it commonly results from the accumulation of earwax that blocks the outer ear canal. Conductive deafness also may result from infection (e.g., otitis media),

and from injury to the eardrum or middle ear (e.g., from barotrauma).

Sensorineural deafness often is incurable. In this type of deafness, sounds that reach the inner ear fail to be transmitted to the brain because of damage to the structures within the ear or to the acoustic nerve, which connects the inner ear to the brain. Sensorineural deafness that is present in early life may be congenital. It also can result from a birth injury or from damage to the developing fetus (e.g., from a mother who has rubella during pregnancy). Sensorineural deafness that occurs in later life may be caused from prolonged exposure to loud noise, disease (e.g., Meniere's disease), tumors, medications, viral infections, or from natural degeneration of the cochlea and/or labyrinth in old age (see Chapter 43).

Special Considerations

Helpful techniques for recognizing a patient with a hearing impairment include noting the presence of hearing aids and observing the patient for poor diction or the inability to respond to verbal communication in the absence of direct eye contact. Accommodations that may be necessary include retrieving the patient's hearing aid and providing paper and pen to aid in communications. (Many persons with hearing impairments use American Sign Language [ASL] and speak with unusual syntax.)

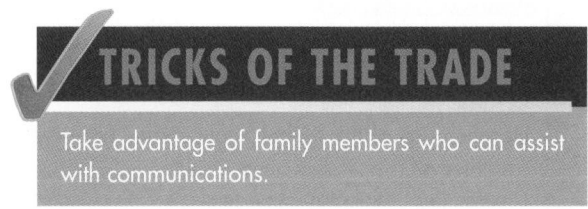

TRICKS OF THE TRADE

Take advantage of family members who can assist with communications.

When providing care to these patients, the paramedic should not shout or exaggerate lip movement. Other methods to aid in communication include speaking softly, directly into the patient's ear canal, and using pictures to illustrate basic procedures. (Some patients may have access to an "amplified" listening device.) It is important to notify the receiving hospital as soon as possible if the patient has severe deafness so that appropriate personnel (e.g., an interpreter) can be made available.

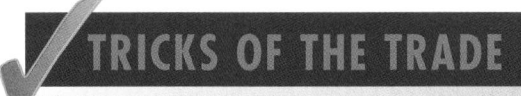

TRICKS OF THE TRADE

Consider carrying a file on the ambulance with pictures of routine medical procedures.

Visual Impairments

Normal vision depends on the uninterrupted passage of light from the front of the eye to the light-sensitive retina at the back. Any condition that obstructs the passage of light from the retina can cause vision loss. Visual impairments may result from a number of causes (Box 45-1), or be present at birth from a congenital disorder.

NOTE

It is estimated that more than 1 million Americans are blind, and 3 million are visually impaired, even with the best correction.[1]

Patients with visual impairments may be totally blind or have a partial loss of vision that affects cen-tral vision, peripheral vision, or both. A patient who has central loss of vision is usually aware of the condition. Those who have a loss of peripheral vision may be more difficult to identify, because the loss often goes unnoticed by the person until it is well advanced.

Special Considerations

Techniques in assessing and managing patients with vision loss are described in Chapter 10. To review, accommodations for these patients that may be necessary include retrieving visual aids, describing all patient care procedures before performing them, and providing sensory information (e.g., location of obstacles) as needed. Ambulatory patients should be guided by "leading" versus "pushing." A guide dog used by the patient should be allowed to accompany the patient to the hospital. Medical direction should be advised of the patient's special needs so that appropriate personnel can be made available.

Speech Impairments

Speech impairments include disorders of language, articulation, voice production, or fluency (blockage of speech), all of which can lead to an inability to communicate effectively (Box 45-2).

Language disorders result from damage to the language centers of the brain (usually from stroke, head injury, or brain tumor). These patients often demonstrate aphasia with a slowness to understand speech and problems with vocabulary and sentence structure. Aphasia can affect both children and adults and may affect their ability to speak and/or to comprehend written or spoken words. Delayed development of language in a child may result from hearing loss, lack of stimulation, or emotional disturbance.

An articulation disorder (sometimes referred to as *dysarthria*) is an inability to produce speech sounds. These disorders result from damage to nerve pathways passing from the brain to the muscles of the larynx, mouth, or lips. Often, the patient's speech will be slurred, indistinct, slow, or nasal. Disorders of articulation may result from brain injury and from diseases such as multiple sclerosis and Parkinson's disease. In children, they commonly are the result of delayed development from hearing problems.

BOX 45-1

CAUSES OF VISUAL IMPAIRMENTS

Cataracts
Degeneration of the eyeball, optic nerve, or nerve pathways
Disease (e.g., diabetes, hypertension)
Eye or brain injury
Infection (e.g., CMV, HSV, bacterial ulcers)
Vitamin A deficiency in children living in developing countries

? CRITICAL THINKING

What may cause a paramedic to become impatient when caring for a patient with this type of disorder?

Voice production disorders are characterized by hoarseness, harshness, inappropriate pitch, and abnormal nasal resonance. They often result from disorders that affect closure of the vocal cords. Some disorders are caused by hormonal or psychiatric disturbances and by severe hearing loss.

Fluency disorders are not well understood. They are marked by repetitions of single sounds or whole words, and by the blocking of speech. An example of a fluency disorder is stuttering.

✓ TRICKS OF THE TRADE

Avoid displays of impatience with someone who stutters. It usually will make things worse.

Special Considerations

Once a speech impairment has been identified, history taking and assessment need to be modified to provide adequate time for the patient to respond to questions. If appropriate, aids such as pen and paper should be made available to assist in communications.

Obesity

Obesity is an abnormal increase in the proportion of fat and cells, mainly in the viscera and the subcutaneous tissues of the body. Although reasons for obesity in some people are unclear, known causes for the condition include the following[2]:

- Caloric intake that exceeds calories burned
- Low basal metabolic rate
- Genetic disposition for obesity

NOTE

Obesity is defined as being 30% above ideal body weight.[3] About one in three Americans meets this definition for obesity.

Complications of obesity are many, and the condition increases a person's chance of becoming seriously ill. For example, obesity is associated with an increased risk for hypertension, stroke, heart disease, diabetes, and some cancers.[4] Osteoarthritis also is aggravated by increased body weight. The condition is treated with weight loss programs, exercise, counseling, medications, and sometimes, surgery. The goal of treatment is permanent weight loss.

? CRITICAL THINKING

How will you respond if a crew member makes an insensitive remark about a patient's obesity within hearing range of the patient or their family?

Special Considerations

Special considerations for caring for an obese patient include the need to obtain a thorough medical history (which often will be extensive). Assessment

---

BOX 45-2

TYPES OF SPEECH IMPAIRMENTS

Language Disorders
Stroke
Head injury
Brain tumor
Delayed development
Hearing loss
Lack of stimulation
Emotional disturbance

Articulation Disorders
Damage to nerve pathways passing from the brain
  to muscles in the larynx, mouth, or lips
Delayed development from hearing problems
Slow maturation of nervous system

Voice Production Disorders
Disorders affecting closure of vocal cords
Hormonal or psychiatric disturbance
Severe hearing loss

Fluency Disorders
Example: stuttering
Patient is not fully understood

may require appropriately sized diagnostic devices (e.g., large blood pressure cuffs), and additional manpower may be needed to assist with moving the patient for ambulance transport. Obese patients often are self-conscious about their weight and may be distraught about the physical hardships they place on the EMS crew. The paramedic should maintain professionalism during these patient care encounters.

Patients with Paraplegia/Quadriplegia

Paraplegia is weakness or paralysis of both legs and sometimes, part of the trunk; **quadriplegia** is weakness or paralysis of all four extremities and the trunk. The conditions result from nerve damage in the brain and spinal cord, usually caused by a motor vehicle crash, sports injury, fall, or gunshot wound. (Medical illnesses also can result in weakness and paralysis.) Both paraplegia and quadriplegia are accompanied by a loss of sensation and urinary control.

Special Considerations

Patients with extremity and trunk paralysis may require accommodations in patient care. For example, the patient may have a halo traction device to stabilize the spine (Fig. 45-1), which may complicate airway management and make patient transport difficult, and ostomies for the trachea, bladder, or colon. (Priapism also may be present in some male pa-

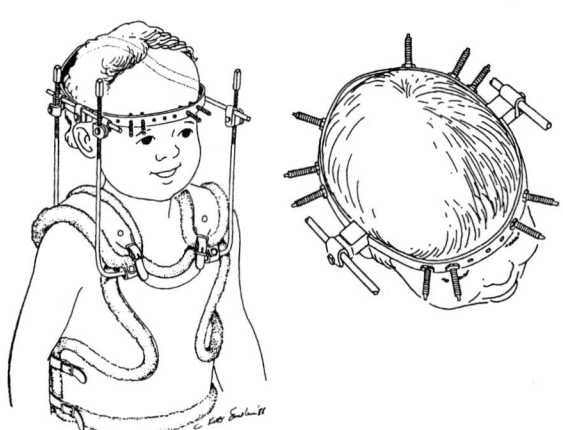

Fig. 45-1 A, Custom halo vest and light superstructure. **B,** Ten pin placement sites for infant halo ring attachment using multiple-pin, low-torque technique. Usually, four pins are placed anteriorly, avoiding temporal area, and remaining six pins are placed in occipital area. (From Mubarak SJ, et al: *J Pediatr Orthop* 9:612, 1989.)

tients.) Patients with paraplegia or quadriplegia often require additional manpower to assist with moving special equipment and to prepare them for ambulance transport.

Mental Challenges

Persons who are mentally challenged have developmental, emotional, behavioral, and psychological/and or psychiatric problems. The specific patient groups presented in this section include those with mental illness, developmental disabilities, emotional impairments, and emotional/mental impairments.

Mental Illness

Mental illness refers to any form of psychiatric disorder. Two broad categories of mental illness are psychoses and neuroses.

Psychoses comprise a group of mental disorders in which the individual loses contact with reality. Psychosis is thought to be related to complex biochemical disease that disorders brain function. Examples include psychoses (e.g., schizophrenia, manic-depressive illness, and organic brain disease) (see Chapter 38).

> **NOTE**
>
> Many patients with psychosis do not know they are ill. Patients with neuroses are generally aware of their disorder.

Neuroses are diseases related to upbringing and personality in which the person remains "in touch" with reality. Neurotic symptoms generally do not limit work or social activity and tend to fluctuate in intensity with stress. Major neurotic disorders include depression, phobias, and obsessive-compulsive behavior.

Special Considerations

Recognizing a patient who is mentally challenged may be difficult, especially when caring for mildly neurotic patients whose behavior may be unaffected. Others with more serious disorders may present with signs and symptoms consistent with mental illness. When obtaining the patient history, the paramedic should not be hesitant to ask about the following:

- History of mental illness
- Prescribed medications
- Compliance with prescribed medications
- Use of over-the-counter herbal products (e.g., St. John's Wort)
- Concomitant use of alcohol or other drugs

NOTE

Patients who are dangerous to themselves or others at the scene may need to be restrained. If a patient demonstrates aggressive or combative behavior, law enforcement personnel should be summoned to the scene to ensure scene safety.

If the patient appears to be paranoid or shows anxious behavior, the paramedic should ask the patient's permission before beginning any assessment or performing any procedure. Once rapport and trust have been established, care should proceed in the same manner as for a patient who does not have mental illness (unless the call is related specifically to the mental illness). These patients will experience illness and injury like all other patient groups.

Developmentally Disabled

A person who is developmentally disabled has impaired or insufficient development of the brain that causes an inability to learn at the usual rate (developmental delay). Developmental delay has numerous causes, including the following:

- Lack of stimulation
- Severe vision or hearing impairment

BOX 45-3

SIGNS OF DEVELOPMENTAL DELAY

Delays may be of varying severity and may affect any or all of the major areas of human achievement, including development of the ability:
- To walk upright
- Of fine hand-eye coordination
- Of listening, language, and speech
- Of social interaction

- Mental retardation
- Brain damage before, during, or after birth, or in infancy
- Severe diseases of body organs and systems

Developmental disability often is evident by signs and symptoms (Box 45-3). Accommodations that may be necessary when providing patient care include allowing adequate time for obtaining a history, performing assessment and patient management procedures, and preparing the patient for transport.

? CRITICAL THINKING

Do you think a patient with developmental delays should have any input into their care? Why?

Down syndrome

Down syndrome results from a chromosomal abnormality that causes mild to severe mental retardation and a characteristic physical appearance (Fig. 45-2). The child with Down syndrome has features that typically include the following:

- Eyes that slope upward at the outer corners
- Folds of skin on either side of the nose that cover the inner corners of the eyes
- A small face and small facial features
- A large and protruding tongue
- Flattening on back of the head
- Hands that are short and broad

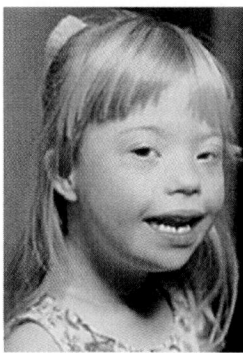

Fig. 45-2 Child with Down syndrome. (From McCance KL, Huether SE: *Pathophysiology: the biologic basis for disease in adults and children*, ed 3, 1998, Mosby.) (Courtesy Drs. A. Olney and M. MacDonald, University of Nebraska Medical Center, Omaha, Neb.)

In most cases, Down syndrome occurs from the failure of the two chromosomes numbered 21 in a parent cell to go into separate daughter cells during the first stage of sperm or egg cell formation. This results in a triplet of chromosomes 21 (trisomy 21) rather than the usual pair. The extra number 21 chromosome is passed on to the child, leading to Down syndrome. The incidence of affected fetuses increases with increased maternal age (mothers over age 35), and those with a family history of Down syndrome.

NOTE

In the general population, trisomy 21 occurs in only 1 of about 600 live births. After age 35, a mother's chances of having a Down syndrome child increases dramatically—to as high as 1 in 80 by age 40.[5] Because of this increased risk, pregnant mothers over age 35 usually are offered chromosome analysis of the fetus to assess for the abnormality. If the fetus is affected, termination of the pregnancy may be an option.

Special considerations. Persons with Down syndrome usually do not survive past their middle years. Many are cared for at home, and others live in long-term nursing care facilities. About 25% of children born with Down syndrome have a heart defect at birth. Many have congenital intestinal disorders, hearing defects, and other illnesses. The degree of mental disability varies with an intelligence quotient (IQ) that ranges from 30 to 80. (An IQ of 80 to 120 is considered average.) Persons with Down syndrome are capable of limited learning, and often are affectionate and friendly. Extra time must be allowed for obtaining a history, and for performing assessment and patient care procedures.

Emotionally Impaired

Persons with emotional impairments include those with neurasthenia (nervous exhaustion), anxiety neurosis, compulsion neurosis, and hysteria (see Chapter 38). All of these disorders can result in a wide range of physical or mental symptoms attributed to mental stress in someone who is not psychotic.

Special Considerations

It may be difficult to distinguish between symptoms produced by stress and those that indicate serious medical illness. Therefore management should always focus on the presenting complaint

---

BOX 45-4

CAUSES OF MENTAL RETARDATION

Genetic Conditions
Phenylketonuria (PKU); a single gene disorder caused by a defective enzyme
Chromosomal disorder (e.g., Down syndrome)
Fragile X syndrome (a single gene disorder on the Y chromosome; the leading inherited cause of mental retardation)

Problems During Pregnancy
Use of alcohol or other drugs by the mother
Use of tobacco
Illness and infection (toxoplasmosis, CMV, rubella, syphilis, HIV)

Problems at Birth
Brain injury
Prematurity
Low birth weight

Problems After Birth
Childhood diseases (whooping cough, chicken pox, measles, Hib disease)
Injury (e.g., head injury, near drowning)
Exposure to lead, mercury, and other environmental toxins

Poverty and Cultural Deprivation
Malnutrition
Disease-producing conditions
Inadequate medical care
Environmental health hazards
Lack of stimulation

From ARC National Headquarters: *Introduction to mental retardation,* Arlington, Tex., 2000, The Association, http://thearc.org/faqs/mrqa.html.

and the most serious etiology should be assumed. As described in Chapter 38, signs and symptoms that may result from emotional impairment include somatic complaints such as chest discomfort, tachycardia, dyspnea, choking, and syncope. It is therefore important to gather a complete history from the patient and to perform a thorough examination to rule out serious illness. Prehospital care for these patients (in the absence of serious illness) primarily is supportive and includes calming measures and transport for physician evaluation.

Emotionally/Mentally Impaired

Emotional/mental impairment (EMI) refers to persons who have impaired intellectual functioning (mental retardation) that results in an inability to cope with normal responsibilities of life. Mental retardation can be further classified with IQ assessment as mild (IQ 50 to 70), moderate (IQ 35 to 59), and profound (IQ less than 20).[6] The more severe grades of EMI usually have a specific physical cause (e.g., brain damage, Down syndrome), whereas mild EMI often has no specific cause, although poverty, malnutrition, and heredity may play a role (Box 45-4).

> **NOTE**
>
> Mild mental retardation is the most common form of EMI, accounting for about 85% of the retarded population.

Special Considerations

Accommodations that may be necessary during patient care will vary by the patient's level of retardation. Many with mild retardation show no psychological symptoms other than slowness in carrying out mental tasks. Others with moderate-to-severe retardation may have limited to absent speech; neurological impairments are common. These patients may require extra time and care in patient assessment, management, and transportation.

Pathological Challenges

Physical injury and disease may result in pathological conditions that require special assessment and management skills. Specific pathological challenges presented in this section include arthritis, cancer, cerebral palsy, cystic fibrosis, multiple sclerosis, muscular dystrophy, poliomyelitis, previous head injury, spina bifida, and myasthenia gravis.

Arthritis

Arthritis is the inflammation of a joint, characterized by pain, stiffness, swelling, and redness. The disease has many forms and varies widely in its effects. Two common forms of arthritis are osteoarthritis that results from cartilage loss and wear and tear of the joints (common in elderly patients), and rheumatoid arthritis (an autoimmune disorder that damages joints and surrounding tissues) (see Chapters 30 and 43).

Special Considerations

Patients with arthritis often have decreased range of motion and mobility that may limit the physical exam. (It is important to ensure patient comfort whenever possible.) The paramedic also should ascertain current medications (e.g., analgesics) before administering drugs to these patients. Transportation strategies must take into account the patient's limited mobility, and the equipment (e.g., backboards, splints) must be adjusted to "fit the patient" (not vice versa) by supplying adequate padding to fill all voids.

Cancer

Cancer is a group of diseases that allow for an unrestrained growth of cells in one or more of the body organs or tissues (see Chapter 35). The malignant tumors most commonly develop in major organs such as the lungs, breasts, intestine, skin, stomach, and pancreas but may also occur in cell-forming tissues of the bone marrow, and in the lymphatic system, muscle, or bone.

Special Considerations

Patients with cancer often are very ill, and the signs and symptoms of their disease depend on

> **NOTE**
>
> Paramedics should consult with medical direction and follow established protocol before accessing a surgically implanted port for fluid or drug therapy.

the cancer's primary site of origin. The paramedic should try to obtain a thorough history from the patient, including a list of all medications. Many cancer patients take anticancer drugs and pain medications through surgically implanted ports (e.g., mediports); transdermal skin patches that contain analgesic agents are common.

Cerebral Palsy (CP)

Cerebral palsy is a general term for nonprogressive disorders of movement and posture. The disease results from damage to the fetal brain during later months of pregnancy, during birth, during the newborn period, or in early childhood. The most common cause of CP is cerebral dysgenesis (abnormal cerebral development) or cerebral malformations.[7] Other less common causes include fetal hypoxia, birth trauma, maternal infection, kernicterus (excessive fetal bilirubin, associated with hemolytic disease), and postpartum encephalitis, meningitis, or head injury. Cerebral palsy often is diagnosed during the child's first year of life when parents notice unusual muscle tone during holding, and sometimes feeding difficulties. Although no cure exists for the disease, those with moderate disability may live with relative independence and have a near-normal life expectancy.

Types of Cerebral Palsy

Three distinct types of cerebral palsy exist: spastic paralysis, athetosis, and ataxia. Spastic paralysis produces abnormal stiffness and contraction of groups of muscles. With this type of CP, the child may be categorized as diplegic (all four limbs are affected, the legs more severely than the arms), hemiplegic (affecting limbs on only one side of the body, the arm usually more severe than the leg), or quadriplegic (all four limbs are severely affected; not necessarily symmetrically). Athetosis produces involuntary writhing movements. Ataxia produces a loss of coordination and balance. Hearing defects, epilepsy, and other CNS disorders are commonly present with the disease.

> **NOTE**
>
> Although some with athetosis and diplegia are highly intelligent, about 60% of all persons with CP have mental retardation.[7] Most with quadriplegia are severely retarded.

> **? CRITICAL THINKING**
>
> *How can you determine the patient's normal level of functioning?*

Special Considerations

Weakness, paralysis, and developmental delay vary by the type and severity of disease. For example, some children with mild cerebral palsy attend regular schools. Others with more severe forms of the disease never learn to walk or effectively communicate and require life-long skilled nursing care. Accommodations that may be required during an emergency call include allowing additional scene time for the physical examination and extra resources and manpower to facilitate transport.

Cystic Fibrosis (CF)

Cystic fibrosis (mucoviscidosis) is an inherited metabolic disease of the lungs and digestive system that manifests in childhood. The disease is caused by a defective, recessive gene that is inherited from each parent. The defective gene causes the glands in the lining of the bronchi to produce excessive amounts of thick mucus, which predisposes the person to chronic lung infections. In addition, the pancreas of a patient with CF fails to produce the enzymes required for the breakdown of fats and their absorption from the intestine. These alterations in metabolism cause classic symptoms of CF that include pale, greasy-looking, and foul-smelling stools (often noticeable soon after birth); persistent cough and breathlessness; and lung infections that often develop into pneumonia, bronchiectasis, and bronchitis. Other features of the disease include stunted growth and sweat glands that produce abnormally salty sweat. In some cases, the child with CF may fail to thrive; many patients survive into adulthood, although poor health is common.

> **NOTE**
>
> If only one defective gene is inherited, that person will be a "carrier" of the disease, but will have no symptoms. Often, these persons are unaware that they carry the defective gene. Genetic counseling and testing are appropriate for persons who have a family history of cystic fibrosis.

Special Considerations

Older patients (and parents of children) with CF generally are aware of their disease. Some may be oxygen-dependent and require respiratory support and suctioning to clear the airway of mucus and secretions. The paramedic should expect a lengthy history and physical exam because of the nature of the disease and associated medical problems. Some patients will have received heart and lung transplants and may require transfer to specialized medical facilities for treatment. If parents are unaware of the possibility of CF in the presence of signs and symptoms described previously, the paramedic should advise the physician at the receiving hospital of his or her suspicions.

Multiple Sclerosis (MS)

Multiple sclerosis is a progressive and incurable autoimmune disease of the CNS, whereby scattered patches of myelin in the brain and spinal cord are destroyed. Scarring and destruction of the tissues cause symptoms that range from numbness and tingling to paralysis and incontinence. The cause of MS is unknown; however, it may have a heritable or viral component. (Many people with MS lead active, normal lives between exacerbations of their illness.) The disease usually begins early in adult life, becomes active for a brief time, and then resumes years later. As described in Chapter 29, the symptoms of MS vary with the affected areas of the CNS and may include the following:

Brain involvement
- Fatigue
- Vertigo
- Clumsiness
- Muscle weakness
- Slurred speech
- Ataxia
- Blurred or double vision
- Numbness, weakness, or pain in the face

Spinal cord involvement
- Tingling, numbness, or feeling of constriction in any part of the body
- Extremities that feel heavy and become weak
- Spasticity

The symptoms of MS may occur singly or in combination and may last from several weeks to several months. Attacks vary in intensity and may be precipitated by injury, infection, or physical or emotional stress. Some patients become disabled, bedridden, and incontinent early in middle life. Disabled patients also often suffer from painful muscle spasms, constipation, urinary tract infection, skin ulcerations, and mood swings. The disease is managed with medications, physical therapy, and counseling.

Special Considerations

Some patients with MS may be difficult to examine and may be unable to provide a complete medical history because of the nature of their illness. The paramedic should allow extra time for patient assessment and to prepare the patient for transport. (The patient should not be expected to ambulate.) In severe cases, respiratory support may be indicated.

Muscular Dystrophy

Muscular dystrophy (see Chapter 29) is an inherited muscle disorder that results in a slow but progressive degeneration of muscle fibers. The disease is classified according to the age that symptoms first appear, the rate at which the disease progresses, and the way in which it is inherited. Muscular dystrophy is incurable.

> **NOTE**
>
> Genetic counseling and testing is appropriate for persons with a family history of muscular dystrophy.

The most common form of the disease is Duchenne muscular dystrophy, caused by a sex-linked, recessive gene that affects only males. Duchenne muscular dystrophy is rarely diagnosed before age 3. Signs and symptoms of the disease include a child who is slow in learning to sit up and walk; an unusual gait; curvature of the spine; and muscles that become bulky as they are replaced by fat. Eventually, most children will be unable to

> **NOTE**
>
> With other less common forms of muscular dystrophy, patients may live well into their middle years with varying degrees of muscle weakness.

TABLE 45-1	BRAIN INJURY DEFICITS		
INJURY	**INJURY DEFICITS**	**INJURY**	**INJURY DEFICITS**
Cerebral Cortex		Temporal lobe	Difficulty in recognizing faces
Frontal lobe	Paralysis of various body parts		Difficulty in understanding spoken words
	Inability to plan a sequence of complex movements		Short-term memory loss
	Inability to focus on tasks		Interference with long-term memory
	Mood changes		Persistent talking
	Personality changes		Aggressive behavior
	Inability to express language		
Parietal lobe	Inability to name an object	**Brain Stem**	Decreased vital capacity in breathing
	Problems with reading and writing		Difficulty in swallowing food and water
	Difficulty in distinguishing right from left		Difficulty with organization
	Difficulty with math skills		Problems with balance and movement
	Difficulty with eye and hand coordination		Dizziness and nausea
			Sleeping difficulties
Occipital lobe	Defects in vision	**Cerebellum**	Loss of ability to coordinate fine movements
	Production of hallucinations		Loss of ability to walk
	Visual illusions		Tremors
	Inability to recognize words		Dizziness
	Difficulties in reading and writing		Slurred speech

walk. Many do not live past their teenage years as a result of chronic lung infections and congestive heart failure.

Special Considerations

Accommodations that may be required during emergency care depend on the person's age, weight, and severity of disease. For example, young children will be relatively easy to examine and prepare for transport. Older patients may require additional manpower and resources to assist with moving the patient to the ambulance. In severe cases, respiratory support may be indicated.

Poliomyelitis

Poliomyelitis (polio) is an infectious disease caused by *Poliovirus hominis*. The virus is spread through direct and indirect contact with infected feces and by airborne transmission. It attacks with variable severity ranging from asymptomatic infection to a febrile illness without neurological sequelae to aseptic meningitis and finally to paralytic disease (including respiratory paralysis) and possible death.

As described in Chapter 29, the incidence of polio has declined since the Salk and Sabin vaccines were made available in the 1950s. The disease may, however, affect nonimmune adults and indigent children. Signs and symptoms of polio in both the nonparalytic and paralytic forms include fever, malaise, headache, and intestinal upset. In the majority of cases, persons with the nonparalytic form of polio recover completely. In the paralytic form, extensive paralysis of muscles of the legs and lower trunk can occur.

Special Considerations

Caring for a patient with paralytic polio who has respiratory paralysis may require advanced airway support to ensure adequate ventilation. If the lower body is paralyzed, catheterization of the bladder may be indicated (see Chapter 46). Additional resources and manpower may be needed to prepare the patient for transport.

Previously Head Injured Patients

Traumatic brain injury can result from many mechanisms of trauma (see Chapter 22). These injuries can affect many cognitive, physical, and psychological skills. Physical deficit can include ambulation, balance and coordination, fine motor skills, strength, and endurance. Cognitive deficits of language and communication, information processing, memory, and perceptual skills are common. Psychological status also is often altered (Table 45-1).

Special Considerations

Depending on the patient's area of brain injury, obtaining a history and performing assessment and patient care procedures may be very difficult. Some patients may require restraint. Family members and other caregivers should be involved in managing the patient (when appropriate), and interviewed to determine if the patient's actions and responses are "normal" for the patient. The paramedic should expect to spend additional time at the scene to provide care to these patients.

? CRITICAL THINKING

> *Why is this group of patients at high risk for injury?*

Spina Bifida

Spina bifida (see Chapter 29) is a congenital defect in which part of one or more vertebrae fails to de-velop, leaving a portion of the spinal cord exposed. The condition ranges in severity from that of minimal evidence of a defect to a child who is severely disabled. In severe cases, the legs of some children may be deformed with partial or complete paralysis and loss of sensation in all areas below the level of the defect. Associated abnormalities may include hydrocephalus with brain damage (Fig. 45-3), cerebral palsy, epilepsy, and mental retardation.

Special Considerations

Because of the varying degrees of spina bifida, pre-hospital care must be tailored to the patient's specific needs. Some patients require no special accommodations. Others need extended on-scene time for assessment and management, and perhaps additional resources and manpower to prepare the patient for transport.

Myasthenia Gravis

Myasthenia gravis is an autoimmune disorder in which muscles become weak and tire easily. The damage occurs to muscle receptors that are responsible for transmitting nerve impulses, commonly affecting muscles of the eyes, face, throat, and extremities. It is a rare disease that can begin suddenly or gradually. Myasthenia gravis can occur at any age but usually appears in women between age

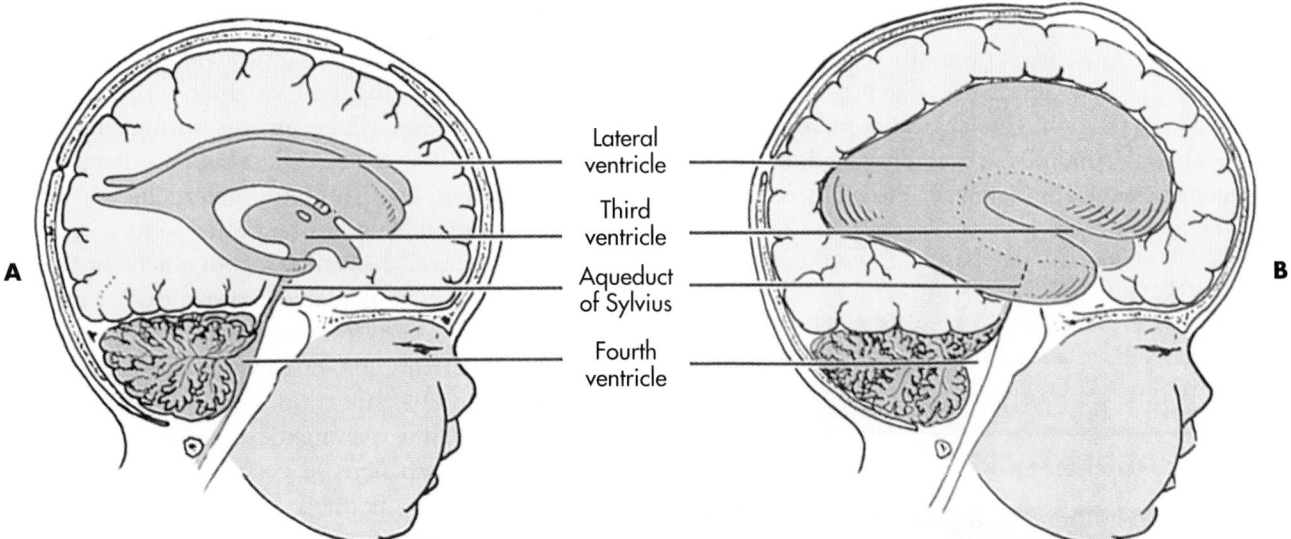

Fig. 45-3 Hydrocephalus: a block in flow of cerebrospinal fluid. **A,** Patent cerebrospinal fluid circulation. **B,** Enlarged lateral and third ventricles caused by obstruction of circulation—stenosis of aqueduct of Sylvius. (From Wong DL: *Nursing care of infants and children,* ed 5, St Louis, 1994, Mosby.)

Labels in figure:
Lateral ventricle
Third ventricle
Aqueduct of Sylvius
Fourth ventricle

20 and 30 and in men between 70 and 80 years of age.[8] Classic signs and symptoms include the following:

- Drooping eyelids, double vision
- Difficulty speaking
- Difficulty in chewing and swallowing
- Difficult extremity movement
- Weakened respiratory muscles

The affected muscles become worse with use but may recover completely with rest. The condition may be exacerbated by infection, stress, medications, and menstruation. Myasthenia gravis often can be controlled with drug therapy to enhance the transmission of nerve impulses in the muscles. (Removal of the thymus gland may improve the condition.) In a small number of patients, the disease will progress to paralysis of the throat and respiratory muscles and may lead to death.

Special Considerations

Accommodations required for care will vary, based on the patient's presentation. In most cases, supportive care and transport will be all that is required. In the presence of respiratory distress, measures should be taken to ensure adequate airway and ventilatory support.

Culturally Diverse Patients

Individuals vary in many ways, and there is enormous diversity in populations of all cultures. **Diversity** (a term once used primarily to describe "racial awareness") now refers to differences of any kind: race, class, religion, gender, sexual preference, personal habitat, and physical ability. Good health care depends on sensitivity toward these differences.

? CRITICAL THINKING

What kinds of diversity is there in your classroom? How do you feel about that diversity?

✓ TRICKS OF THE TRADE

You should become familiar with cultures in your response area.

Experiences of health and illness vary widely as a result of different beliefs, behaviors, and past experiences, and may conflict with learned medical practice of the paramedic. By revealing awareness of cultural issues, the paramedic conveys interest, concern, and respect. When dealing with patients from different cultures, the paramedic should remember the following eight key points:

1. The individual is the "foreground," the culture is the "background."
2. Different generations and individuals within the same family may have different sets of beliefs.
3. Not all people identify with their ethnic cultural background.
4. All people share common problems or situations.
5. Respect the integrity of cultural beliefs.
6. Realize that people may not share your explanations of the causes of their ill health but may accept conventional treatments. (You do not have to "convert" a patient to your way of thinking to get the desired result.)
7. You do not have to agree with every aspect of another's culture nor does the person have to accept everything about yours for effective and culturally sensitive health care to occur.
8. Recognize your personal cultural assumptions, prejudices, and belief systems. Do not let them interfere with patient care.

Special Considerations

Regardless of the patient's cultural background, educational status, occupation, or ability to speak English, most patients will be anxious during an emergency event. The paramedic should attempt to communicate in English first to determine whether the patient understands or speaks some English words or phrases. (Bystanders, co-workers, or family members may be available to provide assistance.) In some areas, special translator devices (e.g., AT&T language line) for non–English-speaking patients are available. If the patient does not speak or understand English, the paramedic should attempt to communicate with signs or gestures. The receiving hospital should be notified as soon as possible so that arrangements for an interpreter can be made.

If time permits, all assessment procedures should be performed slowly and with the patient's permission. The paramedic should be aware that "private space" is culturally defined. It is therefore best to point to the area of the body to be examined before touching the patient. The patient's need for modesty and privacy must be respected at the scene and during transport.

Terminally Ill Patients

As health care professionals, paramedics will care for **terminally ill patients** (patients with advanced stage of disease with an unfavorable prognosis and no known cure). Often, these will be emotionally charged encounters that require a great deal of empathy and compassion for the patient and his or her loved ones. If emotions at the scene are out of control, it will be important for the paramedic to take control and to calm the people involved.

If EMS has been summoned to assess late stages of a patient's terminal illness or a change in the patient's condition, the paramedic should gather a complete history and ask the patient or family about advance directives and the appropriateness of resuscitation procedures (see Chapter 4). Any documentation made available to the paramedic (e.g., a DNR order) should be carefully reviewed and discussed with medical direction so that patient care decisions can be made.

Special Considerations

Care of a terminally ill patient often will be primarily supportive and limited to calming and comfort measures and perhaps transport for physician evaluation. (Many terminally ill patients and their families will be involved in hospice care to help them deal with death and dying.) Pain assessment and the management of pain are important aspects of caring for these patients. The paramedic should attempt to gather a complete pain medication history and examine the patient for the presence of transdermal drug patches or other pain-relief devices. Following an assessment of the patient's vital signs, level of consciousness, and medication history,

medical direction may recommend the administration of analgesics or sedatives (e.g., *morphine, midazolam* [Versed]) to ensure the patient's comfort.

Patients with Communicable Diseases

As described in Chapter 37, exposure to some infectious diseases can pose a significant health risk to EMS providers. It therefore is important to ensure personal protection on *every* emergency response. Required precautions depend on the mode of transmission and the pathogen's ability to create pathological processes. For example, in some cases gloves provide for necessary protection; whereas in other cases, respiratory barriers also will be indicated.

> **NOTE**
> Although paramedics cannot be provided with a totally risk-free environment, simple measures of protection greatly reduce exposure to pathogenic agents.

Special Considerations

Some infectious diseases (e.g., AIDS) take a toll on the emotional well-being of affected patients, their families, and loved ones. The psychological aspects of providing care to these patients include an emphasis on the following:

- Recognizing each patient as an individual with unique health care needs
- Respecting each person's personal dignity
- Providing considerate, respectful care focused upon the person's individual needs

> **? CRITICAL THINKING**
> *How do you think you'll feel when called to care for a patient who is HIV positive or has AIDS?*

Financial Challenges

It is estimated that 41 million Americans and one third of persons living in poverty have no health insurance,[9,10] and insurance coverage held by many others would not carry them through a catastrophic

> **✓ TRICKS OF THE TRADE**
> Remember that culture influences how grief is expressed. This is another reason to become familiar with the different cultures in your response area.

illness. Financial challenges for health care can quickly result from loss of a job and depletion of savings. Financial challenges that are combined with medical conditions that require uninterrupted treatment (e.g., TB, HIV/AIDS, diabetes, hypertension, mental disorders) or that occur in the presence of unexpected illness or injury, can deprive the patient of basic health care services. In addition, poor health is closely associated with homelessness where rates of chronic or acute health problems are extremely high (see the box below).

TRICKS OF THE TRADE

You should be familiar with services for the homeless and know where to refer them for food and shelter.

? CRITICAL THINKING

How do you think that financial pressures influence medication compliance in patients with chronic illness and no insurance?

NOTE

Most medical providers recognize their ethical duty to provide services immediately, without regard to payment, in emergency situations.

HEALTH CARE AND HOMELESSNESS

Many homeless people have multiple health problems. In addition to chronic illness, frostbite, leg ulcers, and respiratory infections are common and often are the direct result of homelessness. Homeless people also are at greater risk for trauma resulting from muggings, beatings, and rape. Homelessness precludes good nutrition, good personal hygiene, and basic first aid. In addition, some homeless people with mental disorders may use alcohol or other drugs to self-medicate, and those with addictive disorders are often at risk of HIV and other communicable diseases.

Special Considerations

Persons with financial challenges often are apprehensive about seeking medical care. Fortunately, the ability to pay for emergency health care generally is not a concern for EMS providers (see Chapter 5). According to *Emergency Medical Services, Agenda for the Future,* "the focus of public access is the ability to secure prompt and appropriate EMS care regardless of socioeconomic status, age, or special need. For all those who contact EMS with a perceived requirement for care, the subsequent response and level of care provided must be commensurate with the situation."[11] When caring for a patient with financial challenges who is concerned about the cost of receiving needed health care, the paramedic should explain the following:

1. The patient's ability to pay should never be a factor in obtaining emergency health care.
2. Federal law mandates that medical screening be provided, regardless of the patient's ability to pay.
3. Payment programs for health care services are available in most hospitals.
4. Government services are available to assist patients in paying for health care.
5. Free (or near-free) health care services are available through local, state, and federally funded organizations.

TRICKS OF THE TRADE

Ask the patients if they know which hospital(s) is covered through their health plan or insurance policy.

In cases in which no life-threatening condition exists, the patient with financial challenges should be counseled about alternative facilities for health care for his or her present condition and future situations that do not require ambulance transport for emergency department evaluation. As an example, the paramedic should provide an approved list of alternative health care sites (e.g., a minor-emergency center, health clinic) that can provide medical care at costs that are much less than those charged by emergency departments.

SUMMARY

- Accommodations that may be necessary for a hearing impaired patient include retrieving the patient's hearing aid, providing paper and pen to aid in communication, speaking softly into the patient's ear, and speaking in clear view of the patient.

- When caring for the visually impaired patient, the paramedic should retrieve visual aids and describe all patient care procedures before performing them.

- Allow extra time for the history of a patient with a speech impairment, and if appropriate provide aids such as a pen and paper to assist in communication.

- When caring for an obese patient, use appropriately sized diagnostic devices, and secure additional manpower if needed to move the patient for ambulance transport.

- Patients with paraplegia or quadriplegia often will require additional manpower to assist with moving special equipment to prepare for ambulance transport.

- Once rapport and trust have been established with a patient who has mental illness, care for physical ailments should proceed in the standard manner.

- When caring for a patient with developmental delays allow enough time to obtain a history, perform an assessment, deliver patient care, and prepare for transport.

- The difficulty in assessing patients with emotional impairments is distinguishing between symptoms produced by stress and those caused by serious medical illness.

- Physical injury and disease may result in pathological conditions that require special assessment and management skills. The paramedic should solicit information about the patient's current medications and normal level of functioning in the history.

- Diversity refers to differences of any kind: race, class, religion, gender, sexual preference, personal habitat, and physical ability. Good health care depends on sensitivity toward these differences.

- Often, calls involving the care of a terminally ill patient will be emotionally charged encounters that require a great deal of empathy and compassion for the patient and his or her loved ones.

- Some infectious diseases will take a toll on the emotional well-being of affected patients, their families, and loved ones. Paramedics should be sensitive to the psychological needs of the patient and their families.

- Financial challenges can deprive a patient of basic health care services. These patients may be reluctant to seek care for illness or injury.

REFERENCES

1. American Academy of Ophthalmology: *Statistics on blindness,* http://upshawinst.org/mehrc/statistics.htm.
2. U.S. Department of Transportation, National Highway Traffic Safety Administration: *EMT-Paramedic national standard curriculum,* Washington, DC, 1998, The Department.
3. Centers for Disease Control and Prevention: *Obesity epidemic increases dramatically in the United States: CDC director calls for national prevention effort,* http://www.cdc.gov/od/oc/media/pressrel/r991026.htm
4. American Heart Association: *Basic life support for healthcare providers,* Dallas, Tex, 1997, The Association.
5. Thibodeau G, Patton K: *Anatomy and physiology,* ed 2, St Louis, 1993, Mosby.
6. *Mental retardation: developmental disability,* PsyWeb.com, http://www.psyweb.com/Mdisord/menret.html
7. Lissauer T, Clayden C: *Illustrated textbook of pediatrics,* St Louis, 1997, Mosby.
8. *Myasthenia gravis: a summary,* Myasthenia Gravis Foundation of America, http://www.myasthenia.org/information/summary.htm

9. Department of Health and Human Services: *Statement by Dr. Claude Earl Fox*, Health Resources and Services Administration on Fiscal Year 1999 President's Budget Request for the Health Resources and Services Administration.

10. National Coalition for the Homeless: *Healthcare and homelessness*, Washington, DC, 1999, The Coalition.

11. U.S. Department of Transportation National Highway Traffic Safety Administration, U.S. Department of Health and Human Services: *Emergency medical services: agenda for the future*, Washington, DC, 1996, The Department.

46 Acute Interventions for the Home Health Care Patient

Upon completion of this chapter, the paramedic student will be able to:

1. **Discuss general issues related to the home care patient.**

2. **Outline general principles of assessment and management of the home health patient.**

3. **Describe medical equipment, assessment, and management of the home health patient with inadequate respiratory support.**

4. **Identify assessment findings and acute interventions for problems related to vascular access devices in the home health setting.**

5. **Describe medical equipment, assessment, and management of the patient with a gastrointestinal (GI) or genitourinary (GU) crisis in the home health setting.**

6. **Identify key assessments and principles of wound care management in the home care patient.**

7. **Outline maternal/child problems that may be encountered early in the postpartum period in the home care setting.**

8. **Describe medical therapy associated with hospice and comfort care in the home health setting.**

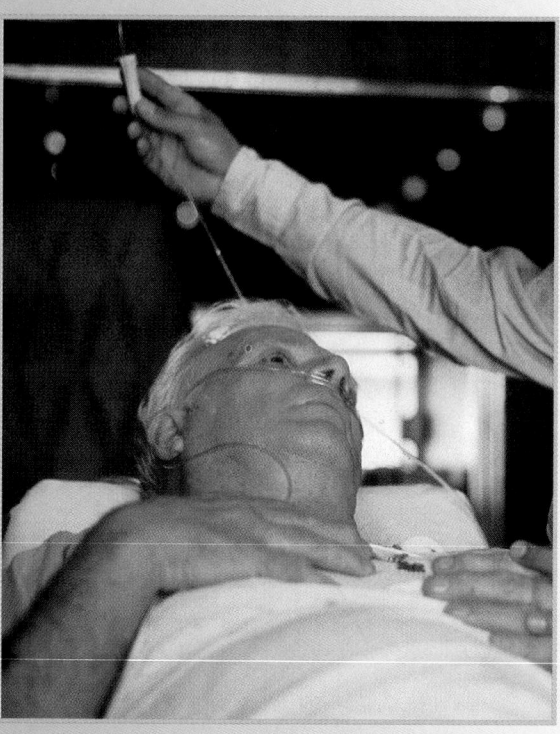

The cost-driven allocation of health care resources and advances in technology have led to shortened hospital stays and allowed many patients to be treated in the home setting. An estimated 8 million people in the United States require home health care services because of acute illness, long-term health conditions, personal preference, permanent disability, or terminal illness.[1] Paramedics will likely play an important role in providing acute interventions to these patients.

KEY TERMS

colostomy: A surgical opening into the large intestine.

failure to thrive: The abnormal retardation of the growth and development of an infant resulting from conditions that interfere with normal metabolism, appetite, and activity.

ileostomy: A surgical opening into the small intestine.

ostomy: An artificial opening into the urinary tract, gastrointestinal tract, or trachea; any surgical procedure in which an opening is created between two hollow organs or between a hollow viscus and the abdominal wall.

palliative care: A unique form of health care primarily directed at providing relief to terminally ill persons through symptom management and pain management; also known as *comfort care*.

Overview of Home Health Care

Home health care started in the United States in the late 1800s as a direct result of rapid city growth and an increase in the number of immigrants moving into large cities.[2] The emphasis of home health care at that time was on personal hygiene and preventive care. The health services were provided by visiting nurses who worked in tenements to assist the poor and also cared for wealthy and middle-class families following births or discharges from hospitals. Initially, few physicians were associated with most of these home health care groups.

> **NOTE**
>
> Medicare is the single largest payer of home care services in the United States. Other funding sources include Medicaid, the Older Americans Act, Title XX Social Services Block Grants, the Veteran's Administration, TRICARE/CHAMPUS for military personnel, private insurance, and managed care organizations.

Until the mid 1960s, home health care continued to focus on the poor, while the rest of the population received care in hospitals and doctors' offices. With the passage of the Social Security Act in 1965, home health became a benefit to older adult patients receiving Medicare and greatly accelerated the industry's growth. (In 1973, these services were extended to certain disabled younger Americans; hospice benefits were added in 1983.) By 1997, an estimated 38.5 million older adult and disabled Americans were enrolled in Medicare programs, and 3.4 million Medicare recipients received home health services.[3] In recent years, federal health care reform has led to the development of managed care services that are provided to members by managed care organizations (see Chapter 1). These plans now cover about 40% of the U.S. population and have greatly influenced methods of health care delivery (including home health care services).

Today, home health care incorporates a wide variety of health and social services. These services are provided at home to recovering, disabled, or chronically ill and terminally ill persons in need of medical, nursing, social, or therapeutic treatment and/or assistance with the essential activities of daily living. A sampling of services provided to home care patients includes:

- Skilled nursing services
- Physical, speech, and occupational therapy
- Medical social services
- Home health aides
- Nutritional counseling

Advanced Life Support Response to Home Care Patients

About 25% of home health patients have conditions related to diseases of the circulatory system as their primary diagnosis.[4] (People with heart disease, including congestive heart failure, make up about half of this group.) Other common diagnoses of home care patients include cancer, diabetes, chronic lung disease, renal failure/dialysis, and hypertension. Therefore emergency responses for acute intervention for home care patients likely will be a

BOX 46-1

EXAMPLES OF HOME CARE PROBLEMS

Home Care Services Requiring Intervention by a Home Health Practitioner or Physician
- Chemotherapy
- Pain management
- Hospice care
- Cardiopulmonary care
- Dermatological and wound care
- Gastroenterological and ostomy care
- Catheter management/IV therapy infusion
- Orthopedic care
- Rehabilitative care
- Urological and renal care
- Specimen collection
- AIDS
- Organ transplantation

Home Care Problems Requiring Acute Intervention
- Inadequate respiratory support
- Acute respiratory events
- Vascular access complications
- Acute cardiac events
- GI/GU crisis
- Acute infections
- Maternal/child conditions
- Hospice/comfort care

common occurrence for emergency medical services (EMS) agencies. Typical responses may include respiratory failure, cardiac decompensation, septic complications, equipment malfunction, and other medical pathologies that worsen in the home care setting (Box 46-1).

Injury Control and Prevention in the Home Care Setting

The scientific approach to illness and injury prevention as a means to minimize morbidity and mortality is discussed in Chapter 3 and the Injury Prevention section in Appendix C. The reader should refer to these areas to review primary prevention, acute care, and rehabilitation (tertiary prevention), their concepts, and their strategies.

Infection Control

As with all other patient encounters, infection control should be practiced in the home care setting. Infection control measures include applying the principles of standard precautions and body substance isolation (BSI, or transmission-based precautions) when indicated. These procedures, along with the philosophy that all patients should be treated as though they have an infectious disease, form the basis for infection control guidelines recommended by the Centers for Disease Control and Prevention (CDC). The Occupational Safety and Health Administration (OSHA), CDC, and Environmental Protection Agency (EPA) recommend the same infection control standards for the treatment of home patients as for acute patients. Equipment set forth by these agencies for infection control in the home setting includes:

? CRITICAL THINKING

What factor(s) decreases the risks of spreading infection within a home care setting versus a hospital?

- Mask
- Gown
- Goggles, glasses, or face shield
- Resuscitation mask
- Specimen bags
- EPA-approved disinfectant effective against hepatitis B virus (HBV), human immunodeficiency virus (HIV), and tuberculosis (TB)
- Soap and water
- Disposable paper towels
- Impervious trash bags and labels

NOTE

This text assumes that appropriate personal protection will be used by paramedics as indicated by the nature of the emergency response and the patient's condition.

BOX 46-2

MAJOR CLASSIFICATIONS OF HOME CARE PATIENTS AND ASSOCIATED COMPLAINTS

Airway Pathologies
Inadequate pulmonary toilet
Inadequate alveolar ventilation
Inadequate alveolar oxygenation

Circulatory Pathologies
Alterations in peripheral circulation

GI/GU Pathologies
Ostomies
Catheters
Home dialysis

Infections
Cellulitis
Sepsis

Wound Care
Surgical wound closure
Decubitus wounds
Drains

Hospice Care

Maternal/Child Care
Apnea monitors
The new parent

Progressive Dementia in the Patient at Home

Psychosocial Support of the Home Care Family

Chronic Pain Management

Home Chemotherapy

The Transplant Candidate

Types of Home Care Patients

Health-cost containment measures and technological advances have allowed many types of patients to receive home care. (Major classifications of home care patients and associated complaints are found in Box 46-2.[5])

NOTE

Some EMS agencies ask their communities to notify them when someone is on a complex home care program. Many of these agencies will make a visit to the home prior to the onset of an emergency to become familiar with the patient's condition and special equipment.

General Principles of Assessment and Management

When arriving at the scene of a home care patient, the scene size-up should include standard precautions, elements of scene safety, and environmental milieu. For example, standard precautions should be employed, and the EMS crew should ensure that any infectious waste found in the home environ-

ment is properly contained and disposed of per protocol. The scene should be evaluated for the presence of dangerous pets, firearms and other home protection devices, and any home hazards. Milieu should be assessed for the patient's ability to maintain a healthy environment; for adequate nutritional support; and to ensure that basic needs of heat, water, shelter, and electricity are available.

The initial patient assessment should focus on life-threatening illness or injury, and appropriate measures should be taken as indicated (see Chapter 14). After the initial assessment, a focused history should be obtained, and a physical examination should be performed. Critical findings should alert the paramedic to forgo a detailed assessment and proceed with resuscitation measures and rapid transport for physician evaluation. If there are no

? CRITICAL THINKING

What feelings may a patient's family member (or caregiver) in the home setting have if there is a problem and the patient's condition worsens?

critical findings, the paramedic should obtain a thorough history and perform a physical examination that considers:

- Medication interactions
- Available home health history
- Compliance issues
- Possibility of dementia

A comprehensive assessment may include a physical examination using inspection, palpation, auscultation, and percussion (as indicated by the patient's condition). The ongoing assessment should evaluate any changes in the patient's status while at the scene or en route to the hospital. These assessment strategies can aid in differential diagnosis, treatment, and direction of patient management.

Management and Treatment Plan

Depending on the patient's condition, home health treatment may need to be replaced with advanced life support treatment modalities, such as airway, ventilatory, and circulatory support, and pharmacological and nonpharmacological interventions (e.g., electrical therapy).

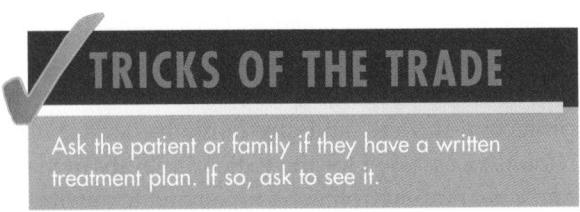

TRICKS OF THE TRADE

Ask the patient or family if they have a written treatment plan. If so, ask to see it.

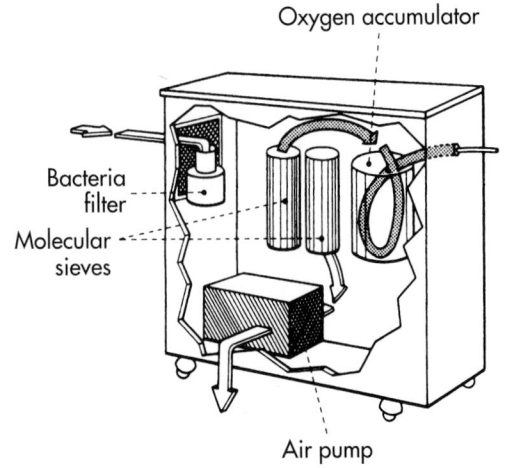

Fig. 46-1 O₂ concentrator. (From Scanlan CL, Wilkins RL, Stoller JK: *Egan's fundamentals of respiratory care*, ed 7, St Louis, 1998, Mosby. Courtesy DeVilbiss Health Care.)

Some patients with acute illness or injury need to be transported to the hospital for physician evaluation. Others only need home care follow-up by home health practitioners or referral to other public service agencies. The paramedic should follow local protocol and consult with medical direction regarding patient referrals and the need for notifying private physicians or home health agencies.

Specific Acute Home Health Interventions

Acute home health situations may occur from equipment failure or malfunction, drug reactions, complications related to home treatment, and worsening medical conditions. This section discusses acute interventions for respiratory support, vascular access devices, GI/GU crisis, acute infections, maternal/child conditions, and hospice/comfort care.

Respiratory Support

More than 600,000 patients are discharged to home care with diseases of the respiratory system each year.[1] These patients are at increased risk for airway infections, and the progression of some respiratory diseases may lead to an increased respiratory demand, making current support inadequate. Examples of chronic pathologies that require home respiratory support include:

- Chronic lung disease
- Asthma
- Bronchopulmonary dysplasia
- Awaiting lung transplant
- Cystic fibrosis
- Sleep apnea
- Infection causing exacerbation of condition

Acute interventions may be required for these patients. Problems that may lead to a request for EMS assistance include increased respiratory demand, increased bronchospasm, increased secre-

NOTE

Any patient with respiratory distress should receive high-concentration oxygen and ventilatory support as priorities in patient care.

tions, obstructed or malfunctioning respiratory devices, or improper application of medical devices to support respirations.

Oxygen Therapy in the Home Setting

There are three common ways to provide oxygen therapy in the home: compressed gas, liquid oxygen, and oxygen concentrators. Compressed gas is oxygen stored under pressure in oxygen cylinders equipped with a regulator that controls flow rate. Liquid oxygen is very cold and stored in a container similar to a thermos. When released, the liquid converts to gas and is used like compressed gas. An oxygen concentrator is an electrically powered device that separates oxygen from air, concentrates it, and stores it (Fig. 46-1). This system does not have to be resupplied and is not as costly as liquid oxygen. A cylinder of oxygen must be available as a backup, however, in case of power failure.

> **? CRITICAL THINKING**
>
> **What safety considerations regarding oxygen administration should you observe for in the home?**

Oxygen is delivered to patients via nasal cannulas, oxygen masks, tracheostomy collars (devices that deliver high humidity and oxygen to patients with surgical airways), and ventilators. Some patients may require continuous positive airway pressure (CPAP) delivered by ventilatory support systems through mask CPAP, nasal CPAP, or bilevel positive airway pressure (BiPAP) (described in Chapter 27). Supportive ventilator management may be indicated to:

- Prevent nocturnal hypoxemia caused by sleep hypoventilation in patients with neuromuscular disorders

> **NOTE**
>
> Obstructive apnea is a form of sleep apnea involving a physical obstruction of the upper airways. The condition usually is marked by recurrent sleep interruptions, choking and gasping spells on awakening, and drowsiness caused by lack of normal sleep. If left uncorrected, this disorder can lead to pulmonary failure, chronic fatigue, and cardiac abnormalities.

- Prevent respiratory fatigue in patients with chronic obstructive pulmonary disease (COPD)
- Improve ventilation and oxygen saturation in patients with obstructive apnea

Home ventilators. Home ventilators can be classified as *volume ventilators, pressure ventilators, and negative pressure ventilators* (Box 46-3). Volume ventilators (volume-preset) deliver a predetermined volume of gas with each cycle, after which inspiration is terminated. These types of ventilators deliver a constant tidal volume regardless of changes in airway resistance or compliance of the lungs and thorax. The volume remains the same unless excessively high peak airway pressures are reached, in which case safety release valves stop the flow (see the box on p. 1342).

Pressure ventilators (pressure-preset) are pressure-cycled devices that terminate inspiration when a preset pressure is achieved. When the preset pressure is reached, the gas flow stops, and the patient passively exhales. These ventilators most commonly are used for patients whose ventilatory resistance is not likely to change.

> **NOTE**
>
> The BiPAP ventilatory support system (designed for mask-applied ventilation in the home) delivers two different levels of positive airway pressure. The system cycles spontaneously between a preset level of inspiratory positive airway pressure (IPAP) and expiratory positive airway pressure (EPAP). The BiPAP ventilatory support system is intended only to augment the patient's breathing; it does not provide for total ventilatory requirements. It is used by some patients with sleep apnea or COPD.

> **BOX 46-3**
>
> **STANDARD INITIAL VENTILATOR SETTINGS**
>
> | | |
> |---|---|
> | FiO_2: | 100% |
> | Tidal volume: | 10 to 15 mL/kg body weight |
> | Respiratory rate: | 10 to 15 breaths/minute |
> | Inspiratory flow: | 40 to 60 L/second |
> | Sensitivity: | 12 cm H_2O |
> | Sigh rate (optional): | 1 to 2/minute |

VENTILATOR ALARMS

Ventilators are equipped with alarms to signal problems with ventilator function, including alarms for loss of power, frequency alarms (indicating changes in respiratory rate), volume alarms (indicating low-exhaled volume or low/high minute-ventilation), and high-pressure alarms. If alarms are sounding, the paramedic should check for the following possible causes:

- Kinks in ET tube
- Disconnected ventilator tubing or poor connections
- Water in ventilator tubing
- Excessive secretions
- Pneumothorax
- Patient anxiety

After consulting with medical direction, acute interventions may include providing temporary ventilation assistance with a bag-valve mask device, repositioning the ET tube, correcting poor ventilator tube connections, emptying water from tube or water traps, suctioning the airway, thoracic decompression, and possible sedation (Table 46-1).

Negative pressure ventilators have settings for the respiratory rate and pressure of the negative force exerted. These devices use negative pressure to raise the rib cage and lower the diaphragm to create negative pressure within the lungs so that air flows into the lungs. Negative pressure ventilators often are used for patients with healthy lungs who have a muscular inability to inhale (e.g., patients with spinal cord injury, neuromuscular disease). Examples of this type of ventilator are the "iron lung" and plastic wrap, or poncho, ventilators.

Assessment Findings

When caring for a patient who requires oxygen therapy, the paramedic should evaluate the patient's work of breathing, tidal volume, peak flow, oxygen saturation, and quality of breath sounds. This assessment can be performed with visual inspection (chest rise and fall), peak flow meters, pulse oximetry, and auscultation (described in Chapter 11 and Chapter 27). The paramedic should be constantly aware of signs and symptoms of hypoxia; these include:

- Restlessness
- Headache
- Confusion and mental status changes
- Hyperventilation
- Tachycardia
- Hypertension
- Dyspnea
- Cyanosis

Management

Management goals for a patient receiving oxygen therapy who requires acute intervention are to improve airway patency, ventilation, and oxygenation.

Improving airway patency. To improve airway patency, the paramedic should first reposition airway devices (e.g., face masks, nasal cannulas) to ensure they are properly applied and well fitted. Secretions that obstruct airflow should be cleared from the airway with suction and from any airway device with sterile water. If necessary, the home airway device should be replaced with a new device. A tracheostomy tube that has become blocked and cannot be cleared may need to be replaced with another tracheostomy tube (or temporarily replaced with an endotracheal [ET] tube) to ensure adequate ventilation.

Improving ventilation and oxygenation. If ventilation does not improve after providing a patent airway, the home care device should be removed, and the patient's ventilations should be assisted with positive-pressure ventilation via a bag-valve mask device and supplemental oxygen. Oxygen saturation should be monitored with pulse oximetry, and supplemental oxygen should be administered as necessary to

NOTE

On some ventilators, inspiratory flow rate is determined by tidal volume, respiratory rate, and the inspiratory:expiratory (I:E) ratio. (The I:E ratio is generally 1:2 to allow for complete exhalation and prevent air trapping.) On other ventilators, flow rate is independently set, which allows adjustment of air flow to the flow wave pattern that is most comfortable for the patient. If the patient is having difficulty with spontaneous breathing, increasing the flow rate may be indicated. However, a higher flow rate means a shorter inspiratory time and usually a higher respiratory pressure secondary to increased resistance, with a lower flow rate requiring a longer inspiratory time with a decreased inspiratory pressure. The paramedic should always consult with medical direction before changing the flow rate on any ventilator device.

TABLE 46-1	VENTILATOR ALARMS	
ALARM TYPE	**CAUSES**	**INTERVENTIONS**
High pressure	Increased secretions	Suction patient
High pressure	Kinked tubing	Unkink tubing
High pressure	Water in tubing	Disconnect tubing and allow it to drain
High pressure	Anxiety	Decrease anxiety by providing a calm environment
Low pressure	Disconnected tubing	Reconnect tubing
Low pressure	Cuff leak	Add 1 mL of air at a time to pilot balloon of tracheostomy tube
Low pressure	Tracheostomy tube out	Reinsert new tracheostomy tube
Oxygen	Insufficient oxygen supply	Manually ventilate patient and prepare for transport
Ventilator not operating	Power failure	Manually ventilate patient and prepare for transport

maintain oxygen saturation at 90% or higher. Medical direction may recommend adjusting the settings of a home care device or changing the flow rate of an oxygen delivery device to improve ventilation and oxygenation. Additional manpower may be needed to assist with moving the patient who has airway devices to the ambulance for transport for physician evaluation.

Psychological Support and Communication Strategies

Respiratory insufficiency can be a horrifying experience for the patient, particularly for a patient who is dependent on a ventilator. The paramedic crew should attempt to calm the patient and family and assure them that respirations will be adequately supported by other means while at the scene and during transport for physician evaluation.

TRICKS OF THE TRADE

Airway insufficiency can be horrifying for the EMS crew as well. Stay calm and remember your *ABCs*: Airway, Breathing, and Circulation!

Loss of verbal communication is a major source of anxiety in patients who have tracheostomies. The ability to communicate with these patients will be based on the patient's cognition, level of consciousness, language, and fine and gross motor skills. Methods of communication may include signing and writing on notepads.

NOTE

Some patients with tracheostomies have special valves attached to the tracheostomy tube ("talking trachs") that redirect exhaled air around the tracheostomy tube, through the vocal cords, and out of the mouth and nose, allowing for normal speech.

TRICKS OF THE TRADE

Enlist the help of family members and other caregivers who may be "experts" in communicating with the patient.

Vascular Access Devices

Many patients in the home care setting will have indwelling vascular access devices (VADs). VADs are used to provide nutritional support and administer medications, and they are used for patients who need long-term vascular access (e.g., patients receiving dialysis, chemotherapy). Those with indwelling vascular devices may experience problems that include:

- Anticoagulation associated with percutaneous or implanted devices
- Embolus formation associated with indwelling devices, stasis, and inactivity
- Air embolus associated with central venous access devices

- Obstructed or malfunctioning VADs
- Infection at the access site
- Infiltration and extravasation
- Obstructed dialysis shunts

Types of VADs

A variety of VADs are encountered in home care patients. These include surgically implanted subcutaneous VADs, medication delivery devices (e.g., Mediports, as described in Chapter 9), peripheral vascular access devices (e.g., peripherally inserted central catheters [PICCs], midline catheters), central venous tunneled catheters (e.g., Hickman, Groshong, Broviac), and dialysis shunts (Fig. 46-2).

Assessment Findings and Acute Interventions for VADs

Assessment findings that may require acute interventions in patients with VADs include infection, hemorrhage, hemodynamic compromise from circulatory overload or embolus, obstruction of the vascular device, catheter breakage, and leakage of medication (e.g., chemotherapeutic agents) (Table 46-2).

Infection. A common problem of VADs is infection near the exit site, tunnel, or port. Signs and symptoms of site infection include pain, redness, warmth, and purulence. Signs and symptoms of systemic infection (which may result from a site infection) include fever, tachycardia, general weakness, malaise, mental status changes, body aches,

and possibly septicemia. General principles in managing the site infection are to:

> **? CRITICAL THINKING**
>
> *Will it always be possible to identify the catheter as the source of sepsis while on the scene?*

1. Ensure aseptic technique when assessing the manipulating line.
2. Clean the site with alcohol and then iodine-povidone solution (per protocol).
3. Apply antimicrobial ointment (per protocol; this is controversial).
4. Cover the site with a transparent, sterile dressing (per protocol).
5. Document the procedure and label the dressing with the date, time, and paramedic's initials.
6. Consult with medical direction.

> **NOTE**
>
> Home patients who have VADs generally are instructed to examine the area for infection and change the dressings around their device frequently. Often this is done by family members and home health practitioners. All types of dressings must be changed immediately if they become wet, soiled, contaminated, or unocclusive.

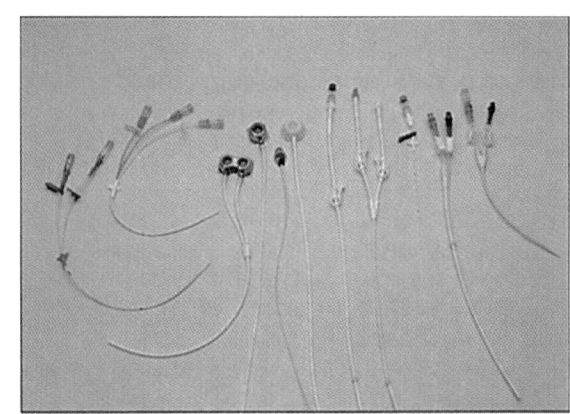 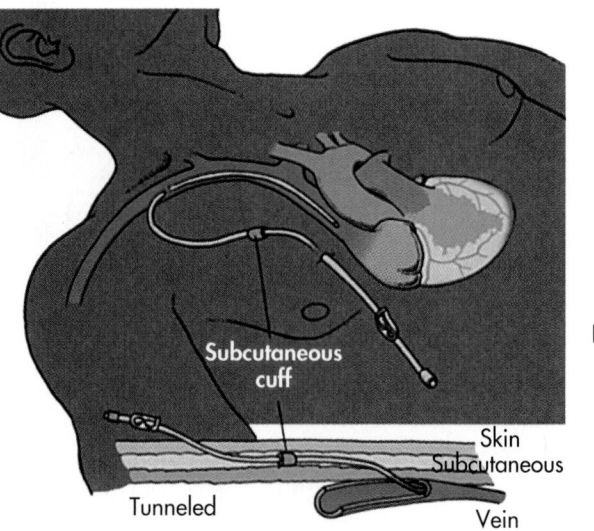

Fig. 46-2 Vascular access devices. **A,** Central venous catheters. **B,** Central venous catheters are inserted into the skin and tunneled through the subcutaneous tissue and into the vein. The distal end of the catheter rests in the superior vena cava.

Hemorrhage. Bleeding at the site of a VAD should be controlled by applying gentle, direct pressure with aseptic technique. These patients need to be transported for physician evaluation. Blood loss from a broken or dislodged VAD can be significant. If blood loss is severe, the patient should be treated for hemorrhagic shock.

Hemodynamic compromise. Hemodynamic compromise may result from circulatory overload or embolus.

Circulatory overload can develop from too much intravenous (IV) fluid delivered too fast. Signs and symptoms of circulatory overload include a rise in blood pressure, distended neck veins, pulmonary congestion (crackles and/or wheezes), and dyspnea. If circulatory overload is suspected, the paramedic should:

1. Slow the infusion to a keep-open rate.
2. Provide high-concentration oxygen.

TABLE 46-2	CORRECTING COMMON PROBLEMS WITH VADs	
COMPLICATION	**SIGNS AND SYMPTOMS**	**PREHOSPITAL INTERVENTIONS**
Mechanical problems		
Clotted IV catheter	Interrupted flow rate, resistance to flushing and blood withdrawal	Attempt to aspirate the clot. If unsuccessful, contact medical direction.
Cracked or broken tubing	Fluid leaking from the tubing	Apply padded hemostat above the break to prevent air from entering the line and change the tubing (with orders from medical direction).
Dislodged catheter	Catheter out of the vein	Apply pressure to the site with a sterile gauze pad.
Too-rapid infusion	Nausea, headache, lethargy, dyspnea	Adjust the infusion rate, and if applicable, check the infusion pump. Contact medical direction about need to transport.
Other problems		
Air embolism	Apprehension, chest pain, tachycardia, hypotension, cyanosis, seizures, loss of consciousness, and cardiac arrest	Clamp the catheter. Place the patient in a steep, left lateral Trendelenburg position. Give oxygen as ordered. If cardiac arrest occurs, begin cardiopulmonary resuscitation.
Extravasation	Swelling and pain around the insertion site	Stop the infusion. Assess the patient for cardiopulmonary abnormalities. Notify medical direction for further advice.
Phlebitis	Pain, tenderness, redness, and warmth	Apply gentle heat to the area; elevate insertion site if possible.
Pneumothorax and hydrothorax	Dyspnea, chest pain, cyanosis, and decreased breath sounds	If signs and symptoms of tension pneumothorax are present, consider needle decompression after consulting with medical direction. Rapid transport is indicated.
Septicemia	Red and swollen catheter site, chills, fever	Transport for physician evaluation.
Thrombosis	Erythema and edema at the insertion site; ipsilateral swelling of the arm, neck, face, and upper chest; pain at the insertion site and along the vein; malaise; fever; tachycardia	Apply warm compresses to insertion site; elevate affected extremity. Transport patient.
Hemorrhage	Bleeding at site of VAD or from broken VAD	Apply pressure to site. Clamp VAD and treat for shock.

3. Elevate the patient's head.
4. Maintain body warmth to promote peripheral circulation and ease the stress on the central veins.
5. Monitor vital signs.
6. Consult with medical direction for patient management and disposition.

? CRITICAL THINKING

What drug(s) may the physician order if this happens?

It is rare for a surgically implanted catheter or port to become displaced. An embolus that occurs from air, thrombus, or plastic or catheter tip entering the circulation, however, can develop (Box 46-4). Signs and symptoms of an embolus include hypotension; cyanosis; weak, rapid pulse; and loss of consciousness. A patient with a suspected embolism should be managed as follows (described in Chapter 9):

1. Stop the IV infusion.
2. Position the patient on the left side with the head down (in an attempt to keep the embolus in the right side of the heart).
3. Administer high-concentration oxygen.
4. Notify medical direction.

NOTE

If a plastic or catheter tip embolism is suspected, medical direction may recommend that a constricting band be applied above a peripheral VAD to stop the embolus from further migration.

BOX 46-4

CAUSES OF EMBOLUS FORMATION

Air Embolism
IV fluid containers that run dry
Air in IV tubing
Loose connections in catheter tubing
Catheter tears and breakage

Thrombus
Clot formation from inactivity or stasis

Plastic or Catheter Tip Migration
Plastic or catheter fragment from tugging or shearing forces
Wire from central line placement

Obstruction of the vascular device. An indwelling vascular device may become obstructed, disrupting the flow of fluids and medications. When this occurs, immediate intervention is required to clear the device by irrigation or administration of thrombolytic agents.

✓ TRICKS OF THE TRADE

Clearing an obstructed VAD requires expertise. The most experienced paramedic should perform this procedure.

NOTE

The paramedic should always consult with medical direction prior to attempting to clear an obstruction from a VAD.

Flushing and irrigation. VADs and medication ports require regular irrigation with normal saline and/or *heparin*, depending on the type of VAD (Table 46-3). The frequency of irrigation depends on the specific device and frequency of medication administration. If a VAD is obstructed, the paramedic should consult with medical direction and follow these steps:

1. Explain the procedure to the patient.
2. Prepare prescribed irrigation solutions (normal saline or normal saline and *heparin*).
3. Clean the injection cap(s) with an antiseptic and alcohol wipe (per protocol) and allow to air-dry.
4. Release the clamp from the catheter (if present).
5. Irrigate the lumen with an appropriate volume of solution using a 10 milliliter (mL) syringe (no faster than 0.5 mL/second). If resistance is persistent, stop the irrigation, or the catheter may rupture.

NOTE

The paramedic must never attempt to force or dislodge a clot or other obstruction. Fibrinolytic agents may be required. The application of force could dislodge the obstruction and cause it to enter the circulatory system.

6. Aspirate blood back into the syringe; this removes clots or fibrin sheaths.
7. Flush with normal saline (10 to 20 mL) to clear system.
8. Use a heparin lock if necessary (e.g., Broviac, Hickman, PICC).
9. Clamp catheter if needed.
10. Loop the catheter with the cap pointing upward on the dressing. Secure with tape.
11. Properly dispose of all equipment.

Anticoagulant therapy. There may be occasions when a medication port or other vascular device will require declotting with fibrinolytic agents. The paramedic should always consult with medical direction prior to administering anticoagulant therapy. Listed here are the steps to follow in declotting a Port-A-Cath device:

1. Explain the procedure to the patient.
2. Prepare the necessary solutions and 1 mL of normal saline solution in a 3 mL syringe with a noncoring (Huber) needle.
3. Using sterile technique, clean the injection cap or area of skin over the Port-A-Cath septum with alcohol followed by a povodine wipe (per protocol) and allow to air dry.
4. Connect the syringe to the integrated extension tubing. Unclamp the tubing.
5. Slowly inject the medication solution into the occluded lumen and port of the Port-A-Cath. Wait 30 minutes.

6. Attempt to aspirate the residual clot.
7. Repeat the procedure with a 15-minute dwell time if patency is not achieved.
8. Notify medical direction if the catheter cannot be aspirated. If patency is achieved, follow the previously described procedure for flushing and irrigation.
9. Properly dispose of all equipment.

Catheter damage. A damaged (e.g., cracked, torn) catheter can allow fluids or medications to infiltrate into the surrounding tissues and lead to an air embolism. Signs and symptoms of a damaged catheter includes leaking fluid, complaint of a burning sensation, or swollen and tender skin near the insertion site. If catheter damage is suspected, the infusion should be stopped immediately, and the catheter clamped between the crack or tear in the catheter and the patient. These patients are managed with high-concentration oxygen, IV access through a peripheral vein, and transport for physician evaluation. A patient who develops an altered level of consciousness (indicating a possible air embolism) should be positioned on the left side with the head slightly lowered to help prevent the embolism from traveling to the brain.

GI/GU Crisis

About 500,000 patients with diseases of the digestive or GU system are discharged to home care each year.[1] Some of these patients have medical devices such as urinary catheters or urostomies,

TABLE 46-3	IRRIGATION FOR VASCULAR ACCESS DEVICES		
DEVICE	**SYRINGE SIZE**	**SOLUTION**	**AMOUNT**
Peripheral access devices			
	3 mL	Heparin flush solution 10 units/mL	2.5-3.0 mL
Central venous access devices (CAVD)			
1. Groshong	10 mL	0.9% sodium chloride (normal saline)	5 mL, 10-20 mL following blood draws
2. Mediports	10 mL	1. Sodium chloride 0.9% (normal saline)	10mL
		2. Heparin 100 units/mL	5 mL
3. Peripherally inserted central catheter (PICC)	10 mL	1. Sodium chloride 0.9% (normal saline)	10 mL
		2. Heparin 100 units/mL	3.0-5.0 mL

Source: Intravenous Therapy-Clinical Principles and Practice, 1995.

indwelling nutritional support devices (e.g., percutaneous endoscopic gastrostomy [PEG] tube, gastrostomy tube [G-tube]), colostomies, and nasogastric (NG) tubes (Box 46-5). Acute interventions that may be required for these patients can result from urinary tract infection (UTI), urosepsis, urinary retention; and problems with gastric emptying or feeding.

Urinary Tract Infection, Urosepsis, and Urinary Retention
UTI is common and occurs in all age groups and both sexes (as described in Chapter 33). The organisms most frequently associated with UTI are gram-negative organisms normally found in the GI tract, including *Escherichia coli, Klebsiella, Proteus, Enterobacter,* and *Pseudomonas.* These frequently are introduced from the hands of health personnel at the time of bladder catheterization.[6] Other factors that increase a person's risk for UTI include:

- Obstructions (e.g., urethral strictures, calculi, tumors, blood clots)
- Trauma (e.g., abdominal injury, ruptured bladder, local trauma related to sexual activity)
- Congenital anomalies (e.g., polycystic kidneys, horseshoe kidney, spina bifida)
- Abdominal or gynecological surgery
- Acute or chronic renal failure
- Immunocompromised state (e.g., patients with HIV, older adults)
- Postpartum state
- Aging changes, particularly in women

> **NOTE**
>
> About 75% of UTIs are the result of urological instrumentation. Sterile technique during these procedures is crucial.

If allowed to progress, UTI may lead to septic complications (urosepsis). This disease is managed with antibiotic therapy.

Urinary retention. Urinary retention may result from urethral stricture, inflammation, enlarged prostate, central nervous system (CNS) dysfunction, foreign body obstruction, and use of certain drugs, such as parasympatholytic or anticholinergic agents. These patients need physician evaluation to determine the cause of urine retention. If the cause is not easily correctable, the patient may require hospitalization. An acute intervention that may be required for some patients is bladder catheterization with an indwelling Foley catheter device. This procedure may be indicated to empty the bladder of a patient with urinary retention or replace a nonfunctioning indwelling urinary catheter device.

> **NOTE**
>
> Bladder catheterization is an invasive procedure that carries some associated risks. These include the introduction of bacteria, which may lead to UTI; hematuria; and the creation of a "false urethral passage," which may result in significant blood loss and the need for surgical repair. Special training and authorization from medical direction is required to perform bladder catheterization.

Indwelling Foley catheter insertion. To insert a Foley catheter, the paramedic should prepare the necessary equipment (e.g., Foley catheter insertion set) and closely follow the recommendations of the manufacturer (Box 46-6). Steps in bladder catheteri-

---

BOX 46-5

MEDICAL THERAPY FOUND IN THE HOME SETTING FOR PATIENTS WITH GI/GU DISEASE

Devices for Gastric/Intestinal Emptying or Feeding
NG tube
Feeding tube
PEG tubes, jejunostomy tubes (J-tubes), G-tubes
Colostomy

Devices for the Urinary Tract
External urinary catheters (e.g., Condom catheter, Texas catheter)
Indwelling urinary catheter (e.g., Foley catheter, Coudé catheter)
Surgical urinary catheters (e.g., suprapubic catheters)
Urostomy

zation for male and female patients are described in this section.

? CRITICAL THINKING

What precaution should you take to protect yourself legally when inserting a Foley catheter in the home care setting?

Male Catheterization (Fig. 46-3)
1. Explain procedure to the patient.
2. Place the patient in supine position and remove the patient's pants and undergarments.
3. Open the catheterization set using sterile technique.
4. Wash hands and don sterile gloves.
5. Place one sterile drape under the patient's penis and another above the penis to cover the abdomen.
6. Open a package of antiseptic solution and saturate sterile sponges (or cotton balls).
7. Attach the syringe to the catheter and test the balloon to make sure it inflates.

8. Open a package of water-soluble lubricant and lubricate the first several inches of the catheter.
9. Grasp the patient's penis with one hand and retract the foreskin (if present).
10. With the other hand, cleanse the glans with a sterile sponge (maintaining hand sterility) and then discard the sponge. Repeat the procedure.
11. Raise the shaft of the penis upright to straighten the penile urethra and pass the tip of the catheter through the meatus.
12. Continue passing the catheter with gentle, steady pressure, advancing the catheter 7 to 9 inches or until urine flows out the distal end of the catheter. Once urine appears, advance the catheter another 2 inches. If mild resistance is felt at the external sphincter, slightly increase traction on the penis and continue with steady, gentle pressure on the catheter. *If significant resistance is met, withdraw the catheter and consult with medical direction.*
13. Attach the syringe to the catheter and inflate the balloon with 3 to 5 mL of sterile saline.
14. Gently pull back on the catheter until the balloon rests against the prostatic urethra. (Resistance will be encountered.) Reposition the retracted foreskin of an uncircumcised patient. Attach the drainage bag to the catheter.
15. Run the catheter tubing along the patient's leg and tape the connecting tubing to the patient's thigh. Do not place any tension on the catheter.
16. Attach the collection bag to the bed or stretcher at a level below that of the patient to facilitate drainage by gravity.

BOX 46-6

NECESSARY EQUIPMENT FOR BLADDER CATHETERIZATION

Personal protective equipment
Urinary catheterization set containing:
- Sterile gloves
- Antiseptic solution
- Sterile cleansing sponges
- Sterile drapes or towels
- Syringe containing 5 mL sterile water
- Connecting tubing and collection bag
- Water-soluble sterile lubricant
Urinary catheter with 5 mL Foley balloon
- Usually a number 16 Foley for males or a 14 Foley for females
- Standard length is 18 inches

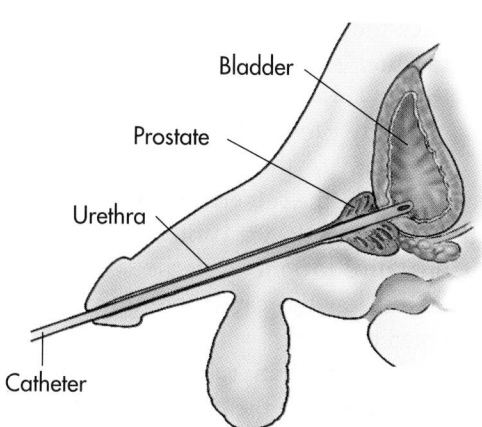

Fig. 46-3 Male catheterization.

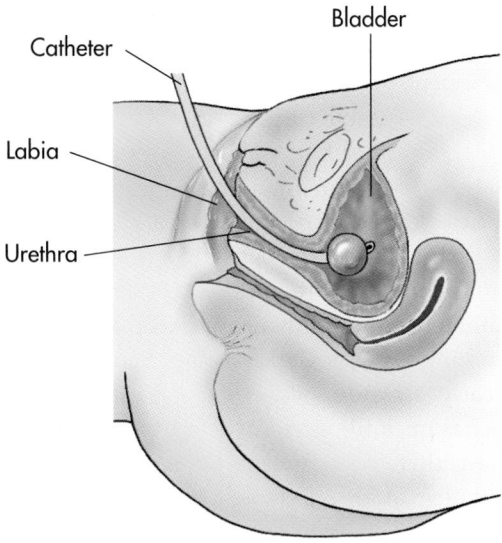

Fig. 46-4 Female catheterization.

TABLE 46-4	FEEDING TUBES: TYPES AND PLACEMENT
TYPE OF TUBE	**PLACEMENT**
NG	Passed via nose into stomach
Nasointestinal	Passed via nose into intestine
Esophagostomy tube	Passed into the esophagus though a surgically created opening in the anterior neck
G-tube	Passed directly into the stomach through an opening created in the abdominal wall
J-tube, PEG tube	Passed into the jejunum through an opening created in the abdominal wall

Female Catheterization (Fig. 46-4)

1. Prepare the patient and equipment as described in steps 1 through 4 and 6 through 8 of the previous procedure. Female patients should be positioned with knees bent, hips flexed, and feet resting about 24 inches apart. The patient should be appropriately draped by placing one sterile drape just under the patient's buttocks; position the fenestrated drape over the perineum, exposing the labia.
2. With one hand, separate the patient's labia to expose the urethral meatus.
3. Cleanse the surrounding area with a sterile sponge or cotton ball (maintaining hand sterility) in downward strokes from anterior to posterior and then discard the sponge. Repeat the procedure.
4. Introduce the tip of the well-lubricated catheter into the urethra using aseptic technique. Continue to advance the catheter 2 to 3 inches with gentle, steady pressure until urine flows out of the distal end of the catheter. Once urine appears, advance the catheter another 2 inches.
5. Attach a syringe to the catheter and inflate the balloon with 3 to 5 mL of sterile saline.
6. Gently pull on the catheter until resistance is encountered.
7. Attach the collection tubing and bag to the catheter and secure the collection tubing to the patient's thigh as described above in 14 and 16 of the previous procedure. Position the collection bag to facilitate drainage.

Problems with Gastric Emptying or Feeding

Gastric tubes found in the home care setting are devices that are inserted into the stomach or intestines for the purpose of removing fluids and gas by suction or gravity, instilling irrigation solutions or medications, and for administering enteral feedings (Table 46-4). Two common problems with gastric tubes are aspiration of gastric contents and malfunction of gastric devices.

Aspiration of gastric contents. Aspiration of gastric contents may occur in the home care patient as a result of a nonpatent gastric tube, improper nutritional support via a feeding tube, or patient positioning with these medical devices. The patients at greatest risk for aspiration of tube feedings are those who:

- Are unconscious
- Are confused
- Are seriously debilitated
- Are older adults
- Have tracheostomies or large-bore feeding tubes
- Have impaired gag reflexes
- Cannot sit upright

Patients with feeding tubes should be closely monitored for respirations that represent minimal respiratory effort and for lung sounds that are clear on auscultation. Respiratory difficulty or tachypnea may indicate developing aspiration pneumonitis. Other problems that can occur in patients with feed-

TABLE 46-5	MANAGING TUBE FEEDING PROBLEMS

The following chart shows some interventions that the nurse, paramedic, patient, or caregiver may try for solving home tube feeding problems.

COMPLICATION	INTERVENTIONS
Aspiration of gastric secretions	Discontinue feeding immediately. Perform tracheal suction of aspirated contents if possible. Notify the doctor. Check tube placement before feeding to prevent complications.
Tube obstruction	Flush the tube with warm water. If necessary, replace the tube. Flush the tube with 50 mL of water after each feeding to remove excess sticky formula, which could occlude the tube.
Nasal or pharyngeal irritation or necrosis	Provide frequent oral hygiene using mouthwash or lemon-glycerin swabs. Use petroleum jelly on cracked lips. Change the tube's position. If necessary, replace the tube.
Vomiting, bloating, diarrhea, or cramps	Reduce the flow rate. Warm the formula. For 30 minutes after feeding, position the patient on the right side with the head elevated to facilitate gastric emptying. Notify the doctor. The doctor may want to reduce the amount of formula being given during each feeding.
Constipation	Provide additional fluids if the patient can tolerate them. Administer a bulk-forming laxative. Increase fruit, vegetable, or sugar content of the feeding.

ing tubes include diarrhea, choking, irritable bowel syndrome, and bowel obstruction.

Obstruction or malfunction of gastric devices. A gastric device may become obstructed or malfunction for reasons such as a kinked or clogged tube or displacement of a surgically implanted feeding tube. Acute interventions that may be required include unkinking a tube, irrigating a clogged tube, and reinserting a displaced tube (per medical direction) (Table 46-5).

NOTE

When transporting a patient with a gastric device, the paramedic must ensure patient comfort and take care in positioning the device to allow for proper drainage and prevent reflux.

Ostomies. An **ostomy** is an artificial opening into the urinary tract, GI tract, or trachea. An ostomy may be temporary or permanent. (An **ileostomy** is an opening into the small intestine. A **colostomy** is an

opening into the large intestine.) The bowel usually discharges liquid or solid feces into the bag (pouch) once or twice a day; the bag is then changed. Potential complications associated with ostomies include:

- Infection
- Hemorrhage
- Obstruction
- Stomal problems (e.g., necrosis, retraction, stenosis, prolapse)

Colostomy irrigation, ostomy care, and pouch changes usually are performed for home care patients by the patients themselves, family members, and home health practitioners. These procedures require special training and usually are not considered an acute intervention for paramedic practice.

NOTE

Bowel perforation and/or significant fluid/electrolyte imbalances may accidentally occur from colostomy irrigation performed by the patient or caregiver.

Assessment and Management of Patients with GI/GU Crisis

A patient who presents with GI/GU complaints should be evaluated by obtaining a focused history and performing a physical examination to determine the need for immediate transport for physician evaluation. Depending on the patient's chief complaint, the physical examination may include assessment for:

- Abdominal pain
- Abdominal distention
- Aspiration
- Intestinal obstruction
- Urinary infection
- Urinary retention
- Fever
- Peritonitis

Acute Infections

More than 160,000 patients with infectious and parasitic diseases are discharged to home care in the United States each year.[1] Home care patients with acute infections have an increased mortality rate from sepsis and severe peripheral infections and may have a decreased ability to perceive pain or perform self-care. Conditions that may result in the need for acute interventions in the home care population include[5]:

- Airway infections in the immunocompromised patient
- Delayed healing and increased peripheral infection from poor peripheral perfusion

- Skin breakdown and peripheral infections from immobility or sedentary lifestyle
- Infection and sepsis from implanted medical devices
- Wounds and incisions
- Abscesses
- Cellulitis

> **NOTE**
>
> Patients with chronic diseases, poor nutrition, or an inability to perform self-care are at increased risk for infection and impaired healing.

Open Wounds

Patients with open wounds who are discharged to home care may have a variety of dressings, wound packings, and drains that permit drainage of fluid or air, as well as a variety of wound closure devices (Box 46-7). (Dressings, packings, and wound closure devices can become contaminated; drains can become occluded or displaced.) Wound healing greatly depends on wound management, and the patient must be made aware of the importance of taking all prescribed medications (especially antibiotics) and completing all wound-care procedures. It generally is believed that wound repair is enhanced by:

- Moist environment
- Wound bed free of necrotic tissue, eschar, and environmental contamination or infection
- Adequate blood supply to meet metabolic demands for tissue generation

---

BOX 46-7

SAMPLING OF WOUND CARE DEVICES FOUND IN HOME CARE PATIENTS

Dressings and Wound Packing Material
Cotton dressings (gauze)
Impregnated cotton dressings
Combination dressings
Paste bandages
Exudate absorptive dressings
Foam dressings
Hydrocolloid dressings
Hydrogel dressings
Hydrophilic powder dressings
Transparent film (adhesive or nonadhesive)

Drains
Penrose drains
Jackson-Pratt drains

Wound Closure Techniques
Sutures
Wires
Staples
Tape
Skin adhesive

- Sufficient oxygen and nutrition for cellular metabolism and tissue generation

General Principles in Wound Care Management

Wound care management requires assessment of the wound and surrounding tissues and evaluation for infection or sepsis. General principles in wound care management include an assessment for[7]:

1. Location and size.
2. Color of the wound bed. A red or pink granular wound bed indicates healing. A green, yellow, or black wound bed suggests infection or necrosis (tissue death).
3. Drainage. Clear or serosanguinous drainage is common in a healing wound. Green or yellow drainage suggests infection.
4. Wound odor. A sweet smell may indicate decay. A foul smell may indicate infection.
5. Surrounding skin. It should be assessed for redness, inflammation, or signs of breakdown.

If the dressing is wet or contaminated, it should be changed (redressed) after wound evaluation. Medical direction may recommend cleaning the wound with normal saline and/or antiseptic solution prior to redressing. Some patients may require transportation for physician evaluation if severe infection or sepsis is suspected.

> **NOTE**
>
> The débridement of necrotic tissue may be required. Mechanical débridement is achieved by gently rubbing the tissue with a gauze pad moistened with sterile, normal saline.

Maternal/Child Conditions

In the early 1990s, many insurance companies began paying only for 24-hour hospital stays for uncomplicated vaginal childbirth ("drive-by deliveries"). In the wake of complaints about inadequate care, states began passing laws in 1995 and 1996 requiring insurance to pay for 48-hour stays. A similar federal law was passed in 1996 that took effect in January 1998. Under this law, health plans must cover hospital stays of at least 48 hours for women who give birth naturally and up to 4 days for those who deliver by cesarean section. Problems that may

be encountered when these patient groups return to the home care setting include:

- Postpartum pathophysiologies (e.g., hemorrhage, infection, pulmonary embolism)
- Postpartum depression
- Septicemia in the newborn
- Infantile apnea
- **Failure to thrive** (FTT)
- Sudden infant death syndrome

Postpartum Pathophysiologies

Postpartum pathophysiologies include hemorrhage, infection, and pulmonary embolism. (Acute interventions for these patients are presented in Chapter 40.) Postpartum hemorrhage occurs in about 5% of all deliveries. It frequently takes place within the first few hours after delivery, but it can be delayed up to 6 weeks.[6] Causes of postpartum hemorrhage include incomplete contraction of uterine muscle fibers, retained pieces of placenta or membranes in the uterus, and vaginal or cervical tears during delivery (which are rare).

Postpartum infection (most commonly endometritis) affects 2% to 8% of all pregnancies. The condition occurs when bacteria proliferate and invade the uterus or other tissues along the birth canal; symptoms usually develop on the second or third day after delivery. Fever and abdominal pain are the most common signs of infection.

Pulmonary embolism during pregnancy, labor, or the postpartum period is one of the most common causes of maternal death. The embolus frequently is the result of a blood clot in the pelvic circulation; it more commonly is associated with cesarean section rather than vaginal delivery.

> **? CRITICAL THINKING**
>
> *What will you do with the baby if the mother is having a postpartum complication that requires urgent transport and they are home alone?*

Postpartum Depression

Postpartum depression affects 10% to 15% of mothers. The depression probably is caused by a combination of sudden hormonal changes and a variety of psychological and environmental factors. The disease ranges from an extremely common and short-lived attack of mild depression ("baby blues") to a depressive psychosis that requires in-hospital supervision. Risk factors for postpartum depression include:

- Low self-esteem
- Anxiety
- Poor marital adjustment
- Adverse socioeconomic conditions
- Previous episodes of depression
- Complicated pregnancy or delivery
- Fetal complications
- Recent life stressors

Recognizing and treating postpartum depression is important because depression can interfere with the bonding between the mother and infant and seriously affect her ability to care for her newborn (Box 46-8). Many women with postpartum depression fear they will harm their babies, and they often feel ashamed and guilty for these feelings. Sensitivity to the possibility of depression is crucial and necessary to successful diagnosis and treatment. (Interventions for depression are presented in Chapter 38.)

Septicemia in the Newborn

Healthy newborns are vulnerable to several conditions that can require hospital treatment (see Chapter 41 and Chapter 42). Examples include jaundice that results from physiological immaturity of bilirubin metabolism, dehydration that can lead to serious electrolyte abnormalities, and sepsis.

NOTE

Neonates are highly susceptible to infection because of diminished nonspecific (inflammatory) and specific (humoral) immunity.

Septicemia in the newborn is usually caused by group B streptococci, *Listeria monocytogenes*, or gram-negative enteric organisms (especially *Escherichia coli*).[8] Signs and symptoms of sepsis may be minimal and nonspecific. ("In the newborn, anything can be a sign of anything.")[5] Examples of signs and symptoms of sepsis in the newborn include:

- Temperature instability
- Respiratory distress
- Apnea
- Cyanosis
- GI changes (e.g., vomiting, distention, diarrhea, anorexia)
- CNS features (e.g., irritability, lethargy, weak suck)

Risk factors for sepsis include prematurity, prolonged rupture of membranes, and chorioamnionitis (an inflammatory reaction in the amniotic membranes caused by bacterial viruses in the amniotic fluid). The diagnosis generally is confirmed by a positive blood, urine, or cerebrospinal fluid (CSF) culture.

BOX 46-8

SIGNS AND SYMPTOMS OF POSTPARTUM DEPRESSION

Severe sleep disturbance
Fear of harming self or baby
Lack of interest in previously enjoyed activities
Anxiety
Forgetfulness or memory loss
Hostility
Unexplainable crying (in joy or sadness)
Desire to leave or feelings of being trapped
Hopelessness
Panic attacks
Change of appetite (either loss of appetite or over-indulgence)

Lack of sexual interest
Excessive concern or lack of concern for baby
Fantasies of disaster or bizarre fears
Rapid mood swings
Irritability
Fatigue or exhaustion
Increased alcohol consumption or other drug use
Difficulty making decisions
Hatred of spouse, self, or baby
Inability to care for baby
Loss of hope

Infantile Apnea

Apnea involves periods of cessation of respirations for more than 10 to 15 seconds with or without cyanosis, pallor, hypotonia (diminished tone), and/or bradycardia, or for less than 10 seconds accompanied by bradycardia.[9] The condition often reflects the immature respiratory control centers in some infants. Other causes of infantile apnea include[10]:

- Metabolic derangements (e.g., hypoglycemia, hypocalcemia, hypothermia)
- Infection (e.g., sepsis, pneumonia, meningitis)
- CNS damage (e.g., hemorrhage, hypoxic injury, seizures)
- Pulmonary disorders (e.g., respiratory distress, hyaline membrane disease, pneumonia, obstruction, upper respiratory abnormalities)
- Intentional poisoning

The presence of apnea must be assessed carefully and documented. Most infants with the presumptive diagnosis of apnea will be hospitalized and observed closely using electronic apnea monitoring devices that detect changes in thoracic or abdominal movement and heart rate. Managing apnea in these patients may include the home care use of apnea monitors, oscillating waterbeds, and CPAP with supplemental oxygen. Some patients also may be prescribed respiratory stimulants (e.g., doxapram, methylxanthines).

Failure to Thrive

FTT is the abnormal retardation of the growth and development of an infant resulting from conditions that interfere with normal metabolism, appetite, and activity. Causative factors include:

- Chromosomal abnormalities
- Major organ system defects that lead to deficiency or malfunction
- Systemic disease or acute illness
- Physical deprivation (primarily malnutrition related to insufficient breast milk, poverty, or poor knowledge of nutrition)
- Various psychosocial factors (e.g., maternal deprivation)

FTT can result in permanent and irreversible retardation of physical, mental, or social development. Any suspicions of FTT should be carefully documented and reported to medical direction.

Well Baby Care

Some infants and children will have periodic health assessments through well baby care programs that specialize in medical supervision and services for healthy infants. Well baby care promotes optimal physical, emotional, and intellectual growth and development. Such health care measures include:

- Routine immunizations to prevent disease
- Screening procedures for early detection and treatment of illness
- Parental guidance and instruction in proper nutrition, injury prevention, and specific care and rearing of the child at various stages of development

The recommended preventative health care schedule for children who are developing normally is monthly for the first 6 months of life, every 2 months until 1 year of age, every 3 months during the second year, and every 6 months during the third year, followed by annual visits. Well baby care may be provided in a clinic ("well baby clinics"), a doctor's office, the office of a community health nursing center, or a school. Nurses or nurse practitioners frequently provide the care in these programs.

Hospice/Palliative Care

In 1996, hospices served nearly 450,000 patients throughout the United States.[11] Hospice services include supportive social, emotional, and spiritual services for the terminally ill, as well as support for the patient's family. Hospice care relies on the combined knowledge and skill of an interdisciplinary team of professionals that includes physicians, nurses, medical social workers, therapists, counselors, chaplains, and volunteers who coordinate an individualized plan of care for each patient and family. The need for hospices will likely continue to rise due to an aging

> **NOTE**
>
> The way people cope with their own death or the death of a loved one depends on their age, maturity, and understanding of death (as described in Chapter 2). The paramedic should be particularly sensitive to the emotional needs of the patient, family, and loved ones.

population, the increasing number of people with acquired immune deficiency syndrome (AIDS), and rising health care costs. Medical professionals and the general public increasingly are choosing hospice care over other forms of health care for terminally ill patients because of its holistic, patient-family, in-home-centered philosophy.

Palliative Care

Palliative care (also called *comfort care*) is a unique form of health care primarily directed at providing relief to terminally ill persons through symptom management and pain management. This specialty focuses on the needs of the patient and family when a life-threatening illness such as cancer or AIDS has reached the terminal stage. A primary goal of palliative care is to improve the quality of a person's life as death approaches and help patients and their families move toward this reality with comfort, reassurance, and strength. Palliative care is not focused on death; it is about specialized care for the

living. Well-rounded palliative care programs also address mental health and spiritual needs. Palliative care may be delivered in hospice, home care settings, and hospitals. Because medical needs vary depending on the disease that is leading toward death, specialized palliative care programs exist for

NOTE

EMS and medical direction should work closely with the families and private physicians of terminally ill patients in private homes and hospice programs so that they will make appropriate use of the EMS system (i.e., knowing when to call 911). Even though resuscitation may not be indicated, EMS may be needed to manage pain, treat acute medical illness or traumatic injury, and provide transportation to a hospital. If the patient is not to receive medical intervention to prolong life, measures of comfort should be provided to the patient, along with emotional support to family members and loved ones.

ESSENTIAL ELEMENTS OF A PALLIATIVE CARE PROGRAM

Palliative care is an accepted specialty of medicine and nursing that concentrates on the total care of patients suffering from any form of terminal illness. Its development, as part of the health care services, is a recognition that dying is a normal consequence of living. The support of health professionals and use of modern medical technology can relieve much of the distress normally associated with dying. Essential elements of a palliative care program are:

1. The coordination of care for patients with a terminal illness, at home or in hospital, by a distinct service.
2. The unit of care is the patient and their family, who have the right to make choices and decisions based on an understanding of their illness and to have those decisions respected.
3. The care is provided by an interdisciplinary team.
4. The care is coordinated and delivered by specifically selected and trained nurses.
5. The service is directed by a physician.
6. The emphasis is on control of symptoms, be they physical, social, or emotional.

7. The services are available on a 24-hours a day/7-days a week/on-call basis.
8. The program must be sensitive to differences in faith and culture and incorporate the patients' beliefs into decisions on their care.
9. Following the death of a patient, the program should ensure that grief support is available for the family. This may be provided by the program itself or by other community services.
10. There is a system of structured staff support and communication.
11. The program is integrated and coordinated with other services, and continuity of care for the patient is provided.
12. There must be regular evaluation of the program and its services. This evaluation may extend into the area of research.
13. The program will provide education for its own staff, other health care providers, and the public.

From *Essential elements of a palliative care program*, Health Canada, Minister of Public Works and Government Services, Canada, 2000.

BILL OF RIGHTS AND RESPONSIBILITIES FOR TERMINALLY ILL PATIENTS

A. Personal Dignity and Privacy

1. You have the right to considerate, respectful service and care, with full recognition of your personal dignity and individuality, without regard to gender, age, ethnicity, income level, lifestyle, educational background, or spiritual philosophy.
2. You have the right to be dressed as you wish and not to be disrobed or uncovered any longer than necessary for your care.
3. You have the right to privacy and the assurance of confidentiality when receiving care, to refuse visitors or persons not directly involved in your care, and to choose who will receive information about your condition.
4. You have the right to request the presence of a person of your choice during interactions with health care professionals.
5. You have the right to experience all emotions, including anger, sadness, confusion, guilt, depression, impatience, fear, and loss.
6. You have the right to have your end-of-life choices respected by health care professionals, including continuing or discontinuing treatment or requesting medications to self-administer for a hastened death.
7. You have the right to die with your loved ones present and to request the presence of a health care professional, if desired.
8. You have the responsibility to treat your caregiver with respect and to follow their directions when consistent with your wishes.
9. You have the responsibility to make certain that your right to privacy and confidentiality is clearly understood by all parties involved in your care and to communicate to your health care providers when you feel that your rights to privacy and confidentiality are in jeopardy.

B. Informed Participation

1. You have the right to honest, accurate, and understandable information about your current diagnosis and prognosis; the recommended treatment and what it is expected to do; the possibility of success; and the possible risks of complications and side effects, including the probability of their occurrence.
2. You have the right to be informed about alternative forms of treatment, including hospice and home care, and to participate in all decisions affecting your care.
3. You have the right to request and receive a second opinion. When curative care is no longer indicated or desired, you have the right to access palliative care, including pain medication in whatever dosage or schedule you deem necessary to alleviate pain and suffering, even at the risk of hastening death.
4. You have the right to make your own decisions regarding what constitutes your human dignity, as long as you are mentally competent and continue to have basic decision-making capacity. You will be considered mentally competent if you can understand the nature of your condition, the treatment alternatives available, the likely outcomes of treatment versus non-treatment, and can accept responsibility for your decisions.
5. You have the right to access information in your medical record and to know if your health care providers believe that your condition or course of disease will result in death. This information may be needed to make informed decisions about your future.
6. You have the right to forgo eating and drinking naturally in order to permit the process of dying to proceed unencumbered.
7. You have the right and responsibility to complete a directive to physicians (Living Will).
8. You have the right and responsibility to execute a Durable Power of Attorney for Health Care so that someone you choose can make health care decisions for you, if needed.

C. Competent Care

1. You have the right to competent medical, nursing, and social services care.
2. You have the right to choose your personal physician and to change your physician at any time.
3. You have the right to know who is responsible for coordinating and supervising your care and to know how to contact that person.
4. You have the right to be informed about who owns and controls the agency or facility involved with your care and the right to referral to institutions, facilities, practitioners who can provide the care you need.
5. You have the responsibility to choose a primary care physician who is able and willing to carry out your wishes.
6. You have the responsibility to communicate your end-of-life wishes to family, friends, and health care providers.

From Compassion In Dying Federation, Portland, Oregon.

common conditions such as cancer and AIDS (see the box on p. 1356).

Hospice Care in the Home Setting

Medical therapy that may be found in the home of patient receiving hospice care includes medication delivery for the relief of pain (e.g., narcotic infusion devices) and medical and legal documents such as Do Not Resuscitate (DNR) orders and advance directives (see Chapter 4). Concerns of the paramedic about effective pain management, overmedication, or interpreting medical or legal documents should be discussed with medical direction (see the box on p. 1357).

SUMMARY

- About 25% of home health patients have conditions related to disease of the circulatory system as their primary diagnosis. Other common diagnoses of home care patients include cancer, diabetes, and hypertension. Typical EMS responses to a home health setting may include respiratory failure, cardiac decompensation, septic complications, equipment malfunction, and other medical problems.

- When arriving at the scene of a home care patient, the scene size-up should include standard precautions, elements of scene safety, and environmental milieu. The initial assessment should focus on life-threatening illness or injury, and appropriate measures should be taken as indicated.

- Patients with diseases of the respiratory system being cared for at home are at increased risk for airway infections, and the progression of their illnesses may lead to increased respiratory demand, making current support inadequate.

- Assessment findings that may require acute interventions in patients with VADs include infection, hemorrhage, hemodynamic compromise from circulatory overload or embolus, obstruction of the vascular device, and catheter damage with leakage of medication.

- Patients with diseases of the digestive or GU system may have medical devices such as urinary catheters or urostomies, indwelling nutritional support devices (e.g., PEG tube, G-tube), colostomies, and NG tubes. Acute interventions required for these patients can result from UTI, urosepsis, urinary retention; and problems with gastric emptying or feeding.

- Home care patients with acute infections have an increased mortality rate from sepsis and severe peripheral infections, and many have a decreased ability to perceive pain or perform self-care.

- Maternal/child conditions that may be encountered in the home care setting during the postpartum period include postpartum hemorrhage, infection, pulmonary embolism, postpartum depression, septicemia in the newborn, infantile apnea, and FTT.

- Hospice services include supportive social, emotional, and spiritual services for the terminally ill, as well as support for a patient's family. Palliative care is primarily directed at providing relief to a terminally ill person through symptom and pain management.

REFERENCES

1. National Association of Home Care: *Basic statistics about home care: 1999 home care stats*, Washington, DC, 1999, http://www.nahc.org/Consumer/hcststs.html.
2. *Home health care: history and philosophy*, Kansas City, Kan, 1997, Spectrum Home Health Agency.
3. Health Care Financing Administration: *Managed care in Medicare and Medicaid*, fact sheet, Washington, DC, 1998, Department of Health and Human Services.
4. National Center for Health Statistics: *An overview of home health and hospice care patients: 1996 national home and hospice care survey*, Hyattsville, Md., 1996.
5. U.S. Department of Transportation National Highway Traffic Safety Administration: *EMT—Paramedic national standard curriculum*, Washington, DC, 1998, The Department.
6. Rosen P, Barkin R: *Emergency medicine: concepts and clinical practice*, ed 4, St Louis, 1998, Mosby.
7. Rice R: *Handbook of home health nursing procedures*, St Louis, 1995, Mosby.
8. Hoekelman R: *Primary pediatric care*, ed 3, St Louis, 1997, Mosby.
9. Polin R, Ditmar M: *Pediatric secrets*, ed 2, Philadelphia, 1997, Hanley & Belfus.
10. Barkin R et al: *Pediatric emergency medicine: concepts and clinical practice*, St Louis, 1992, Mosby.
11. National Association of Home Care: *Basic statistics about hospice: 1998*, Washington, DC, 1999, http://www.nahc.org/Consumer/hcststs.html

Division Seven →

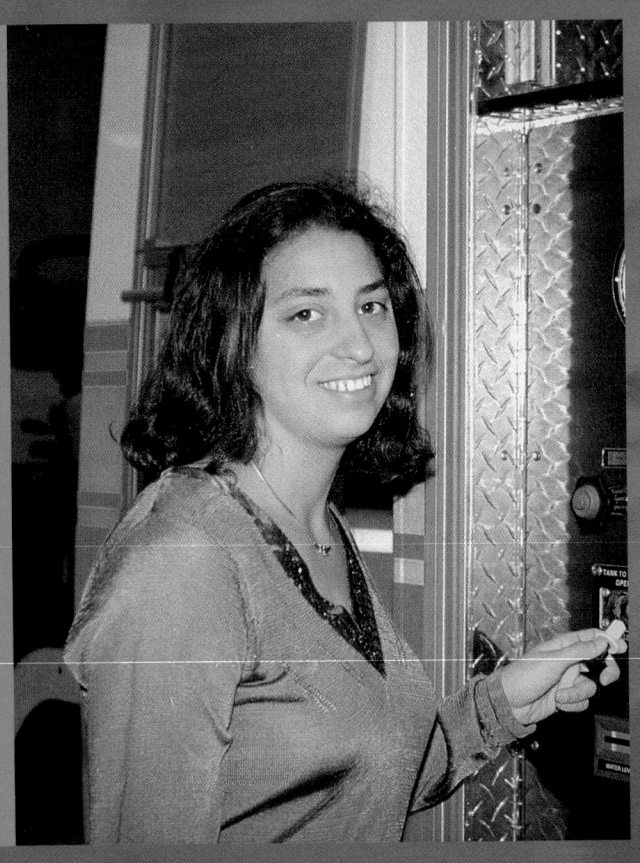

Melissa Napoli, EMT-B,
Paramedic Student
Seminole Community
College
Sanford, Florida

"I've learned that to make a clinical decision, you have to use your experience, what you've been taught, and, ultimately, your gut feelings."

Assessment-Based Management

47 Assessment-Based Management

OBJECTIVES

Upon completion of this chapter, the paramedic student will be able to:

1. **Discuss how assessment-based management contributes to effective patient and scene assessment.**
2. **Describe factors that affect assessment and decision making in the prehospital setting.**
3. **Outline effective techniques for scene and patient assessment and choreography.**
4. **Identify essential take-in equipment for general and selected patient situations.**
5. **Outline strategies for patient approach that promote an effective patient encounter.**
6. **Describe techniques to permit efficient and accurate presentation of the patient.**

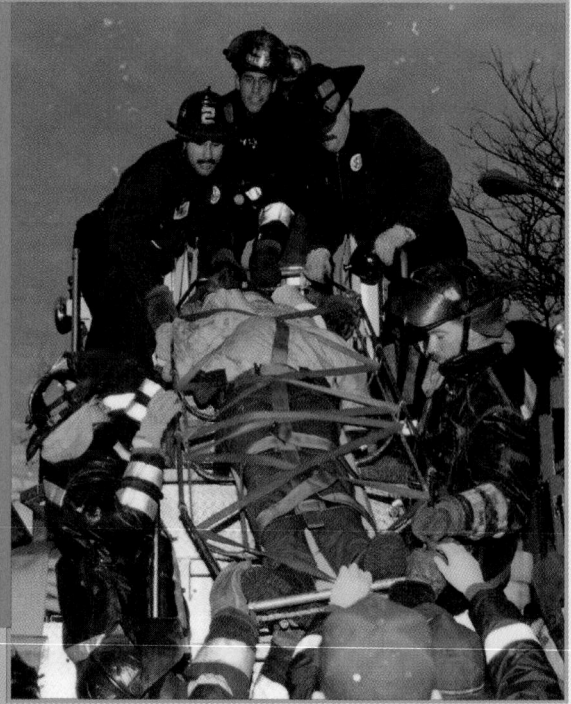

Assessment is the foundation of patient care. To perform an effective assessment, the paramedic must be able to integrate pathophysiological principles and physical examination findings to formulate a field impression and implement a treatment plan for patients with common complaints.

KEY TERMS

NOTE

Assessment-based management "puts it all together" as the paramedic gathers, evaluates, and synthesizes information; makes appropriate decisions based on the information; and takes appropriate actions required for the patient's care.

Effective Assessment

As described throughout this text, effective assessment depends on the patient's history and the physical examination. The paramedic's knowledge of disease allows him or her to maintain a high degree of suspicion for possible illness and focus the history toward the patient's complaint and associated problems. Likewise the paramedic must focus the physical examination toward body systems associated with the patient's complaint. Although some field situations may compromise the thoroughness of the physical examination (e.g., unsafe scenes or entrapment), the paramedic must not overlook the importance of the physical examination nor perform it in a cursory manner.

NOTE

Often as much as 80% of a medical diagnosis is based on the patient's history.[1]

Pattern Recognition

Once paramedics obtain the patient's history and perform the physical examination, they can compare the information gathered with their knowledge base of medical illness and disease. The question then becomes whether the history and physical examination match a recognized pattern of illness. For example, a 55-year-old man with chest pain and shortness of breath "matches" a recognized pattern for acute myocardial infarction (AMI), whereas a 20-year-old female with similar complaints would not match the recognized pattern. Other examples include a 4-year-old child who in is respiratory distress and drooling (matching a recognized pattern for epiglottitis) and an elderly female with distended neck veins and respiratory congestion who produces a pink, frothy sputum upon coughing (matching a recognized pattern for congestive heart failure). **Pattern recognition** makes it possible for the paramedic to form a field impression and implement a treatment plan (Box 47-1).

BOX 47-1

PATTERN RECOGNITION FOR VARIOUS PATIENT PRESENTATIONS

Paramedics are trained in patient assessment and management priorities for patients with the following:

- Chest pain
- Medical and traumatic cardiac arrest
- Acute abdominal pain
- Gastrointestinal bleeding
- Altered mental status
- Dyspnea
- Syncope
- Seizures
- Environmental or thermal problem
- Hazardous material or toxic exposure
- Trauma or multitrauma
- Allergic reactions
- Behavioral problems
- Obstetrical or gynecological problems

The greater the paramedic's knowledge base and the quality of assessment information, the better the probability of accurate assessment and appropriate decision making.

> **NOTE**
>
> Pattern recognition is the process of comparing gathered information with the paramedic's knowledge base of medical illness and disease.

✓ TRICKS OF THE TRADE

The longer you work as a paramedic, the more patterns you will be able to recognize. Remember that every call should be a learning experience.

? CRITICAL THINKING

How can pattern recognition lead you down the wrong path?

Field Impression and Action Plan

The paramedic makes a **field impression** of the patient's condition from pattern recognition and "gut instinct" that results from experience (Fig. 47-1). Once the paramedic makes a field impression, he or she can formulate an **action plan** based on the patient's condition and the environment. Using the previous example of the two patients with chest pain, the field impression of the 55-year-old patient most likely leads to an action plan of administration of oxygen, electrocardiograph (ECG) monitoring, intravenous (IV) therapy, administration of *aspirin*, pain relief, and perhaps drug therapy for dysrhythmias. The 20-year-old patient's action plan most likely includes oxygen administration, ECG monitoring to evaluate paroxysmal supraventricular tachycardia (PSVT), and a more thorough assessment focused on recent respiratory illness to rule out the possibility of pleurisy or pneumonia.

> **NOTE**
>
> The paramedic should not ignore a gut instinct. If something seems wrong, the paramedic should keep looking. Gut instincts often enable the paramedic to identify subtle physical findings that are difficult to quantify (e.g., patient affect or dull and lackluster eyes).

Following the field impression and the formulation of an action plan, the paramedic provides basic life support (BLS) and advanced life support (ALS) treatment based on his or her knowledge of the protocols and judgment (knowing when and how to apply the protocols and knowing when it is appropriate to deviate from the protocols) (Fig. 47-2). For example, administration of concentrated glucose to an unconscious diabetic patient over 50 years of age who may have had a stroke can exacerbate cerebral damage. This cause of altered mental status indicates the need for the paramedic to deviate from a common protocol used to manage patients with suspected hypoglycemia.

? CRITICAL THINKING

How can you continue to improve your patient care judgment?

> **NOTE**
>
> BLS and ALS treatments are driven by knowing which protocols to use, when and how to apply the protocols, and when to deviate from the protocols.

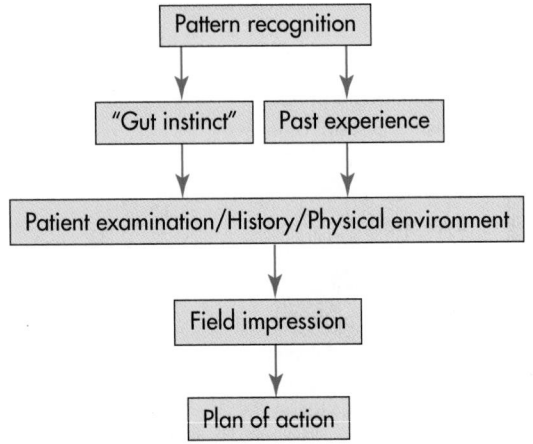

Fig. 47-1 Matrix pattern.

Factors That Affect Assessment and Decision Making

Many factors can affect the quality of assessment and decision making. The following factors are discussed in this section:

- Paramedic's attitude
- Patient's willingness to cooperate
- Distracting injuries
- Labeling and tunnel vision
- Environment
- Patient compliance
- Manpower considerations

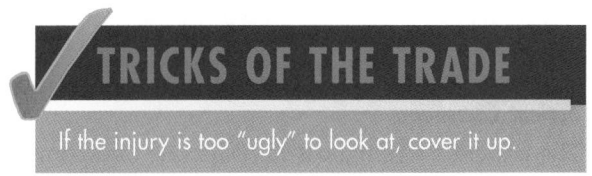

? CRITICAL THINKING

> *Have you ever seen any of these factors affect patient care?*

Paramedic's Attitude

The paramedic must be professional and nonjudgmental to perform an effective assessment. A judgmental or biased attitude can "short-circuit" information gathering, causing the paramedic to overlook important patient data. For example, the paramedic who assumes that an indigent patient is intoxicated may not consider complications from diabetes or hypoxia and hypovolemia from an internal injury.

> **NOTE**
>
> Patients depend on EMS providers for medical assessment and management, not the determination of the patient's social status, worth, or likability.

Patient's Willingness to Cooperate

Uncooperative patients can complicate the patient assessment required for the paramedic to formulate an action plan. The paramedic should evaluate patients who are uncooperative, restless, or belligerent for the following:

- Alcohol or other drug intoxication
- Hypoxia
- Hypovolemia
- Hypothermia
- Hypoglycemia
- Head injury or concussion
- Stroke
- Psychiatric problem

Distracting Injuries

Obvious but non–life-threatening injuries can distract the paramedic from performing a thorough assessment for more serious problems. Examples include open fractures and facial bleeding that appears to be profuse. If necessary, the paramedic should cover these wounds with dressings during the assessment to help him or her focus on the serious problems.

> ✓ **TRICKS OF THE TRADE**
>
> If the injury is too "ugly" to look at, cover it up.

Labeling and Tunnel Vision

Labeling and tunnel vision can lead to an inaccurate assessment and field impression. For example, labeling a patient as "just another drunk" or a "frequent flyer" can sometimes lead to a biased assessment. Likewise, tunnel vision (assuming an incorrect field impression based on gut instinct or focusing on a portion of the presenting illness and thereby missing the "big picture") can result in a rushed judgment early in the patient assessment and an inappropriate action plan.

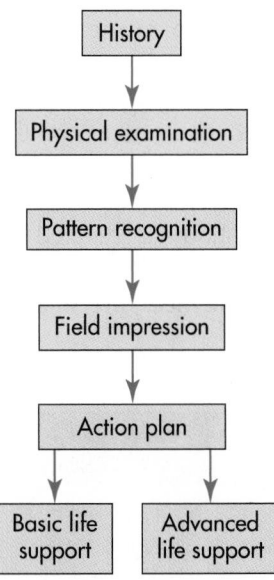

Fig. 47-2 Effective assessment.

Environment

Environmental factors also can adversely affect assessment and decision making at the scene. Examples include scene chaos, violent or dangerous situations, crowds of bystanders or emergency workers, severe weather, and noise levels. After the paramedic ensures personal safety, he or she should quickly establish control of the environment. This can include requesting the help of law enforcement personnel to control the scene so that the paramedic can deliver appropriate assessment and care without distraction.

Patient Compliance

The patient's willingness to cooperate and comply with components of the patient assessment may depend on his or her confidence with the paramedic crew. For example, the patient who perceives the paramedic as competent and professional often will provide a thorough history and agree to a complete physical examination. Other factors that can affect patient compliance include various cultural and ethnic barriers (described in Chapter 45).

Manpower Considerations

Depending on the crew structure of the EMS agency, crews may consist of a single paramedic and an EMT-Basic (EMT-B) or EMT-Intermediate (EMT-I), two paramedics, or multiple responders (e.g., EMS, fire and rescue, and police). In cases where only EMS is involved and there is only one paramedic at the scene, he or she must work with the EMT-B to develop an appropriate sequence for gathering information and providing care. If two paramedics are available, information gathering and treatment often can occur simultaneously, with each paramedic assuming specific responsibilities. If multiple responders and agencies are at the scene, roles and duties should be defined in advance (e.g., one paramedic responsible for history taking and conferring with medical direction, one paramedic

---

TRICKS OF THE TRADE

When multiple agencies manage an emergency call, your involvement as a "team player" often determines the success of the call.

? CRITICAL THINKING

How can too many paramedics on the scene have a negative influence on patient assessment and care?

---

responsible for treatment, fire-rescue members responsible for extrication and/or gathering equipment, and law enforcement personnel responsible for securing the scene).

Assessment and Management Choreography

In cases where multiple responders are present at the scene of an emergency, a coherent assessment can be challenging. This can occur with multiple-tier response systems (e.g., EMS, fire, and police) and often is made more difficult if the responders are trained at the same level (e.g., paramedic) without a clear direction for individual responsibilities. Therefore members of the response team must have a preplan for determining roles. The team can assign these predesignated roles by shift or crew or rotate them among team members.

An example of a preplan for two paramedics is to assign one paramedic as the team leader and one as the patient care person. Although this type of plan must be flexible in dynamic field situations, a basic "game plan" allows others to participate and is important in preventing chaos at the scene. The following are sample responsibilities for each of the paramedics in this type of preplan:

NOTE

Regular partners of a paramedic crew often will develop their own plan and flow for patient care.

---

1. Team leader responsibilities
   a. Accompanies the patient through to definitive care
   b. Establishes contact and a dialogue with the patient
   c. Obtains the history
   d. Performs the physical examination
   e. Presents the patient and gives verbal reports over the radio or at definitive care
   f. Completes all documentation

g. Tries to maintain the overall patient perspective and provides leadership to the team by designating tasks and coordinating transportation

h. Designates and actively participates in critical interventions during the resuscitative phase of initial assessment

i. Acts as initial EMS command in multiple-casualty situations

j. Interprets the ECG, communicates with medical direction and relays drug orders, controls access to the drug box, and documents drug administration and effects during advanced cardiac life support

2. Patient care person responsibilities

a. Provides scene cover (watches the team leader's back)

b. Gathers scene information and talks to family members, bystanders, etc.

c. Obtains vital signs

d. Performs skills and interventions as requested by the team leader (e.g., attaches monitor leads, provides oxygen, initiates IV access, administers drugs, and obtains transportation equipment)

e. Acts as triage group leader in multiple-casualty situations

f. Administers drugs, monitors endotracheal tube placement, and monitors BLS interventions during advanced cardiac life support

The "Right Stuff"

The "right stuff" means carrying the right equipment to the patient's side. Not having the "right stuff" can compromise care and causes pandemonium. The paramedic crew should always be prepared for the worst event and carry essential equipment to manage every aspect of patient care, including cardiac monitoring and defibrillation (Box 47-2).

> **NOTE**
>
> The concept of having the "right stuff" can be compared with backpacking. A person who is backpacking must have essential items that are downsized to facilitate rapid movement with minimum weight and bulk.

BOX 47-2

ESSENTIAL ITEMS FOR ALL ASPECTS OF PATIENT CARE

Personal Protection
Gloves
Eye shields
Masks
Gowns

Airway Control
Oral airways
Nasal airways
Suction (electric or manual)
Rigid Yankauer and flexible suction catheters
Laryngoscope and blades
Endotracheal tubes, stylettes, and tape

Breathing
Mouth-powered ventilation device (pocket mask)
Manual ventilation bag-valve-mask
Spare masks
Oxygen tank and regulator
Oxygen masks, cannulas, and extension tubing

Occlusive dressings
Large-bore IV catheter for thoracic decompression

Circulation
IV fluids, catheters, and tubing
Dressings
Bandages and tape
Infection-control supplies (gloves and eye shields)
Blood pressure cuff and stethoscope
Note pad and pen or pencil

Disability and Dysrhythmia
Rigid collar
Flashlight
Cardiac monitor and defibrillator

Exposure
Scissors
Space blanket or other device to cover and protect the patient

Optional "Take-In" Equipment

In addition to the essential equipment listed in Box 47-2, the paramedic can carry other equipment to the patient's side. For example, most EMS systems, including those that employ paramedic ambulances and those that have nontransporting emergency vehicles staffed by paramedic personnel, require that the paramedic carry portable drug boxes with venous access supplies even though they are not appropriate for every patient contact. Other factors that can affect what optional equipment the paramedic carries to the patient's side depends on the following:

- Local protocol
- Standing order flexibility
- Number of paramedic responders
- Difficulty in accessing patients

Items that are essential on every call include patient care reports or worksheets, pens or pencils, personal wristwatches, flashlights, and portable radios or cellular telephones. Personal protective equipment also should be readily available.

? CRITICAL THINKING

Have you been on ambulance calls when you did not have the "right stuff"? How did it affect patient care?

General Approach to the Patient

Calm and orderly demeanor is essential for the paramedic when approaching a patient. To gain the patient's trust and cooperation, the paramedic must look and act the part of a professional and demon-

TRICKS OF THE TRADE

Most patients do not mind if you take notes during the assessment. They want to be sure that you are listening to them and that you are getting everything down in writing.

strate a caring and confident bedside manner. Patients may not be able to rate medical performance, however, they generally rate "people skills" and service.

As previously described, a preplan should be in effect to prevent confusion at the scene and to improve the accuracy of the assessment. Ideally, one team member should be responsible for talking to the patient using an active and concerned dialogue that allows for careful listening. Taking notes when acquiring the history prevents the paramedic from asking repetitive questions. All essential equipment should be at the patient's side, and the EMS crew should be ready to provide resuscitative care if needed. An initial survey of the scene can provide important clues and help formulate an impression. Initial size-up information that is especially useful in trauma situations includes hazards and potential hazards, mechanism of injury, and the number of patients at the scene.

Setting the Tone for the Patient Encounter

Two approaches in the initial assessment set the tone for the patient encounter: (1) the resuscitative approach and (2) the contemplative approach. The resuscitative approach recognizes the need for immediate intervention for patients who have life-threatening problems, such as the following:

- Cardiorespiratory arrest
- Respiratory distress or failure
- Unstable dysrhythmias
- Seizures
- Coma or altered level of consciousness
- Shock or hypotension
- Major trauma
- Possible cervical spine injury

If a life-threatening problem is present, the paramedic crew should take resuscitative action. The paramedic should postpone history taking and other details until he or she has performed immediate resuscitation measures.

The paramedic uses the contemplative approach in patient assessment when immediate intervention to manage life-threatening problems is not necessary. In these situations the paramedic obtains a patient history and performs a physical examination before providing patient care measures.

In any patient care encounter, it may be necessary for the paramedic to immediately move the patient to the emergency vehicle if any of the following occur:

- The paramedic cannot provide life-saving interventions
- The scene is too unstable or unsafe
- The scene is too chaotic to allow for rational assessment
- Inclement weather hinders assessment and care

"Looking to Find"

Paramedics cannot treat or report anything that is not found, and to find something the paramedic must suspect it. Therefore during the initial assessment the paramedic must actively look for life-threatening problems. He or she must be systematic in the assessment, rapidly determine the patient's chief complaint, assess the degree of distress, obtain baseline vital signs, and stay focused on the patient's history and physical findings.

> **NOTE**
>
> A mental "rule-out list" that considers the most serious problems that could cause the patient's signs and symptoms *first* often is a good approach in "looking to find."

> **NOTE**
>
> The greater the paramedic's knowledge about what he or she is "looking to find," the more productive the line of questioning will be.

Experience assists the paramedic in developing the ability for "multitasking," or being able to ask questions, take notes, and perform skills while listening to the patient's answers. Until the paramedic has gained the level of experience for multitasking, it is best to ask questions and then carefully listen to the patient's response. Important clues are lost by not listening. If a particular task is required while the paramedic is obtaining a patient history, a part-

ner should provide the patient care measure. The patient's ability to describe symptoms and the paramedic's ability to listen may greatly influence the assessment. The severity and location of the patient's pain (e.g., visceral pain) does not always correlate well with some potentially life-threatening conditions. The paramedic's role is to rapidly assess and treat for the worst-case scenario.

Presenting the Patient

Presenting the patient refers to the effective communication and transfer of patient information in the course of out-of-hospital and hospital care. Patient presentation often is a weak link in the chain of emergency care despite its need in every patient encounter. The paramedic routinely provides patient presentation face to face, over the telephone or radio, and in writing. These communication skills are essential for the paramedic to establish trust and credibility with co-workers and other members of the health care team. Good presentations suggest effective patient assessment and care to the listener, and vice versa. Poor presentation also can compromise patient care when the paramedic does not effectively communicate patient needs and status to medical direction. The following are characteristics of an effective patient presentation:

- Is concise, usually lasting less than 1 minute
- Is usually free of extensive medical jargon
- Follows the same basic information pattern
- Generally follows the SOAP format (or some close variation)
- Includes pertinent findings and pertinent negatives

When communicating a patient presentation, the paramedic should begin the report with the end in mind (i.e., he or she should anticipate discrete areas of information that will be asked for and be ready to

> **? CRITICAL THINKING**
>
> *Can you identify any areas for improvement for your skills in "presenting the patient"?*

BOX 47-3

DISCRETE AREAS OF INFORMATION

1. Patient identification, age, sex, and degree of distress
2. Chief complaint
3. Present illness or injury
   a. Pertinent details about the present problem
   b. Pertinent negatives (expected findings that are absent)
4. Medical history, including allergies and medications
5. Physical findings
   a. Vital signs
   b. Pertinent positive findings
   c. Pertinent negative findings
6. Assessment, including paramedic impression
7. Plan
   a. What has been done
   b. Orders requested

provide that information). Until the paramedic is experienced in presenting patients, he or she may elect to use a pre-printed card or other memory device to organize information and assessment findings. Box 47-3 provides discrete areas of an ideal presentation.

SUMMARY

- Assessment-based management "puts it all together" as the paramedic gathers, evaluates, and synthesizes information; makes appropriate decisions based on the information; and takes the appropriate actions required for the patient's care.

- Factors that can affect the quality of assessment and decision making include the paramedic's attitude, the patient's willingness to cooperate, distracting injuries, labeling and tunnel vision, the environment, patient compliance, and manpower considerations.

- To promote a coherent assessment, members of the response team should have a pre-plan for determining roles and responsibilities.

- The paramedic crew should always be prepared for the worst event and carry essential equipment to manage every aspect of patient care.

- Calm and orderly demeanor is essential for the paramedic when approaching a patient. During the initial assessment the paramedic must actively look for life-threatening problems.

- Presenting the patient refers to the effective communication and transfer of patient information in the course of out-of-hospital and hospital care.

REFERENCE

1. U.S. Department of Transportation, National Highway Traffic Safety Administration: *EMT-Paramedic national standard curriculum*, Washington, DC, 1998, The Department.

Division Eight ⟶

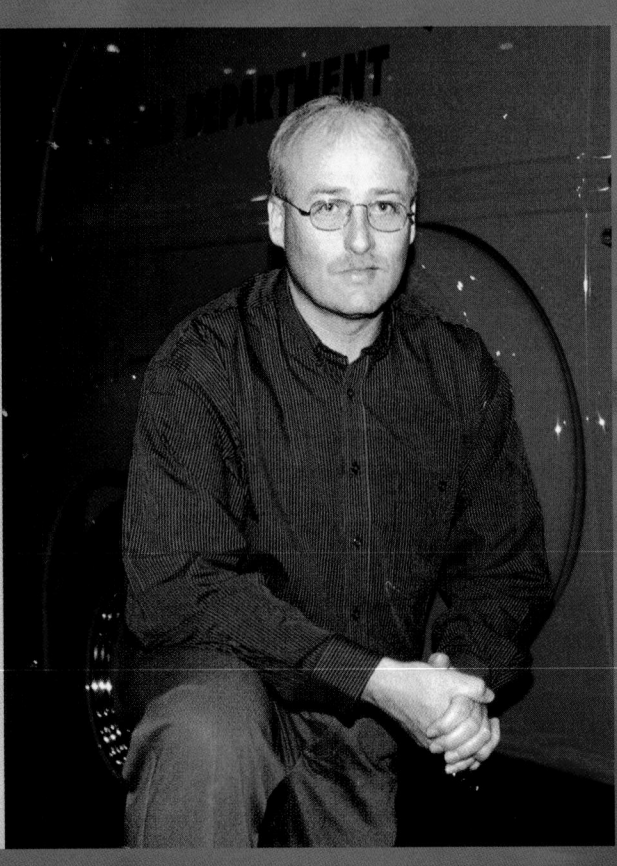

**John MacLean,
Paramedic I
Medical Coordinator –
Training Division
Halifax Regional Fire
and Emergency Service
Halifax, Nova Scotia,
Canada**

*"The most important thing to
remember during a call is that patient
care is our number one priority. It
starts with contact with the patient.
Something as simple as holding a hand
or providing a smiling face at the scene
can be more helpful than all the fancy
equipment we have available."*

Operations

IN THIS DIVISION

48 Ambulance Operations

OBJECTIVES

Upon completion of this chapter, the paramedic student will be able to:

1. *List standards that govern ambulance performance and specifications.*
2. *Discuss the tracking of equipment, supplies, and maintenance on an ambulance.*
3. *Outline the considerations for appropriate stationing of ambulances.*
4. *Describe measures that can influence safe operation of an ambulance.*
5. *Identify aeromedical crew members and training.*
6. *Describe appropriate use of aeromedical services in the prehospital setting.*

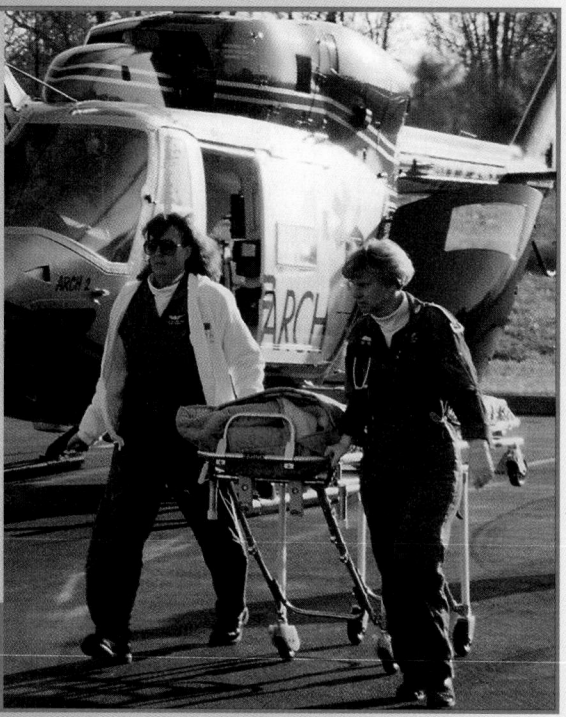

The modern ambulance is more than just a vehicle for transporting a patient to the hospital. Today's ambulance is a well-equipped and efficiently organized vehicle or aircraft with advanced communications and technology that can bring needed medical supplies, personnel, and advanced life support (ALS) care to the emergency scene.

ambulance: A generic term that describes the various land-based emergency vehicles used by EMS personnel.
KKK Standards: The national standards that provide the foundation of uniformity among ambulance vehicles.
landing zone: An area prepared for the landing of an aircraft; generally 100 by 100 feet.

NOTE

This text uses the generic term **ambulance** to describe the various land-based emergency vehicles used by EMS personnel. These emergency vehicles include basic life support (BLS) units, ALS units, paramedic units, mobile intensive care units, and others.

Ambulance Standards

In 1968, the National Academy of Sciences–National Research Council (NAS-NRC) recommended ambulance design standards, including size, shape, color, electrical systems, and emergency equipment, and led to the development of the current federal specifications that many states use for their current ambulance requirements. The national standards developed by NAS-NRC and the National Highway Traffic Safety Administration (NHTSA) are known as the **KKK Standards**. These standards and associated revisions provide the foundation of uniformity among ambulance vehicles. They pertain to the three basic ambulance designs—Type I, Type II, and Type III (Fig. 48-1).

NOTE

In recent years, the extra weight and space requirements of equipment used in rescue and emergency care have led to the development of medium-duty truck chassis for some ambulances. In addition, many fire service apparatuses (e.g., pumpers, rescue units, and fire trucks) carry EMS equipment.

In addition to federal standards of design and performance for ambulance vehicles, other federal standards, state statutes, administrative rules, and city, county, and district ordinances influence ambulance design, equipment, and staffing, including the following:

- Air ambulance standards
- Operational staffing standards
- Operational driver standards
- Operational driving standards
- Operational equipment standards

? CRITICAL THINKING

What do your state or regional standards require for ambulance design, performance, and equipment?

Checking Ambulances

Completing an ambulance equipment and supply checklist at the beginning of every work shift is important for safety, patient care, and risk management issues and for ensuring the appropriate handling and safekeeping of scheduled medications (Fig. 48-2). The paramedic can perform record keeping with pen and paper checklists or with specialized computer software. Some equipment (e.g., glucometers and defibrillators) require routine maintenance, testing, and cleaning to ensure safe and effective operation. The procedure for vehicle maintenance and routine care to improve reliability and extended use of life varies by EMS agency. The paramedic should follow all

✓ TRICKS OF THE TRADE

Never consider checking the ambulance as a "boring part of your job." Your safety and the safety of your co-workers and your patient depend on it.

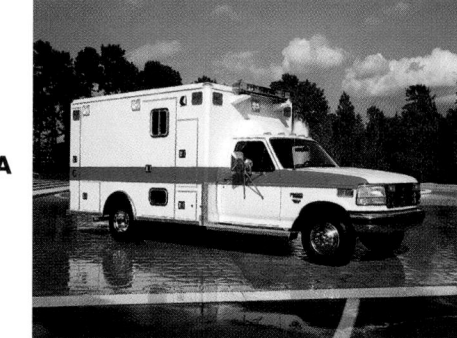
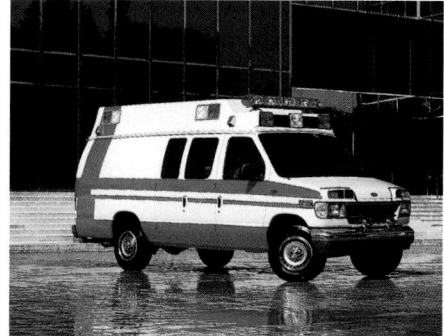
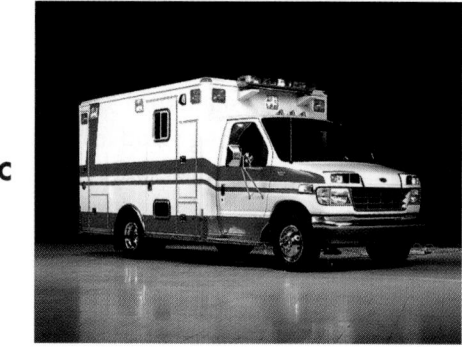

Fig. 48-1 Basic ambulance designs. **A**, Type I. **B**, Type II. **C**, Type III. (Courtesy Wheeled Coach, Orlando, Fla.)

agency guidelines and procedures for checking vehicles, equipment, and supplies.

Ambulance Stationing

In the 1970s, methods for estimating ambulance service needs and stationing in a community were based on ambulance availability and the average response time to the emergency scene. Methods for estimating needs now have shifted toward determining the percentage of compliance in providing EMS services within time frames that meet national standards (e.g., the American Heart Association recommendation that ALS be available at the scene within 8 minutes of a cardiac arrest[1]). The following are factors that affect these estimates:

> ### ? CRITICAL THINKING
> **Why can EMS services not guarantee a definite response time (e.g., less than 8 minutes) 100% of the time?**

- Geographical area
- Population and patient demand
- Traffic conditions
- Time of day
- Appropriate placement of emergency vehicles

Newer strategies for ambulance stationing are based on call volumes and locations and may use computers and other sophisticated technologies to formalize strategic unit deployment and decrease response times. Deployment strategies vary by EMS agency from the simple deployment of one vehicle stationed in the middle of a response area to comprehensive automated deployment plans for each hour of the day and each day of the week, complete with "mini-deployment" plans within each hour, depending on the number ambulances left in the system. The optimal deployment system generally is a compromise between these two extremes.[2]

Safe Ambulance Operations

Safe ambulance operation is crucial for the safety of patients, the EMS crew, and others in the vicinity of an emergency response. Many EMS agencies require personnel to complete an emergency driving course and to participate in periodic evaluations of

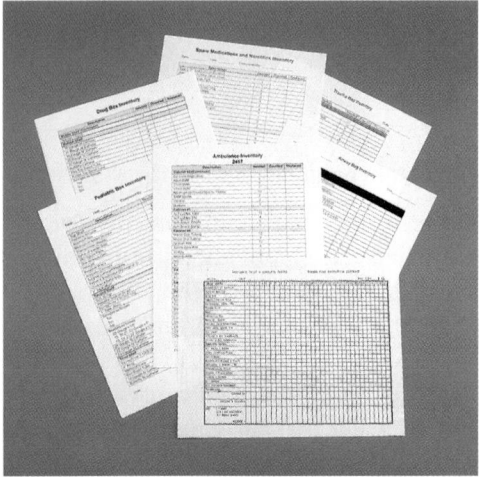

Fig. 48-2 Ambulance checklists.

BOX 48-1

GUIDELINES FOR SAFE AMBULANCE DRIVING

1. Be tolerant and observant of other motorists and pedestrians.
2. Always use occupant safety restraints (both driver and passenger).
3. Be familiar with the characteristics of the emergency vehicle.
4. Be alert to changes in weather and road conditions.
5. Exercise caution in the use of audible and visual warning devices.
6. Drive within the speed limit, except in circumstances allowed by law.
7. Select the fastest and most appropriate route to and from the incident scene.
8. Maintain a safe following distance.
9. Drive with due regard for the safety of all others.
10. Always drive in a manner consistent with managing acceptable levels of risk.

✓ TRICKS OF THE TRADE

When the ambulance is in motion, ensure that all crew members (except the paramedic providing patient care) and passengers have their seat belts securely fastened.

---

their emergency driving skills (Box 48-1). In addition to the size and weight of the emergency vehicle and driver's experience level, factors that influence safe ambulance operations include the following:

- Appropriate use of escorts
- Environmental conditions
- Appropriate use of warning devices
- Proceeding safely through intersections
- Parking at the emergency scene
- Operating with due regard for the safety of others

? CRITICAL THINKING

How do you think you will feel if you strike another vehicle while driving an ambulance?

NOTE

In 1997, more than 4700 ambulances were involved in vehicle collisions in the United States. These crashes were responsible for 31 deaths and more than 3300 injuries.[3]

Appropriate Use of Escorts

Police escorts during an emergency response can be dangerous and should be used sparingly. Collisions can occur as a result of confusion when motorists in the area wrongly assume that only one emergency vehicle is on the roadway. As a rule, the paramedic should only use police escorts when the EMS crew is responding to a scene in an unfamiliar area. Even then the paramedic should maintain a safe distance between the ambulance and police escort. The use of audible and visual warning devices during police escorts should be guided by local protocol. If the paramedic uses audible and visual warning devices,

---

NOTE

Some state motor vehicle laws only grant privileged immunity to drivers of emergency vehicles that respond using *all* available audible and visual warning devices. The paramedic should be familiar with his or her state motor vehicle laws pertaining to emergency response and the use of escorts.

the ambulance and police escort should use different siren tones (per protocol) to alert other motorists that a second emergency vehicle is in the area.

Environmental Conditions

Adverse environmental conditions pose significant dangers when the paramedic is responding to an emergency call. Factors that can affect safe ambulance operation include road and weather conditions, such as fog and heavy rain that decrease visibility, and slippery pavement caused by ice, snow, mud, oil, or water that can cause the ambulance to hydroplane. When adverse environmental conditions are present, the driver of the emergency vehicle should proceed at safe speeds that are appropriate for road and weather conditions. The driver should use low-beam headlights during all emergency responses to increase visibility for the EMS crew and to allow for easier identification of the ambulance by other motorists.

> **? CRITICAL THINKING**
>
> *In what situations do you think that the crew member driving an ambulance may be tempted to drive too fast?*

> **NOTE**
>
> About 69% of all emergency vehicle crashes occur on dry roads, and about 77% occur during clear weather.[4]

Appropriate Use of Warning Devices

As previously stated, the paramedic should use audible and visual warning devices during an emergency response and during patient transportation according to protocol and based on state motor vehicle laws. Most EMS agencies authorize the use of audible and visual warning devices during all emergency responses in which the cause or severity of the emergency is unknown. Use of warning devices during patient transportation generally is reserved for patients with limb- or life-threatening illness or injury.

When audible and visual warning devices are indicated, the paramedic should remember that motorists who drive with the car windows rolled up or who are using an audio, air conditioning, or heating

> **NOTE**
>
> Some communities employ a "tiered response" system whereby multiple units and sometimes multiple agencies respond to emergency calls. The tiered response system allows for a safer emergency response and helps ensure that appropriate resources and personnel are available during an emergency event. For example, a fire service unit staffed with EMT-Bs responds with full use of audible and visual warning devices to a motor vehicle crash. The EMT-Bs determine that the patient's injury is minor. They request a BLS ambulance (either public or private) to respond to the scene in a nonemergency mode (at normal speed and without warning devices) to assume patient care duties and provide transportation to the hospital.

system may not be able to hear the audible devices. Therefore the EMS crew should always proceed with caution and never assume that the vehicle's lights, sirens, and air horns provide an absolute right-of-way or privileged immunity to proceed.

> **? CRITICAL THINKING**
>
> *What situations do you consider serious enough to use audible and visual warning devices?*

> **NOTE**
>
> An effective community education program involves teaching residents "sirens and lights, pull to the right."

> **NOTE**
>
> The paramedic should always use audible and visual warning devices simultaneously. If one is indicated, so is the other.

Proceeding Safely Through Intersections

Approximately 53% of ambulance crashes in the United States occur in intersections when an ambulance goes against a red light.[4] It is important that the driver of an emergency vehicle stop at all controlled intersections and attempt to make eye contact with all drivers before proceeding through it. Other safety precautions for proceeding through intersections include making a secondary stop before crossing the intersection and using the siren's "yelp" mode or air horn to alert nearby traffic.

> **NOTE**
>
> Some emergency vehicles now are equipped with traffic signal preempting devices that change the traffic light at an intersection to green (in the ambulance's direction of travel).

Parking at the Emergency Scene

When parking the ambulance at an accident scene, the paramedic should ensure that the vehicle's location allows for adequate traffic flow around the area. If law enforcement and fire service personnel have secured the scene, the paramedic should position the ambulance about 100 feet past the accident scene (on the same side of the road), uphill (about 200 feet), and upwind if the presence of hazardous materials is suspected. If law enforcement and fire service personnel have not secured the scene, the paramedic should position the ambulance about 50 feet in front of the scene ("fend-off" position) so that it deflects and averts from the scene other vehicles that may strike the ambulance or providers (Fig. 48-3). Other

> **TRICKS OF THE TRADE**
>
> When backing up the ambulance, have someone behind the unit safely guide you, use the mirrors to keep that person in sight, and back up slowly.

> **TRICKS OF THE TRADE**
>
> Always wear reflective gear when working in or near the roadway.

safety precautions for the paramedic parking at an emergency scene include using emergency lighting when the vehicle blocks traffic and setting the parking brake. When choosing an appropriate parking area for the ambulance, the paramedic also should consider the possibility of collapsing structures, fires, explosive hazards, and downed electrical wires.

Operating With Due Regard for the Safety of All Others

Most states allow privileges for drivers of emergency vehicles, such as driving slightly above the speed limit and proceeding through controlled intersections (after a stop) during an emergency

> **TRICKS OF THE TRADE**
>
> Setting the parking brake *before* setting the transmission in "Park" allows the entire weight of the vehicle to be shared between the emergency brake and transmission.

> **TRICKS OF THE TRADE**
>
> Observe the posted speed limit when traveling through school zones, even during an emergency response.

Your unit is the first emergency vehicle on the scene.

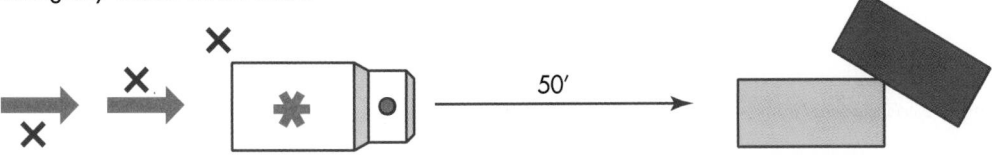

Fig. 48-3 The "fend-off" position.

THE "TWO-SECOND" RULE

Most rear-end collisions are caused by drivers who follow too closely behind the vehicle in front of them. Therefore it is important for the paramedic to ensure that there is sufficient space (following distance) between the emergency vehicle and the vehicle in front to avoid a crash if the car in front brakes suddenly. One method that the paramedic can use to "gauge" the recommended distance required for sufficient space is the "two-second" rule: look at an object by the side of the road (e.g., a tree or sign) that the vehicle ahead will soon pass. Count "one thousand and one, one thousand and two." If you reach the object before you have completed the phrase, you are traveling too close to the vehicle in front of you. This rule applies with good road and weather conditions. If road and weather conditions are not good, the paramedic should increase the following distance to a four- or five-second count.

Braking distance is based on average reaction time, average vehicle weight, average road conditions, and average brakes. Wet roadways, poor brakes, poor tires, heavy vehicle weight, and poor reaction times adversely affect braking distance. The following chart illustrates braking distance at various speeds.

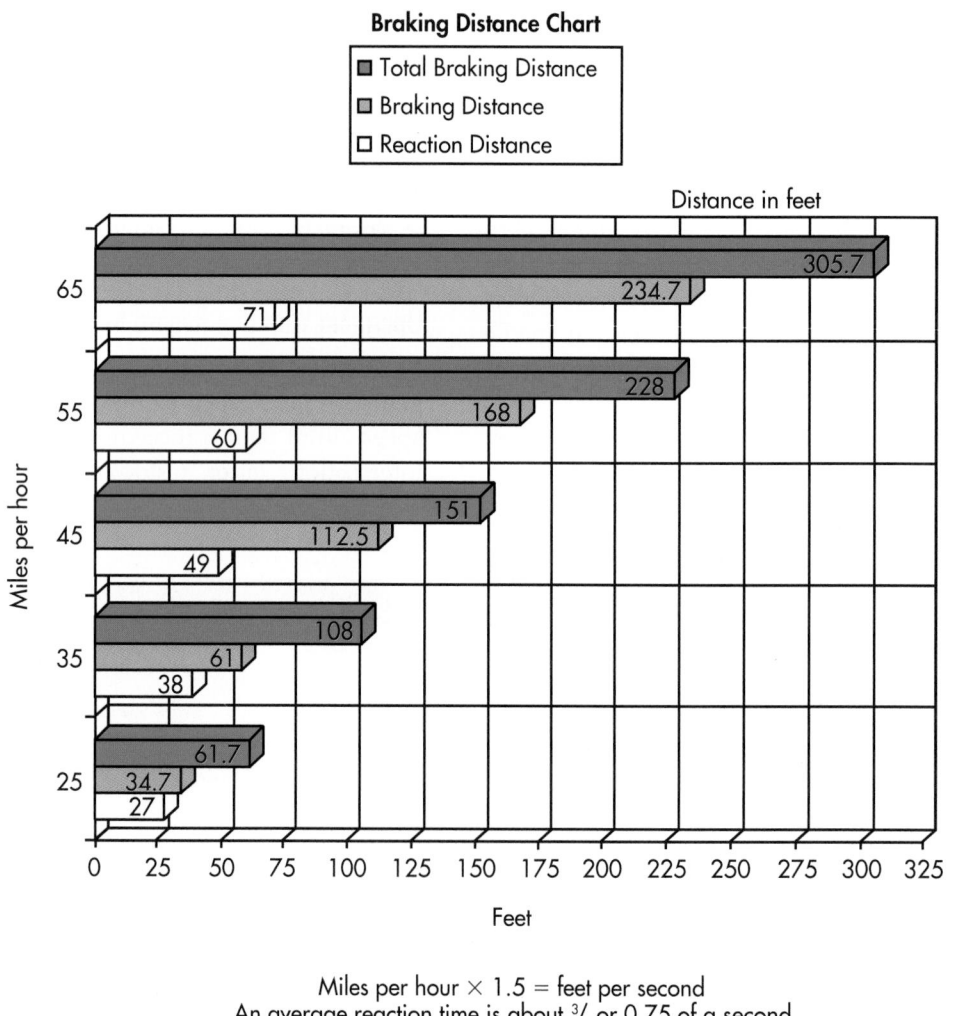

Braking Distance Chart
- Total Braking Distance
- Braking Distance
- Reaction Distance

Miles per hour × 1.5 = feet per second
An average reaction time is about ³/₄ or 0.75 of a second

From http://www.lausd.k12.ca.us/police/traffic/brakgraf.html

NOTE

Larger emergency vehicles (e.g., those mounted on freightliner-type chassis) have different handling characteristics and longer braking and stopping distances than conventional Type I, II, and III emergency vehicles.

response (see the box on p. 1380). However, these privileges must take into consideration the safety of all persons using the roadway. This "due regard for the safety of all others" carries legal responsibility and can result in liability for the paramedic and EMS agency if damage, injury, or death results from its failure. The paramedic should be aware of local and state laws and regulations pertaining to the operation of an emergency vehicle.

Aeromedical Transportation

Air evacuation, like many other aspects of prehospital emergency care, is rooted in military history. During the Prussian siege of Paris in 1870, soldiers and civilians were evacuated by a hot-air balloon, and in 1928 a Marine pilot used an engine-powered aircraft to evacuate the wounded in Nicaragua.[5] However, the first full-scale use of motorized aircraft for medical evacuation did not occur until 1950 during the Korean conflict. The experience gained in Korea was the basis for developing helicopter rescue in Vietnam when nearly 1 million casualties

were transported by air. The most recent military confrontations involving the United States in Panama, Grenada, and the Middle East had massive advanced aeromedical support capabilities and plans onsite before it started. Response times of 25 minutes were achieved for aeromedical evacuation of wounded soldiers in Operation Desert Storm. Field surgical units were set up to handle the estimated 1500 to 3000 casualties occurring within the first 24 hours of the war; most of the injured soldiers arrived by air transportation.[6]

Today there are about 300 civilian EMS flight programs using fixed-wing and/or rotary-wing (helicopter) aircraft throughout the United States.[7] Fixed-wing aircraft services are not usually as high-profile as helicopters and frequently are used for interhospital transfer of patients and vital organ delivery when the distance is greater than 100 miles (Figs. 48-4 and 48-5).

Aeromedical Crew Members and Training

The staffing of air ambulances includes a pilot and various health care professionals (such as EMTs, paramedics, respiratory therapists, nurses, and physicians) with specialized training in flight physiology and advanced medical equipment and procedures. The ACS Committee on Trauma and the Association of Air Medical Services have established guidelines for personnel qualifications. The DOT-NHTSA funded the development of the *Air Medical Crew National Standard Curriculum* in 1988,

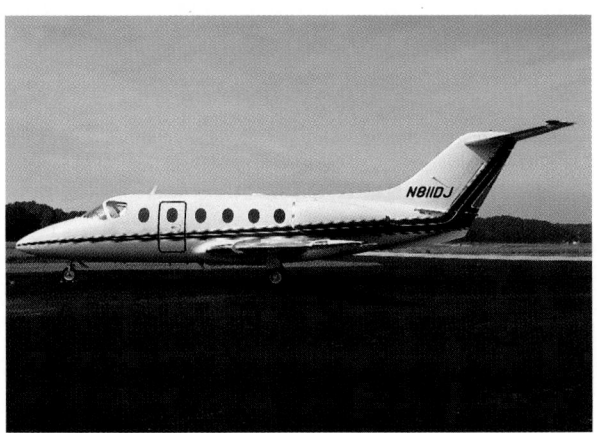

Fig. 48-4 Fixed-wing aircraft. (Courtesy Air Rescue Consortium of Hospitals, St Louis, Mo.)

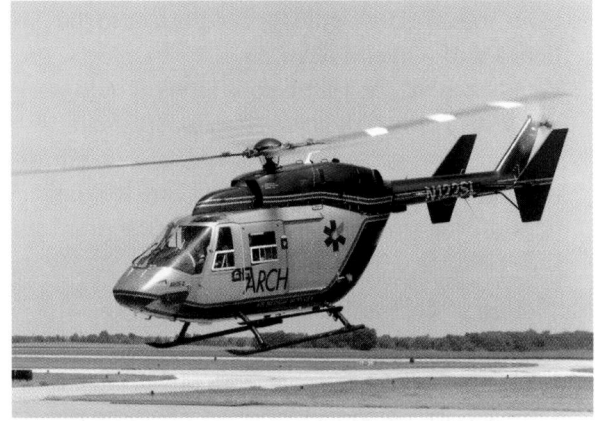

Fig. 48-5 Rotary-wing aircraft. (Courtesy Air Rescue Consortium of Hospitals, St Louis, Mo.)

SAMPLING OF ORGANIZATIONS ASSOCIATED WITH THE AIR MEDICAL INDUSTRY

Air Medical Physicians Association (AMPA)

Association of Air Medical Services (AAMS)

Commission on Accreditation of Air Medical Services (CAAMS)

Commission on the Accreditation of Medical Transport Services (CAMTS)

International Society of Air Medical Services (Australasia) (ISAS)

National Association of Air Medical Communications Specialists (NAACS)

National EMS Pilots Association (NEMSPA)

National Flight Nurses Association (NFNA)

National Flight Paramedics Association (NFPA)

Shock Trauma Air Rescue Society (STARS)

which many flight programs have used to teach flight physiology, aircraft components and construction, safety regulations, aviation and navigation terminology, and operational safety (Box 48-2).

Use of Aeromedical Services

The appropriate authority of the local EMS system develops criteria for requesting aeromedical services to the scene of an emergency. As described in Chapter 18, the paramedic generally should consider air transportation when emergency personnel have found one or more of the following:

1. The time needed to transport a patient by ground to an appropriate facility poses a threat to the patient's survival and recovery.
2. Weather, road, or traffic conditions would seriously delay the patient's access to ALS.
3. Critical care personnel and specialized equipment are necessary to adequately care for the patient during transportation (Box 48-3).

Notification of Aeromedical Services

Most aeromedical transportation providers accept requests for medical services from physicians, EMS and fire service personnel, or other on-scene public service agency personnel. If the paramedic requests air service for medical, trauma, or search and rescue

events, he or she should advise the flight crew of the type of emergency response, number of patients, location of a **landing zone** (LZ), and any prominent landmarks and hazards (e.g., vertical structures or power lines). Direct ground-to-air communications must be available between a designated LZ officer and the aeromedical staff on board the responding aircraft.

NOTE

Local and state guidelines exist for aeromedical activation. The paramedic should consult with medical direction and follow all state statutes, administrative rules, and city, county, and district ordinances and standards when using aeromedical services.

NOTE

On being notified of the probability for an aeromedical response, the flight crews of some services move to the aircraft so that they will be prepared for the flight (placed on "stand-by"). If the paramedic determines that the situation does not require an aeromedical response, he or she should advise the appropriate agency as soon as possible so that the crew can be available for other flights.

Landing Site Preparation

Space requirements for a helicopter LZ generally must be 100 by 100 feet. The ideal LZ should have no vertical structures that can impair takeoff or landing. It should be relatively flat and free of high grass, crops, or other factors that can conceal uneven terrain or hinder access. The LZ also should be free of debris that can injure people or damage structures or the helicopter. If patients are close to the LZ, the paramedic should provide protection by covering wounds and eyes. Rescue personnel close to the landing site should wear protective equipment such as helmets with lowered face shields and safety glasses.

NOTE

If possible, the fire department should be dispatched to the LZ to provide fire-suppression support activities. Law enforcement personnel also should be valuable in securing the scene.

BOX 48-3

ADVANTAGES AND DISADVANTAGES OF AIR MEDICAL SERVICES

Advantages

- Transports are rapid and usually smooth.
- Access to accident sites is quick.
- Traffic, trains, mountains, ship canals, and other barriers can be avoided.
- Travel is still possible when road conditions are unfavorable.
- Sophisticated communication equipment is available.
- Ground ambulances are not detained for long periods.
- Quality of care is improved in rural areas where only BLS is available.
- There are fewer air ambulance crashes than ground ambulance crashes.

Disadvantages

- In urban settings, ground ambulances are usually faster within a 30-mile range.
- If the helicopter is on another flight, no other aircraft may be available.
- Inclement weather may prevent the aircraft from traveling.
- High noise level may limit or prevent communication with the patient or crew.
- Space and weight restrictions may limit access to the patient and restrict the crew, patients, and equipment that can be carried.
- Helicopter transports are more expensive than transports by ground ambulance.
- Helicopter crashes have fewer survivors.

If a nighttime LZ is used, emergency vehicles with lighted bar lights should be situated at the perimeters of the LZ. If white lights are used, they should be directed *down* to the center of the LZ as spotlights because white lights (spotlights or headlights) directed toward the aircraft can temporarily blind the pilot. Traffic cones with reflectors can help identify the LZ. Flares should not be used because the helicopter rotor wash can blow the flares from the site and create a fire hazard. A fire crew should wet down dusty LZs, especially if vehicle traffic is moving in the area. This prevents the pilot and vehicle drivers from being temporarily blinded by the dust.

Helpful radio communications with the pilot include notification of wind direction and any possible obstructions or hazards. Wind direction can be determined by throwing grass or dirt, wetting a finger, or by smoke patterns from smoke canisters. If hazardous materials are present, the paramedic should advise the flight crew of the substance, location of the hazardous materials site, and the possibility of patient contamination. The pilot generally will not land the aircraft until all dangers of fire or explosion are eliminated. After the aircraft is coming in to land, one emergency responder should stand facing the LZ so the pilot can see the landing area. Fig. 48-6 provides LZ hand signals that may be useful to the pilot.

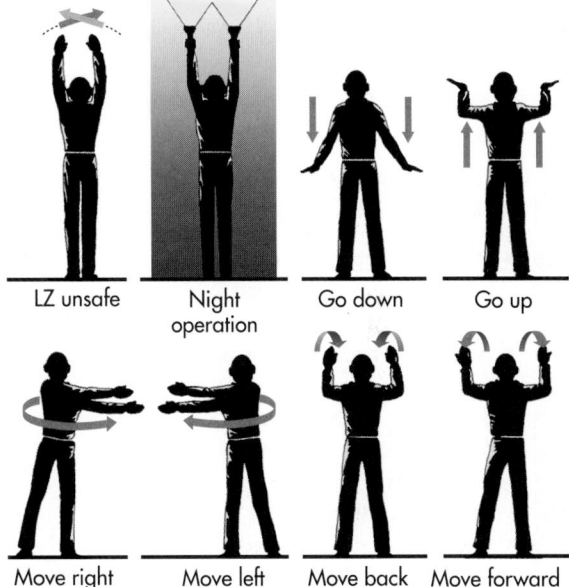

Fig. 48-6 Landing zone hand signals.

Safety Precautions

Everyone should be clear of the landing area during takeoffs and landings. A distance of 100 to 200 feet is best (Fig. 48-7). In addition, the precautions in Box 48-4 should be followed.

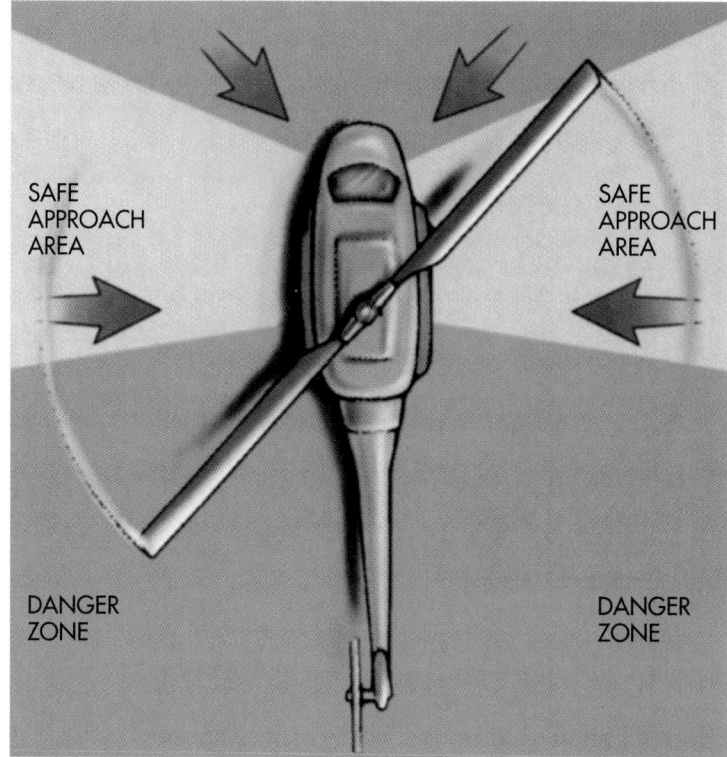

Fig. 48-7 Safe-approach zones. (From American College of Emergency Physicians: *Paramedic field care: a complaint-based approach,* St Louis, 1997, Mosby.)

SAFE APPROACH AREA

SAFE APPROACH AREA

DANGER ZONE

DANGER ZONE

BOX 48-4

SAFETY PRECAUTIONS DURING HELICOPTER LANDING

- Never allow ground personnel to approach the helicopter unless requested to do so by the pilot or flight crew.
- Allow only necessary personnel to help load or unload patients.
- Secure any loose objects or clothing that could be blown by rotor, downwash (e.g., stretcher, sheets, or blankets).
- Allow no smoking.
- After the aircraft is parked, move to the front beyond the perimeter of the rotor blades and *wait for a signal from the pilot* to approach.
- Approach the helicopter in a crouched position staying within view of the pilot or other crew members.
- *Never approach the rear of the aircraft from any direction.* The tail rotors on most aircraft are near the ground and spin at high RPMs, which makes them virtually invisible. Tail rotor injuries are often fatal.
- Carry long objects horizontally and no more than waist high.
- Depart the helicopter from the front and within view of the pilot.

Patient Preparation

Preparing a patient for aeromedical transportation requires the following special considerations:

- The paramedic must establish and secure the patient's airway before loading.
- The paramedic must apply the pneumatic antishock garment (PASG) before loading (per local protocol).
- The paramedic should position external cardiopulmonary resuscitation (CPR) devices according to aircraft configuration.
- Restraints or pharmacological control may be required for combative patients.

? CRITICAL THINKING

How do you think an alert patient will feel when waiting for helicopter transportation?

NOTE

Despite excellent patient assessment and management at the scene, aeromedical crews will perform a brief reassessment before liftoff to verify the patient's condition.

SUMMARY

- The KKK A-1822 standards from the U.S. General Services Administration are the foundation of uniformity among ambulance vehicles.

- Completing an ambulance equipment and supply checklist at the beginning of every work shift is important for safety, patient care, and risk management issues and for ensuring the appropriate handling and safekeeping of scheduled medications.

- Methods for estimating ambulance service needs and stationing in a community have shifted toward compliance in providing EMS services within time frames that meet national standards.

- Factors that influence safe ambulance operation include appropriate use of escorts, environmental conditions, appropriate use of warning devices, proceeding safely through intersections, parking at the emergency scene, and operating with due regard for the safety of all others.

- The staffing of air ambulances includes a pilot and various health care professionals with specialized training in flight physiology and special medical equipment and procedures.

- If the paramedic requests aeromedical service, he or she should advise the flight crew of the type of emergency response, number of patients, location of landing zone, and any prominent landmarks and hazards. The paramedic should always follow strict safety precautions during helicopter landing to prevent injury to air medical crews, ground crews, the patient, or bystanders.

REFERENCES

1. American Heart Association: *Textbook of advanced cardiac life support*, Dallas, 1997, The Association.
2. Fitch J: *Prehospital care administration: issues, readings, cases*, St Louis, 1995, Mosby.
3. National Safety Council: *Injury facts*, Itasca, Ill, 1999, The Council.
4. Kahn C et al: Characteristics of fatal ambulance crashes in the United States: an 11-year retrospective, *Prehospital Emergency Care* 4(1): 2000.
5. U.S. Department of Transportation, National Highway Traffic Safety Administration: *Air medical crew national standard curriculum*, Washington, DC, 1988, The Department.
6. Burkle FM: Emergency medicine in the Persian Gulf. I. Preparations for triage and combat casualty care, *Ann Emerg Med* 23(4):742, 1994.
7. Directory of air medical programs, *AirMed* 6(3):18, 2000.

49 Medical Incident Command

Upon completion of this chapter, the paramedic student will be able to:

1. Identify the components of an effective incident command system.

2. Outline the activities in the preplanning, scene management, and postdisaster follow-up phases of an incident.

3. Identify the five major components of FEMA's incident command system.

4. List command responsibilities during a major incident response.

5. Describe the section responsibilities in the FEMA incident command system.

6. Identify situations that may be classified as major incidents.

7. Describe the steps necessary to establish and operate the incident command system.

8. Given a major incident, describe sectors that would need to be established and the responsibilities of each.

9. List common problems related to the incident command system and to mass casualty situations.

10. Outline the principles and technology of triage.

11. Identify resources for management of critical incident stress.

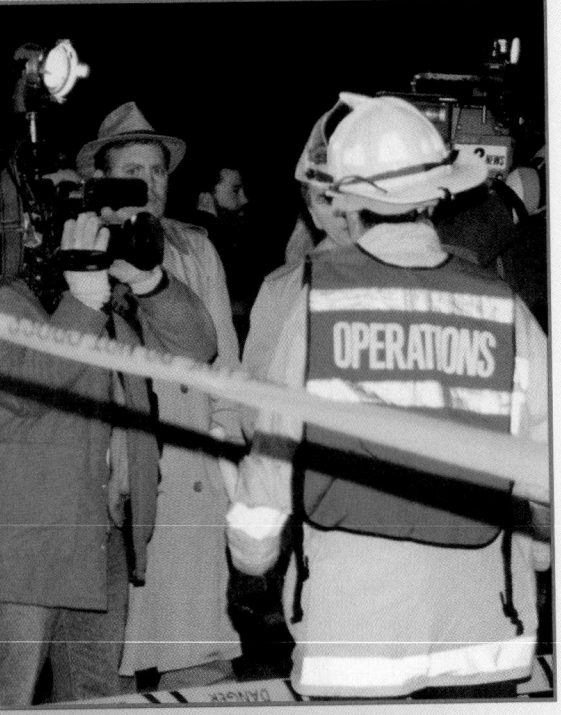

A **major incident** is an event for which available resources are insufficient to manage the number of casualties or the nature of the emergency. Major incidents such as highway accidents, air crashes, major fires, train derailments, building collapses, acts of violence or terrorism, search and rescue operations, hazardous materials releases, and natural disasters stress and may overwhelm local, regional, state, and even national and international resources.

incident command system: A management program designed to control, direct, and coordinate emergency response operations and resources.

major incident: An event for which available resources are insufficient to manage the number of casualties or the nature of the emergency.

mutual aid: An agreement with neighboring emergency agencies that equipment and manpower can be mutually exchanged when necessary.

sectors: Subdivisions of the incident command system that encompass specific areas of responsibility as deemed necessary by the incident commander.

The Incident Command System

Historically, emergency management of major incidents often resulted in the response of several different agencies (EMS, fire service, rescue, law enforcement, and others), each performing activities independently, with little or no interagency organization. This made it difficult to determine who was in charge of the scene and to what extent emergency services were needed or were being provided. The

NOTE

The term *disaster* usually is associated with a man-made or natural event that involves tremendous damage across a large geographical area or to a community's infrastructure (e.g., roads, power, communications, housing). A subset of disaster is a *mass casualty incident* (MCI) in which there are many injuries and/or fatalities. The mobilization of resources and the methods used to meet the needs of a disaster response is called *disaster management.*

? CRITICAL THINKING

What effect do you think lack of organization could have on rescue operations, scene safety, patient care, and transportation in a mass casualty incident?

incident command system (ICS) was developed to address these concerns and to organize interagency functions and responsibilities.

An effective ICS provides for single jurisdiction and single agency involvement, single jurisdiction and multiagency involvement, and multijurisdiction and multiagency involvement. This organizational structure allows the ICS to adapt to any agency or incident for which emergency management would be needed. The ICS also must be able to expand from dealing with a nonmajor incident to a major incident in a logical manner. The practice of using an ICS as standard operating procedure for small incidents permits a smooth transition when a major incident occurs.[1] Other components of an effective ICS include common elements in organization, terminology (Box 49-1), and procedures. The system should be implemented with the least possible disruption to existing systems (EMS, fire, and law enforcement agencies) and should be simple enough to keep operational and maintenance costs to a minimum.

NOTE

ICS is not indicated in a minor incident where the units dispatched to the scene are sufficient to handle the event. If additional units are required (a major incident), ICS should be established. If there is a need for extended operations that will quickly overwhelm the responding units (e.g., a disaster that involves numerous patients or an event that may last several hours to days), ICS should be established.

Declaring a Major Incident

Declaring a major incident is an important phase of the response. If an EMS unit is dispatched to a scene that has this potential, the crew should declare (per established protocol) that they are responding to a possible major incident and will confirm on arrival. This information allows other agencies to be contacted and placed on standby and provides time for the availability of other special resources to be determined. The responding crew (or supervisor) also

BOX 49-1

BOX 49-1

ICS DEFINITIONS

apparatus: A vehicle used for fire suppression or rescue that does not include staff vehicles.

command: The individual in charge of the incident scene (also known as the incident commander).

command post: The area from which command directs operations for an incident.

communications center: A facility used to dispatch emergency equipment and coordinate communications between field units and personnel.

medical direction: A process of ensuring that actions taken on behalf of ill or injured people are medically appropriate, including prospective, concurrent, and retrospective aspects of EMS quality improvement, hiring, and education.

mutual aid: An agreement with neighboring emergency agencies that equipment and personnel can be mutually exchanged when necessary.

sector: A subdivision of the ICS encompassing a specific area of responsibility as deemed necessary by the incident commander.

staging area: A designated area where incident-assigned vehicles are directed and held until needed.

should alert medical direction and area hospitals. Receiving hospitals need information on numbers of patients and severity of injuries as soon as possible to prepare for the patients' arrival. A possible major incident should be declared in the following situations:

- Any situation that requires more than two ambulance units for adequate treatment, particularly in rural areas where communities may have only one ambulance
- Any situation involving hazardous or radioactive materials or chemicals in significant quantity
- Any situation that requires special EMS resources, such as helicopters, rescue teams, or multiple rescue or extrication units
- When in doubt, declare a major incident

TRICKS OF THE TRADE

If you think there is a potential for a major incident, declare it. "It is better to have and not need than to need and not have."

Preparing for a Major Incident

Preparing for a major incident involves three phases: preplanning, scene management, and post-disaster follow-up (or after-action review). A brief description of each phase follows.

Phase 1: The Preplan. Cooperation and preplanning are crucial in managing a major incident. The preplan must be agreed to by all participating emergency response agencies and address common goals and the specific duties of each group. Multi-agency endeavors succeed as a result of frequent meetings and organized practice sessions or exercises (drills or "table-top" exercises). The preplan should include a system of sorting or prioritizing care, treatment, and transportation.

TRICKS OF THE TRADE

Participating in drills and table-top exercises can be a great learning experience.

Other considerations in the preplan include identifying hazards (a risk assessment) within a community, such as manufacturing, storage, and transportation of hazardous materials; fire threats; population base at various times of day; and violence and other potential social problems. An inventory of resources that may be needed during a major incident include the following:

- Shelter and mass feeding
- Air evacuation
- Medical equipment and supplies
- Heavy equipment, power generators, and lighting
- Communications
- Law enforcement
- Specialized rescue services

Phase 2: Scene Management. Phase 2 requires the development of a strategy to manage the emergency scene. Some major incidents can be managed effectively with local resources and personnel (closed or contained incidents). Other incidents, however, may affect geographical and functional jurisdictions (open or uncontained incidents), in which large numbers of federal, state, and local agencies become involved. Regardless of the size of the incident or the number of agencies involved in the response, scene management requires a coordinated effort to ensure an effective response and the efficient and safe use of resources.

Phase 3: Postdisaster Follow-up. Phase 3 includes a post-disaster (or after-action) review of "lessons learned" from the incident and methods of improvement, such as emergency response, planning, and community protection. This phase also should evaluate stress-related anxiety and illness among emergency workers that may have resulted from the incident.

The FEMA Incident Management or Command System

Federal law requires the use of ICS for hazardous materials (Hazmat) incidents, and many states have adopted ICS for responding to all types of incidents. The incident management or command system developed by the Federal Emergency Management Agency (FEMA) is the national standard for incident management.[1] The FEMA ICS is a flexible system used by both public and private sectors in some routine and most large-scale emergencies. Much of the success of ICS has resulted directly from applying a common organizational structure and key management principles in a standardized way. FEMA's ICS organization is built around five major components[2] (Fig. 49-1):

1. Command
2. Planning
3. Operations
4. Logistics
5. Finance/Administration

NOTE

The five major components of ICS, also known as "C-FLOP" (command, finance, logistics, operations, planning), are the foundation on which organization develops. They apply during a major event; in preparing for a major event; or in managing a response to a major event.

Command Function

It generally is agreed that the responsibility of command should belong to *one* person who has the abil-

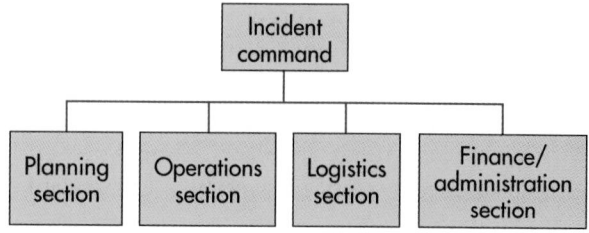

Fig. 49-1 Incident command system structure.

ity to coordinate a variety of emergency activities. This is the cornerstone of the ICS structure.

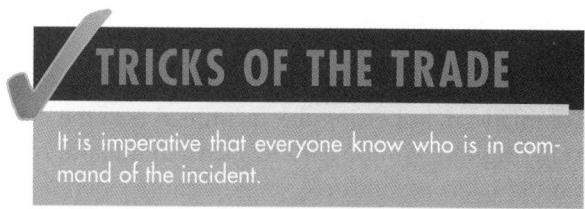

It is imperative that everyone know who is in command of the incident.

Initial command should be determined by a pre-planned system of arriving emergency units and personnel (e.g., the first or second arriving EMS, fire, or law enforcement unit). The person assuming command (the incident commander) must be familiar with the ICS structure and the operating procedures of other responding agencies. It is not necessary that the commander be the individual with the highest rank (although this is common) or most medical training, but rather one who is able to effectively manage the emergency scene.

Command must be established immediately. The commander must be clearly identified, and all others at the scene must be aware of who is in command. As a more qualified individual arrives, command may be transferred per standard operating procedures (SOPs). Once established, command should do the following:

- Assume an effective command mode and position.
- Transmit brief initial radio reports to the communications center and identify the location of the command post.
- Evaluate the situation rapidly.
- Develop a management strategy.
- Request additional resources and provide assignments as necessary.
- Implement a personal accountability system.

- Control and assign **sectors** as required, consistent with the needs of the incident, standard operating procedures, or disaster plans, and provide operating objectives for these sectors.
- Provide continuing effective command and progress reports until relieved by a higher-ranking individual.
- Develop the command organization by delegating authority to subordinates to accomplish incident needs and objectives.
- Review and evaluate the effectiveness of site operations and revise operations as needed.
- Return units to service and terminate command when appropriate.

Types of Command

Command may be singular or unified (see the box in the right column). With singular command, one individual is responsible for the entire operation. This type of command often works well for incidents with limited jurisdictions or responsibilities, and it works best in small events of short duration.

Unified command may be needed in large events or as a small incident evolves. In unified command, specialized organizations are identified (e.g., EMS, fire, police, health department, American Red Cross) and personnel unify to complement command. This type of command stimulates cooperation (the "right" agency leads command at the "right" time)

and provides for balanced decision making. Examples of when unified command may be indicated include incidents (Fig. 49-2) that have the following characteristics:

- Affect more than one political jurisdiction
- Involve multiple agencies within a jurisdiction
- Have an impact on multiple geographic and functional agencies

> **NOTE**
>
> The concept of unified command means that all involved agencies contribute to the command process by:
> - Determining overall objectives
> - Planning jointly for operational activities while conducting integrated operations
> - Maximizing the use of all assigned resources

> **? CRITICAL THINKING**
>
> *Where do you think command should be located in a mass casualty situation that is confined to one area?*

In either type of command, the incident commander may delegate authority for certain activities by activating additional sections (sectors) to meet the needs of the situation. The incident commander

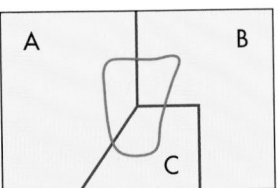
Incidents that affect more than one political jurisdiction

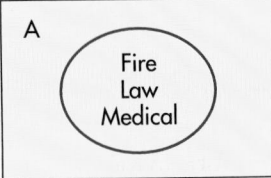
Incidents involving multiple agencies within a jurisdiction

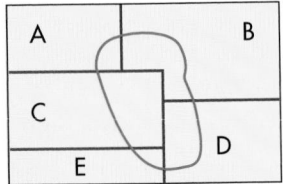
Incidents that have an impact on multiple geographic and functional agencies

Fig. 49-2 Application of unified command.

> **DIFFERENCES BETWEEN SINGLE AND UNIFIED COMMAND**
>
> In a single command structure, a single incident commander is solely responsible (within the confines of authority) to establish objectives and overall management strategy associated with the incident. The incident commander is directly responsible for follow-through to ensure that all functional area actions are directed toward accomplishment of the strategy. The implementation of the planning required to affect operational control will be the responsibility of a single individual (section chief) who will report directly to the incident commander.
>
> In a unified command structure, the persons designated by their jurisdictions (or by departments within a jurisdiction) must jointly determine objectives, strategies, and priorities. As in single command, the section chief will have responsibility for implementation of the plan.

will base the decision to expand (or contract) the ICS organization on three major incident priorities[2]:

1. Life safety. The incident commander's first priority is *always* the safety of the emergency responders and the public.
2. Incident stability. The incident commander is responsible for determining the strategy that will minimize the effect that the incident will have on the surrounding area, and maximize the response effort while using resources effectively.
3. Property conservation. The incident commander is responsible for minimizing damages to property while achieving the incident objectives.

When expansion of command is required, the incident commander will establish the other command staff positions, as shown in Fig. 49-3.

Section Responsibilities

When it has been determined that sections are required to effectively manage an incident, the general staff sections (planning, operations, logistics, and/or finance/administration) are assigned by the incident commander to section chiefs, all of whom report to the incident commander. Section chiefs must be strong supervisors and managers. Their primary role in ICS is to "make things happen" and ensure that all rescuers in their sections are working toward a common goal. The number of sections necessary varies based on the scope of the incident and is determined by the incident commander (Fig. 49-4).

> **NOTE**
>
> In ICS, a manageable span of control (the number of persons one section chief can manage effectively) falls within the range of three to seven, with five being the optimum.[2]

Section chiefs should not become involved in physical tasks (such as carrying litters or operating rescue equipment) so that they can maintain control and supervise the section. General responsibilities of section chiefs include the following:

- Accomplishing objectives provided by command
- Monitoring work progress

- Redirecting activities as necessary
- Coordinating related activities with other sections
- Requesting additional resources as needed for the section
- Monitoring the welfare of personnel from each section
- Providing command with frequent reports
- Reallocating resources within the section

> **NOTE**
>
> The section chief should report to command when a job is assigned, when a job is accomplished, or if a job cannot be accomplished.

Planning Section

Staff functions of the planning section (Fig. 49-5) are to provide past, present, and future information about the incident and the status of resources. This section's responsibilities also can include creation of a written or verbal Incident Action Plan (IAP). The IAP (the need for which is determined by the incident commander) defines the response activities and resource utilization for a specified period. These operational periods can be of various lengths, but they should be no longer than 24 hours. (Twelve-hour operational periods are common for large-scale incidents.) IAPs may be indicated when:

- Resources from multiple agencies are used
- Several jurisdictions are involved
- The incident is complex (e.g., when changes in shifts or personnel are required)

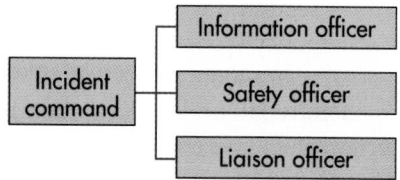

Fig. 49-3 Possible command staff positions. The information officer handles all media inquiries and coordinates the release of information to the media with the public affairs officer at the Emergency Operations Center (EOC). The safety officer monitors safety conditions and develops measures for ensuring the safety of all assigned personnel. The liaison officer is the on-scene contact for other agencies assigned to the incident.

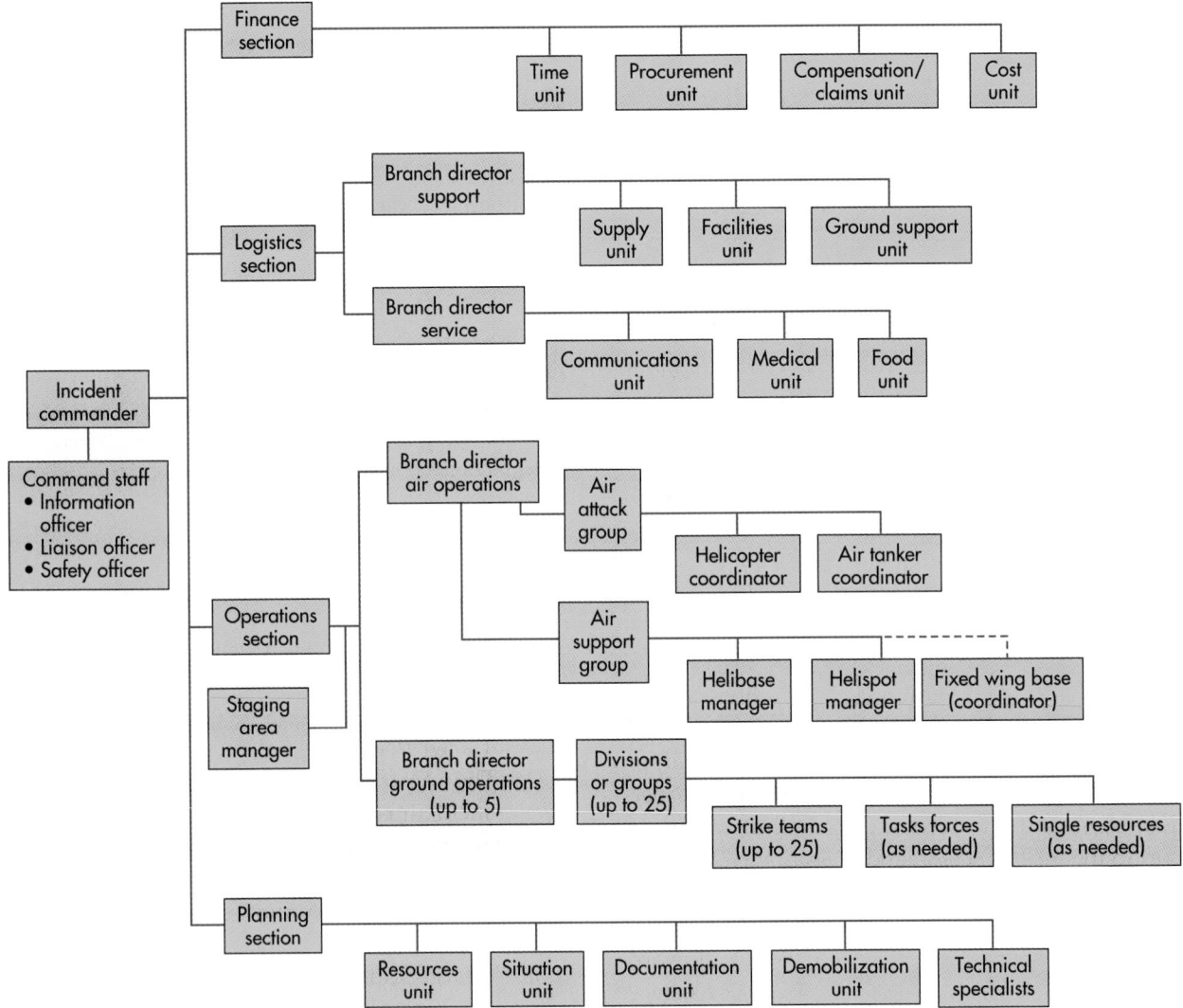

Fig. 49-4 Command section organizational plan.

Operations Section

The operations section (Fig. 49-6) directs and coordinates all emergency scene operations and ensures the safety of all operational personnel. (EMS operation areas generally fall under this section.) The operations section chief is in charge of the actual scene ("ground zero") and is responsible for the following activities:

- Carrying out tactical objectives
- Directing the front-end activities
- Participating in planning
- Modifying action plans as needed
- Maintaining discipline
- Accounting for personnel

Logistics Section

The logistics section (Fig. 49-7) is responsible for providing supplies and equipment (including personnel to operate the equipment), facilities, services, food, and communications support required for the incident. The primary function of this section is to provide gear and support to the incident responders. Essential equipment needed to support a medical incident includes supplies for airway, respiratory, and hemorrhage control; burn management; and pa-

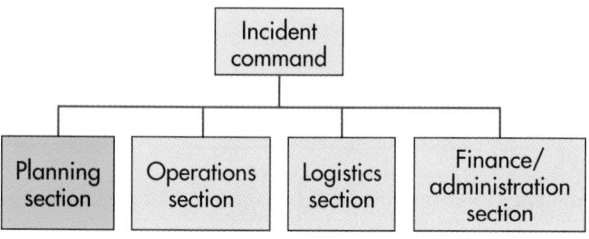

Fig. 49-5 The planning section.

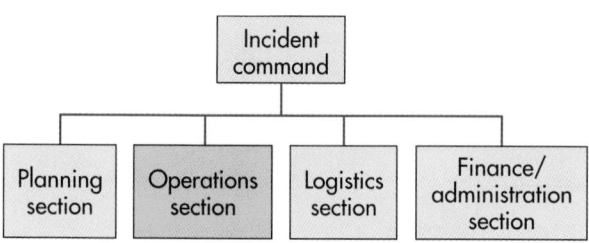

Fig. 49-6. The operations section.

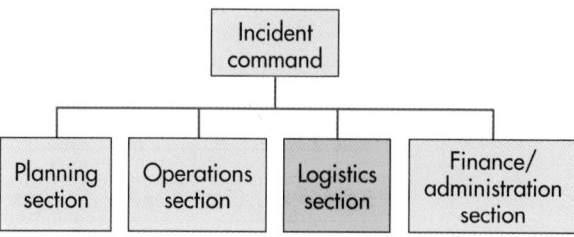

Fig. 49-7. The logistics section.

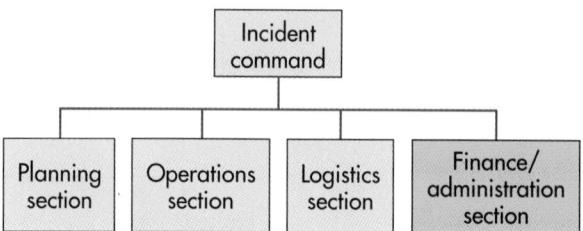

Fig. 49-8. The finance/administration section.

tient packaging and immobilization. The logistics section seldom is used at routine daily incidents.

> **NOTE**
>
> The medical unit of the logistics section cares for the incident responders, not civilian victims.

Finance/Administration Section

The finance/administration section (Fig. 49-8) is important for tracking incident costs and reimbursement accounting. Like the logistics section, the finance/administration section seldom is used in small-scale incidents but is considered essential if the incident grows in magnitude and costs (e.g., a Presidential declaration of a disaster). Functions of the finance/administration section during a major incident may include:

- Time accounting
- Procurement
- Paying claims
- Estimating costs

Major Medical Incidents

The need to establish an ICS at a medical incident is determined by when the number of casualties or

nature of the event will overwhelm available resources ("local/regional threshold"). In communities where the local threshold is low, frequent utilization of ICS for practice purposes is encouraged (e.g., when there are multiple patients).

When the need for ICS is identified, command must be established to determine which groups/sector functions or major functional areas need to be implemented for the size and scope of the incident. Examples of groups and sectors may include support and resources (support sector), helicopter landing zones and vehicle apparatus arrivals (staging sector), and patient care delivery (treatment sector). It also may become necessary to employ a unified command structure comprising EMS, fire, and law enforcement to oversee the various operations (Fig. 49-9).

> **? CRITICAL THINKING**
>
> *How do you think you'll feel when you arrive first on the scene of a major medical incident?*

Scene Assessment

The first EMS unit to arrive at the scene should make a quick and rapid assessment ("windshield assessment") of the situation. A more precise and

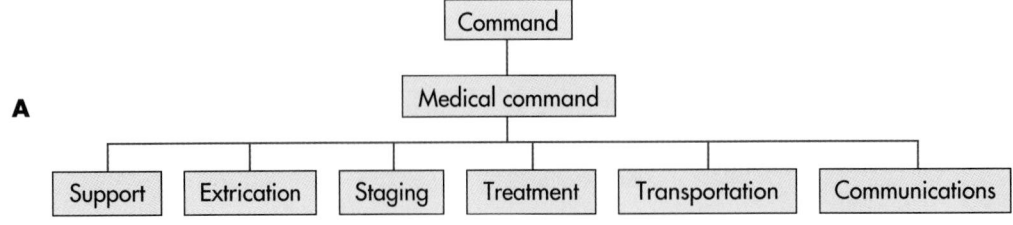

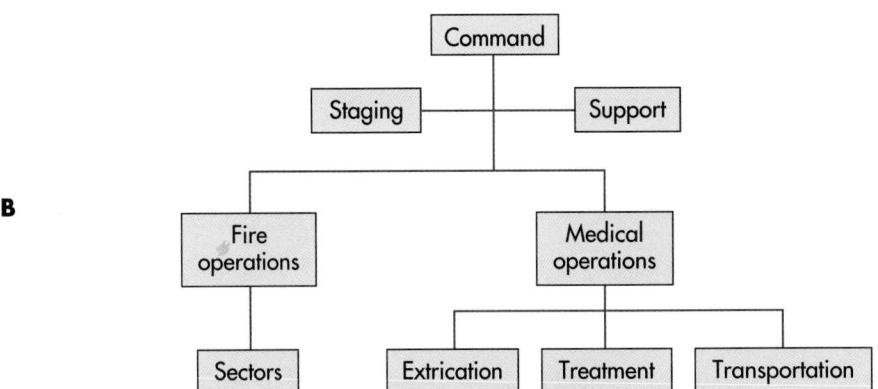

Fig. 49-9 Examples of **(A)** medical ICS and **(B)** ICS with fire operations.

complete assessment should be performed as soon as safety and time permit, including:

- Type of incident and potential duration
- Entrapment or special rescue resources that may be needed
- Number of patients in each triage category (described later in this chapter)
- Any additional resources that may be needed to manage the incident

> **NOTE**
>
> The scene assessment must be continually updated to identify specific needs or changing needs.

Communications

Command must immediately be established over the radio with the communications center or Emergency Operations Center (EOC). Most jurisdictions maintain an EOC as part of their community's preparedness program. An EOC is where department heads, government officers and officials, and volunteer agencies gather to coordinate their response to an emergency event. Command and the EOC share the same goals but function at different levels of responsibility. The incident commander is responsible for on-scene activities, and the EOC is responsible for the entire community-wide response to the event.

> **NOTE**
>
> Radio traffic can be very distracting, and incident personnel must observe strict radio and/or phone procedures, using clear text (plain English). All transmissions should be short and to the point.

Obtaining Resources

Additional units should be requested as soon as the need has been identified or anticipated. (The communications center should have a written SOP for requesting **mutual aid**.) Additional support services may include obtaining food, shelter, and clothing for victims. The incident commander is responsible for instructions for the strategic deployment of resources. (Personnel should stay with their vehicle until instructions are received.) Staging techniques that may be used to deploy resources effectively include the following:

- Lining vehicles up at the scene to facilitate egress
- Staging away from a limited access highway
- Identifying a formal staging area with an assigned staging officer

NOTE

The "tool box" theory for the strategic deployment of resources is to identify the resources ("tools") specific to the incident, use only the needed resources, and issue instructions for deployment of resources.

Group or Sector Functions for a Medical Incident

As previously stated, the number of groups or sectors required at a major medical incident will vary. Common sectors and their responsibilities include extrication/rescue, treatment, transportation, staging, and support.

Extrication Sector

The extrication sector is responsible for managing entrapped patients at the scene. This involves rescue, initial triage, primary treatment, patient categorization, and initial tagging assignments before transfer of the patients to the treatment sector. Patient care activities in this sector should include only assessment and treatment of life-threatening situations, such as securing airways, controlling severe bleeding, and covering open chest wounds. In addition, the extrication sector is responsible for site safety, personnel safety (e.g., supplying self-contained breathing apparatus, protective clothing), and evaluating and directing resources needed for extrication. Extrication sector responsibilities include the following:

- Determining whether triage and the primary treatment will be conducted on site or at the treatment sector
- Attaching tagging assignments to injured patients
- Evaluating resources needed for extrication of trapped patients and for their delivery to the treatment sector
- Providing site safety

- Evaluating resources needed for triage and the primary treatment of patients
- Communicating resource requirements to command
- Allocating assigned resources
- Supervising assigned personnel and resources
- Collecting, assembling, and assessing the "walking wounded"
- Reporting progress to command
- Reporting "all clear" to command when all patients have been extricated and delivered to the treatment sector
- Coordinating with other sectors

? CRITICAL THINKING

What dilemmas might you face when doing triage at a multiple casualty incident situation?

Treatment Sector

The treatment sector works closely with the extrication sector in patient care delivery. As patients are delivered, they are categorized according to their medical needs. This sector provides advanced care and stabilization until the patients are transported to a medical facility. Most paramedics and hospital personnel are assigned to this area. With large numbers of patients, the area usually is further divided into immediate and delayed treatment zones to help determine priorities in patient transportation. Immediate patients include those with life-threatening injuries; delayed patients include the "walking wounded" and those whose care and transport can be delayed if necessary. It should be noted that triage monitoring is a function of all sectors involving ill or injured patients and is a continuing component of the ICS (incident command system). Treatment sector responsibilities include the following:

- Locating a suitable treatment sector area and reporting that location to the extrication sector and command
- Evaluating resources required for patient treatment and reporting these needs to command
- Providing continued triage of patients arriving in the treatment sector
- Providing suitable immediate and delayed treatment areas
- Allocating resources

- Assigning, supervising, and coordinating personnel within the sector
- Reporting progress to command
- Coordinating with other sectors

Rehabilitation Sector

A rehabilitation ("rehab") sector is part of standard operating procedures in many fire and EMS agencies and major incident response plans. This sector usually is set up in a location outside of the operational area and allows rescue personnel to receive physical and psychological rest. (In large-scale incidents, more than one rehab sector may be needed.) Responsibilities of the section chief include ensuring that personnel receive medical evaluation and treatment as needed and keeping accurate logs of persons who enter and exit the area. Records of medical evaluations and treatments are maintained for each person who enters the rehab sector. (Medical monitoring is further addressed in Chapter 51.)

? CRITICAL THINKING

Why do you think a rehab sector is important?

On-Scene Physicians at Multiple Casualty Incidents

Physicians who are on scene can provide valuable help during a multiple casualty incident (MCI). The role of the physician(s) may include providing on-scene medical direction, making difficult triage decisions and secondary triage decisions in a treatment area, and providing emergency surgery to facilitate extrication. Physicians also can perform specialized invasive procedures at the scene and can perform a more detailed assessment and provide direction for specific treatments that may be beyond the scope of normal paramedic practice.

Disposition of the Deceased

Depending on the scale of the incident, personnel may be assigned to disposition of the deceased. Duties of these personnel may include the following:

- Working with the medical examiner, coroner, law enforcement, and other appropriate agencies to coordinate disposition
- Assisting in the establishment of an appropriate and secure area for a morgue, if needed
- Monitoring personnel for signs of stress

NOTE

When possible, the deceased victims should be left in the location in which they were found until a decision and plan for disposition can be determined.

Transportation Sector

The transportation sector communicates with the receiving hospitals, ambulances, and aeromedical services for patient transport. This sector must work closely with the treatment sector to determine appropriate destinations for injured patients. The arrival and departure of transfer vehicles must be coordinated with the staging sector. Transportation sector responsibilities include the following:

- Determining patient transportation needs and obtaining appropriate transportation
- Evaluating resources required to manage patient transportation
- Establishing an ambulance staging area (if command has not already done so) and patient loading areas
- Establishing and operating a helicopter landing zone
- Communicating with hospitals to determine capabilities
- Coordinating patient transportation allocation with the treatment sector and the hospitals
- Tracking patients leaving the site with a written log including patient identification, unit transporting, and destination facility
- Reporting resource requirements to command
- Coordinating with other sectors
- Advising command when the last patient has been transported

Staging Sector

Staging sectors are required for large incidents to prevent vehicle congestion and response delays. All emergency vehicles (fire, police, EMS) should report to this sector for direction. Other agencies, such as disaster-relief services and news media, also should be supervised by the staging sector. Staging sector responsibilities include the following:

- Coordinating with the police department to block streets, intersections, and other areas to facilitate a staging area

- Ensuring that all apparatus is parked in an appropriate manner
- Maintaining a log of all apparatus in the staging area and maintaining an inventory of all specialized equipment and medical equipment that may be needed
- Reviewing with command what resources must be maintained in staging and coordinating this request with the dispatching center
- Assuming a visible position for incoming apparatus (e.g., leaving emergency lights operating on one apparatus and wearing a sector vest)
- Coordinating with other sectors

Support Sector

The support sector coordinates the gathering and distribution of equipment and supplies for all other sectors. This sector may be responsible for procuring medical supplies from area hospitals, rescue supplies, and other equipment needed at the incident. Support sector responsibilities include the following:

- Determining the medical supply needs of other sectors
- Establishing a suitable location for supply operations
- Coordinating procurement of medical supplies from hospitals with the transportation sector
- Coordinating procurement of medical supplies that are not available from hospitals
- Reporting additional resource requirements to command
- Allocating supplies and equipment as needed
- Reporting progress to command
- Coordinating with other sectors

Sector Identification

When an ICS is in place, all emergency responders must know its organizational structure and the lines of radio communications. Although clothing and identification vary by system, the following guidelines usually apply:

- Color-coded vests identify personnel. For example, the commander may wear a white vest; EMS sector managers, blue vests; fire sector managers, red; law enforcement sector managers, green; and so on.

- With the exceptions of command and sector communications, most communications are face to face. Radio use is intended for command operations.
- Radio communications use operation titles instead of personal or unit names: "EMS sector to command" or "fire sector to law-enforcement sector." This system ensures that all participants can reach the appropriate individual by one radio designation.

Radio Communications

A key function during a major incident is communications. Preplanning includes identifying the radio frequencies to be used in major incident responses and ways they are to be used. All responding units, for example, should have multichannel radios using a common frequency and separate frequencies for EMS, fire, and other support operations. Sector officers should have portable radios on a channel that permits direct communications with command. These frequencies may be assigned in advance or by the dispatching agency at the time of the incident. In addition, state, regional, and local communications systems should undergo a periodic review that includes the controls for activating communications, system frequencies, and portable and mobile radio equipment. Other communications considerations are:

- Radio traffic must be clear, concise, and in plain English.
- Messages should be considered and prepared before transmitting.
- The speaker should clearly identify unit number or sector.
- All radio traffic should be minimized.
- Face-to-face communication is preferred and encouraged.

Common Problems at Multiple-Casualty Incidents

In addition to common failures of incident command systems (see the box on p. 1398), there are common problems specific to MCIs. These include[1]:

- Failure to adequately provide widespread notification of the event
- Lack of rapid "initial" stabilization of all patients
- Failure to move, collect, and organize patients rapidly at a treatment area

---

COMMON FAILURES OF INCIDENT COMMAND SYSTEMS

Incident Command Failures
To establish a single, unified command
To establish staging
To request additional resources early
To delegate authority
To wear identification vests

Dispatch Failures
To coordinate the response of on-duty and off-duty emergency personnel to the scene

Communications Failures
To designate a single radio channel for disaster operations
To adopt standard operating procedures that limit radio traffic during incident operations

Staging Operation Failures
To establish a central staging area (command)
To select a large or easily accessible staging area (staging manager)
To frequently inventory specialized equipment and personnel (staging manager)

General Sector Operation Failures
To provide adequate progress reports to command
To become involved in physical tasks (sector manager)

To control the perimeter (law enforcement)
To advise command of available personnel

Extrication or Rescue Sector Failures
To triage and tag patients
To treat patients where they are found rather than stabilizing them and moving them to a treatment area (rescuers)
To provide adequate safety precautions

Treatment Sector Failures
To collect patients into an organized treatment area
To establish a sufficiently large treatment area
To organize the treatment area and monitor patients
To effectively coordinate transportation arrangements with the transportation sector

Transportation Sector Failures
To establish adequate access and egress routes for vehicles
To have adequate personnel to assist in transportation
To alert or update hospitals
To advise hospitals when the last patient is transported

Support Sector Failures
To plan for the medical supply needs of mass-casualty events
To provide rapid transport of supplies to the scene

- Failure to provide proper triage
- Administering overly time-consuming care
- Transporting patients prematurely
- Using personnel improperly in the field
- Failure to properly distribute patients to medical facilities
- Lack of recognizable EMS command in the field
- Lack of communication with local hospitals regarding patient flow and hospital capacity
- Lack of proper preplanning and lack of adequate training of all personnel

Principles and Technology of Triage

Triage is a method used to categorize patients for priorities of treatment. The assessment of patient injury severity is based on abnormal physiological signs, obvious anatomical injury (including mechanism of injury), and concurrent disease factors that might affect the patient's prognosis. It should be stressed that triage is a continuous process during a major incident, and constant monitoring of patient status may indicate a need to change the initial categorization and priority of treatment.

> **NOTE**
>
> The criteria for triage classifications are determined by the size of the incident, the number of injured patients, and the available personnel. At present, no national standards exist for field triage, so the paramedic must be familiar with local methods of patient triage categorization.

Primary Versus Secondary Triage

Triage may be classified as *primary* and *secondary*. Primary triage is used at the site to rapidly categorize patient conditions for treatment. During pri-

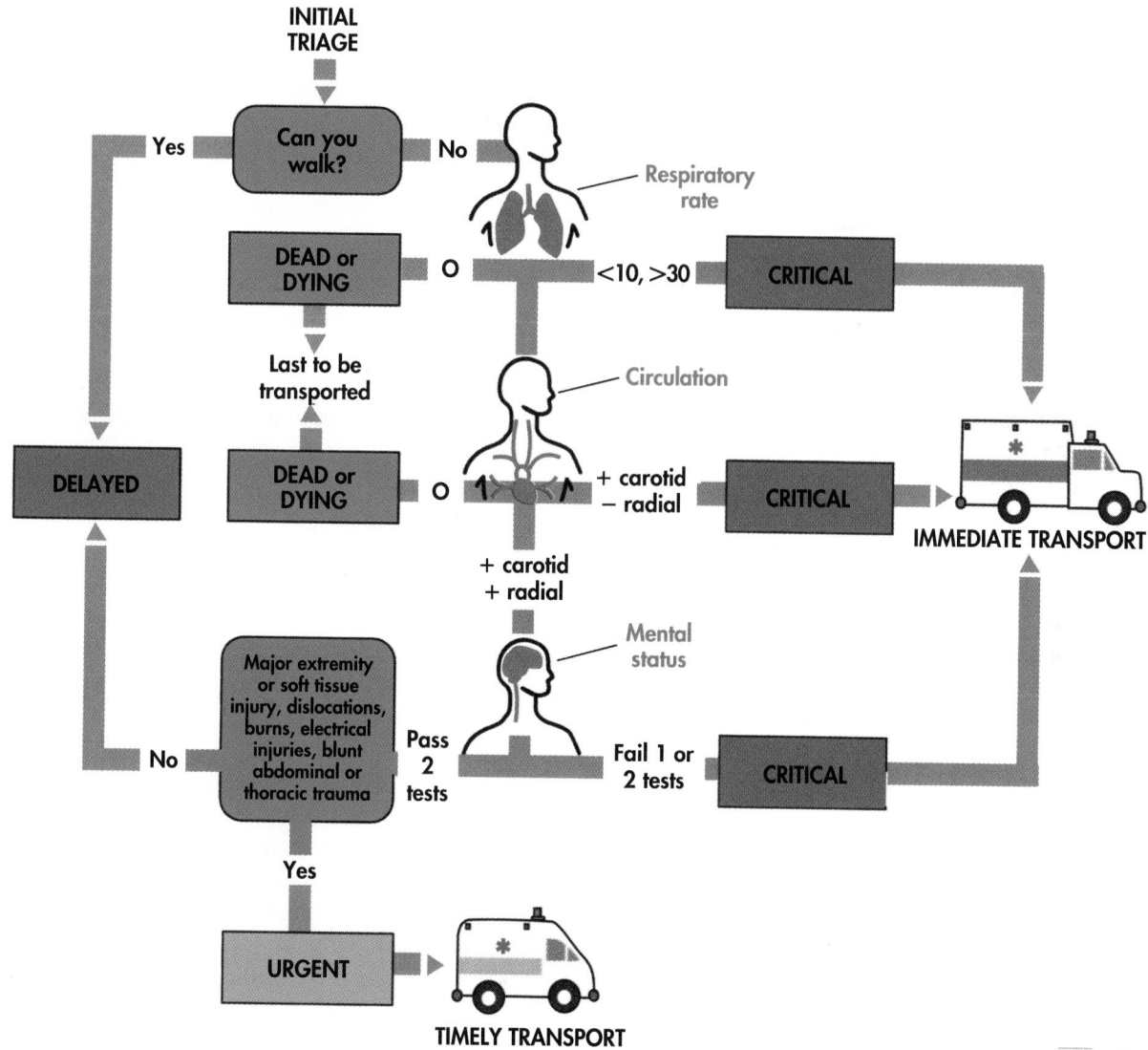

Fig. 49-10 The START triage system sorts patients into critical or delayed categories. Patients are quickly removed from the scene on the basis of the triage group they fall into. (From American College of Emergency Physicians: *Paramedic field care: a complaint-based approach*, St Louis, 1997, Mosby.)

mary triage, the paramedic documents the location of the patient and transport needs. The patient is then labeled with triage labels, tags, or tape. No care (other than immediate life-saving airway or hemorrhage management) is rendered during primary triage. The goal is to sort patients quickly.

Secondary triage is used at the treatment area. During secondary triage, patients are "re-triaged" and labeled (usually with paper tags) to assign priorities of care. Secondary triage often is not indicated at small-scale incidents.

START Technique of Primary Triage

The *START* (Simple Triage and Rapid Treatment) *Field Guide* was developed by Hoag Memorial Hospital in Newport Beach, California. The technique uses a 60-second assessment that focuses on the patient's ability to walk, respiratory effort, pulses/perfusion, and neurological status (Fig. 49-10). This assessment is used to classify victims as urgent, delayed, dead or dying, or critical. The *START Field Guide* allows rescuers to quickly identify victims at greatest risk of early death and advise other rescuers of the patient's need for stabilization by tagging the patient with color-coded disaster tags (described below).

NOTE

START triage requires little knowledge or skill and can be very accurate with practice. Its effectiveness relies on a more thorough assessment performed during the secondary triage.

START Technique

There are four basic assessment steps in START triage. These steps are listed below:

1. Assess the patient's ability to walk. Patients who can walk and understand basic commands are classified as DELAYED (walking wounded). Delayed patients are directed to remain in their location for further assistance or to walk to a treatment or transportation site. If the patient cannot walk, the respiratory rate is assessed (step 2). (Note: The initial triage is directed toward non-walking patients.)
2. Evaluate breathing and rate. If breathing is absent, the patient is classified as DEAD/DYING. A rate of less than 10 or more than 30 breaths per minute in the adult patient indicates CRITICAL status. Based on the respiratory assessment and the paramedic's intuition, these patients also can be classified as URGENT or DELAYED.

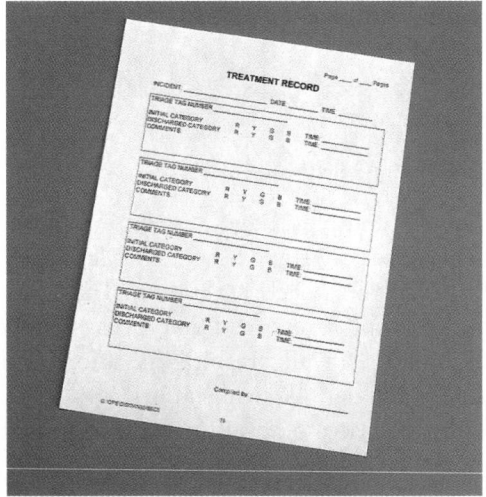

Fig. 49-11 ICS patient log.

---

3. Assess pulses/perfusion. If there is no pulse, the patient is classified as DEAD/DYING. A present carotid pulse and an absent radial pulse indicates CRITICAL status. If both the carotid and radial pulse are present, mental status should be assessed (step 4) before assigning a triage classification.
4. Assess mental status. Mental status can be assessed by asking the patient to perform two simple tasks. Examples include asking the patient to touch his or her nose with the index finger or to stick out the tongue, and assessing orientation with name, date, and year. Patients who can perform both tasks are classified as DELAYED. Those who fail either test are considered CRITICAL patients.

   Repositioning the airway and controlling severe hemorrhage are the only initial treatment efforts in primary triage. In a mass casualty event, however, these measures should not delay the triage of other patients. Depending on circumstances and the number of casualties, the walking wounded can sometimes assist in providing airway support and controlling severe hemorrhage.

Triage Tagging/Labeling

There are many variations of tags, tapes, and labels for categorizing patients during primary and secondary triage. One method is the METTAG system, which uses the international agreement on color cod-

TABLE 49-1	INTERNATIONAL COLOR CODING AND PRIORITIES	
PATIENT STATUS	**COLOR CODE**	**PRIORITY**
Immediate	Red	Priority #1 (P-1)
Delayed	Yellow	Priority #2 (P-2)
Hold	Green	Priority #3 (P-3)
Deceased	Black	Priority #0 (P-0)

ing and priorities to alert emergency care personnel and receiving hospital staffs of patient categorization (Table 49-1). Red identifies the persons who are most critically injured; yellow, those less critically injured; green, those with non–life- or limb-threatening injuries; and black, patients who have died or have injuries that preclude survival (Fig. 49-11).

✓ TRICKS OF THE TRADE

Here's an easy way to remember how to triage a patient: If you find any problem in a patient's airway, breathing, circulation, or level of consciousness, tag the patient RED or URGENT.

NOTE

Triage tags and labels should be used routinely (for practice) so EMS crews become familiar with their use.

Regardless of the labeling system used, categorization must identify the priority of the patient, prevent re-triage of the same patient, and serve as a tracking system during treatment and transport. Therefore all tags and labels should:

- Be easy to use
- Rapidly identify patient priority
- Allow for easy tracking
- Allow room for some documentation
- Prevent patients from "re-triaging" themselves

Tracking Systems for Patients

As previously described, a destination log that integrates the triage tagging system must be maintained by the transportation section officer. In addition, the log should contain the patient's name or triage label ID number. A tracking log (Fig. 49-12) is similar to a shipping manifest and must contain the following information:

- Patient identification
- Transporting unit
- Patient priority
- Hospital destination

? CRITICAL THINKING
Why is it important to track patients?

Transportation of Patients

Methods of transporting patients will be determined by triage priority and situation. Although ambulances are the typical method of transportation, buses may be an appropriate mode for transporting large numbers of patients categorized as priority 3. Air ambulances are most commonly reserved for transporting critical patients.

Critical-Incident Stress Management

As described in Chapter 2, critical-incident stress is a potential hazard for rescue personnel who are exposed to major events. As such, critical-incident stress debriefings should be part of postdisaster standard operating procedures. To review, the basic types of services that should be made available include[3]:

- Preincident stress training to all personnel
- On-scene support for obviously distressed personnel
- Individual consults when only one or two personnel are affected by an incident
- Defusing services immediately after a large-scale incident
- Mobilization services after a large-scale incident

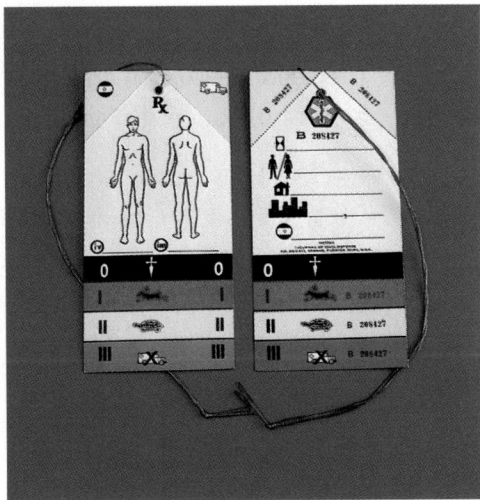

Fig. 49-12 METTAG card. (Courtesy METTAG Products, Starke, Fla.)

- Critical incident stress debriefing 24 to 72 hours after an event for any emergency personnel involved in a stressful incident
- Follow-up services to ensure that personnel are recovering
- Specialty debriefings to nonemergency groups when no other timely resources are available within the community

- Support during routine discussions of an incident by emergency personnel
- Advice to command staff during large-scale events

Other approaches that can help manage stress include employee assistance programs, counseling, spouse support programs, family life programs, pastoral services, and periodic stress evaluations.

SUMMARY

- The ICS organizational structure should be able to adapt to any agency or incident for which emergency management would be needed. The ICS also must be able to expand from dealing with a nonmajor incident to a major incident in a logical manner.

- The ICS preplan (Phase 1) must be agreed to by all participating emergency response agencies and address common goals and the specific duties of each group. Phase 2 requires the development of a strategy to manage the emergency scene. Phase 3 includes a postdisaster review of lessons learned from the incident and methods of improvement.

- The five major components of FEMA's ICS organization are command, planning, operations, logistics, and finance/administration.

- The responsibility of command should belong to one person who can effectively manage the emergency scene.

- The planning section should provide past, present, and future information about the incident and the status of resources. The operations section directs and coordinates all operations and ensures the safety of all operational personnel. The logistics section is responsible for providing supplies and equipment (including personnel to operate the equipment), facilities, services, food, and communications support needed for the incident. The finance/administration section tracks incident costs and reimbursement accounting.

- The need to establish an ICS at a medical incident is determined on the basis of whether the number of casualties or nature of the event will overwhelm available resources.

- The first EMS unit to arrive at the scene should make a quick and rapid assessment of the situation. Command must immediately be established over the radio with the communications center or emergency operations center. Additional units should be requested as soon as the need has been identified.

- Common sectors that may need to be established include extrication/rescue, treatment, transportation, staging, and support. The extrication sector is responsible for managing trapped patients at the scene. The treatment sector provides advanced care and stabilization until the patients are transported to a medical facility. The rehabilitation sector allows rescue personnel to receive physical and psychological rest. The transportation sector communicates with the receiving hospital, ambulances, and aeromedical services for patient transport. The staging sector is used in large incidents to prevent vehicle congestion and response delays. The support sector coordinates the gathering and distribution of equipment and supplies for other sectors.

- Problems of mass casualty incidents and incident command system stem from numerous issues related to communication, resource allocation, and delegation.

- Triage is a method used to categorize patients for priorities of treatment. START triage uses a 60-second assessment that focuses on the patient's ability to walk, respiratory effort, pulses/perfusion, and neurological status. The METTAG system is one of a variety of tapes, tags, and labels used to categorize patients during primary and secondary triage.

- Critical-incident stress debriefing is one component of a critical-incident stress management program. Such debriefing should be part of postdisaster standard operating procedures.

REFERENCES

1. U.S. Department of Transportation, National Highway Traffic Safety Administration: *EMT-Paramedic national standard curriculum,* Washington, DC, 1998, The Department.
2. Federal Emergency Management Agency: *Incident command system for emergency medical services,* 1996, US Fire Administration.
3. Mitchell J, Bray G: *Emergency services stress,* Englewood Cliffs, NJ, 1990, Brady Publishing.

50 Rescue Awareness and Operations

OBJECTIVES

Upon completion of this chapter, the paramedic student will be able to:

1. Describe factors that must be considered to ensure appropriate timing of medical and mechanical skills during rescue.

2. Outline each phase of a rescue operation.

3. Identify appropriate PPE that should be used during rescue situations.

4. Describe considerations during EMS response to surface water rescue situations.

5. Discuss considerations during EMS response to situations associated with hazardous atmospheres, including confined space and trench/cave-in rescues.

6. Describe hazards that may be present during EMS operations on the highway.

7. Describe considerations during EMS response over hazardous terrain.

8. Outline special considerations needed for prehospital assessment and management during rescue.

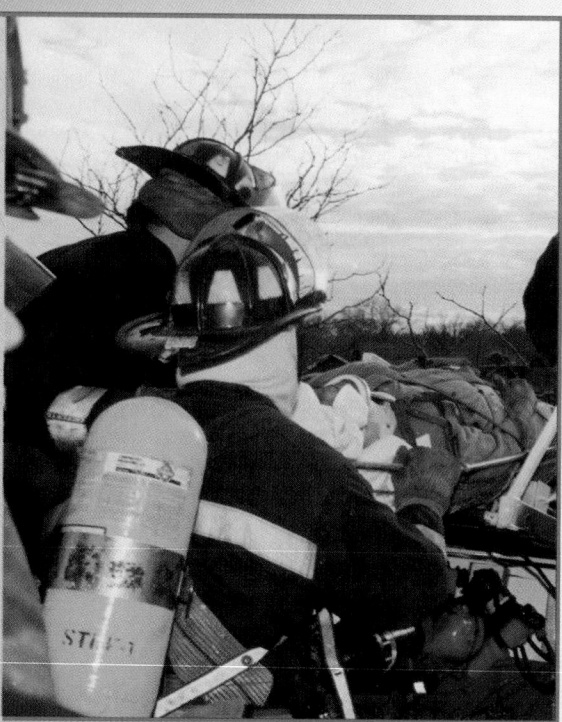

Rescue is defined as "the act of delivery from danger or imprisonment."[1] Many of the day-to-day activities of EMS providers and other public service agencies are embraced by this definition when they are called to care for persons who are traumatized or stranded. Rescue is a patient-driven event (no patient, no rescue) that requires specialized medical and mechanical skills, with the right amount of each being applied at the appropriate time.

KEY TERMS

disentanglement: The process of making a pathway through the wreckage of an accident and removing wreckage from patients.

hazard control: The phase of rescue that includes managing, reducing, and minimizing risks from uncontrollable hazards, ensuring scene safety, and providing PPE that is appropriate for the incident.

patient packaging: The completion of emergency care procedures needed to transfer a patient from the scene to the emergency vehicle.

rescue: The act of delivery from danger or imprisonment.

> **NOTE**
>
> The mechanical skills of rescue have become very specialized (e.g., techniques for farm rescue, high-angle rescue, rescue in confined spaces, search and recovery). Because of the variety of rescue capabilities that may be required within a specific area and the many different techniques involved, this chapter will focus on concepts that are basic to all rescue operations.

Appropriate Training for Rescue Operations

There is no army in the world that does not train and deploy medical people into combat. Like combat, rescue requires training and expertise so that medical and mechanical skills are carefully balanced to ensure that patients obtain effective treatment and timely extrication. The success of a rescue is dependent on a coordinated effort between medical care and specialized rescue effort that allows for:

- Patient access and assessment for treatment needs

> **NOTE**
>
> Rescue effort must be driven by patient needs, both medical and physical.

- Treatment to begin at the site
- Release from entrapment or imprisonment
- Medical care to continue throughout the incident

Role of the Paramedic in Rescue Operations

Most rescue operations in the United States are provided by a systems operations approach. In this form of rescue management, extrication activities are performed by fire service personnel, specialized units, or both, and patient care activities are the responsibility of the EMS provider. A second type of system provides rescue services by fire, EMS, or law-enforcement agencies that have "cross-trained" personnel. In this system, roles and responsibilities for rescue and patient care are shared.

The primary role of the paramedic in rescue operations is to have proper training and appropriate personal protective equipment (PPE) that allow safe access to the patient and the provision of treatment at the site and throughout the incident. Because paramedics often are the first responders to many scenes that require rescue, they should:

- Understand hazards associated with various environments
- Know when it is safe to gain access or attempt rescue
- Have skills to effect a rescue when safe and necessary
- Understand the rescue process and when certain techniques are indicated or contraindicated
- Be skilled in **patient packaging** techniques to allow for safe extrication and medical care

✓ **TRICKS OF THE TRADE**

Don't ignore your own safety. You need and deserve to have adequate PPE from head to toe.

? CRITICAL THINKING

What kind of emotions do you think will be present during a critical life-threatening rescue event?

Safety

Safety during any rescue operation is paramount because of the potential for associated risks. For example, rescues may involve hazardous materials, inclement weather, temperature extremes, fire, electrical hazards, toxic gases, unstable structures, heavy equipment, road hazards, and sharp edges and fragments. Initial scene assessment for hazards, personal protective measures, and constant monitoring throughout the operation are essential for every rescue response.

✔ **TRICKS OF THE TRADE**

"Tombstone courage" and careless heroic efforts have no place in an emergency response.

The priorities for safety in any rescue operation begin with personal safety, followed by the safety of the crew, the safety of bystanders, and, finally, rescue of the trapped and injured. The reasons for this order of priority are:

- When the well-trained and properly equipped rescuer acts safely, remaining vigilant of hazards, he or she minimizes the risk of personal injury and of complicating the scene by becoming another patient who requires care and possibly extrication.
- The crew is the support team for the rescuer. Therefore crew safety is essential to ensure an effective operation and provide mutual support for each member of the team. Operating with disregard for the safety of fellow team members increases risk of injuries and complicates the operation.
- Uninvolved people must be evacuated and kept clear of hazards. Bystanders or untrained "helpers" only increase the risk of additional injuries and complicate the rescue operation.

- Rescue of the trapped or injured is the last priority. These people are already trapped or injured. Carrying out the first three priorities safely maximizes the chance for a successful rescue.

Phases of a Rescue Operation

There are seven phases of a rescue operation.[1] They are arrival and scene size-up, hazard control, gaining access to the patient, medical treatment, disentanglement, patient packaging, and transportation (Box 50-1).

NOTE

As stressed throughout this text, paramedics should not enter a scene until it has been secured and made safe by trained personnel. Personal safety is always a priority.

Arrival and Scene Size-Up

The arrival and scene size-up phase of a rescue requires the paramedic to determine what is needed at a particular emergency event. This involves quickly gathering facts about the situation, analyzing the problems, and determining the appropriate response (Box 50-2). Scene size-up is a continuous evaluation of the emergency scene that begins when the call is received. The paramedic must constantly be alert to situations that may change the needs of a particular incident. If power lines were downed during extrication, for example, electrical utility services may be needed that were not initially required. Three elements of the assessment phase are response, other factors, and resources.

BOX 50-1

SEVEN PHASES OF A RESCUE OPERATION

1. Arrival and scene size-up
2. Hazard control
3. Gaining access to the patient
4. Medical treatment
5. Disentanglement
6. Patient packaging
7. Transportation

Response

During the initial response to an emergency scene, information often is limited. En route, the EMS crew and the dispatcher should gather as much detail about the situation as possible. Essential information includes exact location, type of occupancy (manufacturing, mercantile, residence), number of victims, type of situation, and hazards involved. Weather conditions such as extreme heat or cold, rising water, rain, and high winds also can affect rescue attempts, patient status, and the need to expedite the operation.

Standardized dispatch protocols dictate the initial activation of emergency resources by a predetermined system on the basis of the level of the reported event. If the event is a single-vehicle crash, for example, a first-responder fire company and EMS unit may be dispatched. If the event is a bus accident with multiple patients, several fire companies and EMS units may respond. As the dispatch center receives information indicating that the event is more or less serious, the dispatch protocol upgrades or downgrades the assignment as needed and advises the responding units of the updated reports.

? CRITICAL THINKING

Is there any disadvantage to routinely sending too much emergency equipment to a scene?

Other Factors

Other factors to be considered when one is determining resources for the response are the description of the scene and the time of day. An emergency in a highly populated area such as a high-rise school or shopping mall may require special vehicles and equipment for extrication and fire suppression. An emergency in a rural or wilderness setting may require helicopter rescue or other support resources. If hazardous materials are present, specialized response and decontamination equipment may be needed for bystanders, patients, and rescue personnel.

Time of day may affect scene requirements. There may, for example, be concern about rush-hour traffic and crowd control; additional lighting may be needed for early morning, evening, or night

rescue activities. These and other factors determine the manpower requirements and the scene management operations.

Resources

An important component of any emergency response is available resources. The responding crew may not have the manpower, training, or expertise to handle the event. Resources that may be required include the following:

- Additional emergency vehicles for large numbers of patients
- Area hospital availability and personnel
- Aeromedical services
- Law enforcement
- Fire service for auto extrication, fire suppression, or lighting
- Water rescue, teams with self-contained underwater breathing apparatus (SCUBA), and other specialized rescue units
- Hazardous materials teams
- Urban search-and-rescue teams

NOTE

The ability to quickly and accurately assess an emergency event requires preplanning and the development of a systems approach to the response.

BOX 50-2

ARRIVAL AND SCENE SIZE-UP PHASE OF RESCUE

- Understand the environment and risks
- Establish command and conduct a scene assessment
- Determine the number of patients and triage as necessary
- Determine if the situation is a search, rescue, or body recovery
- Perform a "risk versus benefit" analysis that considers personal safety before attempting rescue
- Request additional resources
- Make a realistic time estimate in accessing and evacuating

Hazard Control

The first-arriving crew should identify and control as many hazards as possible. This phase of rescue includes managing, reducing, and minimizing risks from uncontrollable hazards; ensuring scene safety; and providing PPE that is appropriate for the incident (Box 50-3). **Hazard control** for specific incidents will be discussed throughout this chapter.

? CRITICAL THINKING

What scene factors can interfere with your ability to assess for hazards?

Gaining Access to the Patient

Rapid access to an ill or injured patient requiring extrication or rescue can be critical to the patient's eventual outcome. With patients who have multisystem trauma, assessment, stabilization, and extrication should be rapid. These procedures, however, must be accomplished with the safety of both the patient(s) and the rescue team as a top priority (Box 50-4).

Extrication tools and equipment (Fig. 50-1) can cause injuries. To reduce the risk, the paramedic should use the minimum amount of force needed, clear the area of unnecessary people, and keep extraneous noise to a minimum. In addition, a safety officer should remain alert to the stresses of the operation on the rescuers and rotate personnel to avoid heat exposure disorders and injuries from fatigue. Rescuers should wear approved protective clothing, and protective covering for the patient should be supplied.

Although paramedics may not directly participate in freeing the patient, they have primary responsibility for patient care and serve an important role as observers for potentially hazardous procedures. The "team concept" is the most important element in any rescue system or operation. Teamwork maximizes safety, efficiency, and effectiveness.

✓ TRICKS OF THE TRADE

Teamwork is a fundamental element of prehospital care and has powerful implications for the safety of emergency responders.

Medical Treatment

After the team has gained access to the patient, medical treatment can begin (Box 50-5). The paramedic should perform a rapid initial assessment to identify and manage any life-threatening situations. This may entail opening and maintaining the airway with spinal precautions, stabilizing the cervical spine, and assessing ventilation and circulation. If the paramedic recognizes rapidly fatal or potentially fatal conditions, a "load and go" approach

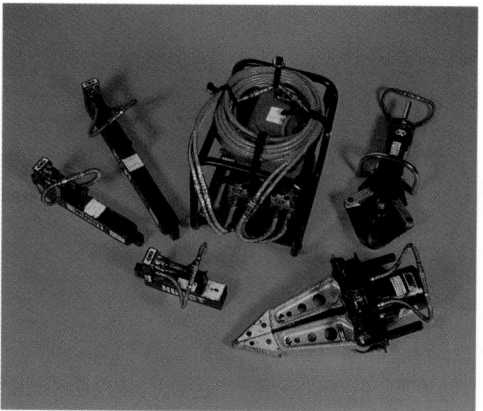

Fig. 50-1 Extrication tools and equipment. (Courtesy Eureka Fire Protection District, Eureka, Mo.)

BOX 50-3

HAZARD CONTROL PHASE OF RESCUE

- Control as many of the hazards as possible
- Manage, reduce, and minimize the risks from uncontrollable hazards
- Make the scene as safe as possible
- Ensure that all personnel are equipped with PPE appropriate for the incident

---

BOX 50-4

GAINING ACCESS TO THE PATIENT

- Determine the best method to gain access
- Deploy personnel to the patient
- Stabilize the physical location of the patient

must be taken. In these situations, expedient extrication and transportation are indicated.

NOTE

Even when patient care activities are limited by circumstances and working area, it may be possible to begin some stabilization procedures, including spinal immobilization, airway management, oxygen administration, and IV fluid therapy.

A physical examination should be performed after the initial assessment is complete and life-threatening conditions have been stabilized. Another crew member may perform the examination simultaneously if it does not interrupt the initial assessment and emergency interventions.

Disentanglement

Disentanglement involves making a pathway through the wreckage of an accident and removing wreckage from patients (Box 50-6). This phase of rescue is driven by patient needs and may require specialized rescue personnel and equipment. Para-

BOX 50-5

MEDICAL TREATMENT PHASE OF RESCUE

Provide medical treatment appropriate for the situation; this may include:
• Spinal immobilization
• Airway management and ventilation
• Oxygen administration
• IV fluid therapy

BOX 50-6

DISENTANGLEMENT PHASE OF RESCUE

• Release the patient from physical entrapment
• Perform a "risk versus benefit" analysis that considers personal safety
• Assess the need for specialized equipment and techniques

medics should be aware of available resources in their area and how to mobilize them.

? CRITICAL THINKING

What specialized rescue teams are accessible to your community?

Patient Packaging

Physical stabilization and preparation for transport (packaging) may require special rescue capabilities, such as moving patients over hazardous terrain or lifting them by hoist to a helicopter. As with all other aspects of rescue operations, coordination of activities and patient care responsibilities among the various agencies offers the greatest chance of a successful outcome (Box 50-7).

It is the paramedic's responsibility to ensure that the patient is ready to be removed from the accident scene and is protected from additional injury during disentanglement and egress. The patient should be covered with blankets or tarpaulins and provided with ear and eye protection. In addition, a face mask with supplemental oxygen or air should be applied to protect the patient from toxic fumes, if present.

The patient's airway and cervical spine must be stabilized, IV lines and oxygen tubing secured, pneumatic antishock garment applied (per protocol), and the patient immobilized on a long spine board as minimum packaging for transport. When time permits, extremity fractures should be immobilized and open wounds covered with sterile dressings and secured with bandages. A scene delay for patients who require rapid stabilization and transport lessens the patient's chances of survival.

Use of other patient care equipment should be considered as the patient is removed from the area of entrapment. Communications and coordination

BOX 50-7

PATIENT PACKAGING PHASE OF RESCUE

• Ensure medical needs are addressed
• Physically secure the patient to prevent further injury

with other rescuers must continue during this process. The exit pathway must be clear and secure, and there should be no additional danger for the patient or the rescuers during the removal phase.

Transportation

If the patient is to be immediately transported to the ambulance, a wheeled stretcher, basket stretcher, or long spine board should be available. While the patient is transported to the emergency vehicle, the terrain, equipment, and personnel requirements for moving the patient should be considered (Box 50-8). The ambulance should be appropriately warmed or cooled based on the needs of the patient and the rescue setting. The rescue is considered complete once the patient is en route to the hospital. As in any other patient transport situation, the EMS crew continues emergency care, and medical direction is advised of the patient's status.

BOX 50-8

TRANSPORTATION PHASE OF RESCUE

- Move the patient to the ambulance
- Consider the need for air evacuation
- Consider the need for specialized resources and additional manpower

---

Rescuer Personal Protective Equipment

PPE for EMS personnel historically has been adapted from other fields (e.g., from fire service). (EMS currently does not have a national, uniform trauma-reporting system to identify potential work-

---

BOX 50-9

OTHER PERSONAL PROTECTIVE EQUIPMENT

Head protection that meets safety standards for the appropriate application
- Compact firefighters' helmet meeting NFPA standards adequate for most vehicle/structural applications
- Climbing helmet for confined space and technical rescue applications
- Padded rafting/kayaking helmet for water rescue

Eye protection
- Adequate face shield (Face shields on most fire helmets are inadequate.)
- ANSI-approved safety glasses/goggles with solid shields preferred

Hearing protection
- Required for high-noise areas
- Ear plugs or ear muffs should be available

Hand protection
- Gloves that allow for adequate dexterity and protection from cuts/punctures

Foot protection
- Gear that provides ankle support to limit range of motion
- Tread that will provide traction and prevent slips
- Insulation from environmental extremes
- Steel toe/shank that meets safety requirements

Flame/flash protection when danger from fire exists
- Nomex/PBI/Flame-retardant cotton to provide limited flash protection, turn-out clothing, jump-suits/flyers/coveralls (NOTE: This clothing does not provide complete protection from punctures or cuts. Thermal protection from turn-out clothing may increase heat stress.)

Personal flotation device (PFD) when operating on or around water
- Must meet Coast Guard standards for flotation
- Type II or III preferred for most water rescue work
- Should have whistle and strobe light attached
- Knife for cutting should be attached

Visibility
- Reflective trim should be on all outerwear
- Orange clothing or safety vests should be used during highway operations

Extended, remote, or wilderness protection
- Additional/different PPE if needed for bad weather conditions not normally encountered (e.g., cold, rain, snow, wind)
- Personal drinking water and snacks
- Possible shelter needs

related exposures. Ideally, risk management and PPE design should be driven by these data.) The standards for protective clothing and PPE established by the National Fire Protection Association[2] and the Occupational Safety and Health Administration[3] have been adopted by many fire and EMS agencies, including a number of municipal and industrial fire services throughout the United States. At a minimum, it generally is agreed that EMS providers involved in rescue and other rescue personnel should have access to the following PPE:

- Impact-resistant protective helmet with ear protection and chin strap
- Safety goggles with elastic strap and vents to prevent fogging
- Lightweight "turn-out" coat that is puncture resistant
- Slip-resistant, waterproof gloves
- Boots with steel insoles and steel toe protection
- Self-contained breathing apparatus (SCBA)

The same PPE is not appropriate in all situations. Adequate protection depends on the level of rescuer involvement and the nature of the incident. Box 50-9 lists other PPE that may be appropriate in some rescue operations.

Personal Protection from Blood-Borne Pathogens

In addition to the PPE described, OSHA has established criteria for workplace protection from blood-borne and air-borne diseases.[4,5] These measures (described in Chapter 37) for personal protection should be observed whenever there is a potential for exposure to communicable diseases.

Surface Water Rescue

People are drawn to moving water for recreation, and many (including rescuers) underestimate the power and hazards of water. The hydraulics of moving water are affected by several variables that

> **NOTE**
>
> Water rescue is very dangerous and requires special training and skills. Water rescue should never be attempted by a single rescuer or by one who is untrained.

include the depth and velocity of water and any obstructions to flow.

Obstructions to Flow

Water that moves over a uniform obstruction can create recirculating currents ("drowning machines") that can trap victims and make escape difficult. Recirculating currents commonly are found in rivers and on "low head" dams, and often appear innocuous. (The height of the dam is no indication of the degree of hazard.) The force of the moving water is very deceptive and makes for a hazardous rescue. Trapped victims often succumb to fatigue, hypothermia, and drowning (Fig. 50-2).

> **? CRITICAL THINKING**
>
> *Can you think of a location in your area where this type of hazard may exist?*

Strainers are obstructions (e.g., trees, grating wire, or mesh) that allow current to flow through, yet can trap objects such as boats or people. The force of the water against the victim makes escape difficult. Rescue teams must cautiously approach strainers to avoid their own entrapment.

Foot/Extremity Pin

It generally is considered unsafe to walk in fast-moving water over knee depth. Doing so may lead to an extremity becoming trapped in a strainer and the victim being dragged under the water's surface. If a foot or extremity pin occurs, it is important to remember that the body part must be extricated from entrapment in the same way it went in.

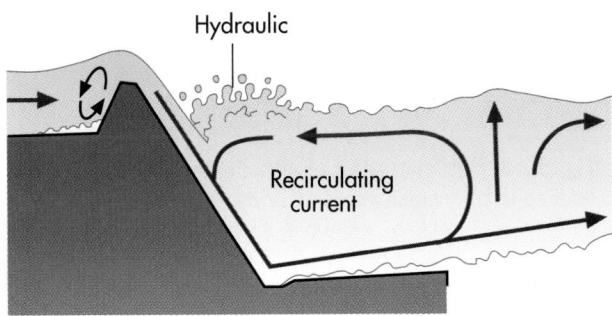

Fig. 50-2 Low-head dams range in height from 6 inches to 10 feet and can create dangerous hydraulics.

Flat Water

About 3900 deaths occur each year in flat (static) water (lakes, ponds, and marsh) as a result of drowning.[6] Factors that contribute to these deaths include alcohol or other drug use, and cool water temperature that leads to hypothermia. Both of these factors can quickly incapacitate a victim and lead to drowning. Personal flotation devices (PFDs) that routinely are worn and fastened properly when one is on or around the water can save lives by decreasing the likelihood of drowning.[1]

> **NOTE**
>
> Most people who drown never planned on being in the water.

> **NOTE**
>
> PFDs are required equipment during water rescue operations. Type I or Type II PFDs are preferred for water rescue work, and specialty Type III PFDs are suitable for some rescue situations.[7]

Water Temperature

As described in Chapter 36, immersion in water that has a temperature lower than 98° F (32° C) can cause hypothermia; a person cannot maintain body heat in water below 92° F (33° C). Water causes heat loss 25 times faster than exposure to air at the same

> **NOTE**
>
> Water temperature varies widely with seasons and runoff. Even on warm days, water temperature can be very low.

temperature. (The colder the water, the faster the rate of heat loss.) A person who experiences a 15- to 20-minute immersion in 35° F (1.6° C) water will likely die from hypothermia and drowning.[1]

Sudden immersion in cold water may trigger laryngospasm, which can lead to aspiration, severe hypoxia, and unconsciousness. If hypothermia develops, the victim often is unable to follow directions (e.g., grab a safety device) or to help himself or herself to safety. PFDs lessen heat loss and the energy required for flotation. If sudden immersion occurs, a single victim should assume the HELP position. Multiple victims should HUDDLE together to decrease heat loss (Fig. 50-3).

Cold Protective Response

The cold protective response, or mammalian diving reflex (described in Chapter 36), increases the chance of a victim's survival in cold water. To review, this protective response includes parasympathetic stimulation from face immersion in cold water that leads to bradycardia, peripheral vasoconstriction that shunts blood to the core, and hypotension. The effectiveness of this protective response is affected by the victim's age, posture in the water, lung volume, and the temperature of the water.

The rapid development of hypothermia sometimes can improve brain viability in patients with prolonged submersion. Therefore, hypothermic patients should be presumed salvageable. ("A victim is never cold and dead—only warm and dead.") The patient must be rewarmed in a hospital before an accurate assessment can be made.

Rescue Versus Body Recovery

In addition to water temperature, other factors that affect the clinical outcome of a patient after a submersion incident include the length of time the victim has been submerged, known or suspected trauma, envi-

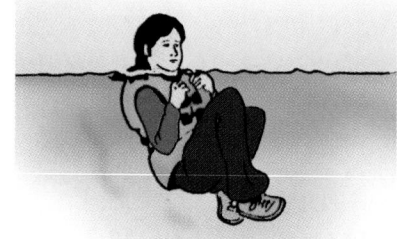
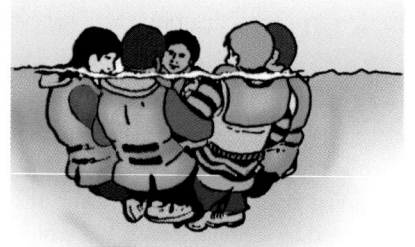

Fig. 50-3 HELP and HUDDLE. When floating in cold water, conserve body heat by using a body position that will reduce the escape of heat. **A,** If alone, use the HELP position. **B,** With other people, HUDDLE together.

ronmental conditions, age and physical condition, and time until rescue or removal has been achieved. Because successful resuscitation with full neurological recovery has occurred in victims with prolonged submersion in extremely cold water, resuscitation should be initiated by rescuers at the scene unless there is obvious physical evidence of death (e.g., putrefaction, dependent lividity, or rigor mortis).[8]

In-Water Spinal Immobilization

In-water spinal immobilization (described in Chapter 23) requires special training. Only rescuers trained in water rescue should enter the water. To review, the steps required for in-water spinal immobilization are:

1. Primary rescuer maintains spinal immobilization and the patient's airway.
2. Second rescuer determines cervical collar size and holds open collar under the victim's neck.
3. Second rescuer brings collar up to back of victim's neck. Primary rescuer allows second rescuer to bring collar around victim's neck and throat while maintaining the airway.
4. Second rescuer secures fastener on collar while primary rescuer maintains the airway.
5. Second rescuer secures victim's hands at victim's waist.
6. The patient is backboarded and extricated.
   a. Submerge the board under the victim at the waist.
   b. Never lift the victim to the board. Allow the board to float up to the victim.
   c. Secure the victim with straps, cravats, or other devices.
   d. Move the victim to an extrication point at shore or boat.
   e. Extricate the victim head first so that body weight will not compress possible spinal trauma.
   f. Avoid extrication of victim through surf because the board could collapse.
   g. Maintain the patient's airway during extrication.

Overview of Rescue Techniques

As previously stated, a rescuer should never underestimate the power of moving water and should never attempt water rescue without highly special-

ized training. The recommended water rescue model is *Reach-Throw-Row-Go*.

> **NOTE**
>
> A shore-based rescue attempt by a first responder, either by coaching the victim in self-rescue or by reaching or throwing, is the method of choice. Boat-based or "go" techniques require specialized training.

1. Reach. If the victim is close to shore, the paramedic should attempt to reach out to the victim with an oar, large branch, pole, or other rescue device. Prior to the rescue attempt, the paramedic should don a PFD and ensure secure footing to avoid being pulled into the water by the victim.

2. Throw. While the paramedic remains on the shore, a flotation device (e.g., a water throw bag attached to polypropylene rope) should be thrown to the victim so that he or she can be pulled to shore.

3. Row. If reach and throw methods are unsuccessful, or if the victim is unconscious, trained rescuers should row out to the victim in a boat (if one is available).

4. Go. If a boat is unavailable and reach and throw methods are not viable options, trained rescuers should go to the patient by wading or swimming.

Self-Rescue Techniques

If the paramedic inadvertently enters dangerous water, he or she should employ the following self-rescue techniques:

1. Cover the mouth and nose during entry.
2. Protect the head and keep the face out of the water.
3. If in flat water, assume the HELP position.
4. If in moving water, do not attempt to stand up.
5. Float on back with feet downstream and head pointed toward the nearest shore at a 45° angle.

Hazardous Atmospheres

Hazardous atmospheres are oxygen-deficient environments that may occur in confined spaces: a space with limited access or egress not designed for human occupancy or habitation. Examples of confined spaces include:

- Grain bins and silos
- Wells and cisterns

- Storage tanks
- Manholes and pumping stations
- Drainage culverts
- Underground vaults
- Trenches and cave-ins

NOTE

The National Institute of Occupational Safety and Health (NIOSH) estimates that 60% of the deaths associated with confined spaces are deaths of people attempting rescue of a victim.[1]

Hazards Associated with Confined Spaces

There are six major hazards associated with confined spaces.[1] These include oxygen-deficient atmospheres, chemical/toxic exposure/explosion, engulfment, machinery entrapment, electricity, and structural concerns.

Oxygen-Deficient Atmospheres

Because oxygen-deficient atmospheres are not a visible problem, rescuers often presume that an atmosphere is safe. The available oxygen in confined spaces must be tested by trained personnel using an atmospheric monitoring meter at the top, middle, and bottom of a confined space before entry. Any confined space that has an oxygen concentration less than 19.5% must be considered an atmospheric hazard.[8] An oxygen level that is too high (above 22%) in a confined space may produce rapid combustion and is also a serious safety hazard.

BOX 50-10

SAMPLING OF TOXIC GASES THAT MAY BE FOUND IN CONFINED SPACES

- Hydrogen sulfide (H_2S)
- Carbon dioxide (CO_2)
- Carbon monoxide (CO)
- Chlorine (Cl)
- Low/high oxygen (O_2) concentrations
- Methane (CH_4)
- Ammonia (NH_3)
- Nitrogen dioxide (NO_2)

NOTE

An increased or decreased oxygen content in a confined space may produce a false reading in monitoring meters.

Chemical/Toxic Exposure/Explosion

Oxygen can be removed from the atmosphere by certain chemical reactions. Examples include chemical reactions that occur during the formation of rust on steel structures and while pouring concrete, and natural decaying processes that displace oxygen by producing dangerous gases (e.g., methane). In addition, the presence of some chemicals and gases can lead to toxic exposure (further described in Chapter 51) and may carry a high risk of explosion (Box 50-10). Some dusts and particulate materials found in grain bins, silos, and storage tanks can be highly explosive when mixed with air. As with oxygen content, trained personnel should monitor the presence of toxic or explosive gases in confined spaces with an appropriate testing device.

? CRITICAL THINKING

Why can workers easily become disabled in these types of situations?

NOTE

Many gases are heavier than air and therefore occur in higher concentration at the bottom of storage vessels.

NOTE

Some silos are specifically designed to produce oxygen-limiting conditions to facilitate fermentation. These structures usually are identified by blue exteriors.

Engulfment

Mechanical entrapment can occur when earth, grain, coal, or any other dry material that can flow engulfs a person in a confined space. Engulfment can produce an oxygen-deficient atmosphere and subsequent suffocation. In addition, persons who are trapped by engulfment may be victims of physical (crushing) injury and are at increased risk for explosive hazards.

Machinery Entrapment

Some structures (e.g., grain bins and silos) often have augers, screws, conveyors, and other machinery to move material stored in them. These and other mechanical devices can entrap a person, necessitating extrication. Before rescue is attempted, trained and experienced personnel should identify and secure all mechanical devices.

Electricity

Electrical hazards from the power supply of motors and materials-management equipment may be present in some situations. Like machinery, all electrical devices (e.g., electrical boxes and switches) must be identified and secured by experienced personnel to help ensure rescuer safety. (This "lock-out process" must prevent any unauthorized person from entering the area or gaining access to the controls that have been shut off.) Motors and other electrical devices can "store" power that can lead to entrapment or injury.

NOTE

Chemical, steam, and water lines also must be secured or "blocked" by trained personnel during all rescue operations.

Structural Concerns

The supporting structures of a confined space must be identified prior to entry to aid in safe rescue and extrication. For example, most cylindrical structures are supported by central I beams that make for relatively easy maneuvering. However, noncylindrical structures may have L-, T-, and X-shaped spaces that can affect entry and rescue procedures and compound the extrication pathway.

Crush Compartment Syndromes Secondary to Entrapment

As described in Chapter 20, compartment syndromes can be caused by crushing mechanisms leading to ischemic muscle damage, tissue necrosis, and crush syndrome. These injuries can be severe and are associated with internal organ rupture, major fractures, and hemorrhagic shock. The degree of injury produced by the crushing force depends on the amount of pressure applied to the body, the length of time the pressure remains in contact with the body, and the specific body region in which the injury occurs. A massive crush injury to vital organs may cause immediate death.

Patients with crush syndrome are victims of compressive forces that crush tissue, causing prolonged hypoxia. (Patients may appear stable for hours or days, as long as the compressive forces remain in place.) When the patient is released from the entrapment, the reperfusion of the trapped body part may lead to detrimental processes that include volume loss into the tissue and the release of myoglobin, lactic acid, and other toxins into the circulation. As described in Chapter 20, these events occur simultaneously and may ultimately lead to death. If the patient's condition or mechanism of injury is suspicious for compartment syndrome or crush injury, the paramedic should consult with medical direction. Management of crush syndrome is controversial, and prehospital care must be supervised through a medical direction physician familiar with this pathological process.

Emergencies in Confined Spaces

OSHA requires a permit process before workers may enter a confined space.[9] As a result, this standard has forced industrial, municipal, and government response teams to be better prepared to manage confined-space incidents. Important elements of this permit process require that:

1. The area must be made safe or workers must don PPE.
2. Fall-arresting and retrieval devices must be in place.
3. Environmental monitoring must be available at the site before entry.

Non-permitted sites that do not perform atmospheric monitoring are likely locations for emergencies. In these operations, entrants may frequently encounter oxygen-deficient atmospheres. Other types of emergencies that can occur in confined spaces (in both permitted and non-permitted locations) include the following:

- Falls
- Medical emergencies
- Explosion
- Entrapment
- Exposure to toxic gases and chemicals

Safe Entry for Rescuers

As previously stated, safe entry for rescuers in a confined space operation requires specialized training. No rescuer should make entry until a rescue team has made the area safe. Safe entry cannot be made without the following[1]:

- Proper and thorough training in confined-space rescue
- Atmospheric monitoring to determine oxygen concentration, hydrogen sulfide level, carbon monoxide, explosive limits, flammable atmosphere, and toxic air contaminants
- Proper ventilation
- Secured electrical systems (lock-out/tag-out of all power)
- Dissipation of stored energy
- Disconnection of all pipes (blinding/blanking) to prevent flow into the site
- Appropriate respiratory protection

✓ TRICKS OF THE TRADE

Resist the urge to "rush in." Rushing can result in serious harm to you and your patient. All patient care activities should be deliberate and cautious.

Supplied-Air Breathing Apparatus Because close quarters make access and extrication difficult in confined-space rescue, use of the typical "bottle-on-back" self-contained breathing apparatus (SCBA) is usually dangerous. The device provides limited air

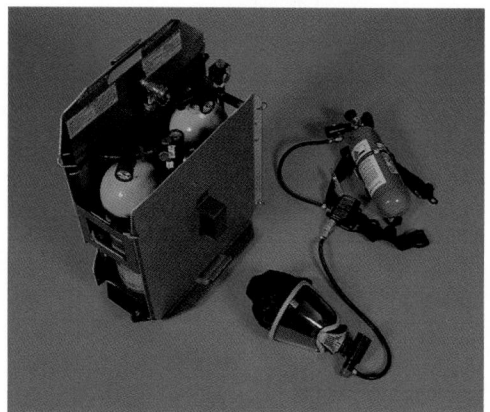

Fig. 50-4 Air in-line SABA. (Courtesy Eureka Fire Protection District, Eureka, Mo.)

supply, can cause entrapment, and may have to be removed to make some entries. The supplied-air (air-line) breathing apparatus (SABA) is preferred in confined space operations (Fig. 50-4). These lightweight devices provide a nearly unlimited supply of air from an air-supply device located outside the confined space.

Potential complications of the SABA include equipment malfunction, damaged or entangled air lines, and limitations imposed by the length of the air hose. Trained rescuers carry a small, personal reserve air supply ("escape bottle") that can be used for a short time if needed.

Arriving at the Scene

An EMS crew that arrives at the scene of a confined-space emergency should proceed as follows:

1. Perform a scene size-up and determine the nature of the emergency by obtaining a copy of the OSHA permit (Fig. 50-5) for the site from the permit/entry supervisor. Determine the number of workers (victims) in the confined space.
2. Request specialized rescue teams.
3. Establish a safe perimeter away from the incident and allow only rescue team members to enter the space.
4. Assist workers at the site with any remote retrieval devices they may be using.

   NOTE: Scene safety is of paramount importance for all involved in the rescue operation. Only specialized rescue personnel should directly perform rescue activities. EMS personnel who are not trained in specialized rescue should assist the rescue team only if they can do so safely without entering the space.

Rescue from Trenches/Cave-Ins

Most trench collapses occur in trenches less than 12 feet deep and 6 feet wide.[1] (Federal law requires either shoring or a "trench box" for evacuations that are 5 feet or deeper.) Often, these collapses occur when contractors forsake safety measures because of the increased costs in providing them. Factors that contribute to collapse include:

- Lips on one or both sides of the trench that cave in
- Walls that shear away and cave in
- Excavated dirt that has been piled too close to the edge, causing collapse

CONFINED SPACE ENTRY PERMIT

SCOPE

Effective date _____ 19 _____ Time _____ [AM / PM] Expiration date _____ Time _____ [AM / PM]

Permit Issued to _____

Description of Work _____

Lease or Area _____ Specific Location _____

PREP

- ☐ Equipment/piping depressurized & vented
- ☐ Powered(forced air) ventilation
- ☐ Other _____
  _____
- ☐ Equipment/piping blinded, blanked, or misaligned
- ☐ Electric, hydraulic,pneumatic & mechanical energy sources shut-off & locked out
- ☐ Vessel/space steamed,cleaned,or washed

ATMOSPHERE TESTING

Type	☐ Flammable		☐ Oxygen		☐ Hydrogen sulfide		☐ Other_____		☐ Continuous Monitoring	
Time									Instrument	
%, LEL or PPM									Most Recent Calibration date	
Tested by		CO. VERIFY		CO. VERIFY		CO. VERIFY		CO. VERIFY	Field Calibration O.K. ☐	
Action Levels	10% L.E.L.	<10% evaluate for toxicity	LESS THAN 19.5% MORE THAN 23%		10 PPM		Carbon Monoxide(35ppm),Aromatic Hydrocarbon(10ppm) Ammonia(25ppm),Mineral Spirits(100ppm),Methanol(200ppm)			

PROTECTIVE EQUIPMENT

OPERATIONAL AND PROTECTIVE EQUIPMENT

- ☐ Warning signs, barricades
- ☐ Barricade tape/cones
- ☐ Ventilation Fan or blower
- ☐ Fire extinguisher
- ☐ Ground fault circuit interupter
- ☐ Lighting(hazardous location rated)
- ☐ Static protection
- ☐ Ladder
- ☐ Other _____

PERSONAL PROTECTIVE EQUIPMENT

- ☐ Self Contained Breathing Apparatus
- ☐ Airline supplied respirator
- ☐ Chemical splash goggles
- ☐ Impervious gloves
- ☐ Impervious clothing
- ☐ Boots
- ☐ Hearing protection
- ☐ Safety glasses
- ☐ Fall protection/arresting equipment
- ☐ Other _____

EMERGENCY ACTION

RESCUE PROCEDURES AND EQUIPMENT

Emergency Phone Number [_____] **Base Station** _____

Location of Phone/Radio _____

RESCUE EQUIPMENT NEEDED

- ☐ Full body harness/lifeline
- ☐ Rescue winch
- ☐ Wristlets
- ☐ Personal motion alarm
- ☐ Davit/Tripod
- ☐ Other _____

CSE COMMUNICATION

- ☐ Radio communication
- ☐ Rope signals
- ☐ Visual hand signals
- ☐ Other _____

POTENTIAL EMERGENCY SITUATION(S) _____
_____

ACTIONS TO BE TAKEN _____
_____

SIGNATURE

CONFINED SPACE ENTRANT(S)   We(I) have reviewed the potential emergency situations and actions to be taken. We(I) are familiar with all rescue equipment, and communication methods.

X _____   X _____   X _____

CONFINED SPACE OBSERVER/STANDBY   I have checked all rescue and communication equipment and reviewed all emergency actions to be taken with entrant personnel. X _____

CONTRACT SUPERVISOR   I have evaluated and completed all portions of this permit. All personnel have reviewed the conditions of the permit and are adequately trained to perform this job. I have reviewed the site to ensure compliance with the requirements of this permit. X _____

MOBIL REPRESENTATIVE   I have evaluated and completed all portions of this permit. All personnel have reviewed the conditions of the permit and are adequately trained to perform this job. I have reviewed the site to ensure compliance with the requirements of this permit. X _____

DEBRIEF

Were any Hazards or Potential Hazards Encountered During the CSE?   NO ☐   YES ☐   If yes, Explain
_____
_____

White - Local Safety Dept.   **Manila Tag - Post at Job Site**

BAKCSE 93

Fig. 50-5 Confined space entry permit sample. (Courtesy Mobil Oil Co.)

- The presence of intersecting trenches
- Ground vibrations
- Water seepage

> **NOTE**
>
> The weight of one cubic foot of soil is 100 pounds; two feet of soil on a person's chest or back is equal to 700 to 1000 pounds of pressure, which can cause burial and rapidly lead to suffocation.[1]

Arriving at the Scene

When arriving at the scene where a collapse has occurred, causing burial, the paramedic should be aware that a second collapse is likely to occur and should not approach the lip. (Rescue attempts by EMS personnel should not be made unless the trench is less than waist deep.) Steps in scene management include:

1. Securing the scene, establishing command, and securing a safe perimeter
2. Shutting down nonessential equipment that can cause vibrations
3. Requesting specialized rescue teams
4. Preventing entry into the trench or cave-in area

> **? CRITICAL THINKING**
>
> *How do you think the EMS and rescue team will feel if, for safety reasons, they are unable to go in after a person who is buried in a trench collapse?*

Access to the patient should be attempted by trained personnel only after proper shoring is in place. The process of shoring and excavating can be labor- and time-intensive. Scene safety is, however, necessary for a successful recovery.

Highway Operations

Traffic flow is the largest hazard in EMS highway operations.[1] Factors that are associated with highway hazards include emergency responses to limited and unlimited access highways, emergency vehicle crashes, and the backup of traffic that impedes flow to and from the scene. Because of the potential problems in traffic flow, EMS personnel must work closely with law enforcement to help ensure a safe response. Techniques to reduce traffic hazards are listed in Box 50-11. Other scene hazards associated with highway operations include:

- Fuel/fire hazards
- Electrical power
- Unstable vehicles
- Airbags/supplemental restraint systems (SRS)
- Hazardous cargoes

Fuel/Fire Hazards

Gasoline spills from automobile crashes are a common fire hazard encountered by EMS providers. The chances that flammable liquids will ignite can be reduced by turning off the vehicle ignition switch, forbidding smoking, and avoiding use of flares near the spill. EMS personnel should approach the scene with fire extinguishers and have the extinguishers ready throughout extrication (see the box on p. 1419). Ideally, a fire apparatus with a charged hose line should be on scene.

> **BOX 50-11**
>
> **TECHNIQUES TO REDUCE TRAFFIC HAZARDS**
>
> 1. Position an apparatus (pumper, rescue, or other emergency vehicle) across the traffic way ("fend-off" position) to protect the scene from traffic hazards.
> 2. Stage unnecessary apparatus off of highway (essential on limited access highway); establish staging area away from scene.
> 3. Position an apparatus to reduce traffic flow and provide for a safe ambulance loading area.
> 4. Use only essential warning lights so that drivers are not distracted or confused. (Consider the use of amber scene lighting.) Turn off headlights that might blind nearby motorists.
> 5. Use traffic cones and flares to redirect traffic away from workers and to create a safe zone. (Use flares safely in proximity to the scene. Do not extinguish once ignited.)
> 6. Be sure that all rescuers wear high-visibility clothing (e.g., orange highway vests, reflective trim).

NOTE

Alternate fuel systems (e.g., natural gas and electrical power) also are capable of producing fire hazards and injury from explosion of high-pressure cylinders and storage cells.

The car battery of a crashed car generally should be left connected in order to operate power electric door locks, windows, seat mechanisms, and trunks. However, if the battery is to be disabled, the ground cable should be disconnected first to reduce the chance of sparking, which may ignite spilled fuel or leaking battery gases. (Most newer American cars have positive ground cables that can be identified by battery markings or by locating the ground wires attached to the frame, engine, or body of the vehicle.) The battery cable can be cut with wire cutters or disconnected with battery pliers. The disconnected cable should be folded back onto itself and securely taped to insulate it from any bare metal contact that might reestablish the electrical ground to the system. Both cables should be disconnected and secured.

Vehicle fires associated with crashes usually are caused by ruptured fuel tanks and fuel lines ignited during the crash. (Catalytic converters are capable of igniting spilled fuel.) Paramedics should not attempt to fight fully-involved vehicle fires unless they have been trained to do so. If the fire service has not arrived and there are victims in a burning vehicle, the EMS crew quickly should determine whether the victims can be safely removed. If the victims are trapped and the vehicle is not completely engulfed by flames, an attempt should be made to stop the fire from spreading by using fire extinguishers.

Burning vehicles present very serious potential hazards and may explode with deadly force at any time. All actions must be directed toward rescuer safety and protection. When approaching a burning vehicle is necessary, the paramedic should crouch low and approach from the side, staying clear of bumpers that may "fly off" during fire conditions. PPE also should be worn to guard against dangerous and caustic smoke.

Electrical Power

Downed electrical wires are dangerous. Modern transformers are programmed to retest broken circuits at certain time intervals, and dead lines can suddenly surge with lethal current. Rescuers must be familiar with the power system in their area and should check with the local power company for in-

NOTE

Victims inside a vehicle that is in contact with downed wires should be advised to remain inside unless they are at additional risk of injury (e.g., explosion, fire). Leaving the vehicle is dangerous and poses a significant risk of electrical injury.

FIRE EXTINGUISHERS

Portable fire extinguishers are classified by their anticipated effectiveness in suppressing four classes of fires: class A, ordinary combustibles; class B, flammable liquids; class C, energized electrical equipment; and class D, combustible metals. ABC-all purpose extinguishers are suitable for more than one class of fire and should be carried by EMS services. These dry chemical extinguishers can be used to suppress fires of ordinary combustible materials, flammable liquids, and electrical equipment. In addition to the letter classifications, class A and B fire extinguishers also receive a numerical rating that designates the size of fire the extinguisher can be expected to suppress. A 20-B extinguisher will generally extinguish 20 times as much fuel as a 1-B extinguisher.

Fire-suppression agents work by reducing heat and eliminating the oxygen necessary to maintain combustion. Eliminating oxygen may present danger to the rescuer and the patient, so caution should be taken when working in confined spaces. In addition, crew members and patients should avoid undue exposure to the fumes of any fire-suppression agent, and all rescuers should use appropriate breathing apparatus.

TRICKS OF THE TRADE

Energy-absorbing bumpers have been in use since the 1970s. Stand clear of them!

formation and the availability of training sessions for the response team. Only utility workers and trained rescuers using proper equipment should secure downed electrical wires.

Rescuers should never approach the patient until the scene is safe. A rescuer who experiences tingling sensations in the soles of the feet, legs, or thorax as he or she enters an area should not proceed. Rather,

the rescuer should retreat from the area. When it is absolutely necessary to touch a patient who is in contact with an electric source, trained personnel may use nonconductive equipment such as leather gauntlets, wooden poles, polypropylene rope, and other specially designed equipment. None of these measures, however, provides absolute safety from electrical injury.

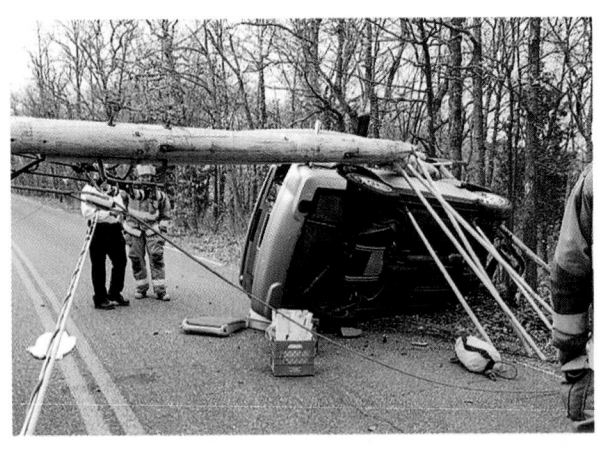
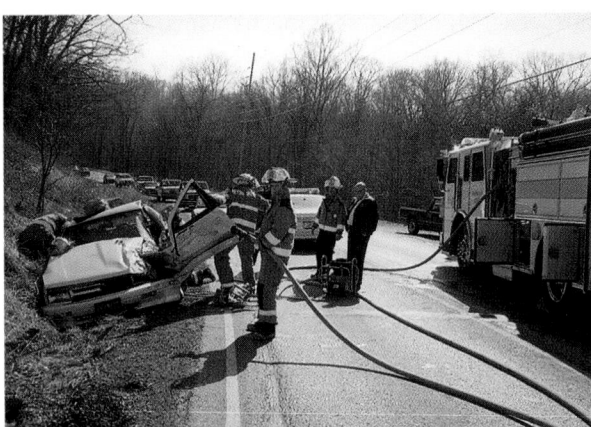
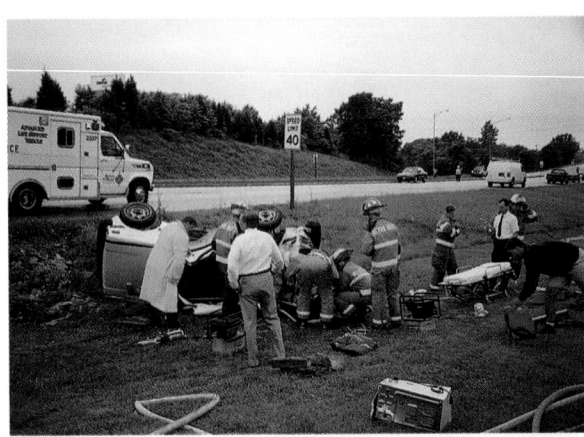
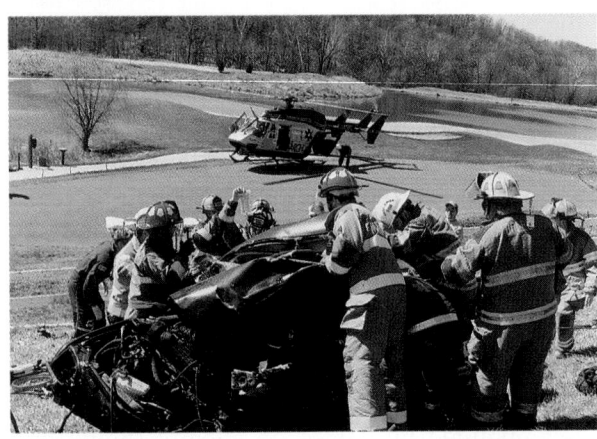
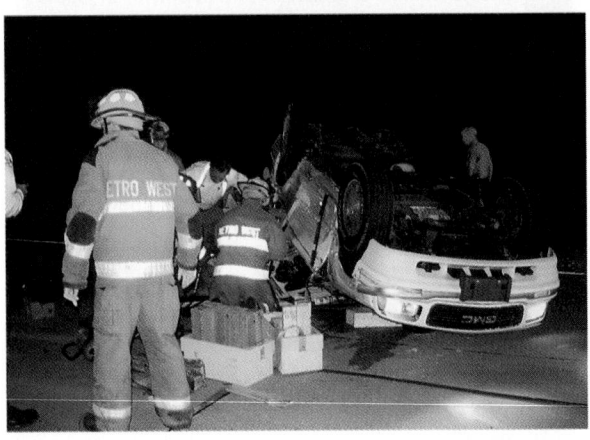
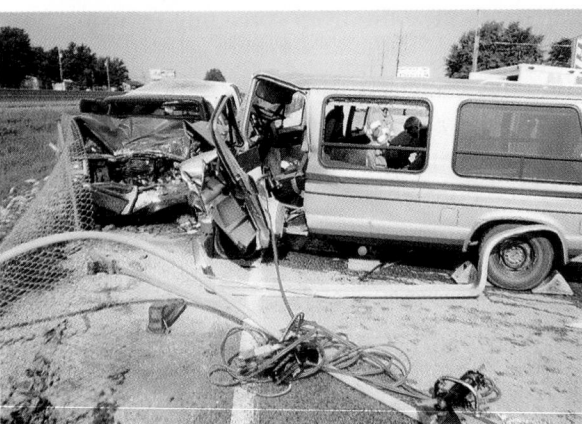

Fig. 50-6 Vehicle stabilization.

Unstable Vehicles

Unstable vehicles are a common hazard in rescue operations, and all unstable vehicles must be stabilized before access is gained. The mechanism of the crash, the position and number of vehicles, and the environment of the scene must all be considered in assessing vehicular stability. Standard methods of stabilizing vehicles include supporting the vehicle with wooden cribbing, wheel chocks, and airbags and securing the vehicle with ropes, cables, and chains to poles, trees, and other vehicles and structures (Fig. 50-6). Fig. 50-7 shows equipment used to stabilize vehicles. Specialized training is required for paramedics involved in this aspect of rescue management.

> ### ✓ TRICKS OF THE TRADE
>
> A crashed vehicle should *always* be stabilized—regardless of its position. Never create additional victims!

> **NOTE**
>
> Some vehicles will be obviously unstable (e.g., a vehicle on its side or on its roof). However, even a car on its wheels that appears to be stable may be unstable from possible movement of the tires and swaying of the vehicle's suspension system. All wrecked vehicles should be approached cautiously.

Airbags/Supplemental Restraint Systems

Airbags as a supplemental restraint system (SRS) have become a required safety feature in the United States from all major automobile manufacturers. The three types of airbags include frontal-impact, side-impact, and head-protection bags. Airbags generally are considered an effective safety device in vehicle crashes. Children and small adults in the passenger seat have, however, been fatally injured after airbag deployment.[10]

Once deployed, airbags are not dangerous, but they do produce a residue that can cause minor skin or eye irritation. Nonhazardous irritation from this residue is temporary and can be avoided by wearing gloves and eye protection; by keeping the residue away from the patient's eyes and wounds and away from the rescuer's eyes; and by thoroughly washing after exposure. Emergency personnel should be trained in detection and scene management of SRS equipment. Rescue guidelines for airbag-equipped cars have been provided by the National Highway Traffic Safety Administration, automobile and airbag manufacturers, and coordinated with the U.S. Fire Administration.[11]

Incident with Fire
- Use the normal fire-extinguishing procedures.
- Although heat may trigger an undeployed airbag, it will not cause the activating canister to explode.

Incident with a Deployed Airbag
- Use normal rescue procedures and equipment.
- Do not delay medical attention.
- Deployed airbags are not dangerous.
- Wear gloves and eye protection.
- Keep residue away from patients' eyes and wounds.
- Remove gloves and wash hands after exposure to residue.

Incident with an Undeployed Airbag
- An undeployed airbag is unlikely to deploy after a crash.

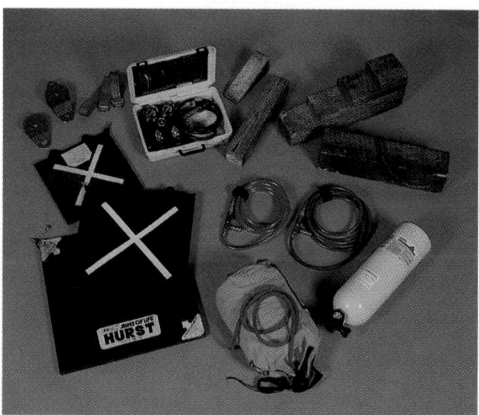

Fig. 50-7 Equipment used to stabilize vehicles. (Courtesy Eureka Fire Protection District, Eureka, Mo.)

- When a patient is pinned directly behind an undeployed airbag, special procedures should be followed:

  Disconnect or cut both battery cables.

  Avoid placing your body or objects in front of the airbag module (the deployment path of the airbag).

  Do not mechanically displace or cut through the steering column until after the system has been fully deactivated.

  Do not cut or drill into the airbag module.

  Do not apply heat in the area of the steering wheel hub.

> **NOTE**
>
> Rescuers should stay clear of the airbag's "strike zone" until it has been disabled. Safe distances generally are considered to be 5 feet from a side airbag; 10 feet from a driver airbag; and 15 feet from a passenger airbag.

Hazardous Cargoes

Most hazardous substances that are transported in the United States travel by road.[1] The paramedic should therefore be suspicious of crashes involving commercial vehicles. Methods that can be used to identify carriers of hazardous cargoes (e.g., UN numbers and placards) and management of hazardous materials incidents will be discussed in Chapter 51.

> **? CRITICAL THINKING**
>
> *What types of vehicles that carry hazardous materials in small quantities may not have external UN numbers or placards?*

Auto Anatomy

A basic understanding of auto anatomy is required during vehicle rescue operations (Fig. 50-8). Several important considerations include the following:

1. Roof and roof support posts (A, B, C, and D posts)
   a. Cutting the supports interrupts the unibody construction

2. Fire wall
   a. Separates single engine and occupant compartment
   b. Frequently collapses onto occupants' legs during high-speed, head-on collisions

3. Engine compartment and power train
   a. Battery usually is in the engine compartment

4. Under-carriage and unibody versus frame construction
   a. Roof posts, floor, fire wall, and trunk support are integral to unibody
   b. Most cars are of unibody construction
   c. Light trucks usually are of frame construction

5. Safety glass versus tempered glass
   a. Safety glass (glass-plastic laminate glass), usually in the windshield, is designed to stay intact when shattered or broken; it fractures into long strands
   b. Tempered glass (high tensile strength) does not stay intact when shattered or broken; it fractures into small pieces

6. Doors
   a. Reinforcing bar in most car doors
   b. Designed to provide structural integrity during front and side collisions
   c. Case hardened steel "Nader" pin/latch is designed to prevent car door from opening during collisions. (If the pin is engaged, it may be difficult to pry the door open; it must be disengaged first.)

Rescue Strategies

Rescue strategies for vehicle crashes should begin during initial scene size-up and can sometimes be based on information provided by the dispatching center prior to arrival. After arriving on the scene, the EMS crew should employ hazard control, establish command, and call for appropriate back-up. Important elements of scene size-up include:

- Scene safety (including protecting the scene from traffic hazards)
- Location of the crash
- Vehicle stability
- Electrical hazards
- Fire hazards
- Hazardous materials
- Special rescue needs
- Number and location of patients

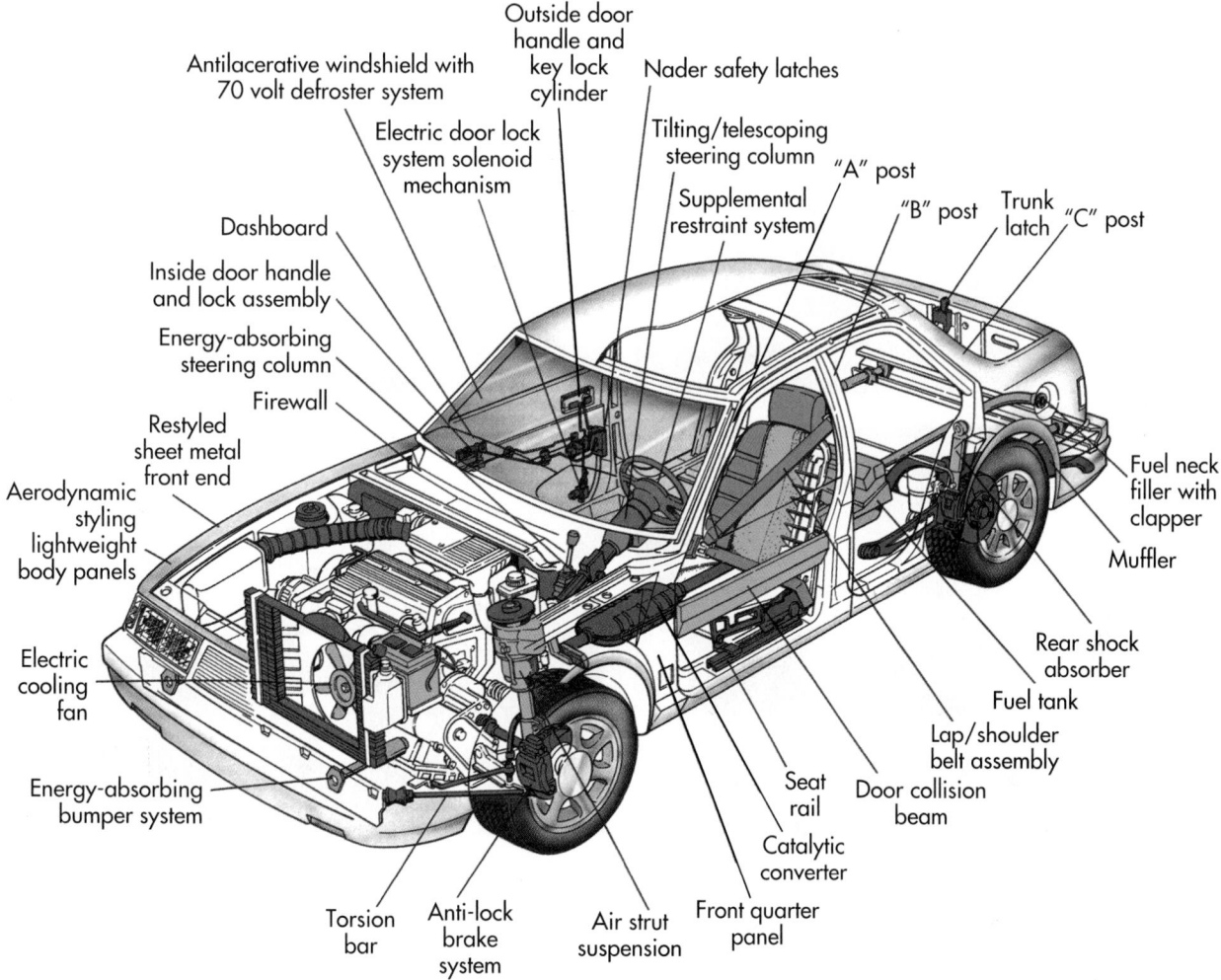

Fig. 50-8 Anatomy of a car. (From Moore RE: *Vehicle rescue and extrication*, St Louis, 1991, Mosby.)

After initial scene size-up and ensuring scene safety, the responding crew should assess the degree of entrapment and the fastest means of extrication. The paramedic should attempt to gain access to trapped victims by first trying to open all car doors. When a door cannot be readily opened by the patient or rescuer, an alternative method to gain access to the patient is through the side windows. (Glass windows can be shattered by striking the glass in a lower corner or by using a spring-loaded center punch.) Initial patient care can then be provided until trained rescue personnel with extrication tools can safely remove the patient from the vehicle by door removal, roof removal, front or rear windshield openings, or a dash roll-up maneuver (Fig. 50-9).

> **NOTE**
>
> Paramedics who are involved in the rescue or who are near the site should wear PPE that provides adequate hand, eye, and body protection. Clothing with reflective striping will provide improved safety during day and night operations.

Hazardous Terrain

Hazardous terrain can pose significant difficulties during rescue operations. Examples include car crashes that occur on embankments and rescues that are required for sport enthusiasts such as rock

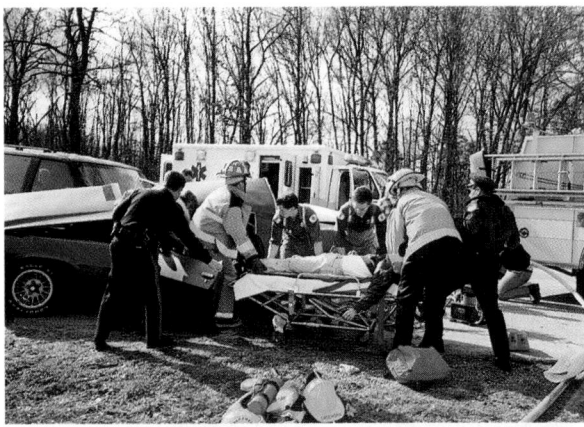
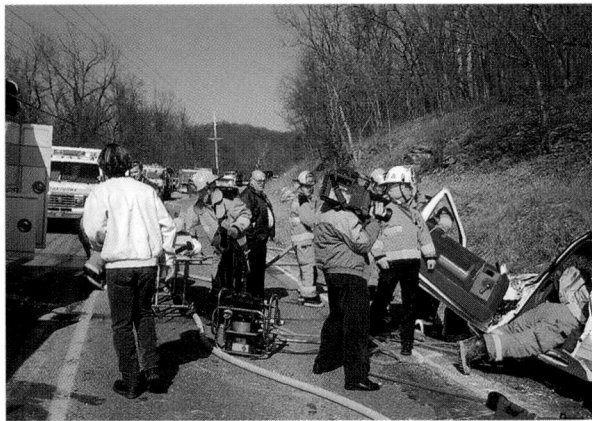
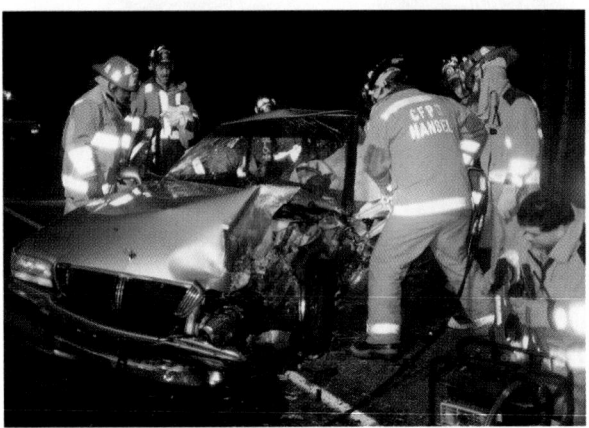
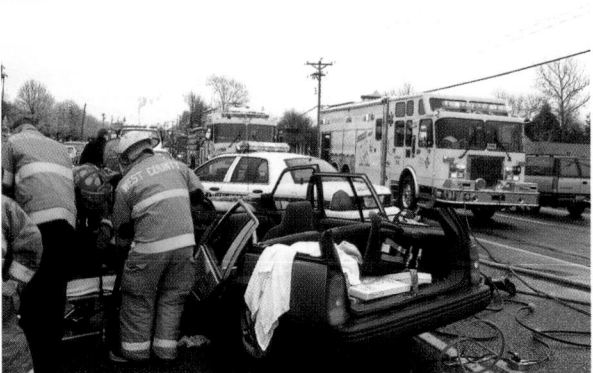

Fig. 50-9 Extrication scenes.

climbers, snow skiers, and mountain bikers. Three common classifications of hazardous terrain are *low-angle, high-angle,* and *flat terrain with obstructions* (Box 50-12).

Low-angle (steep-slope) refers to terrain that is capable of being walked on without the use of

hands. Secure footing may be difficult on steep slopes, making it hazardous to carry a litter even with multiple rescuers. In these situations, low-angle rescue is employed to prevent falls and tumbles by using ropes to counteract gravity during litter carry (Fig. 50-10).

High-angle (vertical) refers to terrain (cliffs, sides of buildings) that is so steep that hands must be used to maintain balance (slopes greater than 40°). In these situations, there will be total dependence on rope or aerial apparatus for litter movement. Rappelling by trained personnel to retrieve victims is required in high-angle rescue. Falls are likely to result in serious injury or death (Fig. 50-11).

Flat terrain may have various obstructions that can make rescue difficult. Examples include level land with large rocks, loose soil (scree), and waterbeds or creeks. In these situations, additional manpower and resources may be needed to safely extricate a victim and ensure safe litter movement.

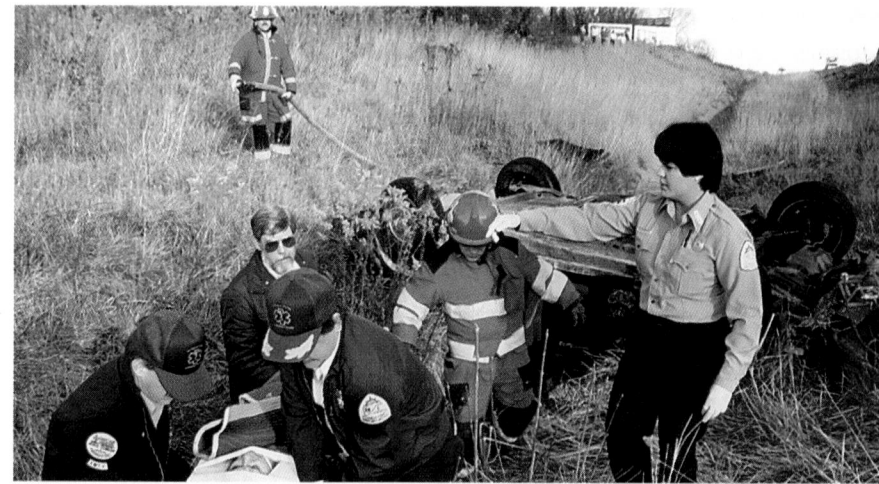

Fig. 50-10 Low-angle rescue.

BOX 50-12

TERMS AND DEFINITIONS RELATED TO RESCUE OVER HAZARDOUS TERRAIN

anchoring: Attaching a high-angle rope to a secure point.

belay: Method of attaching a safety rope and controlling the rope so that if the person or load starts to fall, the belay rope will prevent the fall.

high angle: An environment in which rescuers need to be secured with rope for safety. The majority of the rescue load is supported by the rope system.

low angle: An environment in which the weight of the stretcher is supported primarily by the tender's legs, but rope systems are required to facilitate movement and for fall protection.

rappelling: A method of descent that involves lowering oneself with a rope.

scrambling: Movement over rough terrain that is not steep enough to require the use of a rope.

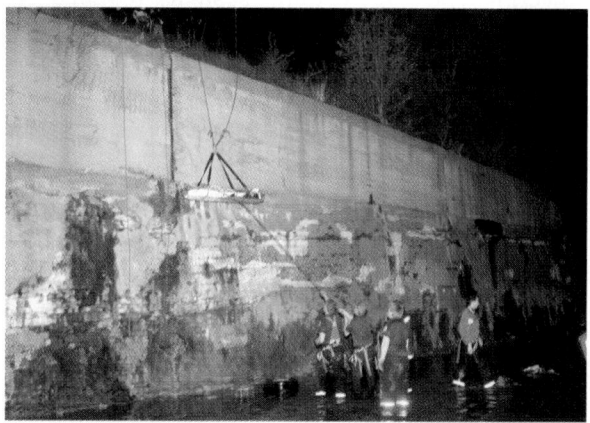

Fig. 50-11 High-angle rescue.

The older "military style" devices do not provide adequate spinal immobilization.)

TRICKS OF THE TRADE

Protect and support your back with proper lifting techniques.

Patient Packaging with Litters

The basket stretcher is the standard for rough terrain evacuation. The rigid frame of this device provides protection for the victim and is relatively easy to carry with adequate personnel. Patients generally are immobilized on a long backboard and secured in the basket. Alternative spinal immobilization devices (e.g., vest-type devices) also can be used in conjunction with the basket stretcher. (Using the basket stretcher itself as a spinal immobilization device should be considered a last resort.

Basket stretchers are of two basic designs: wire mesh ("stokes") and plastic. Wire mesh generally is the strongest of the baskets and is relatively inexpensive. The design allows for air and water to flow through the device, making it ideal in water rescue operations when used with supplemental flotation. Plastic basket stretchers generally are weaker than steel mesh, but provide better protection for the patient. (Plastic bottoms with steel frames are considered superior designs.) Most basket stretchers are equipped with adequate restraints. However, all require additional strapping or lacing (e.g., harness, leg stirrups) to prevent movement, and padding for rough-terrain evacuation or extraction. A plastic helmet or litter shield should be available for patient protection.

Patient Movement

Methods for moving a patient over rough terrain may include nontechnical-nonrope evacuation and litter-carrying over flat terrain, and special rescue equipment such as load-lifting straps, anchors, rope lowering and rope-hauling systems required for

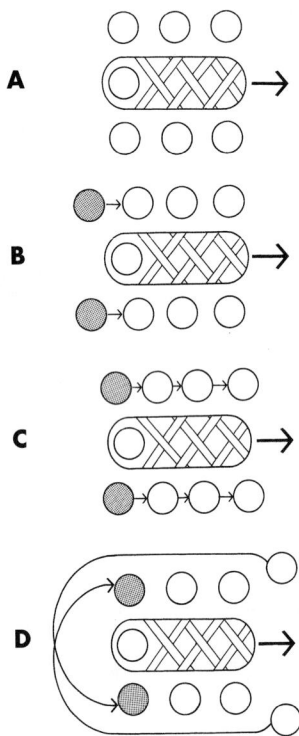

Fig. 50-12 Litter-carrying sequence. **A,** Six rescuers are usually required to carry a litter but may need relief over long distances (greater than ¼ mile). **B,** Relief rescuers can rotate into position while the litter is in motion by approaching from the rear. As relief rescuers move forward, others progressively move forward **(C)** until the forwardmost rescuers can release the litter (peel out) and move to the rear **(D).** Rescuers in the rear can rotate sides so that they can alternate carrying arms. Carrying straps (webbing) can also be used to distribute the load over the rescuers' shoulders. In most cases the litter is carried feet first with a medical attendant at the head monitoring airway, breathing, level of consciousness, and so on.

low-angle and high-angle evacuation. In addition, the use of aerial apparatus (e.g., tower-ladder or bucket trucks, aerial ladders) also may be required in some high-angle rescue operations. Moving a patient during low-angle and high-angle evacuations requires specialized knowledge and skills.

Litter-Carrying Procedures

Carrying a litter across rough, flat terrain requires a minimum of six rescuers—four to carry the litter and two to observe or "scout" for potential hazards (e.g., loose rocks, holes, tree branches). Team members should be matched in height to ensure that equal weight is shared and that the litter remains level. Load-lifting straps sometimes are used to spread the weight of the load over other parts of the rescuer's body (e.g., around the rescuer's shoulders and back). A basic litter-carrying sequence is illustrated in Fig. 50-12.

Helicopter Use in Hazardous-Terrain Rescue

As described in Chapter 48, helicopters can be used for patient transport and for rescue operations. When they are used for rescue, the mission, crew, and capabilities of the helicopter team (civilian and military) are specific for rescue techniques versus providing medical care and transport. The rescue helicopter team has specialized knowledge and skills required to hover or land in tight places and to transport people and equipment. Special rescue techniques that these helicopters employ may include cable hoisting to extract people from the ground, and short-haul ("sling loads") operations that allow personnel and equipment to be carried beneath the helicopter as an external load.

> **NOTE**
> Rescue helicopters have the same safety concerns and limitations as those used in aeromedical transport (described in Chapter 48). All personnel at the scene should be familiar with the elements of scene safety, hazards, and restrictions for helicopter use.

Assessment Procedures During Rescue

Patient assessment during rescue operations often is made difficult by factors such as weather and temperature extremes, available access, equipment limitations, patient entrapment, and cumbersome PPE that affects rescuer mobility (Box 50-13). These and other issues may affect the paramedic's ability to perform a thorough assessment and may result in a compromised physical examination.

> **NOTE**
>
> PPE should never be removed while in the hazardous environment.

Specific Assessment/Management Considerations

During rescue operations, it may be necessary for the paramedic to downsize initial assessment and management equipment from normal boxes and "street packaging" so that it can be transported to the patient. (Ideally, the equipment should be carried hands-free.) In addition to ensuring adequate lighting to perform assessment and treatment, the paramedic should have access to equipment for[1]:

- Airway
  Oral/nasal airways
  Manual suction
  Intubation equipment
- Breathing
  Thoracic decompression
  Small oxygen tank/regulator
  Masks/cannulas
  Pocket mask/BVM
- Circulation
  Bandages/dressings
  Triangular bandages
  Occlusive dressings
  IV fluid administration
  BP cuff and stethoscope
- Disability
  Extrication collars
- Exposure
  Scissors
- Miscellaneous
  Headlamp/flashlight
  Space blanket
  Pneumatic splints
  PPE (e.g., leather gloves, latex gloves, eye shields)

Exposure of Patients

Patients who require rescue may be at high risk for developing hypothermia and should be covered to ensure thermal protection. In addition, the patient should be protected with shields (e.g., backboards or blankets) to prevent injury from equipment and debris during the extrication process.

ALS Skills

ALS skills should only be provided if necessary. (Good BLS skills, however, are mandatory.) As a rule, ALS equipment such as IV lines, ET tubes, and ECG leads will complicate the extrication process. (Definitive airway control and volume replacement may, however, be essential.) Airway control with supplemental oxygen administration must always be a priority throughout the rescue event.

Patient Monitoring

Monitoring the patient's vital signs and level of consciousness is necessary throughout the rescue operation. In high-noise and limited-space environments, it may be necessary to measure blood pressure by palpation and to use compact devices such as a pulse oximeter. The paramedic should establish and continue a rapport with the patient, when possible, and explain what procedures are being done and why. Providing emotional support throughout the rescue operation is essential.

Improvisation

It may be necessary (because of space and equipment limitations) to improvise some patient care procedures during a rescue event. For example, an upper extremity fracture can be temporarily stabilized by tying it to the patient's torso; a lower extremity fracture can be tied to the patient's uninjured leg (buddy splinting). Formable splints (e.g., SAM splint) also can be very useful to secure extremity fractures or dislocations.

BOX 50-13

ENVIRONMENTAL ISSUES AFFECTING PATIENT ASSESSMENT

- Difficulty in completely exposing a patient
- Restrictive clothing and PPE required for personal safety
- Cramped space
- Limited lighting
- Difficulty in transporting medical equipment to the patient

Pain Control

Pain control for patients who require rescue may include both nonpharmacological and pharmacological management. Examples of nonpharmacological pain control include splinting, distraction (talking to the patient and asking questions), and methods such as creating sensory stimuli (e.g., mildly scratching the patient) when a painful procedure or maneuver is performed. Pharmacological therapy may be indicated to control pain that results from trauma. Since pain medication can mask serious injury and alter a patient's level of consciousness, the paramedic should consult with medical direction or follow established protocol regarding the appropriateness of drug therapy in these situations.

SUMMARY

- Rescue is a patient-driven event that requires specialized medical and mechanical skills, with the right amount of each being applied at the appropriate time. The primary role of the paramedic in rescue operations is to have proper training and appropriate PPE that allow safe access to the patient and the provision of treatment at the site and throughout the incident.

- The seven phases of a rescue operation are arrival and scene size-up, hazard control, gaining access to the patient, medical treatment, disentanglement, patient packaging, and transportation.

- The standards for protective clothing and personal protection equipment established by the National Fire Protection Association and OSHA have been adopted by many fire and EMS agencies. Appropriate PPE depends on the level of rescuer involvement and the nature of the incident.

- Water rescue should never be attempted by a single rescuer or one who is untrained.

- Water hazards include obstructions to flow and foot/extremity pins that can trap victims and drag them under water. Factors that contribute to flat-water drowning are alcohol or other drug use and cool water temperature.

- Hazardous atmospheres are oxygen-deficient environments that can occur in confined spaces. The six major hazards associated with confined spaces are oxygen-deficient atmospheres, chemical/toxic exposure/explosion, engulfment, machinery entrapment, electricity, and structural concerns.

- Traffic flow is the largest hazard in EMS highway operations. Other scene hazards associated with highway operations include fuel/fire hazards, electrical power, unstable vehicles, airbags/supplemental restraint systems, and hazardous cargoes.

- Hazardous terrain can pose significant difficulties during rescue operations. Three common classifications of hazardous terrain are low-angle, high-angle, and flat terrain with obstructions.

REFERENCES

1. U.S. Department of Transportation, National Highway Traffic Safety Administration: *EMT-Paramedic national standard curriculum*, 1998, Washington, DC, The Department.
2. National Fire Protection Association: *Standard on protective clothing for structural firefighting (NFPA 1999)*, Quincy, MA, 1992, The Association.
3. Occupational Safety and Health Administration: *Hazardous waste operations and emergency response (HAZWOPER)*, standard 1910.120, Washington, DC, 1990, The Administration.
4. Occupational Safety and Health Administration: *Occupational exposure to bloodborne pathogens*, final rule 29 CFR 1910.1030, Washington, DC, 1992, The Administration.
5. Occupational Safety and Health Administration: *Enforcement policy and procedures for occupational exposure to tuberculosis*, Washington, DC, 1993, The Administration.
6. National Safety Council: *Accident facts*, Itasca, Ill., 1997, The Council.
7. American Academy of Orthopaedic Surgeons: *Basic rescue and emergency care*, Park Ridge, Ill., 1990, The Academy.
8. American Heart Association: A*dvanced cardiac life support*, Dallas, Tex., 1997, The Association.
9. Occupational Safety and Health Administration: *Permit required confined spaces for general industry (29 CFR 1910.146)*, Washington, DC, 1997, The Administration.
10. National Highway Traffic Safety Administration: *Special crash investigation study*, Washington, DC, 1999, The Administration.
11. *Emergency response guidelines for air-bagged equipped cars*, Washington, DC, 1990, US Government Printing Office.

51 *Hazardous Materials Incidents*

OBJECTIVES

Upon completion of this chapter, the paramedic student will be able to:

1. *Define hazardous materials terminology.*

2. *Identify legislation about hazardous materials that influences emergency health care workers.*

3. *Describe resources to assist in identification and management of hazardous materials incidents.*

4. *Identify the protective clothing and equipment needed to respond to selected hazardous materials incidents.*

5. *Describe the pathophysiology and signs and symptoms of internal damage caused by exposure to selected hazardous materials.*

6. *Identify the pathophysiology, signs and symptoms, and prehospital management of selected hazardous materials that produce external damage.*

7. *Outline the prehospital response to a hazardous materials emergency.*

8. *Describe medical monitoring and rehabilitation of rescue workers who respond to a hazardous materials emergency.*

9. *Describe emergency decontamination and management of patients who have been contaminated by hazardous materials.*

10. *Outline the eight steps to decontaminate rescue personnel and equipment at a hazardous materials incident.*

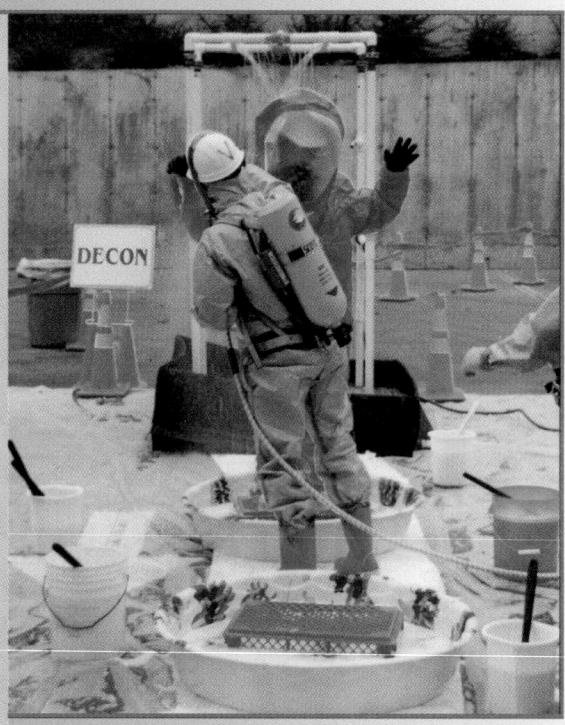

*Hazardous materials (Hazmat) incidents create additional responsibilities for emergency service providers. Large geographical areas covering several political jurisdictions may be involved, and cooperation in mass evacuations and mass **decontamination** procedures may be required. Specialized roles and responsibilities include, among others, recognition and identification of hazardous material, scene safety, containment and cleanup of the material, extrication and decontamination of exposed individuals, provision of emergency care, and continual medical assessment of team members involved in the incident.*

KEY TERMS

decontamination: The process of making patients, rescuers, equipment, and supplies safe by eliminating harmful substances.

placards: Four-sided, diamond-shaped signs displayed on hazardous materials containers that usually are yellow, orange, white, or green. They have a four-digit United Nations identification number and a legend to indicate the contents of the container.

primary contamination: Exposure to a hazardous substance that is harmful only to the person exposed and that poses little risk of exposure to others.

secondary contamination: Exposure to a hazardous substance whereby liquid and particulate substances are easily transferred to others by touching.

shipping papers: Descriptions of the hazardous materials that include the substance name, classification, and United Nations identification number.

NOTE

Not all hazardous materials incidents are large-scale events. A single event involving only one patient may require a full Hazmat response.

Scope of Hazardous Materials

A *hazardous material* is defined as "any substance or material capable of posing an unreasonable risk to health, safety, and property."[1] More than 50 billion tons of hazardous materials are manufactured in the United States each year, and about 4 billion tons are shipped within the United States.[2] It is estimated that 5% to 15% of all trucks on the road at any time carry hazardous materials. Because emergency responses to vehicular crashes are so common, the potential for exposure to hazardous materials is great. Other possible causes of hazardous materials incidents include mishaps in the storage of materials and manufacturing operations and acts of terrorism (see the box below).

Injury or illness also may result from exposure to household chemicals, pesticides, and industrial toxins. The following statistics emphasize the importance of emergency medical service (EMS) personnel knowing how to manage hazardous materials exposure[3]:

- About 9000 deaths occur each year from exposure to poisonous solids, liquids, and gases.
- An estimated 100,000 industrial workers are exposed to respiratory irritants each year.
- Pesticide poisoning accounts for more than 3000 hospitalizations each year.
- Most fire-related deaths result from inhalation of toxic products of combustion.

? CRITICAL THINKING

What industries in your area have the potential for a hazardous materials exposure?

BIOLOGICAL HAZARDS: TOXIN TERRORS

International conventions have long prohibited the use of chemical weapons during war, and they bar any country from making or acquiring biological weapons. A number of countries and some terrorist groups, however, maintain biological weapons that may include anthrax, botulinum toxin ("botox"), ricin, sarin, smallpox, VX, and others. If planes carrying a small payload of some of these agents sprayed a sleeping city on a clear, breezy night, thousands and perhaps millions of people would be killed. For example, 200 pounds of anthrax sprayed over a city the size of Omaha would kill as many as 2.5 million people; 200 pounds of botox could kill as many as 40,000 people in an area the size of the Mall of America; and 200 pounds of VX sprayed over an area the size of Disneyland would kill about 12,500 people.

Modified from The terrors of toxins, *Newsweek*, November 1997.

Laws and Regulations

In recent years much attention has been focused on hazardous materials. Major incidents, such as the Union Carbide disaster in India, the Chernobyl nuclear accident in the Soviet Union, the Three Mile Island accident in the United States, and the need for proper disposal of hazardous wastes have attracted the attention of employee and citizen awareness groups and local, state, and federal officials. This attention has resulted in more laws and regulations to strictly control hazardous materials.

The Superfund Amendments and Reauthorization Act (SARA) of 1986 established requirements for federal, state, and local governments and industry regarding emergency planning and the reporting of hazardous materials–related incidents. This legislation was designed to help communities better meet their responsibilities in the event of chemical emergencies. SARA helped increase the public's knowledge and access to information about hazardous materials in their community. The act required owners and operators of facilities using or storing any of the extremely hazardous substances identified by the Environmental Protection Agency (EPA) to notify the local fire department, the local emergency planning committee, and the state emergency response commission.

In 1989 the Occupational Safety and Health Administration (OSHA) and the EPA published rules to govern training requirements, emergency plans, medical checkups, and other safety precautions for workers at uncontrolled hazardous waste sites and those responding to hazardous chemical releases or spills.[4] SARA mandates that states adopt these rules. The training requirements include the following five categories of individuals who may respond to an emergency involving hazardous materials:

1. *First-responder awareness.* This category pertains to individuals who are likely to witness or discover a hazardous substance release but who do not have emergency response duties pertaining to hazardous materials as part of their job functions. This applies to most law enforcement officers. Individuals in this category must have sufficient training to demonstrate the following:
   a. An understanding of what hazardous materials are and the risks associated with them in an accident
   b. An understanding of the possible outcomes of an emergency in which hazardous materials are present
   c. The ability to recognize the presence of hazardous materials in an emergency
   d. The ability to identify the hazardous materials (if possible)
   e. An understanding of the role of the first responder in the emergency response plan
   f. The ability to recognize the need for additional resources

2. *First-responder operations.* Individuals are included in this category if they respond to hazardous materials incidents to protect nearby people, property, or the environment without trying to stop the hazardous release. Firefighters and EMS personnel are in this category. In addition to the knowledge base of first-responder awareness, these individuals must have training in the following:
   a. Basic hazard and risk assessment techniques
   b. Personal protective clothing and equipment
   c. Basic control, containment, and confinement operations
   d. Basic decontamination procedures

3. *Hazardous material technicians.* Individuals in this category respond to hazardous materials emergencies for the purpose of stopping the release. Hazardous materials technicians usually are considered members of a hazardous materials response team. These individuals have additional training in the following:
   a. Emergency response plans
   b. The use of survey instruments and equipment to identify hazardous materials
   c. Incident command systems
   d. Specialized protective clothing and equipment
   e. Specialized containment and confinement operations

4. *Hazardous materials specialists.* The duties of these individuals require specific knowledge of the various hazardous substances. Hazardous materials specialists respond with and provide support to hazardous materials technicians and act as site liaisons with federal, state, and local government authorities. In addition to the knowledge base of the hazardous materials technician, hazardous materials specialists have training in the following:
   a. The use of advanced survey instruments and equipment
   b. In-depth hazard and risk assessment

c. Implementation of decontamination procedures

d. Site safety and control

e. Chemical, radiological, and toxicological terminology relevant to hazardous substance behaviors

5. *On-scene incident commander.* The on-scene incident commander is trained to assume control of a hazardous materials event. In addition to the first-responder awareness level of training, the on-scene incident commander's responsibilities include the following:

a. Implementation of an incident command system

b. Implementation of emergency response plans

c. Knowledge of both state and federal regional response teams

d. Knowledge of medical hazards and risks for individuals working in protective clothing and equipment

In addition to these training levels outlined by OSHA, the National Fire Protection Association (NFPA) has published standards that address competencies for EMS personnel at Hazmat scenes.[5] According to these standards, paramedics who transport patients who pose no risk of secondary contamination must be trained to NFPA standard 473 Level 1. Paramedics who may have to rapidly decontaminate (decon) or assist in the decontamination area must be trained to NFPA standard 473 Level 2.[6]

Identifying Hazardous Materials

The crux of dealing with hazardous materials is identification of the substance. The two methods used to identify hazardous materials are informal product identification and formal product identification (**placards, shipping papers,** and other hazardous materials information resources).

Informal Product Identification

Arriving emergency personnel may be able to determine the presence and type of hazardous materials at the scene. Informal methods of identification include the following:

- Visual inspection of the scene with binoculars before entering the site

- Verbal reports by bystanders or other responsible individuals
- Occupancy type (intended use of a particular structure such as fuel storage or pesticide plant)
- Incident location (probable location for presence of hazardous materials)
- Location within a building (what is stored in that area)
- Visual indicators (vapor clouds, smoke, leakage)
- Container characteristics (size, shape, color, deformed containers)
- Senses (peculiar smell)
- Signs and symptoms of victims of exposure

Informal methods of product identification should be used only as a temporary means to determine the presence of any hazardous materials. A product should always be identified formally before any activity is undertaken that may pose a threat to the safety of all emergency responders.

> **NOTE**
>
> Personal safety is the number one priority when responding to a hazardous materials incident. If the scene is not safe, the EMS crew should retreat and not enter the scene until it has been made safe by trained personnel.

Formal Product Identification

Traditionally, hazardous materials have been labeled by one or more of the following six systems:

1. The American National Standards Institute uses a label to identify a specific hazard (e.g., explosives, flammable liquids, radioactive materials) rather than a specific chemical.

2. The U.S. Department of Transportation (DOT) uses labels and placards with pictographs and printed hazard categories. In addition, DOT requires specific information on shipping manifests.

3. The United Nations Labeling System uses pictographs, symbols, or both, similar to those used by DOT to identify a specific hazard rather than a specific chemical.

4. The International Air Transport Association uses the United Nations pictographs and indicates written emergency precaution measures in case of an incident.

5. The National Fire Protection Association uses color and a numerical rating scale (NFPA 704 System) to identify the degree of hazard for health, fire, and reactivity. Many state and local fire codes require the diamond-shaped identification symbols on fixed facilities (Fig. 51-1).

6. The U.S. Department of Labor requires Material Safety Data Sheets (MSDSs) for hazardous chemicals that are stored, handled, or used in the workplace.

? CRITICAL THINKING

The next time you are on the highway, see if you can easily spot the placards on large trucks.

Placards and Shipping Papers

Although a variety of identification systems may be used, hazardous materials usually are identified through placards (Fig. 51-2) and shipping papers.

The United Nations class (or division) identification number and North American number (UN/NA number) may be displayed on the bottom of a placard or on the shipping paper after the listed shipping name or names. In certain cases this class or division number may replace the written name of the hazard class in the shipping paper description. The meanings of the class and division numbers are shown in Table 51-1.

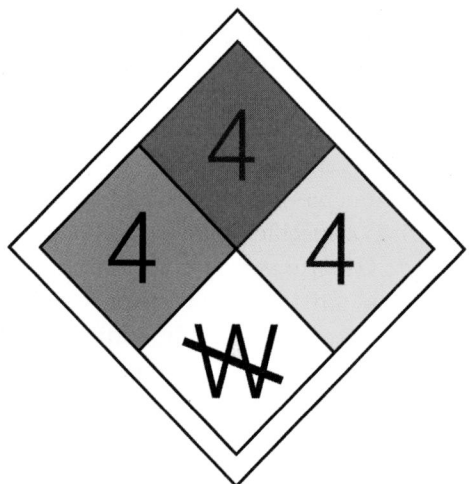

Fig. 51-1 An NFPA placard. The numbers correspond to health, flammability, and reactivity hazards. Anyone using the 704 system to classify chemicals does so at their own risk. (From National Fire Protection Association, Quincy, Mass, 1996.)

NOTE

The location and type of paperwork that identifies hazardous materials varies according to the mode of transport. Most shipping papers are kept near the operator (e.g., driver, pilot, captain) of the vehicle, aircraft, train, or ship.

NOTE

Because several chemical agents may have the same UA/NA number, it is important to refer to specific guidelines for hazardous material by chemical name in addition to this number.

Material Safety Data Sheets

Material Safety Data Sheets (MSDSs) are required by OSHA for each chemical produced, stored, or used in the United States. MSDSs are supplied by the manufacturer and contain information for safe and proper handling and storage of the material, in addition to information on emergency actions. MSDSs also classify the potential of significant health hazards from exposure to a particular substance.

The potential health hazard of a material may be defined in several different ways, depending on the degree of inherent toxicity and type of exposure. Although MSDSs provide useful information, they should not be used as the sole source of chemical information, information on health risks, or treatment recommendations. Paramedics should consult with medical direction, a poison control center, or another appropriate authority.

Other Sources of Information on Hazardous Materials

A number of resources are available for hazardous materials reference. One such reference is the *North American Emergency Response Guidebook* published by DOT, Transport Canada, and the Secretariat of Communications and Transportation of Mexico.

NOTE

Product information should be referenced through more than one source (preferably three) if time and availability permit.

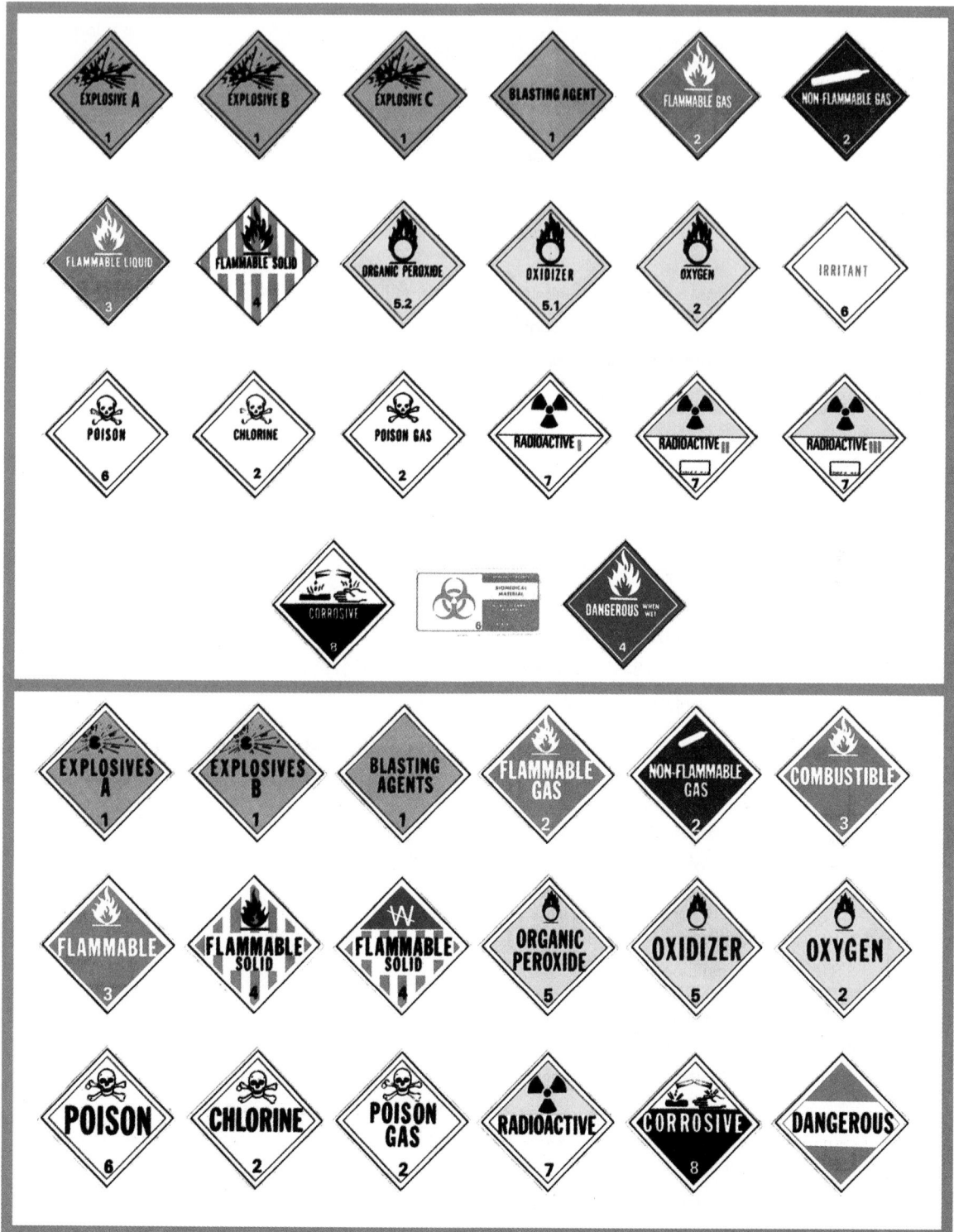

Fig. 51-2 Hazardous materials warning placards and labels. (From Bronstein A: *Mosby's emergency care for hazardous material exposure,* St Louis, 1988, Mosby.)

TABLE 51-1	INTERNATIONAL CLASSIFICATION SYSTEM FOR HAZARDOUS MATERIALS

Class or division numbers may be displayed in the bottom of placards or in the hazardous materials description on shipping papers. In certain cases, a class or division number may replace the written name of the hazard class description on the shipping paper. The class and division numbers have the following meanings:

Class 1   **Explosives**
Division 1.1   Explosives with a mass explosion hazard
Division 1.2   Explosives with a projection hazard
Division 1.3   Explosives with predominantly a fire hazard
Division 1.4   Explosives with no significant blast hazard
Division 1.5   Very insensitive explosives
Division 1.6   Extremely insensitive explosive articles

Class 2   **Gases**
Division 2.1   Flammable gases
Division 2.2   Nonflammable gases
Division 2.3   Poison gases
Division 2.4   Corrosive gases (Canadian)

Class 3   **Flammable Liquids**
Division 3.1   Flashpoint below −18° C (0° F)
Division 3.2   Flashpoint −18° C and above but less than 23° C (73° F)
Division 3.3   Flashpoint of 23° C and up to 61° C (141° F)

Class 4   **Flammable Solids, Spontaneously Combustible Materials, Materials That Are Dangerous When Wet**
Division 4.1   Flammable solids
Division 4.2   Spontaneously combustible materials
Division 4.3   Materials that are dangerous when wet

Class 5   **Oxidizers and Organic Peroxides**
Division 5.1   Oxidizers
Division 5.2   Organic peroxides

Class 6   **Poisonous and Etiological (Infectious) Materials**
Division 6.1   Poisonous materials
Division 6.2   Etiological (infectious) materials

Class 7   **Radioactive Materials**

Class 8   **Corrosives**

Class 9   **Miscellaneous Hazardous Materials**

From *EMT-Paramedic national standard curriculum,* U.S. Department of Transportation National Highway Traffic Safety Administration, Washington D.C., 1997, The Department.

BOX 51-1

SOME AGENCIES THAT ASSIST IN HAZARDOUS MATERIALS INCIDENTS

Federal Agencies
- EPA
- DOT
- National Response Center (NRC)
- United States Coast Guard (USCG)
- Centers for Disease Control (CDC)
- Federal Aviation Administration (FAA)
- United States Armed Forces (Army, Navy, Air Force, Marines)
- U.S. Department of Energy (DOE)

Regional and State Agencies
- State EPA
- State health departments
- National Guard
- State police
- State emergency management agencies

Local Agencies
- Emergency management
- Fire service (Hazmat units)

- Poison control center
- Law enforcement agencies
- Public utilities
- Sewage and treatment facilities

Commercial Agencies
- American Petroleum Institute
- Association of American Railroads (AAR) and Hazardous Materials Systems
- Chemical Manufacturers Association
- HELP (Union Carbide's Emergency Response System for company shipments)
- Chevron (provides assistance with Chevron products)
- Railway industry
- Local industry
- Local contractors
- Local-carriers and transporters

This guidebook lists more than 1000 hazardous materials and appropriate emergency procedures. It includes substance names and identification numbers and is cross-referenced in alphabetical and numerical order. This reference is carried in emergency vehicles by many EMS, fire, and other public service agencies.

Regional poison control centers have been established throughout most of the United States, and they are a valuable asset in any EMS system. Many of these centers are available 24 hours a day. They are staffed with specialists who provide information, consultation, treatment recommendations, patient follow-up, and data collection. Poison control centers are linked to many agencies that deal with toxic substances and are closely tied to all area hospitals. These centers maintain a computerized listing of more than 450,000 drugs, toxic substances, and other products.

The Chemical Transportation Emergency Center *(CHEMTREC)*, a public service of the Chemical Manufacturers Association, provides immediate advice to on-scene personnel about management of hazardous materials. The agency also contacts the shipper of the material for additional assistance and

provides follow-up response when appropriate. CHEMTREC operates 24 hours a day, 7 days a week and can be reached in the United States and Canada through the emergency toll-free number: 1-800-424-9300 (in Alaska 0-202-483-7616). CHEMTREC should be contacted as soon as possible during a hazardous materials incident; it should be supplied with the name of the substance, its identification number, and the nature of the problem. Involving CHEMTREC in management of a hazardous materials incident is usually part of the standard operating procedure of any emergency response team.

CHEMTEL, Inc., is an emergency response communications center that serves the United States and Canada. The office can provide specific product information and referral to appropriate state and federal authorities for incidents that involve radioactive material. CHEMTEL can be reached 24 hours a day, 7 days a week through the toll-free number 1-800-255-3924.

Computer-Aided Management of Emergency Operations *(CAMEO)* systems are designed to quickly assist emergency responders in making operational decisions during release of hazardous materials. The program, which is available to municipalities, uses computer modeling to predict the effects of chemical spills and helps communities prepare emergency response plans. The system currently provides information on more than 83,000 individual chemicals. Other government and private sector agencies that may offer assistance in a hazardous materials incident are listed in Box 51-1.

> **NOTE**
>
> When a hazardous substance cannot be precisely identified, trained personnel may use sophisticated devices to ensure scene safety and to aid in product identification. These devices include air monitoring equipment, gas monitoring equipment, and special equipment for pH testing, chemical testing, and colorimetric tube testing.

Personal Protective Clothing and Equipment

The potential for injury from exposure to hazardous materials is related to the toxicity, flammability, and reactivity of a particular substance. It is important that anyone dealing with hazardous materials take precautionary measures, including the use of appropriate respiratory protection and personal protective equipment (PPE).

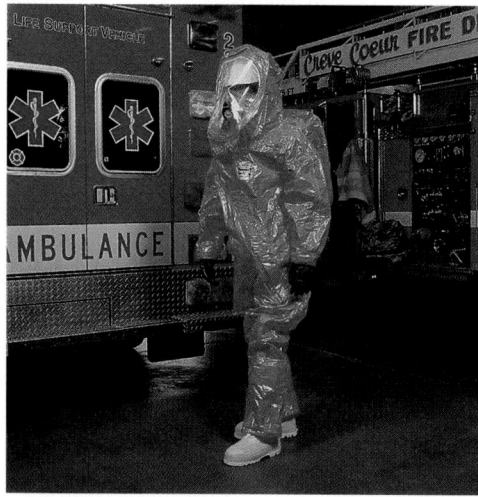

Fig. 51-3 Level A protective clothing. (Courtesy Creve Coeur Fire Protection District, Creve Coeur, Mo.)

> **✓ TRICKS OF THE TRADE**
>
> It is a potentially deadly mistake to enter a Hazmat scene without appropriate PPE.

Protective Respiratory Devices

The potential for exposure of the respiratory system to hazardous materials is of paramount importance to the emergency responder. The respiratory system may be protected by air purification devices and atmosphere supplying respiratory equipment.

Air purification relies on respirators or filtration devices to remove particulate matter, gases, or vapors from the atmosphere. These devices do not use a separate source of air and require constant monitoring for contaminants and oxygen levels. As a rule, they are not recommended for use in a hazardous materials release.

> **NOTE**
>
> Filtration devices are material specific (must match the gas) and are not used in the presence of multiple types of chemicals.

Atmosphere supplying devices rely on a separate source of air and provide the highest level of respiratory protection. The two basic types are the self-contained breathing apparatus (SCBA) and the supplied air breathing apparatus (SABA), or air lines. The use of either requires training, recertification,

> **BOX 51-2**
>
> ### FORMS OF CHEMICAL INTRUSION
>
> **Degredation:** The physical destruction or decomposition of a clothing material caused by exposure to chemicals, use, or ambient conditions.
> **Penetration:** The flow of a hazardous liquid chemical through zippers, stitched seams, pinholes, or other imperfections in a material.
> **Permeation:** The process by which a hazardous liquid chemical moves through a material on a molecular level.

and proper fit-testing as governed by regulations from OSHA.

SCBA provides respiratory protection in oxygen-deficient and toxic atmospheres. Only SCBAs that maintain positive pressure in the face piece during inhalation and exhalation should be used when working with hazardous materials. The SCBA usually is considered an excellent barrier to hazardous environments, but the rescuer should be aware of potential face piece penetration and contamination by certain toxic substances, such as methyl bromide, Telone, and ethyleneimine.

SABAs supply air to the rescuer via an air line hose away from the scene. These devices often are used at hazardous material sites when extended working times are required. SABAs must have an escape capability for operations in atmospheres classified as immediately dangerous to life and health. Respiratory protection devices that combine SCBAs and air line hose units are available.

Classifications of Protective Clothing

Protective clothing is categorized as limited use (disposable) or multiuse (reusable) and is constructed of a variety of materials designed specifically for certain chemical exposures. Examples of this material include Tyvek/Saranex, nitrile rubber, Teflon, and Viton. Because no single material is compatible with all chemicals, the manufacturer's guidelines and recommendations must be followed (Box 51-2). Protective clothing is classified in several ways. The classifications defined by OSHA and the EPA are provided below.[7]

> **NOTE**
>
> Training in the use of personal protective clothing should take place in a safe environment before it is used at emergency scenes.

I. Level A: The greatest level of skin, respiratory, and eye protection (Fig. 51-3)
    Level A equipment constitutes the following:

1. Positive-pressure, full face piece, self-contained breathing apparatus (SCBA) or positive-pressure supplied air respirator with escape SCBA, approved by the National Institute for Occupational Safety and Health (NIOSH)

2. Totally encapsulating (gas tight) chemical protective suit
3. Coveralls (optional)
4. Long underwear (optional)
5. Gloves, outer, chemical resistant
6. Gloves, inner, chemical resistant
7. Boots, chemical resistant, steel toe and shank
8. Hard hat under suit (optional)
9. Disposable protective suit, gloves, and boots (depending on suit construction, may be worn over totally encapsulating suit)

> **NOTE**
>
> Level A provides the highest level of personal protection. It typically is used by Hazmat teams for entry into the incident site.

II. Level B: The highest level of respiratory protection but a lower level of skin protection (Fig. 51-4)
    Level B equipment constitutes the following:

1. Positive-pressure, full face piece, self-contained breathing apparatus (SCBA) or positive-pressure supplied air respirator with escape SCBA (NIOSH approved)
2. Hooded chemical-resistant clothing (overalls and long-sleeved jacket, coveralls, one- or two-piece chemical splash suit, disposable chemical-resistant overalls)

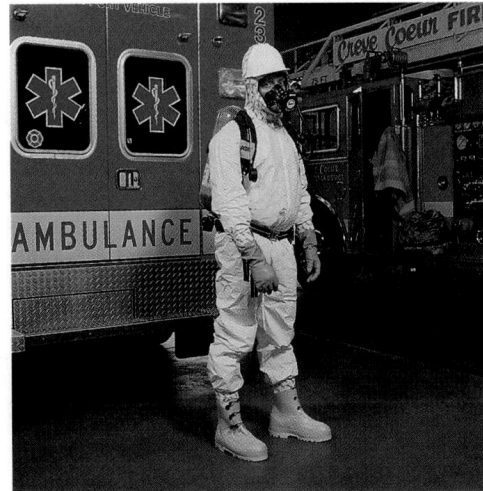

Fig. 51-4 Level B protective clothing. It offers the highest level of respiratory protection and a higher level of skin protection than Level C protective clothing. (Courtesy Creve Coeur Fire Protection District, Creve Coeur, Mo.)

3. Coveralls (optional)
4. Gloves, outer, chemical resistant
5. Gloves, inner, chemical resistant
6. Boots, outer, chemical resistant steel toe and shank
7. Boot covers, outer, chemical resistant (disposable) (optional)
8. Hard hat (optional)
9. Face shield (optional)

> **NOTE**
>
> Level B protection typically is worn by the "decon" team.

III. Level C: Concentration and type of airborne substance (or substances) is known and the criteria for using air-purifying respirators are met Level C equipment constitutes the following:

1. Full face or half mask, air purifying respirators (NIOSH approved)
2. Hooded, chemical-resistant clothing (overalls, two-piece chemical splash suit, disposable chemical-resistant overalls)
3. Coveralls (optional)
4. Gloves, outer, chemical resistant
5. Gloves, inner, chemical resistant
6. Boots, outer, chemical-resistant steel toe and shank (optional)

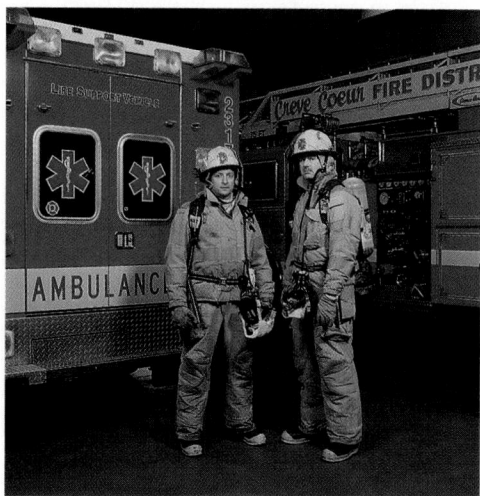

Fig. 51-5 Level D protective clothing. (Courtesy Creve Coeur Fire Protection District, Creve Coeur, Mo.)

7. Boot covers, outer, chemical resistant (disposable) (optional)
8. Hard hat (optional)
9. Escape mask (optional)
10. Face shield (optional)

> **? CRITICAL THINKING**
>
> *Which patient care activities do you think you will be able to provide when wearing each of the levels of Hazmat protective gear?*

> **NOTE**
>
> Level C protection is used during transport of patients who could possibly transfer contamination.

IV. Level D: A work uniform that affords minimal protection, used for nuisance contamination only (Fig. 51-5).
Level D equipment constitutes the following:

1. Coveralls
2. Gloves (optional)
3. Boots or shoes, chemical-resistant steel toe and shank
4. Boots, outer, chemical resistant (disposable) (optional)
5. Safety glasses or chemical splash goggles
6. Hard hat (optional)
7. Escape mask (optional)
8. Face shield (optional)

> **NOTE**
>
> Level D gear is commonly known as firefighter "turn-out" gear. Turn-out gear with SCBA may be considered level B protection for some chemicals that do not pose a risk for skin contact or absorption.

Regardless of the type of PPE used during a Hazmat incident, all avenues through which hazardous materials can enter the body must be protected. The following points should be of particular concern to any rescuer involved in Hazmat response:

- Protective clothing should not be adversely affected by the hazardous materials involved.
- Protective clothing should seal all exposed skin.
- Contact with the hazardous materials should be of the absolute minimal duration required.
- Protective clothing and equipment should be properly decontaminated or properly discarded.
- Safety standards and methods for cleaning and disposing of clothing and equipment should be strictly followed.

Health Hazards

Hazardous materials may enter the human body by inhalation, ingestion, injection, and absorption (see Chapter 34). Entry by means of any of these routes may result in internal and external damage to the rescuer. Exposure to dangerous substances may affect the body in several different ways, producing numerous injuries or illnesses.

> **NOTE**
>
> Exposure to poisons can produce acute toxicity, delayed toxicity, and local and systemic effects. The physiological response or responses depend on the concentration of the chemical at the biological site of action (dose response). The paramedic also should be aware that drug treatment can result in synergistic effects. Therefore all treatment methods must be guided by medical direction, a poison control center, or other appropriate authority.

Internal Damage

Internal damage to the human body from exposure to hazardous materials may involve the respiratory tract, the central nervous system (CNS), or other internal organs. Some substances injure all cells with which they come in contact. Others have a more direct effect on specific organs (target organs), such as the kidneys and liver.

Depending on the hazardous materials, physical injury may range from minor irritation to more serious complications, including cardiorespiratory compromise and death. Chronic illness (e.g., chronic obstructive pulmonary disease [COPD]) and various forms of cancer also may result. Some substances may have teratogenic or mutagenic consequences, causing abnormal fetal development and changes in gene structure. For example, penetrating radiation (described in Chapter 21) can lead to cell and chromosomal changes, subsequent reproductive genetic aberrations, cell death, and sterility.

Irritants

Respiratory problems are a frequent complaint of rescuers and patients exposed to hazardous materials. Chemical irritants emit vapors that affect the mucous membranes of the body, such as the surfaces of the eyes, nose, mouth, and throat. As these irritants combine with moisture, acidic or alkaline reactions may occur. Exposure to these irritants may result in damage to the upper, lower, and deep respiratory tract. Examples of chemical irritants are hydrochloric acid, halogens, and ozone.

Asphyxiants

Asphyxiants are gases that displace the available oxygen required for respiration by diluting the oxygen concentration in the air. Besides simple asphyxiants such as carbon dioxide, methane, and propane, there are also gases that not only displace oxygen in the air but also interfere with tissue oxygenation; these are referred to as *blood poisons* or *chemical asphyxiants* because they tend to interrupt the transport or use of oxygen by tissue cells. Through various mechanisms, these toxic gases deprive body tissue of needed oxygen. Examples include hydrogen cyanide, carbon monoxide, and hydrogen sulfide.

Nerve Poisons, Anesthetics, and Narcotics

Nerve poisons, anesthetics, and narcotics act on the nervous system by affecting either the cardiorespiratory regulating mechanisms of the brain or the ability to transmit impulses required for adequate respiratory and circulatory functions.

Nerve poisons were developed by the military and are commonly referred to as *war gases, nerve gases,* or *nerve agents.* Similar substances are used in solid pesticides, and exposure to these chemicals may result in fatal complications. Examples of these poisons include carbamates, organophosphates, parathion, and malathion. Although anesthetics and narcotics are less hazardous than nerve poisons, continuous exposure or exposure to large concentrations may result in unconsciousness or death. Examples include ethylene, nitrous oxide, and ethyl alcohol.

Hepatotoxins

Hepatotoxins are substances that damage the liver. The poisons accumulate in the body and destroy the liver's ability to function. Examples include chlorinated and halogenated hydrocarbons.

Cardiotoxins

Cardiotoxins are hazardous materials that may induce myocardial ischemia and cardiac rhythm disturbances. Examples of these substances are aliphatic nitrates and ethylene glycol dinitrate. Acute myocardial infarction and sudden death have been reported in healthy young people exposed to these substances. Short-term exposure to fluorocarbons and other halogenated hydrocarbons also has been known to cause cardiac abnormalities.

Nephrotoxins

Nephrotoxins are hazardous materials that are especially destructive to the kidneys. Examples include carbon disulfide, lead, high concentrations of organic solvents, and inorganic mercury. Exposure to carbon tetrachloride used as a solvent or dry-cleaning or fire-extinguishing agent also may have nephrotoxic effects.

Neurotoxins

Neurological and behavioral toxicity may result from exposure to hazardous substances such as arsenic, lead, mercury, and organic solvents. In some cases cerebral hypoxia may occur as a result of cellular respiration impaired by decreased oxygenation of the blood.

Hemotoxins

Hemotoxins are hazardous substances that may cause the destruction of red blood cells, resulting in hemolytic anemia (see Chapter 35). Substances that can produce hemolytic anemia include aniline, naphthol, quinones, lead, mercury, arsenic, and copper. Pulmonary edema and cardiac and liver injury also may be caused by hemotoxin exposure.

Carcinogens

Carcinogens are cancer-causing agents, and many hazardous materials are carcinogenic or suspected carcinogens. Although the precise amount of hazardous materials exposure required for cancer to develop is unknown, it is known that short-term exposure to specific agents can produce long-term ef-

fects. Disease and complications have been reported 20 years after exposure to hazardous materials.

Of particular interest to rescuers involved in fire fighting is that all burning fossil and organic fuels produce dioxins, many of which are carcinogens. (For example, burning wood produces carcinogenic formaldehyde.) A positive-pressure SCBA is the most important piece of protective equipment for use against these carcinogenic vapors and any other respiratory poisons.

General Symptoms of Exposure

Health effects from exposure to hazardous materials vary by individual and depend on the chemical involved, the concentration of the chemical, the duration of exposure, the number of exposures, and the route of entry (inhalation, ingestion, injection, absorption). In addition, personal factors such as an individual's age, gender, general health, allergies, smoking habits, alcohol consumption, and medication use influence how an individual is affected.

Various symptoms may result from exposure to hazardous materials. Some symptoms may be delayed or masked by common illnesses such as influenza or by smoke inhalation. If any of the following symptoms is present after exposure to hazardous materials, the rescuer or patient should seek immediate medical attention:

- Confusion, lightheadedness, anxiety, dizziness
- Chest tightness
- Dim, blurred, or double vision
- Changes in skin color or blushing
- Shortness of breath, burning of the upper airway
- Coughing or painful respiration
- Salivation, drooling, rhinorrhea
- Tingling or numbness of extremities
- Loss of coordination
- Seizure
- Nausea, vomiting, abdominal cramping
- Diarrhea and involuntary urination or defecation (or both)
- Unconsciousness

? CRITICAL THINKING

What actions should be taken immediately if two rescuers complain of similar symptoms on the scene of a rescue that may involve hazardous materials?

NOTE

Multiple simultaneous onset is a critical exposure sign. Any time two or more members of the response team report that they "feel" similar symptoms, a toxic gas or agent should be suspected. EMS responders should always immediately report the onset of symptoms to their crew members.

External Damage

Body surface tissue may be injured by hazardous materials. Many substances have corrosive properties or become corrosive when mixed with water. Exposure to these substances may produce chemical burns and severe tissue damage. Examples include hydrochloric acid, hydrofluoric acid, and caustic soda.

Soft Tissue Damage

Corrosives are acids or bases (alkaline). Exposure to either may cause pain on contact, but alkalis generally burn more extensively than acids. Exposing human tissue to a base corrosive such as lye may result in a breakdown of fatty tissue (liquefaction) that produces a greasy or slick feeling to the skin. These signs should alert the rescuer to immediately decontaminate and seek medical attention. Unless the substance is identified, decontamination should begin by brushing off the powder and flushing the skin with copious amounts of water. Paramedics should never attempt to neutralize an acid or base; doing so could produce great heat and cause further burns. The area should be copiously flushed with water, and the patient should be transported for care.

NOTE

Different areas of the skin absorb chemicals at different rates.

Cryogenics are refrigerant liquid gases that can freeze human tissue on contact. These liquids vaporize as soon as they are released from their containers and may cause tissue damage. Extreme caution should be used when near any refrigerated liquids because they can produce freeze burns, frostbite, and other cold-related injuries. Examples include freon, liquid oxygen, and liquid nitrogen.

Chemical Exposure to the Eyes

Chemical exposure to the eyes (described in Chapter 21) may cause damage ranging from superficial inflammation to severe burns. Patients with these conditions have local pain, visual disturbance, tearing, edema, and redness of surrounding tissues. Basic management guidelines include flushing the eyes with water by using a mild flow from a hose, IV tubing, water from a container, or irrigation lens (per protocol).

NOTE

A rapid assessment of visual acuity is important but should not delay flushing or irrigation of the eyes.

Response to Hazmat Emergencies

When an EMS crew is dispatched to a scene involving hazardous materials, decisions must be made about rescuer safety, the type and degree of the potential hazard, and the involvement of other agencies. As discussed in Chapter 49, preparatory planning and early coordination of activities in these major incidents is imperative. In addition, medical direction should be advised of the incident as soon as possible so that they can prepare personnel and facilities.

Although the first rescue personnel to arrive at the scene of a hazardous materials incident may not be the most qualified, most communities look to these public service agencies to provide immediate safety and direction. Therefore the EMS crew must be knowledgeable and proficient in the initial management of hazardous materials incidents.

Hazard and Risk Assessment

While en route to the emergency scene, EMS personnel should begin to research hazardous materials references and begin a *hazard and risk assessment*. In Hazmat incidents, hazards are the chemical properties of a material that may cause danger or peril (Box 51-3). *Risk* refers to the possibility of suffering harm or loss. Risk levels vary and are influenced by several factors, including the following[8] (Fig. 51-6):

- Hazardous nature of the material involved
- Quantity of the material involved

- Containment system and type of stress applied to the container
- Proximity of exposure
- Level of available resources

A hazard and risk assessment also includes consideration of potential hazards to the public and environment, the potential risk of **primary contamination** to patients, and the potential risk for **secondary contamination** to rescuers (Box 51- 4).

If the product can be identified through hazardous materials references, the EMS crew should familiarize themselves with potential health hazards, recommended personal protective equipment, initial first aid, and the "safe distance" factor as outlined in the reference guides. After the product has been precisely identified, more exact information should be gathered through appropriate Hazmat agencies (e.g., CAMEO, CHEMTREC, poison control).

NOTE

Hazards must be weighed against risks when considering the safety of rescuers, the public, and the environment.

NOTE

Most emergency response guides offer only general management objectives.

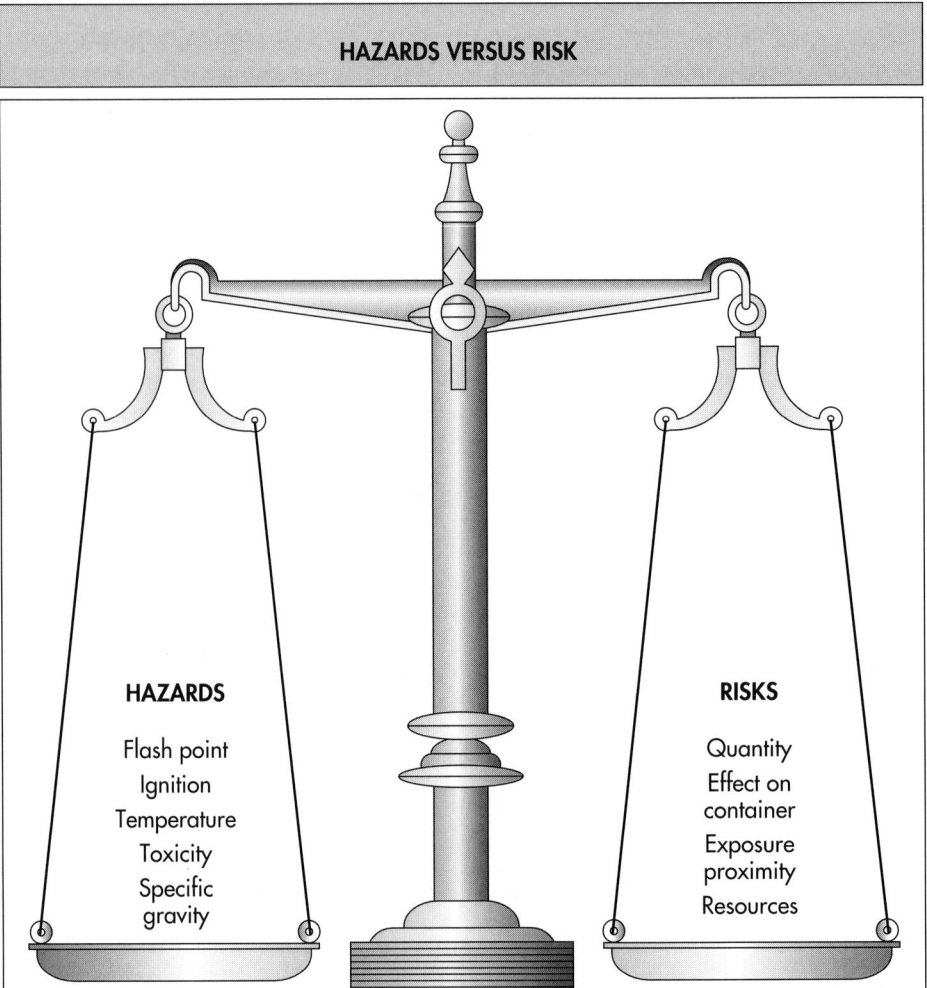

HAZARDS VERSUS RISK

HAZARDS

Flash point
Ignition
Temperature
Toxicity
Specific gravity

RISKS

Quantity
Effect on container
Exposure proximity
Resources

Fig. 51-6 Hazards versus risk. (Redrawn from Noll G et al: *Hazardous materials: managing the incident,* Stillwater, Okla., 1998, Fire Protection Publications.)

Approaching the Scene

The scene should be approached cautiously from uphill and upwind. The EMS crew should be alert to environmental clues such as wind direction, unusual odors, leakage, and vapor clouds. Binoculars can be used to initially observe the scene from a safe distance. Emergency vehicles should never be driven through leakage or vapor clouds, and personnel should not enter the incident area until it has been determined that it is safe. In addition to these guidelines, rescuers should do the following as recommended in the DOT's *Emergency Response Guidebook*[9]:

- Approach cautiously. Resist the urge to rush in; you cannot help others until you know what you are facing.
- Identify the hazards. Placards, container labels, shipping papers, and knowledgeable persons on the scene are valuable information sources. Evaluate all of them and then consult the recommended guide page before you place yourself or others at risk. Do not be alarmed if new information from a CHEMTREC expert changes some of the emphasis or details of the guide page warnings. You must remember that the guide page provides only the most important information for your initial response with a family or class of hazardous materials. As more accurate, material-specific information becomes available, your response becomes more appropriate for the situation.
- Secure the scene. Without entering the immediate hazard zone, do what you can to isolate the area and ensure the safety of people and the environment. Move and keep people away from the scene and the perimeter. Allow enough room to move and remove your own equipment.

BOX 51-3

HAZMAT TERMINOLOGY AND DEFINITIONS

Toxicological Terms Used to Determine Toxicity of a Compound

IDLH (immediately dangerous to life and health): Any atmosphere that poses an immediate hazard to life or produces immediate, irreversible debilitating effects on health.

LD-50 (lethal dose, 50% kill): The amount of a dose that, when administered to laboratory animals, kills 50% of them.

PEL (permissible exposure limit): The maximum time-weighted concentration at which 95% of exposed, healthy adults suffer no adverse effects over a 40-hour workweek.

ppm/ppb: Parts per million/parts per billion.

TLV-C (threshold limit value-ceiling level): The maximum concentration that should not be exceeded even instantaneously.

TLV-STEL (threshold limit value–short-term exposure limit): A 15-minute, time-weighted average exposure that should not be exceeded at any time nor repeatedly more than four times a day, with 60-minute rest periods required between each STEL exposure.

Specific Terminology for Medical Hazmat Operations

Alpha radiation: Large radioactive particles that have minimal penetrating ability.

Beta radiation: Small radioactive particles that can penetrate subcutaneous tissue and usually enter the body through damaged skin, ingestion, or inhalation.

Boiling point: The temperature at which a liquid changes to a vapor or a gas; the temperature at which the pressure of the liquid equals atmospheric pressure.

Flash point: The minimum temperature at which a liquid gives off enough vapors to ignite and flash-over but not to continue to burn without additional heat.

Flammable/exposure limits: The range of gas or vapor concentration that will burn or explode if an ignition source is present.

Gamma radiation: The most dangerous form of penetrating radiation, which can produce both internal and external hazards.

Ignition temperature: The minimum temperature required to ignite gas or vapor without a spark or flame being present.

Specific gravity: The weight of a material as compared with the weight of an equal volume of water.

Vapor density: The weight of a pure vapor or gas compared with the weight of an equal volume of dry air at the same temperature and pressure.

Vapor pressure: The pressure exerted by the vapor within the container against the sides of a container.

Vapor solubility: A vapor's ability to mix with water.

From Noll G et al: *Hazardous materials: managing the incident*, Stillwater, Okla, 1988, Fire Protection Publications.

BOX 51-4

TYPES OF CONTAMINATION

Primary Contamination

Exposure to substance
Substance only harmful to exposed person
Little chance of exposure to others

Secondary Contamination

Exposure to substance
Liquid and particulate substances easily transferred by touching

- Obtain help. Advise your headquarters to notify responsible agencies and call for assistance from trained experts through CHEMTREC and the National Response Center, which can be reached through CHEMTREC or dialed directly.
- Decide on site entry. Any efforts you make to rescue people or protect property or the environment must be weighed against the possibility that you could become part of the problem. Enter the area with the appropriate protective gear (if trained to do so). Above all, *do not walk into or touch spilled material.* Avoid inhaling fumes, smoke, and vapors, even if no hazardous materials are known to be involved. Do not assume that gases or vapors are harmless because of lack of smell.

? CRITICAL THINKING

Which of these guidelines would it be easy for the first arriving crew to miss?

Control of the Scene

The first agency to arrive at the scene has several responsibilities. Its members must detect and identify the materials involved, assess the risk of exposure to rescue personnel and others, consider the potential risk of fire or explosion, gather information from on-site personnel or other sources, and confine and control the incident. In addition, a command post should be established per the preplanned incident command structure, and safety distances and zones must be defined.

Safety Zones

After the presence of hazardous materials has been confirmed, the scene should be separated into hot, warm, and cold zones (Fig. 51-7). These safety zones should be established and enforced early in the incident (Box 51-5).

The *hot zone* is the area of the incident that includes the hazardous material and any surrounding area that may be exposed to gases, vapors, mist, dust, or run-off. All rescue personnel and vehicles should be stationed outside this zone. Anyone entering this zone must wear high-level PPE, and only specially trained EMS personnel should attempt patient care activities in this area. Some EMS agencies and ICS structures refer to the hot zone as the *exclusion zone,* a *restricted area,* or the *red zone.*

✓ TRICKS OF THE TRADE

If you are the first to arrive, make sure you advise the dispatch center and responding units of the location of the hot zone.

The *warm zone* is a larger, buffer area that surrounds the hot zone with "cold" and "hot" end corridors. Although protective clothing is required, it usually is considered a safer environment for workers. However, if the hot zone becomes unstable, the warm zone may be exposed to the hazardous materials. It is in this zone that most EMS activities, such as decontamination and patient care procedures, are performed. Some agencies refer to this zone as the *limited-access zone,* the *containment reduction corridor* (CRC), or the *yellow zone.*

The *cold zone* is the area that encompasses the warm zone. It also is restricted to emergency personnel. This area usually is considered safe, requiring only minimal protective clothing. The cold zone contains the command post and other support agencies necessary to control the incident. This area is referred to by some agencies as a *support zone* or the *green zone.*

Medical Monitoring and Rehabilitation

The safety of rescue personnel is of prime importance in any emergency event. Situations involving

BOX 51-5

HAZMAT ZONES

Hot Zone

Contamination present

Site of incident

Entry with high-level PPE

Entry limited

Warm Zone

Buffer zone outside hot zone

Contains decontamination corridor with "hot" and "cold" end

Cold Zone

Safe area

Staging area for personnel and equipment

Site of medical monitoring

One end of corridor

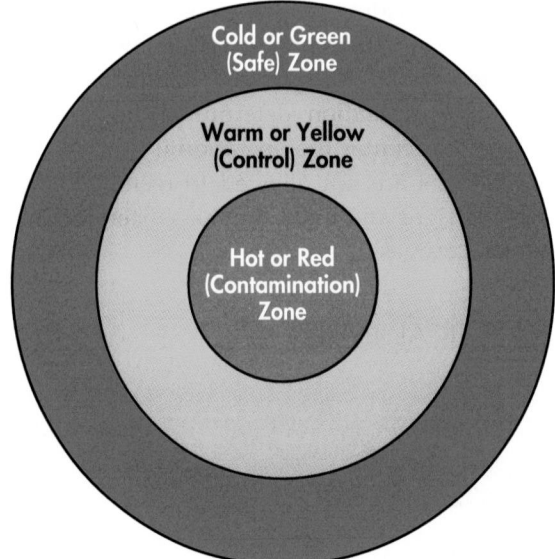

Hot or Red (Contamination) Zone

• Contamination is actually present.
• Personnel must wear appropriate protective gear.
• Number of rescuers limited to those absolutely necessary.
• Bystanders never allowed.

Warm or Yellow (Control) Zone

• Area surrounding the contamination zone.
• Vital to preventing spread of contamination.
• Personnel must wear appropriate protective gear.
• Life-saving emergency care and decontamination are performed.

Cold or Green (Safe) Zone

• Normal triage, stabilization, and treatment are performed
• Rescuers must shed contaminated gear before entering the cold zone.

Fig. 51-7 Zones at a Hazmat incident.

hazardous materials are among the most dangerous. Therefore a medical monitoring program should be part of any EMS/Hazmat system and all hazardous materials incidents.

OSHA requires medical examinations for members of Hazmat response teams and employees who may have been exposed to hazardous substances during an emergency event. Other components of a Hazmat medical monitoring program may include any needed medical care, medical monitoring during a hazardous materials incident, record-keeping, and periodic evaluation of the surveillance program.

Medical monitoring should include assessment protocols that involve a "presuit" medical examination to establish health history and a vital sign baseline for any rescuer who will be exposed to a hazardous substance. Individuals should be advised of the expected symptoms of illness or exposure before entry.

In addition to injury from hazardous materials exposure, emergency responders working in protective clothing and equipment are susceptible to heat illness and dehydration. Rescue protective suits protect, but they also prevent cooling through evaporation, conduction, convection, or radiation. Heat-stress factors are affected by the prehydration of the rescuer, degree of physical fitness, ambient air temperature, and the degree and duration of physi-

cal activity. The parameters of the presuit evaluation should include the following:

• Temperature, pulse, respiration, and blood pressure measurements
• Cardiac rhythm
• Body weight
• Cognitive and motor skills
• Hydration

After entry into the hazardous environment, medical monitoring should include an assessment of the amount of time a rescuer has been in protective clothing. Rescuers should be observed for any signs of heat-related illness or exposure. If illness or injury is detected at any time during the operation, the rescuer should be removed from the hostile environment for appropriate medical treatment.

After the incident, rescue personnel should be reevaluated in the "rehab sector" using the same parameters as in the presuit examination. This postentry examination determines the rescuer's capability to reenter the operation if needed. As a rule, rescuers are not allowed to reenter the site until vital signs and hydration have been returned to normal ranges.

> **? CRITICAL THINKING**
>
> *What might prevent personnel from seeking out EMS for medical monitoring unless there is a strict procedure to ensure this?*

> **NOTE**
>
> Body weight generally is used to estimate fluid loss and the need for oral or intravenous rehydration (per protocol).

Documentation

Thorough documentation is a necessary component of Hazmat medical monitoring and rehabilitation operations. At a minimum, documentation should include the following[6]:

- The hazardous substance
- The toxicity and danger of secondary contamination
- Use of appropriate PPE and any permeation ("breakthrough") that occurred
- The level of decontamination performed or required
- Use of antidotes and other medical treatment
- The method of transportation and destination

Emergency Management of Contaminated Patients

Patient care activities, triage, and evacuation should be part of a preplanned ICS structure. It may take some time to identify a specific hazardous substance, therefore rescue efforts, decontamination, possible evacuation, and timely treatment of toxic exposures are very important. The primary goals of decontamination are to reduce the patient's dosage of material, decrease the threat of secondary conta-

mination, and reduce the risk of rescuer injury.[6] The specific substance and route of contamination affect triage and decontamination methods. The following guidelines for rapid decontamination are general and should not supersede any organizational approach in scene management of hazardous materials incidents or treatment recommendations for chemical exposures:

> **NOTE**
>
> Rapid decontamination is a two-step process: (1) removing the patient from danger and (2) providing gross decontamination.

1. The paramedic should not enter a contaminated area or initiate patient care without adequate PPE and training specific to the incident.
2. Nonambulatory patients should be removed from the hot zone by trained personnel. Removal usually is performed by fire department personnel, specialized Hazmat teams, or both. Patient care activities in the hot zone should be limited to gross airway management, spinal immobilization, and hemorrhage control. Decontamination and additional patient care should be initiated in the warm zone by a properly equipped decontamination team.
3. All patients exposed to the hot zone should be considered contaminated. They should be treated as such until properly assessed and decontaminated.
4. Patient care provisions of airway, breathing, and circulatory support should begin as soon as the patient is contacted and conditions allow. The product-specific information received from Hazmat agencies regarding rescuer safety when initiating basic life support procedures should be applied appropriately.
5. Intravenous therapy should be administered only under a physician's direction. This and other invasive procedures may create a direct route for introducing the hazardous materials into the patient.
6. Decontamination procedures should be initiated without undue exposure to the rescuer. EMS providers assisting in decontamination should be well protected with two or three layers of

gloves, head coverings, positive-pressure SCBA, and proper protective clothing.

7. When the hazardous material is a dry agent, the agent should be removed by lightly brushing the material from patient surfaces, making sure not to introduce the contaminant into the patient's airway. Cutting or removing clothing often removes most of the contaminating material. After the dry agent has been removed, the decontamination should continue as follows:

a. Wash the patient with copious amounts of water (the universal decontamination solution) and mild detergent soap, making sure that all water and run-off is contained in the warm zone. Depending on the exposure, additional patient decontamination procedures may be warranted. Special attention should be paid to irrigation of the eyes, hair, ears, underarms, and pubic areas and thorough cleaning of the body creases of the neck, groin, elbows, and knees. Be careful not to abrade the skin, which may promote absorption of the material involved.

NOTE

Although water is considered the universal decontamination solution to dilute the concentration of a substance, it generally does not alter the chemical structure of a compound. Degradation solutions that may be recommended for some exposures include water and tincture of green soap, isopropyl alcohol, and vegetable oil (among others). These solutions should be used only when prescribed by medical direction or other appropriate authority. They should not be applied directly to the skin.

b. Leave all patient clothing, rescuer clothing, and decontamination equipment in the decontamination area. Safely move the patient to the support zone for further triage, treatment, and transport.

It should be noted that the field decontamination procedures described represent only a gross decontamination. The resources required for complete decontamination usually are unavailable at the emergency scene. Therefore the patient should be isolated from the environment to contain any con-

tamination that has been missed during these procedures. This is accomplished by placing the patient in a body bag to the neck and covering the patient's hair. In the absence of body bags, the victim may be packaged for transport by folding one side of a sheet or blanket over the patient and using the other side to overlap and package the patient. If necessary, the patient's arm may be exposed through an opening in the sheet for vital sign assessment and fluid and drug administration

? CRITICAL THINKING

What type of hazardous materials response resources does your community have?

Decontamination Decision Making

Hazardous materials incidents often are "fast breaking" and may require rapid decision making. For example, a flight of walking, contaminated persons at the scene may be trying to reach rescuers; others "self-rescue" by walking out of the hot zone; and some may become impatient and leave the hot zone while waiting for rescue teams to arrive. In these situations the paramedic crew must be prepared for quick gross decontamination and treatment, rapid application of PPE, and quick transport and isolation procedures.

If the patient's condition is critical (and it is unknown if the exposure involved a life-threatening material), the paramedic should perform decontamination and treatment simultaneously by removing the patient's clothing, treating life-threatening problems, lavaging the patient with copious amounts of water, and providing for isolation and transportation. Patients who are not in critical condition can be managed in the same manner with a more contemplative approach, particularly if the hazardous substance is known.

A hazardous materials incident that is well controlled (not a fast-break event) can be managed over longer duration. In these situations rescue should not be attempted for patients in the hot zone. Rather, the paramedic crew should wait for a Hazmat team and for a decontamination corridor (Fig. 51-8) to be established (which may take an hour or more). Longer duration events allow for more thorough decontamination, better PPE, less chance of secondary contamination, and better environmental protection.

Preparing the Ambulance for Patient Transfer

Contamination of ambulances and equipment can be minimized by preparing the vehicle before transporting a partly decontaminated patient. These protective measures include using as much disposable equipment as possible and removing all items from cabinets that will be required for patient use. Ide-

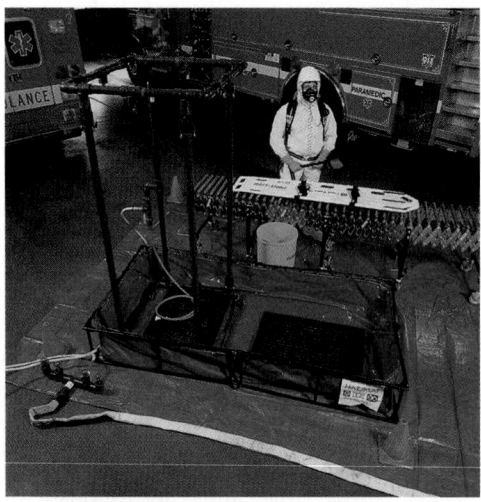

Fig. 51-8 Patient decontamination area. (Courtesy Creve Coeur Fire Protection District, Creve Coeur, Mo.)

ally, the patient should be completely isolated in a stretcher decontamination pool that is covered in plastic and secured to the stretcher.

On arrival at the hospital, the EMS crew should follow the hospital's decontamination protocols. The EMS crew should not return to regular service until rescue personnel, vehicle, and equipment have been monitored for contamination. Equipment decontamination should follow the recommendations of local, state, and federal authorities or medical direction's standard operating procedures. Although specific solutions may be required for a particular hazardous materials exposure, most equipment can be adequately cleaned and made ready for use with soap and water.

Decontamination of Rescue Personnel and Equipment

Decontamination of rescue personnel involves eight steps and begins in the decontamination corridor[6] (Fig. 51-9). These steps include the following:

1. An entry point is established at the "hot" end of the corridor where "dirty" personnel and equipment are set up to start the decontamination process.
2. A tool drop is designated, and outer gloves and boots are removed and placed in a receptacle.
3. Gross surface contamination is removed, generally by washing with copious amounts of water.
4. Contaminated SCBA bottles are removed (doffed) for personnel who must reenter the dirty area; at this step they receive clean SCBA bottles.
5. Protective clothing is removed and handled (stored, decontaminated) as required.
6. Other clothing is removed. This step depends on the seriousness of the hazardous materials involved.
7. Personnel wash their bodies using overhead showers. Usually two washings are required.

Personnel dry off and receive new or clean, uncontaminated clothing.
8. Personnel going through the decontamination system receive medical evaluation. (Medical evaluation continues at a medical facility.)

In addition, the following safety precautions should be followed by any rescuer exposed to hazardous materials:

• Do not touch your face, mouth, nose, or genital area before full body decontamination.
• Shower thoroughly with warm water, surgical soap, sponge, and brush; pay particular attention to hair, body orifices (especially the ears), and any body parts that come in contact with each other (arms and chest, thighs, fingers, toes, and buttocks). Repeat shower and rinse.
• Shampoo hair several times and rinse thoroughly.

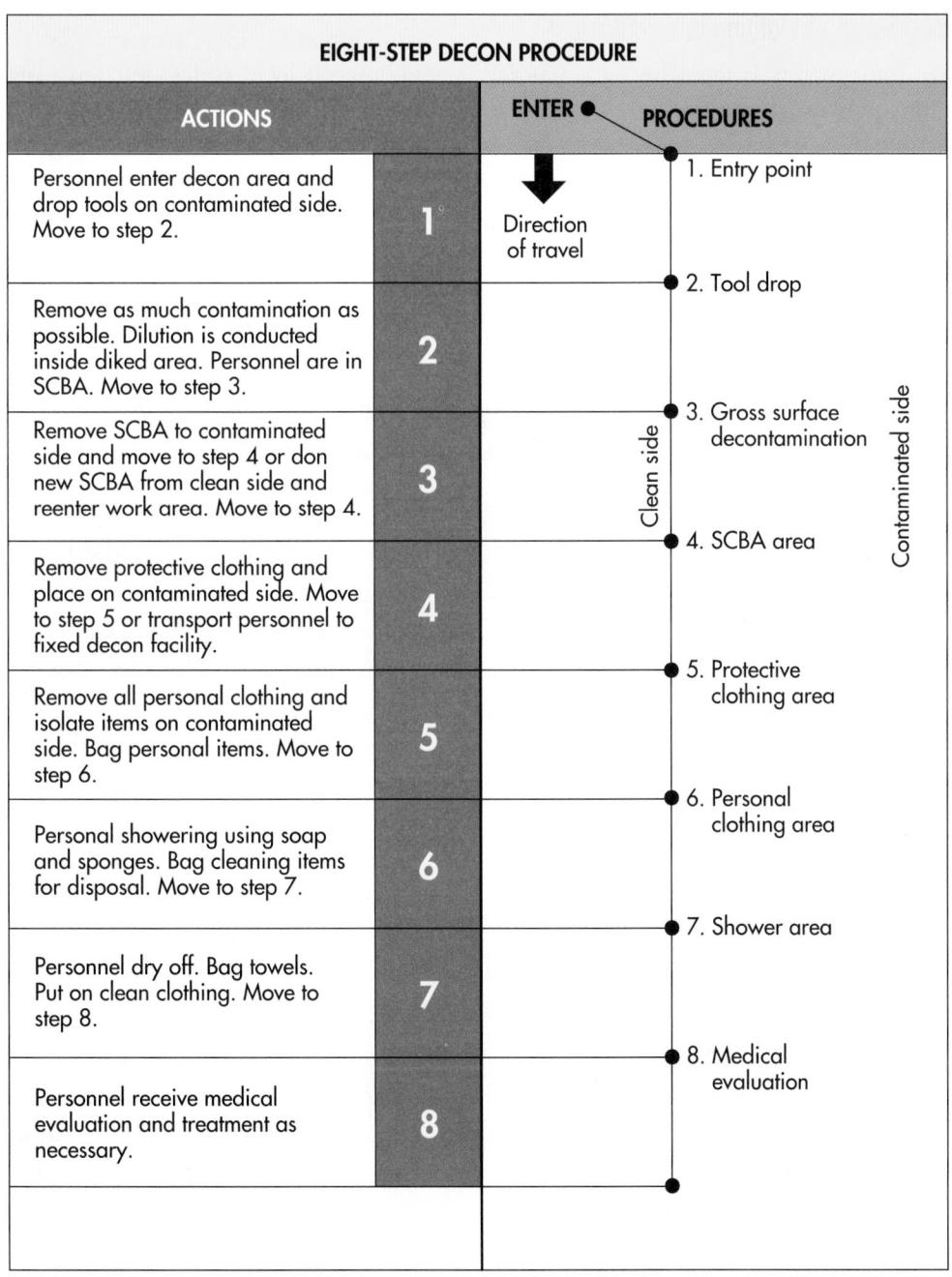

Fig. 51-9 Eight-step decontamination process.

? CRITICAL THINKING

Why do you think that extensive pre-planning and drills are needed to make this system work well?

- Avoid shaving, which might introduce contaminated material through the skin.
- Use clean drying towels after each shower.

Care and Maintenance of Clothing and Equipment

After the hazardous materials incident, the rescuer should take the following precautions:

- Properly dispose of any protective clothing that has been torn or worn through.
- Properly and thoroughly clean all clothing and equipment to avoid the possibility of chemical re-

actions at future incidents and to lessen the potential for chronic exposure to absorbed chemicals. Some hazardous materials cause chemical degradation or permeation of protective clothing and equipment. For this reason, product compatibility tables should be evaluated during the decontamination procedure. Decontamination provides no assurance that protective clothing is clean or that the process of chemical permeation has stopped.

- Do not wash or dispose of clothing or equipment at home to avoid exposing family members and contaminating home articles.
- Follow all local codes and laws regarding disposal or decontamination of equipment and clothing.
- Carefully maintain personal SCBA.

SUMMARY

- A hazardous material is any substance or material capable of posing an unreasonable risk to health, safety, and property.

- The Superfund Amendments and Reauthorization Act of 1986 established requirements for federal, state, and local governments and industry regarding emergency planning and the reporting of hazardous materials–related incidents. In 1989 OSHA and the EPA published rules to govern training requirements, emergency plans, medical checkups, and other safety precautions for workers at uncontrolled hazardous waste sites and those responding to hazardous chemical spills. In addition, the NFPA has published standards that address competencies for EMS personnel at Hazmat scenes.

- The two methods used to identify hazardous materials are informal product identification (visual, olfactory, and verbal clues) and formal product identification (e.g., placards, shipping papers). Resources for hazardous materials reference include the *North American Emergency Response Guidebook,* regional poison control centers, CHEMTREC, CHEMTEL, and CAMEO.

- It is important that anyone dealing with hazardous materials take precautionary measures, including using the appropriate respiratory devices and wearing protective clothing. Because protective clothing is constructed of a variety of materials designed specifically for certain chemical exposures, manufacturers' guidelines and specifications must be followed.

- Hazardous materials may enter the body through inhalation, ingestion, injection, and absorption. Internal damage to the human body from hazardous materials exposure may involve the respiratory tract, CNS, or other internal organs. Chemicals producing internal damage include irritants, asphyxiants, nerve poisons, anesthetics, narcotics, hepatotoxins, cardiotoxins, nephrotoxins, neurotoxins, and carcinogens.

- Exposure to hazardous materials may result in burns and severe tissue damage.

- The first agency to arrive at the scene of a hazardous materials incident must detect and identify the materials involved, assess the risk of exposure to rescue personnel and others, consider the potential risk of fire or explosion, gather information from on-site personnel or other sources, and confine and control the incident.

- A Hazmat medical monitoring program may include medical examination for members of Hazmat response teams, providing medical care, record-keeping, and periodic evaluation of the surveillance program.

- The primary goals of decontamination are to reduce the patient's dosage of material, decrease the threat of secondary contamination, and reduce the risk of rescuer injury.

- Rescuers should follow strict protocols for proper decontamination of themselves, their clothing, and any contaminated equipment.

◼ REFERENCES

1. General Services Administration, National Archives and Records Service, Office of the Federal Register: *Code of federal regulations*, 49 CFR, 173.500, parts 100-177, Washington, DC, 1981, The Administration.
2. Dickinson E: *Fire service emergency care*, International Fire Service Training Association, Upper Saddle River, NJ, 1999, Brady/Prentice Hall.
3. National Safety Council: *Injury facts*, Itasca, Ill, 1999 edition, The Council.
4. *Hazardous waste operations and emergency response standards*, 29 CFR, 1910.120, Washington, DC, 1989, The Administration.
5. National Fire Protection Association: *Standard for competencies for EMS personnel responding to hazardous materials incidents*, NFPA 473 (rev 1997), Quincy, Mass, The Association.
6. U.S. Department of Transportation, National Highway Traffic Safety Administration: *EMT-Paramedic national standard curriculum*, Washington, DC, 1998, The Department.
7. U.S. Department of Health and Human Welfare, Occupational Safety and Health Administration: *General description and discussion of the levels of protection and protective gear*, 20 CFR, 1926.65, App B, Washington, DC, 1994, The Administration.
8. Noll G et al: *Hazardous materials: managing the incident*, Stillwater, Okla, 1988, Fire Protection Publications.
9. U.S. Department of Transportation: *North American emergency response guidebook*, Washington, DC, 1999, The Department.

52 Crime Scene Awareness

OBJECTIVES

Upon completion of this chapter, the paramedic student will be able to:

1. **Describe general techniques for detection of and response to a violent scene.**
2. **Outline techniques for recognizing and responding to potentially dangerous residential calls.**
3. **Outline techniques for recognizing and responding to potentially dangerous calls on the highway.**
4. **Describe signs of danger and EMS response to violent street incidents.**
5. **Identify characteristics of and EMS response to situations involving gangs, clandestine drug labs, and domestic violence situations.**
6. **Outline general safety tactics that EMS personnel may use when a dangerous situation is encountered.**
7. **Describe special EMS considerations when providing tactical patient care.**
8. **Discuss EMS documentation and evidence preservation considerations at a crime scene.**

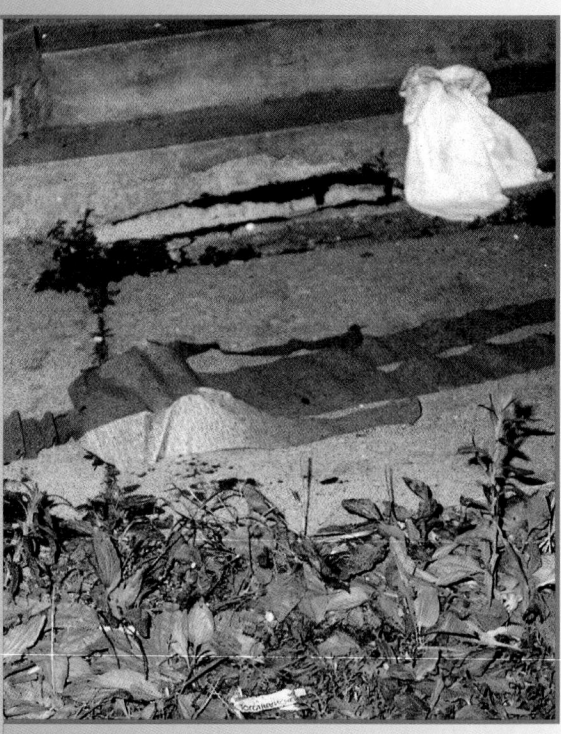

Many violent crimes require an EMS response, and often EMS crews arrive at the scene before law enforcement personnel. Therefore hazard awareness control and avoidance are issues of concern for emergency responders. Although national studies have reported a decline in violent crimes in recent years, violence against EMS personnel that arises from street gangs, threat groups, domestic disputes, and drug users is on the rise.[1,2] Personal safety and crime scene awareness must be the number one priority on every emergency call of this nature.

KEY TERMS

avoidance: The act of keeping away from; requires the paramedic to continually be aware of the scene by being observant and knowledgeable of warning signs that may indicate a dangerous situation.

concealment: To hide or put out of site; provides no ballistic protection.

cover: A type of concealment that hides the body and offers ballistic protection.

crime scene: A location where any part of a criminal act has occurred, or a location where evidence relating to a crime may be found.

distraction: A self-defense measure that creates diversion in a person's attention.

evasive tactics: A self-defense measure in which the moves and actions of an aggressor are anticipated and unconventional pathways are used during retreat for personal safety.

tactical EMS: EMS personnel who are specially trained and equipped to provide prehospital emergency care in tactical environments.

tactical patient care: Patient-care activities that occur inside the scene perimeter or "hot zone."

tactical retreat: Leaving the scene when danger is observed or when violence or indicators of violence are displayed; requires immediate and decisive action.

Approaching the Scene

Determining personal safety is an integral part of analyzing the scene. It begins before arrival at the scene with information provided by a dispatching center (see the box on p. 1456). *A key point in ensuring personal safety is to identify and respond to dangers before they threaten.* Information that may be available from a dispatching center that should alert the EMS crew to possible dangers include known locations of unsafe scenes (e.g., through computer aided dispatch systems) and/or the presence of the following:

- Large crowds
- People under the influence of alcohol or other drugs
- On-scene violence
- Weapons

Other information can sometimes be gathered en route to the scene from crew members and other emergency responders monitoring the call who have had previous experience with a particular area or address. The paramedic also should be aware of additional inherent hazards that may exist at the scene. Examples include downed power lines, busy roadways, toxic substances, the potential for fire, dangerous pets, and vehicle hazards and dangers. If the scene cannot be rendered safe, the EMS crew should retreat and stage at a safe location to await the arrival of law enforcement and/or other rescuers.

TRICKS OF THE TRADE

Dogs are not the only dangerous pets that may be encountered. Venomous snakes, exotic reptiles, and farm animals also can inflict serious injuries.

When responding to a scene with a potential for danger, the EMS crew should begin observation several blocks from the scene and use audible and visual warning devices appropriate for the call. For example, responding with audio and visual warning (AVW) devices to an urban scene may draw a crowd of bystanders; lights generally are required for safety at highway scenes. When possible, joint fire-EMS-law enforcement response postures should be defined with preplanning (e.g., fire-EMS response with full use of AVW devices; law enforcement responding without AVW devices and at normal speed) (see Chapter 48).

Scene safety considerations for all forms of danger must continue throughout the EMS response. A scene that has been made safe can become unsafe (even in the presence of police) if violence resumes, crowds gather or turn violent, or additional persons enter the scene. Violence against EMS personnel also may arise when they are mistaken for police because of uniform colors or badges, or when they exit an

TERRORISM IN THE UNITED STATES

The U.S. Code and the Federal Bureau of Investigation (FBI) define terrorism as "the unlawful use of force or violence against persons or property to intimidate or coerce a government, the civilian population, or any segment thereof, in furtherance of political or social objectives."* Most terrorist incidents in the United States have been bombing attacks, involving detonated and undetonated explosive devices, tear gas, and pipe and fire bombs. The possibility for chemical and biological warfare also is a concern.

In 1997 the FBI recorded 2 terrorist incidents, 2 suspected terrorist incidents, and 21 terrorist preventions. These included letter bombs that were mailed to the United States with Alexandria, Egypt, postmarks in holiday greeting cards; bomb explosions at a women's health facility in Atlanta, Georgia; a bombing at an alternative lifestyle nightclub in Atlanta, Georgia; and planned attacks of terrorism that were thwarted by authorities. Other major incidents in the United States that were thought to result from terrorism in recent years include the following:

1996: A bomb exploded in Atlanta's Centennial Olympic Park, killing one person and injuring 111. Authorities believe the bombing may have been linked to two later attacks in Atlanta (described above).

Federal agents arrested Theodore Kaczynski, a 53-year-old Harvard University graduate and former mathematics professor at the University of California at Berkeley who later confessed to the Unabomber attacks that killed 3 people and wounded 23 others in 16 separate bombing incidents in the United States from 1978 to 1995.

1995: A Minneapolis jury convicted four members of a domestic extremist group of violating the Biological Weapons Anti-Terrorism Act of 1989 for manufacturing the biological agent ricin with the intent to kill law enforcement officers.

1995: A truck bomb destroyed the Alfred P. Murrah Federal Building in Oklahoma City, Oklahoma, killing 168 citizens and injuring hundreds. Timothy McVeigh was convicted of the crime. (This attack was the deadliest terrorist event ever committed on U.S. soil.)

1993: A bombing in the parking garage of the World Trade Center in New York City resulted in the deaths of six people and thousands of injuries. A group of Islamic extremists was later arrested.

The effects of terrorism can vary significantly from loss of life and injuries to property damage and disruptions in services such as electricity, water supply, public transportation, and communications. Public service personnel should learn about the nature of terrorism and prepare to deal with terrorist incidents by adapting many of the same techniques used to prepare for other crises.

* From *Terrorism in the United States,* http://www.fbi.gov/publish/terror/terr97.pdf

emergency vehicle that has AVW devices. The paramedic crew must be familiar with local protocols when intervening in violent situations and have a strategic escape plan ready in case it is needed.

? CRITICAL THINKING

Why isn't it always possible to identify a dangerous scene before arrival?

Known Violent Scenes

If the scene is known to be violent, the EMS crew should remain at a safe and out-of-sight distance from the area until it has been secured ("out of site–out of scene"). Remaining at a safe staging area away from a violent scene is important for several reasons:

- If you can be seen, people will come to you.
- Entering an unsafe scene adds another potential victim(s).
- You may be injured or killed.
- You may become a hostage.
- You may become another patient in a scene that is already a multiple-casualty incident.

NOTE

It must be stressed that if the scene is determined to be unsafe, the EMS crew should retreat to a staging area and wait for adequate resources that can provide scene safety.

The Dangerous Residence

An emergency response to a residence is an everyday occurrence for most EMS providers. However, even calls that appear "routine" require a size-up that begins before exiting the emergency vehicle. Warning signs of danger in residential calls include the following:

- Past history of problems or violence
- Known drug or gang area
- Loud noises (e.g., screams, items breaking, possible gunshots)
- Seeing or hearing acts of violence
- The presence of alcohol or other drug use
- Evidence of dangerous pets (e.g., exotic snakes and reptiles, vicious breeds of dogs)
- Unusual silence or darkened residence

If any of these or other warning signs of danger are present, the EMS crew should retreat from the scene and call for law enforcement assistance.

During an approach to a suspicious residence, the EMS crew should choose tactics that match the threat or situation. For example, avoiding the use of AVW devices, using unconventional pathways (versus a sidewalk, for example) and avoiding a position between the ambulance lights and residence (backlighting) are safety measures that should be considered. In addition, paramedics should listen for signs of danger before announcing their presence or before entering the home, and stand on the side of the entry door opposite the hinges (doorknob side). When actual danger becomes evident, paramedics should immediately retreat from the scene.

TRICKS OF THE TRADE

NEVER stand in front of the door when knocking or ringing the doorbell.

Dangerous Highway Encounters

Like calls to residences, an emergency response to a traffic incident should never be considered routine. In addition to the inherent dangers associated with traffic flow, emergency vehicle positioning, and extrication, a danger of violence may exist. For example, occupants may be armed, wanted, or fleeing felons, intoxicated or drugged, or violent and abusive from an altered mental state.

TRICKS OF THE TRADE

When working in a trafficway, always wear reflective clothing and ensure that you are able to exit the scene quickly and safely if required.

When approaching a vehicle, a one-person approach is recommended.[2] This allows the partner who remains in the ambulance (which is elevated and provides greater visibility), to notify dispatch of the situation, location, license plate number, and state registration of suspicious vehicles. At nighttime, ambulance lights should be used to illuminate the interior of the vehicle and surrounding area.

TRICKS OF THE TRADE

Before approaching a vehicle, consider using the PA system to get a response from passengers in the car.

The paramedic who approaches the car should do so from the passenger side of the vehicle. This provides protection from vehicular traffic and usually is the opposite approach that a driver would expect from law enforcement personnel. Another safety precaution is not to walk between the ambulance and other vehicle (to avoid being trapped and injured if the vehicle backs up) and walking around the rear of the ambulance and then to the passenger side of the vehicle.

TRICKS OF THE TRADE

Open or unlatched trunks may indicate that persons are hiding or have been restrained in the compartment. If the trunk is open, slam it shut without opening it.

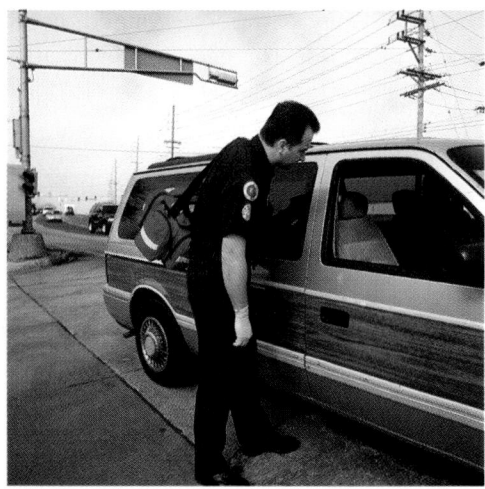

Fig. 52-1 Approach from behind post B.

Car posts A, B, and C (see Chapter 50) may provide the best ballistic protection. The paramedic should observe for unusual activity in the rear seat and not move forward of post nearest the threat unless no threats exist in these areas. The paramedic should observe the front seat from behind post B and move forward only after ensuring safety (Fig. 52-1). If warning signs of danger are present (e.g., weapons, suspicious behavior or movements in the vehicle, arguing or fighting among passengers), the paramedic should immediately retreat to a safe staging area and request law enforcement assistance.

TRICKS OF THE TRADE

If a passenger in the car is adjusting the side or rearview mirror as you approach, retreat to safety. This is a sign of trouble.

? CRITICAL THINKING

What type of EMS calls does law enforcement routinely respond to in your community?

Violent Street Incidents

Murder, assault, and robbery are common occurrences in the United States, and many of these crimes involve dangerous weapons. Violence may be directed toward EMS personnel from perpetrators at the scene (or who return to the scene), and even from injured and distraught patients. In addition, dangerous crowds and bystanders quickly can become large in number and volatile, directing violence toward everyone and everything in the surrounding area. Warning signs of potential danger in violent street incidents include the following:

- Voices that become louder
- Pushing and shoving
- Hostility toward people at the scene (e.g., perpetrator, police, victim)
- A rapid increase in the size of crowds
- The inability of law enforcement personnel to control crowds

NOTE

EMS status does not grant immunity from violent crowds.

Paramedic crews should constantly monitor crowds and retreat from the scene if necessary. When possible and when safe to do so, the patient should be removed from the scene as the crew retreats. (This may eliminate the need to return to the scene.)

Violent Groups and Situations

According to a study completed by the Department of Justice's Office of Juvenile Justice and Delinquency

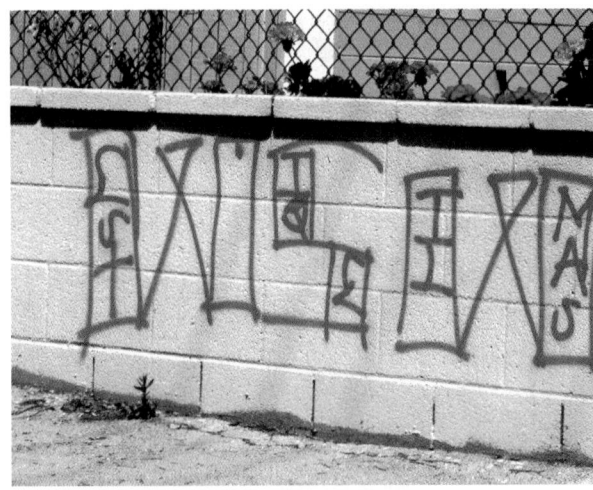

Fig. 52-2 Blood graffiti on a wall in Los Angeles. (Courtesy Lisa Taylor-Austin.)

Prevention (OJJDP), more than 665,000 gang members currently belong to more than 23,000 gangs throughout the United States[3] (see the box above). Most gangs and other threat groups operate on the premise of intimidation and extortion (Box 52-1).

Gang Characteristics

A *gang* can be defined as any group of people who engage in socially disruptive or criminal behavior. They usually are territorial, often but not always of the same gender, and operate by creating an atmosphere of fear in a community. The gang may choose a name, logo, specific color, or method of dress used for purposes of identification for their own members and their counterparts.

Graffiti and Clothing

Graffiti ("tagging") is probably the most visible sign of gang criminal activity. It can be seen in neighbor-

hood parks, the backs and side walls of stores, fences, retaining walls, and any other prominent structure that is paintable (Fig. 52-2). Gang graffiti usually marks territorial boundaries ("turf"). Gang-related clothing often is unique and specific to a group and is worn to identify affiliation and rank. Common, gang-related clothing and styles are listed in Box 52-2.

Safety Issues in Gang Areas

Gangs activities include, but are not limited to, fighting, vandalism, armed robbery, weapon offenses, auto theft, battery, and drug dealing. (Not all

BOX 52-2

Male Clothing and Styles

Shaved, bald head or extremely short hair

Tattoos (variable) and jewelry

Bandanas

White oversized T-shirt creased in the middle

White athletic type undershirt

Polo type knit shirts (oversized) and usually worn buttoned to the top and not tucked in. Oversized Dickie, Ben Davis, or Solos pants

Pants worn low, or "sagging" and cuffed inside at the bottom or dragging on the ground

Baseball caps worn backward (usually black and sometimes with the initials of the gang)

Cut-off, under-the-knee short pants worn with knee-high socks

A predominance of dark or dull clothing, or clothing of one particular color

Black stretch belt with chrome or silver gang initial belt buckle

Oversized shirts

Clothing a mixture of gang colors, black and silver or white

Female Clothing and Styles

Exaggerated use of mousse, gel, or baby oil on hair

Tattoos (variable) and jewelry

Black or dark clothing and shoes

Black oversized jackets, sweatshirts, athletic football jerseys, etc.

Oversized shirts worn outside of pants

Oversized T-shirts

Dark jackets with lettering (cursive or Old English style)

Baggy, long pants dragging on the ground

Heavy make-up, dark and excessive eyeshadow, shaved eyebrows, dark lipstick, dark fingernail polish

Tank tops or revealing blouses

Stretch belt with initial on belt buckle

gang members are engaged in illegal activities.) Criminal activity usually is committed by gang members for monetary benefit to either the gang itself or an individual member. The likelihood for these violent acts and the fact that EMS personnel often "look like" law enforcement officials require that paramedics be extremely cautious about personal safety when working in gang areas.

Clandestine Drug Labs

As described in Chapter 34, the illegal manufacture of drugs can pose significant hazards for emergency providers. Activities that take place in some clandestine drug labs include creating drugs (synthesis) from chemical precursors (e.g., LSD, methamphetamine), and changing a drug's form (conversion)—for example, converting cocaine HCl to a base form. Drug synthesis and conversion can produce oxygen-depleted atmospheres and highly explosive and toxic gases (e.g., phosgene) that can readily be absorbed through the skin in quantities that can be fatal. Toxic solvents involved in drug-making processes also can lead to lab explosions and exposure to dangerous chemicals. Other safety hazards that are associated with clandestine drug labs include "booby traps" that can maim or kill an intruder, and labs with armed or otherwise violent occupants.

> **NOTE**
>
> Clandestine labs usually are located in an area that ensures privacy. The labs generally are well ventilated and have access to water, electric, and gas utilities that are required for drug manufacturing. Suspicious persons, activities, and deliveries are often at the site.

When responding to a scene suspicious for illegal drug manufacture, the EMS crew should be alert for signs such as chemical odors and the presence of chemical equipment (e.g., glassware, chemical containers, heating mantles, burners). If a drug lab is identified, the EMS crew should do the following[2]:

1. Leave the area immediately.
2. Notify law enforcement and request appropriate agencies and personnel (e.g., Hazmat teams, fire service personnel, Drug Enforcement Administration [DEA] personnel, chemistry specialists).
3. Initiate an incident management system and Hazmat procedures (per protocol).
4. Assist law enforcement personnel to coordinate an orderly evacuation of the surrounding area for public safety.

? CRITICAL THINKING

What type of calls might EMS respond to at a drug lab?

Domestic Violence

As described in Chapter 44, *domestic violence* is violence that occurs between persons in a relationship. The perpetrator may be male or female in an opposite-sex or same-sex relationship. Domestic violence results in physical, emotional, sexual, verbal, or economic abuse, and may occur in multiple combinations. To review, many indicators of domestic violence and abuse exist, some of which include the following:

- Apparent fear of a household member
- Different or conflicting accounts by parties at the scene
- One party preventing another from speaking
- A patient who is reluctant to speak
- Injuries that do not match the reported mechanism of injury
- Unusual or unsanitary living conditions or personal hygiene

EMS personnel who respond to a scene of domestic violence should be aware that acts of violence may be directed toward them by the perpetrator and should take all safety precautions. If the scene is considered safe for the EMS crew, the paramedic should treat the patient's injuries and notify medical direction and other authorities consistent with standard operating procedures and protocol. (Mandatory reporting may be required.) To help ensure scene safety for the crew and the abused person, the paramedic should not be judgmental about the relationship nor direct accusations toward the abuser. When appropriate, the paramedic should supply the victim with phone numbers for domestic violence hotlines, community support programs, and available shelters.

Tactics for Safety

Tactics for safety include avoidance, tactical retreat, cover and concealment, and distraction and evasive maneuvers (Box 52-3). Numerous training pro-

BOX 52-3

TACTICAL CONSIDERATIONS FOR SAFETY

Avoidance
Tactical retreat
Cover and concealment
Distraction and evasive maneuvers

grams in the United States specialize in teaching tactical considerations for safety and patient care (see the box on p. 1462). A brief description of these safety tactics is provided in the following section.

Avoidance

Avoidance is always preferable to confrontation. To practice avoidance, paramedics must continually be aware of the scene by being observant and knowledgeable of warning signs that may indicate a dangerous situation. In addition, they must be knowledgeable of tactical responses to avoid danger or to deal with danger that cannot be avoided. An example of avoidance is *staging*, whereby the dispatching center learns of danger and advises the EMS crew not to approach the scene until the danger is handled and the scene is secured by appropriate authorities.

Tactical Retreat

Tactical retreat describes leaving the scene when danger is observed or when violence or indicators of violence are displayed. Tactical retreat requires immediate and decisive action. Retreat on foot or by vehicle (in a calm and safe manner) is possible by choosing the mode and route of retreat that provides the least exposure for danger. During tactical retreat, the EMS crew should be aware that the risks they faced are now located behind them and must stay alert for associated dangers. The required distance from danger for a safe tactical retreat will, of course, be guided by the nature of the incident. In general, a safe distance must accomplish the following:

- Protect the crew from any potential danger
- Keep the crew out of immediate line of sight
- Protect the crew from gunfire (cover)
- Keep the crew far enough away to react if danger reappears

TACTICAL EMS

Tactical EMS (TEMS) refers to EMS personnel who are specially trained and equipped to provide prehospital emergency care in tactical environments, such as hostage-barricaded situations, high-risk search warrants, and other adverse situations involving law enforcement and/or rescue operations where standard EMS units may be inappropriate. The concept of training EMTs and paramedics in TEMS started in the late 1980s and has expanded nationwide. Proactive law enforcement departments have adopted TEMS programs as a way to increase the safety of its Special Weapons and Tactics Team (SWAT) officers, the innocent hostage or bystander, and as a way to address liability exposure. Tactical training for EMS personnel also is recognized as a valuable tool for personal safety when EMS personnel find themselves in an unsafe situation.

A large number of tactical medical teams use the Counter Narcotics Tactical Operations Medical Support (CONTOMS) program to provide fundamental training for their personnel. CONTOMS is a joint federal program supported by the Department of Defense and the Department of Interior, with assistance from the Department of Justice and the Department of Treasury, as well as many state and local law enforcement agencies. The CONTOMS program leads to certification as an EMT-Tactic (EMT-T) or SWAT Medic. The focus of the training is to integrate the following skills to compliment an agency's standard operating procedures:

- Assess and plan for preventive medicine needs in sustained operations.
- Provide preventive medical care in sustained operations.
- Recognize and treat unique wounding patterns resulting from deliberate interpersonal aggression.
- Use medical care skills that are appropriate in hostile and austere environments.
- Explain medical and physiological parameters that lead to performance decrement and implement plans that minimize those effects.
- Develop and apply injury control strategies.
- Access and analyze medical intelligence and execute a medical threat assessment.
- Apply special law enforcement principles to the delivery of medical care.

? CRITICAL THINKING

Could the EMS crew be charged with abandonment if they make a tactical retreat and leave the patient?

Once tactical retreat has been achieved, the EMS crew must notify other responding units and agencies of the danger per interagency EMS/law enforcement standard operating procedures and agreements. (Interagency procedures regarding violent situations should be established in preplanning so that each agency is aware of specific duties and responsibilities.)

Documentation also is essential to reducing liability if injuries or deaths occur. Thorough documentation should include observations of danger at the scene; who was notified of the danger; actions at the scene; and accurate times that retreat or return to the scene occurred.

Cover and Concealment

Cover and **concealment** are means to provide protection from injury. Cover provides ballistic protection by "hiding your body" behind large and heavy structures such as large trees, telephone poles, and the vehicle's engine block. Although concealment

NOTE

Only "cover" provides ballistic protection. Cover and concealment must be used properly to help ensure personal safety.

? CRITICAL THINKING

What parts of your ambulance provide cover?

NOTE

Tactical retreat for appropriate circumstances is not considered patient abandonment.[2]

CLUES FOR VIOLENT AGGRESSION

Warning signs that can indicate impending violence from an aggressor may include a person who:
- Conspicuously ignores emergency responders
- Is verbally abusive
- Invades personal space
- Has a violent history or background
- Shifts weight from side to side or foot to foot ("Boxer stance")
- Has clenched fists
- Has tightened musculature (e.g., stiff arms and/or shoulders)
- Maintains eye contact by staring

SELF-DEFENSE MEASURES

Training in self-defense is probably appropriate for all emergency responders. Although avoidance is always superior to confrontation, some violent scenes may require self-defense. Examples include physical attacks that cannot be avoided, armed confrontation or robbery, hostage situations, and dangerous animals. In addition to methods to control a person with physical or chemical restraint (described in Chapter 38) and the use of equipment (e.g., metal clipboards, jump kits, stretchers) or other items such as furniture to block an aggressor, self-defense measures may include training in the use of pepper sprays or other chemical deterrents and defensive physical maneuvers that can allow escape. If escape cannot be achieved and the paramedic is confined in a dangerous situation (e.g., being held as a hostage), he or she should do the following:
- Remain as calm as possible
- Avoid any confrontation
- Play an active role with the captor in resolving the incident
- Focus on a peaceful resolution and escape

also hides the body, it offers little or no ballistic protection. Examples of concealment include hiding behind bushes, wallboards, and vehicle doors.

Cover and concealment should be integrated in tactical retreat or when the EMS crew is "pinned down" (e.g., by gunfire) or in other dangerous environments. When the need for cover or concealment arises, the paramedic should:

- Constantly be aware of surroundings
- Place as much of the body as possible behind adequate cover
- Constantly look for ways to improve protection and location
- Be aware of reflective clothing (e.g., trim, badges) that may draw attention or serve as a target

Distraction and Evasive Maneuvers

Distraction and **evasive tactics** can be used as self-defense measures during retreat, or when retreat and cover and concealment are not available options (see the box in the right column). For example, using equipment such as wedging a stretcher in a doorway to block an aggressor or throwing equipment to trip or slow an aggressor may provide distraction and enable the EMS crew to make a safe retreat or to gain adequate cover and concealment. Evasive tactics include anticipating moves of the aggressor and using unconventional pathways during retreat (Box 52-4).

Paramedic crews trained in **tactical EMS** often employ preassigned roles for distraction and evasive maneuvers. One paramedic usually is the "contact provider" who initiates and provides direct patient care, including patient assessment and most elements of interpersonal scene contact. Another crew member serves as the "cover provider." In a tactical context, the cover providers' role is to ensure safe cover for the contact providers while they provide patient care and to monitor the scene for danger.

NOTE

The cover provider generally avoids patient-care duties that would prevent observation of the scene. This person also may be responsible for ensuring safe-keeping of equipment, drugs, and supplies while at the scene.

Communication methods between contact and cover providers should be developed in advance that can alert team members of potential dangers without alerting the aggressor(s). This often can be accomplished with subtle verbal and nonverbal signals such as using coded terms, scratching the neck, or rubbing the nose. It is important in these situations to maintain radio contact with the dispatching center and to involve the dispatcher in the danger-signal process. For example, if the dispatcher hears a coded term that indicates danger, a priority response of appropriate personnel can be initiated.

Tactical Patient Care

Tactical patient care refers to patient-care activities that occur inside the scene perimeter or "hot zone." Providing EMS in the hot zone requires special training and authorization, body armor and a tactical uniform, compact and functional equipment, and in some operations, personal defensive weapons. Tactical EMS in the hot zone often requires risks not taken in standard EMS situations.

> **NOTE**
>
> Tactical medics provide immediate medical care to injured persons during a SWAT operation, treating them onsite or stabilizing them and extracting them from the scene. Tactical medics generally work alongside law enforcement officers. Some agencies use persons who are cross-trained in law enforcement and tactical EMS.

Body Armor

As described in Chapter 18, soft body armor (also known as *bullet-proof vests*) offers protection from some blunt and penetrating trauma. These devices are effective for most handgun bullets and most knives. However, they do not provide protection from high-velocity rifle bullets or thin or dual-edged weapons (e.g., ice picks). Like all other protective clothing, body armor is effective only when it is properly worn and when it is in good condition.

> **✓ TRICKS OF THE TRADE**
>
> Body armor is not really "bullet-proof." It provides protection by absorbing and distributing the impact of a ballistic missile or other penetrating object. Don't assume you have complete protection just because you're wearing body armor.

(Vests provide reduced protection when they are wet or worn.) A type III or higher level of protection generally is recommended for tactical EMS providers.

When wearing body armor, the paramedic should remember not to develop a false sense of security from the device. *A general rule is never attempt a maneuver that wouldn't normally be done without body armor.* In addition, the paramedic should be aware that body armor does not cover the entire body, and that severe injury can still result from the forces of cavitation (in the absence of penetration) even when the vest is properly worn.

EMS Care in the Hot Zone

As previously stated, providing EMS care in tactical situations requires special training and authorization. Most tactical medics (EMT-Ts and SWAT medics) are trained in the following[4]:

- Care under fire
- Hostage survival
- Medicine across the barricade
- Medical aspects of extended operations
- Wound ballistics, weapons, and their effects
- Medical threat assessment and medical intelligence
- Clinical forensic medicine and evidence preservation
- Toxic hazards: identification, risks, and management
- Special equipment and medical kits (design, selection, and deployment)

In addition, several hands-on laboratories are included in most training programs. Some of these training exercises include the following:

- Physical assessment under sensory deprivation/overload conditions
- Medical threat assessment
- Advanced medico-tactical techniques
- Field expedient decontamination
- New technologies for safe searches
- Management of dental injuries
- "Officer down" rescue and extraction
- Aeromedical evacuation
- Medical management of clandestine drug laboratory raids
- Safe search techniques
- Remote physical assessment

The differences in delivering patient care in dangerous environments include the frequent need to safely extract a patient(s) from the area; the frequent care of trauma patients; the need for modified care to meet tactical considerations; and medical and transport interventions that must be coordinated with the Incident Commander. Often, tactical EMS providers function under protocols and standing orders that differ from those of more "standard" EMS practice. These medical direction issues regarding patient care are dictated by the nature of the event and the uncontrolled and hazardous scene in which EMS is delivered.

> **NOTE**
>
> Awareness programs for Incident Commanders who supervise or manage personnel assigned to a tactical team and for physicians (and others) who provide medical direction for personnel operating with tactical law enforcement teams are available. Quality assurance mechanisms and direct physician involvement at the local level are recommended.

EMS at Crime Scenes

A **crime scene** can be defined as a location where any part of a criminal act has occurred, or a location where evidence relating to a crime may be found. Important physical evidence that may be found at a crime scene includes fingerprints, footprints, and blood and other body fluids. Fingerprints and footprints are unique to an individual. (No two people have identical prints.) These ridge characteristics often are left behind on a surface along with oil and moisture from the skin. Blood and other body fluids

> ✓ **TRICKS OF THE TRADE**
>
> When at a possible crime scene, *don't touch anything you don't have to.* If you do have to touch or move something to provide patient care, let authorities at the scene know about it.

can be tested for DNA and ABO blood typing and have unique characteristics that may be individual-specific. In addition, particulate evidence (e.g., hair, carpet, and clothing fibers) can provide useful information and is considered valuable at a crime scene.

The paramedic's observations at a crime scene are important and should be documented carefully on the patient care report or other appropriate form. For example, victims' positions, their injuries, and conditions at the scene may be helpful to law enforcement personnel in solving the crime. Documentation also should include any statements made by the patient or other persons at the scene and any dying declarations (see Chapter 4). The paramedic should be careful to record observations objectively; record patient's or bystanders' words in quotes; and avoid personal opinions that are not relevant to patient care. It should be remembered that patient care reports are legal documents that may be used in court.

> **NOTE**
>
> Some crime scenes may have mandatory reporting requirements. Examples include child abuse/elder abuse or neglect, domestic violence, rape, and gunshot wounds. The paramedic should observe all legal requirements and follow policy established by the EMS agency and medical direction.

Preserving Evidence

Patient care is the paramedic's ultimate priority, even at crime scenes. Evidence protection, however, can be performed while caring for the patient by not unnecessarily disturbing the scene or destroying evidence. For example, the paramedic should be observant of the scene and surroundings; touch only what is required for patient care; and wear latex gloves (for infection control and to prevent leaving additional fingerprints at the scene). Other crime scene preservation considerations are listed in Box 52-5.

> **? CRITICAL THINKING**
>
> *If paramedics' primary consideration is patient care, why should they be concerned with evidence preservation?*

BOX 52-5

CRIME SCENE PRESERVATION CONSIDERATIONS

1. Approach no crime scene until it has been secured for your safety.
2. Park your vehicle as far away as conveniently possible to preserve skid marks, tire prints, or other evidence.
3. Survey and assess the scene before proceeding to the victim.
4. Try to approach the victim from a route different from the assailant's probable route.
5. Follow the same path to and from the victim.
6. Avoid stepping on blood stains or spatter if possible.
7. Disturb the victim and the victim's clothing as little as possible while performing your assessment and during treatment.
8. When cutting the clothing from a victim, try to do it in such a manner to preserve the points of wounding.
9. Report your actions and any disturbances you make to the crime scene investigator.
10. Keep all unnecessary people away from the victim.
11. Do not smoke or eat at the crime scene.
12. Do not touch any evidence if at all possible.
13. Make no comments to bystanders about the situation.
14. Save the victim's clothes and personal items in a paper bag. The bag should be labeled, sealed, and turned over to law enforcement personnel.
15. Be aware of any dying declarations made by your patient.
16. Keep accurate, detailed records.
17. Law enforcement personnel are in charge of the crime scene. You are in charge of the patient.

From Vollrath R: Crime scene preservation: it's everybody's concern, *JEMS* 20(1):53, 1995.

SUMMARY

- A key point in ensuring scene safety is to identify and respond to dangers before they threaten. If the scene is known to be violent, the EMS crew should remain at a safe and out-of-sight distance from the area until it has been secured.

- The paramedic should look for warning signs of violence during response to a residence and retreat from the scene if danger becomes evident.

- An emergency response to a highway may present danger from violence as well as other dangers associated with traffic and extrication. Occupants may be armed, wanted or fleeing felons, intoxicated or drugged, or violent/abusive from an altered mental state.

- The paramedic should monitor for warning signs of danger in violent street incidents and retreat from the scene if necessary.

- A gang is any group of people who engage in socially disruptive or criminal behavior. Some gangs are involved in violent criminal activities. Because EMS personnel often look like law enforcement officers, they should be extremely cautious about personal safety when working in gang areas.

- Clandestine lab activities can produce explosive and toxic gases. Other risks include booby traps that can maim or kill an intruder, and armed or violent occupants.

- EMS personnel who respond to a scene of domestic violence should be aware that acts of violence may be directed toward them by the perpetrator; they should take all safety precautions.

- Tactics for safety include avoidance, tactical retreat, cover and concealment, and distraction and evasive maneuvers.

- Tactical patient care refers to patient-care activities that occur inside the scene perimeter or "hot zone." Providing care in this area requires special training and authorization, body armor and a tactical uniform, compact and functional equipment, and in some operations, personal defensive weapons.

- The paramedic's observations at a crime scene are important and should be carefully documented. Evidence protection can be performed while caring for the patient by not unnecessarily disturbing the scene or destroying evidence.

REFERENCES

1. Jacobsen B: Street smarts, *Emergency* 29(11):12, 1997.
2. U.S. Department of Transportation National Highway Traffic Safety Administration: *EMT-Paramedic national standard curriculum*, Washington, DC, 1998, The Department.
3. United States Justice Department: *Justice department helps communities combat youth gang violence*, Washington, DC, 1997, The Department.
4. CONTOMS Programs, Casualty Care Research Center, Department of Military and Emergency Medicine, Uniformed Services University of the Health Sciences, Bethesda, Md, http://www.usuhs.mil/ccr/course.html.

Appendix A
Development Through the Lifespan

Paramedics provide care to patients of all age groups, and patient complaints often are unique to their age group from a developmental standpoint. This appendix outlines norms that are to be expected at different ages in both physiological and psychosocial development.

> **NOTE**
>
> These age classifications and development characteristics defined in the National Standard Curriculum for EMT-Paramedic are "general" descriptions for lifespan development and may differ slightly from other references in this and other textbooks.

Infancy

The term *infant* is used for children 28 days to 1 year of age. For children younger than 28 days of age, the correct term is *neonate*. *Newborn* is used to describe an infant in the first few hours of life.

Vital signs (averages)

- Heart rate
  - First 30 minutes of life: 100 to 200 beats/min
  - By 1 year of age: 120 beats/min
- Respiration
  - At birth: 40 to 60 breaths per minute, dropping to 30 to 40 breaths per minute within a few minutes; tidal volume is 6 to 8 mL/kg.
  - By 1 year of age: 25 breaths per minute; tidal volume is 10 to 15 mL/kg.
  - PCO_2, PO_2, and pH reach normal limits a few hours after birth.
- Temperature: 98° to 100° F (36° C to 37.6° C)
- Blood pressure: Average systolic blood pressure increases from 70 at birth to 90 at 1 year

- Weight
  - Normally 3.0 to 3.5 kg at birth
  - Normally drops 5% to 10 % in the first week of life due to excretion of extracellular fluid
  - Exceed birth weight by second week
  - Grows at approximately 30 g/day during the first month
  - Should double weight by 4 to 6 months
  - Should triple weight at 9 to 12 months
  - Infant's head equal to 25% of the total body weight

Review by body systems

Cardiovascular system

- Soon after birth, systemic vascular resistance increases, and pulmonary vascular resistance decreases.
- During the first year of life, the ductus arteriosus, ductus venosus, and foramen ovale close and the left ventricle becomes stronger.

Respiratory system

- Breathing occurs primarily through the nose during the first month of life.
- The infant's short, narrow airways are less stable than those of adults, and the trachea is bifurcated at a high level.
- Accessory muscles remain underdeveloped. The normal practice of using these muscles for breathing increases the infant's susceptibility to lactic acidosis.
- Collateral ventilation is decreased because the number of alveoli are diminished.
- The principal support for the chest wall comes from muscles rather than bones.
- During infections, the infant breathes more rapidly, quickly losing heat and fluids.

Sensorineural

- During the first 12 months, the infant will suddenly extend and abduct the extremities (Moro reflex) and flex the hands in the palmar grasp response.
- In response to facial stimulation, the infant makes sucking movements (sucking response) and turns the head to one side and sucks (rooting reflex).

Skeletal system

- At infant's head comprises 25% of total body weight, and the muscles comprise 25%.
- Fontanelles close, first the posterior one at 3 months of age and then the anterior one between 9 and 18 months of age. Evaluation of the fontanelles may reveal clues to intracranial events during this time.
- The epiphyseal plate lengthens and bones thicken as new layers are deposited on existing bone.
- Factors influencing bone growth include growth hormone, genetics, thyroid hormone, and the child's general health status.

Immune system

- Passive immunity retained through the first 6 months of life
- Based on maternal antibodies

Nervous system

- Movements
  - Strong, coordinated suck and gag
  - Well-flexed extremities
  - Extremities move equally well when infant is stimulated
- Reflexes
  - Moro reflex
  - Palmar grasp
  - Sucking reflex
  - Rooting reflex
- Fontanelles
  - Posterior fontanelle closes at 3 months
  - Anterior fontanelle closes between 9 to 18 months
  - Fontanelles may provide an indirect estimate of hydration
- Sleep
  - Initially sleeps 16 to 18 hours per day with sleep and wakefulness evenly distributed over 24 hours.
  - Gradually decreases to 14 to 16 hours per day with 9- to 10-hour concentration at night

- Sleeps through the night at 2 to 4 months
- Normal infant is easily arousable

Dental system

- Teeth begin to erupt at 5 to 7 months

Psychosocial development

- Temperament is evident in infants, particularly in the ease or difficulty required to please them. Some may be friendly, and others may warm up to strangers only slowly.
- Infants communicate with different types of cries—a cry to indicate pain, one for anger, and a basic cry used for hunger, discontent, or fatigue.
- Known as reciprocal socialization, relationships are formed between the infant and family members, with secure attachment developing between parents and child.
- Consistency of parental care is the basis for trust versus mistrust issues.
- Situational crises may lead to parental separation reactions, with infants responding in protest, despair, or withdrawal.

Toddlers and Preschoolers

Children 12 to 36 months of age generally are considered toddlers. Those 3 to 5 years of age are preschool-age children.

Vital signs (averages)

- Heart rate
  - Toddlers: 80 to 130 beats/min
  - Preschoolers: 80 to 120 beats/min
- Respiration
  - Toddlers: 20 to 30 breaths/min
  - Preschoolers: 20 to 30 breaths/min
- Temperature: 96.8° to 99.6° F (36° C to 37.6° C)
- Blood pressure
  - Toddlers: 70 to 100 mm Hg systolic
  - Preschoolers: 80 to 100 mm Hg systolic

Review of body systems

Cardiovascular system

- Capillary beds are better developed and able to assist in thermoregulation.
- Hemoglobin levels approach adult levels.

Respiratory system: Ear, nose, and throat structures are similar to those in the infant, but toddlers and preschoolers are less prone to developing infection.

Sensorineural

- Visual acuity is 20/30.
- Hearing is essentially mature by 3 to 4 years of age.
- Brain weight is 90% of adult brain weight.
- Myelination increases cognitive development.

Endocrine system

- Organs become functionally mature.
- Production of growth hormone, insulin, and corticoid increases.
- Toddlers and preschoolers gain an average 6.5 pounds per year.

Excretory system

- Kidneys are well developed.
- Specific gravity and other urinary tract findings are similar to those of adults.

Muscular system

- Walking and other basic motor skills are effortless.
- Fine motor skills develop.

Lymphatic system

- The passive immunity of infancy is lost.
- The child becomes more susceptible to minor respiratory and gastrointestinal infections.

Psychosocial development

Individual development

- Basic language skills are mastered by 3 years of age, with refinement continuing through childhood.
- Toddlers and preschoolers begin to recognize the differences between the sexes and start the process of modeling themselves after persons of their own gender.

Family, peer group, and societal development

- The parents' style of parenting begins to have effects on the child.
- Sibling rivalry begins.
- Firstborn children usually maintain a special relationship with their parents and are expected to exhibit self-control and responsibility when interacting with younger siblings.

- The effects of divorce on toddlers and preschoolers are mediated by several factors, including age, cognitive and social competencies, sense of dependence on or independence from parents, type of day care that they attend, and the parents' ability to respond to the child's needs.
- Within the peer group, interactions with others near the same age and level of maturity occur.
- The peer group provides a source of information about the world outside of the immediate family, exposing the child to other types of families.
- The importance of the peer group increases throughout childhood.
- Toddlers and preschoolers develop the ability to play simple games and follow basic rules.
- Competitiveness in play begins.
- The child may display frustrations during play that are not expressed in other situations.
- Viewing violence on television during this age may cause aggressiveness. Careful parental screening of television shows for children in their toddler or preschool years is recommended.

School-Age Children

Children are considered school-age from 6 to 12 years of age.

Vital signs (averages)

- Heart rate: 70 to 110 beats/min
- Respiration: 20 to 30 breaths/min
- Temperature: 98.6° F (37° C)
- Blood pressure: 80 to 120 mm Hg systolic

Review of body systems

Sensorineural: Brain function increases in both hemispheres.

Reproductive system: The reproductive system becomes active when the child reaches puberty.

Skeletal system: Average gain in height is 2.5 inches per year.

Lymphatic system: Lymphatic tissues are proportionately larger than in adults.

Other: Most bodily functions reach adult levels during this time.

Psychosocial development

Individual development

- As interactions with adults and other children increase, the child begins to compare himself or herself with others, thus developing a self-concept.
- Self-esteem tends to be higher during the early years of school age than during later ones.
- Self-esteem is often based on external characteristics.
- A negative self-esteem at this time can produce damage in later development.
- The child develops moral discrimination using preconventional reasoning, linking punishment with obedience and individualism with purpose.

Family, peer group, and societal development

- In the family setting, the child is allowed more self-regulation in activities, although parents still exercise general supervision.
- Usually parents begin spending less time with the child.
- Self-esteem is affected by popularity with peers, rejection experiences, emotional support, and neglect factors.
- The child uses convention reasoning, developing interpersonal norms for behavior and adopting the morality of the social system.
- Using postconventional reasoning, the child can understand community rights versus individual rights and universal ethical principles.

Adolescents

Adolescents are generally 13 to 18 years of age.

Vital signs (averages)

- Heart rate: 55 to 105 beats/min
- Respiration: 12 to 20 breaths/min
- Temperature: 98.6° F (37° C)
- Blood pressure: 100 to 120 mm Hg systolic

Review of body systems

Cardiovascular system: Blood chemistry values are nearly equal to adult levels.

Endocrine system:

- The amount of body fat decreases early in adolescence and then begins to increase in later years.
- The skin toughens through sebaceous gland activity.

In females:

- Follicle-stimulating hormone and luteinizing hormone are released.
- Gonadotropin promotes estrogen and progesterone production.
- Other biologic changes occur, such as the development of secondary sexual characteristics.
- Before menarche occurs, the girl must have fat levels that are 18% to 20% of her body weight.

In males: Gonadotropin promotes testosterone production.

Reproductive system: The adolescent reaches reproductive maturity.

Muscular system: The growth of muscle mass is nearly complete.

Skeletal system:

- Bone growth is nearly complete.
- There is generally a rapid 2- to 3-year growth spurt during this stage.

Psychosocial development

Individual development

- Development of identity progresses through various stages based on crisis management and other factors.
- Antisocial behavior peaks at about the eighth or ninth grade level.
- Drug use begins.
- Depression and suicide are more common among adolescents than in any other age group.

Family, peer group, and societal development

- Body image is of great concern, with continual comparisons being made among peers.
- Eating disorders are common.
- Ethnic adolescents tend to have more identity crises than do nonethnic adolescents.

Early adulthood

Early adulthood spans from 20 to 40 years of age.

Vital signs (averages)

- Heart rate: 70 beats/min
- Respiration: 16 to 20 breaths/min
- Temperature: 98.6° F (37° C)
- Blood pressure: 120/80 mm Hg

Review of body systems

Reproductive system: Pregnancy is most likely in this age group.

General

- Peak physical condition is achieved between 19 and 26 years of age.
- Lifelong habits and routines develop.
- Body systems are at optimal performance.
- Injuries are the leading cause of death.

Psychosocial development

Individual development: Fewer psychological problems related to well-being exist during this period than during any other.

Family, peer group, and societal development

- The capacity for romantic and affectionate love develops.
- Newly formed families provide new challenges and stress.
- The highest levels of job stress are experienced.

Middle adulthood

Middle adulthood spans from 41 to 60 years of age.

Vital signs (averages)

- Heart rate: 70 beats/min
- Respiration: 16 to 20 breaths/min
- Temperature: 98.6° F (37° C)
- Blood pressure: 120/80 mm Hg

Review of body systems

Cardiovascular system

- Cardiovascular health becomes a concern.
- Cardiac output decreases throughout the period.
- Cholesterol levels increase.

Sensorineural

- Vision changes occur.
- Hearing is less keen.

Endocrine system: Weight control becomes more difficult.

Reproductive system: In women, menopause may occur between the late forties and the early fifties.

Lymphatic system: Cancer strikes frequently in this age group.

Other: Body systems continue to function at a high level, with varying degrees of deterioration.

Psychosocial development

Individual development

- Middle adults are task oriented.
- Middle adults have a sense of time pressure to accomplish lifelong goals.
- Middle adults approach problems more as challenges than as threats.

Family, peer group, and societal development

- Middle adults are concerned with the "social clock."
- The "empty nest" syndrome occurs.
- Common stressors are financial commitments and responsibility for the care of elderly parents and young adult children.

Late adulthood

Persons reach late adulthood at 61 years of age and over.

Vital signs (averages)

- Heart rate, respiration, and blood pressure become dependent on health status.
- Temperature: 98.6° F (37° C)

Review of body systems

Cardiovascular system

Blood vessels

- Functional changes occur as blood vessels thicken and peripheral resistance increases.

- Blood flow to the organs decreases.
- Baroreceptor sensitivity is reduced.
- By 80 years of age, vessel elasticity declines by about 50%.

Heart

- The heart's increased workload causes cardiomegaly, changes in the mitral and aortic valves, and decreased myocardial elasticity.
- The myocardium is less able to respond to exercise.
- Fibrous tissue develops in the sinoatrial node.
- The number of pacemaker cells diminishes, resulting in dysrhythmias.
- Tachycardia is not well tolerated.

Blood cells

- The functional blood volume and platelet count decrease.
- The number of red blood cells diminishes.
- Iron levels are poor.

Respiratory system

- Changes occur in the mouth, nose, and lungs.
- In responses to metabolic changes, lung function decreases and lung capacity diminishes.
- The elasticity of the diaphragm declines.
- The chest wall weakens.
- Diffusion through the alveoli diminishes as a result of lifelong exposure to pollutants.
- Coughing is ineffective because of the weakened chest wall and bone structure.

Gastrointestinal system

- Changes affect the mouth, teeth, and saliva.
- Peristalsis and gastrointestinal secretions decrease.
- The esophageal sphincter is less effective, and internal intestinal sphincters lose tone.
- Vitamin and mineral deficiencies occur.

Sensorineural

- Some taste buds are lost, and the olfactory sense diminishes.
- Pain perception decreases.
- The kinesthetic sense is lessened.
- Visual acuity diminishes.
- Reaction time declines.
- Presbycusis problems with hearing occur.
- Neurons are lost, and neurotransmitters diminish in number.
- The sleep-wake cycle is disrupted.

Endocrine system

- Glucose metabolism and insulin production decreases.
- The thyroid gland shows some diminished T3 production.
- The production of cortisol falls by about 25%.
- The pituitary gland is about 20% less effective than in earlier years.

Reproductive system: Women's reproductive glands atrophy.

Excretory system

- In the kidney, 50% of the nephrons are lost.
- Abnormal glomeruli are more common than at earlier ages.
- The frequency and quantity of elimination decrease.

Other

- The maximum known life span is 120 years.

Psychosocial development

Individual development

- The "terminal drop" hypothesis says that there will be a decrease in cognitive functioning over a 5-year period preceding the individual's death.
- Generally the individual's sense of well-being declines.
- Maintaining a sense of self-worth can be challenging.

Family, peer group, and societal development

- Financial burdens on the family are common.
- The death or dying of companions is a significant issue.
- The societal attitude toward age can either enhance or detract from the individual's sense of self-worth. Some cultures attribute wisdom to age, whereas others feel that the elderly are a burden.
- Approximately 95% of older adults live in communities, with only about 5% in care facilities.

DEVELOPMENTAL MILESTONES (BIRTH THROUGH ADOLESCENCE)

Birth to 12 months: Growth and development should be compared with standard growth charts showing established norms.

2 months
- Tracks object with eyes
- Recognizes familiar faces

3 months: Moves objects to mouth with hands

4 months
- Drools without swallowing
- Reaches out to people

5 months
- Sleeps through the night without food
- Increases to twice birth weight

6 months
- Sits upright in highchair
- Makes one-syllable sounds (ma, mu, da, di)

7 months
- Fears strangers
- Quickly changes from crying to laughing

8 months
- Responds to "no"
- Sits without assistance

9 months
- Responds to adult anger
- Pulls self to standing position
- Explores objects by sucking, chewing, and biting

10 months
- Recognizes own name
- Crawls well

11 months
- Attempts to walk unaided
- Shows frustration at restrictions

12 months
- Walks with assistance
- Increases to three times birth weight

Toddlers and preschoolers
- Is physically capable of being toilet trained by 12 to 15 months of age
- Is psychologically ready for toilet training between 18 and 30 months of age (average age for completion of training is 28 months)

Childhood and adolescence: Individuals move through the developmental stages at different paces.

Appendix B
The Language of Medicine

The Language of Medicine

Most medical terms are derived from Greek, and many have Latin roots. Medical terms are usually composed of a word preceded by a prefix (one or more root syllables at the beginning of a word), followed by a suffix (one or more root syllables at the end of a word), or both. An understanding of the basic prefixes and suffixes promotes ease of communication with medical terminology.

Prefixes

Prefixes appear at the beginning of a medical word and often describe location and intensity. For example, *abnormal* begins with the prefix *ab*, which means "away from," and is followed by *normal*, which means "within a balance." Therefore *abnormal* describes something that is not within balance.

Suffixes

Suffixes appear at the end of a medical word and often describe the patient's condition or diagnosis. For example, *bronchitis* begins with the root word *bronchi*, which refers to a respiratory structure, and is followed by the suffix *itis*, which means "inflammation." Therefore *bronchitis* would describe inflammation of the patient's bronchi.

Root Words

Root words are medical words that may be combined to describe a particular structure or condition. For example, *cardiopulmonary* begins with a root word *cardio*, which means "heart," and is followed by the root word *pulmonary*, which means "lungs." Therefore *cardiopulmonary* refers to the patient's cardiac and respiratory systems.

COMMON PREFIXES

PREFIXES	MEANING	EXAMPLE
a-, an-	without, lack of	Apnea—without breath Anemia—lack of blood
ad-	to, toward	Adhesion—something stuck to or remaining in close proximity to
angio-	vessel	Angiogram—study of vessels
ante-	before, forward	Antenatal—occurring or formed before birth
anti-	against, opposed to	Antipyretic—against fever
arter-	artery	Arteriogram—study of arteries
arthro-	pertaining to a joint	Arthroscopy—inspection of joint
bi-	two	Bilateral—both sides
bio-	life	Biology—study of life
brady-	slow	Bradycardia—slow heart rate
cardi-	pertaining to the heart	Cardiography—recording the movements of the heart
cerebr-	brain	Cerebral—pertaining to the brain
cerv-	neck	Cervical—pertaining to the neck
chole-	pertaining to bile	Cholelithasis—stones in the gallbladder
contra-	against, opposite	Contrastimulant—against stimulating
cost-	pertaining to a rib	Costal margin—margin of lower limit of ribs
cyst-	pertaining to the bladder or any fluid-containing sac	Cystitis—inflammation of the urinary bladder
cyt-	cell	Cytology—study of cells
di-	twice, double	Diplopia—double vision
dys-	with difficulty	Dyspnea—difficulty breathing
ecto-	out from	Ectopic—out of place

COMMON SUFFIXES

SUFFIXES	MEANING	EXAMPLE
-algia	pertains to pain	Neuralgia—pain along a nerve
-centesis	puncturing	Thoracentesis—puncturing of a pleural space
-cyte	cell	Leukocyte—white cell
-ectomy	a cutting out	Tonsillectomy—surgical removal of the tonsils
-emia	blood	Anemia—decrease in blood hemoglobin
-esthesia	sensation	Anesthesia—without sensation
-genic	causing	Carcinogenic—cancer causing
-ology	science of	Psychology—science or study of behavior
-ostomy	creation of an opening	Gastrostomy—artificial opening into the stomach
-osis	condition	Psychosis—condition of the mind
-paresis	weakness	Hemiparesis—one-sided weakness
-phagia	eating	Polyphagia—excessive eating
-pnea	breathing	Dyspnea—difficult breathing
-pathy	disease	Neuropathy—disease of peripheral nerves
-phasia	speech	Aphasia—loss of speech power
-plasty	repair of, tying of	Angioplasty—repair of damaged vessels
-rhythmia	rhythm	Dysrhythmia—variation from a normal rhythm
-rrhagia	bursting forth	Hemorrhage—flowing of blood
-rrhea	flowing	Pyorrhea—discharge of pus
-scopy	examination by inspection	Laparoscopy—examination of the abdominal cavity with a laparoscope
-uria	pertaining to urine	Polyuria—excessive secretion of urine

COMMON ROOT WORDS

ROOT WORDS	MEANING	ROOT WORDS	MEANING
adeno-	gland	mal-	bad
arter-	artery	menigo-	meninges
arthro-	joint	myo-	muscle
asthenia	weakness	nephro-	kidney
bio-	life	neuro-	nerve
bucc-	cheek	noct-	night
burs-	pouch or sac	oculo-	eye
carc-	cancer	orchi-	testicle
cardio-	heart	osteo-	bone
caut-	to burn	oto-	ear
cephalo-	head	ov-	egg
cerv-	neck	pariet-	wall
chole-	bile	phago-	to eat
chondro-	cartilage	pharyngo-	throat
cysto-	bladder	phlebo-	vein
cyto-	cell	photo-	light
dermo-	skin	pneumo-	air
edem-	swelling	procto-	rectum
entero-	intestine	pseud-	false
eryth-	red	psych-	mind
eti-	cause	pyo-	pus
febr-	fever	rhino-	nose
flex-	to bend	sclero-	hardness
gastro-	stomach	sept-	wall
glyco-	sugar	somat-	body
gyn-	female	stern-	chest
hemo-	blood	tact-	to touch
hepato-	liver	thoraco-	chest
hydra-	water	uro-	urinary
iod-	distinct	varic-	dilated vein
leuko-	white	vaso-	vessel

Appendix C

Injury Prevention

Jon A. King, MS, NREMT-P*

Emergency medical services (EMS) traditionally has been a reactionary medical discipline that waits until patients are injured or ill before being used. This is termed the *acute care phase of injury control* or *tertiary injury prevention*. Although EMS excels in acute care, a comprehensive system of injury control is comprised of several facets of which acute care is but one. The injury control strategy of preventing rather than simply treating an injury is known as *primary injury prevention*.

Preventive strategies produce better outcomes than treatment strategies in terms of lives saved and money spent. The success of these strategies depends heavily on data collection and providing injury prevention information to patients. Since communities respect paramedics and generally welcome them into homes and businesses, they have a unique opportunity to identify injury patterns and intervene on behalf of people at risk. The basic concepts of injury prevention and the role that paramedics can play are presented in this appendix.

Injury Concepts

Definition of Injury

A confounding factor that hindered the study of injury and therefore injury prevention was the seeming unrelatedness of different injuries. On the surface, it appeared that there was no relationship between a motor vehicle crash and a poisoning or between a gunshot wound and a drowning. However, it now is known that all injuries are the result of either (1) tissue damage caused by the transfer of energy (mechanical, thermal, electrical, chemical, or

radiation) to the body or (2) tissue damage due to the absence of necessary energy elements, such as heat or oxygen.

Injury Triangle and Haddon's Matrix

Injury is also a disease process. The three factors that are necessary to cause a disease are host, agent, and environment. Together, these factors are known as the *injury triangle*. In the injury triangle, the host is the victim; the agent of injury is energy; and the environment provides a place for the agent and host to come together over time. The actual injury event may take only a fraction of a second, but the events that lead up to an injury and the events that occur as a result of an injury may take place over seconds, minutes, and even months or years.

In the mid-1960s, William Haddon (the "father" of injury prevention) developed an analytical tool (now called *Haddon's matrix*) to aid in understanding the entire injury sequence. The three factors of the injury triangle are placed on a timeline that is divided into three phases: pre-event, event, and post-event. For example, the Haddon's matrix in Table C-1 charts the events that may occur before, during, and after an automobile crash. The table makes it possible to see that injuries often result from a predictable and therefore preventable chain of events and that most injuries are associated with multiple causes.

The *pre-event phase* is the period before the release of injury-causing energy. During this time the person's performance is greater than the task demands and energy is under control. Events in this phase tend to influence the *likelihood* that an injury will occur. Since the injury has yet to occur, primary injury prevention can be successful in this phase. The time frame can be seconds to years, depending on what events come into play to cause the injury.

*Director of EMS Training, Emergency Medicine Research Center, Department of Emergency Medicine, Emory University School of Medicine, Atlanta, GA.

TABLE C-1	HADDON'S MATRIX FOR AUTOMOBILE CRASHES		
	FACTOR		
PHASE	**HOST**	**AGENT**	**ENVIRONMENT**
Pre-Event	Impaired capabilities, age, fatigue, alcohol/drug use, driving experience, adherence to driving laws	Defective equipment, dirty windows, improper maintenance, equipment design	Road shoulder too narrow, poor lighting, weather conditions, highway not divided, inadequate notification signs, road design, and construction
Event	Injury threshold due to aging, chronic disease, alcohol, use of restraints, ejection	Failure of doors, impact with sharp objects in the vehicle, vehicle size	Lack of guardrails, large trees near roadside, oncoming traffic
Post-Event	Type or extent of injury, knowledge of first aid, alcohol	Bursting gas tanks, entrapment	Quality of rescue, EMS, hospitals, rehabilitation

The *event phase* is the period during which the person's performance falls below the demands of the task. The result is the release of uncontrolled energy. The time frame usually is a fraction of a second to very few minutes. Events in this phase affect the transmission of energy. *Secondary injury prevention* recognizes that injuries are going to occur and is centered on reducing the severity of the injury as it is occurring.

The *post-event phase* is the period after the injury has occurred. It can last from a few seconds to years. In this time frame, tertiary injury prevention takes place and traditional EMS exists. Tertiary injury prevention's focus is to lessen the long-term adverse effects of the injury.

Three Es of Injury Prevention

Three broad techniques have traditionally been used to establish injury prevention programs. The three Es of injury prevention are education, enforcement, and engineering. A proactive, prevention-oriented EMS professional can play an important role in all three prevention strategies.

Education

The purpose of education is to persuade high-risk individuals or groups to change hazardous behavior or adopt safety precautions, such as using personal restraints or wearing crash helmets. Education is considered an active countermeasure because it requires the person to do something (change behavior) to take advantage of the knowledge learned. Education is the most commonly used approach in injury prevention and is most effective when used in combination with enforcement and engineering.

Enforcement

Enforcement requires, through force of law, that persons adopt a particular risk-reducing behavior. Mandatory seat belt and motorcycle helmet use laws are examples of this approach. Like education, enforcement is considered an active countermeasure because it requires the person to adhere to the law in order to benefit from it. The effectiveness of this approach depends on compliance of individuals and the ability to enforce these laws. Even so, enforcement is more effective than education alone.

Engineering

Engineering refers to product or environmental design that automatically provides protection or decreases the likelihood that an injury-producing incident will occur. This approach builds safety into a product so that a person does not have to do anything to benefit from it (a passive countermeasure). Examples include air bags in automobiles and sprinkler systems in buildings. Engineering has proven to be the most effective of the three Es but also is the most expensive approach to undertake.

Implementation of Injury Prevention Roles in EMS

A review of medical literature has already identified nine possible EMS-centered injury prevention activities. Others will most certainly be developed as the role of EMS providers expands into injury prevention.

Prevent Injuries in EMS Providers

Organizations should develop formal injury prevention programs for their own employees. Some already employ safety and risk officers whose sole job is to educate, enforce, and engineer injury prevention *within* an EMS organization. Injury prevention must start at home. As stressed throughout this text, no one is more important at the scene of an emergency response than the EMS provider.

Serve as Role Models

A paramedic's appearance and the specialized equipment used in emergency care make the paramedic an expert in many people's eyes. By practicing injury prevention personally (e.g., wearing seat belts or washing hands after every call), the paramedic sets an example for others to follow.

Identify Persons at Risk

When caring for a person in his or her home, the paramedic is in a unique position to recognize persons at risk for injury (or repeat of injury). Programs are available to train providers in identifying high-risk individuals, high-risk behavior, or high-risk environments so that those at risk can be referred to community agencies (e.g., Family and Children's Services or area hospitals) that can help with a particular problem.

Provide Prevention Counseling

Serious and life-threatening calls do not allow for prevention counseling. However, a significant proportion of calls results in nontransport or little or no treatment while en route to the hospital and provides a teachable moment. During these calls, one-on-one prevention counseling lasting 30 to 60 seconds is a possibility.

Collect Injury Data

Paramedics are in an enviable position to gather injury-causing data as part of a scene assessment and patient history. The paramedic can use the documentation of the data in two ways: (1) immediately by other emergency personnel who can reinforce and supplement the paramedic's initial on-scene education and (2) by other community injury prevention professionals as part of their data collection process. Paramedics may be the only ones who can gather certain types of information that are necessary to develop the most beneficial programs.

Survey Residences and Institutions

High-risk environments increase the chance that an injury will occur. Paramedics can perform a quick scene survey to identify hazards that are dangerous to a patient at home. Paramedics also are in a prime position to visit business and industry to perform more detailed surveys as part of an internal injury prevention program.

Conduct Educational Programs and Media Campaigns

Organizations exist in every community (e.g., parent-teacher associations, civic groups, neighborhood associations) that want to hear what medical experts have to say. A speakers' bureau can be set up within an EMS organization to provide prevention information when called upon. It provides a public relations tool for the organization and an opportunity to pass along valuable information to a willing audience.

Advocate Legislative Change

Paramedics can lend their voices as health care experts when a law or regulation is in the discussion and debate process. Paramedics have a place in creating laws and building safety into a product by serving as medical experts and advocates for their patients during development of legal issues that have the opportunity to save lives.

Conclusion

For the most part, injury causation has been tied to the belief that it is the result of "accident" or "bad

BOX C-1

A SAMPLING OF INJURY PREVENTION STRATEGIES*

Children
  Children safety programs
  Safe kids programs
  Child safety seat programs
  EMS-C programs
  Safe schools programs
  Drowning prevention programs
  Parenting classes
  Child abuse prevention programs
  Playground safety programs
  Youth advocacy groups
  Swimming classes
  Baby sitter training classes
Public driving
  Running red light prevention program
  Buckle up programs
  Anti-DWI programs
Elderly
  Reducing elderly fall programs
Trauma
  National trauma awareness month
Poisoning
  National poison prevention week
Bicycle safety
  Bicycle helmet programs
Brain injury
  Brain injury prevention programs
Community safety
  Safe communities programs
Firearm safety
  Gun violence prevention programs
Violence
  Violence prevention programs
  Violence survivors programs
Neurological injury
  Head injury prevention programs
Pedestrian safety
  Pedestrian safety programs
Smoking
  Smoking cessation programs
Substance abuse
  Addiction programs
  Substance abuse prevention programs
  Substance abuse prevention programs for youth
Post-traumatic stress syndrome (PTSS)
  PTSS programs for the community
  PTSS programs for EMS and other public safety
    personnel
Burns
  Fire prevention programs
  Smoke detector programs
Occupational safety
  Occupational illness and injury prevention programs

Home safety
  Home assessment programs
Nutrition
  Proper nutrition programs
Rehabilitation
  Rehabilitation support groups
Research
  Universities all across the United States do research into a multitude of illness and injury prevention strategies. These educational facilities often welcome input from EMS personnel. The input may be in the form of volunteer work in data collection, ride-alongs by the researchers, or assistance in the actual writing of the research documents. EMS personnel should search for injury prevention centers, illness prevention centers, EMS research centers, and schools of public health within colleges and universities in their local area.
Suicide
  Suicide prevention programs
Legal/political
  Being involved as an expert or advisor in the political process during the debate over laws dealing with the following:
    Engineering regulations (building safety into a product)
    Gun legislation
    Helmet laws
    Drunk driving laws
    Child and adolescent safety laws
  Medical sites that contain information on preventing a wide array of medical maladies can be found on the Internet. Many of these sites provide information that can be passed on to the EMS provider's patients either informally or through a formal program with handouts or public service activities. Sites include the following:
    Healthy lifestyle
    Cardiovascular health
    Stroke
    Premenstrual syndrome (PMS)
    Flu
    Acquired immunodeficiency syndrome (AIDS)
    Childhood illnesses
    Senior citizen illnesses
    Parenting
    Cancer
    Heat disorders
    Medical conditions A-Z (CDC site)
  Most local physician offices have brochures that EMS personnel can hand out in cooperation with the local doctor.

*This box should encourage the paramedic student to search for prevention programs that are of interest to him or her since the work will probably be voluntary and will have a better chance of holding his or her interest if the reward is internal rather than external.
This list is compiled from programs already in place. Some of the programs are national, and some are local. The student should be advised to seek those programs that already exist in his or her area. If a program does not exist locally, chances are it exists somewhere in the United States. The student should search the Internet or other sources and find a comparable program to use as a guide for starting a local program.

luck." As long as the public's perception is that injuries are unavoidable or unexpected happenings or acts of divine intervention, it accepts the consequences of injury as an inevitable part of life. The public has long ago rejected that measles and mumps are going to be a major killer of the nation's youth and have accepted vaccines as valuable primary illness prevention strategies. A major role that EMS can play in injury prevention is to work to change the public's perception of accepting injury as an unavoidable fact of life.

Specific Primary Prevention Strategies

EMS can play a major role in improving public health and safety through participating in primary-prevention programs in the community. Box C-1 provides a sampling of these programs. These and other programs currently exist on the national or local level and may exist by different titles throughout the United States. An Internet search may identify injury prevention programs for a specific community.

Suggested Readings

American Heart Association: Guidelines 2000 for cardiopulmonary resuscitation and emergency cardiovascular care, International Consensus on Science, *Circulation* 102(8):77, 2000.

Baker SP, O'Neill B, Ginsburg MJ, Li G: *The injury fact book*, ed 2, New York, 1992, Oxford University Press.

Bonnie RJ, Fulco CE, Liverman CT, editors: *Reducing the burden of injury*, Washington, DC, 1999, National Academy Press.

Butler RN, Todd KH, Kellerman AL, et al: Injury control education in six U.S. medical schools, *Acad Med* 73:524, 1998.

Christoffel T, Gallagher SS: *Injury prevention and public health: practical knowledge, skills, and strategies*, Gaithersburg, Md, 1999, Aspen Publishers.

Garrison HG, Foltin GL, et al: The role of emergency medical services in primary injury prevention, *Ann Emerg Med* 30:80, 1997.

Kellerman AL, Todd KH: Injury control. In Tintinalli JE, Kelen GD, Stapczynski JS, editors: *Emergency medicine: a comprehensive study guide*, New York, 1999, McGraw-Hill.

Kinnane JM, Garrison HG, Coben JH, Alonzo-Serra HM: Injury prevention: Is there a role for out-of-hospital emergency medical services? *Acad Emerg Med* 4:306, 1997.

National Research Council, Commission on Life Sciences, Committee on Trauma Research, Institute of Medicine: *Injury in America: a continuing public health problem*, Washington, DC, 1985, National Academy Press.

National Safety Council: *Injury fact book*, Chicago, 1999, The Council.

U.S. Department of Transportation, National Highway Traffic Safety Administration: *Emergency medical services agenda for the future*, Washington, DC, 1996, GPO. DOT HS-808-441.

U.S. Department of Transportation, National Highway Traffic Safety Administration: *Emergency medical services agenda for the future implementation guide*, Washington, DC, 1998, GPO. DOT HS-808-711.

Waller JA: *Injury control: a guide to the causes and prevention of trauma*, Lexington, Mass, 1985, Lexington Books.

Widome MD, editor: *Injury prevention and control for children and youth*, ed 2, Elk Grove Village, Ill, 1997, American Academy of Pediatrics.

Injury-Related World Wide Websites

URL verified as of June 2001

American Academy of Pediatrics
www.aap.org

American Association of Poison Control Centers
www.aapcc.org

Association for the Advancement of Automotive Medicine
www.carcrash.org

American Trauma Society
www.amtrauma.org/prevent/

Bike Helmet Safety Institute
www.bhsi.org

Brain Injury Association
www.biausa.org

Building Bridges Between Health and Traffic Safety
www.edc.org/HHD/csn/buildbridges

Building Safe Communities
www.edc.org/HHD/csn/bsc

Bureau of Labor Statistics/Safety and Health
  Statistics
www.bls.gov/oshhome.htm

CDC Wonder (CDC searches, queries, guidelines,
  and reports)
http://wonder.cdc.gov

Center for the Advanced Study of Public Safety
  and Injury Prevention
www.albany.edu/sph/injury/injury_3.html

Center for the Study and Prevention of Violence
www.colorado.edu/cspv

Center for Violence Prevention and Control—
  University of Minnesota
www.umn.edu/cvpc

Child Passenger Safety Web
www.childsafety.org/index.html

Colorado Injury Control Research Center
www.ColoState.edu/Orgs/CICRC

Consumer Product Safety Commission
www.cpsc.gov

Creative Partnerships for Prevention—A Drug
  and Violence Prevention Resource
www.CPPrev.org

Early Prevention of Violence Database (Great
  Lakes Area Regional Resource Center)
www.glarrc.org/resources/epvd.cfm

Emergency Medical Services for Children
www.ems-c.org/

Emory Center for Injury Control
www.sph.emory.edu/CIC

Family Health and Safety
www.nsc.org/pubs/fsh.htm

Family Violence Prevention Fund
www.fvpf.org

Fatality Analysis Reporting System (FARS)
www.fars.nhtsa.dot.gov/

Georgia Division of Public Health, Injury
  Prevention

www.ph.dhr.state.ga.us/programs/
  injuryprevention/index.shtml

Gunfree Home (Coalition to Stop Gun Violence)
www.gunfree.org

Handgun Epidemic Lowering Project (HELP
  Network)
www.cphv.org/lifeline.html

Injury Control and Emergency Health Services
  Section of the American Health Association
www.icehs.org

Injury Control Resources Information Network
www.injurycontrol.com/icrin

Institute for Preventive Sports Medicine
http://users.aol.com/wwwipsm/

Insurance Institute for Highway Safety
www.highwaysafety.org

Interdisciplinary Pediatric Injury Control Research
  Center (University of Pennsylvania)
www.upenn.edu/html/vpr/winston.html

Johns Hopkins Center for Injury Research
  and Policy
www.jhsph.edu/Research/Centers/CIRP

JOIN TOGETHER (community substance abuse
  and gun violence programs)
www.jointogether.org

Journal of Trauma
www.jtrauma.com

Kentucky Injury Prevention and Research Center
www.kiprc.uky.edu

Kids Health (Nemours Foundation)
www.kidshealth.org/parent/safety/

Minnesota Center Against Violence and Abuse
www.umn.edu/mincava/

Morbidity and Mortality Weekly report
www.cdc.gov/mmwr

Mothers Against Drunk Driving
www.madd.org

National Association of Governor's Highway
  Safety Representative
www.naghsr.org

National Bicycle Safety Network
www.cdc.gov/ncipc/bike/default.htm

National Center for Health Statistics
www.cdc.gov/nchswww/default.htm

National Center for Injury Control and Prevention (CDC)
www.cdc.gov/ncipc/default.htm

National Center for Statistics and Analysis (NHTSA)
www.nhtsa.dot.gov/people/ncsa

National Clearinghouse for Alcohol and Drug Information
www.health.org

National Data Archive on Child Abuse and Neglect
www.saferide.org

National Fire Protection Association
www.nfpa.org

National Group Rides and Designated Drivers
www.ntlgradd.w1.com/index.shtml

National Health Information Center
www.nhic-nt.health.org

National Highway Traffic Safety Administration
www.nhtsa.dot.gov

National Highway Traffic Safety Administration, Safety City
www.nhtsa.dot.gov/kids

National Institute for Occupational Safety and Health
www.cdc.gov/niosh/homepage.html

National Institute on Disability and Rehabilitation Research
www.ed.gov/offices/OSERS/NIDRR

National Institutes of Health
www.nih.gov

National Network of Violence Prevention Practitioners
www2.edc.org/NVPP/

National Pediatric Trauma Registry
www.nemc.org/rehab/nptrhome.htm

National Program for Playground Safety
www.uni.edu/playground

National Rehabilitation Information Center Home Page
www.naric.com/naric/index.html

National Safety Council
www.nsc.org

Occupational Safety and Health Administration
www.osha.gov

Oklahoma State Department of Health Injury Control Division
www.health.state.ok.us/program/injury/index.html

OSHA Statistics
www.osha.gov/oshstats/

Pacific Center for Violence Prevention
www.pcvp.org

Partnership Against Violence Network
www.pavnet.org

Rehabilitation Services Administration
www.ed.gov/offices/OSERS/RSA/rsa.html#org

Research and Training Center in Rehabilitation and Childhood Trauma
www.nemc.org/rehab/homepg.htm

Safe Communities (WHO)
www.safecommunities.ca/

SafeKids Campaign
www.safekids.org

San Francisco Injury Center
www.surgery.ucsf.edu/sfic/

Scientific Data, Surveillance and Injury Statistics
www.cdc.gov/ncipc/osp/data.htm

Southern California Injury Prevention Research Center
www.ph.ucla.edu/sciprc/sciprc1.htm

State and Territorial Injury Prevention Research Center
www.stipda.org

State Health Departments On-line
www.cdc.gov/epo/mmwr/medassn.html#states

Suicide Awareness: Voices of Education
www.save.org

Texas Department of Health, Injury Prevention
and Control Program
www.tdh.state.tx.us/injury/

THINK FIRST Foundation
www.thinkfirst.org

University of Alabama Injury Control Research
Center
www.uab.edu/icrc/

University of Michigan Transportation Research
Institute
www.umtri.umich.edu/

University of North Carolina Injury Prevention
Research Center
www.sph.unc.edu/iprc/

Violence Against Women Office, U.S. Department
of Justice
www.ojp.usdoj.gov/vawo

WHO Helmet Initiative
www.sph.emory.edu/Helmets

World Health Organization
www.who.int

Best Practices for Youth Violence Prevention
www.cdc.gov/ncipc/dvp/bestpractices.htm

Appendix D
A Brief Overview of Canadian EMS

Darrell Paranich, BSc, EMT-P

The delivery of Canadian emergency medical services is as unique as the country it serves. Canadian EMS regulators, educators, operators, and providers take great pride in meeting the historical, political, cultural, economical, geographical, and environmental challenges that mold and shape the nation and the national Canadian EMS identity.

As the second largest nation in the world, Canadians live in one of the most sparsely populated countries in the world. With an estimated population of 31 million,[1] Canada has a population density of three persons per square kilometer.[1] This is compared with 28.7 in the United States and 242 in the United Kingdom.[2] This fact, in addition to the harsh and varied climate of Canada, makes living, communicating, traveling, working, and surviving prehospital illness and injury a formidable challenge.

Culturally, Canada is the multinational composite of French, British, First Nations, Inuit, and immigrant peoples. Federally, Canada promotes multiculturalism as a way of life. The population is uniquely bilingual, and federal services are provided in the official languages of French and English. Canada is a proud member of the British Commonwealth and recognizes the Queen of England as sovereign and Her representative, the Governor General, as the national head of state. A fundamental part of the Canadian cultural identity is its socialized health care insurance system.

Medicare

Provision of health services is legislated through the Canada Health Act, an act of the Parliament of Canada that was proclaimed into effect in 1984. This Act was the progressive socialization of health insurance and its provisions over 5 decades. Commonly called "Medicare" by Canadians, it is a system of socialized health delivery that is a key source of national pride, strongly supported by all levels of government and Canadians at large. Medicare is a primarily federally financed system of interlaced health insurance programs that are delivered by the ten provinces and three territories of Canada. The constitutional assignment of responsibilities allows for a national structure to Medicare that is jurisdictionally administered by the provincial and territorial governments.

The Canadian Medicare system is based on four key tenets:

1. Medicare must be publicly administered and operated as a nonprofit system that is accountable to each provincial government.
2. The system provides health insurance to 100% of its citizens, including First Nations and Inuit peoples.
3. The Medicare system allows for uniform accessibility regardless of age, race, financial status, or health status and further allows portability within Canada regardless of a person's province of origin.
4. Medicare provides a comprehensive range of medically necessary services that include all in-hospital diagnostic services, procedures, medications, supplies, and outpatient and chronic care services.

Other health-related functions administered by the federal government include disease prevention and health promotion. Canada possesses one of the lowest infant mortality rates and one of the highest life expectancies in the industrialized world.*

Origins of Canadian EMS

Canada lacked a federal act that legislated a national EMS system, such as that enacted in the late 1960s and early 1970s in the United States. Each of Canada's 10 provinces evolved their own unique system of emergency health services that vary widely in a range of delivery models, nomenclature, training, user costs, public access, and levels of care. There were systems in place to transport the sick and injured, but many were poorly integrated for-profit systems, funeral-home operations, or poorly funded and equipped volunteers with little or no standards for attendants or ambulances. The following is a brief overview of current Canadian EMS systems:

- Students graduated from Canada's first advanced life support (ALS) training program at the Southern Alberta Institute of Technology in 1972. This was the first publicly funded training program in Canada and served as a model for the nation. These graduates were called "paramedics." Currently, ALS paramedics serve almost every city in Alberta. The Health Professions Act (1999) of Alberta identifies the Alberta College of Paramedics as a true self-regulating, self-disciplining, and licensure-regulating professional college. This is the only self-regulating EMS provider professional college of its kind in Canada.
- The prairie provinces of Saskatchewan and Manitoba have adopted some of the earlier legislation of Alberta and provide ALS service in most large cities. Air ambulance services to remote communities are either nurse or nurse/paramedic configurations primarily in fixed-wing aircraft.

*The United Nations Human Development Index ranks countries according to their citizens' education, access to health care, and average income. Canada has topped the index for 6 consecutive years (1994-1999). Data from United Nations Development Programme: *Human Development Report,* New York, Oxford University Press.

- The Provincial Government of British Columbia enacted legislation in 1974 to form the British Columbia Ambulance Service. Currently, the service is one of North America's largest EMS systems with about 390,000 ground and 6200 air ambulance runs annually servicing about 4 million people over some of the most challenging mountainous terrain in the world.[2]
- Ontario is the largest and most heavily populated province in Canada. Ontario's provincial EMS system with provincially funded dispatch and air ambulance service staffed with ALS providers began in the 1970s. With a widely varied topography and rugged Canadian shield terrain, the government chose various models of delivery and coordination of activities employed by the EMS systems at municipal and regional levels. Municipalities are currently evaluating the system that best suits their needs at a local level.
- Quebec's EMS system is modeled after European EMS systems with graduate physicians manning the ambulances accompanied by attendants of varied levels of training and capability. The government of Quebec is currently reevaluating the system to closely follow the National Occupational Profile for Paramedicine sponsored by the Paramedic Association of Canada.
- The Canadian Maritime Provinces contain a mixture of EMS systems. Dr. Ron Stewart introduced a provincial EMS system in Nova Scotia combining more than 100 EMS companies into one. Nova Scotia operates a regional ALS air ambulance helicopter system. Prince Edward Island is currently drafting new EMS legislation. Newfoundland currently has intermediate-level practitioners. New Brunswick has adopted a provincial 911 system to assist the approximately 180 communities.
- The Yukon and Northwest Territories have remote, sparsely populated communities served primarily by nursing stations with medivac capabilities to southern centers as the need arises. Three- and four-hour response times in these areas are common and are often followed by long air-medivacs to definitive care in the south.
- Located on Baffin Island in Canada's Eastern Arctic, Iqaluit, is the capital of Canada's newest Territory of Nunavut. Iqaluit has a population of 4700. Average temperatures range from 12° C in the summer to -100° C in the winter, which ex-

tends from mid-October to late May. With a vast north, Canadian EMS has tremendous severity of weather and great distances to overcome.

Canadian EMS Organizations

Canadian national organizations such as Interphase National, Canadian Association of Emergency Physicians, and the Canadian Society of Prehospital Educators have been strong proponents for upgrading, communicating, and integrating Canadian EMS.

In 1988, the Canadian Society of Ambulance Personnel (CSAP) met with practitioners from across Canada to discuss common goals and needs. Renamed the Paramedic Association of Canada (PAC), it is Canada's only EMS organization representing prehospital practitioners in the national forum. The Association has over 16,000 members located in divisional chapters.

Interphase National was founded in Calgary, Alberta, in 1979 to promote interaction and cooperation between all phases of EMS, doctors, nurses, paramedics, firefighters, and others, with the goal of improving the quality of care available to the general public. Interphase National holds yearly conferences across Canada to provide an educational and social environment conducive to these objectives.

Drafting a National EMS Identity

The government of Canada through their branch department of Human Resources Development partnered with the PAC to develop the document *National Occupational Competency Profile for Paramedicine* (NOCPP). The NOCPP was adopted by the PAC in March 2000 and will serve as a template for evaluation criteria for the Canadian Medical Association's Conjoint Committee on Accreditation. The NOCPP is not a standards or licensure document, but rather a national consensus document of key competencies divided into common key areas of paramedic practice. It identifies four levels of care commonly practiced in Canada and several broad areas of competency. The levels of care have been defined as follows:

- Emergency Medical Responder: BLS entry level of practice
- Primary Care Paramedic: Intermediate level of practice, including symptom relief medications
- Advanced Care Paramedic: Advanced airway management and standard ALS medications
- Critical Care Paramedic: Advanced medication regimens, flight and community health care, and advanced procedures

This document will serve as a template to build curriculum blueprinting, essential skills mapping, and regulatory national examination and registration.

About the Author

Darrell Paranich has been working in EMS since 1979 and received his EMT-P diploma from the Southern Institute of Technology, Calgary, Alberta, in 1982. He received his BSc from the University of Alberta in 1985. He was a founding member of the Alberta Prehospital Professions Association, now the Alberta College of Paramedics, and Canadian Society of Ambulance Personnel, now the Paramedic Association of Canada. He has been a paramedic instructor at the Northern Alberta Institute of Technology and works full-time as a ground and air-ambulance paramedic for the City of Edmonton, Alberta. He serves on several committees in the Alberta College of Paramedics and currently sits on the Steering Committee for the Paramedic Association of Canada's NOCPP and National Curriculum Blueprinting and Essential Skills project.

REFERENCES

1. Organization for Economic Co-operation and Development. Labour Force Statistics, 1978-1998, Paris, 1999.
2. BCAS Statistics 1998/99 reporting year.

Emergency Drug Index

Activated Charcoal
Adenosine
Albuterol
Amiodarone
Amrinone
Amyl Nitrite
Aspirin
Atenolol
Atropine Sulfate
Butorphanol
Calcium Chloride
Dexamethasone
Dextrose 50%
Diazepam
Digoxin
Diltiazem
Diphenhydramine
Dobutamine
Dopamine
Droperidol
Epinephrine
Epinephrine Racemic
Etomidate
Fentanyl
Flumazenil
Furosemide
Glucagon
Haloperidol Lactate
Heparin Sodium
Hydralazine
Hydroxyzine
Ibutilide
Insulin
Ipratropium
Isoproterenol
Ketamine
Ketorolac Tromethamine
Labetalol
Lidocaine
Lorazepam
Magnesium Sulfate
Mannitol
Meperidine
Metoprolol
Metaproterenol
Methylprednisolone
Midazolam Hydrochloride
Morphine Sulfate
Nalbuphine
Nalmefene
Naloxone

Nitroglycerin
Nitropaste
Nitrous Oxide:Oxygen
Norepinephrine
Oxygen
Oxytocin
Pancuronium
Phenytoin
Pralidoxime
Procainamide
Promethazine
Propranolol
Reteplase
Sodium Bicarbonate
Streptokinase
Succinylcholine
Syrup of Ipecac
Tetracaine
Thiamine
Tissue Plasminogen Activator
Vasopressin
Verapamil

Drug Identification Guide

The *Emergency Drug Index* is a list of commonly pre-scribed medications that are used in prehospital care; it is not intended to be a complete guide to all emergency medications. For additional drug information, consult other standard references or pharmacology textbooks. Drugs included in this index are listed alphabetically by generic name. The trade name(s) are shown in parentheses following the generic listing.

Activated Charcoal (Aqua, Actidose, Liqui-Char)

Class
Adsorbent, Antidote

Description
Activated charcoal is a fine black powder that binds and adsorbs ingested toxins. Once the drug binds to the activated charcoal, the combined complex is excreted among feces.

Onset and Duration
Onset: Immediate
Duration: Continual while in GI tract

PREGNANCY CATEGORY RATINGS FOR DRUGS

Drugs have been categorized by the Food and Drug Administration (FDA) according to the level of risk to the fetus. These categories are listed for each drug herein under **Pregnancy Safety,** and are interpreted as follows:[1]

Category A: Controlled studies in women fail to demonstrate a risk to the fetus in the first trimester, and there is no evidence of risk in later trimesters; the possibility of fetal harm appears to be remote.

Category B: Either (1) animal reproductive studies have not demonstrated a fetal risk but there are no controlled studies in pregnant women or (2) animal reproductive studies have shown an adverse effect (other than decreased fertility) that was not confirmed in controlled studies on women in the first trimester and there is no evidence of risk in later trimesters.

Category C: Either (1) studies in animals have revealed adverse effects on the fetus and there are no controlled studies in women or (2) studies in women and animals are not available. Drugs in this category should be given only if the potential benefit justifies the risk to the fetus.

Category D: There is positive evidence of human fetal risk, but the benefits for pregnant women may be acceptable despite the risk, as in life-threatening diseases for which safer drugs cannot be used or are ineffective. An appropriate statement must appear in the "Warnings" section of the labeling of drugs in this category.

Category X: Studies in animals or humans have demonstrated fetal abnormalities, there is evidence of fetal risk based on human experience or both; the risk of using the drug in pregnant women clearly outweighs any possible benefit. The drug is contraindicated in women who are or may become pregnant. An appropriate statement must appear in the "Contraindications" section of the labeling of drugs in this category.

Indications

Many oral poisonings and medication overdoses

Contraindications

Corrosives, caustics, petroleum distillates (relatively ineffective, and may induce vomiting), GI bleeding

Adverse Reactions

May indirectly induce nausea and vomiting
May cause constipation or mild, transient diarrhea

Drug Interactions

Syrup of ipecac (adsorbed by activated charcoal, and will result in vomiting of the charcoal)

How Supplied

25 g (black powder)/125 mL bottle (200 mg/mL)
50 g (black powder)/250 mL bottle (200 mg/mL)
Other sizes include 15 g and 30 g, bottles and squeeze tubes. Most products come premixed (not powder) with water (aqueous preparations) or with sorbitol, a cathartic.

Dosage and Administration

Approximately 1-2 g/kg body weight (larger amounts if food is also present), prepared in a slurry and administered PO or slowly via nasogastric or orogastric tube

Adult:	30-100 g
Pediatric (1-12 yrs):	15-30 g
Infant (less than 1 yr):	1 g/kg

Special Considerations

Pregnancy Safety: Category C

Charcoal is frequently administered to pregnant patients and the potential benefit vs. risk is very high. Since charcoal remains within the GI tract, its risk to the fetus is virtually eliminated, unless the charcoal and other stomach contents are aspirated.

Activated charcoal may also be known as "AC"

Is relatively insoluble in water

May blacken feces

Must be stored in a closed container

Different charcoal preparations may have varying adsorptive capacity

Does not adsorb all drugs and toxic substances (e.g., phenobarbital, aspirin, cyanide, lithium, iron, lead, arsenic)

Adenosine (Adenocard)

Class

Endogenous nucleoside, Miscellaneous antidysrhythmic

Description

Adenosine is primarily formed from the breakdown of adenosine triphosphate (ATP). Both ATP and adenosine are found in every cell of the human body, and have a wide range of metabolic roles. Adenosine slows supraventricular tachycardias (SVTs) by decreasing electrical conduction through the AV node without causing negative inotropic effects. It also acts directly on sinus pacemaker cells and vagal nerve terminals to decrease chronotropic (heart rate) activity. Adenosine is recommended as the drug of choice for paroxysmal supraventricular tachycardia (PSVT), and can be used diagnostically for stable, wide-complex tachycardias of unknown type, following two doses of lidocaine.

Onset and Duration

Onset: Immediate

Duration: 10 seconds

Indications

First drug for most forms of narrow-complex PSVT and dysrhythmias associated with bypass tracts such as Wolff-Parkinson-White syndrome, in adults and pediatric patients.

Contraindications

Second- or third-degree AV block, or sick sinus syndrome

Hypersensitivity to adenosine

Atrial flutter, atrial fibrillation, ventricular tachycardia (Adenosine is not effective in converting these rhythms to sinus rhythm)

Adverse Reactions

Lightheadedness

Paresthesias

Headache

Diaphoresis

Palpitations

Chest pain

Hypotension

Shortness of breath

Transient periods of sinus bradycardia, sinus pause, or bradyasystole

Ventricular ectopy (fibrillation, flutter, tachycardia, torsades de pointes)

Nausea

Metallic taste

Drug Interactions

Methylxanthines (e.g., caffeine and theophylline) antagonize the action of adenosine.

Dipyridamole potentiates the effect of adenosine; reduction of adenosine dose may be required.

Carbamazepine may potentiate the AV-nodal blocking effect of adenosine.

How Supplied

Parenteral for IV injection

3 mg/mL in 2 mL and 5 mL flip-top vials

Dosage and Administration

Adult:

Initial dose:	6 mg rapid intravenous bolus over 1-3 seconds, followed by a 20-mL saline flush; elevate extremity
Repeat dose:	If no response is observed after 1-2 min, administer a 12-mg repeat dose in the same manner; may repeat once in 1-2 min (max single dose: 12 mg)
Pediatric:	Initial dose 0.1 mg/kg; may be doubled once (max first dose: 6 mg); rapid IV bolus, followed by a 5 mL saline flush

Special Considerations

Pregnancy Safety: Category C

Place patient in mild reverse Trendelenburg position before drug administration

A brief period of asystole (up to 15 seconds) following conversion, followed by resumption of NSR, is common after rapid administration

Patients taking theophylline may require larger doses of adenosine; cardiac transplant recipients may require only a small dose

May produce bronchoconstriction in patients with asthma and in patients with bronchopulmonary disease

Monitor ECG during administration

Albuterol *(Proventil and others)*

Class

Sympathomimetic, Bronchodilator, Beta$_2$ agonist

Description

Albuterol is a sympathomimetic that is selective for beta$_2$ adrenergic receptors. It relaxes smooth muscles of the bronchial tree and peripheral vasculature by stimulating adrenergic receptors of the sympathetic nervous system.

Onset and Duration

Onset: 5-15 min after inhalation

Duration: 3-4 hr after inhalation

Indications

Relief of bronchospasm in patients with reversible obstructive airway disease

Prevention of exercise-induced bronchospasm

Contraindications

Prior hypersensitivity reaction to albuterol

Cardiac dysrhythmias associated with tachycardia

Adverse Reactions

Usually dose related

Restlessness, apprehension

Dizziness

Palpitations, tachycardia

Dysrhythmias

Drug Interactions

Other sympathomimetics may exacerbate adverse cardiovascular effects

Antidepressants may potentiate effects on the vasculature (vasodilation)

Beta blockers may antagonize albuterol

Albuterol may potentiate diuretic-induced hypokalemia

How Supplied

MDI: 90 mcg/metered spray (17 g canister with 200 inhalations)

Solution for aerosolization: 0.5% (5 mg/mL); 0.083% (2.5 mg) in 3 mL unit dose/nebulizer

Dosage and Administration

Bronchial Asthma

Adult:

MDI:	1-2 inhalations (90-180 mcg) q 4-6 hr (wait five min between inhalations); max 12 inhalation/day
Solution:	2.5 mg (0.5 mL of 0.5% solution) diluted to 3 mL with 0.9% NS (0.083% solution); administer over 5-15 min; 3-4 times/day by nebulizer

Pediatric:

MDI:	Same as for adult
Solution:	0.01-0.03 mL (0.05-0.15 mg)/kg/dose to maximum of 0.50 mL/dose diluted in 2 mL of 0.9% NS; may be repeated q 20 min three times

Special Considerations

Pregnancy Safety: Category C

May precipitate angina pectoris and dysrhythmias

Should be used with caution in patients with diabetes mellitus, hyperthyroidism, prostatic hypertrophy, seizure disorder, or cardiovascular disorder

In prehospital emergency care, albuterol should only be administered via inhalation

Amiodarone (Cordarone)

Class

Class III antidysrhythmic

Description

Amiodarone is a unique antidysrhythmic agent with multiple mechanisms of action. The drug prolongs duration of the action potential and effective refractory period, and when given short term IV, probably include noncompetitive β-adrenoreceptor and calcium channel blockers.

Onset and Duration

Onset:	Within minutes
Duration:	Variable

Indications (IV use)

Initial treatment and prophylaxis of frequently recurring VF and hemodynamically unstable VT in patients refractory to other therapy. Refractory PSVT in conjunction with electrical cardioversion

Contraindications

Pulmonary congestion
Cardiogenic shock
Hypotension
Sensitivity to amiodarone
Bradycardia

Adverse Reactions

Hypotension
Headache
Dizziness
Bradycardia
AV conduction abnormalities
Flushing
Abnormal salivation

Drug Interactions

May potentiate bradycardia and hypotension with beta blocker and calcium channel blockers

May increase risk of AV block and hypotension with calcium channel blockers

May increase anticoagulant effects of warfarin

May decrease metabolism and increase serum levels of phenytoin, procainamide, quinidine, and theophyllines

Routine use in combination with drugs that prolong the QT interval is not recommended

Y-site incompatibilities with furosemide, heparin, and sodium bicarbonate

How Supplied

50-mg/mL vials

Dosage and Administration

Adult:

Pulseless arrest:	300 mg IV push (diluted in 20-30 mL NS or D₅W. Consider repeating 150 mg IV push in 3-5 min (maximum cumulative dose 2 g IV/24 hrs)
Wide-Complex Tachycardia:	May be given as rapid infusion 150 mg IV over first 10 min (15 mg/min) repeated every 10 min as needed; or by slow infusion 360 mg IV over 6 hr (1 mg/min). Maintenance infusion 540 mg IV over 18 hr (0.5 mg/min)

Pediatric:

Pulseless arrest:	5 mg/kg rapid IV bolus
Perfusing tachycardias:	Loading dose 5 mg/kg IV over 20-60 min (maximum dose 15 mg/kg/day)

Special Considerations

Pregnancy Safety: Category D

Continuous ECG monitoring is required

Slow infusion or discontinue if bradycardia or AV block occur

Maintain at room temperature and protect from excessive heat

Amrinone (Inocor)

Class

Inotropic, vasodilator

Description

Amrinone is a rapid-acting inotropic agent that increases cardiac output after IV administration. It is a phosphodiesterase (class III) inhibitor that increases myocardial contractility and produces systemic vasodilation without stimulating either alpha- or beta-adrenergic receptors.

Onset and Duration
Onset: Less than 15 min IV
Duration: 4.5 hr

Indications
Severe congestive heart failure refractory to diuretics, vasodilators, and conventional inotropic agents

Contraindications
Hypotension
Idiopathic hypertrophic subaortic stenosis (IHSS)
Hypersensitivity to amrinone or bisulfite
Valvular obstructive disease

Adverse Reactions
Tachydysrhythmias
Increase in myocardial ischemia
Hypotension
Thrombocytopenia (dose related)
Fever, flulike symptoms
Increase in liver enzyme levels

Drug Interactions
Hypotension may develop when amrinone is used with agents with negative inotropic or vasodilatory effects
Potentiates inotropic, chronotropic, and arrhythmogenic response to catecholamine and theophylline
Incompatible with furosemide

How Supplied
5 mg/mL (20-mL ampules)

Dosage and Administration
Adult: 0.75 mg/kg IV given over 2-3 min; follow with infusion of 5-15 mcg/kg/min titrated to clinical response.
Pediatric: 0.75-1 mg/kg IV/IO over 5 min; may repeat twice (maximum 3 mg/kg); follow with infusion 5-10 mcg/kg/min

Special Considerations
Pregnancy Safety: Category D
Do not mix with dextrose solutions or other drugs
Optimal use requires hemodynamic monitoring

Amyl Nitrite

Class
Coronary vasodilator

Description
Amyl nitrite is chemically related to nitroglycerin and has been used for many years to treat angina pectoris. It is also effective in the emergency management of cyanide poisoning by causing the oxidation of hemoglobin to the compound methemoglobin. Cyanide preferentially binds methemoglobin, thus freeing hemoglobin to react with oxygen.

Onset and Duration
Onset: 30 seconds inhaled
Duration: 3-20 min

Indications
Cyanide poisoning (only until sodium nitrate can be given intravenously)

Contraindications
None when used for cyanide poisoning
Severe anemia
Hypersensitivity to nitrates

Adverse Reactions
Hypotension
Tachycardia
Palpitations
Syncope
Headache
Nausea

Drug Interactions
None significant
Alcohol can increase toxicity

How Supplied
0.3 mL/glass ampule (capsule covered with woven gauze)

Dosage and Administration
Adult: Glass ampule should be broken (crush ampule and hold under patient's nostrils) and inhaled for 30-60 seconds; may be repeated as necessary; 1-6 inhalations from one ampule usually is sufficient
Pediatric: Same as adult

Special Considerations
Pregnancy Safety: Category X
Frequently abused (claimed to be an aphrodisiac)
Also known as "amy"
Cyanide poisoning often produces a bitter almond breath odor (not all persons can detect the odor)
Patient should be supine during administration, and blood pressure should be monitored

Aspirin (ASA, Bayer, Ecotrin, St. Joseph, others)

Class
Analgesic, antiinflammatory, antipyretic, antiplatelet

Description
Aspirin blocks pain impulses in the CNS, dilates peripheral vessels, and decreases platelet aggregation. The use of aspirin is strongly recommended for all acute MI patients.

Onset and Duration

Onset: 15-30 min
Duration: 4-6 hr

Indications

Mild to moderate pain or fever
Prevention of platelet aggregation in ischemia and thromboembolism
Unstable angina
Prevention of myocardial infraction or reinfarction

Contraindications

Hypersensitivity to salicylates
GI bleeding
Active ulcer disease
Hemorrhagic stroke
Bleeding disorders
Children with flulike symptoms

Adverse Reactions

Stomach irritation
Heartburn or indigestion
Nausea or vomiting
Allergic reaction

Drug Interactions

Decreased effects with antacids and steroids
Increased effects with anticoagulants, insulin, oral hypoglycemics, fibrinolytic agents

How Supplied

Tablets (65, 81, 325, 500, 650, 975 mg)
Capsules (325, 500 mg)
Controlled-release tablets (800 mg)
Suppositories (varies from 60 mg to 1.2 g)

Dosage and Administration

Adult:
  Mild pain and fever: 325-650 mg PO every 4 hr
  Myocardial infarction: 160-325 mg PO (chewing is preferable to swallowing)
Pediatric (over 12 years of age):
  Mild pain and fever: 40-100 mg/kg/day in divided doses

Special Considerations

Pregnancy Safety: Category D
Should be given as soon as possible to the patient with AMI

Atenolol *(Tenormin)*

Class

Beta-blocking agent

Description

Atenolol competes with beta-adrenergic agonists for available beta-receptor sites on the membranes of cardiac muscle, bronchial smooth muscle, and the smooth muscle of blood vessels. The Beta1 blocking action on the heart decreases heart rate, conduction velocity, myocardial contractility, and cardiac output. It is used to control ventricular response in supraventricular tachydysrhythmias (PSVT, atrial fibrillation, atrial flutter). It is considered a second-line agent after adenosine, diltiazem, or digitalis derivative.

Onset and Duration

Onset: Within 10 min
Duration: 2-4 hr

Indications

PSVT
Atrial flutter
Atrial fibrillation
To reduce myocardial ischemia and damage in AMI patients

Contraindications

Heart failure
Cardiogenic shock
Bradycardia
Lung disease associated with bronchospasm
Hypersensitivity to atenolol
Hypotension
Second- or third-degree heart block

Adverse Reactions

Bradycardia
AV conduction delays
Hypotension

Drug Interactions

Atenolol may potentiate antihypertensive effects when given to patients taking calcium channel blockers or MAO inhibitors; catecholamine-depleting drugs may potentiate hypotension; sympathomimetic effects may be antagonized; signs of hypoglycemia may be masked.

How Supplied

5 mg in 10-mL ampules

Dosage and Administration

Adult: 5 mg slow IV (over 5 min); wait 10 min then give second dose of 5 mg over 5 min
Pediatric: Not recommended

Special Considerations

Pregnancy Safety: Category C
Must be given slow IV, over 5 min
Concurrent IV administration with IV calcium channel blockers like verapamil or diltiazem can cause severe hypotension
Should be used with caution in persons with liver or renal dysfunction

Atropine Sulfate *(Atropine and others)*

Class

Anticholinergic agent

Description

Atropine sulfate (a potent parasympatholytic), inhibits actions of acetylcholine at postganglionic parasympathetic (primarily muscarinic) receptor sites. Small doses inhibit salivary and bronchial secretions; moderate doses dilate pupils and increase heart rate. Large doses decrease GI motility, inhibit gastric acid secretion, and may block nicotinic receptor sites at the autonomic ganglia and at the neuromuscular junction. Blocked vagal effects result in increased heart rate and enhanced AV conduction with limited or no inotropic effect. In emergency care, it is primarily used to increase the heart rate in life-threatening or symptomatic bradycardia, and to antagonize excess muscarinic receptor stimulation caused by organophosphate insecticides or chemical nerve agents (sarin, soman, etc.).

Onset and Duration

Onset: Rapid
Duration: 2-6 hr

Indications

Hemodynamically significant bradycardia
Asystole
PEA with absolute bradycardia
Organophosphate or nerve gas poisoning
Bronchospastic pulmonary disorders (exercise-induced)

Contraindications

Tachycardia
Hypersensitivity to atropine
Obstructive disease of GI tract
Obstructive uropathy
Unstable cardiovascular status in acute hemorrhage with myocardial ischemia
Narrow-angle glaucoma
Thyrotoxicosis

Adverse Reactions

Tachycardia
Paradoxical bradycardia when pushed too slowly or when used at doses less than 0.5 mg
Palpitations
Dysrhythmias
Headache
Dizziness
Anticholinergic effects (dry mouth/nose/skin, photophobia, blurred vision, urinary retention, constipation)
Nausea and vomiting
Flushed, hot, dry skin
Allergic reactions

Drug Interactions

Use with other anticholinergic agents may increase vagal blockade
Potential adverse effects when administered in conjunction with digitalis, cholinergics, neostigmine
The effects of atropine may be enhanced by antihistamines, procainamide, quinidine, antipsychotics and antidepressants, thiazides
Increased toxicity: Amantadine

How Supplied

Parenteral: There are various injection preparations. In emergency care, atropine usually is supplied in prefilled syringes containing 1 mg in 10 mL of solution.

Dosage and Administration

Bradydysrhythmias
Adult: 0.5-1 mg IV; every 3-5 min for desired response (max total dose 0.04 mg/kg)
Pediatric: 0.02 mg/kg IV, IO, ET (diluted to 3-5 mL); min dose 0.1 mg; maximum single dose of 0.5 mg for a child and 1 mg for an adolescent; may be repeated in 5 min for a maximum total dose 1 mg for a child and 2 mg for an adolescent

Asystole or PEA
Adult: 1 mg IV, ET (2-3 mg diluted to a total of 10 mL of NS); may be repeated every 3-5 min (max 0.03-0.04 mg/kg)
Pediatric: Efficacy has not been established.

Anticholinesterase Poisoning
Adult: 2 mg IV push every 5-15 min to dry secretions (repeat as needed); then every 1-4 hrs for at least 24 hrs
Pediatric: 0.05 mg/kg/dose (usual dose 1-5 mg) IV; may be repeated every 20 min until atropine effect is observed; then 1-4 hrs for at least 24 hrs

Special Considerations

Pregnancy Safety: Category C
Follow ET administration with several positive-pressure ventilations
Atropine causes pupillary dilation rendering the pupils nonreactive; pupil response may not be useful in monitoring CNS status

Butorphanol (Stadol)

Class

Opioid agonist-antagonist analgesic

Description

The exact mechanism of action of opioid agonist-antagonist agents is unknown. They have both agonist and antagonist effects on opioid receptors and have analgesic effects similar to morphine.

Onset and Duration

Onset: 10 min (IM) 1-5 min (IV)
Duration: 3-4 hr

Indications

Relief of moderate-to-severe pain
Preoperative or preanesthetic medication

Contraindications

Head injury
Respiratory depression
Hypersensitivity to butorphanol

Adverse Reactions

Headache
Vertigo
Hallucinations
Palpitations
Increased or decreased blood pressure
Respiratory depression
Possible withdrawal syndrome in narcotic-dependent patients

Drug Interactions

Phenothiazines, droperidol, tranquilizers, and barbiturates may potentiate the actions of butorphanol

How Supplied

1 mg/mL in 1-mL vials; 2 mg/mL in 1-, 2-, and 10-mL vials

Dosage and Administration

Adult: 10-40 mg IM or 0.5-20 mg IV every 3-4 hr as needed to control pain
Pediatric: Safety has not been established

Special Considerations

Pregnancy Safety: Category B
May increase cardiac workload in patients with CHF, AMI, ventricular dysfunction, or coronary insufficiency
Use with caution in patients with end-stage liver disease
Has potential for abuse

Calcium Chloride

Class

Electrolyte

Description

Calcium is an essential component for functional integrity of the nervous and muscular systems, for normal cardiac contractility, and the coagulation of blood. Calcium chloride contains 27.2% elemental calcium. Calcium chloride is a hypertonic solution and should only be administered intravenously (slowly, not exceeding 1 mL/min).

Onset and Duration

Onset: 5-15 min
Duration: Dose dependent (effects may persist for 4 hr after IV administration)

Indications

Hyperkalemia (except when associated with digitalis toxicity)
Hypocalcemia (e.g., after multiple blood transfusions)
Calcium channel blocker toxicity
Hypermagnesemia
To prevent hypotensive effects of calcium channel blocking agents (IV verapamil and diltiazem)

Contraindications

VF during cardiac resuscitation
In patients with digitalis toxicity
Hypercalcemia
Renal or cardiac disease

Adverse Reactions

Bradycardia (may cause asystole)
Hypotension
Metallic taste
Severe local necrosis and sloughing following IM use or IV infiltration

Drug Interactions

Calcium may worsen dysrhythmias secondary to digitalis
May antagonize the peripheral vasodilatory effects of calcium channel blockers

How Supplied

10% solution in 10 mL (100 mg/mL) ampules, vials, and prefilled syringes

Dosage and Administration

Hyperkalemia, Hypocalcemia, Hypermagnesemia and Calcium Channel Blocker Overdose
Adult: 8-16 mg/kg (usually 5-10 mL) of 10% solution slow IV; may be repeated if needed
Pediatric: 20 mg/kg (0.2 mL/kg) IV/IO of 10% solution slow IV (give slowly, no faster than 100 mg/min); may repeat in 10 min if necessary

Special Considerations

Pregnancy Safety: Category C
Calcium may produce vasospasm in coronary and cerebral arteries
Do not use routinely in cardiac arrest
Hypertension and bradycardia may occur with rapid administration
Monitor heart rate during administration

> **NOTE**
>
> It is important to flush IV line between administration of *calcium chloride* and *sodium bicarbonate* to avoid precipitation.

Dexamethasone (Decadron, Hexadrol, and others)

Class

Glucocorticoid

Description

Dexamethasone is a synthetic steroid that is chemically related to the natural hormones secreted by the adrenal cortex. The drug suppresses acute and chronic inflammation, potentiates the relaxation of vascular and bronchial smooth muscle by beta adrenergic agonists, and possibly alters airway hyper-reactivity. In emergency care, dexamethasone is generally used in the treatment of allergic reactions, and asthma.

Onset and Duration
Onset: 4-8 hr after parenteral administration
Duration: 24-72 hr

Indications
Endocrine, rheumatic, hematologic disorders
Allergic states
Septic shock
Chronic inflammation

Contraindications
Hypersensitivity to the product
Active untreated infections (relative)

Adverse Reactions
Hypertension
GI bleeding

Drug Interactions
Barbiturates and phenytoin can decrease dexamethasone effects

How Supplied
Common preparations used in emergency care are for intravenous administration, and are listed below:
4 mg/mL in 1, 5, 10, 25, 30 mL vials
10 mg/mL in 10 mL vials, 1 mL syringe, 1 mL ampule
20 mg/mL in 5 mL vials (IV or IM), 5 mL syringe (IV)
24 mg/mL (IV only) in 5, 10 mL vials

Dosage and Administration
Adult: There is considerable variance in recommended dexamethasone doses. The usual range in emergency care is 4-24 mg IV. Some physicians may prefer significantly higher doses (up to 100 mg) for unusual indications.
Pediatric: 0.25-0.5 mg/kg/dose IV/IO

Special Considerations
Pregnancy Safety: Category C. Crosses the placenta and may cause fetal damage
Medication should be protected from heat
Due to onset of action (4-8 hr), dexamethasone should not be considered a first-line medication for allergic reactions

Dextrose 50%

Class
Carbohydrate, Hypertonic solution

Description
The term "dextrose" is used to describe the six carbon sugar *d-glucose*, the principal form of carbohydrate utilized by the body. 50% dextrose solution (D_{50}) is used in emergency care to treat hypoglycemia, and in the management of coma of unknown origin.

Onset and Duration
Onset: 1 min
Duration: Depends on the degree of hypoglycemia

Indications
Hypoglycemia
Altered level of consciousness
Coma of unknown etiology
Seizure of unknown etiology

Contraindications
Intracranial hemorrhage
Increased intracranial pressure
Known or suspected CVA in the absence of hypoglycemia

Adverse Reactions
Warmth, pain, burning from medication infusion, hyperglycemia, thrombophlebitis

Drug Interactions
None significant

How Supplied
25 g/50 mL prefilled syringe (500 mg/mL)

Dosage and Administration
Adult: 12.5-25 g slow IV; may be repeated once
Pediatric: 0.5 -1 g/kg IV/IO
             1-2 mL/kg 50%
             2-4 mL/kg 25%
             5-10 mL/kg 10%

Special Considerations
Pregnancy Safety: Category C
Draw blood sample prior to administration if possible
Perform blood glucose analysis prior to administration if possible
Extravasation may cause tissue necrosis; use large vein and aspirate occasionally to ensure route patency
D_{50} may sometimes precipitate severe neurological symptoms (Wernicke's encephalopathy) in thiamine deficient patients, for example, alcoholics. (This can be prevented by administering 100 mg of thiamine, IV.)

Diazepam *(Valium and others)*

Class
Benzodiazepine

Description
Diazepam is a frequently prescribed medication to treat anxiety and stress. In emergency care, it is used to treat alcohol withdrawal and grand mal seizure activity. Diazepam acts on the limbic, thalamic, and hypothalamic

regions of the CNS to potentiate the effects of inhibitory neurotransmitters, raising the seizure threshold in the motor cortex. It may also be used in conscious patients during cardioversion and TCP to induce amnesia and sedation. Its use as an anticonvulsant may be short-lived due to rapid redistribution from the CNS. Rapid IV administration may be followed by respiratory depression and excessive sedation, particularly in elderly patients.

Onset and Duration

Onset: (IV) 1-5 min
              (IM) 15-30 min
Duration: (IV) 15 min-1 hr
              (IM) 15 min-1 hr

Indications

Acute anxiety states
Acute alcohol withdrawal
Skeletal muscle relaxation
Seizure activity
Premedication prior to countershock or TCP

Contraindications

Hypersensitivity to the drug
Substance abuse (use with caution)
Coma (unless the patient has seizures or severe muscle rigidity or myoclonus)
Shock
CNS depression as a result of head injury
Respiratory depression

Adverse Reactions

Hypotension
Reflex tachycardia (rare)
Respiratory depression
Ataxia
Psychomotor impairment
Confusion
Nausea

Drug Interactions

Diazepam may precipitate CNS depression and psychomotor impairment when the patient is taking other CNS depressant medications
Should not be administered with other drugs because of possible precipitation (incompatible with most fluids; should be administered into an IV of normal saline solution)

How Supplied

Parenteral: 5 mg/mL vials, ampules, Tubex

Dosage and Administration

Seizure Activity
Adult: 5 mg over 2 min (up to 10 mg for most adults) IV q 10-15 min prn (maximum dose 30 mg)
Pediatric: Dose for infants >30 days to 5 years is 0.2 mg to 0.5 mg slow IV q 2-5 min to max 5 mg; children >5 years is 1 mg q

2-5 min to max 10 mg slow IV
Premedication for Cardioversion or TCP
Adult: 5-15 mg IV, 5-10 min prior to procedure

Special Considerations

Pregnancy Safety: Category D
May cause local venous irritation
Has short duration of anticonvulsant effect
Reduce dose by 50% in elderly patients
Resuscitation equipment should be readily available

Digoxin (Lanoxin)

Class

Cardiac glycoside, Miscellaneous antidysrhythmic

Description

Digoxin (digitalis) is a cardiac glycoside derived primarily from the foxglove plant. Its primary action involves alteration of ion transport across cardiac cell membranes. Increased intracellular calcium improves myocardial contractility. Digoxin increases vagal tone and therefore indirectly decreases sinus node rate, reduces sympathetic tone and decreases AV node conduction velocity (with an increase in AV node refractory period). Sodium pumped out of cells may cause increased automaticity.

Onset and Duration

Onset: (IV) 5-30 min
Duration: 3-4 days

Indications

Supraventricular tachycardias, especially atrial flutter and atrial fibrillation
Congestive heart failure
Cardiogenic shock

Contraindications

Ventricular fibrillation
Ventricular tachycardia
AV block
Digitalis toxicity
Hypersensitivity to digoxin
Second- or third-degree heart block in the absence of artificial pacing

Adverse Reactions *(mostly related to digitalis toxicity)*

Headache
Weakness
Visual disturbances (blurred, yellow or green vision)
Confusion
Seizures
Dysrhythmias (virtually any disturbance, but junctional tachycardias are most common)
Nausea and vomiting
Skin rash

Drug Interactions

Amiodarone, verapamil, and quinidine may increase serum digoxin concentrations by 50%-70%

Concurrent administration of IV digoxin and IV verapamil may lead to severe heart block

Erythromycin and tetracycline may increase serum digoxin concentrations by reducing hepatic breakdown

Diuretics may potentiate digoxin cardiotoxicity via loss of potassium

Sympathomimetics may augment the inotropic and cardiotoxic effects of digoxin

Concomitant administration of kaolin, pectin, and antacids may reduce digoxin absorption from the GI tract

How Supplied

In emergency care, the common form of digoxin is supplied in 2 mL ampules, containing 0.5 mg of the drug (0.25 mg/mL)

Dosage and Administration

Adult: Loading dose 10-15 mcg/kg; maintenance dose affected by body size and renal function

Pediatric: Not recommended in prehospital setting

Special Considerations

Pregnancy Safety: Category C

Patient should be constantly monitored for signs of digitalis toxicity

Patients with myocardial infarction and/or renal failure are prone to developing digitalis toxicity

Digitalis toxicity is potentiated in patients with hypokalemia, hypomagnesemia, and hypercalcemia

Avoid use in patients with WPW syndrome because of possible ventricular dysrhythmias

Diltiazem (Cardizem) Injectable

Class

Slow calcium channel blocker or calcium channel antagonist

Description

Diltiazem is a calcium channel blocking agent that slows conduction, increases refractoriness in the AV node, and causes coronary and peripheral vasodilation. The drug is used to control ventricular response rates in patients with atrial fibrillation or flutter, multifocal atrial tachycardias, and PSVT.

Onset and Duration

Onset: 2-5 min
Duration: 1-3 hr

Indications

Atrial fibrillation
Atrial flutter
Multifocal atrial tachycardias
PSVT

Contraindications

Sick sinus syndrome

Second- or third-degree AV block (except with a functioning pacemaker)

Hypotension (less than 90 mm Hg)

Cardiogenic shock

Hypersensitivity to diltiazem

Atrial fibrillation or atrial flutter associated with WPW syndrome or a short PR syndrome

Concomitant use of IV beta blockers

Ventricular tachycardia

Wide-complex tachycardia of unknown origin

AMI

Adverse Reactions

Atrial flutter
First- and second-degree AV block
Bradycardia
Hypotension
Chest pain
Congestive heart failure
Peripheral edema
Syncope
Ventricular dysrhythmias
Sweating
Nausea and vomiting
Dizziness
Dry mouth
Dyspnea
Headache

Drug Interactions

Caution is warranted in patients receiving medications that affect cardiac contractility and/or SA or AV node conduction

Incompatible with simultaneous furosemide injection

How Supplied

25 mg (5 mL vial); 50 mg (10 mL vial)

Dosage and Administration

Bolus injection: 0.25 mg/kg (15-20 mg for the average patient) IV over 2 min; may be repeated in 15 min (0.35 mg/kg; 20-25 mg for the average patient) IV over 2 min

Maintenance infusion: Dilute 125 mg (25 mL) in 100 mL of solution; infuse 5-15 mg/hr, titrated to heart rate

Pediatric: Similar mg/kg doses as adults (but rarely required in pediatric patients)

Special Considerations

Pregnancy Safety: Category C

Use with caution in patients with impaired renal or hepatic function

Hypotension may occasionally result (carefully monitor vital signs)

PVCs may be present on conversion of PSVT to sinus rhythm

Shelf-life at room temperature is one month

Diphenhydramine (Benadryl)

Class
Antihistamine

Description
Antihistamines prevent the physiologic actions of histamine by blocking H_1 (e.g., diphenhydramine, cimetidine) and H_2 (cimetidine, ranitidine, famodipine, etc.) receptor sites. The effects of antihistamines are short-lived and provide only symptomatic relief. Antihistamines are indicated for conditions in which histamine excess is present (e.g., acute urticaria), but also are used as adjunctive therapy (with epinephrine, for example) in the treatment of anaphylactic shock. Antihistamines also are effective in the treatment of extrapyramidal reactions and for relief of upper respiratory and sinus symptoms associated with allergic reactions.

Onset and Duration
Onset: Maximal effects 1-3 hr
Duration: 6-12 hr

Indications
Moderate to severe allergic reactions (after epinephrine)
Anaphylaxis
Acute extrapyramidal reactions

Contraindications
Patients taking monoamine oxidase (MAO) inhibitors
Hypersensitivity
Narrow-angle glaucoma (relative)
Newborns and nursing mothers

Adverse Reactions
Dose-related drowsiness
Sedation
Disturbed coordination
Hypotension
Palpitations
Tachycardia, bradycardia
Thickening of bronchial secretions
Dry mouth and throat
Paradoxical excitement in children

Drug Interactions
CNS depressants may increase depressant effects
MAO inhibitors may prolong and intensify anticholinergic effects of antihistamines

How Supplied
Parenteral: 10, 50 mg/mL vials, prefilled syringe

Dosage and Administration
Adult: The standard dose of diphenhydramine is 25-50 mg IM, IV every 6-8 hrs (max 300 mg/day)
Pediatric (greater   1.25 mg/kg/dose q 6 hr
than 10 kg):   (max 300 mg/day)

Special Considerations
Pregnancy Safety: Category C
Use cautiously in patients with CNS depression or lower respiratory diseases such as asthma

Dobutamine (Dobutrex)

Class
Sympathomimetic

Description
Dobutamine is a synthetic catecholamine that primarily stimulates $beta_1$ adrenergic receptors, and has much less significant effects on $beta_2$ and alpha adrenergic receptors. The clinical effects of this drug include positive inotropic effects with minimal changes in chronotropic activity or systemic vascular resistance. For these reasons, dobutamine is useful in the management of CHF when an increase in heart rate is not desired.

Onset and Duration
Onset: 1-2 min; peak after 10 min
Duration: 10-15 min

Indications
Inotropic support for patients with left ventricular dysfunction

Contraindications
Tachydysrhythmias (atrial fibrillation, atrial flutter)
Severe hypotension with signs of shock
IHSS
Suspected or known drug-induced shock

Adverse Reactions
Headache
Dose-related tachydysrhythmias
Hypertension
Ventricular ectopy

Drug Interactions
Beta adrenergic antagonists may blunt inotropic responses
Sympathomimetics and phosphodiesterase inhibitors may exacerbate dysrhythmia responses
Incompatible with sodium bicarbonate and furosemide in same IV line; may be given in separate IV lines

How Supplied
12.5 mg/mL injectable

Dosage and Administration
Adult: Usual dose is 2-20 mcg/kg/min IV, based on inotropic effect

Pediatric: 2-20 mcg/kg/min IV/IO, titrated to desired effect

Special Considerations

Pregnancy Safety: Category C

Administer via an infusion pump to ensure precise flow rates

May be administered through a Y-site with concurrent dopamine, lidocaine, nitroprusside, and potassium chloride infusions

Blood pressure should be closely monitored

Increases in heart rate of more than 10% may induce or exacerbate myocardial ischemia

Lidocaine should be readily available

Correct hypovolemia prior to using dobutamine in hypotensive patients

Dopamine *(Intropin)*

Class

Sympathomimetic

Description

Dopamine is chemically related to epinephrine and norepinephrine. It acts primarily on alpha$_1$ and beta$_1$ adrenergic receptors in dose-dependent fashion. At low doses, dopamine acts on dopaminergic receptors causing renal, mesenteric, and cerebral vascular dilation. At moderate doses ("cardiac doses"), dopamine stimulates beta adrenergic receptors causing enhanced myocardial contractility, increased cardiac output, and a rise in blood pressure. At high doses ("vasopressor doses"), dopamine has an alpha-adrenergic effect, producing peripheral arterial and venous constriction. Dopamine is commonly used in the treatment of hypotension associated with cardiogenic shock.

Onset and Duration

Onset: 2-4 min
Duration: 10-15 min

Indications

Hemodynamically significant hypotension in the absence of hypovolemia

Contraindications

Tachydysrhythmias
Ventricular fibrillation
Patients with pheochromocytoma

Adverse Reactions

Dose-related tachydysrhythmias
Hypertension
Increased myocardial oxygen demand (e.g., ischemia)

Drug Interactions

May be deactivated by alkaline solutions (sodium bicarbonate and furosemide)
MAO inhibitors may potentiate the effect of dopamine

Sympathomimetics and phosphodiesterase inhibitors exacerbate dysrhythmia response

Beta adrenergic antagonists may blunt inotropic response

When administered with phenytoin, hypotension, bradycardia and seizures may develop

How Supplied

200 mg, 400 mg, 800 mg in 5 mL prefilled syringe and ampule for IV infusion (IV piggyback)

Dosage and Administration

Adult: Low dose 2-4 mcg/kg/min
            Moderate dose 5-10 mcg/kg/min
              (cardiac doses)
            High dose 10-20 mcg/kg/min
              (vasopressor doses)
Pediatric: 2-20 mcg/kg/min IV/IO, titrated to patient response (not to exceed 20 mcg/kg/min)

Special Considerations

Pregnancy Safety: Category C

Infuse through large, stable vein to avoid the possibility of extravasation injury

Use infusion pump to ensure precise flow rates

Monitor patient for signs of compromised circulation

Correct hypovolemia prior to using dopamine in hypotensive patients

Droperidol *(Inapsine)*

Class

Neuroleptic agent

Description

Droperidol produces dopaminergic and mild alpha-adrenergic blockade. It is used to induce a state of profound analgesia and psychomotor sedation. It also can serve as an antiemetic.

Onset and Duration

Onset: 3-10 min
Duration: 3-6 hr

Indications

Chemical restraint
Intractable vomiting

Contraindications

Hypotension
Tachycardia
Pregnancy
Neuroleptic malignant syndrome
Bronchospasm
Hypersensitivity to droperidol

Adverse Reactions

Hypotension
Hypertension
Tachycardia

Increased excitability
Anxiety
Sweating

Drug Interactions

Respiratory depression may occur when given with other sedatives, tranquilizers, or narcotics
Concurrent use should be avoided

How Supplied

2.5-mg/mL ampules

Dosage and Administration

Adult:	Chemical restraint–5.0 mg slow IV or IM; may be repeated once in 10 to 15 min
	Antiemetic–1.25 mg slow IV or IM
Child (over 2 years of age):	Chemical restraint—not recommended in the prehospital setting
	Antiemetic–0.05-0.1 mg/kg slow IV or IM

Special Considerations

Pregnancy Safety: Category C
Administered only by the IV or IM route
Use with caution in the elderly and in those who have cardiovascular, renal, or liver disease
Rarely, extrapyramidal reactions may occur
Hypotension and tachycardia generally respond well to patient positioning and fluid administration

Epinephrine (Adrenalin)

Class

Sympathomimetic

Description

Epinephrine is an endogenous catecholamine that directly stimulates alpha, beta$_1$, and beta$_2$ adrenergic receptors in dose-related fashion. It is the initial drug of choice for treating bronchoconstriction and hypotension resulting from anaphylaxis as well as all forms of cardiac arrest. It is useful in the management of reactive airway disease, but beta adrenergic agents are usually considered the drugs of choice since they are inhaled and have fewer side effects. Rapid injection produces a rapid increase in blood pressure, ventricular contractility, and heart rate. In addition, epinephrine causes vasoconstriction in the arterioles of the skin, mucosa, and splanchnic areas, and antagonizes the effects of histamine.

Onset and Duration

Onset:	(SQ) 5-10 min
	(IV) (ET) 1-2 min
Duration:	5-10 min

Indications

Bronchial asthma
Acute allergic reaction (anaphylaxis)
Cardiac arrest
   Asystole
   Pulseless Electrical Activity (PEA)
   Ventricular fibrillation and pulseless ventricular tachycardia unresponsive to initial defibrillation
Profound symptomatic bradycardia

Contraindications

Hypersensitivity (not an issue especially in emergencies – the dose should be lowered or given slowly in non-cardiac arrest patients with heart disease)
Hypovolemic shock (as with other catecholamines, correct hypovolemia prior to use)
Coronary insufficiency (use with caution)

Adverse Reactions

Headache
Nausea
Restlessness
Weakness
Dysrhythmias, including ventricular tachycardia and ventricular fibrillation
Hypertension
Precipitation of angina pectoris
Tachycardia

Drug Interactions

MAO inhibitors may potentiate the effect of epinephrine
Beta adrenergic antagonists may blunt inotropic response
Sympathomimetics and phosphodiesterase inhibitors may exacerbate dysrhythmia response
May be deactivated by alkaline solutions (sodium bicarbonate, furosemide)

How Supplied

Parenteral:	1 mg/mL (1:1000), 0.1 mg/mL (1:10,000) ampule and prefilled syringe
	Auto-injector (EpiPen) 0.5 mg/mL (1:2000)

Dosage and Administration

Profound Bradycardia or Hypotension

Adult:	See IV infusion dose
Pediatric:	0.01 mg/kg (1:10,000, 0.1 mL/kg) IV/IO

Pulseless Arrest

Adult:

Initial:	1 mg (10 mL, 1:10,000) IV push or ET (2-2.5 mg diluted in 10 mL of normal saline), repeated every 3-5 min during resuscitation (follow each IV dose with a 20-mL saline flush); higher doses (up to 0.2 mg/kg) may be used if 1 mg doses fail

Pediatric:

First dose: 0.01 mg/kg (1:10,000, 0.1 mL/kg) IV/IO or ET (0.1-0.2 mg/kg of 1:1000 [0.1-0.2 mL/kg]).

Subsequent doses: Repeat initial dose or may increase up to 10 times (0.1 mg/kg, 1:1000, 0.1 mL/kg); administer every 3-5 min; IV/IO/ET doses as high as 0.2 mg/kg of 1:1000 may be effective

Epinephrine infusions for pulseless arrest and symptomatic bradycardia with profound hypotension refractory to other interventions

Adult: Add 30 mg epinephrine (30 mL of 1:1000 solution) to 250 mL of normal saline or D_5W; run at 100 mL/hr and titrate to response

Pediatric: 0.1-1 mcg/kg/min IV/IO; calculate dose by 0.6 × body weight (in kg) equals number of mg diluted to total 100 mL; then 1 mL/hr delivers 0.1 mcg/kg/min

Anaphylactic Reaction or Bronchoconstriction:

Adult: (Mild): 0.3-0.5 mL (1:1000) SQ
(Moderate to Severe): 1-2 mL (1:10,000) slow IV

Pediatric: (Mild): 0.01 mL/kg SQ (1:1000), maximum 0.3 mL
(Moderate to Severe): 0.05-0.15 mcg/kg/min IV infusion

Special Considerations

Pregnancy Safety: Category C
Do not use prefilled syringes for epinephrine infusions
Syncope has occurred following epinephrine administration to asthmatic children
May increase myocardial oxygen demand

> **NOTE**
>
> Complications of IV administration of *epinephrine* are significant and include the development of uncontrolled systolic hypertension, vomiting, seizures, dysrhythmias, and myocardial ischemia. This route should only be used in patients with a critical life-threatening condition. IV administration of *epinephrine* rarely is performed in conscious patients. It is performed with extreme caution in rare circumstances and only with authorization from medical direction.

Epinephrine Racemic (microNEFRIN)

Class

Sympathomimetic

Description

As with other forms of epinephrine, racemic epinephrine acts as a bronchodilator that stimulates $beta_2$ receptors in the lungs, resulting in relaxation of bronchial smooth muscle. This alleviates bronchospasm, increases vital capacity, and reduces airway resistance. It is also useful in treating laryngeal edema. Racemic epinephrine also inhibits the release of histamine.

Onset and Duration

Onset: Within 5 min
Duration: 1-3 hr

Indications

Bronchial asthma
Treatment of bronchospasm
Croup (laryngotracheobronchitis)
Laryngeal edema

Contraindications

Hypertension
Underlying cardiovascular disease
Epiglottitis

Adverse Reactions

Tachycardia
Dysrhythmias

Drug Interactions

MAO inhibitors may potentiate the effect of epinephrine
Beta adrenergic antagonists may blunt the bronchodilating response
Sympathomimetics and phosphodiesterase inhibitors may exacerbate dysrhythmia response

How Supplied

MDI: 0.16-0.25 mg/spray
Solution: 7.5, 15, 30 mL in 1%, 2.25% solution

Dosage and Administration

MDI
  Adult: 2-3 inhalations, repeat once in 5 min prn
Solution
  Adult: Dilute 5 mL (1%) in 5 mL saline, administer over 15 min
  Pediatric: Dilute 0.25 mL (0.1%) in 2.5 mL saline (if less than 20 kg); 0.5 mL in 2.5 mL saline (if 20-40 kg); 0.75 mL in 2.5 mL saline (if greater than 40 kg); administer by aerosolization

Special Considerations

Pregnancy Safety: Category C
May produce tachycardia and other dysrhythmias
Monitor vital signs closely
Excessive use may cause bronchospasm
Rebound exacerbation of severe croup may occur following drug administration
Subcutaneous route typically considered more effective for bronchodilation

Etomidate (Amidate)

Class
Nonbarbiturate hypnotic, Anesthetic

Description
Etomidate is a short-acting drug that acts at the level of the reticular activating system to produce anesthesia. Etomidate may be administered for conscious sedation to relieve apprehension or impair memory prior to tracheal intubation or cardioversion.

Onset and Duration
Onset: Within 30 seconds
Duration: 3-5 min

Indications
Premedication for tracheal intubation or cardioversion

Contraindications
Hypersensitivity to etomidate
Labor/delivery

Adverse Reactions
Nausea and vomiting
Dysrhythmias
Breathing difficulties
Hypotension
Hypertension
Involuntary muscle movement
Pain at injection site

Drug Interactions
Effects may be enhanced when given with other CNS depressants

How Supplied
2 mg/mL vials

Dosage and Administration
Adult: 0.2-0.6 mg/kg IV over
                    30-60 seconds
Pediatric (over   0.2-0.4 mg/kg over 30-60 seconds
10 years of age):

Special Considerations
Pregnancy Safety: Category C
Carefully monitor vital signs
Can suppress adrenal gland production of steroid hormones which can cause temporary gland failure

Fentanyl (Sublimaze)

Class
Opioid analgesic

Description
Fentanyl (like other opioids) combines with receptor sites in the brain to produce potent analgesic effects. The drug usually is given in combination with droperidol for general anesthesia.

Onset and Duration
Onset: 7-8 min
Duration: 0.5-1 hr

Indications
Pain control
Sedation for invasive airway procedures (e.g., RSI)

Contraindications
Respiratory depression
Hypotension
Head injury
Cardiac dysrhythmias
Myasthenia gravis
Hypersensitivity to opiates

Adverse Reactions
Respiratory depression
Bradycardia
Hypotension or hypertension
Nausea and vomiting

Drug Interactions
Effects may be increased when given with other CNS depressants or skeletal muscle relaxants

How Supplied
0.05-mg/mL ampules

Dosage and Administration
Adult: 0.05-0.1 mg IM every 1-2 hr as
                    needed to control pain
Child (over 2 years 0.02-0.03 mg/9 kg IM one time;
of age):   rarely used in the prehospital
                    setting

Special Considerations
Pregnancy Safety: Category C
Fentanyl is a schedule II drug with the potential for abuse
It should be used (if at all) with caution in elderly patients and in those with severe respiratory disorders, seizure disorders, cardiac disorders, or pregnancy
Naloxone or nalmefene should be available to reverse respiratory depression

Flumazenil (Romazicon)

Class
Benzodiazepine receptor antagonist, Antidote

Description
Flumazenil antagonizes the actions of benzodiazepines in the central nervous system. It has been shown to reverse sedation, impairment of recall, and psychomotor impairment produced by benzodiazepines. Flumazenil is not, however, as effective in reversing hypoventilation. Flu-

mazenil does not antagonize CNS effects of ethanol, barbiturates, or opioids.

Onset and Duration

Onset: 1-2 min
Duration: Related to plasma concentration of benzodiazepine

Indications

Reversal of excessive or prolonged benzodiazepine sedation or overdose

Contraindications

Hypersensitivity to flumazenil or to benzodiazepines
Cyclic antidepressant overdose
Cocaine or other stimulant intoxication

Adverse Reactions

Nausea and vomiting
Dizziness
Headache
Agitation
Injection-site pain
Cutaneous vasodilation
Abnormal vision
Seizures

Drug Interactions

Toxic effects of mixed drug overdose (especially cyclic antidepressants) may emerge with the reversal of the benzodiazepine effects

How Supplied

5 and 10 mL vials (0.1 mg/mL)

Dosage and Administration

For suspected benzodiazepine overdose:
Adult: 0.2 mg (2 mL) IV over 15 seconds; an additional dose of 0.3 mg (3 mL) may be given in 30 seconds, followed by 0.5 mg (5 mL) over 30 seconds at 1-minute intervals (maximum dose of 3 mg)
Pediatric: Not recommended

Special Considerations

Pregnancy Safety: Category C
To minimize the likelihood of injection-site pain, administer through an intravenous infusion established in a large vein
Be prepared to manage seizures in patients who are physically dependent on benzodiazepines to control seizures, or who have ingested large doses of other drugs
Flumazenil may precipitate withdrawal syndromes in patients who are dependent on benzodiazepines
Patients should be monitored for possible resedation, respiratory depression, or other residual benzodiazepine effects
Be prepared to establish and assist ventilation

Furosemide (Lasix)

Class

Loop diuretic

Description

Furosemide is a potent diuretic that inhibits the reabsorption of sodium and chloride in the proximal tubule and loop of Henle. Intravenous doses can also reduce cardiac preload by increasing venous capacitance.

Onset and Duration

Onset: (IV) diuretic effects within 15-20 min; vascular effects within 5 min
Duration: 2 hr

Indications

Pulmonary edema associated with CHF, hepatic or renal disease

Contraindications

Anuria (though loop diuretics can be used in patients with reduced creatinine clearance)
Hypersensitivity
Hypovolemia/dehydration
Known hypersensitivity to sulfonamides
Severe electrolyte depletion (hypokalemia)

Adverse Reactions

Hypotension
ECG changes associated with electrolyte disturbances
Dry mouth
Hypochloremia
Hypokalemia
Hyponatremia
Hypercalcemia
Hyperglycemia
Hearing loss can rarely occur after too rapid infusion of large doses especially in patients with renal impairment

Drug Interactions

Digitalis toxicity may be potentiated due to potassium depletion, which can result from furosemide administration
Increases ototoxic potential of aminoglycoside antibiotics
Lithium toxicity may be potentiated due to sodium depletion
May potentiate therapeutic effect of other antihypertensive drugs

How Supplied

Parenteral: 10 mg/mL in 2, 4, 8 mL ampule, 10 mg/mL in 10 mL vial

Dosage and Administration

Adult: 20-40 mg (0.5-1 mg/kg) slow IV over 1-2 min; (not to exceed 20 mg/min); if no response, double dose to 2 mg/kg slow IV over 1-2 min
Pediatric: 1 mg/kg/dose (max 6 mg/kg total dose)

Special Considerations

Pregnancy Safety: Category C

Furosemide has been known to cause fetal abnormalities

Should be protected from light and stored at room temperature; do not use if solution is discolored or yellow

Glucagon

Class

Pancreatic hormone, Insulin antagonist

Description

Glucagon is a protein secreted by the alpha cells of the pancreas. When released, it results in blood glucose elevation by increasing the breakdown of glycogen to glucose (glycogenolysis) and stimulating glucose synthesis (gluconeogenesis). The drug is only effective in treating hypoglycemia if liver glycogen is available, and may therefore be ineffective in chronic states of hypoglycemia, starvation, and adrenal insufficiency. In addition, glucagon exerts positive inotropic action on the heart and decreases renal vascular resistance. For this reason glucagon is also used in managing patients with beta-blocker and calcium channel blocker cardiotoxicity who do not respond to saline infusions or other conventional therapy.

Onset and Duration

Onset: Within 1 min
Duration: 60-90 min

Indications

Persistent hypoglycemia despite glucose supplementation
Calcium channel blocker or β-blocker toxicity

Contraindications

Hypersensitivity (allergy to proteins)

Adverse Reactions

Tachycardia
Hypotension
Nausea and vomiting
Urticaria

Drug Interactions

Effect of anticoagulants may be increased if given with glucagon
Do not mix with saline

How Supplied

Glucagon must be reconstituted (with provided diluent) before administration. Dilute 1 unit (1 mg) white powder in 1 mL of diluting solution (1 mg/mL).

Dosage and Administration

Hypoglycemia
Adult: 0.5-1 mg IM; may repeat in 7-10 min
Pediatric: 0.025-1 mg IM; may repeat in 7-10 min
Calcium channel blocker or β-blocker toxicity
Adult: 1-5 mg over 25 min
Pediatric: Safety and efficacy have not been established

Special Considerations

Pregnancy Safety: Category B

Should not be considered a first-line choice for hypoglycemia

Intravenous glucose will need to be administered if the patient does not respond to a second dose of glucagon

Do not use the provided diluent to mix continuous infusions

Haloperidol Lactate (Haldol)

Class

Antipsychotic/Neuroleptic

Description

Haloperidol has pharmacologic properties similar to those of the phenothiazines. The drug is thought to block dopamine (type 2) receptors in the brain, altering mood and behavior. In emergency care, haloperidol usually is administered IM, but may also be given IV.

Onset and Duration

Onset: (IM) 30-60 min
Duration: 12-24 hr

Indications

Acute psychotic episodes
Emergency sedation of severely agitated or delirious patients

Contraindications

CNS depression
Coma
Hypersensitivity
Pregnancy
Severe liver or cardiac disease

Adverse Reactions

Dose-related extrapyramidal reactions:
    Pseudoparkinsonism
    Akathisia
    Dystonias
Hypotension
Orthostatic hypotension
Nausea, vomiting
Allergic reactions
Blurred vision

Drug Interactions

Other CNS depressants may potentiate effects
May inhibit vasoconstrictor effects of epinephrine

How Supplied
5 mg, 50 mg, 100 mg/mL ampule

Dosage and Administration
Adult: 2-5 mg IM every 4-8 hrs as needed
Pediatric: 0.5 mg IM

Special Considerations
Pregnancy Safety: Category C

Heparin Sodium

Class
Anticoagulant

Description
Heparin inhibits the clotting cascade by activating specific plasma proteins. The drug is used in the prevention and treatment of all types of thromboses and emboli, DIC, arterial occlusion and thrombophlebitis, and prophylactically to prevent clotting before and after surgery. Heparin is also considered part of the "fibrinolytic package" administered to patients with acute myocardial infarction (along with aspirin and fibrinolytic agents) and acute coronary syndromes including unstable angina and non-Q wave myocardial infarction.

Onset and Duration
Onset: (IV) Immediate
          (SQ) 20-60 min
Duration: 4-8 hr

Indications
Acute myocardial infarction
Prophylaxis and treatment of thrombolytic disorders
    (e.g., pulmonary emboli, DVT)

Contraindications
Hypersensitivity
Active bleeding
Recent intracranial, intraspinal, or eye surgery
Severe hypertension
Bleeding tendencies
Severe thrombocytopenia

Adverse Reactions
Allergic reaction (chills, fever, back pain)
Thrombocytopenia
Hemorrhage
Bruising

Drug Interactions
Salicylates, ibuprofen, dipyridamole, hydroxychloroquine
    may increase risk of bleeding

How Supplied
10, 100, and 1000-40,000 U/mL

Dosage and Administration
If used with fibrinolytic therapy, always obtain a blood sample for control of partial thromboplastin time (PTT) before heparin administration. (Heparin along with aspirin is part of the "fibrinolytic package.") Heparin doses range from 100-4000 IU (follow medical direction and local protocol).

Special Considerations
Pregnancy Safety: Category C
Heparin does not lyse existing clots

Hydralazine (Apresoline)

Class
Antihypertensive, Vasodilator

Description
Hydralazine is an arteriolar vasodilating agent that is used in the management of hypertensive crisis. The effects of the drug include a decrease in arterial pressure, a decrease in peripheral resistance, and an increase in cardiac output (as a result of reflex tachycardia).

Onset and Duration
Onset: (IV) 5-30 min
          (IM) 10-40 min
Duration: 2-6 hr

Indications
Hypertensive crisis
Hypertension associated with renal failure, preeclampsia,
    and eclampsia
Primary pulmonary HTN

Contraindications
Compensatory hypertension
Coronary artery disease
Dissecting aneurysm
Hypersensitivity
Mitral valve/rheumatic heart disease

Adverse Reactions
Reflex tachycardia
Palpitations
Hypotension
Facial flushing
Headache
Diaphoresis
Anxiety
Nausea and vomiting
Diarrhea

Drug Interactions
Concurrent use of diazoxide may result in severe
    hypotension
Color changes may occur when given with glucose
    solutions

MAO inhibitors may result in significant hypotension

How Supplied
20 mg in 1 mL ampule (20 mg/mL)

Dosage and Administration
Adult:	10-40 mg IM or IV; may be repeated in 10 min prn
Infusion:	20 mg in 250 mL NS or LR at 5-20 mg/hr
Pediatric:	0.1-0.2 mg/kg/dose q 4-6 hr IM, IV; may be repeated prn
Infusion:	0.75-3 mg/kg q 6-12 hr

Special Considerations
Pregnancy Safety: Category C
Blood pressure and ECG should be continuously monitored

Hydroxyzine (Atarax, Vistaril)

Class
Antihistamine

Description
Hydroxyzine is a H_1 receptor antagonist that is used to treat allergy-induced pruritus, and is used perioperatively for its antiemetic and sedative properties. It is also effective for treatment of anxiety and tension associated with neuroses and alcohol withdrawal. Concomitant use with analgesics may potentiate their effects.

Onset and Duration
Onset:	(IM) 15-30 min
Duration:	4-6 hr

Indications
To potentiate the effects of analgesics
Nausea and vomiting
Anxiety reactions
Motion sickness
Alcohol withdrawal symptoms
Pruritus

Contraindications
Hypersensitivity to hydroxyzine

Adverse Reactions
Dry mouth
Drowsiness

Drug Interactions
The potentiating action of hydroxyzine must be considered when the drug is used in conjunction with CNS depressants such as narcotics, barbiturates, and alcohol, and with anticholinergics.

How Supplied
25, 50 mg/mL in 1 mL vials

Dosage and Administration
Adult:	25-100 mg deep IM
Pediatric:	1 mg/kg/dose, deep IM

Special Considerations
Pregnancy Safety: Category C
Hydroxyzine should be administered by deep IM injection only (not for SC or IV use)
Localized burning at the injection site is a common complaint

Ibutilide (Corvert)

Class
Short-acting antidysrhythmic

Description
Ibutilide prolongs the action potential duration and increases the refractory period of cardiac tissue. It is recommended for acute pharmacological conversion of atrial flutter or atrial fibrillation, or as an adjunct to electrical cardioversion.

Onset and Duration
Onset:	0.5-1.5 hr
Duration:	10-12 hr

Indications
Supraventricular dysrhythmias
Conversion of atrial fibrillation and atrial flutter of brief duration

Contraindications
History of heart failure or VT
Sensitivity to ibutilide

Adverse Reactions
Ventricular dysrhythmias
Hypotension and hypertension

Drug Interactions
Avoid concurrent administration of ibutilide with other antidysrhythmics that prolong the refractory period (e.g., amiodarone) or drugs that induce QT prolongation (e.g., procainamide)

How Supplied
1 mg in 10-mL ampules

Dosage and Administration
Adult (60 kg or more):	1 mg (10 mL) IV over 10 min. A second dose may be administered at the same rate 10 min later. The initial dose for adults who weigh less than 60 kg is 0.01 mg/kg IV.
Pediatric:	Not recommended

Special Considerations

Pregnancy Safety: Category C

Ibutilide must be given slow IV over 10 min. This may make it impractical for use in emergent situations.

Ventricular dysrhythmias develop in 2% to 5% of patients who are given ibutilide; continuous ECG monitoring is essential

Use with caution in patients with impaired LV function

Insulin *(Regular, NPH, Ultralente, and others)*

Class

Antidiabetic agent

Description

Insulin is secreted by the beta cells (islets of Langerhans) of the pancreas and is required for proper glucose utilization by the body. If insulin secretion is diminished (as in diabetes mellitus), supplemental insulin must be obtained by injection. Insulin preparations are classified as *rapid-acting* (Regular), *intermediate-acting* (NPH), and *long-acting* (Ultralente). Insulin is seldom administered in the prehospital setting, and then only when ketoacidosis is confirmed.

Onset and Duration

Onset:	0.5-1 hr (Rapid-Acting)
	1-1.5 hr (Intermediate-Acting)
	4-6 hr (Long-Acting)
Duration:	6-8 hr (Rapid-Acting)
	18-24 hr (Intermediate-Acting)
	More than 36 hr (Long-Acting)

Indications

Type I diabetes mellitus

Type II diabetes mellitus if oral hypoglycemic agents do not adequately control blood glucose

Diabetic ketoacidosis

Nonketotic hyperosmolar coma

Insulin and D_{50} are given together to lower potassium levels in hyperkalemia

Contraindications

Hypoglycemia

Adverse Reactions

Hypoglycemia

Fatigue

Weakness

Confusion

Headache

Tachycardia

Rapid, shallow breathing

Nausea

Diaphoresis

Allergic reaction

Drug Interactions

Corticosteroids, dobutamine, epinephrine, and thiazide diuretics may antagonize (decrease) the hypoglycemic effects of insulin

Alcohol, beta adrenergic blockers, MAO inhibitors, and salicylates may potentiate (increase) the hypoglycemic effects of insulin

How Supplied

100 units/mL in 10 mL vials

Dosage and Administration

Insulin may be administered SQ, IM, or IV, and dosage is governed by the clinical presentation of the patient. A standard dose of insulin administration in diabetic coma is listed below:

Adult:	10-25 units Regular Insulin IV, followed by an infusion of 0.1 units/kg/hr
Pediatric:	0.1-0.2 units/kg/hr IM
Infusion:	50 units of Regular Insulin mixed in 250 mL of NS (0.2 units/mL), infused at a rate of 0.1-0.2 units/kg/hr (use infusion pump)

Special Considerations

Pregnancy Safety: Category B

Insulin is the drug of choice for control of diabetes in pregnancy

Regular insulins are clear, while modified insulins are cloudy

Insulin injected into the abdominal wall is absorbed most rapidly, insulin in the arm is absorbed more slowly, and insulin is absorbed slowest when injected into the thigh

Ipratropium *(Atrovent)*

Class

Anticholinergic, Bronchodilator

Description

Ipratropium inhibits interaction of acetylcholine at receptor sites on bronchial smooth muscle, resulting in decreased cGMP and bronchodilation.

Onset and Duration

Onset:	5-15 min
Duration:	4-6 hr

Indications

Persistent bronchospasm

Contraindications

Hypersensitivity to ipratopium, atropine, alkaloid, soybean protein, peanuts

Adverse Reactions

Nausea and vomiting

Coughing

Headache
Tachycardia
Dry mouth
Blurred vision

Drug Interactions

None reported

How Supplied

Aerosol 18 mcg/actuation

Dosage and Administration

NOTE: When used in combination with beta agonists (e.g., metaproterenol, albuterol), the beta agonist is always administered first with a 5 minute wait before administering ipratropium.

Adult:	1-2 inhalations
Pediatric (over 12 years of age):	Same as adult

Special Considerations

Pregnancy Safety: Category B
Shake well before use
Use with caution in patients with urinary retention

Isoproterenol (Isuprel)

Class

Sympathomimetic

Description

Isoproterenol is a synthetic catecholamine that stimulates both beta$_1$ and beta$_2$ adrenergic receptors (no alpha receptor stimulation). The drug affects the heart by increasing inotropic and chronotropic activity. In addition, isoproterenol causes arterial and bronchial dilation, and is sometimes administered via aerosolization as a bronchodilator to treat bronchial asthma and bronchospasm. (Because of the undesirable beta$_1$ cardiac effects, the use of this drug as a bronchodilator is uncommon in the prehospital setting.)

Onset and Duration

Onset:	1-5 min
Duration:	15-30 min

Indications

Hemodynamically significant bradycardias unresponsive to atropine, TCP, dopamine, and epinephrine
Management of torsades de pointes

Contraindications

Ventricular tachycardia
Ventricular fibrillation
Hypotension (relative)
Pulseless idioventricular rhythm
Ischemic heart disease/angina (relative)
Cardiac arrest

Adverse Reactions

Dysrhythmias
Hypotension
Precipitation of angina pectoris
Facial flushing
Restlessness
Dry throat
Discoloration of saliva (pinkish-red)

Drug Interactions

MAO inhibitors potentiate the effects of catecholamines
Beta adrenergic antagonists may blunt inotropic response
Sympathomimetics and phosphodiesterase inhibitors may exacerbate dysrhythmia response

How Supplied

5 mL (0.2 mg/mL) vial; 0.02 mg/mL in 1 and 10 mL vials

Dosage and Administration

Adult:	Dilute 1 mg in 250 mL of D$_5$W (4 mcg/mL); infuse at 2-10 mcg/min or until the desired heart rate is obtained; in torsades de pointes, titrate to increase heart rate until VT is suppressed
Pediatric:	Not recommended

Special Considerations

Pregnancy Safety: Category C
Isoproterenol increases myocardial oxygen demand, and can induce serious dysrhythmias (including VT and VF)
Administer via infusion pump to ensure precise flow rates
May exacerbate tachydysrhythmias due to digitalis toxicity or hypokalemia
Newer inotropic agents have replaced isoproterenol in most clinical settings
If electronic pacing is available, it should be used instead of isoproterenol, or as soon as possible after the drug has been initiated

Ketamine (Ketalar)

Class

Nonbarbiturate anesthetic

Mechanism of Action

Ketamine acts on the limbic system and cortex to block afferent transmission of impulses associated with pain perception. It produces short-acting amnesia without muscular relaxation. Ketamine is a derivative of the drug of abuse, phencyclidine (PCP).

Indications

Pain control
As an adjunct to nitrous oxide

Contraindications

Stroke
Increased ICP
Severe hypertension
Cardiac decompensation
Hypersensitivity to ketamine

Adverse Reactions

Hypertension
Increased heart rate
Hallucinations, delusions, explicit dreams
Less common side effects include hypotension, bradycardia, and respiratory depression

Drug Interactions

No significant drug interactions have been reported

How Supplied

10-, 50-, and 100-mg/mL ampules

Dosage and Administration

Adult: 1-2 mg/kg IV over 1 min or
                          5-10 mg IM
Child (over 2 years   Same as adult
of age):

Special Considerations

Pregnancy Safety: Category C
May increase blood pressure, muscle tone, and heart rate
Should not be given to patients with kidney or renal failure
As with any anesthetic, the dosage needs to be carefully assessed and individualized
Keep patient in a quiet environment (if possible)

Ketorolac Tromethamine (Toradol)

Class

Nonsteroidal antiinflammatory

Description

Ketorolac tromethamine is an antiinflammatory drug that also exhibits peripherally acting non-narcotic analgesic activity by inhibiting prostaglandin synthesis.

Onset and Duration

Onset: Within 10 min
Duration: 6-8 hr

Indications

Short-term management (less than 5 days) of moderate to severe pain

Contraindications

Hypersensitivity to the drug
Patients with allergies to aspirin or other nonsteroidal antiinflammatory drugs
Bleeding disorders
Renal failure
Active peptic ulcer disease

Adverse Reactions

Anaphylaxis from hypersensitivity
Edema
Sedation
Bleeding disorders
Rash
Nausea
Headache

Drug Interactions

Ketorolac may increase bleeding time when administered to patients taking anticoagulants.
Effects of lithium and methotrexate may be increased.

How Supplied

15 mg or 30 mg in 1 mL
60 mg in 2 mL

Dosage and Administration

Adult: IM: 30-60 mg; then 15-30 mg every 6 hr as
                 needed up to 5 days (max dose:
                 150 mg in 1st 24 hr)
          IV: 30 mg over 1 min (for patients less
                 than 65 years of age); one-half dose
                 (15 mg) for patients over 65 years
                 and in those with renal impairment
Pediatric: Not recommended

Special Considerations

Pregnancy Safety: Category B (diffused in 3rd trimester)
Solution is clear and slightly yellow in color
Use with caution and reduce dose when administering to elderly patients
Ketorolac (30 mg) usually provides analgesia comparable to 12 mg morphine or 100 mg meperidine

Labetalol (Normodyne, Trandate)

Class

Alpha and beta adrenergic blocker

Description

Labetalol is a competitive alpha$_1$ receptor blocker as well as a nonselective beta receptor blocker that is used for lowering blood pressure in hypertensive crisis. Because of alpha and beta blocking properties, blood pressure is reduced without reflex tachycardia, and total peripheral resistance is decreased without a significant alteration in cardiac output. In emergency care, labetalol is administered intravenously.

Onset and Duration

Onset: Within 5 min
Duration: 3-6 hr

Indications

Hypertensive emergencies

Contraindications

Bronchial asthma (relative)
Uncompensated CHF
Second- and third-degree heart block
Bradycardia
Cardiogenic shock
Pulmonary edema

Adverse Reactions

Headache
Dizziness
Edema
Fatigue
Vertigo
Ventricular dysrhythmias
Dyspnea
Allergic reaction
Facial flushing
Diaphoresis
Dose-related orthostatic hypotension (most common)

Drug Interactions

Bronchodilator effects of beta adrenergic agonists may be blunted by labetalol
Nitroglycerin may augment hypotensive effects

How Supplied

5 mg/mL in 4, 8, 20, and 40 mL vials

Dosage and Administration

Adult: 10 mg IV over 1-2 min. May repeat or double labetalol every 10 minutes to a maximum dose of 150 mg.
Infusion: Mix 200 mg in 250 mL D$_5$W (0.8 mg/mL); infuse at a rate of 2-8 mg/min, titrated to supine blood pressure (max 300 mg)
Pediatric: Safety has not been established; initiate cautiously with careful dosage adjustments and blood pressure monitoring.

Special Considerations

Pregnancy Safety: Category C
Blood pressure, pulse rate, ECG should be continuously monitored
Observe for signs of CHF, bradycardia, bronchospasm
Labetalol should only be administered with the patient in a supine position

Lidocaine (Xylocaine)

Class

Antidysrhythmic (Class I-B), Local anesthetic

Description

Lidocaine decreases phase 4 diastolic depolarization (which decreases automaticity), and has been shown to be effective in suppressing premature ventricular complexes. In addition, it is used to treat ventricular tachycardia and some cases of ventricular fibrillation. Lidocaine also raises the ventricular fibrillation threshold.

Onset and Duration

Onset: 30-90 seconds
Duration: 10-20 min

Indications

Ventricular tachycardia
Ventricular fibrillation
Wide-complex tachycardia of uncertain origin
Significant ventricular ectopy in the setting of myocardial ischemia/infarction

Contraindications

Hypersensitivity
Adams-Stokes syndrome
Second- or third-degree heart block in the absence of an artificial pacemaker

Adverse Effects

Lightheadedness
Confusion
Blurred vision
Hypotension
Cardiovascular collapse
Bradycardia
Altered level of consciousness, irritability, muscle twitching, seizures with high doses

Drug Interactions

Metabolic clearance of lidocaine may be decreased in patients taking beta adrenergic blockers or in patients with decreased cardiac output or liver dysfunction
Apnea induced with succinylcholine may be prolonged with large doses of lidocaine
Cardiac depression may occur if lidocaine is given concomitantly with IV phenytoin
Additive neurologic effects may occur with procainamide and tocainide

How Supplied

Prefilled   100 mg in 5 mL of solution
  syringes: 1 and 2 g additive syringes
Ampules: 100 mg in 5 mL of solution
              1 and 2 g vials in 30 mL of solution
              5 mL containing 100 mg/mL

Dosage and Administration

Cardiac Arrest
Adult: 1-1.5 mg/kg IV bolus or ET (at 2-2.5 times the IV dose); consider repeat in 3-5 min (max total dose 3 mg/kg); a single dose of 1.5 mg/kg is acceptable; for refractory VT/VF, an additional bolus of 0.5-0.7 mg/kg can be given; repeat in 5-10 min if necessary
Pediatric: 1 mg/kg IV/IO or ET (diluted to 3-5 mL)

Maintenance infusion after resuscitation from cardiac arrest
Adult: 2-4 mg/min
Pediatric: 20-50 mcg/kg/min (1-2.5 mL/kg/hr)
Wide-Complex PSVT/Wide-Complex Tachycardia of Uncertain Type/Stable VT
Adult: Initial loading dose of 1-1.5 mg/kg IV; if needed, give 0.5-0.75 mg/kg in 5-10 min (max total dose 3 mg/kg); after conversion start a lidocaine drip (2-4 mg/min)
Pediatric: Initial loading dose of 1 mg/kg IV/IO, followed by an infusion of 20-50 mcg/kg/min

Special Considerations

Pregnancy Safety: Category B
A 75-100 mg bolus will maintain adequate blood levels for only 20 min (in absence of shock)
If bradycardia occurs in conjunction with PVCs, always treat the bradycardia first with atropine
Exceedingly high doses of lidocaine can result in coma or death
Decrease dose in the elderly
Avoid lidocaine for reperfusion dysrhythmias following fibrinolytic therapy
Use extreme caution in patients with hepatic disease, heart failure, marked hypoxia, severe respiratory depression, hypovolemia or shock, incomplete heart block or bradycardia and atrial fibrillation

Lorazepam (Ativan)

Class

Benzodiazepine

Description

Lorazepam is a benzodiazepine with antianxiety and anticonvulsant effects. When given by injection, it appears to suppress the propagation of seizure activity produced by foci in the cortex, thalamus, and limbic areas.

Onset and Duration

Onset: 20-30 min
Duration: 6-8 hr

Indications

Agitation requiring sedation
Initial control of status epilepticus or severe recurrent seizures (investigational)

Contraindications

Hypersensitivity to the drug
Substance abuse (relative)
Coma (unless seizing)
Severe hypotension
Shock
Preexisting CNS depression

Adverse Reactions

Respiratory depression
Tachycardia/bradycardia
Hypotension
Sedation
Ataxia
Psychomotor impairment
Confusion

Drug Interactions

Lorazepam may precipitate CNS depression and psychomotor impairment when the patient is taking CNS depressant medications

How Supplied

2 and 4 mg/mL concentrations in 1-mL vials

Dosage and Administration

Prior to IV administration, lorazepam must be diluted with an equal volume of sterile water or sterile saline. When given IM, lorazepam is not to be diluted.
Adult: 1-4 mg slow IM/IV over 2-10 min; may be repeated in 15-20 min to a maximum dose of 8 mg
Pediatric (not   0.05-0.15 mg/kg slow IV/IO/IM
FDA-approved):   over 2 min; may be repeated once in 5-10 min to a maximum dose of 4 mg; 0.1-2 mg/kg (rectal dose)

Special Considerations

Pregnancy Safety: Category D
Monitor respiratory rate and blood pressure during administration
Have suction and intubation equipment available
Inadvertent intraarterial injection may produce arteriospasm, resulting in gangrene that may require amputation
Lorazepam expires in six weeks when not refrigerated; do not use if discolored or if solution contains precipitate

Magnesium Sulfate

Class

Electrolyte, Anticonvulsant

Description

Magnesium sulfate reduces striated muscle contractions and blocks peripheral neuromuscular transmission by reducing acetylcholine release at the myoneural junction. In emergency care, magnesium sulfate is used in the management of seizures associated with toxemia of pregnancy. Other uses of magnesium sulfate include uterine relaxation (to inhibit contractions of premature labor), as a bronchodilator after beta agonist and anticholinergic agents have been used, replacement therapy for magnesium deficiency. Magnesium sulfate is gaining popularity as an initial treatment in the management of various dysrhythmias, particularly torsades de pointes, and dysrhythmias secondary to TCA overdose or digitalis toxicity. The drug also is considered as a Class IIa agent (AHA guidelines; probably helpful) for refractory ventricular fibrillation/ventricular tachycardia after administration of lidocaine doses.

Onset and Duration
Onset: (IV) Immediate
            (IM) 3-4 hr
Duration: 30 min (IV)
            3-4 hr (IM)

Indications
Seizures of eclampsia (toxemia of pregnancy)
Torsades de pointes
Suspected hypomagnesemia
Refractory ventricular fibrillation
Status asthmaticus not responsive to β-adrenergic drugs

Contraindications
Heart block or myocardial damage

Adverse Reactions
Diaphoresis
Facial flushing
Hypotension
Depressed reflexes
Hypothermia
Reduced heart rate
Circulatory collapse
Respiratory depression
Diarrhea

Drug Interactions
CNS depressant effects may be enhanced if the patient is taking other CNS depressants
Serious changes in cardiac function may occur with cardiac glycosides (avoid excess magnesium)

How Supplied
10%, 12.5%, 50% solution in 40 mg, 80 mg, 100 mg, and 125 mg/mL

Dosage and Administration
Seizure activity associated with pregnancy
Adult: 1-4 g (8-32 mEq) IV; max dose of
            1.5 mL/min (max 30-40 g/day)
Pulseless arrest (for hypomagnesemia or torsades de pointes)
Adult: 1-2 g (2-4 mL of a 50% solution) diluted in
            10 mL of D₅W IV push
Pediatric: 25-50 mg/kg (max 2 g) over 10-20 min
Torsades de pointes (not in cardiac arrest) and AMI (if indicated)
Adult: Loading dose of 1-2 g in 50-100 mL of
            D₅W over 5-60 min IV; follow with
            0.5-1 g/hr/IV (titrate dose to control the
            torsades)
Pediatric: Same as pulseless arrest

Special Considerations
Pregnancy Safety: Category B.
Magnesium sulfate is administered for the treatment of toxemia of pregnancy. It is recommended that the drug not be administered in the 2 hr prior to delivery, if possible.
IV calcium gluconate or calcium chloride should be available as an antagonist to magnesium if needed
Convulsions may occur up to 48 hr after delivery, necessitating continued therapy
The "cure" for toxemia is delivery of the baby
Magnesium must be used with caution in patients with renal failure, since it is cleared by the kidneys and can reach toxic levels easily in those patients

Mannitol (Osmitrol)

Class
Osmotic diuretic

Description
Because of mannitol's osmotic properties, it promotes the movement of fluid from the intracellular into the extracellular space. In emergency care, mannitol is used in the treatment of head injury to decrease cerebral edema and intracranial pressure.

Onset and Duration
Onset: 1-3 hr (for diuretic effect)
            Within 15 min (for reduction of intracranial pressure)
Duration: 4-6 hr (for diuretic effect)
            3-8 hr (for reduction of intracranial pressure)

Indications
Cerebral edema
Other causes of increased intracranial pressure (space occupying lesions)
Rhabdomyolysis (myoglobinuria)
Blood transfusion reactions
Promoting urinary excretion of toxic substances

Contraindications
Severe hypotension
Profound hypovolemia
Active intracranial bleeding
Dehydration
Hyponatremia
Severe pulmonary edema or congestion
Profound hypovolemia
Severe renal disease (anuria)

Adverse Reactions
Transient volume overload
Pulmonary edema
Renal failure
CHF
Hypotension (from excessive diuresis)
Sodium depletion

Drug Interactions
When given concurrently with digitalis glycosides, an increase in digitalis toxicity may develop

How Supplied

250 and 500 mL of a 20% solution for IV infusion (200 mg/mL) 25% solution in 50 mL for slow IV push

Dosage and Administration

Adult: 0.5-1 g/kg in a 20% solution over 5-10 min; usual adult dose is 20-200 g/24 hr
Pediatric: 0.2-0.5 g/kg/dose IV infusion over 30-60 min (max 1 g/kg dose) every 4-6 hr

Special Considerations

Pregnancy Safety: Category C
Mannitol may crystallize at low temperatures and may need to be warmed in boiling water until clear (cool to body temperature before use)
In-line filter should always be used
Effectiveness depends on large doses and an intact blood-brain barrier
The use of mannitol and its dosages in emergency care are controversial

Meperidine (Demerol)

Class

Opioid analgesic

Description

Meperidine is a synthetic opioid agonist that works at opioid receptors to produce analgesia and euphoria. Excessive doses can cause respiratory and CNS depression. It has a potential for physical dependence and abuse, and is classified as a Schedule II drug.

Onset and Duration

Onset: (IM) 10-15 min
(IV) within 5 min
Duration: 2-4 hr

Indications

Moderate to severe pain
Preoperative medication
OB analgesia

Contraindications

Hypersensitivity to narcotics
Patients taking MAO inhibitors or selective serotonin reuptake inhibitors
During labor or delivery of a premature infant
Head injury

Adverse Reactions

Respiratory depression
Nausea and vomiting
Euphoria
Delirium
Agitation
Hallucination
Seizures
Headache
Hypotension
Visual disturbances
Coma
Facial flushing
Circulatory collapse
Dysrhythmias
Allergic reaction

Drug Interactions

Respiratory depression, hypotension or sedation may be potentiated by CNS depressants
Therapeutic doses of meperidine have caused fatal reactions in patients taking MAO inhibitors within the previous 14 days
Phenytoin may decrease analgesic effects

How Supplied

Parenteral: 25, 50, 100 mg/mL in 1 and 5 mL prefilled syringe and Tubex

Dosage and Administration

Adult: 50-100 mg IM every 3-4 hr as needed; 15-35 mg IV per hour (dose should be individualized)
Elderly: 25 mg IM every 4 hr as needed
Pediatric: 1-2 mg/kg/dose IM every 3-4 hr as needed

Special Considerations

Pregnancy Safety: Category B (if not used for prolonged periods or in high doses at term)
Use with caution in patients with asthma and COPD
May aggravate seizures in those with convulsive disorders (especially in patients with renal insufficiency)
Use with caution in those susceptible to CNS depression
Naloxone should be readily available
Protect from light and freezing

Metaproterenol (Alupent)

Class

Sympathomimetic, Bronchodilator

Description

Metaproterenol relaxes the smooth muscles of the bronchial tree and peripheral vasculature by stimulating beta$_2$ adrenergic receptors of the sympathetic nervous system.

Onset and Duration

Onset: 1 minute after inhalation
Duration: 3-6 hr

Indications

Bronchial asthma
Reversible bronchospasm (bronchitis, emphysema)

Contraindications

Hypersensitivity
Cardiac dysrhythmias
Tachycardia caused by digitalis toxicity

Adverse Reactions

Restlessness, apprehension
Palpitations
Tachycardia
Dysrhythmias
Decreased blood pressure
Coughing
Tremor
Facial flushing
Diaphoresis

Drug Interactions

Other sympathomimetics may exacerbate adverse cardiovascular effects
TCAs and MAO inhibitors may potentiate hypotensive
effects
Beta blockers may antagonize the effects of metaproterenol

How Supplied

MDI: 0.65/mg/spray (15 mL inhaler)
Solution: 0.4%, 0.6%, and 5%
Syrup: (10 mg/5 mL)

Dosage and Administration

MDI
   Adult: 2-3 inhalations q 3-4 hr (2 min
                               between inhalations); max dose
                               of 12 inhalations/day
   Pediatric (over   Same as adult
    12 years of age):
Solution
   Adult: 5-15 inhalations of 5% solution
   Pediatric (over   Same as adult
    6 yrs of age):

Special Considerations

Pregnancy Safety: Category C
Monitor vital signs for hypotension and tachycardia
Use with caution in patients with coronary artery disease
and diabetes mellitus
Shake well
Do not use if solutions are brown or contain precipitate

Methylprednisolone (Solu-Medrol)

Class

Glucocorticoid

Description

Methylprednisolone is a synthetic steroid that suppresses
acute and chronic inflammation. In addition, it potentiates vascular smooth muscle relaxation by beta adrenergic agonists, and may alter airway hyperactivity. A newer
usage is for reduction of posttraumatic spinal cord
edema.

Onset and Duration

Onset: 1-2 hrs
Duration: 8-24 hr

Indications

Anaphylaxis
Bronchodilator-unresponsive asthma
Shock (controversial)
Acute spinal cord injury

Contraindications

Use with caution in patients with GI bleeding, diabetes
mellitus, severe infection

Adverse Reactions

Headache
Hypertension
Sodium and water retention
Hypokalemia
Alkalosis

Drug Interactions

Hypoglycemic responses to insulin and oral hypoglycemic agents may be blunted
Potassium-depleting agents may potentiate hypokalemia
induced by corticosteroids

How Supplied

20, 40, 80 mg/mL

Dosage and Administration

Adult: Variable; usually within the range of
              40-125 mg IV, except for spinal cord in-
              jury where the initial dose is 30 mg/kg
              IV bolus followed by an IV infusion of
              5.4 mg/kg/hr
Pediatric: 1-2 mg/kg/dose IV

Special Considerations

Pregnancy Safety: Category C

Metoprolol (Lopressor)

Class

Beta-blocking agent

Description

Beta-adrenergic blocking agents compete with beta-
adrenergic agonists for available beta receptor sites on
the membrane of cardiac muscle, bronchial smooth muscle, and the smooth muscle of blood vessels. The beta-1
blocking action on the heart decreases heart rate, conduction velocity, myocardial contractility, and cardiac
output. Metoprolol is used to control ventricular response in supraventricular tachydysrhythmias (PSVT,
atrial fibrillation, atrial flutter). It is considered a second-line agent after adenosine, diltiazem, or a digitalis
derivative.

Onset and Duration

Onset: 1-2 min
Duration: 3-4 hr

Indications

PSVT
Atrial flutter
Atrial fibrillation
To reduce myocardial ischemia and damage in AMI patients

Contraindications

Heart failure
Second- or third-degree block
Cardiogenic shock
Hypotension
Bradycardia
Lung disease associated with bronchospasm
Hypersensitivity to metoprolol

Adverse Reactions

Bradycardia
AV conduction delays
Hypotension

Drug Interactions

May potentiate antihypertensive effects when given to patients taking calcium channel blockers or MAO inhibitors
Catecholamine-depleting drugs may potentiate hypotension
Sympathomimetic effects may be antagonized; signs of hypoglycemia may be masked

How Supplied

1 mg/mL-ampules

Dose and Administration

Adult:　　5 mg slow IV at 5-min intervals to a total of 15 mg
Pediatric:　Safety not established

Special Considerations

Pregnancy Safety: Category C
Must be given slow IV, over 5 min
Concurrent IV administration with IV calcium channel blockers like verapamil or diltiazem can cause severe hypotension
Should be used with caution in persons with liver or renal dysfunction

Midazolam Hydrochloride (Versed)

Class

Short-acting benzodiazepine

Description

Midazolam HCl is a water-soluble benzodiazepine that may be administered for conscious sedation to relieve apprehension or impair memory prior to tracheal intubation or cardioversion.

Onset and Duration

Onset:　　　1-3 min (IV); dose dependent
Duration:　　2-6 hr; dose dependent

Indications

Premedication for tracheal intubation or cardioversion

Contraindications

Hypersensitivity to midazolam
Glaucoma (relative)
Shock
Coma
Alcohol intoxication (relative; may be used for alcohol withdrawal)
Depressed vital signs
Concomitant use of barbiturates, alcohol, narcotics, or other CNS depressants

Adverse Reactions

Respiratory depression
Hiccough
Cough
Oversedation
Pain at the injection site
Nausea and vomiting
Headache
Blurred vision
Fluctuations in vital signs
Hypotension
Respiratory arrest

Drug Interactions

Sedative effect of midazolam may be accentuated by concomitant use of barbiturates, alcohol, or narcotics (and should, therefore, not be used in patients who have taken CNS depressants)

How Supplied

2, 5, 10 mL vials (1 mg/mL)
1, 2, 5, 10 mL vials (5 mg/mL)

Dosage and Administration

Adult:　　　1-2.5 mg slow IV (over 2-3 min); may be repeated if necessary in small increments (total max dose not to exceed 0.1 mg/kg)
Elderly:　　0.5 mg slow IV (max 1.5 mg in a 2-min period)
Pediatric:　Loading dose 0.05-0.2 mg/kg; then continue infusion 1-2 mcg/kg/min

Special Considerations

Pregnancy Safety: Category D
Provide continuous monitoring of respiratory and cardiac function
Have resuscitation equipment and medication readily at hand
Never administer medication as IV bolus

Morphine Sulfate (Astramorph/PF and others)

Class

Opioid analgesic

Description

Morphine sulfate is a natural opium alkaloid that has a primary effect of analgesia. It also increases peripheral venous capacitance and decreases venous return ("chemical phlebotomy"). Morphine sulfate causes euphoria and respiratory and CNS depression. Secondary pharmacologic effects of morphine include depressed responsiveness of alpha adrenergic receptors (producing peripheral vasodilation) and baroreceptor inhibition. In addition, because morphine decreases both preload and afterload, it may decrease myocardial oxygen demand. The properties of this medication make it extremely useful in emergency care. Morphine sulfate is a Schedule II drug.

Onset and Duration

Onset: 1-2 min after administration
Duration: 2-7 hr

Indications

Chest pain associated with myocardial infarction
Pulmonary edema, with or without associated pain
Moderate to severe acute and chronic pain

Contraindications

Hypersensitivity to narcotics
Hypovolemia
Hypotension
Head injury or undiagnosed abdominal pain
Increased ICP
Severe respiratory depression
Patients who have taken MAO inhibitors within 14 days

Adverse Reactions

Hypotension
Tachycardia
Bradycardia
Palpitations
Syncope
Facial flushing
Respiratory depression
Euphoria
Bronchospasm
Dry mouth
Allergic reaction

Drug Interactions

CNS depressants may potentiate effects of morphine (respiratory depression, hypotension, sedation)
Phenothiazines may potentiate analgesia
MAO inhibitors may cause paradoxical excitation

How Supplied

Morphine is supplied in tablets, suppositories, and solution. In emergency care, morphine sulfate is usually administered IV.
Parenteral preparations are available in many strengths. A common preparation is 10 mg in 1 mL of solution, ampules and Tubex syringes.

Dosage and Administration

Adult: 2-4 mg slow IV over 1-5 min every 5-30 min; titrated to effect
Pediatric: 0.1-0.2 mg/kg/dose IV (max 15-mg total dose)

Special Considerations

Pregnancy Safety: Category B (if not used for prolonged periods or in high doses at term); narcotics rapidly cross the placenta
Safety in neonates has not been established
Use with caution in the elderly, those with asthma, and in those susceptible to CNS depression
Should be used with caution in chronic pain syndromes
May worsen bradycardia or heart block in inferior MI (vagotonic effect)
Naloxone should be readily available

Nalbuphine (Nubain)

Class

Opioid analgesic

Description

Nalbuphine is a synthetic analgesic with a potency equivalent to morphine sulfate on a milligram-to-milligram basis. It has both agonist and antagonist properties. Nalbuphine may be used for treating chest pain associated with MI as it reduces oxygen needs of the heart without reducing blood pressure. Nalbuphine is not presently regulated under the Controlled Substance Act.

Onset and Duration

Onset: 2-3 min
Duration: 3-6 hr

Indications

Chest pain associated with myocardial infarction
Moderate to severe acute pain
Pulmonary edema, with or without associated pain (morphine is first-line medication in this class)

Contraindications

Hypersensitivity to narcotics
Hypovolemia
Hypotension
Head injury or undiagnosed abdominal pain

Adverse Reactions

Sedation (most common)
Hypotension
Bradycardia
Facial flushing
Respiratory depression
CNS depression
Euphoria
Paradoxical CNS stimulation
Blurred vision

Drug Interactions

CNS depressants may potentiate effects

How Supplied

10 mg in 1 mL ampule
20 mg in 1 mL ampule

Dosage and Administration

Adult: 2-5 mg slow IV (usual dose 10 mg/70 kg);
          may be augmented with 2 mg doses prn;
          every 3-6 hr (max single dose: 20 mg;
          max daily dose 160 mg)
Pediatric: Not recommended

Special Considerations

Pregnancy Safety: Category B (if not used for prolonged
    periods or in high doses at term)
Use with caution in patients with impaired respiratory
    function or hepatic dysfunction
Has a weak narcotic antagonist effect and may precipitate
    withdrawal syndrome in narcotic-dependent patients
Naloxone should be readily available

Nalmefene (Revex)

Class

Opioid antagonist

Description

Nalmefene is a competitive opioid antagonist used in the
management of known or suspected opioid overdose, including respiratory depression induced by either natural
or synthetic opioids.

Onset and Duration

Onset: Within 2 min
Duration: Up to 8 hr

Indications

For the complete or partial reversal of CNS and respiratory
    depression induced by opioids including propoxy-
    phene, nalbuphine, pentazocine, and butorphanol

Contraindications

Hypersensitivity to nalmefene
Use with caution in narcotic-dependent patients who
    may experience withdrawal syndrome (including neo-
    nates of narcotic-dependent mothers)

Adverse Reactions

Tachycardia
Hypertension
Dysrhythmias
Nausea and vomiting
Diaphoresis
Blurred vision
Withdrawal (opiate)

Drug Interactions

May be an increased risk for seizure with flumazenil

How Supplied

Available in 2 concentrations: Blue label (100 mcg/
    mL) used postoperatively, and Green label (1 mg/
    mL) in 2 mL ampule to manage or reverse narcotic
    overdose

Dosage and Administration (Green Label)

Adult: 0.5-1 mg/70 kg; may be repeated once
          in 2-5 min
Pediatric: Safety not established

Special Considerations

Pregnancy Safety: Category B
Caution should be exercised when administering
    nalmefene to narcotic addicts (may precipitate with-
    drawal with hypertension, tachycardia, and violent
    behavior)

Naloxone (Narcan)

Class

Opioid antagonist

Description

Naloxone is a competitive narcotic antagonist that is used
in the management of known or suspected overdose
caused by narcotics. Naloxone antagonizes all actions of
morphine.

Onset and Duration

Onset: Within 2 min
Duration: 30-60 min

Indications

For the complete or partial reversal of CNS and respi-
    ratory depression induced by opioids including the
    following:
Narcotic agonist
    morphine sulfate
    heroin
    hydromorphone
    methadone
    meperidine
    paregoric
    fentanyl citrate
    oxycodone
    codeine
    propoxyphene
Narcotic agonist/antagonist
    butorphanol tartrate
    pentazocine
    nalbuphine
Decreased level of consciousness
Coma of unknown origin

Circulatory support in refractory shock (investigational)

PCP and alcohol ingestion (investigational)

Contraindications

Hypersensitivity

Use with caution in narcotic-dependent patients who may experience withdrawal syndrome (including neonates of narcotic-dependent mothers)

Adverse Reactions

Tachycardia

Hypertension

Dysrhythmias

Nausea and vomiting

Diaphoresis

Blurred vision

Withdrawal (opiate)

Drug Interactions

Incompatible with bisulfite and alkaline solutions

How Supplied

0.4 mg/mL (1 mL, 10 mL), 1 mg/mL (2 mL) vials

Dosage and Administration

Adult: 0.4-0.8 IM/IV, 0.8 SQ (or ET diluted); may be repeated in 5 min intervals to a maximum of 10 mg

Infusion: Mix 8 mg in 1000 mL of D_5W; infuse at 2/3 of the initial reversal dose titrated to desired effect

Pediatric: 0.1 mg/kg (IV, IO, SQ, ET diluted)

Infusion: If ≤ 5 years old or ≤ 20 kg: 0.1 mg/kg; If > 5 years old or > 20 kg: 2 mg; titrate to desired effect

Special Considerations

Pregnancy Safety: Category B

Seizures have been reported (no causal relationship established)

May not reverse hypotension

Caution should be exercised when administering naloxone to narcotic addicts (may precipitate withdrawal with hypertension, tachycardia, and violent behavior)

Nitroglycerin (Nitrostat and others)

Class

Vasodilator

Description

Nitrates and nitrites dilate arterioles and veins in the periphery (and coronary arteries in high doses). The resultant reduction in preload, and to a lesser extent in afterload, decreases the workload of the heart and lowers myocardial oxygen demand. Nitroglycerin is very lipid soluble and is thought to enter the body from the GI tract through the lymphatics, rather than the portal blood.

Onset and Duration

Onset: 1-3 min

Duration: 30-60 min

Indications

Ischemic chest pain

Pulmonary hypertension

CHF

Hypertensive emergencies

Contraindications

Hypersensitivity

Hypotension

Head injury

Cerebral hemorrhage

Recent Viagra use

Adverse Reactions

Transient headache

Reflex tachycardia

Hypotension

Nausea and vomiting

Postural syncope

Diaphoresis

Drug Interactions

Other vasodilators may have additive hypotensive effects

How Supplied

Tablets: 0.15 mg (1/400 gr), 0.3 mg (1/200 gr), 0.4 mg (1/150 gr), 0.6 (1/100 gr), and extended-release capsules and transdermal preparations

Metered Spray: 0.4 mg per spray

Parenteral: 5 mg/mL, 10, 20, 40 mg/100 mL

Dosage and Administration

Adult: Tablet: 0.3-0.4 mg SL; may repeat twice

Metered spray: Spray onto oral mucosa using a lingual aerosol canister for 0.5-1 second; delivers 0.4 mg/spray

Infusion: 200-400 mcg/mL at a rate of 10-20 mcg/min; increase by 5-10 mcg/min q 5-10 min until desired effect is achieved

Pediatric: Not recommended

Special Considerations

Pregnancy Safety: Category C

Increased susceptibility to hypotension in the elderly

Nitroglycerin decomposes when exposed to light or heat

Must be kept in airtight containers

Active ingredient of nitroglycerin will "sting" when administered SL

Use with caution in patients with inferior AMI

Administer IV nitroglycerin by infusion pump to ensure precise flow rate

PVC tubing may absorb up to 80% of available drug; non-PVC tubing should be used

Nitropaste *(Nitro-Bid Ointment)*

Class
Vasodilator

Description
Nitropaste contains a 2% solution of nitroglycerin in an absorbent paste.

Onset and Duration
Onset: 15-60 min
Duration: 2-12 hr

Indications
Angina pectoris
Chest pain associated with AMI (less easily titratable than IV nitroglycerin)

Contraindications
Hypersensitivity
Hypotension
Head injury
Cerebral hemorrhage

Adverse Reactions
Transient headache
Postural syncope
Reflex tachycardia
Hypotension
Nausea and vomiting
Allergic reaction

Drug Interactions
Other vasodilators may have additive hypotensive effects

How Supplied
20, 60 g tubes of 2% nitroglycerin paste (measuring applicators are supplied)

Dosage and Administration
Adult: Apply 1-2 inches over 2-4 inch area of skin that is free of hair (usually the chest wall); cover with transparent wrap and secure with tape
Pediatric: Not recommended

Special Considerations
Pregnancy Safety: Category C
Wear gloves when applying paste
Do not massage or rub paste (rapid absorption will interfere with the drug's sustained action)
Store paste in a cool place with the tube tightly capped
Although the adverse effects for nitropaste are the same as for SL nitroglycerin, their frequency and severity are usually considerably less with the sustained re-

lease preparations because of the slower absorption and less erratic serum levels

Nitrous Oxide:Oxygen *(50:50)* *(Nitronox)*

Class
Gaseous analgesic/anesthetic

Description
Nitrous oxide:oxygen is a blended mixture of 50% nitrous oxide and 50% oxygen. When inhaled, nitrous oxide/oxygen depresses the central nervous system, causing anesthesia. In addition, the high concentration of oxygen delivered along with the nitrous oxide increases oxygen tension in the blood, thereby reducing hypoxia. Nitrous oxide:oxygen is self-administered.

Onset and Duration
Onset: 2-5 min
Duration: 2-5 min

Indications
Moderate to severe pain
Anxiety
Apprehension

Contraindications
Impaired LOC
Head injury
Chest trauma (pneumothorax)
Inability to comply with instructions
Decompression sickness (nitrogen narcosis, air embolus, air transport)
Undiagnosed abdominal pain or marked distention
Bowel obstruction
Hypotension
Shock
COPD (with history or suspicion of CO_2 retention)

Adverse Reactions
Dizziness
Apnea
Cyanosis
Nausea and vomiting
Malignant hyperthermia (rare but dangerous)

Drug Interactions
None significant

How Supplied
D and E cylinders (blue and white in Canada, blue and green in United States) of 50% nitrous oxide and 50% oxygen compressed gas

Dosage and Administration
Adult: Invert cylinder several times before use; instruct the patient to inhale deeply through a patient-held mask or mouthpiece
Pediatric: Same as adult

Special Considerations

Pregnancy Safety: Nitrous oxide has been shown to increase the incidence of spontaneous abortion

Nitrous oxide is 34 times more soluble than nitrogen and will diffuse into pockets of trapped gas in the patient (intestinal obstruction, pneumothorax, blocked middle ear, etc.). As the nitrogen leaves and is replaced by larger amounts of nitrous oxide, increased pressures or volumes may cause serious damage, for example, intestinal rupture.

Nitrous oxide is a nonexplosive gas

Patient must hold mask and self-administer

NOTE

When delivering nitrous oxide and oxygen from a single tank, it is important to ensure that enough oxygen remains in the tank to provide adequate oxygenation. Inverting the cylinder several times to mix the gases is important for this reason. It is also reasonable to monitor oximetry during administration of nitrous oxide.

Norepinephrine (Levophed)

Class

Sympathomimetic

Description

Norepinephrine is an alpha and beta$_1$ adrenergic agonist. It is a potent vasoconstrictor that also increases myocardial contractility. Because norepinephrine tends to constrict the renal and mesenteric blood vessels, it is rarely used in the prehospital setting.

Onset and Duration

Onset: 1-3 min
Duration: 5-10 min

Indications

Cardiogenic shock
Neurogenic shock
Inotropic support
Hemodynamically significant hypotension refractory to other sympathomimetic amines

Contraindications

Hypotensive patients with hypovolemia

Adverse Reactions

Headache
Dysrhythmias
Tachycardia
Reflex bradycardia
Angina pectoris
Hypertension

Drug Interactions

Can be deactivated by alkaline solutions
MAO inhibitors and bretylium may potentiate the effects of catecholamines
Beta adrenergic antagonists may blunt inotropic response
Sympathomimetics and phosphodiesterase inhibitors may exacerbate dysrhythmia response

How Supplied

1 mg/mL, 4 mL ampule

Dosage and Administration

Adult: Dilute 4 mg in 250 mL of D$_5$W or D$_5$NS (16 mcg/mL); begin infusion at 0.5-1 mcg/min (up to 30 mcg/min) titrated to desired effect (average adult dose is 8-12 mcg/min)
Pediatric: 0.1-2 mcg/kg/min IV/IO

Special Considerations

Pregnancy Safety: Category D
May cause fetal anoxia when used in pregnancy
Infuse norepinephrine through a large stable vein to avoid extravasation and tissue necrosis
Use infusion pump to ensure precise flow rate
Do not administer in same IV line as alkaline solutions

Oxygen

Class

Naturally occurring atmospheric gas

Description

Oxygen is an odorless, tasteless, colorless gas that is present in room air at a concentration of approximately 21%. It is an important emergency drug that is used to reverse hypoxemia; in doing so, it helps oxidize glucose to produce ATP (aerobic metabolism), and helps reduce the size of infarcted tissue during an AMI (in patients who are hypoxemic on room air).

Onset and Duration

Onset: Immediate
Duration: Less than 2 min

Indications

Confirmed or suspected hypoxia
Ischemic chest pain
Respiratory insufficiency
Prophylactically during air transport
Confirmed or suspected carbon monoxide poisoning and other causes of decreased tissue oxygenation (cardiac arrest)

Contraindications

Oxygen should never be withheld in any critical patient

Adverse Reactions

High-concentration oxygen may cause decreased LOC and respiratory depression in patients with chronic carbon dioxide retention

Drug Interactions

None significant

How Supplied

Oxygen cylinders (usually green and white) of 100% compressed oxygen gas

Dosage and Administration

Adult:

High-concentration:	10-15 L/min via nonrebreather mask or high-flow oxygen delivery device
Low concentration:	1-4 L/min via nasal cannula
	Venturi mask concentrations (e.g., 24%, 28%, 32%, 36%) for intermediate rates of oxygen administration in patients with COPD
Pediatric:	Same as for adult

Special Considerations

Pregnancy Safety: NA
Oxygen vigorously supports combustion

Oxytocin (Pitocin)

Class

Pituitary hormone

Description

Oxytocin means "rapid birth," and is a synthetic hormone named for the natural posterior pituitary hormone. It stimulates uterine smooth muscle contractions, and helps expedite the normal contractions of a spontaneous labor. As with all significant uterine contractions, there is a transient reduction in uterine blood flow. Oxytocin also stimulates the mammary glands to increase lactation, without increasing the production of milk. The drug is administered in the prehospital setting to control postpartum bleeding.

Onset and Duration

Onset:	(IV) Immediate
	(IM) Within 3-5 min
Duration:	(IV) 20 min after the infusion is stopped
	(IM) 30-60 min

Indications

Postpartum hemorrhage after infant and placental delivery

Contraindications

Hypertonic or hyperactive uterus
Presence of a second fetus
Fetal distress

Adverse Reactions

Hypotension
Tachycardia
Hypertension
Dysrhythmias
Angina pectoris
Anxiety
Seizure
Nausea and vomiting
Allergic reaction
Uterine rupture (from excessive administration)

Drug Interactions

Vasopressors may potentiate hypertension

How Supplied

10 USP units/1 mL ampule (10 U/mL) and prefilled syringe
5 USP units/1 mL ampule (5 U/mL) and prefilled syringe

Dosage and Administration

Control of postpartum hemorrhage

IM:	3-10 units IM following delivery of placenta

Bleeding following incomplete or elective abortion

IV:	Mix 10 units (1 mL) in 1000 mL NS or LR; infuse at 20-30 drops/min via microdrip tubing, titrated to severity of bleeding and uterine response

Special Considerations

Pregnancy Safety: Category X
Vital signs and uterine tone should be closely monitored
Should only be administered in the prehospital setting after delivery of all fetuses

Pancuronium (Pavulon)

Class

Neuromuscular blocker (nondepolarizing)

Description

Pancuronium produces complete muscular relaxation by binding to the receptor for acetylcholine at the neuromuscular junction, without initiating depolarization of the muscle membrane. As the concentration of acetylcholine rises in the neuromuscular junction, pancuronium is displaced and muscle tone is regained. Neuromuscular blocking agents are used to provide muscle relaxation during surgery (particularly relaxation of the abdominal muscles) without general anesthesia, and to prevent convulsive muscle spasms during electroconvulsive therapy. In emergency care, pancuronium is used to optimize conditions for endotracheal intubation and assisted ventilations.

Onset and Duration

Onset:	Paralysis in 3-5 min
Duration:	45-60 min

Indications

Induction or maintenance of paralysis after intubation to assist ventilations

Contraindications

Known hypersensitivity to the drug
Inability to control airway and/or support ventilations with oxygen and positive pressure
Neuromuscular disease (e.g., myasthenia gravis)

Adverse Reactions

Transient hypotension
Tachycardia
Dysrhythmias
Hypertension
Excessive salivation
Pain, burning at IV injection site

Drug Interactions

Positive chronotropic drugs may potentiate tachycardia

How Supplied

1, 2 mg/mL, 4 mg/2 mL

Dosage and Administration

Adult: 0.04-0.1 mg/kg slow IV; repeat
             q 30-60 min prn
Pediatric: 0.04-0.1 mg/kg slow IV
             (Newborn 0.02 mg/kg/dose)

NOTE

If the patient is conscious, explain the effects of the medication before administration, and always sedate the patient before using a neuromuscular blocking agent.

Special Considerations

Pregnancy Safety: Category C
Patients must be fully sedated with an artificial airway during paralysis
Carefully monitor the patient and be prepared to resuscitate
The effects of pancuronium are antagonized by neostigmine (Prostigmin) 0.05 mg/kg, and should be accompanied by atropine (0.6-1.2 mg IV)
Pancuronium has no effect on consciousness or pain
Will not stop neuronal seizure activity nor decrease CNS damage secondary to seizures
Heart rate, cardiac output, and atrial pressure will be increased
Pancuronium is excreted in the urine; doses should be decreased for patients with renal disease

---

NOTE

Neuromuscular blocking agents produce respiratory paralysis. Therefore intubation and ventilatory support must be readily available.

Phenytoin *(Dilantin)*

Class

Anticonvulsant

Description

Phenytoin (a hydantoin) is a drug of choice in controlling grand mal and focal motor seizure activity. It was developed as an alternative anticonvulsant that would cause less sedation than barbiturates. Phenytoin appears to inhibit the spread of seizure activity by promoting sodium efflux from neurons, thereby stabilizing the neuron's threshold against excitability caused by excess stimulation. Phenytoin has also been used to treat digitalis-induced atrial and ventricular dysrhythmias by stabilizing the sodium influx in Purkinje fibers of the heart, decreasing abnormal ventricular automaticity, and increasing AV node conduction.

Onset and Duration

Onset: 20-30 min for seizure disorder
Duration: As long as 15 days

Indications

Major motor seizures (generalized grand mal, simple partial and complex partial seizures)
Adams-Stokes syndrome

Contraindications

Hypersensitivity
Sinus bradycardia
Second- and third-degree heart block
Sinoatrial block

Adverse Reactions

Hypotension with rapid IV push (greater than 50 mg/min)
Cardiovascular collapse (with rapid IV use)
Dysrhythmias
Bradycardia
Respiratory depression
CNS depression
Ataxia
Nystagmus
Thrombophlebitis
Nausea and vomiting
Pain from injection site

Drug Interactions

Anticoagulants, cimetidine, sulfonamides, and salicylates may increase serum phenytoin levels
Chronic alcohol consumption or use induces metabolism of the drug
Lidocaine, propranolol and other beta blocking agents may increase cardiac depressant effects
Xanthines may result in decreased phenytoin absorption
Precipitation may occur when mixed with D_5W
Incompatible with many solutions and medications
Enhanced anticoagulation with warfarin

How Supplied

50 mg/mL in 2- and 5-mL ampules, 2 mL prefilled syringe

May be diluted in NS (1-10 mg/mL, per protocol); use in-line filter

IV line should be flushed with 0.9% NS before and after the drug is administered

Dosage and Administration

Seizures

Adult: 1000 mg or 15-20 mg/kg (usual loading dose) slow IV; not to exceed 1 g or rate of 50 mg/min; followed by 100-150 mg/dose at 30 min intervals

Pediatric: 10-20 mg/kg slow IV (<0.5 mg/kg/min) loading dose

Special Considerations

Pregnancy Safety: Category D

Phenytoin may normally have slight yellow color

Carefully monitor vital signs

Venous irritation can occur due to alkalinity of the solution

Use with caution in patients with pulmonary, cardiovascular, hepatic, or renal insufficiency

Use large, stable vein for injection (extravasation may cause tissue necrosis)

Pralidoxime *(2-Pam Chloride, Protopam)*

Class

Cholinesterase reactivator and antidote

Description

Pralidoxime reactivates the enzyme acetylcholinesterase, which allows acetylcholine to be degraded, thus relieving the parasympathetic overstimulation caused by excess acetylcholine

Onset and Duration

Onset: Within min
Duration: Variable

Indications

Organophosphate poisoning (after atropine)

Contraindications

Hypersensitivity to pralidoxime

Adverse Reactions

Tachycardia
Hypertension
Laryngospasm
Hyperventilation
Muscle weakness
Nausea

Drug Interactions

Pralidoxime should not be mixed in the same syringe or solution with any other drug

How Supplied

Emergency single-dose kit containing one 20-mL vial of 1 g of the sterile drug, one 20-mL ampule of sterile diluent, and a 20-mL syringe with needle

Dosage and Administration

Adult: 600 mg IM (usually by autoinjector) or 1-2 g IV over 15-30 min

Pediatric: 20-50 mg/kg IV over 15-30 min

Special Considerations

Pregnancy Safety: Category C

Each 1 g of sterile powder is diluted with 20 mL of sterile water for injection

Should be further diluted in 100 mL of normal saline and given as an IV infusion. Use promptly after reconstitution.

Medical direction may recommend the almost simultaneous administration of atropine

Not recommended in carbamate poisoning

Reduce dosage in cases of known renal insufficiency

Procainamide *(Pronestyl)*

Class

Antidysrhythmic (Class I-A)

Description

Procainamide suppresses phase 4 depolarization in normal ventricular muscle and Purkinje fibers, reducing the automaticity of ectopic pacemakers. It also suppresses reentry dysrhythmias by slowing intraventricular conduction. Procainamide may be effective in treating PVCs and recurrent ventricular tachycardia that cannot be controlled with lidocaine.

Onset and Duration

Onset: 10-30 min
Duration: 3-6 hr

Indications

Suppressing PVCs refractory to lidocaine
Suppressing VT (with a pulse) refractory to lidocaine
Suppressing VF refractory to lidocaine
PSVTs with wide-complex tachycardia of unknown origin

Contraindications

Second- and third-degree AV block (without functioning artificial pacemaker)
Digitalis toxicity
Torsades de pointes
Complete heart block
Tricyclic antidepressant toxicity

Adverse Reactions

Hypotension
Bradycardia
Reflex tachycardia
AV block

Widened QRS
Prolonged PR or QT interval
PVCs
VT, VF, asystole
CNS depression
Confusion
Seizure

Drug Interactions
Increases effects of skeletal muscle relaxants
Increases plasma/NAPA (active metabolites) concentrations with cimetidine, ranitidine, beta blockers, amiodarone, trimethoprim, and quinidine

How Supplied
1 g in 10 mL vial (100 mg/mL)
1 g in 2 mL vials (500 mg/mL) for infusion

Dosage and Administration
Adult: 30 mg/min slow IV infusion in recurrent VF/pulseless VT (up to 50 mg/min may be given in urgent situations) (max total 17 mg/kg; max dose usually 1 g)
            Maintenance: Infusion (after resuscitation from cardiac arrest): mix 1 g in 250 mL solution (4 mg/mL), infuse at 1-4 mg/min
Pediatric: Loading dose 15 mg/kg IV/IO; infuse over 30-60 min

Special Considerations
Pregnancy Safety: Category C
Procainamide has potent vasodilating and inotropic effects
Rapid injection may cause procainamide-induced hypotension
Carefully monitor vital signs and ECG (a small amount of QRS widening is expected)
Routine use in combination with other drugs that prolong the QT interval is not recommended
Administer cautiously to patients with asthma, digitalis-induced dysrhythmias, AMI, or cardiac, hepatic, or renal insufficiency

> **NOTE**
>
> Discontinue if the dysrhythmia is suppressed, hypotension develops, the QRS complex is widened by 50% of its original width, or a total of 1 g has been administered.

Promethazine (Phenergan)

Class
Phenothiazine, Antihistamine

Description
Promethazine is an H_1 receptor antagonist that blocks the actions of histamine by competitive antagonism at the H_1 receptor. In addition to antihistaminic effects, promethazine also possesses sedative, antimotion, antiemetic, and considerable anticholinergic activity. It is often administered with analgesics, particularly narcotics, to potentiate their effects, though the occurrence of potentiation is controversial.

Onset and Duration
Onset: IV (rapid)
Duration: 4-6 hr

Indications
Nausea and vomiting
Motion sickness
Pre- and postoperative, obstetric (during labor) sedation
To potentiate the effects of analgesics
Allergic reactions

Contraindications
Hypersensitivity
Comatose states
CNS depression from alcohol, barbiturates, or narcotics
Signs associated with Reye's syndrome

Adverse Reactions
Sedation
Dizziness
May impair mental and physical ability
Allergic reactions
Dysrhythmias
Nausea and vomiting
Hyperexcitability
Dystonias
Use in children may cause hallucinations, convulsions, and sudden death

Drug Interactions
Concomitant use of CNS depressants may have an additive sedative effect
Increased incidence of extrapyramidal effects when given with some MAO inhibitors
Concomitant use of epinephrine (may further decrease blood pressure)

How Supplied
25, 50 mg/mL in 1 mL ampules and Tubex syringes

Dosage and Administration
Adult: 12.5-25 mg IV, deep IM
Pediatric: Not indicated in the prehospital setting

Special Considerations
Pregnancy Safety: Category C (generally considered safe for use during labor)
Use caution in patients with asthma, peptic ulcer, and bone marrow depression
Care must be taken to avoid accidental intraarterial injection

IM injections are the preferred route of administration
Slow IV administration over 1 min

Propranolol (Inderal)

Class
Beta adrenergic blocker, Antidysrhythmic (Class II)

Description
Propranolol is a nonselective beta adrenergic blocker that inhibits chronotropic, inotropic, and vasodilator response to beta adrenergic stimulation. It slows the sinus rate, depresses AV conduction, decreases cardiac output, and reduces blood pressure. In addition, propranolol decreases myocardial oxygen demand, and reduces the risk of sudden death in patients with AMI.

Onset and Duration
Onset: Within 1-2 hr
Duration: 6-12 hr

Indications
Hypertension
Angina pectoris
VT, VF, and rapid supraventricular dysrhythmias refractory to other therapies

Contraindications
Sinus bradycardia
Second- or third-degree AV block
Asthma
Cardiogenic shock
Pulmonary edema
Uncompensated CHF
COPD (relative)

Adverse Reactions
Bradycardia
Heart blocks
Bronchospasm (in susceptible persons)
Dyspnea
Dizziness
Weakness, dizziness
Nausea and vomiting
Visual disturbances

Drug Interactions
Catecholamine-depleting drugs may potentiate hypotension
Sympathomimetic effects may be antagonized
Verapamil may worsen AV conduction abnormalities
Succinylcholine effects may be enhanced
Isoproterenol, norepinephrine, dopamine, and dobutamine may reverse effects of propranolol
Epinephrine may cause a rise in blood pressure, a decrease in heart rate, and severe vasoconstriction
Signs of hypoglycemia may be masked

How Supplied
1 mg/mL vials

Dosage and Administration
Adult: 1-3 mg IV over 2-5 min (not to exceed 1 mg/min); can be repeated after 2 min (total dose of 0.1 mg/kg)
Pediatric: Not recommended.

Special Considerations
Pregnancy Safety: Category C
Propranolol may produce life-threatening side effects; closely monitor patient during administration
Use with caution in elderly patients
Use with caution in patients with impaired hepatic or renal function
Atropine should be readily available

> **NOTE**
>
> Beta$_1$-selective drugs now available are more commonly used for cardiac emergencies.

Reteplase (Retavase)

Class
Fibrinolytic

Description
Reteplase is a recombinant plasminogen activator. Fibrinolytic action occurs by generating plasmin from plasminogen that degrades the fibrin matrix of a thrombus. The drug is used in the management of AMI in adults, for the improvement of ventricular function following AMI, and for a reduction in the incidence of CHF. Treatment with reteplase should be initiated as soon as possible after the onset of AMI symptoms.

Onset and Duration
Onset: Prompt (effecting vessel patency within 90 min for most patients)
Duration: Variable

Indications
Management of AMI in adults (must be confirmed with 12-lead ECG)

Contraindications
Active internal bleeding
History of stroke
Recent intracranial or intraspinal surgery or trauma
Intracranial neoplasm, AV malformation, or aneurysm
Bleeding disorders
Severe uncontrolled hypertension

Adverse Reactions
Bleeding (internal and at superficial sites)
Reperfusion dysrhythmias

Allergic reaction (rare)
Nausea and vomiting
Hypotension

Drug Interactions

Risk of bleeding will be increased if used concurrently with drugs that alter platelet function
Risk of bleeding with concomitant use of heparin, vitamin K antagonist (e.g., warfarin) is markedly increased
Incompatible with heparin; do not administer in the same IV line

How Supplied

Supplied in kit with components for reconstitution: single use reteplase vials (10.8 units each), single use diluent vials of sterile water (10 mL each), sterile 10 mL syringes with 20 gauge needles, sterile dispensing pins, sterile 20 gauge needles for administration, and alcohol swabs. Reconstitute by withdrawing 10 mL of diluent; open the package containing the dispensing pin; remove the needle from the syringe and discard the needle; remove the connective cap from the dispensing pin and connect the syringe to the pin; remove the flip cap from one vial of reteplase; remove the protective cap from the spike end of the dispensing pin and insert the spike into the vial of reteplase; transfer the diluent through the dispensing pin into the vial of reteplase; with the dispensing pin and syringe still attached, swirl (not shake) the vial gently to dissolve the reteplase; withdraw 10 mL of the reconstituted solution back into the syringe; detach the syringe from the dispensing pin, and attach a sterile 20 gauge needle; the 10 mL bolus dose is now ready to administer.

Dosage and Administration

Adult: Administered as 10 + 10 U double-bolus injection. Each bolus is administered IV over 2 min. (The second bolus is given 30 min after the first bolus.) Heparin and aspirin should be administered concomitantly.
Pediatric: Safety not established.

Special Considerations

Pregnancy Safety: Category C
Reteplase should be given in an IV line in which no other medication is being simultaneously injected or infused
Protect contents of package from light

Sodium Bicarbonate

Class

Buffer, Alkalinizing agent, Electrolyte supplement

Description

Sodium bicarbonate reacts with hydrogen ions (H^+) to form water and carbon dioxide and thereby can act to buffer metabolic acidosis. As the plasma hydrogen ion concentration decreases, blood pH rises.

Onset and Duration

Onset: 2-10 min
Duration: 30-60 min

Indications

Known preexisting bicarbonate responsive acidosis
Intubated patient with continued long arrest interval, PEA
Upon return of spontaneous circulation after long arrest interval
Tricyclic antidepressant overdose
Alkalinization for treatment of specific intoxications
Management of metabolic acidosis
DKA

Contraindications

In patients with chloride loss from vomiting and GI suction
Metabolic and respiratory alkalosis
Severe pulmonary edema
Abdominal pain of unknown origin
Hypocalcemia
Hypokalemia
Hypernatremia
When administration of sodium could be detrimental

Adverse Reactions

Metabolic alkalosis
Hypoxia
Rise in intracellular P_{CO_2} and increased tissue acidosis
Electrolyte imbalance (hypernatremia)
Seizures
Tissue sloughing at injection site

Drug Interactions

May precipitate in calcium solutions
Alkalinization of urine may shorten elimination half-lives of certain drugs
Vasopressors may be deactivated

How Supplied

50 mEq in 50 mL, and 0.5, 0.6 mEq/mL

Dosage and Administration

Urgent Forms of Metabolic Acidosis
Adult: 1 mEq/kg IV; repeat with 0.5 mEq/kg q 10 min
Pediatric: Same as adult; infuse slowly and only if ventilations are adequate

Special Considerations

Pregnancy Safety: Category C
When possible, blood gas analysis should guide bicarbonate administration
Bicarbonate administration produces carbon dioxide, which crosses cell membranes more rapidly than

bicarbonate (potentially worsening intracellular acidosis)

May increase edematous or sodium-retaining states

May worsen CHF

Maintain adequate ventilation (gas exchange)

Streptokinase (Streptase)

Class

Fibrinolytic agent

Description

Streptokinase combines with plasminogen to produce an activator complex that converts free plasminogen to the proteolytic enzyme plasmin. The plasmin in turn functions as an enzyme that degrades fibrin threads as well as fibrinogen, causing lysis of the blood clot. Streptokinase is administered to selected patients with acute evolving myocardial infarctions.

Onset and Duration

Onset: 10-20 min (fibrinolysis, 10-20 min; clot lysis, 60-90 min)

Duration: 3-4 hr (prolonged bleeding times up to 24 hr)

Indications

Acute evolving myocardial infarction

Massive pulmonary emboli

Arterial thrombosis and embolism

To clear arteriovenous cannulas

DVT

Contraindications

Hypersensitivity

Active bleeding

Recent surgery (within 2-3 weeks)

Recent CVA

Prolonged CPR

Intracranial or intraspinal surgery

Recent significant trauma (particularly head trauma)

Uncontrolled hypertension (systolic pressure equal to or greater than 180 mm Hg; diastolic pressure equal to or greater than 110 mm Hg)

Adverse Reactions

Bleeding (GI, GU, intracranial, other sites)

Allergic reactions

Hypotension

Chest pain

Reperfusion dysrhythmias

Abdominal pain

Drug Interactions

Acetylsalicylic acid may increase risk of bleeding (may also be beneficial in improving overall effectiveness)

Heparin and other anticoagulants may increase risk of bleeding as well as improve overall outcome

How Supplied

250,000, 750,000, 1.5 million IU vials

Reconstitute by slowly adding 5 mL of sodium chloride or D_5W, directing the stream toward the side of the vial, rather than into the powder. Gently roll—do not shake the vial for reconstitution. Slowly dilute the entire contents of the vial to total of 45 mL.

Dosage and Administration

Evolving acute myocardial infarction

Adult: 1.5 million U diluted to 45 mL (IV) over 1 hr (use infusion pump)

Pediatric: Safety not established

Special Considerations

Pregnancy Safety: Category C

Do not administer IM injections to patients receiving fibrinolytic drugs

Obtain blood sample for coagulation studies prior to administration

Carefully monitor vital signs

Observe the patient for bleeding

Use caution when moving patient to avoid bruising or bleeding

Do not draw arterial blood gas specimens in fibrinolytic therapy candidates

Use one IV line exclusively for fibrinolytic administration

Succinylcholine (Anectine)

Class

Neuromuscular blocker (depolarizing)

Description

Succinylcholine has the quickest onset and briefest duration of action of all neuromuscular blocking drugs, making it a drug of choice for such procedures as endotracheal intubation, electroconvulsive shock therapy, and terminating laryngospasm. Like nondepolarizing blockers, depolarizing drugs also bind to the receptors for acetylcholine. However, because they cause depolarization of the muscle membrane, they often lead to fasciculations and some muscular contractions.

Onset and Duration

Onset: Less than 1 min

Duration: 5-10 min after single IV dose

Indications

To facilitate intubation

Terminating laryngospasm

Muscle relaxation

Contraindications

Acute injuries

Hypersensitivity

Skeletal muscle myopathies

Inability to control airway and/or support ventilations with oxygen and positive pressure
Personal or family history of malignant hyperthermia
Acute rhabdomyolysis

Adverse Reactions

Hypotension
Respiratory depression
Bradycardias
Dysrhythmias
Initial muscle fasciculation
Excessive salivation
Malignant hyperthermia
Allergic reaction
Succinylcholine may exacerbate hyperkalemia in trauma patients (hours post-trauma)

Drug Interactions

Oxytocin, beta blockers, chronic contraceptive use, and organophosphates may potentiate effects
Diazepam may reduce duration of action
Cardiac glycosides may induce dysrhythmias

How Supplied

20, 50, 100 mg/mL, 1 g multidose vial

Dosage and Administration

NOTE

If the patient is conscious, explain the effects of the medication before administration. Premedication with *atropine* should be strongly considered, particularly in the pediatric age group. Premedicating with *lidocaine* may blunt any increase in intracranial pressure associated with intubation. Finally, *diazepam* or another sedative should be used in any conscious patient undergoing neuromuscular blockade.

Adult: 0.3-1.1 mg/kg (25-75 mg) over 10-30 seconds IV; 0.04-0.07 mg/kg to maintain relaxation
Pediatric: 1-2 mg/kg dose rapid IV

Special Considerations

Pregnancy Safety: Category C

NOTE

Neuromuscular blocking agents will produce respiratory paralysis. Therefore intubation and ventilatory support must be readily available.

Carefully monitor the patient and be prepared to resuscitate
Administer with caution to patients with severe trauma, burns, and electrolyte imbalances (high potassium levels)
Brain or spinal cord injury may prolong effects
Patients must have a patent or artificial airway and adequate sedation during paralysis. Children are not as sensitive to succinylcholine on a weight basis as adults and may require higher doses
Succinylcholine has no effect on consciousness or pain
Will not stop neuronal seizure activity
May rarely cause ventricular dysrhythmias/ cardiac arrest in infants and children

Syrup of Ipecac

Class

Emetic, Antidote

Description

Syrup of ipecac acts as a local irritant on the gastric mucosa and on emetic centers of the brain. Vomiting induced by syrup of ipecac occurs in 80%-90% of patients. The drug is available over-the-counter, however, medical direction and/or a poison control center should be consulted prior to administration.

Onset and Duration

Onset: Generally, 15-20 min
Duration: Up to 1-2 hr

Indications

Acute oral drug or toxin overdose in alert patients

Contraindications

Caustics, corrosives, petroleum distillates
TCA overdose
Camphor ingestion
Unprotected airway
Unconscious patient when time elapsed since exposure is greater than 1 hr
Absent gag reflex
Unknown ingestion
Children less than 1 year of age
Rapidly acting CNS depressants (causing decreased level of consciousness faster than ipecac can work), or stimulants (causing seizures)
Upper GI bleeding

Adverse Reactions

Prolonged vomiting
Muscle aching, weakness
Drowsiness

Drug Interactions

Activated charcoal adsorbs ipecac

How Supplied
15, 30 mL vials

Dosage and Administration

Adult:	15-30 mL PO followed by 3-4 glasses of water; may repeat with 15 mL once in 20 min if ineffective
Pediatric (1-12 years):	5-15 mL PO followed by 1½-2 glasses of water; may repeat with 15 mL once in 20 min if ineffective

Special Considerations
Pregnancy Safety: Category C

Carefully monitor patient's airway

90% of patients vomit within one-half hour of administration (average time is 20 min)

Activated charcoal should be administered only after vomiting has ceased for 1-2 hr

A disadvantage of syrup of ipecac is that persistent vomiting may preclude use of activated charcoal

Save emesis sample for evaluation

Patients usually vomit 2-3 times per dose over 1-2 periods. Keep patient awake NPO for 2 hrs

Ipecac should not be given unless OD was witnessed (e.g., acetaminophen ingestion witnessed by parent) and is recommended by medical direction or a poison control center

---

NOTE

Syrup of ipecac is less effective than activated charcoal in decreasing toxin absorption. It is seldom indicated for use in the prehospital setting.

Tetracaine (Pontocaine)

Class
Topical ophthalmic anesthetic

Description
Tetracaine is used for rapid, brief, superficial anesthesia. The agent inhibits conduction of nerve impulses from sensory nerves.

Onset and Duration

Onset:	Within 30 seconds
Duration:	10-15 min

Indications
Short-term relief from eye pain or irritation

Patient comfort before eye irrigation

Contraindications
Hypersensitivity to tetracaine

Open injury to the eye

Adverse Reactions
Burning or stinging sensation

Irritation

Drug Interactions
Incompatible with mercury or silver salts often found in ophthalmic products

How Supplied
0.5% solution

Dosage and Administration

Adult:	1-2 drops
Pediatric:	Same as adult

Special Considerations
Pregnancy Safety: Category C

Can cause epithelial damage and systemic toxicity

Not recommended for prolonged use

Thiamine (Betaxin)

Class
Vitamin (B₁)

Description
Thiamine combines with adenosine triphosphate (ATP) to form thiamine pyrophosphate coenzyme, a necessary component for carbohydrate metabolism. Most vitamins required by the body are obtained through diet, however, certain states such as alcoholism and malnourishment may affect the intake, absorption, and utilization of thiamine. The brain is extremely sensitive to thiamine deficiency.

Onset and Duration

Onset:	Rapid
Duration:	Depends on the degree of deficiency

Indications
Coma of unknown origin (with administration of dextrose 50% or naloxone)

Delirium tremens

Beriberi (rare)

Wernicke's encephalopathy

Contraindications
None significant

Adverse Reactions
Hypotension (from rapid injection or large dose)

Anxiety

Diaphoresis

Nausea and vomiting

Allergic reaction (usually from IV injection; very rare); angioedema

Drug Interactions

None significant

How Supplied

1-,2-mL vials (100 mg/mL)

Dosage and Administration

Adult: 100 mg slow IV or IM
Pediatric: Not recommended in the prehospital setting

Special Considerations

Pregnancy Safety: Category A (Category C if dose exceeds RDA recommendation)
Large IV doses may cause respiratory difficulties
Anaphylactic reactions have been reported

Tissue Plasminogen Activator (t-PA, Activase, Recombinant Alteplase)

Class

Fibrinolytic

Description

Tissue plasminogen activator is a naturally-occurring enzyme derived from DNA technology. The enzyme binds to fibrin-bound plasminogen at the site of an arterial clot, thus converting plasminogen to plasmin. Plasmin digests the fibrin strands of the clot and restores perfusion to the occluded artery. In emergency care, fibrinolytic agents are used in treating selected patients with acute evolving myocardial infarction.

Onset and Duration

Onset: Clot lysis often occurs within 60-90 min
Duration: 30 min (80% cleared in 10 min)

Indications (same as other fibrinolytic agents)

Acute evolving myocardial infarction
Massive pulmonary emboli
DVT
Arterial thrombosis and embolism
To clear arteriovenous cannulas

Contraindications

Active bleeding
Recent surgery (within 2-3 weeks)
Recent CVA
Prolonged CPR
Intracranial or intraspinal surgery
Recent significant trauma (particularly head trauma)
Uncontrolled hypertension

Adverse Reactions

Bleeding (GI, GU, intracranial, other sites)
Allergic reactions
Hypotension

Chest pain
Reperfusion dysrhythmias
Abdominal pain
Active bleeding
Recent CVA
Prolonged CPR
Recent surgery (within 2-3 weeks)
Peptic ulcer disease
Recent intracranial, intraspinal surgery or trauma
Uncontrolled hypertension

Drug Interactions

Acetylsalicylic acid may increase risk of bleeding (may also be beneficial in improving overall effectiveness)
Heparin and other anticoagulants may also increase risk of bleeding and improve overall effectiveness

How Supplied

50, 100 mg/vial with 50, 100 mL of diluent, respectively
May further dilute with equal amounts of 0.9% sodium chloride or D_5W

Dosage and Administration

Adult (for AMI):   Give 15 mg IV bolus, then 0.75 mg/kg over next 30 min (not to exceed 50 mg), then 0.5 mg/kg over next 60 min (not to exceed 35 mg). (Other doses may be prescribed by medical direction.)
Pediatric: Safety not established

Special Considerations

Pregnancy Safety: Category C
Gently roll—do not shake—the vial to mix powder with liquid
Closely monitor vital signs
Observe for bleeding
Obtain blood sample for coagulation studies prior to administration
Do not administer IM injections to patients receiving fibrinolytic drugs
No arterial blood gas specimens should be drawn on potential fibrinolytic therapy candidates due to bleeding tendency
Use caution when moving patient to avoid bleeding or bruising
Use one IV line exclusively for fibrinolytic administration

Vasopressin (Pitressin)

Class

Naturally occurring antidiuretic hormone

Mechanism of Action

Vasopressin acts by direct stimulation of smooth muscle V_1 receptors. When given in extremely high doses, it acts as a nonadrenergic peripheral vasoconstrictor.

Onset and Duration

Onset: Immediate
Duration: Variable

Indications

As an alternative pressor to epinephrine in adult shock-refractory VF
Vasodilatory shock

Contraindications

Responsive patients with coronary artery disease

Adverse Reactions

Ischemic chest pain
Abdominal distress
Sweating
Nausea and vomiting
Tremors
Bronchial constriction
Uterine contraction

Drug Interactions

No significant drug reactions have been reported

How Supplied

5 U/mL

Dosage and Administration

Adult: Cardiac arrest: 40 U IV push
one time
Child and infant: Not recommended

Special Considerations

Pregnancy Safety: Category C
May increase peripheral vascular resistance and provoke cardiac ischemia and angina
Vasopressin may be given IO

Verapamil (Isoptin)

Class

Calcium channel blocker (Class IV antidysrhythmic)

Description

Verapamil is used as an antidysrhythmic, antianginal, and antihypertensive agent. It works by inhibiting the movement of calcium ions across cell membranes. The slow calcium ion current blocked by verapamil is more important for the activity of the SA node and AV node than for many other tissues in the heart. By interfering with this current, calcium channel blockers achieve some selectivity of action. Verapamil decreases atrial automaticity, reduces AV conduction velocity, and prolongs the AV nodal refractory period. In addition, verapamil depresses myocardial contractility, reduces vascular smooth muscle tone, and dilates coronary arteries and arterioles in normal and ischemic tissues.

Onset and Duration

Onset: 2-5 min
Duration: 30-60 min (up to 4 hr is possible)

Indications

PSVTs
Atrial flutter with a rapid ventricular response
Atrial fibrillation with a rapid ventricular response
Vasospastic and unstable angina
Chronic stable angina

Contraindications

Hypersensitivity
Sick sinus syndrome (unless the patient has a functioning pacemaker)
Second- or third-degree heart block
Sinus bradycardia
Hypotension
Cardiogenic shock
Severe CHF
WPW with atrial fibrillation or flutter
Patients receiving intravenous beta blockers
Wide-complex tachycardias (ventricular tachycardia can deteriorate into ventricular fibrillation when calcium channel blockers are given)

Adverse Reactions

Dizziness
Headache
Nausea and vomiting
Hypotension
Bradycardia
Complete AV block
Peripheral edema

Drug Interactions

Verapamil increases serum concentration of digoxin
Beta adrenergic blockers may have additive negative inotropic and chronotropic effects
Antihypertensives may potentiate hypotensive effects

How Supplied

Parenteral: 5 mg/2 mL in 2, 4, 5, mL vials, or
2, 4 mL ampules

Dosage and Administration

Adult:
Initial dose: 2.5- 5 mg IV bolus over 2 min
(1-3 min in elderly patients)
Repeat dose: 5-10 mg in 15-30 min after initial dose; or 5 mg q 15 min until a desired response is achieved (max 30 mg dose)
Pediatric: Not recommended in the prehospital setting

Special Considerations

Pregnancy Safety: Category C

Closely monitor patient's vital signs
Give smaller amounts (2-4 mg) over longer periods of time (3-4 min) when treating the elderly or when the blood pressure is in the lower range of normal
Be prepared to resuscitate
AV block or asystole may occur due to slowed AV conduction

NOTE

Some physicians recommend slow IV administration of 500 mg *calcium chloride* before dose of verapamil to minimize the untoward results of hypotension and bradycardia.

REFERENCES

American Heart Association: *Advanced cardiac life support,* Dallas, 1997, The Association.

American Heart Association: *Pediatric advanced life support,* Dallas, 1997, The Association.

Clark J et al: *Pharmacologic basis of nursing practice,* ed 4, St. Louis, 1993, Mosby.

Gonzalez E et al: Intravenous amiodarone for ventricular arrhythmias: overview and clinical use, *Resuscitation* 39:31, 1998.

Guidelines for cardiopulmonary resuscitation and emergency cardiac care, *JAMA* (16):2171, 1992.

Ryan T et al: *Guidelines for the management of patients with acute myocardial infarction, report of the American College of Cardiology/American Heart Association Task Force on Practice Guidelines (Committee on Management of Acute Myocardial Infarction),* Dallas, 1998, The Association.

Hoekelman R: *Primary pediatric care,* ed 3, St. Louis, 1997, Mosby.

McKenry L, Salerno E: *Mosby's pharmacology in nursing,* ed 18, St. Louis, 1992, Mosby.

Physician's desk reference, ed 53, Oradell, NJ, 1999, Medical Economics Co.

Salerno E: *Pharmacology for health professionals,* St. Louis, 1999, Mosby.

Skidmore-Roth L: *Mosby's 1999 nursing drug reference,* St. Louis, 1999, Mosby.

Am Health Assoc: *2000 Handbook of emergency cardiovascular care for healthcare providers,* Dallas, 2000, The Association.

Resources

EMS Systems: Roles and Responsibilities

American College of Emergency Physicians: *Policy statement on medical direction of prehospital emergency medical services*, Dallas, 1992.

Bledsoe B: *Paramedic emergency care*, ed 3, Englewood Cliffs, N.J., 1996, Prentice-Hall.

Committee on Trauma: *American College of Surgeons: resources for the optimal care of the injured patient*, Chicago, 1993.

Keuhl S: *Prehospital systems and medical oversight*, ed 2, 1994, NAEMSP.

Menegazzi JJ: *Research: the who, what, why, when, and how*, 1993, Ferno-Washington, Inc.

Narad RA: Emergency medical services system design, *Emerg Med Clin North Am* 8:1, 1990.

National Academy of Sciences/Natural Research Council: *Accidental death and disability: the neglected disease of modern society*, Washington, 1966, National Academy of Sciences.

National Association of EMS Physicians: *Prehospital systems and medical oversight*, ed 2, St. Louis, 1994, Mosby.

NHTSA's Air Medical Crew National Standard Curriculum, 1998, ASHBEAMS.

Oregon Health Division-Emergency Medical Services and Systems: *Emergency medical technician EMT: intermediate course curriculum and reference guide*, ed 2, 1998.

Polsky S: *Continuous quality improvement in EMS*, 1992, ACEP.

Steering Committee Project: *Consensus statement on the role of emergency medical services in primary injury prevention*, 1993, NHTSA/MCHB/NAEMSP.

Swor RA et al: *Quality management in prehospital care*, Philadelphia, 1993, Mosby-Lifeline.

The Well-Being of the Paramedic

Emergency Medical Update: *Well-being of EMS, Primedia Workplace Learning*, 1997.

Hoeger W, Hoeger S: *Lifetime physical fitness and wellness*, ed 5, Englewood, Colo., 1998, Morton Publishing.

International Association of Fire Fighters: *International Association of Fire Fighters: infectious diseases and the fire and emergency services*, Washington, D.C., 1992, Department of Occupational Health and Safety, International Association of Fire Fighters.

Internet address: www.cdc.gov, www.maychealth.org, www.nih.gov

Kubler-Ross E: *On death and dying*, New York, 1969, MacMillan.

Mitchell J, Bray G: *Emergency services stress*, Englewood Cliffs, N.J., 1990, Prentice Hall.

U.S. Department of Health and Human Services Public Health Service: *Health people 2000*, 1990, National Health Promotion and Disease Prevention Objectives.

West KH: *Infectious disease handbook for emergency care personnel*, ed 2, Cincinnati, 1994, American Conference of Governmental Industrial Hygienists.

Injury Prevention

Children's Safety Network: *National center for education in maternal and child health, injury prevention professionals: a national directory*, ed 3, Washington, D.C., 1992.

Consensus statement on the role of emergency medical services in primary injury prevention, February 1996.

Prehospital Trauma Life Support Committee of the National Association of Emergency Medical Technicians, Committee on Trauma of the American College of Surgeons, PHTLS: *Basic and advanced prehospital trauma life support*, St. Louis, 1999, Mosby.

Medical/Legal Issues

American College of Emergency Physicians: *DNAR directives in the out-of-hospital setting*, 1994.

Fox E, Seigler M: Redefining the emergency physician's role in do-not-resuscitate decision-making, *Am J Med* 92:125, 1992.

National Association of EMS Physicians: *Prehospital systems and medical oversight*, ed 2, St. Louis, 1994, Mosby.

Ethics

American College of Emergency Physicians: DNAR directives in the out-of-hospital setting, *Ann Emerg Med* 17:1106, 1998.

Emergency Cardiac Care Committee and Subcommittees: *American Heart Association, Advanced Cardiac Life Support*, 1997.

Fox E, Seigler M: Redefining the emergency physician's role in do-not-resuscitate decision-making, *Am J Med* 92:125, 1992.

President's Committee for the Study of Ethical Problems in Medicine and Biomedical and Behavioral Research: *Deciding to forego life-sustaining treatment*, Washington, D.C., 1983, United States Government Printing Office.

Veatch RM: *Medical ethics*, Boston, 1989, Jones and Bartlett.

General Principles of Pathophysiology

Burns MV: *Pathophysiology: a self-instructional program*, Stanford, 1998, Appleton and Lange.

Gould BE: *Pathophysiology for the health related professions*, Philadelphia, 1997, WB Saunders.

Huether SE, McCance KL: *Understanding pathophysiology*, St. Louis, 1996, Mosby.

McCance KL, Huether SE: *Pathophysiology: the biological basis for disease in adults and children*, ed 2, St. Louis, 1994, Mosby-Yearbook.

Scanlon VC, Sanders T: *Essentials of anatomy and physiology*, ed 3, Philadelphia, 1999, FA Davis Company.

Pharmacology

Bledsoe BE, Clayden DE, Papa FJ: *Prehospital emergency pharmacology*, ed 4, Upper Saddle River, N.J., 1996, Prentice Hall.

LaRocca JC, Otto SE: *Intravenous therapy*, ed 3, St. Louis, 1997, Mosby.

Mikolaj AA: *Drug dosage calculations for the emergency care provider*, Upper Saddle River, N.J., 1997, Prentice Hall.

Skidmore-Roth L: *Mosby's 1999 nursing drug reference*, St. Louis, 1999, Mosby.

Wiederhold R: *Dosages and calculations*, Upper Saddle River, N.J., 1992, Prentice Hall.

Therapeutic Communications

Barker L: *Communication*, Prentice Hall.

Jarvis C: *Physical examination and health assessment*, Philadelphia, 1995, WB Saunders.

Othmer E, Othmer S: *The clinical interview, using DSM-IV, fundamentals*, vol 1, 1994, Psychiatric Press.

Samovar L, Mill J: *Oral communication, message and response*, Dubuque, Iowa, 1992, William C. Brown Publishers.

Seidel H et al: *Mosby's guide to physical examination*, ed 3, St. Louis, 1995, Mosby.

Patient Assessment

Bates B: *A guide to physical examination and history taking*, ed 6, Chicago, 1995, JB Lippincott.

Seidel H et al: *Mosby's guide to physical examination*, ed 3, St. Louis, 1995, Mosby.

Communications

Clawson J et al: Effect of a comprehensive quality management process on compliance with protocol in an emergency medical dispatch center, *Ann Emerg Med* 32(5):578, 1998.

Clawson J, Dernocoeur KB: *Principles of emergency medical dispatch*, ed 2, Salt Lake City, 1998, Priority Press.

Clawson J et al: The EMD as a medical professional, *JEMS* 21(5):68, 1996.

NIH Publications: *Emergency medical dispatching: rapid identification and treatment of acute myocardial infarction*, 1994.

Documentation

Dernocoeur K: *Streetsense: communication, safety and control*, ed 3, Redmond, Wash., 1998, Laing Resources.

Head and Facial Trauma

Alexander RH, Proctor HJ: *Advanced trauma life support course for physicians*, ed 5, 1993, The American College of Surgeons Committee on Trauma.

Bullock R: Mannitol and other diuretics in severe neurotrauma, *J Trauma* 3:448, 1995.

Chestnut R: Secondary brain insults after head injury, *J Trauma* 3:366, 1995.

Crooks DA: The pathological concept of diffuse axonal injury: its pathogenesis and the assessment of severity, *J Pathology* 165:5, 1991.

Erhard WL, Chestnut R: Intracranial pressure and cerebral perfusion pressure in severe head injury, *New Horizons* 3:400, 1995.

Guyton AC: *Human physiology and mechanisms of disease*, ed 5, Philadelphia, 1992, WB Saunders.

Hilton G: Diffuse axonal injury, *J Trauma Nurs* 2(1):7, 1995.

Hoff JT: Guidelines for the management of severe head injury, *J Trauma* 40:1048, 1996.

Jacobs BB, Baker P: *Trauma nursing core course*, ed 4, 1995, Emergency Nurses Association.

Rosner MJ, Daughton S: Cerebral perfusion pressure management in head injury, *J Trauma* 30:933, 1990.

Kerr ME, Brucia J: Hyperventilation in the head-injured patient: an effective treatment modality, *Heart & Lung* 22:516, 1993.

Marion DW, Firlik A, McLaughlin MR: Hyperventilation therapy for severe traumatic brain injury, *New Horizons* 3:439, 1995.

McCance KL, Huether SE: *Pathophysiology: the biologic basis for disease in adults and children*, ed 2, St. Louis, 1994, Mosby-Yearbook.

Prendergast V: Current trends in research and treatment of intracranial hypertension, *Critical Care Nursing Quarterly* 17:1, 1994.

Prielipp RC, Coursin DB: Sedative and neuromuscular

blocking drug use in critically ill patients with head injuries, *New Horizons* 3:456, 1995.

Slazinski T, Johnson MC: Severe diffuse axonal injury in adults and children, *J Neuroscience Nur* 26(3):151, 1994.

Spinal Trauma

Goth P: *Spine injury: critical criteria for assessment and management*, Augusta, Ga., 1994, Medical Care Development.

McCance KL, Huether SE: *Pathophysiology: the biologic basis for disease in adults and children*, ed 2, St. Louis, 1994, Mosby-Yearbook.

Thibodeau GA, Patton KL: *Anatomy and physiology*, ed 2, St. Louis, 1993, Mosby-Yearbook.

Thoracic Trauma

American College of Surgeons Committee on Trauma ATLS, Chicago, 1993, ACS.

Guyton A: *Textbook of medical physiology*, ed 7, Philadelphia, 1986, WB Saunders.

Moore KL: *Clinically oriented anatomy*, Baltimore, 1980, Williams and Wilkins.

Pans PT, Honigman B: Prehospital ATLS critical penetrating wounds to the thorax and abdomen, *J Trauma* 25:828, 1985.

PHTLS text, ed 4, St Louis, 1998, Mosby.

Musculoskeletal Trauma

Campbell J: *Basic trauma life support*, ed 2, Englewood Cliffs, N.J., 1998, Prentice Hall.

Crosby L, Lewallen D: *Emergency care and transportation of the sick and injured*, ed 6, American Academy of Orthopaedic Surgeons, Parkridge, Ill.

Limmer D, Elling B, O'Keefe M: *Essentials of emergency care*, ed 2, Upper Saddle River, N.J., 1998, Prentice Hall.

Martini F, Bartholomew E: *Essentials of anatomy and physiology*, Upper Saddle River, N.J., 1997, Prentice Hall.

Environmental Conditions

Generic References

Auerbach PS, Geehr EC: *Management of wilderness and environmental emergencies*, St. Louis, 1989, CV Mosby Company.

Forgey WW: *Wilderness medical society: practice guidelines for wilderness emergency care*, Merrillville, Ind., 1995, ICS Books, Inc.

Stewart CE: *Environmental emergencies*, Baltimore, 1990, Williams and Wilkins.

Immersion Foot and Frostbite

Brown JR: A case of frostbite or "it takes more than two pairs of socks to keep your feet warm," *J R Army Med Corps* 132:93, 1986.

Francis TJR: Nonfreezing cold injury: a historical review, *J Roy Nav Med Serv* 70:134, 1984.

Fuhrman FA, Fuhrman GJ: The treatment of experimental frostbite by rapid thawing: a review and new experimental data, *Medicine* 36:465, 1957.

Haller JS Jr: Trench foot: a study in military-medical responsiveness in the Great War, 1914-1918, *West J Med* 152:729, 1990.

Heggers JP et al: Experimental and clinical observations on frostbite, *Ann Emerg Med* 16:1056, 1987.

Marzella L et al: Morphologic characterization of acute injury to vascular endothelium of skin after frostbite, *Plast Reconstr Surg* 83:67, 1989.

Porter JM et al: Intra-arterial sympathetic blockade in the treatment of clinical frostbite, *Am J Surg* 132:625, 1976.

Hypothermia

Andrew PJ, Parker RS: Treating accidental hypothermia (letter), *BMJ* 2:1641, 1978.

Angelakos ET, Hegnauer AH: Pharmacological agents for the control of spontaneous ventricular fibrillation under progressive hypothermia, *J Pharm Ther* 127:137, 1959.

Bashour TT, Gualberto A, Ryan C: Atrioventricular block in accidental hypothermia: a case report, *Angiology* 40:63, 1989.

Bolte RG et al: The use of extracorporeal rewarming in a child submerged for 66 minutes, *JAMA* 260:377, 1988.

Bristow GK, Giesbrecht GG: Contribution of exercise and shivering to recovery from induced hypothermia (31.2° C) in one subject, *Aviat Space Environ Med* 59:549, 1988.

Budd GM: Accidental hypothermia in skiers, *Med J Aust* 144:449, 1986.

Burton AC, Edholm OC: *Man in a cold environment: physiological and pathological effects of exposure to low temperatures*, Monographs of the Physiological Society, ed 2, New York, 1969, Hafner Publishing Co.

Coleshaw SR et al: Impaired memory registration and speed of reasoning caused by low body temperature, *J Appl Physiol* 44:27, 1983.

Collis ML, Steinman AM, Chaney RD: Accidental hypothermia: an experimental study of practical rewarming methods, *Aviat Space Environ Med* 48(7):625, 1977.

Dannewitz SR, Jilek J, Staten C: Warm intravenous fluid administration using hot packs (letter), *Ann Emerg Med* 13:982, 1984.

Danzl DF, Pozos RS, Hamlet MP: Accidental hypothermia. In Auerbach P, editor: *Management of wilderness and environmental emergencies*, St. Louis, 1989, CV Mosby Co.

Faries G et al: Temperature relationship to distance and flow rate of warmed IV fluids, *Ann Emerg Med* 20:1198, 1991.

Fitzgerald FT, Jessop C: Accidental hypothermia: a report of 22 cases and review of the literature, *Adv Intern Med* 27:128, 1982.

Forgey WW: *Death by exposure: hypothermia*, Merrillville, Ind., 1985, ICS Books.

Gillen JP et al: Ventricular fibrillation during orotracheal intubation of hypothermic dogs, *Ann Emerg Med* 15:412, 1986.

Harari A et al: Pertubations hemodynamiques au cours des hypothermies accidentelles profondes et prolongees, *Nouvelle Presse Medicale* 3:2184, 1974.

Harnett RM, Pruitt JR, Sias FR: A review of the literature concerning resuscitation from hypothermia. I. The problem and general approaches, *Aviat Space Environ Med* 54:425, 1983.

Herr RD, White GL Jr: Hypothermia: threat to military operations, *Milit Med* 156:140, 1991.

Hoffman RG, Pozos RS: Experimental hypothermia and cold perception, *Aviat Space Environ Med* 60:964, 1989.

Keatinge WR: Medical problems of cold weather: the Oliver-Sharpey lecture, *J R Coll Physicians Lond* 20:283, 1986.

Kiss of life for a cold corpse, *Lancet* 335:1435, 1990.

Lathrop TG: *Hypothermia: killer of the unprepared*, Portland, 1975, Mazamas.

LeBlanc J: *Man in the cold: American lectures in environmental studies*, Publication No. 986, Bannerstone Division, Springfield, Ill., 1975, Charles C. Thomas.

Ledingham IM, Mone JG: Treatment of accidental hypothermia: a prospective clinical study, *BMJ* 280:1102, 1980.

Lloyd EL: Airway rewarming in the treatment of accidental hypothermia: a review, *J Wild Med* 1:65, 1990.

Lloyd EL: Hypothermia and cold, *Sci Prog* 73:101, 1989.

Lloyd EL: *Hypothermia and cold stress*, Rockville, Md., 1986, Aspen Systems Corporation.

Lomax P: *Neuropharmacological aspects of thermoregulation: the nature and treatment of hypothermia*, Minneapolis, 1983, University of Minnesota Press.

Lonning PE, Skulberg A, Abyholm F: Accidental hypothermia: review of the literature, *Acta Anaesthesiol Scand* 30:601, 1986.

Maclean D: Emergency management of accidental hypothermia: a review, *J R Soc Med* 79:528, 1986.

Maclean D, Emslie-Smith D: *Accidental hypothermia*, Oxford, 1977, Blackwell Scientific Publications.

Marcus P: The treatment of acute accidental hypothermia: proceedings of a symposium held at the RAF Institute of Aviation Medicine, *Aviat Space Environ Med* 50:834, 1979.

Miller JW, Danzl DF, Thomas DM: Urban accidental hypothermia: 135 cases, *Ann Emerg Med* 9:456, 1980.

Mills WJ Jr: *Accidental hypothermia: the nature and treatment of hypothermia*, vol 2, Minneapolis, 1983, University of Minnesota Press.

Murphy K, Nowak RM, Tomlanovich MC: Use of bretylium tosylate as prophylaxis and treatment in hypothermic ventricular fibrillation in the canine model, *Ann Emerg Med* 15:1160, 1986.

Okada M: The cardiac rhythm in accidental hypothermia, *J Electrocardiol* 17:123, 1984.

Popovic V, Popovic P: *Hypothermia in biology and in medicine*, New York, 1974, Grune & Stratton.

Pozos RS, Wittmers LE: *The nature and treatment of hypothermia: University of Minnesota continuing medical education*, vol 2, Minneapolis, 1983, University of Minnesota Press.

Pugh LG: Accidental hypothermia in walkers, climbers, and campers: report to the medical commission on accident prevention, *Br Med J* 5480:123, 1966.

Savard GK et al: Peripheral blood flow during rewarming from mild hypothermia in humans, *J Appl Physiol* 58:4, 1985.

Sivaloganathan S: Paradoxical undressing and hypothermia, *Med Sci Law* 26:225, 1986.

Treating accidental hypothermia, *Lancet* 1:701, 1978.

Wilkerson JA, Bangs CC, Hayward JS: *Hypothermia, frostbite, and other cold injuries: prevention, recognition, and prehospital treatment*, Seattle, 1986, The Mountaineers.

Heat Illness

Armstrong LE et al: Whole-body cooling of hyperthermic runners: comparison of two field techniques, *Am J Emerg Med* 14:355, 1996.

Szlyk PC et al: Variability in intake and dehydration in young men during a simulated desert walk, *Aviat Space Environ Med* 60:422, 1989.

Tayeb OS, Marzouki ZMH: Tympanic thermometry in heat stroke: is it justifiable? *Clin Physiol Biochem* 7:255, 1989.

Tek DA, Olshaker JS: Hyperthermia, pulmonary edema, and disseminated intravascular coagulation in an 18-year-old military recruit, *Ann Emerg Med* 19:715, 1990.

Yarbrough BE, Hubbard RW: Heat-related illness. In Auerbach PS, Geehr EC, editors: *Management of wilderness and environmental emergencies*, St. Louis, 1989, CV Mosby Co.

Environmental Emergencies

Bartsch P et al: Prevention of high-altitude pulmonary edema by nifedipine, *N Engl J Med* 325:1284, 1991.

Burki NK, Khan SA, Hameed MA: The effects of acetazolamide on the ventilatory response to high altitude hypoxia, *Chest* 101:736, 1992.

Consolazio CF et al: Effects of high-carbohydrate diets on performance and clinical symptomatology after rapid ascent to high altitude, *Federation Proceedings* 28:937, 1969.

Dean AG, Yip R, Hoffmann RE: High incidence of mild acute mountain sickness in conference attendees at 10,000 foot altitude, *J Wild Med* 1:86, 1990.

Evans W et al: Amelioration of the symptoms of acute mountain sickness by staging and acetazolamide, *Aviat Space Environ Med* 47:512, 1976.

Grissom C et al: Acetazolamide in the treatment of acute mountain sickness: clinical efficacy and effect on gas exchange, *Ann Intern Med* 116:461, 1992.

Hackett PH, Rennie D, Levine HD: The incidence, importance, and prophylaxis of acute mountain sickness, *Lancet* 2:1149, 1976.

Hackett PH et al: Dexamethasone for prevention and treatment of acute mountain sickness, *Aviat Space Environ Med* 59:950, 1988.

Hackett PH: High altitude pulmonary edema, *J Wild Med* 1:3, 1990.

King SJ, Greenlee RR: Successful use of the Gamow Hyperbaric Bag in the treatment of altitude illness at Mount Everest, *J Wild Med* 1:193, 1990.

The use of low-dose acetazolamide to prevent mountain sickness (letter), *S Afr Med J* 85:792, 1995.

Oelz O et al: Nifedipine for high altitude pulmonary edema, *Lancet* 2:1241, 1989.

Olson LG, Henslet MJ, Saunders NA: Augmentation of ventilatory response to asphyxia by prochlorperazine in humans, *J Appl Physiol* 53:637, 1982.

Rabold MB: Dexamethasone for prophylaxis and treatment of acute mountain sickness, *J Wild Med* 3:54, 1992.

Schoene RB: Pulmonary edema at high altitude: review, pathophysiology, and update, *Clinics Chest Medicine* 6:491, 1985.

Zafren K, Honigman B: High-altitude medicine, *Emerg Med Clin North Am* 15:191, 1997.

Infections and Communicable Diseases

Infectious disease handbook for emergency care personnel, ed 3, 1999, ACGIH Publishers.

Infectious disease handbook for emergency care personnel, ed 2, 1998, ACGIH Publishers.

Bloodborne pathogens and tuberculosis curriculum guide, OSHA.

Gynecology

Decherney AH: *Current obstetrics and gynecologic diagnosis and treatment*, Norwalk, Conn, 1994, Appleton & Lange.

Seidel H et al: *Mosby's guide to physical examination*, ed 3, St. Louis, 1991, Mosby.

Obstetrics

Apgar BS: Spontaneous abortion, *Prim Care* 20:621, 1993.

Benson RC: *Current obstetric and gynecologic diagnosis and treatment*, Los Altos, Calif., 1992, Lange Medical.

Emergency Cardiac Care Committee and Subcommittee: American Heart Association, Pediatric Advanced Life Support, 1997.

Seidel HM et al: *Mosby's guide to physical examination*, ed 3, St. Louis, 1991, Mosby.

Neonatology

American Heart Association: *Textbook of neonatal resuscitation*, 1995.

American Heart Association: *Textbook of pediatric advanced life support*, 1994.

Cosgriff JH, Anderson DL: *The practice of emergency care*, ed 2, London, 1984, JB Lippincott.

Eichelberger MR et al: *Pediatric emergencies*, Englewood Cliffs, N.J., 1992, Prentice Hall.

Hoekelman RA, Friedman SB, Nelson NM: *Primary pediatric care*, St. Louis, 1992, Mosby-Year Book.

Jaimovich DG, Vidyasagar D: *Handbook of pediatric and neonatal transport medicine*, Philadelphia, 1996, Hanley and Belfus, Inc.

Nelson WE et al: *Textbook of pediatrics*, ed 15, Philadelphia, 1996, WB Saunders.

Simon JE, Goldberg AT: *Prehospital pediatric life support*, St. Louis, 1989, CV Mosby Company.

Acute Interventions for the Home Health Care Patient

Como ND: *Mosby's home health nursing pocket consultant*, St. Louis, 1995, Mosby-Year Book.

Grief J, Golden BA: *AIDS care at home: a guide for caregivers, loved ones, and people with AIDS*, New York, 1994, John Wiley & Sons.

Hatfield MO, Meyer MM, Derr P: *The comfort of home: an illustrated step-by-step guide for caregivers*, 1998, Caretrust Publications Ltd.

Hudak CM, Gallo BM: *Critical care nursing: a holistic approach*, ed 6, Philadelphia, 1994, JB Lippincott.

Kay P, Williams GB: *The caregiver's manual: a guide to helping the elderly and infirmed*, Secaucus, N.J., 1995, Citadel Press.

Rice R: *Handbook of home health nursing procedures*, St. Louis, 1995, Mosby-Year Book.

Rob C, Reynolds J: *The caregiver's guide: helping elderly relatives cope with health and safety problems*, Boston, 1992, Houghton Mifflin Co.

Rovinski CA, Zastocki DK: *Home care: a technical manual for the professional nurse*, Austin, Tex., 1989, Holt, Rinehart & Winston.

Spratt JS, Hawley RL, Hoye RE, editors: *Home health care: principles and practices*, 1996, Saint Lucie Press.

Springhouse Corporation: *Nurse's illustrated handbook of home health care procedures*, Springhouse, Pa., 1998, Springhouse Corporation.

Springhouse Corporation: *Pocket companion for home health nurses*, Springhouse, Pa., 1997, Springhouse Corporation.

Medical Incident Command

Auf der Heide E: *Disaster response: principles of preparation and coordination*, St. Louis, 1989, CV Mosby.

Butman AM: *Responding to the mass casualty incident: a guide for EMS personnel*, Akron, Ohio, 1982, Emergency Training Institute.

Federal Emergency Management Agency (FEMA): *Incident command system for emergency medical services*, 1996, U.S. Fire Administration.

Pediatrics

American Heart Association: *Textbook of neonatal resuscitation*, 1995.

American Heart Association: *Textbook of pediatric advanced life support*, 1994.

Burg FD et al: *Gellis and Kagan's current pediatric therapy*, ed 15, Philadelphia, 1996, WB Saunders Co.

Cosgriff JH, Anderson DL: *The practice of emergency care*, ed 2, London, 1984, JB Lippincott.

Dieckmann R et al: *Pediatric emergencies for paramedics*, 1990.

Eichelberger MR et al: *Pediatric emergencies*, Englewood Cliffs, N.J., 1992, Prentice Hall.

Foltin G et al: *Teaching resource for instructors of prehospital pediatrics*, New York, 1998, Center for Pediatric Emergency Medicine.

Gausche M et al: *Pediatric airway management program*, 1990.

Hoekelman RA et al: *Primary pediatric care*, St. Louis, 1992, Mosby.

Jaimovich DG, Vidyasagar D: *Handbook of pediatric and neonatal transport medicine*, Philadelphia, 1996, Hanley & Belfus, Inc.

Nelson WE et al: *Textbook of pediatrics*, ed 15, Philadelphia, 1996, WB Saunders.

Seidel JS, Henderson DP: *Emergency medical services for children: a report to the nation*, Washington, D.C., 1991, National Center for Education in Maternal and Child Health.

Simon JE, Goldberg AT: *Prehospital pediatric life support*, St. Louis, 1989, CV Mosby.

Tintinalli JE, Ruiz E, Krome RL: *Emergency medicine: a comprehensive study guide*, ed 4, New York, 1996, McGraw-Hill, Inc.

Foundations of EMT-Intermediate

Bledsoe BE: *EMT-Intermediate emergency care*, ed 2, Englewood Cliffs, N.J., 1996, Prentice-Hall.

Consensus statement on the role of emergency medical services in primary injury prevention, 1996.

Emergency medical technician EMT-intermediate course curriculum and reference guide, ed 2, Oregon Health Division-Emergency Medical Services and Systems.

Keuhl S: *Prehospital systems and medical oversight*, ed 2, 1994, NAEMSP.

Menegazzi JJ: *Research: the who, what, why, when, and how*, 1993, Ferno-Washington, Inc.

NHTSA's air medical crew national standard curriculum, 1998, ASHBEAMS.

Polsky SS: *Continuous quality improvement in EMS*, 1992, ACEP.

Shade B et al: *Mosby's EMT-Intermediate textbook*, St. Louis, 1997, Mosby.

Steering Committee Project: *Consensus statement on the role of emergency medical services in primary injury prevention*, 1993, NHTSA/MCHB/NAEMSP.

AIRWAY

Berkow R, Fletcher AJ, Beers MH: *The Merck manual of diagnosis and therapy*, ed 16, Rahway, N.J., 1992, Merck Research Laboratories.

Brashers FL, Davey SS: Structure and function of the pulmonary system. In McCance KL, Heuther SE: *Pathophysiology: the biologic basis for disease in adults and children*, ed 3, St. Louis, 1998, Mosby.

Hastings D, Campbell JE: *Airway management skills, Brady basic trauma life support*, ed 3, Englewood Cliffs, N.J., 1998, Prentice Hall.

Peitzman AB, Rinnert KJ, O'Toole KS: *Prehospital therapy: the trauma manual*, Philadelphia, 1998, Lippincott-Raven.

Stewart RE: *Field endotracheal intubation*, Pittsburgh, 1983, Pittsburgh EMS.

Stewart RD, Campbell JE: *Initial airway management: Brady basic trauma life support*, ed 3, Englewood Cliffs, N.J., 1998, Prentice Hall.

Traynor OT: *Endotracheal intubation and extubation, the streetmedic's handbook*, Philadelphia, 1996, FA Davis Publishing.

Traynor OT, Yee MD: *Obstructed airway: the streetmedic's handbook*, Philadelphia, 1996, FA Davis Publishing.

Whitten CE: *Anyone can intubate*, ed 2, San Diego, 1990, Medical Arts Publishing.

NEONATAL RESUSCITATION

American Heart Association: *Textbook of neonatal resuscitation*, 1995.

American Heart Association: *Textbook of pediatric advanced life support*, 1994.

Cosgriff JH, Anderson DL: *The practice of emergency care*, ed 2, London, 1984, JB Lippincott.

Eichelberger MR et al: *Pediatric emergencies*, Englewood Cliffs, N.J., 1992, Prentice-Hall.

Hoekelman RA et al: *Primary pediatric care*, St. Louis, 1992, Mosby.

Jaimovich DG, Vidyasagar D: *Handbook of pediatric and neonatal transport medicine*, Philadelphia, 1996, Hanley and Belfus, Inc.

Nelson WE et al: *Textbook of pediatrics*, ed 15, Philadelphia, 1996, WB Saunders.

Simon JE, Goldberg AT: *Prehospital pediatric life support*, St. Louis, 1989, CV Mosby Company.

Tintinalli JE, Ruiz E, Krome RL: *Emergency medicine: a comprehensive study guide*, ed 4, New York, 1996, McGraw Hill, Inc.

Pediatric Education for Prehospital Providers (PEPP)

The American Academy of Pediatrics (AAP) has developed an educational program to help prehospital professionals better assess and manage ill or injured children. The course is called Pediatric Education for Prehospital Providers (PEPP).

The PEPP course content addresses the pediatric objectives identified in the National Highway Traffic Safety Administration (NHTSA) National Standard Curricula. The program includes case-based lectures, videos, skill stations, and small group scenarios addressing a broad range of topics geared toward first responders, EMTs and paramedics. For more information, visit the PEPP website at www.peppsite.com or call 800/823-0034.

Emergency Medical Services for Children (EMSC) Program

EMSC is a national initiative designed to reduce infant, child, and adolescent death and disability due to severe illness or injury. Medical personnel, parents, volunteers, community groups, businesses, national organizations, and foundations all contribute to the effort. The EMSC National Resource Center provides technical support and assistance to states on a variety of topics, operates a clearinghouse, and provides information to professionals and the public. The EMSC Web site is located at www.emsc.org, or contact the NRC at (202) 884-4927 for additional information.

Paramedic education products available from the EMSC Clearinghouse:

A Child in Need (version 1)

ALS Airway Management Kit

Children with Special Health Care Needs; Technology Assisted Children (tac)

Course on Pediatric Emergencies (COPE)

Education of Out-of-Hospital Emergency Medical Personnel in Pediatrics: Report of a National Task Force

Emergency Medical Services for Children: Working for Children with Special Health Care Needs (Fact Sheet)

Illinois Prehospital Pediatric Course (disk set)

Office Preparedness for Pediatric Emergencies: Provider Manual

Pediatric Assessment (CD-ROM)

Pediatric Basics: Age and Growth Characteristics/Psychological Aspects–version 1 (CD-ROM)

Pediatric Education for Paramedic Program (PEP) (1997, Combination Set)

Pediatric Respiratory Emergencies (Version 1, CD-ROM)

Pediatric Vascular Assess (CD-ROM)

Risk Watch

Training EMSC Providers in Violence Prevention

TRIPP: Teaching Resource for Instructors in Prehospital Pediatrics (1998 Version 2.0)

TRIPP

About the TRIPP: The Teaching Resource for Instructors in Prehospital Pediatrics was developed to bridge the knowledge gap that exists in the specialized field of prehospital pediatric care. Neither a course nor a curriculum, the TRIPP is an encyclopedic resource that furnishes EMT instructors with fundamental background knowledge about assessing and treating critically ill and injured children so that they can provide more effective teaching to EMT students. While it is intended primarily for instructors who teach the pediatric sections of the revised *EMT-Basic: National Standard Curriculum*, the TRIPP will benefit all emergency medical personnel interested in prehospital care of children.

The TRIPP can be downloaded, at no charge, from the Website at www.cpem.org. Copies are also available (charge for postage only) through the EMSC program:

National MCH Clearinghouse
2070 Chain Bridge Road, Suite 450
Vienna, VA 22182-2536
(703) 902-1203, FAX (703) 821-2098
emse@circsol.com

Websites

NOTE: Below is a sample of U.S., Canadian, and international websites relevant to EMS. Web addresses change frequently. Therefore regular updating of bookmarks may be necessary. In addition, the links listed below are not under the control of the author or the publisher, and we accordingly make no representation concerning the content, quality, or safety of these sites or the suitability of any software found there.

U.S. SITES

American Academy of Pediatrics
www.aap.org

American Association of Critical Care Nurses
www.aacn.org

American Association of Poison Control Centers
www.nlu.edu/aapc

American Burn Association
www.ameriburn.org

American College of Emergency Physicians
www.acep.org

American College of Prehospital Medicine
63.67.198.158/index.shtml

American Heart Association
www.amhrt.org

American Medical Association
www.ama-assn.org

American Red Cross
www.crossnet.org

Association of Air Medical Services
www.aams.org

Association of Emergency Physicians
www.aep.org

Centers for Disease Control and Prevention
www.cdc.gov

Emergency Medical Services for Children
www.ems-c.org

Emergency Nurses Association
www.ena.org

Federal Emergency Management Agency
www.fema.gov

Medline
www.ncbi.nlm.nih.gov/PubMed

Medscape
www.medscape.com

National Associations of EMS Physicians
www.naemsp.org

National Association of EMS Educators
www.naemse.org

National Association of EMTs
www.naemt.com

National Center for Health Statistics
cdc.gov/nchs

National Flight Paramedic Association
www.nfpa.rotor.com

National Heart, Lung and Blood Institute
www.nhlbi.nih.gov

National Highway Traffic Safety Administration
www.nhtsa.gov

National Institute of Emergency Care
www.niec.org

National Institute of Health
www.nih.gov

National Institute of Mental Health
www.nimh.nih.gov

National Library of Medicine
www.nlm.nih.gov

National Registry of EMTs
www.nremt.org

National Safety Council
www.nsc.org

Occupational Safety and Health Administration
www.osha.gov

Society for Academic Emergency Medicine
www.saem.org

CANADIAN SITES

Alberta Health
www.health.gov.ab.ca

Alberta Prehospital Professions Association
www.co-paramedics.com

Ambulance Paramedics of British Columbia
www.paramedicsofbc.com

B.C. Ambulance Service
www.hlth.gov.bc.ca/bcas

Calgary Emergency Medical Services
www.gov.calgary.ab.ca/EMS

Canadian Center for Occupational Health and Safety
www.ccohs.ca

Canadian EMS Directors Website
www.ems-directors.org

Emergency Preparedness Exchange
hoshi.cic.sfu.ca/epix

Manitoba Prehospital Professional Association
www.escape.ca/~mppa

Ontario Paramedic Association
www.paramedic.on.ca

Paramedic Association of Canada
www.paramedic.ca

Paramedic Association of New Brunswick
personal.nbnet.nb.ca/mpharris/panb

Shock Trauma Air Rescue Society of Alberta
www.comcept.ab.ca/stars.air.rescue

Toronto Paramedic Association
www.city.toronto.on.ca/ems/tpa/tpa.htm

INTERNATIONAL SITES

International Association of Fire Chiefs
www.iafc.org

International Association of Fire Fighters
www.iaff.org

International Red Cross
www.icrc.ch/home.nsf/home/icrc-ch

World Association for Disaster and Emergency Medicine
www.pitt.edu/HOME/GHNet/wadem/
wadem.html

World Health Organization
www.who.int

Glossary

abandonment Terminating medical care without legal excuse or turning care over to less qualified personnel, thereby injuring the patient.

abdominal Pertaining to the abdomen.

abdominal aorta The portion of the descending aorta that passes from the aortic hiatus of the diaphragm into the abdomen, where it divides into the two common iliac arteries.

abdominal cavity The space within the abdominal walls between the diaphragm and the pelvic area; it contains the liver, stomach, intestines, spleen, kidneys, and associated tissues and vessels.

abdominopelvic cavity The space between the diaphragm and the groin.

abduction Movement away from the midline.

abnormal Deviating from the normal.

abnormal presentation A type of vaginal delivery in which the newborn's head does not deliver first.

abortion The spontaneous or induced termination of a pregnancy before the fetus has developed into a stage of viability.

abrasion A scraping or rubbing away of a surface of skin by friction.

abruptio placentae Separation of the placenta implanted in a normal position in a pregnancy of 20 weeks or more; occurs during labor or delivery of the fetus.

absolute refractory period The portion of the action potential during which the membrane is insensitive to all stimuli regardless of strength.

absorption The passage of substances across and into tissues, such as the passage of digested food molecules into intestinal cells or the passage of liquids into kidney tubules.

accelerated AV conduction See *anomalous conduction*.

acclimatization Physical adjustment to a different climate or to changes in altitude or temperature.

acetabulum The large, cup-shaped articular cavity at the juncture of the ilium, the ischium, and the pubis that contains the ball-shaped head of the femur.

acetoacetic acid A colorless, oily ketone body produced by the metabolism of lipids and pyruvates; it is excreted in trace amounts in normal urine and in elevated amounts with diabetes mellitus, especially in ketoacidosis.

acetonemia The presence of acetone in the blood, characterized by the fruity breath odor of ketoacidosis.

acetylcholine (ACh) A neurotransmitter, widely distributed in body tissues, with the primary function of mediating the synaptic activity of the nervous system.

acetylcholinesterase (AChE) An enzyme found in the synaptic cleft that causes the breakdown of acetylcholine into acetic acid and choline, thereby limiting the stimulatory effect of acetylcholine.

acid A compound that yields hydrogen ions when dissociated in solution.

acidosis An abnormal increase in the hydrogen ion concentration in the body that results from accumulation of an acid or loss of a base.

acinus A small lobule of a compound gland; the exocrine portion of the pancreas that produces pancreatic juice.

acquired immunodeficiency syndrome (AIDS) A disease that results from infection with the human immunodeficiency virus (HIV); AIDS impairs the immune system, giving rise to opportunistic infections and malignancies.

acromegaly A chronic metabolic condition characterized by a gradual, marked enlargement and elongation of the bones of the face, jaw, and extremities.

acromion process The lateral extension of the spine of the scapula; it gives attachment to the deltoideus and trapezius muscles.

actin A protein found in muscle fibers that acts with myosin to bring about contraction and relaxation.

actinomycosis A chronic systemic disease characterized by deep, lumpy abscesses that extrude a granular pus through multiple sinuses.

action plan A plan of action based on the patient's condition and the environment.

action potential A change in membrane potential in an excitable tissue that acts as an electrical signal and is propagated in an all-or-none fashion.

active transport A carrier-mediated process that can move substances against a concentration gradient.

active tubular secretion Secretion that involves the transport of free drug from the blood across the proximal tubular cell and into the tubular urine by an active process against a concentration gradient.

acute dystonia A sudden impairment of muscle tone; it commonly involves the head, neck, or tongue and often occurs as an adverse effect of medication.

acute mountain sickness (AMS) A common high-altitude illness that results from rapid ascent by an unacclimatized person to altitudes of 8000 feet or higher.

acute pain Severe pain such as may follow trauma or may accompany myocardial infarction or other conditions and diseases.

acute renal failure A clinical syndrome that results from a sudden, marked decrease in filtration through the glomeruli, leading to the accumulation of salt, water, and nitrogenous wastes in the body.

adaptation A cellular response to stress of any kind to escape and protect from injury; a central part of the response to changes in the physiological condition.

addiction Compulsive, uncontrollable dependence on a substance, habit, or practice. See *habituation*.

Addison's disease A life-threatening condition caused by partial or complete failure of adrenocortical function.

adduction Movement toward the midline.

adenohypophysis The anterior lobe of the pituitary gland.

adenoma A tumor of glandular epithelium in which the cells of the tumor are arranged in a recognizable glandular structure.

adenosine A compound derived from nucleic acid, composed of adenine and a sugar.

adenosine diphosphate (ADP) A product of the hydrolysis of adenosine triphosphate.

adenosine monophosphate (AMP) A compound that affects energy release in work done by muscles.

adenosine triphosphate (ATP) Adenosine, an organic base, with three phosphate groups attached to it; ATP stores energy in muscles.

adhesion The quality of remaining in close contact with or stuck to another entity; also, a structure that joins several parts, sometimes abnormally.

adipose tissue A specialized connective tissue that stores lipids; also known as fat tissue.

adrenal gland Either of two secretory glands perched atop the kidneys; each gland consists of two parts, the cortex and medulla, which have independent functions.

adrenal medullary mechanism The mechanism by which epinephrine and norepinephrine are released from the adrenal medulla as a result of the same stimuli that increase sympathetic stimulation of the heart and blood vessels.

Adrenalin Proprietary name for epinephrine.

adrenergic Of or pertaining to sympathetic nerve fibers of the autonomic nervous system that use epinephrine or epinephrine-like substances as neurotransmitters.

adrenocorticotropic hormone (ACTH) A hormone of the anterior pituitary gland that stimulates growth of the adrenal gland cortex and secretion of corticosteroids.

adsorption A substance's capacity to attract and hold other materials or particles on its surface.

adult respiratory distress syndrome (ARDS) A group of symptoms that accompany fulminant pulmonary edema, resulting in acute respiratory failure; also known as noncardiogenic pulmonary edema.

advanced cardiac life support (ACLS) Clinical care or guidelines for care of life-threatening cardiovascular and respiratory disorders.

advanced life support (ALS) Provision of advanced-level care by paramedics or allied health care providers.

aerobic Of or pertaining to the presence of air or oxygen.

aerobic oxidation A biochemical reaction that increases the positive charges on an atom or the loss of negative charges in the presence of oxygen.

aerosol Pressurized gas that contains a finely nebulized medication for inhalation therapy.

affective disorder Any of a group of psychotic disorders characterized by severe and inappropriate emotional responses, prolonged and persistent disturbances of mood and related thought distortions, and other symptoms associated with depressed or manic states.

afferent division Nerve fibers that send impulses from the periphery to the central nervous system.

affinity The propensity of a drug to bind or attach itself to a given receptor site.

afterdrop phenomenon A sudden return of cold blood and waste products to the body's core as a result of rewarming methods used to treat hypothermia.

afterload See *peripheral vascular resistance.*

agglutinated Refers to cells that have clumped together. See *agglutination.*

agglutination A clumping together of cells as a result of their interaction with specific antibodies, called "agglutinins."

agglutinin A kind of antibody; its interaction with antigens is manifested as agglutination.

agonal rhythm A ventricular escape complex or rhythm that occurs when the electrical impulses from the SA node, atria, or AV junction fail to reach the ventricles because of sinus arrest or high-degree AV block; frequently seen as the last rhythm in an unsuccessful resuscitation.

agonist A drug that combines with receptors and initiates a sequence of biochemical and physiological changes; it possesses both affinity and efficacy.

air trapping The result of a prolonged but inefficient expiratory effort, usually caused by chronic obstruction of the pulmonary tree, as is commonly seen in chronic obstructive pulmonary disease (COPD) or asthma.

akathisia An abnormal condition characterized by restlessness and agitation.

albumin A water-soluble protein containing carbon, hydrogen, oxygen, nitrogen, and sulfur.

aldosterone A steroid hormone produced by the adrenal cortex to regulate the sodium and potassium balance in the blood.

alkaline Having the reactions of an alkali.

alkalosis An abnormal condition of body fluids characterized by a tendency toward a pH level above 7.44, as from an excess of alkaline bicarbonate or a deficiency of acid.

aliquot A sample that is representative of the whole.

allergen A substance that can produce a hypersensitivity reaction in the body; it is not necessarily intrinsically harmful.

allergic reaction A hypersensitivity response to an allergen to which a person was previously exposed and to which the person has developed antibodies.

allergy A hypersensitivity reaction to intrinsically harmless antigens, most of which are environmental.

all-or-none principle The principle that when a stimulus is applied to a cell, an action potential either is produced or is not.

alpha adrenergic receptor Any one of the postulated adrenergic components of receptor tissues that responds to norepinephrine and to various blocking agents.

alpha cell A constituent of the islet of Langerhans that produces glucagon.

alveoli Small outpouchings of walls of alveolar space through which gas exchange takes place between alveolar air and pulmonary capillary blood.

alveolar duct Part of the respiratory passages beyond a respiratory bronchiole; alveolar sacs and alveoli arise from it.

alveolus A small cavity; the terminal ending of a secretory gland. Alveoli of the lungs are microscopic, saclike dilations of terminal bronchioles.

Alzheimer's disease A disease characterized by confusion, memory failure, disorientation, speech disturbances, and inability to carry out purposeful movements.

amaurosis fugax Unilateral vision loss as a result of internal carotid artery plaque emboli.

ambulance A generic term that describes the various land-based emergency vehicles used by EMS personnel; the category includes basic life support units, advanced life support units, paramedic units, mobile intensive care units, and others.

amenorrhea The absence of menstruation.

amino acid An organic chemical compound composed of one or more basic amino groups and one or more acidic carboxyl groups.

ammonia A colorless, aromatic gas consisting of nitrogen and hydrogen.

amnestic Causing amnesia.

amniocentesis An obstetrical procedure in which a small amount of amniotic fluid is removed for laboratory analysis; it aids in diagnosis of fetal abnormalities.

amniotic fluid embolism An embolism that occurs when particulate matter in amniotic fluid forms an embolus and gains access to maternal circulation during labor or delivery or immediately after delivery.

amniotic sac A thin-walled bag that contains the fetus and amniotic fluid during pregnancy.

amplitude modulation (AM) A transmitted radio frequency carrier fixed in frequency but increasing or decreasing in amplitude in accordance with the strength of the applied audio.

ampulla A round, saclike dilation of the uterine tube.

amputation The surgical or traumatic removal of a part of a body or a limb or part of a limb.

amylase A starch-splitting enzyme.

amyotrophic lateral sclerosis (ALS) A degenerative disease of the motor neurons, characterized by weakness and atrophy of the muscles of the hands, forearms, and legs that spreads to involve most of the body and face; also known as Lou Gehrig's disease.

anabolic steroid Any of several compounds derived from testosterone or prepared synthetically to promote general body growth, to oppose the effects of endogenous estrogen, or to promote masculinizing effects.

anaerobic Pertaining to the absence of oxygen.

anaerobic metabolism Metabolism that occurs in the absence of oxygen.

anal canal The final portion of the alimentary tract between the rectal ampulla and the anus.

anal fissure A linear ulceration or laceration of the skin of the anus.

anal fistula An abnormal opening of the cutaneous surface near the anus.

anal triangle The posterior portion of the perianal region through which the anal canal opens.

anaphylactic shock Shock that occurs when the body is exposed to a substance that produces a severe allergic reaction.

anaphylaxis An exaggerated, life-threatening hypersensitivity reaction to a previously encountered antigen.

anasarca Generalized, massive edema.

anastomosis The joining of two parts.

anatomical dead space The volume of the conducting airways from the external environment down to the terminal bronchioles.

anatomical position A person standing erect with feet and palms facing the examiner.

androgen Any steroid hormone that increases male characteristics.

anemia A decrease in blood hemoglobin.

aneurysm A localized dilation of a wall of a blood vessel.

anesthesia Without sensation.

angioedema An acute, painless, dermal, subcutaneous or submucosal swelling of short duration involving the face, neck, lips, larynx, hands, feet, genitalia, or viscera.

angiogram A study of vessels.

angioplasty Repair of damaged vessels.

angiotensin I The inactive form of angiotensin, formulated by the stimulation of renin, which is converted to angiotensin II.

angiotensin II A potent vasoconstrictor that also acts to stimulate the secretion of antidiuretic hormone (ADH).

angina pectoris Ischemic chest pain most often caused by myocardial anoxia as a result of atherosclerosis of the coronary arteries.

angioedema A localized edematous reaction of the deep dermal or subcutaneous or submucosal tissues that appears as giant wheals.

angle of Louis See *sternal angle.*

anhedonia The inability to enjoy what is usually pleasurable.

anion An ion with a negative charge.

anisocoria Normal or congenital unequal pupil size.

anomalous conduction A preexcitation syndrome; a clinical condition associated with abnormal conduction pathways between the atria and ventricles that bypass the AV node and bundle of His and allow the electrical impulses to initiate depolarization of the ventricles earlier than usual. Also known as accelerated AV conduction.

anorexia Lack or loss of appetite, resulting in an inability to eat.

anorexia nervosa A disorder characterized by a prolonged refusal to eat, resulting in emaciation, amenorrhea, emotional disturbance concerning body image, and an abnormal fear of becoming obese.

anovulation Failure of the ovaries to produce, mature, or release eggs.

antagonism The opposition between two or more medications; it occurs when the combined (conjoint) effect of two drugs is less than the sum of the drugs acting separately.

antagonist muscle A muscle that works in opposition to another muscle.

antagonist An agent designed to inhibit or counteract effects produced by other drugs or undesired effects caused by normal or hyperactive physiological mechanisms.

antecubital fossa See *antecubital space.*

antecubital space (AC space) The depressed area in front of the elbow or at the bend of the elbow; also known as the antecubital fossa.

antegrade amnesia The loss of memory for events that occurred immediately after recovery of consciousness.

antenatal Occurring or formed before birth.

antepartum The maternal period before delivery.

anterior The front of a structure.

anterior chamber of the eye The chamber of the eye between the cornea and the iris.

anterior communicating artery The artery that connects with the anterior cerebral arteries and completes the circle of Willis.

anterior cord syndrome A spinal cord injury usually seen in flexion injuries; it is caused by pressure on the anterior aspect of the spinal cord by a ruptured intervertebral disk or fragments of the vertebral body that have extruded posteriorly into the spinal canal.

anterior superior iliac spine One of two bony segments that form the iliac crest.

antibody A substance produced by the body that destroys or inactivates a specific substance (antigen) that has entered the body.

anticholinergic Of or pertaining to a blockade of acetylcholine receptors, which results in the inhibition of the transmission of parasympathetic nerve impulses.

anticoagulant A substance that prevents or delays coagulation of the blood.

antidiuretic hormone (ADH) A hormone produced in the posterior pituitary gland to regulate the balance of water in the body by accelerating the resorption of water.

antidote A drug or other substance that opposes the action of a poison.

antigen A substance, usually a protein, that causes the formation of an antibody and reacts specifically with that antibody.

antigenic site A site capable of binding to and reacting with an antibody.

antiplatelet A drug that interferes with platelet aggregation.

antipyretic Something that works against fever.

antivenin A suspension of venom-neutralizing antibodies prepared from the serum of immunized horses.

anuria The inability to urinate; the cessation of urine production; a diminished urinary output of less than 100 to 250 mL per day.

anus The distal end or outlet of the rectum.

anxiety A state or feeling of apprehension, uneasiness, agitation, uncertainty, and fear caused by the anticipation of some threat or danger.

aorta The main and largest artery in the body.

aortic aneurysm A localized dilation of the wall of the aorta.

aortic body Any of the specialized nerve cells located in the arch of the aorta, where they monitor levels of oxygen and hydrogen ions in the cardiovascular system.

aortic semilunar valve A valve that guards the orifice between the left ventricle and the aorta.

apex of the heart The top or tip of the heart opposite the base.

Apgar score A method of evaluating an infant's physical condition, usually performed at 1 minute and again at 5 minutes after birth; evaluation components include heart rate, respiratory effort, muscle tone, reflex irritability, and color.

aphasia Loss of the power of speech.

apical impulse A pulsation of the left ventricle of the heart, palpable and sometimes visible at the fifth intercostal space to the left of the midline.

apnea Without breath.

apneustic center A group of neurons in the pons that has a stimulatory effect on the inspiratory center.

apocrine gland A gland that has cells that contribute cytoplasm to its secretion, such as a mammary gland.

apothecary A system of graduated liquid volumes arranged in order of heaviness; it is based on the "grain."

apparatus A vehicle used for fire suppression or rescue; it does not include staff vehicles.

appendicular region The limbs or extremities.

appendicular skeleton The bones of the upper and lower extremities.

appendix A wormlike, blunt process extending from the cecum; also known as the vermiform appendix.

application of principle A component of critical thinking during which patient care decisions are made based on the examiner's conceptual understanding of the situation and the interpretation of data gathered from the patient.

aqueous humor The clear, watery fluid circulating in the anterior and posterior chambers of the eye.

Arachnida A large class of arthropods that includes spiders, scorpions, mites, and ticks.

arachnoid layer A delicate, weblike middle membrane that covers the brain.

areflexia A neurological condition characterized by absence of the reflexes.

areola The circular, pigmented area surrounding the nipple.

areolar connective tissue A loose tissue that consists of delicate webs of fibers and a variety of cells embedded in a matrix of soft, sticky gel.

areolar gland A gland that forms small, rounded projections from the surface of the areola of the mamma.

arrector pili Smooth muscles of the skin attached to hair follicles; when contraction occurs, the hair rises, resulting in "gooseflesh."

arterial capillary The ends of capillaries closest to arterioles.

arteriogram A study of arteries.

arteriole A small branch of an artery.

arteriovenous anastomosis A vessel that allows blood to flow from arteries to veins without passing through capillaries; also known as an AV shunt.

artery A vessel that carries blood away from the heart.

arthritis An inflammatory condition of the joints, characterized by pain and swelling.

arthroscopy Inspection of a joint.

artifact A deflection on the ECG display or tracing produced by factors other than the heart's electrical activity.

arytenoid cartilages Small, pyramidal laryngeal cartilages that articulate with the cricoid cartilage.

asbestosis A chronic lung disease caused by the inhalation of asbestos fibers; it results in the development of alveolar, interstitial, and pleural fibrosis.

ascending colon The segment of the colon that extends from the cecum in the right lower quadrant of the abdomen to the transverse colon at the hepatic flexure on the right side; usually at the level of the umbilicus.

ascites An abnormal intraperitoneal accumulation of fluid containing large amounts of protein and electrolytes.

aseptic Sterile, without germs.

asphyxiation A state of suffocation, caused by severe hypoxia, that leads to hypoxemia and hypercapnia, loss of consciousness and, if not corrected, death.

aspiration Inhalation of foreign substances into the pulmonary system.

assault Creating apprehension, or unauthorized handling and treatment of a patient.

asthma A respiratory disorder characterized by recurring episodes of paroxysmal dyspnea; wheezing on expiration caused by constriction of the bronchi; coughing; and viscous mucoid bronchial secretions.

asthma exacerbation An aggravation of asthma, usually associated with severe symptoms.

astigmatism An abnormal condition of the eye in which the light rays cannot be focused clearly on a point on the retina because the spherical curve of the cornea is not equal in all meridians.

astrocyte gliosis A tumor composed of glial cells within the nervous system; it may be associated with respiratory center dysfunction and neuroepithelial bodies in the tracheobronchial tree, along with distal atelectasis.

asystole A life-threatening cardiac condition characterized by the absence of electrical and mechanical activity of the heart.

ataxia Failure of muscle coordination.

ataxic breathing A type of cluster or irregular breathing pattern characterized by a series of inspirations and expirations.

atelectasis An abnormal condition characterized by the collapse of lung tissue, preventing respiratory exchange of oxygen and carbon dioxide.

atelectatic breathing A modified respiratory effort thought to be a protective reflex to hyperinflate the lungs and reexpand alveoli that might have been collapsed.

atheroma An abnormal accumulation of fat or lipids as a cyst or a deposit in an arterial wall. A hard, atherosclerotic plaque.

atherosclerosis A common arterial disorder characterized by yellowish plaques of cholesterol, lipids, and cellular debris in the inner layers of the walls of large and medium-sized arteries.

athetosis A neuromuscular condition characterized by slow, continuous, and involuntary movement of the extremities.

atlantooccipital joint One of a pair of condyloid joints formed by the articulation of the atlas of the vertebral column with the occipital bone of the skull.

atlas The first cervical vertebra, which articulates with the occipital bone and the axis.

atom The smallest division of an element that exhibits all the properties and characteristics of the element; atoms comprise neutrons, electrons, and protons.

atmospheric pressure The pressure exerted by the weight of the atmosphere; at sea level this pressure is 760 mm Hg.

atony Weak muscle tone.

atria Chambers or cavities, such as the atria of the heart.

atrial natriuretic factor A peptide released from the atria when atrial blood pressure is increased; it lowers blood pressure by increasing urine production, thus reducing blood volume.

atrial natriuretic hormone (ANH) A hormone secreted by specialized muscle fibers in the atrial wall of the heart that influences water reabsorption in the kidney; it acts as an antagonist of aldosterone.

atrial synchronous ventricular pacemaker An artificial pacemaker synchronized with the patient's atrial rhythm; it paces the ventricles only when an AV block occurs.

atrial-ventricular demand pacemaker An artificial pacemaker that paces either the atria or ventricles when the intrinsic rate of the paced chamber drops dangerously low.

atrioventricular canal The path through which the atria open into the ventricles.

atrioventricular node (AV node) An area of specialized cardiac muscle that receives the cardiac impulse from the sinoatrial node and conducts it to the bundle of His.

atrioventricular valve A valve in the heart through which blood flows from the atria to the ventricles.

atrophy Wasting.

attention deficit disorder (ADD) A syndrome that affects children, adolescents and, in rare cases, adults, characterized by learning and behavioral disabilities.

auditory Of or pertaining to hearing or the organs of hearing.

auditory meatus A tubelike channel of the external ear extending from the auricle to the tympanum of the middle ear.

auditory ossicles The incus, malleus, and stapes; small bones in the middle ear that articulate with each other and the tympanic membrane.

auditory tube The auditory canal; it extends from the middle ear to the nasopharynx. It is also known as the eustachian tube.

aura A sensation that may precede a migraine or seizure activity.

auricle The part of the external ear that protrudes from the head; also known as the pinna.

auscultation The act of listening for sounds within the body.

autoimmune pericarditis Inflammation of the pericardium associated with the production of antibodies directed against one's own tissues.

autoimmunity An abnormal characteristic or condition in which the body reacts against constituents of its own tissues.

autolysis The spontaneous disintegration of tissues or cells by the action of their own autogenous enzymes.

automated external defibrillator (AED) A device used in cardiac arrest to perform a computer analysis of the patient's cardiac rhythm and deliver defibrillatory shocks when indicated.

automatic implanted cardiac defibrillator (AICD) A surgically implanted device that monitors a person's heart rate; it is designed to deliver defibrillatory shocks as needed.

automatic vehicle location (AVL) A radio communications subsystem that uses one or more electronic methods to periodically determine a land, marine, or air vehicle's position and relay that information via radio to a communications center.

automatism Abnormal repetitive motor behavior such as lip smacking, chewing, or swallowing during which the patient is amnestic.

automaticity The ability of a cell to depolarize itself, reach threshold potential, and produce a propagated action potential.

autonomic hyperreflexia syndrome A neurological disorder characterized by a discharge of sympathetic nervous system impulses as a result of stimulation of the bladder, large intestine, or other visceral organs.

autonomic nervous system (ANS) The part of the nervous system that regulates involuntary vital functions, including the activity of cardiac muscle, smooth muscle, and glands; it is subdivided into sympathetic and parasympathetic divisions.

autophagia Nutrition of the body by consumption of its own tissues.

avascular Having blood vessels.

AV dissociation P waves and QRS complexes that occur rhythmically but without a relationship to each other.

Avogadro's number The number of molecules in 1 gram molecule of a substance.

avoidance The act of keeping away from; it requires the paramedic to continually be aware of the scene by being observant and knowledgeable of warning signs that may indicate a dangerous situation.

AV sequential pacemaker An artificial pacemaker that paces the atria first and then the ventricles when spontaneous activity is absent or slowed in both the atria and ventricles.

AV shunt See *arteriovenous anastomosis.*

axial loading Vertical compression of the spine that results when direct forces are transmitted along the length of the spinal column.

axial region The head, neck, thorax, abdomen, and pelvis.

axial skeleton The bones of the head, neck, and torso.

axillae Armpits.

axillary node One of the lymph glands of the axillae that help fight infections in the chest, armpit, neck, and arm and drain lymph nodes from those areas.

axis The second cervical vertebra about which the atlas rotates, allowing the head to be turned, extended, or flexed.

axon The main central process of a neuron that normally conducts action potentials away from the neuron cell body.

azotemia Retention in the blood of excess amounts of nitrogenous compounds; caused by failure of the kidneys to remove urea from the blood and characterized by uremia.

Babinski's sign Plantar reflex; a reflex movement in which the great toe bends upward when the outer edge of the sole of the foot is scratched.

bacteremia The presence of bacteria in the blood.

bacteria Single-celled microorganisms that cause an infection characteristic of that species.

bacterial tracheitis An inflammatory condition of the trachea resulting from bacterial infection.

bacteriocidal Destructive to bacteria.

bacteriostatic Tending to restrain the development or the reproduction of bacteria.

bacteriophage Any virus that causes lysis of host bacteria.

ball-and-socket joint A joint that consists of a ball (head) at the end of one bone and a socket in an adjacent bone into which a portion of the ball fits.

baroreceptor A sensory nerve ending in the walls of the atria of the heart, venae cavae, aortic arch, and carotid sinuses; it is sensitive to stretching of the walls caused by an increase in blood pressure.

barotitis An inflammation of the ear caused by changes in atmospheric pressure.

barotrauma A physical injury sustained as a result of exposure to increased environmental pressure.

Bartholin's gland One of two small, mucus-secreting glands located on the posterior and lateral aspect of the vestibule of the vagina.

Barton's bandage A circumferential head dressing applied to restrict jaw movement and minimize pain.

base A chemical compound that combines with an acid to form a salt; also known as an alkali.

base of the heart The portion of the heart opposite the apex, directed to the right side of the body.

base station A grouping of radio equipment consisting of at least a transmitter, a receiver, a transmission line, and an antenna located at a specific, fixed location.

basilar artery The single arterial trunk formed by the junction of the two vertebral arteries at the base of the skull.

basilar fracture A fracture that may occur when the mandibular condyles perforate the base of the skull but that more commonly results from extension of a linear fracture into the floor of the anterior and middle fossae.

basophil A white blood cell that promotes inflammation; it readily stains with specific dyes.

battery Physical contact with a person without their consent and without legal justification.

Battle's sign Ecchymosis over the mastoid process caused by fracture of the temporal bone.

Beck's triad A combination of three symptoms that characterize pericardial tamponade: increased venous pressure, decreased arterial pressure, and a small, quiet heartbeat.

behavior indicator Nonspecific behavioral changes that may suggest that a child is being maltreated. Behavior indicators for sexual abuse are called "nonspecific" because children may display such behavior changes because of other traumatic conditions as well. Prompt evaluation is warranted when these nonspecific behavior indicators occur to rule out maltreatment and to obtain appropriate assistance for the child.

behavioral emergency A change in mood or behavior that cannot be tolerated by the involved person or others and that requires immediate attention.

Bell's palsy Paralysis of the facial nerve caused by trauma, compression, or an undetected infection.

beta adrenergic receptor Any of the postulated adrenergic components of receptor tissues that respond to epinephrine and various blocking agents.

beta cell A constituent of the islet of Langerhans that produces insulin.

beta-hydroxybutyric acid One of the ketone bodies that occur in abnormal amounts in diabetic ketoacidosis as a result of fatty acid oxidation.

bicarbonate buffer system The principal mechanism for stabilizing acid-base balance.

biceps brachii The biceps muscle of the arm that flexes and supinates the forearm.

bicuspid valve One of the two atrioventricular valves located between the left atrium and ventricle; also known as the mitral valve.

bifurcate To divide into two branches.

bilateral Having or occurring on two sides.

bile A bitter, yellow-green secretion of the liver that is stored in the gallbladder.

bilirubin The orange-yellow pigment of bile, formed principally from the breakdown of hemoglobin in red blood cells after termination of their normal life span.

bioethics The systematic study of moral dimensions of the life sciences and health care, including moral vision, decisions, conduct, and policies.

biological half-life The time required to metabolize or eliminate half the total amount of drug in the body.

biology The study of life.

biosynthesis A chemical reaction that continually occurs throughout the body in which molecules form more complex molecules.

biotransformation The process by which a drug is chemically converted to a metabolite.

Biot's respiration A respiratory pattern consisting of irregular respirations that vary in depth and that are interrupted by intervals of apnea.

biphasic complex A QRS complex that is partly positive and partly negative.

bipolar lead A lead composed of two electrodes of opposite polarity.

bipolar disorder A disorder marked by alternating periods of mania and depression; also known as *manic-depressive disorder.*

blast injury A general term used to describe damage to a person exposed to a pressure field.

blastocyst The stage of mammalian embryos in which the embryo consists of the inner cell mass and a thin trophoblast layer.

bleb An accumulation of fluid under the skin.

blood The fluid and its suspended, formed elements that circulate through the heart, arteries, capillaries, and veins.

blood-brain barrier An anatomical-physiological feature of the brain thought to consist of walls of capillaries in the central nervous system and surrounding glial membranes; its function is to prevent or slow the passage of chemical compounds from the blood into the central nervous system.

blood clot The end result of the clotting process in blood; a blood clot normally consists of red cells, white cells, and platelets enmeshed in an insoluble fibrin network.

blood colloid osmotic pressure Osmotic pressure caused by the presence of plasma proteins (mostly albumin) that are too large to pass through the wall of the capillary; also known as oncotic pressure.

blowout fracture A fracture of the floor of the orbit caused by a blow that suddenly increases the intraocular pressure.

blunt trauma An injury caused by the wounding forces of compression and change of speed, both of which may disrupt tissue.

B lymphocyte A type of lymphocyte responsible for antibody-mediated immunity.

body The largest or main part of any organ or structure.

bone A highly specialized form of hard, connective tissue; it consists of living cells and mineralized matrix.

bone marrow Specialized soft tissue that fills the spaces in the cancellous bone of the epiphyses.

bony labyrinth Part of the inner ear; it contains the membranous labyrinth.

borderline personality disorder A pervasive pattern of instability of interpersonal relationships, self-image, and affect, in addition to marked impulsivity that begins by early adulthood.

botulism An often fatal form of food poisoning caused by an endotoxin produced by the bacillus *Clostridium botulinum.*

bowel obstruction A failure of the contents of the intestines to pass through the lumen of the bowel.

Bowman's capsule The expanded beginning of a renal tubule.

boxer's fracture Fracture of the fifth metacarpal bone from direct trauma to a closed fist.

Boyle's law See *general gas law.*

brachial plexus A network of nerves in the neck that passes under the clavicle and into the axilla, originating in the fifth, sixth, seventh, and eighth cervical nerves and the first two thoracic spinal nerves; the brachial plexus innervates the muscles and the skin of the chest, shoulders, and arms.

bradycardia A heart rate of less than 60 beats per minute.

bradykinin A peptide of nonprotein origin that contains nine amino acid residues; a potent vasodilator.

bradypnea A persistent respiratory rate slower than 12 breaths per minute.

brain stem The midbrain, pons, and medulla.

brand name See *trade name.*

Braxton-Hicks contraction Irregular tightening of the pregnant uterus that begins in the first trimester and increases in frequency, duration, and intensity as pregnancy progresses.

breech presentation The intrauterine position of the fetus in which the buttocks or feet present.

broad ligament A folded sheet of peritoneum draped over the uterine tubes, uterus, and ovaries.

bronchial tree An anatomical complex of the bronchi and bronchial tubes.

bronchiectasis An abnormal condition of the bronchial tree characterized by irreversible dilation and destruction of the bronchial walls.

bronchiole A small branch of a bronchus.

bronchiolitis An acute viral infection of the lower respiratory tract that occurs primarily in infants under 18 months of age; it is characterized by expiratory wheezes, respiratory distress, inflammation, and obstruction at the level of the bronchioles.

Brown-Séquard syndrome A hemitranssection of the spinal cord; pressure on one half of the spinal cord results in weakness of the upper and lower extremities on the ipsilateral side and loss of pain and temperature sensation on the contralateral side.

brow presentation See *face presentation.*

bruit An abnormal sound or murmur heard while auscultating an artery, organ, or gland.

buccal Of or pertaining to the inside of the cheek.

buccal route A route for administering medication in which the agent is placed between the teeth and mucous membrane of the cheek.

bulbourethral glands Small glands located just below the prostate gland that lubricate the terminal portion of the urethra and contribute to seminal fluid; also known as Cowper's glands.

bulimia nervosa A disorder characterized by an insatiable craving for food, often resulting in episodes of binge eating followed by purging (through self-induced vomiting or use of laxatives), depression, and self deprivation.

bullae Thin-walled blisters of the skin or mucous membranes that contain clear, serous fluid.

bullet tumble See *bullet yaw.*

bullet yaw The forward rotation of a bullet around its center of mass, which causes an end-over-end motion, producing a greater energy exchange and greater tissue damage; also known as *bullet tumble.*

bundle of His A band of fibers in the myocardium through which the cardiac impulse is transmitted from the atrioventricular node to the ventricles.

bundle of Kent Fibers that connect atrial muscle to ventricular muscle, bypassing the AV node; also known as *Kent fibers.*

burette An intravenous device used to deliver a wide range of accurate specific volumes.

bursitis An inflammation of the bursa, the connective tissue structure surrounding a joint.

cesarean delivery A surgical procedure in which the abdomen and uterus are incised and the newborn is delivered transabdominally.

calcaneus The heel bone, the largest of the tarsal bones.

calcium (Ca) The fifth most abundant element in the human body; it occurs mainly in bone.

calipers An instrument with two hinged, adjustable legs used to measure components of the electrocardiogram.

canaliculus A very small tube or channel.

cancellous bone Latticelike tissue normally present in the interior of many bones where spaces are usually filled with marrow; also known as spongy bone.

cancer A neoplasm characterized by the uncontrolled growth of anaplastic cells that tend to invade surrounding tissue and to metastasize to distant body sites.

Candida A genus of yeastlike fungi.

candidiasis An infection caused by a species of *Candida* organisms that is characterized by pruritus, exudate, and easy bleeding.

cannulation The insertion of a cannula into a body duct or cavity.

capillary A tiny vessel that connects an arteriole to a venule.

capillary refill test A test used to evaluate the rate of blood flow through peripheral capillary beds.

capitation A method of payment to cover all health care expenses for each member of a managed care organization.

capitulum The lateral aspect of the humerus; it articulates with the head of the radius.

capnography Measuring the proportion of carbon dioxide in expired air.

capsid A protein coat that encloses a virus.

carbaminohemoglobin A chemical complex formed by carbon dioxide and hemoglobin after the release of oxygen by the hemoglobin to a tissue cell.

carbohydrate Any group of organic compounds composed of carbon, hydrogen, and oxygen; it is primarily obtained from plant foods.

carbonic acid An aqueous solution of carbon dioxide.

carbonic anhydrase The enzyme that converts carbon dioxide into carbonic acid.

carboxyhemoglobin A compound produced by the exposure of hemoglobin to carbon monoxide.

carcinogenic Cancer causing.

cardiac cycle The complete round of cardiac systole and diastole.

cardiac muscle A special striated muscle of the myocardium that contains dark, intercalated disks at the junctions of the abutting fibers; cardiac muscle is characterized by special contractile abilities.

cardiac myopathy An abnormal condition of the heart characterized by weakness of the myocardium.

cardiac output The volume of blood pumped by the heart per minute.

cardiac plexus One of several nerve complexes situated close to the arch of the aorta.

cardiac sphincter A ring of muscle fibers at the juncture of the esophagus and stomach.

cardiogenic shock Shock that results when cardiac action is unable to deliver sufficient circulating blood volume for tissue perfusion.

cardiography Recording the movements of the heart.

cardiomyopathy Any disease that affects the myocardium.

cardiopulmonary Of or pertaining to the heart and lungs.

cardiopulmonary resuscitation (CPR) An emergency procedure for life support, consisting of artificial respiration and manual external cardiac massage.

carina of the trachea A downward and backward projection of the lowest tracheal cartilage, forming a ridge between the openings of the right and left primary bronchi.

carotid body A small structure containing neural tissue at the bifurcation of the carotid arteries; it monitors the oxygen content of the blood and helps regulate respiration.

carotid sinus massage See *carotid sinus pressure.*

carotid sinus pressure A technique used to increase vagal tone to convert paroxysmal supraventricular tachycardia to sinus rhythm; also known as *carotid sinus massage.*

carpal Pertaining to the carpus, or wrist.

carpometacarpal joint The joint of the thumb.

carrier A radio signal of specific frequency generated by a transmitter without audio information imposed on it.

carrier molecule A protein that combines with solutes on one side of a membrane, transporting the solute to the other side; it is used in mediated transport mechanisms.

cartilage Firm, smooth, nonvascular connective tissue.

cartilaginous joint See *joint.*

catabolic Pertaining to the destruction of complex substances by living cells to form simple compounds.

cataract An abnormal, progressive condition of the lens of the eye characterized by loss of transparency.

catecholamine Any of a group of sympathomimetic amines, including dopamine, epinephrine, and norepinephrine.

cathartic Causing evacuation of the bowel.

cation An ion with a positive charge.

cavitation A temporary or permanent opening produced by a force that pushes body tissues laterally away from the track of a projectile.

cecum A cul-de-sac constituting the first part of the large intestine.

cell body The part of the cell that contains the nucleus and surrounding cytoplasm, exclusive of any projections or processes; it is concerned more with metabolism of the cell than with a specific function.

cell-mediated immunity Immunity characterized by the formation of a population of lymphocytes that attack and destroy foreign material.

cellular phone An 800- to 900-MHz radio communications system used to gain access to dial-up telephone circuits and vice versa. The system usually is divided into small coverage areas called "cells," which are interconnected via microwave or dedicated telephone circuits.

cellulitis An inflammation of the skin characterized most commonly by local heat, redness, pain, swelling, and occasionally fever, malaise, chills, and headache.

cementum The bonelike connective tissue that covers the roots of the teeth and helps to support them.

centigram A metric unit of mass equal to $\frac{1}{100}$ of a gram.

centimeter (cm) A metric unit of length equal to $\frac{1}{100}$ of a meter, or 0.3937 inches.

central cord syndrome A spinal cord injury commonly seen with hyperextension or flexion cervical injuries; it is characterized by greater motor impairment of the upper extremities than of the lower ones.

central nervous system (CNS) The brain and spinal cord, which are encased in and protected by bone.

central nervous system ischemic response An increase in blood pressure caused by vasoconstriction that occurs when oxygen levels are too low, carbon dioxide levels are too high, or pH is too low in the medulla.

central pain syndrome Infection or disease of the trigeminal nerve (fifth cranial nerve).

central thermoreceptors Nerve endings located in or near the anterior hypothalamus that are sensitive to heat.

centrifugation The process of separating components of different densities contained in a liquid by spinning them at high speeds.

centriole Usually paired organelles lying in the centrosome.

centrosome A specialized zone of cytoplasm close to the nucleus that contains two centrioles.

cephalic presentation A classification of fetal position in which the head of the fetus is at the uterine cervix; also known as vertex presentation.

cephalopelvic disproportion An obstetrical condition in which a newborn's head is too large or a mother's birth canal too small to permit normal labor or birth.

cephalothorax The united head and thorax of a spider.

cerebellar cortex The outer portion of the cerebellum.

cerebellum The second largest part of the brain, which plays an essential role in producing normal movements.

cerebral Pertaining to the brain.

cerebral aqueduct The narrow conduit between the third and fourth ventricles in the midbrain that conveys cerebrospinal fluid.

cerebral cortex A thin layer of gray matter, made up of neuron dendrites and cell bodies, that composes the surface of the cerebrum.

cerebral edema An accumulation of fluid in the brain tissue.

cerebral palsy A motor function disorder caused by a permanent, nonprogressive brain defect or lesion present at birth or shortly thereafter.

cerebral perfusion pressure (CPP) A measure of the amount of blood flow to the brain.

cerebrospinal fluid (CSF) Fluid that fills the subarachnoid space in the brain and spinal cord and in the cerebral ventricles.

cerebral vascular accident (CVA) An abnormal condition of the blood vessels of the brain characterized by occlusion by an embolus, thrombus, or cerebral hemorrhage; also known as *stroke* and *brain attack.*

cerebrum The largest and uppermost part of the brain; it controls consciousness, memory, sensations, emotions, and voluntary movements.

certification (or registration) The process by which an agency or association grants recognition to an individual for meeting specific requirements to participate in an activity.

cerumen A yellowish or brownish waxy secretion produced in the external ear canal; also known as *earwax.*

ceruminous gland The gland that produces a waxy substance, cerumen (earwax).

cervical Pertaining to the neck.

cervical node One of the lymph glands in the neck.

cervical plexus The network of nerves formed by the ventral primary divisions of the first four cervical nerves.

cervical spondylosis A form of degenerative joint and disk disease that affects the cervical vertebrae and results in compression of the associated nerve roots.

cervical vertebrae The first seven segments of the vertebral column, designated C1 to C7.

cervicitis Acute or chronic inflammation of the uterine cervix.

cervix The lower part of the uterus.

Chadwick's sign The bluish coloration of the vulva and vagina that develops after the sixth week of pregnancy as a normal result of local venous congestion; an early sign of pregnancy.

chancre A skin lesion, usually of primary syphilis, that begins at the site of infection as a papule and develops into a red, bloodless, painless ulcer with a craterlike appearance.

channel An assigned frequency or pair of frequencies used to carry voice or data communications or both. In EMS, an ALS "MED" channel is a pair of radio frequencies, one used for transmitting, the other for receiving.

chemical name The exact designation of a chemical structure, determined by the rules of chemical nomenclature.

chemoreceptor A sensory cell stimulated by a change in the concentration of chemicals to produce action potentials.

chemotactic factors Biochemical mediators that are important in activating the inflammatory response.

chemotaxis The response of leukocytes to products formed in immunological reactions; a part of the inflammatory response.

CHEMTREC (Chemical Transportation Emergency Center) A public service of the Chemical Manufacturers Association, the center provides immediate advice to on-scene personnel regarding management of hazardous materials.

Cheyne-Stokes respiration A regular, periodic pattern of breathing with equal intervals of apnea followed by a crescendo-decrescendo sequence of respirations.

chickenpox See *varicella*.

chief complaint A patient's primary complaint.

child abuse The physical, sexual, or emotional maltreatment of a child.

Chlamydia A genus of microorganisms that live as intracellular parasites; a common cause of sexually transmitted diseases and a frequent cause of sterility.

cholecystitis Acute or chronic inflammation of the gallbladder.

cholecystokinin A hormone that stimulates the contraction of the gallbladder and the secretion of pancreatic juice.

cholesterol A fat-soluble compound found in animal fats and oils that is widely distributed in the body.

cholinergic Of or pertaining to nerve fibers that elaborate acetylcholine at the myoneural junctions.

chondrocytes Cartilage cells.

choanal atresia A bony or membranous occlusion that blocks the passageway between the nose and pharynx; it can result in serious ventilation problems in the neonate.

chorioamnionitis An inflammatory reaction in the amniotic membranes caused by organisms in the amniotic fluid.

chorionic gonadotropin A chemical component of the urine of pregnant women.

choroid The portion of the vascular tunic associated with the sclera of the eye.

choroid plexus A network of brain capillaries that are involved in producing cerebrospinal fluid.

chromatin granules The material within the cell nucleus from which chromosomes are formed.

chronic bronchitis Obstructive airway disease of the trachea and bronchi.

chronic obstructive pulmonary disease (COPD) A progressive, irreversible condition characterized by diminished inspiratory and expiratory capacity of the lungs.

chronic pain Pain that continues or recurs over a prolonged period; it is caused by various disease or abnormal conditions.

chronic pulmonary hypertension A condition of abnormally high pressure within the pulmonary circulation.

chronic renal failure A progressive loss of kidney function that leads to an inability of the kidneys to excrete wastes, concentrate urine, and conserve electrolytes.

chronotropic Pertaining to agents that affect the heart rate; a drug that increases the heart rate is said to have a positive chronotropic effect.

chyme The semifluid mass of partly digested food passed from the stomach into the duodenum.

cilia Small, hairlike processes on the outer surfaces of some cells.

ciliary body A structure continuous with the choroid layer that contains smooth muscle cells and that functions in accommodation.

ciliated tissue Any tissue that projects cilia from its surface, such as portions of the epithelium in the respiratory tract.

circadian rhythm A pattern based on a 24-hour cycle applied especially to physiological phenomena, such as eating and sleeping.

circle of Willis The circle of interconnected blood vessels at the base of the brain.

circulatory shock Failure of the cardiovascular system to supply the cells with enough oxygenated blood to meet metabolic demands.

circumduction Movement in a circular motion.

circumflex artery The subdivision of the left coronary artery that feeds the lateral and posterior portions of the left ventricle and part of the right ventricle.

cirrhosis A chronic degenerative disease of the liver.

citrate Any salt or ester of citric acid.

classic heat stroke A severe, sometimes fatal condition resulting from the failure of the temperature-regulating capacity of the body; it is caused by prolonged exposure to the sun or to high temperatures.

claudication Cramplike pains in the calves caused by poor circulation of blood to the leg muscles.

clavicle A long, curved, horizontal bone just above the first rib that forms the ventral portion of the shoulder girdle.

clinical perineum The portion of the perineum between the vaginal and anal openings.

cluster headaches Headaches that occur in bursts (clusters) and often begin several hours after a person falls asleep. The pain usually is located in and around one eye and generally is accompanied by nasal congestion and tearing.

clitoris Erectile tissue located in the vestibule of the vagina.

coagulation Formation of a clot.

coarse ventricular fibrillation Fibrillatory waves greater than 3 mm in amplitude.

coccygeal bone The four segments of the sacral vertebral column that fuse to form the adult coccyx.

coccygeal plexus A network of coccygeal nerves.

cochlea Part of the bony labyrinth of the inner ear.

coitus See *copulation*.

colitis An inflammatory condition of the large intestine characterized by severe diarrhea, bleeding, and ulceration of the mucosa of the intestine.

collagen The ropelike protein of the extracellular matrix.

collecting duct A straight tubule that extends from the cortex of the kidney to the tip of the renal pyramid.

Colles' fracture A fracture of the radius at the epiphysis within 1 inch of the joint of the wrist; it is easily recognized by the resultant dorsal and lateral position of the hand.

colloid A state of matter in which large molecules or aggregates of molecules that do not precipitate are dispersed in another medium.

colon The portion of the large intestine that extends from the cecum to the rectum.

colorectal cancer A malignant disease of the large intestine characterized by a change in bowel habits and the passing of blood.

colostomy Surgical creation of an artificial anus on the abdominal wall.

command (ICS term) The individual in charge of the incident scene; also known as the *incident commander*.

command post (ICS term) The area from which the incident commander directs operations for an incident.

communicability period A stage of infection that begins when the latent period ends and continues as long as the agent is present and has the potential to spread to other hosts.

communications The transmission and reception of information, resulting in common understanding.

communications center A facility used to dispatch emergency equipment and coordinate communication between field units and personnel.

community health assessment An assessment of a target community to identify needs and resources required to provide prevention and wellness promotions.

compact bone Hard, dense bone that usually is found at the surface of skeletal structures, as distinguished from cancellous bone.

compartment syndrome The result of a crush injury usually caused by compressive forces or blunt trauma to muscle groups confined in tight fibrous sheaths with minimal ability to stretch (e.g., below the knee or above the elbow).

competitive antagonist An agent with an affinity for the same receptor site as an agonist. The competition with the agonist for the site inhibits the action of the agonist; increasing the concentration of the agonist tends to overcome the inhibition.

complement One of 11 complex, enzymatic serum proteins; complement causes lysis in an antigen-antibody reaction.

complement system A group of proteins that coat bacteria and help to kill them directly or assist in having them taken up by neutrophils in the blood or by macrophages in the tissues.

complete abortion An abortion in which the patient has passed all the products of conception.

complete breech A delivery presentation that occurs when the fetus has both knees and hips flexed; the buttocks are the presenting part.

compliance A measure of the distensibility of lung volume produced by a unit pressure change.

components of skeletal survey An x-ray study comprising a two-view chest with bone technique, two-view skull technique, views of the lateral lumbar spine and anteroposterior pelvis, and AP views of the upper and lower extremities, including AP views of the feet and PA views of the hands.

computer-aided dispatching (CAD) An enhanced dispatch system in which computerized data is used to assist the dispatcher in selecting and routing emergency equipment and resources.

concealment To hide or put out of site; concealment provides no ballistic protection.

concentration gradient The concentration difference between two points in a solution divided by the distance between the points.

concept formation A component of critical thinking that refers to all elements that are gathered to form a general impression of the patient.

concha The three bony ridges on the lateral wall of the nasal cavity.

concussion A head injury that results from violent jarring or shaking, such as that caused by a blow or explosion.

condyle A rounded projection on a bone, usually for articulation with another bone.

cone A photoreceptor in the retina of the eye; it is responsible for color vision.

confabulation The invention of stories to makeup for gaps in memory.

congenital Present at birth.

congenital rubella syndrome A serious disease that affects approximately 25% of infants born to women infected with rubella during the first trimester of pregnancy; it is associated with multiple congenital anomalies, mental retardation, and an increased risk of death from congenital heart disease and sepsis during the first 6 months of life.

congestive heart failure (CHF) An abnormal condition that reflects impaired cardiac pumping, usually a result of myocardial infarction, ischemic heart disease, or cardiomyopathy.

conjugate gaze Deviation of both eyes to either side at rest; the condition implies a structural lesion.

conjunctiva A mucous membrane that covers the anterior surface of the eyeball and the lining of the eyelids.

conjunctivitis Inflammation of the conjunctiva, caused by bacterial or viral infection, allergy, or environmental factors.

connective tissue Tissue that supports and binds other body tissues and parts.

conservation of energy law The principle that energy can neither be created nor destroyed; it can only change from one form (mechanical, thermal, electrical, or chemical) to another.

continuous quality improvement (CQI) A management approach to customer service and organizational performance that includes constant monitoring, evaluation, decisions, and actions.

constipation Difficulty passing stools, or incomplete or infrequent passage of hard stools.

contact dermatitis Skin rash that results from exposure to an irritant or sensitizing antigen.

contracture deformity An abnormal, usually permanent condition of a joint characterized by flexion and fixation and caused either by atrophy and shortening of muscle fibers or by loss of elasticity of the skin.

contraindication A medical or physiological factor that makes it harmful to administer a medication that would otherwise have therapeutic value.

contrastimulant A factor that works against stimulation.

contrecoup An injury that occurs at a site opposite the side of impact.

contralateral Affecting or originating in the opposite side of the body.

control console Typically, a desk-mounted, enclosed piece of equipment that contains the mechanical and electronic controls used to operate a radio base station.

controlled substance Any drug defined in the five categories of the federal Controlled Substance Act of 1970.

contusion A closed, soft tissue injury characterized by swelling, discoloration, and pain.

copulation The sexual union of two people of the opposite sex in which the penis is introduced into the vagina; also known as *coitus.*

cord presentation A presentation that occurs when the cord slips down into the vagina or appears externally after the amniotic membranes have ruptured.

core body temperature (CBT) The temperature of deep structures of the body.

cornea The convex, transparent, anterior part of the eye.

corneal abrasion The rubbing off of the outer layers of the cornea.

corniculate cartilage A conical nodule of elastic cartilage that surrounds the apex of each arytenoid cartilage.

coronal plane See *frontal plane.*

coronary artery One of two arteries that arise from the base of the aorta and carry blood to the muscle of the heart.

coronary artery disease (CAD) One of several abnormal conditions that affect the arteries of the heart and reduce the flow of oxygen and nutrients to the myocardium.

coronary sinus A short trunk that receives most of the veins of the heart and empties into the right atrium.

cor pulmonale An abnormal cardiac condition characterized by hypertrophy of the right ventricle of the heart as a result of hypertension of the pulmonary circulation.

corpus callosum An arched mass of white matter in the depths of the longitudinal fissure; it is made up of the transverse fibers that connect the cerebral hemispheres.

corpus luteum A yellow endocrine body formed in the ovary at the site of a ruptured vesicular follicle immediately after ovulation.

corpus luteum cyst A type of cyst prone to rupture that forms as a result of hemorrhage in a mature corpus luteum.

cortisol A steroid hormone that occurs naturally in the body.

costal margin The margin of the lower limit of the ribs.

costochondral Pertaining to the junction of the ribs and cartilage.

countershock A high-intensity, short-duration electric shock applied to the area of the heart, resulting in total cardiac depolarization.

coup Local damage that occurs at the site of impact.

couplet Two PVCs in a row.

cover A type of concealment that hides the body and offers ballistic protection.

coverage The area covered by radio communication. The generally accepted national emergency system standard is the "90/90" standard. This means that 90% of the coverage area will have communication 90% of the time. Coverage is usually expressed as dead (no coverage), marginal (spotty), good (few problems), or excellent (no problems).

Cowper's gland See *bulbourethral gland.*

coxae The hip joints; the head of the femur and the acetabulum of the innominate bone.

crackle A fine, bubbling sound heard on auscultation of the lung; it is produced by air entering distal airways and alveoli that contain serous secretions.

cranial nerve One of 12 pairs of nerves that originate from a nucleus within the brain.

cranial vault The eight skull bones that surround and protect the brain; the brain case.

craniectomy Surgical removal of bone fragments from the cranium.

cremaster muscle A thin muscle layer spreading out over the spermatic cord in a series of loops; it functions to draw the testis up toward the superficial inguinal ring in response to cold or stimulation of the nerve.

crenate The shrinking of red blood cells caused by exposure to a hypertonic solution.

crepitus A grating sound associated with rubbing of bone fragments.

cricoid cartilage The most inferior laryngeal cartilage.

cricothyroid membrane The membrane joining the thyroid and cricoid cartilages.

cricothyrotomy An emergency incision into the larynx.

crime scene A location where any part of a criminal act has occurred, or a location where evidence relating to a crime may be found.

Crohn's disease A chronic inflammatory bowel disease that usually affects the ileum or the colon, or both.

croup An acute viral infection of the upper and lower respiratory tract that occurs primarily in infants and young children 3 months to 3 years of age; it is characterized by hoarseness, fever, a harsh, brassy cough, inspiratory stridor, and varying degrees of respiratory distress; also known as *laryngotracheobronchitis.*

crown The portion of the human tooth covered by enamel.

crowning The phase at the end of labor in which the fetal head is seen at the opening of the vagina.

crush injury Injury from exposure of tissue to a compressive force sufficient to interfere with the normal structure and metabolic function of the involved cells and tissues.

crush syndrome A life-threatening and sometimes preventable complication of prolonged immobilization or compression; a pathological process that causes destruction, alteration, or both of muscle tissue.

crystalloid A substance in a solution that can be diffused through a semipermeable membrane.

crystalluria The presence of crystals in the urine.

CSF rhinorrhea Leakage of cerebrospinal fluid (CSF) caused by fracture of the ethmoid cribriform plate.

cubic centimeter (cc) A metric unit of length equal to $\frac{1}{100}$ of a meter.

Cullen's sign The appearance of irregularly formed hemorrhagic patches on the skin around the umbilicus.

cumulative action The effect that occurs when several doses of a drug are administered or when absorption occurs more quickly than removal by excretion, metabolism, or both.

cuneiform cartilage A small rod of elastic cartilage above the corniculate cartilages in the larynx.

CUPS system A method of patient status coding that assigns patients to one of four categories: CPR, unstable, potentially unstable, and stable.

current health status An assessment that focuses on the patient's current state of health, environmental conditions, and personal habits.

Cushing reflex An attempt by the body to compensate for a decline in cerebral perfusion pressure by a rise in mean arterial pressure.

Cushing's disease A metabolic disorder resulting from the chronic and excessive production of cortisol by the adrenal cortex or by the administration of glucocorticoids in large doses for several weeks or longer; also known as *Cushing's syndrome*.

Cushing's syndrome See *Cushing's disease*.

Cushing's triad Increased systolic pressure, widened pulse pressure, and a decrease in the pulse and respiratory rate that result from increased intracranial pressure.

cutaneous Of or pertaining to the skin.

cuticle The skin fold covering the root of the nail.

cyanotic Having bluish discoloration.

cystic medial necrosis Degenerative changes in the connective tissue of the aortic media.

cystitis Inflammation of the urinary bladder and ureters.

cytochrome oxidase A respiratory enzyme that functions in the transfer of electrons from cytochromes to oxygen, thus activating oxygen, which unites with hydrogen to form water.

cytology The study of cells.

cytomegalovirus (CMV) A member of a group of large, species-specific, herpes-type viruses with a wide variety of disease effects.

cytoplasm All of the substance of a cell other than the nucleus.

cytoplasmic membrane The plasma membrane.

cytotoxic Pertaining to a pharmacological compound or other agent that destroys or damages tissue cells.

dartos muscle A layer of smooth muscle in the skin of the scrotum; it raises and lowers the testes in the scrotum in response to changes in ambient temperature.

data interpretation A component of critical thinking whereby the paramedic gathers the necessary data to form a field impression and working diagnosis.

DCAP-BTLS An acronym for wound assessment that includes deformity, contusions, abrasions, penetrations or punctures, burns, tenderness, lacerations, and swelling.

deafness Complete or partial inability to hear.

debriefing An activity in which rescuers and others involved in an emergency event discuss their feelings to relieve emotions and anxiety; it usually takes place 24 to 72 hours after the event.

decerebrate posturing The position of a patient (usually comatose) in which the arms are extended and internally rotated and the legs are extended with the feet in forced plantar position.

deciduous tooth Any of the 20 teeth that appear normally during infancy.

decoding The act of interpreting symbols and format.

decompression sickness A painful, sometimes fatal syndrome caused by the formation of nitrogen bubbles in the tissues of divers, caisson workers, or aviators who move too rapidly from environments of higher atmospheric pressures to those of lower atmospheric pressures.

decontamination The process of making patients, rescuers, equipment, and supplies safe by eliminating harmful substances.

decorticate posturing The position of a comatose patient in which the upper extremities are rigidly flexed at the elbows and the wrists.

dedicated line A special telephone circuit designated for specific point-to-point communication purposes, such as alerting EMS quarters.

deep frostbite A cold injury that results in significant tissue loss even with appropriate therapy; it is associated with subdermal layers and deep tissues.

deep vein thrombosis (DVT) A disorder involving a thrombus in one of the deep veins of the body, most commonly the iliac and femoral veins.

defecation The elimination of feces from the digestive tract through the rectum.

defense mechanism An unconscious, intrapsychic reaction to protect the self from a stressful situation.

defibrillation The delivery of direct electric current in an attempt to terminate ventricular fibrillation or pulseless ventricular tachycardia.

defibrillator A device used to depolarize fibrillating myocardial cells, thus allowing them to repolarize uniformly.

defusing An informal gathering of the people involved in an emergency event to allow an initial release of feelings and an opportunity for people to share their experiences.

degloving injury An injury usually involving the hand or finger in which the soft tissue is removed down to the bone.

degradation The physical destruction or decomposition of clothing material caused by use, ambient conditions, or exposure to chemicals.

degranulation The release of internal substances.

dehydration An excessive loss of water from the body tissues; it may follow prolonged fever, diarrhea, vomiting, acidosis, and other conditions.

delirium An abrupt disorientation for time and place, usually with illusions and hallucinations.

delirium tremens (DTs) An acute, and sometimes fatal psychotic reaction caused by a cessation of excessive alcohol consumption over long periods of time.

delta cell A constituent of the islet of Langerhans; it secretes somatostatin.

delta wave Widened, abnormal slurring or notching of the onset of the QRS complex; it indicates anomalous spread of the impulse and is a diagnostic finding for Wolff-Parkinson-White syndrome.

deltoid muscle A large, thick, triangular muscle that covers the shoulder joint.

dendrite The branching processes of a neuron that receives stimuli and conducts potentials toward the cell body.

dentin The chief material of teeth, surrounding the pulp and situated inside the enamel and cementum.

deoxyribonucleic acid (DNA) A type of nucleic acid that comprises the genetic material of cells.

dependent lividity A red or bluish-purple tissue condition in dependent areas of the body caused by venous congestion.

depersonalization Forced emotional estrangement.

depolarization A change in electrical charge difference across the cell membrane that causes the difference to be smaller or closer to 0 mV; a phase of the action potential in which the membrane potential moves toward zero or becomes positive.

depressant A substance that decreases or lessens a body function or activity.

depressed skull fracture Any fracture of the skull in which fragments are depressed below the normal surface of the skull.

depression A mood disturbance characterized by feelings of sadness, despair, and discouragement that results from and normally is proportionate to some personal loss or tragedy.

dermatitis Inflammation of the skin.

dermatome The skin surface area supplied by a single spinal nerve.

dermis Dense, irregular connective tissue that forms the deep layer of the skin.

descending colon The segment of the colon that extends from the end of the transverse colon at the splenic flexure on the left side of the abdomen down to the beginning of the sigmoid colon in the pelvis.

desensitization Emotional insensitivity.

diabetes insipidus A metabolic disorder characterized by extreme polyuria and polydypsia, caused by deficient production or secretion of antidiuretic hormone (ADH) or inability of the kidney tubules to respond to ADH.

diabetes mellitus A complex disorder of carbohydrate, fat, and protein metabolism that is primarily a result of partial or complete lack of insulin secretion by the beta cells of the pancreas or of defects of the insulin receptors.

diabetic ketoacidosis (DKA) An acute, life-threatening complication of uncontrolled diabetes characterized by hyperglycemia, hypovolemia, electrolyte imbalance, and a breakdown of free fatty acids, causing acidosis; also known as *diabetic coma.*

diad The combination of sarcoplasmic reticulum and T tubules.

diagnosis Identification of a disease or condition by an evaluation of physical signs, symptoms, history, laboratory tests, and procedures.

dialysate A solution used in dialysis.

dialysis fistula An artificial passage, as in an arteriovenous fistula, used to gain access to the patient's bloodstream for hemodialysis.

diaphoresis Profuse secretion of sweat.

diaphragm The dome-shaped, musculofibrous partition that separates the thoracic and abdominal cavities.

diaphragmatic hernia Protrusion of part of the stomach through an opening in the diaphragm.

diaphysis The shaft of a long bone, consisting of a tube of compact bone that encloses the medullary cavity.

diarrhea The frequent passage of loose, watery stools; it is generally the result of increased motility in the colon.

diastolic blood pressure The minimum level of blood pressure measured between contraction of the heart.

diencephalon The parts of the brain between the cerebral hemispheres and the mesencephalon.

differentiation A process in which cells become "specialized" in one type of function or act in concert with other cells to perform a more complex task.

diffusion The process in which solid, particulate matter in a fluid moves from an area of higher concentration to an area of lower concentration, resulting in an even distribution of the particles in the fluid.

diphtheria An acute contagious disease characterized by the production of a systemic toxin and a false membrane lining of the mucous membranes of the throat.

diplopia Double vision.

direct laryngoscopy Visual examination of the larynx with a laryngoscope.

disease period A stage of infection that follows the incubation period and is of variable, disease-specific duration.

disentanglement Systematic removal of a vehicle or structure around a victim.

disequilibrium Unstable equilibrium; motion sickness.

disequilibrium syndrome A group of neurological findings that sometimes occurs during or immediately after dialysis; it is thought to result from a disproportionate decrease in osmolality of the extracellular fluid compared to that of the intracellular compartment in the brain or cerebrospinal fluid.

disoriented Unaware of surroundings.

dispositional hearing The phase of the family court process in which appropriate placement for a child and appropriate treatment, if any, for the parent of a child are determined and ordered.

dissecting aortic aneurysm Localized dilation of the aorta characterized by a longitudinal dissection between the outer and middle layers of the vascular wall.

disseminated intravascular coagulation (DIC) A grave coagulopathy resulting from the overstimulation of the body's clotting and anticlotting processes in response to disease or injury, such as septicemia, acute hypotension, poisonous snakebites, obstetrical emergencies, severe trauma, or hemorrhage.

dissolution The rate at which a solid drug goes into solution after ingestion; the faster the rate of dissolution, the more quickly the drug is absorbed.

distraction A self-defense measure that creates diversion in a person's attention.

distraction injury A spinal injury that occurs if the cervical spine is suddenly stopped while the weight and momentum of the body pull away from it.

distress An emotional or physical state of pain or discomfort.

distribution The transport of a drug through the bloodstream to various tissues of the body and ultimately to its site of action.

disulfiram-ethanol reaction A potentially life-threatening physiological response caused by disulfiram and ethanol that produces ill effects on the gastrointestinal, cardiovascular, and autonomic nervous systems; disulfiram is prescribed to some alcoholic patients to help them maintain abstinence.

diuresis The increased formation and secretion of urine.

diversity Differences of any kind in race, class, religion, gender, sexual preference, personal habitat, and physical ability.

diverticulitis Inflammation of one or more diverticula.

diverticulosis The presence of pouchlike herniations through the muscular layer of the colon.

diverticulum A pouchlike herniation through the muscular wall of a tubular organ; it may be present in the stomach, small intestine or, most commonly, the colon.

do not resuscitate (DNR) A physician order instructing emergency care providers not to attempt resuscitation of a patient in the event of cardiac or respiratory failure; also known as a "no code" order.

dorsal root A sensory component that conveys afferent nerve processes to the spinal cord.

dorsal root ganglia See *spinal ganglia.*

dorsogluteal site An area made up of several gluteal muscles; it is used as an injection site.

Down's syndrome A congenital condition characterized by varying degrees of mental retardation and multiple defects.

dram (dr) A unit of mass equal to an apothecaries' measure of 60 grains or ⅛ ounce.

dromotropic Pertaining to agents that affect conduction velocity through the conducting tissues of the heart; a drug that speeds conduction is said to have a positive dromotropic effect.

drowning Death by asphyxia after submersion.

drug Any substance injected into a muscle, blood vessel, or cavity of the body, taken by mouth, or applied topically to treat or prevent a disease or condition.

drug absorption A process in which drug molecules move from the site of entry into the body to the general circulation.

drug abuse Self-medication or self-administration of a drug in chronically excessive amounts, resulting in psychological or physical dependence (or both), functional impairment, and deviation from approved social norms.

drug allergy A systemic reaction to a drug, resulting from previous sensitizing exposure and the development of an immunological mechanism.

drug dependence A state in which intense physical or emotional disturbance is produced if a drug is withdrawn; previously called *habituation.*

drug interaction The modified effects of one drug caused by prior or concurrent administration of another drug, which increases or decreases either the pharmacological or physiological action of one or both drugs; it may be beneficial or detrimental.

drug-protein complex A complex formed by the attachment of a drug to proteins, mainly albumin.

drug receptor Any part of a cell, usually an enzyme or large protein molecule, with which a drug molecule interacts to trigger its desired response or effect.

ductus arteriosus A vascular channel in the fetus that joins the pulmonary artery directly to the descending aorta.

ductus deferens A thick, smooth muscular tube that allows sperm to exit from the epididymis through the ejaculatory duct; also known as the *vas deferens.*

ductus venosus The continuation of the umbilical vein through the liver to the inferior vena cava.

duodenum The first subdivision of the small intestine.

duplex mode A system that has the ability to transmit and receive traffic simultaneously through two different frequencies, one to transmit and one to receive. Similar in function to telephone communications in that two parties at either end of the communications link can talk simultaneously without blocking either message.

duplex/multiplex system A communications system with the ability to transmit and receive simultaneously with concurrent transmission of voice and telemetry.

dura mater The outermost layer of the meninges.

duration of action The period from the onset of drug action to the time when a drug effect is no longer seen.

dysarthria Difficult and poorly articulated speech resulting from poor control over the muscles of speech.

dysconjugate gaze Deviation of the eyes to opposite sides at rest; it implies a structural brain stem dysfunction in the pathways that traverse the brain stem from the upper midbrain to at least the level of the lower pons.

dyshemoglobinemia Hemoglobin saturated with compounds other than oxygen, such as carbon monoxide or methemoglobin.

dysmenorrhea Pain associated with menstruation.

dyspareunia Pain with intercourse.

dysphagia Inability or difficulty in swallowing due to medical or traumatic causes.

dysphonia An abnormality in the speaking voice, such as hoarseness.

dysplasia Abnormal development of tissue or organs.

dyspnea Difficulty breathing.

dysrhythmia Variation from a normal rhythm.

dystonia Impairment of muscle tone; it may occur as a result of medication use.

EACOM/HEAR Emergency Administrative Communications (EACOM; General Electric), or Hospital Emergency Administrative Radio (HEAR; Motorola). These radio systems use 1500 Hz rotary-pulse dialing, which transmits specific groups of rotary tone pulses for the purpose of selectively addressing hospital-based receivers in particular regions throughout the United States. Most ambulance services have access to this system.

eardrum The cellular membrane that separates the external ear from the middle ear; also known as the *tympanic membrane.*

eating disorders A term referring to anorexia nervosa and bulimia nervosa, conditions in which dissatisfaction with weight and body shape cause an individual to develop disordered eating behaviors.

eclampsia A grave form of pregnancy-induced hypertension, characterized by convulsions, coma, proteinuria, and edema.

ectoparasite An organism that lives on the outside of the body of the host, such as a louse.

ectopic Out of place.

ectopic foci Cardiac dysrhythmias caused by irritation of an excitation impulse at a site other than the sinus node.

ectopic pregnancy An abnormal pregnancy in which the conceptus implants outside the uterine cavity.

eczema Superficial dermatitis of unknown cause.

edema An abnormal accumulation of fluid in interstitial spaces.

effacement The shortening of the vaginal portion of the cervix and the thinning of its walls as it is stretched and dilated by the fetus during labor.

efferent division The nerve fibers that send impulses from the central nervous system to the periphery.

efficacy An intrinsic activity that refers to a drug's ability to initiate biological activity as a result of such binding.

Einthoven's triangle An equilateral triangle formed by the patient's right arm, left arm, and left leg; it is used in electrode sensor placement for ECG monitoring.

ejaculatory duct A duct formed by the joining of the ductus deferens and the duct from the seminal vesicle that allows sperm to enter the urethra.

ejection The forceful expulsion of blood from the ventricle of the heart.

elastin The major connective tissue protein of elastic tissue; it has a structure like a coiled spring.

elder abuse The infliction of physical pain, injury, debilitating mental anguish, or unreasonable confinement on an elderly patient, or the willful deprivation by a caretaker of services necessary to maintain the mental and physical health of an elderly patient.

electroconvulsive therapy Induction of a brief convulsion by passing an electric current through the brain to treat affective disorders.

electrolyte A cation or anion in solution that conducts an electrical current.

elevation Movement of a structure in a superior direction.

ellipsoid joint A modified ball-and-socket joint in which the articular surfaces are ellipsoid rather than spherical in shape.

emaciated To be abnormally lean from disease or lack of nutrition.

embolectomy A surgical incision into an artery for the removal of an embolus or clot.

embryo In human beings, the stage of prenatal development between the time of implantation of the fertilized ovum until the end of the seventh or eighth week.

emergency medical services (EMS) A national network of services coordinated to provide aid and medical assistance from primary response to definitive care; it involves personnel trained in rescue, stabilization, transportation, and advanced treatment of traumatic or medical emergencies.

EMS communications Refers to the delivery of the patient and scene information (either in person, in writing, or through communications technology) to other members of the emergency response team.

Emergency medical technician-paramedic (EMT-P) A person who has completed training based on the *EMT-Paramedic National Standard Curriculum.* A paramedic has advanced training in patient assessment, cardiac rhythm interpretation, defibrillation, drug therapy, and airway management.

emissary veins The small vessels in the skull that connect the sinuses of the dura with the veins on the exterior of the skull through a series of anastomoses.

emotional-mental impairment (EMI) Impairment of intellectual functioning (mental retardation) that results in an inability to cope with normal responsibilities of life.

emphysema An abnormal condition of the pulmonary system characterized by overinflation and destructive changes in the alveolar walls, resulting in a loss of lung elasticity and a decrease in gases.

enamel A hard white substance that covers the dentin of the crown of the tooth.

encephalitis An inflammatory condition of the brain, usually caused by an infection transmitted by the bite of an infected mosquito; it may also result from lead or other poisoning or from hemorrhage.

encoding The act of placing a message in an understandable format, either written or verbal.

endolymph Fluid found within the membranous labyrinth.

endometriosis An abnormal gynecological condition characterized by ectopic growth and function of endometrial tissue; it is thought to result when, during menstruation, fragments of endometrium from the lining of the uterus are regurgitated backward through the fallopian tubes into the peritoneal cavity, where they attach and grow as small cystic structures.

endometritis An inflammatory condition of the endometrium, usually caused by bacterial infection.

endometrium The mucous membrane lining of the uterus; it changes in thickness and structure with the menstrual cycle.

endoplasmic reticulum (ER) A network of connecting sacs or canals that wind through a cell's cytoplasm, serving as a miniature circulatory system for the cell.

endorphin Any of several peptides secreted in the brain that have a pain-relieving effect like morphine.

endotoxin A toxin contained in the cell walls of some microorganisms, especially gram-negative bacteria.

endotracheal intubation An airway management procedure in which an endotracheal tube is inserted through the mouth or nose into the trachea. It is used to maintain a patent airway, to prevent aspiration of material from the digestive tract, to permit suctioning of tracheobronchial secretions, to administer positive-pressure ventilation, and to administer certain medications when other means of vascular access are unavailable.

endotracheal route Refers to drugs administered through an endotracheal tube.

enhanced automaticity The cause of dysrhythmias in Purkinje fibers and other myocardial cells with a high resting membrane potential; it results from an acceleration of phase 4 depolarization commonly caused by abnormally high leakage of sodium ions into the cells, which causes the cells to reach threshold prematurely.

enophthalmos Recessed globe.

enteral route A route of drug administration along any portion of the gastrointestinal tract.

enzyme A protein produced by living cells that catalyzes chemical reactions in organic matter.

eosinophil A white blood cell that inhibits inflammation; it readily stains with acidic dyes.

eosinophil chemotactic factor of anaphylaxis A group of active substances, including histamine and leukotrienes, that are released during an anaphylactic reaction.

epicardium See *visceral pericardium*.

epicondyle A projection on the surface of a bone above its condyle.

epidermis The outer portion of skin; it is formed of epithelial tissue that rests on or covers the dermis.

epididymis A tightly coiled tube that lies along the top of and behind the testes, where sperm mature.

epidural hematoma Accumulation of blood between the dura mater and the cranium.

epidural space The space above or on the dura.

epiglottis A lidlike cartilage that overhangs the entrance to the larynx.

epiglottitis Inflammation of the epiglottis; a severe form of the condition that affects primarily children is characterized by fever, sore throat, stridor, croupy cough, and an erythematous epiglottis.

epilepsy A group of neurological disorders characterized by recurrent episodes of convulsive seizures, sensory disturbances, abnormal behavior, loss of consciousness, or some combination of these.

epinephrine Adrenaline; the secretion of the adrenal medulla.

epiphyseal line A dense plate in a bone that is no longer growing, indicating the former site of the epiphyseal plate.

epiphyseal plate The site of bone elongation; also known as the *growth plate*.

epiphysis The head of a long bone that is separated from the shaft of the bone by the epiphyseal plate until the bone stops growing, the plate is obliterated, and the shaft and the head are united.

epistaxis Bleeding from the nose.

epithelial tissue The cellular covering of internal and external surfaces of the body, including the lining of vessels and other small cavities.

Epstein-Barr virus (EBV) The herpes virus that causes infectious mononucleosis.

erection The condition of hardness, swelling, and elevation observed in the penis and to a lesser degree in the clitoris, usually caused by sexual arousal.

erythrocyte A red blood cell.

escape beat An automatic beat of the heart that occurs after an interval longer than the duration of the dominant heartbeat cycle.

eschar A scab or dry crust resulting from a thermal or chemical burn.

escharotomy Surgical incision into necrotic tissue caused by a severe burn; escharotomy sometimes is necessary to prevent edema from building up sufficient inter-

stitial pressure to impair capillary filling and cause ischemia.

esophagogastric varices See *esophageal varices*.

esophageal reflux A chronic disease manifested by various sequelae associated with reflux of the stomach and duodenal contents into the esophagus.

esophageal stricture An abnormal temporary or permanent narrowing of the esophagus secondary to inflammation, external pressure, or scarring.

esophageal varices A complex of longitudinal, tortuous veins at the lower end of the esophagus that become large and swollen as a result of portal hypertension; these veins are especially susceptible to ulceration and hemorrhage; also known as *esophagogastric varices*.

esophagitis Inflammation of the esophagus.

esophagus The muscular canal extending from the pharynx to the stomach.

estimated date of confinement (EDC) Delivery date for the fetus.

estrogen One of a group of hormonal steroid compounds that promote the development of female secondary sex characteristics.

ethics The discipline relating to right and wrong, moral duty and obligation, moral principles and values, and moral character; a standard for honorable behavior designed by a group with expected conformity.

ethmoid bone The very light, spongy bone at the base of the cranium that forms most of the walls of the superior part of the nasal cavity.

ethmoid sinus One of the numerous small, thin-walled cavities in the ethmoid bone of the skull, rimmed by the frontal maxilla and the lacrimal, sphenoidal, and palatine bones.

ethylene glycol A chemical used in automobile antifreeze preparations.

eukaryote A cell with a true nucleus, found in all higher organisms and in some microorganisms.

eustachian tube See *auditory tube*.

eustress A positive form of stress.

evaluation A component of critical thinking whereby an assessment is made of the patient's response to care.

evasive tactic A self-defense measure where the moves and actions of an aggressor are anticipated and in which unconventional pathways are used during retreat for personal safety.

eversion Turning outward.

evisceration The protrusion of an internal organ through a wound or surgical incision, especially in the abdominal wall.

excitability The property of a cell that enables it to react to irritation or stimulation.

excretion The elimination of toxic or inactive metabolites, primarily by the kidneys; the intestine, lungs, and mammary glands, sweat glands, and salivary glands may also be involved.

excursion Movement from side to side.

exertional heat stroke An abnormal condition characterized by weakness, vertigo, nausea, muscle cramps, and loss of consciousness; caused by depletion of body fluid and electrolytes resulting from exposure to intense heat or inability to acclimatize to heat.

exocrine Secreting into a duct.

exophthalmos An abnormal condition characterized by marked protrusion of the eyeballs.

exothermic Marked or accompanied by the evolution of heat.

exotoxin A toxin secreted or excreted by a living organism.

expiration Breathing out (exhalation), normally a passive process.

expiratory center The region of the medulla that is electrically active during nonquiet expiration.

expiratory reserve volume The maximum volume of air that can be exhaled after a normal expiration.

expressed consent Verbal or written consent to the treatment.

extended scope of practice The expansion of preventative health care services provided by EMTs and paramedics in the prehospital setting.

extension Stretching out.

external anal sphincter A sphincter muscle located at the tip of the coccyx and surrounding fascia; it prevents the movement of feces out of the rectum until it is relaxed.

external auditory canal The passage for sound impulses passing through the ear.

external auditory meatus The canal of the external ear; also known as the *external auditory canal*.

external cardiac pacing The delivery of repetitive electric currents to the heart, substituting for a natural pacemaker that has become blocked or dysfunctional; also known as *transcutaneous cardiac pacing (TCP)*.

external ear The portion of the ear that includes the auricle and external auditory meatus; it terminates at the eardrum.

external jugular vein One of a pair of large vessels in the neck that receive most of the blood from the exterior of the cranium and deep tissues of the face.

external urinary sphincter The smooth muscle that surrounds the urethra as the urethra extends through the pelvic floor; it controls the flow of urine through the urethra.

extracellular Occurring outside of a cell or cell tissues or in cavities or spaces between cell layers or groups of cells.

extracellular fluid (ECF) The portion of the body fluid comprising the interstitial fluid and blood plasma.

extracellular matrix Nonliving chemical substances located between connective tissue cells.

extrapyramidal reaction A response to a treatment or drug characterized by involuntary movement, changes in muscle tone, and abnormal posture.

extravasate The passage or escape of blood, serum, or lymph into the tissues.

extubation Removal of an endotracheal tube.

exudate Fluid, cells, or other substances that have been slowly discharged from cells or blood vessels through small pores or breaks in cell membranes.

face presentation An abnormal presentation in which the brow or forehead of the fetus is the first part of the body to enter the birth canal; also known as *brow presentation*.

facial bones The 14 bones that form the structure of the face in the anterior skull; they do not contribute to the cranial vault.

facial nerve palsy Partial or total loss of the functions of the facial muscles or loss of sensation in the face.

facies A facial expression or appearance.

facilitated diffusion A carrier-mediated process that moves substances into or out of cells from a high to a low concentration.

failure to thrive (FTT) An abnormal retardation of growth and development of an infant resulting from conditions that interfere with normal metabolism, appetite, and activity.

fallopian tube See *uterine tube*.

false imprisonment Intentional and unjustifiable detention of a person.

false movement Unnatural movement of an extremity.

false rib See *rib*.

false vocal cord See *vestibular fold*.

family court Sometimes referred to as juvenile court; it is authorized to handle proceedings involving claims of abuse and neglect, dependency, delinquency, and requests for the termination of parental rights.

fascia The loose areolar connective tissue found beneath the skin or dense connective tissue that encloses and separates muscle.

fascicle A small bundle or cluster of nerve or muscle fibers that provides pathways for impulse conduction.

fasciotomy Incision of a fascia to relieve elevated intracompartmental pressure.

fasciculation A localized, uncoordinated, uncontrollable twitching of a single muscle group that can be palpated and seen under the skin.

family history Illness or disease in a patient's family or a family's background that may be relevant to the patient's complaint.

fat A substance composed of lipids or fatty acids.

febrile seizure A seizure that results from fever.

fecal impaction An accumulation of hardened feces in the rectum or sigmoid colon that the individual is unable to pass.

fecalith A hard, impacted mass of feces in the colon.

feces Waste material discharged from the intestines.

Federal Communications Commission (FCC) A federal agency with jurisdiction over interstate and international telephone and telegraph services and satellite communications.

femoral vein A large vein in the thigh that originates in the popliteal vein and accompanies the femoral artery in the proximal two thirds of the thigh.

femur The thigh bone, which extends from the pelvis to the knee; the largest and strongest bone in the body.

fetal membrane disorder One of several disorders that pertain to the fetus or to the period during its development, including premature rupture of membranes, amniotic fluid embolism, and meconium staining.

fetus Unborn young, from the third month of the intrauterine period until birth.

fibrinogen A soluble blood protein converted into insoluble fibrin during clotting.

fibrocartilage Cartilage that consists of a dense matrix of white collagenous fibers.

fibrosis An abnormal condition in which fibrous connective tissue spreads over or replaces normal smooth muscle or other normal organ tissue.

fibrous connective tissue A connective tissue that consists mainly of bundles of strong, white collagenous fibers arranged in parallel rows.

fibrous joint See *joint*.

fibrous pericardium Fibrous outer layer of the heart.

fibrous tunic The sclera and cornea.

fibula The bone of the leg, lateral to and smaller than the tibia.

Fick principle The principle used to determine cardiac output; that is, the amount of oxygen uptake of each unit of blood as it passes through the lungs equals the oxygen concentration difference between arterial and mixed venous blood.

field impression An impression of the patient's condition formed from pattern recognition and the paramedic's gut instinct that arises from past experience.

filtrate A filtered liquid.

filtration Movement caused by a pressure gradient of a liquid through a filter that prevents some or all of the substances in the liquid from passing through.

fimbria A fringelike structure located at the border of the uterine tube.

fine ventricular fibrillation Fibrillatory waves less than 3 mm in amplitude.

first-degree burn A burn injury in which only a superficial layer of epidermal cells is destroyed.

first-pass metabolism The initial biotransformation of a drug on passage through the liver from the portal vein; it occurs before the drug reaches the general circulation.

first stage of labor The stage of labor that begins with the onset of regular contractions and ends with complete dilation of the cervix.

fistula An abnormal passage from an internal organ to the body surface.

flail chest A chest wall injury in which two or more adjacent ribs are fractured in two or more places.

flat bones Bones that have a thin, flattened shape, such as certain skull bones, the ribs, the sternum, and scapulae.

flatulence Excessive air or gas in the stomach or intestinal tract, causing distention of the organs and in some cases mild to moderate pain.

flexion Bending.

floating rib See *rib*.

flora Microorganisms that live on or in the body to compete with disease-producing microorganisms and provide a natural immunity against certain infections.

flutter waves Abnormal P waves in a "sawtooth" or "picket fence" pattern; they represent atrial depolarization in an abnormal direction followed by atrial repolarization.

focal seizure See *Jacksonian seizure*.

focused history A component of patient assessment to ascertain the patient's chief complaint, history of present illness, past medical history, and current health status.

fontanelle A space covered by a tough membrane between the bones of an infant's cranium.

food poisoning Poisoning that results from food contaminated by toxic substances or by bacteria containing toxins.

foramen ovale An opening in the septum between the right and left atria in the fetal heart; it provides a bypass for blood that would otherwise flow to the fetal lungs.

foramina A passage in the occipital bone through which the spinal cord enters the spinal column.

foreign body airway obstruction A disturbance in normal function or a pathological condition caused by an object lodged in the airway.

formed elements Cells and cell fragments of blood.

formic acid A colorless, pungent liquid found in nature in ants and other insects.

fourth-degree burn A full-thickness burn injury that penetrates the subcutaneous tissue, muscle, fascia, periosteum, or bone.

fourth ventricle The ventricle located in the superior region of the medulla; continuous with the central canal of the spinal cord.

fracture A break in the continuity of a bone.

frank breech See *front breech*.

fraternal twins Two offspring born of the same pregnancy from two ova released simultaneously from the ovary and fertilized at the same time.

French scale system A scale used to denote the size of catheters and other tubular instruments; each unit is roughly equivalent to 0.33 mm in diameter.

frequency The number of repetitive cycles per second completed by a radio wave.

frequency modulation (FM) A deviation of carrier frequency in accordance with the strength of applied audio. FM is less susceptible to some types of interference than AM and is typically used in EMS communications.

frontal bone The single cranial bone that forms the front of the skull.

frontal lobe The largest of the five lobes that comprise each of the two cerebral hemispheres; it significantly influences personality and is associated with higher mental activities such as planning, judgment, and conceptualization.

frontal plane An imaginary plane that divides the body into front and back or anterior and posterior positions; also known as the *coronal plane*.

frontal sinus One of a pair of small cavities in the frontal bone of the skull that communicates with the nasal cavity.

front breech A presentation that occurs when the fetal hips are flexed and the legs extend in front of the fetus, making the buttocks the presenting part; also known as a *frank breech*.

frostbite A localized injury that results from environmentally induced freezing of body tissues.

frostnip The mildest form of cold injury; it may be treated without loss of tissue.

functional residual capacity (FRC) The expiratory reserve volume plus the residual volume; it reflects the amount of gas remaining in the lungs at the end of a normal expiration.

fundus The bottom or rounded end of a hollow organ, such as the fundus of the uterus.

fusion beat A PVC that occurs at approximately the same time that an electrical impulse of the underlying rhythm is activating the ventricles, thereby causing ventricular depolarization to occur simultaneously in two directions; it results in a QRS complex that has the characteristics of both the PVC and the QRS complex of the underlying rhythm.

gag reflex A normal reflex elicited by touching the soft palate or posterior pharynx.

gallbladder A pear-shaped excretory sac on the visceral surface of the right lobe of the liver; it serves as a reservoir for bile.

gallows humor Morbid or cynical humor.

ganglia A group of nerve cell bodies in the peripheral nervous system.

gap junction A small channel between cells that allows the passage of ions and small molecules between cells.

gastric gland A gland located in the stomach mucosa.

gastric lavage The washing out of the stomach with sterile water or normal saline.

gastrin A polypeptide hormone that stimulates the flow of gastric juice and contributes to the stimulus that causes bile and pancreatic enzyme secretion.

gastritis Inflammation of the lining of the stomach; it may be acute or chronic.

gastroenteritis The inflammation of the stomach and intestines that accompanies numerous gastrointestinal disorders.

gastrointestinal Of or pertaining to the organs of the gastrointestinal tract, from mouth to anus.

gastrostomy An artificial opening into the stomach.

gating protein A protein that controls the rate at which ions move through an ion channel.

general gas law The characteristic of gas that it flows from an area of higher pressure or concentration to an area of lower pressure or concentration; also known as *Boyle's law*.

general impression An immediate assessment of the environment and patient's chief complaint; it is used to determine if the patient is ill or injured and the nature of the illness or the mechanism of injury.

generic name The official, established name assigned to a drug; also known as a *nonproprietary name*.

genitalia Reproductive organs.

genitourinary Refers to the genital and urinary systems of the body, the organ structures, functions, or both.

German measles See *rubella*.

gerontology The study of the problems of all aspects of aging.

gestation The period from the fertilization of the ovum until birth.

gestational diabetes mellitus (GDM) A disorder characterized by impaired ability to metabolize carbohydrate, usually caused by a deficiency of insulin; it occurs in pregnancy and disappears after delivery but in some cases returns years later.

gingiva The portion of the oral mucosa surrounding the tooth.

gingival hypertrophy Swelling of the gums; it is often associated with chronic phenytoin therapy.

gingivostomatitis Multiple, painful ulcers on the gums and mucous membranes of the mouth; the result of a herpes virus infection.

Glasgow Coma Scale (GCS) A standardized system for assessing the degree of conscious impairment in the critically ill and for predicting the duration and ultimate outcome of coma.

glia limitans A supporting structure of nervous tissue consisting of large, star-shaped cells.

gliding joint See *plane joint*.

globule A small, spherical mass.

globulin One of a broad category of simple proteins classified by solubility, mobility, and size.

glucagon A hormone produced by the alpha cells in the islets of Langerhans that stimulates the conversion of glycogen to glucose in the liver.

gluconeogenesis The formation of glycogen from fatty acids and proteins rather than carbohydrates.

glomerular filtration rate (GFR) The amount of plasma that filters into Bowman's capsules per minute.

glomerulus The mass of capillary loops at the beginning of each nephron.

glossopharyngeal nerve Either of a pair of cranial nerves essential to the sense of taste, to sensation in some viscera, and to secretion from certain glands.

glottic opening The vocal cords and the space between them.

glottis The space between the vocal cords.

glucocorticoid An adrenocortical steroid hormone that increases glyconeogenesis, exerts an antiinflammatory effect, and influences many body functions.

glucosuria The abnormal presence of glucose in the urine resulting from large amounts of carbohydrate, from kidney disease, or from a metabolic disease such as diabetes mellitus.

gluteus medius muscle The muscle that originates between the anterior and posterior gluteal lines of the ilium and inserts into the greater trochanter of the femur.

glycogenolysis The breakdown of glycogen to glucose.

glycolysis An anaerobic process during which glucose is converted to pyruvic acid.

glycoprotein Any of a large group of conjugated proteins in which the nonprotein substance is a carbohydrate.

goblet cell One of the many specialized cells that secrete mucus and form glands of the epithelium of the stomach, intestine, and parts of the respiratory tract.

goiter A hypertrophic thyroid gland, usually evident as a pronounced swelling in the neck.

golden hour The critical period during which surgical intervention for a trauma patient can enhance survival and reduce complications.

Golgi apparatus Specialized endoplasmic reticulum that concentrates and packages materials for secretion from the cell.

gomphosis An articulation by the insertion of a conic process into a socket, such as the insertion of the root of a tooth into an alveolus of the mandible or maxilla.

gonad A gamete-producing gland, such as an ovary or testis.

gonorrhea A sexually transmitted disease that results from contact with the causative organism *Neisseria gonorrhoeae*.

gout A disease associated with an inborn error of uric acid metabolism that increases production of or interferes with excretion of uric acid; also known as *hyperuricemia*.

gouty arthritis A type of arthritis caused by excess uric acid, which is converted to sodium urate crystals that are deposited in the joints.

graafian follicle See *vesicular follicle*.

grain (gr) The smallest unit of mass in apothecaries' weights equal to 60–65 mg.

gram (g) A metric unit of mass equal to $^1/_{1000}$ of a kilogram.

gram-negative sepsis Sepsis caused by gram-negative bacteria when the bacterium dies and is broken down in the body.

grand mal seizure A seizure characterized by a generalized involuntary muscular contraction and cessation of respiration followed by tonic and clonic spasms of the muscles.

grand multipara A woman who has had seven deliveries or more.

granulosa cell A cell in the layer surrounding the primary follicle.

gravida The number of all current and past pregnancies.

gray matter The gray tissue that makes up the inner core of the spinal column.

great vessels The large arteries and veins entering and leaving the heart; they include the aorta, the pulmonary arteries and veins, and the superior and inferior venae cavae.

growth plate The site of bone elongation; also known as the *epiphyseal plate.*

Guillain-Barré syndrome A relatively rare disease that affects the peripheral nervous system, especially the spinal nerves, but also the cranial nerves; it is associated with a viral infection or immunization.

habituation See *drug dependence.*

hair follicle An invagination of the epidermis into the dermis that contains the root of the hair and receives the ducts of sebaceous and apocrine glands.

hair papilla A small, cup-shaped cluster of cells located at the base of the follicle where hair growth begins.

hair root The part of the hair that lies hidden in the follicle.

hair shaft The visible part of the hair.

half duplex The use of two different frequencies, one to transmit and one to receive, that cannot be used simultaneously.

half-life (t$^1/_2$) The amount of time required to reduce a drug level to one half its initial value.

hallucination The apparent perception of sites, sounds, and other phenomena that are not actually present.

Hantavirus A cause of several different forms of hemorrhagic fever with renal syndrome.

hard palate The floor of the nasal cavity that separates the nasal cavity from the oral cavity.

hazard control The phase of rescue that includes managing, reducing, and minimizing risks from uncontrollable hazards, ensuring scene safety, and providing personal protective equipment that is appropriate for the incident.

head of bone An eminence on a bone by which it articulates with another bone.

heart The muscular, cone-shaped organ that pumps blood throughout the body by coordinated nerve impulses and muscular contractions.

heart murmur An abnormal heart sound caused by altered blood flow into a chamber or through a valve.

heat cramps Brief, intermittent, and often severe muscular cramps that frequently occur in muscles fatigued by heavy work or exercise.

heat exhaustion A form of heat illness characterized by minor aberrations in mental status, dizziness, nausea, headache, and a mild-to-moderate elevation in the core body temperature.

heat stroke A syndrome that occurs when the thermoregulatory mechanisms normally in place to meet the demands of heat stress break down entirely; it results in elevation of the body temperature to extreme levels, producing multisystem tissue damage and physiological collapse.

hemasite A small, button-shaped indwelling vascular device usually placed in the upper arm or proximal, anterior thigh; it is similar to an AV graft but has an external rubber septum sutured to the skin through which a dialysis catheter is inserted for treatment.

hematemesis Vomiting of bright red blood, indicating upper gastrointestinal bleeding.

hematochezia The passage of red blood through the rectum.

hematoma A collection of blood trapped in tissues of the skin or in an organ.

hemiblock Failure in conduction of cardiac impulse in either of two main divisions of the left branch of the bundle of His; interruption may occur in either the anterior (superior) or posterior (inferior) division.

hemiparesis One-sided weakness.

hemiplegia Paralysis of one side of the body.

hemitranssection A cut across the long axis of tissue, such as the spinal cord.

hemoagglutinin An agglutinin that clumps red blood corpuscles.

hemochromatosis A rare disease of iron metabolism characterized by excess deposition of iron throughout the body.

hemodialysis A procedure in which impurities or wastes are removed from the blood; it is used in treating renal insufficiency and various toxic conditions.

hemoglobin A complex protein-iron compound in the blood that carries oxygen to the cells from the lungs and carbon dioxide away from the cells to the lungs.

hemolysis The breakdown of red blood cells and the release of hemoglobin.

hemolytic anemia A condition in which delivery of oxygen to tissues is reduced because of an increase in hemolysis of erythrocytes.

hemopericardium An accumulation of blood within the pericardial sac surrounding the heart.

hemoperitoneum The presence of extravasated blood in the peritoneal cavity.

hemophilia A group of heredity bleeding disorders in which one of the factors necessary for blood coagulation is deficient.

hemophilia A A condition caused by a deficiency of coagulation factor VIII; it is considered the classic type of hemophilia.

hemophilia B A condition caused by a deficiency of coagulation factor IX.

hemopneumothorax See *pneumohemothorax.*

hemopoietic tissue Tissue related to the process of formation and development of various types of blood cells.

hemoptysis Coughing up of blood from the respiratory tract.

hemorrhage Flowing of blood.

hemorrhagic shock Hypoperfusion associated with the sudden and rapid loss of significant amounts of blood.

hemorrhoid A varicosity in the lower rectum or anus caused by congestion in the veins of the hemorrhoidal plexus.

hemostasis The termination of bleeding by mechanical or chemical means or by substances that arrest the blood flow.

hemostatic An agent that reduces bleeding by speeding clot formation.

hemothorax A collection of blood in the pleural space, which causes the lung to collapse.

hemotympanum Blood behind the tympanic membrane from fractures of the temporal bone.

heparin A substance that inhibits blood clotting; it is obtained from the liver.

heparin lock A peripheral vascular access device that has no attached IV tubing; it is used to ensure ready access to peripheral veins for brief administration of medications or when frequent IV therapy is indicated on an outpatient basis (e.g., chemotherapy).

hepatic artery The branch of the aorta that delivers blood to the liver.

hepatic encephalopathy A type of brain damage caused by liver disease and consequent ammonia intoxication.

hepatic portal system The system that transports blood from the digestive tract to the liver.

hepatitis An inflammatory condition of the liver characterized by jaundice, hepatomegaly, anorexia, abdominal and gastric discomfort, abnormal liver function, clay-colored stools, and dark urine. Viruses responsible for hepatitis are hepatitis A virus (HAV), hepatitis B virus (HBV), hepatitis C virus (HCV), hepatitis D virus (HDV), and hepatitis E virus (HEV).

hepatitis A virus (HAV) See *hepatitis.*

hepatitis B virus (HBV) See *hepatitis.*

hepatitis C virus (HCV) See *hepatitis.*

hepatomegaly Enlargement of the liver.

Hering-Breuer reflex A reflex in which afferent impulses from stretch receptors in the lungs arrest inspiration; expiration then occurs.

hernia Protrusion of any organ through an abdominal opening in the muscle wall of the cavity that surrounds it.

herniation A protrusion of a body organ or portion of an organ through an abnormal opening in a membrane, muscle, or other tissue.

herpes Any of several acute inflammatory viral diseases characterized by the eruption of small blisters on the skin and mucous membranes.

herpes simplex virus type 1 (HSV-1) An infection caused by the herpes simplex virus; it tends to occur in the facial area, particularly around the mouth and nose.

herpes simplex virus type 2 (HSV-2) An infection caused by the herpes simplex virus; it usually is limited to the genital region.

hertz (Hz) A unit of frequency equal to 1 cycle per second.

hexaxial reference system The system of intersecting lines of the standard limb leads and three other intersecting lines of reference: aVR, aVL, and aVF leads.

hiatal hernia Protrusion of a portion of the stomach upward through the diaphragm.

Hickman catheter A long, indwelling catheter sometimes used by patients with cancer, gastrointestinal dysfunction, or debilitating disease and by those who need intermittent intravenous administration of antibiotics, nutritional supplements, or other intravenous medications.

high-altitude cerebral edema (HACE) The most severe form of acute high-altitude illness; it is characterized by a progression of global cerebral signs, in addition to acute mountain sickness, that are probably related to increased intracranial pressure.

high-altitude pulmonary edema (HAPE) An illness thought to be related, at least in part, to increased pulmonary artery pressure that develops in response to hypoxia; it results in the release of leukotrienes, which increase pulmonary arteriolar permeability, and in leakage of fluid into extravascular locations.

high-grade AV block Occurs when at least two consecutive AV impulses (atrial P waves) fail to be conducted to the ventricles.

hilum A depression or pit at the part of an organ where the vessels and nerves enter.

hinge joint A joint that consists of a convex cylinder in one bone applied to a corresponding concavity in another bone; this type of joint allows movement in one plane only.

histamine An amine released by mast cells and basophils that promotes inflammation.

history taking Information gathered during an interview with a patient.

Hodgkin's disease A malignant disorder characterized by painless, progressive enlargement of lymphoid tissue, splenomegaly, and the presence of Reed-Sternberg cells.

homeopathic Pertaining to homeopathy, a system of therapeutics in which diseases are treated with small doses of drugs that, in larger doses, are capable of producing in healthy people symptoms like those of the disease to be treated.

homeostasis A state of equilibrium in the body with respect to functions and composition of fluids and tissues.

horizontal plane Any place of the erect body parallel to the horizon; dividing the body into upper and lower parts.

human immunodeficiency virus (HIV) The viral agent responsible for acquired immunodeficiency syndrome (AIDS).

humerus The largest bone of the upper arm, comprising a body, head, and condyle.

humoral immunity One of the two forms of immunity that respond to antigens such as bacteria and foreign tissue.

Huntington's disease A rare, hereditary disease characterized by quick, involuntary movements, speech disturbances, and mental deterioration; it is caused by degenerative changes in the cerebral cortex and basal ganglia; also known as *Huntington's chorea.*

hyaline cartilage Gelatinous, glossy cartilage tissue; it thinly covers the articulating ends of bones, connects the ribs to the sternum, and supports the nose, trachea, and part of the larynx.

hydrocephalus A pathological condition characterized by an abnormal accumulation of cerebrospinal fluid, usually under increased pressure, within the cranial vault, resulting in dilation of the ventricles.

hydrochloric acid (HCl) The acid in gastric juice.

hydrogen ion The acidic element in a solution.

hymen A mucous membrane that may partly or entirely occlude the vaginal outlet.

Hymenoptera A large, highly specialized order of insects that includes wasps, bees, and ants.

hyoid bone The U-shaped bone between the mandible and the larynx.

hyperbilirubinemia Larger than normal amounts of the bile pigment bilirubin in the blood, often characterized by jaundice, anorexia, and malaise.

hypercalcemia A greater than normal concentration of calcium in the blood.

hypercholesterolemia Increased serum cholesterol.

hypercoagulability A tendency of the blood to coagulate more rapidly than normal.

hyperglycemia A greater than normal amount of glucose in the blood.

hyperkalemia A greater than normal concentration of potassium in the blood.

hyperkaluria A high potassium concentration in the urine.

hyperlipidemia An excess of lipids in the plasma.

hypermagnesemia A condition that results from an abnormally high concentration of magnesium in the blood plasma.

hypernatremia A greater than normal concentration of sodium in the blood.

hyperosmolar hyperglycemic nonketotic (HHNK) coma A diabetic coma in which the level of ketone bodies is normal; it is caused by hyperosmolarity of extracellular fluid, resulting in dehydration of intracellular fluid.

hyperparathyroidism A condition of increased parathyroid function.

hyperphosphatemia High levels of alkaline phosphate in the blood.

hyperplasia An increase in the number of cells of a body part.

hyperpolarization An increase in the charge difference across the cell membrane; it causes the charge difference to move away from 0 mV.

hypersensitivity reaction An altered immunological response to an antigen that results in a pathological immune response after reexposure.

hypersomina Excessive drowsiness; a sleep disorder of excessive depth or duration.

hypertension A disorder characterized by elevated blood pressure, which persistently exceeds 140/90 mm Hg.

hypertensive crisis A sudden, severe increase in blood pressure over 200/120 mm Hg.

hypertensive encephalopathy A set of symptoms, including headache, convulsions, and coma, associated with glomerulonephritis.

hyperthermia Abnormal elevation of body temperature.

hyperthyroidism A condition characterized by increased activity of the thyroid gland.

hypertonic A solution that causes cells to shrink.

hyperuricemia See *gout*.

hypertrophy An increase in the size of an organ caused by an increase in the size of the cells rather than the number or cells.

hyperventilation syndrome A persistent, rapid, and deep respiration that often results in hyperpnea.

hyphema A hemorrhage into the anterior chamber of the eye; it usually is a result of blunt trauma.

hypocalcemia A lower than normal concentration of calcium in the blood.

hypocarbia A deficiency of carbon dioxide in the blood; also known as hypocapnia.

hypochlorhydria A deficiency of hydrochloric acid in the stomach's gastric juice.

hypoglycemia A lower than normal amount of glucose in the blood.

hypokalemia A lower than normal concentration of potassium in the blood.

hypomagnesemia A condition that results from an abnormally low concentration of magnesium in the blood plasma.

hyponatremia A lower than normal concentration of sodium in the blood.

hypoparathyroidism A condition of diminished parathyroid function.

hypoperfusion Inadequate circulation that results in insufficient delivery of oxygen and nutrients necessary for normal tissue and cellular function; also known as *shock*.

hypopyon An accumulation of pus in the anterior chamber of the eye.

hypotension An abnormal condition in which the blood pressure is not adequate for normal perfusion and oxygenation of the tissues.

hypopituitarism An abnormal condition caused by diminished activity of the pituitary gland; it is marked by excessive deposits of fat or acquisition of adolescent characteristics.

hypothalamus A portion of the diencephalon of the brain that activates, controls, and integrates the peripheral autonomic nervous system, endocrine processes, and many somatic functions such as body temperature, sleep, and appetite.

hypothermia An abnormal body temperature below 95° F (35° C).

hypothyroidism A condition characterized by decreased activity of the thyroid gland.

hypotonia A condition of diminished tone or tension that may involve any body structure.

hypotonic A solution that causes cells to swell.

hypotonicity of the muscles Decreased muscle tone or tension.

hypovolemia An abnormally low circulating blood volume.

hypovolemic shock A form of shock most frequently caused by hemorrhage but also caused by dehydration.

hypoxia Inadequate, reduced tension of cellular oxygen characterized by cyanosis, tachycardia, hypotension, peripheral vasoconstriction, and mental confusion.

hypoxemia An abnormal deficiency of oxygen in the arterial blood.

hypoxic drive The low arterial oxygen pressure stimulus to respiration that is mediated through the carotid bodies.

I band See *isotropic band.*

iatrogenic Caused by treatment or diagnostic procedures.

identical twins Two offspring born of the same pregnancy and developed from a single fertilized ovum that splits into equal halves during the early phase of embryonic development, giving rise to separate fetuses.

idiopathic epilepsy See *primary epilepsy.*

idiosyncrasy An abnormal or peculiar response to a drug; it is thought to result from genetic enzymatic deficiencies or other unique physiological variables that lead to abnormal mechanisms of drug metabolism or altered physiological effects of the drug.

idioventricular rhythm A ventricular escape rhythm that results when impulses from higher pacemakers fail to reach the ventricles or when the rate of discharge of higher pacemakers become less than that of the ventricles.

ileocecal sphincter The valve between the ilium of the small intestine and the cecum of the large intestine.

ileostomy Surgical formation of an opening of the ileum onto the surface of the abdomen, through which fecal matter is emptied.

ileum The distal portion of the small intestine.

ileus An obstruction of the intestines.

iliac crest The upper free margin of the ilium.

iliac spine A portion of the iliac crest; the flaring portion of the hipbone.

ilium One of the three bones that make up the innominate bone.

immersion hypothermia Hypothermia from immersion in cold water.

immune response A defense mechanism of the body that produces antibodies to destroy invading antigens and malignancies.

immunity Insusceptibility to a particular disease or condition.

immunization The process of rendering a person immune or of becoming immune.

immunogen Any agent or substance capable of an immune response or of producing immunity.

immunoglobulin Any of five structurally and antigenically distinct antibodies present in the serum and external secretions of the body; they are IgA, IgD, IgE, IgG, and IgM.

implied consent The presumption that an unconscious or incompetent person would consent to lifesaving care.

incident command system (ICS) A management program designed to control, direct, and coordinate emergency response operations and resources.

incomplete abortion An abortion in which the patient has passed some but not all of the products of conception.

incomplete breech The presentation that occurs when the fetus has one or both hips incompletely flexed, resulting in the presentation of one or both lower extremities, often a foot.

incubation period A stage of infection during which the organism reproduces; it begins with invasion of the agent and ends when the disease process begins.

incus The middle of the three ossicles in the middle ear.

induced abortion The intentional termination of a pregnancy.

infectious pericarditis Inflammation of the pericardium associated with infection.

inferior Below a given point of reference.

inferior nasal concha bone One of three bony ridges on the lateral wall of the nasal cavity.

inferior vena cava The vein that returns blood from the lower limbs and the greater part of the pelvic and abdominal organs to the right atrium.

infertility The inability to produce offspring.

infiltration The process whereby a fluid passes into tissues.

influenza A highly contagious infection of the respiratory tract transmitted by airborne droplet infection. Researchers have identified three main types of the virus (types A, B, and C).

informed consent Consent obtained from a patient after all facts necessary for the patient to make a reasonable decision have been explained.

inguinal canal The passage through the lower abdominal wall that transmits the spermatic cord in the male and the round ligament in the female.

inguinal node One of approximately 18 nodes in the group of lymph glands in the upper femoral triangle of the thigh.

inhalation injury An upper or lower airway injury (or both) that results from thermal or chemical exposure, or both.

injury risk Actually or potentially hazardous situations that increase the possibility of a person sustaining an injury.

injury surveillance The ongoing, systematic collection, analysis, and interpretation of injury data essential to the planning, implementation, and evaluation of public health practice.

inner ear The part of the ear that contains the sensory organs for hearing and balance.

inotropic Pertaining to the force or energy of muscle contraction, particularly contractions of the heart.

insertion The more movable attachment point of a muscle.

insomina A chronic inability to sleep or to remain asleep throughout the night.

inspection A visual assessment of the patient and surroundings.

inspiration The act of drawing air into the lungs.

inspiratory capacity The sum of the tidal volume and the inspiratory reserve volume.

inspiratory center The region of the medulla that stimulates inspiration.

inspiratory reserve volume The maximum volume of air that can be inspired after a normal inspiration.

insulin A hormone secreted by the pancreatic islets.

integumentary system The largest organ system of the body; it consists of the skin and accessory structures such as hair, nails, and a variety of glands.

interatrial septum Tissue that separates the right and left atria of the heart.

intercalated disk Cell to cell attachment with gap junctions between cardiac muscle cells.

intercellular Occurring between or among cells.

interference Any undesired radio signal on a radio frequency. It may arise from other radio transmitters or other sources of electromagnetic radiation. "Nuisance interference" is interference that can be heard but does not override system signals. "Destructive interference" overrides system signals.

internal anal sphincter A sphincter muscle located at the caudal end of the rectum.

internal carotid artery Each of two arteries that enter the cranial vault through the carotid canals.

internal jugular vein One of a pair of veins in the neck; each collects blood from one side of the brain, the face, and the neck, and both unite with the subclavian vein to form the brachiocephalic vein.

internal mammary artery One of the pair of arteries that arise from the first portions of the subclavian arteries; it supplies the pectoral muscles, breasts, pericardium, and abdominal muscles; also known as the *internal thoracic artery*.

internal thoracic artery See *internal mammary artery*.

internal urinary sphincter The smooth muscle of the bladder located at the junction of the urethra with the urinary bladder; it controls the flow of urine through the urethra.

interneuron See *motor neuron*.

internodal tract Pathways between the segments of a nerve fiber.

interpolated PVC A PVC that falls between two sinus beats without interrupting the rhythm.

interstitial fluid Fluid that occupies the space outside the blood vessels.

interventricular foramen One of two passageways between the two lateral ventricles and the third ventricle.

interventricular septum The tissue that separates the right and left ventricles of the heart.

intervertebral disk One of the fibrous disks between all adjacent spinal vertebrae except the atlas and axis; it serves as a "shock absorber" for the vertebral column and provides additional support for the body; it also prevents the vertebral bodies from rubbing against each other.

intracellular Occurring within cell membranes.

intracellular fluid (ICF) Fluid within cell membranes throughout most of the body.

intracerebral hematoma A collection of blood within the tissues of the brain.

intradermal injection The introduction of a substance (e.g., serum or vaccine) with a hypodermic needle into the dermis.

intramuscular injection The introduction of medication with a hypodermic needle into muscle.

intraocular pressure Pressure within the eye that keeps the eye inflated.

intraosseous injection The introduction of medication or fluid into the bone marrow.

intraosseous infusion (IO infusion) Placement of a rigid needle into a bone and the infusion of fluid and medication directly into the bone marrow.

intrapartum Pertaining to the period of labor and delivery.

intrapleural Within the pleura.

intrapleural pressure See *intrathoracic pressure*.

intrapulmonic pressure The pressure of the gas within the alveoli; it varies slightly above and below 760 mm Hg.

intrathecal injection The introduction of medication with a hypodermic needle into the subarachnoid space.

intrathoracic pressure The pressure in the pleural space; it is usually 751 to 754 mm Hg; also known as *intrapleural pressure*.

intravenous injection The introduction of medication with a hypodermic needle into a vein.

intrinsic factor The factor secreted by the parietal cells of the gastric glands; it is required for adequate absorption of vitamin B_{12}.

invagination Infolding or in-pocketing.

invasion of privacy Making public, without legal justification, details about a person's private life that might reasonably expose that person to ridicule, notoriety, or embarrassment.

inversion Turning inward.

involuntary Occurring without conscious control or direction.

involuntary consent Treatment granted by authority of law.

involuntary muscle A muscle that is not normally consciously controlled; see *smooth muscle*.

ion An atom or group of atoms carrying a charge of electricity by virtue of having gained or lost one or more electrons.

ipsilateral Pertaining to the same side of the body.

iris The colored contractile membrane of the eye that can be seen through the cornea.

iron deficiency anemia Anemia caused by inadequate supplies of iron needed to synthesize hemoglobin.

irregular bones Bones that are not representative of the other three categories (long, short, or flat bones); examples include vertebrae and facial bones.

ischemia A decreased supply of oxygenated blood to a body organ or part, often marked by pain.

ischium One of the three parts of the hipbone, which joins the ilium and the pubis to form the acetabulum.

islets of Langerhans Clusters of cells within the pancreas that produce insulin, glucagon, and pancreatic polypeptide.

isoimmunity An immune response directed against beneficial foreign tissues.

isolette A self-contained incubator unit that provides controlled heat, humidity, and oxygen for the isolation and care of premature and low birth weight neonates.

isometric contraction A muscle contraction in which the length of the muscle does not change, but the tension produced increases.

isotonic solution A solution that causes cells to neither shrink nor swell.

isotonic contraction A muscle contraction in which the tension produced by the muscle stays the same, but the muscle length becomes shorter.

Jacksonian seizure A transitory disturbance in motor, sensory, or autonomic function resulting from abnormal neuronal discharges in a localized part of the brain; also known as a *focal seizure*.

jaundice A yellow discoloration of the skin, mucous membranes, and sclerae of the eyes, caused by a greater than normal amount of bilirubin in the blood.

jejunum One of the three portions of the small intestine.

joint Any one of the connections between bones that are classified according to structure and movability as fibrous, cartilaginous, or synovial. Fibrous joints are immovable, cartilaginous joints are slightly movable, and synovial joints are freely movable.

joint capsule A well-defined structure that encloses a joint.

joint dislocation A displacement of one or more bones that comprise a joint.

Joule's law The principle that the amount of heat produced is directly proportional to the square of the current strength, times the resistance of the tissue, times the duration of the current flow.

J point The point at which the T wave takes off from the QRS complex.

jugular notch The superior margin of the manubrium; it is easily palpated at the anterior base of the neck; also known as the *suprasternal notch.*

jugular vein distention (JVD) Engorgement of jugular veins caused by an increase in central venous pressure; it is estimated by positioning the head of a supine patient at a 45-degree angle and observing the neck veins.

kallikrein/kinin system A proposed hormonal system that functions within the kidneys, mediating production of bradykinin, which acts as a vasodilator peptide.

Kaposi's sarcoma A malignant, multifocal neoplasm of reticuloendothelial cells that begins as soft, brownish or purple papules on the feet and slowly spreads in the skin, metastasizing to the lymph nodes and viscera; it is associated with diabetes, malignant lymphoma, AIDS, and other disorders.

Kehr's sign A common complaint associated with splenic injury in which pain is noted in the left shoulder; it is thought to be caused by referred pain secondary to irritation of the adjacent diaphragm from splenic hematoma or hemoperitoneum.

Kent fibers See *bundle of Kent.*

keratitis Any inflammation of the cornea.

ketoacidosis Acidosis accompanied by the accumulation of ketones in the body, resulting from faulty carbohydrate metabolism.

ketoacids Compounds containing the carbonyl and carboxyl groups.

ketogenesis The formation or production of ketone bodies.

ketone bodies The normal metabolic products of lipid and pyruvate within the liver; excessive production leads to their excretion in urine.

ketonuria Presence in the urine of excessive amounts of ketone bodies.

kidney The organ that cleanses the body of the waste products continually produced by metabolism.

kilogram (kg) A metric unit of mass equal to 1000 grams or 2.2046 pounds.

kilohertz (KHz) A unit of frequency equal to 1000 cycles per second.

kinematics The process of predicting injury patterns that may result from the forces and motions of energy.

kinin Serum protein that causes vasodilation and increases vascular permeability.

KKK standards The national standards that provide the foundation of uniformity among ambulance vehicles.

Koplik's spots Small red spots with bluish white centers on the lingual and buccal mucosa, characteristic of measles.

Korsakoff's psychosis A form of amnesia seen in alcoholics that is characterized by a loss of short-term memory and an inability to learn new skills.

Krebs cycle A sequence of enzymatic reactions involving the metabolism of carbon chains of sugar, fatty acids, and amino acids to yield carbon dioxide, water, and high-energy phosphate bonds.

Kussmaul respiration An abnormally deep, very rapid sighing respiratory pattern characteristic of diabetic ketoacidosis or other metabolic acidosis.

kyphosis An abnormal condition of the vertebral column characterized by increased convexity in the curvature of the thoracic spine as viewed from the side.

labial frenulum A medial fold of mucous membrane connecting the inside of each lip to the corresponding gum.

labia majora Two rounded folds of skin surrounding the labia minora and the vestibule.

labia minora Two longitudinal folds of mucous membrane enclosed by the labia majora and bounding the vestibule.

laceration A torn or jagged wound.

lacrimal bone One of the smallest and most fragile bones of the face; it is located in the anterior part of the medial wall of the orbit.

lacrimal canal The canal that carries excess tears away from the eye.

lacrimal gland The tear gland located in the superolateral corner of the orbit.

lacrimal sac An enlargement of the lacrimal canal that leads into the nasolacrimal duct.

lacrimation Excessive tear production.

lactate A salt of lactic acid.

lactation The secretion of milk from the breasts to nourish an infant or child.

lactic acid A three-carbon molecule derived from pyruvic acid as a product of anaerobic respiration.

lactic acidosis A disorder characterized by an accumulation of lactic acid in the blood, resulting in a lowered pH in muscle and serum.

lactiferous duct The duct that drains the grapelike cluster of milk-secreting glands in the breast.

lactose intolerance A sensitivity disorder resulting in the ability to digest lactose because of a deficiency of or defect in the enzyme lactase.

landing zone (LZ) An area prepared for the landing of an aircraft; it is generally 100 by 100 feet.

lanugo hair Soft, downy hair covering a normal fetus.

laparoscopy Examination of the abdominal cavity with a laparoscope.

large intestine The portion of the digestive tract comprising the cecum, the appendix, the ascending, transverse, and descending colons, and the rectum.

laryngectomy Surgical removal of the larynx, performed to treat cancer of the larynx.

laryngopharynx The lowest part of the pharynx.

laryngoscope An endoscope for visualization of the larynx.

laryngoscopy Examination of the larynx via a laryngoscope.

laryngotracheobronchitis See *croup.*

larynx The voice box, located just below the pharynx.

latent period A stage of infection that begins with pathogenic invasion of the body and ends when the agent can be shed or communicated.

latent period of drug action See *onset of action.*

lateral malleolus The rounded process on the lateral side of the ankle joint.

lateral recumbent position The position in which the patient is lying on his or her right or left side.

lateral ventricle A large, fluid-filled space in each cerebral hemisphere.

laxative A substance that causes evacuation of the bowel by increasing the bulk of the feces, by softening the stool, or by lubricating the intestinal wall.

lead An electrode sensor attached to the body to record electrical activity, especially of the heart and brain.

Le Fort fracture Three patterns of injury that can be produced in the midface region.

left anterior descending artery The subdivision of the left coronary artery that supplies the left auricle and its appendix and supplies branches to both ventricles and numerous small branches to the pulmonary artery and commencement of the aorta.

left coronary artery One of a pair of branches from the ascending aorta that supplies both ventricles and the left atrium.

legend A prescription drug.

Legionnaires' disease See *legionellosis.*

legionellosis An acute bacterial pneumonia caused by infection with *Legionella pneumophila*; it is characterized by an influenza-like illness followed within a week by high fever, chills, muscle aches, and headache.

Lenègre's disease See *Lev's disease.*

lens The crystalline portion of the eye.

lethargy A state of indifference, apathy, or sluggishness.

leukemia A malignant neoplasm of blood-forming organs.

leukocyte White blood cell.

leukocytosis An abnormal increase in the number of circulating white blood cells.

Lev's disease Third-degree block in the elderly from chronic degenerative changes in the conduction system; it is not usually associated with increased parasympathetic tone or drug toxicity; also known as *Lenègre's disease.*

libel Publishing in writing false statements about someone, knowing them to be false, with malicious intent or with reckless disregard for their falsity.

libido The drive associated with sexual desire, pleasure, or creativity.

licensure The process by which a government agency grants permission to an individual to engage in an occupation or profession.

life-threat An illness or injury that threatens survival.

ligament A band of white, fibrous tissue that connects bones.

ligamentum arteriosum A fibrous cord from the pulmonary artery to the branch of the aorta; the remains of the ductus arteriosus of the fetus.

limbic system The parts of the brain involved with emotions and olfaction.

linear fracture A fracture that extends parallel to the long axis of a bone but does not displace the bone tissue.

lingual tonsil A collection of lymphoid tissue on the posterior portion of the dorsum of the tongue.

lipid Any of the free fatty acid fractions in the blood.

lipid bilayer The central layer of the cytoplasmic membrane; it is composed of a double layer of lipid molecules.

lipodystrophy Any abnormality in the metabolism or distribution of fats.

lipoprotein A conjugated protein in which lipids form an integral part of the molecule; it is synthesized primarily in the liver.

liquefaction Conversion of solid tissues to a fluid or semifluid state.

liter (L) A metric unit of capacity equal to 1 cubic decimeter, 61.025 cubic inches, or 1.0567 liquid quarts.

Littre's gland The inner surface of the membrane lining the urethra; it presents the orifices of numerous mucus glands and follicles situated in the submucosal tissue.

loading dose A large quantity of drug that temporarily exceeds the body's capacity to excrete the drug.

lobule A small lobe or subdivision of a lobe.

long bones Bones that are longer than they are wide, such as the humerus, ulna, radius, femur, tibia, fibula, and phalanges.

long saphenous vein See *saphenous vein.*

loop diuretic A group of powerful, short-acting agents that inhibit sodium and chloride reabsorption in the loop of Henle, resulting in an excessive loss of potassium and water and an increase in the excretion of sodium.

loop of Henle The U-shaped portion of the renal tubule.

lordosis An inward curvature in the lumbar spine that is normally present to some degree.

lower esophageal sphincter The ring of muscle located at the inferior end of the esophagus that regulates the passage of materials out of the esophagus.

lucid interval A period of relative mental clarity between periods of decreased consciousness or irrationality.

lumbosacral plexus The combination of all the ventral primary divisions of the lumbar, sacral, and coccygeal nerves.

lumbar vertebrae The five largest segments of the movable part of the vertebral column; they are designated L1 to L5.

lumen A cavity or channel within any organ or structure of the body.

Lund and Browder chart A method used to determine the area of burn injury that assigns specific numbers to each body part; it is often used to measure burns in infants and young children.

lung One of a pair of light, spongy organs in the thorax; the main component of the respiratory system.

lunula The crescent-shaped white area of the nail; it is most visible on the thumbnail.

luxation A complete dislocation.

Lyme disease An acute, recurrent inflammatory infection; it is transmitted by a tick-borne spirochete.

lymph node An encapsulated mass of lymph tissue found among lymph vessels.

lymphangitis An inflammation of one or more lymphatic vessels.

lymphatic system A complex network of capillaries, thin vessels, valves, ducts, nodes, and organs that helps protect and maintain the internal fluid environment of the body.

lymphocyte A type of white blood cell formed in lymphoid tissue.

lymphokine One of the chemical factors produced and released by T lymphocytes that attract macrophages to the site of infection or inflammation.

lymphoma A neoplasm of lymphoid tissue, usually malignant.

lyse To cause decomposition.

lysis The process by which a cell swells and ruptures.

lysosome A membranous-walled organelle that contains enzymes, which enable it to function as an intracellular digestive system.

macrodrip tubing An apparatus used to deliver measured amounts of intravenous solutions at specific flow rates based on the size of drops of the solution. The drops delivered by a macrodrip are larger than those delivered by a microdrip.

macromolecule A molecule of colloidal size, such as a protein, nucleic acid, or polysaccharide.

macrophage A phagocytic cell in the immune system.

macula A small pigmented area that appears separate or different than the surrounding tissue.

maintenance dose The amount of a drug required to keep a desired steady state of drug concentration in the tissues.

major incident An emergency event in which available resources are insufficient to manage the number of casualties or the nature of the emergency.

malaise A vague feeling of weakness or discomfort.

malar eminence The zygomatic bone or cheekbone.

malaria A serious infectious illness caused by one or more of at least four species of the protozoan genus *Plasmodium*; it is characterized by chills, fever, anemia, and an enlarged spleen.

malignant Very dangerous or virulent; likely to cause death.

malleolus A rounded, bony process, such as the protuberance on each side of the ankle.

malleus The largest of the three ossicles in the middle ear.

Mallory-Weiss syndrome A condition characterized by massive bleeding after a tear in the mucous membrane at the junction of the esophagus and the stomach.

mamma The breast; the organ of milk secretion.

mammalian diving reflex A reflex triggered by immersing the face in cold water; it diverts blood from the arms and legs to the central circulation and lowers the heart rate as a result of vagal stimulation.

mammary gland An external accessory sex organ in females; breasts.

managed care Refers to patient care services that are provided to members by managed care organizations.

managed care organization A network that provides patient care services to its members, such as health maintenance organizations (HMOs) and preferred provider organizations (PPOs).

mandible A large bone that constitutes the lower jaw.

mania A phase of bipolar disorder characterized by elation, agitation, hyperexcitability, hyperactivity, and increased speed of thought or speech.

manic Pertaining to a specific psychosis.

manic-depressive disorder See *bipolar disorder.*

manubriosternal junction The point at which the manubrium joins the body of the sternum; the location of the second rib; also known as the sternal angle.

manubrium One of the three bones of the sternum; it has a broad, quadrangular shape that narrows caudally at its articulation with the superior end of the body of the sternum.

Marfan's syndrome An abnormal condition characterized by elongation of the bones, often with associated abnormalities of the eyes and cardiovascular system.

mastectomy Surgical removal of one or both breasts, performed to remove a malignant tumor.

mastication Chewing, tearing, or grinding food with the teeth while it is mixed with saliva.

mastoid air cell One of several spaces within the mastoid process of the temporal bone; it is connected to the middle ear by ducts.

maxilla One of a pair of large bones that form the upper jaw.

maxillary sinus One of the pair of large air cells that form a pyramidal cavity in the body of the maxilla.

McBurney's point A site of extreme sensitivity in acute appendicitis situated in the normal area of the appendix, approximately 2 inches from the right anterior-superior spine of the ilium, on a line between that spine and the umbilicus.

mean arterial pressure (MAP) The arithmetic mean of the blood pressure in the arterial portion of the circulation minus intracranial pressure.

measles An acute, highly contagious viral disease involving the respiratory tract that is characterized by a spreading, maculopapular, cutaneous rash.

meconium aspiration syndrome Inhalation of meconium by the fetus or newborn; the meconium can block the air passages and result in failure of the lungs to expand or cause other pulmonary dysfunction.

meconium staining The presence of fetal stool in amniotic fluid.

medial malleolus The rounded process on the medial side of the ankle joint.

mediastinitis Inflammation of the mediastinum.

mediastinum A portion of the thoracic cavity in the middle of the thorax, between the pleural sacs containing the two lungs; it extends from the sternum to the vertebral column and contains all the thoracic viscera except the lungs.

mediated transport mechanism A mechanism that uses carrier molecules to move large water-soluble molecules or electrically charged molecules across cell membranes.

medical asepsis The removal or destruction of disease-causing organisms or infected material.

medical direction The authority responsible for ensuring that actions taken on behalf of ill or injured people are medically appropriate, including prospective, concurrent, and retrospective aspects of EMS, quality improvement, hiring, and education.

medulla The lowest part of the brain stem, which controls vital functions; an enlarged extension of the spinal cord; also known as the *medulla oblongata*.

medulla oblongata See *medulla*.

medullary cavity A large, marrow-filled cavity in the diaphysis of a long bone.

megahertz (MHz) A unit of frequency equal to 1 million cycles per second; EMS radios transmit and receive on frequencies measured in megahertz.

melanocyte A body cell capable of producing melanin.

melatonin The only hormone secreted in the bloodstream by the pineal gland; it lightens skin pigmentation and may inhibit numerous endocrine functions.

melena Abnormal black, tarry stools containing digested blood.

membrane channel A tunnel through which specific molecules may pass.

membranous labyrinth A membranous structure within the inner ear; it forms the cochlea, vestibule, and semicircular canals.

menarche The first menstruation and the commencement of the cyclic menstrual function.

meninges Fluid-containing membranes surrounding the brain and spinal cord.

meningitis Inflammation of the meninges.

menopause The cessation of menses.

menstruation The periodic discharge through the vagina of a bloody secretion containing tissue debris from the shedding of the endometrium from the nonpregnant uterus.

mental illness A disturbance of emotional equilibrium as manifested in maladaptive behavior and impaired functioning; also known as a mental disorder.

merocrine gland A gland that secretes products with no loss of cellular material, such as a water-producing sweat gland.

mesencephalon See *midbrain*.

mesentery The double layer of peritoneum extending from the abdominal wall to the abdominal viscera; it conveys vessels and nerves.

mesovarium A short peritoneal fold connecting the ovary with the broad ligament of the uterus.

metabolic acidosis A disorder that results when excess acid is added to the body fluids or bicarbonate is lost from them.

metabolic alkalosis A disorder that results from a significant loss of acid in the body or increased levels of base bicarbonate.

metabolism The culmination of all chemical processes that take place in living organisms.

metabolite A substance that is produced by metabolic action or that is necessary for the metabolic process.

metacarpal One of five bones extending from the carpus to the phalanges.

metaplasia The conversion of normal tissue cells into an abnormal form in response to chronic stress or injury.

metarteriole One of the small peripheral blood vessels that contain scattered groups of smooth muscle fibers in their walls; they are located between the arterioles and the true capillaries.

metatarsal Any one of the five bones comprising the metatarsus.

meter (m) A metric unit of length equal to 39.37 inches.

methanol A chemical widely used as a solvent and in the production of formaldehyde.

methemoglobin A form of hemoglobin in which the iron component has been oxidized from the ferrous to the ferric state.

methemoglobinemia The presence of methemoglobin in the blood, causing cyanosis as a result of the red cell's inability to release oxygen.

microdrip tubing An apparatus for delivering relatively small amounts of intravenous solutions at specific flow rates; the drops delivered by a microdrip are smaller than those delivered by a macrodrip.

microgram (μg) A metric unit of mass equal to equal to $^1/_{1,000,000}$ of a gram.

microinfarct A very small infarct caused by obstruction of circulation in capillaries, arterioles, or small arteries.

microorganism Any tiny, usually microscopical entity capable of carry on living processes, such as bacteria, fungi, protozoa, and viruses.

microthrombus A minute thrombus.

microtubule A hollow tube that helps to support the cytoplasm of the cell; a component of certain cell organelles such as centrioles, spindle fibers, cilia, and flagella.

microwave Radio waves with frequencies of 890 MHz and upward. The signals are generated by special equipment that depends on line of sight placement to operate properly. Microwave channels may have a wide band to carry a large number of simultaneous transmissions.

midbrain One of the three parts of the brain stem; also known as the *mesencephalon*.

middle cerebral artery The artery that supplies a large portion of the lateral cerebral cortex.

middle ear An air-filled space within the temporal bone that contains the auditory ossicles.

milliequivalent (mEq) $^1/_{1000}$ of a gram equivalent.

milligram (mg) A metric unit of mass equal to $^1/_{1000}$ of a gram.

milliliter (mL) A metric unit of capacity equal to $^1/_{1000}$ of a liter.

millimeter (mm) A metric unit of length equal to $^1/_{1000}$ of a meter.

mineral An inorganic substance usually referred to by the name of the compound of which it is a part; minerals are important in regulating many body functions.

mineralocorticoid A hormone secreted by the adrenal cortex that maintains normal blood volume, promotes sodium and water retention, and increases urine secretion of potassium and hydrogen ions.

minim (m) A measure of volume in the apothecaries' system, originally 1 drop of water; 60 minims equal 1 fluid dram, and 1 minim equals 0.06 mL.

minimal effective concentration The lowest plasma concentration that produces the desired drug effect.

minute alveolar ventilation The amount of inspired gas available for gas exchange during 1 minute.

minute volume The tidal volume times the respiratory rate, or the amount of gas inhaled or exhaled in 1 minute.

miscarriage See *spontaneous abortion.*

missed abortion The retention of the fetus in utero for 4 or more weeks after fetal death.

mitochondria Small spherical, rod-shaped, or thin filamentous structures in the cytoplasm of cells; a site of ATP production.

mitosis Cell division resulting in two daughter cells with exactly the same number and type of chromosomes as the mother cell.

mitral valve See *bicuspid valve.*

mitral valve prolapse Protrusion of one or both cusps of the mitral valve back into the left atrium during ventricular systole, resulting in incomplete closure of the valve and mitral insufficiency.

mittelschmerz Abdominal pain in the region of the ovary during ovulation; it usually occurs midway through the menstrual cycle.

MMR vaccine The abbreviation for live measles, mumps, and rubella virus vaccine.

mobile data terminal (MDT) A computer connected through a modem ("black box") with a radio that sends and receives pretyped messages to printers, computer screens, or both. Some MDTs have graphics (floor plans) and data base (hazardous materials) capabilities. MDTs rely on a host computer interfaced to a base station.

mobile repeater A mobile radio unit capable of automatically retransmitting any radio traffic originated by a handheld portable, by other mobiles, or by base stations. This repeater may be one-way or two-way and may be known as a PAC-RAT (Motorola) or an extender. Also known as a *vehicle repeater.*

mobile relay station A fixed base station that automatically retransmits mobile or portable radio communications back to the receiving frequency of other portables, mobiles, and base stations operating in the same system; also known as a *"repeater."*

mole A standard unit used to measure the amount of a substance.

monocyte A type of white blood cell found in lymph nodes, spleen, bone marrow, and loose connective tissue.

monomorphic Existing only in one form.

mons pubis The prominence caused by a pad of fatty tissue over the symphysis pubis in the female.

morals Social standards or customs; dealing with what is right or wrong in a practical sense.

morphology The study of the physical shape and size of a specimen, plant, or animal.

motor neuron A neuron that innervates skeletal, smooth, or cardiac muscle fibers; also known as an *interneuron.*

mucin The chief ingredient in mucus.

mucosa Mucous membrane.

mucus The viscous, slippery secretion of mucous membranes and glands.

multifocal PVC A premature ventricular complex that originates from multiple sites in the ventricles.

multigravida A woman who has had two or more pregnancies.

multipara A woman who has had two or more deliveries.

multiple gestation A pregnancy with more than one fetus.

multiple organ dysfunction syndrome (MODS) The progressive failure of two or more organ systems after a very severe illness or injury.

multiple myeloma A malignant neoplasm of the bone marrow.

multiple sclerosis (MS) A progressive disease characterized by disseminated demyelination of nerve fibers of the brain and spinal cord.

multiplex mode A system with the ability to simultaneously transmit two or more different types of information in either or both directions over the same frequency, such as telemetry and voice.

mumps An acute viral disease characterized by swelling of the parotid glands.

muscarinic receptor A class of cholinergic receptor molecule specifically activated by muscarine in addition to acetylcholine.

muscular dystrophy (MD) A group of genetically transmitted diseases characterized by progressive atrophy of symmetrical groups of skeletal muscles without evidence of involvement or degeneration of neural tissue.

muscular tissue A primary tissue type characterized by its contractile abilities.

mutagenic Any chemical or physical environmental agent that induces a genetic mutation or increases the mutation rate.

mutual aid An agreement with neighboring emergency agencies indicating that a mutual exchange of equipment and manpower will be available when called upon.

myalgia Diffuse muscle pain, usually accompanied by malaise; it occurs in many infectious diseases.

myasthenia Muscle weakness.

myasthenia gravis An abnormal condition characterized by chronic fatigue and weakness of muscles, especially in the face and throat; it results from a defect in the nerve impulses at the myoneural junction.

Mycoplasma A genus of microscopic organisms lacking rigid cell walls; they are considered to be the smallest free-living organisms.

myelinated axon A nerve fiber having a myelin sheath.

myeloblast Bone marrow cell.

Mycobacterium leprae A genus of gram-positive bacteria that causes leprosy.

Mycobacterium tuberculosis A genus of gram-positive bacteria that causes tuberculosis.

myocardial hypertrophy An abnormal increase in the size of cardiac muscle.

myocardial infarction (MI) Necrosis of a portion of cardiac muscle caused by obstruction in a coronary artery either from atherosclerosis or an embolus.

myoclonus A spasm of a muscle or group of muscles.

myoepithelium Tissue made up of contractile epithelial cells.

myofibril A slender, striated strand of smooth muscle.

myofilament An extremely fine, molecular, threadlike structure that helps to form the myofibril of muscle; thick myofibrils are formed of myosin, and thin myofilaments are formed of actin.

myoglobinuria The presence of myoglobin in the urine.

myometrium The muscular wall of the uterus.

myosin A cardiac and skeletal muscle protein; it comprises approximately half of the proteins that occur in muscle tissue.

myxedema The severest form of hypothyroidism; it is characterized by swelling of the hands, face, feet, and periorbital tissues.

nail bed The end of a finger or toe covered by the nail; it is abundant in blood vessels.

nail body The visible part of the nail.

narrative The portion of the patient care report that allows for a chronological description of the call.

narcolepsy A syndrome characterized by sudden sleep attacks and visual or auditory hallucinations at the onset of sleep.

nares Nostrils.

nasal bone The bony partition that separates the nasal cavity into left and right parts; also known as the nasal septum.

nasal septum A partition that separates the right and left nasal cavities.

nasogastric decompression The management of gastric distention or emesis control by means of a nasogastric tube.

nasogastric tube (NG tube) Any tube passed into the stomach through the nose.

nasolacrimal duct A duct that leads from the lacrimal sac to the nasal cavity.

nasopharynx The uppermost portion of the pharynx just behind the nasal cavities.

nasotracheal Accessing the trachea through the nasal cavity.

near-drowning Submersion with at least temporary survival.

nebulizer A device for producing a fine spray of medication for inhalation therapy.

necrosis Localized tissue death in response to disease or injury.

negative feedback mechanism Any mechanism that tends to balance a change in a system.

negligence Failure to use such care as a reasonably prudent EMS provider would use in similar circumstances; a deviation from a standard of care.

nematocyst A venomous stinging cell.

neonate An infant in the first 28 days of life.

neoplasia The new and abnormal development of cells.

neoplasm Abnormal growth; a malignant or benign tumor.

nephron The functional unit of the kidney.

nerve A bundle of nerve fibers and accompanying connective tissue located outside the central nervous system.

nerve tract Bundles of parallel axons with associated sheaths in the central nervous system.

nervous tissue A major tissue type characterized by its conductile abilities.

nervous tunic The retina.

neuralgia Pain along a nerve.

neurogenic hypotension Hypotension that occurs secondary to spinal shock; it is caused by a loss of sympathetic tone in the vessels.

neurogenic shock Shock resulting from vasomotor paralysis below the level of injury; also known as *spinal cord shock.*

neuroglia Cells in the nervous system other than neurons.

neurohormone A junction hormone secreted by a neuron.

neuromuscular A specialized synapse between a motor neuron and a muscle fiber.

neuromuscular junction The area of contact between the ends of a large myelinated nerve fiber and a fiber of skeletal muscle.

neuron The functional unit or the nervous system, consisting of the nerve cell body, the dendrites, and the axon.

neuropathy A disease of the peripheral nerves.

neurosis Any faulty or inefficient way of coping with anxiety or inner conflict; it may ultimately lead to a neurotic disorder.

neutrophil A small, phagocytic white blood cell with a lobed nucleus and small granules in the cytoplasm; it stains readily with neutral dyes.

newborn An infant in the first few hours of life.

Newton's first law of motion The principle that an object, whether at rest or in linear motion, remains in that state unless force is applied.

Newton's second law of motion The principle that force is equal to mass times acceleration or deceleration.

nicad batteries Nickel cadmium rechargeable batteries, which are used in portable radios.

nicotinic receptor A class of cholinergic receptor molecules that are specifically activated by nicotine and acetylcholine.

nit The egg of a parasitic insect, particularly a louse.

nitrogen narcosis A condition of depressed central nervous system function brought about by high partial pressure of nitrogen.

nocturia Particularly excessive urination at night.

node of Ranvier The short interval in the myelin sheath of a nerve fiber between adjacent Schwann cells.

noncardiogenic pulmonary edema See *adult respiratory distress syndrome (ARDS).*

noncompensatory pause The pause that occurs when the next expected P wave of the underlying cardiac rhythm appears earlier than it would have if the SA node had not been disturbed by a conduction abnormality.

noncompetitive antagonist An agent that combines with different parts of the receptor mechanism and inactivates the receptor so that the agonist cannot be effective regardless of its concentration.

nonconducted PAC A premature atrial complex blocked at the AV node.

nonelectrolyte A substance with no electrical charge.

nonproprietary name See *generic name.*

nonstriated muscle See *smooth muscle.*

noradrenalin An adrenergic hormone produced by the adrenal medulla, similar in chemical and pharmacological properties to epinephrine. It acts to increase blood pressure by vasoconstriction but does not affect cardiac output; also known as *norepinephrine.*

nuclear membrane A double membrane structure surrounding and enclosing the nucleus; also known as the *nuclear envelope.*

nucleic acids Extremely complex, long-chain compounds of high molecular weight that occur naturally in the cells of all living organisms; they form the genetic material of the cell and direct the synthesis of protein within the cell.

nucleolus Any one of the somewhat rounded, dense, well-defined nuclear bodies with no surrounding membrane; the nucleolus contains ribosomal RNA and protein.

nucleoplasm The protoplasm of the nucleus, as contrasted with that of the cell.

nucleus The central controlling body within a living cell.

nullipara A woman who has never borne a child.

nutrient Any substance that nourishes and aids the growth and development of the body.

nystagmus Involuntary, rhythmic movements of the eyes.

obesity An abnormal increase in the proportion of fat cells, mainly in the viscera and subcutaneous tissues of the body.

obligate Necessary; compulsory.

obsessive compulsive disorder (OCD) A psychiatric disorder in which the person feels stress or anxiety about thoughts or rituals over which he or she has little control.

obtundation A state of being insensitive to unpleasant or painful stimulation associated with a reduced level of consciousness, such as by anesthesia or a strong narcotic analgesic.

obturator foramen A large opening on each side of the lower portion of the hipbone, formed posteriorly by the ischium, superiorly by the ilium, and anteriorly by the pubis.

occipital bone The cuplike bone at the back of the skull, marked by a large opening (the foramen magnum), that communicates with the vertebral canal.

occipital lobe One of the five lobes of each cerebral hemisphere.

occiput posterior presentation An abnormal presentation in which the infant's head is delivered face up instead of face down.

oculomotor nerve The third cranial nerve, which contains both sensory and motor fibers; it provides for movement in most of the muscles of the eye, for constriction of the pupil, and for accommodation of the eye to light.

odontoid process The toothlike projection that rises perpendicularly from the upper surface of the body of the second cervical vertebra or axis, which serves as a pivot point for the rotation of the atlas.

official name Usually the same as the generic name; the official name of a drug is followed by the initials "USP" or "NF," denoting its listing in one of the official publications.

off-line/indirect medical direction The establishment and monitoring of all medical components of an EMS system, including protocols, standing orders, educational programs, and the quality and delivery of on-line/direct medical direction.

olecranon fossa The depression in the posterior surface of the humerus that receives the olecranon of the ulna when the forearm is extended.

olecranon process The large bony process of the ulna; also known as the *olecranon.*

olfactory Of or pertaining to the sense of smell.

olfactory bulb The tissue that receives the olfactory nerves from the nasal cavity.

olfactory membranes Membranes that contain the receptors for the sense of smell; they are located in the roof of the nasal cavity.

olfactory recess The extreme superior region of the nasal cavity.

olfactory tract The nerve tract that projects from the olfactory bulb to the olfactory cortex.

oliguria A diminished capacity to form or pass urine.

omphalocele Congenital herniation of intraabdominal viscera through a defect in the abdominal wall around the umbilicus.

oncotic pressure See *blood colloid osmotic pressure.*

ongoing assessment A repeat of the initial assessment that is performed throughout the paramedic-patient encounter.

on-line/direct medical direction The medical direction physician who directly supervises prehospital care activities via radio or telephone. On-line/direct medical direction is also responsible for the activities of the emergency department staff and other designated physicians at the medical direction hospital.

onset of action The interval between the time a drug is administered and the first sign of its effects; also known as the latent period of drug action.

oocyte An incompletely developed ovum.

open vault fracture A fracture that results in direct communication between a scalp laceration and cerebral substance.

opiate A narcotic drug that contains opium, derivatives of opium, or any of several semisynthetic or synthetic drugs with opium-like activity.

opioid Any synthetic narcotic that has opiate-like activities but is not derived from opium.

opposition Movement of the thumb and little finger toward each other for the purpose of grasping objects.

optic nerve The nerve that carries visual signals from the eye to the crossing of the optic tracts.

orchitis Painful inflammation of the testicle.

organ A structure made up of two or more kinds of tissues, organized to perform a more complex function than any one tissue can manage alone.

organelle Any one of various particles of living substance bound within most cells, such as the mitochondria, the Golgi apparatus, the endoplasmic reticulum, the lysosomes, and the centrioles.

organ of Corti The organ of hearing; it is located in the cochlea and filled with endolymph.

oriented Aware of one's surroundings.

origin The less movable attachment point of a muscle.

orogastric decompression The management of gastric distention or emesis control by means of an orogastric tube.

oropharyngeolaryngeal axis The three axes of the mouth, pharynx, and trachea; a patient position used for direct visualization of the larynx.

oropharynx The portion of the pharynx located behind the mouth.

orthostatic hypotension Abnormally low blood pressure that occurs when an individual assumes the standing posture; also called *postural hypotension.*

orotracheal Gaining access to the trachea through the oral cavity.

osmolality The osmotic concentration of a solution.

osmosis Diffusion of solvent (water) through a membrane from a less concentrated solution to a more concentrated solution.

osmotic pressure The force required to prevent the movement of water across a selectively permeable membrane.

ossified To be changed or developed into bone.

osteoarthritis A form of arthritis in which one or many joints undergo degenerative changes.

osteomyelitis Local or generalized infection of bone and bone marrow, usually caused by bacteria introduced by trauma or surgery.

osteoporosis A disorder characterized by a reduction in bone density; it occurs most often in postmenopausal women.

ostomy Any surgical procedure in which an artificial opening is created between two hollow organs or between a hollow viscus and the abdominal wall.

otorrhea Any discharge from the external ear.

ounce (oz) A unit of weight equal to $1/16$ of a pound or 28.349 grams.

ovarian follicle The spherical cell aggregation in the ovary that contains an oocyte.

ovarian ligament The bundle of fibers that passes to the uterus from the ovary.

ovarian torsion Twisting of an ovary around its vascular pedicle.

ovary One of the pair of female gonads found on each side of the lower abdomen beside the uterus.

ovulation Release of an ovum or secondary oocyte from the vesicular follicle.

oxyhemoglobin Oxygenated hemoglobin.

pacemaker cell Certain myocardial cells capable of initiating an electrical impulse.

packaging See *patient packaging.*

Paget's disease A common, nonmetabolic disease of bone of unknown cause characterized by excessive bone destruction and unorganized bone repair.

paging equipment Equipment typically using tone activation with one-way transmission to receive-only units.

palate A structure that forms the roof of the mouth; it is divided into the hard and soft palates.

palatine bone One of a pair of bones of the skull forming the posterior part of the hard palate, part of the nasal cavity, and the floor of the orbit of the eye.

palatine tonsil One of two large oval masses of lymphoid tissue embedded in the lateral wall of the oropharynx.

palliative care A unique form of health care directed primarily at providing relief to terminally ill individuals through symptom management and pain management; also known as *comfort care.*

palpation A technique used in physical examination in which the examiner feels the texture, size, consistency, and location of certain parts of the body with the hands.

pancreas A fish-shaped nodular gland located across the posterior abdominal wall in the epigastric region of the body; it secretes various substances, including digestive enzymes, insulin, and glucagon.

pancreatic juice The fluid secretion of the pancreas produced by the stimulation of food in the duodenum.

pancreatitis Inflammation of the pancreas; it may be acute or chronic.

para The number of past pregnancies that have remained viable to delivery.

parainfluenza virus One of a group of viruses isolated from patients with upper respiratory tract disease of varying severity in infants and young children; it may cause croup, tracheobronchitis, bronchiolitis, bronchopneumonia, pharyngitis, and the common cold.

paralytic ileus The decrease in or absence of intestinal peristalsis that may occur after abdominal surgery, illness, or injury; the most common cause of intestinal obstruction.

parametritis An inflammatory condition of tissue of the structures around the uterus.

paraplegia Paralysis in the lower limbs and trunk.

parasagittal plane An imaginary vertical plane passing through the body parallel to the medial plane; it divides the body into left and right portions.

parasympathetic Of or pertaining to the craniosacral division of the autonomic nervous system.

parasympathetic nervous system The subdivision of the autonomic nervous system usually involved in activating vegetative functions such as digestion, defecation, and urination.

parasympatholytic agent Anticholinergic; producing effects resembling those of interruption or blockade of the parasympathetic nerve supply to effector organs or tissues.

parasympathomimetic agent An agent with effects that mimic those resulting from stimulation of parasympathetic nerves, especially the effects produced by acetylcholine.

parasystole An independent ectopic rhythm whose pacemaker cannot be discharged by impulses of the dominant rhythm because of an area of depressed conduction surrounding the parasystolic focus.

parenchyma The essential or functional elements of an organ.

parenteral Not in or through the digestive system.

parens patriae A term that refers to the state's authority to intervene over the objections of parents to protect children.

paresthesia A sensation of numbness, tingling, or "pins and needles."

parietal Of or pertaining to the outer wall of a cavity or organ.

parietal bone One of a pair of bones that form the side of the cranium.

parietal lobe The portion of each cerebral hemisphere that occupies the parts of the lateral and medial surfaces covered by the parietal bone.

parietal pericardium The portion of serous pericardium lining the fibrous pericardium.

parietal peritoneum The layer of peritoneum lining the abdominal walls.

Parkinson's disease A slowly progressive, degenerative neurological disorder characterized by resting tremor, loss of postural reflexes, and muscle rigidity and weakness.

parkinsonism A neurological disorder characterized by tremor, muscle rigidity, hypokinesia, a slow shuffling gait, and difficulty in chewing, swallowing, and speaking; it frequently occurs in patients treated with antipsychotic drugs.

parotitis Inflammation or infection of one or both parotid salivary glands.

paroxysm A sudden attack or recurrence of symptoms of a disease.

paroxysmal nocturnal dyspnea A sudden episode of dyspnea that occurs after lying down.

paroxysmal supraventricular tachycardia (PSVT) An ectopic rhythm in excess of 100 beats per minute and usually faster than 170 beats per minute that begins abruptly with a premature atrial or junctional beat and is supported by an AV nodal reentry mechanism or by an AV reentry mechanism involving an accessory pathway.

partial antagonist An agent that has affinity and some efficacy but that may antagonize the action of other drugs that have greater efficacy.

partial pressure The pressure exerted by a single gas; denoted by a P preceding the gas (e.g., PO_2).

partial reabsorption The amount of drug reabsorbed from the renal tubule by passive diffusion.

parturition The process of giving birth.

passive glomerular filtration The renal process where by fluid in the blood is filtered across the capillaries of the glomerulus and into the urinary space of Bowman's capsule.

patella A flat, triangular bone at the front of the knee joint; the kneecap.

patient care report (PCR) A document used in the prehospital setting to record all patient care activities and circumstances related to an emergency response.

patient packaging The completion of emergency care procedures needed to transfer a patient from the scene to the ambulance.

pattern recognition The process of comparing gathered information to the paramedic's knowledge base of medical illness and disease.

patterned injury Injuries that result from an identifiable object.

peak plasma level The highest plasma concentration attained from a dose.

pectoral girdle See *shoulder girdle.*

pectus deformity Malformation of the chest wall.

pediatric trauma score (PTS) An injury severity index that grades six components commonly seen in pediatric trauma patients: size (weight), airway, central nervous system, systolic blood pressure, open wound, and skeletal injury.

pelvic cavity The area of the body enclosed by the bones of the pelvis.

pelvic girdle The encircling bony structure supporting the lower limbs.

pelvic inflammatory disease (PID) Any inflammatory condition of the female pelvic organs, especially one caused by bacterial infection.

penetrating trauma Any wound that enters the body area, organ, or cavity.

penetration The flow of a hazardous liquid chemical through zippers, stitched seams, pinholes, or other imperfections in a material.

penis The external reproductive organ of the male.

pepsin The principal digestive enzyme of gastric juice.

pepsinogen A proenzyme formed and secreted by certain cells of the gastric mucosa.

peptide bond A chemical bond between amino acids.

peptic ulcer A sharply circumscribed loss of the mucous membrane of the stomach, duodenum, or any other part of the GI system.

peptic ulcer disease A condition that results from a complex pathological interaction among the acidic gastric juice and proteolytic enzymes and the mucosal barrier.

percussion A technique in physical examination of tapping the body with the fingertips to evaluate size, borders, and consistency of some of the internal organs and to discover the presence and evaluate the amount of fluid in the cavity of the body.

perfusion The circulation of blood to the tissues.

periappendiceal abscess A cavity containing pus and inflamed tissue around the vermiform appendix.

pericardial cavity The area of the body that surrounds the heart.

pericardial fluid A viscous fluid contained within the pericardial cavity between the visceral and parietal pericardium; it serves as a lubricant.

pericardial friction rub A dry, grating sound heard with a stethoscope during auscultation; suggestive of pericarditis.

pericardial sac The sac that surrounds the heart.

pericardial tamponade Compression of the heart produced by the accumulation of fluid or blood in the pericardial sac.

pericardiocentesis A procedure for withdrawing fluid from the pericardial sac.

pericarditis Inflammation of the pericardium.

pericardium The membrane that surrounds the heart.

perilymph The fluid contained within the bony labyrinth.

perinatal Occurring at or near the time of birth.

perineum The pelvic floor and associated structures occupying the pelvic outlet, bounded anteriorly by the pubic symphysis, laterally by the ischial tuberosities, and posteriorly by the coccyx.

periodontal membrane The membrane that surrounds the root of the tooth.

periosteum Tough connective tissue that covers the bone.

periostitis Inflammation of the periosteum; it is characterized by tenderness and swelling of the affected bone, pain, fever, and chills.

peripheral nervous system (PNS) A major subdivision of the nervous system consisting of nerves and ganglia.

peripheral neuropathy Any functional or organic disorder of the peripheral nervous system.

peripheral thermoreceptors Nerve endings sensitive to heat, located in the skin and some mucous membranes; they usually are categorized as cold or warm receptors.

peripheral vascular disease Any abnormal condition that affects the blood vessels outside the heart and lymphatic vessels.

peripheral vascular resistance (PVR) The total resistance against which blood must be pumped; also known as *afterload*.

peristaltic Pertaining to peristalsis.

peristalsis The coordinated, rhythmic and serial contraction of smooth muscle that forces food through the digestive tract, bile through the bile duct, and urine through the ureters.

peritoneal Pertaining to the peritoneum.

peritoneal cavity The potential space between the parietal and visceral layers of the peritoneum; the two layers normally are in contact.

peritoneal dialysis A procedure performed to correct an imbalance of fluid or electrolytes in the blood or to remove toxins, drugs, or other wastes normally excreted by the kidneys.

peritoneum The serous membrane that covers the abdominal wall of the body and is reflected over the contained viscera.

peritonitis Inflammation of the peritoneum.

peritubular capillary The capillary network located in the cortex of the kidney.

permeable A condition of being pervious so that fluids and other substances can pass through, as occurs in a semipermeable membrane.

permeation The process by which a hazardous liquid chemical moves through a material on a molecular level.

persistent generalized lymphadenopathy (PGL) Enlarged lymph nodes involving two noncontiguous sites other than inguinal nodes; a common feature in early HIV infection.

pertinent negative findings Findings that warrant no medical care or intervention but which, having been sought, show evidence of the thoroughness of the examination and history of the event.

pertussis An acute, highly contagious respiratory disease characterized by paroxysmal coughing that ends in a loud, whooping inspiration; also known as *whooping cough*.

petit mal seizure An epileptic seizure characterized by a sudden, momentary loss of consciousness occasionally accompanied by minor muscle spasms of the neck or upper extremities.

pH An inverse logarithm of the hydrogen ion concentration.

phagocytic Pertaining to phagocytosis.

phagocytosis The process of ingestion by cells of solid substances such as other cells, bacteria, bits of necrosed tissue, and foreign particles.

phalanges Any bone of a finger or toe.

pharmacodynamics The study of how a drug acts on a living organism.

pharmacokinetics The study of the action and effects of drugs within the body, including the routes and mechanisms of absorption and excretion, the rate at which a drug's action begins and the duration of the effect, and biotransformation.

pharmacology The science of drugs used to prevent, diagnose, and treat disease.

pharyngeal tonsil One of two collections of aggregated lymphoid nodules on the posterior wall of the nasopharynx.

pharyngitis Inflammation or infection of the pharynx.

phase 0 The rapid depolarization phase; it represents the very rapid upstroke of the action potential that occurs when the cell membrane reaches the threshold potential (approximately -70 mV).

phase 1 The early rapid repolarization phase; the phase in which the fast sodium channels close, the flow of sodium ions into the cell terminates, and loss of potassium from the cell continues.

phase 2 The plateau phase; the prolonged phase of slow repolarization of the action potential.

phase 3 The terminal phase of rapid repolarization; it results in the inside of the cell becoming markedly negative and the membrane potential returning to approximately -90 mV, or its resting level.

phase 4 The period between action potentials when the membrane has returned to its RMP.

phencyclidine psychosis A true psychiatric emergency with clinical syndromes ranging from a catatonic and unresponsive state to bizarre and violent behavior; it may occur after a single low-dose exposure to phencyclidine and may last several days to weeks.

phlebitis Inflammation of a vein, often accompanied by formation of a clot; also known as thrombophlebitis.

phlebotomy The incision of a vein for the letting of blood.

phobia An anxiety disorder characterized by an obsessive, irrational, and intense fear of a specific object or activity.

phonation The production of speech sounds.

phospholipid One of a class of compounds, widely distributed in living cells, that contains phosphoric acid, fatty acids, and a nitrogenous base.

photophobia Abnormal sensitivity to light.

physical dependence An adaptive physiological state that occurs after prolonged use of many drugs; discontinuation causes withdrawal syndromes that are relieved by readministering the same drug or a pharmacologically related drug.

physiological dead space The sum of the anatomical dead space plus the volume of any nonfunctional alveoli.

pia mater The innermost layer of the meninges that directly covers the brain.

Pickwickian syndrome An abnormal condition characterized by obesity, decreased pulmonary function, somnolence, and polycythemia.

pigmented retina The pigmented portion of the retina.

piloerection Erection of the hairs of the skin in response to cold environment, emotional stimulus, or irritation of the skin.

pineal gland A cone-shaped structure in the brain that secretes the hormone melatonin.

pinna See *auricle.*

pituitary gland A small gland attached to the hypothalamus; it supplies numerous hormones that govern many vital processes.

pivot joint A joint that consists of a relatively cylindrical bony process that rotates within a ring composed partly of bone and partly of ligament.

placard A four-sided, diamond-shaped sign displayed on hazardous material containers; usually yellow, red, orange, white, or green; it contains a four-digit United Nations identification number (UN number) and a legend to indicate the container's contents.

placebo An inactive substance or a less than effective dose of a harmless substance; it is used in experimental drug studies to compare the effects of the inactive substance with those of the experimental drug.

placenta A highly vascular fetal organ through which the fetus absorbs oxygen, nutrients, and other substances and excretes carbon dioxide and other wastes.

placental barrier A protective biological membrane that separates the blood vessels of the mother and fetus; it provides some protection to the fetus by preventing the passage of certain drugs.

placenta previa A condition of pregnancy in which the placenta is implanted abnormally in the uterus so that it impinges on or covers the internal os of the uterine cervix.

plane joint A joint that consists of two opposed flat surfaces that are approximately equal in size; also known as a *gliding joint.*

plasma The fluid portion of blood.

plasma membrane A part of the human cell that encloses the cytoplasm, forming the outer boundary of the cell; also known as the *cytoplasmic membrane.*

plasma-protein binding A type of drug reservoir in which drugs attach to proteins, mainly albumin, and form a drug-protein complex.

plateau phase Prolongation of the depolarization phase of cardiac muscle cell membrane; it results in a prolonged refractory period.

platelet A fragment of a cell; it contains granules in the central part and clear protoplasm peripherally but has no definite nucleus.

pleural cavity The area of the body that surrounds the lungs.

pleural fluid Serous fluid found in the pleural cavity; it helps to reduce friction when the pleural membranes rub together.

pleural friction rub A rubbing or grating sound that occurs as one layer of the pleural membrane slides over the other during breathing.

pleural lavage A rewarming technique that uses warm saline to irrigate the thorax; it is used to treat some patients with severe hypothermia.

pleural space The potential space between the visceral and parietal layers of the pleura.

pleurisy Inflammation of the parietal pleura of the lungs, characterized by dyspnea and stabbing chest pain.

plexus A network of intersecting nerves and blood vessels or lymphatic vessels.

pneumatic antishock garment (PASG) A garment used to manage some forms of hypovolemia and to stabilize some fractures.

pneumococcus A gram-positive diplococcal bacterium of the species *Diplococcus pneumoniae*; the most common cause of bacterial pneumonia.

***Pneumocystis carinii* pneumonia** A bacterial pneumonia caused by infection with the parasite *Pneumocystis carinii*; it is usually seen in infants or debilitated or immunosuppressed people and is characterized by fever, cough, tachypnea and, frequently, cyanosis.

pneumohemothorax A collection of air and blood in the pleural space; also known as a *hemopneumothorax.*

pneumomediastinum The presence of air or gas in the mediastinal tissues.

pneumonia An acute inflammation of the lungs, usually caused by inhaled pneumococci of the species *Streptococcus pneumoniae.*

pneumopericardium The presence of air or gas in the pericardial cavity.

pneumoperitoneum The presence of air or gas within the peritoneal cavity of the abdomen.

pneumotaxic center A group of neurons in the pons that have an inhibitory effect on the inspiratory center.

pneumothorax A collection of air or gas in the pleural space that causes the lung to collapse.

poikilothermy Variation in body temperature according to the ambient temperature.

point of maximum impulse (PMI) The location or area where the apical pulse is palpated the strongest, often in the fifth intercostal space of the thorax just medial to the left midclavicular line.

poison Any substance that produces harmful physiological or psychological effects.

polio See *poliomyelitis.*

poliomyelitis An infectious disease caused by one of three polio viruses; asymptomatic, mild, and paralytic forms of the disease occur.

poliovirus hominis The causative organism of poliomyelitis.

polyarthritis Inflammation of several joints.

polycythemia An abnormal increase in the number of erythrocytes in the blood.

polydipsia Excessive thirst.

polymorphic Occurring in many forms.

polyp A small, tumorlike growth that projects from a mucous membrane surface.

polyphagia Excessive eating.

polysaccharide A carbohydrate that contains three or more molecules of simple carbohydrates.

polyuria Excessive secretion of urine.

pons The part of the brain stem between the medulla and the midbrain.

portal hypertension An increased venous pressure in the portal circulation caused by compression or by occlusion in the portal or hepatic vascular system.

portal vein A vein that ramifies like an artery in the liver and ends in capillary-like sinusoids that convey the blood to the inferior vena cava through the hepatic veins.

positive-end expiratory pressure (PEEP) Ventilation controlled by a flow of air delivered in cycles of constant pressure through the respiratory cycle.

posttraumatic syndrome An anxiety reaction to a severe psychosocial event; also known as posttraumatic stress disorder.

posterior In the back part of a structure.

posterior cerebral artery The artery that supplies the posterior portion of the cerebrum.

posterior chamber of the eye The chamber of the eye between the iris and the lens.

posterior communicating artery The artery that branches off each internal carotid artery and connects with the ipsilateral posterior cerebral artery.

posterior superior iliac spine One of two bony segments that form the iliac crest.

postictal phase The phase that usually follows a seizure in which the person is drowsy and lethargic.

postpartum The maternal period after delivery.

postpartum hemorrhage Blood loss of more than 500 mL after delivery of the newborn.

postsynaptic neuron The membrane of a nerve that is in close association with a presynaptic terminal.

potassium ion The predominate intracellular cation; it helps to regulate neuromuscular excitability and muscle contraction.

potassium-sparing agent A group of medications that promote sodium and water loss without an accompanying loss of potassium.

potential difference The difference in electrical potential, measured as the charge difference across the cell membrane.

potentiation The enhancement of effect caused by concurrent administration of two drugs in which one drug increases the effect of the other drug.

pound (lb) A unit of measure equal to 16 ounces or 0.45359 kilogram.

precapillary sphincter The smooth muscle sphincter that regulates blood flow through a capillary.

precipitous delivery A rapid, spontaneous delivery of less than 3 hours from onset of labor to birth; it results from overactive uterine contractions and little maternal soft tissue or bony resistance. Childbirth that occurs with such speed that usual preparations cannot be made.

precordial thump A CPR technique used to restore circulation in monitored ventricular fibrillation or unstable ventricular tachycardia.

preeclampsia An abnormal condition of pregnancy characterized by the onset of acute hypertension after the twenty-fourth week of gestation.

pregravid Before pregnancy.

preload The amount of blood returning to the ventricle.

premature atrial complex (PAC) A cardiac dysrhythmia characterized by an atrial beat occurring before the expected excitation; it is indicated on the electrocardiogram as an early P wave.

premature birth Refers to an infant who is born before 37 weeks of gestation.

premature junctional complex (PJC) A single contraction that occurs during sinus rhythm earlier than the next expected sinus beat; it is caused by premature discharge of an ectopic focus in the AV junctional tissue.

premature rupture of membranes (PROM) Rupture of the amniotic sac before the onset of labor, regardless of gestational age.

premature ventricular complex (PVC) A cardiac dysrhythmia characterized by a ventricular beat preceding the expected electrical impulse; it is indicated on the electrocardiogram as an early, wide QRS complex without a preceding related P wave.

prenatal Existing or occurring before birth.

prepuce In males, the free fold of skin that covers the glans penis; the foreskin. In females, the external fold of the labia minora that covers the clitoris.

present illness Identifies the chief complaint and provides a full, clear, chronological account of the symptoms.

presenting part The part of the fetus that lies closest to the internal os of the cervix.

presenting the patient The effective communication and transfer of patient information in the course of out-of-hospital and hospital care.

presynaptic neuron The nerve terminal that contains neurotransmitter vesicles.

presynaptic terminal The enlarged axon terminal.

priapism Painful, persistent erection of the penis.

priority patient A patient whose condition warrants immediate care and transport.

primary bronchus One of the two tubes arising at the inferior end of the trachea; each primary bronchus extends into one of the lungs.

primary contamination An exposure to a hazardous substance that is harmful only to the person exposed and that poses little risk of exposure to others.

primary epilepsy Epilepsy for which the cause is unknown; also known as *idiopathic epilepsy.*

primary follicle The ovarian follicle that contains the primary oocyte.

primary injury prevention The practice of preventing an injury from occurring.

primary oocyte The oocyte before the first meiotic division.

primary pulmonary hypertension Abnormally high pressure within the pulmonary circulation.

prime mover A muscle that plays a major role in accomplishing movement.

primigravida A woman who is pregnant for the first time.

primipara A woman who has given birth only one time.

PR interval The time lapse between the beginning of the P wave and the beginning of the QRS complex in the electrocardiogram.

Prinzmetal's angina An atypical form of angina that occurs at rest rather than with effort; it is associated with gross ST elevation in the electrocardiogram that disappears when the pain subsides.

proarrhythmia A serious tachydysrhythmia or bradydysrhythmia seemingly generated by antidysrhythmic agent(s).

prodromal stage The early period of labor before uterine contractions become forceful and frequent enough to result in progressive dilation of the uterine cervix.

progesterone A steroid sex hormone prescribed to treat various menstrual disorders, functional uterine bleeding, and repeated spontaneous abortions.

progestin Any group of hormones secreted by the corpus luteum, placenta, or adrenal cortex that have a progesterone-like effect on the uterus.

prokaryote A cell without a true nucleus and with nuclear material scattered throughout the cytoplasm.

prolapsed umbilical cord An umbilical cord that protrudes beside or ahead of the presenting part of the fetus.

proliferative phase The time between the end of menses and ovulation characterized by rapid division of endometrial cells and the development of follicles in the ovary.

pronation Rotation of the forearm so that the anterior surface is down.

prone position The position in which the patient is lying on his or her stomach (face down).

proprietary name See *trade name.*

proprioception Information about the position of the body and its various parts.

prostaglandin A class of naturally occurring fatty acids that affect body functions such as vasodilation, stimulation and contraction of uterine smooth muscle, and promotion of inflammation and pain.

prostate gland The gland that lies just below the male bladder; its secretion is one of the components of semen.

prostatic hypertrophy Hypertrophy or enlargement of the prostate gland.

prostatitis Acute or chronic inflammation of the prostate gland.

prosthesis An artificial replacement for a missing part of the body, such as an artificial limb.

protein Any of a large group of naturally occurring, complex, organic nitrogen compounds.

prothrombin A chemical that is part of the clotting cascade; the precursor of thrombin.

protoplasm The living substance of a cell.

protraction Movement in the anterior direction

pseudoaneurysm A condition resembling an aneurysm, caused by enlargement and tortuosity of a vessel.

pseudomembranous colitis A life-threatening form of diarrhea caused by *Clostridium difficile.*

psoas muscle A long muscle originating from the transverse processes of the lumbar vertebrae and the fibrocartilage and sides of the vertebral bodies of the lower thoracic vertebrae and the lumbar vertebrae.

psoriasis A common, chronic, inheritable skin disorder characterized by circumscribed red patches covered by thick, dry, adherent scales that result from excessive development of epithelial cells.

psychological dependence Emotional reliance on a drug; manifestations range from a mild desire for a drug to craving and drug-seeking behavior to repeated compulsive use of a drug for its subjectively satisfying or pleasurable effects.

psychology The science or study of behavior.

psychomotor seizure A seizure manifested by impaired consciousness of variable degree; the patient carries out a series of coordinated acts that are inappropriate, bizarre, and serve no useful purpose, about which the patient is amnesic.

psychosis Any major mental disorder of organic or emotional origin characterized by extreme derangement or disorganization of the personality, often accompanied by severe depression, agitation, regressive behavior, illusions, delusions, and hallucinations; the individual loses touch with reality and is incapable of functioning normally in society.

puberty The period of life when the ability to reproduce begins.

"public duty" doctrine or rule The provision that a public official is generally not liable to individuals for his or her negligence in discharging public duties.

public service answering point (PSAP) A communications center that coordinates the deployment of emergency personnel and other resources required for an emergence response.

pubis One of a pair of pubic bones that, with the ischium and the ilium, form the hipbone and join the pubic bone from the opposite side at the pubic symphysis.

pulmonary artery The artery that carries deoxygenated blood from the right ventricle into the lung.

pulmonary capacity The sum of two or more pulmonary volumes.

pulmonary edema The accumulation of extravascular fluid in lung tissues and alveoli.

pulmonary embolism (PE) The blockage of a pulmonary artery by foreign matter such as fat, air, tumor tissue, or a thrombus that usually arises from a peripheral vein.

pulmonary hypertension A condition of abnormally high pressure within the pulmonary circulation.

pulmonary overpressurization syndrome (POPS) A condition that results from expansion of trapped air in the lungs; it may lead to alveolar rupture and extravasation of air into extraalveolar locations.

pulmonary semilunar valve A valve that guards the orifice between the right ventricle and the pulmonary artery.

pulmonary surfactant Certain lipoproteins that reduce the surface tension of pulmonary fluids, allowing the exchange of gases in the alveoli of the lungs and contributing to the elasticity of pulmonary tissue.

pulmonary trunk The large elastic artery that carries blood from the right ventricle of the heart to the right and left pulmonary arteries.

pulmonary vein Any vein that carries oxygenated blood from the lung to the left atrium.

pulmonary ventilation The movement of air in and out of the lungs, bringing oxygen to the lungs and removing carbon dioxide.

pulmonic pressure Right-sided pressure.

pulp The soft, spongy chamber of the tooth.

pulse deficit A condition that exists when the radial pulse is less than the ventricular rate; it indicates a lack of peripheral perfusion.

pulse pressure The difference between systemic and pulmonic pressure.

pulsus paradoxus An abnormal decrease in systolic blood pressure that drops more than 10 to 15 mm Hg during inspiration compared to expiration.

punctate Spotted; marked with points of puncture.

punctum The opening of each lacrimal canal.

puncture wound A traumatic injury caused by the penetration of the skin by a narrow object.

pupil The opening in the center of the iris that regulates the amount of light entering the eye.

purified protein derivative (PPD) A dried form of tuberculin used in testing for past or present infection with tubercle bacilli.

Purkinje fibers Myocardial fibers that are a continuation of the bundle of His and that extend into the muscle walls of the ventricles.

pustule A small, circumscribed elevation of skin containing fluid, which is usually purulent.

P wave The first complex of the electrocardiogram, representing depolarization of the atria.

pyelonephritis An acute infection of the pelvis and parenchyma of the kidney.

pyelolithotomy Removal of a stone from a kidney by surgical incision.

pyloric sphincter A thickened, muscular ring in the stomach that separates the pylorus from the duodenum.

pyorrhea Discharge of pus.

pyrogen Any substance or agent that tends to cause a rise in body temperature.

pyrogenic A substance or agent that produces fever.

pyruvate The end product of glycolysis; it may be metabolized to lactate or acetyl coenzyme A (CoA).

QRS complex The principle deflection in the electrocardiogram, representing ventricular depolarization.

QT interval The time lapse from the beginning of the QRS complex to the end of the T wave, representing the total duration of electrical activity of the ventricles.

quadriplegia Paralysis of the arms, legs, and trunk of the body.

rabies An acute, usually fatal, viral disease of the central nervous system of animals; it is transmitted from animals to people by infected blood, tissue or, most commonly, saliva.

raccoon's eyes Ecchymosis of one or both orbits caused by fracture of the base of the sphenoid sinus.

radial tuberosity A large, oblong elevation at the distal end of the radius.

radioulnar syndesmosis The articulation of the radius and ulna, consisting of a proximal articulation, a distal articulation, and three sets of ligaments.

radius One of the bones of the forearm, lying parallel to the ulna.

range The general perimeter of communications coverage, beyond which coverage is nonexistent or severely degraded to an unusable level; it is measured in miles.

rapid sequence induction (RSI) An airway management technique that involves the virtually simultaneous administration of a potent sedative agent and a neuromuscular blocking agent for the purpose of ET intubation; it provides optimal intubation conditions while minimizing the risk of aspiration of gastric contents.

reabsorption The process of absorbing again that occurs in the kidneys.

reactive airway disease An inflammatory airway condition that develops as a reaction to an antigen.

reactive hyperemia Increased blood flow associated with increased metabolic activity.

receptor molecule A reactive site on the cell surface or within the cell that combines with a drug molecule to produce a biological effect.

reciprocity The practice of granting an individual licensure or certification/registration based on licensure or certification/registration by another state, agency, or association.

rectum The segment of the large intestine continuous with the descending sigmoid colon just proximal to the anal canal.

rectus femoris muscle A muscle of the anterior thigh; one of the four parts of the quadriceps femoris.

red marrow Specialized soft tissue found in many bones of infants and children, in the spongy bone of the proximal epiphyses of the humerus and femur, and in the sternum, ribs, and vertebral bodies of adults. It is essential in the manufacture of red blood cells.

red measles See *rubeola.*

reentry The reactivation of tissue by a returning impulse; the sustaining mechanism in some cases of ventricular bigeminy or trigeminy, ventricular tachycardia, and paroxysmal supraventricular tachycardia.

referred pain Visceral pain felt at a site distant from its origin; for example, pain from a myocardial infarction felt in the patient's arm.

reflection on action A component of critical thinking (usually performed after the event) whereby a patient-care episode is evaluated for possible improvement in future responses of a similar nature.

reflex An automatic response to a stimulus that occurs without conscious thought; produced by a reflex arc.

reflex arc The smallest portion of the nervous system capable of receiving a stimulus and producing a response.

refractory period The period after effective stimulation during which excitable tissue fails to respond to a stimulus of threshold intensity.

refractory shock Shock that is resistant to treatment but is still reversible.

relative hypovolemia Inadequate preload as a result of vasodilation.

relative refractory period The portion of the action potential after the absolute refractory period during which another action potential can be produced with a greater than threshold stimulus strength.

renal calculus Kidney stone.

renal calyx The first unit in the system of the ducts of the kidney carrying urine from the renal pyramid of the cortex to the renal pelvis for excretion through the ureters.

renal capsule The cortical substance that separates the renal pyramids.

renal corpuscle The glomerulus and its enclosing Bowman's capsule.

renal cortex The outer layer of the kidney, which contains approximately 1.25 million renal tubules, which remove body waste in the form of urine.

renal failure Inability of the kidneys to secrete wastes, concentrate urine, and conserve electrolytes; it may be chronic or acute.

renal medulla The inner layer of the kidney.

renal papilla The apex of the renal pyramid.

renal pelvis The funnel-shaped expansion of the upper end of the ureter that receives the calyces.

renal pyramid One of a number of pyramidal masses seen on longitudinal section of the kidney; it contains part of the loop of Henle and the collecting tubules.

renal tubule One of the collecting tubules in the kidney.

renin A proteolytic enzyme that surrounds each arteriole as it enters a glomerulus; it affects blood pressure by catalyzing the change of angiotensin I to angiotensin II.

renin-angiotensin-aldosterone mechanism Renin, released from the kidneys in response to low blood pressure, converts angiotensinogen to angiotensin I. Angiotensin I is converted by angiotensin-converting enzyme to angiotensin II, which causes vasoconstriction, resulting in increased blood pressure. Angiotensin II also increases aldosterone secretion, which increases blood pressure by increasing blood volume.

repolarization The phase of the action potential in which the membrane potential moves from its maximum degree of depolarization toward the value of the resting membrane potential.

reposition To move a structure to its original position.

rescue To free from confinement or danger.

residual volume The volume of air remaining in the lungs after a maximum expiratory effort.

respiration The process of the molecular exchange of oxygen and carbon dioxide within the body's tissues.

respiratory acidosis An abnormal condition characterized by an increased arterial P_{CO_2}, excess carbonic acid, and an increased plasma hydrogen ion concentration.

respiratory alkalosis An abnormal condition characterized by decreased P_{CO_2}, decreased hydrogen ion concentration, and increased blood pH.

respiratory bronchiole The smallest bronchiole that connects the terminal bronchiole to the alveolar duct.

respiratory membrane The membrane in the lungs across which gas exchange occurs with the blood.

respiratory syncytial virus (RSV) A single-strand virus that is a common cause of epidemics of acute bronchiolitis, bronchopneumonia, and the common cold in young children and sporadic acute bronchitis and mild upper respiratory tract infections in adults.

resting membrane potential (RMP) The electrical charge difference inside a cell membrane measured relative to just outside the cell membrane.

reticular Relating to a fine network of cells or collagen fibers.

reticular activating system A functional system in the brain essential for wakefulness, attention, concentration, and introspection.

reticular formation A small, thick cluster of neurons nestled within the brain stem that controls breathing, the heartbeat, blood pressure, level of consciousness, and other vital functions.

retina The nervous tunic of the eye; it is continuous with the optic nerve.

retraction Movement in the posterior direction

retrograde amnesia The loss of memory for events that occurred before the event that precipitated the amnesia.

retroperitoneal Of or pertaining to the organs closely attached to the abdominal wall and partly covered by peritoneum.

retroperitoneum Behind the peritoneum.

retrovirus Any of a family of viruses that converts genetic RNA to DNA after entering the host cell.

revised trauma score (RTS) An injury severity index that uses the Glasgow Coma Scale and measurements for systolic blood pressure and respiratory rate.

Reye's syndrome A combination of acute encephalopathy and fatty infiltration of the internal organs that may follow acute viral infections.

rheumatic fever An inflammatory disease that may develop as a delayed reaction to streptococcal infection of the upper respiratory tract.

rheumatoid arthritis A chronic, sometimes deforming destructive collagen disease that has an autoimmune component.

rheumatoid lungs Rheumatoid arthritis with emphasis on nonarticular changes; for example, pulmonary interstitial fibrosis, pleural effusion, and lung nodules.

rhinitis Inflammation of the mucous membranes of the nose.

rhinorrhea The free discharge of watery, nasal fluid.

Rh factor An antigenic substance present in the erythrocytes of most people; a person lacking the Rh factor is Rh negative.

rhonchi Abnormal sounds heard on auscultation of a respiratory airway obstructed by thick secretions, muscular spasm, neoplasm, or external pressure.

rib One of the 12 pairs of elastic arches of bone forming a large part of the thoracic skeleton. The first seven ribs on each side are called *true ribs* because they articulate directly with the sternum. The remaining five ribs are called *false ribs*; the first three attach ventrally to the ribs and the last two ribs are free at their ventral extremities and are called *floating ribs*.

ribonucleic acid (RNA) A nucleic acid found in both the nucleus and the cytoplasm of cells that transmits genetic instructions from the nucleus to the cytoplasm. In the cytoplasm, RNA functions in the assembly of proteins.

ribosome The "factory" of a cell where protein is synthesized.

right lymphatic duct A vessel that conveys lymph from the right upper quadrant of the body into the bloodstream in the neck at the junction of the right internal jugular and the right subclavian veins.

rigor mortis The rigid stiffening of skeletal and cardiac muscle shortly after death.

Rocky Mountain spotted fever (RMSF) A serious, tick-borne infectious disease caused by *Rickettsia rickettsii* and characterized by fever, chills, severe headache, confusion, and rash.

rod A photoreceptor in the retina of the eye; it is responsible for noncolor vision in low-intensity light.

R-on-T phenomenon The occurrence of a ventricular depolarization during a vulnerable period of relative refractoriness.

root The lowest part of the tooth; it is covered by cementum.

rotation Movement of a structure about its axis.

Rouleau formation An aggregation of red cells in what looks like a stack of coins or checkers.

round ligament The remains of the umbilical vein.

R prime (R′) A subsequent positive deflection in the QRS complex that extends above the baseline and that is taller than the first R wave.

rubella A contagious viral disease characterized by fever, symptoms of mild upper respiratory tract infection, lymph node enlargement, and a diffuse, fine, red maculopapular rash; it is spread by droplet infection; also known as *German measles.*

rubeola An acute, highly contagious viral disease involving the respiratory tract; it is characterized by a spreading, maculopapular, cutaneous rash and occurs primarily in young children who have not been immunized; also known as *red measles.*

ruptured diaphragm A tear or break in the diaphragm, usually as a result of injury.

ruptured ovarian cyst A ruptured globular sac filled with fluid or semisolid material that develops in or on the ovary.

rupture of membranes Rupture of the amniotic sac; it usually occurs toward the end of the first stage of labor.

salpingitis An inflammation or infection of the fallopian tube.

sacral bone Composed of the five segments of the vertebral column that are fused in the adult to form the sacrum; the segments are designated S1 to S5.

sacral promontory The projecting portion of the pelvis at the base of the sacrum.

sacral sparing The preservation of sensory or voluntary motor function of the perineum, buttocks, scrotum, or anus.

sacrum The large, triangular bone at the dorsal part of the pelvis; it is inserted like a wedge between the two hipbones.

saddle joint A joint that consists of two saddle-shaped articulating surfaces oriented at right angles to one another.

sagittal plane An imaginary plane that runs vertically through the middle of the body, producing right and left sections.

salicylate Any one of several widely prescribed drugs derived from salicylic acid (e.g., aspirin).

salivary amylase A digestive enzyme found in saliva that begins the chemical digestion of carbohydrates.

salivary gland One of the three pairs of glands that pour their secretions into the mouth, thus aiding the digestive process.

salpingitis An inflammation or infection of the fallopian tube.

saltatory conduction Conduction in which action potentials jump from one node of Ranvier to the next node of Ranvier.

saphenous vein One of a pair of the longest veins in the body; it begins in the medial marginal vein in the dorsum of the foot and ends in the femoral vein.

sarcoidosis A chronic disorder of unknown origin characterized by the formation of lesions in the lung, spleen, liver, skin, and mucous membranes and in the lacrimal and salivary glands.

sarcolemma Part of a myofibril between adjacent Z lines.

sarcomere The contractile unit of skeletal muscle, which contains thick and thin myofilaments.

sarcoplasmic reticulum Endoplasmic reticulum of the muscle.

scanning A component of attention that refers to one's ability to rapidly review a large amount of sensory input. Different individuals have different capacities for scanning and may use various approaches and styles in their scanning.

scapula One of the pair of large, flat, triangular bones that form the dorsal part of the shoulder girdle.

scene size-up To quickly assess an emergency scene and determine what resources are needed; also known as *size-up.*

schizophrenia Any one of a large group of psychotic disorders characterized by gross distortions of reality, disturbances of language and communication, withdrawal from social interaction, and the disorganization and fragmentation of thought, perception, and emotional reaction.

Schwann cell A cell that forms a myelin sheath around each nerve fiber of the peripheral nervous system.

sciatic nerve A long nerve that originates in the sacral plexus and extends through the muscles of the thigh, leg, and foot with numerous branches.

sciatica Inflammation of the sciatic nerve.

sclera The opaque membrane covering the eyeball.

scoliosis A lateral curvature of the spine.

scrotum The sac of skin that contains the testes.

sebaceous gland A gland of the skin, usually associated with a hair follicle that produces sebum.

sebum The secretion of sebaceous glands; it prevents drying and protects against some bacteria.

second-degree burn A burn injury that extends through the epidermis to the dermis (superficial partial thickness); it is considered a deep partial-thickness injury if it extends to the basal layers of the skin.

secondary bronchus A branch from a primary bronchus that conducts air to each lobe of the lungs.

secondary contamination An exposure to a hazardous substance in which liquid and particulate substances are easily transferred to others by touching.

secondary epilepsy Epilepsy that can be traced to trauma, infection, a cerebrovascular disorder, or another illness that contributes to or causes the seizure disorder.

secondary follicle The follicle in which the secondary oocyte is surrounded by granulosa cells.

second stage of labor The stage of labor measured from full dilation of the cervix to delivery of the newborn.

secretin The hormone that stimulates secretion of pancreatic juice.

secretion A general term for a substance produced inside a cell and released from the cell.

secretory phase The portion of the menstrual cycle extending from the time of formation of the corpus luteum after ovulation to the time when menstrual flow begins.

sector A subdivision of the incident command system that encompasses a specific area of responsibility as deemed necessary by the incident commander.

sedative-hypnotic A drug that reversibly depresses the activity of the central nervous system; these drugs are used chiefly to induce sleep and relieve anxiety.

seizure A hyperexcitation of neurons in the brain that leads to a sudden, involuntary series of skeletal muscle contractions; also known as a *convulsion*.

selectivity A component of attention that refers to a person's ability to pick or chose specific components of the sensory input that the person is reviewing and then focus on that input.

self-contained breathing apparatus (SCBA) A respiratory protection device that provides an enclosed system of air.

self-neglect A type of elder abuse; behaviors of an elderly person that intentionally threaten personal health or safety (e.g., poor nutrition, noncompliance with medication regimens).

Sellick's maneuver Cricoid cartilage pressure directed posteriorly to compress the trachea against the cervical vertebra, thereby occluding the esophagus; this maneuver is useful for limiting the risk of aspiration during an intubation procedure.

semen Male reproductive fluid.

semicircular canal A structure located in the inner ear that generates a nerve impulse when the head moves.

semi-Fowler's position An inclined position with the upper half of the body raised by elevating the head or a stretcher about 30 degrees to prevent reflux of gastric contents.

semilunar valve A valve with a half-moon shape, such as the aortic valve and the pulmonary valve.

seminal vesicle One of two glandular structures that empty into the ejaculatory ducts; its secretion is one of the components of semen.

semipermeable membrane A membrane that is pervious such that fluids and other substances can pass through it.

senile dementia An organic mental disorder of the aged resulting from generalized atrophy of the brain with no evidence of cerebrovascular disease.

sensitization An acquired reaction in which specific antibodies develop in response to an antigen.

sensory Pertaining to a part or all of the body's sensory nerve network.

sensory layer The portion of the retina that contains rods and cones; also known as the *sensory retina*.

sensory retina See *sensory layer*.

sepsis Infection.

septic shock A form of shock that most often results from a serious systemic bacterial infection.

septicemia Systemic infection in which the pathogens are present in the bloodstream, having spread from an infection in any part of the body.

septum A thin wall dividing two cavities or masses of soft tissue.

serotonin A hormone and neurotransmitter released from platelets when blood vessel walls are damaged.

serous membrane One of the many thin sheets of tissue that line closed cavities of the body, such as the pleura lining the thoracic cavity, the peritoneum lining the abdominal cavity, and the pericardium lining the sac that encloses the heart.

serous pericardium The thin inner layer of the pericardium that surrounds the heart.

serum Blood plasma without its clotting factors.

sexual assault A forcible act of sexual contact with the body of another person, male or female, without the person's consent.

shingles An acute infection caused by reactivation of the latent varicella zoster virus (VZV); it is characterized by painful vesicular eruptions that follow the underlying route of cranial or spinal nerves inflamed by the virus; also known as *herpes zoster*.

shipping paper A description of a hazardous material that includes the substance name, classification, and UN identification number; it is generally required to be carried in the transporting vehicle (motor vehicle, train, vessel, or aircraft).

shock An abnormal condition of inadequate blood flow to the body's peripheral tissues associated with life-threatening cellular dysfunction: also known as *hypoperfusion*.

short bones Bones that are approximately as broad as they are long, such as the carpal bones of the wrist and the tarsal bones of the ankle.

shoulder dystocia An obstacle to delivery that occurs when the fetal shoulders press against the maternal symphysis pubis, blocking shoulder delivery.

shoulder girdle The encircling bony structure that supports the upper limbs; also known as the *pectoral girdle*.

shoulder presentation The presentation that results when the long axis of the fetus lies perpendicular to that of the mother; also known as transverse presentation.

shunt A tube or device implanted in the body to redirect the flow of body fluid from one cavity or vessel to another.

shunting The redirection of a flow of body fluid from one cavity or vessel to another.

sickle cell anemia See *sickle cell disease*.

sickle cell crisis An acute episodic condition that occurs in individuals with sickle cell anemia.

sickle cell disease Anemia characterized by the presence of crescent-shaped erythrocytes and excessive hemolysis; an inheritable condition.

side effect An often unavoidable and undesirable effect of using therapeutic doses of a drug; actions or effects other than those for which the drug was originally given.

sighing An occasional deep, audible inspiration that usually is insignificant.

sigmoid colon The segment of the colon that extends from the end of the descending colon in the pelvis to the juncture with the rectum.

significant past medical history A patient's medical background that may offer insight into the patient's current problem.

silicosis A lung disorder caused by continued long-term inhalation of the dust of an inorganic compound, silicon dioxide; the disorder is characterized by dyspnea and the development of nodular fibrosis in the lungs.

simplex mode A system with the ability to transmit or receive in one direction at a time; one party transmits, the other receives. Simultaneous transmission cannot occur without blocking a message.

sinoatrial node (SA node) An area of specialized heart tissue that generates the cardiac electrical impulse.

sinus One of several cavities in the bones of the skull that connect to the nasal cavities by small channels.

sinus headache A headache characterized by pain in the forehead, nasal area, and eyes.

sinusitis Inflammation of one or more paranasal sinuses.

sinusoid A form of terminating blood channel, somewhat larger than a capillary, lined with reticuloendothelial cells.

size-up See *scene size-up*.

skeletal muscle Muscle tissue that appears microscopically to consist of striped myofibrils; also known as striated muscle and voluntary muscle.

Skene's glands The largest of the glands that open into the urethra of women.

skin graft A portion of skin implanted to cover areas where skin has been lost through burns or injury or by surgical removal of diseased tissue.

slander Verbally making false statements to others about a person, knowing that the statements are false, and with malicious intent or reckless disregard for their falsity.

sleep apnea A sleep disorder characterized by periods in which attempts to breathe are absent.

slough To shed or cast off; tissue that has been shed.

slow reactive substance of anaphylaxis A bronchoconstrictor mediator released from mast cells; it increases the production of prostaglandins.

small intestine The longest portion of the digestive tract; it is divided into the duodenum, jejunum, and ileum.

smallpox A highly contagious viral disease characterized by fever, prostration, and a vesicular, pustular rash.

smooth muscle One of two kinds of muscle; it is composed of elongated, spindle-shaped cells in muscles not under voluntary control, such as smooth muscle of the intestines, stomach, and other visceral organs; also known as *visceral muscle* and *nonstriated muscle*.

sniffing position The patient position used during orotracheal intubation in which the patient's neck is flexed at C5 and C6 and the head is extended at C1 and C2.

SOAP format A memory aid used to organize written and verbal patient reports; it includes subjective data, objective data, assessment data, and plan of patient management.

sodium bicarbonate An antacid, electrolyte, and urinary alkalinizing agent.

sodium ions Ions involved in acid-base balance, water balance, nerve impulse transmission, and muscle contraction.

sodium-potassium exchange pump The biochemical mechanism that uses energy derived from ATP to achieve the active transport of potassium ions opposite to that of sodium ions.

soft palate The posterior muscular portion of the palate, which forms an incomplete septum between the mouth and the oropharynx and between the oropharynx and the nasopharynx.

solute A substance dissolved in a solution.

somatic nervous system The part of the nervous system composed of nerve fibers that send impulses from the central nervous system to skeletal muscle.

somatic pain Pain that arises from skeletal muscles, ligaments, vessels, or joints.

somatoform disorder Any of a group of neurotic disorders characterized by symptoms suggesting physical illness or disease, for which there are no organic or physiological causes.

somatomotor Refers to cranial nerves that control the skeletal muscles through motor neurons.

somatomotor nerves Motor nerves to the skeletal muscles.

spasm An involuntary muscle contraction of sudden onset.

spastic colon Abnormally increased motility of the small and large intestines, generally associated with stress; also known as *irritable bowel syndrome*.

special emergency radio service (SERS) A specific group of radio frequencies designated by the FCC for use by emergency agencies.

sperm See *spermatozoon*.

spermatic cord A structure that extends from the deep inguinal ring in the abdomen to the testes; each cord comprises arteries, veins, lymphatics, nerves, and the excretory duct of the testis.

spermatogenesis The process of development of spermatozoa.

spermatozoa See *spermatozoon*.

spermatozoon The male sex cell, composed of a head and tail; it contains genetic information transmitted by the male.

sphenoid bone The bone at the base of the skull anterior to the temporal bones and the basilar part of the occipital bone.

sphenoid sinus One of a pair of cavities in the sphenoid bone that are lined with mucous membrane continuous with that of the nasal cavity.

sphincter Ring-shaped muscle.

sphygmomanometer The device used to measure blood pressure.

spina bifida A congenital neural tube defect characterized by developmental anomaly in the posterior vertebral arch.

spinal cord shock See *neurogenic shock*.

spinal ganglia The structures that contain the cell bodies of sensory neurons; also known as *dorsal root ganglia*.

spinal nerve One of 31 pairs of nerves formed by the joining of the dorsal and ventral routes that arise from the spinal cord.

spinal shock See *neurogenic shock*; also known as *spinal cord shock*.

spinous process A part of the vertebrae that projects backward from the vertebral arch, giving attachment to muscles of the back.

spleen A large, highly vascular lymphatic organ situated in the upper part of the abdominal cavity between the stomach and the diaphragm; it responds to foreign substances in the blood, destroys worn-out erythrocytes, and is a storage site for red blood cells.

splenomegaly An abnormal enlargement of the spleen.

spondylosis A condition of the spine characterized by fixation or stiffness of the vertebral joint.

spontaneous abortion An abortion that usually occurs before the twelfth week of gestation; the lay term is miscarriage.

spontaneous pneumothorax The presence of air or gas in the pleural space as a result of rupture of the lung parenchyma and visceral pleura with no demonstrable cause.

sprain An injury to the tendons, muscles, or ligaments around a joint characterized by pain and swelling.

sputum Material coughed up from the lungs and expectorated from the mouth.

S prime (S′) A subsequent negative deflection in the QRS complex that extends below the baseline.

squelch A radio receiver circuit used to suppress the audio portion of unwanted radio signals or radio noises below a predetermined carrier strength level.

staging area A designated area where incident-assigned vehicles are directed and held until needed.

standing orders Specific treatment protocols that may be used by prehospital emergency care providers in the absence of on-line/direct medical direction when delay in treatment would harm the patient.

stapes The smallest of the three ossicles in the middle ear.

staphylococcal infection An infection caused by any one of several pathogenic species of *Staphylococcus*, commonly characterized by the formation of abscesses of the skin or other organs.

starch The principle molecule used for the storage of food in plants.

Starling's law of the heart A rule that the force of the heartbeat is determined by the length of the fibers comprising the myocardial walls.

stasis A disorder in which the normal flow of fluid through a vessel of the body is slowed or halted.

status asthmaticus A severe, prolonged asthma exacerbation that has not been broken with repeated doses of bronchodilators.

status epilepticus A medical emergency characterized by continual convulsive seizures that occur without intervals of consciousness.

stellate wound A star-shaped wound.

stenosis Abnormal constriction or narrowing of an opening or passageway in a body structure.

sternal angle The point at which the manubrium joins the body of the sternum; also known as the *angle of Louis*.

sternoclavicular joint The double gliding joint between the sternum and the clavicle.

sternomanubrial joint See *angle of Louis;* also known as the *sternal angle.*

sternum The elongated, flattened bone forming the middle portion of the thorax.

steroid A member of a large family of lipids, including some reproductive hormones, vitamins, and cholesterol.

stimulant A drug that enhances or increases body function or activity.

Stokes-Adams syndrome A condition characterized by sudden episodes of loss of consciousness caused by incomplete heart block; seizures may accompany the episodes.

stoma A surgically created artificial opening of an internal organ on the surface of the body.

stomach The major organ of digestion, located in the right upper quadrant of the abdomen.

strain A muscular injury that usually results from physical effort or activity.

stratum basale The innermost layer of the epidermis.

stratum corneum The most superficial layer of the epidermis.

stratum granulosum The layer of the epidermis that lies just beneath the stratum corneum except in the palms of the hands and soles of the feet, where it lies just beneath the stratum lucidum.

stratum lucidum The layer of the epidermis that lies just beneath the stratum corneum; it is present only in the thick skin of the palms of the hands and soles of the feet.

stratum spinosum The layer of the epidermis that lies on top of the stratum basale and beneath the stratum granulosum.

streptococcal infection An infection caused by pathogenic bacteria of one of several species of the genus *Streptococcus* or their toxins.

stress A nonspecific mental or physical strain caused by any emotional, physical, social, economic cause or other factor that initiates a physiological response.

stressor Any factor that causes wear and tear on the body's physical or mental resources.

stretch mark See *stria.*

stria A streak or linear scar that often results from rapidly developing tension in the skin; also known as a *stretch mark.*

striated Having striped or parallel lines, as in skeletal muscle.

striated muscle See *skeletal muscle.*

stridor An abnormal, high-pitched musical sound caused by obstruction in the trachea or larynx.

stroke See *cerebrovascular accident.*

stroke volume (SV) The volume of blood pumped out of one ventricle in a single heartbeat.

ST segment The early part of repolarization in the electrocardiogram of the right and left ventricles.

stupor A state of lethargy and unresponsiveness in which a person seems unaware of his or her surroundings.

stylet A thin metal probe for inserting into or passing through a needle, tube, or catheter; it is sometimes used to change the configuration of an endotracheal tube.

styloid process A bony projection.

subarachnoid hematoma A collection of blood in the subarachnoid space.

subarachnoid space The area below the arachnoid membrane but above the pia matter that contains cerebrospinal fluid.

subclavian vein The continuation of the axillary vein in the upper body; it extends from the lateral border of the first rib to the sternal end of the clavicle, where it joins the internal jugular to form the brachiocephalic vein.

subcutaneous injection The introduction of medicine through a hypodermic needle into the subcutaneous tissue beneath the skin.

subcutaneous tissue The adherent layer of adipose tissue just below the dermal layer; also known as the *hypodermis.*

subdural hematoma A collection of blood in the subdural space.

subdural space The space between the dura matter and arachnoid.

subendocardial infarction See *transmural infarction.*

subgaleal hematoma A collection of blood beneath the strong sheet of fibrous connective tissue that joins the frontal and occipitofrontal muscles.

sublingual route The route of medication administration in which the medication is placed under the tongue so that the tablet dissolves in salivary secretions.

subluxation A partial dislocation.

substrate A substance acted upon and changed by an enzyme in any chemical reaction.

sudden death A death that occurs within the first 2 hours after the onset of illness or injury.

sudden infant death syndrome (SIDS) The unexpected and sudden death of an apparently normal and healthy infant that occurs during sleep and with no physical or autopsic evidence of disease.

sudoriferous gland See *sweat gland.*

summation The combined effect of two drugs that equals the sum of the individual effects of each agent.

superficial frostbite A cold injury with at least some minimal tissue loss; it usually involves the dermis and shallow subcutaneous layers.

superficial pain Pain that arises from the skin or mucous membrane.

superior Situated above or oriented toward a higher place.

superior vena cava The vein that returns blood from the head and neck, upper limbs, and thorax to the right atrium.

supination Rotation of the forearm so that the anterior surface is up.

supine hypotension syndrome Hypotension that occurs in pregnant women who are in a supine position; it results when the uterus compresses the inferior vena cava, decreasing cardiac filling and cardiac output.

supine position The position in which the patient is lying on his or her back (face up).

suprasternal notch The superior margin of the manubrium, which can be easily felt at the anterior base of the neck; also known as the *jugular notch.*

surface tension The tendency of the surface of a liquid to minimize the area of its surface by contracting.

surfactant Lipoproteins that reduce the surface tension of pulmonary fluids.

suspensory ligament The band of peritoneum that extends from the ovary to the body wall; it contains the ovarian vessels and nerves.

suture A border or joint between two bones of the cranium.

sweat gland A structure that produces sweat or viscus organic secretions; also known as a *sudoriferous gland.*

sympathetic nervous system A subdivision of the autonomic nervous system that is usually involved in preparing the body for physical activity.

sympatholytic Antiadrenergic; blocking transmission of impulses from the adrenergic postganglionic fibers to effector organs or tissues.

sympathomimetic A pharmacological agent that mimics the effects of sympathetic nervous system stimulation of organs and structures by acting as an agonist or by increasing the release of the neurotransmitter norepinephrine at postganglionic nerve endings.

symphysis A cartilaginous joint.

symphysis pubis The slightly movable, interpubic joint of the pelvis; it consists of two bones separated by a disk of fibrocartilage and connected by two ligaments; also known as the *pubic symphysis.*

synapse Functional membrane-to-membrane contact of a nerve cell with another nerve cell, muscle cell, gland cell, or sensory receptor; it functions in transmitting action potentials from one cell to another.

synaptic cleft The space between the presynaptic and postsynaptic membranes.

synaptic vesicle A secretory vesicle in the presynaptic terminal that contains neurotransmitter substances.

synchondrosis A cartilaginous joint between two immovable bones, such as the symphysis pubis, the sternum, and the manubrium.

syncope A brief lapse in consciousness caused by transient cerebral hypoxia.

syncytium Cardiac muscle cells that are so tightly bound together and their membranes so permeable to electrical impulse that they act as a mass of merged cells or a single cell.

syndesmosis A fibrous articulation in which two bones are connected by interosseous ligaments.

synergism The combined action of two drugs that is greater than the sum of each individual agent acting independently.

synergist A muscle that works with other muscles to cause movement.

synovial fluid A thin, lubricating film that allows considerable movement between articulating bones.

synovial joint See *joint.*

synovial membrane The inner layer of an articular capsule that surrounds a freely movable joint.

syphilis A sexually transmitted disease characterized by distinct stages of effects over a period of years; any organ system may be involved.

system A group of organs arranged to perform a more complex function than any one organ can perform alone.

systemic circulation Blood flow from the left ventricle to all parts of the body and back to the right atrium.

systemic lupus erythematous (SLE) A chronic inflammatory disease that affects many systems of the body; it is characterized by severe vasculitis, renal involvement, and lesions of the skin and nervous system.

systemic pressure Left-sided pressure.

systolic blood pressure The blood pressure measured during the period of ventricular contraction.

tabes dorsalis An abnormal condition characterized by the slow degeneration of all or part of the body and the progressive loss of peripheral reflexes.

tachycardia A heart rate that exceeds 99 beats per minute.

tachyphylaxis A phenomenon in which the repeated administration of some drugs results in a marked decrease in their effectiveness.

tachypnea A persistent respiratory rate that exceeds 20 breaths per minute.

tactical EMS Refers to EMS personnel who are specially trained and equipped to provide prehospital emergency care in tactical environments.

tactical patient care Patient care activities that occur inside the scene perimeter or "hot zone."

tactical retreat Leaving the scene when danger is observed or when violence or indicators of violence are displayed; it requires immediate and decisive action.

talus The second largest tarsal bone; the ankle bone.

tardive dyskinesia An abnormal condition characterized by involuntary, repetitious movements of the muscles of the face, limbs, and trunk.

tarsal Pertaining to the area of articulation between the foot and the leg.

taste bud Any one of many peripheral taste organs distributed over the tongue and roof of the mouth.

teachable moment The time after an injury has occurred when the patient and observers remain acutely aware of what has happened and may be more receptive to teaching about how the event or injury could be prevented.

telecommunicator A person trained in public safety telecommunications; the term applies to call takers, dispatchers, radio operators, data terminal operators, or any combination of such functions in a public service answering point.

telemedicine Refers to technological communications that allow transmission of photographs, video, and other information directly from the scene to a hospital for physician evaluation and consultation.

telemetry The transmission and reception of physiological data by radio or telephone; for example, electrocardiograms (ECGs).

temporal bone One of a pair of large bones that form part of the lower cranium and that contain various cavities and recesses associated with the ear.

temporal lobe The lateral region of the cerebrum; it contains the center for smell and some association areas for memory and learning.

ten code (10 code) A code sometimes used in radio communications that uses the number 10 plus another number to relay a particular message.

tendon A band or cord of dense connective tissue that connects muscle to bone or other structures; it is characterized by strength and nonstretchability.

tendonitis An inflammatory condition of a tendon, usually caused by a sprain.

tenosynovitis Inflammation of a tendon sheath.

tension headache A headache caused by muscle contractions of the face, neck, and scalp.

tension pneumothorax Accumulation of air or gas within the pleural cavity; if not relieved, it can lead to lung collapse.

teratogenic Any substance, agent, or process that interferes with normal prenatal development.

term A pregnancy that has reached 40 weeks of gestation.

terminal bronchiole The end of the conducting airway.

terminally ill patient A patient with advanced stage of disease with an unfavorable prognosis and no known cure.

termination of action The point at which a drug effect is no longer seen.

tertiary segmental bronchus The bronchus that extends from the secondary bronchus and conducts air to each lobule of the lung.

testes The male gonads, which produce the male sex cells, or sperm.

testicular torsion An axial rotation of the spermatic cord; it occludes the blood supply to the testicle, epididymis, and other structures.

testosterone The male sex hormone.

tetanus An acute, potentially fatal infection of the central nervous system caused by the tetanus bacillus *Clostridium tetani*; it is characterized by muscle spasms and convulsions.

tetralogy of Fallot A congenital cardiac anomaly that consists of four defects: pulmonic stenosis, ventricular septal defect, malposition of the aorta so that it rises from the septal defect or the right ventricle, and right ventricular hypertrophy.

thalamus Tissue located just above the hypothalamus; it helps to produce sensations, associates sensations with emotions, and plays a part in arousal.

therapeutic abortion The legal termination of a pregnancy for reasons of maternal well-being.

therapeutic action The desired, intended action of a drug.

therapeutic index A measurement of the relative safety of a drug.

therapeutic range The range of plasma concentrations that are most likely to produce the desired drug effect with the least likelihood of toxicity; the range between minimal effective concentration and toxic level.

thermogenesis Production of heat, especially by the cells of the body.

thermolysis Dissipation of body heat by radiation, evaporation, conduction, or convection.

thiazide A group of diuretics that are moderately effective in lowering blood pressure.

third-degree burn A burn injury in which the entire thickness of the epidermis and dermis is destroyed.

third stage of labor The stage of labor that begins with delivery of the infant and ends when the placenta has been expelled and the uterus has contracted.

third ventricle The ventricle located in the center of the diencephalon between the two halves of the thalamus.

thoracentesis Puncturing of pleural space.

thoracic aorta The large upper portion of the descending aorta; it supplies many parts of the body such as the heart, ribs, chest muscles, and stomach.

thoracic cavity The area of the body enclosed by the ribs.

thoracic duct The common trunk of all the lymphatic vessels of the body except those on the right side of the head and neck, the thorax, right upper limb, right lung, right side of the heart, and the diaphragmatic surface of the liver.

thoracic vertebrae The 12 bony segments of the spinal column of the upper back, designated T1 to T12.

thoroughfare channel The channel for blood through a capillary bed from an arteriole to a venule.

threatened abortion An abortion diagnosed when a patient has some uterine bleeding with an intrauterine pregnancy in which the internal cervical os is closed; it may stabilize and end in normal delivery or progress to an incomplete or complete abortion.

threshold potential The value of the membrane potential at which an action potential is produced as a result of depolarization in response to a stimulus.

thrill A fine vibration felt by an examiner's hands over the site of an aneurysm or on the pericardium.

thrombectomy The removal of a thrombus from a blood vessel.

thrombin An enzyme formed in plasma as part of the clotting process; it causes fibrinogen to change to fibrin, which is essential in the formation of a clot.

thrombocytes Cell fragments.

thrombocytopenia An abnormal hematological condition in which the number of platelets is reduced; the most common cause is a bleeding disorder.

thromboembolism A condition in which a blood vessel is blocked by an embolus carried in the bloodstream from the site of formation of the clot.

thrombogenesis Clot formation.

thrombolytic agent A drug that dissolves clots after their formation by promoting the digestion of fibrin.

thrombophlebitis See *phlebitis.*

thrombosis An abnormal formation of a thrombus within a blood vessel of the body.

thromboxane An antagonistic prostaglandin derivative that is synthesized and released by degranulating platelets, causing vasoconstriction and promoting the degranulation of other platelets.

thrombus An aggregation of platelets, fibrin, clotting factors, and the cellular elements of the blood attached to the interior wall of a vein or artery, which sometimes occludes the lumen of the vessel.

thymectomy Excision of the thymus.

thymus A single, unpaired gland located in the mediastinum; the primary central gland of the lymphatic system.

thyroid cartilage The largest laryngeal cartilage; it forms the laryngeal prominence, or Adam's apple.

thyroid membrane The fibrous membrane that joins the hyoid and the thyroid cartilages.

thyrotoxicosis Refers to any toxic condition that results from thyroid hyperfunction.

tibia The second longest bone of the skeleton; it is located at the medial side of the leg.

tibial tuberosity A large, oblong elevation at the proximal end of the tibia that attaches to the ligament of the patella.

tick paralysis A rare, progressive, reversible disorder caused by several species of ticks that release a neurotoxin that causes weakness, incoordination, and paralysis.

tidal volume The volume of air inspired or expired in a single resting breath.

tinea A group of fungal skin diseases characterized by itching and scaling and sometimes by painful lesions.

tissue binding A type of drug reservoir in which drug pooling occurs in fat tissue and bone.

T lymphocyte A thymus-derived lymphocyte of immunological importance; it is responsible for cell-mediated immunity.

tolerance A physiological response that requires that a drug dosage be increased to produce the same effect formerly produced by a smaller dose; tolerance exists when there is a decreased physiological response to repeated administration of a drug or chemically related substance.

tone The audio signal or carrier wave of controlled amplitude and frequency used for equipment control purposes or to selectively signal a receiver, such as activating a pager; tones are measured in hertz.

tonsil A large collection of lymphatic tissue beneath the mucous membrane of the oral cavity and pharynx.

tonsillectomy Surgical removal of the tonsils.

tonsillitis Inflammation of the tonsils.

torr A measurement in millimeters of mercury.

torsade de pointes An unusual bidirectional ventricular tachycardia.

total body water All the water within the body, including intracellular and extracellular water plus the water in the GI and urinary tract.

total lung capacity The sum of the inspiratory and expiratory reserve volumes plus the tidal volume and residual volume.

total pressure The combination of pressures exerted by all the gases in any mixture of gas.

Tourette's syndrome An abnormal condition characterized by facial grimaces, tics, and involuntary arm and shoulder movements.

toxic level The plasma concentration at which a drug is likely to produce serious adverse effects.

toxic shock A severe, acute disease caused by infection with strains of *Staphylococcus aureus.*

toxin A poison usually produced by or occurring in a plant or microorganism.

toxoid A toxin that has been treated with chemicals or with heat to reduce its toxic effects but that retains its antigenic power.

trachea A cylindrical tube in the neck composed of cartilage and membrane; it conveys air to the lungs.

tracheal stenosis Constriction of the trachea.

tracheostomy An opening through the neck into the trachea through which an indwelling tube may be inserted.

trade name The copyrighted name of a drug, designated by the drug company that sells the medication; also known as *brand name* or *proprietary name.*

tragus A projection of the cartilage of the auricle at the opening of the external auditory meatus.

transceiver A combination transmitter and receiver with a switching circuit or duplexer to use a single antenna.

transcutaneous cardiac pacing (TCP) The use of an artificial pacemaker to substitute for a natural pacemaker of the heart that is blocked or dysfunctional. In the prehospital setting, a transcutaneous pacemaker is used to treat symptomatic bradycardia; heart block associated with reduced cardiac output that is unresponsive to atropine; pacemaker failure; and asystole.

transsection A complete or incomplete lesion of the spinal cord.

transfusion hepatitis Hepatitis that results from a transfusion with incompatible blood.

transient dysphagia A temporary impairment of speech.

translaryngeal cannula ventilation An advanced airway procedure that provides high-volume/high-pressure oxygenation of the lungs through cannulation of the trachea below the glottis; also known as *needle percutaneous transtracheal ventilation* and *needle cricothyrotomy.*

transmembrane potential The difference in electrical charge between inside and outside the plasma membrane.

transmural infarction A myocardial infarction that extends through the full thickness of the myocardium, including the endocardium and epicardium.

transudate A fluid passed through a membrane as a result of a difference in hydrostatic pressure.

transverse At right angles to the long axis of any common part.

transverse colon The segment of the colon that extends from the end of the ascending colon at the hepatic flexure on the right side across the midabdomen to the beginning of the descending colon at the splenic flexure on the left side.

transverse plane An imaginary plane that divides the body into top and bottom or superior and inferior sections; also known as the horizontal plane.

transverse presentation See *shoulder presentation*.

transverse process The bony segment that extends laterally from each side of the vertebral arch.

trauma An injury caused by a transfer of energy from some external source to the human body.

trauma index (TI) An early measurement that used a numerical injury rating system based on a patient's injured body region, type of injury, and cardiovascular, central nervous system, and respiratory status.

trauma score (TS) An injury severity index used to predict the outcome for patients with blunt or penetrating injuries.

traumatic asphyxia A term used to describe a severe crushing injury to the chest and abdomen that results from an increase in intrathoracic pressure that forces blood from the right side of the heart into the veins of the upper thorax, neck, and face.

traumatic hyphema See *hyphema*.

traumatic iridoplegia Traumatic dilation, or less commonly, constriction, of the pupil.

treatment protocols Guidelines that define the scope of prehospital intervention practiced by emergency care providers.

Trendelenburg position A position in which the head is low and the body and legs are on an inclined plane.

triage A method used to sort or categorize patients according to severity of injury.

triaxial reference system Three intersecting lines of reference used in standard limb leads.

trichomoniasis A vaginal infection caused by the protozoan *Trichomonas vaginalis*; it is characterized by itching, burning, and a frothy, pale yellow to green vaginal discharge.

tricuspid valve The valve located between the right atrium and ventricle.

trigeminal nerve Either of the largest pair of cranial nerves, which are essential for chewing and the general sensibility of the face.

triglyceride A compound consisting of a fatty acid and glycerol.

trigone The triangular smooth area at the base of the bladder between the openings of two ureters and that of the urethra.

trimester One of three periods of approximately 3 months into which pregnancy is divided.

triphosphate bond Energy sources for the body's muscles, nerves, and overall function; an example is adenosine triphosphate (ATP).

triplets Three PVCs in a row.

trochanter One of the two bony projections at the proximal end of the femur that serve as the attachment point for various muscles.

trochlea The medial aspect of the humerus; it articulates with the ulna.

trophoblast A cell layer that forms the outer layer of the blastocyst, which erodes the uterine mucosa during implantation; it contributes to the formation of the placenta.

true rib See *rib*.

true vocal cord See *vocal cord*.

truncal obesity Obesity that preferentially affects or is isolated in the trunk of the body rather than the extremities.

trunking system A radio system consisting of base stations on different channels connected to each other with small computers that work with special mobile and portable signaling to allow multiple simultaneous conversations.

T tubule Tubelike invagination of the sarcolemma that conducts action potentials toward the center of the cylindrical muscle fibers.

tubal ligation One of several sterilization procedures in which both fallopian tubes are blocked to prevent conception from occurring.

tubercle A nodule or small eminence, such as that on a bone or that produced by infection from tubercle bacilli.

tuberculosis (TB) A chronic granulomatous infection caused by *Mycobacterium tuberculosis*; it usually affects the lungs and generally is transmitted by inhalation or ingestion of infected droplets.

tuberosities Elevations or protuberances, especially of bones.

tuboovarian abscess An abscess involving the ovary and fallopian tube.

tunic One of the enveloping layers of a part; one of the coats of a blood vessel; one of the coats of the eye; one of the coats of the digestive tract.

tunica adventitia The outermost fibrous coat of a vessel or an organ that is derived from the surrounding connective tissue.

tunica intima The innermost coat of a blood vessel.

tunica media The middle coat, usually muscular, of an artery or other tubular structure.

turbinate The concha nasalis.

turgor The normal resiliency of the skin caused by the outward pressure of the cells and interstitial fluid.

Turner's sign Bruising of the skin of the flanks or loin in acute hemorrhagic pancreatitis; also known as *Grey Turner's sign*.

Turner's syndrome A chromosomal anomaly characterized by the absence of one X chromosome characterized by short stature, undifferentiated gonads, and various other abnormalities.

T wave Deflection in the electrocardiogram after the QRS complex, representing ventricular repolarization.

tympanic membrane See *eardrum*.

type and crossmatch A test used to determine the patient's ABO group and Rh type.

ulceration The formation of a craterlike lesion on the skin or mucous membranes.

ulna One of the bones of the forearm.

ultra high frequency (UHF) Radio frequency between 300 and 3000 MHz; the 460 MHz range is commonly used for EMS communications.

umbilical cord A flexible structure connecting the umbilicus with the placenta and giving passage to the umbilical arteries and vein.

umbilicus The point on the abdomen at which the umbilical cord joined the fetal abdomen.

unethical Conduct that fails to conform to moral principles, values, or standards.

unifocal PVC A premature ventricular complex that originates from a single ectopic pacemaker site.

unipolar lead A lead composed of a single positive electrode and a reference point.

universal donor A person with blood of type O, Rh factor negative.

universal precautions Infection control practices in health care that are observed with every patient and procedure and that prevents exposure to blood-borne pathogens.

universal recipient A person with blood type AB who can receive any of the four types of blood.

unmyelinated axon A nerve fiber lacking a myelin sheath.

untoward effect A side effect that proves harmful to the patient.

upper esophageal sphincter The ring of muscle located at the superior opening of the esophagus that regulates the passage of materials into the esophagus.

urea A nitrogen-containing waste product.

uremia The presence of excessive amounts of urea and other nitrogenous waste products in the blood, such as occurs in renal failure.

uremic frost A pale, frostlike deposit of white crystals on the skin caused by kidney failure and uremia.

ureter One of a pair of tubes that carry the urine from the kidney into the bladder.

urethra A small tubular structure that drains urine from the bladder; in men, it also serves as a passageway for semen during ejaculation.

urethritis An inflammatory condition of the urethra.

uric acid A product of the metabolism of protein present in the blood and excreted in the urine.

urinary bladder The muscular, membranous sac in the pelvis that stores urine for discharge through the urethra.

urinary retention Incomplete emptying of the bladder; the inability to void or eliminate urine.

urinary tract infection (UTI) An infection of one or more structures of the urinary tract.

urogenital triangle The anterior portion of the perianal region; it contains the openings of the urethra and vagina in the female and the root structures of the penis in the male.

urosepsis A septic complication of urinary tract infection.

urticaria A pruritic skin eruption characterized by transient wheals of various shapes and sizes with well-defined margins and pale centers.

uterine Pertaining to the uterus.

uterine inversion A rare event in which the uterus turns inside out after birth.

uterine rupture A rare event in which the wall of the uterus ruptures when it is unable to withstand the strain placed on it.

uterine tube One of a pair of ducts opening at one end into the uterus and the other end into the peritoneal cavity, over the ovary; also known as a *fallopian tube.*

uterosacral ligament A primary ligament that holds the uterus in place.

uterus The hollow, pear-shaped internal female organ of reproduction.

uvula The cone-shaped process hanging down from the soft palate that helps prevent food and liquid from entering the nasal cavities.

U wave Gradual deviation from the T wave in the electrocardiogram, thought to represent the final stage of repolarization of the ventricles.

vagina The part of the female genitalia that forms a canal from the orifice through the vestibule to the uterine cervix.

vaginitis An inflammation of the vaginal tissues.

vagus nerve Either of the longest pair of cranial nerves essential for speech, swallowing, and the sensibilities and functions of many parts of the body.

vallecula A furrow between the glossoepiglottic folds on each side of the posterior oropharynx.

Valsalva maneuver A vagal maneuver used to slow the heart and decrease the force of atrial contraction by stimulating postganglionic parasympathetic nerve fibers in the wall of the atria and specialized tissues of the SA and AV nodes via the vagus nerve.

varicella An acute, highly contagious viral disease caused by a herpes virus, varicella-zoster virus; it occurs primarily in young children and is characterized by crops of pruritic vesicular eruptions on the skin; also known as *chickenpox.*

varicella-zoster virus (VZV) A member of the herpes virus family that causes the disease varicella (chickenpox) and herpes zoster (shingles).

varicocele A collection of varicose veins in the scrotum.

vasoconstriction A narrowing of the lumen of any blood vessel.

vasodilation An increase in the diameter of a blood vessel caused by inhibition of its constrictor nerves or stimulation of dilator nerves.

vascular tunic The choroid, ciliary body, and iris.

vas deferens See *ductus deferens.*

vasomotor Of or pertaining to the nerves and muscles that control the diameter of the lumen of blood vessels.

vasopressin mechanism The mechanism by which antidiuretic hormone (ADH) secretion increases when blood pressure drops or plasma osmolarity increases; it reduces urine production and stimulates vasoconstriction.

vastus lateralis muscle The largest of the four muscles of the quadriceps femoris; it is situated on the lateral side of the thigh.

vein A vessel that carries blood toward the heart.

venereal disease A contagious disease usually acquired by sexual intercourse or genital contact.

venostasis Retardation of venous flow in a part.

venous capillary The ends of capillaries closest to venules.

venous sinus One of many sinuses that collect blood from the dura mater and drain it into the internal jugular vein.

ventral root The nerve that conveys efferent nerve processes away from the spinal cord.

ventricle A small cavity; it usually refers to the right or left ventricle of the heart.

ventricular bigeminy A cardiac dysrhythmia characterized by two ventricular beats in rapid succession followed by a longer interval.

ventricular fibrillation (VF) A cardiac dysrhythmia marked by rapid, disorganized depolarization of the ventricular myocardium.

ventricular quadrigeminy A cardiac dysrhythmia that occurs when every fourth complex is a PVC.

ventricular tachycardia (VT) Tachycardia that usually originates in the Purkinje fibers.

ventricular trigeminy A cardiac dysrhythmia characterized by three ventricular beats in rapid succession followed by a longer interval.

ventrogluteal muscle The muscle that overlies the iliac crest and the anterior-superior iliac spine.

venule Small blood vessels that collect blood from the capillaries and join to form veins.

vermiform appendix See *appendix.*

vertebra Any one of 33 bones of the spinal column.

vertebral arch The dorsal, bony arch of a vertebra composed of the laminae and pedicles; it protects the spinal cord.

vertebral artery Each of the two arteries branching from the subclavian arteries.

vertebral body A bony disk that serves as the weight-bearing portion of the vertebra.

vertex presentation See *cephalic presentation.*

vertigo A sensation of faintness or an inability to maintain normal balance in a standing or seated position.

very high frequency (VHF) Radio frequencies between 30 and 300 MHz (usually in the 150 MHz range). The VHF spectrum is further divided into "high" and "low" bands.

vesicular Pertaining to a blisterlike condition.

vesicular follicle The secondary follicle in which the oocyte attains its full size; also known as the graafian follicle.

vesiculation The formation of vesicles.

vestibular fold One of two folds of mucous membrane that stretch across the laryngeal cavity; it helps close the glottis; also known as the *false vocal cord.*

vestibule The portion of the inner ear adjacent to the oval window between the semicircular canals and the cochlea.

vestibule of the ear The middle region of the middle ear.

vestibule of the vagina The space behind the labia minora that contains the opening of the vagina, the urethra, and the vestibular glands.

vestibulocochlear nerve The eighth cranial nerve, formed by the cochlear and vestibular nerves; it extends to the brain.

virulence The relative infectiousness of a disease-causing microorganism.

virus A minute, parasitic microorganism without independent metabolic activity that can replicate only within a cell of a living plant or animal host.

visceral Pertaining to internal organs enclosed within a body cavity, primarily the abdominal organs.

visceral pain Deep pain that arises from smooth vasculature or organ systems.

visceral pericardium The portion of the serous pericardium that covers the heart surface; also known as the *epicardium.*

visceral peritoneum The layer of peritoneum that covers the abdominal organs.

vital capacity The volume of gas moved on deepest inspiration and expiration, or the sum of the inspiratory reserve volume, the tidal volume, and the expiratory reserve volume.

vitamin An organic compound essential in small quantities for normal physiological and metabolic functioning of the body.

vitamin D A fat-soluble vitamin essential for the normal formation of bones and teeth and for absorption of calcium and phosphorus from the gastrointestinal tract.

vitamin K A fat-soluble compound essential for the synthesis of several related proteins involved in the clotting of blood.

vitreous humor The transparent, jellylike material that fills the space between the lens and the retina.

vocal cord One of two folds of elastic ligaments covered by mucous membrane that stretch from the thyroid cartilage to the arytenoid cartilage; vibration of the vocal cords is responsible for voice production; also known as a *true vocal cord.*

Volkmann's contracture A serious, persistent flexion contraction of the forearm and hand caused by ischemia.

voluntary Action originated or accomplished by a person's free will or choice.

voluntary muscle A muscle that is consciously controlled; see *skeletal muscle.*

vomer bone The bone forming the posterior and inferior part of the nasal septum.

vulva The external genitals of the female.

wandering atrial pacemaker The passive transfer of pacemaker sites from the sinus node to other latent pacemaker sites in the atria and AV junction.

water vapor pressure The partial pressure exerted by water molecules after they have been converted into a gas.

watt The unit of measurement of a transmitter's power output.

Wenckebach heart block Type I second-degree AV block; a progressive, beat-to-beat prolongation of the PR interval that finally results in a nonconducted P wave; at this point, the sequence recurs.

Wernicke-Korsakoff syndrome A disease that results from chronic thiamine deficiency combined with an inability to utilize thiamine because of a heritable disorder or because of a reduction in intestinal absorption and metabolism of thiamine by alcohol.

Wernicke's encephalopathy A stage of Wernicke-Korsakoff syndrome that usually develops suddenly with the clinical manifestations of ataxia, nystagmus, disturbances of speech and gait, signs of neuropathy, stupor, or coma.

wheeze A form of rhonchus characterized by a high-pitched, musical quality; it is caused by high-velocity airflow through narrowed airways.

windchill chart An index developed to calculate the cooling effects of the ambient temperature based on thermometer readings and the wind speed.

withdrawal syndrome A predictable set of signs and symptoms that occurs after a decrease in the usual dose of a drug or its sudden cessation.

xiphoid process The smallest of three parts of the sternum; it articulates caudally with the body of the sternum and laterally with the seventh rib.

years of productive life The calculation obtained by subtracting the victim's age at death from 65 (the average age of retirement).

yellow fever An acute infection transmitted by mosquitoes; it is characterized by headache, fever, jaundice, vomiting, and bleeding.

yellow marrow Specialized soft tissue (mainly adipose) found in the compact bone of most adult epiphyses.

Z line The delicate, membranelike structure found at either end of a sarcomere.

zone of coagulation In a burn wound, the central area that has sustained the most intense contact with the thermal source; in this area coagulation necrosis of the cells has occurred and the tissue is nonviable.

zone of hyperemia An area in which blood flow is increased as a result of the normal inflammatory response to injury; it lies at the periphery of the zone of stasis.

zone of stasis The area of burn tissue that surrounds the critically injured area; it consists of tissue that is potentially viable despite the serious thermal injury.

zygomatic process See *zygomatic bone.*

zygomatic bone One of a pair of bones that forms the prominence of the cheek, the lower part of the orbit of the eye, and parts of the temporal bone; also known as the *zygomatic process.*

zygote The developing ovum from the time it is fertilized until it is implanted in the uterus as a blastocyst.

Index

References with "t" denote tables; "f" denote figures; "b" denote boxes; "n" denote notes

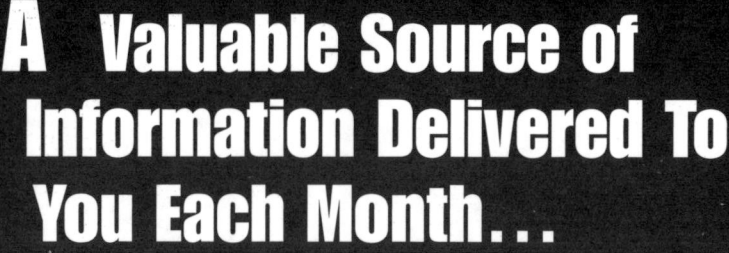
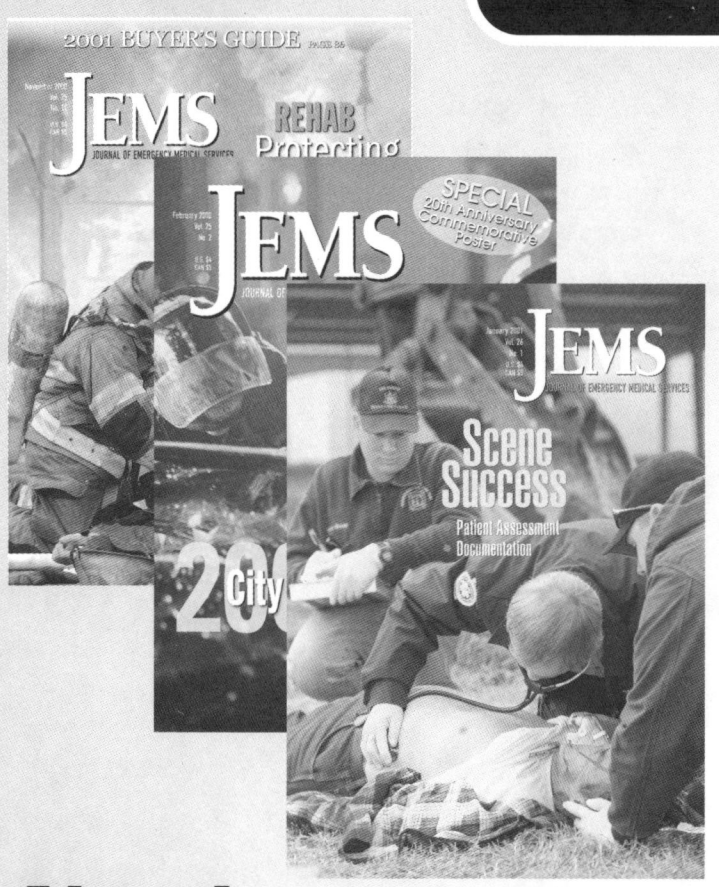

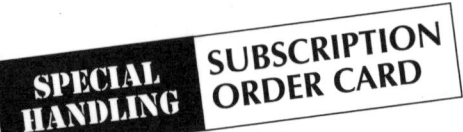 **SPECIAL HANDLING** | **SUBSCRIPTION ORDER CARD**

BUSINESS REPLY MAIL
FIRST-CLASS MAIL   PERMIT NO 806   CARLSBAD CA

POSTAGE WILL BE PAID BY ADDRESSEE

JEMS
PO BOX 469010
ESCONDIDO CA 92046-9976